11/3/97

95 00

CARDIOVASCULAR THERAPEUTICS

A Companion to Braunwald's *Heart Disease*

Edited by

Thomas W. Smith, MD

Chief, Cardiovascular Division
Brigham and Women's Hospital
Boston, Massachusetts

Professor of Medicine
Harvard Medical School
Boston, Massachusetts

Section Editors

Elliott M. Antman, MD

John A. Bittl, MD

Wilson S. Colucci, MD

Antonio M. Gotto, Jr., MD, DPhil

Joseph Loscalzo, MD, PhD

Gordon H. Williams, MD

Douglas P. Zipes, MD

W.B. Saunders Company

A Division of Harcourt Brace & Company

Philadelphia London Toronto Montreal Sydney Tokyo

W.B. SAUNDERS COMPANY
A Division of Harcourt Brace & Company

The Curtis Center
Independence Square West
Philadelphia, Pennsylvania 19106

Library of Congress Cataloging-in-Publication Data

Cardiovascular therapeutics: A companion to Braunwald's *Heart Disease* /
[edited by] Thomas W. Smith.—1st ed.

p. cm.

ISBN 0–7216–5660–9

1. Cardiovascular system—Diseases—Treatment. I. Smith, Thomas Woodward. [DNLM: 1. Cardiovascular Diseases—therapy. WG 166 C2671 1996]

RC671.C37 1996 616.1′06—dc20

DNLM/DLC 95–30947

CARDIOVASCULAR THERAPEUTICS: A Companion to Braunwald's *Heart Disease* ISBN 0–7216–5660–9

Printed in the United States of America.

Last digit is the print number: 9 8 7 6 5 4 3 2

Dedication

To Sherley Goodwin Smith

Julia Goodwin Smith Nelligan

Geoffrey Woodward Smith

Allison Lloyd Smith

Contributors

Elliott M. Antman, MD
Associate Professor of Medicine, Harvard Medical School; Director, Coronary Care Unit, Brigham and Women's Hospital, Boston, Massachusetts
Clinical Trials and Meta-Analysis

Kenneth L. Baughman, MD
Professor of Medicine and Director, Division of Cardiology, The Johns Hopkins University School of Medicine, Baltimore, Maryland
Treatment of Myocarditis

David G. Benditt, BSc (EE), MD
Professor of Medicine, University of Minnesota Medical School; Co-Director, Cardiac Arrhythmia and Syncope Centers, University of Minnesota, Minneapolis, Minnesota
Treatment of Neurally Mediated Syncopal Syndromes

John A. Bittl, MD
Associate Professor of Medicine, Harvard Medical School; Director, Interventional Cardiology, and Associate Director, Cardiac Catheterization Laboratory, Brigham and Women's Hospital, Boston, Massachusetts
Interventional Approaches for Unstable Angina

Bruce H. Brundage, MD
Professor of Medicine and Radiological Sciences, University of California, Los Angeles (UCLA), School of Medicine, Los Angeles; Chief of Cardiology, Harbor-UCLA Medical Center, and Scientific Director, Saint John's Cardiovascular Research Center, Torrance, California
Treatment of Primary Pulmonary Hypertension: Lessons Learned

Robert M. Califf, MD
Professor of Medicine, Duke University School of Medicine; Director of Cardiac Care Unit and Associate Vice Chancellor for Clinical Research, Duke University Medical Center, Durham, North Carolina
Acute Myocardial Infarction
Clinical Trials and Meta-Analysis

Blase A. Carabello, MD
Charles Ezra Daniel Professor of Cardiology, Medical University of South Carolina and the Gazes Cardiac Research Institute; Staff Cardiologist, Ralph H. Johnson Department of Veterans Affairs Medical Center, Charleston, South Carolina
The Timing of Valve Surgery

Jay N. Cohn, MD
Professor of Medicine and Head, Cardiovascular Division, University of Minnesota Medical School; Staff, University of Minnesota Hospital and Clinic, Minneapolis, Minnesota
Long-Term Treatment of the Ambulatory Patient With Heart Failure

Lawrence H. Cohn, MD
Professor of Surgery, Harvard Medical School; Chief, Division of Cardiac Surgery, Brigham and Women's Hospital, Boston, Massachusetts
Coronary Artery Bypass Surgery
Surgical Therapy for Valvular Heart Disease

Wilson S. Colucci, MD
Professor of Medicine and Physiology, Boston University School of Medicine; Associate Chief, Cardiovascular Division, and Director, Cardiomyopathy Program, Boston University Medical Center, Boston, Massachusetts
Pathophysiologic and Clinical Considerations in the Treatment of Heart Failure: An Overview
Management of Patients Hospitalized With Heart Failure

Gregory S. Couper, MD
Assistant Professor of Surgery, Harvard Medical School; Director, Cardiac Surgical Intensive Care Unit, Brigham and Women's Hospital, Boston, Massachusetts
Intra-Aortic Balloon Counterpulsation

Margo A. Denke, MD
Associate Professor, Department of Internal Medicine, Center for Human Nutrition, The University of Texas Southwestern Medical Center at Dallas; Director, Endocrine Clinic, and Attending Physician, Veterans Administration Medical Center, Dallas, Texas
Dyslipoproteinemias/Atherosclerosis: Dietary Therapy

John P. DiMarco, MD, PhD
Julian R. Beckwith Professor of Medicine, and Director, Cardiac Electrophysiology Laboratory, Cardiovascular Division, University of Virginia Health Sciences Center, Charlottesville, Virginia
Drug Treatment of Supraventricular Tachycardias

Robert G. Dluhy, MD
Associate Professor of Medicine, Harvard Medical School; Associate Director, Endocrine Hypertension, Brigham and Women's Hospital, Boston, Massachusetts
Endocrine Causes of Hypertension

Stephen G. Ellis, MD
Professor of Medicine, The Ohio State University, Columbus; Director, Sones Cardiac Catheterization Laboratories, The Cleveland Clinic Foundation, Cleveland, Ohio
Percutaneous Coronary Intervention for Stable Angina

John A. Farmer, MD
Associate Professor of Medicine, Baylor College of Medicine; Chief, Section of Cardiology, Ben Taub General Hospital, Houston, Texas
Dyslipoproteinemias/Atherosclerosis: Introduction
Dyslipoproteinemias/Atherosclerosis: Pharmacologic Therapy

Jonathan C. Fox, MD, PhD
Assistant Professor of Medicine, University of Pennsylvania School of Medicine; Staff Cardiologist, Hospital of the University of Pennsylvania, Philadelphia, Pennsylvania
Gene Therapy for Cardiovascular Disease

Jane E. Freedman, MD
Assistant Professor of Medicine, Boston University School of Medicine, Boston, Massachusetts
Arterial and Venous Thrombotic Disease: Thrombolytic and Antithrombotic Therapies

Ronald Freudenberger, MD
Fellow, Mount Sinai School of Medicine, Cardiovascular Institute, New York, New York
Acute Coronary Syndromes: Thrombosis and Thrombolysis

Peter L. Friedman, MD, PhD
Associate Professor of Medicine, Harvard Medical School; Co-Director, Cardiac Arrhythmia Service and Clinical Electrophysiology Laboratory, Brigham and Women's Hospital, Boston, Massachusetts
Drug Treatment of Ventricular Tachycardias

Victor F. Froelicher, MD
Professor of Medicine, Stanford University; Cardiologist, Palo Alto VA Health Care System, Palo Alto, California
Rehabilitation of the Patient With Cardiovascular Disease

Valentin Fuster, MD, PhD
Dean for Academic Affairs and Arthur M. and Hilda A. Master Professor of Medicine, Mount Sinai School of Medicine; Director, Cardiovascular Institute, and Vice Chairman, Department of Medicine, Mount Sinai Medical Center, New York, New York
Acute Coronary Syndromes: Thrombosis and Thrombolysis

William H. Gaasch, MD
Professor of Medicine, University of Massachusetts Medical School, Worcester; Director of Cardiovascular Research, Lahey Hitchcock Medical Center, Burlington, Massachusetts
Management of Left Ventricular Diastolic Dysfunction

J. Michael Gaziano, MD
Instructor in Medicine, Harvard Medical School; Associate Physician, Divisions of Cardiovascular Disease and Preventive Medicine, Brigham and Women's Hospital, Boston, Massachusetts
Primary Prevention of Ischemic Heart Disease

Bernard J. Gersh, MB ChB, DPhil, FRCP
W. Proctor Harvey Teaching Professor of Medicine and Chief, Division of Cardiology, Georgetown University Medical Center, Washington, D.C.
Ischemic Heart Disease: Surgical Options

Bruce R. Gordon, MD
Associate Professor of Clinical Medicine and Surgery, Cornell University Medical College; Senior Member, The Rogosin Institute, New York, New York
The Steps Beyond Diet and Drug Therapy for Severe Hypercholesterolemia

Antonio M. Gotto, Jr., MD, DPhil
Chairman and Distinguished Professor of Medicine, Department of Medicine, Baylor College of Medicine; Chief, Internal Medicine Service, The Methodist Hospital, Houston, Texas
Dyslipoproteinemias/Atherosclerosis: Introduction
Dyslipoproteinemias/Atherosclerosis: Pharmacologic Therapy

Steven W. Graves, PhD
Assistant Professor of Medicine, Harvard Medical School; Associate Biochemist and Director, The Clinical Endocrine Laboratory, and Director, General Clinical Research Center Core Laboratory, Brigham and Women's Hospital, Boston, Massachusetts
Hypertension During Pregnancy

Scott M. Grundy, MD, PhD
Director, Center for Human Nutrition; Chairman, Department of Clinical Nutrition; and Distinguished Professor of Internal Medicine and Biochemistry, Center for Human Nutrition, The University of Texas Southwestern Medical Center at Dallas; Chief, Metabolic Unit, Veterans Administration Medical Center, Dallas, Texas
Dyslipoproteinemias/Atherosclerosis: Dietary Therapy

William G. Haynes, MBChB, MRCP, MD
Visiting Associate, University of Iowa College of Medicine; Staff, University of Iowa Hospitals and Clinics, Iowa City, Iowa
Treatment of Hypertension in the Patient With Cardiovascular Disease

Charles H. Hennekens, MD
John Snow Professor of Medicine and Professor of Ambulatory Care and Prevention, Harvard Medical School; Chief, Division of Preventive Medicine, Brigham and Women's Hospital, Boston, Massachusetts
Primary Prevention of Ischemic Heart Disease

Jack Hirsh, MD, FRCP(C)
Professor of Medicine, McMaster University; Director, Hamilton Civic Hospitals Research Centre, Henderson General Division, Hamilton, Ontario, Canada
Anticoagulation in Venous Thromboembolism

Norman K. Hollenberg, MD, PhD
Professor of Medicine, Harvard Medical School; Director of Physiologic Research, Radiology Department, Brigham and Women's Hospital, Boston, Massachusetts
Management of Essential Hypertension: An Overview

Mark C. G. Horrigan, MB, FRACP
Senior Fellow, Interventional Cardiology, Department of Cardiology, The Cleveland Clinic Foundation, Cleveland, Ohio
Angioplasty Strategies in Acute Myocardial Infarction

Ralph H. Hruban, MD
Associate Professor of Pathology and Oncology and Assistant Professor of Otolaryngology—Head and Neck, The Johns Hopkins University School of Medicine; Director, Division of Cardiovascular and Respiratory Pathology, The Johns Hopkins Hospital, Baltimore, Maryland
Treatment of Myocarditis

Julie R. Ingelfinger, MD
Associate Professor of Pediatrics, Harvard Medical School; Chief, Pediatric Nephrology, Massachusetts General Hospital, Boston, Massachusetts
Evaluation and Treatment of Hypertension in Children

Adolf W. Karchmer, MD
Professor of Medicine, Harvard Medical School; Chief, Division of Infectious Diseases, New England Deaconess Hospital, Boston, Massachusetts
Treatment of Infective Endocarditis

Clive Kearon, MB, MRCP(I), FRCP(C), PhD
Assistant Professor of Medicine, McMaster University and Henderson General Division, Hamilton Civic Hospital, Hamilton, Ontario, Canada
Anticoagulation in Venous Thromboembolism

Ralph A. Kelly, MD
Assistant Professor of Medicine, Harvard Medical School; Associate Physician, Brigham and Women's Hospital, Boston, Massachusetts
The Pharmacology of Heart Failure Drugs

Lawrence S. Klein, MD
Assistant Professor of Medicine, Indiana University School of Medicine; Research Associate, Krannert Institute of Cardiology, Indiana University Medical Center, Indianapolis, Indiana
Nonpharmacologic Treatment of Supraventricular Tachycardias
Catheter Ablation of Ventricular Tachycardia
Management of Bradyarrhythmias
Use of the Implantable Cardioverter-Defibrillator for Ventricular Arrhythmias

Spencer H. Kubo, MD
Associate Professor of Medicine, University of Minnesota Medical School; Medical Director, Heart Failure–Heart Transplantation Program, University of Minnesota, Minneapolis, Minnesota
Long-Term Treatment of the Ambulatory Patient With Heart Failure

Michael J. Landzberg, MD
Instructor, Internal Medicine and Pediatrics, Harvard Medical School; Director, Boston Adult Congenital Heart Service, Brigham and Women's Hospital and Children's Hospital, Boston, Massachusetts
Interventional Approaches to Congenital Heart Disease and Intracardiac Shunts

Martin M. LeWinter, MD
Professor of Medicine, University of Vermont College of Medicine; Director, Cardiology Unit, Fletcher Allen Health Care, Burlington, Vermont
Chronic Angina: Stable

Wayne Evan Lipson, MS, MD
Clinical Fellow of Surgery, Harvard Medical School; Surgical Resident, Brigham and Women's Hospital, Boston, Massachusetts
Surgical Therapy for Valvular Heart Disease

James E. Lock, MD
Professor of Pediatrics, Harvard Medical School; Chairman, Department of Cardiology, Children's Hospital, Boston, Massachusetts
Interventional Approaches to Congenital Heart Disease and Intracardiac Shunts

J. Antonio G. Lopez, MD
Assistant Professor, University of Iowa College of Medicine; Staff, University of Iowa Hospitals and Clinics, Iowa City, Iowa
Treatment of Hypertension in the Patient With Cardiovascular Disease

Joseph Loscalzo, MD, PhD
Distinguished Professor of Medicine and Biochemistry, Boston University School of Medicine; Chief, Cardiovascular Medicine; Vice Chairman, Department of Medicine; and Director, Whitaker Cardiovascular Institute, Boston University Medical Center, Boston, Massachusetts
Arterial and Venous Thrombotic Disease: Thrombolytic and Antithrombotic Therapies

Keith G. Lurie, MD
Associate Professor of Medicine, University of Minnesota Medical School; Co-Director, Cardiac Arrhythmia and Syncope Centers, University of Minnesota, Minneapolis, Minnesota
Treatment of Neurally Mediated Syncopal Syndromes

JoAnn E. Manson, MD
Associate Professor of Medicine, Harvard Medical School; Associate Physician, Division of Preventive Medicine, Brigham and Women's Hospital, Boston, Massachusetts
Primary Prevention of Ischemic Heart Disease

Allyn L. Mark, MD
Roy J. Carver Professor of Medicine and Associate Dean for Research, University of Iowa College of Medicine; Staff, University of Iowa Hospitals and Clinics; Staff, Veterans Affairs Medical Center, Iowa City, Iowa
Treatment of Hypertension in the Patient With Cardiovascular Disease

William M. Miles, MD
Associate Professor of Medicine, Indiana University School of Medicine; Director, Cardiac Electrophysiology Laboratory, Indiana University Hospital, Indianapolis, Indiana
Nonpharmacologic Treatment of Supraventricular Tachycardias
Catheter Ablation of Ventricular Tachycardia
Management of Bradyarrhythmias
Use of the Implantable Cardioverter-Defibrillator for Ventricular Arrhythmias

Raul D. Mitrani, MD
Assistant Professor of Medicine, University of Miami School of Medicine; Director, Arrhythmia and Pacemaker Center, Jackson Memorial Hospital, Miami, Florida
Nonpharmacologic Treatment of Supraventricular Tachycardias
Catheter Ablation of Ventricular Tachycardia
Management of Bradyarrhythmias
Use of the Implantable Cardioverter-Defibrillator for Ventricular Arrhythmias

Thomas J. Moore, MD
Associate Clinical Professor of Medicine, Harvard Medical School; Physician, Brigham and Women's Hospital, Boston, Massachusetts
Nonpharmacologic and Pharmacologic Treatment of Hypertension

Jonathan N. Myers, PhD
Clinical Assistant Professor of Medicine, Stanford University; Health Research Scientist, Palo Alto VA Health Care System, Palo Alto, California
Rehabilitation of the Patient With Cardiovascular Disease

Lionel H. Opie, MD, PhD
Professor, Department of Medicine, University of Capetown Medical School; Director, Ischemic Heart Disease Research Unit of the Medical Research Council, University of Capetown; Director, Hypertension Clinic, Groot Schuur Hospital, Capetown, South Africa
Pharmacologic Options for Treatment of Ischemic Disease

Joseph K. Perloff, MA (Hon), MD
Streisand/American Heart Association Professor of Medicine and Pediatrics, University of California, Los Angeles, School of Medicine, Division of Cardiology, Los Angeles, California
Medical Management of Adults With Congenital Heart Disease

Marc A. Pfeffer, MD, PhD
Associate Professor of Medicine, Harvard Medical School; Director, Heart Failure/Transplant Center, Brigham and Women's Hospital, Boston, Massachusetts
Prevention of Heart Failure and Treatment of Asymptomatic Left Ventricular Dysfunction

David P. Rardon, MD
Clinical Electrophysiologist, St. Vincent Hospital, Indianapolis, Indiana
Nonpharmacologic Treatment of Supraventricular Tachycardias
Management of Bradyarrhythmias

John T. Repke, MD
Associate Professor of Obstetrics, Gynecology, and Reproductive Biology, Harvard Medical School; Director, Center for Labor and Birth, Brigham and Women's Hospital, Boston, Massachusetts
Hypertension During Pregnancy

Paul M. Ridker, MD
Assistant Professor of Medicine, Harvard Medical School; Associate Physician, Division of Cardiovascular Disease and Preventive Medicine, Brigham and Women's Hospital, Boston, Massachusetts
Primary Prevention of Ischemic Disease

Eric A. Rose, MD
Valentine Mott/Johnson & Johnson Professor and Chairman, Department of Surgery, and Surgeon-in-Chief, Columbia University, College of Physicians and Surgeons, New York, New York
Cardiac Transplantation and Circulatory Assistance

John D. Rutherford, MB, ChB, FRACP, FACC
Professor of Medicine and Gail Griffiths Chair in Cardiology, University of Texas; Associate Chief of Cardiology and Chief of Cardiovascular Disease Service, Southwestern Medical Center at Dallas, Dallas, Texas
Management of Cardiovascular Disease During Pregnancy

Stuart D. Saal, MD
Associate Professor of Clinical Medicine and Surgery, Cornell University Medical College; Senior Member, The Rogosin Institute, New York, New York
The Steps Beyond Diet and Drug Therapy for Severe Hypercholesterolemia

Andrew I. Schafer, MD
The W.A. and Deborah Moncrief, Jr., Professor of Medicine and Vice Chairman, Department of Medicine, Baylor College of Medicine; Chief, Medical Service, Houston Veterans Affairs Medical Center, Houston, Texas
Aspirin and Antiplatelet Agents in Cardiovascular Disease

Edgar C. Schick, MD
Director, Echocardiography Laboratory, Lahey Hitchcock Medical Center, Burlington, Massachusetts
Management of Left Ventricular Diastolic Dysfunction

James A. Schoenberger, MD
Professor of Medicine and Professor of Preventive Medicine, Rush Medical College; Senior Attending Physician, Presbyterian–St. Luke's Hospital, Chicago, Illinois
Evaluation and Treatment of Hypertension in the Elderly Patient

Ellen W. Seely, MD
Assistant Professor of Medicine, Harvard Medical School; Director of Clinical Research, Endocrine-Hypertension Division, and Associate Program Director, General Clinical Research Center, Brigham and Women's Hospital, Boston, Massachusetts
Hypertension During Pregnancy

Ralph Shabetai, MD
Professor of Medicine, University of California, San Diego; Cardiology Section Chief, San Diego VA Medical Center, San Diego, California
Treatment of Pericardial Disease

Thomas W. Smith, MD
Professor of Medicine, Harvard Medical School; Chief, Cardiovascular Division, and Senior Physician, Brigham and Women's Hospital, Boston, Massachusetts
The Pharmacology of Heart Failure Drugs

Burton E. Sobel, MD
E. L. Amidon Professor and Chair, Department of Medicine, University of Vermont College of Medicine; Clinical Leader, Medicine Health Care Service, Fletcher Allen Health Care, Burlington, Vermont
Chronic Angina: Stable

Allen J. Solomon, MD
Assistant Professor in Medicine, Georgetown University School of Medicine; Director, Pacemaker Center; and Co-Director, Coronary Care Unit, Georgetown University Medical Center, Washington, D.C.
Ischemic Heart Disease: Surgical Options

Caren G. Solomon, MD, MPH
Instructor in Medicine, Harvard Medical School; Associate Physician, Brigham and Women's Hospital, Boston, Massachusetts
Endocrine Causes of Hypertension

Lynne Warner Stevenson, MD
Associate Professor of Medicine, Harvard Medical School; Clinical Director, Cardiomyopathy and Transplant Service, Brigham and Women's Hospital, Boston, Massachusetts
Management of Patients Hospitalized With Heart Failure
Cardiac Transplantation and Circulatory Assistance

William G. Stevenson, MD
Associate Professor of Medicine, Harvard Medical School; Co-Director, Cardiac Arrhythmia Service and Clinical Electrophysiology Laboratory, Brigham and Women's Hospital, Boston, Massachusetts
Drug Treatment of Ventricular Tachycardias

Judith L. Swain, MD
Professor of Medicine and Genetics, University of Pennsylvania School of Medicine; Chief, Cardiovascular Division, Hospital of the University of Pennsylvania, Philadelphia, Pennsylvania
Gene Therapy for Cardiovascular Disease

Stephen L. Swartz, MD
Assistant Professor of Medicine, Harvard Medical School; Associate Physician, Brigham and Women's Hospital, Boston, Massachusetts
Nonpharmacologic and Pharmacologic Treatment of Hypertension

Pierre Théroux, MD
Professor of Medicine, University of Montreal; Chief of Coronary Care Unit and Chief of Clinical Research, Montreal Heart Institute, Montreal, Quebec, Canada
Management of Unstable Angina

Eric J. Topol, MD
Professor of Medicine, Ohio State University; Chairman, Department of Cardiology; and Director, Joseph J. Jacobs Center for Thrombosis and Vascular Biology, Cleveland Clinic Foundation, Cleveland, Ohio
Angioplasty Strategies in Acute Myocardial Infarction

Michael L. Tuck, MD
Professor of Medicine, University of California, Los Angeles (UCLA), School of Medicine; Chief, Endocrinology, UCLA San Fernando Valley Medical Program, Sepulvida, California
Hypertension in Diabetes Mellitus and Obesity

Christopher S. Wilcox, MD, PhD
George E. Schreiner Professor of Nephrology, Georgetown University Medical School; Chief, Division of Nephrology and Hypertension, Georgetown University Medical Center, Washington, D.C.
Management of Hypertension in Patients With Renal Disease

David O. Williams, MD
Professor of Medicine, Brown University School of Medicine; Director, Cardiovascular Laboratory and Interventional Cardiology, Rhode Island Hospital, Providence, Rhode Island
Catheterization Interventions for the Treatment of Coronary Artery Disease: Techniques, Results, and Patient Selection

Gordon H. Williams, MD
Professor of Medicine, Harvard Medical School; Director, Clinical

Research Center and Specialized Center of Research in Hypertension, and Chief, Endocrine-Hypertension Division, Brigham and Women's Hospital, Boston, Massachusetts
Secondary Hypertension: Causes and Treatment

Michael R. Zile, MD
Professor of Medicine, Medical University of South Carolina, Charleston, South Carolina
Management of Left Ventricular Diastolic Dysfunction

Douglas P. Zipes, MD
Distinguished Professor of Medicine, Pharmacology and Toxicology, Indiana University Medical Center; Director, Cardiology Division and Krannert Institute of Cardiology, Indiana University School of Medicine, Indianapolis, Indiana
Nonpharmacologic Treatment of Supraventricular Tachycardias
Catheter Ablation of Ventricular Tachycardia
Management of Bradyarrhythmias
Use of the Implantable Cardioverter-Defibrillator for Ventricular Arrhythmias

Randall M. Zusman, MD
Associate Professor of Medicine, Harvard Medical School; Director, Division of Hypertension and Vascular Medicine, Massachusetts General Hospital; Director, Cardiac Rehabilitation and Preventive Cardiology Program, Spaulding Rehabilitation Hospital, Boston, Massachusetts
Treatment of Hypertensive Emergencies

Foreword

As recently as 1960, the treatment options available for patients with cardiovascular disease were quite limited. The major therapeutic measures included bed rest and warfarin for acute myocardial infarction; nitroglycerin for angina pectoris; dietary sodium restriction, bed rest, digitalis, and thiazide diuretics for heart failure; quinidine or procainamide for tachyarrhythmia; large, clumsy first-generation pacemakers for complete heart block; sodium restriction and ganglionic blocking agents for severe hypertension; valvuloplasty for valvular stenosis; and palliative surgery for a limited number of complex congenital cardiac malformations. Mild and even moderate hypertension were not treated, nor were attempts made on a regular basis to lower serum cholesterol in patients with coronary artery disease and hypercholesterolemia. Prosthetic cardiac valves, coronary revascularization, and modern pharmacotherapy of myocardial ischemia had not yet been developed.

No other aspect of medicine has undergone a more radical transformation since then than has cardiovascular therapeutics, and the results have been truly spectacular. Overall mortality rates from heart disease have been declining steadily, and the number of deaths secondary to coronary artery disease, the most common cause of cardiovascular deaths, has been falling at 1% per year since 1966. As we approach the end of the century, effective treatment—albeit, not cure—of almost all forms of heart disease is now possible, allowing the majority of patients with cardiovascular disease to live longer lives of high quality.

Dr. Smith and his Associate Editors, Drs. Antman, Bittl, Colucci, Gotto, Loscalzo, Williams, and Zipes, should be congratulated for providing the most comprehensive, modern text of cardiovascular therapeutics. Instead of focusing narrowly on one or another mode of therapeutics—drugs, interventional cardiology, devices, surgery, and so forth—as has been the custom in this field, this authoritative, scholarly, yet eminently readable book deals with *total* patient management. The several types of therapy that can be brought to bear on patients with specific cardiovascular disorders are presented lucidly and in sufficient detail to serve as the basis for managing the vast majority of patients with cardiovascular disease. This landmark text is of immense value not only to cardiologists but also to internists and primary care physicians, who are shouldering increasing responsibilities for the management of patients with cardiovascular disease.

I am very proud that *Cardiovascular Therapeutics* is a companion to *Heart Disease: A Textbook of Cardiovascular Medicine*. I hope that these two books, along with Marcus et al.'s *Cardiac Imaging* and the other companions currently in preparation, will serve as the basis of a complete cardiovascular library.

EUGENE BRAUNWALD, MD
Boston, Massachusetts

Preface

With the publication of *Cardiovascular Therapeutics,* we intend to fill a long-existing void in the coverage of contemporary therapeutic approaches in the treatment of patients with cardiovascular diseases. Rather than emphasizing a particular drug, catheter-based intervention, or surgical procedure, it provides the clinician with a practical, evidence-based approach to the optimal management of specific clinical problems. The full spectrum from preventive measures to management of advanced and complex disease states is covered in depth, with liberal use of algorithms to guide therapy. The book is organized according to specific clinical problems or disease states, providing the clinician with a highly practical approach to selecting and implementing the most effective therapeutic measures available, in the most appropriate sequence.

Although drawing on mechanistic insights from the fundamental disciplines of pharmacology, physiology, biochemistry, cell and molecular biology, and biophysics, recommended approaches are based first and foremost on data from controlled clinical trials. Chapter 51, by Drs. Antman and Califf, provides an informative overview of the rapidly evolving body of knowledge and experience that underlies the conduct of clinical trials and their meta-analysis and deserves the attention of all who wish to understand the principles according to which evidence-based medicine will increasingly be practiced.

The distinguished Section Editors—Drs. Antman, Bittl, Colucci, Gotto, Loscalzo, Williams, and Zipes—share with the contributors to the 57 chapters in *Cardiovascular Therapeutics* the goal of providing practical and authoritative guidance to primary care physicians and internists as well as cardiologists in the comprehensive management of patients with cardiovascular disease. We have sought to amplify and extend, rather than reiterate, the content of Eugene Braunwald's landmark *Heart Disease,* with which this companion text is extensively cross-referenced. Every effort has been made to provide the reader with up-to-date references to guide further examination of specific topics. We welcome your comments and criticisms.

THOMAS WOODWARD SMITH

Acknowledgments

I welcome this opportunity to acknowledge the debt owed to many inspiring teachers. Among the most important and memorable have been S. James Adelstein, A. Clifford Barger, Edward F. Bland, Eugene Braunwald, George F. Cahill, William B. Castle, Roman W. DeSanctis, Lewis Dexter, Daniel D. Federman, Edgar Haber, James H. Jandl, Alexander Leaf, Samuel Levine, Alexander S. Nadas, Oglesby Paul, Charles A. Sanders, Carl Snyder, Morton N. Swartz, Daniel C. Tosteson, Paul Dudley White, and Peter M. Yurchak. I have admired and learned from many others, both directly and from afar, but those named have exemplified all that medicine and science should be.

I am indebted to the Cardiology Fellows and to my colleagues on the staff and faculty of the Cardiovascular Division at Brigham and Women's Hospital for their dedication to excellence in every facet of patient care, teaching, and research and for their unfailing and thoughtful support in creating and maintaining an environment in which it has been a pleasure to work on this text. Patricia Allen, Ellen J. Edelberg, Ralph A. Kelly, Eva J. Neer, and Patrick T. O'Gara have been helpful in innumerable ways that words cannot capture.

The Section Editors, contributors, and I are grateful to Richard Zorab and his staff at the W.B. Saunders Company for their capable handling of every detail of the preparation of this text.

THOMAS WOODWARD SMITH

Contents

SECTION THREE

SECTION FOUR

SECTION FIVE

SECTION SIX

SECTION SEVEN

SECTION EIGHT

SECTION

ONE Ischemic Disease

1 Primary Prevention of Ischemic Heart Disease

Paul M. Ridker, MD
JoAnn E. Manson, MD
J. Michael Gaziano, MD
Charles H. Hennekens, MD

OVERVIEW

More than a third of all deaths in developed countries are directly attributable to coronary heart disease.[1] In the United States alone, more than 1.6 million myocardial infarctions occur annually, of which 500,000 result in death before hospitalization.[2] Among patients admitted with acute myocardial infarction, approximately 15% die during hospitalization and another 10% die during the ensuing several years.[3] Thus, although worthwhile interventions for coronary heart disease that improve survival by 20% to 25% positively affect tens of thousands of lives, a primary prevention intervention of similar magnitude could, at least in theory, avert more than 100,000 premature deaths each year in the United States alone.[4]

In this opening chapter, the epidemiologic and therapeutic rationales for primary prevention of ischemic heart disease (IHD) are outlined, including clear net benefits of cholesterol reduction, smoking cessation, blood pressure control, and weight reduction, as well as possible net benefits of postmenopausal estrogen replacement, antiplatelet therapy, antioxidant therapy, and a variety of dietary interventions. For each of these, the strength and magnitude of association with coronary heart disease based upon the totality of evidence is summarized. In addition, issues in screening for IHD are discussed as they pertain to emerging hemostatic and thrombotic risk factors such as fibrinogen, endogenous fibrinolytic capacity, homocysteine, and lipoprotein(a), as well as usual coronary risk factors such as total and high-density lipoprotein (HDL) cholesterol. Finally, for interventions on which epidemiologic and clinical consensus exist, guidelines are supplied to direct the physician toward effective cardiovascular disease prevention.

EPIDEMIOLOGY OF PRIMARY PREVENTION

Since 1965, there have been dramatic declines in mortality rates from coronary heart disease and myocardial infarction in both men and women in the United States (Fig. 1–1). In large part, these declines have been the combined result of population-wide behavioral and dietary risk factor modifications, physician-targeted cholesterol and blood pressure interventions, and improved therapies for patients with diagnosed disease. Coronary heart disease, however, remains the leading cause of death in all men and in women over the age of 40 (Fig. 1–2). In fact, diseases of the heart and blood vessels are responsible for almost 1,000,000 American deaths annually, almost as many as from all other causes of death combined.

Successful prevention of cardiovascular disease requires an understanding of epidemiologic principles regarding identification of high-risk persons, differentiation between modifiable and nonmodifiable risk factors, distinction between association and causation, and comprehension of the strengths and limitations of various study designs. In large part, primary prevention guidelines have been based on descriptive and observational analytic studies, as well as on experimental trials.[5]

Descriptive Study Design

Descriptive studies include cross-sectional surveys, cross-cultural comparisons, and studies of temporal trends in selected populations. In cross-sectional surveys, disease prevalence and exposure variables are typically assessed at a single time in a large group of persons. In cross-cultural studies, similar parameters are compared between different populations. Cross-sectional and cross-cultural studies form the basis for much of the understanding of cardiovascular risk. For example, the landmark Seven Countries Study[6] and its World Health

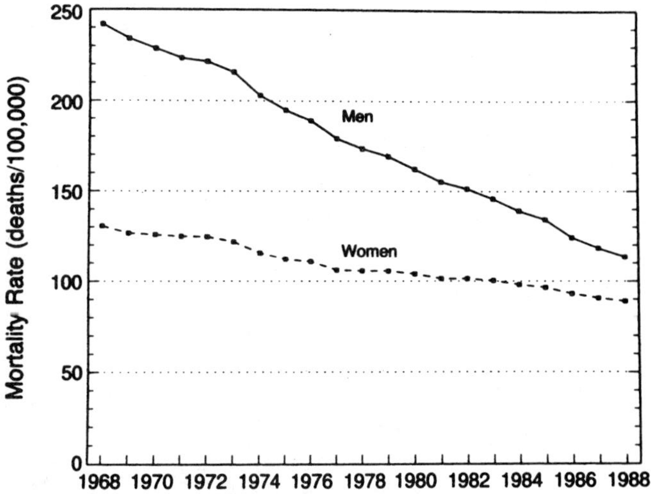

Figure 1–1. Annual mortality rates from acute myocardial infarction among men and women in the United States, 1968–1988. (From Manson JE, Tosteson H, Ridker PM, et al: The primary prevention of myocardial infarction. N Engl J Med 1992; 326:1406–1416.)

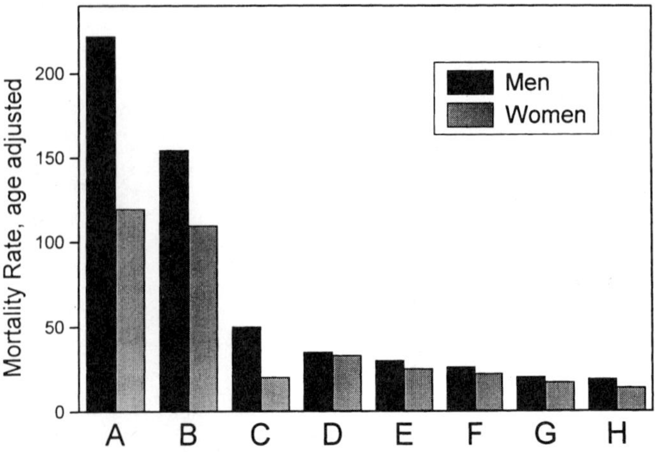

Figure 1–2. Death rates by disease. *Key:* A, heart disease; B, malignancy; C, accidents; D, cerebrovascular disease; E, chronic obstructive pulmonary disease; F, pneumonia; G, liver disease; H, diabetes mellitus. (From the U.S. Public Health Service, National Center for Health Statistics: Vital Statistics of the United States. Washington, DC: U.S. Government Printing Office, 1988.)

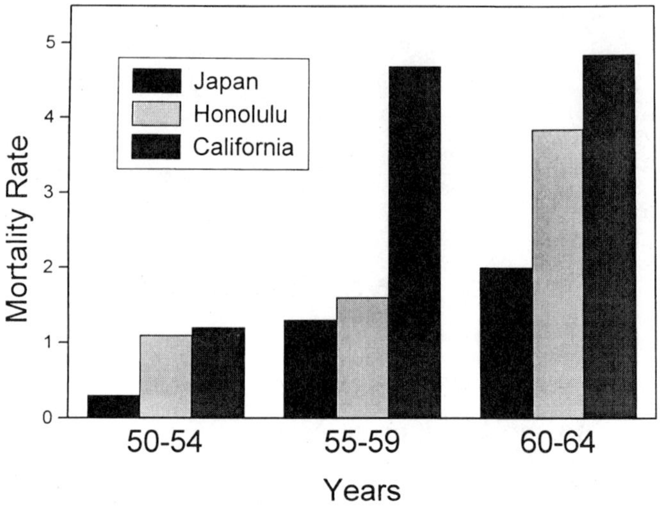

Figure 1–4. Death rates from coronary heart disease in the Ni-Hon-San Study. (From Ockene IS, Ockene JK: Prevention of Coronary Heart Disease. Boston: Little, Brown, 1992.)

Organization (WHO) follow-up[7] clearly demonstrated that regions in which the average cholesterol intake is high, such as Finland, Great Britain, and the United States, have substantially higher incidences of coronary heart disease than do regions in which dietary fat consumption is lower, such as Japan (Fig. 1–3).

Cross-sectional studies have been critical in elucidating differences between genetic and environmental risk factors. For example, migration studies of Japanese men moving to Honolulu and San Francisco,[8] Irish men and women moving to Boston,[9] and Indian men moving to London[10] all indicate that environmental factors are responsible for a major component of cardiovascular risk. The best known migration study is the Ni-Hon-San study,[8] in which rates of mortality from coronary heart disease were lower among Japanese men living in Japan than among Japanese men living in Hawaii. Mortality rates for coronary heart disease for both these groups were lower than mortality rates for genetically similar men living in San Francisco (Fig. 1–4).

Cross-sectional and cross-cultural autopsy studies of patients who died from noncardiovascular causes have also contributed to the understanding of the pathophysiology of atherosclerotic progression. In particular, such studies demonstrate clear associations between plasma lipid levels and severity of atherosclerosis in the aortic and coronary vessels, even among young subjects.[11–13] Cross-cultural studies have also been important in the understanding of geographic differences in the prevalence of aortic and coronary atherosclerosis[14] (Fig. 1–5).

The primary weakness of descriptive studies results from the inability to control for potential factors that may confound apparent associations. In cardiovascular disease epidemiology, known potential confounders include age, sex, smoking status, body mass, genetic background, and a variety of social and behavioral characteristics. Moreover, cross-sectional studies cannot distinguish association from causation. Thus, descriptive studies must generally be viewed as hypothesis generating rather than hypothesis testing.

Analytic Study Designs

Observational Cohort and Case-Control Studies

In contrast to descriptive studies, observational analytic studies allow for substantially improved control of confounding. Analytic studies generally involve a case-control or prospective cohort design. In case-control studies, persons with disease are compared with persons free of disease, and differences in past exposure histories are compared. Case-control studies are efficient and particularly well suited for assessing rare disease states. However, the criteria by which case and control subjects are defined can lead to selection bias, and differences in ability between case and control subjects to

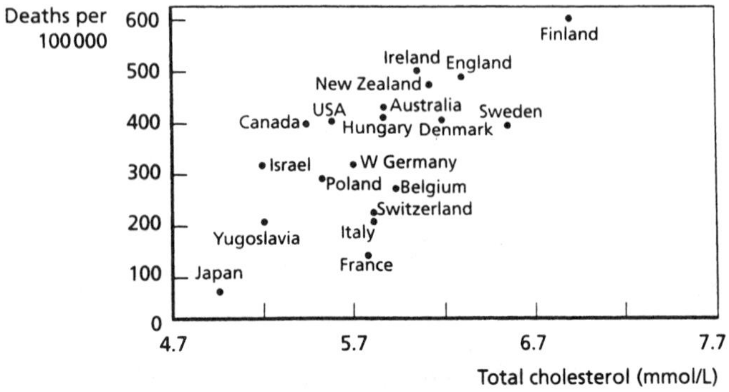

Figure 1–3. Mean total cholesterol level from surveys of various countries plotted against annual coronary mortality. (From Thompson GR, Wilson PW: Coronary Risk Factors and Their Assessment. London: Science Press, 1992.)

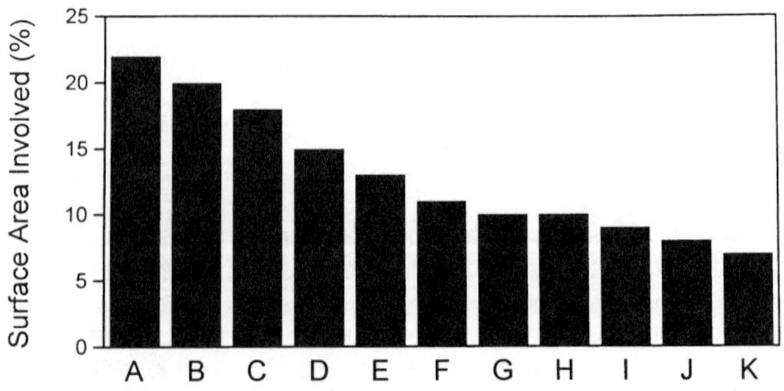

Figure 1–5. International Atherosclerosis Project: extent of aortic and coronary atherosclerosis at autopsy, showing percentage of surface involved by raised lesions for people dying of nonvascular causes. *Key:* A, New Orleans white; B, Oslo; C, Durban Indian; D, New Orleans black; E, Caracas white; F, Puerto Rican white; G, Cali; H, Mexican; I, Sao Paulo black; J, Bogota; K, Durban black.

remember details of exposures can lead to recall bias. These and other epidemiologic limitations can substantially affect results of case-control studies. Nonetheless, case-control studies continue to prove useful in defining new risk factors for IHD. For example, risk factors associated with triggering of acute thrombosis have recently been elucidated with the use of a modification of the case-control design.[15] In addition, unlike purely descriptive analyses, case-control studies allow for the temporal effect of a risk factor to be assessed, because recall of potential exposures occurring before the onset of the disease state is typically sought.

In analytic studies employing a cohort design, exposure status in a given population is typically ascertained at the beginning of the study, and subjects are prospectively observed for the future occurrence of disease. Thus, in contrast to case-control studies, cohort studies select subjects on the basis of exposure. Such studies are particularly well suited for assessing the effects of rare exposures on the risk of future disease. Cohort studies can be *prospective* (in which exposure status is assessed at the time of study initiation), *retrospective* (in which the exposure and disease records used are in existence before study initiation), or *ambispective* (in which existent exposure records are typically combined with further prospective follow-up).

Cohort analyses are less subject to confounding, because a wealth of exposure data can be accumulated for each individual, allowing investigators to stratify analyses for a variety of potential confounding variables. Prospective cohort studies have the further advantage of minimizing recall and selection bias, because exposure is assessed before the development of disease. Furthermore, because exposure data can be obtained on several known and investigational parameters, prospective cohort studies can be used to evaluate interactions between putative risk factors. If appropriately designed, plasma and DNA sampling can be done in prospective cohort studies, allowing for the examination of the effects of biologic parameters many years before the occurrence of overt clinical disease.

It is not surprising that prospective cohort studies have played a major role in describing the epidemiology of IHD and in shaping prevention policies. The Framingham Heart Study among long-term residents of Framingham, Massachusetts,[16] and the Nurses' Health Study[17] of 120,000 female nurses and health professionals are examples of major studies employing prospective cohort designs.

Experimental Study Designs

Analytic studies are particularly useful in developing prevention strategies when the risks associated with a given exposure are moderate to large. However, when the expected benefit of an intervention (or hazard of an exposure) is moderate to small, the uncontrolled confounding inherent in even the best analytic studies has the potential to be as or even more extensive than the effect under evaluation. In this situation, it can be difficult to obtain definitive positive results and/or informative null results. In such situations, experimental studies in which the intervention (or exposure) of interest is allocated by the researcher have particular value.

The most reliable study design in cardiovascular medicine is the randomized clinical trial (see Chapter 51). A fundamental advantage of the randomized trial is that all potential confounding factors—both those known and those unknown—are equally distributed between study groups, provided the cohort is large enough. Furthermore, if efforts are made to render trials double-blind, then all cointerventions occurring after randomization are equally distributed between study groups. Thus, appropriately designed randomized, double-blind, placebo-controlled trials of adequate sample size can minimize confounding and bias to the point where effects as small as 10% to 15% can be accurately assessed. A further advantage of the randomized trial is that both risks and benefits of a given exposure or intervention can be evaluated. This advantage is a major consideration in settings in which a drug with potential benefits but known toxicities is being considered for primary or secondary prevention.

Although they supply the most persuasive data, randomized trials are neither necessary nor desirable for many risk factors of concern; for example, randomized allocation of interventions such as cessation of smoking would likely raise serious ethical concerns. However, in situations in which the true risks and benefits of an intervention are unclear, randomized trials may be the only way to obtain meaningful data; for example, randomized trials are clearly needed to ascertain whether the postulated net benefits of estrogen replacement therapy on cardiovascular disease outweigh its potential and known risks related to cancers of the breast and uterus. Although difficult to render double-blind, randomized trials of weight reduction and physical activity are also useful for confirming findings from observational cohort studies.

EVOLVING CONCEPTS IN ATHEROGENESIS: RELEVANCE FOR PRIMARY PREVENTION

In addition to issues regarding study design, current concepts in the pathogenesis of atherosclerosis are fundamental for physicians concerned with the primary prevention of IHD. In brief, the development and progression of atherosclerosis is now generally believed to occur in two distinct phases. The initial slow, progressive phase of atherosclerosis appears in large part to result from an exaggerated inflammatory response to injury of the arterial wall.[18, 19] This slow phase of atherogenesis was classically believed to progress inevitably toward vascular occlusion. However, abundant data indicate that there exists a second rapid phase of atherosclerotic development, in which established plaque undergoes sudden rupture and the underlying lipid pool is subsequently exposed to the circulation.[20, 21] Such ruptures or fissures can acutely disrupt the intimal surface and lead to rapid platelet aggregation, thrombus formation, and acute ischemia.[22] More often than not, complete occlusion does not ensue, because of the activation of endogenous fibrinolysis. In addition, accumulating data indicate that certain types of plaque are more likely to rupture than others: specifically, plaques prone to rupture tend to be smaller and less fibrotic and to have a softer extracellular lipid matrix.[23] An extensive review of the atherogenic process can be found in other chapters of this text.

Evolving concepts of atherosclerotic development and plaque rupture are important to therapies for primary prevention for several reasons. First, it is now clear that factors involved in the initiation of atherosclerosis are likely to be different from factors involved in the rapid progression of prevalent lesions. Thus the prevention-oriented physician may wish to consider *atherogenic* risk factors, such as total and HDL cholesterol, as being somewhat distinct from *thrombogenic* risk factors, such as plasma fibrinogen, endogenous fibrinolytic capacity, homocysteine, and lipoprotein(a).

Second, recently published data from the Pathological Determinants of Atherosclerosis in Youth[13] Study Group confirm that as early as age 15, a substantial portion of the abdominal aorta is involved with atherosclerotic precursor lesions in persons with coronary risk factors. Moreover, these precursor lesions do not occur randomly; rather, they appear to have predictable topographic distributions, which suggests that local factors such as shear stress may be important in the initiation of vascular injury. Thus prevention-oriented clinicians need to consider whether interventions such as lipid reduction should begin early in life rather than being delayed until substantial atherosclerosis is present.

Third, the fact that acute rupture can lead to complete coronary occlusion greatly helps explain the apparent clinical paradox that myocardial infarction occurs more often in vessels with underlying stenoses of less than 70% than in vessels with tighter obstruction.[24, 25] Indeed, recognition that tight stenoses reliably predict flow-limiting angina but are less reliable as markers for the infarct-related artery has had a major impact on how clinicians think about coronary angioplasty and bypass surgery as revascularization techniques.

Fourth, because one immediate response to plaque rupture is

activation of platelet function with subsequent platelet and fibrin deposition, the plaque fissure hypothesis provides a conceptual framework for understanding in part the efficacy of antiplatelet therapy in both the primary and secondary prevention of myocardial infarction.[26] Moreover, the hypothesis that short-term activation of platelets is a critical process in thrombus formation is consistent with the clinical observation that prophylactic aspirin results in an inhibition of thrombosis but not a slowing of the atherosclerotic process itself.[27]

Finally, the plaque rupture hypothesis also helps explain the fact that acute vascular occlusion is not a random event but one that occurs with a predictable circadian variation in such a way that the onset of symptoms is clustered in the early morning hours.[28] Because several physiologic markers, including catecholamine levels and platelet aggregation, also peak during this time interval, it has been hypothesized that specific "triggers" may exist for thrombus formation and that preventive and therapeutic measures such as beta blockers[29] and antiplatelets[30] may exert much of their beneficial influence by blunting the effect of these circadian stresses.

In addition to evolving theories of plaque rupture, current concepts regarding the role of oxidized low-density lipoprotein (LDL) and dysfunctional endothelium have become important as they too form the basis of several approaches to prevention of cardiovascular disease. Oxidation of LDL appears to be an important mechanism in the initiation and progression of atherosclerosis.[31] In this regard, initial data indicate that oxidative modification of LDL results in enhanced foam cell formation and increased rates of LDL accumulation within developing lesions. However, accumulating data suggest other mechanisms for the atherogenic properties of oxidized LDL, including direct cytotoxicity to the endothelium.[32] At the same time, it is becoming apparent that atherosclerosis alters the normal function of the vascular endothelium, a structure that, in addition to serving as a permeable barrier between the blood elements and the underlying smooth muscle, also has several important antithrombotic and fibrinolytic functions. As discussed later, evolving therapeutic strategies that may be able to reverse and/or inhibit these pathologic processes are becoming available to the prevention-oriented physician.

THERAPEUTIC APPROACHES

Cholesterol Reduction

A series of major case-control and prospective cohort studies have documented that increased levels of serum cholesterol are strongly associated with risk of future coronary heart disease. Overall, this relationship appears remarkably linear in that a 1% increase in total cholesterol is associated with a 2% to 3% increase in risk of coronary heart disease.[33] Overview data indicate that the risk of hypercholesterolemia is even higher at younger ages, in that a 10% increase in total cholesterol was found to be associated with a 54% increase in risk at age 40, a 39% increase in risk at age 50, a 27% increase in risk at age 60, and a 20% increase in risk at age 70.[34, 35] Furthermore, prospective cohort data among patient populations with "low" cholesterol levels suggest that there is unlikely to be a lower threshold to risk. For example, in a study of Chinese men with total cholesterol levels below 190 mg/dL, 10% increases in total cholesterol were associated with approximately 20% increases in risk.[36] Although data are limited, similar associations appear to be present for women. More recent analyses controlling for regression-dilution bias and surrogate-dilution bias indicate that the true association between total cholesterol and coronary heart disease may be even larger than these estimates.[34, 35]

Other abundant data also indicate an important and highly significant inverse association between HDL cholesterol and risk of coronary heart disease.[37, 38] For patient counseling, the ratio of LDL cholesterol to HDL cholesterol may prove to be the most clinically useful lipid parameter. In one large-scale prospective cohort study, a one-unit decrease in this ratio was associated with a 53% decrease in the risk of future myocardial infarction.[39]

A demonstration of association between cholesterol and risk of vascular disease does not on its own imply that levels should be reduced by dietary or pharmacologic means. However, available randomized trial data clearly demonstrate clinically important reductions in risk when LDL cholesterol levels are reduced. Overviews of trials of primary and secondary prevention now include more than 4000 coronary heart disease events among nearly 46,000 participants.[40–43] Overall, 10% reductions in serum cholesterol appear to be associated with reductions in IHD mortality of between 3% and 16% and reductions in IHD events of 13% to 22%. These effects increase with prolonged duration of therapy so that similar reductions in serum cholesterol are associated with a 7% reduction in coronary heart disease events at 2 years, 22% reductions at 5 years, and 25% reductions among those treated for more than 5 years.[34, 35] Although the majority of these data are derived from studies of men, similar data are available for women with regard to secondary prevention.

Epidemiologic findings that cholesterol reduction results in reduced rates of future coronary events has been corroborated by data from several angiographic studies that indicate that initiation of lipid-lowering strategies can lead to a slowing of atherosclerotic progression and, in some cases, to a reduction in the degree of luminal stenosis.[44–49] In an overview of angiographic trials of aggressive lipoprotein management involving more than 2000 subjects, the proportion of patients arteriographically defined as progressing was reduced 24% by lipid intervention. At the same time, the proportion of patients defined as angiographically regressing increased 20%, in comparison with control subjects[50] (Fig. 1–6). These angiographic benefits appear in studies as short as 2 to 4 years. Regression, however, appears less likely to occur among persons with normal cholesterol levels.[51]

Age-stratified population-based distributions of total cholesterol, LDL cholesterol, and HDL cholesterol are provided in Table 1–1. Largely on the basis of data indicating that atherosclerosis can be reversed and that lower levels of total cholesterol may improve mortality, the National Cholesterol Education Program revised the Adult Treatment Panel (ATP-II) guidelines in June 1993 to reflect the high priority of reducing cholesterol in patients with existing coronary disease or established high risk.[52] These revised guidelines further call for screening for HDL cholesterol in all subjects as part of the stratification process. The ATP-II panel also recommended an easing of criteria for primary intervention, particularly among asymptomatic young adults, asymptomatic women of middle age, and the elderly.

Current APT-II algorithms regarding cholesterol reduction for primary and secondary prevention are provided in Figures 1–7 and 1–8. For suitable persons, both algorithms suggest dietary and pharmacologic intervention on the basis of level of LDL cholesterol and risk factors present (including HDL level), as outlined in Table 1–2. Although methods are becoming available to allow for direct assessment of LDL cholesterol, most clinical situations do not require more than a simple fasting cholesterol screen. Provided that the total triglyceride level is less than 400 mg/dL and no abnormal intermediate density lipoproteins are present, LDL cholesterol can be estimated as follows:

$$\text{LDL cholesterol} = \text{total cholesterol} - (\text{HDL cholesterol} + \text{triglycerides}/5).$$

A brief summary of available cholesterol-reducing medications is provided in Table 1–3. These are reviewed in detail in other chapters of this text (see Chapter 25).

Controversy exists in the cholesterol literature regarding potential hazards of nonvascular mortality associated with aggressive cholesterol reduction.[53–55] This controversy has in large part arisen from an apparent excess of traumatic deaths reported in the Helsinki Heart

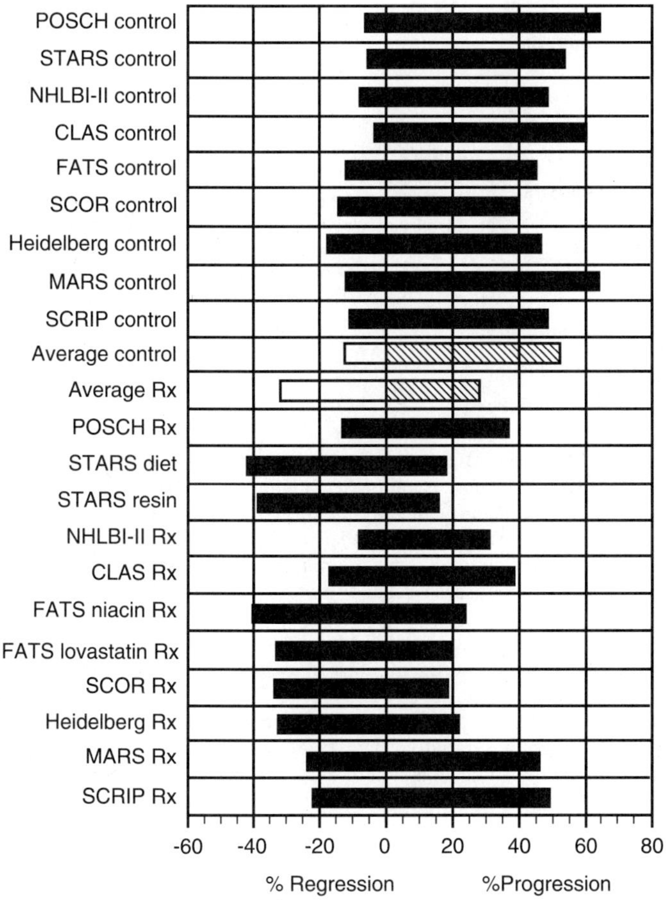

Figure 1–6. Arteriographic evidence of regression and progression in 10 controlled trials of lipid reduction. *Abbreviations:* POSCH, Program on the Surgical Control of the Hyperlipidemias; STARS, St. Thomas Arteriographic Regression Study; NHLBI-II, National Heart, Lung and Blood Institute; CLAS, Cholesterol Lowering Atherosclerosis Study; FATS, Familial Atherosclerosis Treatment Study; SCOR, San Francisco Specialized Center of Research; MARS, Monitored Atherosclerosis Regression Study; SCRIP, Stanford Coronary Risk Intervention Project. (From Superko HR, Krauss RM: Coronary artery disease regression: convincing evidence for the benefit of aggressive lipoprotein management. Circulation 1994; 90:1056–1069.)

Study trial of gemfibrozil[56] and in the Lipid Research Clinics trial of cholestyramine.[57] It is important to note, however, that the total numbers of traumatic events in these trials were exceptionally low and the resultant risk estimates highly unstable. Furthermore, the cause of nonvascular mortality differed in these studies, making it difficult to ascribe any single pathophysiologic process to this potential hazard. Resolving these issues requires the randomization of sufficiently large numbers of patients to accrue adequate numbers of vascular and non–vascular-related deaths. At this time, at least 14 major trials of cholesterol reduction are under way.

The recently reported Scandinavian Simvastatin Survival Study involving 4444 patients with known coronary artery disease has for the first time demonstrated reductions in total mortality with an aggressive lipid-lowering regimen. In this prospective study,[58] the use of a hydroxy-3-methylglutaryl coenzyme A (HMG-CoA) reductase inhibitor over a period of 5 years was associated with a 30% reduction in total mortality, a 42% reduction in cardiovascular mortality, and a 37% reduction in the need for revascularization. Of importance, no excess of non–cardiovascular-related deaths was found in the study.

Population-wide goals for the year 2000 have been established by the U.S. Department of Health and Human Services; they include

TABLE 1–1. GUIDES TO PLASMA CHOLESTEROL AND TRIGLYCERIDE VALUES

Age (Years)	White Males (Percentiles)							White Females (Percentiles)						
	5	10	25	50	75	90	95	5	10	25	50	75	90	95
Plasma Total Cholesterol (mg/dL) (Population Distribution)														
0–4	—	—	—	—	—	—	—	—	—	—	—	—	—	—
5–9	125	131	141	153	168	183	189	131	136	151	164	176	190	197
10–14	124	131	144	160	173	188	202	125	131	142	159	171	191	205
15–19	118	123	136	152	168	183	191	118	126	140	157	176	198	207
20–24	118	126	142	159	179	197	212	121	132	147	165	186	220	237
25–29	130	137	154	176	199	223	234	130	142	158	178	198	217	231
30–34	142	152	171	190	213	237	258	133	141	158	178	199	215	228
35–39	147	157	176	195	222	248	267	139	149	165	186	209	233	249
40–44	150	160	179	204	229	251	260	146	156	172	193	220	241	259
45–49	163	171	188	210	235	258	275	148	162	182	204	231	256	268
50–54	157	168	189	211	237	263	274	163	171	188	214	240	267	281
55–59	161	172	188	214	236	260	280	167	182	201	229	251	278	294
60–64	163	170	191	215	237	262	287	172	186	207	226	251	282	300
65–69	166	174	192	213	250	275	288	167	179	212	233	259	282	291
70+	144	160	185	214	236	253	265	173	181	196	226	249	268	280
Plasma VLDL-Cholesterol (mg/dL) (Population Distribution)														
0–4	—	—	—	—	—	—	—	—	—	—	—	—	—	—
5–9	0	2	4	7	11	15	18	1	1	4	9	13	19	24
10–14	1	2	5	9	13	18	22	2	3	6	10	15	20	23
15–19	2	3	8	12	17	23	26	2	3	6	11	15	22	24
20–24	1	5	8	12	18	24	28	2	4	8	13	18	24	28
25–29	3	6	9	15	22	31	36	2	3	7	11	19	24	29
30–34	1	5	8	11	26	36	48	1	3	6	11	17	21	27
35–39	3	7	12	19	30	46	56	2	3	8	13	21	29	36
40–44	5	8	14	21	30	43	56	3	5	8	13	20	28	32
45–49	5	8	13	20	31	40	51	2	4	9	15	22	33	41
50–54	8	10	14	23	33	49	62	2	5	9	15	23	32	37
55–59	3	6	11	19	28	39	49	2	4	9	18	28	37	49
60–64	3	4	9	16	23	35	44	1	3	6	13	20	29	39
65–69	0	3	8	16	23	40	45	0	3	7	13	21	36	41
70+	0	3	7	15	23	31	38	0	1	6	13	19	32	48
Plasma LDL-Cholesterol (mg/dL) (Population Distribution)														
0–4	—	—	—	—	—	—	—	—	—	—	—	—	—	—
5–9	63	69	80	90	103	117	129	68	73	88	98	115	125	140
10–14	64	72	81	94	109	122	132	68	73	81	94	110	126	136
15–19	62	68	80	93	109	123	130	59	65	78	93	111	129	137
20–24	66	73	85	101	118	138	147	57	65	82	102	118	141	159
25–29	70	75	96	116	138	157	165	71	77	90	108	126	148	164
30–34	78	88	107	124	144	166	185	70	77	91	109	128	147	156
35–39	81	92	110	131	154	176	189	75	81	96	116	139	161	172
40–44	87	98	115	135	157	173	186	74	84	104	122	146	165	174
45–49	98	106	120	141	163	186	202	79	89	105	127	150	173	186
50–54	89	102	118	143	162	185	197	88	94	111	134	160	186	201
55–59	88	103	123	145	168	191	203	89	97	120	145	168	199	210
60–64	83	106	121	143	165	188	210	100	105	126	149	168	191	224
65–69	98	104	125	146	170	199	210	92	99	125	151	184	205	221
70+	88	100	119	142	164	182	186	96	108	127	147	170	189	206
Plasma HDL-Cholesterol (mg/dL) (Population Distribution)														
0–4	—	—	—	—	—	—	—	—	—	—	—	—	—	—
5–9	38	42	49	54	63	70	74	36	38	47	52	61	67	73
10–14	37	40	46	55	61	71	74	37	40	45	52	58	64	70
15–19	30	34	39	46	52	59	63	35	38	43	51	61	68	74
20–24	30	32	38	45	51	57	63	33	37	44	51	62	72	79
25–29	31	32	37	44	50	38	63	37	39	47	55	63	74	83
30–34	28	32	38	45	52	59	63	36	40	46	55	64	73	77
35–39	29	31	36	43	49	58	62	34	38	44	53	64	74	82
40–44	27	31	36	43	51	60	67	34	39	48	56	65	79	88
45–49	30	33	38	45	52	60	64	34	41	47	58	68	82	87
50–54	28	31	36	44	51	58	63	37	41	50	62	73	85	91
55–59	28	31	38	46	55	64	71	37	41	50	60	73	85	91
60–64	30	34	41	49	61	69	74	38	44	51	61	75	87	92
65–69	30	33	39	49	62	74	78	35	38	49	62	73	85	98
70+	31	33	40	48	56	70	75	33	38	48	60	71	82	92

Abbreviations: VLDL, very low density lipoprotein; LDL, low-density lipoprotein; HDL, high-density lipoprotein.

From Expert Panel on Detection, Evaluation, and Treatment of High Blood Cholesterol in Adults: Summary of the Second Report of the National Cholesterol Education Program (NCEP) Expert Panel on Detection, Evaluation, and Treatment of High Blood Cholesterol in Adults (Adult Treatment Panel II). JAMA 1993; 269:3015–3023.

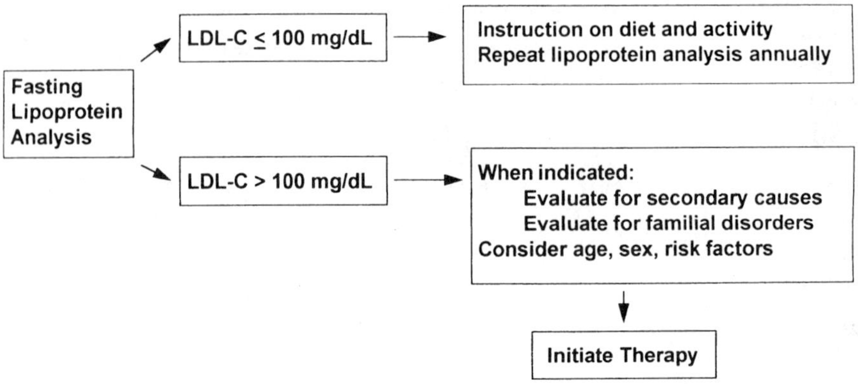

Figure 1–7. Secondary prevention strategy for cholesterol reduction in adults without evidence of coronary artery disease. (Adapted from the Expert Panel on Detection, Evaluation, and Treatment of High Blood Cholesterol in Adults: Summary of the Second Report of the National Cholesterol Education Program [NCEP] Expert Panel on Detection, Evaluation, and Treatment of High Blood Cholesterol in Adults [Adult Treatment Panel II]. JAMA 1993; 269:3015–3023.)

reducing the mean total cholesterol level among U.S. adults to 200 mg/dL or lower and reducing the proportion of U.S. adults with cholesterol levels above 240 to less than 20%. There is accumulating evidence that meeting these goals is within reach and that doing so would represent a major public health achievement. It is important to recall, however, that the relationship between cholesterol level and coronary heart disease risk is graded and that more than one third of all myocardial infarctions occur among persons with "desirable" cholesterol levels.

Smoking Cessation

Cigarette smoking is the most important modifiable risk factor for all forms of coronary heart disease and is directly responsible for more than 115,000 coronary heart disease–related deaths each year in the United States. Landmark epidemiologic studies published in the late 1950s clearly linked smoking with heart disease.[59, 60] Since then, an ever increasing number of case-control and prospective cohort studies in men have demonstrated that smoking increases coronary heart disease–related mortality by over 50%.[61] Among women, smoking accounts for more than half of all myocardial infarctions before age 55.[17, 62] Moreover, a clear dose-response relationship exists between number of cigarettes smoked and risk of coronary heart disease.

Fortunately, the relative risk of myocardial infarction among ex-smokers declines rapidly. Data from both descriptive and analytic studies demonstrate that within 2 to 3 years of smoking cessation, the risk of myocardial infarction for most persons declines to levels

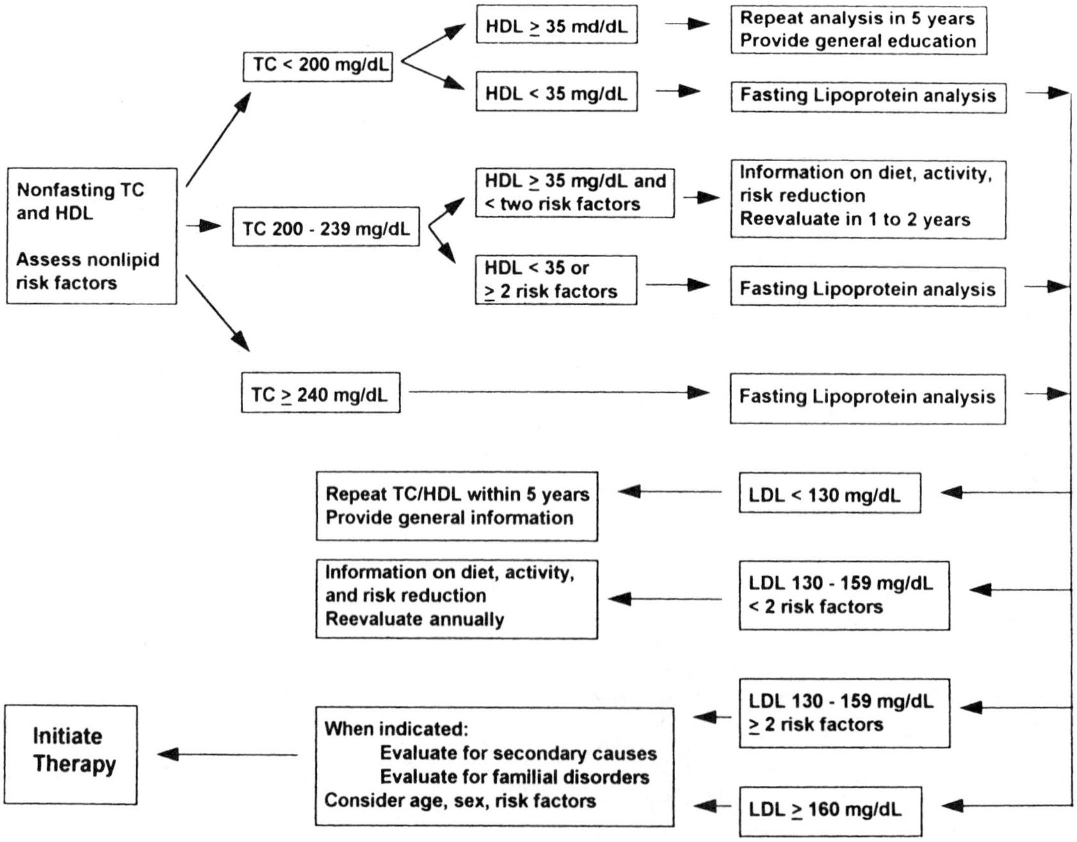

Figure 1–8. Primary prevention strategy for cholesterol reduction in adults with evidence of coronary artery disease. (Adapted from Expert Panel on Detection, Evaluation, and Treatment of High Blood Cholesterol in Adults: Summary of the Second Report of the National Cholesterol Education Program [NCEP] Expert Panel on Detection, Evaluation, and Treatment of High Blood Cholesterol in Adults [Adult Treatment Panel II]. JAMA 1993; 269:3015–3023.)

TABLE 1–2. TREATMENT DECISIONS BASED ON LDL-CHOLESTEROL LEVEL

Patient Category	Initiation Level	LDL Goal
Initiate Dietary Therapy at Designated LDL Level if Patient . . .		
Does not have CAD and has fewer than two risk factors	≥160 mg/dL (4.1 mmol/L)	<160 mg/dL (4.1 mmol/L)
Does not have CAD and has two or more risk factors	≥130 mg/dL (3.4 mmol/L)	<130 mg/dL (3.4 mmol/L)
Has established CAD	≥100 mg/dL (2.6 mmol/L)	≤100 mg/dL (2.6 mmol/L)
Initiate Drug Treatment at Designated LDL Level if Patient. . . .		
Does not have CAD and has fewer than two risk factors	≥190 mg/dL (4.9 mmol/L)	<160 mg/dL (4.1 mmol/L)
Does not have CAD and has two or more risk factors	≥160 mg/dL (4.1 mmol/L)	<130 mg/dL (3.4 mmol/L)
Has established CAD	≥130 mg/dL (3.4 mmol/L)	≤100 mg/dL (2.6 mmol/L)

Abbreviations: CAD, coronary artery disease; LDL, low-density lipoprotein.

Adapted from the Expert Panel on Detection, Evaluation, and Treatment of High Blood Cholesterol in Adults: Summary of the Second Report of the National Cholesterol Education Program (NCEP) Expert Panel on Detection, Evaluation, and Treatment of High Blood Cholesterol in Adults (Adult Treatment Panel II). JAMA 1993; 269:3015–3023.

only slightly higher than that of nonsmokers.[63] For high-risk groups, the elderly, and patients with prevalent coronary disease, studies of smoking cessation have shown more gradual declines in risk in such a manner that risk estimates approach baseline levels after approximately 5 to 7 years.

Although per capita cigarette consumption continues to decline in the United States, cigarette use has actually increased among certain groups, particularly women under the age of 30. Furthermore, smoking rates tend to be inversely related to socioeconomic status and education, which indicates a continued need for targeted public health initiatives. For current smokers, strategies with proven effectiveness in smoking cessation, including nicotine replacement therapy[64, 65] and psychosocial counseling, should be implemented. In general, the efficacy of smoking intervention programs tends to be higher for pharmacologic interventions than for self-help programs. However, most smokers who quit do not use any organized cessation program.

From a primary prevention perspective, a fundamental goal must be to reduce the numbers of people who start smoking. This strategy is effective largely because few people who remain nonsmokers by age 20 ultimately become habitual nicotine consumers. Community-based initiatives to establish smoke-free worksites, public buildings, and entertainment establishments have proved critical in countering aggressive marketing to vulnerable teenagers by the tobacco industry.[66] The wider recognition of passive smoking as a potential cause of heart disease should also help to achieve this goal. In this regard, current data support the conclusion that environmental tobacco smoke appears to increase coronary heart disease–related mortality among nonsmokers[67] and may be responsible for as many as 40,000 IHD deaths in the United States each year.[68]

Blood Pressure Control

Data from a large series of prospective cohort studies indicate that elevated blood pressure is positively associated with risks of myocardial infarction, stroke, and vascular-related death. In an overview, a direct linear relationship was found between usual diastolic blood pressure and risk of all coronary heart disease (Fig. 1–9).[69] No evidence of a threshold effect is apparent in this overview, even at the lower end of the distribution of pressures. Overall, a 7 mm Hg increase in diastolic blood pressure was associated with a 27% increase in coronary heart disease risk and a 42% increase in stroke risk.

For patients with severe elevations of blood pressure, risks of myocardial infarction and stroke are so elevated that interventional

TABLE 1–3. SUMMARY OF LIPID-LOWERING AGENTS

Agents	Mechanism of Action	Biochemical Side Effects	Systemic Side Effects	Daily Dosage Range (Drug)
Bile acid resins	Increases excretion of bile acids in the stool, increases LDL receptor activity	May prevent absorption of fat-soluble vitamins	Constipation, bloating	4–24 g (cholestyramine) 5–30 g (colestipol)
Nicotinic acid	Decreases plasma levels of free fatty acids, possibly inhibits cholesterol synthesis, decreases hepatic VLDL synthesis	Altered liver function test results, increased uric acid, increased glucose intolerance	Cutaneous flushing, pruritus, GI distress	2–6 g (crystalline nicotinic acid) 1–2 g (sustained-release nicotinic acid)
Probucol	Enhances scavenger pathway removal of LDL	Decreased HDL	Diarrhea, nausea, flatulence	1000 mg (probucol)
Fibric acid derivatives	Decreases hepatic VLDL synthesis, increases lipoprotein lipase activity	Altered liver function test results, increased CPK, potentiation of warfarin	Increased incidence of cholelithiasis and perhaps of GI cancer; myositis, diarrhea, nausea, rash (rare)	1200 mg (gemfibrozil) 400 mg (bezafibrate) 100 mg (ciprofibrate) 200 mg (fenofibrate) 2000 mg (clofibrate)
HMG-CoA reductase inhibitors	Inhibits HMG-CoA reductase, increases LDL receptor activity	Elevated transaminase levels, increased CPK	Mild GI symptoms; myositis syndrome	10–80 mg (lovastatin) 10–40 mg (pravastatin) 5–40 mg (simvastatin) 10–40 mg (fluvastatin)

Abbreviations: LDL, low-density lipoprotein; VLDL, very low density lipoprotein; HDL, high-density lipoprotein; GI, gastrointestinal; CPK, creatine phosphokinase; HMG-CoA, 3-hydroxy-3-methylglutaryl–coenzyme A.

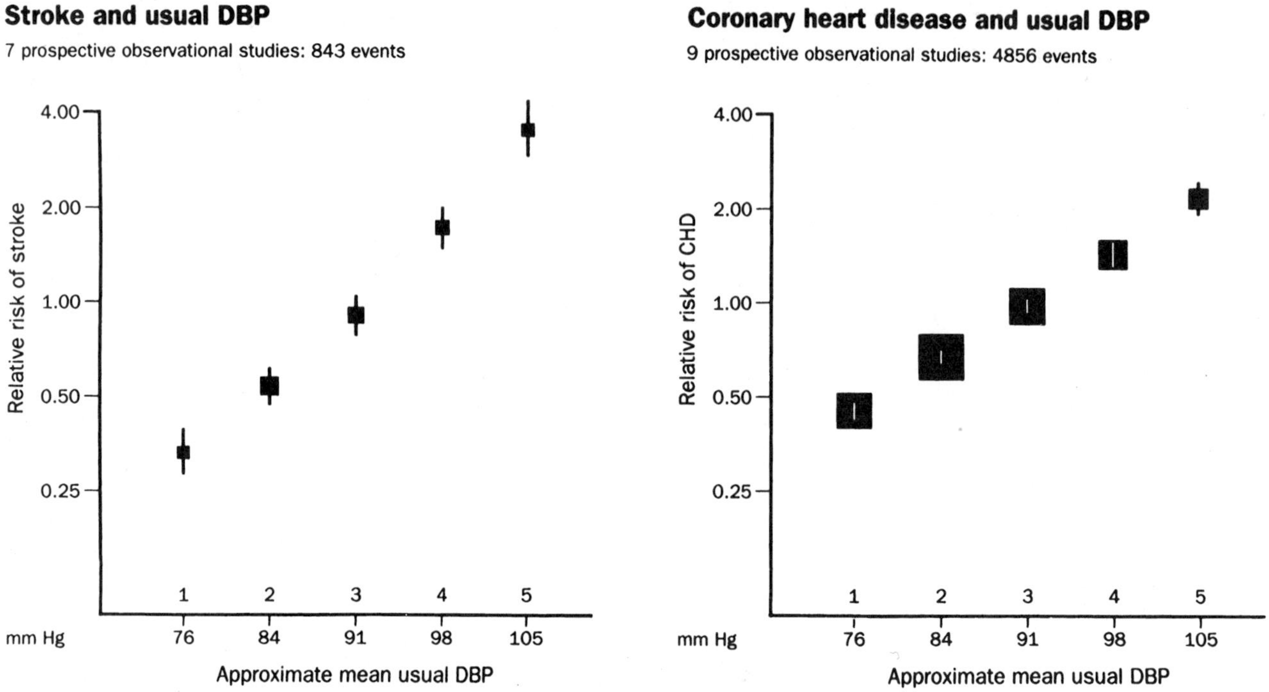

Figure 1–9. Relation between diastolic blood pressure (DBP) and subsequent coronary heart disease and stroke during an average of 10 years' follow-up. (From MacMahon S, Peto R, Cutler J, et al: Blood pressure, stroke, and coronary heart disease. Part 1. Prolonged differences in blood pressure: prospective observational studies corrected for the regression dilution bias. Lancet 1990; 335:765–774.)

trials are neither necessary nor desirable. However, as with cholesterol, the demonstration of association between mild to moderate elevations of diastolic blood pressure and risk of coronary heart disease does not itself imply that levels should be reduced. Nonetheless, abundant data from pharmacologic and nonpharmacologic studies indicate that important risk reductions can be achieved for almost all hypertensive persons. The most precise estimates of risk reductions that can be expected from pharmacologic intervention are derived from a meta-analysis of 14 randomized trials that included more than 37,000 patients treated for up to 5 years.[70] Overall, drug-induced reductions in mean diastolic blood pressure of 5 to 6 mm Hg significantly reduced vascular-related mortality by 21%, stroke by 42%, and myocardial infarction by 14%. In a subsequent overview that included three further interventional trials, the reduction in risk of myocardial infarction associated with diastolic blood pressure control was 17%.[71] Nonpharmacologic interventions such as caloric restriction in overweight subjects and sodium restriction in subjects of normal weight are also effective and are considered a primary step in the treatment of diastolic hypertension.[72–74] Other data also indicate that treatment of isolated systolic hypertension—an increasingly common finding in older persons, especially women—also results in substantial benefit. For example, in the Systolic Hypertension in the Elderly Program,[75] pharmacologic therapy resulted in an 11 mm Hg decline in systolic blood pressure, which was associated with a 36% reduction in stroke and a 27% reduction in nonfatal infarction and coronary death.

The recently released Fifth Report of the Joint Committee on Detection, Evaluation, and Treatment of High Blood Pressure includes current guidelines for hypertension intervention.[76] In general, these guidelines stress nonpharmacologic strategies, including weight loss, limitation of alcohol use, aerobic exercise, and reduction in sodium intake. Unfortunately, nonpharmacologic interventions are associated with poor compliance rates and have proved difficult to maintain over extended periods. Thus many physicians concerned with primary prevention choose to prescribe pharmacologic therapy as initial treatment of patients with mild to moderate hypertension. The choice of agent should most likely be based on the presence of other risk factors, side effect profile, and compliance. Diuretic therapy, if used, should be administered at low doses to avoid risks of chronic hypokalemia. Because of the substantial reductions in risk associated with long-term compliance, the use of antihypertensive medication appears to be cost effective.[77]

Weight Reduction/Physical Activity

Almost 58 million Americans (32 million women and 26 million men) are obese, as defined by having a body weight of 20% or more above the desirable level.[78] Part of the increase in risk of cardiovascular disease associated with obesity relates to the fact that non–insulin-dependent diabetes is common among overweight persons, as are hypertension and lipid abnormalities. However, research indicates that obesity is not only associated with other cardiovascular risk factors but is also an important independent factor on its own. Indeed, because of the high prevalence of obesity, 32% of the population's risk of coronary heart disease can be attributed to obesity.[79]

Data from the Nurses' Health Study provide strong evidence of association between obesity and risk of cardiovascular disease in women. In comparison with lean women (body mass index < 21 kg/m^2), those with body mass index ≥ 29 kg/m^2 had a relative risk of coronary heart disease 3.3 times higher.[80] Similar associations have been found in other large-scale cohort studies, particularly those that controlled for the effects of cigarette smoking. Fat distribution also appears to be an important indicator of risk, wherein abdominal or central obesity is a stronger factor than body mass index or total weight. Several metabolic abnormalities are associated with central obesity, including insulin resistance and frank diabetes.

Fortunately, abundant data indicate that weight reduction, if sustained, can ameliorate many of the adverse cardiovascular effects of obesity. Weight loss is associated with substantial reductions in blood pressure[81] and LDL cholesterol, modest increases in HDL cholesterol, and improved glucose tolerance.[82] Although caloric restriction and increased physical activity remain the primary tools available for intervention in obesity, behavioral modification, drug therapy, and gastric surgery have been used in refractory cases.

Physical activity must also be seen as a primary prevention intervention.[83] In this regard, current levels of physical activity appear to be more closely correlated with a cardioprotective effect than past activity.[84] In a meta-analysis of occupation-based cohort studies, subjects with sedentary professions were found to have a risk of coronary heart disease two times higher than that of subjects employed in active occupations.[85] Similarly, in cohort studies involving men and women undergoing baseline treadmill testing, cardiovascular fitness was inversely correlated with risk of future coronary heart disease.[86] Even modest levels of exercise in these studies have proved superior to no exercise, which is a potentially important consideration because the risk of sudden death may be increased in persons undergoing vigorous exercise.[87] In part reflecting the difficulty of initiating and sustaining a successful life-long physical exercise program, the Centers for Disease Control and Prevention has recommended that all adults sustain at least 30 min of cumulative physical activity daily.[88] It is sobering to consider that this minimal level of exercise is not achieved by more than half of the United States population; for the estimated 60% of U.S. adults who are currently sedentary, physical activity represents a fundamentally important means of reducing cardiovascular risk.[1]

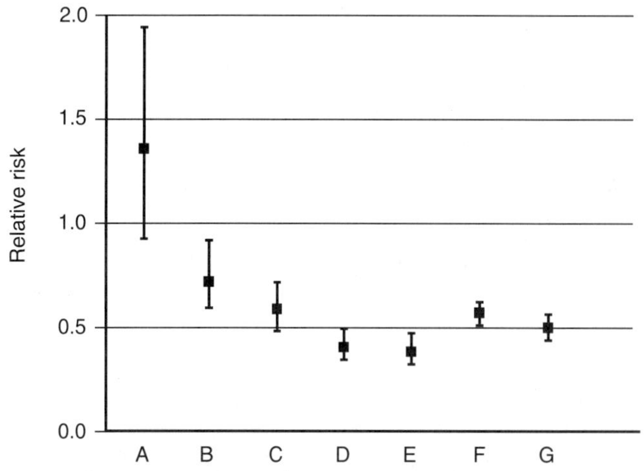

Figure 1–10. Relative risks of coronary heart disease by estrogen use in different study designs. *A,* Hospital-based case-control studies of ever-users. *B,* Population-based case-control studies of ever-users. *C,* Population-based case-control studies of current users. *D,* Cross-sectional studies of ever-users. *E,* Cross-sectional studies of current users. *F,* Prospective internal control studies of ever-users. *G,* All studies. (From Manson JE, Ridker PM, Gaziano JM, Hennekens CH: Primary Prevention of Myocardial Infarction. London: Oxford University Press, 1995.)

Estrogen Replacement Therapy

Risk of coronary heart disease increases dramatically after menopause, so that coronary disease is the leading cause of death in women over age 60.[89] This observation and the association between early age at menopause and subsequent risk of coronary disease have together contributed to the hypothesis that endogenous female hormones are important determinants of coronary risk. Potential mechanisms for this effect include estrogen-associated reductions in LDL cholesterol and increases in HDL cholesterol, as well as beneficial effects of estrogen on coronary vasomotion and endothelial function.[90]

The effect of postmenopausal hormone replacement therapy on risk of coronary disease has been studied in many case-control and cohort studies. Overall, overviews suggest that estrogen replacement may reduce the risk of coronary disease between 40% and 50%.[91] For example, among women in the large prospective Nurses' Health Study who were current users of estrogen, the risk of coronary heart disease was almost half that of nonusers after 10 years of follow-up.[92] These risk reductions were similar for fatal and nonfatal myocardial infarction and persisted after control for numerous risk factors, including smoking, hypertension, diabetes, family history, and obesity. Among women in the same study who underwent early menopause as a result of bilateral oophorectomy and did not receive estrogen replacement, the risk of future coronary heart disease was 1.7 times that of premenopausal women of the same age.

Although the Nurses' Health Study is by far the largest analytic study to address the effects of estrogen replacement therapy, other studies have revealed similar risk reductions, particularly among women with known coronary disease[93, 94] (Fig. 1–10). From a prevention perspective, however, the potential benefits of estrogen must be weighed against possible adverse effects. It is clear that unopposed estrogen use increases the risk of uterine cancer as much as four- to sevenfold, but not if progestin is added. In addition, estrogen use may increase rates of breast cancer, although the increase in risk appears to be small.[95, 96] However, in view of the low rate of occurrence of uterine cancer and its low case-fatality rate, as well as the high prevalence of coronary disease in comparison with breast cancer, many authorities believe it unlikely that the risks of estrogen outweigh its benefit. For example, when the 10-year cumulative mortality risks of coronary heart disease, breast cancer, hip fracture, and uterine cancer for women aged 65 to 74 are compared, the absolute risk that a woman that age will die of coronary disease within the next decade is six times higher than the risk of her dying from breast cancer and 15 times higher than the risk of her dying from uterine cancer.[97]

Despite such data, caution should be used in prescribing hormone replacement therapy. First, the available data concerning the benefits and risks of estrogen use are derived largely from observational case-control and cohort studies. Because coronary heart disease is in many respects preventable, the possibility that women who self-select estrogen replacement therapy also engage in other protective behaviors cannot be excluded. At this time, the National Institutes of Health has initiated a series of studies to evaluate the effects of hormone replacement therapy on total mortality, including a randomized trial of estrogen alone and estrogen plus progestin in comparison with placebo therapy. Such an evaluation is critical because the risk of uterine cancer may be diminished by the addition of progestin. Data also suggest that the formulation of progesterone used in combination with estrogen may be important to consider. In this regard, data from the Postmenopausal Estrogen/Progestin Interventions (PEPI) trial indicate that micronized progesterone in combination with estrogen had greater beneficial effects on HDL cholesterol than did medroxyprogesterone acetate in combination with the same dose of estrogen.[98]

Until randomized trial data are available, the decision to employ hormone replacement therapy should take into account an individual woman's risk factor profile. In this regard, women with a high risk of breast cancer and a low risk of coronary disease may not be optimal candidates for hormonal replacement. However, clinicians should also remember that one in three women dies of coronary heart disease and that in comparison with men, women suffering first myocardial infarctions tend to have substantially higher case-fatality rates. Estrogen replacement therapy should be considered in women with lipid abnormalities, particularly in those with elevated LDL or decreased HDL cholesterol.

Prophylactic Aspirin Use

The potent antiplatelet effects of aspirin have proved highly effective in preventing recurrent myocardial infarction, stroke, and vascular-related death among patients at high risk.[99] Specifically, overview data derived from 25 trials of antiplatelet therapy in the secondary prevention of cardiovascular disease indicate that the use of prophylactic aspirin among subjects with a history of prior infarction, stroke, or unstable angina results in a 32% reduction in recurrent nonfatal myocardial infarction, a 27% reduction in nonfatal stroke, and a 15% reduction in vascular-related death (Table 1–4). When all available trials of antiplatelet agents are pooled, there appears to be a net 27% reduction in the risk of infarction, stroke, or vascular-related death associated with antiplatelet therapy among high-risk patients.[26, 100, 101] On the basis of these secondary prevention data, all high-risk coronary patients—both men and women—without a contraindication to therapy should be considered for chronic aspirin prophylaxis.[102]

With regard to primary prevention, two randomized trials have been completed to date. In the double-blinded and placebo-controlled United States Physicians' Health Study of 22,071 apparently healthy men, the use of 325 mg of aspirin on alternate days was associated with a highly significant 44% reduction in risk of first myocardial infarction.[103] In contrast, in the unblinded British Doctors' Study, no significant reduction in risk was observed to be associated with the use of 500 mg of aspirin daily.[104] Overview analyses of these two primary prevention trials indicate that the use of prophylactic aspirin results in a highly significant 32% reduction in nonfatal myocardial infarction, whereas data on the use of aspirin in the primary prevention of stroke and death from vascular causes are inconclusive (Fig. 1–11). On the basis of these findings, the United States Prevention Services Task Force has recommended that low-dose aspirin therapy be considered for men aged 40 and over who are at increased risk of myocardial infarction and who lack contraindications to the drug.[105] At this time, randomized trial data for women are only being gathered,[106] although observational epidemiologic studies suggest a possible benefit.[107]

As for any prophylactic measure, the decision to use aspirin in the primary prevention of cardiovascular disease must be based on clinical judgment, taking into account the risk profiles of individual patients. The primary risk associated with long-term aspirin use appears to be that of gastrointestinal hemorrhage. Several studies indicate that this risk is dose-related. Thus although the two primary prevention trials assessed 325 mg on alternate days and 500 mg daily, lower doses of aspirin may provide the best risk/benefit ratio. In this regard, laboratory data indicate that aspirin in doses as low as 50 to 75 mg per day, when used on a chronic basis, is adequate to inhibit platelet aggregation and thromboxane production. Enteric-coated formulations may encourage compliance for patients with gastrointestinal intolerance. Few important differences seem to exist between men and women in terms of platelet aggregation, thromboxane inhibition, and prostacyclin sparing. Data suggest that slow delivery of low doses of aspirin may be sufficient to inhibit platelet aggregation in the presystemic portal circulation, which is a potential advantage because this route of administration may leave the systemic endothelial production of prostacyclin intact. Promising findings for controlled-release low-dose aspirin[108] are being tested in large-scale trials. The ongoing Women's Health Study will directly address the issue of low-dose aspirin (100 mg on alternate days) in terms of preventing clinical events in apparently healthy postmenopausal women.

Antioxidant Therapy

Accumulating experimental evidence suggests that dietary antioxidants such as vitamins C and E and beta-carotene may be important in preventing atherosclerotic progression. One mechanism of this effect appears to relate to a slowing of the oxidative modification of LDL cholesterol,[31, 32, 109] although findings from animal models suggest that these antioxidant vitamins may also preserve endothelial function, inhibit platelet aggregation, and reduce atherosclerotic progression.

Several observational, case-control, and blood-based studies indicate inverse associations between dietary antioxidant consumption and risks of coronary disease.[110, 111] In addition, prospective cohort studies suggest that lipid soluble antioxidants such as vitamin E and beta-carotene may have greater effects on atherosclerosis than the water-soluble antioxidant vitamin C. For example, in the Nurses' Health Study, women with the highest intake of beta-carotene had a 22% lower risk of developing future coronary disease than did women with the lowest intake; in women with the highest intake of vitamin E, a 34% reduction in risk was observed; and no reduction was observed with vitamin C.[112] Similar risk reductions have been found for men in studies of vitamin E intake[113] and for elderly persons in studies of beta-carotene.[114]

Until 1992, randomized trial data concerning the effects of antioxidant therapy were limited to small-scale studies of patients with known coronary disease[115–118] (Table 1–5). However, two large-scale prevention trials have since been reported. In the first study, conducted in a poorly nourished population in Linxian, China, a combination of beta-carotene, alpha-tocopherol, and selenium was found to reduce total mortality as a primary result of an effect on gastric cancer.[119] In addition, there appeared to be a small but nonsignificant reduction in risk of cerebrovascular disease. Because coronary heart disease was rare in this population, few data regarding atherosclerotic progression are available from this trial.

The second major antioxidant trial to be reported was conducted in a well-nourished population of Finnish smokers[120] randomized in a factorial design to alpha-tocopherol, beta-carotene, and placebo therapies. In this trial there was no evidence that alpha-tocopherol reduced risks of IHD or ischemic stroke, although the use of this agent was associated with a possible increase in risk of cerebral hemorrhage. For beta-carotene, this trial reported more deaths from IHD in the treatment group than among those randomized to placebo.

TABLE 1–4. OVERVIEW OF 25 TRIALS OF ANTIPLATELET THERAPY IN THE SECONDARY PREVENTION OF CARDIOVASCULAR DISEASE

Endpoint	Prior MI (10 Trials)	Recent UA (2 Trials)	Cardiac History (MI/UA) (12 Trials)	Prior Cerebrovascular Disease (Stroke/TCI) (13 Trials)	Any History (Stroke/TCI/MI/UA) (25 Trials)
Nonfatal MI	31 ± 5	35 ± 17	31 ± 5	35 ± 12	32 ± 5
Nonfatal stroke	42 ± 11	—	40 ± 10	22 ± 7	27 ± 6
Total vascular death	13 ± 5	37 ± 19	14 ± 5	15 ± 7	15 ± 4
Any vascular event	22 ± 4	36 ± 13	26 ± 3	22 ± 5	25 ± 3

Values are percentage ± SD. Patients with prior vascular disease at entry into therapy. Values represent reduction in risk among those assigned antiplatelet therapy.

Abbreviations: MI, myocardial infarction; UA, unstable angina; TCI, transient cerebral ischemia.

From Hennekens CH, Buring JE, Sandercock P, et al: Aspirin and other antiplatelet agents in the secondary and primary prevention of cardiovascular disease. Circulation 1989; 80:749–756.

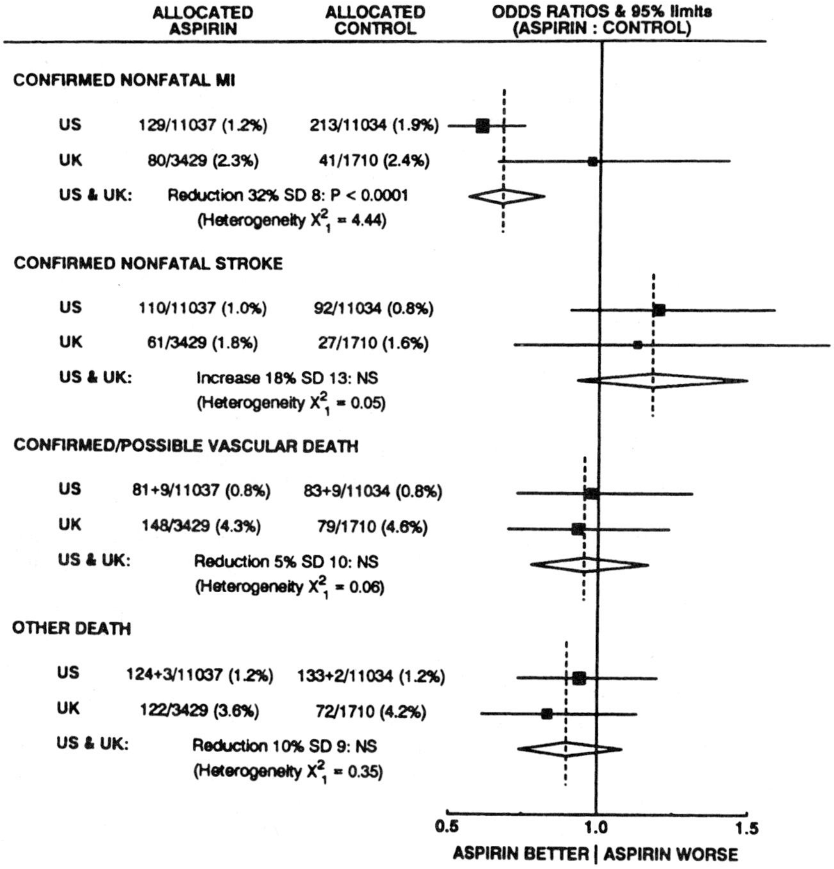

Figure 1–11. Overviews of U.S. and U.K. primary prevention trials of aspirin. (From Hennekens CH, Buring JE, Sandercock P, et al: Aspirin and other antiplatelet agents in the secondary and primary prevention of cardiovascular disease. Circulation 1989; 80:749–756.)

TABLE 1–5. COMPLETED RANDOMIZED, DOUBLE-BLIND, PLACEBO-CONTROLLED TRIALS OF ANTIOXIDANTS IN THE TREATMENT OR PREVENTION OF CARDIOVASCULAR DISEASE

Reference	Study Population	Treatment	Endpoints	Findings
Anderson and Reid, 1974[115]	20 patients with angina pectoris	3200 IU of vitamin E daily for 9 weeks	Angina pain score	Apparent but nonsignificant reduction
Gillilan et al., 1977[116]	52 patients with angina pectoris	1600 IU of vitamin E daily for 6 months	Exercise tolerance, left ventricular function	No significant improvement
Gaziano et al., 1990[117]	333 male physicians with angina pectoris or bypass surgery	50 mg of synthetic beta-carotene on alternate days for 5 years	Major coronary and vascular events	Significant reduction for both endpoints
DeMaio et al., 1992[118]	100 patients after angioplasty	400 IU of vitamin E daily for 4 months	Restenosis by angiogram or exercise test	Nonsignificant trend toward reduction
Blot et al., 1993[119]	29,000 healthy Chinese men and women at high risk for gastric cancer but at low risk for cardiovascular disease	Cocktail of beta-carotene (15 mg), alpha-tocopherol (30 mg), and selenium (50 μg) daily for 5 years	Gastric cancer and cause-specific mortality	Nonsignificant trend toward reduction
The ATBC Lung Cancer Prevention Study Group, 1994[120]	29,000 Finnish male smokers	Factorial design of 20 mg of synthetic beta-carotene daily and 50 mg of synthetic alpha-tocopherol daily for 5–8 years	Lung cancer and cause-specific mortality	No reduction for either antioxidant alone or in combination for mortality from cardiovascular disease

From Gaziano JM, Steinberg D: Prevention of cardiovascular disease by natural antioxidants. *In* Manson JE, Ridker PM, Gaziano JM, Hennekens CH (eds): Primary Prevention of Myocardial Infarction. New York: Oxford University Press, in press.

Because this study was performed among a group of smokers and was primarily designed as a cancer prevention trial, it is difficult to generalize these data, and they should not be construed as a disproof of the antioxidant hypothesis of atherogenesis.[121, 122] Furthermore, the dose of antioxidants tested was very low and may have been inadequate to confer benefit. However, these data do suggest that the potential benefits of antioxidants reported from observational studies may have been overestimated and further raise the possibility that some adverse effects are associated with antioxidant supplementation. At this time, several large-scale trials specifically evaluating the effects of antioxidant therapy on coronary heart disease are under way. Prevention-oriented clinicians should await publication of these studies before making recommendations regarding the use of antioxidant vitamins.

Moderate Alcohol Consumption

Alcohol has complex metabolic, pharmacologic, and psychosocial effects.[123] Alcohol abuse is associated with increased total mortality, in part related to increased rates of myocardial infarction and stroke.[124–127] However, abundant epidemiologic data indicate that mild to moderate levels of alcohol consumption (one to two standard drinks per day) are associated with reduced risks of coronary heart disease. For example, in the prospective Framingham Heart Study, a 30% reduction in risk of myocardial infarction was found among men and women who consumed more than 30 g of alcohol monthly,[128] whereas in the Nurses' Health Study, moderate alcohol consumption was associated with a 40% reduction in risk, in comparison with nondrinkers.[129] Similar reductions have been observed in several other case-control and cohort studies.[130–132] However, the relationship between alcohol use and total mortality is best described by a J-shaped curve because of a positive association between alcohol abuse and deaths not caused by coronary heart disease.[133]

Although much interest has focused on the cardioprotective effects of wine, most studies indicate that risk reductions associated with mild to moderate alcohol use are independent of the type of alcohol consumed. Wine, beer, and distilled liquors have all been shown to increase HDL cholesterol levels, an effect responsible for as much as half of the cardioprotective effect of alcohol.[134, 135] However, even short-term recent alcohol consumption appears to be protective,[136] which suggests the presence of other important mechanisms. In particular, alcohol appears to have potentially beneficial effects on platelet aggregation, endothelial function, and fibrinolytic capacity. In a cross-sectional study, a positive association was found between moderate alcohol intake and plasma level of endogenous tissue plasminogen activator (t-PA) antigen that is independent of HDL cholesterol,[137] a finding that supports the hypothesis that changes in fibrinolytic potential may be an important mechanism whereby moderate alcohol use decreases risk of thrombosis.

Most epidemiologic studies indicate that the maximal cardioprotective effect is achieved with one or two alcoholic beverages per day but that higher levels of consumption are associated with an increase in all-cause mortality. Because heavy consumption of alcohol is associated with a wide variety of medical and social ills, the difference between drinking small to moderate quantities and drinking large amounts may be the difference between preventing and causing disease. Thus any clinical recommendations need to be given with caution and must take into account the full risk profile of a given patient. From a research standpoint, the development of agents that can mimic the beneficial effects of alcohol with an acceptable side effect profile would represent an important new therapeutic modality.

Fatty Acid Intake

In comparison with saturated fats, monounsaturated and polyunsaturated fats tend to produce favorable increases in HDL cholesterol and little change in LDL cholesterol. Thus diets containing primarily monounsaturated and polyunsaturated fats are likely to be more favorable from a prevention perspective than diets in which a similar amount of energy is provided by saturated fat. Standard recommendations for heart-healthy diets therefore include the substitution of olive, sunflower, and corn oils for animal fats, palm oil, and coconut oil. Furthermore, because total fat intake should be limited to less than 30% of total energy intake, most heart-healthy diets encourage the consumption of protein from sources such as fish and chicken, as well as complex carbohydrates from fruits, vegetables, beans, and grains (Table 1–6). More severe dietary restriction has proved feasible in motivated patients.[138]

Unfortunately, in an attempt to avoid animal fats and butter, many people increase the consumption of hydrogenated fat in the forms of vegetable shortening and hard margarine. Hydrogenation of vegetable oils is a common industrial practice used to form margarine from vegetable oils. However, this process produces predominantly trans–fatty acids, which may carry atherosclerotic risks similar to, if not worse than, those of saturated fats. For example, in comparison with a diet based on monounsaturated fat, a diet with 10% energy as trans–fatty acids raises LDL cholesterol and decreases HDL cholesterol.[139] Thus the effect of trans–fatty acid intake on the total cholesterol-to-HDL cholesterol ratio may actually be worse for trans–fatty acids than for saturated animal fat.[140, 141] Cross-sectional,[142] case-control,[143] and prospective cohort studies[144] have all linked increased

TABLE 1–6. THE LIPID-LOWERING DIET

Principle	Amount	Food Sources
Decreased total fat	<30% energy	Avoid butter; hard margarine; whole milk; cream; ice cream; high-fat cheese;
Decreased saturated fat	7%–10% of energy	fatty meats and poultry; sausages; pastries; coffee creamer; products containing hydrogenated oils, palm oil, and coconut oil
Increased use of high protein food (low in saturated fat)		Fish, chicken, and turkey; veal, game, spring lamb
Increased complex carbohydrates; increased fruit and vegetable fiber, increased legumes	About 35 g/day of fiber, one half derived from fruit and vegetables	All fruit, including dried fruit; all fresh and frozen vegetables; lentils, dried beans, chick peas; unrefined cereal foods, including oats
Decreased dietary cholesterol	<300 mg/day	Allowance up to 2 egg yolks per week and liver up to twice monthly; other offal avoided
Moderately increased use of mono- and polyunsaturated oils and products	Mono: 10%–15% of energy Poly: 7%–10% of energy	Olive oil, sunflower oil, corn oil, and products based on these

Adapted from Assmann G: Lipid Metabolism Disorders and Coronary Heart Disease, p 111. Munich: Medizin Verlag, 1993.

intake of trans–fatty acids to elevated risks of IHD. Thus in addition to focusing on monounsaturated and polyunsaturated fats, many researchers have recommended that prevention-conscious diets also include predominantly cis–fatty acids available from liquid vegetable oils rather than trans–fatty acids from processed solid vegetable oils.[145] In this regard, the use of soft margarine is helpful because it typically contains less than 40% of the trans-isomers found in hard stick margarines.

Consumption of Fish Oils and Omega-3 Fatty Acids

Lower rates of coronary heart disease associated with the consumption of fish oil have been observed in several cross-sectional studies and in some, but not all, prospective cohort studies.[146–151] Experimental studies also suggest that omega-3 fatty acids derived from marine fish may reduce very low density lipoproteins (VLDL), inhibit thromboxane production, increase prostacyclin synthesis, enhance fibrinolytic activity, and reduce blood pressure.[152] Taken together, these observations have led many researchers to recommend the use of fish-oriented diets in the prevention of coronary disease and as therapy for regression. However, observations regarding fish consumption and coronary disease have been inconsistent, and the effects of fish oils on hemostatic parameters or blood pressure do not appear significant enough to explain important effects.[153, 154] Furthermore, investigations of the effects of fish oil supplementation on coronary regression are incomplete and do not show consistent effects. Thus, whether increased intake of fish or omega-3 fatty acids reduces the occurrence of IHD is unclear at this time.[145]

Dietary Fiber Intake

Dietary fiber has been shown to improve hyperglycemia and to have mild beneficial effects on plasma lipid profiles. In addition, an inverse relationship between dietary fiber intake and risk of coronary heart disease has been reported in several prospective cohort studies, often after other coronary risk factors are controlled.[9, 155, 156] However, whether these beneficial effects are attributable to fiber intake or to other dietary and lifestyle interventions associated with fiber use is unclear, as is whether specific fibers such as those derived from bran or grain have differential effects. Such data can be generated only from experimental studies. In one randomized trial of a high-fiber diet among patients with prior myocardial infarction, no reduction in risk of recurrent infarction was found. In fact, rates of reinfarction were actually higher in the fiber-enriched group.[157] Thus, although data regarding fiber intake and coronary risk are intriguing, recommendations at this time must be made with appropriate caution.[145]

HEMOSTATIC AND THROMBOTIC RISK FACTORS

The therapeutic interventions discussed so far in this chapter relate primarily to traditional atherosclerotic risk factors. However, there is a growing appreciation that hemostatic and thrombotic risk factors are also present in many persons and that these factors are important in the production of acute thrombi. Knowledge of these factors is important, because traditional markers of atherosclerotic progression and initiation fail to identify most subjects at risk for future coronary occlusion. For example, in two large screening studies, investigators have reported that information on hyperlipidemia, smoking status, blood pressure, and family history predicts less than a third of all future coronary events.[158, 159]

For a few patients, there exist distinct abnormalities of hemostasis and thrombosis that result in a hypercoagulable state and elevated risks of arterial and venous thrombosis (Table 1–7).[160] These inherited defects of coagulation are reviewed elsewhere in this text. Here, the epidemiologic evidence relating several common thrombotic markers of risk are reviewed as they relate to the primary prevention of vascular disease.

TABLE 1–7. THE PRIMARY HYPERCOAGULABLE STATES

State	Deficiency
Antithrombin/heparin disorders	Antithrombin deficiency
	Heparin cofactor II deficiency
Protein C/protein S disorders	Protein C deficiency
	Resistance to activated protein C
	Protein S deficiency
Fibrinolytic disorders	Hypoplasminogenemia
	Dysplasminogenemia
	Plasminogen activator deficiency
	Decreased tissue plasminogen activator
	Increased plasminogen activator inhibitor
	Increased histidine-rich glycoprotein
	Dysfibrinogenemia

Adapted from Schafer AI: Hypercoagulable states: molecular genetics to clinical practice. Lancet 1994; 344:1739–1742.

Plasma Fibrinogen Level and Viscosity

Serum fibrinogen level and plasma viscosity are the two primary determinants of blood rheology. Cross-sectional data indicate that plasma fibrinogen increases with prevalence of coronary artery disease.[161] Furthermore, several well-designed prospective cohort studies demonstrate a positive association between plasma fibrinogen level and cardiovascular risk in that a 1.6-fold increase in incidence of coronary heart disease is present for each standard deviation increase in fibrinogen level.[162–165] For example, in the Northwick Park Heart Study, baseline levels of fibrinogen had predictive value for future IHD similar to that of total cholesterol. In addition, this study demonstrated important relationships between plasma coagulation factor VII and IHD[162] (Fig. 1–12).

More recent data suggest that blood viscosity and fibrinogen are as predictive of future IHD as are a combination of cholesterol, body mass, age, and blood pressure, in that men with the highest levels of either blood viscosity or plasma fibrinogen have risks of coronary

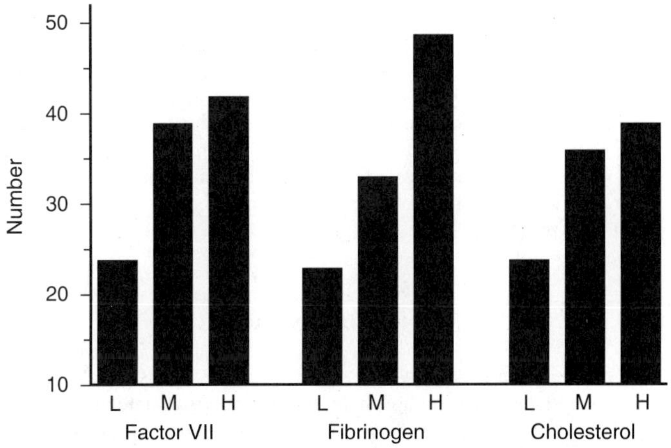

Figure 1–12. Relationships of total cholesterol, fibrinogen, and coagulation factor VII and coronary heart disease in the Northwick Park Heart Study. L, M, and H refer to lowest, middle, and highest tertiles. (Adapted from Meade TW, Mellows S, Brozovic M, et al: Haemostatic function and ischaemic heart disease. Principal results of the Northwick Park Heart Study. Lancet 1986; 2:533–537.)

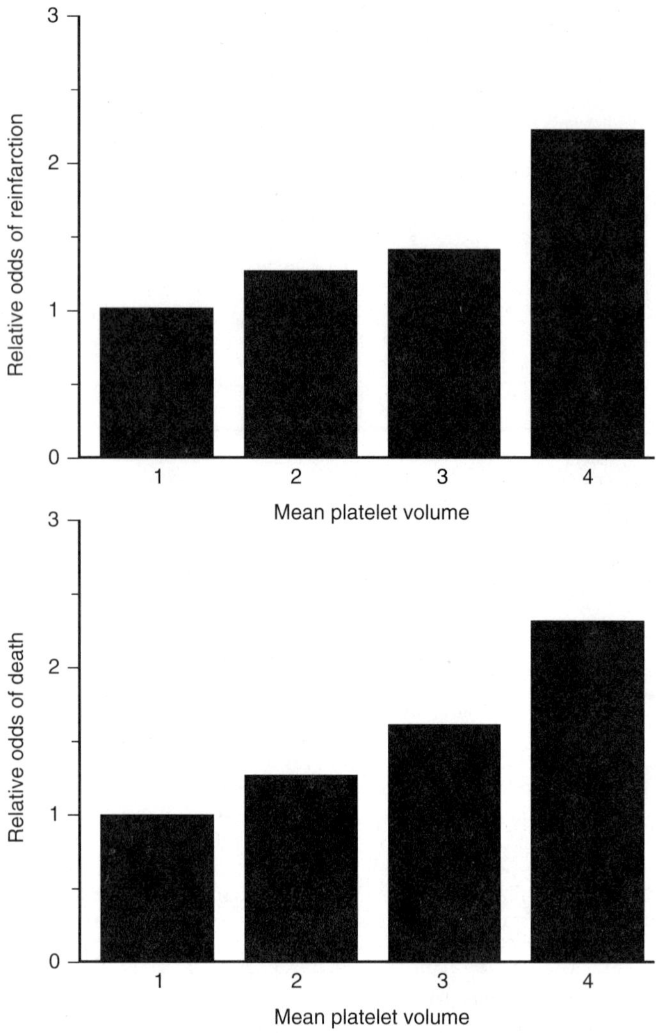

Figure 1–13. Mean platelet volume and risks of death and reinfarction. Numbers refer to increasing quartiles. (Adapted from Martin JF, Bath PMW, Burr ML: Influence of platelet size on outcome after myocardial infarction. Lancet 1991; 338:1409–1411.)

disease four times that of men with lower levels.[166] Blood viscosity also is a potent marker of risk for patients with unstable angina and in healthy subjects.[167, 168]

Smoking cessation and exercise appear to be the most effective means of decreasing fibrinogen level. At this time, no pharmacologic regimen can be recommended to reduce plasma fibrinogen level, and there are no available prospective data from which to assess whether reducing this factor as a prophylactic measure results in any health benefit.

Platelet Size and Activity

Platelet size and activity as assessed by spontaneous platelet aggregation,[169] adenosine diphosphate (ADP)-induced platelet aggregation,[170] platelet volume,[171] or total platelet count[172] appear to be potential independent markers for thrombus formation. Of these, mean platelet volume is the easiest to measure clinically and appears strongly associated with risks of vascular-related death and reinfarction[171] (Fig. 1–13).

The appreciation that platelet function is critical in acute thrombus formation is underscored by the marked efficacy of antiplatelet agents such as aspirin in both the secondary and primary prevention of coronary heart disease.[99, 102] In addition, overviews indicate the efficacy of aspirin in the prevention of deep venous thrombosis and pulmonary embolism as well as in the long-term maintenance of vascular grafts.[100, 101]

Endogenous Fibrinolytic Capacity: t-PA, PAI-1, and D-Dimer

Accumulating evidence suggests that on a population basis, certain people are "prone to thrombosis," whereas others are "prone to hemorrhage." In part, these tendencies appear related to interindividual variation in the level of endogenous fibrinolytic capacity. For example, some work indicates that certain patients with abnormal plasma concentrations of endogenous t-PA or its primary inhibitor, plasminogen activator inhibitor type 1 (PAI-1) may be at substantially increased risk for myocardial infarction. Increased plasma concentrations of PAI-1 have been found in a selected group of young survivors of myocardial infarction,[173] and several investigators have described abnormal levels of PAI-1 among patients with known coronary disease. At the same time, elevated levels of endogenous t-PA antigen (t-PA:ag) appear to be strong predictors of risk for future myocardial infarction[174] and stroke[175] among currently healthy persons (Fig. 1–14) and among patients with angina.[176, 177]

Whether these data indicate that the endogenous fibrinolytic system is activated or inhibited among persons at risk is currently being evaluated. Using a global assay for fibrinolysis, investigators from the Northwick Park Heart Study have suggested that a net inhibition of fibrinolysis is present among high-risk patients.[178] On the other hand, elevated levels of D-dimer, the primary breakdown product of fibrinogen, also are elevated among patients at high risk of future thrombosis, which indicates that activation of the fibrinolytic system may precede vascular occlusion.[179, 180] In this case, rather than being a cause of thrombosis, activation of the endogenous fibrinolytic system may occur as a response to the presence of preclinical atherosclerotic disease (Fig. 1–15).

Preliminary work suggests that alterations in fibrinolytic potential may be possible through the use of angiotensin converting enzyme (ACE) inhibitors, gemfibrozil, and moderate alcohol consumption. Randomized trial data will be required in order to ascertain whether pharmacologic changes in fibrinolytic potential merit consideration as preventive interventions.

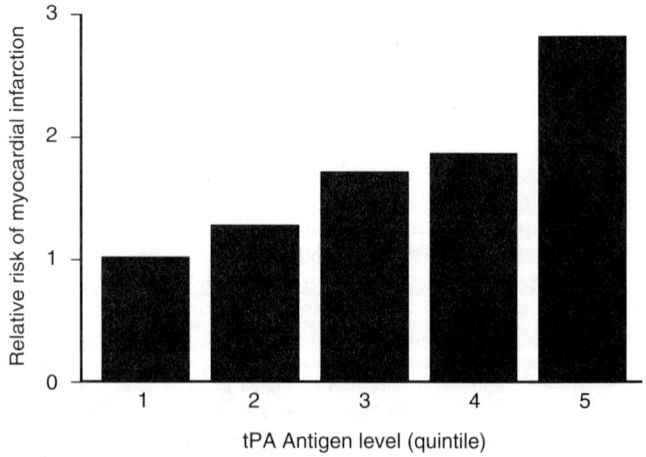

Figure 1–14. Relative risk of future myocardial infarction according to baseline plasma concentration of endogenous tissue plasminogen activator (tPA) antigen. (Adapted from Ridker PM, Vaughan DE, Stampfer MJ, et al: Endogenous tissue–type plasminogen activator and risk of myocardial infarction. Lancet 1993; 341:1165–1168.)

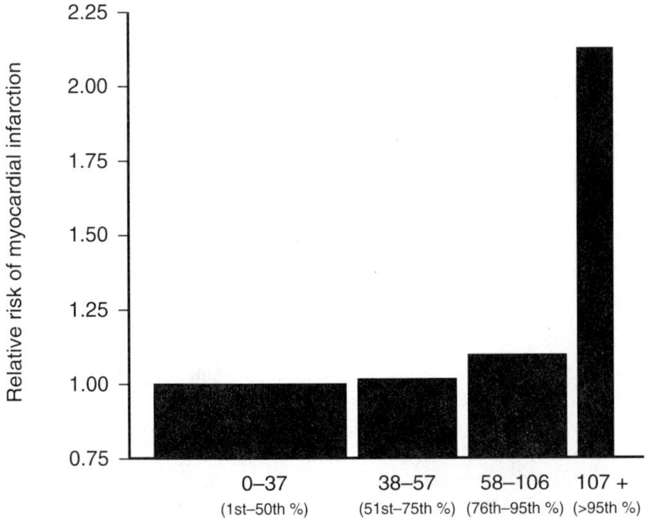

Figure 1–15. Relative risk of future myocardial infarction (MI) according to baseline plasma concentration of D-dimer. (From Ridker PM, Hennekens CH, Cerskus A, Stampfer MJ: Plasma concentration of cross linked fibrin degradation product [D-dimer] and the risk of future myocardial infarction among apparently healthy men. Circulation 1994; 90:2236–2240.)

Homocysteine

Postmortem findings of extensive atherosclerosis among patients with rare genetic causes of homocystinemia have led several investigators to evaluate homocysteine as an independent risk factor for coronary heart disease. Until the early 1990s, evidence linking high-normal blood levels of homocysteine to atherosclerotic disease has been limited to retrospective case-control and cross-sectional studies. However, two prospective studies demonstrated increased risks of future myocardial infarction among subjects with only modest increases in homocysteine level.[181, 182] Furthermore, two large and well-controlled studies demonstrated positive associations between mild increases in homocysteine and the extent of atherosclerosis in the carotid system.[183, 184]

Potential mechanisms linking hyperhomocystinemia and coronary disease include toxic effects of homocysteine on the vascular endothelium, direct prothrombotic effects, and the stimulation of smooth muscle proliferation. Because homocysteine levels are inversely related to folate intake,[185] it is possible that an intervention as simple as the administration of folate and vitamin B_{12} may be sufficient to adequately reduce homocysteine levels among the 40% of the U.S. population with mild to moderate elevations.[186]

Lipoprotein(a)

Several retrospective and cross-sectional studies suggest that plasma levels of lipoprotein(a) (Lp[a]) correlate with prevalent coronary heart disease. Lp(a) levels remain stable over time and appear to be genetically determined. Furthermore, because of sequence homology between the apolipoprotein(a) component of Lp(a) and plasminogen, Lp(a) may compete with plasminogen for binding to fibrin and inhibit endogenous fibrinolysis.[187, 188]

As of this writing, seven prospective cohort studies of plasma Lp(a) and risks of future vascular disease have been presented, four of which suggested a modest association between Lp(a) and future vascular risk, whereas three revealed no evidence of association[189–194, 159] (Table 1–8). One tenable hypothesis for differences between these study findings is that Lp(a) is only a marker of risk among hyperlipidemic subjects. However, the totality of evidence suggests that any true increase in risk of future thrombosis associated with Lp(a) is likely to be of small absolute magnitude. Because the distribution of Lp(a) is markedly skewed in most populations and any postulated association between Lp(a) and vascular risk appears limited to patients with very high levels, most vascular occlusive events will occur among subjects with normal Lp(a) levels.

Genetic Markers of Thrombotic Risk

Finally, genetic markers of thrombotic risk can be expected to play an ever-increasing role in the identification of persons at high risk for vascular occlusion. For example, with regard to arterial thrombosis, data from case-control studies suggest that the genotypic distribution of a common polymorphism in the gene coding for ACE may be associated with increased risks of myocardial infarction,[195] although such findings have been controversial and not corroborated in prospective data.[196]

With regard to venous thrombosis, mutation in coagulation factor V appears to lead to a hypercoagulable state as a result of activated protein C resistance, a phenomenon associated with increased rates of venous thrombosis.[197–199] In a prospective study of primary deep venous thrombosis and/or pulmonary embolism among a cohort of currently healthy men, the presence of mutation in the coagulation

TABLE 1–8. PROSPECTIVE STUDIES OF LIPOPROTEIN(a) AND RISKS OF FUTURE CARDIOVASCULAR DISEASE

Study (Year)	Population	Duration (Years)	Endpoint	Sample Size (Cases)	Relative Risk*	95% CI*
Rosengren et al., 1990[189]	Gothenborg, 50-year-old men	6	MI/fatal coronary heart disease	26	1.36	1.08–1.75
Jauhiainen et al., 1991[190]	Helsinki Heart Study, 40- to 55-year-old men	5	MI/fatal coronary heart disease	138	1.03	0.97–1.09
Ridker et al., 1993[191]	Physicians' Health Study, 40- to 84-year-old men	5	MI	296	1.03	0.95–1.13
Schaefer et al., 1994[192]	Lipid Research Clinics, 35- to 59-year-old hyperlipidemic men	7–10	Coronary heart disease	233	1.12	1.03–1.20
Cremer et al., 1994[194]	Göttingen Risk Study, 40- to 60-year-old men	5	MI	107	NA	NA
Ridker et al., 1995[193]	Physicians' Health Study, 40- to 84-year-old men	7.5	Stroke	198	1.04	0.94–1.15

Abbreviations: CI, confidence interval; MI, myocardial infarction.

*Relative risk and confidence intervals are calculated for a 100 mg/L increase in Lp(a) concentration.

factor V gene resulted in a fourfold increase in risk.[200] Furthermore, mutation in coagulation factor V appears to be an important determinant of venous thrombosis among women taking oral contraception.[201] Because the prevalence of this mutation in the general population is between 5% and 7%, mutation in the factor V gene represents the most common inherited factor predisposing to venous thrombosis recognized so far. Further work will be necessary to discern whether screening for this or other genetic abnormalities will prove efficacious for the primary prevention of thrombosis.

SCREENING FOR CORONARY HEART DISEASE: PUBLIC HEALTH IMPLICATIONS FOR PREVENTION

Preclinical identification of persons at high vascular risk is a major focus of primary prevention efforts. A requirement of any successful screening program is the availability of a sensitive and specific test for a meaningful intermediate endpoint that can be detected before the onset of overt clinical disease. For example, patients with hypertension are typically asymptomatic before the development of major end-organ damage. However, blood pressure measurement is a simple, accurate, and noninvasive method for case identification. Blood pressure screening has, surprisingly, not proved highly successful.

In contrast, persons with preclinical atherosclerosis are also typically asymptomatic and it can be extremely difficult to identify them. At this time, the only widely accepted screening tool for atherosclerotic disease other than blood pressure measurement is assessment of the plasma lipid profile. Screening strategies that have been proposed include mass programs, in which all people are evaluated; opportunistic programs, in which persons presenting for medical attention are evaluated; and targeted programs, in which only selected high-risk subgroups are evaluated. Although targeted screening has intuitive appeal, there is evidence that this method is inefficient. For example, in one study of healthy subjects with a family history of premature coronary heart disease or physical examination findings suggestive of hypercholesterolemia, lipid analysis failed to identify more than two thirds of the subjects at risk.[202]

The availability of rapid and inexpensive tools to measure total cholesterol has led many to endorse a mass screening approach to case identification. It is important to understand, however, that the success of such a program depends greatly on the analytic precision of the cholesterol assay employed. As illustrated in Figure 1–16, small amounts of imprecision in assays used will lead to substantial numbers of false-positive and false-negative screening results. For cholesterol screening in an unselected population, coefficients of variation between 6% and 10% are unacceptable, particularly because

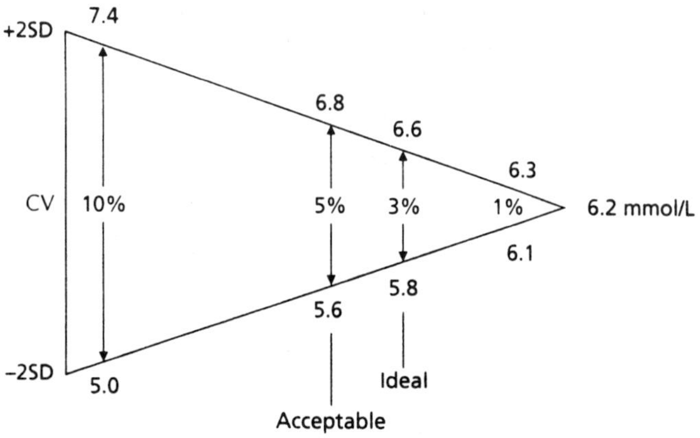

Figure 1–16. The effect of differing degrees of analytic imprecision of cholesterol measurement. *Abbreviations:* CV, coefficient of variations; SD, standard deviation. (From Thompson GR, Wilson PW: Coronary Risk Factors and Their Assessment. London: Science Press, 1992.)

the pretest probability of significant atherosclerotic disease is low. As in any screening test, the positive predictive value increases as the population being screened contains increasing numbers of persons at higher than average risk. However, when combined with assessment of blood pressure, smoking status, electrocardiographic (ECG) criteria for left ventricular hypertrophy, and the presence or absence of diabetes, accurate assessment of blood lipid levels can be used clinically to effectively risk-stratify most patient populations (Fig. 1–17).

Despite favorable trends in smoking cessation, cholesterol reduction, and blood pressure control, major risk factors for IHD remain prevalent in the United States. Published population data indicate that only 18% of U.S. adults are normotensive, nonobese nonsmokers who exercise frequently, have acceptable cholesterol levels, and are free of diabetes mellitus. In contrast, almost half of the adult population has been found to have two or more of these risk factors, 13% to have three risk factors, and 5% to have four to six risk factors.

The public health burden of cardiovascular disease is growing as the population ages. According to the National Center for Health Statistics, 150,000 coronary heart disease deaths in the United States are attributable each year to smoking, 250,000 to hypercholesterolemia, 170,000 to hypertension, 190,000 to obesity, and more than 200,000 to a sedentary lifestyle. Although the remainder of this text deals with the many important therapeutic interventions for patients with clinically apparent disease of the cardiovascular system, clinicians must remain cognizant of the enormous role that prevention must play in the management of all patients with and without known coronary artery disease.[203]

CLINICAL PROFILES IN PRIMARY PREVENTION

Most of the prevention strategies just outlined apply to all people, even those at only moderate risk for coronary heart disease. For the average middle-aged man with one or two conventional risk factors such as hypertension and mild obesity, weight reduction and the institution of a lifelong physical activity plan should be initiated. If there are no contraindications to therapy, low-dose prophylactic aspirin may be employed. If mild hyperlipidemia is present, dietary patterns should be altered so that total fat is reduced, monounsaturated and polyunsaturated fats are substituted for saturated fats, hydrogenated oils and trans–fatty acids are avoided, caloric intake is restricted, and intake of fruits and vegetables is increased. If elevations of blood pressure and/or lipid levels persist, medical therapy for either or both of these disorders may be indicated. Dietary changes to include sources of natural antioxidants should also be encouraged. For postmenopausal women, additional consideration of estrogen replacement therapy should be given. However, all of these interventions are of little value in patients who continue to smoke.

Some people are at substantially high risk and therefore require special attention. For example, management of a young patient with an extensive family history of premature coronary disease or known familial thrombosis may include screening for several of the genetic and thrombotic markers of risk discussed earlier. However, clinicians must be aware that few interventions that specifically target elevations of fibrinogen, t-PA:ag, or Lp(a) are available, although folate therapy can be given to patients with homocystinemia, and warfarin (Coumadin) may be considered in patients with familial thrombotic disorders. However, the preventive management of such patients must begin with aggressive cholesterol and blood pressure reduction, as well as smoking cessation, caloric restriction, increased physical activity, and other lifestyle modifications.

One other group particularly receptive to prevention efforts comprises the offspring of patients who have suffered myocardial infarction, especially at a time when the parents are in the coronary care setting. Prevention-oriented physicians can take advantage of this situation to stress that the risks of future coronary heart disease

Coronary Heart Disease
Risk Factor Prediction Chart

American Heart Association

1. Find Points For Each Risk Factor

Age (If Female)				Age (If Male)			
Age	Pts.	Age	Pts.	Age	Pts.	Age	Pts.
30	−12	47–48	5	30	−2	57–59	13
31	−11	49–50	6	31	−1	60–61	14
32	−9	51–52	7	32–33	0	62–64	15
33	−8	53–55	8	34	1	65–67	16
34	−6	56–60	9	35–36	2	68–70	17
35	−5	61–67	10	37–38	3	71–73	18
36	−4	68–74	11	39	4	74	19
37	−3			40–41	5		
38	−2			42–43	6		
39	−1			44–45	7		
40	0			46–47	8		
41	1			48–49	9		
42–43	2			50–51	10		
44	3			52–54	11		
45–46	4			55–56	12		

HDL-Cholesterol		Total-Cholesterol		Systolic Blood Pressure			
HDL-C	Pts.	Total-C	Pts.	SBP	Pts.	Other	Pts.
25–26	7	139–151	−3	98–104	−2	Cigarettes	4
27–29	6	152–166	−2	105–112	−1	Diabetic-male	3
30–32	5	167–182	−1	113–120	0	Diabetic-female	6
33–35	4	183–199	0	121–129	1	ECG-LVH	9
36–38	3	200–219	1	130–139	2		
39–42	2	220–239	2	140–149	3	0 pts for each NO	
43–46	1	240–262	3	150–160	4		
47–50	0	263–288	4	161–172	5		
51–55	−1	289–315	5	173–185	6		
56–60	−2	316–330	6				
61–66	−3						
67–73	−4						
74–80	−5						
81–87	−6						
88–96	−7						

2. Sum Points For All Risk Factors

_____ + _____ + _____ + _____ + _____ + _____ + _____ = ________

Age + HDL-C + Total-C + SBP + Smoker + Diabetes + ECG-LVH = Point Total

NOTE: *Minus Points Subtract From Total.*

3. Look Up Risk Corresponding To Point Total

Probability			Probability			Probability			Probability		
Pts.	5 Yr.	10 Yr.	Pts.	5 Yr.	10 Yr.	Pts.	5 Yr.	10 Yr.	Pts.	5 Yr.	10 Yr.
≤1	<1%	<2%	10	2%	6%	19	8%	16%	28	19%	33%
2	1%	2%	11	3%	6%	20	8%	18%	29	20%	36%
3	1%	2%	12	3%	7%	21	9%	19%	30	22%	38%
4	1%	2%	13	3%	8%	22	11%	21%	31	24%	40%
5	1%	3%	14	4%	9%	23	12%	23%	32	25%	42%
6	1%	3%	15	5%	10%	24	13%	25%			
7	1%	4%	16	5%	12%	25	14%	27%			
8	2%	4%	17	6%	13%	26	16%	29%			
9	2%	5%	18	7%	14%	27	17%	31%			

4. Compare To Average 10 Year Risk

	Probability	
Age	Women	Men
30–34	<1%	3%
35–39	<1%	5%
40–44	2%	6%
45–49	5%	10%
50–54	8%	14%
55–59	12%	16%
60–64	13%	21%
65–69	9%	30%
70–74	12%	24%

These charts were prepared with the help of William B. Kannel, M.D., Professor of Medicine and Public Health and Ralph D'Agostino, Ph.D., Head, Department of Mathematics, both at Boston University; Keaven Anderson, Ph.D., Statistician, NHLBI, Framingham Study; Daniel McGee, Ph.D., Associate Professor, University of Arizona.

Framingham Heart Study

Figure 1–17. Coronary heart disease risk factor prediction chart. (From the Risk Factor Prediction Kit. Dallas: American Heart Association, 1990.)

for currently healthy people can be substantially modified. Indeed, with lifelong behavioral intervention, children of patients with infarcts may be able to avoid or postpone serious coronary disease later in life.

REFERENCES

1. Manson JE, Tosteson H, Ridker PM, et al: Current concepts: primary prevention of myocardial infarction. N Engl J Med 1992; 326:1406–1416.
2. Heart and Stroke Facts. Dallas: American Heart Association, 1992.
3. Moss AJ, Benhorin J: Prognosis and management after a first myocardial infarction. N Engl J Med 1990; 322:743–753.
4. Manson JE, Ridker PM, Gaziano JM, Hennekens CH (eds): Primary Prevention of Myocardial Infarction. New York: Oxford University Press, in press.
5. Hennekens CH, Buring JE: Epidemiology in Medicine. Boston: Little Brown, 1987.
6. Keys A: Coronary heart disease in seven countries. Circulation 1980; 41:1–19.
7. Simons LA: Interrelations of lipids and lipoproteins with coronary artery disease mortality in 19 countries. Am J Cardiol 1986; 57:5–10.
8. Worth RM, Kato H, Rhoades GG, et al: Epidemiologic studies of coronary heart disease and stroke in Japanese men living in Japan, Hawaii, and California: mortality. Am J Epidemiol 1975; 102:481–490.
9. Kushi LH, Lew RA, Stare FJ, et al: Diet and 20 year mortality from coronary heart disease. The Ireland-Boston Diet Heart Study. N Engl J Med 1985; 312:811–818.
10. Tunstall-Pedoe H, Clayton D, Morris JN, et al: Coronary heart attacks in east London. Lancet 1975; 2:833–838.
11. McNamara JJ, Molot MA, Stremple JF, Cutting RT: Coronary artery disease in combat casualties in Vietnam. JAMA 1971; 216:1186–1187.
12. Enos WF, Holmes RH, Beyer J: Coronary disease among United States soldiers killed in action in Korea: preliminary report. JAMA 1953; 152:1090–1093.
13. PDAY Research Group: Relationship of atherosclerosis in young men to serum lipoprotein cholesterol concentrations and smoking. A preliminary report from the Pathobiological Determinants of Atherosclerosis in Youth (PDAY) Research Group. JAMA 1990; 264(23):3018–3024.
14. Beaglehole R: International trends in coronary heart disease mortality, morbidity, and risk factors. Epidemiol Rev 1990; 12:1–15.
15. Mittelman MA, Maclure M, Tofler GH, et al: Triggering of acute myocardial infarction by heavy physical exertion—protection against triggering by regular exertion. N Engl J Med 1993; 329:1677–1683.
16. Kannel WB, Wolf PA, Castelli WP, D'Agostino RB: Fibrinogen and risk of cardiovascular disease. The Framingham Study. JAMA 1987; 258:1183–1186.
17. Willett WC, Green A, Stampfer MJ, et al: Relative and absolute excess risks of coronary heart disease among women who smoke cigarettes. N Engl J Med 1987; 317:1303–1309.
18. Fuster V, Badimon L, Badimon JJ, Chesebro JH: The pathogenesis of coronary artery disease and the acute coronary syndromes. N Engl J Med 1992; 326:242–250, 310–318.
19. Ross R: The pathogenesis of atherosclerosis: a perspective for the 1990's. Nature 1993; 362:801–809.
20. Davies MJ, Thomas AC: Plaque fissuring: the cause of acute myocardial infarction, sudden ischaemic death, and crescendo angina. Br Heart J 1985; 53:363–373.
21. Davies MJ, Woolf N, Rowles PM, Pepper J: Morphology of the endothelium over atherosclerotic plaques in human coronary arteries. Br Heart J 1988; 60:459–464.
22. DeWood MA, Spores J, Notske R, et al: Prevalence of total coronary occlusion during the early hours of transmural myocardial infarction. N Engl J Med 1980; 303:897–902.
23. Falk E: Morphologic features of unstable atherothrombotic plaques underlying acute coronary syndromes. Am J Cardiol 1989; 63(suppl): 114E–120E.
24. Ambrose J, Tannenbaum M, Alexopoulos D, et al: Angiographic progression of coronary artery disease and the development of myocardial infarction. J Am Coll Cardiol 1988; 12:56–62.
25. Giroud D, Li JM, Urban P, et al: Relation of the site of acute myocardial infarction to the most severe coronary arterial stenosis at prior angiography. Am J Cardiol 1992; 69:729–732.
26. Antiplatelet Trialists' Collaboration: Collaborative overview of randomised trials of antiplatelet therapy—I: Prevention of death, myocardial infarction, and stroke by prolonged antiplatelet therapy in various categories of patients. Br Med J 1994; 308:81–106.
27. Ridker PM, Manson JE, Buring JE, et al: The effect of chronic platelet inhibition with low-dose aspirin on atherosclerotic progression and acute thrombosis: clinical evidence from the Physicians' Health Study. Am Heart J 1991; 122:1588–1592.
28. Muller JE, Stone PH, Turi ZG, et al: Circadian variation in the frequency of onset of acute myocardial infarction. N Engl J Med 1985; 313:1315–1322.
29. Muller JE, Ludmer PL, Willich SN, et al: Circadian variation in the frequency of sudden cardiac death. Circulation 1987; 5:131–138.
30. Ridker PM, Manson JE, Buring JE, et al: Circadian variation of acute myocardial infarction and the effect of aspirin in a randomized trial of physicians. Circulation 1990; 82:897–902.
31. Witztum JL: The oxidation hypothesis of atherosclerosis. Lancet 1994; 344:793–795.
32. Steinberg D, Parthasarathy S, Carew TE, et al: Beyond cholesterol: modifications of low-density lipoprotein that increase its atherogenicity. N Engl J Med 1989; 320:915–924.
33. LaRosa JC, Hunninhake D, Bush D, et al: The cholesterol facts: a summary of the evidence relating dietary fats, serum cholesterol, and coronary heart disease. A joint statement by the American Heart Association and the National Heart Lung and Blood Institute. AHA Medical/Scientific Statement. Circulation 1990; 81:1721–1733.
34. Law MR, Wald NJ, Thompson SG: By how much and how quickly does reduction in serum cholesterol concentration lower risk of ischemic heart disease? Br Med J 1994; 308:367–372.
35. Law MR, Wald NJ, Wu T, et al: Systematic underestimation of association between serum cholesterol concentration and ischemic heart disease in observational studies: data from the BUPA study. Br Med J 1994; 308:363–366.
36. Chen Z, Peto R, Collins R, et al: Serum cholesterol concentration and coronary heart disease in population with low cholesterol concentrations. Br Med J 1991; 303:276–282.
37. Gordon DJ, Rifkind BM: High-density lipoprotein—the clinical implications of recent studies. N Engl J Med 1989; 321:1311–1316.
38. Jacobs DR Jr, Mebane IL, Bangdiwala SI, et al: High density lipoprotein cholesterol as a predictor of cardiovascular disease mortality in men and women: the follow-up study of the Lipid Research Clinics Prevalence Study. Am J Epidemiol 1990; 131:32–47.
39. Stampfer MJ, Sacks FM, Salvini S, et al: A prospective study of cholesterol apolipoproteins and the risk of myocardial infarction. N Engl J Med 1991; 325:373–381.
40. Rossouw JE, Lewis B, Rifkind BM: The value of lowering cholesterol after myocardial infarction. N Engl J Med 1990; 323:1112–1119.
41. Holme I: An analysis of randomized trials evaluating the effects of cholesterol reduction on total mortality and coronary heart disease incidence. Circulation 1990; 82:1916–1924.
42. Muldoon MF, Manuck SB, Matthew KA: Lowering cholesterol concentrations and mortality: a quantitative review of primary prevention trials. Br Med J 1990; 301:309–314.
43. Ravnskov U: Cholesterol lowering trials in coronary heart disease: frequency of citation and outcome. Br Med J 1992; 305:15–19.
44. Blankenhorn DH, Nessim SA, Johnson RL, et al: Beneficial effects of colestipol niacin therapy on coronary atherosclerosis and coronary venous bypass grafts. JAMA 1987; 257:3233–3240.
45. Brensike JF, Levy RI, Kelsey SF, et al: Effects of therapy with cholestyramine on progression of coronary atherosclerosis: results of the NHLBI Type II coronary intervention study. Circulation 1984; 69:313–324.
46. Brown BG, Albers JJ, Fisher LD, et al: Regression of coronary artery disease as a result of intensive lipid-lowering therapy in men with high levels of apolipoprotein B. N Engl J Med 1990; 323:1289–1298.
47. Buchwald H, Varco RL, Matts JP, et al: Effect of partial ileal bypass on mortality and morbidity from coronary heart disease in patients with hypercholesterolemia: report of the program on surgical control of the hyperlipidemias (POSCH). N Engl J Med 1990; 323:946–955.
48. Cashin-Hemphill L, Mack WJ, Pogoda MJ, et al: Beneficial effects of colestipol-niacin on coronary atherosclerosis. JAMA 1990; 264:3013–3017.
49. Kane JP, Malloy MJ, Ports TA, et al: Regression of coronary atherosclerosis during treatment of familial hypercholesterolemia with combined drug regimens. JAMA 1990; 264:3007–3012.
50. Superko HR, Krauss RM: Coronary artery disease regression. Convincing evidence for the benefit of aggressive lipoprotein management. Circulation 1994; 90:1056–1069.

51. Sacks FM, Pasternak RC, Gibson CM, et al: Effect on coronary atherosclerosis of decrease in plasma cholesterol concentrations in normocholesterolaemic patients. Lancet 1994; 344:1182–1186.
52. Expert Panel on Detection, Evaluation, and Treatment of High Blood Cholesterol in Adults: Summary of the Second Report of the National Cholesterol Education Program (NCEP) Expert Panel on Detection, Evaluation, and Treatment of High Blood Cholesterol in Adults (Adult Treatment Panel II). JAMA 1993; 269:3015–3023.
53. Law MR, Thompson SG, Wald NJ: Assessing possible hazards of reducing serum cholesterol. Br Med J 1994; 308:373–379.
54. Oliver MF: Doubts about preventing coronary heart disease. Multiple interventions in middle aged men may do more harm than good. Br Med J 1992; 304:393–394.
55. Oliver MF: Might treatment of hypercholesterolemia increase noncardiac mortality? Lancet 1991; 337:1529–1531.
56. Frick MH, Elo O, Happa K, et al: Helsinki Heart Study: primary prevention with gemfibrozil in middle-aged men with dyslipemia. N Engl J Med 1987; 317:1237–1245.
57. The Lipid Research Clinics Coronary Primary Prevention Trial results: I. Reduction in incidence of coronary heart disease. Lipid Research Clinics (LRC) Program. Lipid Metabolism–Atherogenesis Branch, National Heart, Lung, and Blood Institute. JAMA 1984; 251:351.
58. Scandinavian Simvastatin Survival Study Group: Randomised trial of cholesterol lowering in 4444 patients with coronary heart disease: the Scandinavian Simvastatin Survival Study (4s). Lancet 1994; 344:1383–1389.
59. Doll R, Peto R: Mortality in relation to smoking: 20 year observation on male British doctors. Br Med J 1976; 2:1525–1536.
60. Hammond EC, Horn D: Smoking and death rates: report on forty-four months of follow-up of 187,783 men. II. Death rates by cause. JAMA 1958: 166:1294–1308.
61. U.S. Department of Health and Human Services: Reducing the health consequences of smoking: 25 years of progress. A report of the Surgeon General [DHSS Publication No. (CDC)89–8411]. Washington DC: U.S. Government Printing Office, 1989.
62. Rosenberg L, Palmer JR, Shapiro S: Decline in the risk of myocardial infarction among women who stop smoking. N Engl J Med 1990; 322:213.
63. Rosenberg L, Kaufman DW, Helmrich SP, Shapiro S: The risk of myocardial infarction after quitting smoking in men under 55 years of age. N Engl J Med 1985; 313:1511–1514.
64. Tang JL, Law M, Wald N: How effective is nicotine replacement therapy in helping people to stop smoking? Br Med J 1994; 308:21–26.
65. Silagy C, Mant D, Fowler G, Lodge M: Meta-analysis on efficacy of nicotine replacement therapies in smoking cessation. Lancet 1994; 343:139–142.
66. Breo DL: Kicking butts—AMA, Joe Camel, and the "black-flag" war on tobacco. JAMA 1993; 270:1978–1984.
67. Wells AJ: Passive smoking as a cause of heart disease. J Am Coll Cardiol 1994; 24:546–554.
68. Steenland K: Passive smoking and risk of heart disease. JAMA 1992; 267:94–99.
69. MacMahon S, Peto R, Cutler J, et al: Blood pressure, stroke, and coronary heart disease: prolonged differences in blood pressure—prospective observational studies corrected for the regression dilution bias. Lancet 1990; 335:765–774.
70. Collins R, Peto R, MacMahon S, et al: Blood pressure, stroke, and coronary heart disease II, short-term reductions in blood pressure: overview of randomised drug trials in their epidemiological context. Lancet 1990; 335:827–838.
71. Hebert PR, Moser M, Mayer J, et al: Recent evidence on drug therapy of mild to moderate hypertension and decreased risk of coronary heart disease. Arch Intern Med 1993; 53(5):578–581.
72. Stamler R, Stamler J, Gosch FE, et al: Primary prevention of hypertension by nutritional-hygienic means. JAMA 1989; 262:1801–1807.
73. Hypertension Prevention Trial Research Group: Hypertension Prevention Trial: three-year effects of dietary changes on blood pressure. Arch Intern Med 1990; 150:153–162.
74. Trials of Hypertension Prevention Collaborative Research Group: The effects of nonpharmacologic interventions on blood pressure of persons with high normal levels: results of the Trials of Hypertension Prevention, Phase I. JAMA 1992; 267:1213–1220.
75. SHEP Cooperative Research Group: Prevention of stroke by antihypertensive drug treatment in older persons with isolated systolic hypertension: final results of the Systolic Hypertension in the Elderly (SHEP) Program. JAMA 1991; 265:3255–3264.
76. Joint National Committee on Detection, Evaluation, and Treatment of High Blood Pressure: The Fifth Report of the Joint National Committee on the Detection, Evaluation, and Treatment of High Blood Pressure (JNC V). Arch Intern Med 1993; 153:154–183.
77. Edelson JT, Weinstein MC, Tosteson ANA: The long term cost-effectiveness of various initial monotherapies for mild to moderate hypertension. JAMA 1990; 263:408–413.
78. Kuczmarski RJ, Flegal KM, Campbell SM, Johnson CL: Increasing prevalence of overweight among U.S. adults. The National Health and Nutrition Examination Surveys, 1960 to 1991. JAMA 1994; 272:205–211.
79. Daly PA, Solomon CG, Manson JE: Risk modification in the obese patient. *In* Manson JE, Ridker PM, Gaziano JM, Hennekens CH (eds): Primary Prevention of Myocardial Infarction. New York: Oxford University Press, in press.
80. Manson JE, Colditz GA, Stampfer MJ, et al: A prospective study of obesity and risk of coronary heart disease in women. N Engl J Med 1990; 322:882–889.
81. Tuck ML, Sowers J, Dornfeld L, et al: The effect of weight reduction on blood pressure, plasma renin activity, and plasma aldosterone levels in obese patients. N Engl J Med 1981; 304:930–936.
82. Dattilo AM, Kris-Etherton M: Effects of weight reduction on blood lipids and lipoproteins: a meta-analysis. Am J Clin Nutr 1992; 56:320–328.
83. Paffenbarger RS, Lee IM: Exercise and fitness in the primary prevention of coronary heart disease. *In* Manson JE, Ridker PM, Gaziano JM, Hennekens CH (eds): Primary Prevention of Myocardial Infarction. New York: Oxford University Press, in press.
84. Paffenbarger RS, Hyde RT, Wing AL, Hsieh CC: Physical activity, all-cause mortality, and longevity of college alumni. N Engl J Med 1986; 314:605–613.
85. Berlin JA, Colditz GA: A meta-analysis of physical activity in the prevention of coronary heart disease. Am J Epidemiol 1990; 132:612–628.
86. Ekelund LG, Haskell WL, Johnson JL, et al: Physical fitness as a predictor of cardiovascular mortality in asymptomatic North American men: the Lipid Research Clinics Mortality Follow-Up Study. N Engl J Med 1988; 319:1379–1384.
87. Siscovick DS, Weiss NS, Fletcher RH, Lasky T: The incidence of primary cardiac arrest during vigorous exercise. N Engl J Med 1984; 311:874–877.
88. Pate RR, Pratt M, Blair SN, et al: Physical activity and public health. A recommendation from the Centers for Disease Control and Prevention and the American College of Sports Medicine. JAMA 1995; 273:402–407.
89. Bush TL: The epidemiology of cardiovascular disease in postmenopausal women. Ann N Y Acad Sci 1990; 592:263–271.
90. Eaker ED, Chesebro JH, Sacks FM, et al: Cardiovascular disease in women. Circulation 1993; 88:1999–2009.
91. Stampfer MJ, Colditz GA: Estrogen replacement therapy and coronary heart disease: a quantitative assessment of the epidemiologic evidence. Prev Med 1991; 20:47–63.
92. Stampfer MJ, Colditz GA, Willett WC, et al: Postmenopausal estrogen therapy and cardiovascular disease: ten-year follow-up from the Nurses' Health Study. N Engl J Med 1991; 325:756–762.
93. Bush TL, Cowan LD, Barrett-Connor E, et al: Cardiovascular mortality and noncontraceptive use of estrogen in women: results from the Lipid Research Clinics Program Follow-Up Study. Circulation 1987; 75:1102–1109.
94. Grodstein F, Manson JE, Stampfer M: Postmenopausal hormone therapy. *In* Manson JE, Ridker PM, Gaziano JM, Hennekens CH (eds): Primary Prevention of Myocardial Infarction. New York: Oxford University Press, in press.
95. Colditz GA, Stampfer M, Willett WC, et al: Prospective study of estrogen replacement therapy and risk of breast cancer in postmenopausal women. JAMA 1990; 264:2648–2653.
96. Buring JE, Hennekens CH, Lipnick RJ, et al: A prospective cohort study of postmenopausal hormone use and risk of breast cancer in U.S. women. Am J Epidemiol 1987; 125:939–947.
97. Goldman L, Tosteson A: Uncertainty about postmenopausal estrogen: time for action, not debate. N Engl J Med 1991; 325:800–802.
98. Writing Group for the PEPI Trial: Effects of estrogen and estrogen/progestin regimens on heart disease risk factors in postmenopausal women. The Postmenopausal Estrogen/Progestin Interventions (PEPI) Trial. JAMA 1995; 273:199–208.
99. Hennekens CH, Buring JE, Sandercock P, et al: Aspirin and other antiplatelet agents in the secondary and primary prevention of cardiovascular disease. Circulation 1989; 80:749–756.
100. Antiplatelet Trialists' Collaboration: Collaborative overview of random-

ised trials of antiplatelet therapy—II: Maintenance of vascular graft or arterial patency by antiplatelet therapy. Br Med J 1994; 308:159–168.
101. Antiplatelet Trialists' Collaboration: Collaborative overview of randomised trials of antiplatelet therapy—III: Reduction in venous thrombosis and pulmonary embolism by antiplatelet prophylaxis among surgical and medical patients. Br Med J 1994; 308:235–246.
102. Fuster V, Dyken ML, Vokonos PS, Hennekens CH: Aspirin as a therapeutic agent in cardiovascular disease. Circulation 1993; 87:659–675.
103. Steering Committee of the Physicians' Health Study Research Group: Final report on the aspirin component of the ongoing Physicians' Health Study. N Engl J Med 1989; 321:129–135.
104. Peto R, Gray R, Collins R, et al: A randomised trial of the effects of prophylactic daily aspirin among male British doctors. Br Med J 1988; 296:320–331.
105. U.S. Preventive Services Task Force: Guide to Clinical Preventive Services, chap. 60. Baltimore: Williams & Wilkins, 1989.
106. Buring JE, Hennekens CH: Randomized trials of primary prevention of cardiovascular disease in women: an investigator's view. Ann Epidemiol 1994; 4:111–114.
107. Manson JE, Stampfer MJ, Colditz GA, et al: A prospective study of aspirin use and primary prevention of cardiovascular disease in women. JAMA 1991; 266:521–527.
108. Clarke RJ, Mayo G, Price P, Fitzgerald GA: Suppression of thromboxane A2 but not of systemic prostacyclin by controlled-release aspirin. N Engl J Med 1991; 325:1137–1141.
109. Steinberg D, Workshop Participants: Antioxidants in the prevention of human atherosclerosis: summary proceedings of a NHLBI Workshop: September 5–6, 1991, Bethesda, MD. Circulation 1992; 85:2337–2347.
110. Manson JE, Gaziano JM, Jonas MA, Hennekens CH: Antioxidants and cardiovascular disease: a review. J Am Coll Nutr 1993; 12:426–432.
111. Gaziano JM, Manson JE, Buring JE, Hennekens CH: Dietary antioxidants in cardiovascular disease. Ann N Y Acad Sci 1992; 669:249–258.
112. Stampfer MJ, Hennekens CH, Manson JE, et al: A prospective study of vitamin E consumption and risk of coronary disease in women. New Engl J Med 1993; 328:1444–1449.
113. Rimm EB, Stampfer MJ, Ascherio A, et al: Dietary intake and risk of coronary heart disease among men. N Engl J Med 1993; 328:1450–1456.
114. Gaziano JM, Manson JE, Brnach LG, et al: Dietary beta carotene and decreased cardiovascular mortality in an elderly cohort. J Am Coll Cardiol 1992; 19:377.
115. Anderson TW, Reid W: A double blind trial of vitamin E in the treatment of angina pectoris. Am Heart J 1974; 27:1174–1178.
116. Gillilan RE, Mandell B, Warbasse JR: Quantitative evaluation of vitamin E in the treatment of angina pectoris. Am Heart J 1977; 93:444–449.
117. Gaziano JM, Manson JE, Ridker PM, et al: Beta-carotene therapy for chronic stable angina [Abstract]. Circulation 1990; 82(suppl III):202.
118. DeMaio SJ, King SB, Lembo NJ, et al: Vitamin E supplementation, plasma lipids, and incidence of restenosis after percutaneous transluminal angioplasty. J Am Coll Nutr 1992; 11:131–138.
119. Blot WJ, Li J, Taylor PR, et al: Nutritional intervention trials in Linxian, China: supplementation with specific vitamin/mineral combinations, cancer incidence, and disease-specific mortality in the general population. J Natl Cancer Inst 1993; 85:1483–1492.
120. Alpha-Tocopherol, Beta-Carotene Lung Cancer Prevention Study Group: The effect of vitamin E and beta-carotene on the incidence of lung cancer and other cancers in male smokers. N Engl J Med 1994; 330:1029–1035.
121. Hennekens CH, Buring JE, Peto R: Antioxidant vitamins—benefits not yet proved. N Engl J Med 1994; 330:1080–1081.
122. Gaziano JM, Steinberg D: Prevention of cardiovascular disease by natural antioxidants. *In* Manson JE, Ridker PM, Gaziano JM, Hennekens CH (eds): Primary Prevention of Myocardial Infarction. New York: Oxford University Press, in press.
123. Hennekens CH: Alcohol. *In* Stamler J, Kaplan N (eds): Prevention of Coronary Heart Disease. Practical Management of the Risk Factors, pp 130–138. Philadelphia: WB Saunders, 1983.
124. Klatsky AL, Friedman GD, Siegelaub AB: Alcohol and mortality. A ten-year Kaiser-Permanente experience. Ann Intern Med 1981; 95(2):139–145.
125. Klatsky AL, Armstrong MA, Friedman GD: Risk of cardiovascular mortality in alcohol drinkers, ex-drinkers and nondrinkers. Am J Cardiol 1990; 66:1237–1242.
126. Deutscher S, Rockette HE, Krishnaswami V: Evaluation of habitual excessive alcohol consumption on myocardial infarction risk in coronary disease patients. Am Heart J 1984; 108(4):988–995.
127. Moore RD, Pearson TA: Moderate alcohol consumption and coronary artery disease: a review. Medicine 1986; 65:242–267.
128. Gordon T, Kannel WB: Drinking habits and cardiovascular disease: The Framingham Study. Am Heart J 1983; 105:667–673.
129. Stampfer MJ, Colditz GA, Willett WC, et al: A prospective study of moderate alcohol consumption and the risk of coronary disease and stroke in women. N Engl J Med 1988; 319(5):267–273.
130. Hennekens CH, Rosner B, Cole DS: Daily alcohol consumption and fatal coronary heart disease. Am J Epidemiol 1978; 107:196–200.
131. Buring JE, O'Connor GT, Goldhaber SZ, et al: Decreased HDL_2 and HDL_3 cholesterol, Apo A-I and Apo A-II, and increased risk of myocardial infarction. Circulation 1992; 85:22–29.
132. Rimm EB, Giovannucci EL, Willett WC, et al: Prospective study of alcohol consumption and risk of coronary disease in men. Lancet 1991; 338:464–468.
133. Criqui MH, Ringer BL: Does diet or alcohol explain the French paradox? Lancet 1994; 344:1719–1723.
134. Langer RD, Criqui MH, Reed DM: Lipoproteins and blood pressure as biological pathways for effect of moderate alcohol consumption on coronary heart disease. Circulation 1992; 85:910–915.
135. Gaziano JM, Buring JE, Breslow JL, et al: Moderate alcohol intake, increased levels of high-density lipoprotein and its subfractions, and risk of myocardial infarction. N Engl J Med 1993; 329:1829–1834.
136. Jackson R, Scragg R, Beaglehole R: Does recent alcohol consumption reduce the risk of acute myocardial infarction and coronary death in regular drinkers? Am J Epidemiol 1992; 136:819–824.
137. Ridker PM, Vaughan DE, Stampfer MJ, et al: Association of moderate alcohol consumption and plasma concentration of endogenous tissue–type plasminogen activator. JAMA 1994; 272:929–933.
138. Ornish D, Brown SE, Scherwitz LW, et al: Can lifestyle changes reverse coronary heart disease? Lancet 1990; 336:129–133.
139. Mensink RP, Katan MB: Effect of dietary fats on serum lipids and lipoproteins. Arteriosclerosis Thrombosis 1992; 12:911–919.
140. Zock PL, Katan MB: Hydrogenation alternatives: effects of trans fatty acids and stearic acid versus linoleic acid on serum lipids and lipoproteins in humans. J Lipid Res 1992; 33:399–410.
141. Judd JT, Clevidence BA, Muesing RA, et al: Dietary *trans* fatty acids: Effects on plasma lipids and lipoproteins of healthy men and women. Am J Clin Nutr 1994; 59:861–868.
142. Siguel EN, Lerman RH: *Trans* fatty acid patterns in patients with angiographically documented coronary artery disease. Am J Cardiol 1993; 71:916–920.
143. Ascherio A, Hennekens CH, Buring JE, et al: Trans fatty acid intake and risk of myocardial infarction. Circulation 1994; 89:94–101.
144. Willett WC, Stampfer MJ, Colditz GA, et al: Intake of *trans* fatty acids and risk of coronary heart disease among women. Lancet 1993; 341:581–585.
145. Willett WC, Lenart EB: Diet in the prevention of coronary heart disease. *In* Manson JE, Ridker PM, Gaziano JM, Hennekens CH (eds): Primary Prevention of Myocardial Infarction. New York: Oxford University Press, in press.
146. Kromhout D, Bosscheiter EB, deLezenne Coulander C: The inverse relation between fish consumption and 20-year mortality from coronary heart disease. N Engl J Med 1985; 312:1205–1209.
147. Shekelle RB, Missell L, Paul O, et al: Fish consumption and mortality from coronary heart disease [Letter]. N Engl J Med 1985; 313:820.
148. Norell SE, Ahlbom A, Feychting M, Pedersen NL: Fish consumption and mortality from coronary heart disease. Br Med J 1986; 293:426.
149. Dolecek TA: Epidemiologic evidence of relationships between dietary polyunsaturated fatty acids and mortality in the multiple risk factor intervention trial. Proc Soc Exp Biol Med 1992; 220:177–182.
150. Curb JD, Reed DM: Fish consumption and mortality from coronary heart disease [Letter]. N Engl J Med 1985; 313:821.
151. Hennekens CH, Buring JE, Mayrent SL: Clinical epidemiologic data on the effects of fish oil in cardiovascular disease. *In* Lees R, Karel M (eds): Omega-3 Fatty Acids in Health and Disease, pp 71–86. New York: Marcel Dekker, 1990.
152. Leaf A, Weber PC: Cardiovascular effects of n-3 fatty acids. N Engl J Med 1988; 318:549–557.
153. Morris MC, Sacks FM, Rosner B: Does fish oil lower blood pressure? A meta-analysis of controlled trials. Circulation 1993; 88:523–533.
154. Sassen L, Lamers J, Verdouw P: Fish oil and the prevention and regression of atherosclerosis. Cardiovasc Drugs Ther 1994; 8:179–191.
155. Kromhout D, Bosscheiter EB, deLezenne Coulander C: Dietary fiber and 10-year mortality from coronary heart disease, cancer and all causes: The Zutphen Study. Lancet 1982; 2:518–521.

156. Khaw KT, Barrett-Connor E: Dietary fiber and reduced ischemic heart disease rates in men and women: a 12-year prospective study. Am J Epidemiol 1987; 126:1093–1102.
157. Burr ML, Fehily AM, Gilbert JF: Effects of changes in fat, fish, fibre intakes on death and myocardial infarction: diet and reinfarction trial (DART). Lancet 1989; 2:757–761.
158. Heller RF, Chinn S, Tunstall Pedoe HD, Rose G: How well can we predict coronary heart disease? Findings in the United Kingdom Heart Disease Prevention Project. Br Med J 1984; 288:1409–1411.
159. Wald NJ, Law M, Watt HC, et al: Apolipoproteins and ischaemic heart disease: implications for screening. Lancet 1994; 343:75–79.
160. Schafer AI: Hypercoagulable states: molecular genetics to clinical practice. Lancet 1994; 344:1739–1742.
161. Ernst E: Plasma fibrinogen—an independent cardiovascular risk factor. J Intern Med 1990; 27:365–372.
162. Meade TW, Mellows S, Brozovic M, et al: Haemostatic function and ischaemic heart disease. Principal results of the Northwick Park Heart Study. Lancet 1986; 2:533–537.
163. Wilhelmsen L, Svardsudd K, Korsan-Bengtsen K, et al: Fibrinogen as a risk factor for stroke and myocardial infarction. N Engl J Med 1984; 311:501–505.
164. Kannel WB, Wolf PA, Castelli WP, D'Agostino RB: Fibrinogen and risk of cardiovascular disease. The Framingham Study. JAMA 1987; 258:1183–1186.
165. Stone MC, Thorpe JM: Plasma fibrinogen-A major coronary risk factor. J Roy Coll Gen Pract 1985; 35:565–569.
166. Yarnell JWG, Baker IA, Sweetnam PM, et al: Fibrinogen, viscosity, and white blood cell count are major risk factors for ischemic heart disease. The Caerphilly and Speedwell Collaborative Heart Disease Studies. Circulation 1991; 83:836–844.
167. Neumann FJ, Katus HA, Hoberg E, et al: Increased plasma viscosity and erythrocyte aggregation: Indicators of an unfavourable clinical outcome in patients with unstable angina pectoris. Br Heart J 1991; 66:425–430.
168. Moller L, Kristensen TS: Plasma fibrinogen and ischemic heart disease risk factors. Arteriosclerosis Thrombosis 1991; 11:344–350.
169. Trip MD, Manger Cats V, van Capelle FJL, Vreeken J: Platelet hyperreactivity and prognosis in survivors of myocardial infarction. N Engl J Med 1990; 322:1549–1554.
170. Elwood PC, Renaud S, Sharp DS, et al: Ischemic heart disease and platelet aggregation: the Caerphilly Collaborative Heart Disease Study. Circulation 1991; 83:38–44.
171. Martin JF, Bath PMW, Burr ML: Influence of platelet size on outcome after myocardial infarction. Lancet 1991; 338:1409–1411.
172. Thaulow E, Erikssen J, Sandvik L, et al: Blood platelet count and function are related to total and cardiovascular death in apparently healthy men. Circulation 1991; 84:613–617.
173. Hamsten A, Wiman B, de Faire U, Blombäck M: Increased plasma levels of a rapid inhibitor of tissue plasminogen activator in young survivors of myocardial infarction. N Engl J Med 1985; 313(25):1557–1563.
174. Ridker PM, Vaughan DE, Stampfer MJ, et al: Endogenous tissue–type plasminogen activator and risk of myocardial infarction. Lancet 1993; 341:1165–1168.
175. Ridker PM, Hennekens CH, Stampfer MJ, et al: Prospective study of endogenous tissue plasminogen activator and risk of stroke. Lancet 1994; 343:940–943.
176. Jansson JH, Olofsson BO, Nilsson TK: Predictive value of tissue plasminogen activator mass concentration on long term mortality in patients with coronary artery disease: a seven year follow-up. Circulation 1993; 88:2030–2034.
177. Thompson SG, Kienast J, Pyke SDM, et al: Hemostatic factors and the risk of myocardial infarction or sudden death in patients with angina pectoris. N Engl J Med 1995; 332:635–641.
178. Meade TW, Ruddock V, Stirling Y, et al: Fibrinolytic activity, clotting factors, and long term incidence of ischaemic heart disease in the Northwick Park Heart Study. Lancet 1993; 342:1076–1079.
179. Fowkes FGR, Lowe GDO, Housley E, et al: Cross-linked fibrin degradation products, progression of peripheral arterial disease, and risk of coronary heart disease. Lancet 1993; 342:84–86.
180. Ridker PM, Hennekens CH, Cerskus A, Stampfer MJ: Plasma concentration of cross linked fibrin degradation product (D-dimer) and the risk of future myocardial infarction among apparently healthy men. Circulation 1994; 90:2236–2240.
181. Stampfer MJ, Malinow MR, Willett WC, et al: A prospective study of plasma homocysteine and risk of myocardial infarction in U.S. physicians. JAMA 1992; 268:877–881.
182. Arnesen E, Refsum H, Bonaa KH, et al: The Tromso Study: Serum Total Homocysteine and Myocardial Infarction: A Prospective Study. Presented at the 3rd International Conference on Preventive Cardiology, Oslo, Norway, June 27–July 1, 1993.
183. Malinow MR, Nieto FJ, Szklo M, et al: Carotid artery intimal-medial wall thickening and plasma homocysteine in asymptomatic adults: the Atherosclerosis Risk in Communities Study. Circulation 1993; 87:1107–1113.
184. Selhub J, Jacques PF, Bostom AG, et al: Association between plasma homocysteine concentrations and extracranial carotid-artery stenosis. N Engl J Med 1995; 332:286–291.
185. Selhub J, Jacques PF, Wilson PW, et al: Vitamin status and intake as primary determinants of homocystinemia in an elderly population. JAMA 1993; 270:2693–2698.
186. Stampfer MJ, Malinow MR: Can lowering homocysteine levels reduce cardiovascular risk? N Engl J Med 1995; 332:328–329.
187. Scanu AM: Lipoprotein(a): a genetic risk factor for premature coronary heart disease. JAMA 1992; 267:3326–3329.
188. Loscalzo J: Lipoprotein(a): a unique risk factor for atherothrombotic disease. Arteriosclerosis 1990; 10:671–679.
189. Rosengren A, Wilhelmsen L, Eriksson E, et al: Lipoprotein(a) and coronary heart disease: a prospective case-control study in a general population of middle aged men. Br Med J 1990; 301:1248–1251.
190. Jauhiainen M, Koskinen P, Ehnholm C, et al: Lipoprotein(a) and coronary heart disease risk: a nested case-control study of the Helsinki Heart Study participants. Atherosclerosis 1991; 89:59–67.
191. Ridker PM, Hennekens CH, Stampfer MJ: A prospective study of lipoprotein(a) and the risk of myocardial infarction. JAMA 1993; 270:2195–2199.
192. Schaefer EJ, Lamon-Fava S, Jenner JL, et al: Lipoprotein(a) levels and risk of coronary heart disease in men. The Lipid Research Clinics Coronary Primary Prevention Trial. JAMA 1994; 271:999–1003.
193. Ridker PM, Stampfer MJ, Hennekens CH: Plasma concentration of lipoprotein(a) and the risk of future stroke. JAMA 1995; 273:1269–1273.
194. Cremer P, Nagel D, Labrot B, et al: Lipoprotein Lp(a) as predictor of myocardial infarction in comparison to fibrinogen, LDL cholesterol and other risk factors: results from the prospective Göttingen Risk Incidence and Prevalence Study (GRIPS). Euro J Clin Invest 1994; 24:444–453.
195. Cambien F, Poirer O, Lecerf L, et al: Deletion polymorphism in the gene for angiotensin converting enzyme is a potent risk factor for myocardial infarction. Nature 1992; 359:641–644.
196. Lindpaintner K, Pfeffer MA, Kreutz R, et al: A prospective evaluation of an angiotensin-converting enzyme gene polymorphism and the risk of ischemic heart disease. N Engl J Med 1995; 332:706–711.
197. Zoller B, Dahlback B: Linkage between inherited resistance to activated protein C and factor V gene mutation in venous thrombosis. Lancet 1994; 343:1536–1538.
198. Svensson PJ, Dahlback B: Resistance to activated protein C as a basis for venous thrombosis. N Engl J Med 1994; 330:517–522.
199. Koster T, Rosendaal FR, de Ronde H, et al: Venous thrombosis due to poor anticoagulant response to activated protein C: Leiden Thrombophilia Study. Lancet 1993; 342:1503–1506.
200. Ridker PM, Hennekens CH, Lindpaintner K, et al: Mutation in the gene coding for coagulation factor V and the risk of myocardial infarction, stroke, and venous thrombosis in apparently healthy men. N Engl J Med 1995; 332:912–917.
201. Vandenbroucke JP, Koster T, Briet E, et al: Increased risk of venous thrombosis in oral-contraceptive users who are carriers of factor V Leiden mutation. Lancet 1994; 344:1453–1457.
202. Mann JI, Lewis B, Shephard J, et al: Blood lipid concentrations and other cardiovascular risk factors: distribution, prevalence and detection in Britain. Br Med J 1988; 296:1702–1706.
203. Kannel WB: Contribution of the Framingham Study to the conquest of coronary heart disease. Am J Cardiol 1988; 62:1109–1112.

2 Pharmacologic Options for Treatment of Ischemic Disease

Lionel H. Opie, MD, PhD

NITRATES

Nitrates, although well-established therapeutic agents in the therapy of angina for more than 125 years, act on a messenger system that has only recently come to be recognized for its physiologic importance. In response to a number of physiologic stimuli, the intact vascular endothelium releases nitric oxide, which causes vasodilatation. Nitrates bypass the requirement for a functional endothelium and promote vasorelaxation even when the endothelium is damaged.

Mechanisms of Action of Nitrates

Pharmacodynamics

The most important single property of the nitrates is to cause vasodilatation that occurs especially in the venous capacitance vessels, in the large coronary arteries, and to a lesser extent in the peripheral arterioles.[1] By reduction of preload, the oxygen uptake of the heart is decreased by about 20%–40%.[1] The fall in myocardial oxygen demand reflects reductions in venous return and ventricular volume, along with a modest fall in arterial pressure, although these benefits are to some extent offset by a reflex increase in the heart rate.

Regarding the direct coronary dilator effect, the nitrates dilate large coronary arteries and arterioles greater than 100 μm in diameter. It is not fully understood why they do not dilate the smaller arterioles, but a plausible hypothesis is that the processes converting the nitrates to nitric oxide in the arterial wall are relatively inactive in the coronary arterioles because of the absence of the obligatory sulfhydryl (thiol) groups.[2] By dilating large coronary arteries, the nitrates also (1) redistribute blood flow along collateral channels and from epicardial to endocardial regions and (2) relieve exercise-induced coronary arterial constriction and spontaneous coronary spasm. An important clinical distinction is that agents such as dipyridamole and other vasodilators including sodium nitroprusside that act on small arterioles may induce a "coronary steal" effect.

Vascular Signaling Systems

Although the nitric oxide pathway is now recognized as having an important physiologic messenger role extending beyond the cardiovascular system to, for example, the brain, details of the signals involved are not yet clear. It is uncertain exactly how nitrates promote activity of the nitric oxide pathway. An important step appears to be conversion of the nitrate moiety ($-ONO_2$) to nitric oxide. This biotransformation probably occurs within the vascular smooth muscle cells, although some workers believe that a certain amount of extracellular transformation also takes place. The activity of the enzyme glutathione-*S*–transferase as well as the presence of thiol groups appears to be needed. Not all data are consistent with this hypothesis, and other enzyme systems including an esterase and a microsomal P-450 are reported to produce nitric oxide even in the absence of sulfhydryl groups.[3] The sulfhydryl-independent paths may be important in relation to nitrate tolerance.

Once nitric oxide is produced, the next step is thought to be stimulation of guanylate cyclase to produce cyclic guanosine monophosphate (cGMP), thereby in turn activating a cGMP-dependent protein kinase.[3] It is proposed that activity of this kinase decreases cytosolic calcium ion levels in vascular smooth muscle cells—the "ultimate step" in vascular contraction. The mechanism for this fall in calcium levels is not yet well understood but might involve (1) increased uptake of calcium ions into the sarcoplasmic reticulum (after phosphorylation of phospholamban) or (2) decreased release of calcium from the sarcoplasmic reticulum after a fall of inositol 1,4,5-triphosphate (IP_3); or (3) contraction might be inhibited after decreased phosphorylation of the controlling enzyme in vascular smooth muscle contraction, namely, myosin light chain kinase. cGMP also has direct effects on monovalent cation transport. Furthermore, nitric oxide has effects on potassium channels independently of cGMP. Thus, the pathways involved in nitrate-induced vasodilatation remain uncertain, although those shown in Figure 2–1 may provide a useful model for present concepts.

Why nitrates are more active venous than arterial dilators is not clear. The rate of formation of cGMP is unexpectedly greater in arteries than in veins.[4] It may thus be that the concurrent reduction in preload causes a reflex vasoconstriction that limits the arterial dilatation.

Effects on Platelets

A modest inhibitory effect of nitrates on platelet aggregation can be found in patients with angina or recent acute myocardial infarction. Furthermore, low concentrations of nitroglycerin can partially reverse adenosine diphosphate (ADP)–induced platelet aggregation.[5] The clinical significance of this effect is still unknown. *S*-Nitroso compounds are being developed to have direct specific antiplatelet effects without significant hypotensive effects (see section on antiplatelet agents).

Prostacyclin-Mediated Effects

The late phase of coronary vasodilatation by nitrates is blunted when prostaglandin synthesis is inhibited.[6] This provides a possible explanation for the inability to detect any benefit of nitrates in aspirin-treated patients in the megatrials of acute myocardial infarction. Nonetheless, this possible negative interaction with aspirin is largely inferential.

Direct Effects on Myocardium

It has been suggested that a direct action of NO· on cardiac muscle with a negative inotropic effect[7] may contribute to the anti-ischemic

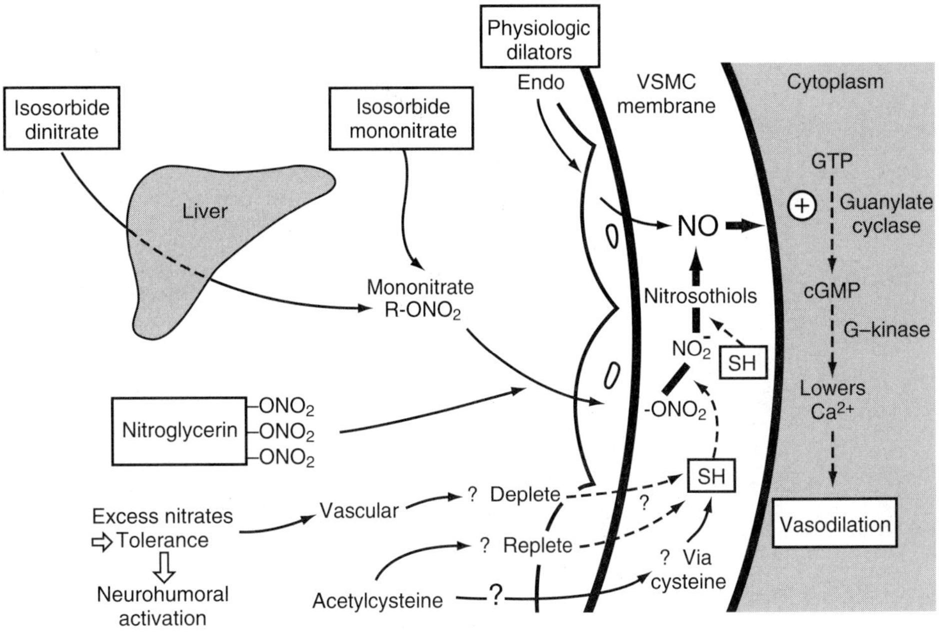

Figure 2–1. Current proposals for the mechanism of nitrate tolerance. Neurohumoral activation is thought to occur as a result of nitrate-induced vasodilatation, possibly involving reflex arterial constriction and impaired renal blood flow. Although nitrate receptors are still hypothetical, downregulated high-affinity receptors (responding to low concentrations of nitrates) and maintained activity of low-affinity receptors (responding to increased concentrations of nitrates) could explain the benefits of dose escalation. *Abbreviations:* VSMC, vascular smooth muscle cell; G-kinase, kinase dependent on cGMP. (Reprinted with permission. Copyright 1996, L.H. Opie.)

protection of nitrates. However, these effects are controversial[3] and may be more obvious in atrial tissue or in neonatal myocytes than in adult ventricular cells.[8] The potential messenger of this protective system may also be cGMP, which by lowering cell calcium levels could theoretically protect against calcium-mediated ischemic damage and arrhythmias.

Comment. The predominant clinically relevant effect of the nitrates is a combination of preload reduction, dilatation of the large coronary arteries (especially at sites of vasoconstriction), and modest reduction of afterload. Other mechanisms of action, such as those on platelets, prostaglandins, and cardiac myocytes, are not yet rigorously established.

Pharmacokinetic Properties of Nitrates

The pharmacokinetic properties of the organic nitrates vary greatly. Plasma levels, difficult to measure, vary from trace and transient concentrations in the case of sublingual nitroglycerin to sustained high blood levels in the case of transdermal patches or certain controlled-release preparations. In the case of nitroglycerin, there is an extensive first-pass hepatic metabolism, so that plasma concentrations are often below the limit of detection. With sublingual administration, plasma nitroglycerin levels transiently increase in the plasma. With transdermal nitroglycerin systems, levels are maintained for a 24-h period with some intraindividual and interindividual variability. In the case of isosorbide dinitrate, hepatic first-pass extraction converts circulating dinitrate to isosorbide-5-mononitrate, the active component, and to a lesser extent to 2-mononitrate. Both of these reach high concentrations in the plasma.

Isosorbide-5-mononitrate is completely absorbed with almost 100% bioavailability. Both standard and controlled-release formulations have been extensively studied for their duration of antianginal effect and with a view to avoiding tolerance.

Whenever blood levels of any of these compounds are maintained for a significant period, the major problem is the development of tolerance. Long-term dose schedules designed to avoid tolerance are at present best established for isosorbide-5-mononitrate[9] when the standard preparation is given as 20-mg tablets 7 h apart or when a controlled-release preparation is given as a large dose once daily.

Indications for Nitrates

Nitrates are used for treatment of a wide variety of anginal syndromes, including acute effort angina (sublingual nitroglycerin and isosorbide dinitrate), angina prophylaxis (particularly the mononitrates in doses designed to avoid tolerance), unstable angina at rest, acute myocardial infarction (intravenous nitroglycerin), and congestive heart failure (intravenous or oral nitrates). Standard doses and preparations are shown in Table 2–1.

Nitrate Tolerance

The phenomenon of nitrate tolerance, once under dispute and ignored by some clinicians, is now established beyond reasonable doubt. The mechanism involved remains unclear (Table 2–2). Nitrate tolerance occurs clinically whenever nitrate blood levels are sustained for many hours without a nitrate-free interval. Tolerance is an established phenomenon in prolonged nitrate treatment of congestive heart failure and stable angina pectoris. There is no definite proof of tolerance when intravenous nitrates are given acutely for unstable angina, although increasing doses are often required.[10] In early acute myocardial infarction, when nitrates are initially infused at low doses, dose escalation is required in about one quarter of patients.[11]

Mechanisms of Tolerance

In vitro, vascular tolerance is accompanied by reduced metabolic conversion of nitrates to the pharmacologically active product, nitric oxide. This concept is supported by in vivo data in which the amount of exhaled nitric oxide decreased as nitrate tolerance developed; with the direct nitric oxide donor sodium nitroprusside, no tolerance developed, nor was there any decrease in exhaled nitric oxide.[12] Hypothetically, excess nitric oxide formation depletes intracellular sulfhydryl groups, which may explain lower platelet cGMP levels in nitrate-tolerant patients.[13] When blood vessels are studied in vitro, there is substantial evidence for the sulfhydryl theory.[10] Whether this concept can be applied to patients is open to question. In isolated vessel experiments, high concentrations of nitroglycerin are used and tolerance is induced within 1 h. Clinically, nanomolar nitrate concentrations are therapeutically effective and the exposure time for tolerance to develop is several hours.

TABLE 2–1. CLINICAL PHARMACOKINETICS OF NITRATE COMPOUNDS

Nitrate Compound	Dose	Plasma Kinetics	Metabolism	Clinical Effects	Comments
NTG sublingual	0.15–1.5 mg Tablets 0.15, 0.3, 0.5, or 0.6 mg; use every 5 min until pain relief, or up to 4–5 tablets	Very low levels* (ng/mL range) Bioavailability about 36% Plasma $t_{1/2}$: few minutes[21]	Very high first-pass hepatic metabolism to dinitrates and then mononitrates, also with short half-life In addition, extensive extrahepatic vascular clearance	Mean time to relief of angina 1.9 min	Best taken before onset of anginal pain
NTG ointment	½ in (7.5 mg) to 2 in (30 mg) spread over 36 sq in (6 × 6 in or 15 × 15 cm)	Blood levels rise to steady state within 1 h of application and wane with half-life of 30 min after removal Plasma $t_{1/2}$ about 3 min	As above	Single application gives antianginal benefit for 7 h 2× daily application for 3 weeks leads to tolerance	Duration of antianginal activity during sustained application not known
NTG transdermal	Should exceed 50 mg/24 h but be applied for only 12 h	Concentrations increase in a period of hours until plateau is reached; then levels may fluctuate, possibly owing to variations in transdermal bioavailability after each application	As above	Rapid development of tolerance within 24 h of first application Effective for 4–8 h during intermittent therapy	Patch on (12 h), then off recommended[36]
NTG intravenous	5–200 μg/min for 24–48 h, occasionally up to 1000 μg/min	Level about 5 ng/mL during prolonged infusion at about 50 μg/min[24]	As above	Unstable angina: titrate dose upward every 5–10 min until relief of chest pain or systolic BP <90 mm Hg or adverse effects; then reduce AMI: control by mean BP, 10% reduction in nonhypertensives and 30% in hypertensives; do not drop below mean BP of 80 mm Hg[11]	Increasing doses may be needed, possibly owing to tolerance[23] Slower than NTG
Isosorbide dinitrate sublingual	2.5–15 mg as needed	Bioavailability about 40%–60% $t_{1/2}$ for active mononitrate metabolite 4 h[21]	Hepatic conversion to isosorbide-5-mononitrate and 2-mononitrate	Mean time to relief of angina 3.4 min	Slower than NTG
Isosorbide dinitrate oral	5–80 mg 1× daily (efficacy for multiple doses not established)	Bioavailability 30% Peak plasma values 30–60 min $t_{1/2}$ 30–50 min	As above	After single dose, antianginal effect maintained for 8 h When 30 mg given 3× daily, antianginal effect declines with each succeeding dose during the day[37]	Need 14–18 h nitrate-free interval to avoid tolerance[9]
Isosorbide dinitrate controlled-release (Tembids)	40 mg controlled-release 1× daily	Bioavailability, as above	As above	Use only 1× daily during long-term dosing, which gives up to 8 h protection	When given 2× daily at 0800 and 1400, not superior to placebo during long-term treatment[36]
Isosorbide-5-mononitrate tablets	20 mg 2× daily 7 h apart	Bioavailability nearly 100% Time to peak level 30–60 min $t_{1/2}$ about 5 h	No first-pass metabolism, then systemic breakdown to inactive glucuronides excreted in urine	Antianginal effect more than 11 h from first dose still maintained at 2–3 weeks; there is a 30%–40% loss of activity due to overall tolerance	Partially prevents nitrate tolerance at this dosage
Isosorbide-5-mononitrate controlled-release	120–240 mg 1× daily	Bioavailability nearly 100% Time to peak levels 4 h	As above	Antianginal effect sustained for a period of 42 days	No tolerance found at tested doses[9]

Abbreviations: AMI, acute myocardial infarction; BP, blood pressure; NTG, nitroglycerin.
*Level = plasma concentration.

TABLE 2–2. NITRATE TOLERANCE: MECHANISMS AND PROPOSED THERAPY

Proposed Mechanism	Proposed Therapy	References
Vascular sulfhydryl depletion	*N*-Acetylcysteine	12, 15
Neurohumoral activation	Angiotensin converting enzyme inhibitors	10
Impaired renal perfusion	Hydralazine	17, 18
Lack of oscillation of nitrate levels	Dose escalation	38

Sulfhydryl donors such as acetylcysteine or methionine (indirect sulfhydryl donor) could theoretically counteract tolerance either by providing sulfhydryl groups within the vascular cells or by forming extracellular thiols (see Fig. 2–1), which could then enter the vascular cells to stimulate guanylate cyclase.[10] In human volunteers, acetylcysteine gives some protection against nitrate tolerance in veins but not in medium-sized arteries.[14] Mehra and colleagues[15] suggested that the best benefit of *N*-acetylcysteine was obtained when it was given before the onset of tolerance in patients with congestive heart failure receiving concurrent isosorbide dinitrate. They suggested that the *N*-acetylcysteine is more effective in increasing extracellular than intracellular sulfhydryl groups. The overall evidence regarding the use of *N*-acetylcysteine to prevent or treat nitrate tolerance remains confusing (see review by Fung and Bauer[10]).

At present, the thiol depletion theory, although well established experimentally, cannot with certainty be applied as the sole explanation of nitrate tolerance.[10] Other mechanisms have been considered and are discussed in the following sections.

Neurohumoral Hypothesis. This hypothesis proposes that venous dilatation leads to preload reduction with reflex activation of the renin-angiotensin and adrenergic systems, with compensatory arteriolar vasoconstriction, which may reduce renal perfusion and function.[10] In congestive heart failure, a prolonged nitroglycerin infusion increases plasma catecholamine and renin activity, whereas the levels of vasodilatory atrial natriuretic peptide decrease.[16] Consequently, there may also be impaired fluid regulation. Concurrent angiotensin converting enzyme (ACE) inhibition may lessen nitrate tolerance in congestive heart failure.[10] There is no proof that the sulfhydryl groups in captopril provide any specific benefit.

Renal Underperfusion Hypothesis. Experimentally, concurrent hydralazine prevents the hemodynamic tolerance found during nitroglycerin infusion alone.[10] In patients, hydralazine helps maintain renal blood flow when it is given with isosorbide dinitrate.[17] Also, in patients with congestive heart failure, concurrent hydralazine helps maintain the hemodynamic effects of infused nitrates.[18] These observations may explain why hydralazine-nitrate therapy was effective in congestive heart failure even when the nitrate was given in doses known otherwise to cause tolerance in many months.[19]

Nitrate Receptors With Varying Affinity. Because it is not the absolute nitrate levels that cause vasodilatation but rather the sudden increase in levels,[20, 21] there is indirect evidence for a model whereby the high-affinity receptors might first be downregulated, leaving low-affinity receptors to interact with the rising blood nitrate levels. Low- and high-affinity components have been found in relation to the effect of nitroglycerin on vascular relaxation.[3]

Prevention of Tolerance

The use of eccentric timing of doses of nitrates is the simplest and most reliable procedure. In effort angina, many studies show that tolerance can be avoided by interval dosing, which has cast doubt on the combined efficacy of nitrate patches continuously releasing nitrates for 24 h.

Dose escalation may be a short-term procedure to bypass tolerance.[20, 21] Even when nitrate tolerance is established, sublingual nitrates still have some, albeit diminished, therapeutic effect.[9, 22] Dose escalation may be useful in congestive heart failure[20] and in unstable angina[23]; in early-phase acute myocardial infarction, modest dose escalation seems to restore efficacy lost in about one quarter of patients given intravenous nitrates.[11] Nevertheless, hard evidence proving this hypothesis is still lacking.

Nitrate Cross-Tolerance

Tolerance to long-acting nitrates should logically cause cross-tolerance to short-acting nitrates, as shown for the capacitance vessels of the forearm, coronary artery diameter, and exercise tolerance during intravenous nitroglycerin therapy.[24] Cross-tolerance to sublingual nitroglycerin (no change in blood pressure or heart rate) has been proposed as a simple clinical test for nitrate tolerance.[25] Nonetheless, because sublingual nitrates so abruptly increase the blood levels, there is also logic in the concept that some acute hemodynamic and antianginal effects may be found despite substantial nitrate tolerance. In contrast, total tolerance is a somewhat different situation in which there is no effect whatsoever of added sublingual nitrates.[9, 24]

Tolerance Versus Resistance

High intravenous nitroglycerin doses (even in excess of 200 μg/min) sometimes have no effect, even when given in the absence of prior nitrate therapy, and there is no point in further dose escalation.[11] Such resistance may occur in congestive heart failure and sometimes even in the absence of congestive heart failure in early acute myocardial infarction. Perhaps intense renin-angiotensin activation in these conditions could predispose to nitrate resistance.[11]

Class Side Effects of Nitrates

Headaches are common and often lead to loss of patient compliance with the prescribed regimen. A decrease in headaches with time is often found and may reflect, in part, subjective adaptation and arterial tolerance. Although many physicians hope that the therapeutic venous effects of nitrates are still maintained even when headaches disappear, solid observations on this point are lacking.

Hypotension is found in about 10% of trials with low-dose intravenous nitroglycerin[11] and can be reversed by discontinuing the infusion or reducing the rate. With oral nitrates, hypotension is seldom found unless there is cotherapy with other drugs, such as beta blockers or especially calcium channel antagonists. Reduction of the interacting drug or a change of drug to one that is less hypotensive would be appropriate.

Another occasional side effect is pulmonary hypoxemia in patients with chronic lung disease due to vasodilatation and increased ventilation-perfusion mismatch. Prolonged high-dose therapy can occasionally cause methemoglobinemia with cyanosis; treatment is by intravenous methylene blue (1% solution given as 1–2 mg/kg for several minutes; repeat 1 h later if needed).

Combination Therapy

Combination Therapy for Anginal Syndromes

Although abundant clinical experience supports the practice of combining nitrates with beta blockers and/or calcium channel antagonists in the therapy of anginal syndromes, there is no rigorous proof for additive antianginal effects.[9] The problem is that the nitrate doses used in past studies have almost all been those subsequently shown to cause tolerance. Thus, new studies are required with, for example, specific nontolerant dose schedules of isosorbide-5-mononitrates to prove an additive antianginal effect with other antianginal drugs.

The combination of beta blockade and nitrates is standard in the therapy of angina. Beta blockers act primarily by decreasing the heart rate and the arterial blood pressure, whereas nitrates act primarily by reducing preload and achieving relief of coronary constriction. Nonetheless, nitrates also decrease blood pressure, so that excess hypotension is the major risk. There appear to be no pharmacokinetic interactions between these two classes of drugs.

Calcium channel antagonists and nitrates are also often combined, yet again without any objective evidence for truly sustained antianginal effect in the absence of nitrate tolerance. Of the calcium channel antagonists, the non-dihydropyridines (verapamil or diltiazem) should theoretically be prescribed in preference to the nifedipine-like dihydropyridines (DHPs) because of the powerful and sometimes excessive afterload reduction achieved by the short-acting DHPs. Verapamil and diltiazem act more like beta blockers, with a negative inotropic effect and a tendency to heart rate reduction, whereas the short-acting DHPs may reflexly increase heart rate.

Triple therapy with nitrates, beta blockers, and calcium channel antagonists combined is frequently thought to be "maximal." Nonetheless, such triple therapy carries the risk of excess hypotension as well as pharmacodynamic interactions between beta blockers and calcium channel antagonists (added negative inotropic effects, added sinoatrial [SA] and atrioventricular [AV] nodal inhibition with verapamil or diltiazem).

Combination Therapy for Congestive Heart Failure

The combination of long-acting nitrates and hydralazine was one of the first regimens to show that vasodilator therapy could influence outcome in chronic heart failure.[19] The isosorbide dinitrate total daily dose was 160 mg/day given in four doses. Timing of the doses was not stated, but assuming that the last dose was given at 8 PM and the first dose at 8 AM, there would have been a 12-h nitrate-free interval with, therefore, recovery of normal response to the first dose of the day. The subsequent doses too may not have evoked as much tolerance as expected because of the cotherapy with hydralazine[18] and its renal vasodilatory effect.[10]

ACE Inhibitors Combined With Nitrates

The combination of an ACE inhibitor with nitrates is theoretically attractive because plasma renin activity increases during the development of nitrate tolerance in patients with heart failure.[26] Nonetheless, benefits of ACE inhibitors are not consistent.[10] In one study in which captopril failed to prevent tolerance, high-dose intravenous nitroglycerin was used; in two other studies, it seemed to prevent tolerance.[10]

The possibility that ACE inhibitors have a more direct vascular effect in preventing nitrate tolerance is raised by a study in which patients with angina pectoris received an infusion of intracoronary nitroglycerin.[27] After 20 h of intravenous nitroglycerin at a mean dose of only 24 μg/min, the coronary vasodilator responses to intracoronary nitroglycerin were attenuated in the placebo but not in the captopril group. The mechanism of this protective effect is not known but is unlikely to involve systemic neurohumoral reactions to the nitroglycerin. By decreasing breakdown of bradykinin, perhaps ACE inhibitors increase the endothelial rates of production of nitric oxide. There is no good evidence that captopril with its sulfhydryl groups is better than other ACE inhibitors in preventing nitrate tolerance.[10]

N-Acetylcysteine

As already reviewed by Fung and Bauer,[10] data with *N*-acetylcysteine are controversial. Because oral *N*-acetylcysteine is not readily available, and ACE inhibitors or hydralazine can be given orally, it is at present more practical to recommend ACE inhibitors or hydralazine as part of combination therapy when the aim is to avoid nitrate tolerance. However, there is no way that is totally sure, short of interval therapy, to avoid nitrate tolerance.

Double-Acting Drug: Nitrate Plus Potassium Channel Opener

Nicorandil is an agent with a double cellular mechanism of action, acting both as a potassium channel activator and as a nitrate. Therefore, it can be expected to cause less tolerance than nitrates do. In Japan, it is a standard antianginal agent in a dose of 10–20 mg every 12 h. Nicorandil has been reported to have antianginal properties in several small trials[28]; nonetheless, in a large American trial, nicorandil 10 or 20 mg twice daily was not superior to placebo in patients with stable effort angina.[29]

Adverse Drug Interactions of Nitrates

The chief drug interactions of nitrates are pharmacodynamic. For example, during triple therapy (nitrates, beta blockers, and calcium channel antagonists) of angina pectoris, efficacy of the combination may be less than expected, probably because of excess hypotension. Even two components of the triple therapy, such as calcium channel antagonists and nitrates, may interact adversely to cause excess hypotension. Excess vasodilatation with alpha-adrenergic blockers and nitrates can also occur.

Direct Nitric Oxide Donors

Sodium Nitroprusside

This drug is the prototype of the direct nitric oxide donors, which can be expected to vasodilate all vessels, both venous and arterial, without differentiation. Because this agent is a direct nitric oxide donor, one of the proposed mechanisms for nitrate tolerance may be bypassed.[1] The general vasodilator effect includes the small coronary arterioles (less than 100 μm in diameter) with risk of coronary steal, as in the case of dipyridamole. In an important study, Mann and coworkers[30] showed that when nitroprusside was given to patients with coronary artery disease, regional myocardial blood flow decreased significantly. In contrast, after sublingual nitroglycerin, regional flow increased. *For that reason, sodium nitroprusside is not the drug of choice when blood pressure reduction is required in the presence of clinical ischemia.* Nonetheless, the drug is still used when coronary artery disease manifests as severe congestive heart failure requiring intravenous afterload reduction.

Nitroprusside is converted to cyanmethemoglobin and free cyanide in red cells; the free cyanide is further converted to thiocyanate in the liver and cleared by the kidneys with a half-life of 7 days. Thus, cyanide may accumulate with prolonged high doses of nitroprusside and produce a lactic acidosis. Inactivation of cyanide by the liver may be limited by the availability of thiol groups, and administration of thiosulfate can protect against nitroprusside toxicity.[31]

An initial infusion of 10 μg/min is increased by 10 μg/min every 10 min up to 40–75 μg/min with a top dose of 300 μg/min.

Although sodium nitroprusside remains the theoretical gold standard for the management of hypertensive emergencies and severe congestive heart failure, in current clinical practice it is used less frequently. It can be given only intravenously, the solution must be protected from light, and care must be taken to avoid extravasation. Exact blood pressure monitoring is required because of the rapid fall in blood pressure and the risk of rebound when therapy ceases. With prolonged infusion, there is the threat of cyanide poisoning, suggested by central nervous symptoms, metabolic acidosis, or methemoglobinemia (the last suggested by the development of cyanosis).

Molsidomine

This drug acts by formation of vasodilatory metabolites such as 3-morpholinosydnonimine (SIN-1, also referred to as linsidomine) formed during first-pass liver metabolism. These metabolites are direct nitric oxide donors and bypass the cysteine-dependent metabolic cascade, which according to the sulfhydryl depletion hypothesis may lessen the risk of nitrate tolerance. However, strict comparative studies are not available. The standard dose is 2 mg three times daily. In the European Study of Prevention of Infarct with Molsidomine (ESPRIM) trial,[32] treatment of patients with early-phase acute myocardial infarction but without overt heart failure was started with linsidomine for 48 h followed by 16 mg molsidomine orally for 12 days. Mortality was unchanged. The reason for the lack of efficacy was not clear, but the authors speculate that the low-risk profile subjects chosen might have limited the power of the study to show a reduction in mortality. A future use of this type of drug may be in lessening the risk of restenosis after angioplasty.[33]

Linsidomine (SIN-1), given intravenously (1–1.6 mg/h), was slightly less effective than intravenous isosorbide dinitrate in the relief of unstable angina.[34]

Nitric Oxide Synthesis in Septic Shock

Endotoxins and cytokines released during septic shock are thought to provoke increased formation of nitric oxide by stimulating in vascular smooth muscle cells the inducible enzyme i-NOS (inducible nitric oxide synthase) to produce large amounts of vasodilatory nitric oxide with excess peripheral vasodilatation and hypotension. (In contrast, it is the endothelial constitutive enzyme, c-NOS, that physiologically produces NO·.) Experimentally, the use of the inhibitor of nitric oxide synthase, *N*-monomethyl-L-arginine, caused a dose-dependent increase in blood pressure and in systemic vascular resistance.[35] Thus, in septic shock, inhibition of i-NOS would be ideal therapy when the appropriate drugs become more widely available. One major problem is the lack of specificity of currently available inhibitors of nitric oxide synthase.

BETA BLOCKERS

Beta-adrenergic receptor blockade is a powerful way of influencing the diseased cardiovascular system, having antianginal, antihypertensive, and antiarrhythmic effects. There has also been keen interest recently in the proposal that beta blockade might beneficially influence the course of congestive heart failure, previously held to be a contraindication rather than an indication.

Fundamental Mechanisms of Beta Blockers

Beta-Adrenergic Receptors

The beta adrenoceptor signal cascade conveys the stimulus applied by the beta agonist to the beta receptor through multiple steps leading to the ultimate change, usually an increase of cell calcium in the myocardium or, conversely, a decrease in cell calcium in vascular smooth muscle. The beta adrenoceptor, chiefly situated on the outer part of the sarcolemma bilayer, was originally divided into β_1 and β_2 receptor types on the basis of pharmacodynamic studies. β_3 adrenoceptors, recently identified, play a role in metabolic regulation of adipose tissue.

β_1 receptors are found in the heart muscle and in the sinus and AV nodes as well as in the conduction system. β_2 receptors are classically found in bronchial and vascular smooth muscle but have now also been identified in the myocardium as well as in the sinus node. It is thought that about 20%–25% of the beta receptors in the myocardium are of the β_2 variety.[39] The proportion of β_2 receptors in the human sinus node is not clear, but for practical purposes, β_1 blockade is as effective in reducing the heart rate as is combined β_1 plus β_2 blockade.[40]

Beta-Adrenergic Receptor Cascade

Stimulation of the beta receptor by agonist molecules, such as the physiologic catecholamines norepinephrine and epinephrine, ultimately leads to increased intracellular formation of the second messenger, cyclic adenosine monophosphate (cAMP), under the influence of adenylate cyclase that converts adenosine triphosphate (ATP) to cAMP. A complex signal transduction system is involved (Figs. 2–2*A*, 2–2*B*). When the receptor is stimulated, multiple molecular changes take place in the G protein system that links the beta receptor to adenylate cyclase. The G proteins cycle between an active guanosine triphosphate (GTP)–liganded form and an inactive guanosine diphosphate (GDP)–liganded form.[41] There are three G protein subunits, alpha, beta, and gamma. The GDP dissociates from the alpha subunit, and GTP binds to it. Thereupon, the α-GTP complex stimulates adenylate cyclase to form cAMP, and simultaneously (some workers propose) the affinity of the beta agonist for its receptor lessens. The α-GTP complex keeps on activating adenylate cyclase until the GTP is broken down by the enzyme GTPase, intrinsic to the alpha subunit, that allows reformation of the original state of the G protein, that is, the inactive alpha-beta-gamma trimeric group with GDP attached to the α_1 subunit. The type of alpha subunit involved in this sequence is called α_S because it stimulates adenylate cyclase when it is combined with GTP. The entire G protein complex, containing α_S and the beta-gamma subunit, is often called G_S.

On the other hand, there is an inhibitory form of the G protein complex, called G_i, that contains the α_i subunit combined with a beta-gamma subunit. In response to vagal muscarinic stimulation, the same α_i detaches from beta-gamma, and it is the beta-gamma complex that lessens the activity of α_S-GTP by enhancing the action of the GTPase. Thus, after this sequence, vagal activity inhibits the formation of cAMP, particularly in the sinus node, atrial tissue, and AV node. In addition, the beta-gamma complex helps open the acetylcholine-dependent potassium channel, thereby hyperpolarizing and slowing the sinus node. The α_1 subunit may not be without activity, because it is proposed that it may activate a potassium channel, K_{ATP}.

cAMP—The Second Messenger

Although cAMP is called the second messenger, in reality it is just one of a long chain of events and is not in itself active. Rather, cAMP activates the enzyme protein kinase A (Fig. 2–3), thereby phosphorylating various crucial proteins that control calcium ion movements and thereby regulating their activity. A prime site of action of protein kinase A is phosphorylation of phospholamban, the key protein that normally strongly inhibits the calcium uptake pump of the sarcoplasmic reticulum. When this inhibition is removed, the activity of the pump is stimulated and calcium is taken up more readily into the sarcoplasmic reticulum. Phosphorylation of phospholamban has an important contribution to the contractile actions of beta stimulation,[42] the concept being that enhanced uptake of calcium ions into the sarcoplasmic reticulum leads not only to enhanced relaxation but also to a subsequent greater release of calcium in response to that calcium that enters through the calcium channel (see

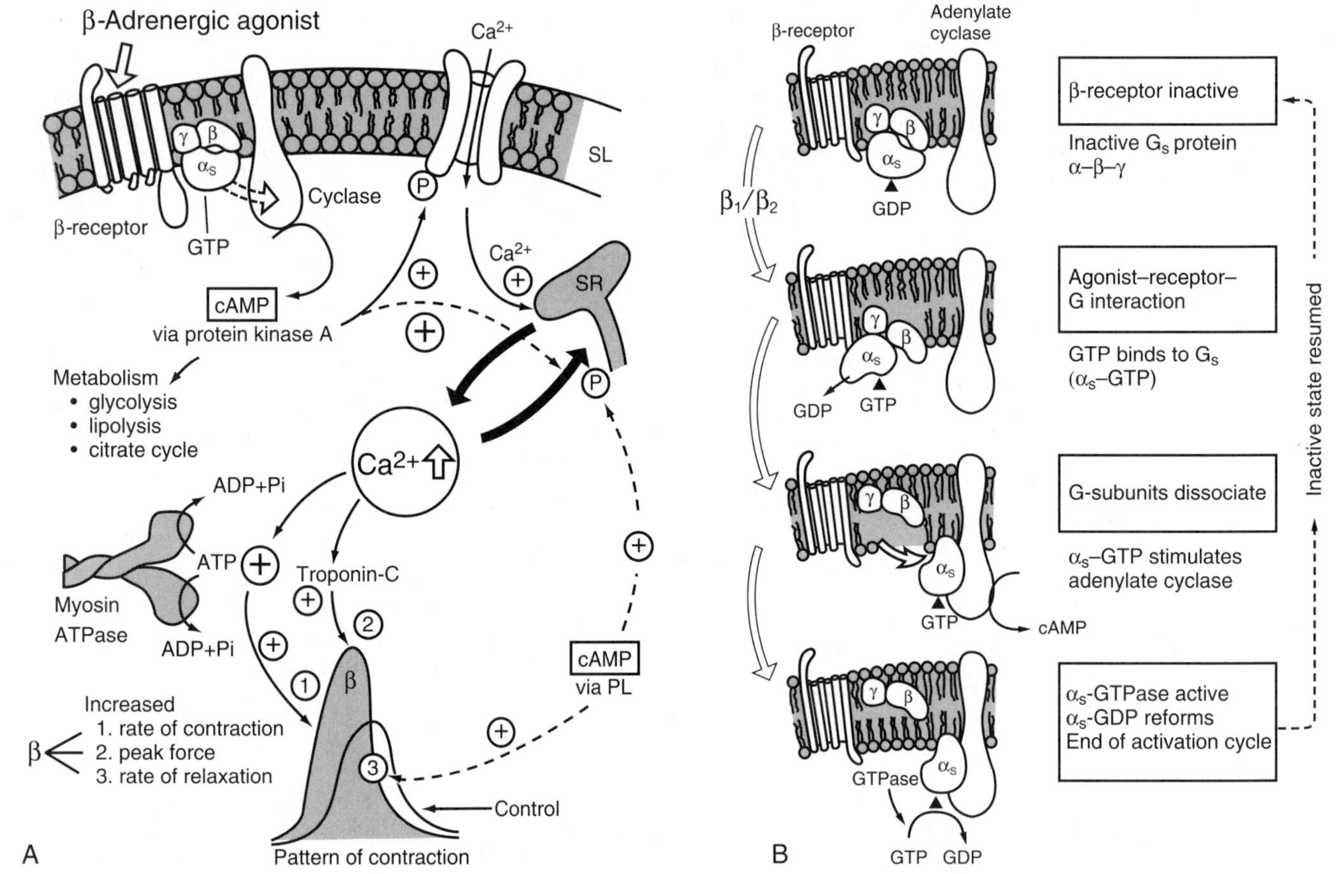

Figure 2–2. *A, B,* Signaling system involved in control of cardiac contraction by beta-adrenergic stimulation. *Abbreviations:* α_S, β, γ, subunits of G_S, stimulatory G protein; P, phosphorylation; PL, phospholamban; SL, sarcolemma; SR, sarcoplasmic reticulum. (Reprinted with permission. Copyright 1996, L.H. Opie.)

Figs. 2–2*A*, 2–2*B*). In addition, protein kinase A activity phosphorylates several sites on the COOH-terminal part of the L-type calcium channel alpha subunit protein to increase the probability of channel opening. A third site of action of protein kinase A is troponin-I. Phosphorylated troponin-I is less sensitive to calcium, and thereby the rate of relaxation may be further enhanced.

Major Effects of Beta Adrenoceptor Agonist Stimulation

The major cardiac effects of beta adrenoceptor agonist stimulation (see Fig. 2–2*A*) are to increase the calcium-dependent pacemaker current in the sinus node (positive chronotropic effect), to enhance the rate of conduction (positive dromotropic effect), to increase the rate and force of contraction (positive inotropic effect), and, finally, to enhance the rate of relaxation (positive lusitropic effect). Logically, beta adrenoceptor blockade should be able to reverse or lessen these effects.

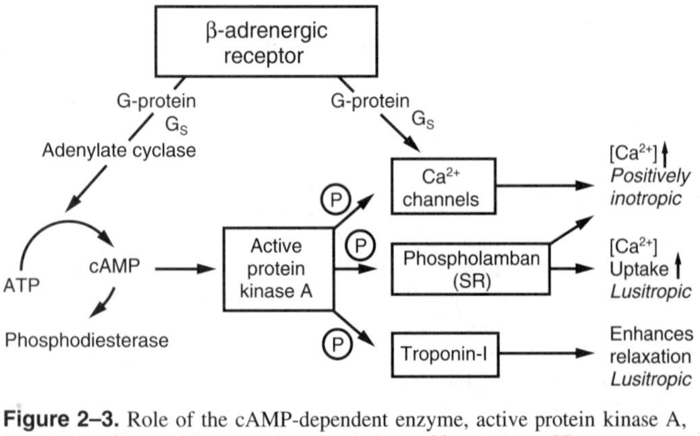

Figure 2–3. Role of the cAMP-dependent enzyme, active protein kinase A, in cellular effects of beta agonist stimulation. *Abbreviations:* SR, sarcoplasmic reticulum; G_S, stimulatory G protein. (Reprinted with permission. Copyright 1996, L.H. Opie.)

Receptor Downregulation

During prolonged beta agonist stimulation, the beta receptors physically leave their standard position on the sarcolemma and move internally to the cytosol. Hypothetically, this process of receptor downregulation is a mechanism of self-protection to avoid overstimulation of contractile cells by excess cAMP and calcium, as may otherwise occur during prolonged and excess catecholamine stimulation. The mechanism of downregulation may involve self-phosphorylation of the receptor, under the influence of a beta adrenoceptor kinase. The phosphorylation may act by changing the physicochemical properties of the receptor.

Receptor downregulation appears to have two clinical correlates. First, during prolonged infusion of a beta agonist, such as dobutamine, there may be a progressive loss or decrease of therapeutic effect, which could theoretically be ascribed to receptor downregulation. Second, in severe congestive heart failure, excess circulating catecholamines by enhanced and prolonged stimulation of β_1 receptors may cause receptor downregulation. β_2 receptors are not downregulated but appear to suffer in another way, becoming uncoupled from the adenylate cyclase system and thereby losing some activity.

Receptor Upregulation

Conversely, during long-term beta blockade therapy, the number of beta receptors increases even though they are still blocked. If beta blockade were suddenly to be withdrawn, the increased receptor density may precipitate an apparently enhanced state of adrenergic stimulation with an increased myocardial oxygen demand[43] and the risk of precipitation of anginal syndromes or even myocardial infarction (the withdrawal syndrome).

Pharmacodynamic and Therapeutic Effects of Beta Blockers

Antianginal Mechanisms

Beta blockers lessen myocardial oxygen demand in several ways (Fig. 2–4). They decrease the heart rate and the force and rate of cardiac contraction by inhibiting the beta receptors in the sinus node and myocardium. Of these effects, the reduction in heart rate may be the most important,[44] especially during exercise. They also reduce afterload by decreasing blood pressure, especially during exercise. Beta blockade is, therefore, able to lessen the myocardial oxygen demand both in effort and in unstable angina at rest.

Does Beta Blockade Cause Coronary Vasoconstriction?

Physiologically, sympathetic stimulation normally decreases distal coronary vascular resistance, so that β_2-mediated vasodilatation offsets alpha-mediated vasoconstriction. Besides containing β_2 receptors, in the small coronary arterioles, the coronary system also has β_1 receptors in the larger arteries, at least in the dog.[40] In humans, combined β_1 and β_2 blockade has a coronary vasoconstrictive effect with a rise in coronary vascular resistance.[45] Although selective β_1 blockade should lessen this problem, there appear to be no data in patients. This tendency to decrease the coronary blood supply is offset by the longer diastolic filling time resulting from the decreased heart rate during exercise, which leads to better diastolic myocardial perfusion.

Antihypertensive Mechanisms

The mechanism of the antihypertensive effect is still under dispute. Initially, beta blockers decrease heart rate, and the cardiac output falls by about 20%. Yet the blood pressure does not fall because the arteriolar resistance reflexly increases. Within 24 h, the peripheral resistance starts to fall, so that arterial pressure declines. The mechanism of this delayed hypotensive effect is unclear but is thought to involve inhibition of prejunctional beta receptors.[46] Alternatively, inhibition of the renin-angiotensin system may explain the delayed vasodilatation.[47] Additional antihypertensive mechanisms may involve a central action and decreased renin release.

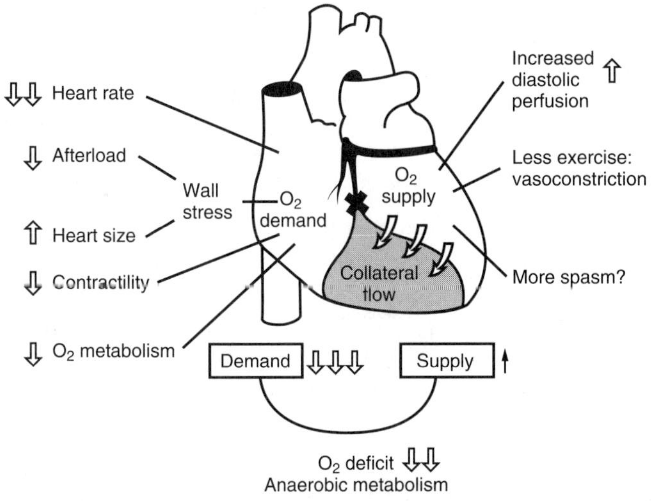

Figure 2–4. Mechanisms whereby beta blockade beneficially alters the demand/supply ratio in the ischemic heart. (Reprinted with permission. Copyright 1996, L.H. Opie.)

Multiple Antiarrhythmic Mechanisms

Beta blockers also have multiple antiarrhythmic mechanisms. The negative dromotropic effect whereby beta blockade strongly inhibits conduction through the AV node accounts for the benefit in supraventricular tachycardias. These include paroxysmal supraventricular nodal reentry tachycardia, the arrhythmias of the Wolff-Parkinson-White syndrome, and a decreased ventricular response rate in atrial fibrillation. The mechanisms underlying the ventricular antiarrhythmic (class II) effects are less clear. In patients with coronary artery disease, the general anti-ischemic effects of beta blockade contribute to an antiarrhythmic effect and may explain the decreased incidence of sudden death in postinfarct patients treated by beta blockade. When there is an enhanced rate of formation of cAMP (i.e., increased adrenergic drive as found during exercise, anesthesia, and early-phase acute myocardial infarction), then calcium-mediated ventricular arrhythmias may occur.[48] Such adrenergic-cAMP-calcium–induced arrhythmias should logically respond to beta blockade. It is less easy to understand why beta blockade should act as an effective ventricular antiarrhythmic in cases of ventricular tachycardia not associated with acute ischemia.[49] Possibly the tachycardia, if prolonged, could invoke a reflex increase in sympathetic activity. Sotalol uniquely has both class II and class III properties, and it compared well with a variety of class I agents in the Electrophysiologic Study Versus Electrocardiographic Monitoring (ESVEM) trial[50] in which patients with significant ventricular tachyarrhythmias were studied.

Specific Pharmacologic Properties of Beta Blocker Subclasses

Beta blockers are sometimes divided into three categories. The first group, with propranolol being the prototype, blocks both β_1 and β_2 receptors. The second includes atenolol, metoprolol, acebutolol, and bisoprolol, which are relatively selective for β_1 receptors when given in low doses. The third type has added vasodilatory effects.

Nonselective Agents (β_1 Plus β_2 Blockers)

Propranolol decreases heart rate, conduction, and contractility largely by blocking β_1 receptors, and it therefore has the full spectrum of cardiovascular benefits. Blockade of β_2 receptors also plays a role in the negative inotropic effect. β_2 receptor blockade in smooth muscle promotes contraction and may precipitate bronchospasm and peripheral or coronary vasoconstriction. Other nonselective blockers are nadolol, sotalol, oxprenolol, timolol, and penbutolol.

Relatively β_1-Selective Blockers

These agents should have two theoretical benefits. First, by exerting relatively less β_2 blockade, bronchospasm should be decreased. Second, by similar reasoning, peripheral and coronary constriction at the level of the resistance peripheral and coronary arterioles should also be less. Nonetheless, it should be recalled that such selectivity is lost at high doses. Thus, only low-dose β_1-selective agents can be used and only with care in patients with bronchospasm or chronic lung disease or chronic smoking. No beta blocker, including the β_1-selective agents, can be regarded as safe in asthmatics. Some of the new beta blockers, such as bisoprolol and celiprolol (the latter is not available in the United States), are claimed to be more selective than earlier drugs such as atenolol and metoprolol.

Vasodilatory Beta Blockers

Beta Blockers With Added Intrinsic Sympathomimetic Activity (Partial Agonist Activity). Beta blockers with added intrinsic sympathomimetic activity (ISA) are typified by pindolol, whose properties have been thoroughly investigated. Despite the added peripheral vasodilatory qualities, there are no good data showing that pindolol or similar agents would be more effective than standard beta blockers in the therapy of hypertension. During exercise, the beta-blocking qualities are strong enough to decrease the heart rate. Nonetheless, agents with ISA remain poorly tested for angina and are not approved for that purpose by the Food and Drug Administration (FDA). A potential disadvantage of ISA is stimulation of the central nervous system at night, when sympathetic tone is low, causing sleep impairment.[51] Potential but not proven advantages are in elderly patients in whom fatigue might be avoided by better maintenance of heart rate and cardiac output, in black patients in whom vasodilatation may improve the antihypertensive effect, and in patients with hyperlipidemias in whom concurrent ISA may disturb the lipid profile less. Thus, in general, ISA remains an attractive property but with ill-defined therapeutic benefits.

Additional Alpha-Blocking Activity. The two chief representatives of this category are labetalol, approved by the FDA in both its oral and intravenous formulations for use in hypertension, and carvedilol. Carvedilol is approved for the treatment of hypertension and is under consideration for congestive heart failure. Such combined alpha-beta blockers can acutely reduce blood pressure in contrast to exclusively beta-blocking drugs. There are no long-term studies establishing whether added vasodilatation from alpha blockade gives superior antihypertensive control compared with pure beta blockade.

Other Vasodilatory Beta-Blocking Molecules. Bucindolol, another drug used in trials in patients with congestive heart failure, has a hydralazine-like moiety in its molecule.

Pharmacokinetic Properties of Beta Blockers

Lipid Solubility and Hepatic Metabolism

Lipid-soluble hydrophilic compounds such as atenolol, sotalol, and nadolol are excreted virtually exclusively by renal mechanisms, have a low brain penetration, and as a group have low rates of hepatic metabolism and protein binding. Highly lipid-soluble compounds represented by propranolol and labetalol have high rates of first-pass liver metabolism that vary greatly between patients and alter the dose required for a given therapeutic effect. Hepatic metabolism is also important in the case of acebutolol, bisoprolol, metoprolol, and timolol, agents that have only modest lipid solubility. Acebutolol produces large amounts of diacetolol, which like the parent is cardioselective with ISA but has a longer half-life, is excreted chiefly by the kidneys, and is more water soluble.

Half-Lives

These are shown in Table 2–3. In addition, esmolol is an intravenous β_1 blocker with a "biologic" half-life of only 9 min because of rapid inactivation by blood esterases. This short half-life is an attractive feature allowing esmolol to be given even when there is hemodynamic instability; in the case of any adverse effects, the infusion (50–300 μg/kg/min) can be terminated. Recovery from beta blockade by esmolol usually occurs within 30 min.

Indications for Beta Blockade

Angina Pectoris

In effort angina, the oxygen-sparing quality of beta blockers means that they are often part of standard therapy. All beta blockers are potentially equally effective. Conventionally, the dose is adjusted to secure a resting heart rate of about 50–60 beats per minute and an exercise heart rate not exceeding 100 beats per minute. With vasodilatory alpha-beta blockers, the heart rate is higher for an equivalent antianginal effect, at least in hypertensive patients also with angina.[52] When beta blockers are ineffective in effort angina, the explanations may include (1) severe obstructive coronary artery disease, (2) an increase in left ventricle chamber size after the negative inotropic effect, and (3) promotion of coronary vasoconstriction.

In mixed angina (combined effort and rest angina), several studies have suggested that an increased heart rate is important in precipitating angina even when it occurs at rest. Correspondingly, beta blockers may be strikingly effective in this situation.[53]

In silent myocardial ischemia or in patients with predominant silent changes (ambulatory electrocardiographic ST segment), beta blockers have established efficacy.[54]

In unstable angina with threat of myocardial infarction, therapy by beta blockade is conventional, and beta blockers that reduce the heart rate are logically preferred (see Chapter 6). Nonetheless, the objective evidence favoring the use of beta blockers in unstable angina is limited to one placebo-controlled trial.[55] There was only a trend to improvement in those treated by beta blockade compared with control subjects. Conceivably, the small number of patients might have masked any potential benefit.

In Prinzmetal variant angina, drugs with exclusive beta blockade are usually avoided to obviate enhanced coronary spasm as a result of inhibition of the vasodilatory β_1 and β_2 receptors. Agents with additional vasodilatory properties may be useful, although no large-scale clinical trials are available to confirm this concept.

In cold-induced angina, beta blockade appears to be less effective than calcium antagonism.[56]

Acute Myocardial Infarction

Initial Stages. There are good theoretical reasons to use beta blockade early in acute myocardial infarction because of increased catecholamine secretion with adverse effects, including increased myocardial oxygen demand, a proclivity to severe and potentially lethal ventricular arrhythmias,[48] and enhanced pain sensitivity. For prophylaxis against ventricular fibrillation and ventricular tachycardia, the evidence is best for intravenous propranolol[57] or metoprolol.[58] In the United States, metoprolol and atenolol[59] are licensed for intravenous use in acute myocardial infarction.

Postinfarct Follow-Up. Beta blockade is now standard therapy and reduces the risk of sudden death and reinfarction by about 25%. The subclass of beta blocker used seems not to matter. Of interest is the finding that it is particularly the high-risk patients who appear to benefit most and, specifically, those with a clinical diagnosis of heart failure.[60, 61] The reduction in mortality associated with beta blockade is most evident in the first 6 months after infarction and in high-risk patients.[62]

Hypertension

The antihypertensive effects of beta blockers are not under dispute, nor is their ability to reduce stroke. Hence, they are recommended

TABLE 2–3. PROPERTIES OF VARIOUS ORALLY ACTIVE BETA-ADRENOCEPTOR ANTAGONIST AGENTS, NONSELECTIVE VERSUS CARDIOSELECTIVE AND VASODILATORY AGENTS

Generic Name (Trade Name)	ISA	Plasma Half-Life (h)	Cleared by Liver (L) or Kidney (K)	Usual Dose for Angina (Other Indications in Parentheses)	Usual Doses as Sole Therapy for Mild/Moderate Hypertension (US)
Noncardioselective					
Propranolol*† (Inderal)	–	1–6	L	40–80 mg 2–4× daily usually adequate (may give 160 mg 2×)	Start with 10–40 mg 2× daily Mean 160–320 mg/day, 1–2 doses
(Inderal LA)	–	8–11	L	80–320 mg 1× daily	80–320 mg 1× daily
Carteolol* (Cartrol)	+	5–6	K	(Not studied)	2.5–10 mg single dose
Nadolol*† (Corgard)	–	20–24	K	40–80 mg 1× daily; up to 240 mg	40–80 mg/day 1× daily; up to 320 mg
Penbutolol* (Levatol)	+	20–25	L	(Not studied)	10–20 mg daily
Sotalol‡ (Betapace)	–	7–18 (mean 12)	K	(240–480 mg/day in 2 doses for arrhythmias)	80–320 mg/day; mean 190 mg
Timolol* (Blocadren)	–	4–5	L, K	(post-AMI: 10 mg 2× daily)	10–30 mg 2× daily
Cardioselective					
Acebutolol* (Sectral)	+ +	8–13 (diacetolol)	L, K	(400–1200 mg/day in 2 doses for PVCs)	400–1200 mg/day; can be given as a single dose
Atenolol*† (Tenormin)	–	6–7	K	50–200 mg 1× daily	50–100 mg/day 1× daily
Betaxolol* (Kerlone)	–	14–22	L, then K	10–20 mg 1× daily (use pending approval)	10–20 mg 1× daily
Bisoprolol* (Zebeta)	–	9–12	L, K	10 mg 1× daily (not in US)	2.5–40 mg 1× daily
Metoprolol*† (Lopressor)	–	3–7	L	50–200 mg 2× daily	50–400 mg/day in 1–2 doses
Vasodilatory Beta Blockers, Nonselective					
Labetalol* (Trandate) (Normodyne)	–	6–8	L, some K	As for hypertension	300–600 mg/day in 2–3 doses; top dose 2400 mg/day
Pindolol* (Visken)	+ + + $\beta_1\beta_2$	4	L, K	2.5–7.5 mg 3× daily (in UK, not US)	5–30 mg/day 2× daily
Carvedilol* (Coreg)	–	6	L	25–50 mg 2× daily (in UK, not US)	25–50 mg 1× daily
Vasodilatory Beta Blockers, Selective					
Celiprolol (Celectol in UK; not in US)	+β_2	6–8	Chiefly K, also L	400 mg once daily	400 mg once daily

Abbreviations: AMI, acute myocardial infarction; ISA, intrinsic sympathomimetic activity; PVCs, premature ventricular contractions; US, United States; UK, United Kingdom.
*Approved by FDA for hypertension.
†Approved by FDA for angina pectoris.
‡Approved for life-threatening ventricular tachyarrhythmias.
For further details of lipid solubility, first-pass effect, plasma protein binding, and intravenous use, see Opie et al.[85]

among first-line therapy by the American Joint National Committee.[63] Yet beta blockers are not equally effective in all subgroups of patients.

In elderly white patients, beta blockade is nearly as effective as in the young in reducing blood pressure, at least in men.[64] In contrast, in elderly black men, beta blockade was not impressively better than placebo. In left ventricular hypertrophy, beta blockade might be less effective than ACE inhibition, although conflicting data exist in the literature.[65, 66]

Despite a reduction in stroke, a corresponding fall in coronary mortality has not been found in some studies.[67] In the Swedish Trial in Old Patients (STOP) study[68] in elderly hypertensives, beta blockade was used as a first-line agent but often combined with a diuretic to reduce blood pressure. There was an overall reduction in mortality and in stroke, yet the effect on myocardial infarction was only marginal. In systolic hypertension in the elderly, in the Systolic Hypertension in the Elderly Program (SHEP) study,[69] atenolol 25–50 mg daily was the second agent used after a low-dose diuretic (chlorthalidone 15 mg daily). In this study, there was a major effect on stroke, but also coronary heart disease was reduced by about 25%. It is not clear what percentage of these patients received combination therapy.

Arrhythmias

Beta blockers appear to be among the few antiarrhythmic agents that may prolong rather than decrease life expectancy, especially in postinfarct patients.[70]

Hypertrophic Cardiomyopathy

In this condition, the negative inotropic effect of propranolol is the basis of its use in therapy, particularly in the presence of outflow tract obstruction. However, there are no long-term comparative studies with other agents such as verapamil.

Congestive Heart Failure

The initial rationale for prescribing beta blockers to patients with congestive heart failure was that the β_1 receptors were downregulated. However, benefit has also been found in conditions in which β_1 downregulation appears to be of lesser importance, and one current proposal is that the decreased heart rate allows better left ventricular filling.[71] Alternatively, excess catecholamines cause cellular damage and necrosis (catecholamine toxicity), a process that might be halted by beta blockade.

Class Side Effects of Beta Blockers

These are an exaggeration of the normal cardiac therapeutic effects resulting in excess bradycardia, AV block, and excess negative inotropic effect.

All beta blockers tend to promote bronchospasm, with low doses of β_1-selective agents being least harmful. Cold extremities occur with both selective and nonselective agents,[72] yet agents containing ISA may give a slightly better skin temperature than propranolol, at least during an acute study.[73] The adverse effects of all beta blockers on the peripheral circulation may be less marked than previously thought.[74, 75]

Fatigue is a frequent side effect, again found particularly with propranolol, with less of an effect when a β_1-selective or vasodilatory blocker is used, so that both central and peripheral hemodynamic mechanisms may be involved. Although one double-blind study shows no difference between the effects of the β_1-selective agent atenolol and placebo,[72] exercise physiologists find that there is some impairment in peak exercise with all beta blockers.

Impotence is often reported by patients receiving beta blockers who are, however, usually middle-aged men, often with atherosclerotic arterial disease. In one study, erectile dysfunction occurred in 11% of patients given a beta blocker for hypertension, compared with 26% of those given a diuretic and 3% of placebo-treated patients.[76]

An impaired quality of life found especially with propranolol[77] is theoretically ascribed to its lipid solubility and brain penetration. Yet a variety of beta blockers other than propranolol and with different properties leave the quality of life intact in hypertensives.[78] Central effects of beta blockers are often subtle and not always explicable by the lipid-penetration hypothesis.[79]

Contraindications to Beta Blockers

There are several absolute contraindications. Cardiovascular contraindications include severe bradycardia, pre-existing high-degree AV block, overt left ventricular failure (except when beta blockade is given initially in low doses and under supervision to patients already receiving diuretics, digoxin, and an ACE inhibitor), and active peripheral vascular disease with rest ischemia. Severe asthma or severe bronchospasm is an absolute contraindication, even to β_1-selective agents. Severe psychologic depression is an important relative contraindication, particularly for propranolol.

Drug Combinations With Beta Blockers

Beta Blockers With Calcium Channel Antagonists

Hemodynamically, these two types of agents have different effects on the circulation (Fig. 2–5), leading to the possibility of therapeutic combination. Of the combinations, beta blockade plus a DHP, such as nifedipine, is likely to be simplest. The DHPs do not inhibit the sinus or the AV node and can therefore more readily be combined with a beta blocker than can the non-DHPs, such as verapamil and diltiazem. Because the tendency to tachycardia with the DHPs is antagonized by the beta blocker, there are no additive effects on the sinus or the AV node, and the DHPs can by vasodilatation, including coronary vasodilatation, contribute to the antianginal effect. Beta blockade should only cautiously be combined with the non-DHPs such as verapamil and diltiazem. With non-DHP calcium antagonists, there is risk of extreme bradycardia, AV block, or a marked negative inotropic effect.[80]

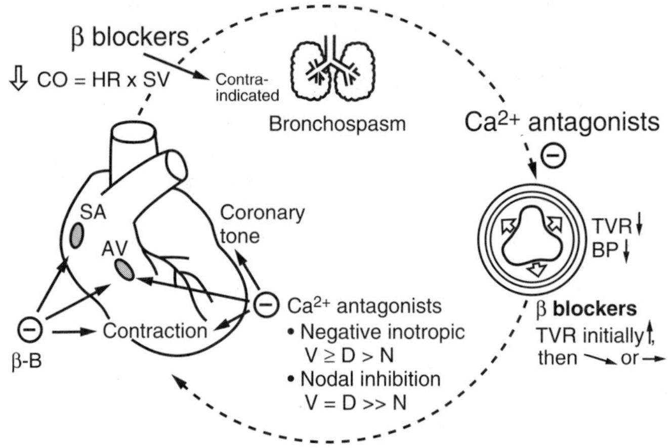

Figure 2–5. Comparison of hemodynamic effects of beta blockers (β-B) and calcium channel antagonists and possibilities for combination therapy. *Abbreviations:* CO, cardiac output; HR, heart rate; SV, stroke volume; SA, sinoatrial node; AV, atrioventricular node; TVR, total vascular resistance; BP, blood pressure; V, verapamil; D, diltiazem; N, nifedipine. (Reprinted with permission. Copyright 1996, L.H. Opie.)

Second-generation calcium antagonists, such as the DHPs amlodipine, felodipine, isradipine, and nicardipine, can as readily be combined with beta blockade as nifedipine.

Besides evidence that these combinations improve symptoms in effort angina, a preliminary report from the TIBET study[81] suggests that the combination of beta blockade by atenolol and calcium antagonism by nifedipine lessens hard endpoints (such as acute myocardial infarction, unstable angina, or death) in patients with effort angina.

Beta Blockers With Nitrates

Reference has already been made to their complementary antianginal properties.

Beta Blockers With Antihypertensive Therapy

Beta blockers have been combined in many studies with diuretics, calcium channel antagonists, alpha blockers, or centrally active agents to achieve a greater reduction of blood pressure. In general, adverse pharmacodynamic interactions have been few. For example, most of the adverse effects of combination with calcium channel antagonists have been described in patients with clinical ischemic heart disease.

Beta Blockers With ACE Inhibition

In patients with postinfarct left ventricular dysfunction treated by captopril,[82] the rate of development of heart failure was reduced, and the benefits of captopril were still found in the presence of beta blockade. Because beta blockade has its maximal beneficial effect within the first year[62] and because the effect of captopril became evident only after a delay of months, the mechanisms involved might be different and could be additive. In fact, the decrease in mortality achieved by captopril was highest in patients also given beta blockade, although these differences were probably not statistically significant. A concept that appears to be gaining ground is that in postinfarct patients with added left ventricular dysfunction, both beta blockade and ACE inhibition are desirable. A possible negative pharmacodynamic interaction is excess hypotension.

Beta Blockers With Class IC Antiarrhythmics

Beta blockade may help lessen the proarrhythmic side effects of the class IC agents, such as flecainide. Experimentally, the proarrhythmic effects of flecainide can be reversed by propranolol.[83] In the Cardiac Arrhythmia Suppression Trial (CAST),[84] in patients with asymptomatic or mildly symptomatic ventricular arrhythmias who had survived myocardial infarction, the use of class IC agents alone was harmful and increased mortality (proarrhythmic effect). Retrospectively, those receiving concurrent beta blocker therapy had enhanced survival compared with those who did not, and there was a one-third reduction in arrhythmic deaths or cardiac arrest. Furthermore, in patients with a history of heart failure, beta blocker therapy prolonged the time to new or worsened heart failure.[61]

Drug Interactions of Beta Blockers

Beta blockers are subject to a number of hemodynamic, electrophysiologic, hepatic, and antihypertensive interactions (Table 2–4).[85, 86]

CALCIUM CHANNEL ANTAGONISTS

Calcium channel antagonists (calcium blockers, calcium entry blockers) are agents that tend to inhibit certain calcium-dependent functions in the cardiovascular system. By decreasing vascular smooth muscle contraction and tone, they achieve peripheral and coronary vasodilatation. By inhibiting myocardial contraction, there is a negative inotropic effect, sometimes undesired. Certain specific agents inhibit calcium-dependent AV nodal conduction. It is these actions that explain the use of calcium channel antagonists in hypertension, angina pectoris, and supraventricular tachycardias.

These drugs bind to the calcium channel subunits, to lessen the probability of calcium channel opening, so they can correctly be called calcium channel antagonists. Because channel block is never complete, the term calcium blocker is less ideal—but neither this term nor the companion term beta blocker is likely to disappear.

Fundamental Mechanisms of Calcium Channel Antagonists

The Calcium Channel as a Site of Action

By definition, calcium channel antagonists are agents that interfere with the entry of calcium ions into cells through the voltage-dependent calcium channels. For cardiologists, the major sites of action are (1) vascular smooth muscle cells, (2) cardiac myocytes, and (3) nodal cells. By binding to specific sites in the protein of the calcium channel, these agents are able to diminish the degree to which the calcium channel pores open in response to voltage depolarization (Fig. 2–6).

Molecular Structure. The calcium channel consists of four high-molecular-weight subunits, namely the α_1, α_2, beta, and gamma. Of these, it is the α_1 subunit that contains the calcium channel pores and the binding sites for the calcium channel antagonist drugs. The α_1 subunit in turn consists of four major domains (see Fig. 2–6), each one with six transmembrane units. The calcium channel pore is thought to be located between S5 and S6, and studies by Schwartz' group have identified a glutamine structure that may regulate the opening of the pore.[87] The voltage sensor is thought to be located on S4. Four of the α_1 units, when united in a circular pattern, each contribute their S5/S6 pore units to the overall entry channel for the calcium ions.[88]

There are two other regulatory aspects. First, when cAMP activates protein kinase A to phosphorylate the calcium channel, there are a number of phosphorylation sites on the COOH-terminal portion of each of the α_1 subunits. Such phosphorylation allows the channel to stay in a more open state. Second, the beta subunit binds to the cytoplasmic link between the domains I and II of the α_1 subunit[89]

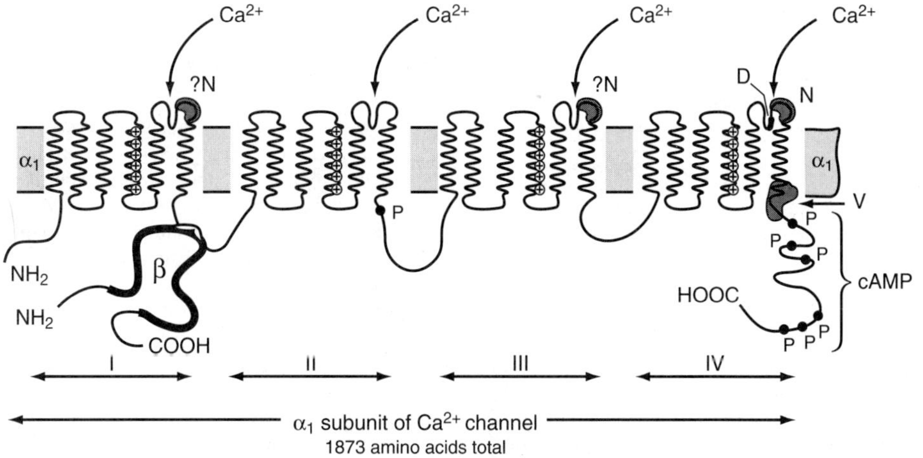

Figure 2–6. Molecular structure of L-type calcium channel with sites of calcium ion entry through the four pores, one in each of the four domains (I to IV). The positive voltage signs indicate the sites at which voltage sensing may take place. The beta subunit (β) binds to a cytoplasmic loop between domains I and II and acts to promote calcium pore opening. The site of action of binding of the nifedipine-like compounds (N), verapamil (V), and diltiazem (D) is shown. Nifedipine may bind to more than one domain. cAMP, by phosphorylating the one terminal loop derived from the fourth domain, phosphorylates certain critical amino acids. Thereby, the state of opening of the calcium channel pore is enhanced. *Abbreviations:* P, phosphorylation. (Reprinted with permission. Copyright 1996, L.H. Opie.)

TABLE 2–4. PHARMACODYNAMIC AND PHARMACOKINETIC INTERACTIONS OF BETA-ADRENERGIC BLOCKING AGENTS

Cardiac Drug	Interacting Drugs	Mechanism	Consequence	Prophylaxis
		Hemodynamic Interactions		
All beta blockers	Calcium antagonists, especially nifedipine	Added hypotension	Risk of myocardial ischemia	Blood pressure control, adjust doses
	Verapamil or diltiazem	Added negative inotropic effect	Risk of myocardial failure	Check for CHF, adjust doses
	Flecainide	Added negative inotropic effect	Hypotension	Check LV function, flecainide levels
		Electrophysiologic Interactions		
All beta blockers	Verapamil	Added inhibition of SA and AV nodes	Bradycardia, asystole, complete heart block	Exclude "sick sinus" syndrome, AV nodal disease; adjust dose; exclude predrug LV failure
	Diltiazem	Added negative inotropic effect	Excess hypotension	
		Hepatic Interactions		
Propranolol (P)	Cimetidine (C)	C decreases P metabolism	Excess P effects	Reduce both drug doses
	Lidocaine (L)	Low hepatic blood flow	Excess L effects	Reduce L dose
Metoprolol (M)	Verapamil (V)	V decreases M metabolism	Excess M effects	Reduce M dose
	Cimetidine (C)	C decreases M metabolism	Excess M effects	Reduce both drug doses
Labetalol (L)	Cimetidine (C)	C decreases L metabolism	Excess L effects	Reduce both drug doses
		Antihypertensive Interactions		
All beta blockers	Indomethacin (I), other NSAIDs	I inhibits vasodilatory prostaglandins	Decreased antihypertensive effect	Avoid NSAIDs; use alternative drugs
		Immune-Interacting Drugs		
Acebutolol	Other drugs altering immune status: procainamide, hydralazine, captopril	Theoretical risk of additive immune effects	Theoretical risk of lupus or neutropenia	Check antinuclear factors and neutrophils; low doses during cotherapy

Abbreviations: AV, atrioventricular; CHF, congestive heart failure; LV, left ventricular; NSAIDs, nonsteroidal anti-inflammatory drugs; SA, sinoatrial.
From Opie LH: Adverse cardiovascular drug interactions. *In* Schlant RC, Alexander RW (eds): The Heart, 8th ed, pp 1971–1985. New York: McGraw-Hill, 1994.

and thereby enhances calcium channel opening. Activity of the beta subunit may also alter the binding of calcium channel antagonists to the α_1 subunit.[90] Species specificity may lie here. For example, the human heart beta subunit has a molecular pattern different from that of the rabbit or rat.[91] In the future, there may be drugs modulating calcium ion entry by altering the properties of the beta subunit. At present, the only agents available all bind to the α_1 unit in the neighborhood of the S5/S6 pore.

Drug Binding Sites. It is now known that there are at least three binding sites for drugs. These have been simplified into the V, N, and D binding sites, because the prototype agents are verapamil, nifedipine, and diltiazem, respectively. More correctly, the N-binding site is termed the DHP site, to which all DHPs are thought to bind. The DHP or N-binding site is on the outer portion of the S5/S6 pore of the fourth domain of the α_1 subunit, but DHPs possibly also bind to two other domains.[92] The verapamil binding site[93] is deep within the S6 subunit of the fourth domain and could be thought of as binding to the inner opening of the calcium channel pore.[94] Regarding the third binding site, that for diltiazem, this site had been thought to be close to that of verapamil. Nonetheless, the most recent molecular structures identify a more superficial site in the calcium channel pore,[95] physically removed from the verapamil site.

The critical issue is that each of these different types of agents binds to specified sites on the various domains, and none binds to all the pores in all the domains. Thus, clinically, calcium channel block can never be complete.

Calcium Channels: L- and T-Types

The most important property of all calcium channel antagonists is selectively to inhibit the inward flow of charge-bearing calcium ions when the calcium channel becomes permeable or is "open." The term "slow channel" was previously used, but now it is realized that the calcium current travels much faster than previously believed and that there are at least two types of calcium channels, the L and T. The conventional calcium channel, which is termed the L-type (long-acting) channel, is blocked by calcium channel antagonists and increased in activity by catecholamines. The function of the L-type channel is to admit the substantial amount of calcium ions required for initiation of contraction by calcium-induced calcium release from the sarcoplasmic reticulum.

The T-type (transient) channel appears at more negative potentials than the L-type and probably plays an important role in the initial depolarization of sinus and AV nodal tissue. A relatively selective blocker for T-type calcium channels is now under investigation; it could be expected (1) to inhibit the spontaneous contractions in vascular smooth muscle initiated by local pacemaker activity[96] and (2) to slow the firing rate of the sinus node. Of interest is that T-

TABLE 2–5. RELATIVE EFFECTS OF THE THREE PROTOTYPICAL CALCIUM ANTAGONISTS IN EXPERIMENTAL PREPARATIONS COMPARED WITH THERAPEUTIC LEVELS IN HUMANS

	Verapamil	Diltiazem	Nifedipine
Therapeutic level in humans			
ng/mL	80–400	50–300	15–100
Molecular weight	455	415	346
Molar value*	$2–8 \times 10^{-7}$ M	$1–7 \times 10^{-7}$ M	$0.3–2 \times 10^{-7}$ M
Protein binding	About 90%	About 85%	About 95%
Molar value, corrected for protein binding	$2–8 \times 10^{-8}$ M	$1–5 \times 10^{-8}$ M	$0.3–1 \times 10^{-8}$ M
Slowing of sinus rate by 20% (isolated atria)	10^{-6} M	10^{-8} M	10^{-5} M
Negative inotropic effect, isolated human papillary muscle	6×10^{-7} M	6×10^{-7} M	10^{-7} M
Human coronary artery contraction, 50% inhibition	Similar to papillary muscle	Similar to papillary muscle	10^{-8} M
K^+ contracture, pig coronary strips, 50% inhibition	About 10^{-7} M	About 10^{-7} M	About 10^{-8} M
Vascular smooth muscle contraction (portal vein)	4×10^{-7} M	6×10^{-7} M	4×10^{-8} M
Vascular selectivity			
Animals	1.4	7	14
Humans	1.0	1.0	10

*All concentrations (e.g., 10^{-7}) in molar units, that is, moles per liter.

For data sources, see Opie LH: Clinical Use of Calcium Antagonist Drugs, pp 50–51. Boston: Kluwer Academic, 1990. Vascular selectivity data from Stone et al[98] and Godfraind et al.[99]

type activity seems relatively more important in the hypertrophied myocardium and in a model of cardiomyopathy.[97]

Pharmacologic Properties of Calcium Channel Antagonists

Pharmacodynamic Effects

Despite their structural diversity and binding differences, calcium channel antagonists display common pharmacologic actions that differ between the DHPs and non-DHPs only in the degree of expression (Table 2–5):

1. a negative inotropic effect;
2. negative chronotropic and dromotropic effects on the SA node and AV nodal conducting tissue;
3. vasodilatation; this effect is more marked on arteriolar than on venular vessels and includes the coronary vasculature.

The first two effects (negative inotropic and nodal inhibitory effects) are especially evident in the case of diltiazem and verapamil. The reason is that these two agents more powerfully and specifically inhibit nodal tissue. Experimentally, high concentrations of nifedipine also have inhibitory effects on the nodes, but depression is clinically relevant only during overdose or when there is pre-existing myocardial depression.

Classification of Calcium Channel Antagonists

The pharmacodynamic effects lead to classification of the calcium channel antagonists. The DHPs all bind to the same sites on the α_1 subunit and exert a greater inhibitory effect on vascular smooth muscle than on the myocardium, which explains their common property of vascular selectivity (Fig. 2–7). Thus, their major therapeutic effect is peripheral and coronary vasodilatation.

Nifedipine is the prototype DHP. The fast-acting capsular form, originally the only preparation available, rapidly produces vasodilatation, relieves severe hypertension, and terminates attacks of coronary spasm. However, the brisk peripheral vasodilatation leads to rapid reflex adrenergic activation with tachycardia and stimulation of the

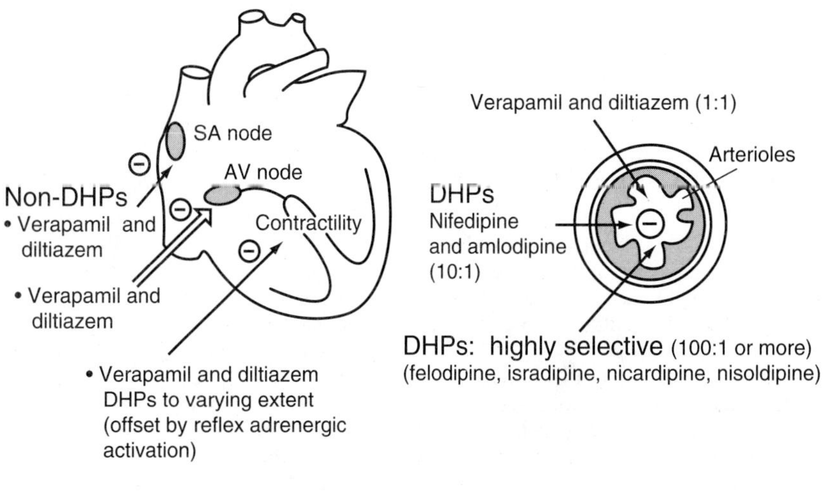

Figure 2–7. Relative sites of action of non-dihydropyridines non-DHPs, verapamil and diltiazem) and dihydropyridines (DHPs). As a group, the DHPs can be divided into the modestly selective (nifedipine and amlodipine) and the highly selective (felodipine, isradipine, lacidipine, nicardipine, and nisoldipine). Antianginal efficacy does not correlate simply with the degree of vascular selectivity. Rather, a certain degree of inhibition of contractility may also be required for an optimal antianginal effect. (Reprinted with permission. Copyright 1996, L.H. Opie.)

renin-angiotensin system. The introduction of truly long-acting compounds, such as amlodipine, or sustained-release formulations of nifedipine, felodipine, or isradipine has led to substantially fewer symptomatic side effects.

The second-generation DHPs are distinguished by a longer half-life, as in the case of amlodipine, or by a greater vascular selectivity.

The non-DHPs, verapamil and diltiazem, although binding to different sites on the α_1 subunit, have many properties in common. Both act on nodal (SA and AV) tissue and both are therapeutically effective in supraventricular tachycardias. Both tend to decrease the sinus rate and inhibit myocardial contraction more than the DHPs do (i.e., are less vascular selective). Pharmacologically, the nodal blocking and negative inotropic effects are closer in position to vasodilatation on the dose-response curve, whereas in the case of the DHPs, the vasodilating property is to the left of the other two. It can therefore be anticipated that these agents would act in angina through mechanisms somewhat different from those invoked by the DHPs. The overall therapeutic spectrum of the non-DHPs is closer to that of the beta blockers with, however, an important exception in that there is no effect on the usual types of ventricular tachycardia for which these agents are strongly contraindicated because of the risk of excess hypotension. This stricture does not apply to nonischemic-mediated ventricular tachycardia arising in the right ventricular outflow tract in young individuals.

Both these agents appear to have major effects on the AV rather than on the SA node, but the explanation may be frequency dependence. Thus, there is better access to the binding sites when the calcium channel pore is open. During supraventricular tachycardia, the calcium channel of the AV node opens more frequently, so that the drug binds more avidly and hence more specifically inhibits the AV node to interrupt the reentry circuit.

Regarding side effects, non-DHPs, being less active than vascular smooth muscle, also have fewer vasodilatory consequences than DHPs. Sinus tachycardia is uncommon because of the inhibitory effects on the SA node. High-degree AV block is a risk with preexisting disease or during cotherapy with nodal depressant drugs. Non-DHPs have a more marked depressive effect on ventricular function. It is often thought that verapamil is more powerful in this respect than diltiazem,[98] but strict comparative clinical data are lacking. Constipation occurs as a side effect with verapamil but seldom with diltiazem for reasons that are not readily apparent.

Vascular Selectivity

The mechanisms of vascular contraction differ from that of the myocardium. Although contraction is ultimately still calcium dependent, it is the myosin light chain kinase that is activated by calcium-calmodulin (Fig. 2–8). In the case of the human myocardium, Godfraind and associates[99] proposed that the ratios of vasodilatation to negative inotropy for the prototype calcium channel antagonists were nifedipine 10:1, diltiazem 1:1, and verapamil 1:1. Some more recent DHP compounds have even greater vascular selectivity, up to 1000:1.[99] In terms of clinical application, these observations provide the basis for considering a clinical division of the calcium channel antagonists into two groups, the DHPs (i.e., nifedipine and its analogues) and the non-DHPs (verapamil and diltiazem and their derivatives).

Noncardiovascular Effects

Although highly active on vascular smooth muscle, calcium channel antagonists have little or no effect on other smooth muscle such as that of the bronchi or gut. This difference probably reflects variations between tissues in either the structure or function of their calcium channels. Also crucial to the therapeutic applicability of calcium channel antagonists is the fact that skeletal muscle does not react to conventional calcium channel antagonists. As a result, skeletal muscle weakness is not an undesired side effect of their administration. In skeletal muscle, depolarization-activated calcium release from the sarcoplasmic reticulum is the principal source of the myoplasmic calcium rise. *Thus, only the myocardium and not skeletal muscle responds to calcium entry through the voltage-dependent calcium channels, and only the myocardium has its rise in contractile calcium inhibited by calcium channel antagonists.*

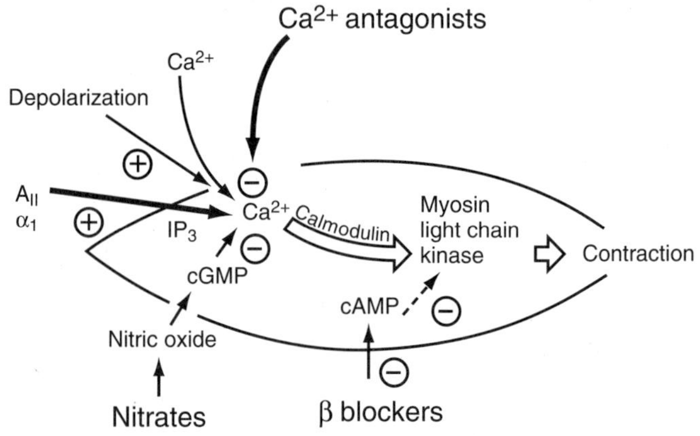

Figure 2–8. Mechanism of action of calcium channel antagonists in comparison with nitrates and with inhibitory effects of beta blockers. Note that in vascular smooth muscle, contraction is calcium dependent as in the myocardium but is activated by myosin light chain kinase in response to calcium-calmodulin. *Abbreviations:* A_{II}, angiotensin II; α_1, α_1-adrenergic activity; IP_3, inositol 1,4,5-triphosphate. (Reprinted with permission. Copyright 1996, L.H. Opie.)

Pharmacokinetics

From the point of view of drug interactions, all these drugs are metabolized in the liver by an enzyme system that is inhibited by cimetidine or liver-disease and increased in activity by anticonvulsants.

Major Indications for Calcium Channel Antagonists

Hypertension

All calcium channel antagonists act on peripheral arterioles, although with a different potency relative to that of the effect on the heart (see Fig. 2–8). They are excellent antihypertensive agents and effective in the "low-renin" groups, such as elderly black men. All DHPs decrease peripheral vascular resistance and appear to have an additional ill-understood diuretic effect. Verapamil and diltiazem are less powerful vasodilators, and a negative inotropic effect may contribute to their antihypertensive mechanism. Calcium channel antagonists have not yet been used in any long-term outcome study. In the Treatment of Mild Hypertension (TOMH) study,[100] which lasted 4 years, amlodipine was as effectively antihypertensive as four other agents of different antihypertensive categories and, furthermore, was the best tolerated of the agents. Nitrendipine is the calcium channel antagonist chosen for the SystEur outcome study on elderly hypertensives in Europe.

Angina Pectoris

Although the antianginal mechanisms of the different types of agents appear to vary, nonetheless common properties are (1) coronary vasodilatation, especially in relation to exercise-induced coronary constriction, and (2) afterload reduction due to decreased blood pressure. Furthermore, in the case of verapamil and diltiazem, slowing of the sinus node, a decrease in exercise heart rate, and a negative inotropic effect may all contribute.

As coronary dilators, the calcium channel antagonists have a site of action on the coronary tree different from that of the nitrates (Table 2–6). The calcium channel antagonists act more specifically on the coronary resistance vessels, where the tone is higher and the calcium inhibitory effect more marked.

Calcium channel antagonists are specifically effective in those types of angina caused by coronary spasm, such as Prinzmetal variant angina, cold-induced angina, and that induced by hyperventilation.

Studies on silent electrocardiographic ischemia and on patients with mixed (effort and rest) angina have not shown any specific role for calcium channel antagonists in the therapy of these conditions in which it is now suspected that a tachycardia plays a precipitating role even in the absence of effort.

Supraventricular Tachycardia

Verapamil and diltiazem, through their inhibitory effect on the AV node, interrupt the reentry circuit in supraventricular tachycardias. The DHPs are ineffective.

Postinfarct Protection

Verapamil is licensed in Scandinavian countries for postinfarct protection in patients in whom beta blockers are contraindicated.

Specific Calcium Channel Antagonists

Verapamil

After peripheral vasodilatation, the cardiac output and left ventricular ejection fraction do not increase as expected, probably the result of the negative inotropic effect.

Pharmacokinetics. The elimination half-life of standard verapamil tablets is usually 3–7 h but increases significantly during long-term administration and in patients with liver or advanced renal insufficiency. Bioavailability is only 10%–20% (high first-pass liver metabolism). The parent compound and the active hepatic metabolite norverapamil are excreted 75% by the kidneys and 25% by the gastrointestinal tract. Verapamil is 87%–93% protein bound.

Dose

1. *Oral preparations.* The usual dose of the standard preparation is 80–120 mg three times daily. During long-term oral dosing, less frequent daily doses are needed (norverapamil metabolites). *Slow-release preparations* (doses 240–480 mg daily) are Calan SR and Isoptin SR (once or twice daily) and Verelan (once daily).
2. *Intravenous use* (caution: only in monitored patients). For supraventricular reentry tachycardias, when there is no myocardial depression, a bolus of 5–10 mg (0.1–0.15 mg/kg) can be given in 1 min and repeated 10 min later if needed. After a successful bolus, the dose is 0.005 mg/kg/min for about 30–60 min, decreasing thereafter. When used for uncontrolled atrial fibrillation, verapamil may be given at 0.005 mg/kg/min, increasing as needed, or as an intravenous bolus of 5 mg followed by double the dose if needed.[101] In the presence of myocardial disease or interacting drugs, a very low dose (0.0001 mg/kg/min) is infused and titrated upward against the ventricular response.

Side Effects. Class side effects include headaches, facial flushing, dizziness, and ankle edema—all lower in frequency than with the DHPs. Constipation occurs in up to one third of patients. A negative inotropic effect sometimes precipitates congestive heart failure. When intravenous verapamil is used, the risk of hypotension is high if there is prior beta blockade, myocardial disease, or disopyramide therapy. Pre-treatment with calcium gluconate 90 mg as a slow intravenous injection should be given before the infusion.[102]

Contraindications. Sick sinus syndrome and pre-existing AV nodal block are contraindications to intravenous verapamil. Use of oral preparations in these conditions may require a pacemaker. In the Wolff-Parkinson-White syndrome with atrial fibrillation, intravenous verapamil may promote forward conduction of impulses along the bypass tract with risk of ventricular fibrillation. In wide QRS complex ventricular tachycardia, verapamil is *absolutely contraindicated* because the combined negative inotropic and peripheral vasodilatory effects can be fatal; furthermore, verapamil is unlikely to terminate the arrhythmia.

Pregnancy: category C (use only if potential benefit justifies potential risk to fetus). No well-controlled trials are available.

Diltiazem

Diltiazem is used for the same spectrum of diseases as verapamil: hypertension, angina pectoris, and supraventricular arrhythmias. The side effect profile is similar except that constipation is much less common.

Pharmacokinetics. More than 90% of oral diltiazem is absorbed,

TABLE 2–6. EFFECTS OF CALCIUM CHANNEL ANTAGONISTS AND OTHER VASODILATORS ON LARGE CORONARY ARTERIES AND CORONARY RESISTANCE VESSELS AND ON EFFORT ANGINA

	Large Epicardial Conductance Vessels*	Coronary Resistance Vessels*	Effort Angina†
Nitrates‡	+ + +	+	+ + +
Nifedipine + dihydropyridines§	+ +	+ +	+ +
Diltiazem	+ +	+ +	+ +
Verapamil	+ +	+ +	+ +
Dipyridamole	0	+ + +	0, −

*For vessels: + + + = marked dilatation; + + = moderate dilatation; + = mild dilatation; 0 = no dilatation.
†For angina: + + + = highly effective; + + = effective; 0 = ineffective; − = may be harmful.
‡Poor effect of nitrates on coronary resistance vessels may be related to lack of available sulfhydryl groups in the arterioles.[2]
§Mechanism of action on large coronary arteries may be in part through flow-dependent dilatation.
Modified from Schwartz JS, Bache RJ: Pharmacologic vasodilators in the coronary circulation. Circulation 1987; 75(suppl I):162–167.

with about 45% bioavailability (first-pass hepatic metabolism). Onset of action is within 15–30 min; peak effect occurs at 1–2 h. Elimination half-life is 4–7 h. Protein binding is 80%–86%. Diltiazem is acetylated in the liver to deacyldiltiazem (40% of the activity of the parent compound), which accumulates with long-term therapy. Only 35% of diltiazem is excreted by the kidneys (65% by the gastrointestinal tract; note differences from verapamil).

Dose. The standard oral dose of diltiazem is 120–360 mg, usually in four daily doses of the short-acting formulation. Of the *slow-release preparations,* Cardizem SR is given twice daily. Dilacor XR is given once daily and is licensed in the United States for hypertension, whereas Cardizem CD (once daily) is licensed for hypertension and angina. *Intravenous diltiazem* (approved for arrhythmias, not hypertension) is given as 0.25 mg/kg in 2 min with electrocardiographic and blood pressure monitoring; if the response is inadequate, the dose is then repeated as 0.35 mg/kg in 2 min. Acute therapy is usually followed by an infusion of 5–15 mg/h. (For cautions, see intravenous verapamil.)

Side Effects. With the standard preparation, these are few and limited to headaches, dizziness, and ankle edema in about 6%–10% of patients. With extended- or slow-release preparations used for hypertension, the side effect profile is similar to placebo. With use for angina, bradycardia and first-degree AV block are more commonly found. Exfoliative dermatitis occurs occasionally. Side effects of intravenous diltiazem resemble those of intravenous verapamil.

Contraindications. Contraindications are similar to those of verapamil: pre-existing marked depression of the sinus or AV node, hypotension, myocardial failure, and the Wolff-Parkinson-White syndrome. Postinfarct left ventricular failure with an ejection fraction below .40 is a clear contraindication.[103]

Pregnancy: category C (see verapamil).

Nifedipine—The Prototypical Dihydropyridine

The major therapeutic action of the DHPs is by arteriolar dilatation, which explains their use in hypertension, Prinzmetal variant angina, Raynaud phenomenon, and cold-induced angina. The direct negative inotropic effect is usually overcome by simultaneous arteriolar unloading, except in patients with congestive heart failure. There is no clinically significant effect against the AV node, so that it is not used against supraventricular arrhythmias, and it can be better combined than non-DHPs with beta blockers with less fear of added nodal side effects.

Pharmacokinetics. Nifedipine in *capsule form* is most rapidly absorbed after bite-and-swallow ingestion; peak blood values occur within 20–45 min, with a half-life of 3 h and a duration of action of 4–8 h. The hypotensive and antianginal effect starts within 20 min of swallowing a capsule and within 5 min of a bite-and-swallow dose. Hepatic metabolism (P-450) inactivates almost all circulating nifedipine (high first-pass metabolism) to metabolites that are excreted renally. A *slow-release preparation* (Procardia XL) and a *core-coat system* (Adalat CC) give sustained 24-h blood levels within the therapeutic range.

Dose. In *effort angina,* the dose of nifedipine capsules is 30–60 mg daily (i.e., 1–2 capsules three times daily). Concerns about higher doses have been raised[104] and refuted.[105] Gradual dose increases avoid precipitation of ischemic pain. Similar doses are used for *cold-induced angina.* Higher doses may be needed for *coronary spasm.* For *angina,* the dose of Procardia XL is 30–90 mg once daily. In hypertension, doses are 30–60 mg of Procardia XL or Adalat CC once daily. In severe hypertension, one 10-mg capsule (bite-and-swallow) frequently works within 20–60 min, although the drug is not licensed in the United States for this purpose, nor is such a rapid blood pressure reduction necessarily desirable.

Contraindications and Cautions. These are the danger of exaggerated pressure gradients in tight aortic stenosis or obstructive hypertrophic cardiomyopathy. In pre-existing myocardial depression, the added negative inotropic effect may precipitate clinical heart failure. In unstable angina, in the absence of concurrent beta blockade, the outcome is adverse.[55] Nifedipine should not be given in the acute phase of myocardial infarction. Relative contraindications are subjective intolerance to nifedipine, previous adverse reactions, and pre-existing hypotension or tachycardia.

Pregnancy: category C (see verapamil).

Side Effects. Overall, the drug is safe when the contraindications are observed. Especially with capsules, abrupt vasodilatation may cause flushing, dizziness, headaches, and palpitations as a result of reflex adrenergic discharge. After a dose, angina may be caused by reflex tachycardia or coronary underperfusion. Ankle edema is not due to cardiac failure. Rather, nifedipine itself has a mild diuretic effect and occasionally causes hypokalemia. With extended- or slow-release nifedipine preparations, the low frequency of acute vasodilatory side effects appears to reflect the slow rate of rise of blood DHP levels. The other side effects of this preparation are restricted to headache (nearly double that found in control subjects) and ankle edema (dose-dependent, 10% with 30 mg daily, 30% with 180 mg daily; manufacturer's information). In patients with left ventricular depression, the direct negative inotropic effect can be a serious problem. Occasionally, side effects compatible with the effects of excess hypotension and organ underperfusion have been reported: myocardial ischemia or even infarction, retinal and cerebral ischemia, and renal failure.

Second-Generation Calcium Channel Antagonists

Theoretically, the more vascular selective agents, such as felodipine, isradipine, and nicardipine, should be better in the management of angina or hypertension when there is prior impairment of left ventricular function. Proof of benefit of such agents in congestive heart failure has been difficult to obtain, and none of these drugs is yet licensed for that purpose. An extreme degree of vascular selectivity as found in nisoldipine is not necessarily beneficial because, by intense peripheral vasodilatation, there is reflex adrenergic and renin-angiotensin activation. Contrary to common opinion, amlodipine is no more vascular selective than nifedipine, but it has unusual aspects to its kinetics, including slow onset and offset of binding to the calcium channel site and a prolonged elimination half-life. Doses, pharmacokinetics, side effects, and interactions of these agents are shown in Table 2–7.

Combined Sodium-Calcium Blockade by Bepridil

Bepridil (Vascor) is a nonspecific calcium channel antagonist[93] with added sodium channel inhibition and hence with a class I antiarrhythmic effect. It differs from the other calcium channel antagonists in having only mild antihypertensive properties. Inhibition of repolarizing potassium currents may explain QT interval prolongation and risk of torsades. Bepridil is very long acting (elimination half-life, 42 h). The antianginal mechanisms remain unclear but may include a reduction of the rate-pressure product on exercise.[106] It is approved for use in angina (200–400 mg once daily) when conventional treatment has failed. It may be combined with propranolol.[107] To lessen torsades, avoid hypokalemia and cotherapy with other cardiac drugs that may prolong the QT interval, such as quinidine, sotalol, and amiodarone, as well as certain noncardiac drugs such as erythromycin and terfenidine.

Contraindications are previous serious ventricular tachycardia or

TABLE 2–7. SECOND-GENERATION DIHYDROPYRIDINE CALCIUM CHANNEL ANTAGONISTS: SALIENT FEATURES FOR CARDIOVASCULAR USE

Agent	Dose	Pharmacokinetics and Metabolism	Side Effects and Contraindications	Interactions and Precautions
Amlodipine	5–10 mg once daily	t max 6–12 h Extensive but slow hepatic metabolism, 90% inactive metabolites, 60% renal $t_{1/2}$ 35–50 h; steady state in 7–8 days	As for nifedipine XL (see text) In congestive heart failure, amlodipine does not lead to deterioration in New York Heart Association class II or III	Reduce dose in liver failure and with cimetidine Increase dose with hepatic enzyme inducers (barbiturates, phenytoin, rifampin)
Felodipine SR	5–10 mg once daily Reduce dose in elderly	t max 3–5 h Complete hepatic metabolism (P-450) to inactive metabolites, 75% renal loss $t_{1/2}$ 22–27 h	As for nifedipine XL May directly stimulate myocardium	As for amlodipine
Isradipine	2.5–10 mg 2× daily	t max 2 h Complete hepatic metabolism to inactive metabolites, 75% renal, 25% gastrointestinal loss $t_{1/2}$ 8.4 h Food delays absorption	As for nifedipine Also, animal data show inhibitory effect on sinus node so that tachycardia should be less C/I: sick sinus syndrome	As for amlodipine
Nicardipine				
Capsules	20–40 mg 3× daily	Rapid absorption High first-pass saturable effect; plasma clearance may be limited by hepatic blood flow Peak time 1 h Hepatic metabolites 60% renal, 35% gastrointestinal Increasing dose disproportionately increases blood level	As for nifedipine, except for less cardiodepression	As for amlodipine
SR	30–60 mg 2× daily	As above; $t_{1/2}$ 9 h	As above	As for amlodipine
Intravenous	5–15 mg/h	High first-pass metabolism inactivates drug, possibly in proportion to liver blood flow Blood pressure starts to fall within 10 min	Excess hypotension if beta blockade plus anesthesia C/I: severe aortic stenosis, obstructive cardiomyopathy	As for amlodipine

Abbreviations: t max, time to peak blood level; $t_{1/2}$, plasma elimination half-life; SR, slow release; C/I, contraindication.
Modified from Opie LH: Drugs for the Heart, 4th ed, pp 74–75. Philadelphia: WB Saunders, 1995. See also references 104 and 105.

congenital QT prolongation. Thus far, its antiarrhythmic potential has received less attention than its proarrhythmic risks.

Drug Interactions of Calcium Channel Antagonists

Verapamil (Table 2–8)

Beta Blockers. Verapamil either may give added SA, AV, or myocardial depression or may interact at a hepatic metabolic level with those beta blockers metabolized by the liver, such as propranolol and metoprolol. Although verapamil has been successfully combined with beta blockade in the therapy of angina or hypertension, clinicians should monitor patients for possible adverse effects.

Digoxin. Verapamil increases blood digoxin levels by decreasing the renal excretion of digoxin. Enhancement of AV block can be fatal when intravenous verapamil is given to patients with digitalis poisoning.

Diltiazem

In general, drug interactions of diltiazem are similar to those of verapamil, yet diltiazem has a slight or negligible effect on blood digoxin levels. Although diltiazem may be cautiously combined with beta blockade, the combination was no more effectively antianginal in some studies than high-dose diltiazem itself.

Dihydropyridines

Combination of DHPs with beta blockers is simpler than with non-DHPs (absence of nodal interaction). When there is pre-existing left ventricular depression, the added negative inotropic effects of the beta blocker and DHP may precipitate overt heart failure.

In therapy of hypertension, nifedipine has been combined with diuretics, beta blockers, methyldopa, and ACE inhibitors. Combination with prazosin may lead to adverse hepatic interactions with hypotensive consequences. Drugs such as cimetidine, which inhibit the hepatic P-450 enzyme system, increase blood nifedipine levels (see Table 2–8).

TABLE 2–8. KINETIC AND DYNAMIC INTERACTIONS OF NITRATES AND CALCIUM CHANNEL ANTAGONISTS

Cardiac Drug	Interacting Drugs	Mechanism	Consequence	Prophylaxis
Nitrates				
All nitrates	Calcium antagonists	Excess vasodilatation	Syncope, dizziness	Monitor BP
	Prazosin (PZ)	Excess vasodilatation	Syncope, dizziness	Monitor BP and start with low PZ dose
Calcium Antagonist Drugs				
Verapamil (V)	Beta blockers	SA and AV nodal inhibition Myocardial failure	Added nodal and negative inotropic effects	Care during cotherapy Check ECG, BP, heart size
	Cimetidine	Hepatic metabolic interaction	Blood V rises	Adjust dose
	Digitalis poisoning	Added SA and AV nodal inhibition	Asystole; complete heart block after intravenous V	Avoid intravenous V in digitalis poisoning
	Digoxin (D)	Decreased D clearance	Risk of D toxicity	Halve D dose; blood D level
	Disopyramide	Pharmacodynamic	Hypotension, constipation	Check BP, LV, and gut
	Flecainide (F)	Added negative inotropic effect	Hypotension	Check LV; F levels
	Prazosin	Hepatic interaction	Excess hypotension	Check BP during cotherapy
	Quinidine (Q)	Added alpha receptor inhibition; V decreases Q clearance	Hypotension; increased Q levels	Check Q levels and BP
	Theophylline (T)	Inhibition of hepatic metabolism	Increased blood T levels	Reduce T, check levels
Nifedipine (N)	Beta blockers	Added negative inotropism	Excess hypotension	Check BP, use test dose of N
	Cimetidine	Hepatic metabolic interaction	Increased blood N levels	Decreased N dosage by 40%
	Digoxin (D)	Minor/modest changes in D	Increased D levels	Check D levels
	Prazosin (PZ)	PZ blocks alpha reflex of N	Postural hypotension	Test dose of N or PZ
	Propranolol (P)	N and P have opposite effects on blood liver flow	N decreases P levels; P increases N levels	Readjust P and N doses if needed
	Quinidine (Q)	N improves poor LV function; Q clearance faster	Decreased Q effect	Check Q levels
Diltiazem (D)	Beta blockers	Added SA and AV nodal inhibition; negative inotropism	Bradycardia, hypotension	Check ECG and LV function
	Cimetidine	Hepatic metabolic interaction	Increased D levels	Reduce D dose by one third
	Cyclosporine (C)	Hepatic metabolism of C inhibited	Increased blood C levels	Decrease C dose
	Digoxin (D)	Some fall in D clearance	Only in renal failure	Check D levels
	Flecainide (F)	Added negative inotropic effect	Hypotension	Check LV; F levels
Nicardipine (see also nifedipine)	Cyclosporine (C)	Hepatic metabolism of C inhibited	Increased blood C levels	Decrease C dose
	Digoxin (D)	Decreased D clearance	Blood D doubles	Decrease D, D levels

Abbreviations: AV, atrioventricular node; BP, blood pressure; ECG, electrocardiogram; LV, left ventricle; SA, sinoatrial node.
Modified from Opie LH: Adverse cardiovascular drug interactions. *In* Schlant RC, Alexander RW (eds): The Heart, 8th ed, pp 1971–1985. New York: McGraw-Hill, 1994.

ANTIPLATELET AGENTS

Antiplatelet agents have now become part of the standard armamentarium used in the overall attack against arterial disease and thrombosis.[108] Aspirin, the prototype antiplatelet agent, has beneficial effects in a wide spectrum of arterial and even venous diseases. Several other agents are available in case of aspirin intolerance. Antiplatelet agents act to modify the physiologic role of platelets in the thrombotic process.

Platelet Structure and Function

For platelets to participate in the thrombotic process requires their activation, a process in which an increase of cytosolic calcium plays a crucial role (Fig. 2–9). Once calcium rises, strands of actin and myosin in the platelets contract and surface receptors are expressed, allowing platelets to link together with the aid of certain circulating factors such as fibrinogen and the von Willebrand factor. Therefore, avoidance of such thrombogenic activation requires careful and continuous control of cytosolic calcium. Such control of calcium is achieved chiefly by regulation of the rate of calcium release from the endoplasmic reticulum (also called the dense tubules), a process that is stimulated by IP_3 and inhibited by cAMP (Fig. 2–10). *Thus, for practical clinical purposes, attempted control of platelet calcium ion entry by calcium channel antagonists does not work.*[109] Rather, an intact endothelium, by release of prostacyclin and nitric oxide, plays an important indirect role in achieving control of platelet calcium (see Fig. 2–9).

Calcium Release From the Endoplasmic Reticulum. The endoplasmic reticulum of platelets is the major site of storage of calcium within these cells. There are both calcium release and calcium uptake channels, as in the case of cardiac myocytes. Calcium release is, however, largely under the control of IP_3, which in turn is a messenger of the phosphatidylinositol 4,5-bisphosphate (PIP_2) pathway (Fig. 2–11). PIP_2 is stimulated by the activity of the membrane-bound enzyme phospholipase C, which in turn is activated by a variety of platelet receptors, including those for serotonin, thrombin, and ADP; these receptor agonists are formed in response to tissue injury. (This path is akin to that stimulated by alpha-adrenergic receptor activity or angiotensin II in cardiac myocytes.)

Calcium Uptake Into Endoplasmic Reticulum. cAMP is the other major messenger controlling release of calcium from the endoplasmic reticulum. cAMP, by enhancing the uptake of calcium into the endoplasmic reticulum, decreases cytosolic calcium. The inhibitory G protein, G_i, is stimulated in response to thromboxane A_2 (TXA_2), thrombin, or epinephrine and decreases cytosolic cAMP concentrations. Thereby, these agents lessen the uptake of calcium into the endoplasmic reticulum and increase platelet calcium (see Fig. 2–10).

Thus, platelet calcium is under regulation of counteracting signal systems. Calcium increases in response to IP_3, part of the signal system involving phospholipase and activated by the products of tissue injury such as ADP, thrombin, and serotonin. Conversely, platelet calcium falls when cAMP rises in response to prostacyclin, or platelet calcium falls when cAMP is inhibited by G_i during receptor stimulation by TXA_2, thrombin, or epinephrine. Thus, in sum, there are five stimuli to an increase in platelet calcium and only one (prostacyclin) leading to a decrease. Whenever calcium increases, actin-myosin interaction is promoted and platelet activation becomes more likely.

Role of Thromboxane A_2. TXA_2 interacts with a platelet surface receptor linked to G_i (see Fig. 2–10). It is formed by platelets when either the cell membrane or the endoplasmic reticulum is damaged.[110] A rising cystolic calcium concentration also helps activate phospholipase A_2,[110] which is involved in steps in the initial pathway of TXA_2 synthesis. The TXA_2 thus formed diffuses out of the cell to interact with its platelet receptor. Thus, a self-perpetuating platelet activation circle leads from membrane damage to cytosolic calcium to an even greater activation of TXA_2. Another powerful effect of TXA_2 is vasoconstriction, which in turn slows platelet flow and therefore increases the probability of platelet-platelet interaction. When, however, the endothelium is intact, then thrombin can induce the release of nitric oxide through the same receptor mechanism.[111]

Platelet Glycoprotein Receptors (IIb/IIIa and Ia/IIa). During platelet damage, several receptors (membrane glycoproteins) are activated. The mechanisms are twofold: (1) activation by protein kinase C action in response to membrane damage, and (2) molecular rearrangement of the receptors during the configurational changes of platelet activation. Activated receptors allow macromolecules such as the circulating von Willebrand factor (a high-molecular-weight protein) and fibrinogen to "chain" receptors together and thereby to promote interplatelet adhesion. Second, they help the process of platelet activation by releasing calcium from the endoplasmic reticulum. Thrombin, although a protease in the coagulation process, also activates the platelet thrombin receptor by cleaving a specific extracellular amino acid domain, thereby exposing the active ligand.[112] The activated thrombin receptor raises platelet calcium levels both by inhibiting adenylate cyclase and by stimulating phospholipase C (see Fig. 2–11).

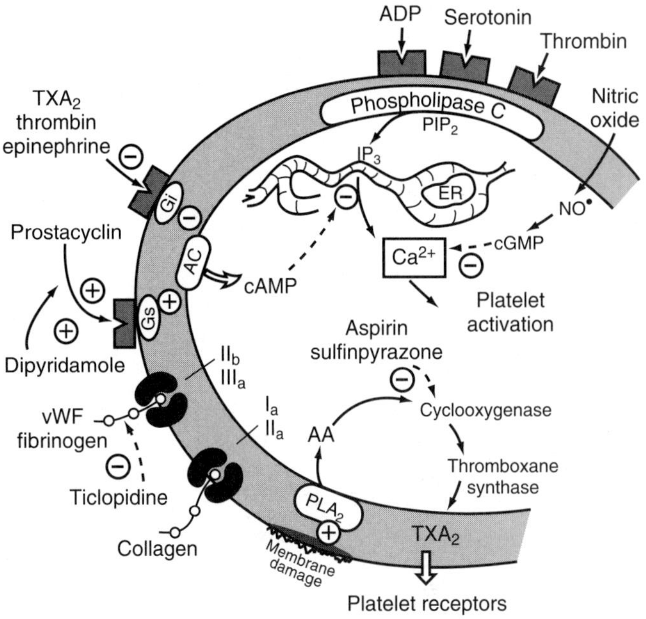

Figure 2–10. Role of platelet receptors in regulating internal platelet calcium and thereby platelet activation. All factors increasing internal calcium (Ca^{2+}) concentration promote platelet activation (see Fig. 2–9). Proposed sites of action of antiplatelet agents are shown. Inhibitory effects are indicated by broken arrows. Note opposing roles of inositol 1,4,5-triphosphate (IP_3) and cAMP in respectively mobilizing and inhibiting release of calcium from the endoplasmic reticulum (ER). Adenosine diphosphate (ADP), serotonin, collagen, and thrombin all promote formation of IP_3. Thromboxane A_2 (TXA_2), formed when membrane damage increases activity of phospholipase A_2 (PLA_2), is released externally to interact with the signal system that inhibits cAMP and increases platelet calcium (see also Fig. 2–11). *Abbreviations:* AA, arachidonic acid; AC, adenylate cyclase; G_i, G protein inhibiting adenylate cyclase; G_S, G protein stimulating adenylate cyclase; Gp, glycoprotein; PIP_2, phosphatidylinositol 4,5-bisphosphate; vWF, von Willebrand factor. (Reprinted with permission. Copyright 1996, L.H. Opie.)

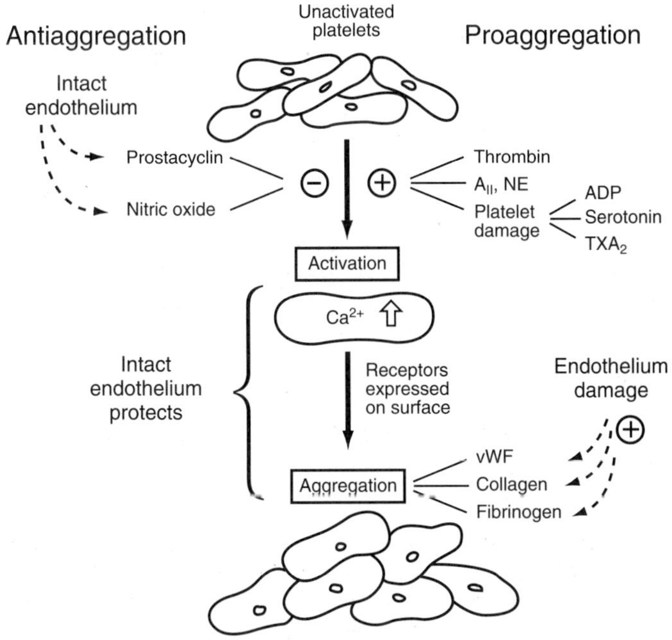

Figure 2–9. Schematic representation of the balance between factors inhibiting and promoting platelet aggregation. Note important role of an intact endothelium. *Abbreviations:* A_{II}, angiotensin II; NE, norepinephrine; ADP, adenosine diphosphate; TXA_2, thromboxane A_2; vWF, von Willebrand factor. (Reprinted with permission. Copyright 1996, L.H. Opie.)

Platelet Aggregation. After the critical rise in intracellular platelet calcium concentration, the interaction of platelet actin and myosin follows to cause platelet contraction. The latter event and/or mechanical shear stress[113] exposes the glycoprotein receptor IIb/IIIa, which mediates the final common path in platelet aggregation by allowing a greater rate of interaction with various macromolecules, including the von Willebrand factor, fibrinogen, and thrombin. These macromolecules bind the platelets to each other and to those platelets already adhering to the vessel wall.

von Willebrand Factor and Platelet Aggregation. von Willebrand factor is a multimeric high-molecular-weight glycoprotein synthesized by endothelial cells and secreted by them during vascular injury.[114] Functional binding domains for the glycoproteins Ib and IIb/IIIa platelet receptors have been identified. During high shear stress, as in atherosclerotic vessels with turbulent blood flow, von Willebrand factor binds to IIb/IIIa and promotes platelet aggregation; by contrast, in low stress, platelet aggregation is promoted by fibrinogen binding to IIb/IIIa.

Platelets and Vascular Contraction. During and after platelet

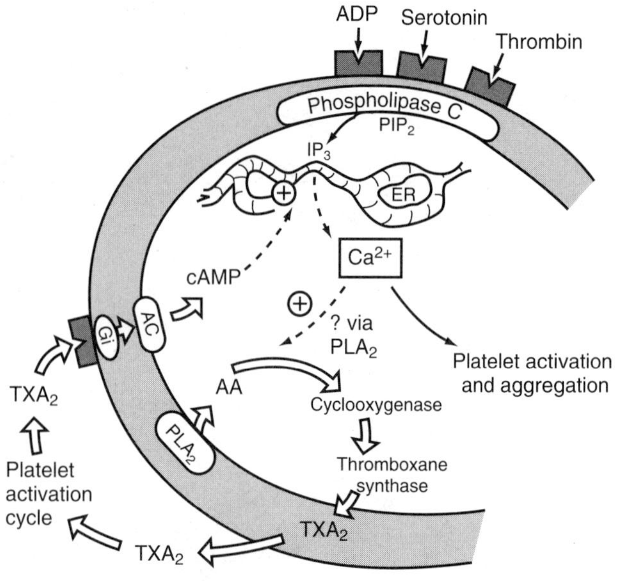

Figure 2–11. Proposed platelet activation cycle. Role of formation of thromboxane A_2 (TXA_2) in increasing platelet calcium concentration, thereby activating phospholipase A_2 (PLA_2) and promoting further formation of TXA_2, which diffuses out of the platelet to interact with the external receptor and thereby promotes a platelet activation cycle. For abbreviations, see Figure 2–10. (Reprinted with permission. Copyright 1996, L.H. Opie.)

aggregation, platelets release 5-hydroxytryptamine (serotonin) and other potentially important products, such as platelet factor 4 and β-thromboglobulin, that may help in the formation of the hemostatic plug and/or cause vasoconstriction. For example, serotonin normally causes vasodilatation in the presence of an intact vascular endothelium. In contrast, when the endothelium is damaged, serotonin causes vasoconstriction that may promote vascular stasis, enhanced platelet interaction, and thrombosis.

Platelets and Atheroma. Platelets may also have much longer lasting effects. They are thought to play an important role in atheroma by interacting with damaged arterial walls and, therefore, releasing substances such as platelet-derived growth factor (PDGF). PDGF may also stimulate smooth muscle cell proliferation and migration into the subintimal layer with subsequent synthesis of connective tissue and intimal hyperplasia, thereby promoting the development of atheroma.

Platelet Adhesion to the Vessel Wall. Activated platelets adhere not only to each other but also to the injured vessel wall (see Figs. 2–9, 2–10). First, release from the endothelium of von Willebrand factor promotes platelet interaction and platelet adhesion to the damaged endothelium. Second, microfibrils of collagen from the deeper layers of the vessel become exposed as a result of endothelial injury, thereby promoting platelet adhesion.

Antiaggregatory Factors. Just as a damaged endothelium by release of von Willebrand factor and exposure of collagen promotes platelet interaction, so does an intact endothelium protect against platelet aggregation. Such protection is achieved first by production of prostacyclin, a compound that decreases platelet calcium, and second by nitric oxide, whose antiaggregatory effect has only recently been inferred.[115] Therefore, an intact endothelium is antiaggregatory (see Fig. 2–9).

Platelets and Thrombosis. Finally, platelets stimulate the intrinsic path of coagulation whereby prothrombin is converted to thrombin. *Hence, antiplatelet agents are indirectly also antithrombotic, adding to their marked effectiveness in ischemic heart disease.*

Aspirin—The Prototypical Antiplatelet Agent

Pharmacologic Properties of Aspirin

Platelet Inhibition by Aspirin. Aspirin (acetylsalicylic acid) irreversibly acetylates platelet cyclooxygenase, more correctly called type I prostaglandin-GH synthase.[116] It is the standard antiplatelet agent (Table 2–9). Platelets, being primitive cells, cannot synthesize new proteins, so that aspirin removes all the platelet cyclooxygenase activity for the life span (8–10 days) of the platelet. Therefore, aspirin stops the production of the proaggregatory TXA_2 and is also an indirect antithrombotic agent. Aspirin also has important nonplatelet effects because it likewise inactivates cyclooxygenase in the vascular endothelium and thereby diminishes formation of antiaggregatory prostacyclin. Why in clinical practice the antithrombotic effects predominate is still not clear.[117] One difference is that the vascular cyclooxygenase can be resynthesized within hours, so that low doses of aspirin may preferentially act on platelets. Second, aspirin may be most active in the portal circulation, before aspirin is metabolized in the liver. Any effects of aspirin on the portal vascular bed and its endothelium are probably not of importance. Third, in high-risk patients, the TXA_2 pathway is activated (see Fig. 2–11), so that the effects of its inhibition are relatively more beneficial.

Aspirin Pharmacokinetics. Aspirin undergoes substantial presystemic hydrolysis to form salicylic acid, which is only a weak inactivator of cyclooxygenase with a longer half-life of 2–3 h versus 15–20 min for aspirin. Although even very low doses of aspirin, such as 20 mg, have a documented platelet inhibitory effect and may selectively inhibit the formation of TXA_2 rather than prostacyclin,[117] the problem with such doses is that the full antithrombotic effect takes up to 48 h or longer to be manifested.[116] In contrast, with higher doses, the effect is seen within hours. Thus, full-dose aspirin (160–320 mg) should be given at the start of symptoms of acute myocardial infarction.[118]

Aspirin Indications and Doses

Indications for Aspirin (see Table 2–9). Judging by the recent meta-analysis of about 100,000 patients,[108] aspirin protects against a spectrum of vascular events such as recurrent thrombosis or embolization, especially in patients who are regarded as being at high risk (see Fig. 51–9). These include those with unstable angina, suspected acute myocardial infarction, a past history of myocardial infarction or of stroke, or transient ischemic attacks. Other high-risk patients include those who have had coronary bypass (aspirin may lessen saphenous vein graft closure), patients who have had angioplasty, patients with stable angina, those with atrial fibrillation, and those with prior valve surgery.

Medium- Versus Low-Dose Aspirin. The doses of aspirin used to prevent cardiovascular complications have gradually decreased from initially 1300 mg daily for prevention of transient ischemic attacks to 30 mg daily for the same purpose.[119] Other workers proposed that standard (medium) doses are 160–320 mg daily, with low doses being regarded as 80 mg or less daily.[108, 120] The concept is that the lower doses have fewer side effects, yet according to the existing data and the meta-analyses, they still maintain efficacy. When there is risk of gastrointestinal bleeding, there is support for the benefit of only small doses, such as 30 mg daily.[119]

At the start of acute myocardial infarction, 160–320 mg is preferred[116] and first principles argue for the higher dose. Thereafter, following the information from the Second International Study of

TABLE 2–9. ORAL ANTIPLATELET AGENTS: INDICATIONS, DOSE, SIDE EFFECTS, AND CONTRAINDICATIONS

Agent	Indications	Dose (Daily)	Side Effects (S/E) and Contraindications (C/I)
Aspirin	Start of AMI[116] AMI[108, 116, 121] Postinfarct[108] Unstable angina[108, 132] TIA prevention[108, 119] With low-dose warfarin (warfarin 3 mg daily[120]) Other uses including prevention of bypass graft vein occlusion[108]	325 mg once 160–325 mg 75–325 mg 75–325 mg 30–325 mg 60 mg 75–325 mg	S/E: GI including bleeding; gout; hemorrhagic stroke (rare) C/I: Aspirin intolerance; hemophilia; GI or GU bleeds; untreated severe hypertension
Ticlopidine	Prevention of thrombotic stroke or unstable angina whenever aspirin cannot be used	250 mg 2× with food; takes several days to work	S/E: Neutropenia, must do blood count every 2 weeks for first 3 months; minor bleeds; skin rashes; increased serum cholesterol and triglyceride levels C/I: Whenever aspirin can be used; acute thrombotic events
Dipyridamole	Sometimes for mechanical valves (with warfarin)	75–100 mg 4×/day	S/E: GI; headaches; hypotension; coronary steal C/I: Whenever aspirin can be used
Sulfinpyrazone	Prophylaxis of gout Hyperuricemia (no evidence of added antiplatelet effect with aspirin)	200–800 mg in 2 doses with meals, gradually increasing Reduce when blood urate controlled	S/E: GI including ulcer activation and bleeding C/I: Peptic ulcer, renal failure, renal stones, AMI (renal risk)

Abbreviations: AMI, acute myocardial infarction; GI, gastrointestinal; GU, genitourinary; TIA, transient ischemic attacks.

Infarct Survival (ISIS-2), the dose can be decreased to 160 mg daily.[121]

Side Effects, Contraindications, and Drug Interactions

Side Effects. Gastrointestinal side effects (dyspepsia, nausea, vomiting) may be dose limiting in about 10%–20% of patients. The most important measure in reducing side effects is to reduce the daily dose. The second most important step is to use buffered or enteric-coated aspirin (avoiding preparations containing high sodium contents) or to take aspirin with food (e.g., in the middle of the evening meal). Nonetheless, gastrointestinal bleeding may still occur, and frank melena can be expected in about 1% of patients per year and hematemesis in about 0.1%. When the aspirin dose is very low (30 mg daily), there is a substantial reduction in the frequency of such serious bleeding, but subjective gastrointestinal side effects are virtually unchanged.[119] Gout, although uncommon, may be precipitated because aspirin impairs urate secretion. The possibility that hemorrhagic stroke may be a side effect in those taking aspirin at standard doses for primary prevention[108] has led several authorities including the FDA to warn against self-administration of aspirin for this purpose.

Contraindications. These include aspirin intolerance, hemophilia, history of gastrointestinal bleeds or of active peptic ulcer, or other potential sources of gastrointestinal or genitourinary bleeding. Untreated hypertension (risk of cerebral bleed) and active retinal bleeding are also contraindications.

Relative Contraindications. These include dyspepsia, iron deficiency anemia (risk of added gastrointestinal bleed), gout, and the perioperative period unless the dose is very low. In patients with hypertensive or diabetic retinopathy without active bleeding, aspirin prophylaxis is often thought to confer more benefit than harm, provided that the blood pressure is controlled.

Drug Interactions. Drug interactions are shown in Table 2–10.

Pharmacologic Properties of Other Antiplatelet Agents

Ticlopidine

This agent acts at a site different from that of aspirin, and its advantages in clinical trials must be balanced against the greater risk of potentially serious side effects.

Mechanism of Action. Ticlopidine (Ticlid) inhibits the transformation of the glycoprotein IIb/IIIa receptor into its high-affinity ligand-binding state. Therefore, it inhibits platelet aggregation. This effect is irreversible and lasts for the duration of the life of the platelet.

Pharmacokinetics. Ticlopidine has nonlinear kinetics, and the clearance from plasma decreases after repeated dosing. ADP-induced platelet aggregation is reduced after 4 days, with a maximal effect after 8–11 days of dosage (manufacturer's data).

Indications. Ticlopidine is indicated to reduce the risk of thrombotic stroke (fatal or nonfatal) in patients who have experienced stroke precursors and in patients who have had a completed thrombotic stroke. In patients with unstable angina, an Italian trial showed a striking fall in total coronary events,[122] and this drug may be considered if aspirin is thought to be inadequate or ineffective. Because of the time delay to the onset of action, ticlopidine is not suited for use at the onset of acute myocardial infarction and cannot replace aspirin in the acute phase. Because ticlopidine is associated with a risk of neutropenia/agranulocytosis, which may be life-threatening, it should be reserved for patients who are intolerant of aspirin therapy but need an antiplatelet agent to prevent stroke[123] or threat of acute myocardial infarction.

Dose. A standard dose is 250 mg twice daily taken with food (to lessen gastric intolerance).

TABLE 2–10. DRUG INTERACTIONS OF ANTIPLATELET DRUGS

Drug	Interacting Drug	Mechanism	Consequence	Prophylaxis
Aspirin (A)	Hepatic P-450 enzyme inducers (barbiturates, phenytoin, rifampin)	Increased A metabolism	Decreased A effect	Adjust A dose Check A side effects
	Sulfinpyrazone (S), probenecid (P)	A decreases urate excretion	Decreased uricosuric effect of S or P	Increase dose of S or P or avoid combination
	Thiazide diuretics	A decreases urate excretion	Hyperuricemia, risk of gout	Check blood urate
	Warfarin (W)	A is antithrombotic	Excess bleeding	Check INR; low doses[120]
	ACE inhibitors	? less vasodilatory PGs	CHF worse	Reduce aspirin dose
Ticlopidine (T)	Aspirin	T potentiates A effect on platelet aggregation	Excess bleeding	Avoid combination
	Cimetidine	T clearance reduced by 50%	Excess bleeding	Reduce T dose
	Hepatic enzyme inducers (barbiturates, phenytoin, rifampin)	Increased T metabolism	Decreased T effect	Avoid combination
Dipyridamole	Adenosine	Decreases adenosine removal	Excess hypotension during treatment of SVT	Reduce adenosine dose to about 1/9
Sulfinpyrazone (S)	Warfarin (aspirin, see above)	S displaces W from plasma proteins	Excess bleeding	Check INR

Abbreviations: ACE, angiotensin converting enzyme; CHF, congestive heart failure; INR, International Normalized Ratio (see text); PGs, prostaglandins; SVT, supraventricular tachycardia.

Side Effects. The major problem with ticlopidine is neutropenia (2.4%), the subject of a boxed warning in the package insert. Neutropenia occurs within the first 3 months of treatment. There may also be minor bleeding (up to 10%), skin rash (up to 15%), toxic liver effects (4%), and diarrhea (ticlopidine 22%, placebo 0%)—which, however, are all reversible.[124] Serum cholesterol concentration increases by about 8%–10%, and serum triglyceride levels rise (package insert).

Precautions. It is, therefore, essential that a complete blood count and white cell differential count be performed every 2 weeks until the end of the third month (manufacturer's information), when the danger of neutropenia passes. Ticlopidine should be discontinued 10–14 days before elective surgery.

Drug Interactions. These may be with aspirin, cimetidine, and phenytoin (see Table 2–10).

Comment. Ticlopidine is a promising drug, but on meta-analysis its benefits cannot be distinguished from those of aspirin.[108] In view of its potentially serious side effects, it cannot be recommended above aspirin unless aspirin fails[125] or is contraindicated.

Clopidogrel

This ticlopidine analogue has a number of similarities to ticlopidine yet has a rapid onset of action and can be given intravenously. It also prevents the transformation of the glycoprotein IIb/IIIa receptor into its high-affinity state. In addition, it appears to promote formation of platelet cAMP and therefore lowers platelet calcium.[109] Clinical trials are still under way in, for example, acute unstable angina, in which ticlopidine is not suitable because of its delayed onset of action.

Dipyridamole

Dipyridamole (Persantine) is now used less frequently.

Mechanism of Action. In comparison with aspirin, dipyridamole has far more inhibitory effect on platelet adhesion to the vessel wall and much less on platelet aggregation. Dipyridamole has two other effects. First, there are the well-known coronary vasodilator effects mediated by inhibition of adenosine transport, which is the basis of the dipyridamole-thallium stress test. Second, at high and supraclinical doses, dipyridamole enhances platelet cAMP formation by inhibiting the phosphodiesterase breaking down cAMP and thereby inhibits platelet aggregation in vitro but not in vivo at standard doses.[109] Thus, whether it has any clinically relevant platelet antiaggregatory effect is doubtful.[109]

Indications. In general, dipyridamole has been tested for the same indications as aspirin. In 10 trials on vascular events using dipyridamole alone, an insignificant reduction of 23% was found, whereas in 34 trials, aspirin and dipyridamole combined gave a highly significant reduction of 28%, but no different from the 28% fall in vascular events achieved by aspirin alone at a dose of 160–320 mg/day.[108] Thus, there is no convincing evidence that dipyridamole is additive to the benefits obtained by aspirin alone. Furthermore, after coronary bypass surgery, dipyridamole added to low-dose aspirin adversely increased the clinical event rate.[126] *At present, the only specific indication for dipyridamole is aspirin intolerance.* In patients with prosthetic mechanical valves, dipyridamole may be added to aspirin and warfarin if thromboembolism persists.

Dose. Most trials have used 75 mg three times daily. The manufacturers recommend 75–100 mg four times daily.

Side Effects. Gastrointestinal irritation is common. Vasodilatory and hypotensive effects include intractable headache, dizziness, flushing, syncope, and occasional angina pectoris (coronary steal).

Relative Contraindications. Whenever clinical judgment indicates that aspirin can be used, dipyridamole should not be preferred.

Drug Interactions (see Table 2–10). Because dipyridamole leads to accumulation of adenosine, the potential hypotensive effects of *adenosine* given intravenously for supraventricular tachycardia may become serious, and the dose of adenosine must be reduced to about 1/9 of normal.[127]

Sulfinpyrazone

Sulfinpyrazone (Anturane) appears to have clinical activity comparable to that of aspirin, yet without any proof of superiority.[108] There is no evidence that sulfinpyrazone added to aspirin achieves any greater clinical benefit.

Mechanism of Action. Sulfinpyrazone also inhibits cyclooxygenase, decreasing the production of TXA_2 and prostacyclin. The mechanism of action on the cyclooxygenase is different from that of aspirin in that sulfinpyrazone competitively and reversibly *inhibits* the enzyme, whereas aspirin *inactivates* it, so that sulfinpyrazone is much weaker. In addition, it is an effective uricosuric agent.

Indications. In the United States, the only licensed indication is gouty arthritis, chronic or intermittent. By inference, it may be used for hyperuricemia. In mitral stenosis, however, a prospective blinded study for a 4-year period showed that sulfinpyrazone (200 mg four times daily) decreased thromboembolism and reverted the shortened platelet survival time toward normal.[128]

Drug Interactions. Drug interactions are shown in Table 2–10.

New Antiplatelet Agents

Monoclonal Antibody c7E3 Against Platelet IIb/IIIa Integrin Receptor

A final common path in platelet aggregation is the interaction of fibrinogen and the von Willebrand factor with the exposed IIb/IIIa receptors. Such binding plays a crucial role in thrombus formation. A monoclonal antibody to this receptor, called 7E3, has been developed. Experimentally, 7E3 is highly effective in preventing thrombosis in stenosed coronary arteries and gives better protection than other antiplatelet agents do in a model of coronary cyclic flow reduction.[109] For clinical testing, a chimeric version has been evolved (c7E3), and this appears to be less immunogenic but as effective. In clinical trials, this antibody, which can be given only intravenously, helps inhibit restenosis after revascularization.[129] In unstable angina, a bolus dose of c7E3 followed by an infusion was strikingly effective, with a reduction in myocardial infarction and late death.[130] The FDA has now approved c7E3 Fab for use in angioplasty in patients thought to be at high risk for ischemic complications.

S-Nitrosoglutathione

This compound is an *S*-nitrosothiol from which NO• is released by platelet-bound membranes to stimulate platelet guanylate cyclase with formation of cGMP. cGMP decreases platelet calcium to prevent activation and aggregation after coronary angioplasty.[131] Clinical trials in the prevention of restenosis are now under way.

ANTITHROMBOTIC AGENTS (ANTICOAGULANTS)

As already outlined in the previous section, platelets play a pivotal role in thrombus formation by undergoing activation and aggregation and by simultaneously promoting the conversion of prothrombin to thrombin. The latter step is crucial for thrombosis, and antithrombotic agents either inhibit the activity of thrombin (heparin and heparinoids) or decrease the formation of prothrombin (warfarin). Antiplatelet agents are indirect thrombolytics.

Physiologic Functions of Thrombin

Role in Thrombogenesis

Thrombin is a protease (glycosylated, trypsin-like) that splits fibrinogen to fibrin.[132] Generation of thrombin from prothrombin requires prothrombinase activity, which in turn depends on factor Xa (Fig. 2–12). Furthermore, it activates factor XIII to produce XIIIa, which (1) causes the fibrin to cross-link and (2) activates factors V and VIII, which in turn promote more formation of Xa and thereby enhance prothrombin generation. Thus, the process is self-perpetuating (Fig. 2–13).

Role in Platelet Aggregation. Thrombin furthermore acts as an agonist to the platelet thrombin receptor, thereby activating phospholipase C by a G protein and hence ultimately elevating platelet calcium concentration and promoting platelet activation and aggregation.[132] During the latter processes, thromboplastin is generated and the extrinsic path stimulated so that more prothrombin is formed (see Fig. 2–13).

Counterregulation. By binding to thrombomodulin, thrombin stimulates protein C, which together with protein S promotes inactivation of factors Va and VIIIa (see Fig. 2–12). Thus, formation of factor Xa is lessened, and there is a self-regulating antithrombotic mechanism.

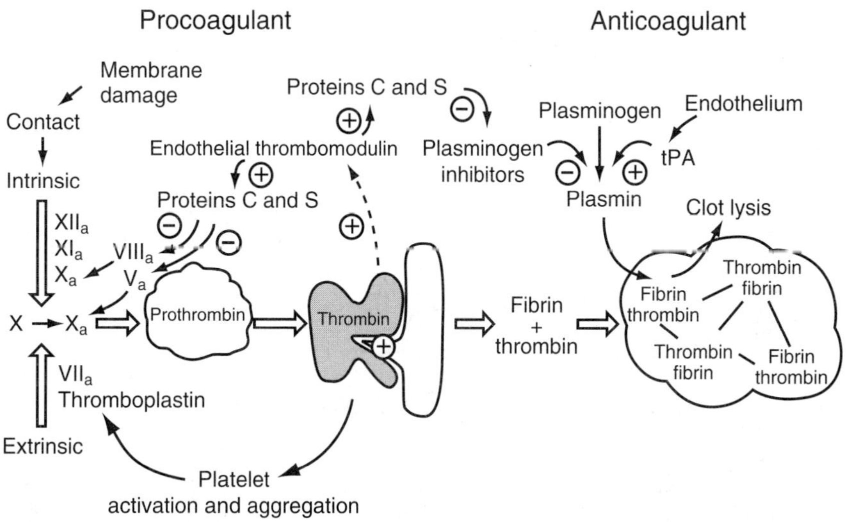

Figure 2–12. There is a balance physiologically between the procoagulant and fibrinolytic tendencies, so that major clot formation does not occur. *Abbreviation:* tPA, tissue plasminogen activator. (Reprinted with permission. Copyright 1996, L.H. Opie.)

Endothelial Interaction. Thrombin is one of several substances (including acetylcholine) that in the presence of endothelial damage change their normal vasodilatory effect to that of vasoconstriction. The vasoconstriction is thought to occur by release of endothelin. Furthermore, thrombin can stimulate growth of endothelium and vascular smooth muscle cells, perhaps in part through release of PDGF from platelets. Further actions may include promotion of leukocyte adhesion to the endothelium and release of interleukin-1 from monocytes.[133]

Thrombin Structure. The molecular structure of thrombin is complex and has at least five binding sites (Fig. 2–14): (1) the catalytic site, a "deep narrow canyon"[133]; (2) a substrate recognition site, to which fibrinogen binds to increase the specificity of thrombin for fibrinogen and hence to promote catalytic activity; (3) a fibrin binding site, so that as fibrinogen is converted to fibrin, the thrombin molecules become bound together; (4) the heparin binding site to which heparin binds by 13 of its saccharide structural units to prevent the further binding of fibrinogen to its site on thrombin; and (5) the platelet binding sites, for glycoprotein Ib and for a specific thrombin platelet receptor.

Other Events in Thrombus Formation. Thrombin is thus involved in the last of the three crucial steps in thrombus formation, which are (1) exposure of the circulating blood to a thrombogenic surface, such as a damaged vascular endothelium resulting from a ruptured atherosclerotic plaque; (2) a sequence of platelet-related events involving platelet adhesion, platelet activation, and platelet aggregation, with release of agents further promoting aggregation and causing vasoconstriction; and (3) triggering of the clotting mechanism with an important role for thrombin in the formation of fibrin, the latter cross-linking to form the backbone of the thrombus. Thrombin is in itself a powerful stimulator of platelet adhesion and aggregation. Once formed, the thrombus may be broken down by plasmin-stimulated fibrinolysis. Current antithrombotic medications include those inhibiting platelets (antiplatelet agents, see previous section) and those preventing coagulation (antithrombotics or anticoagulants).

Heparin

Mechanism of Action of Heparin

Heparin is a heterogeneous mucopolysaccharide (glycosaminoglycan) with extremely complex effects on the coagulation mechanism

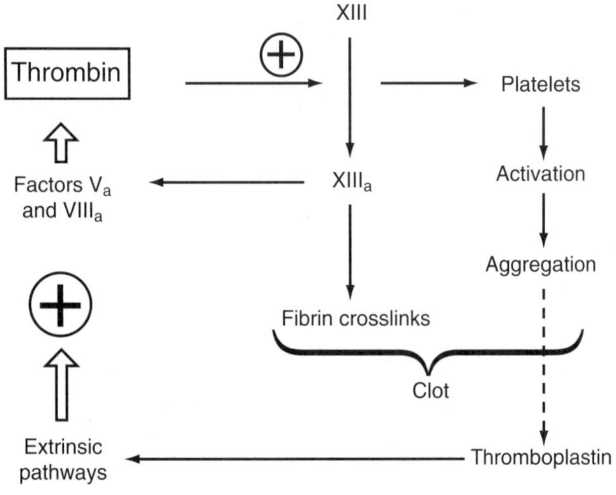

Figure 2–13. Thrombin has at least two self-promoting mechanisms whereby its rate of formation can be accelerated. (Reprinted with permission. Copyright 1996, L.H. Opie.)

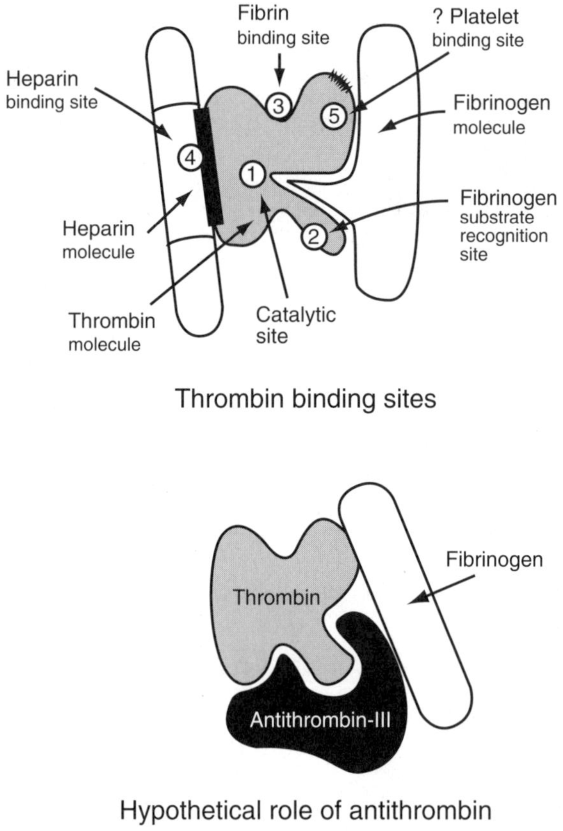

Figure 2–14. Five proposed binding sites or receptors on thrombin. Hypothetically, antithrombin prevents fibrinogen from reacting to its catalytic and substrate recognition sites. (Reprinted with permission. Copyright 1996, L.H. Opie.)

and on blood vessels. Heparin also exerts direct antiplatelet (antiaggregatory) effects by binding to and inhibiting the von Willebrand factor. Heparin, therefore, inhibits the thrombin-induced platelet aggregation that initiates unstable angina and venous thrombosis. Furthermore, long-term heparin administration has ill-understood effects in lessening experimental atheroma and in promoting angiogenesis.[134] The major effect of heparin is interaction with antithrombin III and thrombin. Inhibition of thrombin by heparin requires (1) binding of heparin to antithrombin III and (2) simultaneous binding of heparin to thrombin.[135] The complex of heparin with antithrombin III also inhibits factor Xa and a number of other clotting factors.

Dose-Effect Relationship. This is difficult to predict because heparin is a heterogeneous group of molecules extracted by a variety of procedures and having variable potency from batch to batch. Heparin also variably binds to plasma proteins, endothelial cells, and macrophages. The binding to these cells inactivates some of the heparin; the rest leaves the circulation by the renal route. These complexities, added to the difficulty of controlling the dose, mean that heparin is far from ideal as an intravenous anticoagulant and explain why fixed-dose regimens are not optimal for serious disease.

Clinical Use of Heparin

Doses. Doses of heparin are shown in Table 2–11.

Control of the Dose of Intravenous Heparin. When heparin is given in acute myocardial infarction or unstable angina, meticulous laboratory control of the heparin dose is required (activated partial thromboplastin time [aPTT] of 1.5–2.5 times normal, up to 60–85

TABLE 2–11. ANTITHROMBOTIC AGENTS: INDICATIONS, DOSE, SIDE EFFECTS, AND CONTRAINDICATIONS

Drug	Indications	Dose	Side Effects (S/E) and Contraindications (C/I)
Heparin	AMI, with t-PA Proximal DVT	5000 U bolus; then 1000 U/h for 48 h (dose-adjusted to aPTT 1.5–2.5× normal) May also be given intravenously every 4–6 h	S/E: Bleeding, thrombocytopenia, thrombosis, allergy, osteoporosis after prolonged use C/I: Bleeding state or source, care in uncontrolled hypertension, hypersensitivity to heparin *Caution:* Platelet counts required if heparin is given for more than 5 days
	DVT treatment (nonproximal)	SC 10,000–15,000 U/12 h for 3–5 days until warfarin effective	S/E: As for heparin C/I: As for heparin
	Prevention of DVT, postoperative or during acute myocardial infarction	Ultralow dose IV 1 U/kg/h for 3–5 days *or* SC 5000 U 2–8 h preoperatively and then every 12 h for 7 days	S/E: As for heparin C/I: As for heparin but safer than high dose if bleeding source
	AMI with SK	IV or SC optional Dose not established	S/E: As for heparin
	AMI without lytics	300 U/kg bolus (with aspirin),* then infused to aPTT 2.0–2.5× normal	S/E: As for heparin
Low-molecular-weight heparin (under study)	When heparin is contraindicated Note there may be cross-reactivity in case of thrombocytopenia	SC: 200 U/kg/day or 15,000–20,000 U/day or 75 U/kg/day for prophylaxis Start about 25 h preoperatively and then continue for 14 days thereafter	S/E: As for heparin, may cause less thrombocytopenia (cross-reactivity a possibility)
Heparinoids (under study)	Heparin-induced thrombocytopenia (caution) Prevention of DVT	Danaparoid sodium: for DVT prevention, 750 U 1–4 h preoperatively, then 2× daily for 7–10 days	S/E and C/I: As for heparin but cause less thrombocytopenia (cross-reactivity a possibility)
Hirudin (under study)	Unstable angina and other acute ischemic syndromes (under test) Coronary angioplasty (under study)	0.1 mg/kg bolus followed by 0.1 mg/kg/h	S/E: IC hemorrhage when combined with thrombolytics

Abbreviations: AMI, acute myocardial infarction; aPTT, activated partial thromboplastin time; DVT, deep venous thrombosis; IC, intracranial; IV, intravenous; SC, subcutaneous; SK, streptokinase; t-PA, tissue plasminogen activator.

*See Verheugt FWA, Marsh RC, Veen G, et al: High-dose bolus heparin alone as primary reperfusion therapy for acute transmural myocardial infarction: preliminary results of the ongoing angiographic HEAP pilot study [Abstract]. Circulation 1994; 90(I, pt 2):563.

sec with monitoring at 6, 12, and 24 h).[136] Although this test is not ideal,[133] it is the best currently available. If the aPTT rises above 85 sec, the risk of hemorrhage is too high.[137] Patients with optimal heparinization and an aPTT of twice normal have greater coronary artery patency than others do.[138] A new bedside device gives the aPTT within 3 min,[139] which with the use of a nomogram[140] should facilitate management (Table 2–12). An inherent limitation to the aPTT is that different commercial reagents give different aPTT values,[135] especially the portable device, which gives readings about 10 sec longer than those of standard laboratories.[133]

TABLE 2–12. SUGGESTED HEPARIN NOMOGRAM

If Activated Partial Thromboplastin Time (aPTT) Is	Make This Adjustment
3× control value	Decrease infusion by 50%
2–3× control value	Decrease infusion by 25%
1.5–2× control value	No change
<1.5× control value	Increase infusion by 25% (maximal rate, 2500 U/h)

From Flaker GC, Bartolozzi J, Davis V, et al, for the TIMI-4 Investigators: Use of a standardized heparin nomogram to achieve therapeutic anticoagulation after thrombolytic therapy in myocardial infarction. Arch Intern Med 1994; 154:1492–1496.

Indications. Early-phase acute myocardial infarction, unstable angina, thromboembolism, left ventricular thrombus,[141] and temporary anticoagulation during percutaneous transluminal coronary angioplasty[142] are indications for the use of heparin. Logically, because heparin and aspirin have different and additive antithrombotic mechanisms, the combination should be better than either alone in unstable angina. This simple supposition has been difficult to prove and more trials are needed.[117]

Pregnancy Anticoagulation. Heparin is the anticoagulant of choice in pregnancy. Yet, if it is given in doses greater than 20,000 U daily for more than 5 months, it can cause osteoporosis.[135]

Precautions and Side Effects. An increased danger of heparin-induced hemorrhage exists in patients with subacute bacterial endocarditis, hematologic disorders including hemophilia, hepatic disease, and gastrointestinal or genitourinary ulcerative lesions. There is only a narrow therapeutic window for heparin plus thrombolytic therapy,[137, 143] so that the recommended doses of heparin should not be exceeded to avoid intracerebral hemorrhage. Platelet plugs are the main hemostatic defense of heparinized patients; the coadministration of aspirin, sulfinpyrazone, dipyridamole, or indomethacin may predispose to bleeding.

Heparin-induced thrombocytopenia occurs in about 10% of patients after heparin use for 5 days or more, is usually asymptomatic, and is reversible on heparin withdrawal. If continued intravenous anticoagulation is essential, a heparinoid (danaparoid sodium,

Orgaran) may be used (dose: 750 U subcutaneously twice daily up to 14 days).

Platelet abnormalities may also, paradoxically, and by a poorly understood mechanism, predispose to heparin thrombosis characterized by a "white clot."[144] Heparin hemorrhage may occur in clinically inapparent sites such as the adrenal glands, which is potentially life-threatening and demands immediate cortisol replacement. Some patients have heparin resistance, and high-dose heparin with aPTT monitoring every 4 h is advised. Heparin is derived from animal tissue and occasionally causes allergy; a trial dose of 100–1000 U is required in allergic patients.

Contraindications. The following are contraindications to the use of heparin: clinically overt bleeding; known potential source of bleeding; excess thrombolytic treatment; during thrombolytic therapy of early acute myocardial infarction when aPTT cannot be measured; thrombocytopenia; and uncontrolled hypertension (care required).

Heparin Overdose. This is treated by stopping the drug and, if clinically required, giving protamine sulfate (1% solution) as a very slow infusion at no more than 50 mg in any 10-min period. Each 1 mg of protamine sulfate neutralizes about 90 U lung-derived heparin or 100 U intestine-derived heparin.

Low-Molecular-Weight Heparins and Heparinoids

Low-molecular-weight heparins constitute about one third of the molecular weight of heparin and are less heterogeneous in size. Approximately 25%–30% of the molecules of various preparations contain the crucial 18 or more saccharide units to bind to both antithrombin III and thrombin. The remaining molecules of low-molecular-weight heparin bind only to factor Xa. Low-molecular-weight heparins, still under evaluation, have better bioavailability and a longer plasma half-life than standard heparin. They are usually given subcutaneously in a fixed dose once daily[145] because they are cleared more slowly, having lower affinity than heparin for endothelial cells and for plasma proteins. They are at least as effective as and possibly better than standard aPTT-monitored unfractionated heparin when given intravenously for prophylaxis and treatment of deep venous thrombosis.[145, 146] At present, they are the agents of choice when heparin is contraindicated by nonavailability of aPTT measurements, but the disadvantage is expense.[147] Yet, time of skilled personnel is saved by having to avoid aPTT tests, dose adjustments, and an intravenous infusion. In the future, the convenience and simplicity of administration will probably make these more popular agents, especially if the price decreases.

Heparinoids are similar in properties to low-molecular-weight heparin but consist chiefly (80%) of heparan sulfate (for danaparoid sodium, see earlier).

Direct Specific Thrombin Inhibitors

Hirudin

The prototype of these agents is hirudin, which is a 65–amino acid peptide derived from the leech salivary gland but also synthesized as recombinant hirudin (r-hirudin). Hirudin blocks both the catalytic and substrate recognition sites of thrombin (sites 1 and 2, see Fig. 2–14). It binds directly with high affinity to thrombin[145] and can inactivate thrombin already bound to fibrin (clot-bound thrombin), which unfractionated heparin cannot do as effectively.[148] Hirudin does not require endogenous cofactors such as antithrombin III for its activity. Also, unlike heparin, hirudin can inhibit thrombin-induced platelet aggregation.[149] Hirudin will be compared with heparin in early unstable angina in 8000 patients in the Canadian Organization to Assess Strategies for Ischemic Syndromes (OASIS) trial. The role of hirudin in coronary angioplasty has been evaluated in a large European trial known as HELVETICA. Intracranial or other hemorrhage has been a serious side effect with the higher doses used in three trials of thrombolytic therapy for acute myocardial infarction,[137, 143, 150] necessitating a reduction in dose (see Chapter 7).

Other Thrombin Inhibitors

New molecular techniques have led to other agents that inhibit activated factor X (i.e., factor Xa). Two examples are antistasin, derived from the Mexican leech, and a tick anticoagulant peptide derived from the soft tick. Another approach is to activate protein C, thereby promoting a powerful antithrombotic activity that destroys factors Va and VIIIa; the possibility of infusing activated protein C as an adjuvant to thrombolysis is now being explored.

Hirugen is a synthetic hirudin derivative but binds to site 2 and not site 1; it is also weaker than hirudin and therefore not under clinical tests. Hirulog, like hirudin, binds to sites 1 and 2 (see Fig. 2–14). Argatroban inactivates the catalytic site (site 1, see Fig. 2–14) by binding to an adjacent site. The agent is promising and the subject of early clinical trials.[151]

Oral Anticoagulation by Warfarin

Warfarin (coumarin, Coumadin, Panwarfin) is the most commonly used oral anticoagulant. A single dose causes a stable anticoagulation as a result of the excellent oral absorption and a long circulating half-life. Apart from bleeding, warfarin also has remarkably few side effects. The major defect is its susceptibility to many drug interactions.[152]

Mechanism of Action. Warfarin and other coumarins inhibit the formation of reduced vitamin K in hepatic microsomes (Fig. 2–15). The result is decreased hepatic carboxylation of glutamyl residues in the molecules of the vitamin K–dependent clotting factors including prothrombin and factors VII, IX, and X. The incompletely carboxylated molecules are deprived of calcium-binding activity.

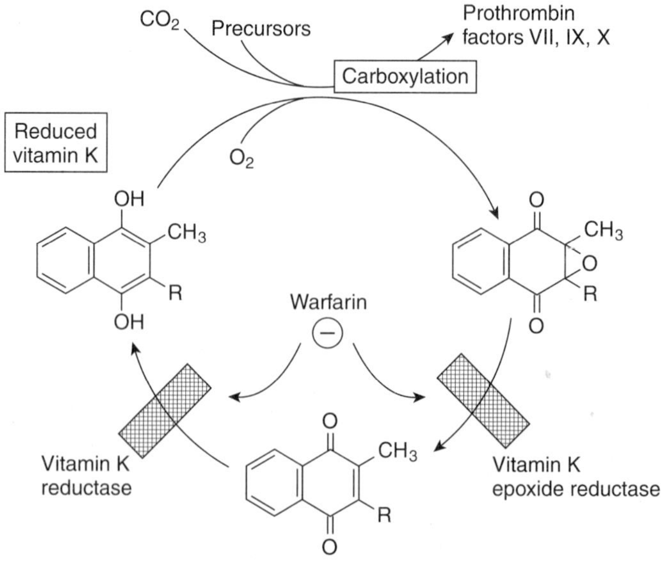

Figure 2–15. Schematic for site of action of warfarin. By inhibiting formation of reduced vitamin K in the liver, it lessens the rate of carboxylation of the glutamyl residues of the precursors (proenzymes) of prothrombin and factors VII, IX, and X. (Modified from Furie B, Furie BC: Molecular basis of vitamin K–dependent gamma-carboxylation. Blood 1990; 75:1753–1762.)

Pharmacokinetics. Oral warfarin is rapidly and completely absorbed. In the circulation, it is almost totally bound to plasma albumin. The half-life is 37 h. It is metabolized by hepatic microsomes to inactive metabolites excreted in urine and stool. There is a delay in onset of clinical action of 2–7 days.[153]

Dose (Table 2–13). A standard procedure is to give warfarin 5 mg/day for 5 days or 10 mg/day for 3 days, checking the International Normalized Ratio (INR) daily until the therapeutic range is reached, thereafter three times weekly for up to 2 weeks, and then weekly until stabilized. Large initial doses may provoke an excess fall of prothrombin with increased risk of skin necrosis in those predisposed (see side effects). The maintenance dose cannot be predicted; it may be 4–9 mg daily or may vary from 1–20 mg and must be individualized according to the INR (next section).

International Normalized Ratio Versus Prothrombin Time. The INR is the prothrombin time ratio (PTR) that would be obtained if the international reference thromboplastin, as approved by the World Health Organization, were used. This thromboplastin, by definition, has an International Sensitivity Index (ISI) of 1. With other ISI values, the formula becomes

$$\text{INR} = \text{PTR}^{\text{ISI}}$$

where the PTR is raised to the power of the ISI of the thromboplastin actually used. Although the INR is far more reliable than the PTR,[154] it is still not universally used, and some laboratories persist in giving the prothrombin time. Yet standardization of thromboplastin is also required for an accurate interpretation of the prothrombin time (see Table 4 of reference 153). Such laboratory inaccuracies can impair the clinical efficacy of warfarin.[154]

Therapeutic Range for INR Values. Currently, two levels of intensity of warfarin therapy are usually recommended: a medium dose with an INR of 2.0–3.0, and a higher dose with an INR of 2.5–3.5.[153] Prosthetic heart valves require the highest safe INR values within the latter range, that is, about 3.0 (corresponding roughly to a PTR of 1.5). Higher values greatly increase the risk of bleeding.[153] Less intense anticoagulation (medium dose) is appropriate with an INR of 2.0–3.0 for deep venous thrombosis with pulmonary embolism, for acute myocardial infarction in the early stages or with risk of thromboembolism, and for patients with thromboembolism thought to be at high risk for stroke. In patients with atrial fibrillation without valvular heart disease, the lower limits may be less, for example, an INR of only 1.5 and a PTR of about 1.2.[155] For such patients, a fixed low-dose combination of aspirin 80 mg and warfarin 3 mg is under test.[120] Once the steady-state warfarin requirement is known, the INR is checked only once every 4–6 weeks.

Concurrent Disease and Dose. Reduction of warfarin dose is required in the presence of decreased liver blood flow (congestive heart failure), liver damage (alcohol, malnutrition), or renal impairment (may decrease plasma protein binding). Thyrotoxicosis enhances (and myxedema decreases) the catabolism of vitamin K to decrease (or increase) the dose of warfarin needed. Increased dietary vitamin K (green salads) antagonizes warfarin. Fad diets with alternate high and low salad periods may correspondingly change the INR.

Elderly Patients. The response to warfarin is greater,[156] so that the dose is relatively lower. Age brings with it a greater risk of various conditions predisposing to bleeding.[157] When added to problems of compliance, increasing age is a relative contraindication to the use of warfarin.

Contraindications. The following are contraindications to the use of warfarin: recent stroke; recent surgery; uncontrolled hypertension; hepatic cirrhosis; and potential gastrointestinal and genitourinary bleeding points, such as hiatal hernia, peptic ulcer, gastritis, colitis, proctitis, and cystitis. (For cardiac surgery, see section on side effects.) If anticoagulation is deemed essential, the risk/benefit ratio must be evaluated carefully.

Pregnancy: category X (contraindicated, embryopathic, do not use unless judged absolutely essential for the mother's health; consider termination of pregnancy). Warfarin is contraindicated in the first trimester (teratogenic) and also in the last (risk of fetal bleeding). Consider long-term subcutaneous heparin for valve prophylaxis against thromboembolization in pregnant patients who require continuous anticoagulation.

Drug Interactions. These are many (more than 80), the most important of which are shown in Table 2–14.

TABLE 2–13. WARFARIN: INDICATIONS, DOSE, SIDE EFFECTS, AND CONTRAINDICATIONS

Drug	Indications	Dose	Side Effects (S/E) and Contraindications (C/I)
Warfarin	AMI to prevent thromboembolism	5 mg/day for 5 days or 10 mg/day for 3 days; monitor INR (2.0–3.0)[153]	S/E: Bleeding, skin necrosis, prothrombotic after cardiac surgery, numerous drug interactions (e.g., amiodarone, aspirin, sulfinpyrazone)
	Early post-AMI in large anterior infarct	As above*	C/I: Uncooperative patient, recent stroke, uncontrolled hypertension, gastrointestinal or genitourinary bleeding, hemophilia, pregnancy first and third trimesters
	Pulmonary embolism and venous thromboembolism	As above	*Caution:* Elderly patients, concurrent aspirin, drug interactions; delayed onset of action (2–7 days)
	Atrial fibrillation with valve disease	As above but INR 1.5 or more	
	Atrial fibrillation, lone		
	Age younger than 65 years	No warfarin	
	Age older than 65 years or other risk factors†	INR 1.5 or more	
	Mechanical prosthetic valves	INR 2.5–3.5 with aspirin 100 mg daily[159] or with ticlopidine 100–200 mg 2× daily[158]	
	Bioprosthetic valves	INR 2.0–3.0 for 3 months	

Abbreviations: AMI, acute myocardial infarction; INR, International Normalized Ratio (see text).
*Under test in CARS study: fixed-dose warfarin 3 mg plus aspirin 80 mgdaily.[120]
†For risk factors in atrial fibrillation, see text.

TABLE 2–14. CARDIAC AND OTHER DRUG INTERACTIONS WITH WARFARIN

Cardiac Drug	Interacting Drug	Mechanism	Consequence	Prophylaxis
Warfarin (W)	**Potentiating Drugs**			
	Allopurinol	Mechanism unknown	Excess bleeding	Check INR
	Amiodarone	Mechanism unknown, may decrease metabolism	Sensitizes to W for 1–2 months	Avoid combination
	Anti-infectives (erythromycin, chloramphenicol, metronidazole, trimethoprim and sulfamethoxazole)	Decrease metabolism	Sensitizes to W	Check INR
	Aspirin	Added bleeding tendency	Excess bleeding	Check INR; low doses[120]
	Cimetidine	Decreased W degradation	Increased blood W	Check INR
	Quinidine	Hepatic interaction	Excess bleeding	Check INR
	Sulfinpyrazone	Displaces W from plasma proteins	Excess bleeding	Check INR
	Inhibitory Drugs			
	Cholestyramine	Less W absorption	Decreased W effect	Check INR
	Colestipol	Less W absorption	Decreased W effect	Check INR

Abbreviation: INR, International Normalized Ratio (see text).

Side Effects. Besides bleeding, warfarin occasionally promotes thrombosis after cardiac surgery. The mechanism may be by inhibition of protein C, which is also the proposed explanation for skin necrosis. Cardiopulmonary bypass lowers protein C levels. Hence, after cardiac surgery, warfarin should be started in very low doses while heparin is being administered. Release of atheromatous plaques may be enhanced with risk of microembolization, including "purple toes syndrome."

Warfarin Overdose. The risk of bleeding is considerably decreased by targeting an INR of 2.0–3.0 rather than 3.0–4.5. This can generally be achieved by a small reduction in the warfarin dose by only 1 mg daily.[153] An excessively high INR without bleeding or with only minor bleeding requires dose reduction or discontinuation of warfarin, bearing in mind that its half-life is about 37 h. If bleeding is serious, oral or subcutaneous vitamin K_1 (phytonadione) 2–5 mg may be required. Vitamin K_1 does not act at once but takes several hours, so that an overdose should be avoided. In patients with prosthetic valves, vitamin K_1 is contraindicated, unless there is a life-threatening intracranial bleed, because of the risk of rebound valve thrombosis. When there is no response to vitamin K_1, appropriate therapy includes (1) transfusion of a concentrate of the prothrombin group of coagulation factors, including II, IX, and X; (2) fresh frozen plasma 15 mL/kg; and (3) transfusion of fresh, whole blood.

THROMBOLYTIC AGENTS

Natural Fibrinolytic Systems

There is normally a fine balance between prothrombotic and thrombolytic forces. When vascular damage occurs, the balance is swung toward thrombosis, as outlined in Figures 2–9 and 2–12. The thrombotic system is normally sufficiently active to counterbalance any attempts at thrombosis caused, for example, by minor vascular damage. Such physiologic fibrinolysis occurs by the activity of natural enzymes, the plasminogen activators that promote the fibrinolytic system. Thus, recombinant tissue plasminogen activator converts plasminogen into the active enzyme plasmin, which in turn digests the fibrin component of a thrombus.

Therapeutically, the five major current thrombolytic agents are recombinant tissue-type plasminogen activator (rt-PA, alteplase), streptokinase, anisoylated plasminogen streptokinase activator complex (APSAC, anistreplase), two-chain urokinase-type plasminogen activator (tcu-PA, urokinase), and recombinant single-chain urokinase-type plasminogen activator (rscu-PA, prourokinase, saruplase). Of these five, only the last is not approved by the FDA for use.[160] Streptokinase, APSAC, and two-chain urokinase extensively activate the fibrinolytic system, which degrades fibrinogen, factor V, and factor VIII. The physiologic plasminogen activators, rt-PA and rscu-PA, have a relative specificity for fibrin so that plasminogen is preferentially activated at the fibrin surface. Plasmin thus formed is associated with the fibrin surface and hence is protected from rapid inhibition by antiplasmin.

Recombinant Tissue-Type Plasminogen Activator

Tissue plasminogen activator (rt-PA, alteplase, Activase) binds to fibrin with a relatively greater affinity than does streptokinase. Fibrin-bound rt-PA converts plasminogen to plasmin on the fibrin surface. Although it is "clot selective," some systemic effects including delayed bleeding do occur when clinical doses are used (Fig. 2–16).

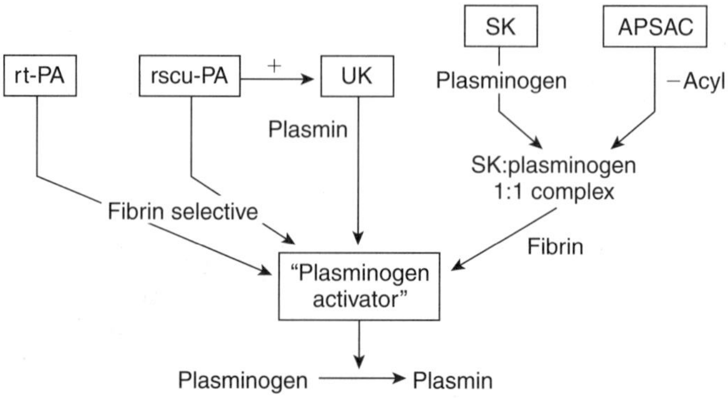

Figure 2–16. Therapeutic thrombolytics act by promoting the conversion of plasminogen to plasmin, the latter being fibrinolytic. "Plasminogen activator" refers to the effect of the complex between plasminogen and the agent given (e.g., rt-PA or streptokinase) in catalyzing the conversion of plasminogen to plasmin. For abbreviations of fibrinolytics, see Table 2–15. (Modified from Gersh BJ, Opie LH: Antithrombotic agents: platelet inhibitors, anticoagulants, and fibrinolytics. *In* Opie LH [ed]: Drugs for the Heart, 4th ed, pp 247–285. Philadelphia: WB Saunders, 1995.)

Indications. In acute myocardial infarction, rt-PA induces more rapid clot lysis at 90 min than does streptokinase or other major agents available (Table 2–15). Other indications are acute pulmonary embolism, thrombosed arteriovenous shunts, and thrombosed mechanical valves.[161] It should also be effective for arterial thromboembolism and deep venous thrombosis, but data are lacking. Unstable angina is clearly not an indication.[162, 163]

Dose. "Front-loading," as used in the Global Utilization of Streptokinase and Tissue Plasminogen Activator for Occluded Coronary Arteries (GUSTO) trial,[136] gives two thirds of the total standard dose of 100 mg in the first 30 min, starting with an initial bolus of 15 mg, then 50 mg in 30 min, followed by 35 mg in 1 h. Correcting for body weight, the doses used in the GUSTO trial[136] were 0.75 mg/kg for a 30-min period after the initial bolus, and then 0.5 mg/kg for 1 h. Splitting the standard dose of 100 mg into two bolus injections spaced by 30 min seems simpler and gives a patency rate at 90 min of 88%.[164] A higher total dose (150 mg) leads to no greater benefit and an increased risk of cerebral hemorrhage.[165] Heparin cotherapy is standard because (1) rt-PA does not cause marked systemic fibrinolytic states, as does streptokinase, and (2) rt-PA is short acting, and the prothrombin system is rapidly reactivated to increase the risk of rethrombosis. Chewable aspirin (160–320 mg) is started as soon as possible in patients with acute myocardial infarction treated by rt-PA.

Contraindications. Hemorrhage is the greatest risk. Concurrent heparin must be strictly controlled with an aPTT of no more than 85 sec.[137] Any recent hemorrhage or cerebrovascular accident, uncontrolled hypertension, advancing age with fear of intracranial hemorrhage, coagulation defects, and hemorrhagic retinopathy are all contraindications (see Chapter 7). Other contraindications are potential sources of microemboli (such as enlarged left atrium and ventricular or aortic aneurysms) and potential bleeding sites (recent surgery, peptic ulcer, or pregnancy). Menstruation is not a contraindication with only the disadvantage of increased vaginal bleeding. Gentamicin sensitivity is a specific exclusion, because gentamicin is used in the preparation of rt-PA. Previous streptokinase therapy within the past 12 months is an indication for rt-PA (because of the antigenicity of streptokinase).

Cost Effectiveness. To offset its therapeutic superiority, the major disadvantage of rt-PA remains the greatly increased cost compared with streptokinase; both the cost of the agent and the cost of repeated heparin dose monitoring by the aPTT (time of personnel, laboratory costs) must be taken into account. With streptokinase, dose-adjusted heparin is not essential.

Cotherapy With Heparin. rt-PA has a very short half-life caused by rapid hepatic metabolism. This necessitates adjunctive therapy with heparin as discussed in Chapters 7 and 29.

Streptokinase

Streptokinase itself has no direct effect on plasminogen. It binds with plasminogen to form a 1:1 complex, which becomes an active enzyme to convert another molecule of plasminogen to plasmin.[166] In addition, streptokinase may increase circulating levels of activated protein C, which enhances clot lysis.[167] Finally, streptokinase activates systemic lytic systems to degrade fibrinogen (blood levels fall) and also factors V and VIII.[168]

Indications. Streptokinase is indicated to achieve clot lysis in acute myocardial infarction, acute pulmonary embolism, acute deep venous thrombosis, and arterial thrombosis or embolism.

Dose. In several megatrials in acute myocardial infarction, the infusion rate has been 1.5 million U in 100 mL of physiologic saline in 1 h. A higher dose (3 million U) can achieve a higher patency rate at 2.8 h after the start[169] but is seldom used. For conditions other than acute myocardial infarction, streptokinase is infused as 250,000 U in 30 min, then 100,000 U every hour for about 72 h.

Contraindications. These are similar to those for rt-PA, excluding

TABLE 2–15. PHARMACOLOGIC PROPERTIES OF MAJOR THROMBOLYTIC AGENTS

	rt-PA	SK	APSAC	UK	rscu-PA
Fibrin-selective	Yes	No	No	No	Partially (also forms UK)
Plasminogen binding	Direct	Indirect	Indirect	Direct	Direct
Half-life (min)	6	20	70	4*	4
Fibrinogen breakdown†	1–2+	4+	4+	3+	2–3+
Duration of infusion (min)	180 or less	60 or less	2–5	5–15	60
Dose for acute myocardial infarction	15 mg bolus, then 50 mg/30 min, then 35 mg/30 min *or* 50 mg bolus repeated 30 min later	1.5 MU infused in 1 h or less	30 U as bolus or in 4–5 min	3 MU in 45–90 min	20 mg bolus, then 60 mg in 60 min *or* 12 mg bolus with 48 mg in 60 min[185]
Early heparin required	Yes	No	No	?No	?Yes
Hypotension	No	Yes	Yes	No	No
Allergic reactions	No	Yes	Yes	No	No
Approximate cost/dose	$2300/100 mg	$300/1.5 MU	$1200/30 mg	$2200/3 MU	High
Patency at 90 min	81[187]–88[164] (75)‡	53[188]–65[184] (53)‡	55[188]–65[189]	66[190]	71[184]–73[185]
Patency at 2–3 h	73[192]–76[187]	70[192]–73[187]	No data	No data	No data
Patency at 24 h	78[190]–86[187]	80[187]–88[184]	88[188]–92[189]	73[190]	85[184]

Abbreviations: APSAC, anisoylated plasminogen streptokinase activator complex (anistreplase); MU, million units; rscu-PA, single-chain urokinase (prourokinase) plasminogen activator; rt-PA, recombinant tissue plasminogen activator; SK, streptokinse; UK, urokinase.

*Apparent clearance.[176]

†Fibrinogen breakdown arbitrarily graded; 4+ = maximum, patency = grade 2 and 3 combined.

‡Mean value of 11 earlier trials for streptokinase and 13 for rt-PA.[191]

For other data sources, see Marder and Sherry.[193]

Modified from Gersh BJ, Opie LH: Antithrombotic agents: platelet inhibitors, anticoagulants, and fibrinolytics. *In* Opie LH (ed): Drugs for the Heart, 4th ed, pp 247–285. Philadelphia: WB Saunders, 1995.

gentamicin sensitivity. Additional contraindications are (1) recent streptococcal infections, because bacterial toxins induce resistance to streptokinase, and (2) previous treatment by streptokinase or anistreplase, because the induced antibodies diminish efficacy and increase the risk of allergic reactions.[170] Hypertension may be less of a contraindication to streptokinase than to rt-PA because of the lower risk of intracerebral bleeding with streptokinase, especially in thin elderly women.[171]

Side Effects and Complications. Allergic reactions include fever or rashes (in about 10%) and rarely (0.1%) anaphylactoid reactions. Minor bleeding requires local measures, not cessation of lytic therapy, because of the dangers of rebound or a persistent excess lytic state. Poststreptokinase bleeding diathesis is a risk especially with combined heparin therapy, arguing against the use of this combination. For control of major bleeding, see rt-PA.

Anistreplase

Anistreplase (APSAC, anisoylated plasminogen streptokinase activator complex, Eminase) is a stoichiometric combination of streptokinase and plasminogen, stabilized by the addition of an anisoyl group that is bound to the catalytic center of plasminogen. Once injected, anistreplase is deacylated at a controlled rate, so that it releases the streptokinase-plasminogen complex relatively slowly. The fibrinolytic activity has a half-life of 90–110 min, which coincides with the deacylation rate of 105–120 min. Thus, the drug can be given as a single intravenous dose, which is its major advantage. Prehospital use is more feasible than with rt-PA or streptokinase, although this advantage seems not to have been fully exploited. Such prehospital administration of anistreplase could lead to more patients being treated within the "golden" first 70 min.[172, 173]

Dose. In the European Myocardial Infarction Project (EMIP) study,[174] anistreplase was given as a single intravenous injection of 30 U in 4–5 min. Linderer and coworkers[175] preceded this injection with 100 mg methylprednisolone to avoid allergy.

Side Effects. Most common is hypotension, with some fall in blood pressure in about 60% of patients and a severe fall in 7%.[176] This effect is treated as an allergic reaction, and hydrocortisone and an antihistaminic are given. Hemorrhagic stroke may occur as with streptokinase.

Contraindications. These are similar to those for streptokinase, including the loss of efficacy after prior use of streptokinase or anistreplase.

Cotherapy With Heparin. Withholding heparin reduces bleeding complications without changing the outcome.[177]

Urokinase

This agent has indications, contraindications, and effects similar to those of streptokinase. However, it is prepared from human renal tissue, so allergic effects are minimal. Furthermore, because of its short half-life of only 3 min, it causes less sustained systemic fibrinolysis than does streptokinase. The specific indication is for intraocular clot lysis (chosen because of absence of allergic properties). When it is used for acute myocardial infarction, the dose is 3 million U in 45–60 min.[178] It is not licensed for this purpose in the United States but only for pulmonary embolism and intravenous catheter clearance.

Combinations of Therapy

In the GUSTO trial,[136] rt-PA 90 mg with 1 million U streptokinase, and with intravenous heparin, fared worse than rt-PA alone and was similar to streptokinase alone.

Beta Blockade. In view of the proven benefits of both early beta blockade and early thrombolysis in acute myocardial infarction, it is logical to consider this combination. In phase II of the Thrombolysis In Myocardial Infarction (TIMI-II) trial,[179] there were fewer reinfarctions and recurrent ischemic episodes in patients receiving intravenous metoprolol, although there were few long-term benefits.[165] Beta blockade, by reducing blood pressure, may reduce intracerebral bleeding. Thus, in acute myocardial infarction with hypertension, intravenous esmolol (although not formally tested) becomes an option for rapid control of blood pressure before thrombolytic therapy. Controlled studies are lacking, however. Furthermore, lytic therapy in the presence of hypertension, even when treated, is debatable.

Nitrates. An oral mononitrate was combined with streptokinase in the Fourth International Study of Infarct Survival (ISIS-4). Intravenous followed by transdermal nitroglycerin was used in the Third Italian Study of Streptokinase in Myocardial Infarction (GISSI-3). Neither nitrate gave any added benefit beyond that achieved by the fibrinolytic. In hypertensives with acute myocardial infarction, intravenous nitroglycerin is one of several options to control blood pressure.

ACE Inhibitors. The benefit achieved by early oral captopril added to streptokinase in ISIS-4 was slight. In GISSI-3, early lisinopril reduced mortality by 11%. In the Survival of Myocardial Infarction Long-Term Evaluation (SMILE) study,[180] an ACE inhibitor given within 24 h of onset to patients with anterior acute myocardial infarction who did not receive thrombolysis improved mortality, so that the use of an ACE inhibitor could be encouraged when thrombolysis is either contraindicated or not achieved. Judging by the Acute Infarction Ramipril Efficacy (AIRE) study,[181] in which the ACE inhibitor was added 3–10 days after the onset of acute myocardial infarction, it is likely that ACE inhibition would be particularly effective in a subgroup of patients with left ventricular failure or threatened left ventricular failure.

ACE Inhibitors With Intravenous Nitrates. This combination reduced mortality by 17% in streptokinase-treated patients in GISSI-3 without causing further hypotension. There is a possible double benefit: first, left ventricular enlargement could have been lessened by combined preload and afterload reduction; second, the ACE inhibitor could have prevented nitrate tolerance.[27]

Magnesium. ISIS-4 decisively showed that intravenous magnesium started *after* fibrinolysis gave no added benefit, possibly because of the low control mortality rate.[182] The possible benefit of intravenous magnesium administered before thrombolysis requires further study.

New Fibrinolytics or Lesser Used Agents

"All currently available thrombolytic agents suffer from a significant number of limitations"[160] that include (1) an early patency rate of less than 100% (see Table 2–15), (2) the risk of coronary reocclusion with a lower patency rate at 2–3 h than at 90 min (see Table 2–15), and (3) the risk of bleeding, especially in combination with intravenous heparin. Hence, there is a quest for better and more specific agents.

New Types of rt-PA

The standard formulation of rt-PA consists predominantly of two-chain molecules. In development are mutant (e.g., BM 06.022 that contains two of the rt-PA domains) and chimeric rt-PAs (e.g., one involving the kringle 1 and 2 domains and the serine protease domain). These may have longer half-lives, be more resistant to the effects of plasminogen activator inhibition, and have increased thrombolytic efficacy. They are still at the stage of early clinical trials.[160] One agent, reteplase, is claimed to achieve greater arterial patency than a standard regimen of rt-PA.[183]

Prourokinase

Recombinant single-chain urokinase plasminogen activator (saruplase, rscu-PA) is rapidly cleared from the blood in two phases with half-lives of 4–8 min and 48 min, respectively, so that this agent must be continuously infused.[160] Once plasmin forms, rscu-PA is rapidly converted to urokinase; thus, there is an added fibrinolytic activation as for urokinase and streptokinase. In 401 patients with early acute myocardial infarction, in a direct double-blind comparison between intravenous saruplase (80 mg in 60 min) and streptokinase (1.5 million U in 60 min), there was less bleeding and less transfusion requirement in the saruplase versus the streptokinase group.[184] The circulating fibrinogen levels fell marginally less in those patients treated by saruplase. Patency at 90 min was 71% with saruplase versus 73% in another study using a different prourokinase preparation.[185]

Staphylokinase

This agent, purified from *Staphylococcus aureus,* induces relatively fibrin-specific clot lysis in vitro. Clot specificity may be ascribed to the binding of staphylokinase-plasminogen complex to fibrin, thereby reducing by about 130 times the normal affinity of antiplasmin for staphylokinase.[160] It acts more on platelet-rich fibrin-containing clots and is less immunogenic than streptokinase.[160]

Future Prospects

As thrombolytic agents become more and more clot specific and added antithrombin therapy moves from standard unfractionated heparin to specific thrombin inhibitors, it is likely that future measurable but rather small decreases in the mortality of acute myocardial infarction will occur. It will be difficult to demonstrate superiority over rt-PA and unfractionated heparin with early patency rates of about 75%. Thus, the major emphasis should be on the speed of reperfusion rather than on the agent used to achieve reperfusion. The "pain-to-needle" time must be reduced by an organized community approach to chest pain.[152, 186]

REFERENCES

1. Anderson TJ, Meredith IT, Ganz P, et al: Nitric oxide and nitrovasodilators: similarities, differences and potential interactions. J Am Coll Cardiol 1994; 24:555–566.
2. Kurz MA, Lamping KG, Bates JN, et al: Mechanisms responsible for the heterogeneous coronary microvascular response to nitroglycerin. Circ Res 1991; 68:847–855.
3. Torfgard KE, Ahlner J: Mechanisms of action of nitrates. Cardiovasc Drugs Ther 1994; 8:701–717.
4. Tadjkarimi S, O'Neil GS, Luu TN, et al: Comparison of cyclic GMP in human internal mammary artery and saphenous vein: implications for coronary artery bypass graft patency. Cardiovasc Res 1992; 26:297–300.
5. Chirkov YY, Naujalis JI, Barber S, et al: Reversal of human platelet aggregation by low concentrations of nitroglycerin in vitro in normal subjects. Am J Cardiol 1992; 70:802–806.
6. Trimarco B, Cuocolo A, Van Dorne D, et al: Late phase of nitroglycerin-induced coronary vasodilatation blunted by inhibition of prostaglandin synthesis. Circulation 1985; 71:840–848.
7. Balligand J-L, Kelly RA, Marsden PA, et al: Control of cardiac muscle cell function by an endogenous nitric oxide signaling system. Proc Natl Acad Sci USA 1993; 90:347–351.
8. Weyrich AS, Ma X, Buerke M, et al: Physiological concentrations of nitric oxide do not elicit an acute negative inotropic effect in unstimulated cardiac muscle. Circ Res 1994; 75:692–700.
9. Thadani U, Lipicky RJ: Short- and long-acting oral nitrates for stable angina pectoris. Cardiovasc Drugs Ther 1994; 8:611–623.
10. Fung H-L, Bauer JA: Mechanisms of nitrate tolerance. Cardiovasc Drugs Ther 1994; 8:489–499.
11. Jugdutt BI: Nitrates in myocardial infarction. Cardiovasc Drugs Ther 1994; 8:635–646.
12. Husain M, Adrie C, Ichinose F, et al: Exhaled nitric oxide as a marker for organic nitrate tolerance. Circulation 1994; 89:2498–2502.
13. Watanabe H, Kakihana M, Ohtsuka S, et al: Platelet cyclic GMP. A potentially useful indicator to evaluate the effects of nitroglycerin and nitrate tolerance. Circulation 1993; 88:29–36.
14. Boesgaard S, Iversen HK, Wroblewski H, et al: Altered peripheral vasodilator profile of nitroglycerin during long-term infusion of *N*-acetylcysteine. J Am Coll Cardiol 1994; 23:163–169.
15. Mehra A, Shotan A, Ostrzega E, et al: Potentiation of isosorbide dinitrate effects with *N*-acetylcysteine in patients with chronic heart failure. Circulation 1994; 89:2595–2600.
16. Dupuis J, Lalonde G, Lemieux R, Rouleau JL: Tolerance to intravenous nitroglycerin in patients with congestive heart failure: role of increased intravascular volume, neurohumoral activation and lack of prevention with *N*-acetylcysteine. J Am Coll Cardiol 1990; 16:923–931.
17. Leier CV, Magorien RD, Desch CE, et al: Hydralazine and isosorbide dinitrate: comparative central and regional hemodynamic effects when administered alone or in combination. Circulation 1981; 63:102–109.
18. Gogia H, Mehra A, Parikh S, et al: A randomized study to evaluate the effect of hydralazine on the development of nitrate tolerance in patients with heart failure [Abstract]. Circulation 1994; 90(pt 2):I-601.
19. Cohn JN, Archibald DG, Ziesche S, et al: Effect of vasodilator therapy on mortality in chronic congestive heart failure. Results of a Veterans Administration Cooperative Study. N Engl J Med 1986; 314:1547–1552.
20. Mehra A, Ostrzega E, Shotan A, et al: Overcoming early nitrate tolerance with escalating oral dose of isosorbide dinitrate in chronic heart failure [Abstract]. J Am Coll Cardiol 1993; 21:252A.
21. Bogaert M: Clinical pharmacokinetics of nitrates. Cardiovasc Drugs Ther 1994; 8:693–699.
22. Rudolph W, Dirschinger J, Reiniger G, et al: When does nitrate tolerance develop? What dosages and which intervals are necessary to ensure maintained effectiveness? Eur Heart J 1988; 9(suppl A):63–72.
23. Thadani U, Opie LH: Nitrates for unstable angina. Cardiovasc Drugs Ther 1994; 8:719–726.
24. Zimrin D, Reichek N, Bogin KT, et al: Antianginal effects of intravenous nitroglycerin over 24 hours. Circulation 1988; 77:1376–1384.
25. Amidi M, Shaver JA: Sublingual NTG test for detection of nitrate tolerance in patients with coronary artery disease [Abstract]. Circulation 1989; 80(suppl II):II-214.
26. Ghio S, Poli A, Ferrario M, et al: Differential tolerance to the hemodynamic effects of nitroglycerin in heart failure patients [Abstract]. J Am Coll Cardiol 1993; 21:252A.
27. Meredith IT, Alison JF, Zhang F-M, et al: Captopril potentiates the effects of nitroglycerin in the coronary vascular bed. J Am Coll Cardiol 1993; 22:581–587.
28. DiSomma S, Liguori V, Pettito M, et al: A double-blind comparison of nicorandil and metoprolol in stable effort angina pectoris. Cardiovasc Drugs Ther 1993; 7:119–123.
29. Thadani U, Strauss W, Glasser SP, et al, for the Nicorandil Study Group: Evaluation of antianginal and anti-ischemic efficacy of nicorandil: results of a multicenter study [Abstract]. J Am Coll Cardiol 1994; 23:267A.
30. Mann T, Cohn PF, Holman L, et al: Effect of nitroprusside on regional myocardial blood flow in coronary artery disease. Results in 25 patients and comparison with nitroglycerin. Circulation 1978; 57:732–758.
31. Murphy J, Lavie CJ, Bresnahan D: Arteriolar and venous vasodilators. *In* Messerli FH (ed): Cardiovascular Drug Therapy, pp 861–870. Philadelphia: WB Saunders, 1990.
32. ESPRIM (European Study of Prevention of Infarct with Molsidomine) Group: The ESPRIM trial: short-term treatment of acute myocardial infarction with molsidomine. Lancet 1994; 344:91–97.
33. ACCORD Study Investigators: Nitric oxide donors reduce restenosis after coronary angioplasty: the ACCORD Study [Abstract]. J Am Coll Cardiol 1994; 23:59A.
34. Giraud T: Unstable angina: a multicenter comparative study of linsidomine and isosorbide dinitrate [Abstract]. J Am Coll Cardiol 1994; 23:289A.
35. Petros A, Bennett D, Vallance P: Effect of nitric oxide synthase inhibitors on hypotension in patients with septic shock. Lancet 1991; 338:1557–1558.

36. Thadani U, Lipicky RJ: Ointments and transdermal nitroglycerin patches for stable angina pectoris. Cardiovasc Drugs Ther 1994; 8:625–633.
37. Bassan MM: The daylong pattern of the antianginal effect of long-term three times daily administered isosorbide dinitrate. J Am Coll Cardiol 1990; 16:936–940.
38. Thadani U, Bittar N: Effects of 8:00 a.m. and 2:00 p.m. doses of isosorbide-5-mononitrate during twice-daily therapy in stable angina pectoris. Am J Cardiol 1992; 70:286–292.
39. Murphree SS, Saffitz JE: Delineation of the distribution of beta-adrenergic receptor subtypes in canine myocardium. Circ Res 1988; 63:117–125.
40. McLeod AA, Brown JE, Kuhn C, et al: Differentiation of hemodynamic, humoral and metabolic responses to $beta_1$- and $beta_2$-adrenergic stimulation in man using atenolol and propranolol. Circulation 1983; 67:1076–1084.
41. Neer EJ, Clapham DE: Signal transduction through G-proteins in the cardiac myocyte. Trends Cardiovasc Med 1992; 2:6–11.
42. Luo W, Grupp IL, Harrer J, et al: Targeted ablation of the phospholamban gene is associated with markedly enhanced myocardial contractility and loss of beta-agonist stimulation. Circ Res 1994; 75:401–409.
43. Frishman WH: Beta-adrenergic blocker withdrawal. Am J Cardiol 1987; 59:26F–32F.
44. Guth BD, Heusch G, Seitelberger R, et al: Mechanism of beneficial effect of beta-adrenergic blockade on exercise-induced myocardial ischemia in conscious dogs. Circ Res 1987; 60:738–746.
45. Wolfson S, Gorlin R: Cardiovascular pharmacology of propranolol in man. Circulation 1969; 40:501–511.
46. Majewski H, Rand MJ, Tung LH: Activation of prejunctional beta-adrenoceptors in rat atria by adrenaline applied exogenously or released as co-transmitter. Br J Pharmacol 1981; 73:669–679.
47. Van den Meiracker AH, Man in't Veld AJ, Ritsema van Eck HJ, et al: Hemodynamic and hormonal adaptations to beta-adrenoceptor blockade. A 24-hour study of acebutolol, atenolol, pindolol, and propranolol in hypertensive patients. Circulation 1988; 78:957–968.
48. Lubbe WF, Podzuweit T, Opie LH: Potential arrhythmogenic role of cyclic AMP and cytosolic calcium overload: implications for antiarrhythmic effects of beta-blockers and proarrhythmic effects of phosphodiesterase inhibitors. J Am Coll Cardiol 1992; 19:1622–1633.
49. Steinbeck G, Andresen D, Bach P, et al: A comparison of electrophysiologically guided antiarrhythmic drug therapy with beta-blocker therapy in patients with symptomatic, sustained ventricular tachyarrhythmias. N Engl J Med 1992; 327:987–992.
50. Mason JW, for the Electrophysiologic Study Versus Electrocardiographic Monitoring Investigators: A comparison of seven antiarrhythmic drugs in patients with ventricular tachyarrhythmias. N Engl J Med 1993; 329:452–458.
51. Kostis JB, Rosen RC: Central nervous system effects of beta-adrenergic blocking drugs: the role of ancillary properties. Circulation 1987; 75:204–212.
52. Jee LD, Opie LH: Double-blind trial comparing labetalol with atenolol in the treatment of systemic hypertension with angina pectoris. Am J Cardiol 1985; 56:551–554.
53. Quyyumi AA, Crake T, Wright CM, et al: Medical treatment of patients with severe exertional and rest angina: double-blind comparison of beta-blocker, calcium antagonist, and nitrate. Br Heart J 1987; 57:505–511.
54. Pepine CJ, Cohn PF, Deedwania PC, et al, for the ASIST Study Group: Effects of treatment on outcome in mildly symptomatic patients with ischemia during daily life. Circulation 1994; 90:762–768.
55. HINT Research Group (Holland Interuniversity Nifedipine/Metoprolol Trial): Early treatment of unstable angina in the coronary care unit: a randomised double-blind placebo-controlled comparison of recurrent ischaemia in patients treated with nifedipine or metoprolol or both. Br Heart J 1986; 56:400–413.
56. Peart I, Bullock RE, Albers C, Hall RJC: Cold intolerance in patients with angina pectoris: effect of nifedipine and propranolol. Br Heart J 1989; 61:521–528.
57. Norris RM, Brown MA, Clarke ED, et al: Prevention of ventricular fibrillation during acute myocardial infarction by intravenous propranolol. Lancet 1984; 2:883–886.
58. Hjalmarson A, Elmfeldt D, Herlitz J, et al: Effect on mortality of metoprolol in acute myocardial infarction. Lancet 1981; 2:823–827.
59. ISIS-1 (First International Study of Infarct Survival) Collaborative Group: Randomized trial of intravenous atenolol among 16,027 cases of suspected acute myocardial infarction: ISIS-I. Lancet 1986; 2:57–66.
60. Lichstein E, Hager WD, Gregory JJ, et al, for the Multicenter Diltiazem Post-Infarction Research Group: Relation between beta-adrenergic blocker use, various correlates of left ventricular function and the chance of developing congestive heart failure. J Am Coll Cardiol 1990; 16:1327–1332.
61. Kennedy HL, Brooks MM, Barker AH, et al, for the CAST Investigators: Beta-blocker therapy in the Cardiac Arrhythmia Suppression Trial. Am J Cardiol 1994; 74:674–680.
62. Viscoli CM, Horwitz RI, Singer BH: Beta-blockers alter myocardial infarction: influence of first year clinical course on long-term effectiveness. Ann Intern Med 1993; 118:99–105.
63. Joint National Committee: The fifth report of the Joint National Committee on detection, evaluation, and treatment of high blood pressure (JNC V). Arch Intern Med 1993; 153:154–183.
64. Materson BJ, Reda DJ, Cushman WC, et al: Single-drug therapy for hypertension in men. A comparison of six antihypertensive agents with placebo. N Engl J Med 1993; 328:914–921.
65. Dahlof B, Hansson L: Regression of left ventricular hypertrophy in previously untreated essential hypertension: different effects of enalapril and hydrochlorothiazide. J Hypertens 1992; 10:1513–1524.
66. Senior R, Imbs JL, Bory M, et al: Comparison of the effects of indapamide with hydrochlorothiazide, nifedipine, enalapril and atenolol on left ventricular hypertrophy in hypertension: a double-blind parallel study [Abstract]. J Am Coll Cardiol 1993; 21:57A.
67. Medical Research Council Working Party: Medical Research Council trial of treatment of hypertension in older adults: principal results. Br Med J 1992; 304:405–412.
68. Dahlof B, Lindholm LH, Hansson L, et al: Morbidity and mortality in the Swedish Trial in Old Patients with Hypertension (STOP-Hypertension). Lancet 1991; 338:1281–1285.
69. SHEP Cooperative Research Group: Prevention of stroke by antihypertensive drug treatment in older persons with isolated systolic hypertension. Final results of the Systolic Hypertension in the Elderly Program (SHEP). JAMA 1991; 265:3255–3264.
70. Teo KK, Yusuf S, Furberg D: Effects of prophylactic antiarrhythmic drug therapy in acute myocardial infarction. An overview of results from randomized controlled trials. JAMA 1993; 270:1589–1595.
71. Asseman P, McFadden E, Bauchart JJ, et al: Why do beta-blockers help in idiopathic dilated cardiomyopathy—frequency mismatch? Lancet 1994; 344:803–804.
72. Simpson WT: Nature and incidence of unwanted effects with atenolol. Postgrad Med J 1997; 53(suppl 3):162–167.
73. Vandenburg MJ, Conlon C, Ledingham JM: A comparison of the effects of propranolol and oxprenolol on forearm blood flow and skin temperature. Br J Clin Pharmacol 1981; 11:485–490.
74. Hiatt WR, Stoll S, Nies AS: Effect of beta-adrenergic blockers on the peripheral circulation in patients with peripheral vascular disease. Circulation 1985; 72:1226–1231.
75. Thadani U, Whitsett TL: Beta-adrenergic blockers and intermittent claudication. Arch Intern Med 1991; 151:1705–1707.
76. Wassertheil-Smoller S, Oberman A, Blaufox MD, et al: The Trial of Antihypertensive Interventions and Management (TAIM) study. Final results with regard to blood pressure, cardiovascular risk, and quality of life. Am J Hypertens 1992; 5:37–44.
77. Croog SH, Levine S, Testa MA, et al: The effect of antihypertensive therapy on the quality of life. N Engl J Med 1986; 314:1657–1664.
78. Beto JA, Bansal VK: Quality of life in treatment of hypertension. A metaanalysis of clinical trials. J Hypertens 1992; 5:125–133.
79. Streufert S, DePadova A, McGlynn T, et al: Impact of beta-blockade on complex cognitive functioning. Am Heart J 1988; 116:311–315.
80. Strauss WE, Parisi AF: Combined use of calcium channel and beta-adrenergic blockers for the treatment of chronic stable angina. Ann Intern Med 1988; 109:570–581.
81. Dargie HJ, for the TIBET Study Group: Medical treatment of angina can favourably affect outcome [Abstract]. Eur Heart J 1993; 14(abstr suppl):304.
82. Pfeffer MA, Braunwald E, Moye LA, et al: Effect of captopril on mortality and morbidity in patients with left ventricular dysfunction after myocardial infarction. Results of the Survival and Ventricular Enlargement Trial. N Engl J Med 1992; 327:669–677.
83. Myerburg RJ, Kessler KM, Cox MM, et al: Reversal of proarrhythmic effects of flecainide acetate and encainide hydrochloride by propranolol. Circulation 1989; 80:1571–1579.
84. The Cardiac Arrhythmia Suppression Trial II Investigators: Effect of the antiarrhythmic drug moricizine on survival after myocardial infarction. N Engl J Med 1992; 327:227–233.

85. Opie LH, Sonnenblick EH, Frishman W, Thadani U: Beta-blocking agents. *In* Opie LH (ed): Drugs for the Heart, 4th ed, pp 1–30. Philadelphia: WB Saunders, 1995.
86. Opie LH: Adverse cardiovascular drug interactions. *In* Schlant RC, Alexander RW (eds): The Heart, 8th ed, pp 1971–1985. New York: McGraw-Hill, 1994.
87. Yatani A, Bahinski A, Mikala G, et al: Single amino acid substitutions within the ion permeation pathway alter single-channel conductance of the human L-type cardiac Ca^{2+}-channel. Circ Res 1994; 75:315–323.
88. Hullin R, Biel M, Flockerzi V, Hofmann F: Tissue-specific expression of calcium channels. Trends Cardiovasc Med 1993; 3:48–53.
89. Pragnell M, De Waard M, Mori Y, et al: Calcium channel beta-subunit binds to a conserved motif in the I-II cytoplasmic linker of the $alpha_1$-subunit. Nature 1994; 368:67–70.
90. Lory G, Varadi G, Schwartz A: The beta-subunit controls the gating and dihydropyridine sensitivity of the skeletal muscle Ca^{2+} channel. Biophys J 1992; 63:1421–1424.
91. Collin T, Wang J-J, Nargeot J, Schwartz A: Molecular cloning of three isoforms of the L-type voltage-dependent calcium channel beta-subunit from normal human heart. Circ Res 1993; 72:1337–1344.
92. Striessnig J, Murphy BJ, Catterall WA: Dihydropyridine receptor of L-type Ca^{2+} channels: identification of binding domains for [^{3}H](+)-PN200-110 and [^{3}H]azidopine within the $alpha_1$-subunit. Proc Natl Acad Sci USA 1991; 88:10769–10773.
93. Spedding M, Paoletti R: Classification of calcium channels and calcium antagonists: progress report. Cardiovasc Drugs Ther 1992; 6:35–39.
94. Striessnig J, Glossmann H, Catterall WA: Identification of a phenylalkylamine binding region within the $alpha_1$-subunit of skeletal muscle Ca^{2+} channels. Proc Natl Acad Sci USA 1990; 87:9108–9112.
95. Watanabe K, Kalasz H, Yabana H, et al: Azidobutyryl clentiazem, a new photoactivatable diltiazem analog, labels benzothiazepine binding sites in the $alpha_1$-subunit of the skeletal muscle calcium channel. FEBS Lett 1993; 334:261–264.
96. Mishra SK, Hermsmeyer K: Selective inhibition of T-type Ca^{2+}-channels by Ro 40-5967. Circ Res 1994; 75:144–148.
97. Sen LS, Smith TW: T-type Ca^{2+} channels are abnormal in genetically determined cardiomyopathic hamster hearts. Circ Res 1994; 75:149–155.
98. Stone PH, Antman EM, Muller JE, Braunwald E: Calcium channel blocking agents in the treatment of cardiovascular disorders. Part II. Hemodynamic effects and clinical applications. Ann Intern Med 1980; 93:886–904.
99. Godfraind T, Salomone S, Dessy C, et al: Selectivity scale of calcium antagonists in the human cardiovascular system based on in vitro studies. J Cardiovasc Pharmacol 1992; 20(suppl 5):S34–S41.
100. Neaton JD, Grimm RH, Prineas RJ, et al, for the Treatment of Mild Hypertension Study Research Group: Treatment of Mild Hypertension Study. Final results. JAMA 1993; 270:713–724.
101. Talano JV, Tommaso C: Slow channel calcium antagonists in the treatment of supraventricular tachycardia. Prog Cardiovasc Dis 1982; 25:141–156.
102. Weiss AT, Lewis BS, Halon DA, et al: Use of calcium with verapamil in the management of supraventricular arrhythmias. Int J Cardiol 1983; 4:274–280.
103. Multicenter Diltiazem Postinfarction Trial Research Group: The effect of diltiazem on mortality and reinfarction after myocardial infarction. N Engl J Med 1988; 319:385–392.
104. Furberg CD, Psaty BM, Meyer JV: Nifedipine. Dose-related increase in mortality in patients with coronary heart disease. Circulation 1995; 92:1326–1331.
105. Opie LH, Messerli FH: Nifedipine and mortality. Grave defects in the dossier. Circulation 1995; 92:1068–1073.
106. Singh BN, for the Bepridil Collaborative Study Group: Comparative efficacy and safety of bepridil and diltiazem in chronic stable angina pectoris refractory to diltiazem. Am J Cardiol 1991; 68:306–312.
107. Frishman WH: Comparative efficacy and concomitant use of bepridil and beta-blockers in the management of angina pectoris. Am J Cardiol 1992; 69:50D–55D.
108. Antiplatelet Trialists' Collaboration: Collaborative overview of randomised trials of antiplatelet therapy. I. Prevention of death, myocardial infarction, and stroke by prolonged antiplatelet therapy in various categories of patients. Br Med J 1994; 308:81–106.
109. Folts JD: Drugs for the prevention of coronary thrombosis: from an animal model to clinical trials. Cardiovasc Drug Ther 1995; 9:31–43.
110. Brass LF, Hoxie JA, Manning DR: Signaling through G proteins and G protein–coupled receptors during platelet activation. Thromb Haemost 1993; 70:217–223.
111. Ku DD, Zaleski JK: Receptor mechanism of thrombin-induced endothelium-dependent and endothelium-independent coronary vascular effects in dogs. J Cardiovasc Pharmacol 1993; 2:609–616.
112. Coughlin SR: Thrombin receptor function and cardiovascular disease. Trends Cardiovasc Med 1994; 4:77–83.
113. Kroll MH, Hellums JD, Guo Z, et al: Protein kinase C is activated in platelets subjected to pathological shear stress. J Biol Chem 1993; 268:3520–3524.
114. Wu KK, Phillips M, D'Souza D, Hellmus JD: Platelet activation and arterial thrombosis. Lancet 1994; 344:991–995.
115. Rovin JD, Stamler JS, Loscalzo J, Folts JD: Sodium nitroprusside, an endothelium-derived relaxing factor congener, increases platelet cyclic GMP levels and inhibits epinephrine-exacerbated in vivo platelet thrombus formation in stenosed canine coronary arteries. J Cardiovasc Pharmacol 1993; 22:626–631.
116. Patrono C: Aspirin as an antiplatelet drug. N Engl J Med 1994; 330:1287–1294.
117. Fuster V, Dyken ML, Vokonas PS, Hennekens C: Aspirin as a therapeutic agent in cardiovascular disease. Circulation 1993; 87:659–675.
118. Ridker PM, Hebert PR, Fuster V, Hennekens CH: Are both aspirin and heparin justified as adjuncts to thrombolytic therapy for acute myocardial infarction? Lancet 1993; 341:1574–1577.
119. Dutch TIA Trial Study Group: A comparison of two doses of aspirin (30 mg vs. 283 mg a day) in patients after a transient ischemic attack or minor ischemic stroke. N Engl J Med 1991; 325:1261–1266.
120. Goodman SG, Langer A, Durica SS, et al, for the Coumadin Aspirin Reinfarction (CARS) Pilot Study Group: Safety and anticoagulation effect of a low-dose combination of warfarin and aspirin in clinically stable coronary artery disease. Am J Cardiol 1994; 74:657–661.
121. ISIS-2 (Second International Study of Infarct Survival) Collaborative Group: Randomised trial of intravenous streptokinase, oral aspirin, both, or neither among 17187 cases of suspected acute myocardial infarction: ISIS-2. Lancet 1988; 2:350–360.
122. Balsano F, Risson P, Violi F, et al: Antiplatelet treatment with ticlopidine in unstable angina. A controlled multicenter clinical trial. Circulation 1990; 82:17–26.
123. Feinberg WM, Albers GW, Barnett HJM, et al: Guidelines for the management of transient ischemic attacks. From the Ad Hoc Committee on Guidelines for the Management of Transient Ischemic Attacks of the Stroke Council of the American Heart Association. Circulation 1994; 89:2950–2965.
124. Ticlopidine [Editorial]. Lancet 1991; 337:459–460.
125. Manson JE, Stampfer MJ, Colditz GA, et al: A prospective study of aspirin use and primary prevention of cardiovascular disease in women. JAMA 1991; 266:521–527.
126. Van der Meer J, de la Riviere AB, van Gilst WK, et al: Effects of low-dose aspirin (50 mg/day), low-dose aspirin plus dipyridamole, and oral anticoagulant agents after internal mammary artery bypass grafting: patency and clinical outcome at 1 year. J Am Coll Cardiol 1994; 24:1181–1188.
127. Watt AH, Webster BJ, Passani SL, et al: Intravenous adenosine in the treatment of supraventricular tachycardia: a dose-ranging study and interaction with dipyridamole. Br J Clin Pharmacol 1986; 21:227–230.
128. Steele P, Rainwater J: Favorable effect of sulfinpyrazone on thromboembolism in patients with rheumatic heart disease. Circulation 1980; 62:462–465.
129. Topol EJ, Califf RM, Weisman HF, et al, on behalf of the EPIC Investigators: Randomised trial of coronary intervention with antibody against platelet IIb/IIIa integrin for reduction of clinical restenosis: results at six months. Lancet 1994; 343:881–886.
130. Lincoff AM, Califf RM, Anderson K, et al, for the EPIC Investigators: Striking clinical benefit with platelet GP IIb/IIIa inhibition by c7E3 among patients with unstable angina: outcome in the EPIC trial [Abstract]. Circulation 1994; 90:I-21.
131. Langford EJ, Brown AS, Wainwright RJ, et al: Inhibition of platelet activity by *S*-nitrosoglutathione during coronary angioplasty. Lancet 1994; 344:1458–1460.
132. Stubbs MT, Bode W: Structure and specificity in coagulation and its inhibition. Trends Cardiovasc Med 1995; 5:157–166.
133. Lefkovitz J, Topol EJ: Direct thrombin inhibitors in cardiovascular medicine. Circulation 1994; 90:1522–1536.
134. Sasayama S: Effect of coronary collateral circulation on myocardial ischemia and ventricular dysfunction. Cardiovasc Drugs Ther 1994; 8:327–334.

135. Hirsh J, Fuster V: Guide to anticoagulant therapy. Part 1. Heparin. Circulation 1994; 89:1449–1468.
136. GUSTO (Global Utilization of Streptokinase and Tissue Plasminogen Activator for Occluded Coronary Arteries) Investigators: An international randomized trial comparing four thrombolytic strategies for acute myocardial infarction. N Engl J Med 1993; 329:673–682.
137. The Global Use of Strategies to Open Occluded Coronary Arteries (GUSTO) IIa Investigators: Randomized trial of intravenous heparin versus recombinant hirudin for acute coronary syndromes. Circulation 1994; 90:1631–1637.
138. Arnout JEF, Simoons M, de Bono D, et al: Correction between level of heparinization and patency of the infarct-related coronary artery after treatment of acute myocardial infarction with alteplase (rt-PA). J Am Coll Cardiol 1992; 20:513–519.
139. Becker RC, Corrao JM, Ball SP, Gore JM: A comparison of heparin strategies after thrombolytic therapy. Am Heart J 1993; 126:750–752.
140. Flaker GC, Bartolozzi J, Davis V, et al, for the TIMI-4 Investigators: Use of a standardized heparin nomogram to achieve therapeutic anticoagulation after thrombolytic therapy in myocardial infarction. Arch Intern Med 1994; 154:1492–1496.
141. Heik LCW, Kupper W, Hamm C, et al: Efficacy of high dose intravenous heparin for treatment of left ventricular thrombi with high embolic risk. J Am Coll Cardiol 1994; 24:1305–1309.
142. Friedman HZ, Cragg DR, Glazier SM, et al: Randomized prospective evaluation of prolonged versus abbreviated intravenous heparin therapy after coronary angioplasty. J Am Coll Cardiol 1994; 24:1214–1219.
143. Antman EM, for the TIMI-9A Investigators: Hirudin in acute myocardial infarction. Safety report from the Thrombolysis and Thrombin Inhibition in Myocardial Infarction (TIMI) 9A trial. Circulation 1994; 90:1624–1630.
144. Hunter JB, Lonsdale RJ, Wenham PW, Frostick SP: Heparin induced thrombosis: an important complication of heparin prophylaxis for thromboembolic disease in surgery. Br Med J 1993; 307:53–55.
145. Leizorovicz A, Simonneau G, Decousus H, Boissel JP: Comparison of efficacy and safety of low molecular weight heparins and unfractionated heparin in initial treatment of deep venous thrombosis: a meta-analysis. Br Med J 1994; 309:299–304.
146. Hull RD, Raskob GE, Pineo GF, et al: Subcutaneous low-molecular-weight heparin compared with continuous intravenous heparin in the treatment of proximal-vein thrombosis. N Engl J Med 1992; 326:975–982.
147. Salzman EW: Low-molecular-weight heparin and other new antithrombotic drugs. N Engl J Med 1992; 326:1017–1019.
148. Fuster V: Coronary thrombolysis—a perspective for the practicing physician. N Engl J Med 1993; 329:723–725.
149. Topol EJ, Fuster V, Harrington RA, et al: Recombinant hirudin for unstable angina pectoris. A multicenter, randomized angiographic trial. Circulation 1994; 89:1557–1566.
150. Hirayama A, Adachi T, Asada S, et al: Late reperfusion for acute myocardial infarction limits the dilatation of left ventricle without the reduction of infarct size. Circulation 1993; 88:2565–2574.
151. Willerson JT, Casscells W: Thrombin inhibitors in unstable angina: rebound or continuation of angina after argatroban withdrawal? J Am Coll Cardiol 1993; 21:1048–1051.
152. Gersh BJ, Opie LH: Antithrombotic agents: platelet inhibitors, anticoagulants, and fibrinolytics. *In* Opie LH (ed): Drugs for the Heart, 4th ed, pp 247–285. Philadelphia: WB Saunders, 1995.
153. Hirsh J, Fuster V: Guide to anticoagulant therapy. Part 2. Oral anticoagulants. Circulation 1994; 89:1469–1480.
154. Eckman MH, Levine HJ, Pauker SG: Effect of laboratory variation in the prothrombin-time ratio on the results of oral anticoagulant therapy. N Engl J Med 1993; 329:696–702.
155. Singer DE: Randomized trials of warfarin for atrial fibrillation. N Engl J Med 1992; 327:1451–1453.
156. Fihn SD, McDonell M, Martin D, et al, for the Warfarin Optimized Outpatient Follow-up Study Group: Risk factors for complications of chronic anticoagulation. A multicenter study. Ann Intern Med 1993; 118:511–520.
157. Gurwitz JH, Goldberg RJ, Holder A, et al: Age-related risks of long-term oral anticoagulant therapy. Arch Intern Med 1988; 148:1733–1736.
158. Hayashi J-I, Nakazawa S, Oguma F, et al: Combined warfarin and antiplatelet therapy after St. Jude medical valve replacement for mitral valve disease. J Am Coll Cardiol 1994; 23:672–677.
159. Turpie AFF, Gent M, Laupacis A, et al: A comparison of aspirin with placebo in patients treated with warfarin after heart-valve replacement. N Engl J Med 1993; 329:524–529.
160. Verstraete M, Lijnen HR: Novel thrombolytic agents. Cardiovasc Drugs Ther 1994; 8:801–812.
161. Silber H, Khan SS, Matloff JM, et al: The St. Jude valve. Thrombolysis as the first line of therapy for cardiac valve thrombosis. Circulation 1993; 87:30–37.
162. Neri Serneri GG, Gensini GF, Poggesi L, et al: Effect of heparin, aspirin, or alteplase in reduction of myocardial ischaemia in refractory unstable angina. Lancet 1990; 335:615–618.
163. TIMI-IIIB Investigators: Effects of tissue plasminogen activator and a comparison of early invasive and conservative strategies in unstable angina and non–Q-wave myocardial infarction. Results of the TIMI-IIIB Trial. Circulation 1994; 89:1545–1556.
164. Purvis JA, McNeill AJ, Siddiqui RA, et al: Efficacy of 100 mg of double-bolus alteplase in achieving complete perfusion in the treatment of acute myocardial infarction. J Am Coll Cardiol 1994; 23:6–10.
165. TIMI Study Group: Comparison of invasive and conservative strategies after treatment with intravenous tissue plasminogen activator in acute myocardial infarction. Results of the Thrombolysis in Myocardial Infarction (TIMI) phase II trial. N Engl J Med 1989; 320:618–627.
166. Anderson HV, Willerson JT: Thrombolysis in acute myocardial infarction. N Engl J Med 1993; 329:703–708.
167. Gruber S, Pal A, Kiss RG, et al: Generation of activated protein-C during thrombolysis. Lancet 1993; 342:1275–1276.
168. Collen D, Lijnen HR: Thrombolytic agents. *In* Singh BN, Dzau VJ, Vanhoutte PM, Woosley RL (eds): Cardiovascular Pharmacology and Therapeutics, pp 267–279. New York: Churchill Livingstone, 1994.
169. Six AJ, Louwerenburg HW, Braams R, et al: A double-blind randomized multicenter dose-ranging trial of intravenous streptokinase in acute myocardial infarction. Am J Cardiol 1990; 65:119–123.
170. Buchalter MB: Are streptokinase antibodies clinically important? Br Heart J 1993; 70:101–102.
171. Simoons ML, Maggioni AP, Knatterud G, et al: Individual risk assessment for intracranial haemorrhage during thrombolytic therapy. Lancet 1993; 342:1523–1528.
172. Weaver WD, Cerqueira M, Hallstrom AP, et al, for the Myocardial Infarction Triage and Intervention Trial: Prehospital-initiated vs hospital-initiated thrombolytic therapy. JAMA 1993; 270:1211–1216.
173. Fath-Ordoubadi F, Al-Mohammad A, Huehns TY, Beatt KJ: Meta-analysis of randomised trials of prehospital versus hospital thrombolysis [Abstract]. Circulation 1994; 90(pt 2):I-325.
174. EMIP (The European Myocardial Infarction Project) Group: Prehospital thrombolytic therapy in patients with suspected acute myocardial infarction. N Engl J Med 1993; 329:383–389.
175. Linderer T, Schroder R, Arntz R, et al: Prehospital thrombolysis: beneficial effects of very early treatment on infarct size and left ventricular function. J Am Coll Cardiol 1993; 22:1304–1310.
176. GREAT (Grampian Region Early Anistreplase Trial) Group: Feasibility, safety, and efficacy of domiciliary thrombolysis by general practitioners: Grampian Region Early Anistreplase Trial. Br Med J 1992; 305:548–553.
177. O'Connor CM, Meese R, Carney R, et al, for the DUCCS Group: A randomized trial of intravenous heparin in conjunction with anistreplase (anisoylated plasminogen streptokinase activator complex) in acute myocardial infarction: The Duke University Clinical Cardiology Study (DUCCS) 1. J Am Coll Cardiol 1994; 23:11–18.
178. Wall TC, Phillips HR, Stack RS, et al: Results of high-dose intravenous urokinase for acute myocardial infarction. Am J Cardiol 1990; 65:124–131.
179. Mueller HS, Cohen LS, Braunwald E, et al: Predictors of early morbidity and mortality after thrombolytic therapy in acute myocardial infarction: analyses of patient subgroups in the Thrombolysis In Myocardial Infarction (TIMI) trial, phase II. Circulation 1992; 85:1254–1264.
180. Borghi C, Ambrosioni E, Magnani B, on behalf of SMILE Investigators: Effects of early ACE inhibition on long-term survival in patients with acute anterior myocardial infarction [Abstract]. Circulation 1994; 90(pt 2):I-18.
181. Acute Infarction Ramipril Efficacy (AIRE) Study Investigators: Effect of ramipril on mortality and morbidity of survivors of acute myocardial infarction with clinical evidence of heart failure. Lancet 1993; 342:821–828.
182. Antman EM, Lau J, Berkey C, et al: Large versus small trials of magnesium for acute myocardial infarction: big numbers do not tell the whole story [Abstract]. Circulation 1994; 90(pt 2):I-325.
183. Smalling RW, Bode C, Kalbleisch J, et al: Improvement of global and regional LV function by the bolus administration of recombinant plasminogen activator (r-PA) in acute myocardial infarction: a compari-

son with standard dose alteplase [Abstract]. Circulation 1994; 90(pt 2):I-562.
184. PRIMI Trial Study Group: Randomised double-blind trial of recombinant pro-urokinase against streptokinase in acute myocardial infarction. Lancet 1989; 1:863–865.
185. Weaver WD, Hartmann JR, Anderson JL, et al: New recombinant glycosylated prourokinase for treatment of patients with acute myocardial infarction. J Am Coll Cardiol 1994; 24:1242–1248.
186. Gersh BJ, Opie LH: Antithrombotic agents: platelet inhibitors, anticoagulants, and fibrinolytics. *In* Opie LH (ed): Drugs for the Heart, 4th ed, pp 248–287. Philadelphia: WB Saunders, 1995.
187. GUSTO Angiographic Investigators: The effects of tissue plasminogen activator, streptokinase, or both on coronary artery patency, ventricular function, and survival after acute myocardial infarction. N Engl J Med 1993; 329:1615–1622.
188. Hogg KJ, Gemmill JD, Burns JMA, et al: Angiographic patency study of anistreplase versus streptokinase in acute myocardial infarction. Lancet 1990; 335:254–258.
189. Pacouret G, Charbonnier B, for the IRS II Study: Multicentre European randomized trial of anistreplase versus streptokinase in acute myocardial infarction [Abstract]. Circulation 1989; 80(suppl II):II-420.
190. Neuhaus K-L, Feuerer W, Jeep-Tebbe S, et al: Improved thrombolysis with a modified dose regimen of recombinant tissue-type plasminogen activator. J Am Coll Cardiol 1989; 14:1566–1569.
191. Collen D: Coronary thrombolysis: streptokinase or recombinant tissue-type plasminogen activator? Ann Intern Med 1990; 112:529–538.
192. Granger CB, Califf RM, Topol EJ: Thrombolytic therapy for acute myocardial infarction. Drugs 1992; 44:293–325.
193. Marder VJ, Sherry S: Thrombolytic therapy: current status. N Engl J Med 1988; 318:1512–1520.

3 Catheterization Interventions for the Treatment of Coronary Artery Disease: Techniques, Results, and Patient Selection

David O. Williams, MD

OVERVIEW

Cardiovascular Therapeutics devotes several chapters to catheter-based interventional techniques for the treatment of patients with coronary artery disease. Most focus on a specific technique or device and include detailed descriptions of the design, mechanism of action, and results of each. The goal of this chapter is to provide a more global view of interventional cardiology with an emphasis on the selection of patients and devices in clinical practice. Issues to be addressed include the relative merits and limitations of specific interventional techniques, when techniques might be used in combination, and unique applications of these techniques for specific clinical subsets.

ASSESSMENT OF PATIENTS FOR CORONARY INTERVENTION (Fig. 3–1)

History and Physical Examination

Although findings obtained from the diagnostic cardiac catheterization contribute substantially to deciding whether a specific patient is suitable for coronary intervention, information from the history and physical examination is of considerable importance. First, the symptomatic status of the patient must be determined to establish not only the presence of symptoms but also their severity. Particularly significant is the extent to which symptoms are responsive to optimal medical therapy and to what degree they limit quality of life. Such information is essential for developing a risk/benefit profile for each patient.

The magnitude of symptoms often does not correlate with the extent or severity of coronary artery disease. For example, two patients might demonstrate a 90% narrowing of the mid–left anterior descending coronary artery. One patient might experience severe angina pectoris at rest despite medical therapy, whereas the other could be completely asymptomatic with ischemia that is detectable only by noninvasive stress testing.[1] In this situation, the risks associated with intervention are more justifiable in the severely symptomatic patient than in the asymptomatic patient.

Second, certain noncoronary medical factors can influence the outcome of the interventional procedure, and these must be identified. They include presence of fever, active infection, severe anemia, active bleeding or a bleeding diathesis, uncontrolled hypertension, digitalis toxicity, metabolic derangements, severe peripheral vascular disease, active cerebrovascular disease, hypersensitivity to radiographic contrast agents, arrhythmia, generalized debility or cachexia, and severe pulmonary disease.[2] The history and physical examination are essential for identifying and determining the presence and severity of these disorders. Their impact on the patient's welfare must also be considered in the risk/benefit analysis.

Role of Noninvasive Testing

Noninvasive testing serves several purposes in assessing patients for coronary interventional procedures. First, noninvasive testing can confirm the presence of myocardial ischemia. This concern is of importance for patients who exhibit "borderline" lesions on coronary angiography, on which it is unclear whether the magnitude of narrowing is sufficient to compromise coronary artery blood flow.

Second, noninvasive testing may help identify, from among two or more diseased coronary arteries, the one responsible for the greatest degree of ischemia. This application of noninvasive testing is most informative in patients with unstable angina and multivessel coronary artery disease. Frequently in this setting, a single coronary artery or lesion is identified as the "culprit."[3] Successful treatment of only the culprit lesion can result in substantial clinical improvement.

Third, noninvasive testing can determine whether myocardium in

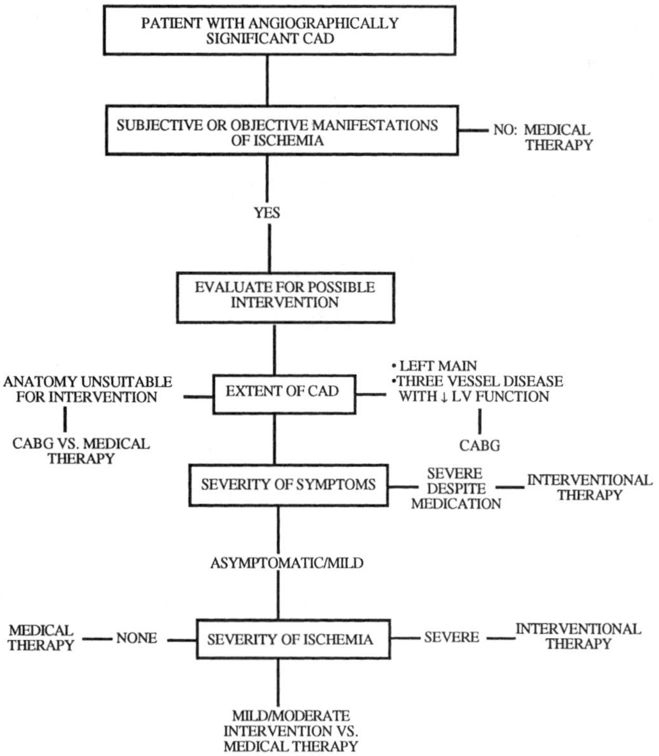

Figure 3–1. Decision tree describing the process of evaluating a patient for coronary intervention.

the distribution of a narrowed coronary artery is viable, as opposed to infarcted. This concern arises frequently in patients who have experienced a myocardial infarction and in whom the artery responsible for the infarction is shown to be patent but substantially narrowed. Evidence of viable but jeopardized myocardium in the distribution of the narrowed artery has been considered as a justification for revascularization.[4]

Finally, noninvasive testing is of great value in assessing the effectiveness of the coronary intervention. Noninvasive testing can objectively confirm relief of pre-existing induced ischemia. During later follow-up, noninvasive testing may be helpful in evaluating patients who develop recurrent symptoms suggestive of ischemia.

Role of Diagnostic Cardiac Catheterization

The information obtained from diagnostic cardiac catheterization, including coronary angiography and left ventriculography, is essential for determining the suitability of coronary interventional therapy. The coronary arteriogram answers several critical questions.

Does the Patient Have Significant Coronary Artery Disease? The angiogram is reviewed to identify whether an area of narrowing is present and of sufficient severity to reduce the diameter of the arterial lumen by at least 50% of normal.[5] In cases in which narrowings are of borderline severity, additional tests of coronary circulatory function may be helpful. Regional measurement of coronary flow reserve can be performed at the time of diagnostic catheterization.[6] Also, the use of intracoronary ultrasonography has provided assistance as an alternative technique for quantitating the degree of coronary narrowing. Evaluation of the left ventriculogram may also provide evidence of the functional significance of coronary narrowing. Presence of a regional systolic contractile abnormality in the area of myocardium supplied by the diseased coronary artery supports the ischemic potential of the lesion.

Is the Patient a Suitable Candidate for Coronary Intervention? For coronary bypass surgery, few patients are not candidates for treatment because of coronary anatomic characteristics; in contrast, a significant proportion of patients requiring revascularization may not be candidates for catheter-based interventions. For example, only 30%–40% of patients with multivessel disease may be suitable, primarily because the other 60%–70% demonstrate chronic coronary artery occlusion.[7] Other coronary anatomic features that may limit the application of catheter-based interventions include marked coronary artery tortuosity or angulation, distorted aortic anatomy, and diffuse coronary atherosclerosis.

Findings from left ventriculography may also influence the decision of whether to perform a catheter-based intervention. Impaired left ventricular systolic function enhances the risk of hemodynamic deterioration during coronary interventions. Of particular concern is the patient with prior infarction and in whom the remaining viable myocardium is supplied by a single coronary artery that requires revascularization. Sustained or even transient occlusion of this artery as a consequence of the coronary intervention can result in further loss of left ventricular systolic function and the development of cardiogenic shock.

Which Intervention Is the Most Appropriate? As will be discussed, catheter-based interventions differ as to how the obstructive atherosclerotic plaque is treated. Such differences have led to the concept that for certain types of plaques, one interventional technique may be superior to another. For example, if a plaque is heavily calcified, it may not yield to the dilating force of a balloon angioplasty catheter; because of its drilling capability, rotational atherectomy can be successful in this situation. As might be expected, information from the coronary angiogram is critical for characterizing lesions with regard to location, artery diameter, lesion length, severity, calcification, eccentricity, or ulceration and the presence of thrombus or vessel angulation. Once the lesion is characterized, a hierarchy of device preference can be developed (Fig. 3–2). Furthermore, there are circumstances wherein it is advantageous to use devices in combination to treat a single lesion. The synergistic use of devices is most sensible when each device provides a unique and necessary benefit for achieving a successful outcome. Of importance, however, is that in many instances, one device may be just as effective and safe as another. In such situations, other factors—for example, the physician's experience or preference—may influence device selection.

Alternative Therapies

An important component in the process of evaluating a patient for any therapy is to compare its value with that of alternative therapies.

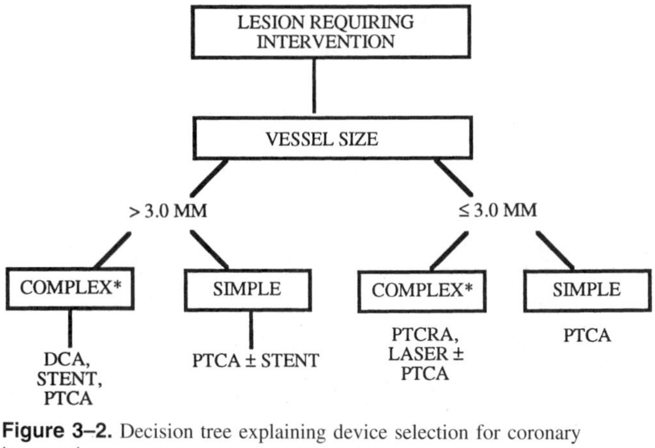

Figure 3–2. Decision tree explaining device selection for coronary intervention.

In the case of coronary interventions, alternative therapies are medical therapy and coronary bypass surgery. The advantages of medical therapy are ease of administration, low toxicity from the pharmacologic agents, and reasonable efficacy for relief of angina. For many patients with mild, stable angina, medical therapy provides results similar to those of coronary bypass in terms of survival and freedom from myocardial infarction.[8–12] In one randomized clinical trial, medical therapy was compared with balloon angioplasty for patients with stable angina and evidence of exercise-induced myocardial ischemia.[13] The results indicated that angioplasty was superior to medical therapy in relieving exercise-induced ischemia and the severity of angina. Balloon angioplasty has been compared with thrombolytic medical therapy in patients with acute myocardial infarction. Balloon angioplasty consistently reduces the frequency of recurrent angina after infarction, and there are trends toward a significant survival benefit, particularly for certain patient subsets.[14]

Balloon angioplasty has been extensively compared with coronary bypass surgery for patients with multivessel coronary artery disease and clinical indications for coronary revascularization. Several randomized clinical trials have reported equivalent outcomes with regard to rates of infarction or death over 1 and 3 years of follow-up.[15–18] Recurrent angina, repeat angioplasty procedures, crossover to coronary bypass surgery, and hospitalizations occur more commonly during follow-up among patients initially treated with balloon angioplasty.

When alternative treatment is considered, it is important to note that for some patients there is little choice. Many patients referred for catheter interventional therapy are those in whom medical therapy has been tried but has failed. Some form of revascularization is required for these patients. For patients with single-vessel disease, bypass surgery is rarely the initial choice. On the other hand, many patients with multivessel disease are excluded from catheter interventions for technical reasons, as noted earlier. In such situations, coronary artery bypass graft (CABG) is clearly the preferred means of revascularization.

Potential Benefits and Risks

By reducing the severity of coronary narrowing, each of the coronary interventional techniques has the potential of relieving myocardial ischemia. As a consequence, benefits for patients may include alleviation of angina and of objective manifestations of ischemia such as impaired flow reserve, disordered myocardial metabolism, and abnormal findings on electrocardiography (ECG), thallium imaging, or studies of left ventricular wall motion.[19–21] Balloon angioplasty has been evaluated extensively in patients with acute myocardial infarction. Angioplasty has been demonstrated to reestablish blood flow, relieve chest pain, improve cardiovascular hemodynamics, reduce infarct size, and augment survival.[14, 22–26]

The potential adverse effects of a catheter-based coronary intervention include complications known to be associated with cardiac catheterization. Death and the very serious complications of myocardial infarction and stroke, although rare (<0.5%), can result from coronary angiography alone without any coronary intervention. Less severe but more common complications that are associated with any invasive procedure include allergic reactions to contrast agents, renal failure, bleeding, and peripheral vascular damage or obstruction.

Certain complications occur more commonly with interventional techniques than with diagnostic invasive procedures. Because coronary interventions by nature involve placement of a device into a coronary artery, there is potential for trauma or damage to the artery targeted for therapy. Coronary arterial trauma can result in dissection of the coronary arterial wall and development of an intramural hematoma that can compress the arterial lumen. Luminal narrowing can also occur if thrombus forms at the site of trauma or if trauma results in an obstructive intimal flap. Exacerbation of luminal narrowing as a result of catheter intervention can cause abrupt total coronary occlusion and acute myocardial infarction. Fortunately, the incidence of complete coronary occlusion as a result of catheter intervention is typically less than 5%. The overall risk of acute infarction is approximately 4%, and that of death is 1%.[27] Furthermore, strategies such as prolonged balloon inflation, intracoronary stents, and coronary bypass surgery have been developed for managing abrupt closure. It follows that current guidelines limit the performance of coronary interventional procedures to facilities capable of providing immediate emergency coronary bypass surgery. *It is essential that the physician performing a catheter-based coronary intervention must always consider the possible consequences of acute coronary occlusion when considering patients for this therapy.* In certain circumstances, acute coronary occlusion would likely be fatal: for example, if the lesion targeted for intervention is in the only patent coronary artery supplying blood to the heart. Catheter intervention is attempted in such patients only in unusual circumstances in which other reasonable treatment options do not exist, and the patient and family are appraised of the potential consequences.

Peripheral arterial complications are more common after coronary interventional procedures than after invasive diagnostic ones. Because the dimensions of the catheters utilized for coronary intervention are larger than those used in diagnostic catheterization, the potential for damage of a peripheral artery is greater. The potential consequences of arterial trauma include obstruction, bleeding, and incomplete healing of the entry site wound. Also, coronary interventions require a greater intensity of anticoagulation, which further increases the incidence of bleeding, than do invasive diagnostic procedures.

Certain interventional procedures are associated with unique complications. For example, angioplasty balloon catheters can rupture and on occasion inject radiographic contrast into the arterial wall. Other specific complications include failure of the balloon to deflate or loss of a part of the balloon catheter system, such as fracture of the intracoronary guide wire. Fortunately, such complications have become exceedingly rare (<1%) as technology in balloon catheter design and manufacture have become more refined. Directional atherectomy has been associated with a higher incidence of arterial dissection, acute arterial closure, and myocardial infarction than has balloon angioplasty.[28–30] Rotational atherectomy can result in a decrease in or a transient cessation of coronary blood flow, owing to embolization in the distal coronary arterial microcirculation of debris that is created in the drilling process.[31–33] Each of the atherectomy procedures, as well as laser angioplasty, can cause perforation of a coronary artery and hemopericardium. This complication seems to be most common with laser angioplasty[34–36] and the extraction atherectomy device.[37, 38] Intracoronary stents do not cause direct coronary arterial trauma but can cause coronary thrombosis or embolization into the systemic arterial circulation.[39–42] Fortunately, these unique complications are uncommon but nevertheless are considered in the overall evaluation of the risk/benefit assessment for each coronary interventional device.

In the final analysis, judgment of patient suitability for catheter-based coronary intervention involves considering the answers to two questions: (1) What type and magnitude of improvement in the clinical status of the patient could be reasonably expected if each lesion targeted for revascularization is treated successfully? (2) What is the likely consequence if any artery targeted for intervention becomes occluded during the procedure? The responses to these questions need to be weighed together, along with consideration of the patient's clinical status and preference for a particular lifestyle and the relative value of alternative therapies, in arriving at a recommendation of whether to proceed with a coronary intervention.

CATHETER-BASED CORONARY ARTERY INTERVENTIONS

General Comments

Although the various coronary interventions differ in the approach for relieving coronary narrowing, they share certain features. Each is performed in the catheterization laboratory and requires all of the resources normally used for cardiac angiography and catheterization. The demands for coronary artery imaging exceed those of routine diagnostic cineangiography because on-line decisions, based on the appearance of lesions undergoing treatment, are made during the procedure. These added requirements necessitate upgrading of conventional radiographic imaging techniques with the addition of sophisticated videographic capability and of digitization and processing of videographic images.

Before the procedure, patients are premedicated with a sedative, an antihistamine, aspirin, and a calcium antagonist. Once arterial and venous access are obtained, intravenous heparin is used to achieve full anticoagulation. the dosage is adjusted to prolong the activated partial thromboplastin time to 300–350 sec. Results of investigations suggest that the addition of newer antiplatelet and antithrombin agents may further improve the results of coronary interventions in patients who are at increased risk for abrupt closure.[43–46]

Cineangiograms of the arteries targeted for treatment are then performed with the use of special "guiding" catheters that have lumen large enough to accommodate passage of the interventional device. Typically, a small (0.010- to 0.018-inch) flexible-tipped guide wire is next advanced under fluoroscopic guidance into the targeted coronary artery and across the lesion. This wire acts as a rail for placement of the interventional device into the coronary artery and across the lesion. The universal goals of each interventional device are to enlarge the narrowed arterial lumen to its normal diameter and not cause significant coronary arterial damage.

Once the lesion targeted for angioplasty is successfully treated (lesion obstruction causing <50% diameter reduction with normal anterograde flow), coronary cineangiography is repeated to document the outcome of the procedure. This aspect of coronary intervention—namely, that the results of the intervention are known immediately to the physician and patient—is unique to catheter-based revascularization procedures. Such information is not available for coronary artery bypass grafting.

For the majority of coronary interventions, access is obtained from the femoral artery and vein by means of vascular sheaths. These sheaths are removed at the bedside once the anticoagulant effects of heparin have diminished. For uncomplicated cases, patients are usually discharged the day after sheath removal. Discharge medications typically include an antiplatelet agent such as aspirin. Some physicians prescribe a calcium antagonist for 1 month to reduce the likelihood of postprocedural coronary spasm, although no available large-scale randomized trial results support this practice. A noninvasive stress test 2–4 weeks after the procedure aids in objectively evaluating the functional outcome of the procedure.

Balloon Angioplasty

Coronary balloon angioplasty was the first nonsurgical catheter-based technique capable of relieving atherosclerotic coronary narrowing in humans.[47] This procedure involves the use of a small balloon tipped catheter that dilates the diseased coronary artery segment. The balloon is cylindric and can vary in inflated diameter from 1.5 to 4.0 mm, and balloon lengths typically range from 10 to 40 mm. The balloon catheter includes a lumen for the coronary guide wire. As the catheter is advanced, it tracks over the wire until it straddles the narrowed region. Once properly positioned, the balloon is inflated by a hand-held inflation device to a pressure ranging from 1 to 20 bar (15–300 psi). The inflated balloon transiently obstructs coronary blood flow and, unless a well-developed coronary collateral circulation is present, results in myocardial ischemia. The duration of balloon inflation typically ranges from 60 to 180 sec. Manifestations of ischemia, such as chest pain and ECG repolarization abnormalities, usually resolve promptly when the balloon is deflated. Longer inflations without ischemia are possible in some patients with the use of balloon catheters that permit some degree of blood flow through the catheter itself.

Balloon inflation results in an increase in the internal and external diameters of the artery by stretching the artery and by compression, splitting, and remodeling of the plaque.[48] Microscopic dissection probably occurs in each instance of balloon angioplasty. Small degrees of macroscopic dissection, visible by coronary angiography, are detectable in many patients and are usually without any clinical consequences.

As balloon angioplasty technique and equipment have become more refined and physicians have become more knowledgeable about which patients are the most suitable candidates for the procedure, the success rate of balloon angioplasty has risen since its inception. Angiographic success, defined as achieving a residual narrowing of less than 50% with normal anterograde blood flow, is now achieved in 85%–95% of patient cohorts.[27, 28]

The incidence of abrupt coronary artery closure in the course of balloon angioplasty ranges from 3% to 10%; in about half of these instances, abrupt closure can be successfully treated with repeat but prolonged balloon inflation. Placement of an intracoronary stent (vida infra) is a very effective means of treating abrupt closure in patients in whom the target artery exceeds 3 mm in diameter and is not exceedingly tortuous. Overall, for patients with angina pectoris, balloon angioplasty is currently associated with a periprocedural mortality rate of 0%–1%, an acute myocardial infarction rate of 2%–4%, and an emergency CABG rate of 1%–3%.[26–28]

A major shortcoming of balloon angioplasty and of other coronary interventional techniques is the attrition that has been observed in clinical outcome after an initial successful procedure. Up to 35%–50% of patients in whom angioplasty is initially successful demonstrate recurrent narrowing, or "restenosis," of the treated lesion. Usually this recurrence develops within 6 months of the initial procedure. Approximately half the patients with restenosis experience angina pectoris again. Repeat angioplasty is feasible in such patients and is usually recommended before resorting to coronary bypass surgery.[49]

A limited number of randomized clinical trials have compared balloon angioplasty with alternative therapies for coronary artery disease. For patients with stable angina and evidence of exercise-induced ischemia, balloon angioplasty is superior to contemporary medical therapy with regard to the relief of exercise-induced ischemia assessed at 6-month follow-up.[13] Comparisons of the results of angioplasty with those of medical therapy in patients with multivessel coronary artery disease are lacking.

Several randomized clinical trials have compared angioplasty with CABG in selected patients with multivessel disease.[15–18] As of this writing, either procedure selected as the initial technique for revascularization has provided comparable results at 1- to 3-year follow-up with regard to the occurrence of death or myocardial infarction. Patients initially treated by angioplasty, however, are more likely to experience angina, require a subsequent hospitalization for additional revascularization, and cross over to the alternate therapy. The rate of repeat percutaneous transluminal coronary angioplasty (PTCA) is approximately 20%–40%, and that of subsequent CABG is about 20%. Approximately 50% of patients initially treated with PTCA are managed successfully with just the one initial procedure.

New Devices

In comparison with other catheter-based interventions, balloon angioplasty is technically simpler, is less expensive, and has had opportunities for procedural and equipment refinement. Certain new techniques such as stents complement rather than substitute for balloon angioplasty. In selected patients, stents increase the success rate of angioplasty, improve its safety profile, and enhance its durability. Other techniques, such as directional or rotational atherectomy and laser angioplasty, treat arterial narrowing by mechanisms different from those of balloon angioplasty. Nevertheless, they may be used in conjunction with angioplasty in greater numbers of coronary patients or to enhance the outcome over that achieved by angioplasty alone.

Directional Atherectomy

The principle underlying directional coronary atherectomy (DCA) is to shave off and extract layers of the coronary plaque. A unique catheter has been designed for this purpose, and after its evaluation in pathologic specimens, it was successfully utilized in patients.[50–52] The catheter includes a soft, tapered, flexible nose cone; a metal housing that contains a high-speed spinning cylindric cutter; and a long flexible shaft for delivery. Once the open "window" of the housing is positioned over the plaque, a balloon is inflated to further approximate the plaque into the window and stabilize or fix the device within the artery. The spinning cutter is then advanced across the plaque to shave or slice off a strip of the plaque. This tissue is trapped in the forward section, or nose cone, of the device. The balloon is then deflated, and the device is repositioned or rotated in such a way that additional radial or longitudinal plaque removal is possible.

An important feature of directional atherectomy is that sections of the plaque are removed. Thus this device can "debulk" plaque, which may be of special importance in instances when plaque volume is large. Also, the extracted sections are often large enough to allow histologic examination. Accordingly, an added benefit of directional atherectomy is the ability to analyze the pathologic composition of the tissue that causes coronary obstruction.

DCA has been demonstrated to reduce the severity of coronary narrowing with angiographic success rates varying from 83% to 91%.[28–30, 50, 51] Initial reports indicated the periprocedural rate of death was 1%; the rate of myocardial infarction, 2%; and need for emergency CABG, 4%.

Three randomized clinical trials have compared DCA with conventional balloon angioplasty.[28–30] The largest trial focused on patients with native vessel coronary artery disease.[28] This trial demonstrated that DCA resulted in an initial greater relief of coronary narrowing than did PTCA. The mean value of minimal lumen diameter after DCA was 2.02 mm, in comparison with 1.80 mm in PTCA-treated patients. During the initial hospitalization, however, DCA-treated patients were more likely to experience myocardial infarction. At 6-month follow-up, DCA patients had experienced a greater loss in the extent of initial improvement. The final lumen diameter of DCA-treated patients was slightly greater than that of PTCA-treated patients, and fewer DCA-treated patients experienced restenosis. The need for subsequent revascularization procedures, however, was similar in both groups. At 1 year of follow-up, however, the total mortality rate for directional atherectomy–treated patients was 2.2%, in comparison with 0.2% in patients assigned to balloon angioplasty.[52] Similar results were reported from a trial performed in Canada, in which only patients with lesions of the left anterior descending coronary artery were included in the investigation.[29] A more recent trial compared DCA and PTCA for patients with lesions within saphenous vein bypass grafts.[30] DCA resulted in a better angiographic outcome than did PTCA but was associated with more distal embolization. Criticisms of the initial trials of DCA have been that patients with excessively small arteries were included and that DCA was not performed in its most optimal manner. Additional trials comparing DCA with PTCA are now being conducted.

In view of the unique ability for DCA to actually remove plaque, there are several subsets of patients whose coronary lesions appear to be well suited for DCA. First, patients with lesions of large volume may be better treated with DCA than with PTCA.[53] Second, lesions at the origins of coronary arteries or of vein grafts or at bifurcations do not respond well to PTCA because of elasticity or plaque shifting. Debulking such lesions with DCA before PTCA appears to provide better results. Third, lesions that are eccentric can be selectively treated by DCA without excessive disruption of the nondiseased opposite arterial wall.

DCA does have certain limitations. Because of the large physical dimensions and rigidity of the DCA catheter, the use of DCA is limited to larger coronary arteries and vein grafts without acute angulations. Also, a substantial component of the mechanism by which DCA relieves narrowing cannot be ascribed to plaque removal. The "Dottering" effect of displacing the lesion by simply advancing the catheter through it and the consequences of inflating the balloon that is attached to the DCA catheter are likely responsible in part for its effectiveness.[54]

Rotational Atherectomy

Rotational atherectomy is based on the concept of debulking the atheromatous plaque by a process of drilling. Although different devices have been developed for this purpose, only one employing high speeds of rotation has gained clinical acceptance.[31–33] Like directional atherectomy and balloon angioplasty, the device, commercially known as the Rotablator, includes a central lumen to enable over-the-wire performance. Atherectomy is accomplished by advancing a small (1.25–2.50 mm), high-speed spinning bur into and through the plaque. The leading edge of the bur is coated with diamond microchips that ablate the plaque into minute particles that can pass through the coronary microcirculation. Sequential use of burs of increasing diameter results in stepwise enlargement of the coronary lumen while minimizing the embolic debris. Some patients may achieve adequate relief of coronary narrowing with rotational atherectomy alone, whereas others need supplemental balloon angioplasty. The optimal technique of performing this new procedure is the subject of investigation.

Initial observational reports indicate that rotational atherectomy alone can reduce coronary narrowing from 78% to 40%.[33] Supplementing rotational atherectomy with balloon angioplasty results in further improvement and a final result better than that achievable by balloon angioplasty alone. In this regard, rotational atherectomy and balloon angioplasty might be considered complementary or even synergistic procedures.

Rotational atherectomy is of special value for certain lesions known to be problematic for balloon angioplasty. Such lesions include those that are rigid or hard, wherein the balloon catheter cannot cross the narrowing. Also, lesions located at osteal sites and lesions that are long respond particularly well to rotational atherectomy but poorly to balloon angioplasty. Eccentric lesions also appear well suited for rotational atherectomy as the device preferentially ablates plaque rather than normal arterial wall tissue.

Results of early observational investigations suggested that rotational atherectomy followed by balloon angioplasty can achieve larger lumens with less arterial wall disruption and trauma than can balloon angioplasty alone.[55] This benefit of rotational atherectomy has been confirmed by a recent randomized clinical trial.[56] In this investigation, rotational atherectomy achieved a higher initial success rate than did balloon angioplasty. To date, no differences between the two approaches have been noted in the rates of lesion recurrence.

The complications that may be experienced with rotational atherectomy are similar to those associated with balloon angioplasty. There are two concerns, however, that are more specific to rotational atherectomy than to PTCA. The debris that is generated from plaque ablation can cause obstruction of the coronary microcirculation. The mechanism of obstruction appears to be a combination of mechanical blockade in addition to intense vasospasm. Obstruction can be severe enough to cause both complete termination of anterograde coronary blood flow and significant myocardial ischemia. Typically, this no-flow phenomenon is transient and can be attenuated by careful attention to technique, appropriate selection of patients, and the use of potent vasodilating pharmacologic agents.[57] This potential for embolization has discouraged the use of rotational atherectomy in coronary venous bypass grafts, in which obstructions are commonly composed of very friable tissue. An uncommon but possible consequence of rotational atherectomy is coronary arterial perforation, which has been reported in 1.5% of patients. Again, with attention to technique, the incidence of this undesirable complication can be minimized but not eliminated.

The exact role of rotational atherectomy in relation to other coronary interventions remains to be clarified. For type B and C lesions—that is, those with complex anatomic features—employing rotational atherectomy as the initial treatment may offer an advantage over balloon angioplasty. It is unquestionable that rotational atherectomy allows successful catheter-based treatment of the very complex coronary lesions that have been untreatable by balloon angioplasty alone.

Because the maximum bur size is 2.5 mm, rotational atherectomy is therapy largely directed to coronary arterial segments 3.25 mm in length and less. Directional atherectomy and the use of intracoronary stents are more suitable for arterial or vein grafts 3.5 mm and larger.

Extraction Atherectomy

The transluminal extraction catheter (TEC) has a forward-facing rotating blade that cuts tissue. Fragments are aspirated into the catheter and captured in a vacuum bottle. As in other devices, the catheter is advanced over a guide wire. The device ranges in diameter from 5.5 to 7.5 French. Because the device cannot distinguish nondiseased from diseased arterial wall, it has the potential of cutting either. To prevent coronary perforation, the TEC catheter must be undersized in relation to the normal diameter of the vessel to be treated. Additional balloon angioplasty is thus required in order to maximize relief of coronary narrowing.

Thus far, the utility of extraction atherectomy can be judged only from observational reports.[37, 38, 58] Extraction atherectomy can reduce the degree of stenosis to about 50%–60%. Rates of success range from 30% to 50%. Complications include myocardial infarction (2%) and death (2%). As might be anticipated, the rate of arterial perforation is higher with the TEC in extraction atherectomy than with devices used in other therapies.

Because of the unique ability of the device to extract substantial quantities of tissue and its forward-cutting ability, its use has been directed to the treatment of saphenous vein aortocoronary bypass grafts.[37, 38] Atherosclerotic disease in grafts frequently takes the form of a loose grumous material often associated with substantial amounts of thrombus. Although the results of TEC use in this setting have been mixed, it may offer an advantage in comparison with other devices.

Treatment of degenerated aortocoronary bypass grafts has been the primary indication for the TEC. Some investigators have proposed its use in native coronary arteries, particularly in the presence of intraluminal thrombus.[59] No comparative clinical trials, however, have yet defined a superior role of the TEC over other available devices.

Laser Angioplasty

The transmission of laser energy to the tip of a catheter enables vaporization of atherosclerotic coronary arterial lesions. In the most frequently used catheter, pulsed excimer laser is used for tissue ablation. The laser catheter is advanced over a coronary guide wire up to the area of narrowing. Laser energy is then applied as the catheter is intermittently advanced through the plaque. With currently available equipment, laser angioplasty is highly successful in increasing the arterial intimal lumen diameter, but the magnitude of this improvement is limited. Thus in contrast to balloon angioplasty and atherectomy devices, use of laser alone seldom results in a residual stenosis of less than 50% diameter reduction. Consequently, balloon angioplasty is required in most cases.[34, 35] When laser is coupled with balloon angioplasty, success rates may exceed 90%. The frequency and types of complications associated with laser angioplasty are similar to those of balloon angioplasty except that the incidence of arterial dissection and perforation are slightly higher (16% and 1%, respectively).[36]

Osteal, long, and rigid lesions may be well suited for laser angioplasty.[60, 61] The development of an eccentric laser may be of value for eccentric and bifurcation lesions. The greatest contribution of laser angioplasty may be the successful treatment of chronic total coronary occlusions. Preliminary reports support the feasibility of a laser wire for this purpose but suggest that further refinements will be required in order to enhance efficacy and reduce the risk of perforation.[62]

Intracoronary Stents

Intracoronary stents are cylindric metallic permanent prostheses that are placed into a narrowed coronary segment. The scaffolding effect of a stent increases the dimension of the arterial lumen and makes the lumen more circular than would be achieved otherwise. Two additional consequences of stents are noteworthy: First, stents effectively treat intimal flaps that normally result from balloon angioplasty and protrude into the arterial lumen; these small tissue fragments are sandwiched between the stent and the arterial wall. Furthermore, a stent can seal fissures and dissections of the arterial wall that might otherwise lead to the formation of an intramural hematoma. Both these actions contribute to decreasing the incidence of abrupt coronary closure after PTCA.

Most stents require an angioplasty balloon catheter for deployment. These stents are mounted on the balloon either by the manufacturer or by the physician operator. The stent/balloon catheter is advanced to the lesion to be stented, and when in position, the stent delivery balloon is inflated. Usually, lesions are pre-dilated with a traditional angioplasty balloon catheter before stent delivery in order to facilitate passage and positioning of the stent-delivering catheter. Appropriate apposition of the stent to the arterial wall is achieved by a subsequent inflation of a high-pressure angioplasty balloon within the stent. Some stents are self-expanding, and with others, a different type of stent delivery system is used.

Currently, all stents are made of metal and thus create a potential nidus for thrombus formation. Stent thrombosis has been observed and can progress to complete coronary artery occlusion and myocardial infarction. Typically, this process is rapid, and abrupt closure often results in acute myocardial infarction. Because of this thrombotic potential, current recommendations are that patients receiving stents should undergo full anticoagulation with heparin and then warfarin for at least 2 months in addition to treatment with antiplatelet agents such as aspirin and dipyridamole. The use of intensive anticoagulant therapy increases the risk for bleeding and incomplete wound healing after the coronary interventional procedure. Also, the length of hospital stay is longer after stent placement than after other interventions. Results of investigations have suggested that the incidence of stent thrombosis may be effectively minimized with the use of ticlopidine instead of warfarin anticoagulation.[63] A formal randomized trial testing this hypothesis has not been completed, and concerns about the safety profile of ticlopidine exist.

Stents are usually used, not for the primary treatment of coronary narrowing, but rather as an adjunct to achieve an improved acute and long-term result. Consequently, stent placement typically follows the initial use of balloon angioplasty or atherectomy. Another limitation of stents is that their use is currently limited to coronary arteries 3 mm or larger in diameter. Stent placement into smaller arteries is feasible, but the incidence of stent thrombosis is higher than observed in larger arteries.

In two randomized clinical trials, a strategy of balloon angioplasty alone has been compared with balloon angioplasty followed by stent placement.[64, 65] Results of both strategies indicated convincingly that the routine use of stents resulted in an increase in the minimal lumen diameter immediately after the procedure, a lower rate of acute coronary occlusion, and, at 6-month follow-up, a larger minimal lumen diameter. Also, fewer patients experienced lesion recurrence or needed to repeat revascularization procedures. These two randomized clinical trials evaluated the same stent (Palmaz-Schatz Balloon Expandable Stent, Johnson and Johnson). Although other stents are available for use, each differs in design and potentially in performance.[66] Accordingly, it may be inappropriate to extrapolate the results of one stent to another. Although stents are also deployed for lesions located within aortocoronary vein grafts, confirmation of benefit from stents in these conduits is not yet available.

MATCHING THE LESION WITH THE PATIENT

Consideration of Specific Lesion Features

The concept of lesion specific therapy is based on the principle that certain interventional devices have functional or physical characteristics that render them particularly suitable for certain types of coronary lesions. For example, rotational atherectomy is the procedure of choice for significantly calcified lesions. The bur is capable of drilling through calcium, whereas other devices may be unable to cross such lesions. Rotational atherectomy also is particularly well suited for treating long lesions, diffuse disease, and ostial lesions. Laser angioplasty may also be effective for such lesions. Certain lesions can be crossed with a balloon catheter but do not respond well to balloon dilation because of excessive plaque volume or elasticity. Lesions of this type need to be debulked, and atherectomy devices appear to be most efficacious. Certain ostial and bifurcation lesions fall into this category. As noted previously, directional atherectomy and stents are well suited for large vessels and may be used in combination in this setting.

Influence of the Extent of Coronary Artery Disease

Treatment strategies for patients with coronary artery disease fall into three main categories: medical therapy, catheter-based interventions, and coronary bypass surgery. The extent of coronary disease influences the selection among these options. Coronary bypass surgery is rarely the initial treatment choice for patients with single-vessel disease. In most such patients, medical therapy or catheter-based interventions are usually effective. Furthermore, with the exception of left main coronary artery disease, there are no convincing data that indicate that bypass surgery confers a survival benefit for such patients. Thus the issue of treatment selection for patients with single-vessel disease focuses on a choice between medical therapy and a coronary interventional procedure. At this point, the magnitude of symptoms and ischemia, the response to medical initial therapy, and coronary and left ventriculographic features are each considered. If medical therapy has been unsuccessful in restoring the patient to an acceptable quality of life, catheter interventions should certainly be considered. However, if the coronary disease present does not put at risk a substantial area of myocardium, if the magnitude of ischemia is small, and if symptoms do not significantly disrupt patient activities, medical therapy may be most appropriate. Under certain circumstances, coronary intervention may be appropriate in asymptomatic patients who demonstrate substantial ischemia on noninvasive testing. Examples of such patients include those who have experienced a recent myocardial infarction and those who, because of the nature of their work, cannot be employed if they demonstrate even silent ischemia.

Patients with multivessel coronary disease who demonstrate significant symptoms or ischemia are considered candidates for revascularization. Those with left main disease and those with three-vessel disease with impaired left ventricular function are selected for bypass surgery on the basis of the improved survival known to be associated with that therapy. As noted previously, a substantial proportion of patients with multivessel disease demonstrate chronic total occlusion of at least one coronary artery, which warrants revascularization. In view of the limited ability of catheter-based interventions to treat such lesions successfully, surgery is selected for these patients. For the remaining patients, current information suggests that either catheter-based intervention or surgery is an acceptable choice.

Considerations of Clinical Presentation

Patients with coronary artery disease can vary considerably in clinical presentation. At one extreme are patients who are asymptomatic, and at the other extreme are patients who present with acute myocardial infarction or sudden death. As noted previously, the severity of symptoms and the prognosis associated with the specific clinical presentation are significant factors in the assessment of the appropriateness of catheter-based interventional therapy.

Certain coronary syndromes have unique influences on the outcome of coronary interventions. Early reports of balloon angioplasty indicated that immediate and late procedural outcomes were less favorable for patients with unstable angina than for patients with stable angina.[67, 68] The incidence of initial procedural success was lower and that of complications was higher in patients with at-rest angina. Also, unstable angina was recognized as a risk factor for developing restenosis. More recently, the results of balloon angioplasty for patients with unstable angina have matched or exceeded those of patients with stable angina, probably as a result of refinements in technique and equipment coupled with the more aggressive use of heparin anticoagulation therapy. Additional benefits may be derived from the adjunctive use of new antiplatelet and antithrombin agents.

Coronary interventional therapy may play a special role for patients with acute myocardial infarction. Information gained from emergency coronary angiograms demonstrated that the mechanism of acute myocardial infarction is acute coronary occlusion with fresh thrombus superimposed on a fissured atherosclerotic plaque.[69] In this setting, coronary intervention, particularly balloon angioplasty, has the ability not only to relieve plaque narrowing but to restore coronary blood flow. The magnitude of flow improvement appears to be greater than that which can be achieved by thrombolytic therapy. Furthermore, if resources are available, flow may be restored more rapidly by balloon angioplasty than by medical therapy. Coronary bypass surgery has also been shown to be feasible in the setting of acute myocardial infarction.[70] Under usual clinical circumstances, however, the time required for surgery to be initiated and completed is too long to achieve any significant degree of myocardial salvage.

REFERENCES

1. Parmley WW: Prevalence and clinical significance of silent myocardial ischemia. Circulation 1989; 80:IV-68–IV-73.
2. Pepine CJ, Allen HD, Bashore TM, et al: ACC/AHA guidelines for cardiac catheterization and cardiac catheterization laboratories. Circulation 1991; 84:2213–2247.
3. Wohlgelernter D, Cleman M, Highman HA, Zaret BL: Percutaneous transluminal coronary angioplasty of the "culprit lesion" for management of unstable angina pectoris in patient with multivessel coronary artery disease. Am J of Cardiol 1986; 58:460–464.
4. The TIMI Study Group: Comparison of invasive and conservative strategies after treatment with intravenous tissue plasminogen activator in acute myocardial infarction. Results of the Thrombolysis in Myocardial Infarction (TIMI) II Trial. N Engl J Med 1989; 310:618–627.
5. Gould KL, Hamilton GW, Lipscomb K, et al: Method for assessing stress-induced regional malperfusion during coronary arteriography. Experimental validation and clinical application. Am J Cardiol 1974; 34:557–563.
6. Segal J, Kern MJ, Scott NA, et al: Alterations in phasic coronary artery flow velocity in humans during percutaneous coronary angioplasty. J Am Coll Cardiol 1992; 20:276–286.

7. Rogers WJ, Alderman EL, Chaitman BR, et al: Bypass Angioplasty Revascularization Investigation (BARI): Baseline Clinical and Angiographic Data. Am J Cardiol 1995,75:9C–17C.
8. Alderman EL, Bourassa M, Cohen LS, et al: Ten-year follow-up of survival and myocardial infarction in the randomized Coronary Artery Surgery Study. Circulation 1990; 82:1629–1646.
9. The Veterans Administration Coronary Artery Bypass Surgery Cooperative Study Group: Eleven-year survival in the Veterans Administration randomized trial of coronary bypass surgery for unstable angina. N Engl J Med 1984; 311:1333–1339.
10. The VA Coronary Artery Bypass Surgery Cooperative Study Group: Eighteen-year follow-up in the Veterans Affairs Cooperative Study of Coronary Artery Bypass Surgery for Stable Angina. Circulation 1992; 86:121–130.
11. Yusuf S, Zucker D, Peruzzi P, et al: Effect of coronary artery bypass graft surgery on survival: Overview of 10-year results from randomized trials by the Coronary Artery Bypass Graft Trialist Collaboration. Lancet 1994; 344:563–570.
12. Varnauskas E: Twelve-year follow-up of survival in the Randomized European Coronary Surgery. N Engl J Med 1988; 319:332–337.
13. Parisi AF, Folland ED, Harrigan P: A comparison of angioplasty with medical therapy in the treatment of single vessel coronary artery disease. N Engl J Med 1991; 326:10–16.
14. Michaels KB, Yusuf S: Does PTCA in acute myocardial infarction affect mortality and reinfarction rates? A quantitative overview (meta-analysis) of the randomized clinical trials. Circulation 1995; 91:476–485.
15. King SB, Lembo JN, Weintraub WS, et al: A randomized trial comparing coronary angioplasty with coronary bypass surgery. N Engl J Med 1944; 331:1044–1050.
16. Coronary angioplasty versus coronary artery bypass surgery: The Randomized Intervention Treatment of Angina (RITA) Trial. Lancet 1993; 341:573–580.
17. Rodriguez A, Boullon F, Perez-Balino N, et al: Argentine randomized trial of percutaneous transluminal coronary angioplasty versus coronary artery bypass surgery in multivessel disease (ERACI): In-hospital results and 1-year follow-up. J Am Coll Cardiol 1993; 22:1060–1067.
18. Hamm CW, Reimers J, Ischinger T, et al: A randomized study of coronary angioplasty compared with bypass surgery in patients with symptomatic multivessel coronary disease. German Angioplasty Bypass Surgery Investigation (GABI). N Engl J Med 1994; 331:1037–1043.
19. Williams DO, Riley RS, Singh AK, Most AS: Coronary circulatory dynamics before and after successful coronary angioplasty. J Am Coll Cardiol 1983; 1:1268–1272.
20. Irzel HO, Nuesch K, Gruntzig AR, Luetolt UM: Short and long-term changes in myocardial perfusion after percutaneous transluminal coronary angioplasty assessed by thallium-201 exercise scintigraphy. Circulation 1981; 63:1001–1007.
21. Fioretti PM, Pozzoli MM, Ilmer B, et al: Exercise echocardiography versus thallium-201 SPECT for assessing patients before and after PTCA. Eur Heart J 1992; 13:213–219.
22. O'Keefe JH Jr, Rutherford BD, McLonahay DR, et al: Early and late results of coronary angioplasty without antecedent thrombolytic therapy for acute myocardial infarction. Am J Cardiol 1989; 64:1221–1230.
23. Lee L, Bates ER, Pitt B, et al: Percutaneous transluminal coronary angioplasty improves survival in acute myocardial infarction complicated by cardiogenic shock. Circulation 1988; 78:1245–1251.
24. Williams DO, Ruocco NA, Formans and TIMI Investigators: Coronary angioplasty following recombinant tissue-type plasminogen activator in acute myocardial infarction: A report from the Thrombolysis in Myocardial Infarction Trial. J Am Coll Cardiol 1987; 10:45B–50B.
25. Gibbons R, Holmes DR, Reeder GS, et al: Immediate angioplasty compared with administration of a thrombolytic agent followed by conservative treatment for myocardial infarction. N Engl J Med 1993; 328:685–691.
26. O'Neill W, Timmis GC, Bourdillon PD, et al: A prospective randomized clinical trial of intracoronary streptokinase versus coronary angioplasty for acute myocardial infarction. N Engl J Med 1986; 314:812–818.
27. Detre K, Holubuv R, Kelsey S, et al: Percutaneous transluminal coronary angioplasty in 1985–1986 and 1977–1981. The National Heart, Lung, and Blood Institute Registry. N Engl J Med 1988; 318:265–270.
28. Topol EJ, Leya F, Pinkerton CA, et al: A comparison of directional atherectomy with coronary angioplasty in patients with coronary artery disease. The CAVEAT Study Group. N Engl J Med 1993; 329:221–227.
29. Adelman AG, Cohen EA, Kimball BP, et al: A comparison of directional atherectomy with balloon angioplasty for lesions of the left anterior descending coronary artery. N Engl J Med 1993; 329:228–233.
30. Holmes DR Jr, Topol EJ, Califf RM, et al: A multicenter, randomized trial of coronary angioplasty versus directional atherectomy for patients with saphenous vein bypass graft lesions. Circulation 1995; 91:1966–1974.
31. Warth DC, Leon MB, O'Neill W, et al: Rotational atherectomy multicenter registry: acute results, complications and 6-month angiographic follow-up in 709 patients. J Am Coll Cardiol 1994; 24:641–648.
32. Ellis SG, Popma JJ, Burchbinder M, et al: Relation of clinical presentation stenosis morphology and operator technique to the procedural results of rotational atherectomy and rotational atherectomy–facilitated angioplasty. Circulation 1994,89:882–892.
33. Safian RD, Niazi KA, Strzelecki M, et al: Detailed angiographic analysis of high-speed mechanical rotational atherectomy in human coronary arteries. Circulation 1993; 88: 961–968.
34. Litvack F, Eigler N, Margolis J, et al: Percutaneous excimer laser coronary angioplasty: results in the first consecutive 3,000 patients. J Am Coll Cardiol 1994; 23:323–329.
35. Bittl JA, Ryan JJ Jr, Keany JF Jr, et al: Coronary artery perforation during excimer laser coronary angioplasty. The percutaneous excimer laser coronary angioplasty registry. J Am Coll Cardiol 1993; 21:1158–1165.
36. Gnazzal ZM, Hearn JA, Litvack F, et al: Morphologic predictors of acute complications after percutaneous excimer laser coronary angioplasty. Results of a comprehensive angiographic analysis: importance of the eccentricity index. Circulation 1992; 86:820–827.
37. Twidale N, Barth CW III, Kipperman KM, et al: Acute results and long-term outcome of transluminal extraction catheter atherectomy for saphenous vein graft stenoses. Cathet Cardiovasc Diag 1994; 31:187–191.
38. Safian RD, Grines CL, May MA, et al: Clinical and angiographic results of transluminal coronary atherectomy in saphenous vein bypass grafts. Circulation 1994; 84:302–312.
39. Eeckhout E, Goy JJ, Vogt P, et al: Complications and follow-up after intracoronary stenting: critical analysis of a 6-year single-center experience. Am Heart J 1994; 172:262–272.
40. Berder V, Bedossa M, Gras D, et al: Retrieval of lost coronary stent from the descending aorta using a PTCA balloon and biopsy forceps. Cathet Cardiovasc Diagn 1993; 28:351–353.
41. Nath FC, Muller DW, Ellis SG, et al: Thrombosis of a flexible coil coronary stent: frequency, predictors and clinical outcome. J Am Coll Cardiol 1993; 21:622–627.
42. Haude M, Erbel R, Issa M, et al: Subacute thrombotic complications after intracoronary implantation of Palmaz-Schatz stents. Am Heart J 1993; 126:15–22.
43. The EPIC Investigators: Use of monoclonal antibody directed against the platelet glycoprotein IIb/IIIa receptor in high-risk coronary angioplasty. N Engl J Med 1994:330:956–961.
44. Tcheng JE, Harrington RA, Kottke-Marchant K, et al: Multicenter, randomized, double-blind, placebo-controlled trial of the platelet integrin glycoprotein IIb/IIIa blocker Integrelin in elective coronary intervention. Circulation 1995; 91:2151–2157.
45. Topol EJ, Bonan R, Jeritt D, et al: Use of a direct antithrombin hirulog, in place of heparin during coronary angioplasty. Circulation 1993; 87:1622–1629.
46. Van den Bos AA, Deckers JW, Hegndrickx GR, et al: Safety and efficacy of recombinant hirudin (CGP 39 393) versus heparin in patients with unstable angina undergoing coronary angioplasty. Circulation 1993; 88:2058–2066.
47. Gruntzig A, Senning A, Siegenthaler W: Nonoperative dilation of coronary artery stenosis. N Engl J Med 1979; 301:61–68.
48. Faxon DP, Sanborn TA, Haudenschild CC: Mechanism of angioplasty and its relation to restenosis. Am J Cardiol 1987; 60:5B–9B.
49. Williams DO, Gruntzig AR, Kent KM, et al: Efficacy of repeat percutaneous transluminal coronary angioplasty for coronary restenosis. Am J Cardiol 1984; 53:32B–35B.
50. Baim DS, Hinohara T, Holmes D, et al: Results of directional coronary atherectomy during multicenter preapproval testing. The U.S. Directional Coronary Atherectomy Investigator Group. Am J Cardiol 1993; 72:6E–11E.
51. Popma JJ, Mintz GS, Satler LF, et al: Clinical and angiographic outcome after directional coronary atherectomy. A qualitative and quantitative analysis using coronary arteriography and intravascular ultrasound. Am J Cardiol 1993; 72:55E–64E.
52. Elliot JM, Berdan LG, Holmes DR, et al: One-year follow-up in the Coronary Angioplasty versus Excisional Atherectomy Trial (CAVEAT I). Circulation 1995; 91:2158–2166.

53. Holmes DR Jr, Topol EJ, Adelman AG, et al: Randomized trials of directional coronary atherectomy: implications for clinical practice and future investigation. J Am Coll Cardiol 1994; 24:431–439.
54. Braden GA, Herrington DM, Downes TR, et al: Qualitative and quantitative contracts in the mechanisms of lumen enlargement by coronary balloon angioplasty and directional coronary atherectomy. J Am Coll Cardiol 1994; 23:40–48.
55. Burkey DC, Sharaf BL, Miele NJ, Williams DO: Superior outcome with rotational atherectomy combined with balloon angioplasty compared to balloon angioplasty along: Results of a case control study. Am J Coll Cardiol 1995; 25:96A.
56. Vandormel M, Reifart N, Preuster W, et al: Six month follow-up results following excimer laser angioplasty, rotational atherectomy and balloon angioplasty for complex lesions: ERBAC Study. Circulation 1994; 90:213.
57. Piana RN, Paik GY, Mosucci M, et al: Incidence and treatment of "no-reflow" after percutaneous coronary intervention. Circulation 1994; 89:2514–2518.
58. Popma JJ, Leon MD, Mintz GS, et al: Results of coronary angioplasty using the transluminal extraction catheter. Am J Cardiol 1992; 27:1526–1532.
59. Lasorda DM, Incorrati DL, Randall RR: Extraction atherectomy during myocardial infarction in a patient with prior coronary artery bypass surgery. Cathet Cardiovasc Diagn 1992; 26:117–121.
60. Cook SL, Eigler NL, Shefer A, et al: Percutaneous excimer laser coronary angioplasty of lesions not ideal for balloon angioplasty. Circulation 1991; 84:632–643.
61. Lawson CS, Cooper IC, Webb-Peploe MM: Initial experience with excimer laser angioplasty for coronary osteal stenoses. Br Heart J 1993; 69:255–259.
62. Henson KD, Leon MD, Pepma JJ, et al: Treatment of refractory coronary occlusions with a new excimer laser catheter: preliminary clinical observations. Coron Artery Dis 1993; 4:1001–1006.
63. Morice MC: Advances in post stenting medication protocol. J Invasive Cardiol 1995; 7:32A–35A.
64. Fischman DL, Leon MB, Baim DS, et al: A randomized comparison of coronary stent placement and balloon angioplasty in the treatment of coronary artery disease. N Engl J Med 1994; 331:496–501.
65. Serruys PW, deJaegere P, Kiemeneij F, et al: A comparison of balloon expandable stent implantation with balloon angioplasty in patients with coronary artery disease. N Engl J Med 1994; 331:489–495.
66. Serruys PW, Strauss BH, Beatt KJ, et al: Angiographic follow-up after placement of a self expanding coronary artery stent. N Engl J Med 1991; 324:13–17.
67. Bentivoglio LG, Holubkov R, Kelsey SF, et al: Short and long term outcome of percutaneous transluminal coronary angioplasty in unstable vs. stable angina pectoris: a report from the 1985–1986 NHLBI PTCA Registry. Cath and Cardiovasc Diag 1991; 23:227–238.
68. Kamp O, Beatt KJ, de Feyter PJ, et al: Short-, medium-, and long-term follow-up after percutaneous transluminal coronary angioplasty for stable and unstable angina pectoris. Am Heart J 1989; 117:991–996.
69. Fuster V, Badimon JJ, Chesebro JH: The pathogenesis of coronary artery disease and the acute coronary syndromes. N Engl J Med 1992; 326:242–225, 310–318.
70. DeWood MA, Notske RN, Berg R Jr, et al: Medical and surgical management of early Q wave myocardial infarction. 1. Effects of surgical reperfusion on survival, recurrent myocardial infarction, sudden death and functional class at 10 or more years of follow-up. J Am Coll Cardiol 1989; 14:65–77.

4 Ischemic Heart Disease: Surgical Options

Allen J. Solomon, MD
Bernard J. Gersh, MB ChB, DPhil, FRCP

Since its introduction in the 1960s, coronary bypass graft (CABG) surgery has undergone intense scrutiny.[1] In the 1970s, three large multicenter randomized trials evaluated the role of initial CABG compared with initial medical therapy in the treatment of chronic stable angina.[2–6] The decade of the 1980s saw more widespread use of the internal thoracic artery graft and improved myocardial preservation as well as improvements in cardiac anesthesia, preoperative care, and postoperative care. In the 1990s, six randomized clinical trials have been completed comparing the efficacy of CABG with percutaneous transluminal coronary angioplasty (PTCA) in patients with single-vessel and multivessel coronary artery disease.[7–12]

Currently, nearly 1 in every 1000 persons in the United States undergoes CABG each year.[13] The patient population undergoing CABG in the 1990s is changing in comparison with earlier cohorts. Specifically, they are older; they are more likely to be women; and they frequently have impaired left ventricular function, previous cardiovascular surgery, or multiple comorbid conditions (peripheral vascular disease, cerebrovascular disease, or diabetes mellitus). Despite this, the operative mortality is unchanged or only slightly increased.

As the population undergoing coronary bypass surgery changes, a marked regional variability in rates of use has been observed.[14] Specifically, the age-adjusted rate of coronary artery bypass graft surgery in 1989 in California was 27% higher than in New York and 80% higher than in three Canadian provinces combined. Moreover, women are less likely to undergo coronary bypass than are men, although it has not been clearly established whether this reflects overuse in men or underuse in women.[15, 16] In addition, rates of surgery are higher for whites than for blacks, even within the same system of health care delivery.[17] The explanations are multifactorial and include access to health care, socioeconomic status, and the patient's and physician's attitudes and expectations.

COMPARISON WITH MEDICAL THERAPY

In the 1970s, three large multicenter randomized trials compared a strategy of initial CABG surgery with initial medical therapy[2–6] (Table 4–1). Although much has been made about the differences between these trials, their consistencies deserve greater emphasis. Specifically, the sicker the patient (based on the severity of ischemia,

TABLE 4–1. PATIENT DEMOGRAPHICS FROM THE THREE RANDOMIZED TRIALS OF CORONARY ARTERY BYPASS GRAFT SURGERY

	Veterans Administration Cooperative Study	European Coronary Surgery Study	Coronary Artery Surgery Study
Enrollment	1972–1974	1973–1976	1975–1979
Number of patients	686	767	780
Age (years)	No limit	<65	≤65
Gender	100% male	100% male	90% male
Number of discussed vessels	≥1	≥2	≥1
Ejection fraction	≥0.25	≥0.50	≥0.35
Class III–IV angina	58%	42%	0%

the number of vessels diseased, and the presence of left ventricular dysfunction), the greater the survival benefit of surgery over medical therapy. The relevance of these trials to current practice has been questioned, because by and large these trials antedated the use of the internal thoracic artery, platelet inhibitor therapy, aggressive risk factor modification, and comprehensive medical therapy. Moreover, few women were included. Nonetheless, it is unlikely that coronary bypass surgery will ever again be subjected to a randomized trial in comparison with medical therapy alone. Therefore, although surgical and medical therapy have changed considerably since the completion of these trials, their results still provide a reference standard and a qualitative approach to the indications for coronary revascularization.

The Veterans Administration Cooperative Study (VACS)[2] randomized 686 male patients, with at least 6 months of stable angina, between 1972 and 1974. Patients had evidence of coronary artery disease in one or more vessels and a left ventricular ejection fraction greater than or equal to 25%. The severity of angina was New York Heart Association (NYHA) class III or class IV in 58% of the population studied. Patients with a recent myocardial infarction, diastolic hypertension, uncompensated congestive heart failure, unstable angina, or left ventricular aneurysm were excluded from the trial.

After 11 years of follow-up, no significant difference in overall mortality was observed in patients treated with initial CABG compared with medical therapy.[18] However, a mortality advantage with surgery was observed in specific subsets. Patients with left main coronary artery disease or three-vessel coronary artery disease with impaired left ventricular function had an improved survival when randomized to an initial surgical approach (Fig. 4–1). The survival advantage decreased, however, between the 7th and 11th postoperative years.

From 1973 to 1976, the European Coronary Surgery Study (ECSS) Group[4] randomized 767 men younger than 65 years, with more than 3 months of angina, to initial surgery or initial medical treatment. Patients were included if they had at least two-vessel coronary artery disease and an ejection fraction of at least 50%. Forty-two percent of the patients had Canadian Cardiovascular Society (CCS) class III angina.

Unlike the VACS and the Coronary Artery Surgery Study (CASS), the ECSS resulted in an overall survival advantage for patients randomized to an initial surgical approach[19] (Fig. 4–2). In addition, new subsets of patients yielded a survival advantage. Patients with three-vessel coronary artery disease and normal left ventricular func-

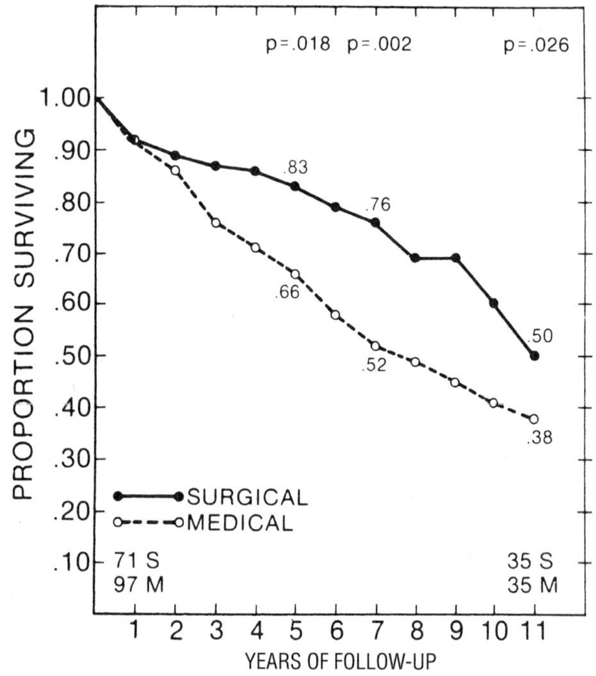

Figure 4–1. Eleven-year cumulative survival in the Veterans Administration Cooperative Study according to angiographic risk. Angiographic high risk was defined as three-vessel coronary artery disease plus left ventricular dysfunction. *Abbreviations:* S, surgical treatment; M, medical treatment. (From the Veterans Administration Coronary Artery Bypass Surgery Cooperative Study Group: Eleven-year survival in the Veterans Administration Randomized Trial of Coronary Bypass Surgery for Stable Angina. N Engl J Med 1984; 311:1333–1339.)

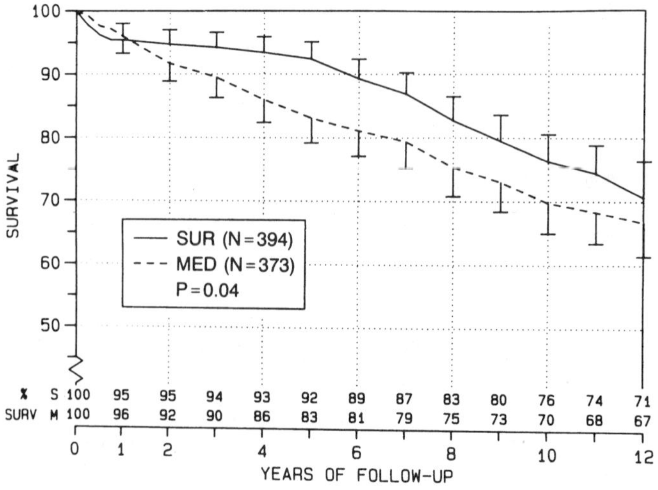

Figure 4–2. Twelve-year cumulative survival in the European Coronary Surgery Study for all patients randomized to initial surgical treatment (SUR, S) or initial medical treatment (MED, M). (From Varnauskas E, European Coronary Surgery Study Group: Twelve-year follow-up of survival in the randomized European Coronary Surgery Study. N Engl J Med 1988; 319:332–337.)

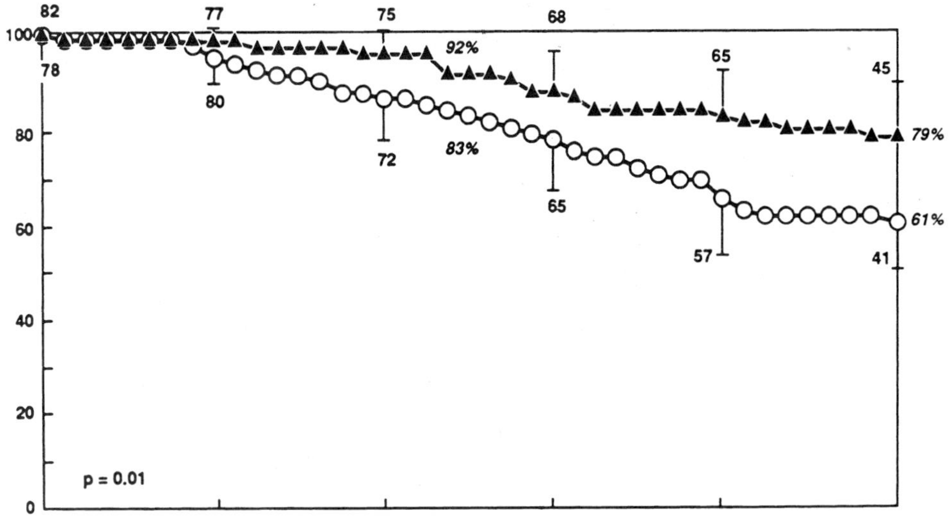

Figure 4–3. Ten-year cumulative survival in the Coronary Artery Surgery Study for patients with an ejection fraction of less than 0.50 randomized to an initial surgical strategy (▲) or initial medical strategy (○). (From Alderman EL, Bourassa MG, Cohen LS, et al: Ten-year follow-up of survival and myocardial infarction in the randomized Coronary Artery Surgery Study. Circulation 1990; 82:1629–1646.)

tion, a stenosis in the proximal left anterior descending coronary artery, an abnormal resting electrocardiogram, ST segment depression of 1.5 mm or more during an exercise treadmill test, peripheral vascular disease, and increasing age all had a survival advantage with surgery. Explanations for the difference in results between the two studies may involve the relatively high operative mortality (5.8%) in the VACS and the inclusion of relatively low-risk patients in the CASS.

Finally, the CASS[5] enrolled 780 patients (90% male) younger than 65 years between 1975 and 1979. Although the lower limit of left ventricular ejection fraction was 35%, this cohort of patients had the least severe angina. Twenty-two percent of the patients had no angina, and patients with CCS class III and class IV angina were excluded.

As in the VACS, there was no long-term (10 years) survival advantage for the group of patients treated with CABG.[20] However, in patients with an ejection fraction of less than 50%, a marked survival advantage with an initial surgical strategy was observed (Fig. 4–3). The greatest comparative advantage for surgical therapy was found in patients with three-vessel coronary artery disease and an ejection fraction of less than 50%. There was also a progressively increasing benefit for surgery in years 3 through 10.

Yusuf and colleagues[21] reviewed data from seven randomized trials that compared a strategy of initial surgical therapy with initial medical therapy. The CABG group had a significantly lower mortality than that of the medical group at 5, 7, and 10 years. Surgical revascularization resulted in the greatest benefit in patients with the highest preoperative risk. Specifically, patients with the most severe symptoms, ischemia, extent of coronary artery disease, and left ventricular dysfunction derived the greatest comparative benefit. In all of these trials, left main coronary artery disease and three-vessel coronary artery disease with moderately depressed left ventricular dysfunction were the clearest indications for a surgical approach.

Surgical treatment of these subsets initially resulted in a marked improvement in symptoms and survival. However, the comparative benefit of bypass surgery over medical therapy lessened during the long-term follow-up. This should not come as a surprise if one considers the design of these trials. In the three studies, 36% to 38% of medically treated patients "crossed over" to surgical therapy during follow-up, and 6% to 8% of surgically treated patients never underwent coronary artery surgery (Fig. 4–4). Thus, analysis of the data on the basis of the "intention to treat" diluted any apparent benefit from surgery over time. Therefore, these trials compared two different treatment "strategies" rather than two different treatments. Specifically, an initial surgical strategy was compared with an initial medical therapy, with surgery reserved for pharmacologic failures.

Results of these trials also do not accurately reflect current surgical practice in several important ways. These studies antedated the widespread use of internal thoracic artery grafts, which have dramatically improved long-term graft patency. When the left internal thoracic artery is used to bypass a proximal stenosis in the left anterior descending coronary artery, patency rates of approximately 95% are observed at 10 years.[22] This contrasts markedly with saphenous vein grafts, in which only 50% to 60% are patent at 10 years.[23, 24] Patency rates of saphenous vein grafts can be improved, however, by the administration of antiplatelet agents, which also were not used exclusively in these trials.[25] Surgical results would also be expected to improve as a result of improvements in preoperative care, cardiac anesthesia, myocardial preservation, and postoperative care. Finally, few data were obtained on subsets of patients who commonly undergo bypass surgery today. Two of the three trials excluded women, and only 10% of the patients in the CASS trial were women. Similarly, the three trials provide few data regarding the prognostic importance of age older than 65 years or reoperation.

Medical therapy has also changed since these trials were performed. It is now understood that aggressive risk factor modification and the use of aspirin will result in a decrease in cardiac events. Although beta blockers were available during these trials, the full benefit of these agents in secondary prevention after a myocardial infarction had not been documented, and their use was low. Widespread use of calcium channel antagonists did not occur until after these trials were completed.

The randomized trials and numerous registry and database studies have provided us with a large body of carefully collected evidence, which provides the basis for an informed opinion on the indications for coronary revascularization in the individual patient. Although there have been recent advances in surgical and medical therapy, the major conclusions from these trials can be applied to current clinical practice. Current experience reveals that bypass surgery clearly relieves symptoms and decreases mortality in high-risk patients. In patients at lower risk, a trial of initial medical therapy followed by revascularization in patients who fail pharmacologic management is reasonable. The explosion of PTCA over the last decade has brought to the forefront the question of which method of revascularization is preferable, and in which patients. Nonetheless, this debate of the 1990s should not allow us to forget the lessons of the 1970s, in which the indications for coronary revascularization were established.

COMPARISON WITH PERCUTANEOUS TRANSLUMINAL CORONARY ANGIOPLASTY

The VACS, ECSS, and CASS trials have established the role of revascularization in the treatment of chronic stable angina.[2–6] Six

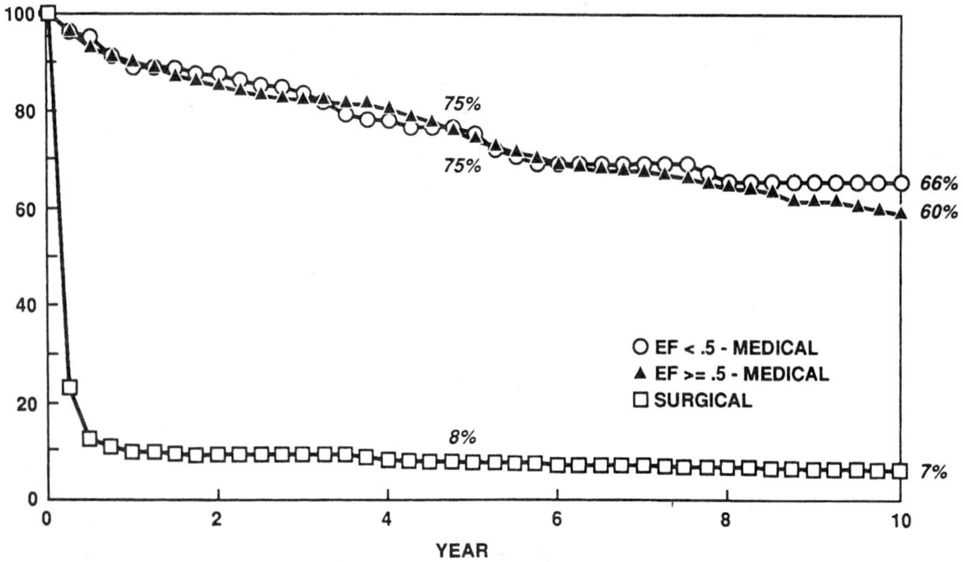

Figure 4–4. Patients in the Coronary Artery Surgery Study who have not undergone coronary artery bypass graft surgery in 10 years of follow-up. This represents medical patients who have "crossed over" to surgical therapy and surgical patients who never underwent surgery. *Abbreviation:* EF, ejection fraction. (From Alderman EL, Bourassa MG, Cohen LS, et al: Ten-year follow-up of survival and myocardial infarction in the randomized Coronary Artery Surgery Study. Circulation 1990; 82:1629–1646.)

large randomized studies have compared surgical and percutaneous revascularization. The Randomised Intervention Treatment of Angina Trial (RITA), the German Angioplasty Bypass Surgery Investigation (GABI), the Emory Angioplasty versus Surgery Trial (EAST), and the Argentine Randomized Trial of Percutaneous Transluminal Coronary Angioplasty versus Coronary Artery Bypass Surgery in Multivessel Disease (ERACI) have all been completed.[7–10] The Coronary Angioplasty Bypass Revascularization Investigation (CABRI) and the Bypass Angioplasty Revascularization Investigation (BARI) have completed enrollment, but final results are pending.[11, 12] Each of these studies randomized patients with coronary artery disease to treatment with CABG or PTCA.

It is crucial to emphasize the highly selective nature of patients included in these trials, because the data should not be extrapolated to other subsets of patients. Approximately two thirds of patients found to be clinically eligible were excluded for angiographic reasons, including the inability to dilate occluded vessels or to achieve complete revascularization. Moreover, these were trials of patients with well-preserved left ventricular function, which excluded many patients in whom surgical revascularization would probably be most beneficial (i.e., patients with compromised left ventricular function and multivessel disease).

Given the differences between the studies, it is reassuring to note that the results are remarkably consistent with previously published data and among the trials themselves. In these highly selective subsets of patients, after a 1- to 3-year period of follow-up, the outcome in regard to the end points of death and myocardial infarction was similar between the two treatment strategies. Not unexpectedly, however, the need for repeated revascularization procedures was much higher in the PTCA group, of whom approximately 40% underwent repeated PTCA or bypass surgery within the period of follow-up. Initially, the recurrence of angina was substantially greater in the angioplasty group, although these differences diminished over time. Another understandable finding was the lower in-hospital costs in patients undergoing PTCA. However, the need for repeated revascularization procedures and recurrent hospitalizations in the angioplasty group over the subsequent period of follow-up contributed to an increase in postdischarge costs, such that overall costs were similar between the two strategies after 2 to 3 years.[10, 26]

The RITA trial randomized 1011 patients (3% of patients registered) who were thought to be candidates for PTCA or CABG and in whom revascularization was deemed to be "equivalent" with either technique.[7] Single-vessel coronary artery disease was present in 45% of patients; three-vessel disease was present in only 12%. After 2.5 years of follow-up, there was no difference in the predefined combined end point of death or myocardial infarction (Fig. 4–5). Bypass surgery patients had a longer initial hospital stay, whereas PTCA patients required more revascularization procedures, experienced more angina, and took more antianginal agents. As a result, the initial cost of randomizing a patient to PTCA was 52% of CABG.[26] However, the increased rate of subsequent revascularization procedures, coronary arteriograms, and pharmacologic therapy greatly diminished this initial cost advantage (Fig. 4–6).

In the ERACI study, 127 patients (9% of those undergoing angiography) were randomized.[8] In this population with multivessel coronary artery disease, 83% had "unstable" angina. After 1 year of follow-up, there was no difference in mortality or nonfatal myocardial infarction between patients undergoing PTCA and those having CABG surgery. However, in the surgical group, there was less angina and need for repeated revascularization procedures. This benefit, however, was associated with a doubling of costs.

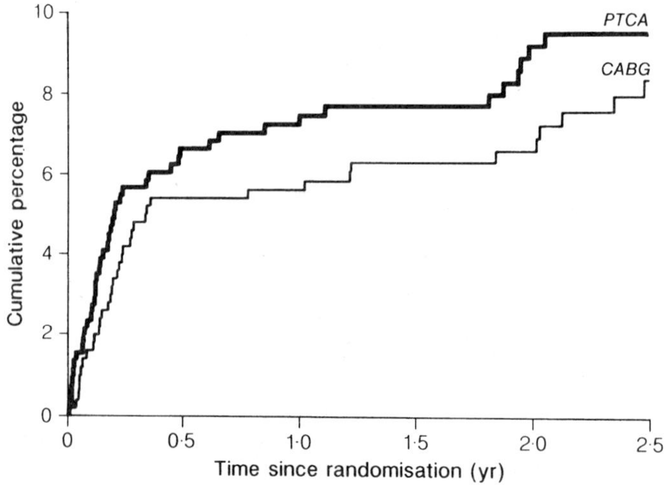

Figure 4–5. Cumulative risk of death or myocardial infarction by treatment group in the Randomised Intervention Treatment of Angina (RITA) Trial. *Abbreviations:* PTCA, percutaneous transluminal coronary angioplasty; CABG, coronary artery bypass graft. (From RITA Trial Participants: Coronary angioplasty versus coronary artery bypass surgery: the Randomised Intervention Treatment of Angina [RITA] Trial. Lancet 1993; 341:573–580.)

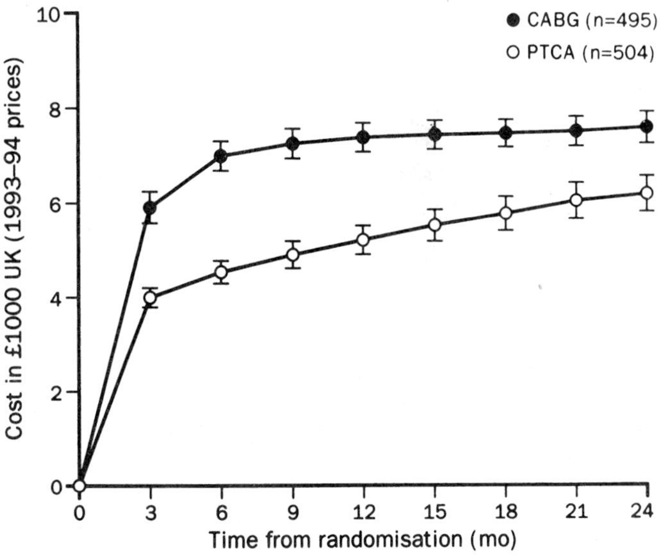

Figure 4–6. Mean cost by treatment group in the RITA trial. *Abbreviations:* PTCA, percutaneous transluminal coronary angioplasty; CABG, coronary artery bypass graft. (From Sculpher MJ, Seed P, Henderson RA, et al: Health service costs of coronary artery bypass surgery: the Randomised Intervention Treatment of Angina [RITA] Trial. Lancet 1994; 344:927–930.)

The GABI trial studied 359 patients (4% of those screened) with multivessel disease.[9] The primary end point was freedom from angina at 1 year of follow-up. As opposed to other studies, this trial resulted in a decrease in the combined end point of mortality and major cardiac events, after 1 year, in the PTCA cohort. With regard to the primary end point, however, there was no difference in freedom from angina at 1 year. As in other trials, PTCA patients underwent a significantly greater rate of repeated revascularization procedures (44% versus 6%).

The EAST trial randomized 392 patients with multivessel disease (8% of those screened) to treatment with PTCA or CABG.[10] Once again, there was no difference in the combined primary end point of death, Q wave myocardial infarction, or large ischemic defect on thallium imaging. In addition, surgical patients had less angina, took less antianginal medicines, and underwent fewer revascularization procedures compared with percutaneous revascularization at 3 years of follow-up. The impact of repeated procedures in the angioplasty group is illustrated by the similarity in overall costs between the two groups at 3 years.

Two additional studies are in progress. The National Heart, Lung, and Blood Institute is directing the largest trial, BARI, which has enrolled nearly 2000 patients.[12] Patients were included if they had unstable angina, a recent myocardial infarction, severe angina or ischemia, and multivessel coronary artery disease. The 5-year follow-up data are expected to be announced in late 1995. The CABRI trial is a European study; preliminary results, after 1 year of follow-up, also show no change in mortality or nonfatal myocardial infarction as well as an increased frequency of repeated revascularization procedures in the PTCA group.[11]

The results of these six trials are remarkably consistent and are unlikely to initiate the level of controversy that followed publication of the early trials of CABG compared with medical therapy. With the exception of RITA, these trials studied patients with multivessel coronary artery disease who were good candidates for either CABG or PTCA. For the most part, patients had good left ventricular function and no evidence of left main coronary artery disease, previous revascularization procedures, or recent myocardial infarction. Thus, these patients were often "ideal" candidates for revascularization.

Summary

Despite the imperfections of the randomized trials comparing coronary bypass surgery with medical therapy, they have provided us with invaluable information from which to define the indications for coronary revascularization. No trial has shown a survival advantage for patients with single-vessel disease. In addition, there are subsets of patients with multivessel disease and mild angina or ischemia, and well-preserved left ventricular function, in whom a survival advantage from surgery over medical therapy has not been documented. On the other hand, there are anatomic subsets of patients in whom bypass surgery does improve survival compared with medical therapy. These include patients with left main coronary artery disease and patients with multivessel coronary artery disease, particularly in association with disease of the proximal left anterior descending coronary artery and impaired left ventricular function. Surgical revascularization, with a goal of symptomatic relief, is clearly indicated in patients with severe symptoms or ischemia. One could make a case for coronary revascularization in patients with severe ischemia, irrespective of left ventricular function, with the intent of improving survival. Registry studies and a meta-analysis of the randomized trials suggest that the presence of multivessel disease and severe ischemia is associated with an improved survival from surgery compared with medical therapy.[21]

The current debate is over the preferred method of revascularization. However, we should continue to heed the lessons of the 1970s regarding the indications for revascularization. In patients with single-vessel disease in whom revascularization is deemed necessary on the basis of symptoms or ischemia, PTCA is generally preferred to coronary bypass surgery. In patients with multivessel disease referred for revascularization, the decision to perform PTCA or coronary bypass surgery will be based on the angiographic characteristics of the lesion, the number of lesions, the diffuseness of disease, the presence or absence of left ventricular dysfunction, and an assessment of the likely consequences in the event that PTCA fails. Among patients with severe ischemia, multivessel disease, and left ventricular dysfunction, complete revascularization is usually required. This will not be achieved by PTCA in the majority of patients with use of current technology.

On the other hand, in patients with preserved left ventricular function and milder degrees of ischemia, "incomplete" revascularization may suffice, and PTCA could be the appropriate initial therapy in such patients. The decision whether to perform PTCA or bypass surgery needs to be individualized, and the patient's preference is crucial and appropriate. Among many patients who need coronary revascularization, PTCA is a reasonable initial therapeutic strategy, provided that the patient understands the strong likelihood of the need for a repeated procedure within the next 1 to 3 years. The decision to undergo angioplasty initially is not associated with an increase in mortality or late myocardial infarction.

In the current era, coronary bypass surgery will remain the treatment of choice for most patients with triple-vessel disease, left ventricular dysfunction, and diffuse disease and for patients with unfavorable angiographic anatomy (e.g., complete occlusion). Nonetheless, there is a role for PTCA in patients with multivessel disease, but this will tend to be in patients with two-vessel disease, relatively well preserved left ventricular function, and suitable anatomy (Table 4–2).

INDICATIONS FOR CORONARY ARTERY BYPASS GRAFT SURGERY

Since the initiation of coronary bypass surgery in the 1960s, the indications have been expanded to a diversity of clinical syndromes and anatomic subsets of patients with ischemic heart disease. These include patients with stable and unstable angina pectoris, patients

TABLE 4–2. FACTORS INFLUENCING THE METHOD OF REVASCULARIZATION

Coronary Artery Bypass Graft Surgery	Percutaneous Transluminal Coronary Angioplasty
Left main or three-vessel coronary artery disease	One- or two-vessel coronary artery disease
Involvement of proximal left anterior descending coronary artery	Normal left ventricular function
Diffuse coronary artery disease	Mild to moderate ischemia
Occluded coronary artery	
Left ventricular dysfunction	
Poor prognosis if percutaneous transluminal coronary angioplasty fails	
Severe ischemia	

with acute myocardial infarction, patients with "silent" ischemia, survivors of sudden cardiac death, patients with congenital coronary anomalies, and patients presenting with congestive heart failure secondary to reversible ischemia. Although the initial objective of coronary bypass surgery was to relieve the symptoms of angina pectoris, lessons learned from the randomized trials and database studies of the late 1960s and 1970s identified additional subgroups of patients in whom coronary bypass surgery appeared to improve survival compared with medical therapy.

Stable Angina Pectoris

The VACS, ECSS, and CASS trials have established the role of surgical revascularization in the treatment of stable angina pectoris.[2–5] A clear mortality advantage has been observed when patients with left main coronary artery disease undergo coronary bypass surgery. Improved survival with surgery is also seen in patients with three-vessel coronary artery disease and impaired left ventricular function as well as two-vessel coronary artery disease with involvement of the proximal left anterior descending coronary artery (Fig. 4–7).

Coronary bypass surgery also results in a marked decrease in anginal symptoms and an improvement in exercise capacity compared with medical therapy. In the three large randomized trials, 60% to 70% of the surgical group was free of angina at 1 year, compared with 10% to 20% of the medically treated patients. The number of surgically treated patients who were free of angina decreased to 50% to 60% at 5 years, and the results of medical and surgical therapy converged after 10 years of follow-up.[6, 27, 28] This is undoubtedly a result of crossover to surgical therapy, graft stenosis, and progression of native vessel atherosclerosis (Fig. 4–8).

A greater improvement in exercise capacity was also observed in the surgically treated patients. This was most likely a result of improved myocardial blood flow after CABG. A study by Hossack and colleagues[29] demonstrated an improvement in maximal oxygen consumption, cardiac index, and maximal rate-pressure product in patients with complete revascularization.[29] These changes were not observed postoperatively in patients with incomplete revascularization.

Despite the marked symptomatic improvement observed in patients with stable angina after surgical revascularization, left ventricular function is usually unchanged.[30] However, in patients with left ventricular dysfunction associated with chronic ischemia, bypass surgery may improve contractility in these patients with "hibernating" myocardium.[31] Finally, none of the three major trials has shown a decrease in subsequent myocardial infarctions in surgically treated patients. The rate of nonfatal myocardial infarctions was 2% to 3% per year in both the surgically and medically treated patients.[32, 33] However, data from the CASS Registry document a reduction in new myocardial infarctions with surgical revascularization.[34]

Unstable Angina Pectoris

Ischemic discomfort is defined as unstable if it is new, occurs at rest, or changes in frequency or severity.[35] It is usually the result of fixed atherosclerotic coronary artery disease with superimposed plaque rupture, platelet activation, and thrombus formation. Initial therapy is medical and consists of bed rest, oxygen, sedation, aspirin, heparin, nitrates, beta blockers, and sometimes calcium channel antagonists. In refractory cases, an intra-aortic balloon pump may be effective. All patients should also be evaluated early for the presence of precipitating factors, such as anemia, hyperthyroidism, hypoxemia, infection, uncontrolled hypertension, arrhythmias, valvular heart disease, or hypertrophic cardiomyopathy.

The role of coronary angiography in patients with unstable angina is controversial.[36] On the basis of results of the Thrombolysis in Myocardial Ischemia (TIMI-III) trial, a case can be made to perform coronary angiography in all patients who present with unstable angina. However, this trial also supports a conservative approach, with angiography reserved for those who have spontaneous ischemia or a positive stress test result while receiving medical therapy. Although there was no difference in mortality when a conservative approach was compared with an "aggressive" strategy, the conservative approach resulted in an increase in recurrent angina and future hospital-

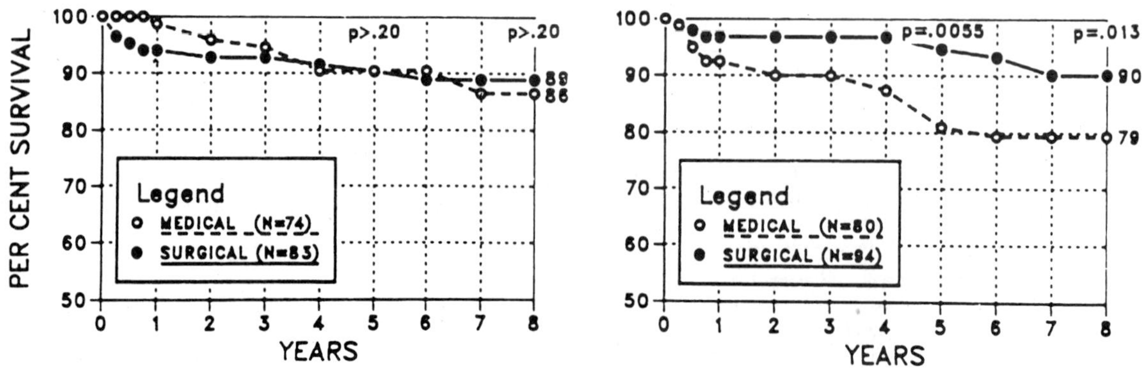

Figure 4–7. Cumulative survival in the European Coronary Surgery Study for patients with two-vessel coronary artery disease randomized to initial medical (○) or surgical (●) therapy. A significant difference favoring surgery was observed in patients with a stenosis greater than 75% in the proximal left anterior descending coronary artery *(right panel)* compared with patients with a stenosis less than 75% *(left panel).* (From Varnauskas E, European Coronary Surgery Study Group: Survival, myocardial infarction, and employment status in a prospective randomized study of coronary bypass surgery. Circulation 1985; 72[suppl V]:90–101.)

izations. Angiography will reveal significant coronary artery disease in 80% to 90% of patients studied.[37]

The choice of medical therapy, PTCA, or CABG depends on the patient's clinical status, the results of angiography, and an assessment of left ventricular function. The National Cooperative Study Group[38] compared medical therapy with CABG in 288 patients with unstable angina pectoris from 1972 to 1976. Patients with left main coronary artery disease, a recent myocardial infarction, and poor left ventricular function were excluded from the study. During this trial, there was no difference in hospital mortality. However, at a mean follow-up of 2 years, there was a higher rate of myocardial infarctions in the surgical group, whereas NYHA class III or class IV angina was more common in medically treated patients. The VACS trial also compared medical and surgical therapy in the treatment of unstable angina pectoris.[39] There was no significant difference in survival or nonfatal myocardial infarction at 2 years. However, in patients with impaired left ventricular function (ejection fraction of 0.30 to 0.59), a survival advantage was demonstrated for surgically treated patients (Fig. 4–9). Both of these studies were associated with a high rate of crossover to surgical therapy (34% to 36% at 24 to 30 months).

There are no large randomized trials of PTCA versus medical therapy or CABG in patients with unstable angina pectoris. However, many patients in the six randomized trials comparing surgical and percutaneous revascularization had a diagnosis of unstable angina.[7–12] Therefore, it is reasonable to conclude that both therapies would have similar in-hospital mortality rates in patients with good left ventricular function. Recurrent angina, the need for antianginal medications, and repeated revascularization procedures would be expected to be higher in the PTCA group.

In summary, initial medical therapy is the treatment of choice for unstable angina pectoris. Patients who continue to have ischemia despite optimal medical management and patients with "high-risk" coronary anatomy are candidates for myocardial revascularization. When cardiac catheterization demonstrates left main coronary artery disease, three-vessel coronary artery disease with impaired left ventricular function, or multivessel disease involving the proximal left anterior descending coronary artery, surgical revascularization is the preferred strategy. In patients with ongoing ischemia and one- or two-vessel coronary artery disease with normal left ventricular function, percutaneous revascularization is a reasonable approach. The most critical question is the timing of revascularization. In patients with unstable angina, acute revascularization (surgical or percutaneous) results in increased mortality and nonfatal myocardial infarctions, in comparison with patients with stable angina. In addition, the frequency of abrupt closure and the need for urgent CABG is increased in the PTCA patients. For these reasons, a strong case can be made to delay revascularization until the patient is clinically stable, which may require intra-aortic balloon counter-pulsation. This approach suffices for the majority of patients, and emergency revascularization can be reserved for the relatively few patients in whom symptoms are refractory to medical therapy.

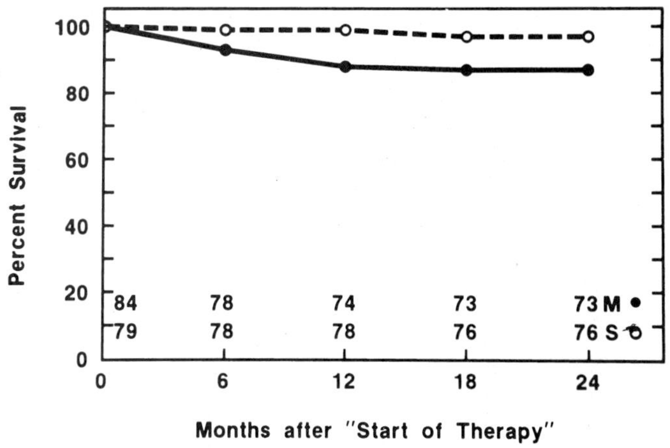

Figure 4–9. Cumulative survival in patients with unstable angina and an ejection fraction of 0.30 to 0.59 in patients randomized to surgical treatment (S, ○) or medical treatment (M, ●). (From Luchi RJ, Scott SM, Deupree RH, et al: Comparison of medical and surgical treatment for unstable angina pectoris. Results of a Veterans Administration Cooperative Study. N Engl J Med 1987; 316:977–984.)

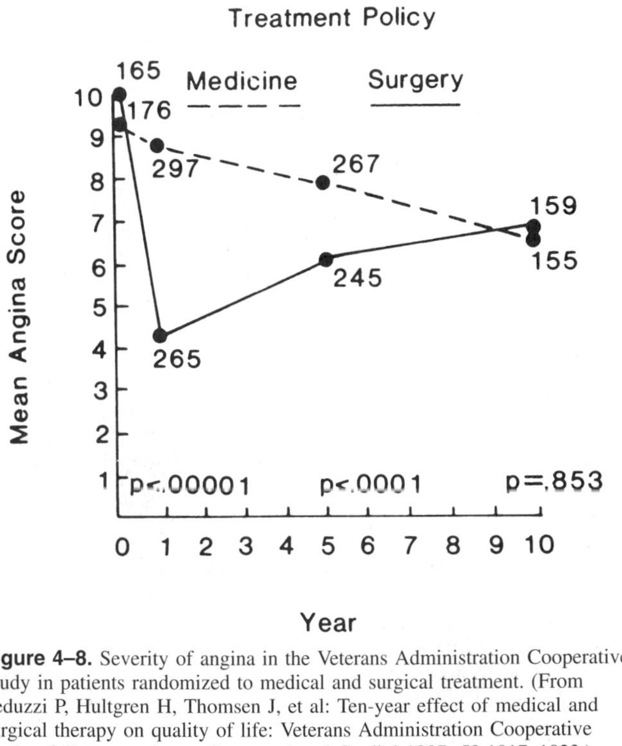

Figure 4–8. Severity of angina in the Veterans Administration Cooperative Study in patients randomized to medical and surgical treatment. (From Peduzzi P, Hultgren H, Thomsen J, et al: Ten-year effect of medical and surgical therapy on quality of life: Veterans Administration Cooperative Study of Coronary Artery Surgery. Am J Cardiol 1987; 59:1017–1023.)

Silent Ischemia

The indications for surgery in patients with silent ischemia are less clear-cut, as is its impact on prognosis. The prognosis is dependent on the definition of silent ischemia. Ischemia may be considered silent after an asymptomatic but electrically positive stress test result in a patient who has angina at other times. In contrast, other patients are completely asymptomatic and have no prior history of angina, but ischemia is detected during Holter monitoring or stress testing. The majority of patients with silent ischemia have symptomatic ischemia at other times, and in these patients the indications for coronary bypass surgery are the same as in patients with overt angina pectoris. Among asymptomatic patients, the prognostic impact of "true" silent ischemia on ambulatory electrocardiography is unknown and warrants further testing.

The CASS Registry included 53 asymptomatic patients with left main coronary artery disease.[40] In this cohort, the 5-year surgical survival of 88% was significantly better than the 57% survival in the medical group. In contrast, a small randomized trial in asymptomatic patients after myocardial infarction failed to show a difference in survival between medically and surgically treated patients.[41] The impact of this trial, however, is diminished by the lengthy 2-month delay between the myocardial infarction and entry into the trial. It would be expected that a majority of postinfarction deaths in patients receiving medical therapy occur within this 2-month period.

Weiner and colleagues[42] reviewed the experience of 692 patients from the CASS Registry with silent ischemia during their initial exercise test. A marked survival benefit was observed in patients with three-vessel coronary artery disease and impaired left ventricular function undergoing surgical revascularization. After 7 years of follow-up, survival was 90% in the surgically treated patients and 37% in the medically treated patients ($p < .001$). This study was limited by its nonrandomized study design and the high prevalence of symptomatic ischemia in treated patients. A nonrandomized study by Tyras and coworkers[43] retrospectively analyzed data on 447 patients with coronary artery disease and minimal or absent angina. At a mean follow-up of 38.6 months, there was a significant improvement in survival in surgically treated patients.

Although bypass surgery is effective in relieving angina, its effect on silent ischemia is more controversial. In a study by Egstrup,[44] the frequency and severity of silent ischemia surprisingly increased after CABG. Conversely, Droste and associates[45] observed a decrease in both symptomatic and asymptomatic ischemia after CABG, when patients were observed with serial ambulatory electrocardiographic monitoring. Weiner and colleagues[46] reported prospective results from 174 patients in the CASS Registry who had exercise treadmill testing before and 6 months after CABG. Although symptomatic ischemia decreased significantly after surgery (52% to 6%), there was no change in the prevalence of silent ischemia (30% to 29%). The long-term prognosis was significantly better for patients with no ischemia (80% survival at 12 years) compared with that for patients with silent ischemia (68%) or symptomatic ischemia (45%).

Although it would be logical to assume that the total "ischemic" burden should be the target of therapy, there is no definitive evidence to suggest that the elimination of silent in addition to symptomatic ischemia provides any added benefit.[47] Nonetheless, the current role of bypass surgery for patients with silent ischemia remains somewhat controversial. It is reasonable to recommend angiography in patients with evidence of severe ischemia based on the extent of ST segment depression during exercise, exercise-induced hypotension, or a large area of reversible ischemia on scintigraphic imaging or stress echocardiography. If coronary angiography documents an anatomic subset shown in previous studies to benefit from bypass surgery, coronary bypass surgery is appropriate, particularly when left ventricular dysfunction is present.

Acute Myocardial Infarction

The most important goal in the treatment of an acute myocardial infarction is the rapid restoration of antegrade blood flow. Multiple, large, randomized, placebo-controlled trials have unequivocally established the benefit of thrombolytic agents.[48–51] However, thrombolysis may be ineffective in more than 20% of patients, whereas others have contraindications to its use, which has prompted the use of alternative reperfusion strategies. Both surgical and percutaneous revascularization have been used as primary therapies and in conjunction with thrombolytic agents. No matter which method is chosen, the degree of myocardial salvage and the subsequent reduction in mortality are directly proportional to the speed of reperfusion.

Several recently completed, large, randomized trials have compared the use of immediate angioplasty of the infarct-related coronary artery with thrombolytic therapy.[52–55] These studies have clearly established the technical feasibility of this strategy, with success rates of 93% to 98%. The major disadvantage of primary angioplasty is the lack of accessibility of a cardiac catheterization laboratory for the majority of patients who present with an acute myocardial infarction. However, when a catheterization laboratory equipped to perform primary angioplasty is available, it appears to be the treatment of choice for patients with contraindications to thrombolytic therapy, for patients in cardiogenic shock, and for patients undergoing PTCA for an acute chest pain syndrome in which the typical electrocardiographic indications for thrombolysis are absent.[56–59]

Although the logistic constraints associated with coronary artery surgery for acute myocardial infarction are even more formidable than for angioplasty, this strategy has been used successfully for more than 20 years.[60] It has the advantage of providing the most complete revascularization in patients with multivessel coronary artery disease. In addition, surgical reperfusion by use of cardiopulmonary bypass may result in a reduction in reperfusion injury. Full cardiopulmonary bypass results in an improved myocardial oxygen supply-demand relationship.[61] Decompression of the left ventricle lowers preload and afterload; metabolic demands are reduced by hypothermia and complete sedation.

Early studies have demonstrated that acute surgical revascularization is safe and technically feasible. DeWood and colleagues[62] reported a 4.4% mortality rate in 701 patients undergoing CABG for acute myocardial infarction. However, this study was limited by its nonrandomized study design and the inclusion of mostly low-risk patients. Specifically, 84% of patients were NYHA class I or class II, 85% had no prior history of myocardial infarction, and 29% had single-vessel coronary artery disease. A second study by Phillips and coworkers[63] reported an operative mortality of 1.3% in 75 patients undergoing emergency CABG.

A randomized study by Koshal and colleagues[64] compared surgical and medical therapy in 68 patients presenting within 4 hours of a myocardial infarction. However, medically treated patients received neither thrombolytic agents nor PTCA, and data on the use of beta blockers were not provided. As a result, the mortality rate was 2.9% in patients undergoing surgical revascularization compared with an extraordinarily high mortality rate of 20.6% in medically treated patients.

The increasing use of thrombolytic agents in the treatment of acute myocardial infarction has created two new subsets of patients for surgical revascularization. First, thrombolysis may be unsuccessful in opening an occluded coronary artery. In this case, bypass surgery is performed on an emergency basis to achieve reperfusion and limit infarct size. Although emergency coronary bypass surgery is effective, this is achieved at the price of an increased morbidity and mortality. In the TIMI trial, 1.6% of the patients underwent emergency bypass surgery within 24 hours of entry into the trial. This was associated with a perioperative mortality of 16.7% and a major surgical hemorrhage in 74.1% of patients.[65] Second, thrombolysis may be successful in achieving reperfusion, but a residual high-grade coronary stenosis may remain, resulting in spontaneous or provokable ischemia. The choice between PTCA and CABG, however, needs to be individualized.

Cardiovascular surgery may be life-saving in patients with mechanical complications of a myocardial infarction. Papillary muscle rupture, ventricular septal defects, and left ventricular free wall perforations carry an extraordinarily high short-term mortality rate. Management of these patients should include a diagnostic cardiac catheterization, insertion of an intra-aortic balloon pump, and surgical intervention. The major objective of surgical intervention is to correct the mechanical complication, but concomitant coronary bypass surgery is usually performed, particularly in patients with multivessel disease. Although there are no definitive data to support the use of bypass grafting in this setting, its use is logical.

In summary, surgical revascularization appears to be safe and effective in the treatment of acute myocardial infarction. However, its routine use is markedly limited by the lack of access to emergency CABG in most hospitals and the proven benefits of thrombolytic therapy and primary angioplasty. Subsets of myocardial infarction patients may benefit from a surgical strategy. Patients with left main or three-vessel coronary artery disease discovered at initial presentation or during postinfarction angina may be ideal candidates. Unstable patients with lesions unsuitable for angioplasty, or after failed angioplasty, may be candidates for surgery. Among patients undergoing surgery for the repair of the mechanical complications of acute myocardial infarction, concomitant coronary revascularization for patients with multivessel disease is logical, but its added benefits are unproven. Thus, there are reasonable indications for coronary bypass surgery among subsets of patients in the setting of acute myocardial infarction, but a randomized trial of this approach in comparison with thrombolytic therapy or primary angioplasty would be difficult to undertake.

Aborted Sudden Cardiac Death

Sudden cardiac death is the most common cause of mortality in patients with ischemic heart disease, affecting up to 400,000 persons annually in the United States alone.[66] In the majority, death is due to a ventricular tachyarrhythmia, although some events are the result of a bradydysrhythmia or a nonarrhythmic cause. The most common patient profile is a man with multivessel coronary artery disease, a remote myocardial infarction, and impaired left ventricular function. Sudden cardiac death is associated with an acute myocardial infarction in a minority of cases. In a study by Baum and associates,[67] only 17% of cardiac arrest survivors had a new Q wave myocardial infarction.

There is little doubt that ventricular arrhythmias occur as the result of acute myocardial ischemia, but its frequency in the overall spectrum of sudden cardiac death is uncertain. Nonetheless, there is a considerable body of circumstantial evidence to suggest that ischemia may provide the substrate for ventricular arrhythmias, either reentrant or automatic, leading to sudden cardiac death. Data from the Framingham Heart Study[68] have shown that the incidence of sudden death is increased in patients with symptomatic ischemic heart disease. This study also revealed a circadian variation associated with episodes of sudden cardiac death that correlated with variations in autonomic tone and platelet aggregability as well as with acute ischemic events.[69] Anti-ischemic therapy with beta-blocking agents or CABG surgery leads to a reduction in the incidence of sudden cardiac death.[70–72] On the other hand, conflicting data suggest that acute ischemia does not play a primary role in causing sudden cardiac deaths. It is well established that most victims do not experience angina immediately preceding the event, and there is a dearth of clinical or pathologic evidence of acute myocardial necrosis in patients dying of sudden cardiac death.

Sudden cardiac death probably occurs as a result of a complex interplay between a fixed anatomic substrate and dynamic changes in the myocardial milieu. The combination of myocardial ischemia in concert with an electrolyte disturbance, hypoxemia, acidosis, changes in autonomic tone, or the addition of cardiac or noncardiac drugs may facilitate the development of ventricular fibrillation. Thus, the treatment should be directed at both the substrate and the more dynamic factors.

Surgical revascularization has been shown to play an important role in the prevention of sudden cardiac death. Data from the CASS trial revealed a 5.2% incidence of sudden cardiac death in medically treated patients, compared with 1.8% in the surgical cohort[71] (Fig. 4–10). This difference was even greater in patients with a history of congestive heart failure or impaired left ventricular function.[71, 72] The ECSS trial provided further support in that sudden cardiac deaths occurred in 9% of medically treated patients and in only 3% of surgically treated patients after 8 years of follow-up.[33]

Coronary artery surgery has also been suggested to reduce the incidence of sudden cardiac death in survivors of an out-of-hospital cardiac arrest. Every and colleagues[73] observed 265 patients who experienced an aborted cardiac arrest between 1970 and 1988. Both the 1- and 5-year survival in the approximately one third who underwent surgical revascularization was superior to those treated medically. However, this study was limited by its nonrandomized design, which was reflected in the fact that surgical patients had better left ventricular function, less prior congestive heart failure, and more angina preceding the initial cardiac arrest.

Additional information implying that patients resuscitated from an out-of-hospital cardiac arrest would benefit from coronary revascularization is provided by a series of electrophysiologic studies in 50 survivors of out-of-hospital cardiac arrest.[74] Preoperatively, 80% of the patients had inducible ventricular arrhythmias, but among patients in whom this was ventricular tachycardia, only 20% of the patients were rendered noninducible after bypass surgery. In contrast, of the patients in whom the initial arrhythmia was ventricular fibrillation, none was inducible after bypass surgery. These data suggest that sustained monomorphic ventricular tachycardia is due to a fixed substrate in the majority, whereas ventricular fibrillation is primarily ischemic in origin and thus amenable to coronary revascularization.

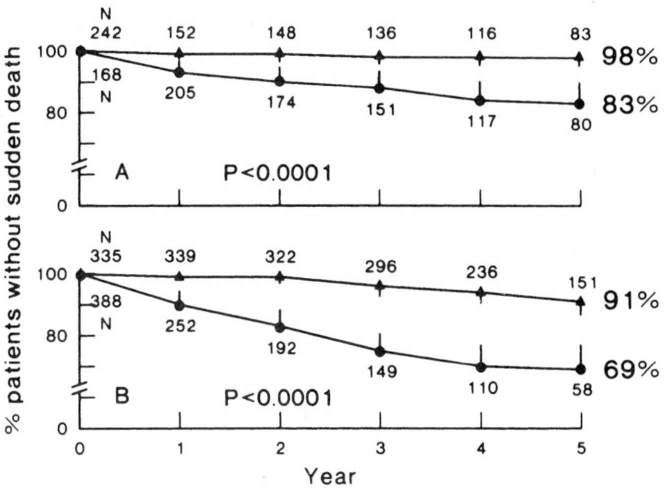

Figure 4–10. Coronary Artery Surgery Study patients without sudden cardiac death when randomized to surgical treatment (▲) or medical treatment (●). *A,* Patients with two-vessel coronary artery disease and a history of congestive heart failure. *B,* Patients with three-vessel coronary artery disease and a history of congestive heart failure. (From Holmes DR, Davis KB, Mock MB, et al: The effect of medical and surgical treatment on subsequent sudden cardiac death in patients with coronary artery disease: a report from the Coronary Artery Surgery Study. Circulation 1986; 73:1254–1263.)

In summary, sudden cardiac death is usually the result of a combination of fixed anatomic substrate and more transient precipitating factors. Acute myocardial ischemia may be the trigger in some cases, but definitive proof is difficult to establish. Nonetheless, coronary artery bypass surgery is an important therapeutic tool and should be performed in the patient with evidence of ischemia, especially with multivessel coronary artery disease and left ventricular dysfunction. Additional antiarrhythmic therapy with an implantable cardiac defibrillator, subendocardial resection, aneurysmectomy, or antiarrhythmic drugs is almost always required. In the occasional patient with well-preserved left ventricular function, single-vessel disease, and exercise-induced ventricular fibrillation, it is logical to presume that coronary revascularization without any additional therapy will suffice. This is particularly true in the case of patients in whom exercise-induced ventricular fibrillation is preceded by evidence of ischemia on exercise testing. In contrast, coronary revascularization in the patient with sustained monomorphic ventricular tachycardia is unlikely to prevent recurrences in the absence of additional therapy.

Congestive Heart Failure

Over the past 2 decades, left ventricular dysfunction has changed from a contraindication to an indication for coronary artery surgery. Early studies often excluded patients with marked left ventricular dysfunction. The CASS trial excluded patients with an ejection fraction of less than 35%, whereas the ECSS trial excluded ejection fractions of less than 50%.[4, 5] However, more recent data have shown marked improvements in left ventricular function after coronary revascularization in patients with congestive heart failure and coronary artery disease.[75, 76] Debate continues over the preferred approach to the patient with severe left ventricular dysfunction and evidence of ischemia, particularly in the absence of pain.

Improvements in ventricular function after revascularization may occur as the result of hibernating myocardium, in which chronically ischemic myocardium remains viable but its function is markedly reduced.[31, 77] Controversy exists as to whether hibernation is the result of diminished contractility in an effort to conserve metabolic demands in response to a reduction in regional blood flow or the consequence of "stunning" due to repeated cycles of ischemia and reperfusion injury.[78] Regardless of the cause, revascularization increases myocardial blood flow, with a subsequent improvement in regional ventricular function. Although positron emission tomography is the "gold standard" for detecting myocardial viability, quantitative thallium scintigraphy incorporating reinjection and delayed redistribution imaging may provide the clinically relevant data.[79–82]

The VACS and CASS trials demonstrated an improvement in survival in patients with three-vessel coronary artery disease and an ejection fraction of 0.35 to 0.50.[5, 18] However, there are no randomized controlled trials of coronary revascularization in patients with left ventricular ejection fractions of less than 35%. Thus, we are left with a series of nonrandomized studies with several limitations. In general, surgical patients in these trials were healthier than their medically treated counterparts. In addition, surgical patients usually had more angina, less symptoms of congestive heart failure, and more extensive coronary artery disease.

Several individual series have documented that coronary bypass surgery in patients with severe left ventricular dysfunction may improve both systolic and diastolic function.[76, 83] Elefteriades and associates[76] evaluated the safety and efficacy of CABG in 83 consecutive patients with a left ventricular ejection fraction of 30% or less. Although the in-hospital mortality rate was high (8.4%), long-term survival was 87% at 1 year and 80% at 3 years. This was associated with an improvement in ejection fraction from 24.6% to 33.2% as well as a marked improvement in symptoms. In addition, Humphrey and colleagues[83] were able to show an improvement in diastolic function after bypass surgery.[83]

An extensive literature review by Baker and colleagues[84] examined the role of revascularization in the treatment of patients with moderate to severe left ventricular systolic dysfunction. The perioperative mortality was 2.5 times greater in patients with congestive heart failure than in those without heart failure, and mortality continued to increase as ejection fraction decreased. Despite this increased perioperative mortality rate, surgical revascularization improved long-term survival by 30% to 50% compared with medical therapy in patients with moderate to severe systolic dysfunction and angina. Therefore, although the perioperative and late mortality is higher than in patients with preserved left ventricular function, there does appear to be a survival benefit of surgery over medical therapy, especially in patients in whom the primary symptom is angina as opposed to patients in whom the dominant presentation is that of chronic heart failure.

In summary, in many patients with moderate to severe left ventricular dysfunction and coronary artery disease, some of the decrement in left ventricular function is a result of hibernating myocardium rather than of fibrosis. The optimal approach to the evaluation and treatment of these patients is hampered by the paucity of data on the prevalence of silent ischemia in patients with congestive heart failure. In addition, there is a lack of randomized trials comparing coronary bypass surgery, cardiac transplantation, or pharmacologic therapy. In patients with congestive heart failure and unequivocal angina pectoris, a recent myocardial infarction, or multiple risk factors for coronary artery disease, a physiologic test should be performed to uncover severe ischemia or hibernating myocardium. When it is present, coronary angiography should follow with an eye toward revascularization. An important focus of investigation for this decade is on improving methods of detecting myocardial viability and to establish the degree of ischemia that would justify the risk of revascularization in hopes of improving long-term prognosis.

Failed Percutaneous Transluminal Coronary Angioplasty

The expansion of an angioplasty balloon within a coronary artery results in localized trauma. In a minority of cases, this can lead to a coronary artery dissection with an occlusive intimal flap or thrombus formation, which in turn can result in severe myocardial ischemia, myocardial infarction, hemodynamic deterioration, or death. Newer catheter-based interventions including perfusion balloons, intracoronary stents, and repeated balloon inflations have reduced the frequency of emergency coronary bypass surgery. Nonetheless, the need for emergency coronary bypass surgery has not been eliminated, and it is unlikely to decline further as the pool of sick patients with complex anatomy amenable to transcatheter techniques is expanded in concert with the development of new devices.

The National Heart, Lung, and Blood Institute Registry reported a 3.4% incidence of emergency coronary artery surgery after PTCA.[85] This occurred in 2.9% of single-vessel angioplasties, 3.7% of two-vessel angioplasties, and 4.3% of three-vessel angioplasties. An elective CABG was required in another 2.2% of patients. In this registry, PTCA resulted in a mortality rate of 1.0% and an incidence of nonfatal myocardial infarction of 4.3%.

Because of this risk of abrupt closure of a coronary artery, surgical back-up from an experienced cardiovascular surgical team has been deemed mandatory by the American College of Cardiology/American Heart Association Task Force for all elective angioplasty procedures.[86] However, this remains an area of emotional and occasionally heated debate. Emergency surgical revascularization is indicated in patients with a failed PTCA resulting in severe ischemia, hemodynamic deterioration, cardiogenic shock, or ventricular tachyarrhythmias. An intra-aortic balloon pump should be placed immediately in hopes of decreasing the severity of myocardial ischemia. Emergency CABG should then be performed as soon as possible. However, even with emergency surgery, 25% to 40% will have a new Q wave myocardial infarction.[87, 88]

Congenital Coronary Artery Anomalies

Coronary artery anomalies can be asymptomatic, or they can result in ischemia, myocardial infarction, or sudden cardiac death. Asymptomatic lesions usually require no specific treatment; however, symptomatic lesions frequently require surgical revascularization. Click and associates[89] reported a 0.3% prevalence of coronary artery anomalies after reviewing 24,959 coronary angiograms. The most common lesions that resulted in symptoms and required surgical treatment were a left main coronary artery arising from the right sinus of Valsalva or proximal right coronary artery, a right coronary artery arising from the left sinus of Valsalva or proximal left coronary artery, coronary arteries arising from the pulmonary artery, or coronary artery aneurysms.

The congenital anomaly with the highest frequency of sudden cardiac death and myocardial infarction is a left main coronary artery that originates from the right sinus of Valsalva or right coronary artery and passes between the proximal aorta and the pulmonary trunk. Roberts[90] performed a necropsy study in 43 patients with this anomaly and found that death was related to the coronary anomaly in 79% of cases. In patients younger than 20 years, 5 of the 26 had evidence of a myocardial infarction. A right coronary artery that originates from the left sinus of Valsalva and passes between the aorta and pulmonary trunk can also result in sudden cardiac death and myocardial infarction, but the frequency appears to be less than with a left main coronary artery that originates from the right sinus of Valsalva.[91]

The mechanisms whereby these anomalies cause ischemia are speculative. The acute angle of take-off of the aberrant coronary artery may result in a slitlike orifice. Exercise then results in dilatation of the aorta and pulmonary trunk, further increasing the acute angle of the coronary artery take-off and compromising coronary blood flow.[92] In addition, dilatation of the aorta and pulmonary trunk may compress the aberrant coronary artery between the two great vessels. Finally, the acute angle of take-off of the coronary artery may predispose to early atherosclerosis.[93]

Although coronary artery fistulas may be acquired as a consequence of trauma or invasive cardiovascular procedures, the majority are probably congenital communications between a coronary artery and a cardiac chamber or other vascular structure. Coronary artery fistulas may cause angina, congestive heart failure, or rarely death because of rupture. Symptomatic or large hemodynamically significant fistulas warrant surgical ligation and bypass.[94] The approach to small asymptomatic fistulas is generally conservative, although a clear consensus or definitive data to justify this approach are not available.

Coronary artery anomalies may result in acute myocardial ischemia and subsequent myocardial infarction or death. CABG is an effective treatment of each of these anomalies and represents the procedure of choice.

SPECIAL CONSIDERATIONS

The Elderly

In 1990, more than 28 million people were older than 65 years and more than 7 million people were older than 80 years in the United States alone.[95] The morbidity and mortality of coronary artery disease in the elderly is substantial. In general, the elderly are at higher risk because of an increased prevalence of severe symptoms, left main coronary artery disease, multivessel disease, and compromised left ventricular function.[96] This is the crux of a clinical dilemma in that the potential for gain is enhanced, but so are the risks entailed in trying to achieve this. On one hand, the sicker nature of the elderly patient strengthens the case for revascularization over medical therapy. However, the morbidity and mortality of both PTCA and bypass surgery are increased owing to the combination of older age and increased comorbid conditions, especially peripheral vascular and cerebrovascular disease.

Although surgical revascularization is now routinely performed in the elderly, it carries an increased morbidity and mortality compared with that in younger patients (Fig. 4–11). In the CASS Registry, the perioperative mortality rate was 5.2% in 1086 patients older than 65 years but only 1.9% in 7827 patients younger than 65 years.[96] Five-year survival was 84% in patients 65 to 69 years old, 80% in patients

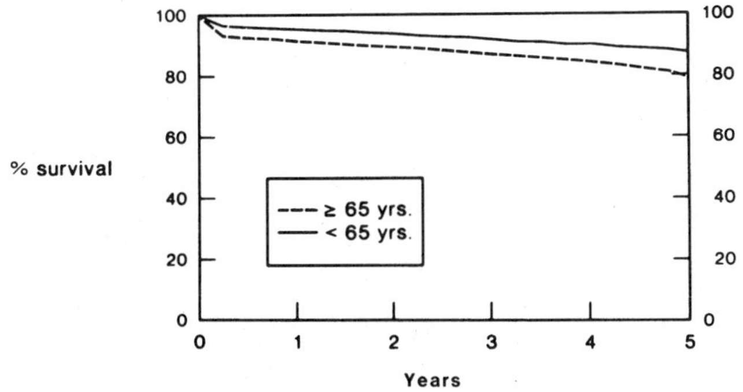

	% (No.)	% (No.)	% (No.)	% (No.)	% (No.)	% (No.)
---	100(1086)	93(1013)	91(992)	89(894)	87(729)	83(471)
——	100(7827)	97(7595)	96(7384)	95(6759)	93(5456)	91(3646)

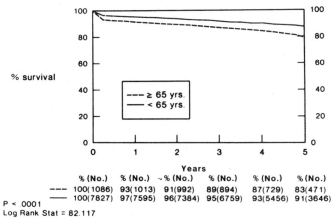

P < .0001
Log Rank Stat = 82.117

Figure 4–11. Comparison of cumulative 5-year survival of patients 65 years old or older versus those younger than 65 years undergoing surgical revascularization. (From Gersh BJ, Kronmal RA, Schaff HV, et al: Long-term [5 year] results of coronary bypass surgery in patients 65 years of age or older. A non-randomized study from the Coronary Artery Surgery Study [CASS] registry. N Engl J Med 1985; 313:217–224.)

70 to 74 years old, and 70% in patients older than 75 years. This was compared with a 91% 5-year survival in patients younger than 65 years.[97] However, despite this decrease in survival in the elderly, they received an equivalent symptomatic benefit.[98] In a more contemporary series at the Cleveland Clinic, an in-hospital mortality rate of 1.4% was reported for patients younger than 70 years, compared with 3.5% for patients 70 years old or older.[99]

The results of coronary artery surgery in octogenarians has also been addressed. Edmunds and colleagues[95] studied 100 consecutive patients, 80 years of age or older, undergoing open heart surgery. The risk factors for early death in this study included NYHA class IV disease, prior myocardial infarction, cachexia, and an emergent procedure. Freeman and associates[100] also reviewed the results of coronary artery bypass surgery in octogenarians. The total hospital mortality was 12.9%; however, this rate was only 5.6% in patients undergoing an elective operation. The greatest perioperative mortality was observed in patients with congestive heart failure, a left ventricular ejection fraction of less than 0.50, and functional class IV symptoms and in those undergoing an emergency procedure.

In a large series of isolated coronary bypass surgery in octogenarians from the Mayo Clinic, the overall perioperative mortality rate was a creditable 10.4%, given the high proportion of patients with class III or class IV symptoms who required urgent surgery.[101] In patients with isolated coronary artery disease, the perioperative mortality was approximately 4%, but this increased by approximately fourfold in patients with associated peripheral vascular disease. The remarkable adverse impact of peripheral vascular disease on outcome is probably the consequence of diffuse atheromatous emboli, which increase with age and in the presence of peripheral vascular disease.[102] Nonetheless, long-term outcome in perioperative survivors is excellent, particularly in patients with well-preserved left ventricular function, and the symptomatic benefit is equivalent to that achieved in younger patients.[101]

Perioperative morbidity is also increased in elderly patients. Loop and colleagues[103, 104] documented an increase in perioperative strokes, renal failure, respiratory complications, bleeding, and atrial fibrillation leading to an increased length and cost of hospital stay. Neurocognitive dysfunction, which fortunately is usually transient, is also more frequent in the elderly.

That coronary bypass surgery has an established role in the therapeutic armamentarium of the elderly is not in dispute. Moreover, the demographic tide in the United States will inevitably be accompanied by an increased use of invasive cardiovascular procedures in older patients. Improved surgical techniques and perioperative care continue to expand the upper age limit for bypass surgery. This raises new issues that are social, ethical, and economic. The key to an optimal surgical result in the elderly is careful attention to the overall assessment of the patient, with a meticulous approach to defining or excluding comorbid conditions that may complicate not only the perioperative outcome but the long-term expectations of quality and quantity of life. A rigorous evaluation, which goes beyond the cardiovascular system, is essential for the physician to provide the patient with a well-informed opinion. Although much of the increased mortality in older patients can be accounted for on the basis of the increased prevalence of multivessel disease, left ventricular dysfunction, and comorbid conditions, age remains an independent predictor of an adverse outcome. Coronary bypass surgery is a proven and worthwhile approach to patients of advanced age with symptomatic coronary artery disease; however, careful selection is essential.

Women

Although coronary artery disease develops in men at an earlier age than in women, the frequency of ischemic heart disease accelerates in women after menopause, and it is the leading cause of death in women as well as in men in the United States. That there are differences in men and women in the diagnosis, evaluation, and treatment of coronary artery disease is unequivocal. Whether these are due to bias or clinical judgment, and whether clinical judgment is appropriate or not, is more controversial. Rates of use of coronary angiography and bypass surgery are substantially less in women than in men.[15, 16] Whether this represents overuse in men or underuse in women has not been clearly established. The higher rate of referral for angiography after an abnormal stress test result in men, compared with women, has been documented, but the reasons are unclear.[105] In contrast, women undergoing angiography are more likely to have normal coronary arteries.[106] Once angiography has been performed, however, subsequent revascularization rates in men and women are almost identical.[107]

Compared with men, women undergoing coronary bypass surgery are sicker, as defined by age, the prevalence of diabetes and hypertension, and the severity of angina.[108–110] The distribution of coronary artery disease and left ventricular dysfunction is similar, however, with a trend toward a higher ejection fraction and less triple-vessel disease in women. In the CASS Registry, female patients had an operative mortality of 4.6%, compared with 2.0% in men.[111] In the Cleveland Clinic experience, female patients also had more than double the operative mortality of men (2.9% versus 1.3%).[108] However, female gender did not result in an increased mortality when adjustments were made for the patient's size and clinical variables.[112] Therefore, the smaller stature of women, as well as their smaller coronary arteries, may explain the differences in mortality.

After the initial postoperative period, the survival curves for men and women are identical.[108, 111] Loop and colleagues[108] reported no gender differences in long-term survival at 5 and 10 years. However, there was a difference observed in symptomatic relief. Female patients had significantly less relief of angina at 5 and 10 years after CABG. Women also had lower saphenous vein graft patency rates at 2 years (73% versus 79%), although there was no difference in the patency of internal mammary artery grafts.[108]

The increased mortality in women is probably the result of an older age, increased comorbidity, more severe symptoms, and perhaps as yet unidentified variables associated with female gender. None of these data should, however, lead to a delay in referral. The issue is not whether the perioperative mortality of women is higher than that of men, but whether the long-term outcome of women with coronary artery surgery is better than that of women treated medically. In this regard, the randomized trials are of limited help. Only 10% of patients in the CASS trial were women, and in the VACS and the ECSS trials, women were not included. Therefore, many of our conclusions on the relative merits of bypass surgery versus medical therapy in women are extrapolated from results obtained from men. Given the demographic and physiologic differences between the sexes, this may or may not be appropriate.

Reoperation

Because graft and native vessel atherosclerosis is a progressive process, it is not surprising that the frequency of repeated coronary revascularization is increasing. Initially, progression of atherosclerosis in native coronary arteries was the most common indication for repeated CABG (55%). However, more recent experience has revealed a change in the spectrum of indications. Graft failure is the indication for reoperation in 85% of cases; graft failure alone is the indication in 25%; and graft failure in combination with progressive native vessel atherosclerosis is the indication in 60%.[113] The risk of requiring a reoperation is increased in patients who are young, have good left ventricular function, or have incomplete revascularization at the time of their first coronary surgery.[114] The use of an internal thoracic artery graft decreases reoperations and increases the length of time between a first and second CABG.

Coronary reoperations are associated with a higher operative risk and decreased long-term survival compared with primary revascularization. Most of this increased risk, however, is the result of a higher prevalence of preoperative risk factors.[113] Lytle and coworkers[115] reviewed the results in 1500 consecutive patients undergoing a first reoperation. The overall mortality was 3.4% in this series, which was approximately three times the rate for first coronary revascularization procedures. The major risk factors for operative mortality were left main coronary artery disease, class III or class IV symptoms, and advanced age. Schaff and colleagues[116] reported a 2.8% mortality rate in 106 consecutive reoperations. This was associated with an actuarial survival rate of 94% at 5 years and 89% at 7 years for hospital survivors.

The morbidity of a reoperation is also increased. The procedure is complicated by a perioperative myocardial infarction in 4% to 7.5% of patients.[113, 116] Repeated bypass surgery also carries an increased risk due to reentry through a median sternotomy, which increases the rate of bleeding complications as well as the chance of injury to a cardiac chamber or graft. Symptomatic relief is not as good as after the primary operation. Schaff and colleagues[116] reported that only 28% of hospital survivors were free from recurrent angina, a third CABG, a myocardial infarction, or death at 5 years. In a report from the Cleveland Clinic,[115] only 57% of patients were without symptoms at 5 years. However, most of the patients with symptoms had only mild (class II) symptoms. Up to 89% of patients with severe angina before reoperation had either no angina or only mild angina postoperatively.[103]

The expanding population of patients who have undergone coronary bypass surgery will continue to increase the volume of patients needing reoperation. These patients compose a subgroup who are older and sicker and in whom coronary anatomy is complex. Although coronary bypass surgery and PTCA are often considered competitive procedures, they frequently complement each other. Therefore, PTCA and other catheter-based interventions are being increasingly applied to patients with bypass grafts and recurrent angina.

Peripheral Vascular Disease With Coronary Artery Disease

Because atherosclerosis is a systemic process, a significant number of patients with coronary artery disease also have peripheral vascular disease, and vice versa. Tomatis and colleagues[117] performed coronary arteriograms in 100 consecutive patients admitted for evaluation of symptomatic peripheral vascular disease and found that 50% had a significant stenosis in one or more coronary arteries. Hertzer and coworkers[118] investigated the presence of coronary artery disease in 1000 consecutive patients with peripheral vascular disease. Of the 554 patients with clinically suspected coronary artery disease, 78% had a greater than 70% stenosis in one or more coronary arteries. Of the 446 without clinical coronary artery disease, 37% were still found to have significant coronary disease. Furthermore, most patients with coronary artery disease had multivessel disease.

Cardiac death accounts for a majority of the early and late mortality after peripheral vascular surgery. This risk is highest in patients with known coronary artery disease preoperatively. A comprehensive analysis by Hertzer[119] revealed that perioperative cardiac events occurred in 11% of patients with clinically suspected coronary artery disease but in only 1.7% of patients without. Raby and colleagues[120] found that preoperative ambulatory myocardial ischemia was present in 92% of patients with postoperative cardiac events (cardiac death, myocardial infarction, unstable angina, or pulmonary edema) but in only 12% of patients without postoperative events.

Because the presence of critical coronary artery disease is associated with a greater frequency of perioperative cardiac morbidity and mortality, preoperative risk assessment is warranted. Eagle and coworkers[121] described five useful clinical variables for stratifying risk of peripheral vascular surgery patients. These variables included

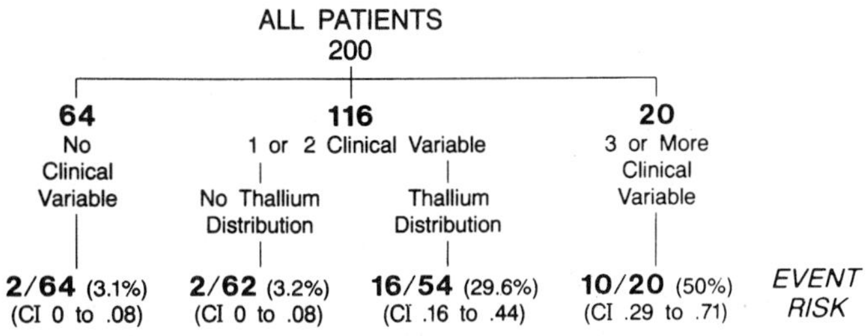

Figure 4–12. Algorithm for using clinical variables and the results of dipyridamole-thallium imaging to stratify cardiac risk in 200 patients undergoing peripheral vascular surgery. Events are unstable angina, ischemic pulmonary edema, myocardial infarction, or cardiac death. *Abbreviation:* CI, cardiac index. (From Eagle KA, Coley CM, Newell JB, et al: Combining clinical and thallium data optimizes preoperative assessment of cardiac risk for major vascular surgery. Ann Intern Med 1989; 18:203–214.)

age older than 70 years, the presence of Q waves on electrocardiogram, a history of angina, a history of ventricular arrhythmia requiring treatment, and diabetes mellitus requiring treatment (Fig. 4–12). If no clinical variables were present, only 3% of patients had postoperative cardiac ischemic events, and these patients could be classified as low risk. In contrast, if three or more clinical variables were present, 50% of the patients had a postoperative ischemic event and were considered high risk. Therefore, both of these groups could be risk-stratified by clinical variables alone. However, the intermediate-risk group required further stratification. In this group, the absence of thallium redistribution on dipyridamole-thallium testing stratified patients to a low-risk group, whereas the presence of thallium redistribution defects identified a high-risk subset.

Surgical revascularization does play a role in the preoperative evaluation of patients before peripheral vascular surgery. Hertzer[119] reported an operative mortality of 1.5% in vascular surgery patients with prior CABG. This compared favorably with a 1.3% operative mortality in vascular surgery patients without clinically suspected coronary artery disease and with a 6.8% operative mortality in patients with unbypassed but clinically suspected coronary artery disease (Table 4–3). When these same groups were observed after 5 years, the long-term mortality rate was 21% in patients with a prior CABG, 20% in patients without clinically suspected coronary artery disease, and 41% in those with unbypassed but suspected coronary artery disease.[119]

Despite the improved survival in vascular surgery patients with prior coronary bypass surgery, this strategy carries significant risks. The mean age of patients undergoing peripheral vascular surgery is approximately 65 years.[122] In the CASS Registry and in the Cleveland Clinic experience, the operative mortality rate for coronary bypass surgery is approximately three times greater in patients older than 65 years.[96, 103] Mullany and coworkers[101] presented data on coronary artery bypass graft surgery in 159 octogenarians. They reported an operative mortality of 16.7% in patients with concomitant peripheral vascular disease compared with 4% in patients without other medical conditions.

TABLE 4–3. MORTALITY IN PATIENTS UNDERGOING OPERATION FOR VASCULAR DISEASE

	Operative Mortality*		5-Year Mortality†	
Cardiac Status	**Number**	**(%)**	**Number**	**(%)**
Overall	14,180	(3.3)	7,805	(31)
No "overt" CAD	1,782	(1.3)	1,185	(20)
Suspected CAD	1,337	(6.8)	1.092	(41)
Prior CABG	1,237	(1.5)	1,172	(21)

Abbreviations: CABG, coronary artery bypass grafting; CAD, coronary artery disease.

*Based on 29 reported series representing 14,180 patients.

†Based on 23 reported series representing 7805 patients (53% of deaths were cardiac related).

Data from Hertzer NR: Basic data concerning associated coronary disease in peripheral vascular patients. Ann Vasc Surg 1987; 1:616–620.

The protective shield of coronary bypass surgery in patients with peripheral vascular disease comes at a price in terms of an increase in perioperative morbidity and mortality and a poorer late outcome than in patients without coronary artery disease. On the other hand many patients with peripheral vascular disease have high-risk coronary artery anatomy and as such would be expected to experience a survival benefit from bypass surgery over medical therapy. In the CASS Registry, coronary artery bypass surgery resulted in a marked improvement in long-term survival, compared with medical therapy, despite a higher perioperative morbidity and mortality.[123] However, the beneficial effects of bypass surgery were concentrated in patients with three-vessel coronary artery disease and impaired left ventricular function. Therefore, the clinical questions are analogous to those posed by the elderly. The early and late risks of the procedure are increased, but so is the potential for gain. The physician must carefully tailor therapy to the individual, knowing that the presence of peripheral vascular disease markedly enhances the complexity of the decision-making process.

In summary, patients with coronary artery disease are at increased risk when they undergo peripheral vascular surgery, and patients with peripheral vascular disease are at increased risk during CABG. Thus, the decision to perform coronary angiography should depend on several clinical variables as well as functional testing in patients at intermediate risk. Peripheral vascular surgery is not an indication for "prophylactic" coronary bypass surgery, but the presence of peripheral vascular disease does identify an individual in whom coronary artery disease may have a substantial adverse impact on perioperative and long-term outcomes. The indications for coronary bypass surgery are similar to those in patients without vascular disease and are based on the expectations of an effect on symptoms and late prognosis. The scope and the magnitude of the proposed peripheral vascular procedure, however, influence the timing of coronary bypass surgery but not its indications.[122]

Cerebrovascular Disease With Coronary Artery Disease

As is the case with peripheral vascular disease, cerebrovascular disease also frequently occurs in combination with coronary artery disease. The prevalence of severe cerebrovascular disease in patients undergoing coronary artery bypass surgery has been reported to be between 2% and 20%.[124, 125] In addition, up to 50% of patients with cerebrovascular disease will have concomitant symptomatic coronary artery disease.[126] This combination of vascular diseases results in a therapeutic dilemma. If coronary artery surgery is performed first, the risk of a postoperative stroke increases. In contrast, if carotid endarterectomy is performed first, the risk of myocardial infarction increases.

The incidence of perioperative stroke in patients undergoing elective coronary artery bypass surgery ranges from 1% to 2%.[127, 128] However, in patients with a prior history of stroke or transient ischemic attacks, this rate increases to almost 9%.[128] When patients undergoing an elective CABG complicated by a perioperative stroke were compared with patients without this complication, specific risk factors were identified. Patients with perioperative strokes were older, had more atherosclerotic disease in the ascending aorta, and were more likely to have a cervical bruit.[128]

The presence of coronary artery disease also dramatically affects the long-term outcome after carotid endarterectomy. Rihal and coworkers[129] examined the prognostic importance of coronary artery disease in 177 Olmsted County residents undergoing carotid endarterectomy. When patients with and without overt coronary artery disease were compared, there was no significant difference in mortality, myocardial infarction, or stroke 30 days after carotid endarterectomy. However, the cumulative incidence of a cardiac event 8 years after surgery was 61% in patients with overt coronary artery disease and 25% in those without overt coronary artery disease. Almost 50% of the total deaths were cardiac in origin, whereas only 7% were due to a stroke.

As a result of the high incidence of cardiac events after carotid endarterectomy and of perioperative strokes in CABG patients with symptomatic cerebrovascular disease, a combined surgical approach is advocated by some. This combined approach to the treatment of carotid and coronary artery disease was first described by Bernhard and colleagues.[130] A meta-analysis reported a perioperative mortality rate of 4.6% and a stroke rate of 3.2% for this combined operation.[124] This compared favorably with a group of patients undergoing a staged procedure in which the carotid endarterectomy was done first. In this cohort, the perioperative mortality rate was 7.5%, and the stroke rate was 3.2%.[124] Finally, the Cleveland Clinic performed a trial in which patients were prospectively randomized to the combined approach or a staged procedure with coronary revascularization done first.[131] In patients randomized to the combined approach, the mortality rate was 4.2%, with a stroke rate of 2.8%. In the cohort undergoing a staged procedure, the combined mortality rate was 5.3%, which was not significantly different from the combined approach. However, the incidence of stroke totaled 14% after coronary artery surgery followed by carotid endarterectomy, which was significantly worse ($p = .04$) than the combined approach.

Therefore, in patients with symptomatic cerebrovascular disease and stable coronary artery disease, carotid endarterectomy should be performed as a single procedure. However, because coronary artery disease is the most common cause of late morbidity and mortality, a thorough cardiac evaluation should be performed at some point. In patients with unstable coronary artery disease and asymptomatic cerebrovascular disease, a staged procedure can be performed with coronary revascularization done first, followed by carotid endarterectomy when indicated.[129] Finally, in the uncommon situation of both unstable coronary artery disease and cerebrovascular disease, a combined surgical procedure should be advocated.

PREOPERATIVE EVALUATION

The goal of the preoperative evaluation is to optimize the patient's clinical status. This involves correcting hemodynamic perturbations, electrolyte disturbances, and hypoxemia and maximizing anti-ischemic therapy. The coronary angiogram must be carefully reviewed to ensure that complete revascularization will occur. Prophylactic antibiotics are required and should be continued for 48 hours postoperatively.

Anti-ischemic therapy should be titrated to allow coronary revascularization to be performed as an elective procedure. It may take the form of pharmacologic therapy or an intra-aortic balloon pump. Pharmacologic therapy with oral or intravenous nitrates, beta blockers, calcium channel antagonists, or heparin may be helpful alone or in combination. The dose should be individualized to prevent symptomatic as well as silent ischemia while an adequate blood pressure is maintained. Pharmacologic therapy should be continued into the operating room, particularly in patients with unstable angina.

If moderate to severe ischemia continues despite maximal medical therapy, an intra-aortic balloon pump is indicated.[132] This will increase diastolic blood pressures to maximize coronary blood flow and decrease systolic blood pressure to decrease afterload. The most common scenarios in which intra-aortic balloon counterpulsation is required are medically refractory ischemia, profound left ventricular dysfunction, left main coronary artery disease, failed thrombolytic therapy, mechanical complications of an acute myocardial infarction, ischemic complications of a failed angioplasty, and refractory ventricular arrhythmias. However, an intra-aortic balloon pump should be used only in selected cases because of the risks of peripheral vascular complications.

POSTOPERATIVE MANAGEMENT

After successful aortocoronary bypass surgery, the major objective of early postoperative management is to ensure hemodynamic stability. Low cardiac output states can be treated with pacing, correction of intravascular volume status, inotropes, vasodilators, vasoconstrictors, or intra-aortic balloon pump. Symptomatic bradyarrhythmias should be treated with pacing therapy. In addition, sustained or symptomatic atrial and ventricular tachyarrhythmias as well as systemic and pulmonary hypertension should be treated.

Subsequent management is directed at the prevention of early vein graft thrombosis with antiplatelet agents, risk factor modification, and prophylaxis against atrial arrhythmias. The harvesting of saphenous veins results in endothelial damage, platelet deposition, and thromboxane production.[133] This combination of factors provides a substrate for early graft thrombosis, which occurs in approximately 10% of patients within the first month of surgery.[134] Therefore, it was logical to begin a series of trials on the use of platelet inhibitors.

The first prospective, randomized, double-blind study to define the role of antiplatelet therapy was conducted by Chesebro and associates.[135] Patients were given dipyridamole preoperatively and aspirin plus dipyridamole postoperatively. Within 1 month of CABG, 8% of the patients in the treated group had an occluded graft, compared with 21% in the placebo arm. There was no significant increase in blood loss, transfusions, or reoperation in the treated group. This benefit was maintained for the first postoperative year.[136] Repeated coronary angiography at 11 to 18 months after surgery revealed an occluded graft in 22% of the treated patients and in 47% of the placebo group.

A VACS trial compared several different antiplatelet regimens.[137, 138] In this trial, 555 patients were randomly assigned to receive aspirin (325 mg daily), aspirin (325 mg three times daily), aspirin plus dipyridamole, sulfinpyrazone, or placebo. All aspirin-containing regimens were started 12 hours before surgery. Coronary angiography was performed within 60 days of surgery and resulted in a graft patency rate of 93.5% with aspirin daily, 92.3% with aspirin three times daily, 91.9% with aspirin plus dipyridamole, 90.2% with sulfinpyrazone, and 85.2% with placebo. Although aspirin-containing regimens improved graft patency over placebo ($p < .05$), these regimens also resulted in increased blood loss and reoperations.[137] When angiography was repeated after 1 year, the graft occlusion rate in all of the aspirin groups combined was 15.8% versus 22.6% for the placebo group ($p < .03$). The major benefit observed at 1 year, however, appeared to be confined to grafted vessels of less than 2.0 mm in diameter.[138] Therefore, preoperative aspirin therapy, at a dose of 325 mg daily, resulted in improved graft patency; however, postoperative bleeding was increased.

The VACS group then compared early postoperative aspirin therapy (started 6 hours after surgery) with preoperative therapy.[139] When cardiac catheterization was performed at an average of 8 days after CABG, the saphenous vein graft occlusion rate was 7.4% in the preoperative aspirin group and 7.8% in the postoperative aspirin group (p = NS). In contrast, the preoperative aspirin group had an increased requirement for blood transfusions and an increased reoperation rate. Thus, aspirin therapy begun 6 hours after surgery offered maximal early vein graft patency with decreased bleeding complications. It should be continued for at least 1 year, but it does not seem to improve saphenous vein graft patency when it is continued for more than 1 year.[140] More recent data show that smaller doses of aspirin (80 to 100 mg) may be equally effective.[141] There appears to be no advantage to the routine use of dipyridamole alone or in combination with aspirin.

Risk factor management is another critical aspect of postoperative care.[142] Cigarette smoking, hyperlipidemia, hypertension, obesity, physical inactivity, and diabetes mellitus adversely affect prognosis. The goals of risk factor modification are to slow the progression or cause regression of atherosclerosis and the stabilization of plaques within bypass grafts as well as in native coronary arteries.

The cessation of cigarette smoking has been shown to decrease morbidity and mortality after coronary revascularization (Fig. 4–13). In patients randomized to the surgical arm of the CASS, survival at 10 years was 84% among those who smoked at entry but quit, compared with 68% among those who continued to smoke.[143] In addition, smokers were more likely to have angina, be unemployed, and be readmitted to the hospital.

Long-term bypass graft patency has been correlated with high levels of high-density lipoprotein (HDL) cholesterol and low levels of low-density lipoprotein (LDL) cholesterol and Lp(a).[144, 145] Therefore, dietary and pharmacologic interventions directed at these abnormalities are warranted. All patients should be counseled about a low-fat, low-cholesterol diet, with a goal of therapy to achieve an LDL cholesterol level of less than 100 mg/dL.[146] If this cannot be achieved, pharmacologic therapy should be instituted. The Cholesterol Lowering Atherosclerosis Study (CLAS) randomized hyperlipidemic men with previous bypass surgery to a combination of colestipol hydrochloride and niacin or placebo.[147] Treatment resulted in a 43% reduction in LDL cholesterol and a 37% increase in HDL cholesterol, which was associated with a reduction in the progression of atherosclerosis in both native coronary arteries and venous bypass grafts.

Along with smoking cessation and the control of serum lipid levels, postoperative management should include the treatment of hypertension, diabetes mellitus, and obesity. A comprehensive cardiac rehabilitation program can be helpful. A meta-analysis by Oldridge and associates[148] reported a 25% risk reduction for mortality in patients participating in cardiac rehabilitation.

Another important component of postoperative management is the prevention of atrial fibrillation. This is one of the most frequent complications of cardiac surgery, occurring in up to 40% of patients.[149] Its frequency increases with advancing age and most commonly occurs 24 to 60 hours after surgery. The development of atrial fibrillation usually does not result in long-term sequelae; however, potential complications include embolic phenomena, hemodynamic compromise, sustained atrial fibrillation, and increased length and cost of hospital stay.

A number of different agents have been investigated in the prevention of postoperative atrial fibrillation. Studies of beta blockers, including propranolol, timolol, and acebutolol, have uniformly shown them to be efficacious.[150–153] These trials used low doses of beta blockers, which effectively blocked the effects of excess catecholamines and the subsequent development of atrial fibrillation. In contrast, the data on digoxin, verapamil, and magnesium are more controversial. Some studies using perioperative digoxin show a decreased frequency of postoperative atrial fibrillation, whereas others show an increased frequency.[154, 155] This is also true of trials using magnesium.[156, 157] The use of verapamil results in no change in the overall frequency of atrial fibrillation; however, the ventricular response is controlled when it does occur.[158]

Therefore, all patients without contraindications should receive aspirin and beta blocker therapy in the immediate postoperative period. This significantly decreases the occurrence of early vein graft occlusion and postoperative atrial fibrillation. In addition, all patients should be counseled about the importance of risk factor modification before discharge. Finally, patients should be entered into a cardiac rehabilitation program shortly after discharge from the hospital.

VEIN GRAFT PATENCY

Despite the widespread use of the internal thoracic artery, the saphenous vein remains the conduit preferred to the right and left circumflex coronary arteries. Angelini and Newby[159] have reported that approximately two thirds of grafts to the left anterior descending artery were performed with the internal thoracic artery, whereas only 4% of the grafts to the right and left circumflex coronary arteries were done with an arterial graft. The saphenous vein is usually the conduit of choice in emergency situations. Therefore, improving the long-term patency rates of saphenous vein grafts is an important but formidable objective.

The patency rates of saphenous vein grafts are directly related to symptom relief and survival and have thus been the subject of multiple studies.[160, 161] In the early postoperative period, 8% to 12% of saphenous vein grafts are found to be occluded.[134, 162] This number increases to 10% to 20% by the end of the first postoperative year.[134, 162] After the first year, the occlusion rate decreases to an annual rate of 2% per year, so that at 5 years, the occlusion rate is 20% to 30%.[134, 163] However, between the 6th and 10th postoperative years, the attrition rate increases to 5% per year. Therefore, 10 years after coronary artery bypass surgery, only approximately 50% of vein grafts are patent.[24, 164]

The pathologic features of saphenous vein graft attrition have been well described.[165, 166] The first stage occurs in the early postoperative period and is characterized by thrombotic occlusion.[167–169] The next stage is fibrous intimal hyperplasia.[170] This occurs within the first postoperative year and, unlike the first stage, is not prevented by platelet inhibition. This process appears to represent an adaptation of the vein to its new function and probably has little effect on graft patency. The third stage occurs in the latter half of the first postoperative year and consists of increased fibrous intimal hyperplasia with superimposed thrombi. The final pathologic stage is vein graft athero-

Figure 4–13. Ten-year survival in surgically treated patients in the Coronary Artery Surgery Study. Patients who quit smoking (▲) had an improved survival over those who continued to smoke (●). (From Cavender JB, Rogers WJ, Fisher LD, et al: Effects of smoking on survival and morbidity in patients randomized to medical or surgical therapy in the Coronary Artery Surgery Study [CASS]: 10-year follow-up. J Am Coll Cardiol 1992; 20:287–294.)

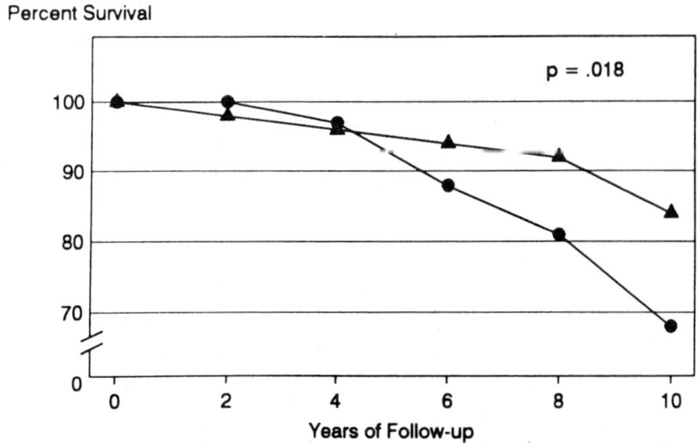

sclerosis, which is histologically distinct from the process that occurs in native coronary arteries. The atherosclerosis that occurs in saphenous vein grafts is diffuse, concentric, unencapsulated, and friable.[171] Risk factor modification is crucial in inhibiting this process.

Campeau and colleagues[160, 161] have correlated symptom relief and survival with graft patency. Approximately 6 years after coronary bypass surgery, graft occlusion or stenosis was found in 27% of patients with symptomatic deterioration but in only 5% of symptomatically improved patients.[160] In addition, 82% of patients with a patent graft at 1 year were alive at 12 years, compared with 42% in the group with no patent grafts.[161]

Progression of atherosclerosis in native coronary arteries is also seen during long-term follow-up. In an angiographic study by Hwang and associates,[172] 94% of grafted coronary arteries exhibited disease progression compared with 59% of nongrafted arteries at 10 years. In grafted vessels, disease progression was more common proximally (84%) than distal to the anastomoses (16%). Once again, symptoms could be correlated with disease progression.

INTERNAL THORACIC ARTERY PATENCY

The internal thoracic artery has become the preferred conduit for myocardial revascularization as a result of its relative immunity to atherosclerosis. Although the early patency rates for the left internal thoracic artery are only slightly superior to saphenous vein grafts, long-term patency rates are dramatically improved over vein grafts (Fig. 4–14). Lytle and colleagues[164] demonstrated an early patency rate of 97% at a mean of 14 months after surgery and a patency rate of 93% at a mean of 88 months after surgery. This group also reported patency rates dependent on the coronary artery grafted.[99] Patency rates of 95% to the left anterior descending coronary artery, 88% to the left circumflex coronary artery, and 76% to the right coronary artery were reported. Patency rates for free internal thoracic artery grafts were only slightly lower than those reported for in situ grafts. Long-term data on right internal thoracic artery grafts have also been presented. Huddleston and coworkers[173] found patency rates of 90% for left internal thoracic artery grafts compared with 79% for right internal thoracic artery grafts at 5 years after surgery.

There were several possible explanations for these improved patency rates observed with arterial grafts. Chaikhouni and associates[169] have shown that the intact endothelium of the internal thoracic artery produces significantly more prostacyclin than saphenous veins do. Prostacyclin acts as a potent vasodilator and platelet inhibitor, which should improve patency rates. Luscher and colleagues[174] have also demonstrated improved endothelium-dependent relaxation in internal thoracic artery grafts compared with saphenous vein grafts. Other factors that may contribute to its greater patency rate include a uniform internal elastic lamina and its ability to obtain nourishment from the lumen rather than the vasa vasorum.[175]

This superior patency rate of the left internal thoracic artery, especially when it is grafted to the left anterior descending coronary artery, has been shown to result in an improved clinical status. Loop and coworkers[22] compared the 10-year actuarial survival rates of patients receiving a left internal thoracic artery graft to their left anterior descending coronary artery with survival rates of patients receiving only saphenous vein grafts. In the cohort receiving an internal thoracic artery graft, there was a decreased risk of death, late myocardial infarction, cardiac events, and reoperations. This clinical advantage has been maintained throughout a follow-up period of 20 years.[176] Although patency rates and survival are better with a single internal thoracic artery graft than with vein grafts alone, it is still controversial whether bilateral internal thoracic artery grafts produce better long-term results.

ALTERNATIVE SURGICAL STRATEGIES

Although most patients with medically refractory ischemia are candidates for CABG surgery or PTCA, some patients are not amenable to coronary revascularization. For these patients, alternative surgical strategies, such as transmyocardial laser revascularization and cardiac transplantation, have been developed. Both of these treatment modalities have important limitations, however.

The technique of transmyocardial laser revascularization involves the creation of transmural laser channels in the left ventricular myocardium. These channels permit blood in the left ventricular cavity to directly perfuse the adjacent myocardium. Mirhoseini and Cayton[177] used a carbon dioxide laser in a canine model of left anterior descending coronary occlusion. Laser revascularization, from the epicardial surface, resulted in a dramatic and surprising reduction in mortality (from 83% to 0%). Horvath and associates[178] also used a carbon dioxide laser to the epicardium to study regional contractility in an ovine infarct model. They were able to demonstrate short- and long-term improvements in regional contractility as well as a reduction in myocardial necrosis, compared with control subjects. Yano and coworkers[179] were able to perform laser revascularization from the endocardial surface, using holmium:yttrium-aluminum-garnet laser energy. This technique also resulted in the preservation of regional myocardial function. Furthermore, this endocardial approach may lend itself to percutaneous therapy in the future.

Horvath and associates[180] have also reported early results in patients with medically refractory angina who were not candidates for surgical or percutaneous revascularization. Transmyocardial channels

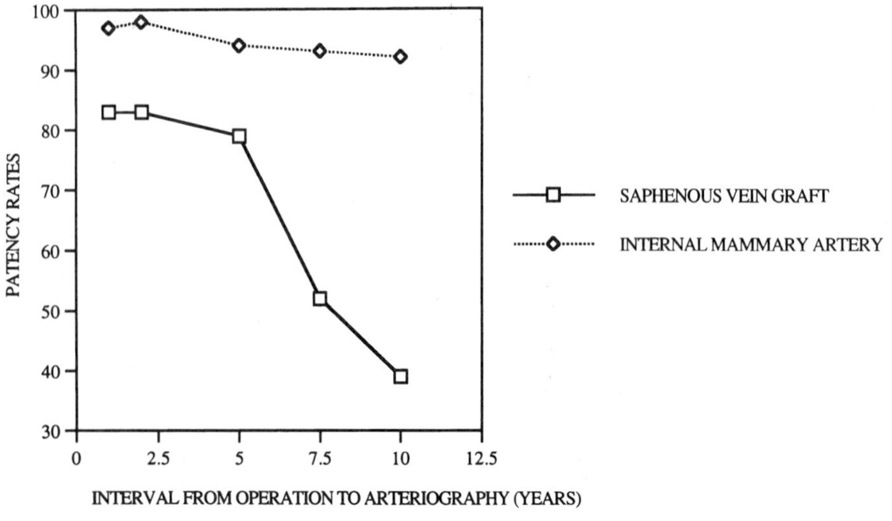

Figure 4–14. Long-term patency rates of internal mammary artery and saphenous vein bypass grafts. (Adapted from Lytle BW, Loop FD, Cosgrove DM, et al: Long term [5 to 12 years] serial studies of internal mammary and saphenous vein coronary bypass grafts. J Thorac Cardiovasc Surg 1985; 89:248–258.)

were created with a carbon dioxide laser to the epicardial surface corresponding to regions where technetium-99m sestamibi perfusion defects were identified. Laser revascularization resulted in a significant reduction in anginal class as well as a reduction in the size of fixed and reversible technetium-99m sestamibi perfusion defects. Although early results with this procedure are promising, this is still an investigational technique. Whether this technique will find an established place among the surgical approaches to coronary artery disease or whether this will be added to the list of innovative techniques that were initially promising but ultimately doomed to obscurity remains to be proven.

Orthotopic heart transplantation represents another treatment strategy for patients with medically refractory ischemic heart disease and contraindications to coronary revascularization (see Chapter 15). Briefly, this technique is indicated for patients with intractable angina and no potential for revascularization and for patients with end-stage ischemic cardiomyopathy without evidence of significant amounts of hibernating myocardium.[181] Important contraindications include systemic diseases that are likely to limit survival or increase the risk of death from rejection or from complications of immunosuppression, irreversible pulmonary hypertension, age, and unresolved pulmonary infarctions. Currently, the 1-year survival rate after cardiac transplantation is 85% to 90%, and the 5-year survival rate is almost 70%.[182] Despite the success of orthotopic heart transplantation, the most serious limitation of this technique continues to be an inadequate donor supply.

The success of the internal thoracic artery has led to the use of other arterial grafts. Both the right gastroepiploic and inferior epigastric arteries have been used as free (aorta to coronary) grafts with a great deal of success.[183, 184] The right gastroepiploic artery can be used as an in situ graft, like the internal thoracic artery. The radial artery has also been used as an aortocoronary bypass graft; however, the 1-year patency rates are lower.[185]

REFERENCES

1. Favaloro RG: Saphenous vein graft in the surgical treatment of coronary artery disease: operative technique. J Thorac Cardiovasc Surg 1969; 58:178–185.
2. Murphy ML, Hultgren HN, Detre K, et al: Treatment of chronic stable angina: a preliminary report of survival data of the randomized Veterans Administration Cooperative Study. N Engl J Med 1977; 297:621–627.
3. Takaro T, Hultgren HN, Lipton MJ, et al: The VA cooperative randomized study of surgery for coronary arterial occlusive disease. II. Subgroup with significant left main lesions. Circulation 1976; 54(suppl III):III-107–III-117.
4. European Coronary Surgery Study Group: Prospective randomized study of coronary artery bypass surgery in stable angina pectoris: second interim report. Lancet 1980; 2:491–495.
5. CASS principal investigators and their associates: Coronary Artery Surgery Study (CASS): a randomized trial of coronary artery bypass surgery; survival data. Circulation 1983; 68:939–950.
6. CASS principal investigators and their associates: Coronary Artery Surgery Study (CASS): a randomized trial of coronary artery bypass surgery; quality of life in patients randomly assigned to treatment groups. Circulation 1983; 68:951–960.
7. RITA Trial Participants: Coronary angioplasty versus coronary artery bypass surgery: the Randomised Intervention Treatment of Angina (RITA) Trial. Lancet 1993; 341:573–580.
8. Rodriguez A, Boullon F, Perez-Balino N, et al: Argentine randomized trial of percutaneous transluminal coronary angioplasty versus coronary artery bypass surgery in multivessel disease (ERACI): in-hospital results and 1-year follow-up. J Am Coll Cardiol 1993; 22:1060–1067.
9. Hamm CW, Reimers J, Ischinger T, et al: A randomized study of coronary angioplasty compared with bypass surgery in patients with symptomatic multivessel coronary disease. N Engl J Med 1994; 331:1037–1043.
10. King SB, Lembo NJ, Weintraub WS, et al: A randomized trial comparing coronary angioplasty with coronary bypass surgery. N Engl J Med 1994; 331:1044–1050.
11. Protocol for the Bypass Angioplasty Revascularization Investigation. Circulation 1991; 84(suppl V):V-1–V-27.
12. BARI, CABRI, EAST, GABI, RITA: Coronary angioplasty on trial. Lancet 1990; 335:1315–1316.
13. Lytle BW, Cosgrove D, Loop FD: Future implications of current trends in bypass surgery. Cardiovasc Clin 1991; 21:265–278.
14. Anderson GM, Grumbach K, Luft HS, et al: Use of coronary artery bypass surgery in the United States and Canada. Influence of age and income. JAMA 1993; 269:1661–1666.
15. Ayanian JZ, Epstein AM: Differences in the use of procedures between women and men hospitalized for coronary heart disease. N Engl J Med 1991; 325:221–225.
16. Steingart RM, Packer M, Hamm P, et al: Sex differences in the management of coronary artery disease. N Engl J Med 1991; 325:226–230.
17. Whittle J, Congliaro J, Good CB, Lofgren RP: Racial differences in the use of invasive cardiovascular procedures in the Department of Veteran's Affairs medical system. N Engl J Med 1993; 329:621–627.
18. The Veterans Administration Coronary Artery Bypass Surgery Cooperative Study Group: Eleven-year survival in the Veterans Administration Randomized Trial of Coronary Bypass Surgery for Stable Angina. N Engl J Med 1984; 311:1333–1339.
19. Varnauskas E, European Coronary Surgery Study Group: Twelve-year follow-up of survival in the randomized European Coronary Surgery Study. N Engl J Med 1988; 319:332–337.
20. Alderman EL, Bourassa MG, Cohen LS, et al: Ten-year follow-up of survival and myocardial infarction in the randomized Coronary Artery Surgery Study. Circulation 1990; 82:1629–1646.
21. Yusuf S, Zucker D, Peduzzi P, et al: Effect of coronary artery bypass graft surgery on survival: overview of 10 year results from randomised trials by the Coronary Artery Bypass Graft Surgery Trialist Collaboration. Lancet 1994; 344:563–570.
22. Loop FD, Lytle BW, Cosgrove DM, et al: Influence of the internal-mammary-artery graft on 10-year survival and other cardiac events. N Engl J Med 1986; 314:1–6.
23. Bourassa MG, Fischer LD, Campeau L, et al: Long-term fate of bypass grafts: the Coronary Artery Surgery Study (CASS) and Montreal Heart Institute experiences. Circulation 1985; 72:V-71–V-78.
24. Grondin CM, Campeau L, Lesperance J, et al: Comparison of late changes in internal mammary artery and saphenous vein grafts in two consecutive series of patients 10 years after operation. Circulation 1984; 70(suppl I), I-208–I-1212.
25. Sanz G, Pajaron A, Alegria E: Prevention of early aortocoronary bypass occlusion by low-dose aspirin and dipyridamole. Circulation 1990; 82:765–773.
26. Sculpher MJ, Seed P, Henderson RA, et al: Health service costs of coronary angioplasty and coronary artery bypass surgery: the Randomised Intervention Treatment of Angina (RITA) Trial. Lancet 1994; 344:927–930.
27. Hultgren HN, Peduzzi P, Detre K, et al: The 5-year effect of bypass surgery on relief of angina and exercise performance. Circulation 1985; 72:V-79–V-83.
28. Peduzzi P, Hultgren H, Thomsen J, et al: Ten-year effect of medical and surgical therapy on quality of life: Veterans Administration Cooperative Study of Coronary Artery Surgery. Am J Cardiol 1987; 59:1017–1023.
29. Hossack KF, Bruce RA, Ivey TD, et al: Improvement in aerobic and hemodynamic responses to exercise following aorta-coronary bypass grafting. J Thorac Cardiovasc Surg 1984; 87:901–907.
30. Arbogast R, Solignac A, Bourassa MG: Influence of aortocoronary saphenous vein bypass surgery on left ventricular volumes and ejection fraction. Am J Med 1973; 54:290–296.
31. Braunwald E, Rutherford JD: Reversible ischemic left ventricular dysfunction: evidence for the "hibernating myocardium." J Am Coll Cardiol 1986; 8:1467–1470.
32. CASS principal investigators and their associates: Myocardial infarction and mortality in the Coronary Artery Surgery Study (CASS) randomized trial. N Engl J Med 1984; 310:750–758.
33. Varnauskas E, and the European Coronary Surgery Study Group: Survival, myocardial infarction, and employment status in a prospective randomized study of coronary bypass surgery. Circulation 1985; 72(suppl V):V-90–V-101.
34. Myers WO, Gersh BJ, Fisher LD, et al: Time to first new myocardial infarction in patients with mild angina and three-vessel disease comparing medicine and early surgery: a CASS Registry study of survival. Ann Thorac Surg 1987; 43:599–612.

35. Unstable Angina: Diagnosis and Management. Rockville, MD: Agency for Health Care Policy and Research, Number 10, May 1994. AHCPR publication 94–0602.
36. The TIMI IIIB Investigators: Effects of tissue plasminogen activator and a comparison of early invasive and conservative strategies in unstable angina and non Q wave myocardial infarction: results of the TIMI IIIB Trial. Circulation 1994; 89:1545–1556.
37. Alison HW, Russel RO, Mantle JA, et al: Coronary anatomy and arteriography in patients with unstable angina pectoris. Am J Cardiol 1978; 41:204–209.
38. Unstable angina pectoris: National Cooperative Study Group to compare surgical and medical therapy. II. In-hospital experience and initial follow-up results in patients with one, two, and three vessel disease. Am J Cardiol 1978; 42:839–848.
39. Luchi RJ, Scott SM, Deupree RH, et al: Comparison of medical and surgical treatment for unstable angina pectoris. Results of a Veterans Administration Cooperative Study. N Engl J Med 1987; 316:977–984.
40. Taylor HA, Deumite NJ, Chaitma BR, et al: Asymptomatic left main coronary artery disease in the Coronary Artery Surgery Study (CASS) registry. Circulation 1989; 79:1171–1179.
41. Norris RM, Agnes TM, Brandt PWT, et al: Coronary surgery after a recurrent myocardial infarction: progress of a trial comparing surgical with non surgical management for asymptomatic patients with advanced coronary disease. Circulation 1981; 63:785–792.
42. Weiner DA, Ryan TJ, McCabe CH, et al: Comparison of coronary artery bypass surgery and medical therapy in patients with exercise-induced silent myocardial ischemia: a report from the Coronary Artery Surgery Study (CASS) registry. J Am Coll Cardiol 1988; 12:595–599.
43. Tyras DH, Barner HB, Kaiser GC, et al: Coronary artery disease with minimal angina: medical versus surgical therapy. J Thorac Cardiovasc Surg 1981; 82:699–705.
44. Egstrup K: Asymptomatic myocardial ischemia as a predictor of cardiac events after coronary artery bypass grafting for stable angina pectoris. Am J Cardiol 1988; 61:248–252.
45. Droste C, Lemmen S, Nitsche R, et al: ST-segment monitoring before, three weeks, and six months after aortocoronary bypass surgery. Eur Heart J 1988; 9(suppl N):169–175.
46. Weiner DA, Ryan TJ, Parsons L, et al: Prevalence and prognostic significance of silent and symptomatic ischemia after coronary bypass surgery: a report from the Coronary Artery Surgery Study (CASS) randomized population. J Am Coll Cardiol 1991; 18:343–348.
47. Pepine CJ, Geller NL, Knatterud GL, et al: The Asymptomatic Cardiac Ischemia Pilot (ACIP) Study: Design of a randomized clinical trial, baseline data and implications for a long-term outcome trial. J Am Coll Cardiol 1994; 24:1–10.
48. Gruppo Italiano per lo Studio della Streptochinasei nell'Infarto Miocardio (GISSI): Effectiveness of intravenous thrombolytic treatment in acute myocardial infarction. Lancet 1986; 1:397–402.
49. ISIS-2 (Second International Study of Infarct Survival) Collaborative Group: Randomized trial of intravenous streptokinase, oral aspirin, both, or neither among 17,187 cases of suspected acute myocardial infarction: ISIS-2. Lancet 1988; 2:349–360.
50. ISIS-3 (Third International Study of Infarct Survival) Collaborative Group: ISIS-3: a randomized comparison of streptokinase vs. tissue plasminogen activator vs. anistreplase and of aspirin plus heparin vs. aspirin alone among 41299 cases of suspected acute myocardial infarction. Lancet 1993; 339:753–770.
51. The GUSTO Investigators: An international randomized trial comparing four thrombolytic strategies for acute myocardial infarction. N Engl J Med 1993; 329:673–682.
52. Grines CL, Brown KF, Marco J, et al: A comparison of immediate angioplasty with thrombolytic therapy for acute myocardial infarction. N Engl J Med 1993; 328:673–679.
53. Zijlstra F, Jan De Boer M, Hoorntje JLA, et al: A comparison of immediate coronary angioplasty with intravenous streptokinase in acute myocardial infarction. N Engl J Med 1993; 328:680–684.
54. Gibbons RJ, Holmes DR, Reeder GS, et al: Immediate angioplasty compared with the administration of a thrombolytic agent followed by conservative treatment for myocardial infarction. N Engl J Med 1993; 328:685–691.
55. de Boer JM, Hoorntje JCA, Ottervanger JP, et al: Immediate coronary angioplasty versus intravenous streptokinase in acute myocardial infarction: left ventricular ejection fraction, hospital mortality and reinfarction. J Am Coll Cardiol 1994; 23:1004–1008.
56. Himbert D, Juliard JM, Steg G, et al: Primary coronary angioplasty for acute myocardial infarction with contraindications to thrombolysis. Am J Cardiol 1993; 71:377–381.
57. Lee L, Bates ER, Pitt B, et al: Percutaneous transluminal coronary angioplasty improves survival in acute myocardial infarction complicated by cardiogenic shock. Circulation 1988; 78:1345–1351.
58. Moosvi AR, Khaja F, Villaneuva L, et al: Early revascularization improves survival in cardiogenic shock complicating myocardial infarction. J Am Coll Cardiol 1992; 19:907–914.
59. Hibbard MD, Holmes DR, Bailey KR, et al: Percutaneous transluminal coronary angioplasty in patients with cardiogenic shock. J Am Coll Cardiol 1992; 19:639–646.
60. Keon WJ, Abbas SZ, Shankar KR, Nino AF: Emergency aortocoronary bypass grafting: cardiogenic shock. Can Med Assoc J 1971; 105:1291–1296.
61. Lee KF, Mandell J, Rankin JS, et al: Immediate versus delayed coronary grafting after streptokinase treatment: post-operative blood loss and clinical results. J Thorac Cardiovasc Surg 1988, 95:216–222.
62. DeWood MA, Spores J, Berg R, et al: Acute myocardial infarction: a decade of experience with surgical reperfusion in 701 patients. Circulation 1983; 68(suppl II):II-8–II-16.
63. Phillips SJ, Kongtahworn C, Skinner D: Emergency coronary artery reperfusion: a choice of therapy for evolving myocardial infarction. J Thorac Cardiovasc Surg 1983; 86:679–688.
64. Koshal A, Beanlands DS, Davies RA, et al: Urgent surgical reperfusion in acute evolving myocardial infarction: a randomized controlled study. Circulation 1988; 78(suppl I):171–178.
65. Gersh BJ, Chesebro JH, Braunwald E, et al: Coronary artery bypass graft surgery after thrombolytic therapy in the Thrombolysis In Myocardial Infarction trial, phase II (TIMI II). J Am Coll Cardiol 1995; 25:395–402.
66. Kuller LH: Sudden death—definition and epidemiologic considerations. Prog Cardiovasc Dis 1980; 23:1–12.
67. Baum RS, Alvarez H, Cobb LA: Survival after resuscitation from out-of-hospital ventricular fibrillation. Circulation 1974; 50:1231–1235.
68. Kannel WB, Thomas HE: Sudden cardiac death: the Framingham Study. Ann N Y Acad Sci 1982; 382:3–20.
69. Willich SN, Levy D, Roco MB, et al: Circadian variation in the incidence of sudden cardiac death in the Framingham Heart Study Population. Am J Cardiol 1987; 60:801–806.
70. Beta Blocker Heart Attack Trial Research Group: A randomized trial of propranolol in patients with acute myocardial infarction: I. Mortality results. JAMA 1982; 247:1707–1714.
71. Holmes DR, Davis KB, Mock MB, et al: The effect of medical and surgical treatment on subsequent sudden cardiac death in patients with coronary artery disease: a report from the Coronary Artery Surgery Study. Circulation 1986; 73:1254–1263.
72. Passamani E, Davis KB, Gillespie MJ, et al: A randomized trial of coronary artery bypass surgery: survival of patients with a low ejection fraction. N Engl J Med 1985; 312:1665–1671.
73. Every NR, Fahrenbruch CE, Hallstrum AP, et al: Influence of coronary bypass surgery on subsequent outcome of patients resusicitated from out of hospital cardiac arrests. J Am Coll Cardiol 1992; 19:1435–1439.
74. Kelly P, Ruskin JN, Vlahakes GJ, et al: Surgical coronary revascularization in survivors of prehospital cardiac arrest: its effect on inducible arrhythmias and long-term survival. J Am Coll Cardiol 1990; 15:267–273.
75. Topol EJ, Weiss JL, Guzman PA, et al: Immediate improvement of dysfunctional myocardial segments after coronary revascularization: detection by intraoperative TEE. J Am Coll Cardiol 1984; 4:1123–1134.
76. Elefteriades JA, Tolis G, Levi E, et al: Coronary artery bypass grafting in severe left ventricular dysfunction: excellent survival and improved ejection fraction and functional state. J Am Coll Cardiol 1993; 22:1411–1417.
77. Rahimtoola SH: The hibernating myocardium. Am Heart J 1989; 117:211–213.
78. Vanoverschelde JLJ, Wijns W, Depre C, et al: Mechanisms of chronic regional postischemic dysfunction in humans: new insights from the study of noninfarcted collateral-dependent myocardium. Circulation 1993; 87:1513–1523.
79. Schelbert HR, Phelps ME, Hoffman E, et al: Regional myocardial blood flow, metabolism, and function assessed noninvasively with positron emission tomography. Am J Cardiol 1980; 80:1269–1277.
80. Tillisch JH, Brunken R, Marshall R, et al: Reversibility of cardiac wall-motion abnormalities predicted by positron tomography. N Engl J Med 1986; 314:884–888.

81. Bonow RO, Dilsizian V, Cuocolo A, et al: Identification of viable myocardium in patients with chronic coronary artery disease and left ventricular dysfunction. Comparison of thallium scintigraphy with reinjection and PET imaging with 18F-fluorodeoxyglucose. Circulation 1991; 83:26–37.
82. Kayden DS, Sigal S, Soufer R, et al: Thallium-201 for assessment of myocardial viability: quantitative comparison of 24-hour redistribution imaging with imaging after reinjection at rest. J Am Coll Cardiol 1991; 18:1480–1486.
83. Humphrey LS, Topol EJ, Rosenfeld GI, et al: Immediate enhancement of left ventricular relaxation by coronary artery bypass grafting: intraoperative assessment. Circulation 1988; 77:886–896.
84. Baker DW, Jones R, Hodges J, et al: Management of heart failure. III. The role of revascularization in the treatment of patients with moderate or severe left ventricular systolic dysfunction. JAMA 1994; 272:1528–1534.
85. Detre K, Holubkov R, Kelsey S, et al: Percutaneous transluminal coronary angioplasty in 1985–1986 and 1977–1981. The National Heart, Lung, and Blood Institute Registry. N Engl J Med 1988; 318:265–270.
86. Ryan TJ, Bauman WB, Kennedy JW, et al: Guidelines for percutaneous transluminal coronary angioplasty. A report of the American College of Cardiology/American Heart Association Task Force on assessment of diagnostic and therapeutic cardiovascular procedures (committee on percutaneous transluminal coronary angioplasty). J Am Coll Cardiol 1993; 22:2033–2054.
87. Golding LAR, Loop FD, Hollman JL, et al: Early results of emergency surgery after coronary angioplasty. Circulation 1986; 74(suppl III):III-26–III-29.
88. Ullyot DJ: Surgical standby for percutaneous coronary angioplasty. Circulation 1987; 76(suppl III):III-149–III-152.
89. Click RL, Holmes DR, Vlietstra RE, et al: Anomalous coronary arteries: location, degree of atherosclerosis and effect on survival—a report from the Coronary Artery Surgery Study. J Am Coll Cardiol 1989; 13:531–537.
90. Roberts WC: Major anomalies of coronary arterial origin seen in adulthood. Am Heart J 1986; 111:941–963.
91. Roberts WC, Siegel RJ, Zipes DP: Origin of the right coronary artery from the left sinus of Valsalva and its functional consequences: analysis of 10 necropsy patients. Am J Cardiol 1982; 49:863–868.
92. Virmani R, Chun PKC, Goldstein RE: Acute takeoffs of the coronary arteries along the aortic wall and congenital coronary ostial valve-like ridges. Association with sudden death. J Am Coll Cardiol 1984; 3:766–771.
93. Hutchins GM, Miner MM, Boitnott JK: Vessel caliber and branch-angle of human coronary artery branch-points. Circ Res 1976; 38:572–576.
94. Urrutia-S CO, Falaschi G, Ott DA, Cooley DA: Surgical management of 56 patients with congenital coronary artery fistulas. Ann Thorac Surg 1983; 35:300–307.
95. Edmunds LH, Stephenson LW, Edic RN, et al: Open-heart surgery in octogenarians. N Engl J Med 1988; 319:131–136.
96. Gersh BJ, Kronmal RA, Frye RL, et al: Coronary arteriography and coronary bypass surgery: morbidity and mortality in patients 65 years of age and older. A report from the Coronary Artery Surgery Study. Circulation 1983; 67:483–491.
97. Gersh BJ, Kronmal RA, Schaff HV, et al: Long-term (5 year) results of coronary bypass surgery in patients 65 years old or older: a report from the Coronary Artery Surgery Study. Circulation 1983; 68(suppl II):II-190–II-199.
98. Gersh BJ, Kronmal RA, Schaff HV, et al: Comparison of coronary artery bypass surgery and medical therapy in patients 65 years of age or older. A non-randomized study from the Coronary Artery Surgery Study (CASS) registry. N Engl J Med 1985; 313:217–224.
99. Lytle BW, Cosgrove DM: Coronary artery bypass surgery. Curr Probl Surg 1992; 29:735 807.
100. Freeman WK, Schaff HV, O'Brien PC, et al: Cardiac surgery in the octogenarian: perioperative outcome and clinical follow-up. J Am Coll Cardiol 1991; 18:29–35.
101. Mullany CJ, Darling GE, Pluth JR, et al: Early and late results after isolated coronary artery bypass surgery in 159 patients aged 80 years and older. Circulation 1990; 82(suppl IV):IV-229–IV-236.
102. Blauth CI, Cosgrove DM, Webb BW, et al: Atheroembolism from the ascending aorta; an emerging problem in cardiac surgery. J Thorac Cardiovasc Surg 1992; 103:1104–1112.
103. Loop FD, Lytle BW, Cosgrove DM, et al: Coronary artery bypass graft surgery in the elderly. Indications and outcome. Cleve Clin J Med 1988; 55:23–34.
104. Rahimtoola SH, Grunkemeier GL, Starr A: Ten year survival after coronary artery bypass surgery for angina in patients aged 65 years and older. Circulation 1986; 74:509–517.
105. Tobin JN, Smoller SW, Wexler JP, et al: Sex bias in considering coronary bypass surgery. Ann Intern Med 1987; 107:19–25.
106. Chaitman BR, Bourassa MG, Davis K, et al: Angiographic prevalence of high-risk coronary artery disease in patient subsets (CASS). Circulation 1981; 64:360–367.
107. Bell MR, Berger PB, Holmes DR, et al: Referral for coronary artery revascularization procedures after diagnostic coronary angiography: evidence for a gender bias? J Am Coll Cardiol 1995; 25:1650–1655.
108. Loop FD, Golding LR, MacMillan JP, et al: Coronary artery surgery in women compared with men: analysis of risks and long-term results. J Am Coll Cardiol 1983; 1:383–390.
109. King KB, Clark PC, Hicks GL: Patterns of referral and recovery in women and men undergoing coronary artery bypass grafting. Am J Cardiol 1992; 69:179–182.
110. Gardner TJ, Horneffer PJ, Gott VL, et al: Coronary artery bypass grafting in women: a ten-year perspective. Ann Surg 1985; 201:780–784.
111. Myers WO, Davis K, Foster ED, et al: Surgical survival in the Coronary Artery Surgery Study (CASS) registry. Ann Thorac Surg 1985; 40:245–260.
112. Fischer LD, Kennedy JW, Davis KB, et al: Association of sex, physical size, and operative mortality after coronary artery bypass in the Coronary Artery Surgery Study (CASS). J Thorac Cardiovasc Surg 1982; 84:334–341.
113. Loop FD, Lytle BW, Cosgrove DM, et al: Reoperation for coronary atherosclerosis. Changing practice in 2509 consecutive patients. Ann Surg 1990; 212:378–386.
114. Cosgrove DM, Loop FD, Lytle BW, et al: Predictors of reoperation after myocardial revascularization. J Thorac Cardiovasc Surg 1986; 92:811–821.
115. Lytle BW, Loop FD, Cosgrove DM, et al: 1500 coronary reoperations—results and determinants of early and late survival. J Thorac Cardiovasc Surg 1987; 93:847–859.
116. Schaff HV, Orszulak TA, Gersh BJ, et al: The morbidity and mortality of reoperation for coronary artery disease and analysis of late results with use of actuarial estimate of event-free interval. J Thorac Cardiovasc Surg 1983; 85:508–514.
117. Tomatis LA, Fierens EE, Verbrugge GP: Evaluation of surgical risk in peripheral vascular disease by coronary arteriography: a series of 100 cases. Surgery 1972; 71:429–435.
118. Hertzer NR, Beven EG, Young JR, et al: Coronary artery disease in peripheral vascular patients: a classification of 1000 coronary angiograms and results of surgical management. Ann Surg 1984; 199:223–233.
119. Hertzer NR: Basic data concerning associated coronary disease in peripheral vascular patients. Ann Vasc Surg 1987; 1:616–620.
120. Raby KE, Goldman L, Creager MA, et al: Correlation between preoperative ischemia and major cardiac events after peripheral vascular surgery. N Engl J Med 1989; 321:1296–1300.
121. Eagle KA, Coley CM, Newell JB, et al: Combining clinical and thallium data optimizes preoperative assessment of cardiac risk for major vascular surgery. Ann Intern Med 1989; 110:859–866.
122. Gersh BJ, Rihal CS, Rooke TW, et al: Evaluation and management of patients with both peripheral vascular and coronary artery disease. J Am Coll Cardiol 1991; 18:203–214.
123. Rihal CS, Eagle KA, Mickel MC, et al: Surgical therapy for coronary artery disease among patients with combined coronary artery and peripheral vascular disease. Circulation 1995; 91:46–53.
124. Cosgrove DM, Hertzer NR, Loop FD: Surgical management of synchronous carotid and coronary artery disease. J Vasc Surg 1986; 3:690–693.
125. Carrel T, Stillhard G, Turina M: Combined carotid and coronary artery surgery: early and late results. Cardiology 1992; 80:118–125.
126. Ennix CL, Lawrie GM, Morris GC, et al: Improved results of carotid endarterectomy in patients with symptomatic coronary artery disease: an analysis of 1546 consecutive carotid operations. Stroke 1979; 10:122–130.
127. Cosgrove DM, Loop FD, Lytle BW, et al: Primary myocardial revascularization: trends in surgical mortality. J Thorac Cardiovasc Surg 1984; 88:673–684.
128. Jones EL, Craver JM, Michalik RA, et al: Combined carotid and coronary operations: when are they necessary? J Thorac Cardiovasc Surg 1984; 87:7–16.

129. Rihal CS, Gersh BJ, Whisnant JP, et al: Influence of coronary heart disease on morbidity and mortality after carotid endarterectomy: a population-based study in Olmsted County, Minnesota (1970–1988). J Am Coll Cardiol 1992; 19:1254–1260.
130. Bernhard JM, Johnson WD, Peterson JJ: Carotid stenosis. Association with surgery for coronary artery disease. Arch Surg 1972; 105:837–842.
131. Hertzer NR, Loop FD, Beven EG, et al: Surgical staging for simultaneous coronary and carotid disease: a study including prospective randomization. J Vasc Surg 1989; 9:455–463.
132. McEnany MT, Kay HR, Buckley MJ, et al: Clinical experience with intraaortic balloon pump support in 728 patients. Circulation 1978; 58(suppl I):I-124–I-132.
133. Fuster V, Dewanjee MK, Kaye MP, et al: Noninvasive radioisotopic technique for detection of platelet deposition in coronary artery bypass grafts in dogs and its reduction with platelet inhibitors. Circulation 1979; 60:1308–1312.
134. FitzGibbon GM, Leach AJ, Keon WJ, et al: Coronary bypass graft fate: angiographic study of 1179 vein grafts early, one year, and five years after operation. J Thorac Cardiovasc Surg 1986; 91:773–778.
135. Chesebro JH, Clements IP, Fuster V, et al: A platelet-inhibitor–drug trial in coronary-artery bypass operations: benefit of preoperative dipyridamole and aspirin therapy on early postoperative vein-graft patency. N Engl J Med 1982; 307:73–78.
136. Chesebro JH, Fuster V, Elveback LR, et al: Effect of dipyridamole and aspirin on late vein-graft patency after coronary bypass operations. N Engl J Med 1984; 310:209–214.
137. Goldman S, Copeland J, Moritz T, et al: Improvement in early saphenous vein graft patency after coronary artery bypass surgery with antiplatelet therapy: results of a Veterans Administration Cooperative Study. Circulation 1988; 77:1324–1332.
138. Goldman S, Copeland J, Moritz T, et al: Saphenous vein graft patency 1 year after coronary artery bypass surgery and effects of antiplatelet therapy: results of a Veterans Administration Cooperative Study. Circulation 1989; 80:1190–1197.
139. Goldman S, Copeland J, Moritz T, et al: Starting aspirin therapy after operation: effects on early graft patency. Circulation 1991; 84:520–526.
140. Goldman S, Copeland J, Moritz T, et al: Long-term graft patency (3 years) after coronary artery surgery. Effects of aspirin: results of a VA Cooperative Study. Circulation 1994; 89:1138–1164.
141. Lorenz RL, Schacky CV, Weber M, et al: Improved aortocoronary bypass patency by low dose aspirin (100 mg daily): effects on platelet aggregation and thromboxane formation. Lancet 1984; 1:1261–1264.
142. Pearson T, Rapaport E, Criqui M, et al: Optimal risk factor management in the patient after coronary revascularization. A statement for healthcare professionals from an American Heart Association Writing Group. Circulation 1994; 90:3125–3133.
143. Cavender JB, Rogers WJ, Fisher LD, et al: Effects of smoking on survival and morbidity in patients randomized to medical or surgical therapy in the Coronary Artery Surgery Study (CASS): 10-year follow-up. J Am Coll Cardiol 1992; 20:287–294.
144. Campeau L, Enjalbert M, Lesperance J, et al: The relation of risk factors to the development of atherosclerosis in saphenous-vein bypass grafts and in the progression of disease in the native circulation: a study 10 years after aortocoronary bypass surgery. N Engl J Med 1984; 311:1329–1332.
145. Hoff HF, Beck GJ, Skibinski CI, et al: Serum Lp(a) level as a predictor of a vein graft stenosis after coronary artery bypass surgery in patients. Circulation 1988; 77:1238–1244.
146. Summary of the second report of the National Cholesterol Education Program (NCEP) expert panel on detection, evaluation, and treatment of high blood cholesterol in adults (Adult Treatment Panel II). JAMA 1993; 269:3015–3023.
147. Blankenhorn DH, Nessim SA, Johnson RL, et al: Beneficial effects of combined colestipol-niacin therapy on coronary atherosclerosis and coronary venous bypass grafts. JAMA 1987; 257:3233–3240.
148. Oldridge NB, Guyatt GH, Fischer ME, Rimm AA: Cardiac rehabilitation after myocardial infarction: combined experience of randomized clinical trials. JAMA 1988; 260:945–950.
149. Lauer MS, Eagle KA, Buckley MJ, DeSanctis RW: Atrial fibrillation following coronary artery bypass surgery. Prog Cardiovasc Dis 1989; 31:367–378.
150. Matangi MF, Neutze JM, Graham IC, et al: Arrhythmia prophylaxis after aorta-coronary bypass: the effects of minidose propranolol. J Thorac Cardiovasc Surg 1985; 89:439–443.
151. White HD, Antman EM, Glynn MA, et al: Efficacy and safety of timolol for prevention of supraventricular tachyarrhythmias after coronary artery bypass surgery. Circulation 1984; 70:479–484.
152. Daudon P, Corcos T, Gardjbakah I, et al: Prevention of atrial fibrillation or flutter by acebutolol after coronary bypass grafting. Am J Cardiol 1986; 58:933–936.
153. Andrews TC, Reimold SC, Berlin JA, Antman EM: Prevention of supraventricular arrhythmias after coronary bypass surgery. A meta-analysis of randomized control trials. Circulation 1991; 84(suppl III):III-236–III-244.
154. Johnson LW, Dickstein RA, Freuhan CT, et al: Prophylactic digitalization for coronary artery bypass surgery. Circulation 1976; 53:819–822.
155. Tyras DH, Stothert JC, Kaiser GC, et al: Supraventricular tachyarrhythmias after myocardial revascularization: a randomized trial of prophylactic digitalization. J Thorac Cardiovasc Surg 1979; 77:310–314.
156. Fanning WJ, Thomas CS, Roach A, et al: Prophylaxis of atrial fibrillation with magnesium sulfate after coronary artery bypass grafting. Ann Thorac Surg 1991; 52:529–533.
157. Parikka H, Toivonen L, Pellinen T, et al: The influence of intravenous magnesium sulfate on the occurrence of atrial fibrillation after coronary artery by-pass operation. Eur Heart J 1993; 14:251–258.
158. Davison R, Hartz R, Kaplan K, et al: Prophylaxis of supraventricular tachyrhythmia after coronary bypass surgery with oral verapamil: a randomized, double-blind trial. Ann Thorac Surg 1985; 39:336–339.
159. Angelini GD, Newby AC: The future of saphenous vein as a coronary artery bypass conduit. Eur Heart J 1989; 10:273–280.
160. Campeau L, Lesperance J, Hermann J, et al: Loss of the improvement of angina between 1 and 7 years after aortocoronary bypass surgery: correlation with changes in vein grafts and in coronary arteries. Circulation 1979; 60(suppl I):I-1–I-5.
161. Campeau L, Enjalbert M, Bourassa MG, et al: Improvement of angina and survival 1 to 12 years after aortocoronary bypass surgery: correlation with changes in grafts and in the native coronary circulation. J Heart Transplant 1984; 3:220–223.
162. Grondin CM, Lesperance J, Bourassa MG, et al: Serial angiographic evaluation in 60 consecutive patients with aortocoronary artery vein grafts 2 weeks, 1 year, and 3 years after operation. J Thorac Cardiovasc Surg 1974; 67:1–6.
163. Grondin CM, Lesperance J, Solymoss BC, et al: Atherosclerotic changes in coronary grafts six years after operation. J Thorac Cardiovasc Surg 1979; 77:24–31.
164. Lytle BW, Loop FD, Cosgrove DM, et al: Long term (5 to 12 years) serial studies of internal mammary and saphenous vein coronary bypass grafts. J Thorac Cardiovasc Surg 1985; 89:248–258.
165. Fuster V: Drugs interfering with platelet function: mechanisms and clinical relevance. *In* Verstraete M (ed): Thrombosis and Hemostasis. Leuven, Belgium: Leuven University Press, 1987.
166. Solymoss BC, Leung TK, Pelletier LC, et al: Pathologic changes in coronary artery saphenous vein grafts and related etiologic factors. Cardiovasc Clin 1991; 21:45–65.
167. Fuchs JCA, Mitchener JS, Hagen PO: Postoperative changes in autologous vein grafts. Ann Surg 1978; 188:1–15.
168. Unni KK, Kottke BA, Titus JL, et al: Pathologic changes in aortocoronary saphenous vein grafts. Am J Cardiol 1974; 34:526–532.
169. Chaikhouni A, Crawford FA, Kochel PJ, et al: Human internal mammary artery provides more prostacyclin than saphenous vein. J Thorac Cardiovasc Surg 1986; 92:88–91.
170. Brody WR, Kosek JC, Angell WW: Changes in vein grafts following aortocoronary bypass induced by pressure and ischemia. J Thorac Cardiovasc Surg 1972; 64:847–854.
171. Ratliff NB, Myles JL: Rapidly progressive atherosclerosis in aortocoronary saphenous vein grafts: possible immune mediated disease. Arch Pathol Lab Med 1989; 113:772–776.
172. Hwang MH, Meadows WR, Palac RT, et al: Progression of native coronary artery disease at 10 years: insights from a randomized study of medical versus surgical therapy for angina. J Am Coll Cardiol 1990; 16:1066–1070.
173. Huddleston CB, Stoney WS, Alford WC, et al: Internal mammary artery grafts: technical factors influencing patency. Ann Thorac Surg 1986; 42:5–13.
174. Luscher TF, Diederich D, Siebenmann R, et al: Difference between endothelium-dependent relaxation in arterial and in venous coronary bypass grafts. N Engl J Med 1988; 319:462–467.
175. Ferro M, Conti M, Novero D, et al: The thin intima of the internal mammary artery as the possible reason for freedom from atherosclerosis and success in coronary bypass. Am Heart J 1991; 122:1192–1195.

176. Cameron AAC, Green GE, Brogno DA, et al: Internal thoracic artery grafts: 20-year clinical follow up. J Am Coll Cardiol 1995; 25:188–192.
177. Mirhoseini M, Cayton MM: Revascularization of the heart by laser. J Microsurg 1981; 2:253–260.
178. Horvath KA, Smith WJ, Laurence RG, et al: Recovery and viability of on acute myocardial infarct after transmyocardial laser revascularization. J Am Coll Cardiol 1995; 25:258–263.
179. Yano OJ, Bielefeld MR, Jecvanandem V, et al: Prevention of acute regional ischemia with endocardial laser channels. Ann Thorac Surg 1993; 56:46–53.
180. Horvath KA, Mannting F, Cohn LH: Improved myocardial perfusion and relief of angina after transmyocardial laser revascularization [Abstract]. Circulation 1994; 90:I-640.
181. Copeland JG, Emery RW, Levinson MM, et al: Selection of patients for cardiac transplantation. Circulation 1987; 75:2–9.
182. Kriett JM, Kaye MP: The registry of the International Society for Heart Transplantation: Seventh official report—1990. J Heart Transplant 1990; 9:323–330.
183. Lytle BW, Cosgrove DM, Ratliff NB, et al: Coronary artery bypass grafting with the right gastroepiploic artery. J Thorac Cardiovasc Surg 1989; 97:826–831.
184. Puig LB, Ciongolli W, Cividanes GUL, et al: Inferior epigastric artery as a free graft for myocardial revascularization. J Thorac Cardiovasc Surg 1990; 99:251–255.
185. Fisk RL, Brooks CH, Calaghan JC, et al: Experience with the radial artery graft for coronary artery bypass. Ann Thorac Surg 1976; 21:513–518.

5 Chronic Angina: Stable

Martin M. LeWinter, MD
Burton E. Sobel, MD

INTRODUCTION

Effective treatment of angina pectoris is predicated on accurate categorization of pathophysiology and risk in the individual patient. Although angina is a manifestation of an intermittent imbalance between myocardial oxygen requirements and supply, underlying pathophysiologic mechanisms are diverse, and prognosis is variable. Accordingly, the characterization of patients with regard to underlying pathophysiologic mechanisms and risk is discussed first; treatment modalities are described next; and treatment is subsequently related to specific categories of both.

In contrast to *unstable angina* (a term embracing new-onset and crescendo angina, angina exhibiting a rapid change in frequency or severity despite no change in physical activity, and preinfarction angina[1]), the term *stable angina* is applied to a syndrome of intermittent discomfort (usually substernal) attributable to transitory myocardial ischemia with reasonably consistent clinical manifestations, including the intensity at which activity initiates discomfort and the prompt disappearance of discomfort with cessation of activity and/or administration of nitroglycerin. The frequency of occurrence of stable angina and the level of activity required to produce it are relatively constant, but the definition encompasses symptoms that become worse over time. Despite the apparent simplicity of this definition, the initial episode can obviously qualify as "unstable" until the clinical features of the underlying syndrome have been clarified. Furthermore, some patients with angina that is stable, in the sense of a clinically consistent syndrome, have episodic angina at rest that can be construed as unstable when it first appears. Treatment options for patients with stable angina or angina of gradually progressive severity and/or frequency of symptoms differ markedly from those for patients in whom an abrupt change in clinical course characterizes the disorder as being unstable angina, a syndrome typically occurring with the onset of episodes at rest.

CATEGORIZATION OF PATIENTS WITH STABLE ANGINA PECTORIS

Pathophysiology

Stable angina in most patients is attributable to fixed coronary artery stenoses, physiologically inappropriate coronary vasoconstriction or failure of dilatation, or both ("mixed" angina). Following is a brief description of pathophysiology. The reader is referred to Chapters 36 and 38 of *Heart Disease*, 5th Edition (edited by E. Braunwald, published by W.B. Saunders, 1996), for a more extensive discussion.

Angina Attributable to Fixed Coronary Artery Stenoses

The most common cause of fixed coronary artery stenoses responsible for chronic, stable angina is the advanced, complex, relatively lipid-poor atheromatous lesion with a fibrous cap that compromises the lumen of medium-sized to large coronary arteries.[2] Rare causes, such as vasculitis and congenital abnormalities, are discussed in detail in Chapters 29, 30, 38, and 56 of *Heart Disease*, 5th Edition.

Fixed stenoses generally result in effort, or "demand," angina, which reflects limitation of the augmentation of myocardial perfusion that ordinarily accompanies increased physical activity and other stresses. The result is an imbalance between myocardial oxygen delivery and requirements.[3] In addition to physical activity, a variety of other factors such as mental and emotional stress,[4] exposure to cold,[5] and increased circulatory stress secondary to the postprandial state[6] can increase myocardial oxygen demands sufficiently to cause angina in patients with fixed coronary stenoses. Although in most patients with fixed stenoses and predominantly effort angina the level of myocardial oxygen demand at which ischemia appears is predictable, the threshold is markedly variable in other patients, sometimes as a result of physiologically inappropriate coronary vasomotor responses[3, 7–9] (Fig. 5–1). Finally, some patients with fixed stenoses have ischemia without chest discomfort per se but with angina "equivalents," including dyspnea, nausea, and diaphoresis.[10]

Angina Attributable to Coronary Vasospasm

Angina attributable to inappropriate intense coronary vasospasm was first recognized in 1959 by Prinzmetal,[11] who described patients in whom the pattern of angina was consistent but atypical. Such patients, said to have Prinzmetal or variant angina, exhibit angina at rest associated with elevation of the ST electrocardiographic segment. Subsequently, the mechanism responsible was confirmed to be severe focal vasospasm of a large or medium-sized coronary artery.[12] Patients with variant angina frequently have angiographically normal (or near normal) coronary arteries in the absence of ischemia.

Mechanisms responsible for inappropriate coronary vasomotor tone in variant angina have not been delineated definitively, but a variety of paradoxical or exaggerated responses consistent with endothelial dysfunction have been described.[13–16] The endothelial dysfunction thought to underlie many cases of variant angina may actually be an early manifestation of atherosclerosis, with functional impairment of endothelial cells preceding major luminal obstruction by atheroma (see Chapters 34, 36, and 38 of *Heart Disease,* 5th Edition). Other causes of vasospasm (and even frank myocardial infarction) include cocaine or amphetamine abuse[17, 18] and, possibly, abnormal magnesium metabolism.[19]

Variant angina is a heterogeneous syndrome (for a detailed discussion, see Chapters 36 and 38 of *Heart Disease,* 5th Edition). Attacks typically occur at rest, without any obvious provocation. However, specific provocative factors are sometimes identified, including exposure to cold, emotional stress, and cigarette smoking. In rare instances, attacks can be provoked by exercise. Concomitant ventricular arrhythmias, conduction abnormalities, and even syncope are relatively common.

The hallmark of variant angina is reversible ST segment elevation. Provocative diagnostic testing is sometimes performed by inducing hyperventilation[20] or administering intracoronary acetylcholine[13, 14] or ergonovine,[16] which typically precipitate an attack of variant angina associated with focal coronary spasm.

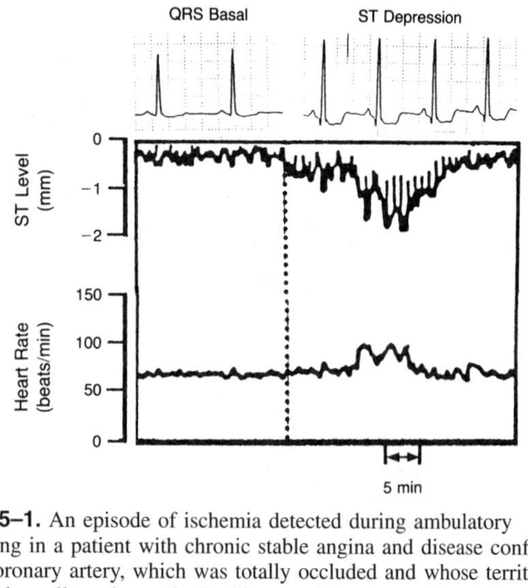

Figure 5–1. An episode of ischemia detected during ambulatory monitoring in a patient with chronic stable angina and disease confined to a single coronary artery, which was totally occluded and whose territory was supplied by collateral vessels. In this case, ST segment depression occurs in the absence of a preceding increase in heart rate, implying a primary change in oxygen supply rather than demand. Because of the complete occlusion, the presumed mechanism is vasoconstriction of either distal or collateral vessels. (From Pupita G, Maseri A, Kaski JC, et al: Myocardial ischemia caused by distal coronary-artery constriction in stable angina pectoris. N Engl J Med 1990; 323:514.)

Angina Attributable to Fixed Stenoses Accompanied by Increased Coronary Vasomotor Tone

Some patients with fixed stenoses and effort angina also manifest signs or symptoms consistent with vasospasm and/or inadequate coronary flow reserve (i.e., abnormal vasomotor tone) and are categorized as having *mixed angina.*[21] (In this context, vasospasm does not imply total occlusion of a conductance coronary artery as in variant angina.) The clinical picture comprises typical effort angina, episodic nocturnal angina, angina accompanying emotional stress or exposure to cold, or angina with no apparent provocation. A hallmark of angina caused by abnormal vasomotor tone is that it is not preceded by identifiable increases in myocardial oxygen requirements[7–9] (Fig. 5–2). Patients with mixed angina usually exhibit ST segment depression during ischemic episodes that are presumably caused by abnormal vasomotor tone[7–9, 21] (see Figs. 5–1, 5–2). Episodes of ischemia in these patients often reflect an interaction between relatively modest increases in myocardial oxygen demands and inappropriate or inadequate coronary vasomotor responses, as is likely the case in patients with predominantly effort angina but a variable anginal threshold[7–9, 21] (Fig. 5–3). In the case of provocation by factors such as emotional stress or exposure to cold, it may be very difficult in an individual patient to delineate whether the underlying mechanism is an increase in oxygen demand, reduced flow reserve, or a combination of the two.

Silent Ischemia

Patients with angina may have objective evidence of ischemia in the absence of discernible symptoms.[22–24] In some cases, this so-called *silent ischemia* represents subclinical effort angina in association with increased oxygen demands; in others, it is a manifestation of abnormal vasomotor tone; and in still others, it may be an indication of an abnormal visceral pain threshold. Silent ischemia is more common among smokers,[25] patients with diabetes mellitus (in whom pain perception may be altered by neuropathy),[26] and perhaps also stoic persons.[4, 27]

Angina Ascribable to Coexisting Cardiac Disorders in the Absence of Angiographically Detectable Fixed Stenoses or Vasospasm

Angina can occur with dynamic impairment of myocardial perfusion that is attributable to factors other than fixed stenoses or coronary vasospasm. The most common cause is valvular aortic stenosis, in which the combination of high myocardial compressive forces, a relatively low pressure distal to the stenotic aortic valve, and high left ventricular diastolic pressures together with concentric hypertrophy of the left ventricle can result in an imbalance between myocardial oxygen requirements and oxygen supply, particularly in the subendocardium (see Chapters 32 and 36 of *Heart Disease,* 5th Edition). Aortic insufficiency can also cause angina but less commonly than aortic stenosis.

Angina is not uncommon among patients with hypertrophic cardiomyopathy (see Chapter 41 of *Heart Disease,* 5th Edition), in whom myocardial oxygen delivery cannot keep pace with augmented requirements, perhaps because of subendocardial hypoperfusion related to marked ventricular hypertrophy.[28] Severe pulmonary hypertension of any cause can be associated with chest pain that may be attributable to oxygen supply/demand imbalance in the right ventricle (see Chapter 25 of *Heart Disease,* 5th Edition). Chest pain may occur with the syndrome of mitral valve prolapse, but its nature is highly

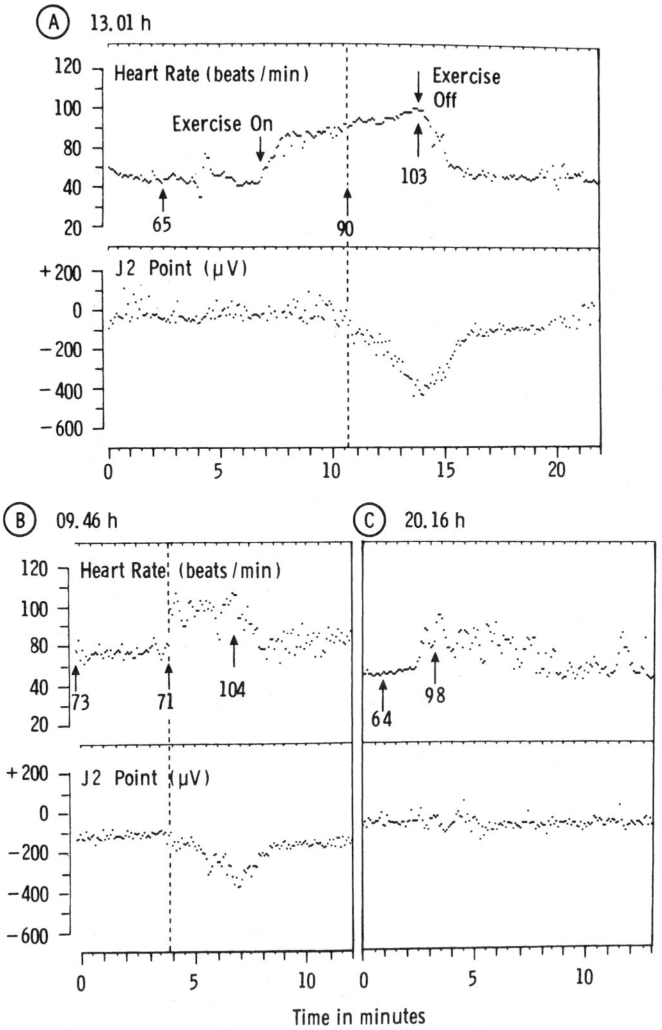

Figure 5–2. An example of two mechanisms of ischemia in a patient with chronic stable angina. *A,* Heart rate and ST segments (J2 point) during an exercise test. Increases in heart rate precede ST depression; that is, increased demand precedes onset of ischemia. *B,* Heart rate and ST segment are shown during ambulatory monitoring. In this case, ischemic ST depression is not preceded by an increase in heart rate, which implicates a decrease in supply as the initiating event. In contrast, during ambulatory monitoring *(C),* a period of tachycardia occurs without ST segment depression, which indicates that increased demand has not exceeded this patient's ischemic threshold. (From Chierchia S, Gallino A, Smith G, et al: Role of heart rate in pathophysiology of chronic stable angina. Lancet 1984; 2:1353.)

variable and the mechanisms uncertain. One possibility is excessive tension in or ischemia of the posterior papillary muscle related to excessive stretching,[29] but in most patients there is no objective evidence of ischemia. Finally, paroxysmal tachycardia can cause angina by increasing myocardial oxygen requirements, decreasing coronary perfusion pressure secondary to impaired ventricular filling and cardiac output, or both.

"Microvascular" Angina

A number of patients with symptoms consistent with angina do not have angiographically demonstrable coronary stenoses, evidence of focal coronary spasm, or any of the coexisting cardiac disorders mentioned earlier. A minority of this group manifest objective signs of myocardial ischemia during symptoms[30, 31] and have been considered to have a condition called Syndrome X (a term that should be discarded because it is also applied to an independent entity: insulin resistance, hypertension, hypertriglyceridemia, obesity, and type II diabetes mellitus, which may in turn predispose to coronary artery disease with fixed stenoses). Moreover, patients with diabetes or hypertension may have coronary disease exclusively at the microvascular level.[32] Microvascular angina is thought to reflect impaired coronary vasodilator reserve associated with microvascular disease.[30, 31, 33–35] It is more common among women than among men and generally carries a good prognosis.[30, 31, 33, 36]

Syndromes Simulating Angina Pectoris

Despite vigorous investigation, a cardiac basis for intermittent chest discomfort is not discernible in many subjects. Some of these patients may have a poorly understood hypersensitivity to various cardiac stimuli.[37] Alternative disorders that may be responsible include pleural or pericardial based pain, esophagitis, gastroesophageal reflux, cholecystitis or cholelithiasis, musculoskeletal disorders (including costochondritis), and herpes simplex (before the appearance of an eruption). Angina can also be simulated by psychogenic discomfort with or without hyperventilation.

Concomitant Conditions Influencing Management

Consideration of concomitant conditions that can worsen angina and/or modify the efficacy of treatment regimens is essential. A number of commonly encountered medical conditions can manifest as progressive angina in the absence of a change in the underlying coronary disease; these include anemia, weight gain, hypertension, congestive heart failure, and increased sympathoadrenal stimulation, each of which augments myocardial oxygen requirements. Acceleration of heart rate in patients with atrial fibrillation, in whom the ventricular rate may be well controlled at rest but becomes excessively high with even mild physical exertion or emotional stress, can also cause progressive angina. In more rare instances, occult thyrotoxicosis, infection, or poor control of chronic conditions such as diabetes mellitus may be implicated. Psychosocial stress with occult physiologic consequences, as well as changes in habits (such as resumption of smoking with consequent vasoconstriction[38]), acceleration of heart rate, hypoxemia, and increased concentrations of carbon monoxide in the blood (all of which can exacerbate angina), must also be kept in mind. Failure to recognize these conditions can lead to misguided therapy that not only will fail to relieve symptoms but also can precipitate adverse consequences.

Delineation of Risk

Risk assessment is the other key element in the evaluation of patients with angina pectoris. It guides selection of initial treatment, provides a baseline against which the clinical course can be characterized objectively, and constitutes a framework for determining whether a change in therapy is indicated over time. Risk assessment is particularly important in deciding whether a revascularization procedure is indicated.

Natural History of Stable Angina Pectoris

In general, the underlying coronary disease in patients presenting with stable angina is slowly progressive (see Chapters 34, 35, 38, 39, and 40 of *Heart Disease,* 5th Edition). The clinical course can wax or wane over long periods of time without the intercession of major coronary events. Nevertheless, the annual overall coronary-related mortality rate is approximately 2%–3%, the risk being higher in men than in women (Fig. 5–4). In addition to rate of progression of the underlying coronary disease, prognosis is related to diverse

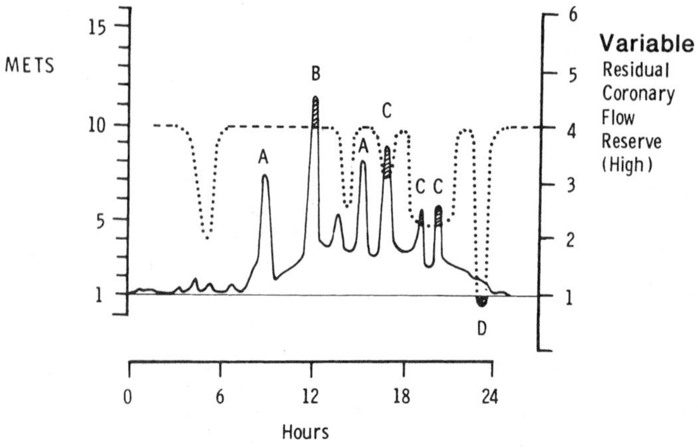

Figure 5–3. Schematic to explain variability of anginal threshold and the occurrence of rest angina in patients with a mixed anginal pattern. Dashed line represents coronary flow reserve, which varies below a maximal level when factors such as alterations in coronary vasomotor tone change. Solid line represents oxygen demand, represented as the level of physical activity in metabolic equivalents (METs). When demand exceeds reserve, angina occurs (shaded areas). With coronary flow reserve at its maximum, anginal threshold is also at its maximum (point B). Anginal threshold is reduced when coronary flow reserve decreases (points C). When flow reserve is severely reduced, rest angina occurs (point D). As long as exercise is below the threshold set by coronary flow reserve, ischemia does not occur (points A). (From Maseri A, Chierchia S, Kaski JC: Mixed angina pectoris. Am J Cardiol 1985; 56:30E.)

clinical and angiographic factors, including severity of disease,[39, 41] extent of ventricular functional impairment,[39] and exercise capacity[42] (which is often inversely related to impaired ventricular performance with stress). Accordingly, a single, static risk assessment may not suffice. On average, patients with stable angina and single-vessel disease with normal left ventricular function and good exercise capacity have an overall annual mortality rate of about 1%, only modestly worse than that of the general population.[39]

Surprisingly, the severity of angiographic disease per se has a relatively modest effect on prognosis when ventricular function is normal and symptoms are mild.[39] Thus the overall mortality rate among patients with two-vessel disease and well-preserved ventricular function is only slightly worse than that among patients with single-vessel disease: about 2% per annum. Even three-vessel disease with well-preserved ventricular function and mild symptoms entails a favorable long-term outlook, with an annual mortality rate of 4%–5%.[39] A major exception is left main coronary stenosis, an ominous prognostic finding even with normal ventricular function and mild symptoms.[39, 41] The significance of ventricular dysfunction is underscored by data from the Coronary Artery Surgery Study (CASS),[39] in which a depressed ejection fraction was associated with an approximate doubling of mortality for any level of severity of angiographic disease.

The relatively low mortality rate and reasonably good prognosis associated with stable angina in comparison with acute coronary syndromes may reflect fundamental differences in the underlying nature of the vascular disease. Stable angina is generally a manifestation of diffuse coronary disease with multiple lesions of varying severity and a relative absence of thrombosis.[43] Sequential angiographic analyses have demonstrated that the rate of progression of a specific stenosis in patients with stable angina is highly variable.[44] Approximately 3% of lesions exhibit significant progression annually, whereas 1% exhibit spontaneous regression (Fig. 5–5). Approximately 15% of patients exhibit a new stenotic lesion each year, the majority of which are not associated with acute myocardial infarction. Angiographic progression of disease in patients with stable angina is accelerated by cigarette smoking, hypercholesterolemia, and possibly the concomitant presence of insulin resistance.[44, 45] In contrast, acute coronary syndromes, manifested by unstable angina or acute infarction, are associated with active vascular lesions, sometimes modest in number but commonly associated with thrombosis.[2, 43, 46] Predisposition to thrombotic events is associated with lipid-rich atheroma, as opposed to fibrocalcific lesions.[2]

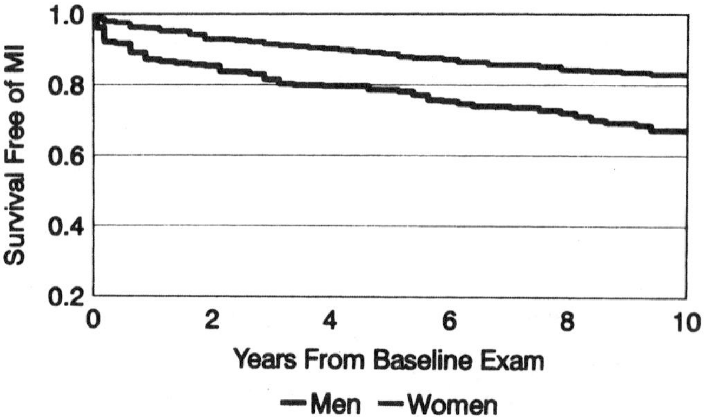

Figure 5–4. Kaplan-Meier age-adjusted myocardial infarction (MI)–free survival in subjects whose initial presentation of coronary artery disease is angina. Note the relatively high chance of MI-free survival; women have a better outlook than do men. (From Murabito JM, Evans JC, Larson MG, et al: Prognosis after the onset of coronary heart disease. Circulation 1993; 88:2548.)

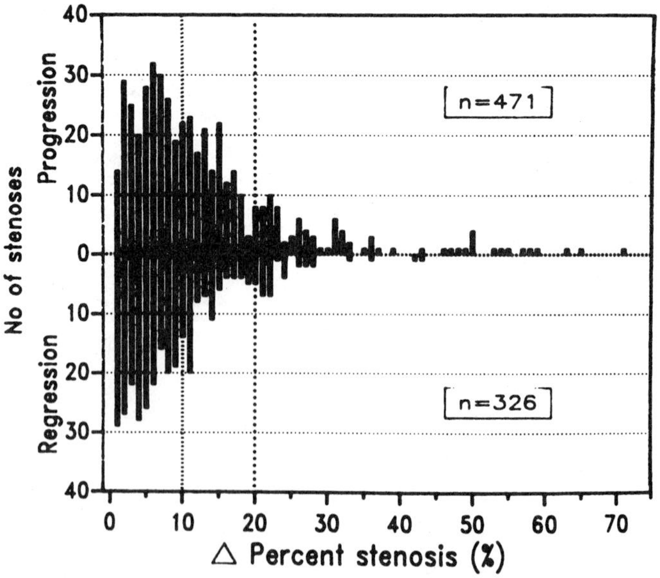

Figure 5–5. Data obtained during coronary angiography and 3 years later from patients with stable coronary disease. The change in 471 separate stenoses present on initial angiogram is plotted by number of stenoses, showing progression vs. regression, with percentage of change on the abscissa. For lesions demonstrating insignificant changes (<10%), numbers of lesions progressing and regressing are about equal. For stenoses with larger changes, the number of progressing lesions is greater than that of those regressing. (From Lichtlen PR, Nikutta P, Josh S, et al: Anatomical progression of coronary artery disease in humans as seen by prospective, repeated, quantitated coronary angiography. Circulation 1992; 86:828.)

Despite the overall favorable prognosis associated with stable angina, a proportion of patients are at substantially higher risk. Those with impaired ventricular function, left main coronary lesions, severe three-vessel coronary stenoses, and certain types of two-vessel coronary stenoses in association with specific clinical features are subject to higher rates of acute myocardial infarction, sudden cardiac arrest, and overall mortality.[39, 41, 47, 48] Identification of patients with these risk factors depends on careful acquisition of history, noninvasive assessment of cardiac performance, and stress testing designed to detect manifestations of severe disease. Among patients judged to be at high risk, coronary arteriography and left ventriculography remain the gold standards for delineation of the distribution and severity of coronary arterial lesions and ventricular function. Because of its importance, specific aspects of risk stratification merit attention.

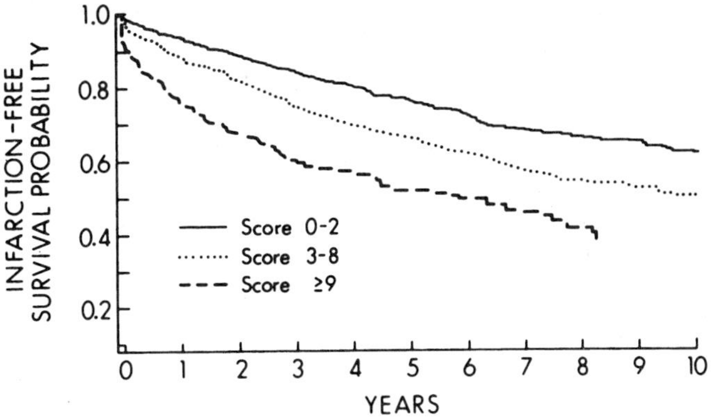

Figure 5–6. Use of a clinical angina score to determine prognosis in a group of patients with stable angina pectoris. The score includes weighted factors based on angina frequency, presence of ST-T changes, and rate of progression of symptoms. Inclusion of rate of progression substantially improves predictive value. (From Califf RM, Mark DB, Harrell FE Jr, et al: Importance of clinical measures of ischemia in the prognosis of patients with documented coronary artery disease. J Am Coll Cardiol 1988; 11:20.)

The Nature of Symptoms

Severe symptoms, especially when they occur at low levels of physiologic stress, are generally associated with severe angiographic coronary disease and poorer prognosis.[42, 49–51] Progression of symptoms may be at least as important as absolute severity. Thus an angina score such as that proposed by Califf and coworkers,[49] which includes both absolute frequency and trends in the severity of symptoms, along with the presence or absence of ST-T wave abnormalities, is an excellent prognostic tool (Table 5–1, Fig. 5–6). When symptoms of heart failure occur in association with ischemic chest discomfort or in the form of angina "equivalents," the underlying coronary disease is often severe. Although silent ischemia was traditionally believed to be a particularly ominous prognostic sign, current evidence suggests that it does not constitute a major independent risk factor.[52–54] In fact, the differentiation between silent and clinically manifest ischemia may relate more to the duration of the ischemic episode (episodes typically being silent initially), to factors that influence the duration of ischemia (such as exercise duration), to the intensity of ischemia in absolute terms, and to the presence or absence of abnormal coronary vasomotor tone (a component of mixed angina that may convert a silent episode to a clinically manifest one).

Physical Findings

Assessment of ventricular function by physical examination is a valuable tool in risk stratification (see Chapters 2 and 38 of *Heart Disease,* 5th Edition). Cardiomegaly, dyskinesia of the left ventricle, a third heart sound, a mitral regurgitant murmur indicative of papillary muscle dysfunction, and signs of heart failure (rales, elevated jugular venous pressure) all portend a poor outlook.

Physical examination at the time of an episode of suspected angina can be particularly enlightening. The appearance of dyskinesia, a third heart sound, paradoxical splitting of the second heart sound as a result of prolongation of the pre-ejection period and abbreviation of left ventricular ejection time, pulsus alternans, transient rales, and a murmur indicative of mitral insufficiency and papillary muscle dysfunction are hallmarks of severe coronary artery disease associated with left ventricular functional impairment during the attack.

TABLE 5–1. COMPONENTS OF AN ANGINAL SCORE

Component	Points*
Course	
Unstable or variant angina	3
Progressive (with nocturnal episodes)	2
Progressive (without nocturnal episodes)	1
Nonprogressive	0
Frequency (per day)	0–5
ST-T abnormalities present	0–6

*Score = course × (1 + frequency) + ST-T abnormalities (possible range, 0–24).
Adapted from Califf RM, Mark DB, Harrell FE Jr, et al: Importance of clinical measures of ischemia in the prognosis of patients with documented coronary artery disease. J Am Coll Cardiol 1988; 11:20.

Rest and Exercise Electrocardiographic Criteria

Survival is worse in patients whose resting electrocardiograms (ECGs) show evidence of previous Q wave myocardial infarction or ST-T wave abnormalities in the absence of Q wave infarction.[47, 55]

Stress electrocardiography (treadmill or bicycle exercise with multilead recording and blood pressure monitoring) remains a reliable, easily performed, and relatively inexpensive risk stratification tool in patients with stable angina (see Chapter 5 of *Heart Disease,* 5th Edition).[42, 49–51] Inducible ST segment depression actually correlates more closely with impaired coronary flow reserve than with the magnitude of angiographically defined coronary stenosis.[51]

The sensitivity of exercise electrocardiography for detecting single-vessel coronary disease is approximately 50% when 1 mm of flat ST segment depression in lead V5 is the diagnostic criterion.[56] Radionuclide perfusion imaging or echocardiography used in conjunction with electrocardiographic monitoring is more sensitive for detection of single-vessel disease (see Chapters 5 and 9 of *Heart Disease,* 5th Edition). In contrast, ST segment depression during exercise electrocardiography has a sensitivity of approximately 80%–90% for severe multivessel and/or left main artery disease.[56] This level of sensitivity is only slightly less than that afforded by perfusion imaging (see Chapters 5 and 9 of *Heart Disease,* 5th Edition).[57, 58] Thus the absence of ST depression in a patient with stable angina provides considerable reassurance.

Other features of exercise electrocardiography, in addition to whether the ST segment shifts, provide additional incremental prognostic information (Table 5–2). Duration of exercise is an especially important prognostic criterion. Patients with stable angina who can exercise to at least stage III (Bruce protocol) have a much better prognosis than do those who cannot continue beyond stage I or II.[42, 49–51] The magnitude of ST segment depression during exercise is generally correlated with the severity and prognosis of the underlying coronary disease (see Chapter 5 of *Heart Disease,* 5th Edition).[50, 56] Thus ST depression exceeding 1.5–2 mm, particularly at a relatively low workload or heart rate, portends a poor prognosis. Signal averaging, electronic filtration of repolarization wave forms, and quantifi-

TABLE 5–2. EXERCISE ELECTROCARDIOGRAPHY: FEATURES ASSOCIATED WITH INCREASED MORTALITY AND OTHER MORBID EVENTS

>1.5- to 2.0-mm ST segment depression (≤Stage II, Bruce protocol)
ST segment depression at low workload (≤Stage II, Bruce protocol)
Poor exercise tolerance (≤Stage II, Bruce protocol)
>5-min postexercise ST segment depression
Impaired blood pressure response during exercise (≥20-mm Hg drop after initial rise or drop below rest value)
Abnormal blood pressure response after exercise (increase or abnormally small decrease)
Chronotropic incompetence (peak heart rate below 2 standard deviations from the mean)
Ventricular arrhythmias
Bundle branch block

cation of the slope and area of ST segment deviation from baseline may facilitate more accurate delineation of prognosis.[59]

One of the most significant adverse prognostic signs elicited by exercise testing is exercise-induced hypotension, or simply failure of the anticipated physiologic augmentation of systemic arterial blood pressure.[60] Interestingly, an increase or retarded decrease in blood pressure during exercise recovery is also associated with more severe disease.[61] Failure of acceleration of heart rate to the level anticipated with a given workload (chronotropic incompetence) in the absence of medications that diminish the positive chronotropic response to exercise and the appearance of ventricular arrhythmias or bundle branch block are additional manifestations of severe, as opposed to mild, coronary disease.[62–64]

Despite the powerful diagnostic and prognostic information provided by exercise electrocardiography, several limitations must be kept in mind. In patients with resting intraventricular conduction abnormalities, particularly bundle branch block and/or baseline repolarization abnormalities, who are being treated with cardiac medications (such as digitalis) that can alter the electrocardiographic response to exercise, as well as in those whose exercise is limited because of medications or noncardiac conditions, exercise electrocardiography has reduced sensitivity and/or specificity for both diagnosis and risk stratification.

Exercise Myocardial Scintigraphy and Echocardiography

Both radionuclide perfusion imaging (thallium-201 [^{201}Tl] or technetium-99m methoxy isobutyl isonitrile [^{99m}Tc-Sestamibi]) and echocardiography provide valuable prognostic information in patients with stable angina (see Chapters 3 and 9 of *Heart Disease,* 5th Edition).[58, 65–69] Both are employed in conjunction with physiologic or pharmacologic stress. Agents causing pharmacologic stress (e.g., dipyridamole or dobutamine) are helpful in patients who have difficulty exercising. However, in comparison with conventional exercise electrocardiography, the incremental information provided by these imaging modalities is relatively modest in high-risk patients with multivessel and/or left main coronary artery disease who can exercise and who do not have any of the other factors noted earlier that reduce the utility of the ECG.

Imaging procedures (radionuclide or echocardiographic) provide important incremental information with regard to considerations other than prognosis. They help define the specific region and distribution of coronary vascular disease and may thus be helpful in determining which vessels and lesions require mechanical intervention and/or the hemodynamic significance of a coronary arterial stenosis detected at angiography. ^{201}Tl imaging is helpful in differentiating zones of previous infarction from those in which myocardial ischemia is induced. The former produce defects at rest, and the latter produce defects evident with stress that subsequently reverse at rest ("filling in" with tracer as a result of "redistribution" attributable to continued but slow uptake into jeopardized tissue of tracer circulating in the blood pool, to diminished washout of tracer from ischemic zones, or to both). For patients with left ventricular dysfunction, the techniques of imaging after reinjection of ^{201}Tl[70] or late reimaging after a resting injection of ^{201}Tl[71] are useful in distinguishing viable from nonviable regions of myocardium.

Exercise ^{201}Tl or ^{99m}Tc-Sestamibi imaging yields positive results in approximately 80% of patients with single-vessel disease and in more than 90% of patients with multivessel disease.[57, 58] However, obfuscation attributable to variable attenuation (particularly from overlying breast tissue in women), global depression of perfusion limiting delineation of abnormal from normal regions, and superimposition of tracer from overlapping regions of myocardium can decrease sensitivity and specificity. Some of these deficiencies can be overcome by single-photon emission computed tomography (SPECT) imaging and the use of dynamic data processing (quantifying rates of washout of tracer from diverse regions of the heart), as opposed to static, planar imaging.

Multivessel disease is suspected when ^{201}Tl images show multiple perfusion defects. Left ventricular dilatation and increased tracer uptake by the lungs are nonspecific signs of severe disease that may be evident during ^{201}Tl exercise imaging.[72, 73] Sestamibi is superior to ^{201}Tl with respect to dosimetry and image contrast. In contrast to ^{201}Tl, it undergoes little redistribution and thus must be administered both during stress and during rest. Its capacity to represent ventricular wall motion is superior to that of ^{201}Tl, however.[57]

Radioventriculography (i.e., imaging of the left ventricular blood pool with radionuclides in either a first pass, multiple-gated acquisition [MUGA] or equilibrium mode) has been used to detect impaired ventricular performance with exercise and to identify patients at particularly high risk.[74, 75] These techniques are significantly less expensive than radionuclide perfusion imaging.

Exercise echocardiography has been used to assess severity of coronary disease and provides information approximately comparable with that provided by radionuclide imaging (see Chapter 5 of *Heart Disease,* 5th Edition).[66] Its major disadvantage is the difficulty in obtaining excellent-quality images in significant numbers of patients. However, it is also less expensive than myocardial perfusion imaging.

Positron emission tomography (PET) with tracers of metabolism (^{18}F-fluorodeoxyglucose [FDG] and carbon-11–labeled palmitate) and tracers of perfusion (oxygen-15–labeled H_2O and nitrogen-15 ammonia) can quantitatively delineate ischemic regions at rest or during physiologic and pharmacologic stress. PET has been most useful in identifying subjects who may benefit from coronary revascularization by defining jeopardized but still viable regions of myocardium.[76] Its widespread use is limited by the necessity for complex and expensive instrumentation and radiochemical and data processing support systems and personnel and by the desirability of an on-site cyclotron.

Pharmacologic Stress Testing

When exercise cannot be employed to induce physiologic stress, ECGs and image-based stress tests can nonetheless be implemented by performance of diagnostic procedures with concomitant pharmacologic stress. The vasodilator dipyridamole (Persantine) has been used extensively in conjunction with ^{201}Tl myocardial scintigraphy.[58, 65] Dipyridamole-induced coronary vasodilation increases perfusion, particularly in zones subserved by relatively normal vessels, and accentuates the disparity in perfusion between them and zones perfused by vessels with stenoses. Because of the vasodilator effects of dipyridamole and secondary tachycardia, there may be a modest increase in double product that may induce an episode of angina, seen in approximately 10% of patients studied. This adverse effect may also reflect "coronary steal" and interdicts continuation of infusion of dipyridamole.[77] Theophylline and other xanthines inhibit the pharmacologic effects of dipyridamole. Their use must be discontinued before testing, and they may be used to pharmacologically reverse effects of dipyridamole if untoward side effects are encountered during testing.

Pharmacologic stress can be induced by increasing myocardial oxygen demands, most commonly with dobutamine administered intravenously to patients undergoing stress echocardiography.[68] The appearance of new regional wall motion abnormalities is a hallmark of severe coronary stenoses. In contrast, improvement of a hypokinetic region with dobutamine testing suggests the presence of "hibernating" myocardium, which is viable but poorly contracting as a result of low perfusion pressure.

Left Ventricular Performance

Depressed ejection fraction at rest and/or a large area of abnormal wall motion are often hallmarks of severe coronary disease and signify a poor prognosis.[39, 55, 57, 66, 72–75] Even when ventricular function is normal at rest, impairment during exercise portends a poor prognosis.[75, 76] Accordingly, patients with angina and impaired ventricular performance usually merit angiographic evaluation and consideration for revascularization. Impairment of ejection fraction at rest is rare in patients with entirely normal 12-lead ECGs. When electrocardiographic abnormalities are present (Q waves, repolarization abnormalities, bundle branch block, and intraventricular conduction abnormalities) or when other features of the initial evaluation suggest impaired ventricular function, noninvasive confirmation is indicated and can be obtained with echocardiography or radionuclide ventriculography. As mentioned earlier, ^{201}Tl reinjection and/or dobutamine echocardiography can be useful in identifying viable myocardium in patients with depressed ventricular function.

Invasive Assessment

Delineation of coronary arterial lesions, distribution, severity, and impact on ventricular performance is accomplished most definitively by cardiac catheterization, coronary angiography, and contrast ventriculography—procedures that are indicated for patients suspected of being at high risk who are being considered for revascularization procedures. Among all patients with stable angina, cardiac catheterization as an initial risk assessment procedure is required in only a very small minority. However, when noninvasive assessments suggest a poor prognosis, invasive evaluation is appropriate. For patients with multiple or particularly impressive risk factors for coronary disease and those for whom a cardiac event could pose a hazard for others, cardiac catheterization may be undertaken relatively early in the course of risk assessment. The same can be said for very young subjects with stable angina, on the basis of the presumption that the rate of progression of the underlying coronary disease has been unusually rapid or that an unusual form of coronary disease is present (e.g., congenital abnormalities). A history of recent progression of symptoms or the presence of angina equivalents also may be an indication for early invasive risk assessment. Although silent ischemia per se does not seem to constitute an independent risk factor, a change in the frequency and/or severity of silent ischemia likely has the same significance as a change in symptomatic ischemia.

SPECIFIC TREATMENT MODALITIES

General Principles

The treatment of patients with stable angina is directed at both the underlying coronary artery disease and its consequences. Arrest of progression of coronary atherosclerosis or induction of regression should be a primary objective. Accordingly, treatment of hyperlipidemia occupies a central role and is discussed in detail in Chapters 23–26. A few salient principles are outlined here. Although improved overall survival in prospective studies of patients without overt coronary disease has not yet been demonstrated,[78] secondary prevention trials have demonstrated reduction of cardiovascular morbidity and mortality among patients with overt coronary artery disease treated with lipid-lowering regimens.[76] Most recently, the Scandinavian trial of pravastatin has shown substantial improvement in overall mortality among patients with both angina and myocardial infarction.[80] The relatively greater efficacy of secondary prevention may simply reflect the value of interdicting progression to lethality of an already advanced atherosclerotic process, as opposed to retardation of less advanced disease, for which the survival benefit may not become evident for decades.

Lipid lowering arrests progression of obstructive coronary disease delineated angiographically.[79] In fact, actual regression has been demonstrated with diverse lipid-lowering regimens.[79] Reduction in adverse clinical events (exacerbation of angina, recurrent myocardial infarction, sudden cardiac arrest) is markedly greater than the modest regression of lesions would imply (on the order of 10ths of millimeters in some studies). This may reflect conversion of potentially hazardous atheromatous plaques, characterized by high lipid and thrombogenic activity, to more inactive, fibrous, relatively lipid-poor, calcified, and capped lesions.

Lipid lowering, specifically directed at low-density lipoprotein (LDL) cholesterol, is appropriate for patients with overt coronary artery disease even when the baseline LDL level is not markedly elevated. The consensus of the National Cholesterol Education Program Adult Treatment Panel II is that the target LDL cholesterol level in such patients should be 100 mg/dL.[81] Thus many patients with "normal" LDL levels should be treated to achieve a target of 100 mg/dL or less.

Strategies for lipid lowering for patients with overt coronary disease are identical to those for primary prevention except for the more aggressive approach indicated.[81] Thus implementation of a rigorous diet (American Heart Association Step 1, Step 2 if necessary) should be followed by use of pharmacologic agents to lower the LDL cholesterol level to 100 mg/dL or less. For postmenopausal women, a powerful approach is hormone replacement therapy. Often, this lowers the LDL cholesterol level markedly without the need for specific lipid-lowering agents. The choice of the pharmacologic lipid-lowering regimen to be used when dietary and hormone replacement therapy is insufficient depends, of course, on the nature of the hyperlipidemia (relative or absolute). However, because of the urgency of aggressive lipid lowering for patients with overt coronary disease, use of hydroxy-3-methyglutaryl coenzyme A (HMG CoA) reductase inhibitors (the statins) is often indicated (see Chapter 25).

Correction of other identified risk factors is imperative as well. Thus, vigorous treatment of hypertension, cessation of smoking, control of carbohydrate intolerance in patients with overt diabetes mellitus, and weight reduction are all major treatment goals. Risk factor modification also constitutes therapy that frequently directly improves the balance between myocardial oxygen supply and demand (for example, control of hypertension) and can therefore be expected to contribute to immediate symptomatic improvement.

Although the underlying vascular disease typically associated with stable angina pectoris is not characterized primarily by thrombotic events, derangements of the hemostatic and fibrinolytic systems have nonetheless been implicated in young survivors of acute myocardial infarction, including elevation of plasminogen activator inhibitor type-1 (PAI-1) in plasma.[82] Reduction of acute coronary events in diverse settings has been documented to result from administration of antiplatelet agents, particularly aspirin (see Chapter 27).[83] Accordingly, treatment of patients with stable angina should include administration of aspirin (80–300 mg/day) coupled with surveillance for toxicity, particularly gastrointestinal tract bleeding. For patients who are intolerant of aspirin, alternative antiplatelet agents, including dipyridamole (a less powerful antiplatelet agent than aspirin), 300–

400 mg/day in three to four divided doses, or ticlopidine, 250 mg twice per day, can be substituted.

Treatment also includes correction of the underlying, sometimes subtle conditions discussed earlier that may exacerbate angina, including thyrotoxicosis, hypertension, weight gain or obesity, anemia, poorly controlled heart failure, fever caused by occult infection or other conditions, and tachycardia at rest or with exertion as well as other arrhythmias.

An important issue for patients with angina is compliance with sometimes complicated medical regimens that can often cause side effects. Noncompliance results not only in difficulty in initial control of symptoms but also can account for worsening of symptoms that may be mistakenly ascribed to progression of underlying disease. Compliance is maximized by careful patient education and simplifying therapeutic regimens whenever possible.

Results of several studies of coronary patients subjected to prolonged endurance exercise indicate salutary effects on exercise performance and quality of life (see Chapter 56).[84] Both cardiac and peripheral mechanisms have been implicated. Thus the magnitude of electrocardiographic ST segment deviation in response to a given workload is reduced, skeletal muscle blood flow and left ventricular performance at a given workload is improved, and indirect indexes suggest enhanced development of collateral vessels and improved myocardial perfusion after prolonged endurance exercise training. Organized, carefully monitored cardiac rehabilitation programs are therefore useful in motivated patients.

Antianginal Drugs

Organic Nitrates

Mechanism of Action. Nitrates have been used for the treatment of angina since the 1880s.[85] Sublingual nitroglycerin, 0.3–0.6 mg, administered for treatment of a single attack, remains a cornerstone. Long-acting nitrate preparations are useful for prophylaxis of effort, vasospastic, and mixed angina.[85–87] As discussed in Chapter 2, nitroglycerin and its congeners (the organic nitrates) are endothelial-independent vasodilators;[86, 87] thus they dilate vascular smooth muscle even in vessels in which the endothelium has been denuded. This class of agents, which includes other nitrovasodilators such as nitroprusside, differs from so-called endothelium-dependent vasodilators such as acetylcholine, which induce relaxation of vascular smooth muscle secondary to elaboration of endothelial cell–derived relaxing factor (EDRF), shown to be nitric oxide (see Chapter 2).[85–87] In contrast, organic nitrates are converted directly to nitric oxide as a result of reactions requiring sulfhydryl group donors such as methionine and cysteine. Ultimately, nitric oxide exerts its effects by increasing intracellular levels of cyclic guanosine monophosphate (cGMP).

At conventional therapeutic doses, organic nitrates exert their most prominent vasodilatory effects on systemic veins (see Chapter 2).[86] Conductance arteries are dilated as well. Dilatation of arterial resistance vessels is much more modest.[88, 89] The vasodilator effects result in improvement of the balance between myocardial oxygen supply and demand. Venodilatation diminishes diastolic filling, first in the right side of the heart and subsequently, because of decreased pulmonary blood flow, in the left ventricle. The decreased left ventricular volume diminishes systolic wall stress and myocardial oxygen requirements and is a major mechanism underlying the antianginal effects of organic nitrates.

Systemic blood pressure is typically mildly reduced by organic nitrates primarily because of diminution of left ventricular diastolic pressure and volume rather than by the direct, modest effect on systemic arterial resistance. The double product is relatively unchanged at rest and with physical activity because modest decreases in blood pressure are offset by reflex tachycardia.[85–87] However, the double product does not adequately represent myocardial oxygen requirements under these circumstances because it fails to accurately reflect changes in wall stress.

Despite the limited vasodilatory reserve in coronary arteries with fixed stenoses, administration of nitrates to patients with stable angina pectoris may directly improve blood flow to ischemic regions as a result of several possible mechanisms. Nitrates have been shown to cause modest stenosis dilatation with potentially important effects on post-stenosis perfusion pressure.[88] They relieve coronary vasoconstriction related to endothelial dysfunction.[85–87] Blood flow to ischemic regions may be increased by organic nitrates as a result of dilatation of collateral vessels.[90] Thus patients with well-developed collateral vessels are particularly responsive to organic nitrates.[91] Reduction of diastolic ventricular pressure may increase myocardial perfusion pressure, particularly in the subendocardium. The anginal threshold during atrial pacing is improved by systemic but not intracoronary nitrates.[92] This observation suggests that in some patients with effort angina, direct effects on the coronary circulation are relatively unimportant.

The response of a patient to nitrates depends on multiple factors, including the severity and distribution of specific coronary arterial lesions, the extent to which altered coronary vasomotor tone contributes to symptoms, the presence or absence of collateral vessels, and whether dilatation of conductance vessels influences post-stenotic perfusion pressure. Effects on wall stress (and their salutary clinical consequences) depend on the extent to which wall stress is elevated before treatment. Thus patients with significant left ventricular dilatation, poorly controlled congestive heart failure, and high ventricular diastolic pressure may exhibit especially favorable responses to administration of nitrates as a result of relatively large decreases in myocardial oxygen demand.[85, 86] Effects of nitrates are also dependent upon posture. When they are given to patients in an upright position, effects on venous return and wall stress are more prominent.

Clinical Pharmacology. A detailed review of the clinical pharmacology of organic nitrates is presented in Chapter 2. The following discussion is focused on issues that have particular clinical relevance to patients with chronic stable angina.

In addition to its utility in treatment of specific attacks, sublingual nitroglycerin (0.3–0.6 mg) is effective for short-term prophylaxis of angina. Because of its pharmacokinetics, with dissipation of effects within 30 minutes or less, it cannot be used for long-term suppression of angina.[93] Aerosolized nitroglycerin sprays (0.4–0.8 mg) have an onset and duration of action similar to those of sublingual nitroglycerin[94] and are useful for patients with dry mucous membranes.

When administered orally, most organic nitrates undergo extensive first-pass conversion by the liver to inactive metabolites in reactions catalyzed by glutathione organic nitrate reductase (see Chapter 2).[85, 93] Accordingly, relatively large doses are required in order to elicit therapeutic effects. For example, 2.5–5 mg of isosorbide dinitrate administered sublingually is ordinarily effective, whereas a minimum of 20–30 mg administered orally is usually required. When sufficiently large doses are employed, oral "long-acting" nitrates such as isosorbide dinitrate exert prolonged therapeutic effects.[95, 96] Because of the marked first-pass hepatic conversion after oral organic nitrate administration, formulations with alternative routes of administration have been developed (see Chapter 2), including ointments,[97] 7.5–30 mg twice per day 6 h apart; transdermal patches,[98, 99] 0.2–0.8 mg/h for 10–12 h; transmucosal (buccal),[95] 3 mg three times per day; and sublingual isosorbide dinitrate preparations, 2.5–10 mg two or three times per day.

Prolongation of effects after oral administration has been the objective of development of long-acting, slow-release preparations of substances such as isosorbide dinitrate (40–80 mg once per day). An alternative is isosorbide 5-mononitrate (20 mg two times per day or 30–120 mg once per day of the long-acting preparation), an orally administered agent with minimal first-pass hepatic effects and relatively prolonged and consistent bioavailability.[99, 100]

Nitrate Tolerance. Long-lasting therapeutic efficacy of organic nitrates is compromised by the development of tolerance, a problem that is particularly significant in chronic angina as opposed to acute ischemic syndromes. This phenomenon is virtually universal and constitutes a major limitation in the use of long-acting nitrates for prophylaxis of angina pectoris[85, 87, 95–98, 102, 103] (Fig. 5–7). One mechanism of tolerance appears to be reduced generation of nitric oxide over time, ascribed to depletion of sulfhydryl donor groups needed to convert organic nitrates into nitric oxide.[85, 103–108] Alternatively, counterregulatory responses activated as a result of prolonged exposure to nitrates may be involved.[85, 103–105] Hypotension induced by nitrates can reflexively activate the sympathetic nervous system[109] and attenuate therapeutic effects as a result of increased heart rate and systemic vascular resistance. Neurohumoral activation may underlie rebound phenomena, worsening of symptoms when nitrates are discontinued or near the conclusion of a nitrate-free interval (the so-called zero h phenomenon).[103] Concomitant administration of beta-adrenergic blocking agents may diminish both the rebound phenomenon and nitrate tolerance. Although angiotensin converting enzyme (ACE) inhibitors can reduce tolerance to nitrates,[111] the mechanism may not be attenuation of counterregulatory activation of the renin-angiotensin system per se because only ACE inhibitors containing sulfhydryl groups have been shown to be effective.

Tolerance to nitrates may also occur as a result of plasma volume expansion,[104, 105, 110] in turn a consequence of neurohumoral activation and possibly altered venous hemodynamics. Although volume expansion has been implicated as a cause, it occurs relatively slowly and is not well correlated temporally with the appearance of tolerance. Its persistence even after tolerance has appeared is consistent with retention of vasodilatory properties of administered nitrates despite a decreased therapeutic response.[112] Concomitant diuretic therapy may not diminish tolerance despite diminishing plasma volume.[113] Tolerance to nitrates is generally partial. Thus most patients who become tolerant continue to exhibit therapeutic responses to sublingually administered nitroglycerin[95] (see Fig. 5–7).

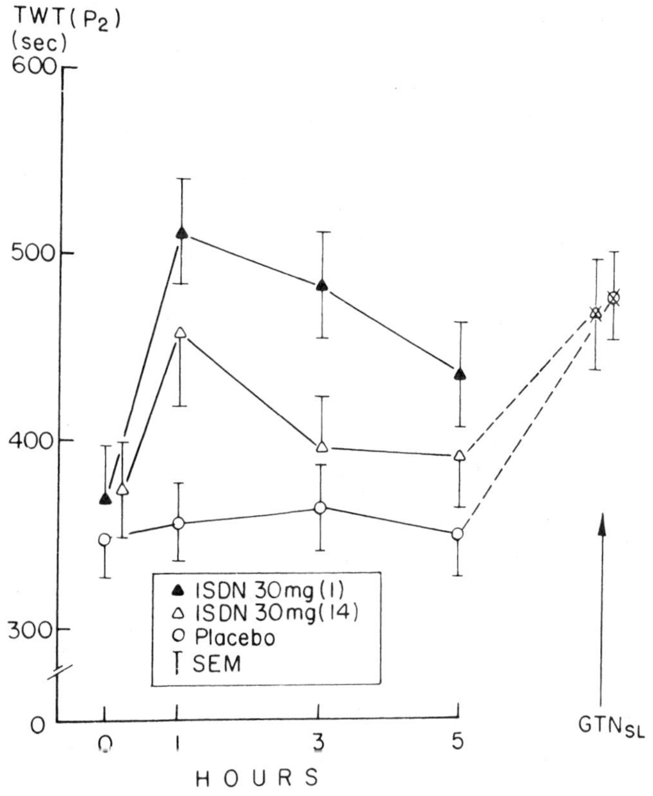

Figure 5–7. Improvement in treadmill walking time (TWT) after a first 30-mg dose of isosorbide dinitrate (ISDN), in comparison with responses after placebo and after 14 d of treatment with 30 mg of ISDN q.i.d. Note appearance of tolerance after 14 days, with reduced improvement in TWT in comparison with performance after the first dose. In addition, note that sublingual nitroglycerin (GTN) response is unaltered after 14 days of ISDN treatment. *Other abbreviation:* SEM, standard error of the mean. (From Parker JO, VanKoughnett KA, Farrell B: Comparison of buccal nitroglycerin and oral isosorbide dinitrate for nitrate tolerance in stable angina pectoris. Am J Cardiol 1985; 56:724.)

The rapid appearance of tolerance after exposure to organic nitrates (seen as early as the end of the first dose interval with preparations that provide constant and high blood levels, such as transdermal patches) is striking. If exposure is uninterrupted, loss of most or all of the therapeutic effect of the agent is usually evident within 24–48 h. Tolerance develops most rapidly when high doses of organic nitrates are used, when blood levels are relatively constant, and when dosing schedules do not permit a substantial nitrate-free interval on a regular basis.[95–98, 102–104] As a result, smaller doses of long-acting nitrates are sometimes more effective than larger doses.

The most important therapeutic maneuver in avoiding tolerance is ensuring a substantial nitrate-free interval daily.[114] In general, such an interval or intervals must last at least 10–12 h. Dosing schedules that markedly reduce or eliminate tolerance have been developed. For example, use of buccal nitroglycerin, 3 mg three times per day, has been reported not to result in tolerance.[95] Similarly, in a very small study, a three-times-a-day schedule of nitroglycerin ointment (average dose, 5 mg) did not result in tolerance.[97] Asymmetric dose intervals with drug administered twice a day within a relatively short time (for example, at 8:00 AM and 3:00 PM) reduce or minimize tolerance.[85, 100, 101, 103] Even with a relatively long-acting drug such as isosorbide mononitrate (20-mg doses), this approach has been successful.[100, 101]

In view of these considerations, tolerance in patients with chronic angina can be minimized with oral long-acting nitrate preparations such as isosorbide dinitrate by administering the agent twice a day and providing a nitrate-free interval during the night. One dose (20–40 mg) is administered when the patient awakens, resulting in high blood levels during the morning hours when the frequency of angina is maximal.[9, 115] A second dose is administered in the mid-afternoon. The asymmetry of dosing can be modified for patients with specific temporal patterns of angina to optimize therapeutic effects while minimizing tolerance. When nitroglycerin transdermal patches (0.2–0.8 mg/h) are used, the duration of application of the patch should not exceed 12 h per 24-h interval because of the prolonged, high, steady-state blood levels present while the patch is in place. Even with such a regimen, substantial loss of efficacy occurs rapidly, probably because of the constancy of the high blood levels during the 12 h in which the patch is applied.[98, 99] Accordingly, transdermal patch administration of nitrates, despite being convenient, is generally less desirable than administration of nitrates by other routes.

Because of the need for nitrate-free intervals, patients with chronic angina given long-acting nitrates in dosing schedules that minimize tolerance do not experience antianginal protection all day. When angina is confined to a specific time of day, this is not a problem. However, for most patients, treatment with nitrates should be combined with other antianginal agents to avoid protracted intervals during which no pharmacologic protection is present. In many patients with variant or mixed angina, the timing of episodes is unpredictable. Accordingly, monotherapy with long-acting nitrates is generally insufficient.

Unfortunately, determination of whether tolerance is present is often difficult. When the patient with chronic angina exhibits clear reduction of symptoms initially after onset of treatment but therapeutic benefit is transient, tolerance can certainly be suspected. A decrease in the augmentation of platelet cGMP activity after administration of nitrates has been reported to be an objective marker of the presence of tolerance,[106] as has diminished exhalation of nitric oxide.[116] However, these indexes have not yet been validated clinically and are not currently recommended for routine management of patients with stable angina.

Adverse Effects of Organic Nitrates. The most common and troublesome adverse effects of organic nitrates are direct extensions of their pharmacologic properties: namely, headache, flushing, and hypotension. A complete discussion of these and other adverse effects is presented in Chapter 2. When troubling side effects occur, they can usually be managed with appropriate dose reduction and/or analgesics.

Selection of Patients for Treatment With Nitrates. Virtually all patients with stable angina can benefit from occasional use of a rapid-acting nitrate preparation: sublingual preparations of nitroglycerin, isosorbide dinitrate or comparable polynitrates, or aerosolized or buccal nitroglycerin. The usual dose of sublingual nitroglycerin is 0.3–0.6 mg. Typically, an attack is terminated within a few minutes. In rare instances, for severe attacks, a second or third dose may be required. If more than two or three doses are needed, the patient should seek medical attention for suspected unstable angina or myocardial infarction. The most common cause of failure to elicit a therapeutic effect with sublingual nitroglycerin is use of an old preparation that has deteriorated.

Sublingual nitroglycerin can be used effectively prophylactically when the duration of protection required is brief. Thus it is particularly helpful in preventing postprandial angina, nocturnal angina that occurs early after retiring, angina associated with brief intervals of relatively high-level physical exertion that cannot be avoided, or angina induced by sexual intercourse.

As indicated earlier, long-acting nitrates are effective in patients with effort, mixed, and variant angina. They may be useful in microvascular angina, although little systematic experience in these patients has been published. They are particularly helpful in patients with underlying left ventricular dysfunction because of their favorable effects on loading conditions. In contrast, beta-adrenergic blocking agents and calcium channel blockers, to be discussed, must be used more cautiously in such patients and may exacerbate symptoms of heart failure.

When angina is attributable to etiologies other than fixed or dynamic coronary stenoses, the efficacy of nitrates is less predictable, and their use may be deleterious; for example, in some patients with aortic stenosis, peripheral vasodilatation and systemic arterial hypotension may compromise coronary perfusion.

Beta-Adrenergic Blocking Drugs

Effects of Beta-Adrenergic Blockade. Beta-adrenergic blocking drugs exert therapeutic effects in effort angina by diminishing increased heart rate and contractility accompanying stress (see Chapter 2).[117, 118] The resulting decrease in double product is indicative of decreased myocardial oxygen demand at a given level of stress. Slower heart rate also increases the diastolic time available for coronary perfusion, which is of particular importance for patients with fixed coronary stenoses in whom the ratio of systolic to diastolic perfusion is abnormally high. The attenuated heart rate and contractility are associated with increased ventricular volume that may increase myocardial oxygen demand. However, in most patients this effect is much less striking than the decreased demand related to the negative chronotropic and inotropic effects. Beta-adrenergic blockers can adversely influence coronary vasomotor tone, in part because of unopposed alpha-adrenergic mediated vasoconstriction.[119] Conversely, some patients with angina exhibit exercise-induced vasoconstriction that may be relieved by beta-adrenergic blockade, because of reduction of endogenous sympathoadrenal stimulation induced by ischemia.[120, 121]

Beta-adrenergic blockade decreases blood flow to most organs because of unopposed alpha-adrenergic vasoconstriction and blockade of vascular β_2 receptors.[122] However, initial increases in vascular resistance typically vanish with long-term use,[123] and effects on peripheral perfusion are generally unimportant even in patients with peripheral vascular disease.[124] Because of the decreased blood flow to skeletal muscle, beta-adrenergic blockade can reduce maximal exercise capacity, an effect that is less prominent with β_1-selective drugs.[125] Blockade of β_2 receptors in bronchial smooth muscle may precipitate bronchoconstriction in asthmatic patients, an adverse effect of considerable clinical importance.

As discussed in detail in Chapter 2, beta-adrenergic blockade impairs glycogenolysis and can prolong recovery from hypoglycemic episodes in insulin-dependent diabetics, and augments plasma concentrations of triglycerides with secondary decreases in high-density lipoprotein (HDL) levels. The central nervous system depressant effects of beta-adrenergic blockade account for common adverse reactions.

Utility of Beta-Adrenergic Blockers in Chronic Stable Angina. Beta-adrenergic blockers constitute primary pharmacologic treatment for effort angina. They increase exercise tolerance and time to ischemia assessed by standardized exercise testing, and reduce the frequency of anginal attacks.[117, 118] Even when fixed coronary stenoses are present in conjunction with abnormal coronary vasomotor tone (mixed angina), beta-adrenergic blockade is usually effective, especially when ischemic episodes are associated with increased heart rate and blood pressure.[126] Beta-adrenergic blockers are very effective in suppressing episodes of silent ischemia even when they occur in the absence of increased heart rate, perhaps because of a decrease in average heart rate and blood pressure with consequent diminution of the effects of abnormal vasomotor tone.[127–129] Nevertheless, they are not generally indicated for patients with pure variant angina, in whom they may occasionally exacerbate symptoms.

Chronic beta-adrenergic blockade unequivocally reduces long-term mortality rates among patients who have survived acute myocardial infarction and is indicated for patients with stable angina who have suffered infarction. It is possible that agents with intrinsic sympathomimetic activity may not offer this benefit.[130] However, survival effects in patients with stable angina without a history of myocardial infarction have not yet been demonstrated.

Clinical Pharmacology of Beta-Adrenergic Blockers. In contrast to calcium channel blockers, which differ considerably amongst themselves, all beta-adrenergic blockers exhibit essentially identical mechanisms of antianginal action.[117, 118] Accordingly, differences in clinical pharmacology constitute a main reason to select one beta-adrenergic blocker over another. A detailed discussion of clinical pharmacology and a list of currently available drugs are provided in Chapter 2. Features of clinical pharmacology of major relevance in chronic angina are as follows:[131, 132]

1. Absorption and disposition: Beta-adrenergic blocker solubility profiles (lipophilic vs. hydrophilic) are important determinants of absorption, disposition, and bioavailability. Orally administered beta-adrenergic blockers exhibit considerable variation in bioavailability, but this is more prominent with lipophilic agents. For example, an oral dose of the highly lipophilic drug propranolol can result in a 20-fold variation in plasma levels. The half-life of hydrophilic beta-adrenergic blockers exceeds that of lipophilic agents. However, active metabolites with long half-lives may prolong the effects of lipophilic drugs.

   Lipophilic beta-adrenergic blockers are usually administered every 6–8 h. Hydrophilic blockers can be administered less often (once or twice per day). Availability of slow release preparations of drugs such as propranolol (80–320 mg once per day) and metoprolol (100–400 mg once per day) has reduced the need for frequent administration of some agents, helping to improve compliance by patients with chronic angina.

Although rational selection of a beta-adrenergic blocking drug for patients with chronic angina and coexisting renal or hepatic insufficiency can be based on solubility and disposition characteristics, from a practical standpoint such considerations are not critical because of the large difference between plasma concentrations at which beta-adrenergic blockade occurs and those at which non–beta-adrenergic blockade–dependent toxic effects are observed. It is judicious, however, to initiate therapy at relatively low doses in situations in which drug effects may be more prolonged or prominent than usual in order to minimize beta-adrenergic blockade–related adverse effects.

Although oral administration is the rule, an intranasal propranolol spray preparation (5-mg puff) has been developed to rapidly induce beta-adrenergic blockade,[133] an approach potentially useful for the treatment of individual episodes of angina and for more consistent bioavailability.

2. Receptor specificity: Beta-adrenergic blockers differ with regard to receptor specificity (i.e., β_1 or cardioselective, as opposed to nonselective, with equivalent blockade of both β_1 and β_2 receptors). At relatively high doses (which are routinely administered clinically), β_1-selective drugs such as atenolol, metoprolol, and acebutolol lose this property. Thus these drugs cannot be administered freely to patients with a predisposition to unwanted β_2 blocking effects.
3. Intrinsic sympathomimetic activity (ISA): Some beta-adrenergic blockers exhibit weak agonist activity, a property that can be advantageous. They function as competitive blockers because they are much less potent agonists than endogenous catecholamines. At rest, most subjects have low levels of endogenous beta-adrenergic stimulation. The net result of use of an agent with appreciable ISA may therefore be no alteration in resting heart rate or blood pressure. If the patient with stable angina has resting bradycardia and/or conduction system disease, weak β_1 agonist activity may be useful in avoiding adverse effects on heart rate and rhythm. β_2 agonist activity may be useful for patients predisposed to bronchospasm and in those benefiting from peripheral arterial vasodilatation. ISA-mediated effects are generally not marked enough to substantially interfere with therapeutic efficacy during stress in patients with effort angina.

Practical Considerations in the Use of Beta-Adrenergic Blockers for Patients With Stable Angina. All beta-adrenergic blockers for treatment of chronic angina are comparable in efficacy because their mechanism of action is the same.[117, 118] Accordingly, selection of an agent should be based on side effect profile, convenience, and cost. Once- or twice-a-day dosing is available with hydrophilic drugs such as nadolol or atenolol or with lipophilic drugs available in long-acting preparations, such as propranolol or metoprolol. In the authors' view, hydrophilic agents are somewhat preferable for patients with stable angina because of their more consistent bioavailability and lack of direct central nervous system depressant effects. In the case of atenolol, the authors recommend an initial dose of 50 mg once per day, increasing to 100 mg if therapeutic response is inadequate. Some patients may require as much as 200 mg to achieve an optimal response. In the authors' experience, twice-a-day dosing of atenolol (to the same total daily dose) is sometimes preferable. In the case of nadolol, they recommend an initial dose of 40 mg once per day, increasing to 80 mg if necessary. The recommended regimen for propanolol is 30–60 mg three or four times per day for the regular preparation and 80–320 mg once per day for the long-acting preparation; for metoprolol, 50–200 mg twice per day for the regular preparation and 100–400 mg once per day for the long-acting preparation. Relatively cardioselective beta-adrenergic blockers are preferred for patients predisposed to undesirable effects of β_2 blockade. An alternative is an agent with significant ISA—for example, pindolol (5–20 mg twice per day).

Beta-adrenergic blockers are not ordinarily indicated for patients with purely vasospastic angina unless substantial increases in heart rate and blood pressure occur in association with attacks. In this circumstance, they may be useful in combination with calcium channel blockers (to be described). They are highly effective in suppressing silent ischemia[127–129] and are a logical choice for patients with stable angina and atrial fibrillation in whom control of ventricular rate associated with stress is critical.

In some patients with chronic angina and significant ventricular dysfunction, beta-adrenergic blockade can precipitate or exacerbate heart failure. In such patients, fatigue may replace angina as the factor limiting physical activity with little overall change in exercise tolerance.[134] However, beta-adrenergic blockers are often well-tolerated by patients with ventricular dysfunction if they are administered initially at relatively low doses. Indeed, there is considerable evidence that beta-adrenergic blockade is effective treatment for ischemic and nonischemic dilated cardiomyopathy.[135]

Because of marked individual variation in sensitivity and endogenous sympathoadrenal activity coupled with variable bioavailability, it is sometimes difficult to ascertain whether clinically significant beta-adrenergic blockade has been induced in response to a given dose of a specific agent. Blood levels of beta-adrenergic blockers are not correlated strongly enough with extent of beta-adrenergic blockade to be a useful measurement in individual patients. Proof of beta-adrenergic blockade in patients with effort angina can be acquired by comparing pre- and post-treatment responses to standardized exercise testing (i.e., suppression of increases in heart rate and blood pressure).[136] An unequivocal decrease in resting heart rate measured under consistent conditions is a reliable marker as well, but in general, at least a 10-beat-per-minute decrease is required. Furthermore, a patient may be well protected by beta-adrenergic blockade and yet have minimal or no change in resting heart rate, especially when the beta-adrenergic blocker being used has ISA. Clinical response (reduction of frequency and severity of angina) is directly related to induction of adequate beta-blockade. Unfortunately, placebo effects can sometimes simulate therapeutic benefit, at least initially, thereby rendering clinical response only partially reliable as an indication of the adequacy of beta-adrenergic blockade. Bedside maneuvers such as the heart rate response to standing or to handgrip exercise may be helpful in defining extent of beta-adrenergic blockade, but variability of responses limits their utility. Mild, semiquantitative bouts of exercise that can be performed easily in an office setting before and after starting a drug (e.g., a timed walk in a hallway or up and down stairs) are practical and can be quite useful in assessing beta-adrenergic blockade. Because of the wide toxic-to-therapeutic ratio, patients without contraindications to beta-adrenergic blockers can usually be given generous doses safely.

Sudden discontinuation of beta-adrenergic blockers can induce rebound effects, including unstable angina and even myocardial infarction.[137] Usually these reactions reflect withdrawal of previously effective therapy that suppresses symptoms and/or unmasking of progression of underlying disease. In rare instances, true pharmacologic rebound—that is, an exaggerated response to catecholamines—may occur. Rebound can be minimized by gradual withdrawal and adjustment of other antianginal therapy.

Adverse Effects. These are discussed in detail in Chapter 2. Those that are especially pertinent for patients with chronic angina are mentioned briefly here. Adverse effects related to central nervous system depression (lack of energy, depression, loss of libido, confusion, nightmares) are common. Such effects can be direct (with lipophilic drugs), indirect and secondary to decreased cardiac output (with lipophilic and hydrophilic drugs), or both. Gastrointestinal side effects including constipation, diarrhea, and nausea can occur. Monitoring of lipids in hyperlipidemic patients with adjustment of management as needed is appropriate.

In insulin-requiring diabetic patients, metabolic effects can potentiate hypoglycemia and suppress its signs and symptoms, many of which are secondary to activation of the sympathetic nervous system. Beta-adrenergic blockers can be used successfully in such patients, but they must be administered very cautiously, and blood glucose must be monitored. β_1-selective agents are preferable.

Untoward cardiac effects include worsening of heart failure and bradycardia secondary to depression of sinus node function and/or atrioventricular block. Most patients with mild conduction system disorders, including modest first-degree heart block, can tolerate cautious use of beta-adrenergic blockers, but these drugs are contraindicated in the presence of higher grade atrioventricular block. As a practical matter, the authors would withhold beta-adrenergic blockers from patients with PR intervals >.24 sec, with the exception that drugs with substantial ISA may be used, albeit cautiously, in such patients.

For patients with stable angina and relative contraindications to beta-adrenergic blockers in whom their use is deemed to be worthy of a trial, the authors favor beginning treatment with half the usual recommended starting dose and then gradually increasing the dose every 2–3 days with monitoring of appropriate parameters (e.g., the PR interval; signs and symptoms of heart failure) until a desired therapeutic effect and/or a usual clinical dose is achieved, provided that untoward effects do not occur.

Calcium Channel Blocking Drugs

Spectrum of Activity. Calcium channel blocking drugs are all therapeutically active as virtually pure arterial (including coronary) vasodilators, with variable effects on cardiac conduction and contractility. Their mechanisms of action are discussed in detail in Chapter 2. Specific aspects of their spectrum of activity pertinent to patients with stable angina are considered here.

Currently available calcium channel blockers for management of stable angina include the dihydropyridines, phenylalkylamines, and benzothiazepines (see Chapter 2).[138] Dihydropyridines, the prototype of which is nifedipine, have little or no direct effects on myocardium in vivo. Dihyropyridines are more potent vasodilators than the phenylalkylamines, which in turn are more potent than the benzothiazepines (see Chapter 2).[138, 139] Second-generation dihydropyridines (nicardipine, felodipine, isradipine, amlodipine) have been developed to provide even greater vascular selectivity, to have longer half-lives, and to produce less variability in blood levels.[139] The phenylalkylamine prototype is verapamil, a drug with prominent effects on myocardium and on the conduction system in vivo. The benzothiazepine prototype is diltiazem, which also has significant effects on myocardium and on the conduction system.[138, 140, 141] Its negative inotropic and dromotropic effects are somewhat less prominent than those of verapamil.

In patients with stable angina and normal ventricular function at rest, negative inotropic effects of calcium channel blockers are clinically insignificant.[142–144] By contrast, in patients with depressed ventricular function, calcium channel blockers can precipitate heart failure. Verapamil is the most common offender, but even dihydropyridines can occasionally be problematic.[142–144]

In addition to those in the major classes, several other agents that block L-type calcium channels have been developed and used in chronic angina. Bepridil (200–400 mg once per day) acts at the dihydropyridine binding site but exerts blocking effects on the fast sodium channel as well.[145] This drug exhibits favorable antiarrhythmic properties but also causes QT prolongation and the risk of proarrhythmic effects. Perhexiline maleate, a relatively nonspecific calcium channel antagonist, has also been used in the treatment of angina.[146] Its mechanism of action is poorly understood but probably involves alterations in myocardial cellular energy sources. Dosage is highly variable (25–300 mg per day in two divided doses to achieve therapeutic blood levels that should be monitored on a regular basis).

Antianginal Effects. When administered to patients with chronic effort angina, calcium channel blockers do not reduce the double product at peak exercise because endogenous neurohumoral mechanisms—adrenergic stimulation and parasympathetic withdrawal—usually overcome direct negative chronotropic and inotropic effects.[147–149] Instead, phenylalkylamines and benzothiazepines retard the increase in myocardial oxygen demand at submaximal workloads sufficiently to increase the anginal threshold and are the most effective calcium channel blockers for the treatment of effort angina.[149, 150] With dihydropyridines, little or no decrease in double product occurs at any level of exercise, inasmuch as lowering of blood pressure tends to be offset by an increase in heart rate. Nevertheless, ischemia is reduced and exercise tolerance is usually improved.[147, 151] It has been proposed that the mechanism is increased coronary blood flow,[150] perhaps as a result of stenosis dilatation, as seen with nitrates. Calcium channel blockers may attenuate or reverse exercise-induced vasoconstriction, thereby improving collateral flow, and enhance myocardial relaxation, reducing ventricular diastolic pressures and improving effective coronary perfusion pressure.

Because they are powerful coronary vasodilators, calcium channel blockers are particularly effective in the treatment of patients with vasospasm and variant angina,[152–155] especially the dihydropyridines.[152, 155] They also may be effective in patients without fixed stenoses of epicardial coronary arteries in whom angina is associated with reduced vasodilator reserve.[156]

Calcium channel blockers slow the progression of atherosclerosis in studies of cholesterol-fed rabbits.[157] Although calcium channel blockers do not exert major effects on serum lipids, they may diminish proliferative processes within atherosclerotic lesions. In two clinical trials[157] that have assessed nifedipine with respect to angiographic progression of atherosclerosis, modest but significant favorable effects were seen.

Selection of a Calcium Channel Blocker. The clinical pharmacology and dosage regimens of calcium channel blockers are described in Chapter 2. A few points pertinent to patients with chronic stable angina are mentioned here. All three prototypic calcium channel blockers (verapamil, nifedipine, and diltiazem) exhibit comparable pharmacokinetics when administered orally, with good absorption via the gastrointestinal tract, substantial first-pass metabolism in the liver and consequently reduced bioavailability, a time to onset of action of 30 to 60 minutes, and appreciable binding to plasma proteins with pharmacologic half-lives from 1.3 to 5 h.[138, 139] Slow-release preparations of each of these three drugs are now available, facilitating twice- or, in some cases, once-a-day dosing. An oral osmotic pump preparation of nifedipine has also been developed,[158] which is potentially useful as part of a maintenance regimen for patients with chronic angina. Second-generation dihydropyridines have longer half-lives, smoother onset of action, reduced fluctuations of blood levels, and greater vasodilator and particularly coronary arterial selectivity. However, their efficacy in effort angina has reportedly been mixed.[159–161] Because of the relative comparability of pharmacokinetics, factors such as spectrum of activity in relation to pathophysiology of angina and side effect profile are usually more important in the selection of a calcium channel blocker in a patient with chronic stable angina (to be described).

Calcium channel blockers are the treatment of choice for patients with chronic angina caused by coronary vasospasm who do not have fixed coronary stenoses. All these drugs are highly effective. They also appear to be effective in patients with presumed microvascular angina.[156] In patients with effort or mixed angina, verapamil and diltiazem are effective as monotherapy. Dihydropyridines suppress symptoms as well but should be avoided as monotherapy because they increase the risk of exacerbating ischemia as a result of reflex sympathetic nervous system activation. Beta-adrenergic blockers appear to be significantly more effective than either nifedipine or diltiazem in suppressing silent ischemia detected by ambulatory monitoring.[127–129]

Calcium channel blockers are not first-line drugs for the treatment of angina in patients with significant systolic ventricular dysfunction and/or heart failure, although they can be used when symptoms cannot be controlled with other antianginal drugs.

Adverse Effects and Contraindications to Calcium Channel Blockers. A detailed side effect profile is presented in Chapter 2. Of special pertinence for patients with chronic angina are the following side effects: Signs and symptoms related to excessive peripheral vasodilatation can occur with all of the calcium channel blockers, particularly the dihydropyridines; these include headaches, flushing, postural hypotension, dysesthesias, and, in rare instances, consequences of worsening of myocardial ischemia secondary to sympathetic nervous system activation and attendant increases in myocardial oxygen demand (see Chapter 2).[151, 160] Hypotension with reduced coronary perfusion pressure and/or coronary steal may also contribute. In rare instances, exacerbation of myocardial ischemia has caused death; because of their depressant effects on the conduction system, the benzothiazepines and phenylalkylamines are less likely than the dihydropyridines to exacerbate ischemia through increased myocardial oxygen demand. Clinically significant myocardial depression has been seen with all types of calcium channel blockers, but it is usually seen only in patients with underlying ventricular dysfunction. In patients with angina and severe, chronic contractile dysfunction, calcium channel blockers may adversely affect long-term prognosis.[162] Because of their negative dromotropic effects, benzothiazepines and phenylalkylamines should be used very cautiously or not at all in patients with coexistent conduction system disease.

Calcium channel antagonists are generally contraindicated in patients with angina secondary to aortic valve disease. In contrast to the beta-adrenergic blockers, they can be employed without difficulty in patients with angina and peripheral vascular disease or Raynaud's phenomenon. They should be avoided when hyperthyroidism or severe anemia is present because vasodilation and sympathoadrenal activation are likely to be prominent in these conditions.

A number of drug interactions can occur with calcium channel blockers (see Chapter 2). A few of particular relevance for patients with stable angina are briefly mentioned here. Combined use of verapamil and beta-adrenergic blocking drugs is ordinarily contraindicated because of the potential summation of negative inotropic, dromotropic, and chronotropic effects. Verapamil and digoxin should be used very carefully in combination because of potential toxic effects on the conduction system. Monitoring serum digoxin levels may be helpful in such patients. Calcium channel blockers in combination with alpha-adrenergic blockers or peripheral vasodilators such as quinidine can induce severe hypotension. Calcium antagonists prescribed in combination with type I antiarrhythmics can occasionally result in symptomatic bradycardia. Accordingly, dose reduction may be necessary when calcium channel blockers are employed in combination with this class of drugs. Careful monitoring of the ECG (sinus rate, PR interval) during the first 2 weeks of combined therapy is recommended.

Other Antianginal Drugs

Numerous agents besides nitrates, beta-adrenergic blockers, and calcium channel blocking drugs have been used to treat stable angina. These drugs may be employed when conventional antianginals are ineffective, are contraindicated, or cause unacceptable side effects. A few are considered briefly.

Molsidomine (N-ethoxycarbonyl-3-morpholino-sydnonimine), a sydnonimine, exerts hemodynamic effects similar to those of the organic nitrates.[163] Its mechanism of action involves activation of guanylate cyclase without conversion of the drug to nitric oxide. N-nidroso-N-morpholino-acetonitrite (SIN 1A) is the primary metabolite, an active vasodilator that is formed in the liver. The dose is 2 mg three times per day. Molsidomine is an appropriate alternative to long-acting nitrates.

Perhexiline maleate,[146] a nonspecific calcium channel blocker introduced in the 1970s, produces marked hepatic and neurologic toxicity. Its mechanism of action in angina is not necessarily calcium channel blockade and may be related to a shift of substrate metabolism from fatty acid to glucose oxidation. Perhexiline has been used successfully in patients with angina refractory to other drugs. The dose range is 25–300 mg, administered twice per day in a divided dose. Because toxicity is related to blood level, which can now be monitored, interest in this agent has resurfaced, but perhexiline remains an agent that should be reserved for patients with angina that is refractory to other agents.

Nicorandil,[163] a nicotinamide derivative, is both an arterial dilator and a venodilator. Its arterial dilator activity is thought to be attributable to potassium channel activation, and its venodilator activity to the nitrate group that it contains. Side effects (seen in 20%–50% of patients), mainly headache and postural hypotension, are similar to those seen with other vasodilators. Nicorandil can be considered as an alternative to either long-acting nitrates or calcium channel blockers. The usual dose is 10–20 mg, administered twice per day.

Theophylline and related compounds have venodilator properties but do not dilate coronary arteries. They exert antianginal effects secondary to blockade of adenosine A_1 receptors and cause relatively selective inhibition of adenosine-induced coronary vasodilation in nonischemic regions, thereby increasing distribution of coronary blood flow to ischemic zones.[165] Even though theophylline increases cardiac work, it increases the double product at which ischemia occurs, which is consistent with augmentation of delivery of oxygen to ischemic myocardium. Theophylline has been used in doses of 400 mg twice per day.[166] Although there is little clinical experience with theophylline as an antianginal drug, it may be considered as an adjunctive treatment for patients with angina that is refractory to other agents.

Catheter-Based Revascularization

The reader is referred to Chapter 3 of this volume and Chapter 39 of *Heart Disease,* 5th Edition, for detailed considerations of technical aspects of interventional cardiology, short- and long-term anatomic and mortality results, complications, and restenosis. This section focuses on the aspects of catheter-based revascularization that are most pertinent to patients with stable angina. The discussion is confined to the role of routine angioplasty in management.

Percutaneous Transluminal Coronary Angioplasty (PTCA): Nonrandomized Studies

The National Heart, Lung & Blood Institute (NHLBI) PTCA Registry has been an important source of information on the results of PTCA, but it is not restricted to patients with chronic stable angina. The most recent reports[167, 169] revealed an overall 1-year mortality rate of 3.2%, a 1-year myocardial infarction rate of 7.2%, and a 1-year coronary bypass surgery rate of 13.2%. About 18.5% of patients require repeat PTCA during the first year. An impressive finding, especially considering that these data were gathered in 1988, is that 75% of survivors were angina-free at 1 year.

In a 10-year follow-up of patients treated originally by Gruntzig and coworkers,[170] most of whom had stable angina, the overall survival rate was 89.5%. Late restenosis with reappearance of symptoms was rare among patients who underwent a single successful dilatation procedure for single-vessel disease. In a larger group of patients treated by the same group for whom 5-year follow-up data are available,[171] 85% of patients were asymptomatic, 20% required additional PTCA, 94% were free from myocardial infarction, and 84% did not require bypass surgery. The overall cardiac mortality rate was a remarkably low 1.9%. However, these data reflect results in a patient population comprising a large number of subjects with initial single-vessel disease and relatively "ideal" lesions.

Initially, PTCA was not considered to be a procedure of choice for patients with multivessel disease. However, patients with stable angina and certain types of two-vessel disease, patients with multivessel disease in whom one specific lesion appears to be the culprit, and patients for whom the risk of bypass surgery is unusually high may be good candidates for catheter-based revascularization.[168, 172–174] Complete revascularization need not be the goal.[175–178] In fact, PTCA may be preferable to bypass surgery in treating a young patient with angina in whom such a procedure, even though it does not result in complete revascularization, is sufficient to alleviate symptoms and delay surgery that will be needed ultimately and can be performed at a time when multiple lesions have evolved and can be attacked simultaneously. Survival after PTCA among patients with multivessel disease is remarkably good: as high as 88% after 5 years.[168, 172–174, 179] Nevertheless, the incidence of late adverse events (myocardial infarction, need for bypass surgery) is greater than among patients with single-vessel lesions. Most patients are angina-free in follow-up intervals ranging from 1 to 5 years. Late outcome in patients with multivessel disease may be determined more by the severity and rate of progression of the underlying disease than the extent of revascularization achieved during the initial procedure.[173, 174, 177, 179] Thus in some studies, the 2-year outcome is not very different between patients with complete and those with incomplete revascularization.

Prospective Randomized Trials of PTCA Compared With Medical Therapy or Surgery

To study patients with single-vessel disease, the randomized Angioplasty Compared With Medicine (ACME) study is being performed as of this writing by a consortium of Veterans Administration (VA) hospitals in 212 men with stable angina (most patients), a markedly positive result on an exercise tolerance test, or a recent myocardial infarction.[180] The angiographic procedural success rate has been relatively low (82%). The complications seen in this study were consistent with those seen generally. Interim results indicate that in the first 6 months, 10% of patients who were randomly chosen for medical therapy crossed over to PTCA, and 15% of PTCA patients required a second PTCA. At 6-month follow-up, a statistically significant advantage was evident among patients treated with PTCA: 64% were angina-free, in comparison with 46% of medically treated patients. Exercise test performance was also more improved with PTCA. Three infarctions and one death occurred in the medical group, in comparison with none in the PTCA group, but the difference was not statistically significant. At 3-year follow-up, PTCA patients exhibited better exercise capacity, fewer subsequent catheterizations and late interventions, and fewer hospitalizations, but the proportion of angina-free patients was no longer significantly larger than that in the medical management group.

The ACME study provides the only currently available prospective data comparing medical management with PTCA in patients with stable angina and single-vessel disease. It is difficult to draw firm conclusions at this time because the study is incomplete and relatively small in size. The procedural success rate has been relatively low, and advances in interventional techniques such as coronary stents were not incorporated. These points bias the results toward medical management. The results do provide an objective quality-of-life rationale for recommending PTCA to patients with single-vessel disease and chronic stable angina. However, because there remain considerable gaps in our knowledge—for example, whether there are subgroups of patients who benefit more or less from PTCA, whether similar results pertain in women, long-term cost-benefit comparisons—recommendations in such patients are still largely empirical. Stenoses in the left anterior descending coronary artery tend to cause more concern than those in other vessels, sometimes resulting in a more aggressive management approach. However, there is little objective evidence that this is the correct approach for patients with chronic stable angina, independent of the extent to which these lesions result in a larger amount of myocardium at risk.

A number of trials of PTCA compared with surgery, predominantly in patients with multivessel disease, are in progress.[181–185] Patients for whom bypass surgery has been shown unequivocally to improve survival are not included; nor are those who have lesions that are unsuitable for PTCA. These trials are not restricted to chronic stable angina, although they include large numbers of such patients. (The Randomised Intervention Treatment of Angina [RITA] trial[182] is most heavily weighted toward patients with stable angina.) The aggregate, incomplete results available to date (Table 5–3) in general indicate that complete revascularization is more frequent with bypass surgery than with PTCA. The in-hospital mortality rate is not significantly different. Periprocedural infarction rates appear higher with surgery.

As expected, initial costs are higher with surgery. At 3-year follow-up, the overall incidences of myocardial infarction and death for the two approaches appear to be comparable. However, the combination of less complete initial revascularization and the usual incidence of restenosis with PTCA is associated with a much greater need for repeat angiography and repeat revascularization procedures for patients randomized initially to PTCA (Fig. 5–8). Thus, subsequent costs are higher for PTCA. At early follow-up, the percentage of patients with angina appears to be somewhat higher after PTCA. However, at later follow-up (2–3 years), symptomatic status appears to be similar in the PTCA and surgical groups. Although it is premature to define the precise role of PTCA versus surgery for patients with stable angina and multivessel disease, it appears likely, on the basis of results to date, that interventional technology will eventually assume an important place in the therapeutic armamentarium available to these patients.

Selection of Patients With Chronic Angina for Catheter-Based Revascularization

The following are general guidelines. In the last section of this chapter, they are incorporated in a decision tree format and integrated with medical and surgical management options.

Referral of a patient with stable angina for catheter-based revascularization usually begins with a decision to perform cardiac catheterization and coronary angiography because of a suspicion of high risk, based on noninvasive stratification and/or unacceptably severe symptoms. If angiography confirms that a patient belongs in a high-risk subgroup (to be described), bypass surgery is usually preferred unless coronary anatomy precludes complete revascularization. In

TABLE 5–3. PTCA VERSUS CORONARY BYPASS SURGERY*

	Advantage of PTCA	Advantage of Surgery	No Difference
Complete revascularization		X	
Early mortality rate			X
Early myocardial infarction rate		X	
3-year follow-up:			
Mortality			X
Myocardial infarction			X
Angina		X	
Initial costs	X		
Subsequent catheterization/revascularization/costs		X	

*Aggregate results, references 181–185. Long-term cost-effectiveness advantage is unknown.

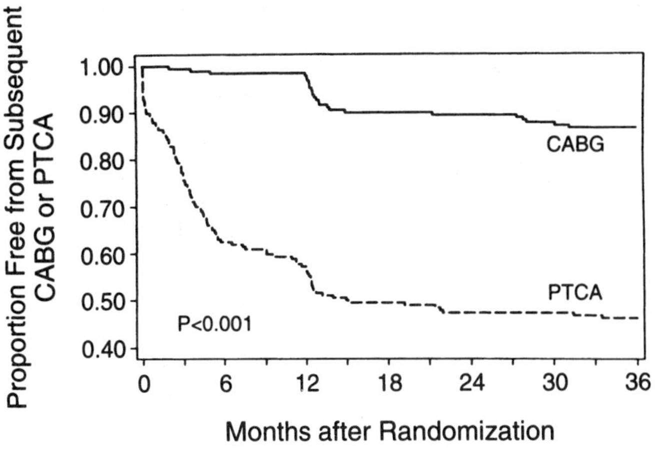

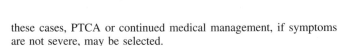

	No. of Patients/Proportion Free from Subsequent Procedure						
CABG	194	188/0.98	186/0.97	168/0.90	164/0.89	161/0.87	158/0.87
PTCA	198	122/0.62	110/0.56	95/0.49	90/0.47	88/0.47	84/0.46

Figure 5–8. Cumulative event rates for the 2½ years after randomization to percutaneous transluminal coronary angioplasty (PTCA) or coronary artery bypass surgery (CABG) in the Randomised Intervention Treatment of Angina (RITA) trial. Note that cumulative event rates for death and myocardial infarction are not significantly different. With addition of CABG and PTCA, the event rate is significantly higher after PTCA randomization than after CABG. (From RITA Trial Participants: Coronary angioplasty versus coronary artery bypass surgery: the Randomised Intervention Treatment of Angina [RITA] trial. Lancet 1993; 341:573.)

these cases, PTCA or continued medical management, if symptoms are not severe, may be selected.

For patients with symptoms that are refractory to medical management who are not in a high-risk subgroup as judged angiographically, PTCA is generally preferred because of lower initial cost and morbidity in comparison with surgery. However, if PTCA results can be anticipated to be suboptimal because of lesion characteristics (eccentricity, extensive calcification, tortuosity; see Chapter 3) or concerns about extent of revascularization (e.g., a high likelihood that a functionally important stenosis will not be successfully dilated in a patient with multivessel disease), bypass surgery may be preferred. In the latter circumstance, myocardial perfusion imaging during stress may be a helpful adjunct in defining the relative significance of myocardial stenoses and guiding therapy in these difficult cases.

For patients whose symptoms can be adequately managed medically who are not at high risk according to noninvasive testing, medical management is generally preferred. (It is difficult to extrapolate from the ACME results to all patients with mild symptoms because of reasons cited previously and lack of a favorable effect of PTCA on event rates or mortality despite the modest improvement in exercise capacity.) An exception is the patient with mild symptoms but severe ischemia with routine stress testing, in whom PTCA for single-vessel disease or low-risk two-vessel disease may be justified despite the present lack of proof of conferral of a survival advantage. This is a category of patients in whom radionuclide or echocardiographic imaging with stress is especially helpful in defining myocardium at risk.

Coronary Bypass Surgery

History

Surgical revascularization is highly effective in ameliorating symptoms in appropriately selected patients with stable angina.[186, 187] It became established as the preferred treatment for angina that is refractory to medical management as a result of three major randomized studies conducted in the 1970s (to be described). Coronary bypass surgery (CBS) was soon shown to improve survival among patients with left main coronary disease,[188] but delineation of the effect of CBS on survival in other patients required much more long-term follow-up data. The reader is referred to Chapters 4 and 46 for additional detailed discussion of CBS.

Influence of Coronary Bypass Surgery on Survival: Randomized Studies

The major randomized trials of CBS in comparison with medical management were the Veterans Administration Cooperative Study,[55, 189, 190] the European Cooperative Surgery Group Study (ECSG),[47, 191, 192] and the NIH-sponsored CASS.[193–197] Several detailed reviews of these studies are available.[198–200] Randomization features and baseline characteristics are summarized in Table 5–4. The VA study included patients with severe angina, abnormal ventricular function, and all grades of angiographic severity of disease. The ECSG excluded patients with single-vessel disease, more than moderate angina, and ejection fractions less than .50. The CASS included patients with all grades of disease severity but excluded those with ejection fractions below .35. It also included asymptomatic patients with a history of recent myocardial infarction in addition to those with angina. Most patients enrolled in these studies indeed had chronic stable angina.

In aggregate, the results of these studies established the following points that are relevant to the choice of therapeutic options for patients with chronic angina: (1) patients with single-vessel disease do not exhibit a survival benefit with CBS, perhaps because the prognosis of single-vessel disease treated medically is excellent, with 5-year survival of 90%–95%; (2) survival is enhanced with CBS in patients with three-vessel disease and abnormal ventricular function; (3) survival benefit is not seen in patients with two-vessel disease, regardless of ventricular function, unless the proximal segment of the left anterior descending artery is involved, especially if concomitant proximal left circumflex obstruction is present as well (so-called left main equivalent); and (4) survival benefit is directly related to the extent of impairment of ventricular function (probably because additional myocardial damage is more likely to be lethal when superimposed on extensive prior infarction). Moreover, left ventricular function improves after CBS in some patients,[201] possibly becaue of recovery of "hibernating" myocardium.

Additional clinical descriptors identifying enhanced survival with CBS include ST segment depression on resting ECG (VA study); history of myocardial infarction, hypertension, or more than 1.5-mm ST segment depression during exercise testing (ECSG); angina during exercise testing (CASS);[202] concomitant peripheral vascular disease (ECSG); and advanced age (ECSG). Thus CBS survival benefit is greatest in patients in whom prognosis, as judged from clinical descriptors and results of noninvasive testing, is now known to be poor with medical management alone.

TABLE 5–4. RANDOMIZATION AND BASELINE FEATURES OF RANDOMIZED TRIALS OF CORONARY BYPASS SURGERY

Feature	VA	ECSG	CASS
Recruitment period	1/72–12/74	9/73–3/76	8/75–5/79
Number randomized	686	768	780
Age	≤67	<65	≤65
% male	100	100	90
Angina class (%)			
None	0	0	22
II	42*	57†	74†
III	58‡	42	0
IV		0	0
Nonexertional			5
% stenosis threshold	≥50	≥50	≥70; left main, ≥50, <70
Left ventricular function			
Normal (%)	45	100	74
Abnormal (%)	55	0	21§
Operative mortality (%)	5.6	3.6	1.4
5-year crossover rate (medicine to surgery) (%)	17	24	24

Abbreviations: VA, Veterans Administration; ECSG, European Coronary Surgery Group; CASS, Coronary Artery Surgery Study.

Adapted from Nwasokwa ON, Koss JH, Friedman GH, et al: Bypass surgery for chronic stable angina: Predictors of survival benefit and strategy for patient selection. Ann Intern Med 1991; 114:1035.

*New York Heart Association.

†Canadian Cardiovascular Society.

‡Combined classes III and IV.

§Not measured in 6 subjects.

Survival benefit attributable to CBS in patients with chronic coronary disease peaks 5–8 years after surgery. It is reduced after 10–12 years and, in the VA study, absent after 18 years because of graft deterioration, progression of underlying vascular disease, and the increasing chance of noncardiovascular-related death as the population ages (Fig. 5–9).

Limitations of the Randomized Coronary Bypass Surgery Studies

Despite their impressive design and long-term follow-up, some features of these studies limit applicability to current management of patients with stable angina. Because maximal ages were 65 (ECSG and CASS) and 67 (VA), the magnitude of surgical survival benefit conferred to septuagenarians and octogenarians was not delineated. Because more than 90% of the patients were male, extrapolation of results to women may not be straightforward. Subsequent studies have delineated the importance of objective estimation of the extent of ischemia (not generally appreciated when the three initial studies were done) in predicting surgical survival advantage. Surgical techniques have improved considerably since the three studies were completed.[48] Cardioplegia is now more sophisticated, and internal thoracic and other arterial conduits have been shown to be superior to veins for grafting. Perioperative infarction and mortality rates have declined, as have early graft closure and late stenosis. Moreover, the value of postoperative antiplatelet agents has been established. Thus surgical survival benefit may be greater than initially recognized.

On the basis of these considerations and results of the nonrandomized studies to be discussed, indications for CBS according to survival advantage have been liberalized. However, it should be kept in mind that medical management has also evolved. The use of beta-adrenergic blockers, calcium channel blockers, long-acting nitrates, and aggressive risk factor modification has probably improved outcome in medically managed patients, potentially reducing the relative survival benefit conferred by surgery. Finally, in part because it became clear early on that CBS was successful in relieving symptoms in appropriately selected patients, the focus of these studies in general was on survival rather than on quality-of-life comparisons. Thus there is relatively little long-term information available from these studies with regard to objective assessment of exercise tolerance and residual or recurrent ischemia, return-to-work status, and cost/benefit analyses. Obviously, the last item is a key element in clinical decision making for patients with chronic angina.

Influence of CBS on Survival: Nonrandomized Studies

A number of CBS registries have provided continuing, updated information, including the CASS, Duke University, the University of Alabama, the Cleveland Clinic, and the Northern New England group. In contrast to the original randomized studies, however, registry data are much more heterogeneous with respect to clinical presentation; in particular, they contain larger numbers of patients with acute ischemic syndromes. With this caveat in mind, registry data in general indicate the following:[48, 203–210] (1) outcome after CBS has continued to improve, which is consistent with technical advances, including cardioplegia; (2) use of internal thoracic and other arterial conduits has contributed to greater long-term patency, especially of left anterior descending coronary artery grafts; (3) the incidence of perioperative myocardial infarction has been substantially reduced; (4) the operative mortality rate among patients younger than 65 with normal ventricular function is now approximately 1%–2% (<1% in many centers); (5) even when ventricular function is substantially impaired, perioperative mortality is generally ≤5%; (6) the long-term 7-year survival rates are as high as 87% with three-vessel disease, 93% with two-vessel disease, and 94% with single-vessel disease (Duke); and (7) the 7-year survival rates are as high as 94% with initial ejection fraction >.50, 90% with ejection fraction .35–.50, and 80% with ejection fraction <.35 (Duke).

Although the importance of previous myocardial infarction and an abnormal resting ECG as predictors of surgical survival benefit has been reconfirmed, it has become clear that the extent of myocardium at risk is probably the most important determinant of the potential for surgical enhancement of survival. This provides a rationale for a more liberal application of imaging techniques in conjunction with stress testing when there is doubt as to the most appropriate therapeutic recommendation. Correspondingly, the magnitude of deterioration

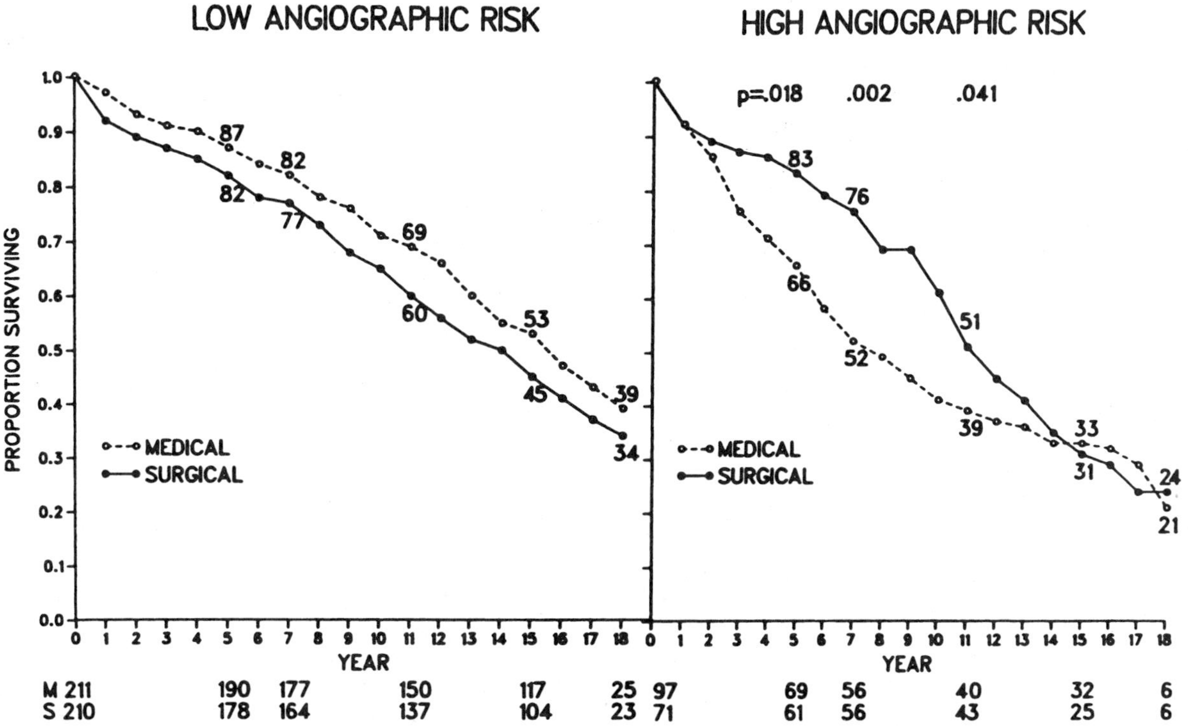

Figure 5–9. Eighteen-year follow-up data from the Veterans Administration Coronary Artery Bypass Graft Study Group. Patients in the high-angiographic-risk group had three-vessel coronary disease and abnormal ventricular function. This group demonstrated improved survival with surgery for about 11 years, but the benefit disappeared subsequently. The low-angiographic-risk group contained all other patients and demonstrated longer survival with medical management, but the difference was not statistically significant. (From The Veterans Administration Coronary Artery Bypass Surgery Cooperative Study Group: 18-year follow-up in the Veterans Affairs Cooperative Study of Coronary Artery Bypass Surgery for Stable Angina. Circulation 1992; 86:121.)

of ventricular function during exercise before surgery, assessed by radionuclide ventriculography, is a powerful descriptor of enhanced survival.[211] It is also now understood that patients at highest risk with medical management, who tend to have the greatest long-term CBS survival benefit, also have the highest perioperative mortality rate. Thus although CBS can now be performed with acceptable mortality rates among patients with low ejection fractions, the benefits of CBS are, at some currently uncertain level of depressed function, probably offset by an unacceptably high perioperative mortality rate. Because this level is unknown, it is unwise to be dogmatic about the often very difficult decision to recommend CBS to patients with stable angina and markedly depressed ventricular function.

The authors' current practice is to use an ejection fraction of .20–.25 as a cutoff, below which they would not ordinarily recommend CBS. However, this recommendation should be tempered by consideration of the patient's age and general condition, the presence of overt heart failure with circulatory congestion, the completeness of revascularization that can be anticipated, and the knowledge that ventricular function can improve after revascularization. Use of imaging techniques such as reinjection ^{201}Tl, late reimaging with ^{201}Tl injection after rest, dobutamine echocardiography, and PET scanning (if available), which assist in identifying viable myocardium, may be of considerable utility in decision making in these patients. Finally, if angina is truly refractory and severely disabling, situations will arise in which a high perioperative mortality rate resulting from depressed ventricular function is an unavoidable and yet acceptable risk.

Registry data indicate that CBS enhances survival in patients with three-vessel disease and normal ventricular function if angina is severe or evidence of moderate to severe ischemia is evident with stress testing.[48, 204, 207, 211, 212] The same holds for patients with three-vessel disease that includes proximal obstruction of the left anterior descending artery, regardless of whether it is symptomatic. In virtually all patients with two-vessel disease involving the proximal left anterior descending artery, surgery confers a survival advantage if angina is present or if ischemia can be documented by stress testing.[213] Of patients with coronary anatomy as described earlier, those with ventricular dysfunction continue to exhibit even greater improvement in survival with CBS. Major angiographic and clinical features that are now recognized as conferring a surgical survival advantage are summarized in Table 5–5; consensus CBS indications are delineated in an American College of Cardiology/American Heart Association Task Force Report.[214]

Other Factors Contributing to Outcome After CBS

In general, results in women may be slightly worse than those in men with regard to perioperative mortality and long-term survival,[215] probably because of smaller vessels and other factors related to body size. However, the differences are too small to constitute a barrier to the use of CBS in women.

TABLE 5–5. SELECTED ANGIOGRAPHIC AND CLINICAL FEATURES INDICATING IMPROVED SURVIVAL AFTER CORONARY BYPASS SURGERY

Left main stenosis
Three-vessel disease combined with
Proximal LAD stenosis
Reduced LV function
Severe and/or progressive symptoms
Severe ischemia with stress testing
Resting ST-T changes
Two-vessel disease (including proximal LAD stenosis) combined with any of above

Abbreviations: LAD, left anterior descending (coronary artery); LV, left ventricular.

The perioperative mortality rate is increased in elderly patients (in the CASS registry, 1.9% among patients <65 and 5.2% in those ≥65). Nevertheless, the relative survival advantage attributable to CBS may well be greater in the elderly, and properly selected older patients have an excellent functional result.[216] There is, of course, some age at which the relative survival benefit is lost because of limited life expectancy and high risk of surgery, but this age has not yet been defined. Therefore, as with depressed ventricular function, it is unwise to be dogmatic about age and recommendations for CBS. For patients with truly disabling, refractory angina who are not good candidates for PTCA and who do not have comorbid conditions such as pulmonary and renal insufficiency, diabetes, severe hypertension, and peripheral or cerebral vascular disease (all of which decrease short- and long-term survival and increase perioperative morbidity), there is no medical reason to withhold CBS on the basis of age alone, provided that the patient understands the age-related increased risk. If the indication for CBS is a survival advantage over medical management, the authors use an arbitrary age range of 75–80 as a cutoff, above which they generally do not recommend CBS. The presence to a significant extent of any of the comorbidities just described in an elderly patient has such a marked negative effect on perioperative morbidity and mortality that CBS should ordinarily be avoided.

Finally, mortality rates among patients requiring repeat CBS are two- to threefold higher,[48, 208, 209, 214] and clinical benefit is not as striking (see Chapters 4 and 46).

Selection of Patients for Bypass Surgery

The following recommendations are also incorporated in a treatment decision tree in the last section of this chapter. As with catheter-based revascularization, candidates for CBS with chronic stable angina generally represent two groups: patients with severe symptoms and those with milder symptoms in whom noninvasive testing indicates a relatively high risk with medical management alone. (Severe angina itself is predictive of a greater survival advantage with CBS if angiographic anatomy is appropriate.) All patients with left main coronary disease and three-vessel disease with abnormal ventricular function should be considered candidates for CBS, as should those with three-vessel disease and moderate to severe symptoms or moderate to severe ischemia detected during noninvasive stress testing. Patients with two- or three-vessel disease, including proximal stenosis of the left anterior descending artery, should be managed surgically regardless of symptoms and regardless of the presence or absence of stress-induced ischemia. Those with three-vessel disease, mild symptoms, no inducible ischemia, and no stenosis in the proximal left anterior descending artery have a good prognosis and are usually not ideal candidates for PTCA. The 1991 consensus report[214] concluded that in patients with stable angina and single-vessel disease with a severe proximal stenosis of a large left anterior descending coronary artery, CBS provided an advantage over medical management, regardless of severity of symptoms. However, this conclusion is not supported by results of the three randomized trials and is difficult to glean from registry data. Accordingly, although the authors believe that this is a sensible recommendation, this is a somewhat controversial area.

For patients in whom severity of symptoms is the indication for cardiac catheterization and in whom angiographic variables do not identify a surgical survival benefit, the choice of treatment (PTCA or surgery) depends largely on the details of coronary anatomy. All else being equal, the authors prefer PTCA because of the possibility of complete revascularization and/or substantial relief of symptoms without a surgical procedure, at a lower initial cost. For patients with single-vessel disease in whom symptoms are refractory to medical management, PTCA is ordinarily preferred, with the aforementioned possible exception of a severe, proximal lesion in a large left anterior descending coronary artery.

In patients with mild symptoms in whom stress testing indicates an extensive amount of jeopardized myocardium, a survival advantage is conferred by surgery if coronary anatomy is as described earlier. An interesting group of patients consists of those with high-risk features, as judged from noninvasive testing, in whom the angiographic findings do not, in fact, confirm a high risk. Included are patients with mild symptoms and two-vessel disease without proximal left anterior descending stenosis and those with single-vessel disease. Although the discrepancy is unusual, angiographic findings should take precedence with regard to whether CBS offers a survival advantage.

In some patients with chronic stable angina and severe ventricular dysfunction, the question of whether regions with abnormal contraction patterns are viable and may therefore improve after revascularization may arise in the course of decision making. (This is a somewhat more common problem among patients with acute ischemic syndromes, in whom the presence of stunned and/or "hibernating" myocardium is more prevalent.) As indicated earlier, modalities such as reinjection ^{201}Tl imaging, late ^{201}Tl injection reimaging after rest, dobutamine echocardiography, and PET scanning (if available) are useful adjuncts in these situations.

As stated earlier, CBS relieves symptoms in properly selected patients with chronic stable angina.[217] Most become angina free or exhibit only very mild symptoms for 5 years or more after surgery. Many remain angina free for 10–15 years. The use of internal thoracic and other arterial conduits has increased the duration of relief. The most common cause of lack of adequate relief of symptoms is distal stenosis or any other feature that compromises the extent of revascularization.

MANAGEMENT OF PATIENTS IN SPECIFIC CATEGORIES

Patients With Effort or Mixed Angina and Fixed Coronary Stenoses

This category includes patients with a history of effort or mixed angina who are judged to have fixed coronary stenoses on clinical grounds and/or on the basis of results of stress testing or cardiac catheterization. Their management entails initial pathophysiologic categorization, identification of any associated conditions that may exacerbate angina, and risk stratification. As discussed previously, routine exercise electrocardiography in conjunction with a noninvasive assessment of left ventricular function, if there is a reason to suspect an abnormality, is generally adequate for risk stratification. Myocardial stress or pharmacologic imaging (radionuclide or echocardiographic) is indicated when the exercise ECG is unreliable or ambiguous. These studies are also useful for assessing myocardium at risk when the hemodynamic significance of a lesion detected on coronary angiography is uncertain and for delineating viable myocardium in patients with global or regional ventricular dysfunction. However, in view of their additional cost, the incremental information provided by these studies, especially for patients at high risk, is insufficient to recommend their routine use in the average patient. A summary of indications and recommendations for imaging studies for patients with stable angina is provided in Table 5–6.

In general, the authors do not strongly favor radionuclide as opposed to echocardiographic imaging approaches for patients with stable angina. Cost, convenience, and local expertise should all be considered when more than one option is available. For purposes of risk stratification, the authors prefer exercise over pharmacologic stress because of the incremental information provided by exercise (see earlier discussion). For reasons cited earlier, they do not recommend routine ambulatory electrocardiographic monitoring in the initial assessment of this group of patients.

TABLE 5–6. MYOCARDIAL IMAGING STUDIES IN PATIENTS WITH STABLE ANGINA AND FIXED CORONARY STENOSES: INDICATIONS AND RECOMMENDATIONS

Risk Stratification (Before Catheterization)	
Suspicion of depressed ventricular function	
	Echocardiogram, radionuclide ventriculography
Exercise ECG unreliable or ambiguous (resting ST-T abnormalities, drugs, borderline responses)	
	Exercise ^{201}Tl, Sestamibi, or echocardiography
Inability to exercise	
	Persantine ^{201}Tl or Sestamibi
	Dobutamine echocardiography
Assessment of Myocardial Viability (Before or After Catheterization)	
Severe global ventricular dysfunction in patients who are possible CBS candidates (EF < ~.25)	
	Reinjection ^{201}Tl
	Late ^{201}Tl injection reimaging after resting
	Dobutamine echocardiography
	PET scanning (if available)
Regional dysfunction (to determine whether revascularization of a specific stenosis will result in return of function)	
	Same as for severe dysfunction
Assessment of Stenosis Significance (After Catheterization)	
Borderline angiographic stenoses, identification of culprit lesion in multivessel disease	
	Exercise or persantine ^{201}Tl/Sestamibi
	Exercise or dobutamine echocardiography

Abbreviations: ECG, electrocardiogram; ^{201}Tl, thallium-201; CBS, coronary bypass surgery; EF, ejection fraction; PET, positron emission tomography.

Role of Cardiac Catheterization

A fundamental decision is whether and when the need for cardiac catheterization and coronary angiography exists. Catheterization is indicated if symptoms cannot be managed adequately medically or if the patient may be in a high-risk category according to noninvasive assessment (Table 5–7). Severe symptoms (New York Heart Association or Canadian Cardiovascular Association class III or IV) per se are associated with high risk, as is progressive worsening of symptoms. Nonetheless, catheterization may be inappropriate or best deferred for extremely elderly patients and for patients with important comorbidities or associated untreated conditions that exacerbate angina.

For patients with mild symptoms, noninvasive high-risk criteria argue for cardiac catheterization, particularly when ventricular dysfunction (verified by echocardiography or radionuclide techniques) is present or stress testing results indicate a substantial amount of myocardium at risk. Q wave infarction noted on the ECG should prompt noninvasive assessment of left ventricular function because of the possibility of an extensive wall motion abnormality or diminished overall systolic function. Resting ST and T wave abnormalities are good predictors of survival benefit from CBS, as are stress imaging studies that demonstrate extensive myocardium at risk.

TABLE 5–7. INDICATIONS FOR CARDIAC CATHETERIZATION IN PATIENTS WITH STABLE ANGINA

Failure of medical management
Severe/progressive symptoms
Left ventricular dysfunction (verify noninvasively)
High-risk exercise electrocardiography and/or stress imaging
Special situations
Young age of patients
Family history of premature death
"Need to know" situations

Findings during exercise electrocardiography that indicate a poor prognosis and should prompt consideration of catheterization include a markedly abnormal ST segment response (>1.5- to 2-mm depression), abnormal blood pressure (lack of rise or decrease) or heart rate responses, appearance of angina and ST segment abnormalities at very low workloads, and ventricular arrhythmias. Less common indications for catheterization include very young age of patients, a strong family history of premature death, and "need to know" situations, such as occupations in which patients require the most definitive evaluation possible (pilots, truck drivers). The decision to manage a patient medically is based on either lack of an indication for cardiac catheterization or, conversely, results of catheterization that indicate that medical management is most appropriate.

Goals of Therapy

The objectives of treatment are relief of symptoms and, when coronary anatomy is appropriate, prolongation of survival. With regard to symptom relief, it is now possible, by medical management and/or revascularization, to achieve a quality of life in many if not most patients that is largely or completely unrestricted by angina with no more than minimal adverse effects of therapy. This level of therapeutic success is an appropriate and realistic goal and should dictate management decisions. Obviously, these expectations can and should be modified for certain patients, especially the elderly and those with major comorbidities. With regard to overall costs, there is no current evidence that setting such a goal is more expensive than a less ambitious approach.

Symptomatic therapy is best monitored with careful follow-up histories to establish levels of activity that are well tolerated. Regularly repeated exercise testing or ambulatory monitoring are generally not needed to assess treatment efficacy unless the response to therapy is ambiguous. However, repeated exercise testing may be useful in tracking the progression of disease and determining whether the patient's risk profile has changed. Because there is currently no evidence that treatment designed to suppress silent ischemia improves prognosis, specific treatment of silent ischemia alone is not justified.

Medical Management

General Measures. Patients with chronic stable angina should be encouraged to engage in regular physical activity but to discontinue such activities when symptoms develop. They should avoid unusually stressful, uncontrolled situations in which they could be called upon to exert themselves physically. All should receive low-dose aspirin (80–300 mg per day) unless a contraindication is present and should carry sublingual nitroglycerin (0.3–0.6 mg) or another rapid-acting nitrate preparation. The authors recommend that patients take sublingual nitroglycerin whenever they have angina unless symptoms disappear extremely rapidly with cessation of activity or if a patient has severe headache and/or other side effects with administration of rapid-acting nitrates. Nitroglycerin should always be employed for symptoms that occur at rest, even as part of a stable pattern, and for symptoms that are unusual, such as with a provocation that usually does not cause angina. If a first nitroglycerin tablet fails to provide relief, one or two more may be taken at 5- to 10-min intervals. The patient should be advised to seek emergency care if symptoms persist after three nitroglycerin tablets spaced 5 min apart or recur soon thereafter.

Risk factor modification is essential. Smoking cessation, control of hypertension and diabetes, weight loss, and, most important, treatment of hyperlipidemia may modify progression of the underlying atherosclerotic process. However, it has not been rigorously shown that comprehensive strategies aimed at regression of atherosclerosis that include extensive lifestyle modification and stress management offer significant additional benefits beyond those attributable to lipid lowering per se.[82]

Pharmacologic Therapy. The following approach is outlined in Fig. 5–10 with the use of a decision tree algorithm. For patients with fixed stenoses and exclusively or predominantly effort angina, the cornerstone of treatment is a beta-adrenergic blocking agent. In the authors' view, a second drug is useful in most patients. Certain potentially deleterious effects of beta-adrenergic blockers, especially increases in wall stress and unopposed alpha-adrenergic vasoconstriction, can be offset by the use of either a long-acting nitrate or calcium channel blocker. Moreover, improved efficacy has been demonstrated when either a long-acting nitrate or a calcium channel blocker is added to a beta-adrenergic blocker.[218–224] In general, a long-acting nitrate is adequate and can be administered in such a way that additional antianginal protection is provided during the times of day when angina is most likely to occur. Calcium channel blockers may be equally effective.[218, 220, 224] However, in some studies, calcium channel blockers in combination with a beta-adrenergic blocker have resulted in increased side effects without improved efficacy.[225–227] Because of the potential for adverse conduction system effects, verapamil should not be combined with a beta-adrenergic blocker. In contrast, dihydropyridines should usually be administered to these patients in conjunction with a beta-adrenergic blocker.

For patients in whom two-drug therapy is inadequate and who are not candidates for revascularization procedures, a third drug of a different class should be added. However, additional benefit may be modest, and deleterious effects may occur.[228]

For some patients with fixed stenoses, a beta-adrenergic blocker may not necessarily be the drug of choice for prophylaxis of angina. Included among such patients are those with frequent rest angina, in whom a calcium channel blocker (diltiazem or verapamil) as primary therapy may be more advisable. For many elderly patients, use of a single drug—a beta-adrenergic blocker, a non-dihydropyridine calcium channel blocker, or a long-acting nitrate—is prudent for minimizing side effects. In the authors' experience, long-acting nitrates alone are often an excellent choice for elderly patients. For patients with effort angina who cannot take beta-adrenergic blockers because of adverse effects or contraindications, verapamil and diltiazem are alternatives that provide the advantages of a calcium channel blocker and effects on the double product at submaximal workloads comparable with those of beta-adrenergic blockers.

These drugs must be used in effective doses. This may occasionally require increases in doses until side effects first occur. In occasional patients who are difficult to manage medically and who are not candidates for revascularization procedures, a spinal cord stimulator[229] may be helpful by reducing myocardial oxygen demands and increasing the angina threshold through mechanisms that are not well understood. Such patients should also be considered for treatment with one of the miscellaneous antianginal drugs mentioned earlier. Unfortunately, the only ones that are readily available in the United States at present are bepridil and theophylline and related compounds.

Revascularization Procedures. Patients with mild symptoms who undergo catheterization because noninvasive evaluation suggests high risk may have disease that is, in fact, angiographically mild. Medical management is then indicated. PTCA should not be performed simply because a stenosis is present unless its functional significance is clearly demonstrable and its severity marked. Patients with distal disease are poor candidates for revascularization and are often best managed medically. Much more typically, however, the choice following catheterization is between catheter-based revascularization and CBS. The relative cost effectiveness of different treatment strategies is presently controversial. As discussed earlier, CBS is associated with higher initial costs. However, because of restenosis and initially less complete revascularization, the cost of PTCA increases in relation to the cost of surgery over time.

A decision tree incorporating clinical features and keyed to results

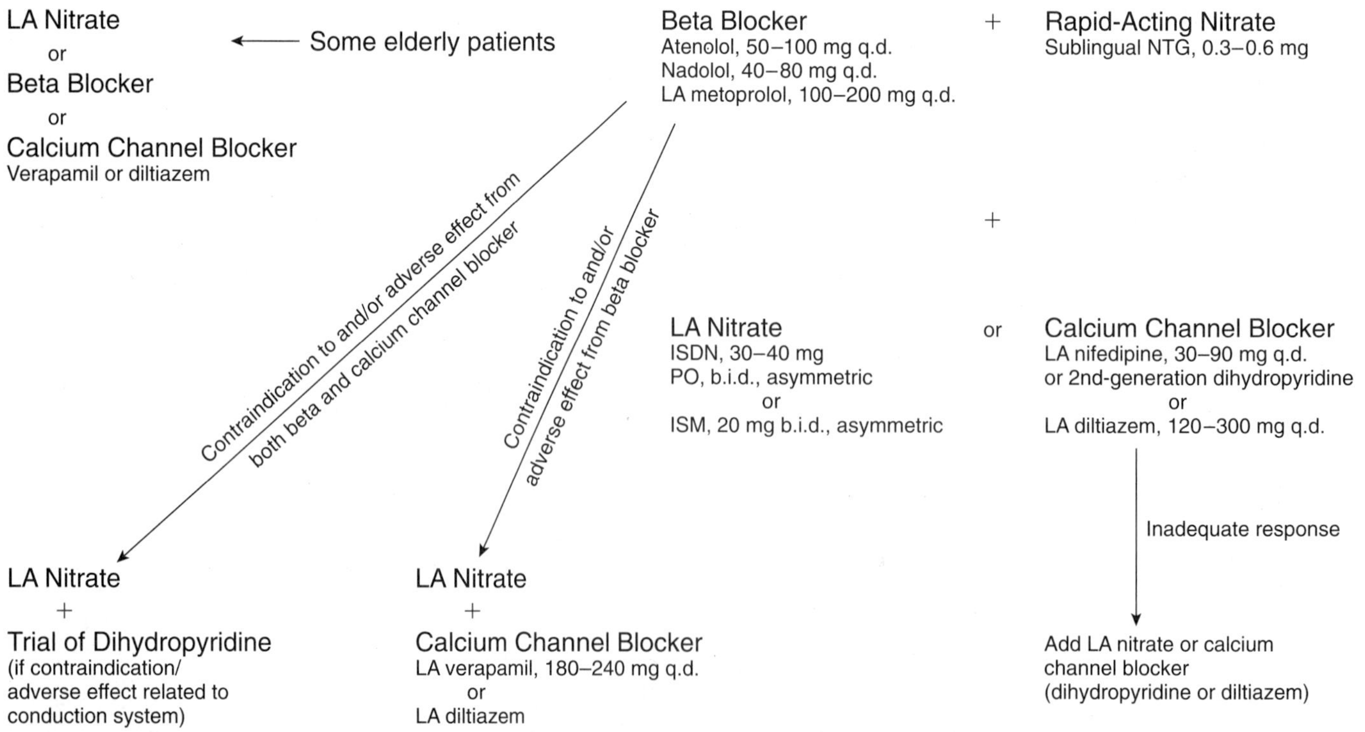

Figure 5–10. Decision tree algorithm for pharmacologic management of stable angina resulting from fixed coronary stenoses. Rapid-acting and long-acting nitrates and beta blockers other than those named may be used with comparable efficacy. Doses represent typical ranges. *Abbreviations:* LA, long-acting; NTG, nitroglycerin; ISDN, isosorbide dinitrate; ISM, isosorbide mononitrate.

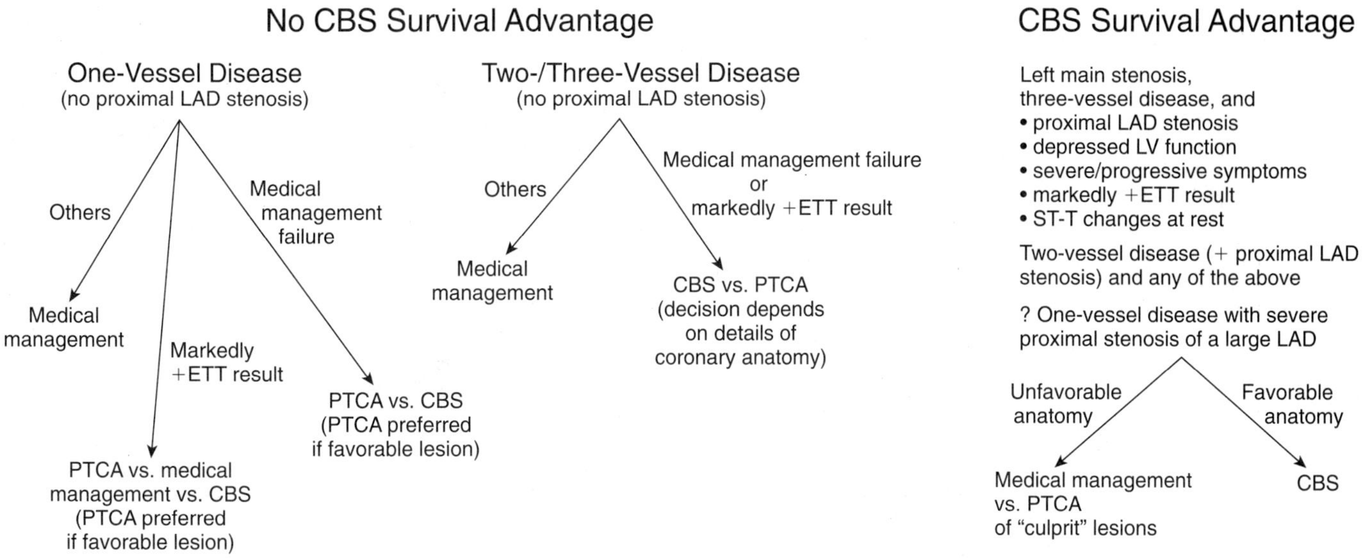

Figure 5–11. Decision tree algorithm for recommendations after cardiac catheterization. *Abbreviations:* CBS, coronary bypass surgery; LAD, left anterior descending coronary artery; ETT, exercise or other stress test; PTCA, percutaneous transluminal coronary angioplasty.

at catheterization is presented in Fig. 5–11. When a survival benefit of CBS in comparison with medical management is present, CBS is favored unless the anatomy is clearly unfavorable for revascularization, in which case medical management and PTCA of specific culprit lesions are the remaining options. Because long-term data demonstrating a survival benefit for PTCA in comparison with medical management are not yet available, PTCA should not be substituted for CBS unless patient preference dictates it or comorbidities reduce potential advantages of surgery. On the sole basis of angiographic findings, all patients with left main coronary disease, three-vessel disease with depressed ventricular function, three-vessel disease with involvement of the proximal left anterior descending artery (regardless of ventricular function), and two-vessel disease involving the proximal left anterior descending artery (also regardless of ventricular function) are candidates for CBS. As indicated earlier, there may be a CBS survival advantage in patients with severe proximal stenosis of a large left anterior descending coronary artery.[168, 214] The authors view this as an uncertain situation, in which recommendations must be highly individualized. In general, the authors certainly favor revascularization in such patients, but the choice between CBS and PTCA is a difficult one. Relatively young patients may perhaps be best managed with PTCA, whereas older patients may benefit from the relative certainty of long-term patency of an internal mammary graft.

Patients with three-vessel disease without involvement of the proximal left anterior descending artery and normal ventricular function are candidates for surgery or PTCA if poorly controlled symptoms are present or a stress test result is strongly positive. When such patients have mild symptoms and no indication of severe inducible ischemia, they may ordinarily be managed medically. For patients with two-vessel disease in whom the proximal left anterior descending artery is not involved, PTCA or medical management is usually the preferred approach, depending on the level of symptoms and/or severity of inducible ischemia.

With the exception of severe proximal left anterior descending lesions (described earlier), the choice for patients with single-vessel disease is usually between medical management and PTCA, except in the case of lesions that are not amenable to PTCA in patients who cannot be managed medically. For patients with mild symptoms, medical management is usually indicated.

Additional factors that must be considered in decision making are the technical feasibility and likelihood of success of PTCA and CBS in a given case. Except in cases of distal coronary disease or when bypassable vessels clearly supply areas of scar tissue, CBS predictably and consistently improves nutritive flow. In contrast, PTCA is more problematic. Thus although PTCA or medical management is preferred for many patients with two-vessel disease and for most with single-vessel disease, CBS is entirely appropriate when symptoms are refractory to medical management and PTCA is considered to be a less-than-optimal procedure from a technical standpoint.

It is not unusual to employ more sophisticated (and expensive) stress-imaging studies to assist in decision making after cardiac catheterization (see Table 5–6) in order to guide revascularization procedures, especially PTCA. These are indicated when there is uncertainty as to the hemodynamic significance of a stenosis detected angiographically (radionuclide perfusion or echocardiography), delineation of viable myocardium when there is either globally or regionally depressed wall motion (reinjection ^{201}Tl, late ^{201}Tl injection reimaging after resting, PET, and dobutamine echocardiography), and identification of culprit lesions in patients with multivessel disease who are candidates for catheter-based revascularization (radionuclide perfusion or echocardiography).

Patients who have undergone revascularization procedures for stable angina (either CBS or PTCA) are always at risk for recurrent angina. In the case of restenosis after initial PTCA, repeat PTCA is often required. Decision making becomes more difficult when a second or third restenosis supervenes, at which time CBS may be the best option. Ordinarily, patients with recurrent symptoms late after PTCA or CBS should be risk-stratified and evaluated angiographically if their symptoms are severe or if they are at high risk. In these patients, myocardial perfusion imaging is especially useful for risk stratification because of the possibility of complex coronary flow patterns. If repeat CBS is ultimately undertaken, risk is higher and potential benefit somewhat lower than with an initial procedure (see Chapter 4).[46] Nonsurgical revascularization is often preferable, if technically feasible, especially if there is a clearly discernible new culprit lesion in a native vessel or in the distal portion of a graft (see Chapter 3).

Patients With Variant Angina

The common denominators in these patients are an exclusive or predominant pattern of angina unrelated to increases in myocardial oxygen demand and the presence of documented coronary spasm reflected by transient ST segment elevation either with attacks or at the time of cardiac catheterization. Cardiac catheterization is indicated in virtually all such patients to determine whether significant, fixed coronary stenoses are present, as well as to demonstrate provokable spasm. Management of patients without fixed stenoses or only mild luminal irregularities at catheterization (a common finding) should include calcium channel blockers as the mainstay of prophylaxis. In contrast to nitrates, these agents provide round-the-clock therapeutic effects. Of the calcium channel blockers, the dihydropyridines (long-acting nifedipine, 30–90 mg per day, or a second-generation agent) are the most powerful coronary vasodilators and exert minimal effects on the conduction system in vivo. Individual attacks can be treated with sublingual nitroglycerin (0.3–0.6 mg) or sublingual nifedipine (10 mg).

For prophylaxis, addition of long-acting nitrates or the concurrent use of two classes of calcium antagonists may sometimes be required. In occasional patients with variant angina and significant fixed coronary stenoses, addition of a beta-adrenergic blocker is helpful if a component of effort angina is present as well. In such patients, it may be useful to undergo exercise testing to document that effort angina (i.e., demand ischemia) is present, as opposed to the occasional finding of effort-induced coronary vasospasm with ST segment elevation. Low-dose aspirin (80–300 mg per day) is appropriate because of the risk of thrombosis implicitly associated with the endothelial dysfunction thought to be present in these patients.

Revascularization has no demonstrated role for patients with pure, vasospastic angina who do not have significant (>50%) fixed coronary obstructions. For patients with vasospastic angina, ambulatory monitoring is useful in assessing therapy if episodes of silent ischemia are present at baseline.

Patients With Angina Attributable to Coexisting Cardiac Disorders

The most common setting in which this occurs is aortic valve disease, usually aortic stenosis. The appearance of angina is ordinarily considered to be an indication for aortic valve replacement. Thus in the majority of cases, medical management of angina is only a short-term consideration. Medical management is difficult because of the substantial risk of adverse effects of antianginal drugs. For patients without coexisting fixed coronary artery stenoses, beta-adrenergic blocking drugs are generally contraindicated because of potential depression of cardiac function and increases in wall stress related to increased diastolic volume. Calcium channel blockers are also problematic because they can decrease coronary perfusion pressure, thereby exacerbating angina. Those that depress myocardial performance can elicit adverse effects similar to those of beta-adrenergic blockers. Nitrates are useful, despite their risks, because of their beneficial effects on the distribution of myocardial blood flow and the fact that in usual doses they do not decrease and may even increase coronary perfusion pressure. However, nitrates can cause profound decreases in cardiac output by reducing preload coupled with physiologically inappropriate intraventricular baroreceptor activation.[230]

For patients awaiting valve replacement, the most reasonable treatment for angina is, therefore, often simply restriction of physical activities. In patients with aortic stenosis who do have coexisting fixed coronary stenoses, the same potential problems with the use of antianginal drugs exist. However, it is reasonable to be more liberal in using such drugs, especially if restriction of activities is insufficient to prevent symptoms. The authors again recommend long-acting nitrates as a first choice, with cautious use of a beta-adrenergic blocker as a second choice. In this situation, a drug with significant ISA (e.g., pindolol, 5–20 mg twice per day) should be considered. Results of aortic valvuloplasty for relief of symptoms of aortic stenosis have been disappointing. However, in rare patients with aortic stenosis and angina who are not candidates for valve replacement, it may be palliative.

For patients with hypertrophic cardiomyopathy as the cause of angina, treatment is of the underlying cardiomyopathy (see Chapter 13 of this volume and Chapter 41 of *Heart Disease,* 5th Edition). Current medical management centers on the use of verapamil (180–360 mg per day), although beta-adrenergic blockers are also effective. In patients with refractory symptoms, atrioventricular sequential pacing has largely supplanted septal myotomy as an alternative to medical management,[231] although the long-term relative efficacy of pacing and myotomy has not been delineated.

Chest pain syndromes in patients with mitral valve prolapse do not necessarily reflect myocardial ischemia and do not constitute a risk factor for morbid events. Accordingly, treatment is not essential unless symptoms are severe or disabling. Beta-adrenergic blockers may be helpful.[232] Responses to nitrates or calcium channel blockers are variable and unpredictable.

In rare patients with angina attributable to pulmonary hypertension, a trial of nitrates is reasonable because of their venodilator properties and reduction of right ventricular oxygen demands. However, reliable data regarding efficacy are not available. When angina is caused by tachyarrhythmia, the treatment, of course, is of the underlying rhythm disturbance.

Patients With "Microvascular" Angina

Patients without significant coronary stenosis demonstrable on angiograms or without vasospasm of epicardial coronary arteries are a heterogeneous group, regardless of whether objective criteria of ischemia are present. Treatment is entirely empirical. Calcium channel blockers are sometimes effective.[156] Other antianginals may certainly be employed, but efficacy is uncertain. Some patients respond to imipramine (50 mg once per day), which is thought to block visceral pain impulses.[233] The value of aspirin has not been established.

Patients With Concomitant Conditions That Influence Management

Patients with poorly controlled heart failure should be treated conventionally with vasodilators, diuretics, and digitalis, as outlined in Chapters 8, 9, and 11. At present, calcium channel blockers should probably be avoided unless required for relief of angina. Treatment with beta-adrenergic blockers must be carefully individualized but need not necessarily be discontinued. The cautious use of beta-adrenergic blocking drugs is indicated for patients with angina pectoris in association with hyperthyroidism and other conditions with increased adrenergic stimulation such as anemia, volume depletion or blood loss, and infection. In these circumstances, relatively rapid-acting, short half-life drugs are often appropriate, at least as initial therapy, in order to quickly assess therapeutic effects (e.g., decreases in heart rate) and promptly manipulate dosing. Thus propranolol at an initial dose of 30–40 mg every 6 h is a reasonable choice, with subsequent increases in dose as necessary. The guiding precepts are individualization of management, careful monitoring for adverse effects, and aggressive treatment of the coexistent problem.

REFERENCES

1. Braunwald E: Unstable angina: a classification. Circulation 1989; 80:410.
2. Fuster V, Badimon L, Badimon JJ, et al: The pathogenesis of coronary artery disease and the acute coronary syndromes. N Engl J Med 1992; 326:242.
3. Selwyn AP, Yeung AC, Ryan TJ Jr, et al: Pathophysiology of ischemia in patients with coronary artery disease. Progr Cardiovasc Dis 1992; 35:27.
4. Davies RF, Linden W, Habibi H, et al: Relative importance of psy-

chologic traits and severity of ischemia in causing angina during treadmill exercise. J Am Coll Cardiol 1993; 21:331.
5. Marchant B, Donaldson G, Mridha K, et al: Mechanisms of cold intolerance in patients with angina. J Am Coll Cardiol 1994; 23:630.
6. Colles P, Juneau M, Grégoire J: Effect of a standardized meal on the threshold of exercise-induced myocardial ischemia in patients with stable angina. J Am Coll Cardiol 1993; 21:1052.
7. Deanfield JE, Selwyn AP, Chierchia S, et al: Myocardial ischemia during daily life in patients with stable angina: its relation to symptoms and heart rate changes. Lancet 1983; 2:753.
8. Chierchia S, Smith G, Morgan M, et al: Role of heart rate in pathophysiology of chronic stable angina. Lancet 1984; 2:1353.
9. Rocco MB, Barry J, Campbell S, et al: Circadian variation of transient myocardial ischemia in patients with coronary artery disease. Circulation 1987; 75:395.
10. Cook DG, Shaper AG: Breathlessness, angina pectoris and coronary artery disease. Am J Cardiol 1989; 63:921.
11. Prinzmetal M, Kennamer R, Merliss R, et al: Angina pectoris: I. A variant form of angina pectoris. Am J Med 1959; 27:375.
12. Oliva PB, Potts DE, Pluss RG: Coronary arterial spasm in Prinzmetal angina: documentation by coronary arteriography. N Engl J Med 1973; 288:745.
13. Okumura K, Yasu H, Matsuyama K, et al: A study on coronary hemodynamics during acetylcholine-induced coronary spasm in patients with variant angina: endothelium-dependent dilation in the resistance vessels. J Am Coll Cardiol 1992; 19:1426.
14. Vita JA, Treasure CB, Yeung AC, et al: Patients with evidence of coronary endothelial dysfunction as assessed by acetylcholine infusion demonstrate marked increases in sensitivity to constrictor effects of catecholamines. Circulation 1992; 85:1390.
15. McFadden EP, Clarke JG, Davies GJ, et al: Effect of intracoronary serotonin on coronary vessels in patients with stable angina and patients with variant angina. N Engl J Med 1991; 324:648.
16. Schroeder JS, Bolen JL, Quint RA, et al: Provocation of coronary spasm with ergonovine maleate: new test with results in 57 patients undergoing coronary angiography. Am J Cardiol 1977; 40:487.
17. Lange RA, Cigarroa RG, Yancy CW, et al: Cocaine-induced coronary artery vasoconstriction. N Engl J Med 1989; 321:1557.
18. Smith HWB III, Liberman HA, Brody SL, et al: Acute myocardial infarction temporally related to cocaine use. Ann Int Med 1987; 107:13.
19. Myagi H, Yasu H, Okumura K, et al: Effect of magnesium on anginal attack induced by hyperventilation in patients with variant angina. Circulation 1989; 79:597.
20. Prentali M, Ardissino D, Barberis P, et al: Hyperventilation and ergonovine tests in Prinzmetal's variant angina pectoris in men. Am J Cardiol 1989; 63:17.
21. Maseri A, Chierchia S, Kaski JC: Mixed angina pectoris. Am J Cardiol 1985; 56:30E.
22. Deedwania PC, Carbajal EV: Prevalence and patterns of silent myocardial ischemia during daily life in stable angina patients receiving conventional antianginal drug therapy. Am J Cardiol 1990; 65:1090.
23. Borzak S, Fenton T, Glasser SP, et al: Discordance between effects of anti-ischemic therapy on ambulatory ischemia, exercise performance and anginal symptoms in patients with stable angina pectoris. J Am Coll Cardiol 1993; 21:1605.
24. Hecht HS, Debord L, Sotomayor N, et al: Truly silent ischemia and the relationship of chest pain and ST segment changes to the amount of ischemic myocardium: evaluation by supine bicycle stress echocardiography. J Am Coll Cardiol 1994; 23:369.
25. Deanfield JE, Shea MJ, Wilson RA, et al : Direct effects of smoking on the heart: silent ischemic disturbances of coronary flow. Am J Cardiol 1986; 57:1005.
26. Langer A, Freeman MR, Josse RG, et al: Detection of silent myocardial ischemia in diabetes mellitus. Am J Cardiol 1991; 67:1073.
27. Falcone C, Sconocchia R, Guasti L, et al: Dental pain threshold and angina pectoris in patients with coronary artery disease. J Am Coll Cardiol 1988; 12:348.
28. Cannon RO, Schenke WH, Mann BJ, et al: Differences in coronary flow and myocardial metabolism at rest and during pacing between patients with obstructive and patients with nonobstructive cardiomyopathy. J Am Coll Cardiol 1987; 10:53.
29. LeWinter MM, Hoffman JR, Shell WE, et al: Phenyleprine-induced atypical chest pain in patients with prolapsing mitral valve leaflets. Am J Cardiol 1974; 34:12.
30. Maseri A, Crea F, Kaski JC: Mechanisms of angina pectoris in Syndrome X. J Am Coll Cardiol 1991; 17:499.
31. Cannon RO III, Camici P, Epstein SE: Pathophysiological dilemma of Syndrome X. Circulation 1992; 85:883.
32. Fuh MM-T, Jeng C-Y, Young MM-S, et al: Insulin resistance, glucose intolerance, and hyperinsulinemia in patients with microvascular angina. Metabolism 1993; 42:1090.
33. Cannon RO III: Angina pectoris with normal coronary angiograms. Cardiol Clinics 1991; 9:157.
34. Quyyumi AA, Cannon RO III, Panza JA, et al: Endothelial dysfunction in patients with chest pain and normal coronary arteries. Circulation 1992; 86:1864.
35. Bugiardini R, Pozzati A, Ottani F, et al: Vasotonic angina: a spectrum of ischemic syndromes involving functional abnormalities of the epicardial and microvascular coronary circulation. J Am Coll Cardiol 1993; 22:417.
36. Opherk D, Schuler G, Wetterauer K, et al: Four-year follow-up study in patients with angina pectoris and normal coronary arteriograms ("Syndrome X"). Circulation 1989; 80:1610.
37. Cannon RO, III, Quyyumi AA, Schenke WH, et al: Abnormal cardiac sensitivity in patients with chest pain and normal coronary arteries. J Am Coll Cardiol 1990; 16:1359.
38. Winniford MD, Jansen DE, Reynolds GA, et al: Cigarette smoking–induced coronary vasoconstriction in atherosclerotic coronary artery disease and prevention by calcium antagonists and nitroglycerin. Am J Cardiol 1987; 59:203.
39. Mock MB, Ringqvist I, Fisher LD, et al: Survival of medically treated patients in the coronary artery surgery study (CASS) registry. Circulation 1982; 66:562.
40. Murabito JM, Evans JC, Larson MG, et al: Prognosis after the onset of coronary heart disease. Circulation 1993; 88:2548.
41. Conley MJ, Ely RL, Kisslo J, et al: The prognostic spectrum of left main stenosis. Circulation 1978; 57:947.
42. Weiner DA, Ryan TJ, McCabe CH, et al: Prognostic importance of a clinical profile and exercise test in medically treated patients with coronary artery disease. J Am Coll Cardiol 1984; 3:772.
43. Bogaty P, Brecker SJ, White SE, et al: Comparison of coronary angiographic findings in acute and chronic first presentation of ischemic heart disease. Circulation 1993; 87:1938.
44. Lichtlen PR, Nikutta P, Jost S, et al: Anatomical progression of coronary artery disease in humans as seen by prospective, repeated, quantitated coronary angiography. Circulation 1992; 86:828.
45. Wang XL, Tam C, McCredie RM, et al: Determinants of severity of coronary artery disease in Australian men and women. Circulation 1994; 89:1974.
46. Mizuno K, Satomura K, Miyamoto A, et al: Angioscopic evaluation of coronary artery thrombi in acute coronary syndromes. N Engl J Med 1992; 326:287.
47. European Coronary Surgery Study Group: Long-term results of prospective randomized study of coronary artery bypass surgery in stable angina pectoris. Lancet 1982; 2:1173.
48. Califf RM, Harrell FE Jr, Lee KL, et al: The evolution of medical and surgical therapy for coronary artery disease. JAMA 1989; 261:2077.
49. Califf RM, Mark DB, Harrell FE Jr, et al: Importance of clinical measures of ischemia in the prognosis of patients with documented coronary artery disease. J Am Coll Cardiol 1988; 11:20.
50. Bogaty P, Dagenais GR, Cantin B, et al: Prognosis in patients with a strongly positive exercise electrocardiogram. Am J Cardiol 1989; 64:1284.
51. Wilson RF, Marcus ML, Christensen BV, et al: Accuracy of exercise electrocardiography in detecting physiologically significant coronary arterial lesions. Circulation 1991; 83:412.
52. Pepine CJ: Is silent ischemia a treatable risk factor in patients with angina pectoris? Circulation 1990; 82(suppl II):135.
53. Mulcahy D, Parameshwar J, Holdright D, et al: Value of ambulatory ST segment monitoring in patients with chronic stable angina: does measurement of the "total ischaemic burden" assist with management. Br Heart J 1992; 67:47.
54. Ghandhi MM, Wood DA, Lampe FC: Characteristics and clinical significance of ambulatory myocardial ischemia in men and women in the general population presenting with angina pectoris. J Am Coll Cardiol 1994; 23:74.
55. The Veterans Administration Coronary Artery Bypass Surgery Cooperative Study Group: Eleven-year survival in the Veterans Administration Randomized Trial of Coronary Bypass Surgery for Stable Angina. N Engl J Med 1984; 311:1333.
56. Detrano R, Froelicher VF: Exercise testing: uses and limitations considering recent studies. Progr Cardiovas Dis 1988; 31:173.

57. Iskandrian AS, Heo J, Kong B, et al: Use of technetium-99m isonitrile (RP-30A) in assessing left ventricular perfusion and function at rest and during exercise in coronary artery disease and comparison with coronary arteriography and exercise thallium-201 SPECT imaging. Am J Cardiol 1989; 64:270.
58. Brown KA: Prognostic value of thallium-201 myocardial perfusion imaging: a diagnostic tool comes of age. Circulation 1991; 83:363.
59. Hollenberg M, Budge R, Wisneski JA, et al: Treadmill score quantifies electrocardiographic response to exercise and improves test accuracy and reproducibility. Circulation 1980; 61:276.
60. Dubach P, Froelicker VF, Klein J, et al: Exercise-induced hypotension in a male population. Circulation 1988; 78:1380.
61. Hoshimoto M, Okamoto M, Yamagata T, et al: Abnormal systolic blood pressure response during exercise recovery in patients with angina pectoris. J Am Coll Cardiol 1994; 22:659.
62. Wiens RD, Lafia P, Marder CM: Chronotropic incompetence in clinical exercise testing. Am J Cardiol 1984; 54:74.
63. McHenry PL, Morris SN, Kavalier M, et al: Comparative study of exercise-induced ventricular arrhythmias in normal subjects and patients with documented coronary artery disease. Am J Cardiol 1976; 37:609.
64. Williams MA, Esterbrooks DJ, Nair CK, et al: Clinical significance of exercise-induced bundle branch block. Am J Cardiol 1988; 61:346.
65. Hendel RC, Layden JJ, Leppo JA: Prognostic value of dipyridamole thallium scintigraphy for evaluation of ischemic heart disease. J Am Coll Cardiol 1990; 15:109.
66. Quiñones MA: Technical considerations in exercise echocardiography: preference of exercise methodology, imaging approach, and comparison with radionuclide techniques. Coronary Art Dis 1991; 2:536.
67. Iskandrian AS, Chae SC, Heo J, et al: Independent and incremental prognostic value of exercise single-photon emission computed tomographic (SPECT) thallium imaging in coronary artery disease. J Am Coll Cardiol 1993; 22:665.
68. Marwick T, D'Hondt A-M, Baudhuin T, et al: Optimal use of dobutamine stress for the detection and evaluation of coronary artery disease: combination with echocardiography or scintigraphy, or both? J Am Coll Cardiol 1993; 22:159.
69. Stratmann HG, Williams GA, Wittry MD, et al: Exercise technetium-99m Sestamibi tomography for cardiac risk stratification of patients with stable chest pain. Circulation 1994; 89:615.
70. Bonow RO, Dilsizian V, Cuocolo A, Bacharach SL: Identification of viable myocardium in patients with chronic coronary artery disease and left ventricular dysfunction. Comparison of thallium scintigraphy with reinjection and PET imaging with 18F-fluorodeoxyglucose. Circulation 1991; 83:26.
71. Udelson JE, Coleman PS, Metherall J, et al: Predicting recovery of severe regional ventricular dysfunction. Circulation 1994; 89:2552.
72. Weiss AT, Berman DS, Lew AS, et al: Transient ischemic dilation of the left ventricle on stress thallium-201 scintigraphy: a marker of severe and extensive coronary artery disease. J Am Coll Cardiol 1987; 9:752.
73. Gill JB, Ruddy TD, Newell JB, et al: Prognostic importance of thallium uptake by the lungs during exercise in coronary artery disease. N Engl J Med 1987; 317:1485.
74. Iskandrian AS, Hakki A-H, Goel IP, et al: The use of rest and exercise radionuclide ventriculography in risk stratification in patients with suspected coronary artery disease. Am Heart J 1985; 110:864.
75. Lee KL, Pryor DB, Pieper KS, et al: Prognostic value of radionuclide angiography in medically treated patients with coronary artery disease. Circulation 1990; 82:1705.
76. Eitzman D, Al-Aouar Z, Kanter HL, et al: Clinical outcome of patients with advanced coronary artery disease after viability studies with positron emission tomography. J Am Coll Cardiol 1992; 20:559.
77. Chambers CE, Brown KA: Dipyridamole-induced ST segment depression during thallium-201 imaging in patients with coronary artery disease. Angiographic and hemodynamic determinants. J Am Coll Cardiol 1988; 12:37.
78. Holme I: An analysis of randomized trials evaluating the effect of cholesterol reduction on total mortality and coronary heart disease incidence. Circulation 1990; 82:1916.
79. Vos J, deFeyter PJ, Simoons ML, et al: Retardation and arrest of progression or regression of coronary artery disease: a review. Progr Cardiovasc Dis 1993; 35:435.
80. Scandinavian Simvastatin Survival Study Group: Randomized trial of cholesterol lowering in 4444 patients with coronary heart disease: the Scandinavian Simvastatin Survival Study. Lancet 1994; 344:1383.
81. Grundy SM, Bilheimer D, Chait A, et al: 2nd Report of the Expert Panel on Detection, Evaluation and Treatment of High Blood Cholesterol in Adults (Adult Treatment Panel II). Bethesda, MD: National Cholesterol Education Program, National Institutes of Health, 1993.
82. Hamsten A, Wiman A, deFaire U, et al: Increased plasma levels of a rapid inhibitor of tissue plasminogen activator in young survivors of myocardial infarction. N Engl J Med 1985; 313:1557.
83. Ridker PM, Manson JE, Gaziano M, et al: Low-dose aspirin therapy for chronic stable angina: a randomized, placebo-controlled clinical trial. Ann Intern Med 1991; 114:835.
84. Ades PA, Waldmann ML, Poehlman EP, et al: Exercise conditioning in older coronary patients: submaximal lactate response and endurance capacity. Circulation 1993; 88:572.
85. Abrams J: Nitrates. Med Clin North Am 1988; 72:1.
86. Cohn JN: Pharmacologic mechanisms of nitrates in myocardial ischemia. Am J Cardiol 1992; 70:38G.
87. Parker JO: Nitrates and angina pectoris. Am J Cardiol 1993; 72:3C.
88. Brown BG, Bolson E, Petersen RB, et al: The mechanisms of nitroglycerin action: stenosis vasodilatation as a major c component of the drug response. Circulation 1981; 64:1089.
89. Sudhir K, MacGregor JS, Barbant SD, et al: Assessment of coronary conductance and resistance vessel reactivity in response to nitroglycerin, ergonovine and adenosine: in vivo studies with simultaneous intravascular two-dimensional and Doppler ultrasound. J Am Coll Cardiol 1993; 21:1261.
90. Cohn PF, Maddox D, Holman BL, et al: Effect of sublingually administered nitroglycerin on regional myocardial blood flow in patients with coronary artery disease. Am J Cardiol 1977; 39:672.
91. Ohno A, Fujita M, Miwa K, et al: Importance of coronary collateral circulation for increased treadmill exercise capacity by nitrates in patients with stable effort angina pectoris. Cardiology 1991; 78:323.
92. Ganz W, Marcus HS: Failure of intracoronary nitroglycerin to alleviate pacing-induced angina. Circulation 1972; 46:880.
93. Fung H-L: Clinical pharmacology of organic nitrates. Am J Cardiol 1993; 72:9C.
94. Parker JO, VanKoughnett KA, Farrell B: Nitroglycerin lingual spray: clinical efficacy and dose-response relation. Am J Cardiol 1986; 57:1.
95. Parker JO, VanKoughnett KA, Farrell B: Comparison of buccal nitroglycerin and oral isosorbide dinitrate for nitrate tolerance in stable angina pectoris. Am J Cardiol 1985; 56:724.
96. Parker JO, Farrell B, Lahey KA, et al: Effect of intervals between doses on the development of tolerance to isosorbide dinitrate. N Engl J Med 1987; 316:1440.
97. Reichek N, Goldstein RE, Redwood DR, et al: Sustained effects of nitroglycerin ointment in patients with angina pectoris. Circulation 1974; 50:348.
98. DeMots H, Glasser SP: Intermittent transdermal nitroglycerin therapy in the treatment of chronic stable angina. J Am Coll Cardiol 1989; 13:786.
99. Rossetti E, Luca C, Bonetti F, et al: Transdermal nitroglycerin reduces the frequency of anginal attacks but fails to prevent silent ischemia. J Am Coll Cardiol 1993; 21:337.
100. Abshagen UWP: Pharmacokinetics of isosorbide mononitrate. Am J Cardiol 1992; 70:61G.
101. Thadani U, deVane PJ: Efficacy of isosorbide mononitrate in angina pectoris. Am J Cardiol 1992; 70:676.
102. Bassan MM: The daylong pattern of the antianginal effect of long-term three times daily administered isosorbide dinitrate. J Am Coll Cardiol 1990; 16:936.
103. Frishman WH: Tolerance, rebound, and time-zero effect of nitrate therapy. Am J Cardiol 1992; 70:43G.
104. Packer M: What causes tolerance to nitroglycerin? The 100-year-old mystery continues. J Am Coll Cardiol 1990; 16:932.
105. Elkayam U, Mehra A, Shotan A, et al: Possible mechanisms of nitrate tolerance. Am J Cardiol 1992; 70:496.
106. Watanabe H, Kakihana M, Ohtsuka S, et al: Platelet cyclic GMP: a potentially useful indicator to evaluate the effects of nitroglycerin and nitrate tolerance. Circulation 1993; 88:29.
107. May DC, Popma JJ, Black WH, et al: In vivo induction and reversal of nitroglycerin tolerance in human coronary arteries. N Engl J Med 1987; 317:805.
108. Levy WS, Katz RJ, Wasserman AG: Methionine restores the venodilative response to nitroglycerin after the development of tolerance. J Am Coll Cardiol 1991; 17:474.
109. Boesgaard S, Aldershvile J, Poulsen HE: Preventive administration of intravenous N-acetylcysteine and development of tolerance to isosorbide dinitrate in patients with angina pectoris. Circulation 1992; 85:143.

110. Dupuis J, Lalonde G, Lemieux R, et al: Tolerance to intravenous nitroglycerin in patients with congestive heart failure: role of increased intravascular volume, neurohumoral activation and lack of prevention with N-acetylcysteine. J Am Coll Cardiol 1990; 16:923.
111. Metelitsa VI, Martsevich SY, Kozyreva MP, et al: Enhancement of the efficacy of isosorbide dinitrate by captopril in stable angina pectoris. Am J Cardiol 1992; 69:291.
112. Stewart DJ, Elsner SS, Sommer D, et al: Altered spectrum of nitroglycerin action in long-term treatment: nitroglycerin-specific venous tolerance with maintenance of arterial vasodepressor potency. Circulation 1986; 74:573.
113. Parker JD, Farrell B, Fenton T, et al: Effects of diuretic therapy on the development of tolerance during continuous therapy with nitroglycerin. J Am Coll Cardiol 1992; 20:616.
114. Amsterdam EA: Rationale for intermittent nitrate therapy. Am J Cardiol 1992; 70:55G.
115. Parker JD, Testa MA, Jimenez AH, et al: Morning increase in ambulatory ischemia in patients with stable coronary artery disease. Circulation 1994; 89:604.
116. Husain M, Adrie C, Ichinose F, et al: Exhaled nitric oxide as a marker for organic nitrate tolerance. Circulation 1994; 89:2498.
117. Thadani U, Davidson C, Singleton W, et al: Comparison of five β-adrenoceptor antagonists with different ancillary properties during sustained twice daily therapy in angina pectoris. Am J Med 1980; 68:243.
118. Kostis JB, Lacy CR, Krieger SD, et al: Atenolol, nadolol, and pindolol in angina pectoris on effort: effect of pharmacokinetics. Am Heart J 1984; 108:1131.
119. Kerm MJ, Ganz P, Horowitz JD, et al: Potentiation of coronary vasoconstriction by beta-adrenergic blockade in patients with coronary artery disease. Circulation 1983; 67:1178.
120. Gaglione A, Hess OM, Corin WJ, et al: Is there coronary vasoconstriction after intracoronary beta-adrenergic blockade in patients with coronary artery disease. J Am Coll Cardiol 1987; 10:299.
121. Chierchia S, Muiesan L, Davies A, et al: Role of the sympathetic nervous system in the pathogenesis of chronic stable angina. Circulation 1990; 82(suppl II):71.
122. Nies AS, Evans GH, Shand DG: Regional hemodynamic effects of beta-adrenergic blockade with propranolol in the unanesthetized primate. Am Heart J 1973; 85:97.
123. Mimran A, Ducailar G: Systemic and regional haemodynamic profile of diuretics and alpha- and beta-blockers. A review comparing acute and chronic effects. Drugs 1988; 35(suppl 6):60.
124. Hiatt WR, Stoll S, Nies AS: Effect of β-adrenergic blockers on the peripheral circulation in patients with peripheral vascular disease. Circulation 1985; 72:1226.
125. Kaiser P, Tesch PA, Frisk-Holmberg M, et al: Effect of beta and nonselective beta-blockade on work capacity and muscle metabolism. Clin Physiol 1986; 6:197.
126. Chierchia S, Glazier JJ, Gerosa S: A single-blind, placebo-controlled study of effects of atenolol on transient ischemia in "mixed" angina. Am J Cardiol 1987; 60:36A.
127. Imperi GA, Lambert CR, Coy K, et al: Effects of titrated beta-blockade (metoprolol) on silent myocardial ischemia in ambulatory patients with coronary artery disease. Am J Cardiol 1987; 60:519.
128. Stone PH, Gibson RS, Glasser SP, et al: Comparison of propranolol, diltiazem, and nifedipine in the treatment of ambulatory ischemia in patients with stable angina. Circulation 1990; 82:1962.
129. Ardissino D, Savonitto S, Egstrup K, et al: Transient myocardial ischemia during daily life in rest and exertional angina pectoris and comparison of effectiveness of metoprolol versus nifedipine. Am J Cardiol 1991; 67:946.
130. Yusuf S, Peto R, Lewis J, et al: Beta-blockade during and after myocardial infarction: an overview of the randomized trials. Progr Cardiovasc Dis 1985; 27:335.
131. Drayer DE: Lipophilicity, hydrophilicity, and the central nervous system side effects of beta-blockers. Pharmacotherapy 1987; 7:87.
132. McDevitt DG: Comparison of pharmacokinetic properties of beta-adrenoceptor blocking drugs. Eur Heart J 1987; 8(suppl M):9.
133. Landau AJ, Frishman WH, Alturk N, et al: Improvement in exercise tolerance and immediate beta-adrenergic blockade with intranasal propranolol in patients with angina pectoris. Am J Cardiol 1993; 72:995.
134. Crawford MH, LeWinter MM, O'Rourke RA, et al: Combined propranolol and digoxin therapy in angina pectoris. Ann Intern Med 1975; 83:399.
135. Waagstein F, Bristow MR, Swedberg K, et al: Beneficial effects of metoprolol in idiopathic dilated cardiomyopathy. Lancet 1993; 342:1441.
136. Thadani U: Assessment of "optimal" beta blockade in treating patients with angina pectoris. Acta Med Scand 1984; 694(suppl):178.
137. Miller RR, Olson HG, Amsterdam EA, et al: Propranolol withdrawal rebound phenomenon. Exacerbation of coronary events after abrupt cessation of antianginal therapy. N Engl J Med 1975; 293:416.
138. Wood AJJ: Calcium antagonists. Pharmacologic differences and similarities. Circulation 1989; 80(suppl IV):184.
139. Opie LH: Calcium channel antagonists. Part V. Second generation agents. Cardiovasc Drugs Ther 1988; 2:191.
140. Lathrop DA, Valle-Aquilera JR, Millard RW, et al: Comparative electrophysiologic and coronary hemodynamic effects of diltiazem, nisoldipine and verapamil on myocardial tissue. Am J Cardiol 1982; 49:613.
141. Mitchell LB, Schroeder JS, Mason JW: Comparative clinical electrophysiologic effects of diltiazem, verapamil and nifedipine: a review. Am J Cardiol 1982; 49:629.
142. Hurwitz L, Partridge LD, Leach JK (eds): Calcium channels: their properties, functions, regulation and clinical relevance. Boca Raton, FL: CRC Press, 1991.
143. Boden WE, Bough EW, Reichman MJ, et al: Beneficial effects of high-dose diltiazem in patients with persistent effort angina on beta-blockers and nitrates: a randomized, double-blind, placebo-controlled crossover study. Circulation 1985; 71:1197.
144. Elkayam U, Amin J, Mehra A, et al: A prospective, randomized, double-blind crossover study to compare the efficacy and safety of chronic nifedipine therapy with that of isosorbide dinitrate and their combination in the treatment of chronic congestive heart failure. Circulation 1990; 82:1954.
145. Hollingshead LM, Faulde D, Fitton A: Bepridil. A review of its pharmacological properties and therapeutic use in stable angina pectoris. Drugs 1992; 44:835.
146. Cote PL, Beamer AD, McGowan N, et al: Efficacy and safety of perhexiline maleate in refracting angina: a double-blind placebo-controlled clinical trial of a novel antianginal agent. Circulation 1990; 81:1260.
147. Mueller HS, Chahine RA: Interim report of multicenter double-blind, placebo-controlled studies of nifedipine in chronic stable angina. Am J Med 1981; 71:645.
148. Hossack KF, Bruce RA: Improved exercise performance in persons with stable angina pectoris receiving diltiazem. Am J Cardiol 1981; 47:95.
149. Subramanian VB, Bowles MJ, Davies AB, et al: Calcium channel blockade as primary therapy for stable angina pectoris. Am J Cardiol 1982; 50:1158.
150. Subramanian VB, Bowles MJ, Khurmi NS, et al: Rationale for the choice of calcium antagonists in chronic stable angina. An objective double-blind placebo-controlled comparison of nifedipine and verapamil. Am J Cardiol 1982; 50:1173.
151. Yokota M, Takashi M, Iwase M, et al: Hemodynamic mechanisms of antianginal action of calcium channel blocker nisoldipine in dynamic exercise-induced angina. Circulation 1990; 81:1887.
152. Antman E, Maller J, Goldberg S, et al: Nifedipine therapy for coronary artery spasm. N Engl J Med 1980; 302:1269.
153. Rosenthal SJ, Ginsburg R, Lamb IH, et al: Efficacy of diltiazem for control of symptoms of coronary arterial spasm. Am J Cardiol 1980; 46:1027.
154. Johnson SM, Mauritson DR, Willerson JT, et al: A controlled trial of verapamil for Prinzmetal's variant angina. N Engl J Med 1981; 304:862.
155. Chahine RA, Feldman RL, Giles TD, et al: Randomized placebo-controlled trial of amlodipine in vasospastic angina. J Am Coll Cardiol 1993; 21:1365.
156. Cannon RO, Watson RM, Rosing DR, et al: Efficacy of calcium channel blocker therapy for angina pectoris resulting from small-vessel coronary artery disease and abnormal vasodilator reserve. Am J Cardiol 1985; 56:242.
157. Waters D, Lespérance J: Interventions that beneficially influence the evolution of coronary atherosclerosis. The case for calcium channel blockers. Circulation 1992; 86(suppl III):111.
158. Parmley WW, Nesto RW, Singh BN, et al: Attenuation of the circadian patterns of myocardial ischemia with nifedipine GITS in patients with chronic stable angina. J Am Coll Cardiol 1992; 19:1380.
159. Thadani U, Zellner SR, Glasser S, et al: Double-blind, dose response, placebo-controlled multicenter study of nisoldipine. A new second-generation calcium channel blocker in angina pectoris. Circulation 1991; 84:2398.

160. DiBianco R, Schoomaker FW, Singh JB, et al: Amlodipine combined with beta-blockade for chronic angina. Results of a multicenter, placebo-controlled, randomized double-blind study. Clin Cardiol 1992; 15:519.
161. Deedwania P, Cheitlin MD, Das SK, et al: Amlodipine once a day in stable angina: double-blind crossover comparison with placebo. Clin Cardiol 1993; 16:599.
162. Packer M: Pathophysiological mechanisms underlying the adverse effects of calcium channel–blocking drugs in patients with chronic heart failure. Circulation 1989; 80(suppl IV):59.
163. Pirzada AM, DeFeyter PJF, Van der Wall EE, et al: Molsidomine in the treatment of patients with angina pectoris. Acute hemodynamic effects and clinical efficacy. N Engl J Med 1980; 302:1.
164. Frampton J, Buckley MM, Fitton A: Nicorandil. A review of its pharmacology and therapeutic efficacy in angina pectoris. Drugs 1992; 44:625.
165. Crea F, Galassi AR, Kaski JC, et al: Effect of theophylline on exercise-induced myocardial ischaemia. Lancet 1989; 1:683.
166. Crea F, Pupita G, Galassi AK, et al: Effects of theophylline, atenolol and their combination on myocardial ischemia in stable angina pectoris. Am J Cardiol 1990; 66:1157.
167. Detre K, Holubkov R, Kelsey S, et al: Percutaneous transluminal coronary angioplasty in 1985–1986 and 1977–1981: The National Heart, Lung and Blood Institute Registry. N Engl J Med 1988; 318:265.
168. Ryan TJ, Bauman WB, Kennedy JW, et al: Guidelines for percutaneous transluminal coronary angioplasty. A report of the American College of Cardiology/American Heart Association Task Force on Assessment of Diagnostic and Therapeutic Cardiovascular Procedures (Committee on Percutaneous Transluminal Coronary Angioplasty). J Am Coll Cardiol 1993; 22:2033.
169. Detre K, Holubkov R, Kelsey S, et al: One-year follow-up results of the 1985–1986 National Heart, Lung and Blood Institute's Percutaneous Transluminal Coronary Angioplasty Registry. Circulation 1989; 80:421.
170. King SB III, Schlumpf M: Ten-year completed follow-up of percutaneous transluminal coronary angioplasty: the early Zurich experience. J Am Coll Cardiol 1993; 22:353.
171. Talley JD, Hurst JW, King SB III, et al: Clinical outcome 5 years after attempted percutaneous transluminal coronary angioplasty in 427 patients. Circulation 1988; 77:820.
172. O'Keefe JH Jr, Rutherford BD, McConahay DR, et al: Multivessel coronary angioplasty from 1980 to 1989: procedural results and long-term outcome. J Am Coll Cardiol 1990; 16:1097.
173. Ellis SG, Vandormael MG, Cowley MJ: Coronary morphologic and clinical determinants of procedural outcome with angioplasty for multivessel coronary disease. Implications for patient selection. Circulation 1990; 82:1193.
174. Faxon DP, Ghalilli K, Jacobs AK, et al: The degree of revascularization and outcome after multivessel coronary angioplasty. Am Heart J 1992; 123:854.
175. Reeder GS, Holmes DR Jr, Detre K, et al: Degree of revascularization in patients with multivessel coronary disease: a report from the National Heart, Lung and Blood Institute Percutaneous Transluminal Coronary Angioplasty Registry. Circulation 1988; 77:638.
176. Samson M, Meester HJ, deFeyter PJ, et al: Successful multiple segment coronary angioplasty: effect of revascularization in single-vessel multilesions and multivessels. Am Heart J 1990; 120:1.
177. Bell MR, Bailey KR, Reeder GS, et al: Percutaneous transluminal angioplasty in patients with multivessel coronary disease: how important is complete revascularization for cardiac event–free survival? J Am Coll Cardiol 1990; 16:553.
178. Bourassa MG, Holubkov R, Yeh W, et al: Strategy of complete revascularization in patients with multivessel coronary artery disease (a report from the 1985–1986 NHLBI PTCA Registry). Am J Cardiol 1992; 70:174.
179. Thomas ES, Most AS, Williams DO: Coronary angioplasty for patients with multivessel coronary artery disease: follow-up clinical status. Am Heart J 1988; 115:8.
180. Parisi AF, Folland ED, Hartigan P: A comparison of angioplasty with medical therapy in the treatment of single-vessel coronary artery disease. N Engl J Med 1992; 326:10.
181. Protocol for the Bypass Angioplasty Revascularization Investigation. Circulation 1991; 84(suppl V):1.
182. RITA Trial Participants: Coronary angioplasty versus coronary bypass surgery: the Randomised Intervention Treatment of Angina (RITA) Trial. Lancet 1993; 341:573.
183. Rodriguez A, Boullon F, Perez-Baliño N, et al: Argentine randomized trial of percutaneous transluminal coronary angioplasty versus coronary bypass surgery in multivessel disease (ERACI): in-hospital results and 1-year follow-up. J Am Coll Cardiol 1993; 22:1060.
184. Hamm CW, Reimers J, Ischinger T, et al: A randomized study of coronary angioplasty compared with bypass surgery in patients with symptomatic multivessel coronary disease. N Engl J Med 1994; 331:1037.
185. King SB III, Lembo NJ, Weintraub WS, et al: A randomized trial comparing coronary angioplasty with coronary bypass surgery. N Engl J Med 1994; 331:1044.
186. CASS Principal Investigators and Their Associates: Coronary Artery Surgery Study (CASS): a randomized trial of coronary artery bypass surgery. Quality of life in patients randomly assigned to treatment groups. Circulation 1983; 68:951.
187. Hultgren HM, Peduzzi P, Detre K, et al: The 5-year effect of bypass surgery on relief of angina and exercise performance. Circulation 1985; 72(suppl V):79.
188. Takaro T, Pifarre R, Fish R: Left main coronary artery disease. Progr Cardiovasc Dis 1985; 28:229.
189. Detre K, Peduzzi P, Murphy M, et al: Effect of bypass surgery on survival in patients in low- and high-risk subgroups delineated by the use of simple clinical variables. Circulation 1981; 63:1329.
190. The VA Coronary Artery Bypass Surgery Cooperative Study Group: Eighteen-year follow-up in the Veterans Affairs Cooperative Study of Coronary Artery Bypass Surgery for Stable Angina. Circulation 1992; 86:121.
191. Varnauskas E, the European Coronary Surgery Study Group: Survival, myocardial infarction, and employment status in a prospective randomized study of coronary bypass surgery. Circulation 1985; 72(suppl V):90.
192. Varnauskas E, the European Coronary Surgery Study Group: Twelve-year follow-up of survival in the randomized European Coronary Surgery Study. N Engl J Med 1988; 319:332.
193. Alderman EL, Fisher LD, Litwin P, et al: Results of coronary artery surgery in patients with poor left ventricular function (CASS). Circulation 1983; 68:785.
194. CASS Principal Investigators and Their Associates: Coronary Artery Surgery Study (CASS): a randomized trial of coronary artery bypass surgery. Survival data. Circulation 1983; 68:939.
195. Passamani E, Davis KB, Gillespie MJ, et al: A randomized trial of coronary artery bypass surgery. Survival of patients with a low ejection fraction. N Engl J Med 1985; 312:1665.
196. Killip T, Passamani E, Davis K, et al: Coronary Artery Surgery Study (CASS): a randomized trial of coronary bypass surgery. Eight years follow-up and survival in patients with reduced ejection fraction. Circulation 1985; 72(suppl V):102.
197. Alderman EL, Bourassa MG, Cohen LS: Ten-year follow-up of survival and myocardial infarction in the randomized coronary artery surgery study. Circulation 1990; 82:1629.
198. Rahintoola SH: A perspective on the three large multicenter randomized clinical trials of coronary bypass surgery for chronic stable angina. Circulation 1985; 72(suppl V):123.
199. Detre K, Peduzzi P, Scott SM, et al: Long-term survival results in medically and surgically randomized patients. Progr Cardiovasc Dis 1985; 28:235.
200. Nwasokwa ON, Koss JH, Friedman GH, et al: Bypass surgery for chronic stable angina: predictions of survival benefit and strategy for patient selection. Ann Intern Med 1991; 114:1035.
201. Kronenberg MW, Pederson RW, Harston WE, et al: Left ventricular performance after coronary artery bypass surgery. Prediction of functional benefit. Ann Intern Med 1983; 99:305.
202. Ryan TJ, Weiner DA, McCabe CH, et al: Exercise testing in the Coronary Artery Surgery Study randomized population. Circulation 1985; 72(suppl V):31.
203. Picott JD, Kouchoukos NT, Oberman A, et al: Late results of surgical and medical therapy for patients with coronary artery disease and depressed left ventricular function. J Am Coll Cardiol 1985; 5:1036.
204. Myers WO, Gersh BJ, Fisher LD, et al: Medical versus early surgical therapy in patients with triple-vessel disease and mild angina pectoris: a CASS Registry study of survival. Am Thorac Surg 1987; 44:471.
205. Vigilante GJ, Weintraub WS, Klein LW, et al: Improved survival with coronary bypass surgery in patients with three-vessel coronary disease and abnormal left ventricular function. Am J Med 1987; 82:697.
206. Bounous EP, Mark DB, Pollock BG, et al: Surgical survival benefits for coronary disease patients with left ventricular dysfunction. Circulation 1988; 78(suppl I):151.
207. Myers WO, Schaff HV, Gersh BJ, et al: Improved survival of surgically

treated patients with triple vessel coronary artery disease and severe angina pectoris. A report from the Coronary Artery Surgery Study (CASS) Registry. J Thorac Cardiovasc Surg 1989; 97:487.
208. Muhlbaier LH, Pryor DB, Rankin JS, et al: Observational comparison of event-free survival with medical and surgical therapy in patients with coronary artery disease. 20 years of follow-up. Circulation 1992; 86(suppl II):198.
209. Rahimtoola SH, Fessler CL, Grunkemeier GL, et al: Survival 15 to 20 years after coronary bypass surgery for angina. J Am Coll Cardiol 1993; 21:151.
210. O'Connor GT, Plume SK, Olmstead EL: A regional prospective study of in-hospital mortality associated with coronary artery bypass grafting. JAMA 1991; 266:803.
211. Jones RH, Floyd RD, Austin EH, et al: The role of radionuclide angiocardiography in the preoperative prediction of pain relief and prolonged survival following coronary artery bypass grafting. Ann Surg 1983; 197:743.
212. Kaiser GC, Davis KB, Fisher LD, et al: Survival following coronary artery bypass grafting in patients with severe angina pectoris (CASS). An observational study. J Thorac Cardiovasc Surg 1985; 89:513.
213. Mock MB, Fisher LD, Holmes DR, et al: Comparison of effects of medical and surgical therapy on survival in severe angina pectoris and two-vessel coronary artery disease with and without left ventricular dysfunction: a Coronary Artery Surgery Registry Study. Am J Cardiol 1988; 61:1198.
214. A report of the American College of Cardiology/American Heart Association Task Force on Assessment of Diagnostic and Therapeutic Cardiovascular Procedures (Subcommittee on Coronary Artery Bypass Graft Surgery): ACC/AHA Guidelines and indications for coronary artery bypass graft surgery. Circulation 1991; 83:1125.
215. Rahimtoola SH, Bennett AJ, Grunkemeier GL, et al: Survival at 15 to 18 years after coronary bypass surgery for angina in women. Circulation 1993; 88(part 2):71.
216. Ko W, Gold JP, Lazzaro R, et al: Survival analysis of octogenarian patients with coronary artery disease managed by elective coronary artery bypass surgery versus conventional medical treatment. Circulation 1992; 86(suppl II):191.
217. Gersh BJ, Califf RM, Loop FD, et al: Coronary bypass surgery in chronic stable angina. Circulation 1989; 79(suppl I):46.
218. Lynch P, Dargie H, Krikler S: Objective assessment of antianginal treatment: a double-blind comparison of propranolol, nifedipine and their combination. Br Med J 1980; 2:184.
219. Bassam MM, Weiler-Ravell D: The additive antianginal action of oral isosorbide dinitrate in patients receiving propranolol. Magnitude and duration of effect. Chest 1983; 83:233.
220. Morse JR, Nesto RW: Double-blind crossover comparison of the antianginal effects of nifedipine and isosorbide dinitrate in patients with exertional angina receiving propranolol. J Am Coll Cardiol 1985; 6:1395.
221. Strauss WE, Parisi AF: Combined use of calcium channel and beta-adrenergic blockers for the treatment of chronic stable angina. Rationale, efficacy, and adverse effects. Ann Intern Med 1988; 109:570.
222. Stone PH, Ware JH, DeWood MA, et al: The efficacy of the addition of nifedipine in patients with mixed angina compared to patients with classic exertional angina: a multicenter, randomized double-blind placebo-controlled clinical trial. Am Heart J 1988; 116:961.
223. Meluzín J, Zeman K, Stetka F, et al: Effects of nifedipine and diltiazem on myocardial ischemia in patients with severe stable angina pectoris treated with nitrates and β-blockers. J Cardiovasc Pharmacol 1992; 20:864.
224. Kawanishi DT, Reid CL, Morrison EE, et al: Response of angina and ischemia to long-term treatment in patients with chronic stable angina: a double-blind randomized individualized dosing trial of nifedipine, propranolol and their combination. J Am Coll Cardiol 1992; 19:409.
225. Hung J, Lamb IH, Connolly SJ, et al: The effect of diltiazem and propranolol alone and in combination on exercise performance and left ventricular function in patients with stable effort angina: a double-blind, randomized, and placebo-controlled study. Circulation 1983; 68:560.
226. Packer M: Combined beta-adrenergic and calcium-entry blockade in angina pectoris. N Engl J Med 1985; 320:709.
227. El-Tamimi H, Davies GJ, Kaski J-C, et al: Effects of diltiazem alone or with isosorbide dinitrate or with atenolol both acutely and chronically for stable angina pectoris. Am J Cardiol 1989; 64:717.
228. Tolins M, Weir EK, Chesler E, et al: "Maximal" drug therapy is not necessarily optimal in chronic angina pectoris. J Am Coll Cardiol 1984; 3:1051.
229. de Jongste MJL, Hautvast RWM, Hillege HL, et al: Efficacy of spinal cord stimulation as adjuvant therapy for intractable angina pectoris: a prospective, randomized clinical study. J Am Coll Cardiol 1994; 23:1592.
230. Grech ED, Ramsdale DR: Exertional syncope in aortic stenosis: evidence to support inappropriate left ventricular baroreceptor response. Am Heart J 1991; 121:603.
231. Fananapazir L, Cannon RD III, Tripodi D, et al: Impact of dual-chamber permanent pacing in patients with obstructive hypertrophic cardiomyopathy with symptoms refractory to verapamil and beta-adrenergic blocker therapy. Circulation 1992; 85:2149.
232. Winkle RA, Harrison D: Propranolol for patients with mitral valve prolapse. Am Heart J 1977; 93:422.
233. Cannon RO III, Quyyumi AA, Mincemoyer R, et al: Imipramine in patients with chest pain despite normal coronary angiograms. New Engl J Med 1994; 330:1411.

6 Management of Unstable Angina

Pierre Théroux, MD

Through decades of medical observations and more recent basic investigation and clinical research, unstable angina has become a well-defined clinical entity, rich in therapeutic options. Selection of treatment requires clinical experience and knowledge both of the pharmacologic actions of various drugs and of the potential of a variety of intervention procedures. The syndrome is challenging for the clinician; it allows recognition and treatment of a disease before more severe complications and irreversible myocardial damage occur. The initial goal of therapy is to control the acute disease process; the second is to orient the long-term management of the underlying coronary artery disease.

PATHOPHYSIOLOGIC MECHANISMS AND THERAPEUTIC IMPLICATIONS

Coronary artery disease is most often a chronic and diffuse disease, but unstable angina, like myocardial infarction, is an acute syndrome caused by the focal disease of one plaque, the so-called culprit coronary lesion.[1–3] Figures 29–1 to 29–3 summarize the process of activation of an atherosclerotic plaque after a fissure or rupture that exposes the subendothelial adhesive proteins to flowing blood. Circulating platelets adhere rapidly to these proteins and more specifically to collagen and von Willebrand factor via, respectively, the integrin membrane receptor glycoproteins I_a and I_b. The consequences are an increase in the free cytosolic content of calcium in platelets, cytoskeleton contraction, and shape change and the release of potent proaggregant substances (such as thromboxane A_2, adenosine diphosphate, and serotonin) and of procoagulants (such as fibrinogen and factor V).

Tissue factor, exposed from monocytes and from the endothelium, combines with factor VII to stimulate the coagulation cascade. At the platelet surface, activated factor X forms with factor V the prothrombinase complex, generating thrombin. Thrombin, in vivo, is the most potent stimulant for platelet aggregation. Its receptor has been identified and cloned.[4] Thrombin binds its receptor via the anion-binding exosite and cleaves it, unmasking a new amino acid terminus that acts as a tethered ligand that activates an as-yet-undefined domain of the receptor. Synthetic peptides, the thrombin receptor agonist peptides, can mimic the effects of the tethered ligand.

The many pathways leading to platelet aggregation converge to activate the integrin platelet receptor, glycoprotein II_b/III_a. A single platelet contains more than 50,000 expressions of this receptor in a nonactive state. Once activated, the receptor is recognized by a dodecapeptide sequence on the gamma chain of fibrinogen and by a tripeptide sequence on the alpha chain, the Arg-Gly-Asp (RGD) sequence.[5] The dodecapeptide sequence is specific for fibrinogen whereas the RGD sequence is also present in other adhesive proteins. Although GP II_b/III_a is the specific receptor for fibrinogen, it binds von Willebrand factor at high shear rates and also fibronectin, vitronectin, and thrombospondin.[6] The GP II_b/III_a receptor is of critical importance, being the common and obligatory pathway to platelet aggregation. The subsequent steps to intravascular blood clot formation lead to formation of the fibrin network. Thrombin cleaves fibrinopeptides A and B from fibrinogen, forming fibrin monomers that subsequently polymerize in soluble fibrillar strands of fibrin. Crosslinking of the fibrin strands produces the insoluble three-dimensional blood clot matrix.

Blood clot formation is modulated by endogenous inhibitors. The intact endothelium produces nitric oxide and prostacyclin, stimulating the formation of cyclic guanosine monophosphate (cGMP) and cyclic adenosine monophosphate (cAMP), respectively. Both decrease cytosolic calcium content to produce vasodilatation and stabilize platelets.[7, 8] Other important natural anticoagulants are antithrombin III, heparin cofactor II, the tissue factor pathway inhibitor, and activated protein C and protein S (see Chapters 28 and 29). Antithrombin III inhibits thrombin, factors X_a and IX_a, and also factors XI_a and XII_a. Antithrombin II specifically inhibits thrombin in the endothelium with dermatan sulfate as a cofactor. The tissue factor pathway inhibitor first binds and inactivates factor X_a to subsequently inactivate factor VII_a.[9] Protein C, activated by the complex formed by thrombin and thrombomodulin on the endothelium, inhibits factors V_a and VIII_a and stimulates the production of tissue plasminogen activator.[10]

This description oversimplifies the complex mechanisms involved in endovascular thrombus formation. It is provided to help the reader understand how current treatments and treatments under investigation might be of clinical benefit (Fig. 6–1). Some other pathophysiologic mechanisms may also have a major role and become targets for new effective interventions. Thus platelet-leukocyte interactions, tissue factor release by monocytes, and inflammatory and growth factor mediators may play an important etiologic role in unstable angina. Critical evaluation by clinical trials of any new intervention remains the key to defining the usefulness of the intervention and also to understanding more completely the mechanisms of the disease.

GOALS OF TREATMENT

Appropriate treatment of unstable angina covers a large spectrum of options from minimal to very aggressive therapy. It requires individualization of treatment to patient symptoms and to severity of disease. Risk evaluation in unstable angina is a continuous process: it begins at hospital admission and is updated as the clinical course evolves and the results of various diagnostic procedures become available; long-term prognosis is evaluated before hospital discharge.[11] A higher risk of an adverse clinical outcome is present in patients with prolonged chest pain, hemodynamic disturbances with chest pain, and the presence of either electrocardiographic ST segment depression, 1-mm or more, or deeply inverted T waves on the admission electrocardiogram (ECG) or on an ECG obtained during or close to an episode of chest pain. Lower risk patients are those who lack clearly accelerating symptoms or new onset exertional angina and have a normal ECG.[12–16]

The immediate goal of treatment in unstable angina is to stabilize

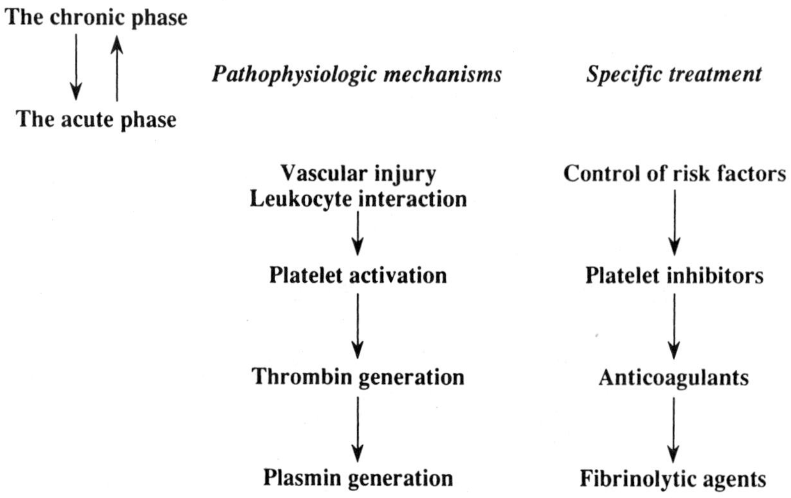

Figure 6–1. Mechanisms involved in unstable angina with specific therapeutic strategies (see text for discussion).

the thrombotic process to prevent more severe complications and myocardial infarction. Because myocardial infarction may lead to death or permanent disability, more subtle preceding endpoints are needed in clinical practice in order to evaluate success or failure of treatment. Recurrence of chest pain during treatment marks incomplete control and a presumably persistent active disease.[12–17] Of patients who develop an early myocardial infarction, 85% manifest recurrent ischemic symptoms.[15] In asymptomatic patients, an ischemic response to a provocative test indicates significant coronary stenosis, related either to the thrombogenic process itself or to more severe and extensive coronary artery disease.[18–22] Therapy cannot be considered optimal in patients with spontaneous or inducible ischemia at a low threshold of exercise. These patients remain at higher risk, their quality of life is impaired, and they require more aggressive therapy. In this situation, the need for an intervention is a marker of treatment failure and is therefore a useful endpoint in clinical trials. An intervention performed electively on the basis of the findings of a coronary angiogram or stable symptoms is probably less meaningful and more related to the severity of the underlying coronary artery disease. The timing of a stress ECG is critical; negative results of tests performed acutely can be misleading because they may not detect imminent thrombus formation. Provocative tests should therefore be delayed a few days, until the disease process is clinically controlled. Figure 6–2 suggests general guidelines for progression to less aggressive and to more aggressive treatment after risk evaluation.

DIAGNOSTIC TOOLS

The 12-lead ECG helps diagnose the presence, severity, extent, and site of ischemia. A non–Q wave myocardial infarction is usually associated with more persistent ST segment depression. Transient elevations of creatine kinase (CK) and of its MB fraction confirm the diagnosis of myocardial infarction. Coronary angiography documents the presence, severity, and extent of coronary artery disease and adds information on the morphology of the culprit lesion for a better understanding of pathophysiology and prognosis.[23–25] Coronary angioscopy enhances the sensitivity of angiography for detecting an intravascular thrombus, and endovascular ultrasonography allows definition of the characteristics of the plaque and of the vessel wall. New diagnostic tests marking an ongoing intravascular thrombotic and inflammatory process and myocardial cell damage are now under investigation with a potential for more objective evaluation of diagnosis, severity, and prognosis of the disease. These tests need more validation before their widespread use is recommended.

Troponin T and troponin I are cardiac specific proteins released in the circulation after the loss of the integrity of the myocardial cell membrane; they are sensitive and specific markers of myocardial cell injury associated with severe ischemia and necrosis; and their release in the circulation may signify the presence of microinfarction.[26] In one study, elevated levels of troponin T could be detected in 39% of patients admitted for unstable angina in blood samplings obtained 8 h to 2 days after admission. Thirty percent of those patients experienced a myocardial infarction during hospitalization, in comparison with only 2% of the patients with normal troponin T serum levels.[27] Other studies have also documented a worse prognosis when plasma levels of troponin T were elevated.[28]

C-reactive protein and serum amyloid A are acute-phase reactants reflecting cytokine-mediated hepatic production triggered by inflammation, infection, and tissue injury. Increased concentrations have been documented in many patients with unstable angina.[29, 30] In one study, elevated levels at admission predicted a worse prognosis; myocardial infarction occurred in 25% of affected patients, death in 10%, and ischemic events in 90%. The predictive value was additive to the value of plasma levels of troponin T.[30]

Activation of platelets and the coagulation system are also found in many patients with coronary artery disease. The urinary levels of 2–3 dinor thromboxane B_2 are elevated with peaks corresponding to episodes of chest pain, which is suggestive of episodic platelet activation.[31] The prothrombin fragment F_{1+2} and the fibrinopeptide A plasma levels are also high during the acute phase; persistent elevation is associated with an increased risk of recurrent coronary events.[32–34]

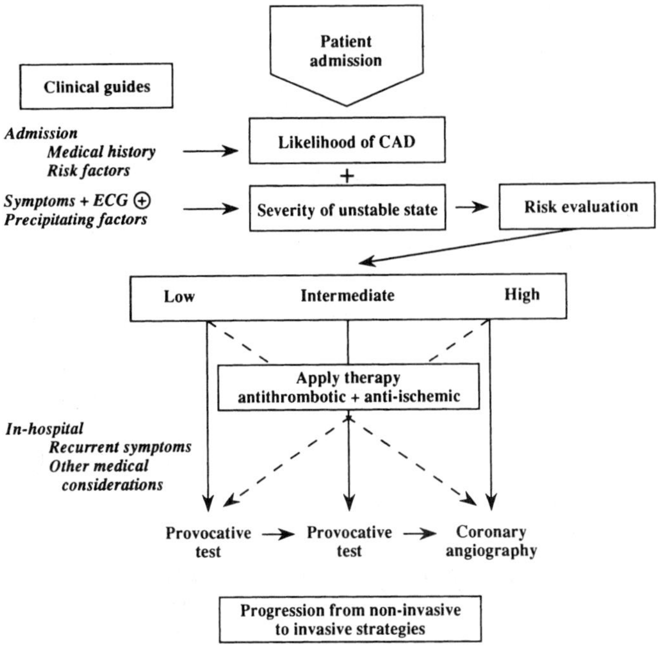

Figure 6–2. Diagnosis of unstable angina, early management, and risk stratification. The clinical history, including risk factors, and the electrocardiogram (ECG) at admission and during pain help the physician obtain an initial risk evaluation that is rapidly updated to the clinical course on treatment, within the first 12–48 h. Patients at high risk are usually catheterized, and others may be rapidly risk-stratified through the use of one of the many available provocative tests. The *dashed arrows* represent alternative pathways as indicated by specific local practice, other medical considerations, and additional information on patients. Certain low-risk patients may be candidates for bypassing the provocative tests and proceeding directly to coronary angiography (*dashed arrow,* left to right); such patients might include those who specifically request diagnostic arteriography, persons who are in a job in which the health and safety of other individuals may be at risk (e.g., airline pilot, bus driver). Alternatively, certain high-risk patients who ordinarily would be referred for coronary angiography may be referred for a provocative test first (*dashed arrow,* right to left); such patients might include those who have complicating additional medical illnesses such as severe chronic obstructive pulmonary disease or malignancy and patients who are reluctant to undergo angioplasty or revascularization surgery because of personal preference. Subsequent management decisions are described in Figure 6–8. *Other abbreviation:* CAD, coronary artery disease.

INTERVENTIONS TO STABILIZE THE PLAQUE AND THE DISEASED ENDOTHELIUM

Factors influencing plaque rupture have been extensively studied.[3] They include plaque geometry associated with higher wall stress,[35, 36] frailty of a thinly capped lipid-rich plaque,[37–39] and an abnormal response of the diseased endothelium.[40, 41] The depth of plaque rupture also influences host reaction and subsequent clinical evolution.[39] It is therefore possible to conceive of interventions that would stabilize the ruptured plaque to attenuate the severity of the insult and modulate thrombus formation. Intervention trials with lipid-lowering drugs in patients with stable coronary artery disease have documented a striking reduction in clinical events, exceeding the modest improvement observed in the severity of stenosis, which suggests that modification of the plaque content in lipids could reduce the frequency or consequences of a rupture.[36, 42] Control of risk factors can restore a normal response in the diseased endothelium.[43, 44] Use of aspirin can also reduce the rate of clinical events[45] and their severity[46] and prevent the development of new lesions.[47] The magnitude of long-term benefits that result from this multifactorial approach of plaque stabilization is still unknown but may be substantial and rewarding. Interventions on various selectin and integrin platelet receptors, on leukocyte membrane receptors, and on adhesive proteins may also modulate the release of cytokines, mitogens, and growth factors and prevent the rapid progression of atherosclerosis.

In this chapter, treatment to prevent fatal and nonfatal myocardial infarction is reviewed first, followed by treatments to prevent recurrent ischemia. Finally, treatment aimed at secondary prevention and improving quality of life is discussed.

PREVENTION OF DEATH AND OF MYOCARDIAL INFARCTION: ANTITHROMBOTIC THERAPY

Nonfatal myocardial infarction and myocardial infarction progressing to death are the most serious complications of unstable angina. They mark an evolutionary disease and a high-likelihood of progression to complete occlusion of the culprit coronary artery. These events can be objectively diagnosed; and they represent hard endpoints in clinical trials. The amounts of new and prior left ventricular damage determine the immediate and subsequent prognoses.

Thrombolytic Therapy

The role of intermittent thrombotic coronary occlusion in unstable angina, combined with the striking benefits of thrombolysis in acute myocardial infarction, has stimulated the investigation of thrombolytic therapy in unstable angina. Early angiographic studies suggested benefit in some thrombolytic-treated patients who experienced less frequent thrombotic occlusion and less severe residual stenosis.[48–50] In the Thrombolysis in Myocardial Ischemia (TIMI) 3A angiographic study, recombinant tissue plasminogen activator (rt-PA) was more successful than placebo in improving TIMI flow by two grades or more or reducing stenosis severity by 20% or more.[51] In the Thrombolysis in Patients with Unstable Angina (UNASEM) study, 12 of the 17 patients with an occluded artery who received anistreplase experienced flow restoration, in comparison with none of the 11 patients who received placebo; more patients receiving treatment, however, experienced recurrent angina (27% vs. 12%; p = .06).[52] The largest trial in unstable angina, TIMI 3B, enrolled 1473 patients; death or myocardial infarction occurred in 8.8% of patients treated with rt-PA and in 6.2% of patients treated with placebo.[55] Figure 6–3 summarizes the results of seven randomized, placebo-controlled clinical trials that have enrolled 100 patients or more.[52–58]

The pooled analysis of these data reveals a 39% increase in the risk of fatal or nonfatal myocardial infarction with fibrinolytic therapy. Various thrombolytic agents, administered for a variable period of time, were used in these studies. Other studies have shown larger resting thallium-201 defects and longer duration of ST segment shifts on Holter recording in patients who received rt-PA than in patients who received placebo[59] and more frequent need for an urgent intervention because of refractory angina.[60] Analyses of subsets of patients with ST segment depression enrolled in the mega-trials that have established the benefits of thrombolysis in acute myocardial infarction, Gruppo Italiano per lo Studio della Streptochinasi nell'Infarto Miocardico (GISSI) and International Study of Infarct Survival (ISIS-2), also failed to show a benefit in non–Q wave myocardial infarction.[61, 62] In these two trials, death occurred in 153 of the 795 patients treated (19%) and in 142 of the 793 placebo patients (17%).

Possible reasons for the failure of thrombolysis in unstable angina include the facts that (1) the clot is not completely occlusive in most patients with unstable angina, as opposed to patients with ST elevation myocardial infarction, (2) the composition of the clot differs with more platelets and less fibrin, and (3) thrombolysis does not correct the underlying disease process that remains active with the potential of exacerbation by thrombin and platelet stimulation induced by fibrinolysis.[63, 64] Thrombolysis is therefore not indicated in unstable angina and in myocardial infarction occurring with ST segment depression. An exception is true posterior wall myocardial infarction with ST segment depression in the right precordial leads.

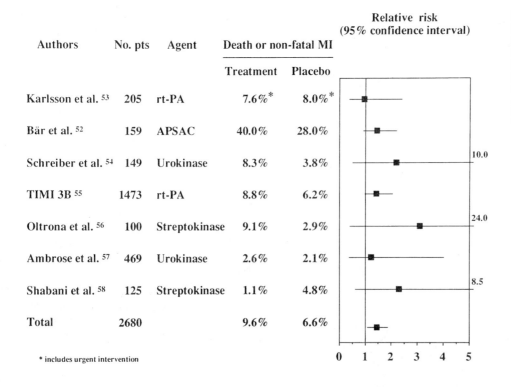

Authors	No. pts	Agent	Death or non-fatal MI: Treatment	Death or non-fatal MI: Placebo
Karlsson et al. [53]	205	rt-PA	7.6%*	8.0%*
Bär et al. [52]	159	APSAC	40.0%	28.0%
Schreiber et al. [54]	149	Urokinase	8.3%	3.8%
TIMI 3B [55]	1473	rt-PA	8.8%	6.2%
Oltrona et al. [56]	100	Streptokinase	9.1%	2.9%
Ambrose et al. [57]	469	Urokinase	2.6%	2.1%
Shabani et al. [58]	125	Streptokinase	1.1%	4.8%
Total	2680		9.6%	6.6%

* includes urgent intervention

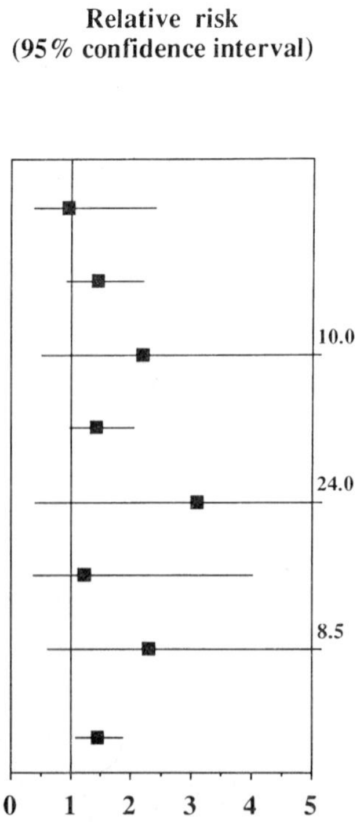

Figure 6–3. Results of clinical trials with thrombolysis in unstable angina. The pooled analysis shows an increase in death and myocardial infarction (MI) with thrombolytic therapy in comparison with placebo. *Other abbreviations:* rt-PA, recombinant tissue plasminogen activator; APSAC, anisoylated plasminogen-streptokinase activator complex; TIMI, Thrombolysis in Myocardial Ischemia.

Aspirin

In contrast with the failure of thrombolysis, randomized and controlled trials with aspirin in patients with unstable angina have consistently shown benefits of aspirin, with a more than 50% reduction in the risk of fatal or nonfatal myocardial infarction.[65–68] The Veterans Administration study randomized 1266 men within 48 h of admission to 324 mg of aspirin in an effervescent buffered powder or the buffer alone for a period of 12 weeks. Death and myocardial infarction were study endpoints.[65] The Canadian Multicenter trial evaluated 555 men and women randomly allocated, within 8 days of admission, to placebo, 325 mg of aspirin four times a day, 200 mg of sulfinpyrazone four times a day, or the combination of sulfinpyrazone and aspirin. The mean follow-up period was 18 months, and the endpoints were cardiac death and nonfatal myocardial infarction.[66] In the Montreal study, 479 patients of either sex were randomized, within 12 h of admission, to 325 mg of aspirin twice a day, intravenous heparin titrated to an activated partial thromboplastin time (aPTT) 1.5 to 2.5 × control, the combination of aspirin and heparin, or equivalent placebos. Endpoints were measured in the hospital after a mean of 5 days, before the discontinuation of the study drugs; they included death, myocardial infarction, and the recurrence of severe ischemia.[67] The fourth trial was published by a group of investigators from southeastern Sweden. A total of 796 men were enrolled in this placebo-controlled trial with a 2 × 2 factorial design; a low dose of 75 mg of aspirin a day was used, and heparin was administered as intravenous boluses of 5000 units every 6 h for 24 h, followed by 3750 units for 4 days. The endpoints of death and myocardial infarction were measured at 5 days, 1 month, and 3 months.[68]

The relative risk of death and nonfatal myocardial infarction observed in these four trials are shown in Figure 6–4. The reduction in the incidence of death and nonfatal myocardial infarction with aspirin was homogeneous in all trials and independent of the differences in protocols, such as doses of aspirin, time of initiation of treatment, and duration of follow-up. Initiation of the drug early after admission was more effective than later initiation.

Aspirin was also beneficial in reducing the incidence of refractory ischemia during the acute phase from 23% to 16% of patients in one study[67] and from 2.8% to 0.8% in another study.[68] Over the long term, the need for angiography because of severe angina was less frequent with aspirin therapy; risk ratios were 0.59 at 3 months (95% confidence limits 0.42–0.84, $p < .0001$), and 0.71 at 1 year (95% confidence limits 0.56–0.91, $p < .0001$). This benefit was additive to the reduction of death and nonfatal myocardial infarction.[69]

The collaborative overview of randomized trials of antiplatelet therapy by the Oxford group included 100,000 subjects from 145 trials, 70,000 of whom were patients with at least one high-risk condition. Antiplatelet therapy resulted in reductions in nonfatal myocardial infarction by one third, in nonfatal stroke by one third, and in vascular-related death by one sixth ($p < .00001$) in all high-risk categories. Low and higher doses of aspirin were equally effective.[70]

Maintenance doses of 80–160 mg daily are recommended; higher doses offer no additional benefits but are associated with more frequent side effects.[71] However, the loading dose should probably be higher, in the range of 160–360 mg of a nonenteric formulation, to rapidly achieve full inhibition of thromboxane A_2 formation.[72]

Other Antiplatelet Agents

Sulfinpyrazone, evaluated in the Canadian Multicenter Trial, showed no trend to better results in comparison with placebo, and the combination of sulfinpyrazone with aspirin showed no significant additional benefit in comparison with aspirin alone.[66] Cardiac death or myocardial infarction occurred in 21 patients (15%) randomized to sulfinpyrazone alone, in 20 patients (14%) randomized to placebo, in 13 (9%) of patients who received the combination of sulfinpyrazone and aspirin, and in 16 (12%) with aspirin alone.

Ticlopidine was evaluated in one study from Italy.[73] This open-label trial randomized 652 patients of either sex with unstable angina, excluding non–Q wave myocardial infarction, to standard therapy or to standard therapy plus ticlopidine within 48 h of admission. No patients received aspirin. The rate of fatal or nonfatal myocardial infarction and of vascular death was reduced at 6 months with ticlopidine from 13.6% to 7.3%, corresponding to the same risk reduction as observed with aspirin (see Fig. 6–4). The benefits of ticlopidine appeared, however, only after 15 days of treatment, which is consistent with the delayed onset of action of the drug. Ticlopidine is therefore not appropriate for acute management but can be used for the long-term management of patients intolerant of aspirin. The dose is 250 mg twice per day.

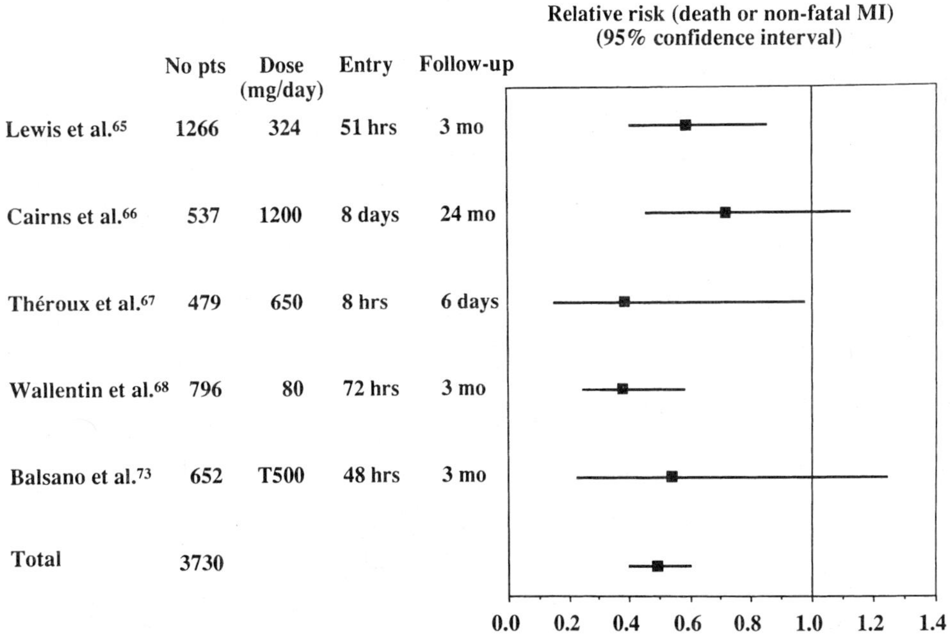

Figure 6–4. Relative risk of fatal and nonfatal myocardial infarction (MI) in randomized, placebo-controlled trials of aspirin in unstable angina. The benefits observed with aspirin are homogeneous and independent of doses used, time of initiation of therapy after the acute episode, and duration of follow-up. The results of one trial with ticlopidine are also included: T500 = ticlopidine 250 mg b.i.d.

Heparin

A trial published in 1982 by Telford and Wilson suggested that heparin could be useful for the management of the acute phase of unstable angina.[74] The authors studied 214 patients randomized at hospital admission to 100 mg of atenolol per day, 5000 units of heparin intravenously every 6 h at fixed doses, the combination of the same doses of atenolol and heparin, or placebo. The study was criticized because of the exclusion from analysis of a large proportion of enrolled patients. Its results nevertheless suggested a significant benefit of heparin: the incidence of death and myocardial infarction was reduced from 17% without heparin to 3%; the relative risk was 17%. No aspirin was used in this study.

Two studies from Montreal subsequently documented the benefits of heparin. The first included 479 patients randomized to aspirin, heparin, both, or neither.[67] With heparin, titrated to an aPTT twice that of the control aPTT, the rate of myocardial infarction and death was reduced from 7.5% to 1.0% (relative risk, 0.15; $p = .0007$); with aspirin, it was reduced from 6.4% to 2.5% (relative risk, 0.37; $p = .04$). The rates were similar with heparin alone (0.8%) and the combination of heparin plus aspirin (1.6%). To further investigate the relative benefits of heparin and of aspirin, the study was extended to include a total of 488 patients randomized to heparin alone or to aspirin alone.[75] This extension trial confirmed a statistically significant reduction in the risk of myocardial infarction from 3.7% with aspirin to 0.8% with heparin; the absolute risk difference of 2.9% favored heparin (relative risk, 0.23; 95% confidence limits, 0.05–0.90; $p = .035$) (Fig. 6–5).

Heparin was also effective in preventing refractory angina in the Montreal studies, decreasing the incidence from 23% to 0.6% (relative risk, 0.43; $p = .002$).[67] In a study from Italy, 90 patients with demonstrable recurrent ischemia on Holter monitoring and receiving triple antianginal therapy with a nitrate, a beta blocker, and a calcium channel antagonist were randomized to heparin boluses of 6000 units every 6 h, to an infusion of heparin titrated to an aPTT 1.5 to 2.0 times higher than the control aPTT, or to 325 mg of aspirin per day.[76] Only the intravenous infusion of heparin significantly reduced the numbers of anginal attacks and episodes of silent ischemia detected by continuous electrocardiographic monitoring; angina occurred in 19% of patients who received the heparin infusion and in 89% of patients who received aspirin. The authors subsequently compared the intravenous infusion of heparin to an infusion of rt-PA over a 12-h period; again, a significant reduction in ischemic events was observed only with heparin.

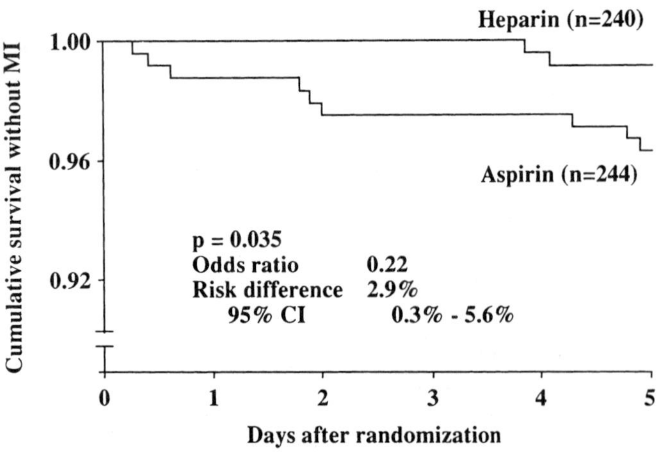

Figure 6–5. Cox survival curves of patients randomized to aspirin or to heparin during the acute phase of unstable angina. The use of heparin resulted in a significant early absolute decrease of 2.9% in the rate of fatal and nonfatal myocardial infarction. (From Théroux P, Waters D, Qiu S, et al: Aspirin versus heparin to prevent myocardial infarction during the acute phase of unstable angina. Circulation 1993; 88[part 1]:2045.)

Full therapeutic intravenous doses of heparin are recommended: a bolus injection of 5000 units, followed by an infusion titrated to achieve an aPTT 1.5 to 2.5 times higher than the control aPTT. An algorithm for dose titration is provided in Table 28–2.

Rebound After the Discontinuation of Heparin

A rebound reactivation of disease after the discontinuation of heparin in unstable angina has been recognized.[77] The manifestations include myocardial infarction or severe ischemic pain that necessitates an urgent intervention. This rebound effect was observed in 13% of patients and clustered a median of 9.5 h after the discontinuation of the drug (range, 3–18 h). Concomitant aspirin treatment could attenuate it, which may explain the better longer term benefit of aspirin used alone[67] or in combination with heparin.[68] Tapering the heparin infusion rather than discontinuing it abruptly could be one method of preventing rebound; the benefits remain to be determined.

The possible mechanisms explaining the rebound effect have been reviewed.[78] Depletion of antithrombin III after prolonged heparin use is a potential[79] but unlikely mechanism.[80] Heparin can also downregulate the responsiveness of the thrombomodulin–protein C system. Reactivation can also result from the continuous generation of coagulation substrates in the proximal portion and midportion of the coagulation cascade, resulting in thrombin generation after the discontinuation of heparin.[78] The most likely mechanism causing the rebound effect, however, is a persisting active state of the disease, reflecting the inability of heparin to inactivate thrombin bound to fibrin.[81] Bound thrombin continues to activate platelets and generate new thrombin by activating factors V and VIII to cause thrombus growth.[81] Entrapped factor X_a is also inaccessible to heparin and may facilitate reactivation of disease. Some evidence of this rebound reactivation of thrombin was also described after the discontinuation of argatroban, a direct thrombin inhibitor, although after a very short, 4-h duration of treatment.[82]

Discontinuation of heparin is associated with an increase in fibrinopeptide A and prothrombin fragment$_{1+2}$ plasma levels.[83]

Low-Molecular-Weight Heparins

Heparin is a mixture of sulfated polysaccharides with an average molecular weight of 15,000 D. Low-molecular-weight heparins are depolymerized fragments of heparin with molecular weights varying between 4000 and 6500 D. Shorter-chain fragments have a reduced ability to inhibit thrombin but are capable of inhibiting factor X_a.[84] The various commercially available low-molecular-weight heparins inhibit factor X_a in relation to thrombin in ratios varying between 4:1 to 2:1. Also, low-molecular-weight heparins bind less avidly to plasma proteins and endothelial cells, thereby providing greater bioavailability and a longer plasma half-life and resulting in a more predictable anticoagulant response and fewer hemorrhagic complications. This allows once- or twice-a-day subcutaneous injections; because of the favorable antithrombotic-to-hemorrhagic ratio, little or no monitoring is required.

The low-molecular-weight heparins have shown advantages over unfractioned heparins for the prevention and management of venous thrombosis.[84] Experience with their use in treating arterial thromboembolic disease is limited. In a single-blind randomized study of 219 patients with angina at rest in the previous 24 h, recurrent angina occurred in 21% of patients treated with low-molecular-weight heparins plus aspirin, in comparison with 44% of patients treated with standard heparin plus aspirin and 59% of patients treated with aspirin alone ($p = .002$); and myocardial infarction in 0% vs. 6% and 9.5%, respectively.[85] Other pilot trials using low-molecular-weight heparins in unstable angina are near completion as of this writing and should provide important information on the usefulness of low-molecular-weight heparins in treating unstable angina. The potential benefit of enoxaparin is being investigated by the TIMI group.

Oral Anticoagulants

Oral anticoagulants are inappropriate for acute use because of their delayed onset of action. Over the long term, they have been

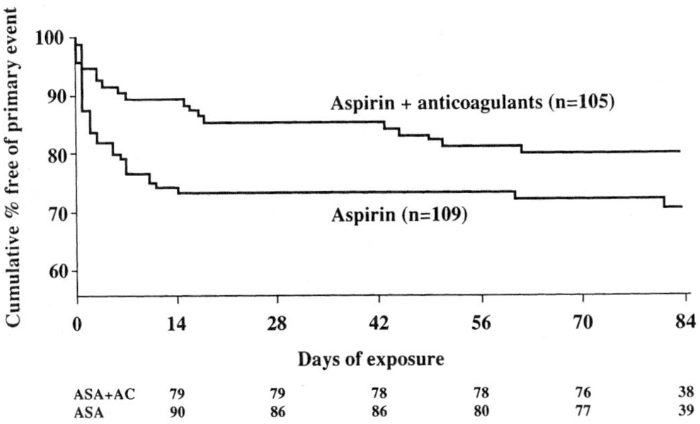

Figure 6–6. Cumulative percentages of patients receiving aspirin alone (ASA) or aspirin plus anticoagulation (ASA + AC) who were free from death, myocardial infarction, and recurrent ischemia. (From Cohen M, Adams PC, Parry G, et al: Combination antithrombotic therapy in unstable rest angina and non–Q-wave infarction in nonoption aspirin users. Primary end points analysis from the ATACS trial. Circulation 1994; 89:81–88.)

proven useful for secondary prevention of acute myocardial infarction.[86, 87] For unstable angina, only a few studies with small sample sizes have been carried out.[88–90] Wood, in 1961, published the results of a trial in which alternate patients received anticoagulants.[88] The study was stopped prematurely after enrollment of the first 40 patients because of striking benefits observed with anticoagulants; subsequent control patients were enrolled on the basis of a contraindication to the use of anticoagulants. After 2 months, myocardial infarction had occurred in 3% and death in 2% of the 100 patients who received anticoagulants and in 22% and 16%, respectively, of the 50 control patients. In an early observational study of 360 patients, the mortality rate at 3 months was 9.5% in patients treated with anticoagulants and 23.7% in other patients.[89] A report on the use of anticoagulants in an open-labeled, randomized study was published in 1986. Cardiac events at 6 months occurred in 12% of the patients who received anticoagulants, in comparison with 34% of controls ($p < .05$).[90] The use of warfarin titrated to an international normalized ratio (INR) of 2.0 to 3.0 is a rational long-term therapeutic alternative for patients intolerant to aspirin.

Combination of Aspirin and Anticoagulants

In a study published in 1994, patients admitted for unstable angina or non–Q wave myocardial infarction with no previous aspirin use were randomized to aspirin alone or to the combination of aspirin and heparin.[91] Heparin was administered intravenously and discontinued once adequate oral anticoagulation to an INR of 2.0 to 3.0 with warfarin (Coumadin) was achieved. No clinical reactivation was observed with this therapeutic regimen, and after 14 days, there was a significant reduction in the combined endpoint of death, myocardial infarction, and recurrent ischemia with the combination treatment versus aspirin alone (10.5% vs. 27%; $p = .004$). The benefits were maintained after 12 weeks (Fig. 6–6). A pooled analysis of the three studies in which aspirin was compared with aspirin plus heparin revealed a significant reduction in fatal and nonfatal myocardial infarction to a relative risk of 0.44 with 95% confidence limits of 0.21–0.93 (Fig. 6–7).[6]

Another trial published in 1994 provided data inconsistent with the event rate usually observed in unstable angina. In this trial, 285 patients were randomized to aPTT-titrated heparin plus aspirin, 150 mg a day, or to aspirin alone.[92] The total ischemic time determined by Holter recording was reduced by 41% with the combination treatment; this difference was not statistically significant. Death or myocardial infarction occurred in 82 patients (29%), in a similar disproportionately high rate in the two study groups, probably in relation to non–Q wave myocardial infarction already present at admission.

In ongoing trials, the potential benefits of the combination of low-dose oral anticoagulant and low-dose aspirin are being compared with the benefits of aspirin alone. Many studies address secondary prevention of acute myocardial infarction, and one, the Organization to Assess Strategies for Ischemic Syndromes (OASIS), assesses long-term management after an episode of unstable angina. In one trial (platelet-thrombin), the investigators are also studying the combination of therapeutic doses of warfarin (Coumadin) and low-dose aspirin vs. aspirin alone or warfarin alone, in higher risk patients with unstable angina who have previously undergone coronary arterial or venous bypass graft surgery.

Except in high-risk patients in whom prior treatment has failed, the combination of aspirin and warfarin is not recommended until the results of ongoing investigations are known.

ANTI-ISCHEMIC THERAPY

The clinical course of unstable angina is often marked by recurrent symptoms despite therapy. These recurrent symptoms have a wide range of manifestations, including atypical chest pain, typical angina, and angina with objective evidence of myocardial ischemia manifested by transient ST-T wave changes during pain or rapid hemodynamic deterioration. Recurrent chest pain can occur as an isolated event or can be repetitive. These events often cannot be assessed as

Authors	No. pts	MI / death: Aspirin	MI / death: Aspirin + heparin
Théroux et al.[67]	243	3.3%	1.6%
RISC [68]	399	3.7%	1.4%
ATACS [91]	214	8.3%	3.8%
Total	856	4.8%	2.1%

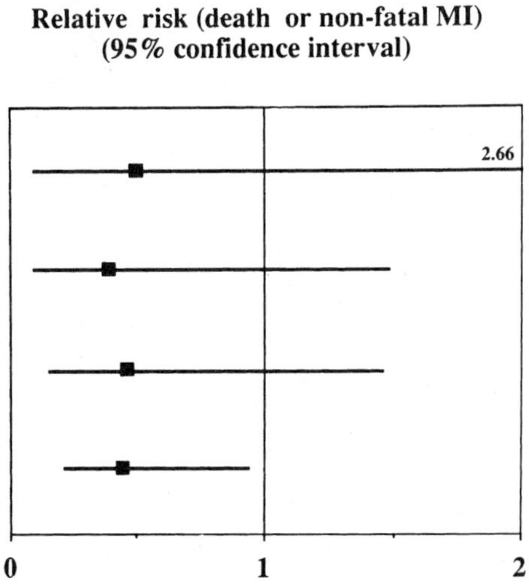

Figure 6–7. Pooled analysis of relative risk and 95% confidence limits of the risk of death and myocardial infarction (MI) with aspirin plus heparin versus aspirin alone. (Adapted from Cohen M, Adams PC, Parry G, et al: Combination antithrombotic therapy in unstable rest angina and non–Q-wave infarction in nonprior aspirin users. Primary end points analysis from the ATACS trial. Circulation 1994; 89:81–88.)

TABLE 6–1. GRADING SYSTEM FOR THE EVALUATION OF THE SEVERITY OF RECURRENT CHEST PAIN

Class 0	No recurrent angina or angina equivalents
Class 1	Occasional pain that does not necessitate modification of treatment
Class 2	Recurrent pain and/or ischemia that necessitates intensification of medical treatment
Class 3	Recurrent angina/ischemia that persists despite intensive medical treatment
Class 4	Increasingly severe chest pain or hemodynamic deterioration, which necessitates intervention

Adapted from Théroux P, Waters D: Diagnosis and management of patients with unstable angina. *In* Schlant RC, Alexander RW (eds): Hurst's The Heart, 8th ed, pp 1083–1106. New York: McGraw-Hill, 1994.

objectively as death and myocardial infarction; they are nevertheless clinically relevant because they mandate more intensive treatment. A gradation in severity can also be described, the most severe being manifested by hemodynamic deterioration and transient ischemic electrocardiographic changes. A classification that can be useful in clinical practice and in clinical trials is described in Table 6–1.[93] Classes III and IV in this schema represent recurrent and refractory ischemia, are important predictors of a worse prognosis, and mandate more aggressive management. As previously discussed, clinical manifestations of unstable angina can be controlled by heparin during the acute phase[67] and by aspirin during and after the acute phase.[69]

The antianginal therapy currently available includes nitroglycerin, beta blockers, and calcium channel antagonists. These drugs act by favorably influencing the balance between myocardial oxygen supply and myocardial oxygen needs. They are described in more detail in Chapter 2. Their discussion in this section is limited to the specific applications in unstable angina.

Nitroglycerin

Nitroglycerin has been used increasingly since the mid-1980s for the management of acute coronary syndromes.[94] Its mechanism of action was elucidated with the recognition of the physiologic effects of nitric oxide to produce venous and arterial dilatation and to inhibit platelet aggregation.[8, 95] Nitroglycerin is exogenous nitric oxide with arterial and venous dilatory properties that can be useful in the treatment of stable angina by reducing the loading conditions on the heart and by producing coronary arterial dilatation. Additional benefit can be obtained in unstable angina, in which variable degrees of coronary constriction and vasospasm are found.[96] The antiplatelet effects of nitroglycerin may also be additive to those of aspirin, but to what extent they translate into clinical benefit is still unclear.[97–99]

Nitroglycerin is now commonly used in the management of unstable angina. It was also widely used during the acute phase of myocardial infarction; the ISIS-4,[100] GISSI-3,[101] and the Enquête de Prévention Secondaire de l'Infarctus du Myocarde (ESPRIM) trials[102] could not, however, document that oral nitrates resulted in improved survival. Large clinical trials in unstable angina are lacking; the existing trials have been limited to a few early uncontrolled studies, involving fewer than 100 patients and various dose regimens administered for variable periods of time (Table 6–2).[103–109] The results of these trials have been inconsistent, although most suggested a moderate reduction in the incidence of recurrent ischemia.[110] None, however, showed that nitroglycerin could reduce death or myocardial infarction. Despite this paucity of investigation, the clinical experience with nitroglycerin is favorable, and side effects are self-limited. Caution is needed to avoid bradycardia and hypotension, particularly in patients with hypovolemia, right ventricular infarction, or pericardial disease. Nitroglycerin is indicated for the immediate relief of chest pain, prophylactically when the clinical presentation is more severe, and when angina recurs. The medication can be administered intravenously, transdermally, or orally. The superiority of one form of administration over others in unstable angina has not been demonstrated. Intravenously, nitroglycerin is initiated at a rate of 5–15 μg/min. The infusion is increased by 5–10 μg/min every 5–10 minutes until relief of symptoms, side effects, or hypotension develops. Transdermally, it is applied by systems delivering 0.4–0.8 mg/h.

Tolerance of the hemodynamic effects of nitroglycerin rapidly develops within 12–24 h.[111, 112] For this reason, it is recommended that the patch application be discontinued for 8–12 h per day and that increasing the rate of an intravenous infusion every 12–24 h be considered. Paradoxically, despite the development of tolerance in many patients, the discontinuation of nitroglycerin can be associated with a recurrence of symptoms and of ischemia.[113]

Beta Blockers

Of the antianginal drugs, beta blockers reduce myocardial oxygen needs most reproducibly; they slow heart rate and decrease myocardial contractility. These drugs reduce mortality in myocardial infarction, both during the acute phase and during follow-up.[114–116] By extension, it can be assumed that beta blockers help patients with unstable angina and no contraindication to their use. A review of five trials totaling 4700 patients with "threatened myocardial infarction" revealed a 13% relative reduction in the risk of developing myocardial infarction, from 32% to 29% ($p < .04$), which suggests that patients with prolonged chest pain or non–Q wave myocardial infarction could benefit from beta blockers.[117] Results of a subset analysis in one trial suggested protection against myocardial infarction in patients who had not previously received beta blockade therapy.[118] Beta blockers were also prescribed in most patients en-

TABLE 6–2. INTRAVENOUS NITROGLYCERIN IN UNSTABLE ANGINA*

Authors	Year	No. Patients	Dose (mg/min)	Pain Relief: Complete	Pain Relief: Partial (% Patients)	Pain Relief: None	Duration (Days)
Dauwe et al[103]	1979	14	9–180	—	—	—	6.7
Mikolich et al[104]	1980	45	5–267	0	89	11	—
Page et al[105]	1981	67	12–50	63	32	5	7.4
DePace et al[106]	1982	20	15–326	70	15	15	—
Squire et al[107]	1982	42	225–390	0	45	55	4.3
Roubin et al[108]	1982	16	85–1020	38	62	0	3.2
Kaplan et al[109]	1983	35	50–350	71	23	6	5.5

*Review of some clinical studies published on the use of intravenous nitroglycerin in unstable angina.
From American Journal of Cardiology Supplement 1987; 60(15):31H–34H.

rolled in the clinical trials that have documented the efficacy of aspirin and heparin in unstable angina. A definitive, large placebo-controlled trial in unstable angina is, however, lacking. In the study by Telford and Wilson, heparin, but not atenolol, significantly reduced death and myocardial infarction.[74] The benefits of beta blockers in preventing recurrent ischemia, however, were documented in most trials.[119–120] Impressive results are at times observed in patients presenting with chest pain and a hyperadrenergic state with sinus tachycardia and hypertension. Intravenous beta blockade can then result in prompt relief of symptoms, which stresses the importance of an excess in oxygen demand in some patients with compromised supply.

Contraindications to beta blockers are bronchial asthma, congestive heart failure, hypotension, sinus bradycardia, and atrioventricular block. Oral administration is adequate in the majority of patients, but intravenous administration (see Chapter 2) is preferred when severe chest pain and tachycardia are present at rest. The initial dose is adjusted to the clinical situation, and the clinical response is used to guide subsequent titration. Metoprolol (50–200 mg/day) and atenolol (50–200 mg/day) are most frequently prescribed because of the experience gained in clinical trials. Other beta blockers without intrinsic sympathetic activity are also probably adequate. Esmolol (50–250 μg/kg/min), because of its short half-life, can be useful when side effects are of concern.

Calcium Channel Antagonists

Calcium channel antagonists possess negative chronotropic and inotropic effects and are peripheral arterial and coronary vasodilators. The magnitude of these effects varies with the different agents. Dihydropyridines are more potent vasodilators and can lead to a reflex tachycardia.[121] The initial enthusiasm manifested for calcium channel antagonist in the treatment of unstable angina, based on the role of vasospasm in this disease[96] and documented benefit in Prinzmetal variant angina,[122] was not supported by the results of clinical trials. Trials performed with nifedipine were interrupted prematurely because of an excess of cardiac events in treated patients; for example, Muller and associates reported 7 deaths among 89 patients treated for 2 weeks, in comparison with none of 82 patients who received placebo ($p = .02$).[123] In the Holland Interuniversity trial, nifedipine alone increased the risk of myocardial infarction or recurrent ischemia in relation to placebo by 16%, metoprolol decreased it by 24%, and the combination decreased it by 20%.[118] The addition of calcium channel antagonists to the treatment of symptomatic patients despite the use of nitrates and beta blockers can help prevent symptoms. Diltiazem and propranolol, directly compared in a randomized trial, achieved similar results with regard to recurrent ischemia, the need for surgery, myocardial infarction, and death.[124] Intravenous diltiazem at a dose of 10 mg per h in two small studies resulted in less frequent ST segment depression than did intravenous nitroglycerin.[125, 126] The new generation of calcium channel antagonists has not been evaluated in the treatment of unstable angina.

In summary, nitroglycerin, calcium channel antagonists, and beta blockers are useful in unstable angina for preventing recurrent angina with additive benefit when patients receive double- and triple-drug therapy. Dihydropyridines used alone have a deleterious effect. Beta blockers can be useful in the treatment of impending myocardial infarction by providing myocardial protection through prevention of tachycardia and hypertension. The benefit of nitroglycerin remains to be investigated more thoroughly.

REVASCULARIZATION PROCEDURES

Coronary Angiography

The use of coronary angiography in the evaluation of unstable angina varies widely among countries, hospitals, and physicians. The extent of use is notably influenced by the availability of a cardiac catheterization laboratory. Angiography is indicated in patients with persisting symptoms who are receiving medical therapy, in order to investigate the possibility of coronary angioplasty or bypass surgery. Other higher risk situations with hemodynamic instability, left ventricular dysfunction, extensive ST-T changes, and ischemia at low-level exercise testing are also indications. Patients with symptoms suggesting restenosis after coronary angioplasty are also catheterized with a view to redilatation of the culprit lesion. Other indications such as previous bypass surgery and non–Q wave myocardial infarction necessitate individualized patient assessment. Coronary angiography is also indicated for diagnostic purposes in some patients and for evaluating prognosis in others (see Fig. 6–8). The most extreme situation is routine catheterization for all patients except when a contraindication is present or the coronary anatomy is already known. Routine catheterization leads to more frequent use of interventional procedures.

Interventional Procedures

By angiographic criteria, most patients with unstable angina would be eligible for a revascularization procedure. Representative statistics suggest that one third of patients are referred for angioplasty, one third for bypass surgery, and one third for medical therapy. The choice between balloon angioplasty and surgery is influenced by many factors, including locations and shapes of lesions, number of diseased vessels, left ventricular function, risk of the respective procedures, and often by the patient's or the doctor's preference. Determining the appropriateness of the indications for these interventions in individual patients, as well as their timing, requires discrimination and judgment.

The indication can be based on symptoms or on anatomy. The distinction is important from both a clinical and an investigational perspective. Refractory angina and ischemia are markers of a worse prognosis and should be corrected whenever possible to improve prognosis and relieve symptoms. Lesions at risk that create a large area of ischemic myocardium and are accompanied by symptomatic left ventricular dysfunction necessitate treatment. Surgery is also indicated when it can prolong life, such as in patients with left main artery disease or three-vessel disease with left ventricular dysfunction.

Only a few trials have compared bypass surgery with medical treatment, and coronary angioplasty has not been directly compared with medical therapy. The TIMI 3B trial compared an early invasive strategy with an early conservative strategy (see pp. 120–121).[55]

Coronary Bypass Surgery

In an early pilot study published in 1978, Pugh and colleagues randomized 27 patients to medical or surgical treatment; the results, 1.5 years later, were similar except for more frequent relief of symptoms with surgery.[127] The National Cooperative Study Group enrolled 288 patients in a randomized study; the in-hospital mortality rates were 5% in the surgical group and 3% in the medical group (nonsignificant), and myocardial infarction rates were 17% and 8%, respectively ($p < .05$).[128] Severe angina during the first year was more common among medically treated patients and resulted in a crossover to surgery in 19% of patients at 1 year. The mortality rates at 1 year were the same in the two groups.

The most recent and largest trial was the Veterans Administration Cooperative Study.[129] It involved 468 men, excluding patients with myocardial infarction within the previous 3 months, previous bypass surgery, left main artery disease, and ejection fraction below 30%. Events were counted from the day of surgery performed 9.3 days after randomization. After 2 years, nonfatal myocardial infarction had occurred in 11.7% of patients treated surgically and in 12.2% of patients treated medically (nonsignificant); the survival rates were

TABLE 6–3. RESULTS OF CORONARY ANGIOPLASTY IN UNSTABLE ANGINA

			Major Complications			Follow-Up Events		
Clinical Status	**No. Patients**	**Success Rate (%)**	**Death (%)**	**MI (%)**	**Acute Surgery (%)**	**Death (%)**	**MI (%)**	**Angina (%)**
Initially stabilized	1036	89	0.3	5.1	5.8	0.7	1.4	27
Refractory ischemia	1438	85	1.3	6.3	6.8	2.7	2.9	28
Early post-infarction angina	634	88	1.1	6.3	6.5	1.3	2.5	22
Stable angina	10,129	92	0.7	1.6	2.5	—	—	—

Abbreviation: MI, myocardial infarction.

Adapted from de Feyter PJ, Serruys PW: Percutaneous transluminal coronary angioplasty for unstable angina. *In* Topol EJ (ed): Textbook of Interventional Cardiology, 2nd ed, pp 274–291. Philadelphia: WB Saunders, 1994.

also the same. Subset analyses, however, revealed a favorable trend for better survival with surgery among patients with three-vessel disease and significant improvement in patients with abnormal left ventricular function. The 5-year survival rates with three-vessel disease were 89% with surgery and 75% with medical treatment ($p <$ .02). A lower ejection fraction analyzed as a continuous variable negatively influenced survival in the medical cohort ($p = .004$) but not in the surgical cohort. Survival rates among patients with ejection fractions between .30 and .58 were 86% with surgery and 73% without; patients with higher ejection fractions tended to do better with medical therapy. In this study, as in others, crossover to surgery was common: 34% of patients at 2 years. The perioperative mortality rates were higher among the crossover patients (10.3%) than among patients randomized to surgery (3.1%). Other benefits of surgery in this trial included a better quality of life, as assessed by subjective evaluation, by exercise tolerance, and by cardiac medication used.[130] The working status, however, did not differ between the two groups, and the less common need for rehospitalization observed early among patients undergoing surgery disappeared with time.

Kaiser and coworkers reviewed 14 reports of patients who underwent operations for unstable angina.[131] The operative mortality rate was 3.7%, and the rate of perioperative myocardial infarction was 9.9%. Angina relief was excellent, and by 7–10 years, 80% of patients were asymptomatic or had only minimal symptoms. The annualized rate of myocardial infarction was 3%–4%. In this review, risk factors for morbidity and mortality were the same as for stable angina.

Coronary Angioplasty

De Feyter and Serruys reviewed the published results on coronary angioplasty in unstable angina (Table 6–3).[132] Although the success rate approached 90%, which was close to the rate observed in stable angina, acute complications (including myocardial infarction, need for emergency surgery, in-hospital mortality, and need for repeat angioplasty) occurred two to four times more frequently. The risk for these events may reach 10% and extend through the follow-up period; 31% of patients with unstable angina experienced an event by 12 months, in comparison with 16% of patients with stable angina. The best results were obtained in patients with stabilized angina. The higher complication rate correlated with the presence of an intracoronary thrombus.[133, 134] Myler and associates reported both Q and non–Q wave myocardial infarction in 6.5% of patients, emergency surgery in 9.4%, and follow-up mortality in 5.8% with the procedure performed early (within 1 week), as opposed to respective rates of 1.6%, 4.8%, and 1.7% when angioplasty was deferred 2–4 weeks after the acute episode.[133]

The TIMI 3B study randomized patients to rt-PA or placebo and to early invasive or early conservative strategy.[55] All patients received intravenous heparin at therapeutic doses. The protocol-dictated angioplasty was performed 18–48 h after randomization. The complication rates of early procedures were similar to the complication rates associated with delayed procedures in patients randomized to the conservative strategy and catheterized because of recurrent ischemia, ST segment depression on a 24-h ECG monitor, or unsatisfactory

TABLE 6–4. EVENT RATES IN THE TIMI 3B TRIAL AT 42 DAYS

Variable Studied	**Early Invasive Strategy (*n*=740) (%)**	**Early Conservative Strategy (*n*=733) (%)**
No patients catheterized	98	64
Revascularization	61	49
PTCA	38	26
CABG	25	24
Results of PTCA		
Improved artery	96	96
Nonfatal infarction	2.9	3.6
Abrupt closure	2.2	4.1
Emergency CABG	0.7	0.5
Death within 24 h	0.4	0.5
Endpoints at 42 days		
Angina class III or IV	7.6	9.5
Myocardial infarction	5.1	5.7
Death	2.4	2.5
Readmission	7.8	14.1

Abbreviations: TIMI, Thrombolysis in Myocardial Ischemia (study); PTCA, percutaneous transluminal coronary angioplasty; CABG, coronary artery bypass graft.

From TIMI 3B Investigators: Effects of tissue plasminogen activator and a comparison of early invasive and conservative strategies in unstable angina and non–Q-wave myocardial infarction. Circulation 1994; 89:1545–1556.

results on a predischarge stress thallium exercise test. The event rates of this trial are shown in Table 6–4. Early invasive therapy resulted in a higher rate of interventions (by protocol design) (61% vs. 49%) but did not significantly influence the endpoints of death and myocardial infarction. Rehospitalization, residual angina, and the use of antianginal drugs were all more common in the conservative group.

On the basis of these observations, an initial period of stabilization is recommended for 24–72 hours after admission with administration of aspirin and intravenous heparin. Catheterization is then performed or the patient is risk-stratified, through the use of a provocative test for ischemia. Medical therapy is intensified if symptoms recur. Refractory angina and ischemia during medical treatment are indications for more urgent catheterization, as is hemodynamic deterioration. Balloon counterpulsation is recommended in a more unstable state as a bridge procedure to cardiac catheterization, balloon angioplasty, and bypass surgery. In view of the higher rate of rehospitalization and greater use of antianginal drugs in the early conservative strategy in TIMI 3B, many clinicians believe that it is more cost effective to pursue an early invasive strategy even in patients whose symptoms are initially controlled medically.

Significant progress has been made in high-risk angioplasty with the addition of c7E3 (ReoPro, the Fab fragments of a chimeric monoclonal antibody to the platelet membrane receptor GP II_b/III_a) used in conjunction with aspirin and heparin. The Evaluation of c7E3 in the Prevention of Ischemic Complications (EPIC) trial randomized 2097 patients to c7E3 administered as a bolus, c7E3 administered as a single bolus followed by an infusion for 12 h, or placebo.[135] The acute complications of death, myocardial infarction, and the need for a reintervention procedure occurred in 12.8% of control patients and 11.4% of patients administered the single bolus but in only 8.3% of patients administered the bolus plus infusion; the relative risk was 0.62 (95% confidence limits, 0.44–0.87). The benefits were greater when the indication for angioplasty was unstable angina.[136] ReoPro has been approved for clinical use in high-risk angioplasty. The definition of high risk in the EPIC trial included (1) acute evolving myocardial infarction within 12 h after the onset of symptoms that necessitated direct or rescue percutaneous intervention; (2) early postinfarction angina or unstable angina with at least two episodes of angina at rest associated with changes on the resting ECG during the previous 24 h, despite medical therapy; and (3) angiographic characteristics indicating high risk. The dose of ReoPro in EPIC was a bolus of 0.25 mg/kg followed by an infusion of 10 μg/min for 12 h. Heparin was discontinued after 12 h. It is likely that earlier discontinuation of heparin could have reduced the high local bleeding rate observed in this study.

NEW ANTITHROMBOTIC THERAPEUTIC APPROACHES

c7E3 is one of the new antithrombotic agents being developed for clinical use in acute coronary syndromes that may offer advantages over current treatment. Aspirin does not block platelet adhesion and platelet aggregation and is ineffective against thrombin, which is the most potent stimulant to platelet aggregation in acute coronary syndromes. Heparin has a narrow risk/benefit ratio[137] and limited efficacy on the prothrombinase complex and on thrombin bound to fibrin, to fibrin degradation products, and to the extracellular matrix.[81] It is also inhibited by acute-phase proteins and platelet-released factors. Ticlopidine and oral anticoagulants have delayed onset of action, which limits their usefulness.

The two new classes of thromboactive drugs now being evaluated in acute coronary syndromes are the direct thrombin inhibitors, of which hirudin is the prototype,[138] and the inhibitors of the platelet membrane receptor GP II_b/III_a, of which c7E3 is the prototype.[139] Recombinant hirudin and a synthetic peptide composed of 21 amino acids, Hirulog,[140] block both the anion-binding site and the catalytic site of thrombin. Argatroban, derived from L-arginine, and efegatran and inogatran, two small peptides, block the catalytic site. The phase 2 trials with this class of drugs have yielded interesting results.[141–144] Recombinant hirudin is now being studied in the Global Utilization of Streptokinase and Tissue Plasminogen Activator for Occluded Arteries (GUSTO 2) trial, which involves over 10,000 patients with acute myocardial infarction or unstable angina. Synthetic inhibitors of the platelet membrane receptors that possess the RGD sequence that interferes with the binding of fibrinogen to the platelet receptor GPIIb/IIIa have been introduced. Integrelin is a cycloheptapeptide, and tirofiban (MK-383) and lamifiban (RO 44-9883) are nonpeptidic tyrosine-like compounds. The results of phase 2 trials with these drugs have been promising, with 75% reductions in the risk of fatal and nonfatal myocardial infarction[145] and in the risk of refractory and recurrent ischemia.[145, 146] The safety profile of these new inhibitors also appears favorable. A phase 3 trial in high-risk percutaneous transluminal coronary angioplasty (PTCA) has been completed with integrelin, and phase 3 trials are now ongoing with lamifiban in acute myocardial infarction and unstable angina and with tirofiban in unstable angina and coronary angioplasty.

Global Strategy

General Measures

Extensive practical guidelines on diagnosis and management of unstable angina have been published by a panel of experts convened by the Agency for Health Care Policy and Research and by the National Heart, Lung, and Blood Institute.[147] Patients presenting with chest pain or new symptoms are first evaluated for low, intermediate, or high likelihood of coronary artery disease, on the basis of the medical history and the characteristics of the symptoms, and for short-term risk of the disease, on the basis of the momentum of symptoms, the ECG, and the hemodynamic stability (see Fig. 6–2). Patients with a low likelihood of coronary artery disease and low risk are rapidly investigated in the emergency room or on an outpatient basis. Patients with a high probability of disease or definitive evidence of coronary artery disease are best evaluated in the hospital, preferably in the coronary care unit when adverse risk features such as frequent or prolonged bouts of chest pain and hemodynamic compromise are present. Patients are considered high risk during this initial evaluation until shown otherwise. General measures to ensure well-being of patients are applied, such as relief of pain, control of anxiety, adequate oxygenation, and attention to other problems such as constipation and insomnia.

Figure 6–8, adapted from these guidelines, proposes a progression from noninvasive to invasive strategies on the basis of risk appraised by clinical characteristics, early response to treatment, and markers of myocardial ischemia.

Drug Therapy

The administration of aspirin is an immediate measure when an acute coronary syndrome is suspected. There exist very few contraindications to its use, at least acutely. The initial bolus dose is 160–360 mg orally of a nonenteric formulation for rapid and complete inhibition of thromboxane A_2 generation. Subsequent doses depend on the formulations available. Low doses of 80 mg per day are as effective as high doses and cause fewer side effects. Heparin is also indicated in hospitalized patients unless the diagnosis is unlikely or the patient's angina abates rapidly and does not recur. An initial bolus of 5000 units is administered, followed by an intravenous infusion of 1000 units per hour, titrated after 6 h to achieve aPTTs 1.5 to 2.5 times higher than the control values. The

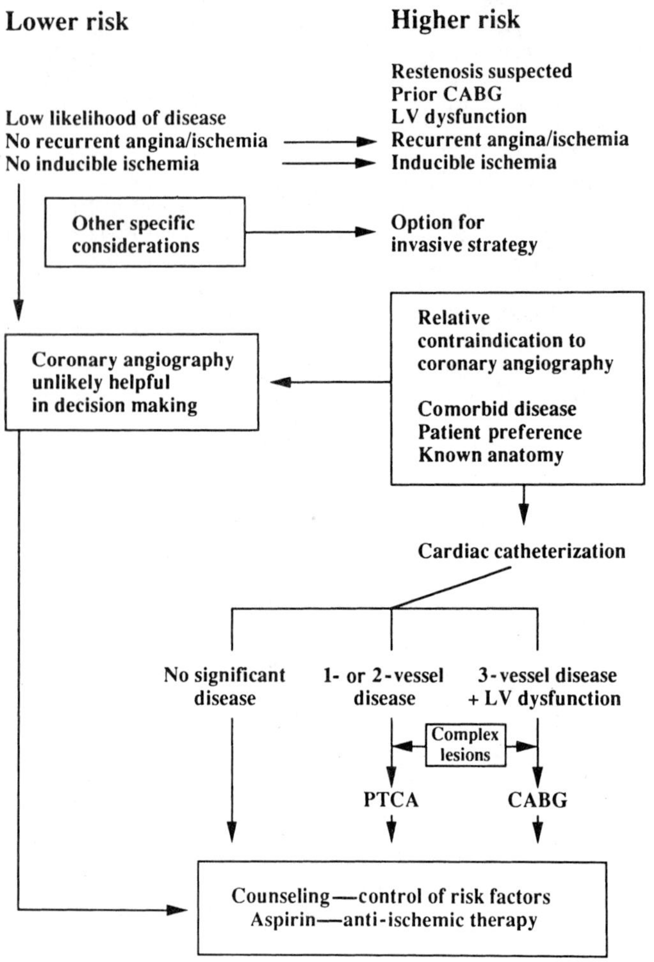

Figure 6–8. Progression from noninvasive to invasive strategy. The original recommendations propose an immediate orientation to early noninvasive and early noninvasive strategy with crossover between the two strategies, depending on various influences. (Modified from the U.S. Department of Health and Human Services, Public Health Service: Unstable Angina: Diagnosis and Management. Clinical Practice Guideline Number 10 [AHCPR Publication No. 94-0602]. Washington, DC: Agency for Health Care Policy and Research, 1994.)

aPTT should be rechecked 6 h after changes in the infusion rate. The achievement of optimal hemodynamic conditions is also an early goal of therapy. Sinus tachycardia and hypertension are corrected by the administration of an oral or intravenous beta blocker, in the absence of a contraindication. Nitroglycerin is indicated when chest pain is present, and intravenous morphine is indicated if the pain persists despite the administration of nitroglycerin. Congestive heart failure is treated by a diuretic and by intravenous nitroglycerin. These general measures are promptly instituted while a general patient work-up is conducted, including complete medical history, physical examination, and laboratory tests to rule out a cause that could have provoked or aggravated angina.

Close follow-up in the hospital is critical for the management of patients; the recurrence of chest pain is an indication for the intensification of medical treatment. A 12-lead ECG is obtained if chest pain recurs, to help evaluate the presence, severity, and extent of ischemia. The aPTT may then also be rechecked to ensure adequate anticoagulation. If the chest pain is prolonged, serum cardiac markers

TABLE 6–5. ASSESSMENT OF RISK FACTORS IN THE PATIENT UNDERGOING SURGICAL OR NONSURGICAL REVASCULARIZATION

Risk Factor	Assessment	Therapeutic Goal
Elevated LDL cholesterol	Fasting lipid profile	<100 mg/dL (<2.6 mmol/L)
Decreased HDL cholesterol	Fasting lipid profile	>35 mg/dL (>0.9 mmol/L)
Hypertension	Blood pressures confirmed on two visits	<140/90 mm Hg
Physical inactivity	Interview	>20 minutes of physical activity or level walking, 1½–2 miles/day, 3 times per week as a minimum
Smoking	Interview	Complete cessation
Obesity	Body weight for height	<130% of ideal body weight
Diabetes	Fasting blood glucose	<140 mg/dL
Stress	Interview	Improved coping skills

Abbreviations: LDL, low-density lipoprotein; HDL, high-density lipoprotein.

From Pearson T, Rapaport E, Criqui M, et al: Optimal risk factor management in the patient after coronary revascularization. A statement for healthcare professionals from the American Heart Association Writing Group. Circulation 1994; 90:3125–3133.

are measured to exclude a myocardial infarction. Refractory angina during medical therapy prompts cardiac catheterization and possibly subsequent interventional procedures, if indicated. Patient counseling is an important part of the medical strategy, and the control of risk factors is an essential component of treatment. Over the long term, the medical strategy includes secondary prevention of recurrent unstable angina, myocardial infarction, and progression of coronary artery disease.

Long-Term Management and Secondary Prevention After Myocardial Revascularization

Although myocardial revascularization procedures are very effective in relieving symptoms and are sometimes life-saving, the interventions are not without risk and may be beneficial only transiently. They can also create a new disease, and they do not modify the basic mechanisms of atherosclerosis. The occlusion rates of vein grafts are 10% at 1 month, 20% at 1 year, and 50% at 10 years.[148] Acute occlusion associated with venous graft angioplasty occurs three times as frequently when the procedure is performed during the acute phase of unstable angina or myocardial infarction than in a more stable state,[132] and the restenosis rate after 6 months may also be higher (>40%) in these circumstances.[149, 150]

Aspirin prevents early graft thrombosis and the thrombotic complications associated with coronary angioplasty and coronary artery bypass graft surgery. The drug should be initiated before or within 48 h after surgery.[151–153] Aspirin doses of 100 mg per day have been shown to be as effective as higher doses.[153] Preoperative aspirin is safe but associated with increased hemorrhagic complications and with more frequent need for reintervention because of tamponade.[152] Ticlopidine, 250 mg per day, is also effective and is a valid alternative to aspirin.[154] Aspirin, used before angioplasty, reduces the incidence of acute occlusion and of periprocedural Q and non–Q wave myocardial infarction. It does not, however, prevent restenosis.

Because patients undergoing revascularization have coronary artery disease, an aggressive program to control risk factors is indicated, to prevent progression of the disease. The presence of risk factors has a negative impact on subsequent morbidity and mortality. Continued smoking after the intervention doubles the risk of death 10 years later.[155] Other lifestyle modification measures such as exercise programs and behavioral modifications are associated with a 25% reduction in subsequent coronary events. Interventions to reduce high levels of blood cholesterol delay progression of coronary artery disease and decrease the risk of fatal and nonfatal myocardial infarction by as much as 25%. The program recommended by the American Heart Association for the control of risk factors in patients undergoing revascularization is described in Table 6–5.[156]

REFERENCES

1. Falk E: Unstable angina with fatal outcome. Dynamic coronary thrombosis leading to infarction and/or sudden death: autopsy evidence of recurrent mural thrombosis with peripheral embolization culminating in total vascular occlusion. Circulation 1985; 71:699-708.
2. Davies MJ, Thomas AC: Thrombosis and acute coronary-artery lesions in sudden ischemic death. N Engl J Med 1984; 310:1137–1140.
3. Fuster V, Badimon L, Badimon JJ, et al: The pathogenesis of coronary artery disease and the acute coronary syndromes. N Engl J Med 1992; 326:310–318.
4. Vu TK, Wheaton VI, Hung DT, et al: Domains specifying thrombin-receptor interaction. Nature 1991; 353:674–677.
5. Ginsberg MH, Loftus JC, Plow EF: Cytoadhesins, integrins, and platelets. Thromb Haemost 1988; 59:1–6.
6. Plow EF, Srouji AH, Meyer D, et al: Evidence that three adhesive proteins interact with a common recognition site on activated platelets. J Biol Chem 1984; 259:5388–5391.
7. Moncada S, Vane JP: Arachidonic acid metabolites and the interaction between platelets and blood-vessel wall. N Engl J Med 1979; 300:1142–1147.
8. Palmer RMJ, Ferrige AG, Moncada S: Nitric oxide release accounts for the biological activity of endothelium-derived relaxing factor. Nature 1987; 327:524–526.
9. Broze GJ, Warren LA, Novotny WF, et al: The lipoprotein-associated coagulation inhibitor that inhibits the factor VII–tissue factor complex also inhibits factor X_a: Insights into its possible mechanism of action. Blood 1988; 71:335–343.
10. Esmond CT: Protein C: biochemistry, physiology, and clinical implications. Blood 1983; 62:1155–1158.
11. Braunwald E, Jones RH, Mark DB, et al: Diagnosing and managing unstable angina. Circulation 1994; 90:613–622.
12. Gazes PC, Mobley EM Jr, Faris HM Jr, et al: Preinfarctional (unstable) angina: a prospective study—ten year follow-up: prognostic significance of electrocardiographic changes. Circulation 1973; 48:331–337.
13. Mulcahy R, Daly L, Graham I, et al: Unstable angina. Natural history and determinants of prognosis. Am J Cardiol 1981; 48:525–528.
14. Betriu A, Heras M, Cohen M, et al: Unstable angina: outcome according to clinical presentation. J Am Coll Cardiol 1992; 19:1659–1663.
15. Théroux P, Ouimet H, Latour JG, et al: Prediction and prevention of myocardial infarction during the acute phase of unstable angina [Abstract]. J Am Coll Cardiol 1989; 13:192A.
16. ECLA 3: Clinical predictors of in-hospital prognosis in unstable angina [Abstract]. Circulation 1993; 88:I-608.
17. Castaner A, Roig E, Serra T, et al: Risk stratification and prognosis of patients with recent onset angina. Eur Heart J 1990; 11:868–875.
18. Gibson RS, Beller GA, Gheorghiade M, et al: The prevalence and clinical significance of residual myocardial ischemia 2 weeks after uncomplicated non–Q wave infarction: a prospective natural history study. Circulation 1986; 73:1186–1198.
19. Severi S, Orsini E, Marracini P, et al: The basal electrocardiogram and the exercise stress test in assessing prognosis in patients with unstable angina. Eur Heart J 1988; 9:441–446.
20. Madsen JK, Thomsen BL, Mellemgaard K, et al: Independent prognostic risk factors for patients referred because of suspected acute myocardial infarction without confirmed diagnosis. Prognosis after discharge in relation to medical history and non-invasive investigations. Eur Heart J 1988; 9:611–618.
21. Nyman I, Areskog M, Areskog NH, et al: The predictive value of silent ischemia at an exercise testing in men with suspected unstable coronary artery disease. J Intern Med 1993; 234:293–301.
22. Moss AJ, Goldstein RE, Hall WJ, et al: Detection and significance of myocardial ischemia in stable patients after recovery from an acute coronary event. Multicenter Myocardial Ischemia Research Group. JAMA 1993; 269:2379–2385.
23. Ambrose JA, Winters SI, Arora RR, et al: Coronary angiographic morphology in myocardial infarction: a link between the pathogenesis of unstable angina and myocardial infarction. J Am Coll Cardiol 1985; 6:1233–1238.
24. Williams AE, Freeman MR, Chislholm RJ, et al: Angiographic morphology in unstable angina pectoris. Am J Cardiol 1988; 62:1024–1027.
25. Lespérance J, Théroux P, Hudon G, et al: A new look at coronary angiography: plaque morphology as a help to diagnosis and to evaluate prognosis. Intern J Cardiac Imaging 1994; 10:75–94.
26. Katus HA, Kubler W: Detection of myocardial cell damage in patients with unstable angina by serodiagnostic tools. *In* Bleifeld W, Hamm CW, Braunwald E (eds): Unstable Angina, pp 92–100. Berlin: Springer-Verlag, 1990.
27. Hamm CW, Ravkilde J, Gerhardt W, et al: The prognostic value of serum troponin T in unstable angina. N Engl J Med 1992; 327:146–150.
28. Ravkilde J, Nissen H, Horder M: Independent prognostic value of serum creatine kinase isoenzyme MB mass, troponin T and myosin light chain levels in suspected acute myocardial infarction. Analysis of 28 months of follow-up in 196 patients. J Am Coll Cardiol 1995; 25:574–581.
29. Berk BC, Weintraub WS, Alexander RW: Elevation of C-reactive protein in "active" coronary artery disease. Am J Cardiol 1990; 65:168–170.
30. Liuzzo G, Biasucci LM, Gallimore JR, et al: The prognostic value of C-reactive protein and serum amyloid A protein in severe unstable angina. N Engl J Med 1994; 331:417–424.
31. Fitzgerald DJ, Roy L, Catella F, et al: Platelet activation in unstable coronary disease. N Engl J Med 1986; 315:983–989.
32. Neri Serneri GG, Gensini GF, Carnovali M, et al: Association between

time of increased fibrinopeptide A levels in plasma and episodes of spontaneous angina: a controlled prospective study. Am Heart J 1987; 113:672–678.
33. Théroux P, Latour JG, De Lara J, et al: Fibrinopeptide A and platelet factor levels in unstable angina. Circulation 1987; 75:156–162.
34. Merlini PA, Bauer KA, Oltrona L, et al: Persistent activation of coagulation mechanism in unstable angina and myocardial infarction. Circulation 1994; 90:61–68.
35. Taeymans Y, Théroux P, Lespérance J, et al: Quantitative angiographic morphology of the coronary artery lesions at risk of thrombotic occlusion. Circulation 1992; 85:78–85.
36. Brown BG, Zhao X-Q, Sacco DE, et al: Lipid lowering and plaque regression: new insights into prevention of plaque disruption and clinical events in coronary disease. Circulation 1993; 87:1781–1791.
37. Davies MJ: A macro and micro view of coronary vascular insult in ischemic heart disease. Circulation 1990; 82:II-38–II-46.
38. Hangartner JRW, Charleston AJ, Davies MJ, et al: Morphological characteristics of clinically significant coronary artery stenosis in stable angina. Br Heart J 1986; 56:501–508.
39. Fuster V: Mechanisms leading to myocardial infarction: insights from studies of vascular biology. Circulation 1994; 90:2126–2146.
40. Furchgott RF, Zawadzki JV: The obligatory role of endothelial cells in the relaxation of arterial smooth muscle by acetylcholine. Nature 1980; 299:373–376.
41. Shimokawa H, Vanhoutte PM: Impaired endothelium-dependent relaxations to aggregating platelets and related vasoactive substances in hypercholesterolemic and atherosclerotic porcine coronary arteries. Circ Res 1989; 64:900–914.
42. Waters D: Plaque stabilization: a mechanism for the beneficial effect of lipid-lowering therapies in angiographic studies. Prog Cardiovasc Dis 1994; 37:107–120.
43. Treasure CB, Talley JD, Stillabower ME, et al: Coronary endothelial responses are improved with aggressive lipid lowering therapy in patients with coronary atherosclerosis [Abstract]. Circulation 1993; 88(part 2):I-368.
44. Anderson TJ, Meredith IT, Yeung AL, et al: Cholesterol lowering therapy improves endothelial function in patients with coronary atherosclerosis [Abstract]. Circulation 1993; 88(part 2):I-368.
45. The Steering Committee of the Physicians' Health Study Research Group: Final report on the aspirin component of the ongoing Physicians' Health Study. N Engl J Med 1989; 321:129–135.
46. Garcia-Dorado D, Théroux P, Tornos P, et al: Previous aspirin use attenuates the severity of the manifestation of acute ischemic syndromes. Circulation 1995; 92:1743–1748.
47. Chesebro JH, Webster MWI, Smith HC, et al: Antiplatelet therapy in coronary artery disease progression: Reduced infarction and new lesion formation [Abstract]. Circulation 1989; 80:II-266.
48. Freeman MR, Langer A, Wilson RF, et al: Thrombolysis in unstable angina. Randomized double-blind trial of t-PA and placebo. Circulation 1992; 85:150–157.
49. de Zwaan C, Bär FW, Janssen JHA, et al: Effects of thrombolytic therapy in unstable angina: clinical and angiographic results. J Am Coll Cardiol 1988; 12:301–309.
50. Gold HK, Johns JA, Leinbach RC, et al: A randomized, placebo-controlled trial of recombinant human tissue-type plasminogen activator in patients with unstable angina pectoris. Circulation 1987; 75:1192–1199.
51. The T-3A Investigators: Early effects of tissue plasminogen activator, added to conventional therapy, on the culprit coronary lesion in patients presenting with unstable angina: results of the Thrombolysis in Myocardial Ischemia (T-3A) Trial. Circulation 1993; 87:38–52.
52. Bär FW, Verheugt FW, Col J, et al: Thrombolysis in patients with unstable angina improves the angiographic but not the clinical outcome: results of UNASEM, a multicenter, randomized, placebo-controlled, clinical trial with anistreplase. Circulation 1992; 86:131–137.
53. Karlsson JE, Berglund U, Bjorkholm A, et al: Thrombolysis with recombinant tissue-type plasminogen activator during instability in coronary artery disease: effect on myocardial ischemia and need for coronary revascularization. TRIC Study Group. Am Heart J 1992; 124:1419–1426.
54. Schreiber TL, Rizik D, White C, et al: Randomized trial of thrombolysis versus heparin in unstable angina. Circulation 1992; 86:1407–1414.
55. TIMI 3B Investigators: Effects of tissue plasminogen activator and a comparison of early invasive and conservative strategies in unstable angina and non–Q-wave myocardial infarction. Circulation 1994; 89:1545–1556.
56. Oltrona L, Merlini PA, Spinola A, et al: A randomized trial on prolonged streptokinase infusion with concomitant heparin administration in unstable angina pectoris [Abstract]. Circulation 1993; 88(part 2):I-608.
57. Ambrose JA, Almeida OD, Sharma SK, et al: Adjunctive thrombolytic therapy during angioplasty for ischemic rest angina. Results of the TAUSA trial. Circulation 1994; 90:69–77.
58. Shabani F, Theroux P, de Guise P, Thibault B: A randomized, double-blind trial of streptokinase versus placebo for the management of unstable angina and non–Q wave myocardial infarction in patients with previous coronary artery bypass surgery [Abstract]. J Am Coll Cardiol 1995; (special issue):421A.
59. Freeman MR, Williams AE, Chrisholm RJ, et al: Role of resting thallium-201 perfusion in predicting coronary anatomy, left ventricular wall motion, and hospital outcome in unstable angina pectoris. Am Heart J 1989; 117:306–314.
60. Topol EJ, Nicklas JM, Kander NH, et al: Coronary revascularization after intravenous tissue plasminogen activator for unstable angina pectoris: results of a randomized double-blind, placebo-controlled trial. Am J Cardiol 1988; 62:368–371.
61. Gruppo Italiano per lo studio della Streptokinase nell'Infarto Miocardico (GISSI): Effectiveness of intravenous thrombolytic treatment in acute myocardial infarction. Lancet 1986; 1:397–402.
62. ISIS-2 (Second International Study of Infarct Survival) Collaborative Group: Randomised trial of intravenous streptokinase, oral aspirin, both, or neither among 17187 cases of suspected acute myocardial infarction: ISIS-2. Lancet 1988; 2:349–360.
63. Rapold HJ, Kuemmerli H, Weiss M, et al: Monitoring of fibrin generation during thrombolytic therapy of acute myocardial infarction with recombinant tissue-type plasminogen activator. Circulation 1989; 79:980–989.
64. Fitzgerald DJ, Wright F, Fitzgerald GA: Increased thromboxane biosynthesis during coronary thrombolysis: evidence that platelet activation and thromboxane A_2 modulate the response to tissue-type plasminogen activator in vivo. Circ Res 1989; 65:83–95.
65. Lewis HDJ, Davis JW, Archibald DG, et al: Protective effects of aspirin against acute myocardial infarction and death in men with unstable angina. Results of a Veterans Administration Cooperative Study. N Engl J Med 1983; 309:396–403.
66. Cairns JA, Gent M, Singer J, et al: Aspirin, sulfinpyrazone, or both in unstable angina. Results of a Canadian Multicenter Trial. N Engl J Med 1985; 313:1369–1375.
67. Théroux P, Ouimet H, McCans J, et al: Aspirin, heparin, or both to treat acute unstable angina. N Engl J Med 1988; 319:1105–1111.
68. The RISC Group: Risk of myocardial infarction and death during treatment with low dose aspirin and intravenous heparin in men with unstable coronary artery disease. Lancet 1990; 336:827–830.
69. Wallentin LC, the Research Group on Instability in Coronary Artery Disease in Southeast Sweden: Aspirin (75 mg/day) after an episode of unstable coronary artery disease: long-term effects on the risk for myocardial infarction, occurrence of severe angina and the need for revascularization. J Am Coll Cardiol 1991; 18:1587–1593.
70. Antiplatelet Trialists' Collaboration: Collaborative overview of randomized trials of antiplatelet therapy: I. Prevention of death, myocardial infarction, and stroke by prolonged antiplatelet therapy in various categories of patients. Br Med J 1994; 308:81–106.
71. Patrono C: Aspirin as an antiplatelet agent. N Engl J Med 1994; 330:1287–1294.
72. FitzGerald GA, Oates JA, Harviger J, et al: Endogenous biosynthesis of prostacyclin and thromboxane and platelet function during chronic administration of aspirin in man. J Clin Invest 1983; 71:676–688.
73. Balsano F, Rizzon P, Violi F, et al: Antiplatelet treatment with ticlopidine in unstable angina. A controlled multicenter clinical trial. Circulation 1990; 82:17–26.
74. Telford AM, Wilson C: Trial of heparin versus atenolol in prevention of myocardial infarction in intermediate coronary syndrome. Lancet 1981; 1:1225–1228.
75. Théroux P, Waters D, Qiu S, et al: Aspirin versus heparin to prevent myocardial infarction during the acute phase of unstable angina. Circulation 1993; 88(part 1):2045–2048.
76. Serneri GGN, Gensini GF, Poggesi L, et al: Effect of heparin, aspirin, or alteplase in reduction of myocardial ischaemia in refractory unstable angina. Lancet 1990; 1:615–618.
77. Théroux P, Waters D, Lam J, et al: Reactivation of unstable angina after the discontinuation of heparin. N Engl J Med 1992; 327:141–145.
78. Becker RC: The heparin rebound phenomenon—does it offer insights

toward understanding the pathobiology of coronary thrombosis and its treatment? J Thromb Thrombolysis 1995; 1:157–161.
79. Marcianak E, Gockerman JP: Heparin-induced decrease in circulating antithrombin III. Lancet 1977; 2:581–584.
80. Lidón RM, Théroux P, Robitaille D: Antithrombin-III plasma activity during and after prolonged use of heparin in unstable angina. Thromb Res 1993; 72:23–32.
81. Weitz JJ, Hudoba M, Massel D, et al: Clot-bound thrombin is protected from inhibition by heparin–antithrombin III but is susceptible to inactivation by antithrombin III–independent inhibitors. J Clin Invest 1990; 86:385–391.
82. Gold HK, Torres FW, Garabedian HD, et al: Evidence for a rebound coagulation phenomenon after cessation of a 4-hour infusion of a specific thrombin inhibitor in patients with unstable angina pectoris. J Am Coll Cardiol 1993; 21:1039–1047.
83. Granger CB, Miller JM, Bovill EG, et al: Rebound increase in thrombin generation and activity after cessation of intravenous heparin in patients with acute coronary syndromes. Circulation 1995; 91:1929–1935.
84. Hirsh J, Levine MN: Low molecular weight heparin. Blood 1992; 79:1–17.
85. Gurfinkel EP, Manos EJ, Mejaíl RI, et al: Low molecular weight heparin versus regular heparin or aspirin in the treatment of unstable angina and silent ischemia. J Am Coll Cardiol 1995; 26:313–318.
86. Smith P, Arnesen H, Holme I: 1. The effect of warfarin on mortality and reinfarction after myocardial infarction. Lancet 1990; 323:147–152.
87. Anticoagulant in the Secondary Prevention of Events in Coronary Thrombosis (ASPECT) Research Group: Effect of long-term oral anticaogulant treatment on mortality and cardiovascular morbidity after myocardial infarction. Lancet 1994; 343:499–503.
88. Wood P: Acute and subacute coronary insufficiency. Br Med J 1961; 1:1779–1782.
89. Vakil RJ: Intermediate coronary syndrome. Circulation 1961; 24:557–571.
90. Williams DO, Kirby MG, McPherson K, et al: Anticoagulant treatment in unstable angina. Br J Clin Pract 1986; 40:114–116.
91. Cohen M, Adams PC, Parry G, et al: Combination antithrombotic therapy in unstable rest angina and non–Q-wave infarction in nonoption aspirin users. Primary end points analysis from the ATACS trial. Circulation 1994; 89:81–88.
92. Holdright D, Patel D, Cunningham D, et al: Comparison of the effect of heparin and aspirin versus aspirin alone on transient myocardial ischemia and in-hospital prognosis in patients with unstable angina. J Am Coll Cardiol 1994; 24:39–45.
93. Théroux P, Waters D: Diagnosis and management of patients with unstable angina. *In* Schlant RC, Alexander RW (eds): Hurst's The Heart, 8th ed, pp 1083–1106. New York: McGraw-Hill, 1994.
94. Abrams J: The role of nitrates in coronary disease. Arch Int Med 1995; 155:357–364.
95. Moncada S, Higgs A: The *l*-arginine-nitric oxide pathway. N Engl J Med 1993; 329:2002–2012.
96. Maseri A, L'Abbate A, Baroldi G, et al: Coronary vasospasm as a possible cause of myocardial infarction: conclusion derived from the study of "pre-infarction angina." N Engl J Med 1978; 299:1271–1277.
97. Diodati J, Théroux P, Latour JG, et al: Effects of nitroglycerin at therapeutic doses on platelet aggregation in unstable angina pectoris and acute myocardial infarction. Am J Cardiol 1990; 66:683–687.
98. Folts JD, Stamler J, Loscalzo J: Intravenous nitroglycerin infusion inhibits cyclic blood flow response caused by periodic platelet thrombus formation in stenosed coronary arteries. Circulation 1991; 83:2122–2127.
99. Stamler JS, Loscalzo J: The antiplatelet effects of organic nitrates and related nitroso compounds in vitro and in vivo and their relevance in cardiovascular disorders. J Am Coll Cardiol 1991; 18:1529–1536.
100. ISIS-4. Randomised study of oral isosorbide mononitrate in over 50,000 patients with suspected acute myocardial infarction. ISIS Collaborative Group [Abstract]. Circulation 1993; 88(part 2):I-394.
101. Gruppo Italiano per lo Studio della Sopravvivenza nell'Infarto Miocardico (GISSI-3): Effects of lisinopril and transdermal glyceryl trinitrate singly and together on 6-week mortality and ventricular function after acute myocardial infarction. Lancet 1994; 343:1115–1122.
102. ESPRIM Group: Can NO donors improve the prognosis of acute M.I. patients? Results from a large scale placebo controlled study [Abstract]. Circulation 1993; 88(part 2):I-394.
103. Dauwe F, Affaki G, Waters DD, et al: Intravenous nitroglycerin in refractory unstable angina [Abstract]. Am J Cardiol 1979; 43:416.
104. Mikolich JR, Nicoloff NB, Robinson PH, et al: Relief of refractory angina with continuous intravenous infusion of nitroglycerin. Chest 1980; 77:375–379.
105. Page A, Gateau P, Ohayon J, et al: Intravenous nitroglycerin in unstable angina. *In* Lichtlen PR, Engel HJ, Schrey A, Swan JHC (eds): Nitrates III Cardiovascular Effects, pp 371–376. Berlin: Springer-Verlag, 1981.
106. DePace NL, Herling IM, Kotler MN, et al: Intravenous nitroglycerin for rest angina. Potential pathophysiologic mechanisms of action. Arch Intern Med 1982; 142:1806–1809.
107. Squire A, Cantor R, Packer M: Limitations of continuous intravenous nitroglycerin prophylaxis in patients with refractory angina at rest [Abstract]. Circulation 1982; 66:II-120.
108. Roubin GS, Harris PJ, Eckhardt I, et al: Intravenous nitroglycerin in refractory unstable angina. Aust N Z J Med 1982; 12:598–602.
109. Kaplan K, Davison R, Parker M, et al: Intravenous nitroglycerin for the treatment of angina at rest unresponsive to standard nitrate therapy. Am J Cardiol 1983; 51:694–698.
110. Conti RC: Use of nitrates in unstable angina pectoris. Am J Cardiol 1987; 60:31H–34H.
111. May DC, Popma JJ, Black WH: In vivo induction and reversal of nitroglycerin tolerance in human coronary arteries. N Engl J Med 1987; 317:805–809.
112. Horowitz JD: Role of nitrates in unstable angina pectoris. Am J Cardiol 1992; 70:64B–71B.
113. Figueras J, Lidón RM, Cortadellas J: Rebound myocardial ischemia following abrupt interruption of intravenous infusion in patients with unstable angina at rest. Eur Heart J 1991; 12:405–411.
114. ISIS-I Collaborative Group: A randomized trial of intravenous atenolol among 16,027 cases of suspected myocardial infarction. Lancet 1986; 2:57–66.
115. The MIAMI Trial Research Group: Metoprolol in acute myocardial infarction (MIAMI): A randomized placebo-controlled international trial. Eur Heart J 1985; 6:199–226.
116. Yusuf S, Wittes J, Friedman L: Overview of results of randomized clinical trials in heart disease: 1. Treatments following myocardial infarction. JAMA 1988; 260:2088–2093.
117. Yusuf S, Wittes J, Friedman L: Overview of results of randomized clinical trials in heart disease: 2. Unstable angina, heart failure, primary prevention with aspirin, and risk factor modification. JAMA 1988; 260:2259–2263.
118. Holland Interuniversity Nifedipine-Metoprolol Trial (HINT) Research Group: Early treatment of unstable angina in the coronary care unit: a randomised, double-blind, placebo-controlled comparison of recurrent ischemia in patients treated with nifedipine, metoprolol or both: Report of the Holland Interuniversity Nifedipine/Metoprolol Trial (HINT) Research Group. Br Heart J 1986; 56:400–413.
119. Gerstenblith G, Ouyang P, Achuff SC, et al: Nifedipine in unstable angina: a double-blind randomized trial. N Engl J Med 1982; 306:885–889.
120. Gottlieb SO, Weisfeldt ML, Ouyang P, et al: Effect of the addition of propranolol to therapy with nifedipine for unstable angina pectoris: a randomized, double-blind, placebo-controlled trial. Circulation 1986; 73:331–337.
121. Théroux P, Taeymans Y, Waters DD: Calcium antagonists: clinical use in treating angina. Drugs 1983; 25:178–195.
122. Waters DD, Théroux P, Szlachcic J, Dauwe F: Provocative testing with ergonovine to assess the efficacy of treatment with nifedipine, diltiazem and verapamil in variant angina. Am J Cardiol 1981; 48:123–130.
123. Muller JE, Turi ZG, Pearle DL, et al: Nifedipine and conventional therapy for unstable angina pectoris: a randomized, double-blind comparison. Circulation 1984; 69:728–739.
124. Théroux P, Taeymans Y, Morissette D, et al: A randomized study comparing propranolol and diltiazem in the treatment of unstable angina. J Am Coll Cardiol 1985; 5:717–722.
125. Fang ZY, Picart N, Abramovicz M, et al: Intravenous diltiazem versus nitroglycerin for silent and symptomatic myocardial ischemia in unstable angina pectoris. Am J Cardiol 1991; 68:42C–46C.
126. Göbel EJ, Spanjaard JN, Hautvast RW, et al: Intravenous diltiazem in patients with unstable angina: a randomized, double blind comparison with nitroglycerin. First results [Abstract]. Circulation 1994; 90(part 2):I-232.
127. Pugh B, Platt MR, Mills LJ, et al: Unstable angina pectoris: a randomized study of patients treated medically or surgically. Am J Cardiol 1978; 41:1291–1298.
128. Russell RO, Moraski RE, Kouchoukos N, et al: Unstable angina pecto-

ris: National Cooperative Study Group to compare surgical and medical therapy: II. In-hospital experience and initial follow-up results in patients with one, two and three vessel disease. Am J Cardiol 1978; 42:838–848.

129. Luchi RJ, Scott SM, Deupree RH, and the Principal Investigators and their Associates of Veterans Administration Cooperative Study No. 28: Comparison of medical and surgical treatment for unstable angina pectoris. N Engl J Med 1987; 316:977–984.
130. Booth DC, Deupree RH, Hultgren HM, et al: Quality of life after bypass surgery for unstable angina: 5-year follow-up results of a Veterans Affairs Cooperative Study. Circulation 1991; 83:87–95.
131. Kaiser GC, Schaff HV, Killip T: Myocardial revascularization for unstable angina pectoris. Circulation 1989; 79:I-60–I-67.
132. de Feyter PJ, Serruys PW: Percutaneous transluminal coronary angioplasty for unstable angina. *In* Topol EJ (ed): Textbook of Interventional Cardiology, 2nd ed, pp 274–291. Philadelphia: WB Saunders, 1994.
133. Myler RK, Shaw RE, Stertzer SH, et al: Unstable angina and coronary angioplasty. Circulation 1990; 82:II-88–II-95.
134. de Guise P, Théroux P, Bonan R, et al: Rethrombosis after successful thrombolysis and angioplasty in acute myocardial infarction [Abstract]. J Am Coll Cardiol 1988; 11:192A.
135. The EPIC Investigators: Use of a monoclonal antibody directed against the platelet glycoprotein II_b/III_a receptor in high-risk coronary angioplasty. N Engl J Med 1994; 330:956–961.
136. Lincoff AM, Califf RM, Anderson K, et al: Striking clinical benefit with platelet GP II_b/III_a inhibition by c7E3 among patients with unstable angina: Outcome in the EPIC trial [Abstract]. Circulation 1994; 90:I-21.
137. Hirsh J: Heparin. N Engl J Med 1991; 324:1565–1574.
138. Markwardt F, Kaiser B, Novak G: Studies on antithrombotic effects of recombinant Hirudin. Thromb Res 1989; 54:377–388.
139. Coller BS: A new murine monoclonal antibody reports on activation-dependent change in the conformation and/or microenvironment of the platelet glycoprotein II_b/III_a complex. J Clin Invest 1985; 76:101–108.
140. Maraganore JM, Bourdon P, Jablonski J, et al: Design and characterization of Hirulogs: a novel class of bivalent peptide inhibitors of thrombin. Biochemistry 1990; 29:7095–7101.
141. Gold HK, Gimple LW, Yasuda T, et al: Pharmacodynamic study of F(ab′)2 fragments of murine monoclonal antibody 7E3 directed against human platelet glycoprotein II_b/III_a in patients with unstable angina. J Clin Invest 1990; 86:651–659.
142. Simoons ML, de Boer MJ, van den Brand MJBM, et al: Randomized trial of GP II_b/III_a platelet blocker in refractory unstable angina. Circulation 1990; 89:593–603.
143. Lidón RM, Théroux P, Juneau M, et al: Initial experience with a direct antithrombin, Hirulog, in unstable angina. Anticoagulant, antithrombotic and clinical effects. Circulation 1993; 88:1495–1501.
144. Cannon CP, McCabe CH, Henry TD, et al: A pilot trial of recombinant desulfatohirudin compared with heparin in conjunction with tissue-type plasminogen activator and aspirin for acute myocardial infarction: results of the Thrombolysis in Myocardial Ischemia (TIMI) 5 trial. J Am Coll Cardiol 1994; 23:993–1003.
145. Théroux P, White H, David D, et al: A heparin-controlled study of MK-383 in unstable angina [Abstract]. Circulation 1994; 90(part 2):I-231.
146. Théroux P, Kouz S, Knudtson ML, et al: A randomized double-blind controlled trial with the non-peptidic platelet GP II_b/III_a antagonist RO 44-9883 in unstable angina [Abstract]. Circulation 1994; 90(part 2):I-232.
147. U.S. Department of Health and Human Services, Public Health Service: Unstable Angina: Diagnosis and Management. Clinical Practice Guideline, Number 10 (AHCPR Publication No. 94-0602). Washington, DC: Agency for Health Care Policy and Research, 1994.
148. Campeau L, Enjalbert M, Lespérance J, et al: The relation of risk factors to the development of atherosclerosis in saphenous-vein bypass grafts and the progression of disease in the native circulation: a study 10 years after aortocoronary bypass surgery. N Engl J Med 1984; 311:1329–1332.
149. Rupprecht HJ, Brenneke R, Rottmeyer M, et al: Short- and long-term outcome after PTCA in patients with stable and unstable angina. Eur Heart J 1990; 11:964–973.
150. Bauters C, Khanoyan P, McFadden EP, et al: Restenosis after delayed coronary angioplasty of the culprit vessel in patients with a recent myocardial infarction treated by thrombolysis. Circulation 1995; 91:1410–1418.
151. Chesebro JH, Clements IP, Fuster V, et al: A platelet-inhibitor-drug trial in coronary-artery bypass operations: benefit of perioperative dipyridamole and aspirin therapy on early postoperative vein-graft patency. N Engl J Med 1982; 307:73–78.
152. Goldman S, Copeland J, Moritz T, et al: Saphenous vein graft patency 1 year after coronary artery bypass surgery and effects of antiplatelet therapy: results of a Veterans Administration Cooperative Study. Circulation 1989; 80:1190–1197.
153. Lorenz LR, Schacky CV, Weber M, et al: Improved aortocoronary bypass patency by low-dose aspirin (100 mg daily). Effects on platelet aggregation and thromboxane formation. Lancet 1984; 1:1261–1264.
154. Limet R, David JL, Magotteaux P, et al: Prevention of aorto-coronary bypass graft occlusion: beneficial effect of ticlopidine on early and late patency rates of venous coronary bypass grafts: a double blind study. J Thorac Cardiovasc Surg 1987; 94:773–783.
155. Cavender JB, Rogers WJ, Fisher LD, et al: Effects of smoking on survival and morbidity in patients randomized to medical and surgical therapy in the Coronary Artery Surgery Study (CASS): 10-years follow-up. J Am Coll Cardiol 1992; 20:287–294.
156. Pearson T, Rapaport E, Criqui M, et al: Optimal risk factor management in the patient after coronary revascularization. A statement for healthcare professionals from the American Heart Association Writing Group. Circulation 1994; 90:3125–3133.

7 Acute Myocardial Infarction

Robert M. Califf, MD

Perhaps no human condition has been studied in as much detail in so many patients as acute myocardial infarction. Randomized clinical trials involving more than 500,000 patients have been reported in the literature, and many more trials are currently in progress or in planning phases. This rich database presents an interesting dilemma for clinicians: the possibility of practicing medicine on the basis of empirical evidence offers a dramatic gain for patients, but the techniques for interpretation of the information are unfamiliar to many practicing physicians and raise difficult questions about the extrapolation of data from large trials to the care of an individual patient.

This chapter provides an overview of routine therapies for acute myocardial infarction and then focuses on specific problems that commonly recur in the care of these patients. The material on each complication or problem may be thought of as a guide to an episode of clinical care that might be necessary at any point in a patient's course. As much as possible, an effort has been made to orient the chapter to the time frame of a patient going through a typical hospital course. When the information available allows for a clear recommendation that is based on empirical evidence from clinical trials data, it is so denoted (see Chapter 51). In several situations, however, in view of many possible justifiable choices, the approach used in the author's Cardiac Care Unit is outlined, along with the rationale for the decisions.

PATHOPHYSIOLOGY

Acute myocardial infarction is precipitated by a series of events that is discussed in more detail in E. Braunwald's *Heart Disease* (5th ed; Philadelphia: WB Saunders, 1995). Most acute events are caused by disruption of an atherosclerotic plaque in an epicardial coronary vessel, followed by complete occlusion of the vessel by thrombosis.[1, 2] The atherosclerotic plaque that most often causes symptomatic myocardial infarction is lipid-rich and in most cases does not significantly limit coronary blood flow before the acute event.[3, 4] These less stenotic "vulnerable" plaques are frequently characterized by infiltration of the fibrous cap of the plaque by macrophages[5] and are often located at branch points or bends in the arterial tree. In combination with heightened vulnerability of the individual plaque, systemic activation of the sympathetic nervous system and the coagulation system provide an immediate trigger for the acute event.[6, 7] Once the surface of the plaque fissures, the circulating blood is exposed to tissue factors, the coagulation cascade is activated, and platelet aggregation is initiated.[2] If the vessel becomes totally occluded and there is no extensive collateral supply, a wavefront of myocardial necrosis begins within 15 min and spreads from the endocardium toward the epicardium.[8] The lethal sequelae of myocardial infarction (sudden arrhythmia, cardiogenic shock, myocardial rupture) are predominantly related to the extent of myocardial necrosis. From this perspective, the major goals of therapy are to restore blood flow as quickly as possible, to prevent lethal consequences of necrosis, and to react quickly with therapeutic maneuvers when life-threatening events occur. A final medical goal is to create an environment that promotes healing of the damaged myocardium while maximizing the social and functional recovery of the patient.

CLINICAL EPIDEMIOLOGY

The American Heart Association has estimated that 1.5 million acute myocardial infarctions occur in the United States each year,[9] that approximately one third of the patients with these events die, and that half the deaths occur before the patients can receive medical attention. A convenient classification from previous textbooks stressed the diagnosis of myocardial infarction on the basis of enzymatic measurements of myocardial necrosis and serial evaluation of the electrocardiogram (ECG) to determine whether the myocardial infarction was to be classified as a Q wave or non–Q wave infarction. From the point of view of current therapeutic decisions, this classification is inadequate, predominantly because the most important interventions need to be made before the serum cardiac markers can be determined or definitive ECG abnormalities denoting Q wave or non–Q wave infarction appear.

A conceptual framework for this chapter is outlined in Figure 7–1. Patients are considered to have an acute coronary syndrome until they reach a facility where a 12-lead ECG can be obtained. At this point patients are categorized as either those with ST segment elevation or those without ST segment elevation, because of the critical importance of reperfusion therapy in lowering the chances of mortality and morbidity of the patients with ST segment elevation. Among patients without ST segment elevation, serial electrocardiography and measurement of serum cardiac markers are used to determine whether myocardial necrosis has occurred. Throughout the course, the patient is constantly evaluated with an integrated assessment of overall risk and a specific assessment of complications that necessitate particular diagnostic techniques and therapeutic modalities. Specific evaluations are performed sequentially in the emergency department, the cardiac care unit (CCU) (after 24 h of stability), and the hospital ward (after 4 days of stability).

PREHOSPITAL PHASE

Diagnostic Methods

Many patients experience symptoms that could be interpreted as characteristic of an acute coronary syndrome. A critical initial component of coronary care is to perform the evaluation in a facility that has the capability of obtaining and interpreting an ECG and, if possible, the full capability of initiating reperfusion therapy (thrombolysis or angioplasty), monitoring the patient, and providing advanced cardiac life support.[10] These recommendations stem from the observations that the risk of catastrophic arrhythmia is highest immediately after coronary occlusion and declines as a function of time, that the delay between onset of symptoms and treatment is an important mediator of mortality, and that proper interpretation of the

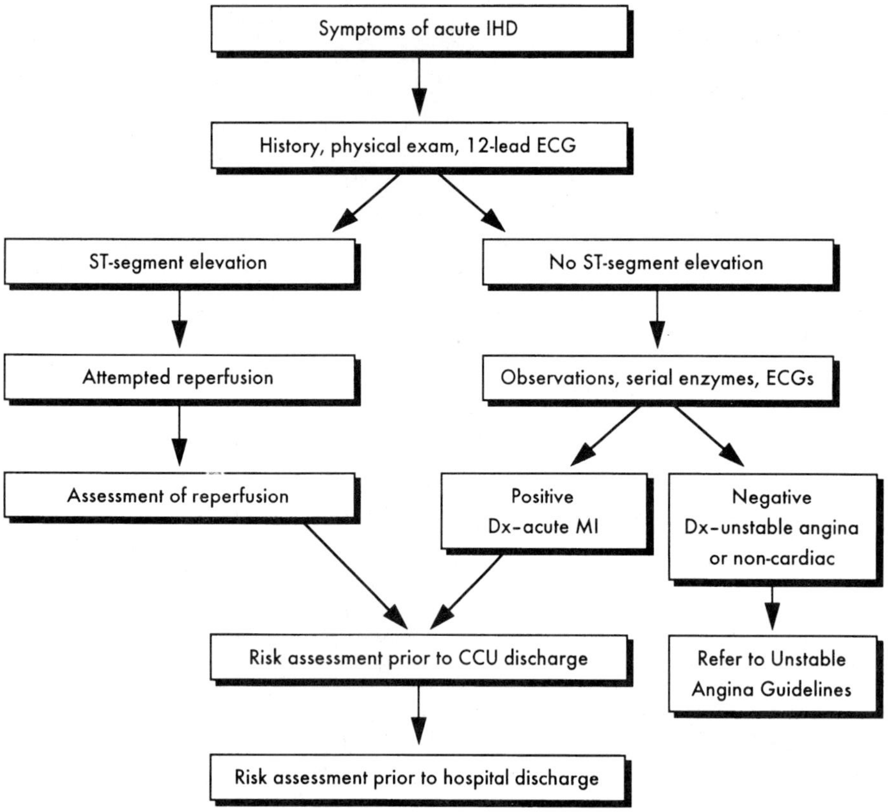

Figure 7–1. Diagram of major stratification criteria in patients with acute symptoms of ischemic heart disease (IHD). By focusing initially on whether ST segment elevation is present on the electrogram (ECG), the practitioner can identify candidates for acute reperfusion. Subsequent orderly stratification of risk can lead to effective determination of which patients need particular therapies and the intensity and duration of high-level medical care. *Abbreviations:* Dx, diagnosis; MI, myocardial infarction; CCU, cardiac care unit.

ECG is a critical element of the evaluation. Because the allocation of resources is in question in this era of cost-conscious medicine, these seem to be the minimal requirements for facilities to evaluate acute ischemic symptoms.

Prehospital Electrocardiogram

Evaluation of the patient in the prehospital phase should include a checklist oriented toward identifying patients with likely myocardial infarction, other common diagnoses, and risk factors for poor outcome.[11] Several studies have indicated that a 12-lead ECG obtained by emergency medical technicians in the field substantially speeds the treatment of the patient upon arrival at the hospital.[12] Data from the Myocardial Infarction Triage and Intervention (MITI) study[13] and other reports[14] of prehospital thrombolytic therapy suggest that a thorough prehospital evaluation saves enough time by speeding the initiation of emergency department therapy that prehospital thrombolysis is unnecessary. In areas where the nearest hospital is more than 60 min away, prehospital thrombolysis may still be advantageous.[15]

Treatment

The extent to which prehospital services can be offered is a function of the public tax base and the presence of community support. Because the efficacy of most interventions is assumed to be greatest when they are undertaken soon after coronary occlusion, it is reasonable to assume that ideal decision making and treatment should take place at the first point of contact with the medical care system. The substantial costs of equipment, education, and personnel and the risk of misdiagnosis or inappropriate treatment must be weighed against the potential advantage of speed.

At a minimum, it is assumed that emergency medical services should have access to rapid defibrillation for patients in whom cardiac arrest develops and that cardiac rhythm monitoring should be available en route. In addition, it is reasonable for most emergency medical service systems to offer sublingual nitroglycerin for pain relief; many offer morphine sulfate.

Prehospital thrombolysis has been the source of considerable interest. Trials in Seattle,[11, 13] the United Kingdom,[16] and Central Europe[15, 17] all showed a benefit of earlier treatment; the magnitude of the advantage of prehospital treatment was approximately proportional to the time between the cardiac event and treatment in the hospital for the control group. None of the trials individually was convincing, but a systematic overview showed a 17% reduction in mortality (95% confidence interval, 2%–29%). Although prehospital thrombolysis is clearly feasible and probably beneficial in systems with experienced, highly trained personnel or in countries with physicians on the cardiac ambulances, the author and colleagues believe that for the most part in the United States, a focus on early identification and reduced time to treatment in the emergency department seems to be a more effective approach.

EMERGENCY DEPARTMENT PHASE

Early Diagnosis

Monitoring/Defibrillation

All patients with a suspected acute coronary syndrome should be maintained on a cardiac monitor until that diagnosis is effectively ruled out. An intravenous line should be started for access and for the rapid delivery of cardiac medications. The author and colleagues believe that the emergency facility should have an established record of an interval between ventricular fibrillation and defibrillation of less than 1 min. Advance directives should be clarified very early after patients' arrival in the emergency department, particularly for extremely elderly patients, to prevent them from being treated in a manner contrary to their wishes.

Oxygen

The use of oxygen has been a standard procedure for all patients with suspected acute myocardial ischemia or necrosis. The rationale for routine use of oxygen stems from the recognition that hypoxemia is detrimental in patients with ongoing myocardial necrosis and that ventilation-perfusion mismatches are common among patients with acute myocardial infarction, particularly after heparin administration.[18] However, the empiric basis for routine use of oxygen is not firmly established. Experimental data support the concepts that normal levels of oxygen reduce infarct size[19] and that hyperbaric oxygen may be beneficial.[20] Alternatively, a high oxygen concentration has been shown to increase coronary vasomotor tone. The cost of administering oxygen via nasal prongs is $70/day. Until further data are available, routine use of oxygen at 2–4 L/min by nasal cannulae for 6–12 h is recommended so as to ensure adequate oxygenation. In patients with known chronic lung disease, measurement of blood gases is recommended so as to detect carbon dioxide retention. It is likely that as pulse oximetry becomes more widespread, oxygen will be reserved for patients who have documented hypoxemia or physical signs or symptoms of heart failure.

Pain Relief

Patients with acute myocardial infarction are in a hyperadrenergic state, and pain is commonly severe in the acute phase of the event. The clinician should focus on two aspects of pain management: acute relief of symptoms of ongoing myocardial ischemia and necrosis and general relief of anxiety and apprehension, which frequently exacerbate pain. These issues have become important particularly with increasing evidence that surges of catecholamines are implicated in the genesis of plaque fissuring and thrombus propagation.

Morphine sulfate has remained the standard drug for relieving pain and anxiety from acute myocardial ischemia. The drug is administered in incremental doses of 2–4 mg intravenously every 5–10 min while the level of pain and anxiety, the blood pressure, heart rate, and respiration are monitored. Although concern regarding depression of respiration and hypotension with morphine is justifiable, the most common error is not administering enough to make the patient comfortable; doses of 10–30 mg are often required in the acute phase of the infarction. Naloxone in doses of 0.4 mg intravenously every 3 min for up to three administrations can be used to reverse the effects of morphine if respiratory compromise occurs. Although other narcotics have been investigated, none has supplanted morphine as a more effective agent. Some interest has been raised about the use of patient-controlled administration and thoracic epidural anesthesia,[21, 22] but adequate clinical trials are not available to justify widespread use, and their additional cost is substantial. Rather, the frequent, direct observation of the patient with acute ischemia makes the traditional administration of morphine by the confident and reassuring health care provider an attractive approach to analgesia.

Electrolytes

Since the mid-1970s, interest in electrolytes as a correctable risk factor for arrhythmia has waxed and waned. The measurement of serum electrolytes has become a routine practice in patients with suspected acute ischemia, and considerable resources are expended in the supplementation of potassium and magnesium in many emergency departments and CCUs.

Hypokalemia has been identified as an "arrhythmogenic" factor for many years, and studies have shown low serum potassium levels in survivors of sudden cardiac arrest. Several studies have documented that patients with acute myocardial infarction who have a low serum potassium concentration have an increased risk of primary ventricular fibrillation.[23–25] However, these potassium levels may be low as a result of confounding factors rather than primary risk factors; for example, larger infarctions are associated with higher adrenergic levels, which cause an influx of potassium into cells, and thus the lower potassium level may simply be a reflection of a larger infarction with its attendant risk. No clinical trial data concerning the effect of supplementation of potassium on the risk of ventricular fibrillation are available. Nevertheless, it seems prudent to measure serum potassium and to supplement it to a level above 4.0 mEq/L in patients with suspected acute myocardial infarction.

In the setting of life-threatening ventricular arrhythmias, potassium is generally given as intravenous doses of 10 mEq over a period of 1 h for a potassium level between 3.5 and 4.0 mEq/L; 20 mEq over a period of 1 h for a potassium level below 3.5 mEq/L; and up to 40 mEq over a period of 1 h for potassium levels below 2.5 mEq/L. Infusions at rates greater than 10 mEq/h must be given via central access because of the caustic effect of concentrated potassium on veins. Serum potassium levels should be rechecked 2 h after administration. In the presence of a serum creatinine level above 1.5 mg/dL, a lower rate of potassium infusion is used for hypokalemic patients. For the entirely stable patient with hypokalemia, a less aggressive approach with oral supplementation or slower rates of intravenous infusion is appropriate.

Similar studies of serum magnesium levels have failed to demonstrate a relationship with primary ventricular fibrillation, despite evidence that low magnesium levels are generally associated with more ambient arrhythmias.[25] The ongoing controversy about magnesium repletion is discussed in the next section. In the absence of definitive information, the policy at the author's institution is to measure serum magnesium levels upon admission and to proceed with magnesium repletion if the level is below 2.0 mg/dL. For patients with low magnesium concentrations, magnesium is administered as an infusion of 2 g in 100 mL of intravenous fluid over a period of 2 h. Particular concern must be present for patients with hypokalemia because magnesium levels must be repleted to allow rapid normalization of potassium concentration.

Reperfusion Therapy

Thrombolysis

Thrombolytic Agents (see Chapters 2 and 29)

Thrombolytic agents act by converting plasminogen to plasmin, which then lyses the fibrin-enmeshed clot.[26] The drugs can be divided into fundamental classes on the basis of relative fibrin specificity and half-life. Currently, streptokinase, urokinase, alteplase (tissue plasminogen activator [t-PA]), and anisoylated plasminogen streptokinase activator complex (APSAC) are commercially available (Table 7–1). Because of the higher cost and the inferior clinical outcome profiles of urokinase and APSAC, streptokinase and alteplase are the current choices. Streptokinase must create a systemic fibrinolytic state in order to lyse coronary thrombi and has a relatively long half-life, whereas alteplase is relatively fibrin-specific, which means that it preferentially activates plasminogen on the surface of the clot. This fibrin specificity is only relative, however, and some systemic fibrinogen depletion is the rule rather than the exception with alteplase.[27, 28] Several new thrombolytic agents are to undergo large-scale testing with the common theme of greater fibrin specificity (bat-PA),[29] a longer half-life allowing bolus administration (reteplase [r-PA]),[30] or both (TNK t-PA).[31, 32]

General Results

Thrombolytic agents reduce mortality, improve left ventricular function, reduce the incidence of congestive heart failure, and generally reduce complications of infarction emanating from extensive left ventricular damage, including ventricular fibrillation, atrial fibrillation, and heart block. The mechanism of these beneficial effects is

TABLE 7–1. COMPARISON OF U.S. FOOD AND DRUG ADMINISTRATION–APPROVED THROMBOLYTIC AGENTS

Characteristic	Streptokinase	APSAC	Alteplase
Dose	1.5 million units (30–60 min)	30 mg (5 min)	Weight-adjusted (90 min)*
Circulating half-life (min)	20	100	6
Antigenic	Yes	Yes	No
Allergic reactions	Yes	Yes	No
Systemic fibrinogen depletion	Substantial	Substantial	Moderate, variable
Intracerebral hemorrhage	~0.4%	~0.6%	0.6%
90-min recanalization rate†	~40%	~63%	~79%
TIMI-2 and TIMI-3 combined‡	60%	NA	81%
TIMI-3‡	32%	NA	54%
Lives saved per 100 treated	~2.5	~2.5	~3.5§
Cost per dose (approximate U.S. dollars)	200	1700	2200
Cost per life saved (approximate U.S. dollars)	8000	68,000	62,857
Cost per year of life saved (approximate U.S. dollars)	<1000	NA	25,000–35,000¶

Abbreviations: APSAC, anisoylated plasminogen streptokinase activator complex; TIMI, Thrombolysis in Myocardial Infarction; GUSTO, Global Utilization of Streptokinase and t-PA for Occluded Coronary Arteries.

*Accelerated alteplase is given as follows: 15 mg bolus, then 0.75 mg/kg over 30 min (maximum, 50 mg), then 0.50 mg/kg over 60 min (maximum, 35 mg).

†Based on published data and under assumption that 20% of arteries are already open before therapy.

‡These data are from the GUSTO-I angiographic substudy.[33]

§Based on the finding from the GUSTO-I trial that accelerated alteplase saves one more additional life per 100 treated than does streptokinase.

¶Incremental cost per year of life saved for alteplase in comparison with streptokinase.

restoration of coronary blood flow, and the benefit is specifically related to the occurrence of Thrombolysis in Myocardial Infarction (TIMI) grade 3 flow.[33, 34] As far as currently known, all of these beneficial effects correlate with the reduction in mortality; no trials have shown a dissociation between mortality reduction and pump failure or arrhythmic events. The major toxic effect of thrombolytic therapy is intracranial bleeding, although systemic bleeding, allergic reactions (with streptokinase and APSAC), and myocardial rupture in patients treated late[35] must be considered.

An extensive compilation of experience with thrombolysis has been accomplished with the use of individual patient records in a database known as the Fibrinolytic Therapy Trialists' Collaboration (FTT), which included clinical trials of more than 1000 patients.[36] This resource has allowed a complete evaluation of the results of multiple clinical trials that collectively enrolled more than 58,500 patients randomized to thrombolytic therapy or to control therapy with either placebo or conservative care. The results demonstrate an 18% reduction in short-term mortality overall and a 25% reduction in short-term mortality among patients with ST segment elevation or bundle branch block shown on the ECG who were treated within 12 h of symptom onset. These results were maintained for 1 year in a large number of studies[37–39] and for 5 years in selected studies.[40] Furthermore, the benefits are evident across a wide variety of subgroups (Fig. 7–2).

Considerable discussion has centered around the evaluation of patient characteristics and the question of whether individual characteristics can be used to identify patients without a substantial likelihood of benefit.[41] Initial concern arose about patients with inferior infarction and about elderly patients. The FTT analysis clearly demonstrates that among patients with ST segment elevation or bundle branch block, the proportional reduction in risk is constant across individual patient characteristics and that the number of patients needed to treat is inversely proportional to the underlying risk of death without thrombolytic therapy (Fig. 7–3). Randomized trial evidence in more than 6000 patients fails to show any evidence of benefit in patients without ST segment elevation or bundle branch block on the ECG.

The critical markers of risk in ST elevation infarction include advanced age, decreased blood pressure, increased heart rate, anterior infarction location, and advanced Killip class.[42] More detailed analysis of ECG data indicates that the extent (number of leads) and height (peak) of ST segment elevation[43] are much stronger predictors of mortality than is infarct location. The presence of a conduction disturbance (i.e., heart block, bundle branch block) is also associated with a high rate of mortality. Thus patients with one or more of these characteristics should be considered to have the most to gain from efforts at reperfusion.

Age is one of the most interesting individual patient characteristics.[44–46] The tendency of physicians is to assume that younger patients achieve the greatest benefit with very little risk of bleeding. Indeed, the empiric data support the low risk of bleeding; intracranial bleeding is particularly rare in patients under age 55. However, these same young patients have a very low risk of death, and therefore the absolute gain in lives saved from thrombolytic treatment is less. Despite the lack of significant gain with regard to mortality in younger patients given thrombolytic therapy, the preservation of left ventricular function may decrease significant morbidity in this group. The FTT analysis demonstrates a constant proportional improvement in risk as a function of age, possibly with some deterioration in relative benefit in patients over the age of 75 years.[36] Because of the direct relationship between age and underlying risk of death, the absolute benefit (lives saved per 100 patients treated) increases as a function of age until age 75, when it levels off as a result of the fall in the relative benefit (see Fig. 7–3).

Patients with inferior infarction have been a source of controversy, and concern has been expressed anew with the publication of the FTT data because the confidence limits for the effect on mortality barely include the possibility of no treatment effect. However, the point estimate for benefit in inferior myocardial infarction is approximately a 15% reduction in the risk of death and a savings of approximately 9 lives per 1000 patients treated. Substantial extant information supports the concept that without thrombolytic therapy and thus a greater expected benefit of treatment, mortality rates are higher among patients with inferior myocardial infarction and concomitant right ventricular infarction[47]; patients with precordial ST segment depression[48]; and patients with ST segment elevation in

Presentation features	Percent of patients dead: Fibrinolytic	Percent of patients dead: Control	Stratified statistics: O-E	Stratified statistics: Variance	Chi-square test of odds ratios in different patient categories: Heterogeneity	Trend
ECG					21.28 on 6 df (P<.01)	
BBB	18.7%	23.6%	-24.5	83.3		
ST elev, anterior	13.2%	16.9%	-122.0	420.6		
ST elev, inferior	7.5%	8.4%	-27.1	237.4		
ST elev, other	10.6%	13.4%	-42.1	159.6		
ST depression	15.2%	13.8%	12.9	108.7		
Other abnormality	5.2%	5.8%	-9.6	103.2		
Normal	3.0%	2.3%	3.4	12.9		
Hours from onset					9.69 on 4 df (P<.05)	9.55 on 1 df (2P=0.002)
0-1	9.5%	13.0%	-29.3	83.3		
2-3	8.2%	10.7%	-100.2	354.8		
4-6	9.7%	11.5%	-78.5	387.6		
7-12	11.1%	12.7%	-51.5	336.7		
13-24	10.0%	10.5%	-11.1	212.6		
Age (years)					8.27 on 3 df (P<.05)	6.58 on 1 df (2P=0.01)
<55	3.4%	4.6%	-45.9	155.6		
55-64	7.2%	8.9%	-86.3	360.0		
65-74	13.5%	16.1%	-113.7	533.0		
75+	24.3%	25.3%	-12.6	266.6		
Gender					1.99 on 1 df (NS)	
Male	8.2%	10.1%	-208.1	928.0		
Female	14.1%	16.0%	-62.2	436.8		
Systolic BP (mm Hg)					1.31 on 3 df (NS)	0.68 on 1 df (NS)
<100	28.9%	35.1%	-38.7	132.2		
100-149	9.6%	11.5%	-168.9	850.0		
150-174	7.2%	8.7%	-59.2	290.0		
175+	7.2%	8.2%	-10.8	74.1		
Heart rate					0.51 on 2 df (NS)	0.31 on 1 df (NS)
<80	7.2%	8.5%	-83.2	464.9		
80-99	9.2%	11.3%	-65.8	287.2		
100+	17.4%	20.7%	-51.7	238.6		
Prior MI					2.09 on 1 df (NS)	
Yes	12.5%	14.1%	-43.7	322.4		
No	8.9%	10.9%	-228.5	1001.9		
Diabetes					1.57 on 1 df (NS)	
Yes	13.6%	17.3%	-41.4	145.7		
No	8.7%	10.2%	-142.6	830.4		
ALL PATIENTS	2820/29315 9.6%	3357/29285 11.5%	-269.5	1377.4		

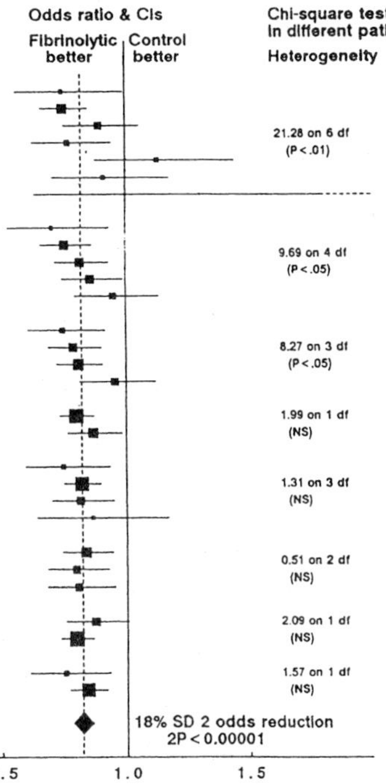

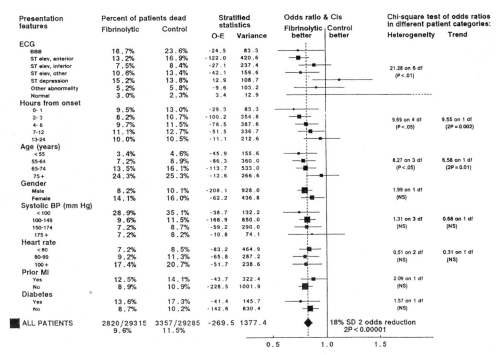

Figure 7–2. Proportional effects of fibrinolytic therapy on mortality during days 0–35, subdivided by presentation features. "Observed minus expected" (O − E) number of events among fibrinolytic-assigned patients (and its variance) is given for subdivisions of presentation features, stratified by trial. This is used to calculate odds ratios (ORs) of death among patients assigned to fibrinolytic therapy vs. those assigned to control treatment. ORs (*black squares* with areas proportional to amount of "statistical information" contributed by the trials) are plotted with their 99% confidence intervals [CIs] (*horizontal lines*). *Squares* to left of the solid vertical line indicate benefit (significant at $2p < .01$ only where entire CI is to the left of the vertical line). Overall result and 95% CI is represented by the diamond; overall proportional reduction in the odds of death and statistical significance are given alongside. Chi-square tests for evidence of heterogeneity of, or trends in, size of ORs in subdivisions of each presentation feature are also given. *Abbreviations:* ECG, electrocardiogram; BBB, bundle branch block; NS, not significant; BP, blood pressure; MI, myocardial infarction. (From Fibrinolytic Therapy Trialists' [FTT] Collaborative Group: Indications for fibrinolytic therapy in suspected acute myocardial infarction: collaborative overview of early mortality and major morbidity results from all randomised trials of more than 1000 patients. Lancet 1994; 343:311–322.)

leads V_5, V_6, I, or aV_L. Even for an isolated inferior infarction, it seems prudent to assume that the benefit, although small, exceeds the risk unless a strong relative contraindication exists.

The reason for the failure of thrombolytic therapy to improve outcome in patients without ST segment elevation is unknown. The leading concepts are that either these patients have extensive multivessel disease, with little to gain from lysis of the thrombus component in only one of the involved vessels, or they have a patent vessel, in which case lytic therapy serves only to cause paradoxical thrombosis as a result of the exposure of clot-bound thrombin. In the former situation, a high mortality rate would be expected with or without thrombolytic therapy; in the latter situation, a low mortality rate would be expected in either case, although there would be concern about an increased risk of reinfarction.[49] One situation that provokes concern about withholding thrombolytic therapy is the presence of "mirror-image" ST segment depression in leads V_1, V_2, and V_3, representing circumflex occlusion. Although it is reasonable to expect that the mortality reduction achieved in these patients might be the same as that achieved in other patients with ST segment elevation representing epicardial injury, a subset of these patients has not been rigorously identified from the clinical trials.

Substantial research has provided a comprehensive view of the risk of intracranial hemorrhage with thrombolytic therapy and the patient characteristics associated with specific risk.[50–53] In descending order of importance, the most significant risk factors include a history of stroke or transient ischemic attack, advanced age, higher diastolic and systolic blood pressures, lower body weight, and history of hypertension. Multiple other factors have been identified in individual studies (Table 7–2). The same risk factors are the most important pretreatment risk factors for extracranial bleeding, although vascular procedures also account for substantial risk in thrombolytic patients. Overall, 35%–45% of strokes are fatal; more than 60% of intracranial hemorrhages are fatal, whereas only 20% of nonhemorrhagic strokes result in death. Treatment with alteplase is associated with a higher risk of hemorrhagic stroke than is treatment with streptokinase, particularly when intravenous heparin is not used with streptokinase. In the Global Use of Streptokinase and t-PA for Occluded Coronary Arteries (GUSTO-I) trial, an accelerated course of alteplase was associated with a 0.70% risk of intracranial hemorrhage, in comparison with 0.57% for streptokinase and intravenous heparin and 0.46% for streptokinase and subcutaneous heparin (Fig. 7–4).[54]

Inclusion and Exclusion Criteria

A simple approach to thrombolytic therapy is to assume that all patients with ST segment elevation on the 12-lead ECG should be treated unless a contraindication is evident. Table 7–3 lists the commonly accepted indications for and contraindications to thrombolytic therapy. Unfortunately, all of the contraindications are only relative, inasmuch as in certain situations, any one of them might be ignored if the patient is not close to invasive facilities to achieve reperfusion. Several of these contraindications merit special consideration. When a history of stroke is elicited, careful documentation that a stroke has actually occurred is desirable, because patients are often uncertain about the exact diagnosis. When the suspicion of a stroke is

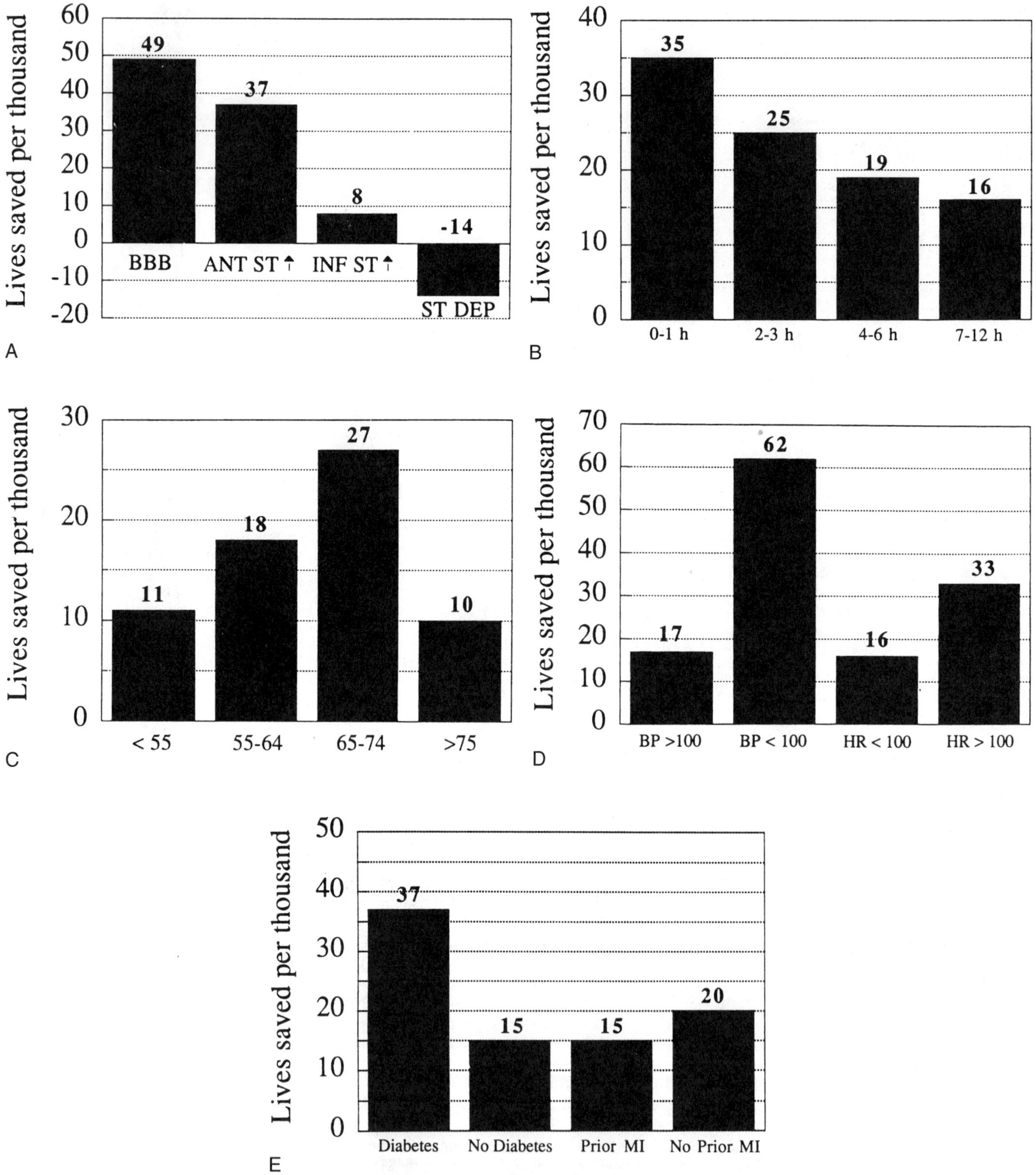

Figure 7–3. The effect of thrombolytic therapy on mortality in various patient subsets classified according to the admission ECG (A), the time from symptom onset to treatment (B), age (C), the blood pressure (BP) (D), and heart rate (HR) (D), and the presence or absence of diabetes or prior myocardial infarction (MI) (E). Patients with bundle branch block (BBB) and anterior ST segment elevation (ANT) derive the most benefit from thrombolytic therapy; effects in patients with inferior ST segment elevation (INF) are much less, while patients with ST segment depression (ST DEP) do not benefit. Patients treated early derive the most benefit. Despite a higher overall risk of death, patients over the age of 75 years do not derive a greater absolute benefit than do younger patients. Patients with hypotension or tachycardia benefit the most, and patients with diabetes are more likely to benefit than nondiabetic patients. The presence of prior infarction does not predict a greater benefit. (From Martin GV, Kennedy JW: Choice of thrombolytic agent. *In* Julian DG, Braunwald E [eds]: Management of Acute Myocardial Infarction, pp 90–91. Philadelphia: WB Saunders, 1994.)

TABLE 7–2. RISK FACTORS FOR STROKE AFTER THROMBOLYTIC THERAPY IN ACUTE MYOCARDIAL INFARCTION*

Risk Factor	Cerebral Infarction	Intracranial Hemorrhage
Age	+ + +	+ + +
Head trauma		+
Elevated systolic and diastolic blood pressures		+ + +
History of cerebral vascular disease	+ + +	+ + +
Lower body weight		+ + +
History of hypertension	+ + +	+ + +
Dementia		+
Thrombolytic agent (alteplase and APSAC carry more risk than streptokinase)		+ + +
Heparin		+ +
Elevated pulse pressure		+ +
Thrombolytic therapy dose		+ + +
Calcium channel blocker		+
Female sex		+
Diabetes mellitus		+
Atrial fibrillation	+ + +	
History of anticoagulation		+
Hemodynamic compromise	+ + +	
Anterior myocardial infarction	+ + +	
Higher Killip class	+ + +	

Symbols: + + +, definite risk factor identified in multiple studies; + +, likely risk factor; +, questionable risk factor; needs verification. *Abbreviation:* APSAC, anisoylated plasminogen streptokinase activator complex.

*Listed in order of importance for risk of intracranial hemorrhage.

Adapted with permission from O'Connor CM: Stroke during acute myocardial infarction. *In* Califf RM, Mark DB, Wagner GS (eds): Acute Coronary Care, 2nd ed, pp 635–650. St. Louis: Mosby–Year Book, 1995.

high, especially if it was recent, thrombolysis should be avoided unless the myocardial infarct is large and there is no immediate access to an interventional catheterization laboratory. Patients with systolic (>200 mm Hg) or diastolic (>100 mm Hg) hypertension have a substantially increased risk of intracranial hemorrhage, but many of these patients also have a substantial expected benefit. The practice at the author's institution is to use percutaneous transluminal coronary angioplasty (PTCA) in patients with acute hypertension unless a catheterization laboratory is more than 1 h away. Minor trauma or surgery should not be considered an absolute contraindication, although preference should be given to PTCA if a major question about localized bleeding exists. Many patients have a diagnosis of peptic ulcer disease, and some of them have endoscopic documentation. Although the risk of bleeding is certainly increased in these patients, the author and colleagues have considered this to be only a minor contraindication. The more recent and definitive the diagnosis and the lower risk the infarction, the more likely the author and colleagues are to avoid thrombolytic therapy.

Choice of Agent

Because thrombolytic therapy is planned, the physician must select a thrombolytic regimen, and because the different regimens have different associated costs and outcomes, the trade-off between cost and expected benefit should be considered. Data from the GUSTO trial provide evidence that the marginal incremental cost for using alteplase in an accelerated dosing regimen in comparison with standard streptokinase (associated with a savings of 10 lives per 1000 patients treated) is $25,000–$35,000 per year of life saved, a value that is well within the accepted cost-effectiveness ratios for other therapies commonly used in the United States.[55] Further evaluation of the patient population revealed a familiar theme: the patient characteristics that carried higher risk were associated with more benefit from an accelerated regimen of alteplase. In fact, the degree of benefit was directly proportional to the degree of underlying risk (Fig. 7–5). Therefore, older patients and patients with large infarcts or previous events received more benefit with accelerated alteplase. The expected benefit can be calculated according to the nomogram in Figure 7–6.

Direct PTCA

General Results

Because of the well-known limitations of thrombolytic therapy, including failure to reperfuse in many patients, reocclusion in others, long delay in reperfusion time, and risk of bleeding, direct coronary angioplasty has a number of theoretical advantages. It offers the opportunity to confirm the diagnosis, identify high-risk subgroups of patients who may benefit from surgical intervention, and achieve reperfusion without the hemorrhagic risk of thrombolysis. In addition, successful direct PTCA typically results in restoration of complete reperfusion (TIMI grade 3 flow); this may render it superior

TABLE 7–3. CRITERIA FOR THROMBOLYSIS IN ACUTE MYOCARDIAL INFARCTION

Indications
Chest pain or equivalent symptoms consistent with acute myocardial infarction
Electrocardiographic changes
  ST-segment elevation ≥0.1 mV in at least two contiguous leads
  New or presumably new left bundle branch block
Time from onset of symptoms
  <3 h: most beneficial
  <6 h: lesser but still important benefits
  6–12 h: diminishing benefits but still useful
  >12 h: benefit uncertain

Substantial Contraindications
Active internal bleeding
Suspected aortic dissection
Recent head trauma or known intracranial neoplasm
Pregnancy
History of stroke known to be hemorrhagic
Any stroke within 1 year
Previous allergic reaction to the thrombolytic agent (streptokinase or APSAC)

*Relative Contraindications**
Recent trauma or surgery more than 2 weeks previously; trauma or surgery within previous 2 weeks, which could be a source of rebleeding, is an absolute contraindication
History of chronic, severe hypertension with or without drug therapy or recorded blood pressure >180/110
History of stroke
Known bleeding diathesis
Significant liver dysfunction
Prior exposure to streptokinase or APSAC (this contraindication is particularly important in the initial 6–9 months after streptokinase or APSAC administration and applies to reuse of any streptokinase-containing agent but does not apply to rt-PA or urokinase)
Prolonged (>10 min) cardiopulmonary resuscitation

Abbreviations: APSAC, anisoylated plasminogen streptokinase activator complex; rt-PA, recombinant tissue plasminogen activator.

*These should be considered on a case-by-case analysis or risk/benefit. These contraindications (particularly the first five) are of paramount importance, such as more recent trauma or surgery or active peptic ulcer with history of bleeding, when weighed against a less-than-life-threatening, evolving acute myocardial infarction.

Adapted from AHA Medical/Scientific Statement Special Report: ACC/AHA guidelines for the early management of patients with acute myocardial infarction, Circulation 1990; 82:664–707; and from Anderson HV, Willerson JT: Thrombolysis in acute myocardial infarction, N Engl J Med 1993; 329:703–709.

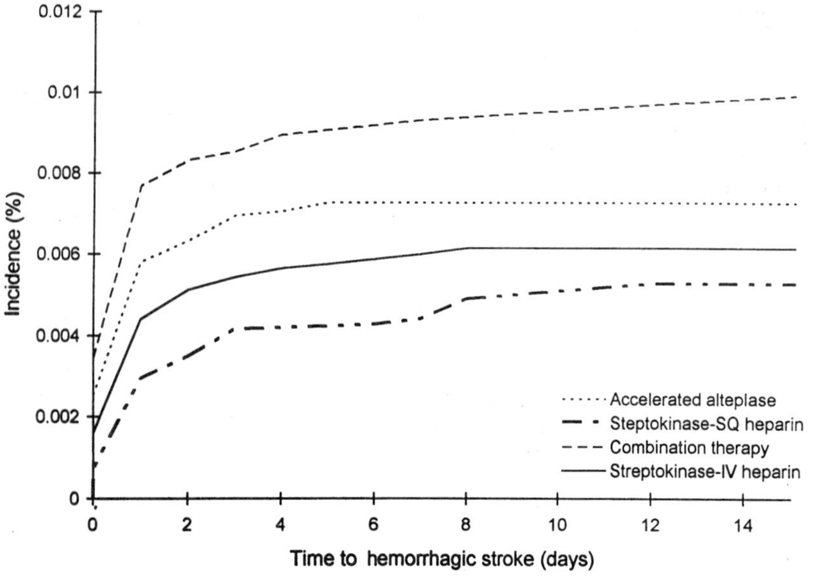

Figure 7–4. Timing of primary hemorrhagic stroke per treatment assignment in GUSTO-I. *Abbreviations:* SQ, subcutaneous; IV, intravenous. "Combination therapy" = streptokinase and alteplase plus intravenous heparin. (Adapted from Gore JM, Granger CB, Sloan MA, et al: Stroke after thrombolysis: mortality and functional outcomes in the GUSTO-I trial. Circulation 1995; 92:2811–2818.)

to thrombolysis. Indeed, a number of observational studies have demonstrated that direct angioplasty can be performed with a very high coronary perfusion rate and low rates of mortality, stroke, and reinfarction. In the Primary Angioplasty Registry of 271 patients enrolled in the emergency department, 245 underwent attempted angioplasty; in 238, the procedure was successful.[56] Of the 26 patients not undergoing angioplasty, 12 had already achieved reperfusion at the time of the diagnostic injection, 3 had no myocardial infarction or no significant stenosis, and 5 had left main stenosis. The attempted procedure was unsuccessful in only seven patients, and four patients were treated medically because significant stenoses could not be approached with angioplasty. This prospective registry thus provides convincing evidence that the procedure can be performed, with the achievement of reperfusion and less than 50% residual stenosis, in most patients identified in the emergency department.

Several trials have compared direct angioplasty with thrombolytic therapy in the acute myocardial infarction setting.[57–59] These trials have shown dramatic differences in the rates of death, reinfarction, recurrent ischemia, and stroke in the patients treated with direct angioplasty in comparison with patients treated with thrombolytic therapy (Table 7–4).[57, 58, 220–225] Bleeding rates have not been different. These studies, combined with early observational studies and the prospective PAR study, provide both convincing evidence that direct angioplasty is at least as beneficial as thrombolysis and initial evidence that it may be better.

These trials have several limitations that are to be expected in early studies of new technologies. The clinical sites were experienced centers with a particular interest in the procedure, and almost all were high-volume angioplasty centers by U.S. standards. Whether the same results will be transferable to lower volume centers remains uncertain, especially in view of the evidence that mortality rates among patients with myocardial infarction treated with angioplasty in the Medicare registry are much higher in low-volume sites.[60] In addition, the outcomes in the thrombolytic-treated patients in these trials have been worse than observed in trials comparing one thrombolytic regimen with another. Regardless of whether this stems from enrollment of higher risk patients into trials of direct angioplasty or from chance, future trials comparing direct angioplasty with thrombolysis through the use of accelerated regimens of alteplase will provide more insight into indications for each treatment.

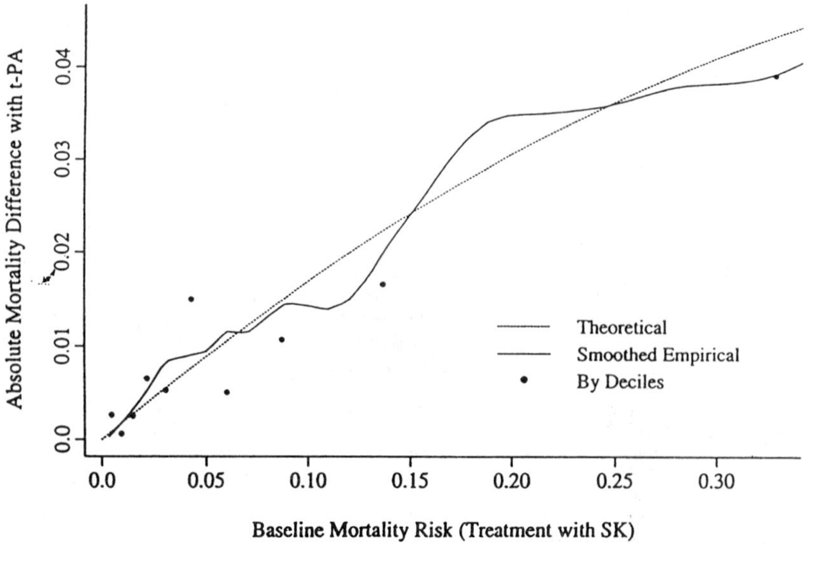

Figure 7–5. Plots of absolute mortality decrease with accelerated tissue plasminogen activator (t-PA, alteplase) treatment vs. baseline mortality risk (assuming streptokinase treatment). The "Theoretical" series represents expected mortality as a function of underlying patient risk, generated from the statistical model developed from all available baseline characteristics. "By Deciles" reflects the difference in the proportions of patients who died in each decile of predicted risk for patients who received alteplase vs. streptokinase. The "Smoothed Empirical" series represents a nonparametric estimate of the relationship between predicted patient risk and the observed mortality in the alteplase group vs. the combined streptokinase group.

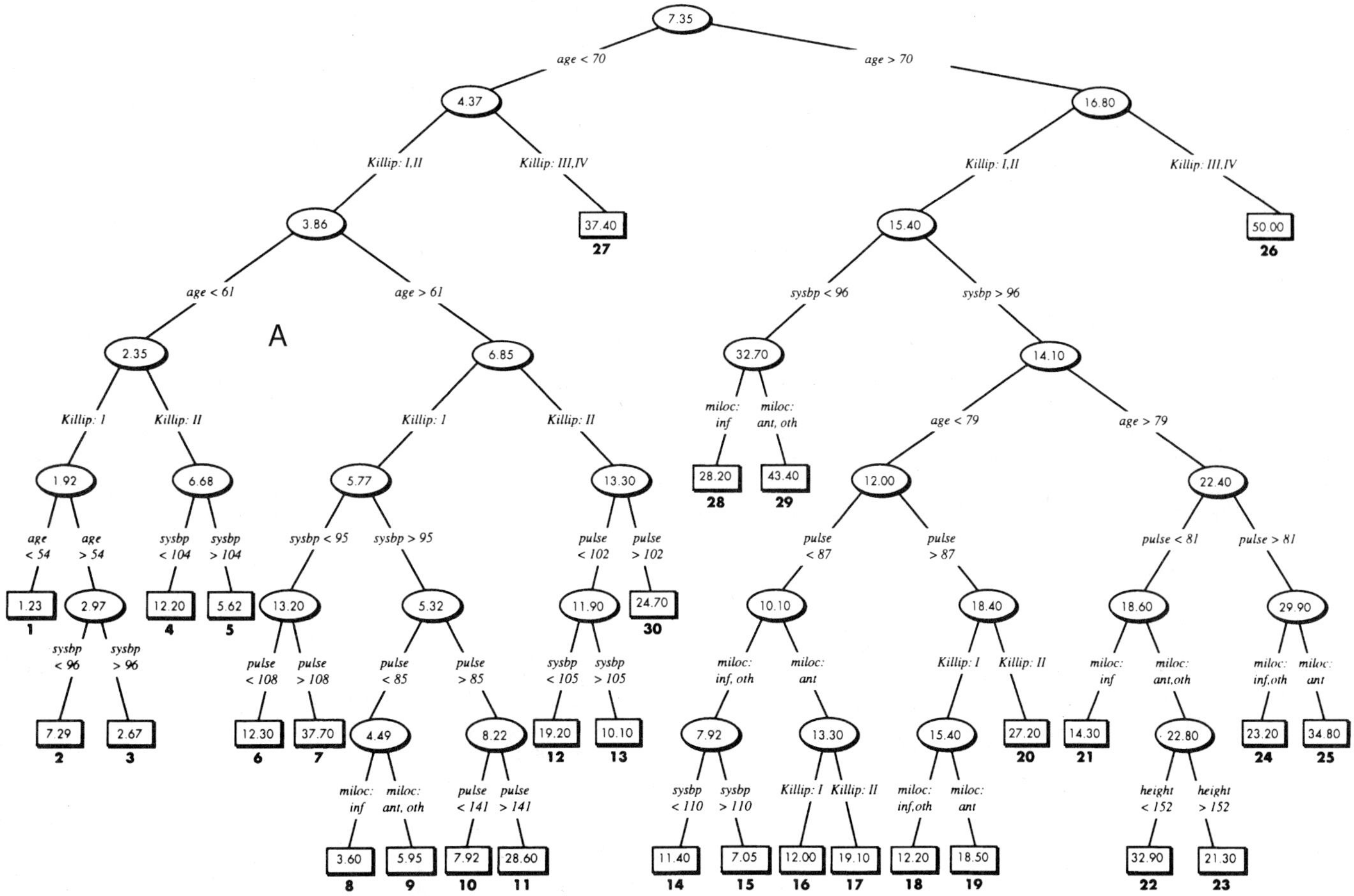

Figure 7–6. This figure depicts the results of a statistical analysis of the GUSTO-I data in which patients were split into groups on the basis of estimation of risk of death if treated with streptokinase (the numbers in the ovals and rectangles are the mortality rates at each point). Because the degree of benefit with alteplase was directly related to the extent of underlying risk with streptokinase, the illustration also points out the patients who receive the most benefit when alteplase is chosen rather than streptokinase. The most important determinants are age, Killip class, systolic blood pressure (sysbp), heart rate, and myocardial infarct location (miloc): anterior (ant) vs. inferior (inf) or other (oth).

TABLE 7–4. OUTCOMES IN RANDOMIZED TRIALS OF DIRECT PTCA VS. THROMBOLYTIC THERAPY

	Deaths				Deaths or Nonfatal Reinfarction			
	At 6 Weeks		At 1 Year		At 6 Weeks		At 1 Year	
Trials	*Inv*	*Cons*	*Inv*	*Cons*	*Inv*	*Cons*	*Inv*	*Cons*
O'Neill et al.[220]	2/29*	1/27*	NA	NA	3/29*	2/27*	NA	NA
DeWood and Fisher[221]	3/46	2/44	4/46	2/44	3/46	2/44	4/46	2/44
Grines et al. (PAMI)[57]	5/195*	13/200*	NA	NA	10/195*	24/200*	NA	NA
Zijlstra et al.[222]	3/152*	11/149*	NA	NA	5/152*	23/149*	NA	NA
Gibbons et al.[58]	2/47*	2/56*	3/47	2/56	2/47*†	2/56*†	3/47	4/56
Ribeiro et al.[223]	3/50	1/50	3/50	2/50	5/50	2/50	4/50	3/50
Elizaga et al.[224]	3/52	7/48	3/52	8/48	7/52	8/48	7/52	11/48
Total	21/571	37/574	13/195	14/198	35/571	63/574	18/195	20/198
	(3.7%)	(6.4%)	(6.7%)	(7.1%)	(6.1%)	(11.0%)	(9.2%)	(10.1%)

Abbreviations: PTCA, percutaneous transluminal coronary angioplasty; Inv, invasive: Cons, conservative; PAMI, Primary Angioplasty in Myocardial Infarction.
*At hospital discharge.
†Only data on mortality were available.
Adapted from Michels KB, Yusuf S: Does PTCA in acute myocardial infarction affect mortality and reinfarction rates? A quantitative overview (meta-analysis) of the randomized clinical trials. Circulation 1995; 91:476–485.

Because the amount of randomized trial data is limited, the decision about when to use thrombolytic therapy and when to use direct angioplasty is somewhat subjective. The first principle is that direct angioplasty should be considered only by an experienced operator and support staff. Second, direct angioplasty requires efficiency and planning in order to bring the patient and the staff to the angiographic laboratory in a timely manner. Third, direct angioplasty (when performed efficiently by experienced operators) appears to provide superior reperfusion and better outcomes, according to available data. The policy at the author's institution is to perform direct angioplasty when the angiographic laboratory and an experienced support staff are available within 1 h of a patient's arrival at the emergency department.

Cardiogenic shock is a special situation in which the observational evidence that direct angioplasty is superior to thrombolysis is most convincing.[61] However, because of the absence of randomized trial information, the results of the Should We Emergently Revascularize Occluded Coronaries for Cardiogenic Shock (SHOCK) trial may alter this view.[62] Because multiple observational studies have shown a better outcome among patients treated with direct coronary angioplasty than among those treated with conservative care, and because results with thrombolytic treatment have been disappointing, the author and colleagues will continue to refer patients with cardiogenic shock for PTCA until the results of the SHOCK study are available.

Patients with ST segment elevation infarction and a strong relative contraindication to thrombolytic therapy constitute an important group. For the most part, these patients have much to gain by myocardial reperfusion but have a substantial risk of intracranial or systemic bleeding. In the author's practice, patients with minor head trauma, which frequently happens with transient syncope during inferior myocardial infarction or after resuscitated ventricular fibrillation, are referred for direct angioplasty.[63] Similarly, patients with substantial hypertension (systolic pressure > 180 and diastolic pressure > 110 mm Hg) are taken to direct angioplasty. Patients with a history of definite stroke have a marked increase in the risk of stroke during thrombolytic therapy.[52, 63] Patients who have recently undergone surgery or trauma similarly have a markedly enhanced risk of systemic bleeding, and direct angioplasty should be associated with a reduction in this risk.

Practical issues in the performance of direct angioplasty center on the maintenance of a protocol dictating a common approach to maintaining an experienced and competent staff. Close collaboration with the emergency department can allow the patient to be prepared for the procedure while the staff is preparing the laboratory. In addition to a call system to prevent delays in starting treatment, a carefully planned surgical backup system is needed.[64] Every effort is made to give enough heparin to keep the activated clotting time at >300–350 sec so as to reduce the risk of ischemic complications during the procedure. The noninfarcted vessels are imaged first, unless the patient is in extremis, to ensure that if emergency surgery is needed during attempted revascularization of the infarcted vessel, the nonculprit anatomy is known. Adjunctive pharmacotherapy after the procedure is the same as that for patients treated with thrombolytic therapy.

The author's current approach to the choice of reperfusion method in patients with ST segment elevation accompanying myocardial infarction is shown in Figure 7–7. Patients with cardiogenic shock or large infarcts are treated with direct coronary angioplasty if an interventional facility is available within 1 h of arrival at the emergency department. All other patients are treated with an accelerated course of alteplase, although patients with an underlying mortality

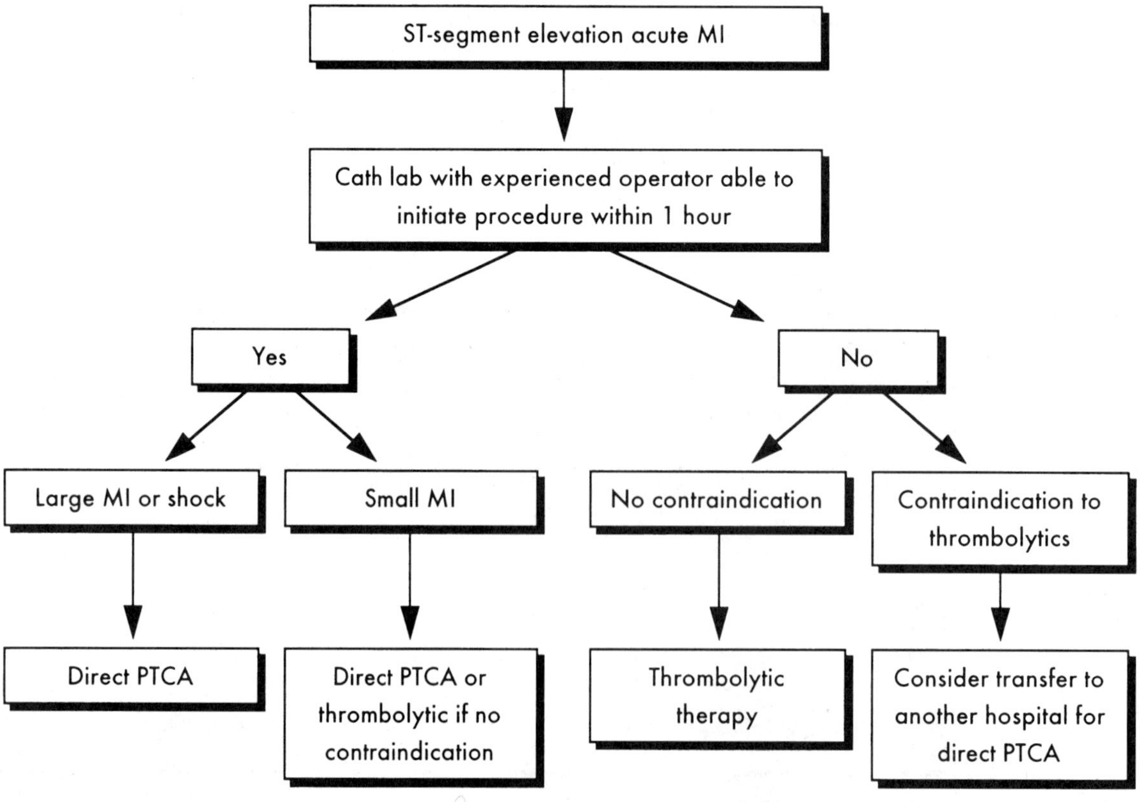

Figure 7–7. Suggested approach to the decision about the use of direct coronary angioplasty vs. thrombolytic therapy in patients with acute ST segment elevation during myocardial infarction (MI) or acute MI associated with left bundle branch block. If the patient can have an angioplasty procedure by a high-volume operator in a high-volume center with good results within 1 h of arrival, direct angioplasty is chosen. If the time elapsed is expected to exceed 1 h, thrombolytic therapy is chosen. Of the patients who must be transferred, only those with cardiogenic shock are considered for direct coronary angioplasty. *Other abbreviation:* PTCA, percutaneous transluminal coronary angioplasty.

risk of less than 5% can be treated with streptokinase, with only a small difference in expected mortality.

Digitalis (see Chapter 9)

The role of digitalis is still a matter of some controversy. On the one hand are concerns about increased risk of mortality after its long-term use (according to observational studies), and on the other hand are studies that suggest a neutral effect with regard to mortality.[65, 66] Digitalis has been shown to improve symptomatic status and have a favorable effect on the neurohormonal system in patients with definite systolic left ventricular dysfunction. The mortality issue will be resolved when a large trial by the Digitalis Investigators Group concludes. At this time, the author and colleagues reserve digitalis for patients with proven systolic left ventricular dysfunction and symptomatic heart failure. They use a loading dose of 12–15 μg/kg of lean body weight, giving half the dose acutely and the other half in 25% increments 6 h apart. A maintenance dose of 0.125–0.375 mg/day is given, depending on renal function and lean body weight.

Heparin (see Chapter 28)

Thrombin is thought to play a major role in the pathogenesis and clinical outcomes of myocardial infarction through a variety of mechanisms.[67] As the key component in the conversion of fibrinogen to fibrin, thrombin plays a central role in the initial process of coronary thrombosis. Thrombin is also a key activator of platelets, and its effects on platelet activation are not totally inhibited by aspirin. Active thrombin is bound to the propagating clot so that as lysis occurs, clot-bound thrombin is exposed to the circulating blood, creating a thrombogenic state.

Heparin, discovered in 1916, is a complex polysaccharide consisting of a mixture of molecules with a variety of molecular weights ranging from 5000 to 20,000; each component has a different effect on the coagulation system. Anticoagulation is achieved by the inactivation of thrombin and factor X through complexing with antithrombin III (AT-III). The variable effect of a given dose of heparin on the thrombotic system is believed to result from a variety of factors, including fluctuating levels of AT-III, inactivation of heparin by platelet factor IV, binding of heparin to other plasma proteins, and the inability of heparin to inactivate clotbound thrombin.[67] In addition, the clinical effect of heparin is directly related to weight (6-sec lower activated partial thromboplastin time [aPTT] for each 10-kg increase in weight), age (5-sec lower aPTT for each 10 years younger), and sex (11-sec higher aPTT for women than for men).[68]

Nonthrombolytic Patients

Before the thrombolytic era, patients treated with heparin were compared with a control group in a series of randomized trials. A systematic overview demonstrated a 17% reduction in mortality and a 22% reduction in the risk of reinfarction with heparin (Fig. 7–8).[69] These studies were done before aspirin, beta blockers, and nitrates were routine therapy, and thus clinicians are somewhat uncertain about whether this effect is as strong today. Nevertheless, because this evidence is the best available, the author and colleagues currently use intravenous heparin as routine therapy in patients with myocardial infarction who are not candidates for reperfusion, unless a strong contraindication to anticoagulation is present.

Thrombolysis

Streptokinase and APSAC. When a patient is to be treated with streptokinase or APSAC, substantial information now points to the lack of need to treat with heparin. The third International Study of Infarct Survival (ISIS-3)[70] and the second Gruppo Italiano per lo Studio della Sopravvivenza nell'Infarto Miocardico (GISSI-2)[71] studies randomized a total of more than 60,000 patients to subcutaneous heparin or no subcutaneous heparin with thrombolytic therapy. No differences were observed in rates of mortality in either trial; ISIS-3 found a slightly elevated risk of intracranial hemorrhage, whereas GISSI-2 did not, and an excess rate of systemic bleeding was observed with subcutaneous heparin in both trials. The GUSTO-I trial randomized more than 20,000 patients to intravenous or subcutaneous heparin with streptokinase, and no differences were observed in rates of mortality, reinfarction, or nonhemorrhagic stroke,[72] but an excess of hemorrhagic stroke and systemic bleeding did appear in the intravenous heparin–treated patients. The Duke University Clinical Cardiology Study (DUCCS) 1 randomized a small cohort of patients to APSAC with or without intravenous heparin.[73] The heparin-treated patients had no advantage on a composite clinical endpoint of death, reinfarction, stroke, or heart failure or on a careful measurement of left ventricular function, but they experienced a significant increase in the risk of bleeding. The summary of these studies provides no empiric rationale for the use of heparin in combination with non–fibrin-specific thrombolytic agents such as streptokinase and APSAC.

Alteplase. Alteplase most often does not produce a profound sys-

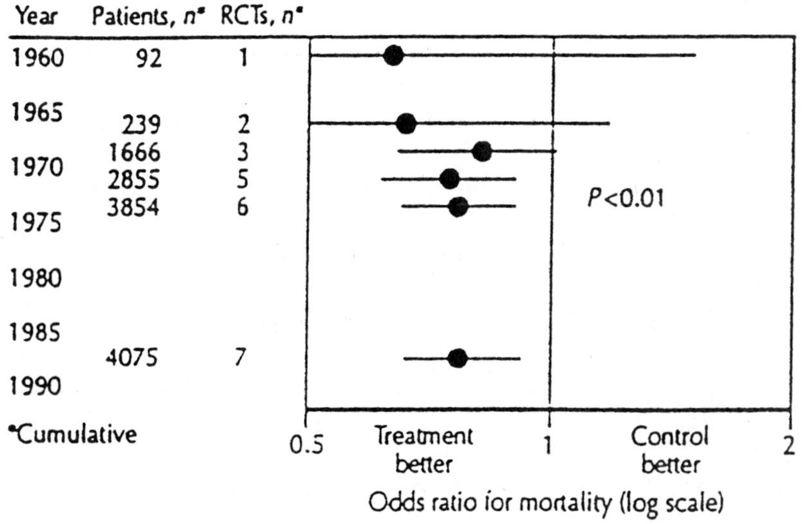

Figure 7–8. Meta-analysis of results from seven randomized controlled trials (RCTs) of heparin after acute myocardial infarction. All these trials were conducted in the prethrombolytic era (1960–1990) and indicate a reduction of approximately 17%–25% in the odds ratio for mortality among patients receiving active therapy. (From Antman E, Lau J, Kupelnick B, et al: A comparison of results of meta-analyses of randomized control trials and recommendations of clinical experts: treatments for myocardial infarction. JAMA 1992; 268:240–248.)

temic fibrinolytic state; thus the rationale for antithrombin therapy is stronger than it is for non–fibrin-specific lytic agents. A number of angiographic trials have demonstrated that intravenous heparin resulted in a higher rate of perfusion of the infarcted artery than did control therapy[74–76] and that this rate was directly proportional to the aPTT.[75, 76] However, according to a systematic overview of the clinical outcomes from these studies, the rate of mortality was decreased by 11% with broad confidence limits, including the possibility of no treatment effect, and the rates of bleeding are significantly increased with heparin, with nonsignificant increases in reinfarction and hemorrhagic and nonhemorrhagic stroke (Fig. 7–9).[77] This paradoxical trend toward more thrombotic events in the heparin-treated patients is disconcerting, but in view of the pathophysiologic rationale, the reperfusion data, and the trend toward mortality reduction in the heparin-treated patients, the author and colleagues continue to use heparin in alteplase-treated patients.

Uncertainty About Dosing

According to the arterial perfusion data just described, the therapeutic range for heparin in coronary arterial thrombosis should presumably be higher than generally recommended for venous thrombosis. Other information, however, strongly supports an aPTT target of 1.5–2.0 times higher than the control value. Analyses of the GUSTO-I[78] and TIMI[79] data indicate that the best outcome with regard to mortality, reinfarction, stroke, and bleeding is in patients with an aPTT of 50–70 sec, as measured by standard assays (Fig. 7–10). Furthermore, when the dose of heparin was increased to achieve an aPTT of 60–85 sec in GUSTO-IIa and 60–90 sec in TIMI 9a, an unacceptable rate of intracranial hemorrhage ensued. The current algorithm for intravenous heparin dosing is displayed in Figure 7–11.

Studies have demonstrated a delay of several hours in the reporting of aPTT values from the typical hospital laboratory. In view of the information now demonstrating the risk of intracranial hemorrhage and systemic bleeding from high aPTT values with heparin therapy, rapid reporting of the aPTT value is critical for the thrombolytic-treated patient. In the GUSTO-I trial it was demonstrated that bedside aPTT monitoring, although not providing exactly the same value as standard laboratory reagents,[80] led to equivalent or better outcomes in comparison with central laboratory monitoring.[81] The most important point is that each hospital should have a validated system that will lead to turnaround times of less than 1 hour from when the sample is drawn to when the value is returned to the patient's bedside; reporting time can be <30 sec with bedside monitoring.

Left Ventricular Thrombus and Large Anterior Infarction

In most studies the occurrence of a large anterior myocardial infarction has been associated with an increased risk of embolic events, including strokes. Because the author and colleagues routinely treat patients with aspirin and heparin unless the patient is treated with a non–fibrin-specific thrombolytic agent, such as streptokinase or APSAC, this issue does not arise. When a patient with a large anterior infarction is treated with a non–fibrin-specific fibrinolytic agent, it is reasonable, on the basis of current evidence, to initiate therapy with subcutaneous or intravenous heparin.[82] The decision about the duration of anticoagulation is discussed in the section on oral antithrombotic therapy.

Aspirin

Aspirin appears to exert its antiplatelet effects by acetylating cyclooxygenase and thereby inhibiting the formation of thromboxane A_2, a coronary vasoconstrictor and platelet activator. When aspirin is ingested, acetylation of platelets occurs before systemic absorption; this phenomenon is believed to occur in the portal circulation.[83] A linear relationship exists between dose of aspirin and inhibition of thromboxane B_2, whereas doses of less than 50 mg of aspirin have little effect on prostacyclin inhibition. Water-soluble aspirin is much more rapidly absorbed than enteric-coated aspirin,[84] although chewing enteric-coated aspirin does lead to absorption within 20–30 min. Collagen-induced aggregation of platelets is inhibited for the life of the platelets, and with typical dosing of 160–235 mg/day, values for platelet aggregation normalize about 1 week after the last dose.

Clinical Trials Results. Aspirin is truly the "wonder drug" of cardiology, leading to a 25% reduction in rates of mortality, reinfarction, and stroke in patients with myocardial infarction; the mortality effect is in addition to the effect of thrombolytic therapy (Fig.

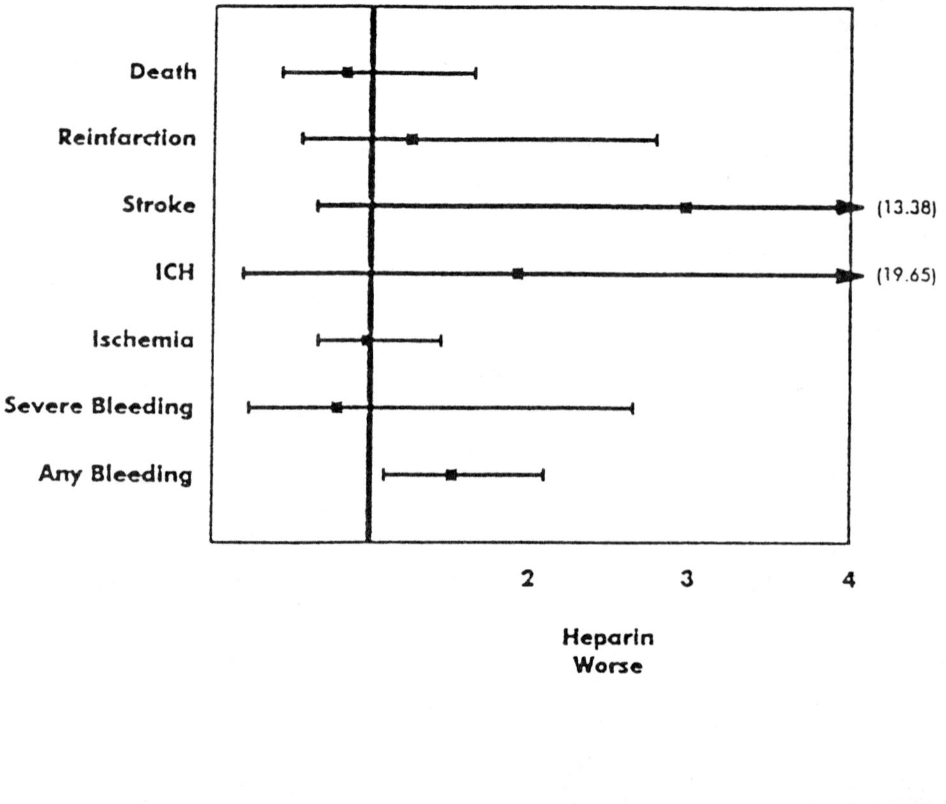

Figure 7–9. Odds ratios (and 95% confidence intervals) for intravenous heparin in comparison with no heparin for major clinical outcome events in trials using tissue plasminogen activator (t-PA) (alteplase). *Abbreviation:* ICH, intracranial hemorrhage. "Severe bleeding" = bleeding associated with hemodynamic compromise or necessitating blood transfusion. (From Mahaffey KW, Granger CB, O'Connor CM, et al: Overview of randomized trials of intravenous heparin in patients with acute myocardial infarction treated with thrombolytic therapy. Am J Cardiol, in press.)

7–12).[85–88] This benefit is achieved at the price of only a modest increase in the risk of significant bleeding or intracranial hemorrhage in the setting of thrombolytic therapy. The optimal dose of aspirin remains highly controversial; advocated doses range from 30 to 325 mg/day for acute myocardial infarction and even higher for secondary prevention in cerebrovascular disease (see Chapters 1 and 27). The only clear information about dosing is that gastrointestinal side effects and bleeding are dose-related. A reasonable approach in acute myocardial infarction is to use a dose of 160 mg, since this dose was used in the ISIS-2 study and is in the midrange of dosing recommendations. In the acute phase, chewing aspirin is recommended because of concern about absorption during the nausea that frequently accompanies the acute event.

When a patient reports an allergy to aspirin, it is important to scrutinize the history, because most often the "allergy" is simply gastrointestinal upset, which should not be an absolute contraindication to its use. True aspirin intolerance is present in fewer than 5% of patients.[89] If a true allergy manifested by hives, nasal polyps, bronchospasm, or anaphylaxis has occurred, the current recommendation is to treat with ticlopidine. Ticlopidine inhibits adenosine diphosphate (ADP)–induced platelet aggregation, and although the mechanism is not entirely clear, it may be that the drug inhibits fibrinogen binding to the glycoprotein IIb/IIIa (GpIIb/IIIa) receptor on the platelet surface.[90] Given at a dose of 250 mg b.i.d., it has been shown to reduce rates of mortality, myocardial infarction, and stroke in several clinical trials, although the patient cohorts had a primary diagnosis of cerebrovascular disease or unstable angina.[91–93] Unfortunately, the antiplatelet effect may require 3–5 days to peak, and severe neutropenia (which occurs in 1% of patients), rash (14%), and gastrointestinal upset or diarrhea (20%) are limiting factors. Some evidence suggests that a more rapid antiplatelet effect can be achieved through bolus dosing with 1000 mg of ticlopidine given orally.[94]

Glycoprotein IIb/IIIa Inhibitors (see Chapter 27)

A variety of approaches have been developed for inhibition of the predominant final common pathway of platelet aggregation, the GpIIb/IIIa receptor. Although a number of peptide and nonpeptide compounds are currently in clinical trials, only abciximab, the Fab fragments of a humanized monoclonal antibody, is currently available for routine clinical use. When PTCA is attempted during or shortly after an acute myocardial infarction, a bolus of 0.25 mg/kg, followed by an infusion of 10 μg/min over a period of 12 h, has been shown to reduce the incidence of ischemic events during and after the procedure by 35% (Fig. 7–13).[95] Furthermore, events during the period up to 6 months after the initial procedure are also reduced,[96] resulting in a cost savings (excluding the price of the drug) of $1200 per patient.[97] These benefits were achieved at a price of doubling the risk of bleeding that necessitated transfusion.[98] More recent work has indicated that a lower heparin dose with abciximab may nullify the increase in bleeding risk.[99] Because only a small segment of the Evaluation of 7E3 for the Prevention of Ischemic Complications (EPIC) trial participants were in the throes of an acute myocardial infarction, the author and colleagues do not use abciximab routinely in primary PTCA (a clinical trial addressing this specific issue is under way). They currently use abciximab routinely in patients undergoing PTCA during the same hospitalization as for the index myocardial infarction who have either recurrent ischemia or unfavorable anatomic characteristics that would place the patients at high risk.[100]

Beta Blockers

The decision about whether to administer a beta blocker in the setting of acute myocardial infarction has been a point of considerable discussion. Small studies have demonstrated convincingly that beta blockers relieve ischemic discomfort and reduce electrocardiographic evidence of extent of infarction.[101] More than 30 randomized trials with almost 30,000 patients demonstrate without doubt that the initiation of beta blockade in the hospital reduces the risk of death, reinfarction, and serious ventricular arrhythmias.[102] Significant improvements in the rates of reinfarction, cardiac arrest, and progression to definite myocardial infarction also have been demonstrated (Fig. 7–14). Small but measurable increases in the risks of early heart block, heart failure, and shock have also been demonstrated.

In all these trials, a regimen of early intravenous followed by oral beta blockade was compared with no beta blockade. The major issue confronting the clinician is whether to initiate intravenous beta blockade or whether to start with a more "gentle" approach of using only oral beta blockade on the first day. No trials have specifically compared early intravenous and oral beta blockade against oral beta blockade alone. In the largest trial, ISIS-1 randomized 16,027 patients to an open control group or to intravenous atenolol followed by oral atenolol.[103] More than half of the mortality difference occurred on the first day, which implies that the early intravenous beta blockade was critical. In the TIMI-II trial, which was not powered to evaluate mortality effects, the risk of death or reinfarction and recurrent ischemia were substantially reduced among patients treated within the first 2 h of symptom onset with intravenous metoprolol in addition to alteplase.[104]

A complete evaluation of the GUSTO-I database indicated that the mortality rate among patients treated with a beta blocker is lower than that among patients treated without a beta blocker.[105] However, it was higher among patients treated with intravenous beta blockade followed by oral beta blockers than among patients treated with oral beta blockers alone. Whether these findings represent selection bias and confounding remains unclear in that most of the contraindications to beta blockade also denote a high risk of death. After attempts to use statistical methods of adjustment to control for differences in underlying characteristics, the apparent negative effect of intravenous beta blockers was mostly, but not entirely, accounted for by differences in baseline characteristics, whereas the positive effect of any beta blocker vs. none remained substantial.

On the basis of this information, it is recommended that intravenous followed by oral beta blockade should be used in patients without a major contraindication, including pulmonary edema (rales found in more than one third of lung fields), bronchospasm, PR interval of more than 0.24 sec or advanced atrioventricular (AV) block, heart rate of less than 60 beats per minute, or systolic blood pressure of less than 100 mm Hg. Both metoprolol and atenolol have been adequately studied to justify their use in the emergency department. Atenolol is given in two 5-mg doses intravenously 5 min apart, followed by 50–100 mg orally each day, started 1 h after the second intravenous dose. Metoprolol is administered in three 5-mg doses intravenously at 5-min intervals, followed by 50–100 mg orally b.i.d., started 1 h after the last intravenous dose. During and shortly after administration, careful monitoring for hypotension, heart block, bronchospasm, and heart failure is necessary. The author and colleagues generally believe that the use of intravenous beta blockade allows the astute clinician to rapidly determine whether a patient will tolerate beta blockade at a time when the biologic effect of the drug is short-lived; although initiating low-dose oral beta blockade seems "safe," the effect will remain for a longer time if a complication occurs. As discussed later, patients with a contraindication should be continuously evaluated throughout the hospitalization so that beta blockade can be instituted when the contraindications have cleared.

Nitrates (see Chapter 2)

Nitrates have been identified for many years as effective agents for relief of myocardial ischemia and as prophylactics against future ischemic episodes.[106] The physiologic effects of nitrates include re-

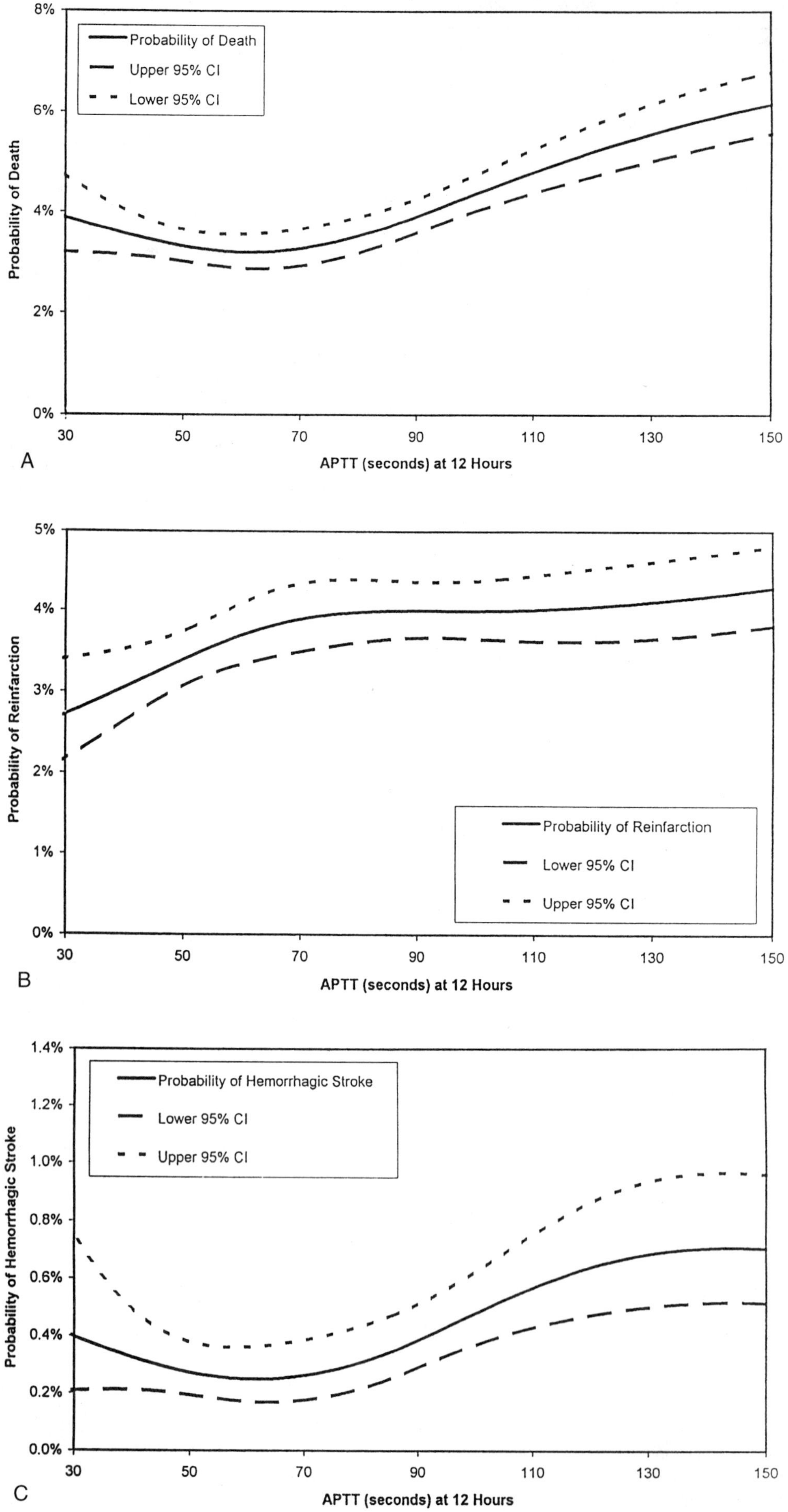

Figure 7–10. Composite of five relationships between activated partial thromboplastin time (APTT) measured 12 h after initiation of treatment in GUSTO I and clinical outcome events, including *(A)* death, *(B)* reinfarction, *(C)* hemorrhagic stroke,

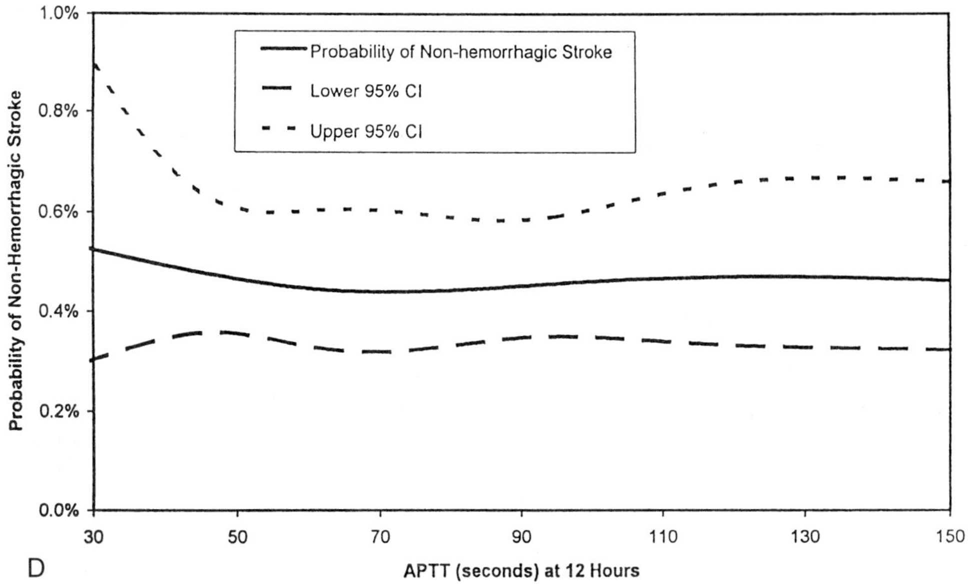

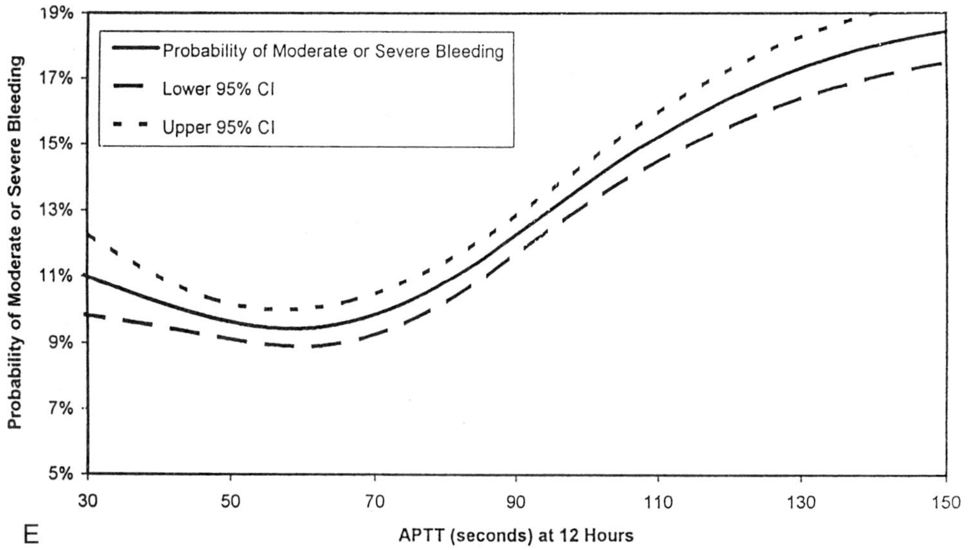

Figure 7–10 *Continued (D)* nonhemorrhagic stroke, and *(E)* major bleeding. In no case did an APTT longer than 70 sec relate to a better clinical outcome. *Other abbreviation:* CI, confidence interval. (From Granger CB, Hirsh J, Califf RM, et al: Activated partial thromboplastin time and outcome after thrombolytic therapy for acute myocardial infarction: results from the GUSTO-I trial. Circulation 1996; 93:870–878.)

ducing preload and afterload through peripheral arterial and venous dilation, relaxation of epicardial coronary arteries to improve coronary flow, and dilation of coronary collateral vessels, thus creating a more favorable subendocardial/epicardial flow ratio. Nitrates may also have a platelet-inhibiting effect. The question of whether they should be used routinely—intravenously, orally, or topically—remains unsettled, however, because of conflicting clinical trial reports.

Early small clinical trials suggested evidence of reduced infarct size and more favorable left ventricular remodeling. A systematic overview demonstrated a 35% reduction in mortality among patients routinely treated with intravenous nitrates and a less striking mortality reduction but an intriguing favorable trend in patients treated with oral nitrates (Fig. 7–15).[107] Two large trials seem to provide evidence to the contrary, however. The GISSI-3 trial randomized more than 19,000 patients to an infusion of intravenous nitroglycerin followed by topical nitrates for 6 weeks or to a control group that received no nitrates.[108] The group randomized to nitrates was started within 24 h of the onset of symptoms of infarction, and a nitrate-free interval was used for patients already receiving chronic therapy. No significant difference in mortality was observed at 6 weeks (6.52% of the nitrate-treated group and 6.92% of the control group). However, half the control group was treated with nitrates within the first several days. The 6-month follow-up from this study demonstrated an interesting trend toward a favorable mortality effect from the combination of nitrates and angiotensin converting enzyme (ACE) inhibitors. The ISIS-4 trial randomized more than 58,000 patients to oral, controlled-release isosorbide mononitrate or to placebo and also found no significant effect on survival, again with a high use of nitrates in the control group.[109] A meta-analysis that included the ISIS-4 and GISSI-3 trials demonstrated a very modest effect of nitrates on mortality ($5.5\% \pm 2.6\%$ reduction, $2p = 0.03$).[109]

The author and colleagues usually initiate nitrate therapy with intravenous nitroglycerin in a bolus of 10 μg, followed by 10 μg/min by continuous infusion with an increase of 5–10 μg/min every 5–10 min until symptoms resolve and the mean arterial pressure is lowered by 10% in normotensive patients and 30% in hypertensive patients or until the heart rate increases by more than 10 beats per minute. The dose can thus range from 20 μg/min to well over 200 μg/min, depending on the hemodynamic state and nitrate responsiveness of the patient. If the blood pressure suddenly drops, the

HEPARIN ADJUSTMENT NOMOGRAM

For a mean control aPTT of **26–36** seconds
Highest reportable aPTT **> 150** seconds
50 units/mL of heparin

Goal of therapy = therapeutic aPTT of 50–75 seconds

	aPTT (seconds)	**Bolus Dose** (units)	**Stop Infusion** (minutes)	**Rate Change** (mL/hour)	**Repeat aPTT**
	<40	3000	0 min.	+ 2 mL/hour	6 hours
	40 – 49	0	0 min.	+ 1 mL/hour	6 hours
TARGET →	50 – 75	0	0 min.	0 (no change)	next AM
	76 – 85	0	0 min.	– 1 mL/hour	next AM
	86 – 100	0	30 min.	– 2 mL/hour	6 hours
	101 – 150	0	60 min.	– 3 mL/hour	6 hours
	>150	0	60 min.	– 6 mL/hour	6 hours

• The bolus dose in this chart is based on a concentration of 1000 units/mL of heparin.
• The infusion is based on a concentration of 50 units/mL of heparin.

For aPTTs obtained before 12 hours post initiation of thrombolytic therapy:

1. Do NOT discontinue or decrease the infusion unless significant bleeding occurs or the aPTT is >150 seconds.

2. Adjust the infusion upward if the aPTT is <50 seconds.

For aPTTs obtained ≥12 hours post initiation of thrombolytic therapy, use the entire nomogram.

Deliver the bolus, stop the infusion, and/or change the rate of infusion based on the aPTT, as noted on the appropriate line of the nomogram.

Figure 7–11. Algorithm for intravenous heparin dosing.

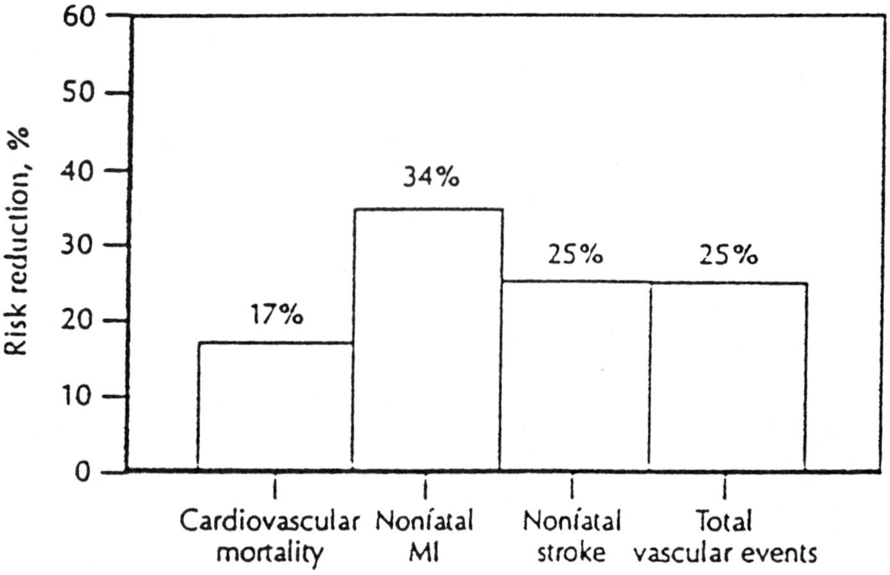

Figure 7–12. The results of antiplatelet therapy after myocardial infarction (MI) in the Antiplatelet Trialists' Collaboration extended the meta-analytic observations regarding the beneficial effects of such therapy. Patients given active antiplatelet therapy after MI not only achieved a lower rate of cardiovascular mortality but also had fewer recurrent nonfatal MIs, strokes, and total vascular events. (From Antman E: Medical therapy for acute coronary syndromes: an overview. *In* Califf RM [ed]: Acute Myocardial Infarction and Other Acute Ischemic Syndromes. Philadelphia: Current Medicine, in press.)

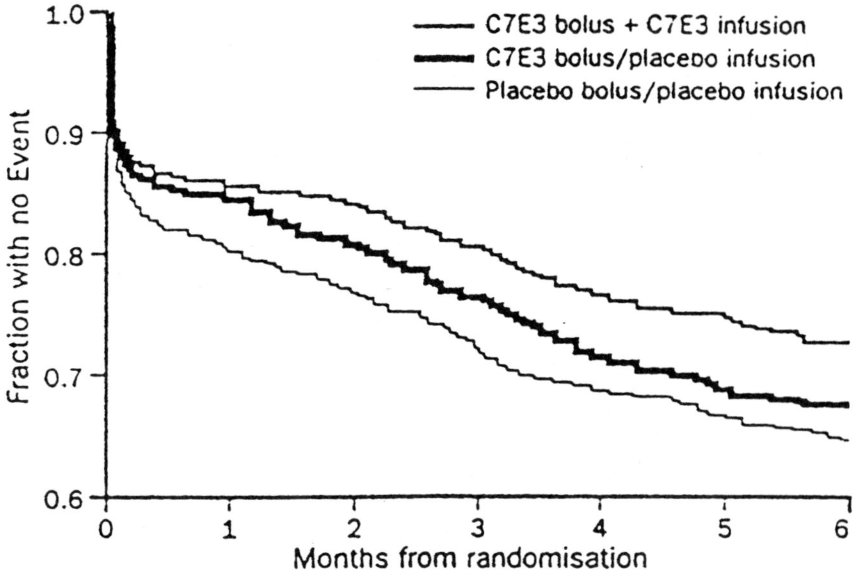

Figure 7–13. Kaplan-Meier curve of all events (death, myocardial infarction, coronary revascularization) for all patients enrolled in the EPIC Trial. There was a significant reduction of events for the c7E3 (abciximab) bolus/c7E3 infusion group compared with the active bolus only or placebo treatments (p = .001). A substantial proportion of events occurred after 1 month. (From Topol EJ, Califf RM, Weisman HF, et al: Randomised trial of coronary intervention with antibody against platelet IIb/IIIa integrin for reduction of clinical restenosis: results at six months. Lancet 1994; 343:881–886.)

infusion is slowed or discontinued while fluids are given; this action almost always rapidly raises the blood pressure.

The most common side effect of nitrates is headache, which occurs commonly but is usually short-lived as the patient becomes tolerant of the drugs. With the first dose of nitrates, some patients develop sudden hypotension and bradycardia, a syndrome that can be reversed by giving fluids, raising the legs, or using atropine if these maneuvers fail. Hypotension is particularly likely in patients with right ventricular infarction, although right ventricular infarction is not an absolute contraindication to nitrate therapy.

Magnesium

Considerable enthusiasm developed for the routine use of magnesium on the basis of the results of seven clinical trials that were combined into a systematic overview.[110] These results were confirmed by the second Leicester Intravenous Magnesium Intervention Trial (LIMIT-2), which evaluated 2300 patients randomized to placebo or to a 24-h magnesium infusion. Mortality, 10.3% in the control group, was reduced to 7.8% in the treated group.[111] The pathophysiologic explanations for the beneficial effect of magnesium included prevention of arrhythmia, antiplatelet effect, prevention of reperfusion injury, and coronary vasodilation.[112]

Just as routine magnesium was being added to the orders in many practices, the ISIS-4 trial was completed.[109] This study randomized more than 58,000 patients to routine intravenous magnesium or to control therapy and found a small, insignificant trend towards *excess* mortality with magnesium. This direct contradiction of the findings from previous studies sparked vigorous debate about the interpretation of the results. The ISIS group argued that the previous results lacked adequate numbers and may have suffered from positive reporting bias. Authors who remain optimistic about the positive role of magnesium have mounted a series of arguments to counter the

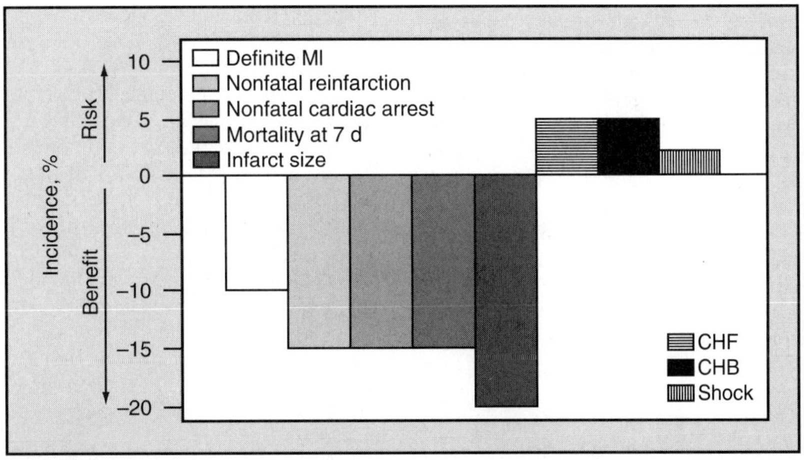

Figure 7–14. Results of intravenous beta blockade in acute myocardial infarction (MI): acute phase of treatment. The benefits of beta blockers given intravenously followed by oral administration for 1 week in patients with suspected acute MI include reductions in the rate of development of definite MI, the incidence of nonfatal reinfarction and cardiac arrest, mortality at 7 days, and infarct size. In appropriately selected patients—that is, those with a heart rate of 55 beats per minute or higher, systolic blood pressure of 100 mm Hg or more, PR interval of less than 0.24 sec, rales in less than one third of the lung field, and no history of bronchospastic lung disease—the risks for congestive heart failure (CHF), complete heart block (CHB), and cardiogenic shock are acceptably low. (From Antman E: Medical therapy for acute coronary syndromes: an overview. *In* Califf RM [ed]: Acute Myocardial Infarction and Other Acute Ischemic Syndromes. Philadelphia: Current Medicine, in press.)

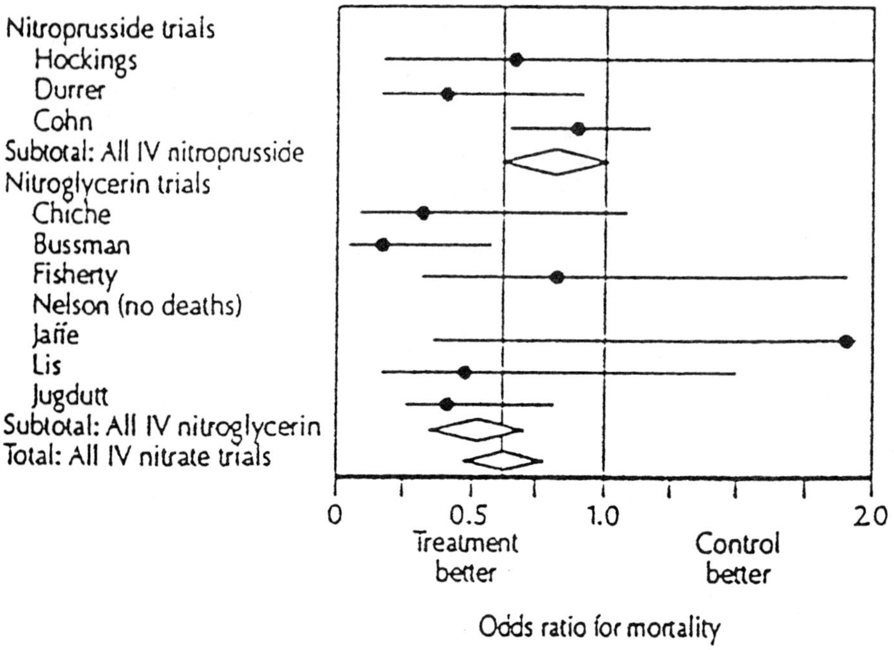

Figure 7–15. A meta-analysis of 10 trials from the prethrombolytic era indicated a favorable effect of nitrate-like compounds in the acute phase of myocardial infarction. *Abbreviation:* IV, intravenous. (From Yusuf S, Collins R, MacMahon S, Peto R: Effect of intravenous nitrates on mortality in acute myocardial infarction: an overview of the randomised trials. Lancet 1988; 1:1088–1092.)

ISIS results: first, the ISIS patients were treated relatively late after the onset of symptoms; second, the underlying mortality rate in the ISIS-4 trial was relatively low, perhaps because the high-risk patients were excluded. Antman demonstrated that when regression analysis is applied to the cumulative results of previous magnesium intervention trials, the results of ISIS-4 are actually consistent with those of previous studies because of the delayed time to treatment and low underlying risk.[113] Until this controversy is resolved, the general policy at the author's institution is to reserve magnesium therapy for patients with magnesium depletion on admission to the CCU.

Special Considerations

Cardiogenic Shock

Patients in whom cardiogenic shock develops have a dismal prognosis. Clinically, cardiogenic shock can be defined by the presence of a systolic pressure below 90 mm Hg or more than 30 mm Hg below the usual pressure, by evidence of peripheral hypoperfusion (oliguria, cyanosis, or altered mental status), and by persistence of this state after correction of extramyocardial factors such as fluid status and arrhythmias. When this diagnosis is established, the physician must be careful to understand the preferences of the patient. The therapy of cardiogenic shock involves a complex series of maneuvers that require intense coordination of the medical system. Because the prognosis of these patients is poor regardless of the approach, and because even with a good outcome the duration of hospitalization is long and the cost is high, the wishes of the patient with regard to aggressive care must be considered early in the hospital course. Patients desiring nonaggressive care should be treated with comfort measures.

In the GUSTO-I trial, cardiogenic shock was present in 0.7% of patients on arrival and later developed in 6%; these figures are consistent with the 6%–19% incidence rates in multiple previous reports.[61] The clinician should keep in mind that in the majority of patients with cardiogenic shock, this condition develops over the course of the first 24 h, but shock is generally not discernible on admission.

General Management

When a patient with cardiogenic shock is initially evaluated, supportive and resuscitative efforts must be swift and definitive to maximize the possibility of survival. Among the most important focal points of therapy are restoration of sinus rhythm, ventilation, correction of acid-base abnormalities, and relief of psychologic distress from pain and poor perfusion. Nasal intubation should be avoided if thrombolytic therapy is contemplated because of the excess risk of abrasions that lead to hemorrhage into the lungs. Once it has been demonstrated through the physical examination and/or chest radiograph that the patient has excess intravascular volume and persistent cardiogenic shock, inotropic support should begin immediately with the goals of achieving a systolic blood pressure >90 mm Hg and adequate tissue perfusion.

Inotropic and Vasopressor Agents. A variety of pharmacologic agents are considered in the attempt to enhance tissue perfusion (see Chapter 9). In general clinical terms, the author and colleagues find it useful to consider these agents in three classes: predominant vasoconstrictors with inotropic properties, inotropic catecholamines without predominant vasoconstrictive properties, and phosphodiesterase inhibitors. The selection of an agent depends on the clinical circumstances.

Dopamine and norepinephrine represent the available vasoconstrictor inotropic agents. Dopamine is generally the agent of choice in cardiogenic shock because it combines the properties of vasoconstriction, inotropy, and short half-life, allowing rapid dose titration. By directly stimulating alpha- and beta-adrenergic receptors and releasing norepinephrine from nerve endings, dopamine increases contractility and heart rate, causes vasoconstriction, and, at low to moderate doses, increases renal blood flow. One of the most interesting characteristics of dopamine is its differential physiologic effect depending on dosing. At low doses (1–3 μg/kg/min) it predominantly affects dopaminergic receptors with differential renal vascular vasodilation. At doses of 5–10 μg/kg/min, inotropic (β_1) effects predominate, whereas at higher doses, vasoconstrictor (alpha) effects are more dominant.

Dobutamine is a beta agonist with a predominant effect on β_1 receptors; it thus was designed to produce the same increase in contractility as that of dopamine without causing substantial vasoconstriction and with less tachycardia and arrhythmogenesis. Its effects on pulmonary resistance are variable.[114] In practice, dobutamine usually has little effect on peripheral vascular resistance and increases cardiac output.[115] However, it does frequently produce tachycardia and arrhythmia, although no more frequently than does dopamine. Dobutamine is usually given in a starting dose of 2.5–5 μg/kg/min and increased to 20 μg/kg/min as dictated by the hemodynamics and heart rate.

Norepinephrine is sometimes used because of its predominant vasoconstrictive effect, when maintenance of blood pressure is the goal. Although definitive comparative studies for arrhythmia outcomes with the various inotropic agents have not been performed, norepinephrine may be used to maintain cardiac output when dopamine or dobutamine causes unacceptable tachycardia.

The phosphodiesterase inhibitors, amrinone and milrinone, were developed because of their "nonreceptor" mechanism of action. These agents have both inotropic and vasodilatory properties with a more profound effect on preload than do beta agonists. Of importance is that the inotropic effect appears to add to that of beta agonists. During development, these agents were particularly promising because of their oral bioavailability. Unfortunately, amrinone has an unacceptable side effect profile, and milrinone was associated with excess mortality when given orally.[116] Excretion of these drugs is predominantly renal, and they have relatively long half-lives.

The author and colleagues generally choose dopamine as the intravenous inotropic agent when the patient has substantial hypotension (systolic blood pressure < 90 mm Hg) and dobutamine when an adequate blood pressure is present but augmentation of cardiac output is needed. When a patient is receiving a high dose ($>$15 μg/kg/min) of dopamine, norepinephrine is generally substituted in doses of 2–20 μg/min. In all other situations, the author and colleagues prefer dobutamine as the agent of first choice. The major advantage of the beta agonists is their short half-life; in essence, the drugs can be titrated in a matter of minutes to the desired effect. In addition, these agents are considerably less expensive than the phosphodiesterase inhibitors. During the titration, the heart rate and rhythm must be carefully monitored. If maximal doses are reached, milrinone can be added in an effort to gain additional effect. Particular caution must be exerted in using milrinone for patients with significant renal dysfunction, because drug accumulation will occur and the half-life will increase.

Intra-Aortic Balloon Pumping

The intra-aortic balloon pump (IABP) improves both coronary blood flow by diastolic augmentation and cardiac output by afterload reduction. Early studies in cardiogenic shock demonstrated improvement in hemodynamics and short-term outcome but no improvement in long-term outcome before the reperfusion era. However, two small randomized trials failed to show a benefit by reducing infarct size or mortality. Observational studies have supported a role for the IABP in patients undergoing reperfusion therapy with PTCA,[117] and one randomized clinical trial has demonstrated a beneficial effect of balloon pumping in preventing reocclusion after successful reperfusion in patients without shock.[118] Vascular complications have been reported in 5%–20% of patients, but these complications are usually managed with conservative measures.[119] Early insertion of the IABP is thus considered standard therapy when a patient with cardiogenic shock is being treated aggressively.

Intra-Aortic Balloon Pump Management. The IABP has uses in the care of acute myocardial infarction beyond the treatment of cardiogenic shock. Patients with acute mechanical complications, including ventricular septal defect and mitral regurgitation, and patients with postinfarction unstable angina refractory to medical therapy benefit from use of the IABP. In addition, studies have indicated that after rescue coronary angioplasty, the IABP can improve persistent coronary patency rates[120] and clinical outcomes.[118]

The IABP can be inserted safely percutaneously at the bedside. Operator experience is critical to successful placement and management. The most important contraindications to placement of the IABP are aortic regurgitation and severe peripheral vascular disease. The most common complication is loss of pulse at the site of insertion (10% of cases). More severe thrombotic complications may also occur, necessitating careful evaluation of peripheral pulses, including Doppler ultrasound examination. Hemorrhage at the site of insertion, particularly after removal, is also relatively common. Platelet counts routinely drop with the IABP in place, although rarely does this become a clinical problem.

Meticulous maintenance of the insertion site, physical examinations of the lower extremities, and attention to the timing and characteristics of balloon inflation are necessary. The standard routine for maintenance of the IABP in the Duke University Medical Center CCU is illustrated in Table 7–5.

Thrombolytic Therapy

Despite the overwhelming evidence of the benefit of thrombolytic therapy in patients with ST segment elevation during myocardial infarction and the demonstration that patients at highest risk derive the greatest benefit,[36] the results in patients with cardiogenic shock have been disappointing. Mortality rates for patients treated with thrombolytic therapy vs. placebo or with one thrombolytic agent vs. another have been almost identical, although it is interesting that two trials (GUSTO-I and GISSI-2) found a trend toward a benefit of streptokinase over alteplase in patients with cardiogenic shock.[71, 72] Although these results are not definitive because of the broad confidence limits on the observations, angiographic evidence supports a low reperfusion rate in patients with cardiogenic shock in comparison with other patients with ST elevation during myocardial infarction.[121] For this reason, the author and colleagues currently reserve thrombolytic therapy for patients for whom an angiographic suite is not immediately accessible.

TABLE 7–5. DUKE UNIVERSITY MEDICAL CENTER CCU MANAGEMENT PROCEDURE FOR IABP

Management of the Patient with IABP

1. Monitor pulses distal to insertion site every hour
2. Observe site and affected extremity for skin color and integrity, hematoma formation, blanching, temperature, and sensation every hour
3. Change dressing every 24 h or as needed (more frequently if site is oozing blood)
4. Monitor IABP timing and calibrate/rezero every 4 h or as needed
5. Assess vital signs and chest pain hourly
6. Assess and respond to anxiety levels of patient/family
7. For patient comfort, turn side to side every 2 h

IABP Removal

1. The IABP is usually removed by the physician who inserted it
2. Administer medication (usually meperidine [Demerol] and promethazine [Phenergan]) before removal of IABP
3. Discontinue heparin before removal and ensure that results of coagulation studies are within desired limits (PTT normal or heparin discontinued for at least 4–6 h)
4. Monitor vital signs frequently (q 15 min four times, then hourly for 6 h)
5. Offer pain medication and comfort measures

Miscellaneous

1. Blood is not to be drawn through IABP catheter, except in an emergency
2. Ensure that air bubbles do not enter the closed tubing system
3. An extra console should be located on the unit as a backup
4. Head of bed should not be elevated more than 30 degrees
5. In the event of cardiac arrest, turn trigger element of IABP to "internal trigger"

Abbreviations: CCU, cardiac care unit; IABP, intra-aortic balloon pump; PTT, partial thromboplastin time.

Percutaneous Transluminal Coronary Angioplasty

Multiple observational studies have demonstrated that patients treated with direct PTCA have better survival rates than do historical and contemporary controls treated without direct PTCA.[121–123] These data, coupled with the observation from randomized trials of PTCA vs. thrombolysis that PTCA has a greater benefit in sicker patients, have led to the widescale recommendation of direct PTCA for patients with cardiogenic shock. However, several studies have shown that patients selected for catheterization have better survival rates regardless of whether PTCA is performed.[62, 124] These observations have resulted in some caution in making the recommendation for direct PTCA in patients with cardiogenic shock, and a randomized trial is now ongoing.

Other Approaches

Substantial experience has been gained with surgical revascularization, with generally excellent results in comparison with historical or contemporary controls.[61] Unfortunately, no substantial randomized trials or observational studies using detailed statistical adjustments have been published. Percutaneous bypass[125] and other methods of mechanical assistance[126] may be used in younger patients who would be candidates for cardiac transplantation. The criteria for use of these devices are not well established.

Regionalization

In view of the resources required for aggressive management of cardiogenic shock, transfer of patients to a medical center that has the capability of providing angioplasty, surgery, and intensive care seems appropriate. Each hospital should have a plan for transferring such patients immediately if it lacks such facilities. A protocol for initiating volume repletion, inotropic support, and mechanical ventilation should be developed and rehearsed with appropriate staff.

Right Ventricular Infarction

Although pathologic evidence of right ventricular infarction is common among patients with inferior or posterior myocardial infarcts, hemodynamic evidence of right ventricular involvement occurs in less than 20% of cases, and serious hemodynamic instability is observed in less than 10%. Nonetheless, careful attention to the specific issues involved in hemodynamically significant right ventricular infarction can improve patient outcome. As with pericardial effusion, the triad of elevated jugular venous pressure, systemic hypotension, and clear lung fields in the presence of an inferior or posterior infarct should alert the clinician to this possibility, although elevated jugular venous pressure and the Kussmaul sign were found to be the best markers of right ventricular infarction in the most thorough study of physical findings.[127] The ECGs commonly show >1 mm of ST segment elevation in the right precordial lead V_3R or V_4R, but these findings subside in more than half of the patients within 24 h.[128] Noninvasive imaging with echocardiography, radionuclide ventriculography, or technetium pyrophosphate can provide interesting information, but rarely are these methods needed.

When hypotension occurs with right ventricular infarction, the initial approach to therapy is to ensure that an adequate filling pressure is present. If initial efforts with boluses of 1–2 L of normal saline are unsuccessful, right-sided heart catheterization is indicated. The diagnosis is confirmed by giving volume to achieve a right atrial pressure of ≥10 mm Hg with a ratio of right atrial pressure to pulmonary capillary wedge pressure of ≥0.85. The initial goal is to raise the right atrial pressure to 10–14 mm Hg, because this maneuver has been shown almost uniformly to increase cardiac output.[129] If the pulmonary capillary wedge pressure is brought up to 15–20 mm Hg and the cardiac output remains low, dobutamine should be added. Finally, all efforts should be made to achieve and maintain AV synchrony. When sinus bradycardia or heart block is present, dobutamine alone is often sufficient, but temporary dual chamber pacing may be necessary.[130]

Common complications of right ventricular infarction include AV block, tricuspid regurgitation, and cardiogenic shock. Although tricuspid regurgitation is common, it is rarely a hemodynamically limiting factor.[131] One study found right ventricular infarction to be a risk factor for ventricular fibrillation during right-sided heart catheterization.[132] An unusual but important complication of right ventricular infarction is right-to-left interatrial shunting, which can cause refractory hypoxemia because of a shunt across a patent foramen ovale.[133] Finally, after successful treatment of a hemodynamically significant right ventricular infarction, it is common for mobilization of sequestered fluid to lead to pulmonary edema several days after admission.

Chest Pain Unit

Of all patients presenting to an emergency department with chest pain, only 10%–15% ultimately receive a diagnosis of acute myocardial infarction. As discussed earlier, as many as half of these patients do not exhibit ST segment elevation on the ECG. Furthermore, over half have negative initial serum creatine kinase (CK) or CK-MB concentrations, and more than one quarter have neither a diagnostic ECG nor elevated serum levels of cardiac enzyme markers. Most early catastrophic outcomes are concentrated in patients with ongoing myocardial necrosis, including patients without ST segment elevation. As a result, a number of hospitals have sought efficient methods for assessing these patients and administering beneficial therapy before the diagnosis is established, while at the same time avoiding unnecessary CCU or ward admissions for the majority who do not have myocardial infarctions. In most patients, this assessment can be accomplished with 12–24 h of careful physiologic monitoring with protocol-driven physical assessments, electrocardiography, and serum cardiac marker determinations. The routine orders for the Chest Pain Observation Unit at Duke University Medical Center are displayed in Figure 7–16.

Evaluations by Gaspoz and colleagues have demonstrated that acute myocardial infarction can be excluded as a diagnosis within 12 h of admission under such a program.[134] In an evaluation of 592 patients, the likelihood of acute myocardial infarction was less than 1% in patients with negative cardiac enzymes, no new symptoms of ischemia, and no new electrocardiographic changes during a 12-h observation period. Furthermore, in a cost model, this approach saved $7274 in comparison with admission to a CCU and $2785 over admission to the wards.[134]

CARDIAC CARE UNIT PHASE

General Measures

Diet

Much mythology has existed about the preferred in-hospital diet of patients with acute myocardial infarction. Because the risk of sudden catastrophic events declines exponentially with time, most admission orders call for clear liquids only during the first 12–24 h after admission. This recommendation also seems reasonable because of the frequent occurrence of nausea in the early hours of the acute event. However, this general guideline is based on common sense, which would also dictate that the guideline could be altered when circumstances dictate. After the acute phase, the patient should be introduced to the low-fat, low-cholesterol diet that will be a fundamental component of the discharge program. There is no rational basis for excluding caffeine except for patients who have a known sensitivity to it.[135]

7300 Outpatient Observation Chest Pain Unit Orders

ALLERGIES: ______________________

VS q4hr

Saline lock with routine flushes

Continuous telemetry

Bedrest with bathroom privileges

Diet—Step I AHA, No caffeine

O_2 2 liters NC to keep O_2 sat > 92%

LABS: **Nurse to draw and leave at HUC desk to send STAT**

CK/CKMB: __________ (Timed 4 hours from ED admission)
CK/CKMB: __________ (Timed 8 hours from ED admission)
CK/CKMB: __________ (Timed 12 hours from ED admission)

ECG: **Nurse to order stat at times indicated below:**

ECG: __________ (Timed 4 hours from ED admission)
ECG: __________ (Timed 8 hours from ED admission)
ECG: __________ (Timed 12 hours from ED admission)

ECG prn with chest pain—STAT

MEDICATIONS: **NTG sl 0.4 mg prn**
Tylenol 650 mg po q4h prn
Chloral Hydrate 500 mg po qhs prn
Aspirin

OTHER MEDS: ______________________

Physician's Signature: ______________________

ID #: ______________________

Figure 7–16. Routine orders for Chest Pain Unit in the Duke Hospital.

Activity

For the first 24 h, bed rest with bedside commode privileges is recommended in order to reduce myocardial oxygen consumption. The bedside commode has been demonstrated to cause less tachycardia than does use of the bedpan.[136] As with diet, these guidelines are based on common sense rather than on empiric testing, and they can be altered to allow earlier ambulation by appropriate patients.

Visitation

Intensive care units have traditionally limited visitation in order to allow the unimpeded medical care of the patient. This practice has been frustrating to patients and families, often causing unnecessary anxiety for the patient and suspicion on the part of the family. An alternative approach is to establish specific quiet times during changes of shifts for nursing, when the status of the patient can be reviewed and physical findings can be confirmed, and otherwise to allow free visitation as deemed reasonable by the bedside nurse responsible for the patient's care.

Anxiety and Delirium

The occurrence of an acute myocardial infarction is an anxiety-provoking event. This observation has led some authorities to recommend benzodiazepines as a routine therapy, even in uncomplicated cases. Animal models have shown a reduction in infarct size and arrhythmia with treatment with benzodiazepines. The author and colleagues currently do not use this class of drugs routinely, but they do carefully evaluate each patient with a low threshold for anxiolytics. Lorazepam (Ativan) may be used to reduce anxiety in doses of 1–2 mg every 6 h orally or 1–2 mg intravenously every 4 h as needed. In elderly patients, 0.5 mg intravenously is initially used because of the sensitivity of such patients to the hypnotic effects of benzodiazepines. The author and colleagues prefer lorazepam because of its short half-life (10 h), its lack of active metabolites, and its ability to be given orally or intravenously.

Agitation and delirium are extremely common in the CCU setting; reported incidences range from 7% to 57%. The most important risk factors for "ICU [intensive care unit] psychosis" include older age, pre-existing central nervous system dysfunction, and idiosyncratic drug reactions (Table 7–6). Preventive measures include keeping the CCU stay as short as possible, allowing frequent visitation, and interrupting the sleep/wake cycle as little as necessary. Evaluation of acute delirium should begin with a thorough neurologic examination. A focal deficit should prompt a brain imaging study, but in the absence of focality, electrolytes and thyroid function should be checked and the patient's medications should be reviewed. A history indicative of substance abuse should be sought.

Substance Abuse

All patients admitted to the CCU should be queried about frequency and amount of alcohol and other drug use. In patients with significant use of psychotropic drugs or pain medication, the medications are continued throughout the acute phase of the hospitalization. When a history of more than several drinks per day is obtained,

TABLE 7–6. RISK FACTORS AND TREATMENT FOR ICU DELIRIUM

Risk Factors
Patient Factors
Pre-existing central nervous system dysfunction
Prior stroke
Dementia
Low cardiac output
Hypoxemia
Renal failure
Drugs, including alcohol
Drug withdrawal
Environmental Factors
Sleep deprivation
Undue noise
Treatment
Environment
Cycle lighting to keep day-night awareness
Liberal visitation
Reduction of noise
Prevention
Maintain home sedative or narcotic regimen
Lorazepam, 1–2 mg orally or IV every 4 h
Acute Delirium: Haloperidol
1–3 mg IV for mild agitation
5–7 mg IV for moderate agitation
10 mg IV for severe agitation
Double dose every 20 min as needed to control delirium

Abbreviations: ICU, intensive care unit; IV, intravenously.

prophylactic benzodiazepines are prescribed (lorazepam, 3–5 mg orally every 4–6 h) and alcohol is offered with meals in a quantity of at least half of the patient's routine intake. It is stressed to the patient and the staff that the intent is not to reinforce the drinking habit but to prevent the hyperadrenergic state of substance withdrawal in the presence of acute ischemia when the patient is at risk of reinfarction, sudden arrhythmia, and infarct expansion. Formal evaluation by substance abuse counselors is a routine practice before discharge.

If a patient develops acute delirium, haloperidol is preferred, mostly because it has been used extensively with documented salutary results. Intravenous haloperidol has a peak effect within 10 min and often results in control of delusion and hallucinations without further impairment of higher cognitive functions. The commonly used ICU protocol calls for intravenous haloperidol at doses of 1–3 mg for mild agitation, 5–7 mg for moderate agitation, and 10 mg for severe agitation. In a protocol that has been tested in several environments, the dose has been doubled every 20 min until the agitation is controlled.[137, 138] When extrapyramidal side effects occur, diphenhydramine, 25–50 mg intravenously, can rapidly reverse these findings.

General Treatment

Aspirin

Aspirin should be continued in all patients in the CCU except those who are actively bleeding; when aspirin hypersensitivity occurs in the absence of bleeding, ticlopidine is recommended. A dose of aspirin between 80 and 325 mg/day is acceptable, although the author and colleagues recommend 160 mg/day, as in ISIS-2.

Beta Blockers

If intravenous beta blockers have been initiated and no adverse effects have been observed, this therapy should be continued. Many patients do not start treatment with beta blockers in the emergency phase because of concern about relative or absolute side effects. The Beta-Blocker Heart Attack Trial (BHAT) demonstrated with considerable certainty that patients with transient pump dysfunction or electrical instability achieve the most benefit from long-term beta blockade.[139] A reasonable general rule is to initiate beta blockade after 24 h of freedom from a relative contraindication. For example, patients with transient pulmonary edema in the acute phase may safely start receiving beta blockers 24 h after the lungs have cleared. When heart block has been the contraindication, waiting 48 h after freedom from heart block seems prudent because this rhythm tends to recur unpredictably.

ACE Inhibitors (see Chapters 9 and 34)

The use of ACE inhibitors has become a topic of great interest as a result of a variety of studies demonstrating a beneficial effect of these agents. Most of these studies have initiated therapy well after hospital admission. In patients with documented left ventricular dysfunction, the value of ACE inhibitors in reducing mortality and admissions for congestive heart failure has been confirmed in multiple studies, both in the post–myocardial infarction setting[141] and in the chronic heart failure setting.[141] Interestingly, these studies also demonstrated a reduction in new ischemic events,[140, 142] which raises the question of whether ACE inhibitors may be beneficial in all patients with ischemic heart disease.

Because of substantial experimental evidence that acute use of ACE inhibitors might maximize left ventricular recovery, as well as promising early clinical study results, the second Cooperative North Scandinavian Enalapril Survival Study (CONSENSUS II) evaluated more than 6000 patients randomized either to immediate intravenous enalaprilat followed by oral enalapril or to placebo. This trial was discontinued early because of an adverse mortality trend.[143] There is controversy over whether the study should be considered definitive about a detrimental effect of very early ACE inhibition or whether further studies are needed.

The Acute Infarction Ramipril Efficacy (AIRE) study randomized more than 2000 patients with symptoms or signs of heart failure to ramipril or to placebo, beginning 3–10 days after myocardial infarction.[144] A substantial reduction in mortality and other morbid endpoints was observed, which demonstrates that quantitative measurement of left ventricular dysfunction is not necessary before a decision to begin ACE inhibitor therapy after myocardial infarction.

Three very large studies evaluating early initiation of ACE inhibitors in patients with acute myocardial infarction have been reported.[108, 109, 145] All showed evidence of benefit in the short term, with a savings of 5 lives per 1000 patients treated. Unfortunately, information about the magnitude of benefit from these trials is sketchy in available reports, but it appears that the benefit is proportional to the severity of the acute event; benefit was concentrated in patients with anterior infarction and prior infarction. Table 7–7 lists the available evidence about ACE inhibitors after myocardial infarction.

In practical terms, the author and colleagues use ACE inhibitor therapy on the day of admission in all patients with clinical evidence of substantial left ventricular dysfunction, as evidenced by anterior location, extensive prior infarction, or pulmonary edema. For every patient, they obtain a measure of systolic left ventricular function before discharge and begin ACE inhibitors in patients with an ejection fraction of <40%. In patients started on ACE inhibitors early who have a later measurement of ejection fraction of >40%, ACE inhibitors are generally continued because of the evidence that they prevent new ischemic events.

The most common serious side effects of ACE inhibitors are hypotension and hyperkalemia. On the first day of the acute event, the author and colleagues withhold ACE inhibitors from patients with a systolic blood pressure below 110 mm Hg. If by the second day the blood pressure is stable, even if it is below 110 mm Hg, and the patient has evidence of substantial left ventricular dysfunction, ACE inhibitors are carefully initiated. Serum potassium levels should be checked daily for the first several days of therapy, and supplemental potassium should be used cautiously. Uncommon but important side effects include angioedema and dose-related agranulocytosis.

The serum creatinine concentration frequently increases marginally when ACE inhibitors are begun. An effort should be made to ensure that the patient has adequate volume status and that other causes of renal dysfunction are ruled out. If the serum creatinine concentration rises by more than 1 mg/dL, the author and colleagues usually discontinue the ACE inhibitor until stability is reached.

Cough, rash, and dysgeusia are more common but less serious side effects. Although it is unclear whether angiotensin II blockers have the same beneficial effects on clinical outcomes, it is reasonable to consider such therapy when one of these side effects becomes unbearable to the patient.[146]

The selection of a particular ACE inhibitor is based on opinion only. The author and colleagues prefer to start with captopril, which has a short half-life, at a dose of 12.5 mg three times per day, doubling the dose at each interval with a goal of 50 mg t.i.d. because this dose was shown to lower mortality in clinical trials. After the patient has reached stability, the regimen is changed to an ACE inhibitor that can be given once a day. Any of the choices in Table 7–7 are acceptable, and the choice should depend on ease of administration and cost in the local environment.

Heparin

The duration of heparin therapy remains uncertain because only one study has randomly assigned patients to discontinuation before

TABLE 7–7. CLINICAL TRIALS OF ANGIOTENSIN CONVERTING ENZYME INHIBITORS

Trial	*N*	Comparison Group	Characteristics	Significant Difference	Mortality Reduction	Combined Endpoint Reduction	Comments
VHEFT I (1986)	642	Hydralazine (270 mg) + ISDN (135 mg) vs. Prazosin (11 mg)	Patients with CHF	Hydralazine-ISDN: Yes Prazosin: No	Hydralazine-ISDN: 1 year, 28%; 2 year, 34% Prazosin: 0%	Hydralazine-ISDN: improvement in LVEF	
VHEFT II (1991)	804	Hydralazine (199 mg) + ISDN (100 mg) vs. enalapril (25 mg)	Patients with CHF, mean LVEF 29%	Enalapril: Yes	Enalapril: 2 years, 28% Hydralazine: 0%	Improvement in exercise performance in hydralazine-ISDN	Lower mortality in enalapril arm attributable to a reduction in sudden death
CONSENSUS (1987)	253	Enalapril (18 mg) vs. placebo	Patients with NYHA class IV heart disease	Yes	6 months: 40% 1 year: 3%	Improvement in NYHA class	Lower mortality because of a reduction in progressive CHF
SOLVD Treatment Trial (1991)	2569	Enalapril (17 mg) vs. placebo	90% with NYHA class II or III heart disease, LVEF ≤ 35%	Yes	16%	Death or hospitalization: 25%	Reduction in mortality with enalapril caused by a reduction in progressive CHF
SOLVD Prevention Trial (1992)	4228	Enalapril (17 mg) vs. placebo	Asymptomatic patients; 33% NYHA class II heart disease, LVEF ≤ 35% Patients not taking digoxin, diuretics, or vasodilator	No for death; Yes for death or hospitalization for CHF	0%	Death or hospitalization for CHF	
CONSENSUS II (1992)	6090	IV → PO enalapril vs. placebo	Patients treated within 24 h of an acute MI	6 mos mortality: No			Trial terminated early because of adverse hypotension effect in elderly patients
SAVE (1992)	2231	Captopril (150 mg) vs. placebo	3–16 days post-MI, LVEF < 40%	Yes for morbidity and mortality			
AIRE (1993)	2006	Ramipril (5 mg) vs. placebo	Day 3–10 post-MI CHF	Yes for death, severe CHF or stroke Yes for death alone	27%	Death, severe CHF, stroke, MI: 19%	This benefit was apparent as early as 30 days
GISSI-3 (1994)	19,394	4 Treatment Groups for 6 wks: Lisinopril (5 → 10 mg), GTN (IV → Transdermal 10 mg) combination therapy vs. placebo	Acute MI	Lisinopril: yes for death and combined mortality and severe left ventricular dysfunction GTN: No Magnesium: No			Combined therapy also produced significant reduction in overall mortality and in combined endpoint The favorable effect of lisinopril alone or with GTN was clear in high-risk subsets (i.e., elderly, women) for combined endpoint
SMILE (1995)	1556	6 weeks of Zofenopril (7.5 → 30 mg b.i.d. vs. placebo	Acute anterior MI ineligible for thrombolytic therapy	Yes for death and combined death or severe CHF	6 weeks: 25% 1 year: 29%	6 weeks death or CHF: 34% 6 weeks CHF: 46%	
ISIS-4 (1995)	58,050	1 month captopril (PO 6.25 → 50 mg b.i.d.) vs. placebo 1 month CR mononitrate (PO 30 → 60 mg) vs. placebo 24-h IV magnesium sulfate (8 mmol bolus → 72 mmol) vs. placebo	Suspected acute MI	Captopril: Yes Mononitrate: No Magnesium: No	Captopril: 5 weeks, 7%; 1 year, 5.4 fewer deaths/1000		For captopril, the absolute benefits appear to be larger in certain high-risk groups (i.e., previous MI or CHF)
CCS-1 (1995)	13,634	1 month captopril (PO 6.25 → 12.5 mg t.i.d.) vs. placebo	Suspected acute MI	4 week mortality: no			

Abbreviations: VHEFT, Vasodilator Heart Failure Trial; ISDN, isosorbide dinitrate; CHF, congestive heart failure; LVEF, left ventricular ejection fraction; CONSENSUS, Cooperative North Scandinavian Enalapril Survival Study; NYHA, New York Heart Association; SOLVD, Studies of Left Ventricular Dysfunction; IV, intravenous; PO, per os (oral); MI, myocardial infarction; SAVE, Survival and Ventricular Enlargement; AIRE, Acute Infarction Ramipril Efficacy; GISSI, Gruppo Italiano per lo Studio della Sopravvivenza nell'Infarto Miocardico; GTN, glyceryl trinitrate; SMILE, Survival of Myocardial Infarction Long-Term Evaluation; ISIS, International Study of Infarct Survival; CR, controlled-release; CCS, Chinese Cardiac Study.

several days of treatment. Conceptually, it is attractive to assume that 3–5 days of heparin are required to allow healing of the disrupted endothelium, and this concept has been the basis for the duration of dosing in most studies. However, the one randomized trial, although substantially underpowered to detect differences in clinical outcomes, showed no beneficial effect of continued heparin after the first 24 h.[147]

As in the acute phase, the therapeutic target remains an aPTT in the range of 1.5–2.0 times higher than the control range. The aPTT should be checked every 6 h until a stable dose is reached and then it can be checked once daily. If the dose must be adjusted (see nomogram in Fig. 7–11), the aPTT should be measured 6 h later.

There is considerable accumulating evidence that when heparin is discontinued, a clustering of clinical events occurs in association with "rebound" thrombin activity.[148] This finding has led to a policy at the author's institution of carefully monitoring patients shortly after heparin is discontinued. Several ongoing protocols are evaluating the use of heparin tapering or subcutaneous heparin at the usual time of heparin discontinuation.

Platelet counts should be measured daily during heparin therapy because heparin-induced thrombocytopenia has been associated with serious thrombotic events.[149] If the platelet count drops below 100,000, a heparin-associated platelet aggregation study is obtained,[149] and heparin is transiently discontinued. Often, the initial test result is negative, but if the platelet count continues to drop, the result eventually becomes positive.

Nitrates

If intravenous nitrates have been initiated in the early phase of the infarction, a decision must be made about dosing and continuation during the CCU phase. Increasing concern has been raised about nitrate tolerance with the information that prolonged continuous exposure to nitrates leads to a loss of effect on arterial and venous vasodilation and exercise tolerance, presumably through a mechanism of depletion of sulfhydryl groups in the vessel wall. Patients with ongoing hemodynamic or ischemic instability can be maintained on increasing doses of intravenous nitroglycerin titrated to blood pressure and heart rate parameters. The decision about when to use nitrates beyond the acute phase is based on incomplete information. Although the ISIS-4 trial showed no significant benefit of nitrates, the GISSI-3 trial showed a modest benefit at 6-month follow-up, especially when ACE inhibitors were also used.[108, 109] Accordingly, the author and colleagues continue nitrates for several days in the hospital and then discontinue them except in patients with left ventricular dysfunction, extensive unrevascularized myocardium, or ongoing symptoms of ischemia. During the transition phase in the stable patient, their practice is to convert to topical nitrates within 24 h. A strategy of discontinuing nitroglycerin after 24–48 h without a transition to oral or topical nitrates is also reasonable. Conversion from intravenous to topical nitrates is done by adding 1 inch of nitroglycerin ointment for every 50 μg/min of nitroglycerin infusion before the infusion is discontinued. The nitrate-free interval has become standard practice, generally observed at bedtime. Concern has arisen about this schedule because of growing evidence that the incidence of acute ischemic events is highest in the early morning hours. Whether the nocturnal nitrate-free interval exposes patients to increased risk during this time has not been addressed.

Calcium Channel Blockers (see Chapter 2)

Calcium channel blockers were developed with considerable theoretical rationale for providing a beneficial effect in patients with acute myocardial infarction.[150] By reducing blood pressure and providing afterload reduction, they have the theoretical potential to improve hemodynamic balance. Coronary vasodilation, enhanced collateral vessel flow, and reduced platelet aggregation have been documented, and prevention of reperfusion injury has been suggested by animal models. Unfortunately, the great promise of calcium channel blockers has not been realized in controlled clinical trials; indeed, increasing concern has arisen about the clinical effects of these compounds, particularly when heart rate is not slowed.

When used as routine therapy for acute myocardial infarction, calcium channel blockers as a whole have been associated with an increase in mortality; in ischemic heart disease as a whole, some evidence for a detrimental effect has been generated. This evidence has been most striking for nifedipine,[151] although the effect also appears to be present for diltiazem[152] and verapamil[153, 154] in patients with left ventricular dysfunction. Because each of the calcium channel blockers has a distinct profile, the question about whether they should be considered as a class has also been raised. Figure 7–17 presents the evidence for each calcium channel blocker in graphic format. Although the evidence for nifedipine is particularly negative and the evidence for prevention of reinfarction with verapamil and diltiazem tends to be positive, none of the available information provides a rationale in the author's opinion for using calcium channel blockers routinely. Only amlodipine has withstood a controlled clinical trial in patients with left ventricular dysfunction without evidence for a detrimental effect, but this trial had limited power to prove equivalence (upper 95th percentile confidence limit for increased mortality among patients with ischemic heart disease = 1.29), and the population did not include patients who had suffered recent myocardial infarction (Christopher M. O'Connor, personal communication, 1995).

These considerations have led the author and colleagues to avoid calcium channel blockers in the acute phase of myocardial infarction and to use them in the CCU phase only for patients with recurrent ischemia and either with a contraindication to beta blockers or

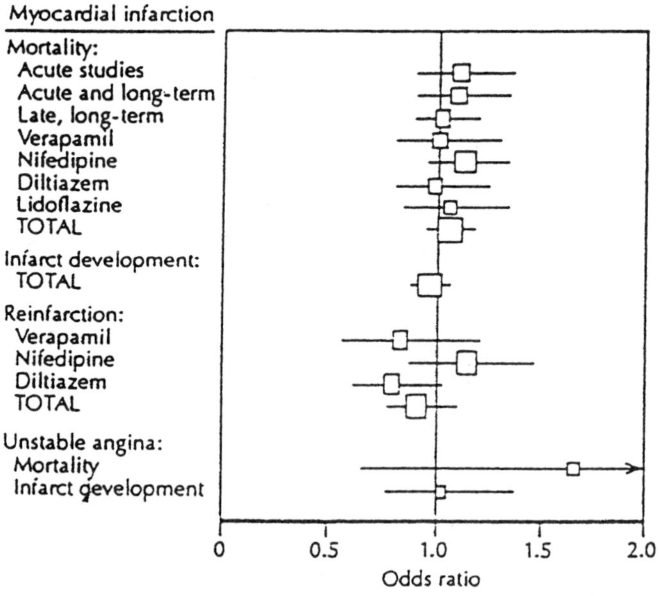

Figure 7–17. Results of therapy with calcium channel antagonists in acute coronary syndromes. This meta-analysis indicates that calcium channel antagonists have no significant beneficial effect on mortality in patients with acute myocardial infarction and may even be associated with a trend toward an increase in mortality; no evidence of a beneficial effect was detected in patients with unstable angina, either. Reinfarction rates tended to be lower in the patients treated with verapamil or diltiazem, but these values did not achieve statistical significance (confidence intervals overlap vertical line). On the basis of these observations, calcium channel antagonists cannot be recommended as primary therapy for unstable angina or acute myocardial infarction. (From Held PH, Yusuf S, Furberg CD: Calcium channel blockers in acute myocardial infarction and unstable angina: an overview. Br Med J 1989; 299:1187–1192.)

already receiving a maximal dose of beta blockers. The author and colleagues choose amlodipine, starting with a dose of 5 mg/day orally and increasing to 10 mg/day if needed, as the agent of preference because of the clinical trial data that indicate no increase in mortality among patients with left ventricular dysfunction and because of the reasonable side effect profile.

Hemodynamic Status

In a series of observations that have formed the basis for conceptualizing hemodynamic status, Forrester and colleagues evaluated 200 patients with myocardial infarction soon after admission to the hospital.[155] Patients with a high pulmonary capillary wedge pressure and a low cardiac index had the highest risk of death, whereas patients with a high cardiac index and a low wedge pressure had the lowest risk of death. This empiric finding confirmed the clinical observations of Killip and Kimball,[156] who devised the Killip classification by combining evidence of peripheral perfusion on the physical examination with evidence of pulmonary congestion (Table 7–8).

Killip Class I

Patients who remain in Killip class I throughout the hospitalization generally have uncomplicated courses, and the mortality rate is low. These patients should receive the routine therapies outlined earlier. The length of stay in the CCU can be 24 h unless a nonhemodynamic complication occurs, and the total length of stay in the hospital can be less than 7 days.

Killip Class II

Patients classified as Killip class II have no or mild pulmonary congestion (rales over <50% of the lungs) and evidence of peripheral hypoperfusion (diastolic blood pressure < 90 mm Hg or systolic blood pressure > 30 mm Hg below the usual level). The clinician should immediately evaluate such patients for likely causes of hypovolemia. Drug effect (nitrates, morphine, ACE inhibitors, beta blockers) should be considered, and acute bleeding, especially in the thrombolytic-treated patient, must be ruled out. Inferior infarction with the Bezold-Jarisch reflex should be considered, and right ventricular infarction in particular should be suspected. In most situations, administration of intravascular volume expanders rapidly restores adequate peripheral perfusion. A common error is to administer fluid too cautiously; in a patient with hypotension or poor peripheral perfusion, a 500-mL bolus of normal saline should be administered over a period of 15 min, and the patient's heart rate, blood pressure, and respiratory function should be monitored every 15 min until the patient is stable.

If the patient's blood pressure or perfusion does not respond to volume expanders, or if pulmonary congestion develops, additional therapy is indicated. An indwelling arterial line may be needed, and sequential considerations of inotropic or vasopressor support and right-sided heart catheterization should be contemplated.

Inotropic and Vasopressor Support. In most patients who are hemodynamically stable or have only transient hypotension, automatic blood pressure cuff monitors can provide ample monitoring capability. When patients have persistent hypotension despite corrective maneuvers, indwelling arterial pressure monitoring is indicated. Percutaneous insertion via the radial artery after the Allen test is performed is preferred,[157] although in patients with profound hypotension, femoral insertion is sometimes necessary because of peripheral vasoconstriction. Inotropic or vasopressor support may be required in order to maintain an adequate systolic blood pressure while the underlying etiology of profound hypotension is determined. If adequate intravascular volume is achieved and pulmonary edema develops while the patient remains hypotensive with hypoperfusion, the patient has reached Killip class IV (cardiogenic shock).

Killip Class III

The patient with acute pulmonary edema without hypoperfusion presents an interesting clinical challenge. When pulmonary edema initially develops, careful evaluation for recurrent infarction, recurrent ischemia, or a mechanical complication of the myocardial infarction is required. Mitral regurgitation may be an especially important mechanical complication of acute myocardial infarction in this setting. A common cause of pulmonary edema several days after myocardial infarction is mobilization of fluid in patients with right ventricular infarction as right ventricular function improves.

The mainstays of therapy for patients in Killip class III include nitrates, diuretics, and ACE inhibitors. Adequate oxygenation should be ensured through supplemental oxygen administration, and morphine may be used acutely to reduce preload, afterload, and anxiety. Nitrates may be initiated in the same manner as described for routine therapy. The dose of diuretic should depend on the severity of the pulmonary edema, the presence and extent of underlying renal disease, and the estimated degree of reserve; furosemide is used in doses of 10–40 mg with incremental doses up to 160 mg as needed to produce diuresis. ACE inhibitors are generally started after the patient has become comfortable, hemodynamic stability is achieved, and intravascular volume is adequate.

The occurrence of acute pulmonary edema, even in the absence

TABLE 7–8. HEMODYNAMIC CLASSIFICATIONS OF PATIENTS WITH ACUTE MYOCARDIAL INFARCTION

Based on Clinical Examination				Based on Invasive Monitoring		
Class	Definition	Mortality (%)	GUSTO-I Mortality (%)	Subset	Definition	Mortality (%)
I	Rales and S_3 absent	8	5.1	I	Normal hemodynamics PCWP < 18, CI > 2.2	2
II	Rales over <50% of lung	30	13.6	II	Pulmonary congestion PCWP > 18, CI < 2.2	10
III	Rales over >50% of lung fields (pulmonary edema)	44	32.2	III	Peripheral hypoperfusion PCWP < 18, CI > 2.2	22
IV	Shock	80–100	57.8	IV	Pulmonary congestion and peripheral hypoperfusion PCWP > 18, CI < 2.2	56

Abbreviations: GUSTO, Global Utilization of Streptokinase and t-PA for Occluded Coronary Arteries; PCWP, pulmonary capillary wedge pressure; CI, cardiac index.
Adapted from Rabbani LE, Antman EM: Acute myocardial infarction. *In* Rakel RE (ed): Conn's Current Therapy. Philadelphia: WB Saunders, 1993.

of peripheral hypoperfusion, is an emergency that heralds a grave long-term prognosis. Consequently, the author and colleagues aggressively treat pulmonary edema while carefully monitoring the patient's heart rate and blood pressure and performing a physical examination every 15 min; if the situation does not rapidly improve, right-sided heart catheterization is performed so that therapy can be tailored to the hemodynamics. Should ongoing ischemia be evident, IABP insertion should be considered. The echocardiogram is a useful tool for evaluating systolic and diastolic function and for ruling out valvular lesion or septal rupture.

Disorders of Heart Rhythm During Acute Myocardial Infarction

Sinus Rhythm

The general goal of therapy is to achieve a hemodynamic state in which the patient has a heart rate between 60 and 80 beats per minute. Figure 7–18 demonstrates the relationship between heart rate and mortality after adjustment for other factors in patients with ST elevation during infarction. Both sinus bradycardia and sinus tachycardia are associated with excess mortality. Heart rates between 60 and 70 are associated with improved diastolic filling time and produce less myocardial oxygen demand than do higher rates. Profound sinus bradycardia can be associated with decreased tissue perfusion and a progressive spiral of deterioration.

Sinus Tachycardia

A number of studies have demonstrated that patients with sinus tachycardia have an increased risk of death.[158] The diagnosis of sinus tachycardia is made by demonstrating a heart rate over 100 beats per minute with association of the P wave with each QRS complex. When the rate is over 120 beats per minute, the clinician must be careful not to overlook paroxysmal atrial tachycardia or atrial flutter as the diagnosis. Carotid sinus massage is a helpful maneuver for providing evidence that another mechanism is involved, although this maneuver often fails.

In the hemodynamically stable patient, adenosine can be used to provide a diagnostic challenge. A dose of 6 mg is given intravenously, and if no effect is observed after 1 min, a 12-mg dose can be given. Over 90% of supraventricular arrhythmias respond either by termination of the arrhythmia or by a short-lived increase in the level of AV block. Transient side effects, including chest pain, bronchospasm, heart block, and flushing, may occur but are short-lived.

When the clinician detects sinus tachycardia, a thorough evaluation of the patient is recommended in order to attempt to determine the underlying cause. Most commonly the patient will be in a state of low cardiac output. If the output is low as a result of volume depletion, the tachycardia can be readily controlled by volume infusion, unless the patient is actively bleeding. However, the patient with low output and adequate volume has a seriously compromised situation and requires urgent attention. Another common cause of sinus tachycardia is simply anxiety; if a state of low cardiac output has been dismissed as an underlying cause or corrected by volume repletion, beta blockade should be initiated or increased. Clinical assessment of the hemodynamic state in this situation is critical because acute administration of a beta blocker in a patient with low output can be devastating. The next most common causes of sinus tachycardia are fever and hypoxemia, which should be treated.

Sinus Bradycardia

Traditional teaching has been that when the heart rate falls below 60 beats per minute, the physician should not become concerned unless signs or symptoms of myocardial or systemic hypoperfusion develop. This rhythm disturbance occurs most commonly in the first several hours after infarction in patients with inferior and especially right ventricular infarcts. When profound symptomatic bradycardia or sinus arrest occurs, the initial treatment is to give 0.5 mg of atropine intravenously; lower doses have been associated with paradoxical sinus slowing. If the first dose fails, it can be repeated to a total dose of 2 mg. If the patient remains in distress, a beta agonist agent (isoproterenol) should be administered intravenously while external pacing is established and preparations are made to institute temporary transvenous pacing.

Atrial Fibrillation/Flutter

Acute atrial fibrillation occurs in over 10% of patients with acute myocardial infarction. Its occurrence is associated with an increased risk of death and stroke, particularly embolic stroke.[159] Although most of this adverse prognosis appears to be related to the fact that the arrhythmia occurs more often in older patients and in patients with larger infarctions, atrial fibrillation and flutter are arrhythmias of concern for any patient because of both prognosis and the obvious physiologic advantage of slower heart rate and synchronized atrial contraction afforded by conversion to sinus rhythm. As in ventricular arrhythmia, the stability of a patient in whom atrial fibrillation or flutter develops should be assessed by measuring blood pressure and

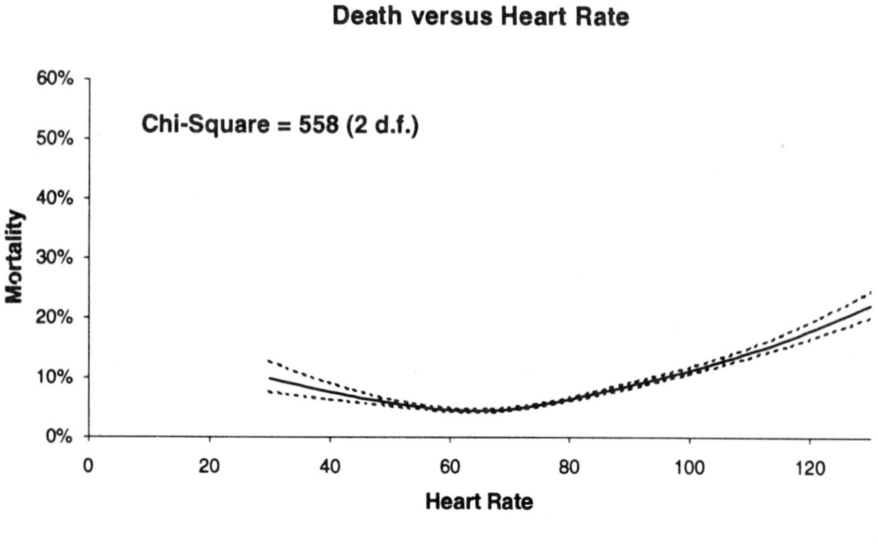

Figure 7–18. Plot of results from the GUSTO-I Trial showing unadjusted (univariate) relation between heart rate per minute and 30-day mortality based on logistic regression. Two linear splines were used to model the relation. *Abbreviation:* d.f., degrees of freedom.

performing a brief directed examination of mental status, the heart, and the lungs. If the patient is hypoperfused or experiencing exacerbated myocardial ischemic symptoms, cardioversion is indicated. Synchronized cardioversion can generally be initiated at 100 joules for atrial fibrillation and 50 joules for atrial flutter.

When the patient is not immediately compromised, initial attention should be focused on slowing the ventricular response. Digoxin has traditionally been the drug of choice for this indication because it does not have negative inotropic effects. When the author and colleagues use digoxin acutely, they give an intravenous dose of 12–15 μg/kg of lean body weight; half the dose is given initially, and 25% is given in two doses at 6-h intervals. An oral dose is then given, calculated as the percentage lost per day multiplied by the loading dose. The percentage lost per day can be calculated by the formula [(CrCl/5) + 14], where CrCl is creatinine clearance. However, multiple studies have demonstrated that digoxin does not reach its peak effect for 6–12 h and that its AV nodal blocking effects can be easily overcome by the adrenergic stimulation that frequently accompanies myocardial infarction. Beta blocking agents provide an effective means of blocking the AV node in patients with stable left ventricular function while providing the other benefits of beta blockade in the setting of acute myocardial infarction.[160] Metoprolol in a dose of 5 mg intravenously every 5 min for three doses as needed in conjunction with standard oral dosing provides a reasonable regimen. Calcium channel blockers, especially diltiazem, have become popular for atrial fibrillation/flutter because of their rapid onset of action and the ability to titrate the dose.[161] Diltiazem can be given in 0.25 mg/kg intravenously, followed by 60 mg orally every 6 h. If the desired ventricular response is not reached with the first bolus, a second bolus of 0.35 mg/kg can be given after 15 min followed by 90 mg (instead of 60 mg) orally every 6 h.

When the AV node is effectively blocked, traditional teaching has included use of a type I antiarrhythmic drug to convert the patient or to prevent recurrence after successful spontaneous or electrical cardioversion. Evidence of excessive mortality with long-term post-infarction treatment with encainide, flecainide, and moricizine (Fig. 7–19),[162] coupled with meta-analysis data of excessive mortality with chronic treatment of atrial fibrillation outside the setting of myocardial infarction,[163] have caused considerable caution in using type I agents in acute or chronic atrial fibrillation. If a decision is made to use a type I agent, the author and colleagues use procainamide in a loading dose of 17 mg/kg intravenously over a period of 1 h, followed by an infusion dose of 3 mg/kg/h if the creatinine clearance is >60 mL/min. Procainamide is avoided in patients with renal dysfunction unless the dose is carefully adjusted.[164]

One of the most difficult post–myocardial infarction situations is atrial fibrillation combined with known substantial left ventricular dysfunction or symptomatic heart failure. Assuming that efforts to convert to sinus rhythm have failed, one of several difficult choices must be made. Beta blockade is relatively contraindicated if the patient is symptomatic from heart failure. This situation represents the major indication for esmolol, a beta blocking agent with a short half-life (2–5 min). A loading dose of 0.5 mg/kg over 2–5 min can be given, followed by an infusion of 0.05 mg/kg/min titrated upward as needed to a maximal dose of 0.2 mg/kg/min. If symptomatic heart failure develops or progresses, the infusion can be rapidly discontinued. Intravenous diltiazem has the same problem in that deterioration in left ventricular function can occur in patients with known left ventricular dysfunction, and an increase in mortality with long-term oral therapy has been reported. Nevertheless, if used in a continuous intravenous infusion under careful supervision, rapid control of the ventricular response can be gained, although the cost of the intravenous infusion is substantial.

Because of the increased risk of embolic stroke in patients with atrial fibrillation, the author and colleagues attempt to maintain intravenous anticoagulation in these patients unless a contraindication exists.

After the acute phase of the arrhythmia, a decision must be made about long-term therapy. In patients with continued atrial fibrillation, the author's preference is to use an oral beta blocking agent to control the ventricular response unless the patient has symptomatic heart failure. In the case of heart failure in association with atrial fibrillation, the author and colleagues use chronic oral digoxin to control the ventricular response. Attempts are increasingly being made to use short-term oral amiodarone to convert these patients or to effectively block the AV node, maintain sinus rhythm, and prevent ventricular arrhythmias.[165] Patients with greater degrees of left ventricular dysfunction may be treated with 200–400 mg/day of amiodarone. Type I antiarrhythmic agents are not recommended until definitive outcome studies are available.

All of these patients undergo anticoagulation with warfarin (Coumadin) unless a contraindication exists. For patients who have converted to sinus rhythm after only one bout of atrial fibrillation, the author and colleagues simply maintain a regimen of an oral beta blocking agent and instruct the patients to report any palpitations. Currently, these patients do not undergo anticoagulation. Patients with multiple recurrences of atrial fibrillation in the acute phase are treated with amiodarone at a dose of 200 mg/day for 6 weeks in an effort to maintain sinus rhythm after a loading dose of approximately 6 g, given as 800 mg orally every 12 h. If no recurrences are noted at 6-week follow-up, the amiodarone is discontinued. In general, these patients undergo anticoagulation unless a strong relative contraindication exists.

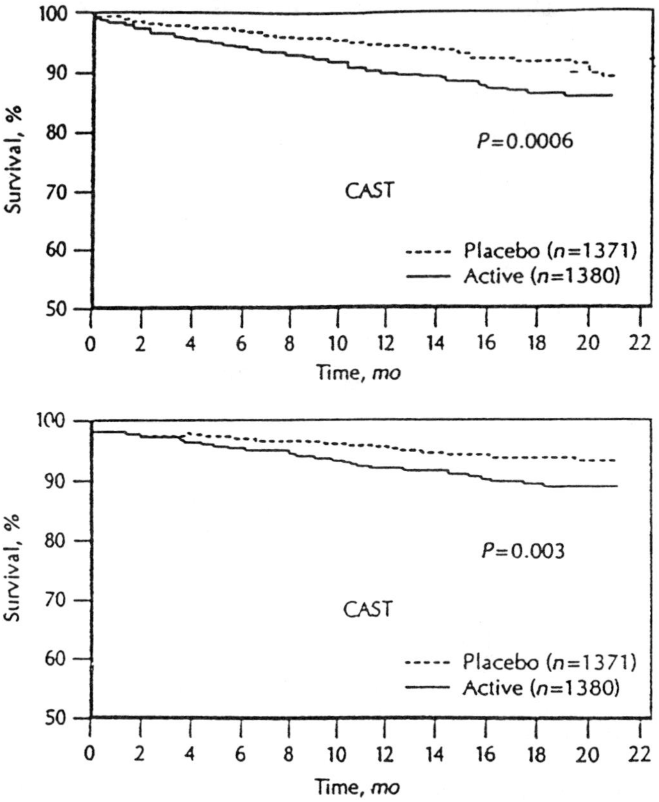

Figure 7–19. Results of the Cardiac Arrhythmia Suppression Trial (CAST), demonstrating an increase in the risk of long-term total mortality (top panel) and sudden death (bottom panel) in post–myocardial infarction patients treated with encainide, flecainide, or moricizine. (From Epstein AE, Hallstrom AP, Rogers WJ, et al: Mortality following ventricular arrhythmia suppression by encainide, flecainide, and moricizine after myocardial infarction. JAMA 1993; 270:2451–2455.)

Premature Ventricular Beats

During the 1970s and 1980s, an argument was developed for the concept that the frequent ventricular arrhythmias that accompany

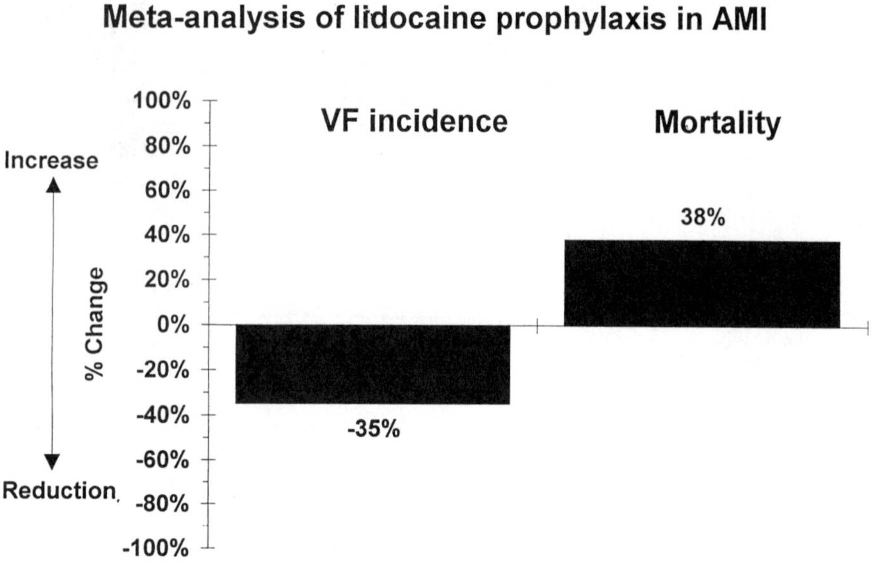

Figure 7–20. Although prophylactic lidocaine was clearly beneficial in reducing the risk for primary ventricular fibrillation (VF) in the absence of congestive heart failure or cardiogenic shock in the prethrombolytic era, its use was associated with a trend toward increased mortality, probably from fatal bradycardia and asystolic arrest. *Other abbreviation:* AMI, acute myocardial infarction. (Based on data from MacMahon S, Collins R, Peto R, et al: Effects of prophylactic lidocaine in suspected acute myocardial infarction. JAMA 1988; 260:1910–1916.)

acute myocardial infarction should be suppressed. Early in the evolution of CCUs, an association between "warning arrhythmias" and the risk of sudden ventricular fibrillation was described.[166] These observations were confirmed in a number of studies, and experimental work led to the concept that suppressing these arrhythmias with lidocaine could prevent ventricular fibrillation. A series of small randomized trials confirmed that lidocaine prevents sudden ventricular fibrillation. However, as described later, the overall effect of lidocaine on mortality rates is negative because of the increase in deaths from bradyarrhythmia, and suppression of premature ventricular beats did not result in less mortality after myocardial infarction (Fig. 7–20).[167] On the basis of this evidence, the author and colleagues have concluded that the most important therapeutic maneuver in the post-myocardial infarction patient is to ignore these arrhythmias short of sustained or hemodynamically significant ventricular tachycardia or fibrillation. As described earlier, the use of available antiarrhythmic agents except for amiodarone has no empiric basis other than to suppress symptomatic, immediately life-threatening arrhythmias. Beta blockers should be used routinely, and the results with amiodarone are currently ambiguous.

Several studies have suggested that amiodarone may be an effective therapy for preventing ventricular fibrillation after hospital discharge. In doses ranging from 200 to 400 mg, four different pilot studies have shown favorable trends.[168–171] One trial evaluating amiodarone in patients with left ventricular dysfunction, the majority of whom had ischemic heart disease, found no effect on mortality.[172] Two large trials, one in Canada (Canadian Amiodarone Myocardial Infarction Arrhythmia Trial [CAMIAT]) and one in Europe (European Myocardial Infarction Amiodarone Trial [EMIAT]), are evaluating the routine use of amiodarone in post–myocardial infarction patients with adequate sample sizes to detect an effect on mortality.

Nonsustained Ventricular Tachycardia

As the spectrum of clinical significance moves from isolated premature beats toward nonsustained ventricular tachycardia, the issue of risk and benefit of antiarrhythmic agents becomes more complex. Particularly in patients with multiple runs of nonsustained ventricular arrhythmia, the risk of sudden hemodynamic collapse is substantial. Yet to date, demonstration of an effective antiarrhythmic treatment in terms of prevention of death is lacking. Because of the certainty of high risk for sudden death among these patients but the uncertainty about effective treatment, a randomized trial comparing electrophysiology-guided therapy with conservative management is ongoing (Multicenter UnSustained Tachycardia Trial [MUSTT]). When multiple bouts of nonsustained ventricular tachycardia are observed, the level of surveillance should be intensified, electrolytes should be checked, and the patient's hemodynamic status should be evaluated, initially through the physical examination and then through the use of right-sided heart catheterization if necessary, in addition to ensuring that ongoing ischemia is not present.

Accelerated Idioventricular Rhythm

Accelerated idioventricular rhythm, characterized by a wide QRS rhythm with the ventricular rate faster than the atrial rate and <150 beats per minute, is commonly present in the early stages of myocardial infarction. This rhythm occurs somewhat more often in patients with early reperfusion, although it is neither sensitive nor specific enough to merit consideration as a marker of reperfusion. Because of the wide complex nature of the rhythm and AV dissociation, it can be mistaken for bundle branch block; temporary pacing is not indicated, however, unless the AV dissociation leads to a substantial drop in blood pressure. Suppression of the rhythm with antiarrhythmic therapy also is not beneficial and may cause hemodynamic compromise.

Sustained Ventricular Tachycardia

Sustained monomorphic ventricular tachycardia generally is defined as a wide complex tachycardia with a heart rate of >100 beats per minute with documentation of AV dissociation or a constellation of QRS duration of >140 msec with right bundle branch block or >160 msec with left bundle branch block and positive or negative concordance of the QRS complex in all of the precordial leads.

The most important initial maneuver is to ensure that vital signs are stable. If the patient is severely hypotensive (blood pressure < 90 or there is evidence of peripheral hypoperfusion), direct-current cardioversion is indicated. If the vital signs are reasonably stable, documentation of the rhythm is critical because supraventricular rhythms are frequently mistaken for ventricular tachycardia and the converse occurs even more commonly. A 12-lead ECG can be invaluable in this situation to observe for the hallmark finding of AV dissociation.

After sustained ventricular tachycardia is initially terminated by cardioversion, the author and colleagues recommend treatment with either intravenous procainamide or intravenous lidocaine, although intravenous amiodarone is a reasonable alternative. Procainamide is an effective short-term agent that carries significant risk of proarrhythmic effect or myocardial depression, especially in patients with renal insufficiency. The efficacy of lidocaine remains somewhat in question because of the lack of properly controlled randomized clinical trials. Lidocaine is given in an intravenous loading dose of 75 mg, followed by three 50-mg doses at 5-min intervals. A maintenance dose of 2 mg/min is typical. Patients over 75 years of age, patients with heart failure, and patients with liver disease are given half the maintenance dose. For incessant ventricular tachycardia, a rare but distinctive situation, the author and colleagues usually insert atrial and ventricular wires in an effort to electrically convert the patient.

Ventricular Fibrillation

Ventricular fibrillation is a medical emergency necessitating immediate defibrillation according to advanced cardiac life support protocol. The one potential new approach is to use intravenous amiodarone, although controlled clinical trial results are not available (see Chapter 18). Every acute care environment should have documented proficiency in defibrillation and a measured time to defibrillation of less than 1 min.

As discussed earlier, pharmacologic prevention of ventricular fibrillation other than beta blockade has been a disappointing effort. After the first bout of ventricular fibrillation, however, most authorities recommend initiating a lidocaine infusion, although no definitive data confirm its ability to prevent a second episode of ventricular fibrillation. As discussed, lidocaine must be carefully administered according to guidelines based on hepatic function, age, and estimated cardiac output. Lidocaine is discontinued after 12–24 h. When patients require multiple bouts of defibrillation, external patch electrodes are helpful and pacing should be considered, especially when the ventricular fibrillation appears to be bradycardia- or tachycardia-dependent.[173]

Asystole

Asystole occurs in 5%–10% of patients, most often in patients with inferior myocardial infarcts. Treatment should consist of discontinuation of drugs affecting the sinus node, including beta blockers, digoxin, amiodarone, and calcium channel blockers. Care must be taken to avoid the common errors of mistaking fine ventricular fibrillation or lack of systolic data as a result of lead detachment or inappropriate lead placement as asystole. Emergency treatment consists of administration of atropine, starting with 1 mg and repeating the dose to a total of 3 mg, and epinephrine in doses of 1 mg or more. Care must be taken to ensure that the patient is adequately ventilated during the resuscitative effort. Temporary pacing is required unless the asystole is brief and a reversible precipitating cause is not found.

Atrioventricular Block

AV block may result from increased vagal tone, especially in inferior myocardial infarction, in addition to the effects of ischemia on the conduction system. This common complication of acute myocardial infarction has been characterized in a number of studies; the prognosis and appropriate therapy are dependent on the severity of the conduction disturbance and the setting in which it occurs. The characteristics of AV block as a function of location of the block are reviewed in Table 7–9.

First-degree AV block, characterized by lengthening of the PR interval (beyond 0.20 sec), is extremely common in inferior myocardial infarction and very rarely results in symptoms. No treatment is indicated, although a markedly prolonged PR interval is a contraindication to beta blockade.

Second degree AV block is commonly divided into Mobitz type I and type II AV block. In Mobitz type I 2° AV block, the PR interval is variable and QRS complexes do not follow every P wave; in Mobitz type II AV block, the PR interval is constant despite the skipped QRS complexes. This distinguishing feature is important, because Mobitz type I AV block rarely leads to hemodynamic collapse and usually does not necessitate placement of a pacemaker even if it progresses to complete heart block. In contrast, Mobitz type II does necessitate pacemaker placement, regardless of whether it progresses to complete heart block. Mobitz type I is generally caused by failure of conduction at the level of the AV node; Mobitz type II results from ischemia in the conduction system below the AV node. Mobitz type I is usually self-limited and progresses from first-degree AV block; Mobitz type II generally progresses from a premonitory intraventricular conduction block.

In both situations, the mortality rate is substantially increased in comparison with patients not experiencing AV block. In the TIMI[174] and Thrombolysis and Angioplasty in Myocardial Infarction (TAMI)[175] trials, in patients with inferior myocardial infarction and therefore a predominantly Mobitz type I mechanism, mortality was increased threefold among patients with AV block. Mortality rates exceed 40% in patients with anterior myocardial infarction and high-degree AV block. Interestingly, in modern CCUs, AV block itself is rarely the cause of death; rather, the occurrence of AV block in a patient with a larger infarct implies a higher risk of death from ventricular arrhythmias or sudden death.

Criteria for temporary pacing have been developed from a series of observational studies. Pacing is rarely necessary in Mobitz type I second-degree AV block in which complete heart block does not develop via that mechanism. The occurrence of hypotension or bradycardia-dependent ventricular arrhythmia would merit temporary pacing. However, temporary pacing followed by permanent pacing is recommended for patients with high-degree AV block that develops via the Mobitz type II mechanism.

A number of studies have evaluated risk profiles of patients in whom serious AV block develops. Patients with bilateral bundle branch block or first-degree AV block with bundle branch block have a risk of more than 25% of developing serious AV block and thus are thought to merit prophylactic temporary pacing. Patients with simple new bundle branch block without first-degree AV block have a risk of 10%–20%, which exceeds the threshold for some practitioners and not for others. Lamas and colleagues[176] developed a useful risk score, giving one point for every risk factor (first-degree AV block, Mobitz type I second-degree AV block, Mobitz type II second-degree AV block, hemiblock, and either right or left bundle branch block). A point score of ≥ 3 was associated with a 36% risk of developing complete heart block, a score of 2 with a 25% risk, and a score of 0–1 with a risk of $<1.5\%$.

The availability of reliable transcutaneous pacing has provided a less invasive route for temporary prophylactic pacing, but when symptoms are present or the risk of hemodynamic collapse is high, transvenous pacing is preferred.[177] Emergency treatment as pacing is initiated includes atropine, 0.5 mg intravenously; failure of atropine on repeated dosing should prompt isoproterenol infusion, starting with 1 μg/min with escalation of the infusion until hemodynamic stability is achieved. The author and colleagues therefore use prophylactic standby transcutaneous pacing in high- and medium-risk patients. Even high-risk patients are treated with prophylactic transcutaneous pacing after thrombolytic therapy.

Recurrent Symptoms

Recurrent symptoms after myocardial infarction that could represent recurrent ischemia or infarction pose a clinical dilemma. In the GUSTO-I and GUSTO-II trials, recurrent ischemia was diagnosed in 20% and 23%, respectively, of patients initially with ST segment elevation during infarction, in comparison with 31% of patients in

TABLE 7–9. FEATURES OF AV CONDUCTION DISTURBANCES IN ACUTE MYOCARDIAL INFARCTION

Feature	Location of AV Conduction Disturbance: Proximal	Distal
Site of block	Intranodal	Infranodal
Site of infarction	Inferoposterior	Anteroseptal
Compromised arterial supply	RCA (90%), LCX (10%)	Septal perforators of LAD
Pathogenesis	Ischemia, necrosis, hydropic cell swelling, excess parasympathetic activity	Ischemia, necrosis, hydropic cell swelling
Predominant type of AV nodal block	First degree (PR > 200 msec) Mobitz type I second degree	Mobitz type II second degree Third degree
Common premonitory features of third-degree AV block	First degree progressing to second-degree AV block Mobitz type I pattern	Intraventricular conduction block Mobitz type II pattern
Features of escape rhythm following third degree block		
Location	Proximal conduction system (His bundle)	Distal conduction system (bundle branches)
QRS width	<0.12 sec*	>0.12 sec*
Rate	45–60 per minute but may be as low as 30 per minute	Often <30 per minute
Stability of escape rhythm	Rate usually stable; asystole uncommon	Rate often unstable with moderate to high risk of ventricular asystole
Duration of high-grade AV block	Usually transient (2–3 days)	Usually transient, but some form of AV conduction disturbance and/or intraventricular defect may persist
Associated mortality rate	Low unless associated with hypotension and/or congestive heart failure	High because of extensive infarction associated with power failure or ventricular arrhythmias
Pacemaker therapy		
Temporary	Rarely required; may be considered for bradycardia associated with left ventricular power failure, syncope, or angina	Indicated in patients with anteroseptal infarction and acute bifascicular block
Permanent	Almost never indicated, because conduction defect is usually transient	Indicated for patients with high-grade AV block with block in His-Purkinje system and those with transient advanced AV block and associated bundle branch block

Abbreviations: AV, atrioventricular; RCA, right coronary artery; LCX, left circumflex coronary artery; LAD, left anterior descending coronary artery.

*Some studies suggest that a wide QRS escape rhythm (>0.12 sec) after high-grade AV block in inferior infarction is associated with a worse prognosis.

Based on information from Antman EM, Rutherford JD: Coronary Care Medicine: A Practical Approach, Boston: Martinus Nijhoff, 1986; and Dreifus LS, Fisch C, Griffin JC, et al: Guidelines for implantation of cardiac pacemakers and antiarrhythmia devices. J Am Coll Cardiol 1991; 18:1–13.

TABLE 7–10. OUTCOMES OF PERCUTANEOUS INTERVENTION IN PATIENTS WITH STABLE AND UNSTABLE ANGINA

Angina Type	No. of Patients	Success Rate (%)	Major Complication Rate: Death (%)	Myocardial Infarction (%)	Acute Surgery (%)
Stable	10,129	92	0.7	1.6	2.5
Unstable					
Stabilized	1036	89	0.3	5.1	5.8
Refractory	1438	85	1.3	6.3	6.8
Post–myocardial infarction	634	88	1.1	6.3	6.5

From deFeyter PJ, Serruys PW: Percutaneous transluminal coronary angioplasty for unstable angina. *In* Topol EJ (ed): Textbook of Interventional Cardiology, 2nd ed, vol 1, pp 274–291. Philadelphia: WB Saunders, 1994.

GUSTO-II with non–ST segment elevation during infarction. The goal of the evaluation is to distinguish among reinfarction, recurrent ischemia, pericarditis, pulmonary embolism, and noncardiac causes of chest pain. The time course of reinfarction demonstrates that the risk declines exponentially after the initial myocardial infarction event.

Recurrent Ischemia

Most bouts of recurrent ischemia do not result in a re-elevation of serum cardiac markers. Rather, these episodes may be considered a warning in that they are associated with an increased risk of adverse outcomes, including death, arrhythmias, pump dysfunction, and additional cost.[178] Indeed, when patients with recurrent ischemia are stratified as a function of new ECG changes, hypotension, and pulmonary edema, there is a marked gradient of risk according to the number of these factors that is observed.[179]

Diagnostic Algorithm and Treatment

When patients are admitted to the CCU, frequent observation for signs and symptoms of recurrent ischemia is warranted. The recurrence of chest discomfort should prompt measurement of vital signs, cardiopulmonary auscultation, and electrocardiography. Rapid acquisition of the ECG is critical for detecting definitive occurrences of ischemia. Common problems in diagnosis are the nonspecific nature of the symptomatic discomfort and the pre-existing ECG abnormality. Many patients have mild residual discomfort for the first 24 h after an acute myocardial infarction, and the majority of patients become acutely aware of fleeting discomfort. Others enter a stage of denial, making ascertainment of symptoms impossible. Baseline ECG abnormalities frequently cause uncertainty about whether a change in the ECG represents evolution of the previous event or a new event.

If myocardial ischemia is suspected or proved, sublingual nitroglycerin should be given in a dose of 0.4 mg and repeated every 5 min; blood pressure and heart rate should be checked every 10–15 min. Serum cardiac markers should be measured if the episode lasts longer than 15 min or if recurrent ST segment elevation is observed. The clinician should review the medications to ensure that the patient is treated with aspirin and beta blockers unless a contraindication is present, and the beta blocker should be titrated to the appropriate heart rate (in general, 55–70 beats per minute at rest unless pump dysfunction or pulmonary disease is a limiting factor). Nitrates should be instituted if the patient is not currently being treated with them, or the dose of nitrates should be increased with special attention to the potential problem of tolerance.

If recurrent ST segment elevation is documented in the absence of another cause (pericarditis), the patient should be presumed to have a reinfarction. Controlled studies are not available, but serious consideration should be given to the repeated administration of thrombolytic therapy or attempted mechanical revascularization. Repeated thrombolytic administration for reinfarction has been reported in four series with a total of 139 patients.[180–183] Major bleeding occurred in 4%–12% of patients, patency was documented in 54%–73%, and the mortality rates ranged from 6% to 17%. In the absence of a control group, the benefit of therapy cannot be determined. If reinfarction is suspected, care should be taken not to readminister streptokinase within 6 h of its previous administration; indeed, most authorities recommend not repeating streptokinase under any circumstances. The dose of alteplase should be reduced to <100 mg. In GUSTO-I, 43% of patients with suspected reinfarction were treated with repeat thrombolytic therapy; the mortality rate was 11% in comparison with 24% among patients who were not treated. Ellis and colleagues reported a single series in which 74 patients with recurrent ischemia were treated with aggressive angiography and revascularization.[184] When patency could not be achieved with angioplasty, a 32% rate of mortality was observed. These studies may be biased by selection of lower risk patients for intervention, whereas patients who died before an attempt could be made to reestablish patency were counted in the conventional treatment group.

In the absence of definitive clinical trial data, the author and colleagues recommend angioplasty in patients with suspected reinfarction, with therapy guided by the combined clinical and angiographic findings. The sicker the patient or the larger the infarct, the more the cardiologist should be inclined to attempt to open the infarcted artery with percutaneous technology. When facilities or expertise is not readily available, repeated thrombolytic therapy is recommended. If streptokinase was used initially, alteplase is used because of the report by White and colleagues[180] of 50% allergic reactions with readministration of streptokinase.

The appropriate treatment of recurrent ischemia without reocclusion remains controversial. Post–myocardial infarction angina is generally considered to be an indication for angiography because it is a high-risk marker. Indications for revascularization are then based on the standard criteria for choosing coronary artery bypass grafting (CABG) or PTCA[185] and the suitability of the lesion for intervention. An interesting study in Denmark (DNAMI) is comparing a strategy of angiography and revascularization after recurrent post–myocardial infarction ischemia with a strategy of intensified medical therapy, wherein angiography is reserved only for "breakthrough" symptoms occurring during maximal medical therapy. After 2½ years of a 5-year follow-up, no difference was discerned in mortality (the primary endpoint) in the two groups, but secondary endpoints of recurrent myocardial infarction, hospitalization for unstable angina, or the need for increased antianginal medications were dramatically reduced in patients in the angiography group.

The major difficulty with percutaneous revascularization in patients with post–myocardial infarction angina is the documented hazard of the procedure, which is directly related to the time elapsed since the index event. The acutely disrupted atherosclerotic plaque poses a higher risk of abrupt closure, repeated myocardial necrosis, and death. In an overview, deFeyter and Serruys reported a twofold increase in mortality and a substantially increased risk of recurrent myocardial infarction and acute surgery in patients undergoing revascularization with refractory unstable angina or post–myocardial infarction angina in comparison with stable angina and stabilized unstable angina (Table 7–10).[186]

Considerable insight into recurrent ischemia and reinfarction came from detailed angiographic studies evaluating coronary reocclusion after thrombolysis. Reocclusion is associated with a doubling of mortality[187] and a substantial increase in arrhythmia and pump dysfunction complications. Unfortunately, the propensity for reocclusion is difficult to predict, although lower initial TIMI grade flow, 3-h administration of alteplase, infarction of the right coronary artery, and bradycardia were found to be predictive in one model.[187] In studies using systematic angiography, approximately half of the episodes of reocclusion have been clinically silent.

Reinfarction

Reinfarction is defined as a repeated episode of myocardial necrosis; the diagnosis is complex in the first 24 h after the index infarction. In a patient whose serum cardiac markers have not yet returned to the normal range, the diagnosis is made by a significant (usually twofold) elevation beyond the previous nadir. It is readily apparent that the reported rate of reinfarction is directly proportional to the frequency of sampling of serum cardiac markers and to the intensity of symptomatic and electrocardiographic surveillance. Of routine therapies for myocardial infarction, beta blockers have been shown to reduce the risk of reinfarction, whereas thrombolytic therapy is associated with a slight excess in reinfarction.[188] Heart rate–slowing calcium channel blockers may reduce the rate of reinfarction among patients with normal left ventricular function after myocardial infarction, whereas the role of heparin is controversial (see the heparin section).

Before the elucidation of the primary acute coronary occlusion in the pathogenesis of acute myocardial infarction, the term *reinfarction* was often used synonymously with the term *extension,* which referred to a repeated necrotic event after 24 h from hospital presentation and before hospital discharge. Now that the relevant pathophysiologic process is thought to be thrombotic reocclusion, the term *reinfarction* is commonly used to describe any repeated episode of myocardial necrosis after the initial infarction. The therapy of reinfarction is reviewed in previous sections.

Structural Defects

Ventricular Septal Defect

Rupture of the ventricular septum is a devastating complication of acute myocardial infarction, occurring in 2%–4% of cases. Risk factors for acute ventricular septal defect (VSD) include first infarction, history of hypertension, and female gender.[189] This complication should be suspected in a patient with hypotension, poor perfusion, and a new pansystolic murmur. Frequently, evidence of pulmonary congestion is minimal because of the shunt. Despite earlier pathologic observations that VSD most often occurred more than 4 days after the acute event, clinical observations demonstrate that the highest risk is in the first 24 h.

Patients with acute VSD should be treated with an IABP and invasive hemodynamic monitoring (Fig. 7–21). Vasodilator therapy with nitroprusside should be initiated to optimize hemodynamic parameters. Renal dysfunction is common and frequently worsens despite efforts to stabilize the hemodynamics with medical therapy. In fact, acute deterioration can be sudden and unpredictable, making the urge to "stabilize" the patient a logically flawed approach.

Definitive treatment is surgical repair. Unfortunately, the rate of operative mortality is high, ranging from 20% to 70%. Preoperative shock and inferoposterior infarction, especially right ventricular dysfunction, are the key cardiac risk factors for poor outcome with surgery. The most common dilemma concerning surgical therapy is in elderly patients with moderate renal insufficiency. Operative mortality and morbidity can be expected to be very high in this population. Aggressive and early surgery leads to the highest survival rates, although many patients have prolonged hospital stays with costs in excess of $100,000.

When a VSD is suspected, echocardiography with color-flow Doppler imaging should be done as soon as possible. This procedure confirms the diagnosis, establishes the coexistence of other cardiac problems such as mitral regurgitation, and provides estimates of right and left ventricular function. If a decision is made to proceed with surgical therapy, coronary angiography should be done to identify vessels in need of CABG. Left ventriculography may not be necessary when echocardiographic imaging provides adequate information about left ventricular performance.

Mitral Regurgitation

Mitral regurgitation is a very high-risk indicator in patients with acute myocardial infarction.[190, 191] Among patients with documented moderate to severe mitral regurgitation, the 1-year survival rate is only approximately 50%. The diagnosis is generally made by detection of a new systolic murmur. The murmur may be pansystolic or may be delayed in onset until well after the first heart sound. Unfortunately, as many as half of the patients with severe mitral regurgitation do not have an audible murmur. Although on average patients with mitral regurgitation have a later onset murmur, more pulmonary edema, and less neck vein distention than do patients with an acute VSD, in practice both conditions necessitate emergency stabilization and echocardiography for diagnosis. Because of the frequency of "silent" mitral regurgitation, the clinician must suspect this etiology in any patient with unexplained hypotension or pulmonary edema.

The outcome and therapy depend to a great extent upon the etiology of the mitral regurgitation. Papillary muscle dysfunction resulting from ischemia and/or infarction of the adjacent ventricular wall is the most common cause; this condition carries an intermediate prognosis and may be improved by medical therapy, percutaneous revascularization, or surgery. When global left ventricular dilatation causes failure of the mitral leaflets to coapt and the mitral regurgitation is severe, the prognosis is grim because surgical therapy is unlikely to improve the problem. The etiology with the greatest potential for successful surgical intervention is papillary muscle or chordal rupture, which accounts for fewer than 5% of cases of acute mitral regurgitation; the patient generally does well with prompt valve replacement.

Developing guidelines for the management of acute mitral regurgitation is challenging. Initial reports enthusiastically endorsed reperfusion with thrombolytic therapy and direct angioplasty as a means of restoring valvular competence. Unfortunately, the majority of patients continue to suffer from mitral regurgitation despite prompt reperfusion. In a patient with significant hemodynamic compromise, the clinician should pursue vasodilator therapy with nitroglycerin or nitroprusside,[192] IABP placement,[193] and hemodynamic monitoring to allow vigorous diuresis while maintaining adequate tissue perfusion. Within the first 12 h of the onset of symptoms of acute myocardial infarction, the ideal place for carrying out this therapeutic plan is the cardiac catheterization laboratory. The approach should be to ensure reperfusion of the infarcted artery while assessing the extent of anatomic disease and left ventricular dysfunction. Serial echocardiography can be used to assess whether reperfusion alone is adequate to ameliorate the mitral regurgitation. If moderate to severe mitral regurgitation remains, surgical therapy should be recommended. Data continue to indicate that valve repair with the assistance of intraoperative transesophageal echocardiography, if the repair can be accomplished technically, yields better results at a lower risk than does valve replacement. The patient and family must be informed, however, that concomitant coronary bypass and mitral valve surgery continue to be associated with a very high mortality rate.

Pseudoaneurysm and Free Wall Rupture

Rupture of the left ventricular free wall is generally thought of as sudden and catastrophic. However, the astute clinician may be able to detect early and intermediate signs and symptoms that can lead to successful intervention. Although the definitive clinical epidemiologic process is elusive because of the incomplete nature of autopsy series, free wall rupture is thought to occur in 2%–4% of cases and to produce 10%–20% of the deaths in acute myocardial infarction. Similar to acute ventricular septal rupture, the key risk factors are older age, female gender, hypertension, first myocardial infarction, and transmural infarction in the absence of collateral vessel flow.

Often the initial event is heralded by chest pain and sudden hypotension. The patient may then have a transient period of stability, perhaps representing thrombosis of the communication between the ventricle and the pericardium. If the rupture site remains sealed, the patient can survive for a long term with a left ventricular pseudoaneurysm. However, pseudoaneurysms may also rupture catastrophically and should therefore generally be repaired.

The relationship between thrombolytic therapy and rupture has been a topic of interest. Honan and colleagues demonstrated that early thrombolysis decreased the risk of rupture by limiting the amount of damage or necrosis, whereas late thrombolysis increased the risk, presumably as a result of dissection of necrotic myocardial tissue by intramyocardial hemorrhage.[35] This phenomenon is thought to explain at least a portion of the early hazard of thrombolytic therapy.

When a patient has sudden unexplained hypotension, especially with the risk factors for cardiac rupture, the physical examination should include careful evaluation for evidence of pericardial tampon-

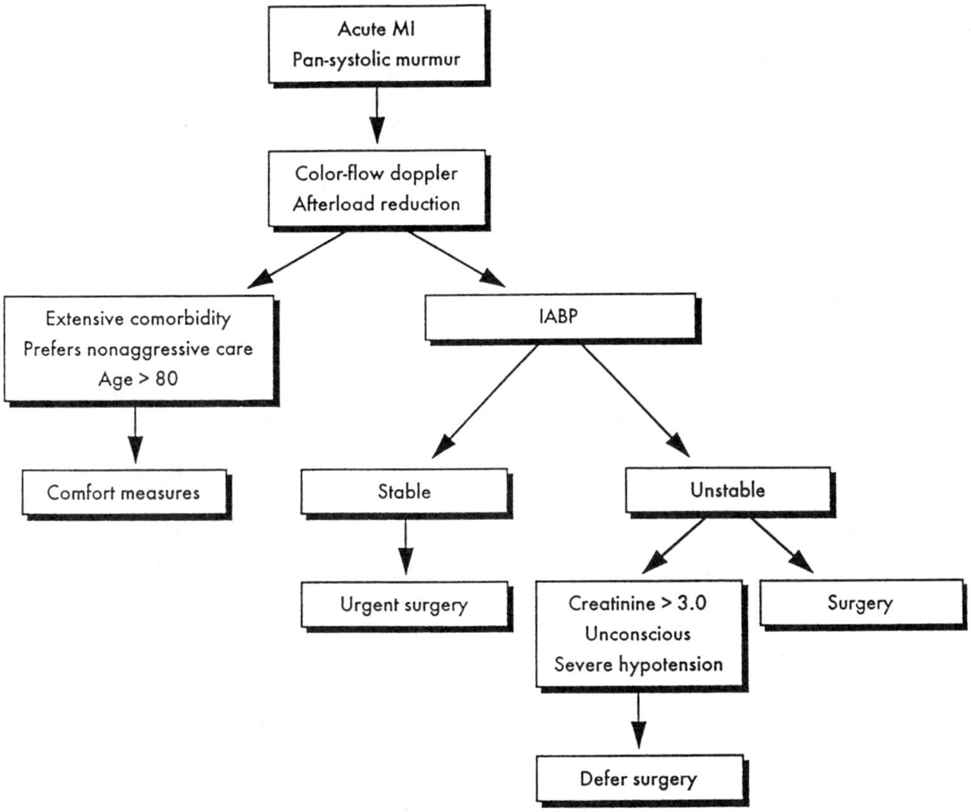

Figure 7–21. Flow diagram for management of patients with post–myocardial infarction (MI) ventricular septal defect. Patients who are hemodynamically stable should undergo surgery immediately; patients with multiple comorbid factors, especially those with renal failure or extensive right ventricular dysfunction and advanced age, are at very high risk and require careful consideration of risks and benefits with substantial uncertainty. Patients preferring conservative care should not undergo surgical therapy. *Other abbreviation:* IABP, intra-aortic balloon pump.

ade (especially elevated right-sided heart pressure, pulsus paradoxicus, sinus tachycardia, and low voltage). An emergency echocardiogram should be performed, and if the diagnosis is confirmed, an immediate decision about cardiac surgery is required. In the few case reports of surviving patients, simultaneous pericardiocentesis and replacement of volume through central lines have been used to maintain viability until the operation could be initiated.

Pericarditis

Pericarditis that follows myocardial infarction is a common clinical problem, but the diagnosis is dependent on the auscultatory skill of the clinician. Before the advent of thrombolytic therapy, the reported incidence was 7%–20%, but in the thrombolytic era, the reported rate has been 5% or less. Signs and symptoms generally appear between the second and sixth days after the acute myocardial infarction. The diagnosis is made by auscultation of a friction rub, and often patients have pleuritic chest pain made worse by changing position or coughing and eased by sitting up. The ECG may demonstrate persistent diffuse ST segment elevation or re-elevation in the area of initial injury and PR interval depression.

It is tempting to order an echocardiogram in patients with a clinical diagnosis of post–myocardial infarction pericarditis, but the echocardiogram frequently fails to demonstrate a pericardial effusion. For this reason, the echocardiogram should not be ordered routinely but should be reserved for patients with evidence of hemodynamic compromise (tachycardia, hypotension, pulsus paradoxicus, distended neck veins) or when assessment of left ventricular function is needed.

Distinguishing post–myocardial infarction pericarditis from recurrent ischemic discomfort can be quite difficult, because the chest discomfort can be vague and difficult to describe. Patients with post–myocardial infarction pericarditis have larger infarcts and can be expected to have worse outcomes.[194] The myocardial infarct extends in a more transmural manner in these patients. Pericardial tamponade is rare, even among patients treated with thrombolytic therapy and anticoagulation. Nevertheless, when post–myocardial infarction pericarditis is initially diagnosed, the patient should be observed more carefully for at least 24 h or until the signs and symptoms improve. There is a small but finite risk of hemodynamically significant pericardial effusion or tamponade. Although it is not mandatory to discontinue anticoagulation when a rub is heard, the onset of pericarditis should prompt reconsideration of the overall risk and benefit of anticoagulation.

The preferred therapy for post–myocardial infarction pericarditis is continued observation and aspirin in higher doses (650 mg orally every 4–6 h); excellent results have been reported with this approach.[195] Morphine sulfate or oral analgesia can be used for pain relief. In patients with ongoing symptoms that are severe, nonsteroidal anti-inflammatory agents (ibuprofen, indomethacin) have been effective in relieving symptoms. Unfortunately, these agents have been associated with an increased risk of unfavorable remodeling and myocardial rupture.[196] Similarly, intravenous or oral steroids can be quite effective in relieving pain, but these agents also have been associated with thinning and rupture.[197] If nonsteroidal anti-inflammatory agents or steroids are used, therapy should be continued only until the patient is comfortable.

Risk Stratification

Risk stratification is discussed traditionally in terms of a predischarge evaluation after myocardial infarction. Current thinking is evolving, however, to the concept that the physician should stratify risk from admission throughout the hospitalization so that the benefits and risks of interventions and commitments of resources can be compared. For convenience, the clinician can consider four phases of the course of acute myocardial infarction: the acute evaluation, the CCU phase, the convalescent (hospital) phase, and the predischarge evaluation.

The Acute Evaluation

The initial evaluation of a patient with symptoms of acute ischemic heart disease includes the history, a brief directed physical examination, and the 12-lead ECG and measurement of serum cardiac markers. Of these, if the history is suggestive, the presence of ST segment changes on the ECG and an elevated cardiac-specific troponin or CK-MB provide the most important information. The finding of ST segment elevation in particular heralds the need to attempt immediate acute reperfusion. Several predictive instruments are available to provide quantitative estimates of the risk of myocardial infarction.[198] In the patient with ST segment elevation, age, systolic blood pressure, Killip class, heart rate, amount and height of ST segment elevation, presence of a conduction disturbance, and infarct location provide the bulk of prognostic information.

The CCU Phase

After a decision has been made to admit the patient to the CCU, constant surveillance is needed in order to identify complications of the infarction. Particularly in patients treated with thrombolytic therapy, a 12-lead ECG and symptom assessment should be performed 60–90 min after the initiation of the infusion. If the ST segment has not resolved more than 50% from its peak value in the lead with the maximal ST-segment elevation, especially if ischemic symptoms continue, it should be assumed that reperfusion has been unsuccessful.[199] When the infarct is estimated to be large, "rescue" angioplasty should be considered.

In patients who have had no evidence of recurrent ischemia, electrical instability (frequent nonsustained or sustained ventricular tachycardia or ventricular fibrillation, high-degree AV block, asystole), or clinical pump dysfunction (pulmonary edema, sinus tachycardia, prolonged hypotension) after 24 h in the CCU, the disease process should be considered uncomplicated and the patients transferred from the CCU. In general, any of these complications connotes higher risk and merits additional CCU stay. Newby and Califf demonstrated a very low mortality rate among patients without these complications through the first 4 days of hospitalization; in the GUSTO-I trial, these patients constituted more than 55% of patients with myocardial infarction; the 30-day mortality rate was 1% and the 1-year mortality rate was 3.6%.[200]

The Hospital Phase

As in the CCU phase, the major goal of risk stratification in patients during the hospital phase is to identify clinical findings indicative of increased risk so that more aggressive evaluation and treatment can ensue. The converse of this goal, to identify candidates for early discharge, has taken on increasing importance because of the preeminence of cost as an issue in medical practice. Fundamentally, the absence of the complications listed earlier indicates that the patient is at low risk and may be discharged on days 4 to 5.

The Predischarge Phase

By hospital day 4 or 5, 50% of patients will have had a clinical complication identifying them as being at higher risk. Among the remaining 50% of patients, provocative testing might be used to identify relatively high-risk and low-risk patients. Multiple methods of provoking and measuring myocardial ischemia and assessing left ventricular function have been developed. Unfortunately, comparative studies have not been done to guide the clinician in choosing a particular test for an individual patient. The issues to be addressed by predischarge testing include left ventricular function, inducible ischemia, electrical instability, and secondary prevention.

Left Ventricular Function

Measurement of left ventricular function provides general information about prognosis[201, 202] and also provides critical information that can identify candidates for ACE inhibitors and CABG. The shape of the relationship between left ventricular ejection fraction and mortality has been confirmed in multiple studies (Fig. 7–22).[203] Overviews by Yusuf and colleagues[204] provided definitive evidence that impaired left ventricular function is a major predictor of the benefit of bypass surgery, and the *proven* mortality reduction with ACE inhibitors is confined to patients with ejection fractions of <35% (although benefit may yet exist in patients with ejection fractions of >35%).[205] For these reasons, the author and colleagues recommend quantitative assessment of left ventricular function in all patients after myocardial infarction.

A simple noninvasive assessment to estimate ejection fraction has been proposed by Silver and colleagues.[206] In their experience, the absence of prior Q wave infarction, prior heart failure, and current conduction disturbance and the presence of a non–anterior index infarction had a positive predictive value of .98 for ejection fractions of >40%. Radionuclide angiography is another method with substantial validation of prognostic capability. Echocardiography provides simultaneous information about valvular function and thrombus in the left ventricle, which makes it attractive in relation to other procedures. The final decision about the method to be chosen depends on both the method chosen to evaluate inducible ischemia and the timing (patients with early complicated courses often need echocardiography to guide therapy). When a decision has already been made to proceed with cardiac catheterization, other ventricular function estimates are superfluous.

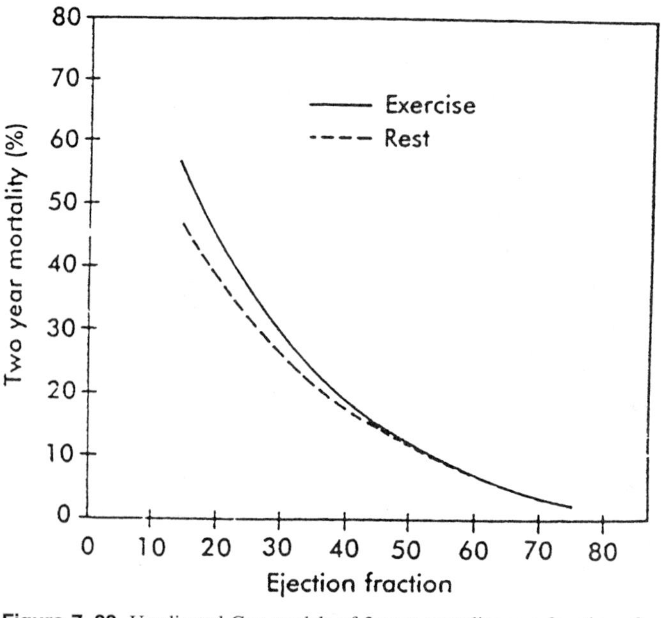

Figure 7–22. Unadjusted Cox models of 2-year mortality as a function of rest and exercise ejection fraction. (From Morris KG: Use of radionuclide angiography following acute myocardial infarction. *In* Califf RM, Mark DB, Wagner GS [eds]: Acute Coronary Care, 2nd ed, pp 797–813. St. Louis: Mosby–Year Book, 1995.)

Inducible Ischemia

Routine clinical practice includes an exercise test when possible not only because of the need to assess ischemia but also to provide a basis for advice about physical exertion after discharge. The choice of which test to perform depends on local expertise and cost factors, because adequate-sized populations have not been directly compared to determine which tests actually yield superior information.

In an overview of 29 studies with 15,526 patients and 541 (5%) follow-up deaths, the author and colleagues evaluated the prognostic significance of findings on the routine treadmill exercise test.[207] ST segment depression was found to be predictive of death in 43% of studies, in comparison with angina that was predictive in 27%, impaired systolic blood pressure in 54%, impaired exercise duration in 75%, and ventricular arrhythmia in 18%. The operating characteristics of each of the findings is displayed in Table 7–11. The major message is that impaired exercise performance and hypotension are more powerful indicators of poor prognosis than is ST segment depression.

Myocardial Perfusion Imaging. Myocardial perfusion imaging with thallium or sestamibi has more favorable operating characteristics than does routine treadmill testing. Multiple perfusion defects are associated with multivessel disease and an even higher risk.[208] The incremental value of perfusion imaging appears to be particularly enhanced when the ECG has substantial resting abnormalities; in the absence of these, perfusion imaging did not add to standard exercise testing.[209] Although arguments have been mounted on both sides, the choice between thallium and sestamibi remains unclear (Tables 7–12, 7–13).

Stress Ventricular Function Imaging. The exercise ejection fraction is one of the most powerful prognostic measures in cardiology.[210] Substantially more data currently exist to support the use of multigated or single-pass nuclear imaging. The echocardiography literature is relatively new and scanty in this area, but the available information is promising.

Pharmacologic Stress Testing. In patients who cannot exercise because of comorbidity, pharmacologic stress with dipyridamole, adenosine, or dobutamine has been shown to be feasible and can be combined with the imaging methods just delineated. The combined literature to date includes only 894 patients and 53 deaths. Nevertheless, the predictive ability of pharmacologic stress appears to be similar to that of exercise. Interestingly, even with a negative result of a test for ischemia, patients undergoing pharmacologic stress have a high event rate, which raises the question of whether more of them should be undergoing catheterization early.

Electrical Instability

The risk of sudden cardiac death after myocardial infarction remains a major concern. A number of technologies have been employed to identify patients at increased risk. The presence of frequent premature ventricular beats and nonsustained ventricular tachycardia on ambulatory monitoring is associated with increased risk.[211] Similarly, the signal-averaged ECG has been shown to be highly specific but only modestly sensitive in predicting risk of sudden cardiac death.[212] The combination of frequent ectopy on ambulatory monitoring, a positive signal-averaged ECG, and left ventricular dysfunction connotes particularly high risk. Heart rate variability and baroreceptor sensitivity, which are measures of autonomic tone, have been shown to detect patients at high risk.[213] Despite the success in identifying high-risk patients, the absence of a specifically effective therapy that would lower the risk precludes recommending these methods of identifying patients at high risk of sudden death other than clinical observation for the presence of sustained ventricular tachycardia.

Secondary Prevention

Before discharge, the physician and patient should review specific modifiable risk factors and medications that are known to have a beneficial effect. A plan for treatment should be formulated and agreed to before discharge. This plan should be reviewed with the patient and family to ensure that it is understood.

Ample evidence exists to support aggressive therapy to lower low-density lipoprotein (LDL) cholesterol levels in patients with known ischemic heart disease. Although LDL and high-density lipoprotein (HDL) cholesterol levels drop with hospitalization for acute myocardial infarction, values within the first 24 h are reflective of the baseline state.[214] The author and colleagues therefore check a lipid panel (total cholesterol, LDL cholesterol, HDL cholesterol, and triglycerides) within the first 24 h of admission. An LDL cholesterol

TABLE 7–11. PREDISCHARGE RISK STRATIFICATION BY EXERCISE TESTING

	Sensitivity		Specificity		Positive Predictive Value		Negative Predictive Value	
	Cardiac Death	Cardiac Death/MI	Cardiac Death	Cardiac Death/MI	Cardiac Death	Cardiac Death/MI	Cardiac Death	Cardiac Death/MI
Exercise ECG								
ST depression > 1 mm	.38	.44	.79	.70	.05	.16	.98	.91
Impaired systolic BP	.46	.23	.74	.87	.05	.21	.98	.88
Limited duration of exercise	.60	.53	.61	.65	.03	.18	.98	.91
Chest pain during exercise	.27	.29	.82	.82	.05	.19	.97	.89
Myocardial Perfusion Imaging								
Reversible ^{201}Tl defect	.89	.80	.38	.48	.07	.16	.98	.95
Multiple ^{201}Tl defects	.64	.75	.71	.76	.07	.17	.98	.97
Ventricular Function Imaging								
Peak EF < 30%–40%	.63	.60	.77	.75	.27	.31	.94	.91
Blunted EF	.80	.55	.67	.74	.15	.18	.98	.94
New/worsening WMA	*	.78	*	.50	*	.17	*	.94

Abbreviations: MI, myocardial infarction; ECG, electrocardiography; BP, blood pressure; EF, ejection fraction; WMA, wall motion abnormality.
*Not available.

Table 7–12. PREDICTIVE VALUE OF MYOCARDIAL PERFUSION IMAGING IN THE POST–MYOCARDIAL INFARCTION PATIENT

					Deaths		Death or MI		Predictors of Cardiac Death/Nonfatal MI*	
Study	*N*	% Tested	Protocol	Imaging	*N*	%	*N*	%	Reversible ^{201}Tl Defect	Size of Perfusion Defect
Hung (1984)[226]	117	†	Submaximal Naughton	Qualitative planar ^{201}Tl	2	1.7	8	6.8	Yes	Yes
Leppo (1984)[227]	51	39	IV dipyridamole	Semi-quantitative planar ^{201}Tl	8	15.7	15	29.4	Yes	No
Gibson (1986)[228]	241	67	Submaximal	Quantitative planar ^{201}Tl	21	8.7	47	2.4	Yes for death; for MI, only NQMI	†
Abraham (1986)[229]	103	53	Submaximal Upright bicycle or modified Bruce	Qualitative planar ^{201}Tl	4	3.9	8	7.8	No (soft)	†
Gimple (1989)[230]	40	†	IV dipyridamole	Qualitative planar ^{201}Tl	1	2.5	3	7.5	Yes (soft)	†
Tilkemeier (1990)[231]	171	83	Maximal modified Bruce	Qualitative planar ^{201}Tl	5	2.9	12	7.0	Yes (soft)	†
Hendel (1991)[232]	71	†	IV dipyridamole	Qualitative planar ^{201}Tl	2	2.8	10	14.1	No	†
de Cock (1992)[233]	100	80	Maximal Bruce	Qualitative planar ^{201}Tl	10	10.0	20	20.0	Yes	†
Total *N*	894				53					
Average	112	64.4			7	6.0	15	11.9	50%	50%

Abbreviations: MI, myocardial infarction; IV, intravenous; NQMI, non–Q wave myocardial infarction.
*Yes, univariate or multivariable predictor of cardiac death or MI; No, not a univariate predictor of cardiac death or MI; soft, indicates univariate or multivariable predictor only when soft endpoints were used.
†Not available.

level of <100 mg/dL is the current target, although further information may alter this target as lipid subfractions become better understood. The author's practice is to begin lipid-lowering therapy in most patients with LDL cholesterol levels of <100 mg/dL rather than simply relying on diet.

Counseling to discontinue smoking is one of the most cost-effective interventions during an admission for acute myocardial infarction. Multiple studies have documented the increased risk of recurrent events in patients who continue to smoke after discharge. Among those who stop smoking, however, the risk of recurrence falls within 3 years to a level similar to that among patients who have never smoked. An overview of available data with a decision model provided substantial evidence that nurse-based intervention saves substantial lives at a low cost.[215]

Although in many cases the occurrence of a myocardial infarction reduces the subsequent ambient blood pressure, 30%–40% of stricken patients have hypertension. Because of the secondary prevention information currently available, the author and colleagues emphasize the use of beta blockers and ACE inhibitors and the avoidance of calcium channel blockers in the treatment of hypertension.

Diabetes is also a common condition in patients with myocardial infarction. Because of the understanding that insulin is a growth factor and because of the absence of significant outcome data on the degree of glucose control that would be best for clinical outcomes, the most appropriate regimen for patients with diabetes remains uncertain. The Diabetes Control and Complications Trial indicated that tight control of insulin-dependent diabetes was associated with a reduction in "macrovascular" events from 0.84 events per 100 patient years to 0.49 events per 100 patient years.[216] Of 12 major cardiovascular events, 9 occurred in the conservatively treated group and 3 occurred in the intensively treated group. Unfortunately, when all-cause mortality was considered, seven deaths were observed with intensive treatment, in comparison with four deaths among the conservatively treated patients. Until further results are available, the author and colleagues continue to advocate moderately tight control of diabetes.

In addition to modification of risk factors, it is imperative to ensure that patients understand the medical regimens that are associated with improved outcomes. Aspirin should be taken by every patient at the time of discharge unless a true allergy or bleeding tendency is present. Similarly, beta blocking medications have been shown to be effective in preventing death, reinfarction, and ventricular fibrillation in long-term follow-up. ACE inhibitors in doses that have been shown to be beneficial are mandatory in patients with ejection fractions of <35% unless a specific contraindication is present.

The indications for long-term anticoagulation remain controversial. The routine use of warfarin (Coumadin) for secondary prevention after myocardial infarction was recently approved by the U.S. Food and Drug Administration on the basis of a series of clinical trials culminating with the Anticoagulants in the Secondary Prevention of Events in Coronary Thrombosis (ASPECT) trial, which randomized more than 3000 patients to warfarin or placebo after myocardial infarction. A cumulative meta-analysis of 15 randomized trials showed a relative risk of death of 0.87, a relative risk of recurrent myocardial infarction of 0.59, and a relative risk of stroke of 0.59.[217] Unfortunately, these studies did not include aspirin in the control group. Despite a cost/benefit analysis showing favorable cost-effectiveness ratios for routine warfarin use when compared with other standard treatments,[218] the even more favorable cost-effectiveness profile of aspirin renders it the antithrombotic of choice.[219]

Among the possible indications for warfarin instead of aspirin are left ventricular thrombus, large anterior infarction or aneurysm, and persistent atrial fibrillation. Despite a number of observational studies demonstrating better outcome in patients treated with warfarin after echocardiographic detection of left ventricular thrombus, adequately controlled studies have not been performed. Similarly, the presence of a large anterior infarct as a risk factor for stroke has been demonstrated, but no controlled trials have been completed to assess the benefit and risk of anticoagulation. The indication for warfarin in the setting of atrial fibrillation is much firmer, in view of the substantial randomized trial evidence in its favor.

TABLE 7–13. PREDICTIVE VALUE OF VENTRICULAR FUNCTION IMAGING IN THE POST–MYOCARDIAL INFARCTION PATIENT

					Deaths		Deaths or MI		Predictors of Cardiac Death or Nonfatal MI*		
Study	*N*	% Tested	Protocol	Imaging	*N*	%	*N*	%	New or Worsening WMA	Peak Exercise EF	EF Change < ±5%
Nicod (1983)[234]	42	†	Supine bicycle at 25–50 w/4 min.	Multigated equilibrium blood pool imaging	7	16.7	11	26.2	No	Yes for MVD (EF < 40%)	†
Dewhurst (1983)[235]	100	†	Maximal bicycle at 60–70 w/3 min.	RNV	11	11.0	17	17.0	†	Trend	Yes (soft)
Hung (1984)[226]	117	†	Maximal bicycle	RNV	2	1.7	8	6.8	†	Yes	Yes
Morris (1985)[236]	106	64	Submaximal upright bicycle at 17 w/min.	Multigated equilibrium blood pool imaging	12	11.3	16	15.0	Yes for MI	Yes for Death	No
Fioretti (1986)[237]	351	50	Maximal bicycle	RNV	70	19.9	†	†	†	Yes	†
Ryan (1987)[238]	40	†	Submaximal TM at 1.5 METs/3 min.	2-Dimensional echocardiography	3	7.5	6	15.0	Yes (soft)	†	†
Kuchar (1987)[239]	153	73	Maximal semi-supine bicycle at 15 w/min.	Multigated equilibrium blood pool imaging	11	6.2	24	13.4	Yes	Yes (EF < 30%)	Yes
Applegate (1987)[240]	67	74	Maximal upright bicycle	2-Dimensional echocardiography	3	4.5	11	16.4	Yes	†	Yes
Abraham (1987)[241]	75	42	Maximal semi-supine bicycle at 15 w/min.	Multigated equilibrium blood pool imaging	6	8.0	8	10.7	†	Yes (soft) (EF < 50%)	Yes (soft)
Bolognese (1992)[242]	217	94	High-dose (0.84 mg/kg) dipyridamole	2-Dimensional echocardiography	5	2.3	12	5.5	Yes (soft)	†	†
Sclavo (1992)[243]	107	†	High-dose (0.84 mg/kg) dipyridamole	2-Dimensional echocardiography	2	1.9	1	0.9	Yes (Soft)	†	†
Picano (1993)[244]	925	94	High-dose (0.84 mg/kg) dipyridamole	2-Dimensional echocardiography	34	3.2	71	6.6	Yes	†	†
Total *N*	2,300				166						
Average	209	70			15	8.6	19	13.4	37.5	71.4	50.0

Abbreviations: MI, myocardial infarction; WMA, wall-motion abnormality; EF, ejection fraction; MVD, multivessel disease.

*Yes, univariate or multivariable predictor of cardiac death or MI; No, not a univariate predictor of cardiac death or MI; Soft, indicates univariate or multivariable predictor only when soft endpoints were used.

†Not available.

REFERENCES

1. Falk E: Coronary thrombosis: pathogenesis and clinical manifestations. Am J Cardiol 1991; 68:28B–35B.
2. Fuster V, Steele PM, Chesebro JH: Role of platelets and thrombosis in coronary atherosclerotic disease and sudden death. J Am Coll Cardiol 1985; 5:175B–184B.
3. Little WC, Constantinescu M, Applegate RJ, et al: Can coronary angiography predict the site of a subsequent myocardial infarction in patients with mild to moderate coronary artery disease? Circulation 1988; 78:1157–1166.
4. Falk E: Plaque rupture with severe pre-existing stenosis precipitating coronary thrombosis: characteristics of coronary atherosclerotic plaques underlying fatal occlusive thrombi. Br Heart J 1983; 50:127–134.
5. Davies MJ, Woolf N, Rowles PM, Pepper J: Morphology of the endothelium over atherosclerotic plaques in human coronary arteries. Br Heart J 1988; 60:459–464.
6. Muller JE, Ludmer PL, Willich SN, et al: Circadian variation in the frequency of sudden cardiac death. Circulation 1987; 75:131–138.
7. Rocco MB, Barry J, Campbell S, et al: Circadian variation of transient myocardial ischemia in patients with coronary artery disease. Circulation 1987; 75:395–400.
8. Reimer KA, Lowe JE, Rasmussen MM, Jennings RB: The wave-front phenomenon of ischemic cell death: 1. Myocardial infarct size versus duration of coronary occlusion in dogs. Circulation 1977; 56:786–794.
9. American Heart Association: Heart and Stroke Facts. Dallas: American Heart Association, 1993.
10. Braunwald E, Mark DB, Jones RH, et al: Unstable Angina: Diagnosis and Management. Rockville, MD: Agency for Health Care Policy and Research, 1994.
11. Weaver WD, Cerquerira M, Hallstrom AP, et al: Prehospital-initiated vs hospital-initiated thrombolytic therapy: the Myocardial Infarction Triage and Intervention trial. JAMA 1993; 270:1211–1216.
12. Gibler WB, Kereiakes DJ, Dean EN, et al: Prehospital diagnosis and treatment of acute myocardial infarction: a north-south perspective. The Cincinnati Heart Project and the Nashville Prehospital TPA Trial. Am Heart J 1991; 121:1–11.
13. Weaver WD, Eisenberg MS, Martin JS, et al: Myocardial Infarction Triage and Intervention project—phase I: patient characteristics and feasibility of prehospital initiation of thrombolytic therapy. J Am Coll Cardiol 1990; 15:925–930.
14. Kereiakes DJ, Weaver WD, Anderson JL, et al: Time delays in the diagnosis and treatment of acute myocardial infarction: a tale of eight cities. Am Heart J 1990; 120:773–779.
15. European Myocardial Infarction Project (EMIP) Subcommittee: Potential time saving with pre-hospital intervention in acute myocardial infarction. Eur Heart J 1988; 9:118–124.
16. GREAT Group: Feasibility, safety, and efficacy of domiciliary thrombolysis by general practitioners: Grampian Region Early Anistreplase Trial. Br Med J 1992; 305:548–553.
17. European Myocardial Infarction Project Group: Prehospital thrombolytic

therapy in patients with suspected acute myocardial infarction. N Engl J Med 1993; 329:383–389.
18. Fillmore SJ, Shapiro M, Killip T: Arterial oxygen tension in acute myocardial infarction: serial analysis of clinical state and blood-gas exchanges. Am Heart J 1970; 79:620–629.
19. Maroko P, Radvany P, Braunwald E, Hale S: Reduction of infarct size by oxygen inhalation following acute coronary occlusion. Circulation 1975; 52:360–368.
20. Sterling DL, Thornton JD, Swafford A, et al: Hyperbaric oxygen limits infarct size in ischemic rabbit myocardium in vivo. Circulation 1993; 88:1931–1936.
21. Blomberg S, Emanuelsson H, Ricksten S: Thoracic epidural anesthesia and central hemodynamics in patients with unstable angina pectoris. Anesth Analg 1989; 69:558–562.
22. Kock M, Blomberg S, Emanuelsson H, et al: Thoracic epidural anesthesia improves global and regional left ventricular function during stress-induced myocardial ischemia in patients with coronary artery disease. Anesth Analg 1990; 71:625–630.
23. Nordrehaug JE, Johannessen KA, von der Lippe G: Serum potassium concentration as a risk factor of ventricular arrhythmias early in acute myocardial infarction. Circulation 1985; 71:645–649.
24. Dyckner T, Helmers C, Lundman T, Wester PO: Initial serum potassium level in relation to early complications and prognosis in patients with acute myocardial infarction. Acta Med Scand 1975; 197:207–210.
25. Higham PD, Adams PC, Murray A, Campbell RWF: Plasma potassium, serum magnesium and ventricular fibrillation: a prospective study. Q J Med 1993; 86:609–617.
26. Granger CB, Califf RM, Topol EJ: Thrombolytic therapy for acute myocardial infarction. A review. Drugs 1992; 44:293–325.
27. Stump DC, Califf RM, Topol EJ, et al: Pharmacodynamics of thrombolysis with recombinant tissue-type plasminogen activator. Correlation with characteristics of and clinical outcomes in patients with acute myocardial infarction. The TAMI Study Group. Circulation 1989; 80:1222–1230.
28. Mueller HS, Roberts R, Teichman SL, Sobel BE: Thrombolytic therapy in acute myocardial infarction: part II—rt-PA. Med Clin North Am 1989; 73:387–407.
29. Gardell SJ, Ramjit DR, Stabilito II, et al: Effective thrombolysis without marked plasminemia after bolus intravenous administration of vampire bat salivary plasminogen activator in rabbits. Circulation 1991; 84:244–253.
30. Smalling RW, Bode C, Kalbfleisch J, et al: More rapid, complete, and stable coronary thrombolysis with bolus administration of reteplase compared with alteplase infusion in acute myocardial infarction. Circulation 1995; 91:2725–2732.
31. Keyt BA, Paoni NF, Refino CJ, et al: A faster-acting and more potent form of tissue plasminogen activator. Proc Natl Acad Sci USA 1994; 91:3670–3674.
32. Collen D, Stassen JM, Yasuda T, et al: Comparative thrombolytic properties of tissue-type plasminogen activator and of a plasminogen activator inhibitor-1–resistant glycosylation variant, in a combined arterial and venous thrombosis model in the dog. Thromb Haemost 1994; 72:98–104.
33. The GUSTO Angiographic Investigators: The effects of tissue plasminogen activator, streptokinase, or both on coronary-artery patency, ventricular function, and survival after acute myocardial infarction. N Engl J Med 1993; 329:1615–1622.
34. Reddy KNN: Mechanism of activation of human plasminogen by streptokinase. *In* Kline DL, Reddy KNN (eds): Fibrinolysis, pp 71–94. Boca Raton: CRC Press, 1980.
35. Honan MB, Harrell FE Jr, Reimer KA, et al: Cardiac rupture, mortality and the timing of thrombolytic therapy: a meta-analysis. J Am Coll Cardiol 1990; 16:359–367.
36. Fibrinolytic Therapy Trialists' (FTT) Collaborative Group: Indications for fibrinolytic therapy in suspected acute myocardial infarction: collaborative overview of early mortality and major morbidity results from all randomised trials of more than 1000 patients. Lancet 1994; 343:311–322.
37. van der Laarse A, Kerkhof PL, Vermeer F, et al: Relation between infarct size and left ventricular performance assessed in patients with first acute myocardial infarction randomized to intracoronary thrombolytic therapy or to conventional treatment. Am J Cardiol 1988; 61:1–7.
38. Bar F, Vermeer F, de Zwaan C, et al: Value of admission electrocardiogram in predicting outcome of thrombolytic therapy in acute myocardial infarction. Am J Cardiol 1987; 59:6–13.
39. Kaplan EL, Meier P: Nonparametric estimation from incomplete observations. J Am Stat Assoc 1958; 53:457–481.
40. Simoons ML, Vos J, Tijssen JG, Vermeer F, et al: Long-term benefit of early thrombolytic therapy in patients with acute myocardial infarction: 5 year follow-up of a trial conducted by the Interuniversity Cardiology Institute of the Netherlands. J Am Coll Cardiol 1989; 14:1609–1615.
41. Vermeer F, Simoons ML, Bar FW, et al: Which patients benefit most from early thrombolytic therapy with intracoronary streptokinase? Circulation 1986; 74:1379–1389.
42. Lee KL, Woodlief LH, Topol EJ, et al: Predictors of 30-day mortality in the era of reperfusion for acute myocardial infarction: results from an international trial of 41,021 patients. Circulation 1995; 91:1659–1668.
43. Zabel KM, Hathaway WR, Peterson ED, et al: Baseline electrocardiogram predicts 30-day mortality among 32,812 patients with acute myocardial infarction treated with thrombolysis [Abstract]. J Am Coll Cardiol 1995; 25:342A.
44. White HD, Granger C, Gore J, Barbash G, for the GUSTO Investigators: Older age is associated with a large increase in mortality and total stroke, but not non-fatal disabling stroke: results of the GUSTO trial [Abstract]. Circulation 1994; 90(suppl I):563.
45. Maggioni AP, Maseri A, Fresco C, et al: Age-related increase in mortality among patients with first myocardial infarctions treated with thrombolysis. N Engl J Med 1993; 329:1442–1448.
46. Weaver WD, Litwin PE, Martin JS, et al: Effect of age on use of thrombolytic therapy and mortality in acute myocardial infarction: the MITI Project Group. J Am Coll Cardiol 1991; 18:657–662.
47. Isner JM, Roberts WC: Right ventricular infarction complicating left ventricular infarction secondary to coronary heart disease: frequency, location, associated findings, and significance from analysis of 236 necropsy patients with acute or healed myocardial infarction. Am J Cardiol 1978; 42:885–894.
48. Peterson ED, Hathaway WR, Zabel KM, et al: The prognostic importance of anterior ST-segment depression in inferior myocardial infarctions: results in 16,185 patients [Abstract]. J Am Coll Cardiol 1995; 25:342A.
49. TIMI Study Group: Early effects of tissue-type plasminogen activator added to conventional therapy on the culprit coronary lesion in patients presenting with ischemic cardiac pain at rest. Results of the Thrombolysis in Myocardial Ischemia (TIMI IIIA) Trial. Circulation 1993; 87:38–52.
50. Califf RM, Massey EW: Myocardial infarction and stroke in the thrombolytic era. *In* Califf RM, Mark DB, Wagner GS (eds): Acute Coronary Care in the Thrombolytic Era, pp 539–547. Chicago: Year Book Publishers, 1988.
51. Maggioni AP, Franzosi MG, Farina ML, et al: Cerebrovascular events after myocardial infarction: analysis of the GISSI trial. Br Med J 1991; 302:1428–1431.
52. Gore JM, Sloan M, Price TR, et al: Intracerebral hemorrhage, cerebral infarction, and subdural hematoma after acute myocardial infarction and thrombolytic therapy in the Thrombolysis In Myocardial Infarction study: Thrombolysis In Myocardial Infarction, Phase II, pilot and clinical trial. Circulation 1991; 83:448–459.
53. Longstreth WT Jr, Litwin PE, Weaver WD, the MITI Project Group: Myocardial infarction, thrombolytic therapy, and stroke. A community-based study. Stroke 1993; 24:587–590.
54. Gore JM, Granger CB, Sloan MA, et al: Stroke after thrombolysis: mortality and functional outcomes in the GUSTO-I trial. Circulation 1995; 92:2811–2818.
55. Mark DB, Hlatky MA, Califf RM, et al: Cost effectiveness of thrombolytic therapy with tissue plasminogen activator as compared with streptokinase for acute myocardial infarction. N Engl J Med 1995; 332:1418–1424.
56. O'Neill WW, Brodie BR, Ivanhoe R, et al: Primary coronary angioplasty for acute myocardial infarction (the Primary Angioplasty Registry). Am J Cardiol 1994; 73:627–634.
57. Grines CL, Browne KF, Marco J, et al: A comparison of immediate angioplasty with thrombolytic therapy for acute myocardial infarction. The Primary Angioplasty in Myocardial Infarction Study Group. N Engl J Med 1993; 328:673–679.
58. Gibbons RJ, Holmes DR, Reeder GS, et al: Immediate angioplasty compared with the administration of a thrombolytic agent followed by conservative treatment for myocardial infarction. The Mayo Coronary Care Unit and Catheterization Laboratory Groups. N Engl J Med 1993; 328:685–691.
59. Zijlstra F, de Boer MJ, Moorntje JC, et al: A comparison of immediate coronary angioplasty with intravenous streptokinase in acute myocardial infarction. N Engl J Med 1993; 328:680–684.

60. Jollis JG, Peterson ED, DeLong ER, et al: The relation between the volume of coronary angioplasty procedures at hospitals treating Medicare beneficiaries and short-term mortality. N Engl J Med 1994; 331:1625–1629.
61. Califf RM, Bengtson JR: Cardiogenic shock. N Engl J Med 1994; 330:1724–1730.
62. Hochman JS, Boland J, Sleeper LA, et al: Current spectrum of cardiogenic shock and effect of early revascularization on mortality: results of an international registry. Circulation 1995; 91:873–881.
63. Granger C, White H, Simoons M, et al: Risk factors for stroke following thrombolytic therapy: case-control study from the GUSTO trial [Abstract]. J Am Coll Cardiol 1995; 25:232A.
64. Weaver WD, Litwin EP, Martin JS: Use of direct angioplasty for treatment of patients with acute myocardial infarction in hospitals with and without on-site cardiac surgery. The Myocardial Infarction, Triage, and Intervention Project Investigators. Circulation 1993; 88:2067–2075.
65. Byington R, Goldstein S: Association of digitalis therapy with mortality in survivors of acute myocardial infarction: observations in the Beta-Blocker Heart Attack Trial. J Am Coll Cardiol 1985; 6:976–982.
66. Bigger JT Jr, Fleiss JL, Rolnitzky LM, et al: Effect of digitalis treatment on survival after acute myocardial infarction. Am J Cardiol 1985; 55:623–630.
67. Hirsh J: Heparin. N Engl J Med 1991; 324:1565–1574.
68. Granger CB, Hirsh J, Califf RM, et al: Activated partial thromboplastin time and outcome after thrombolytic therapy for acute myocardial infarction: results from the GUSTO-I trial. Circulation 1996; 93:870–878.
69. MacMahon S, Collins R, Knight C, et al: Reduction in major morbidity and mortality by heparin in acute myocardial infarction [Abstract]. Circulation 1988; 78(suppl II):98.
70. ISIS-3 (Third International Study of Infarct Survival Collaborative Group): ISIS-3: a randomised comparison of streptokinase vs tissue plasminogen activator vs anistreplase and of aspirin plus heparin vs aspirin alone among 41,299 cases of suspected acute myocardial infarction. Lancet 1992; 339:753–770.
71. Gruppo Italiano per lo Studio della Sopravvivenza nell'Infarto Miocardico: GISSI-2: A factorial randomised trial of alteplase versus streptokinase and heparin versus no heparin among 12,490 patients with acute myocardial infarction. Lancet 1990; 336:65–71.
72. The GUSTO Investigators: An international randomized trial comparing four thrombolytic strategies for acute myocardial infarction. N Engl J Med 1993; 329:673–682.
73. O'Connor CM, Meese R, Carney R, et al: A randomized trial of intravenous heparin in conjunction with anistreplase (anisoylated plasminogen streptokinase activator complex) in acute myocardial infarction: the Duke University Clinical Cardiology Study (DUCCS) 1. J Am Coll Cardiol 1994; 23:11–18.
74. Bleich SD, Nichols TC, Schumacher RR, et al: Effect of heparin on coronary arterial patency after thrombolysis with tissue plasminogen activator in acute myocardial infarction. Am J Cardiol 1990; 66:1412–1417.
75. de Bono DP, Simoons ML, Tijssen J, et al: Effect of early intravenous heparin on coronary patency, infarct size, and bleeding complications after alteplase thrombolysis: results of a randomised double blind European Cooperative Study Group trial. Br Heart J 1992; 67:122–128.
76. Hsia J, Hamilton WP, Kleiman N, et al: A comparison between heparin and low-dose aspirin as adjunctive therapy with tissue plasminogen activator for acute myocardial infarction. Heparin-Aspirin Reperfusion Trial (HART) Investigators. N Engl J Med 1990; 323:1433–1437.
77. Mahaffey KW, Granger CB, O'Connor CM, et al: Overview of randomized trials of intravenous heparin in patients with acute myocardial infarction treated with thrombolytic therapy. Am J Cardiol in press.
78. Granger C, White HD, Hirsh J, et al: Relationship of APTT to outcome after thrombolysis: results from the GUSTO trial [Abstract]. Circulation 1993; 88(suppl I):200.
79. Cannon CP, Becker RC, Loscalzo J, et al: Usefulness of APTT to predict bleeding for hirudin (and heparin). Circulation 1994; 90(pt 2):I-563.
80. Becker RC, Cyr J, Corrao JM, Ball SP: Bedside coagulation monitoring in heparin-treated patients with active thromboembolic disease: a coronary care unit experience. Am Heart J 1994; 128:719–723.
81. Zabel KM, Granger CB, Becker RC, et al: Bedside aPTT monitoring is associated with less bleeding among GUSTO patients receiving IV heparin following thrombolytic administration [Abstract]. Circulation 1994; 90(suppl I):553.
82. The SCATI (Studio sulla Calciparina nell'Angina e nella Trombosi Ventricolare nell'Infarto) Group: Randomised controlled trial of subcutaneous calcium-heparin in acute myocardial infarction. Lancet 1989; 2:182–186.
83. Pedersen AK, Fitzgerald GA: Dose-related kinetics of aspirin. N Engl J Med 1984; 311:1206–1211.
84. Ross-Lee LM, Elms MJ, Cham BE, et al: Plasma levels of aspirin following effervescent and enteric coated tablets, and their effect on platelet function. Eur J Clin Pharmacol 1982; 23:545–551.
85. ISIS-2: Randomised trial of intravenous streptokinase, oral aspirin, both, or neither among 17,187 cases of suspected acute myocardial infarction: ISIS-2. Lancet 1988; 2:349–360.
86. Antiplatelet Trialists' Collaboration: Secondary prevention of vascular disease by prolonged antiplatelet treatment. Br Med J 1988; 296:320–331.
87. Baigent C, Collins R, for the ISIS Collaborative Group: ISIS-2: 4-year mortality follow-up of 17,187 patients after fibrinolytic and antiplatelet therapy in suspected acute myocardial infarction [Abstract]. Circulation 1993; 88(suppl I):291.
88. Roux S, Christeller S, Ludin E: Effects of aspirin on coronary reocclusion and recurrent ischemia after thrombolysis: a meta-analysis. J Am Coll Cardiol 1992; 19:671–677.
89. Settipane GA: Aspirin sensitivity and allergy. Biomed Pharmacother 1988; 42:493–498.
90. Jugdutt BI, Warnica JW: Intravenous nitroglycerin therapy to limit myocardial infarct size, expansion, and complications: effect of timing, dosage, and infarct location. Circulation 1988; 78:906–919.
91. Balsano F, Rizzon P, Violi F, et al: Antiplatelet treatment with ticlopidine in unstable angina: a controlled multicenter clinical trial. The Studio della Ticlopidina nell'Angina Instabile Group. Circulation 1990; 82:17–26.
92. Gent M, Blakely JA, Easton JD, et al: The Canadian American ticlopidine study (CATS) in thromboembolic stroke. Lancet 1989; 1:1215–1220.
93. Hass WK, Easton JD, Adams HP Jr, et al: A randomized trial comparing ticlopidine hydrochloride with aspirin for the prevention of strokes in high risk patients. N Engl J Med 1989; 321:501–507.
94. Bauman RP, Harrington RA: Adjunct pharmacologic support during an interventional procedure. *In* Roubin GS, Califf RM, O'Neill WW, et al (eds): Interventional Cardiovascular Medicine: Principles and Practice, pp 593–600. New York: Churchill Livingstone, 1994.
95. The EPIC Investigators: Use of a monoclonal antibody directed against the platelet glycoprotein IIb/IIIa receptor in high-risk coronary angioplasty. N Engl J Med 1994; 330:956–961.
96. Topol EJ, Califf RM, Weisman HF, et al: Randomised trial of coronary intervention with antibody against platelet IIb/IIIa integrin for reduction of clinical restenosis: results at six months. Lancet 1994; 343:881–886.
97. Mark DB, Talley JD, Lam LC, et al: Reduced restenosis from aggressive platelet inhibition reduces costs of high risk angioplasty: results from the EPIC randomized trial [Abstract]. Circulation 1994; 90(suppl I):44.
98. Aguirre F, Topol EJ, Ferguson JJ, et al: Bleeding complications with the chimeric antibody to platelet glycoprotein IIb/IIIa integrin in patients undergoing percutaneous coronary intervention. Circulation 1995; 91:2882–2890.
99. Lincoff AM, Tcheng JE, Bass TA, et al: A multicenter, randomized, double-blind pilot trial of standard versus low dose weight-adjusted heparin in patients treated with the platelet Gp IIb/IIIa receptor antibody c7E3 during percutaneous coronary revascularization [Abstract]. J Am Coll Cardiol 1995; 25:80A–81A.
100. Tenaglia AN, Fortin DF, Califf RM, et al: Predicting the risk of abrupt vessel closure after angioplasty in an individual patient. J Am Coll Cardiol 1994; 24:1004–1011.
101. Yusuf S, Sleight P, Rossi P, et al: Reduction in infarct size, arrhythmias, chest pain, and morbidity by early intravenous beta blockade in suspected myocardial infarction. Circulation 1983; 67(suppl I):32–41.
102. Yusuf S, Peto R, Lewis J, et al: Beta blockade during and after myocardial infarction: an overview of the randomized trials. Prog Cardiovasc Dis 1985; 27:335–371.
103. ISIS-1 (First International Study of Infarct Survival) Collaborative Group: Randomised trial of intravenous atenolol among 16,027 cases of suspected acute myocardial infarction: ISIS-1. Lancet 1986; 2:57–66.
104. TIMI Study Group: Comparison of invasive and conservative strategies after treatment with intravenous tissue plasminogen activator in acute

myocardial infarction: results of the Thrombolysis In Myocardial Infarction (TIMI) phase II trial. The TIMI Study Group. N Engl J Med 1989; 320:618–627.
105. Brener SJ, Cox JL, Pfisterer ME, et al: The potential for unexpected hazard of intravenous beta-blockade for acute myocardial infarction: results from the GUSTO trial [Abstract]. J Am Coll Cardiol 1995; (special issue):5-A–6-A.
106. Brunton TL: Lectures on the actions of medicines. New York: Macmillan, 1867.
107. Yusuf S, Collins R, MacMahon S, Peto R: Effect of intravenous nitrates on mortality in acute myocardial infarction: an overview of randomised trials. Lancet 1988; 1:1088–1092.
108. Gruppo Italiano per lo Studio della Sopravvivenza nell'Infarto Miocardico: GISSI-3: effects of lisinopril and transdermal glyceryl trinitrate singly and together on 6-week mortality and ventricular function after acute myocardial infarction. Lancet 1994; 343:1115–1121.
109. ISIS-4 (Fourth International Study of Infarct Survival) Collaborative Group: ISIS-4: A randomised factorial trial assessing early oral captopril, oral mononitrate, and intravenous magnesium sulphate in 58,050 patients with suspected acute myocardial infarction. Lancet 1995; 345:669–685.
110. Teo KK, Yusuf S, Collins R, et al: Effects of intravenous magnesium in suspected acute myocardial infarction: overview of randomised trials. Br Med J 1991; 303:1499–1503.
111. Woods KL, Fletcher S, Roffe C, Haider Y: Intravenous magnesium sulphate in suspected acute myocardial infarction: results of the second Leicester Intravenous Magnesium Intervention Trial (LIMIT-2). Lancet 1992; 339:1553–1558.
112. Yusuf S, Teo K, Woods K: Intravenous magnesium in acute myocardial infarction. An effective, safe, simple, and inexpensive intervention. Circulation 1993; 87:2043–2046.
113. Antman E: Randomized trials of magnesium in acute myocardial infarction: big numbers do not tell the whole story. Am J Cardiol 1995; 75:391–393.
114. Sonnenblick EH, Frishman WH, LeJemtel TH: Dobutamine: a new synthetic cardioactive sympathetic amine. N Engl J Med 1979; 300:17–22.
115. Goldstein RA, Passamani ER, Roberts R: A comparison of digoxin and dobutamine in patients with acute infarction and cardiac failure. N Engl J Med 1998; 303:846–850.
116. Packer M, Carver JR, Rodeheffer RJ, et al: Effect of oral milrinone on mortality in severe chronic heart failure. N Engl J Med 1991; 325:1468–1475.
117. DeWood MA, Notske RN, Hensley GR, et al: Intraaortic balloon counterpulsation with and without reperfusion for myocardial infarction shock. Circulation 1980; 61:1105–1112.
118. Ohman EM, George BS, White CJ, et al: Use of aortic counterpulsation to improve sustained coronary artery patency during acute myocardial infarction: results of a randomized trial. Circulation 1994; 90:792–799.
119. Goldberger M, Tabak SW, Shah PK: Clinical experience with intraaortic balloon counterpulsation in 112 consecutive patients. Am Heart J 1986; 111:497–502.
120. Ohman EM, Califf RM, George BS, et al: The use of intraaortic balloon pumping as an adjunct to reperfusion therapy in acute myocardial infarction. The Thrombolysis and Angioplasty in Myocardial Infarction (TAMI) Study Group. Am Heart J 1991; 121:895–901.
121. Bengtson JR, Kaplan AJ, Pieper KS, et al: Prognosis in cardiogenic shock after acute myocardial infarction in the interventional era. J Am Coll Cardiol 1992; 20:1482–1489.
122. Lee L, Erbel R, Brown TM, et al: Multicenter registry of angioplasty therapy of cardiogenic shock: initial and long-term survival. J Am Coll Cardiol 1991; 17:599–603.
123. Lee L, Bates E, Pitt B, et al: Percutaneous transluminal coronary angioplasty improves survival in acute myocardial infarction complicated by cardiogenic shock. Circulation 1988; 78:1345–1351.
124. Holmes DR Jr, Bates ER, Kleiman NS, et al: Contemporary reperfusion therapy for cardiogenic shock: the GUSTO-I trial experience. J Am Coll Cardiol 1995; 26:668–674.
125. Shawl FA, Domanski MJ, Hernandez TJ, Punja S: Emergency percutaneous cardiopulmonary bypass support in cardiogenic shock from acute myocardial infarction. Am J Cardiol 1989; 64:967–970.
126. Gacioch GM, Ellis SG, Lee L, et al: Cardiogenic shock complicating acute myocardial infarction: the use of coronary angioplasty and the integration of the new support devices into patient management. J Am Coll Cardiol 1992; 19:647–653.
127. Dell'Italia LJ, Starling MR, O'Rourke RA: Physical examination for exclusion of hemodynamically important right ventricular infarction. Ann Intern Med 1983; 99:608–611.
128. Braat SH, Brugada P, den Dulk K, et al: Value of lead V_4R for recognition of the infarct coronary artery in acute inferior myocardial infarction. Am J Cardiol 1984; 53:1538–1541.
129. Berisha S, Kastrati A, Goda A, Popa Y: Optimal value of filling pressure in the right side of the heart in acute right ventricular infarction. Br Heart J 1990; 63:98–102.
130. Topol EJ, Goldschlager N, Ports TA, et al: Hemodynamic benefit of atrial pacing in right ventricular myocardial infarction. Ann Intern Med 1982; 96:594–597.
131. Korr KS, Levinson H, Bough EW, et al: Tricuspid valve replacement for cardiogenic shock after acute right ventricular infarction. JAMA 1980; 244:1958–1960.
132. Lopez-Sendon J, Lopez de Sa E, Gonzalez Maqueda I, et al: Right ventricular infarction as a risk factor for ventricular fibrillation during pulmonary artery catheterization using Swan-Ganz catheters. Am Heart J 1990; 119:207–209.
133. Bansal RC, Marsa RJ, Holland D, et al: Severe hypoxemia due to shunting through a patent foramen ovale: a correctable complication of right ventricular infarction. J Am Coll Cardiol 1985; 5:188–192.
134. Gaspoz JM, Lee TH, Weinstein MC, et al: Cost-effectiveness of a new short-stay unit to ''rule out'' acute myocardial infarction in low risk patients. J Am Coll Cardiol 1994; 24:1249–1259.
135. Lynn LA, Kissinger JF: Coronary precautions: should caffeine be restricted in patients after myocardial infarction? Heart Lung 1992; 21:365–371.
136. Winslow EH: Cardiovascular consequences of bed rest. Heart Lung 1985; 14:236–246.
137. Crippen DW: The role of sedation in the ICU patient with pain and agitation. Crit Care Clin 1990; 6:369–392.
138. Clinton JE, Sterner S, Stelmachers Z, Ruiz E: Haloperidol for sedation of disruptive emergency patients. Ann Emerg Med 1987; 16:319–322.
139. Beta-Blocker Heart Attack Research Group: A randomized trial of propranolol in patients with acute myocardial infarction: I. Mortality results. JAMA 1982; 247:1707–1714.
140. Pfeffer MA, Braunwald E, Moye LA, et al: Effect of captopril on mortality and morbidity in patients with left ventricular dysfunction after myocardial infarction. N Engl J Med 1992; 327:669–677.
141. The SOLVD Investigators: Effect of enalapril on mortality and the development of heart failure in asymptomatic patients with reduced left ventricular ejection fractions. N Engl J Med 1992; 327:685–691.
142. Yusuf S, Pepine CJ, Garces C, et al: Effect of enalapril on myocardial infarction and unstable angina in patients with low ejection fractions. Lancet 1992; 340:1173–1178.
143. Swedberg K, Held P, Kjekshus J, et al: Effects of the early administration of enalapril on mortality in patients with acute myocardial infarction. N Engl J Med 1992; 327:678–684.
144. The Acute Infarction Ramipril Efficacy (AIRE) Study Investigators: Effect of ramipril on mortality and morbidity of survivors of acute myocardial infarction with clinical evidence of heart failure. Lancet 1995; 342:821–828.
145. Chinese Cardiac Study Collaborative Group: Oral captopril versus placebo among 13,634 patients with suspected acute myocardial infarction: interim report from the Chinese Cardiac Study (CCS-1). Lancet 1995; 345:686–687.
146. Weber MA: Clinical experience with the angiotensin II receptor antagonist losartan. A preliminary report. Am J Hypertens 1992; 5(12, pt 2):247S–251S.
147. The Australian National Heart Study Trial: A randomized comparison of oral aspirin/dipyridamole versus intravenous heparin after rt-PA for acute myocardial infarction [Abstract]. Circulation 1989; 80(suppl II):114.
148. Granger CB, Miller JM, Bovill EG, et al: Rebound increase in thrombin generation and activity after cessation of intravenous heparin in patients with acute coronary syndromes. Circulation 1995; 91:1929–1935.
149. Warkentin TE, Levine MN, Hirsh J, et al: Heparin-induced thrombocytopenia in patients treated with low-molecular-weight heparin or unfractionated heparin. N Engl J Med 1995; 332:1330–1335.
150. Braunwald E: Mechanism of action of calcium-channel blocking agents. N Engl J Med 1982; 307:1618–1627.
151. Wilcox RG, Hampton JR, Banks DC, et al: Trial of early nifedipine in acute myocardial infarction: the TRENT study. Br Med J 1986; 293:1204–1208.

152. The Multicenter Diltiazem Postinfarction Trial Research Group: The effect of diltiazem on mortality and reinfarction after myocardial infarction. N Engl J Med 1988; 319:385–392.
153. The Danish Study Group on Verapamil in Myocardial Infarction: Verapamil in acute myocardial infarction. Eur Heart J 1984; 5:516–528.
154. The Danish Study Group on Verapamil in Myocardial Infarction: Effect of verapamil on mortality and major events after acute myocardial infarction (the Danish Verapamil Infarction Trial II–DAVIT II). Am J Cardiol 1990; 66:779–785.
155. Forrester JS, Diamond G, Chatterjee K, Swan HJ: Medical therapy of acute myocardial infarction by application of hemodynamic subsets [first of two parts]. N Engl J Med 1976; 295:1356–1362.
156. Killip T, Kimball J: Treatment of myocardial infarction in a coronary care unit. A two year experience with 250 patients. Am J Cardiol 1967; 20:457–464.
157. Liebowitz RS, Rippe JM: Arterial line placement and care. *In* Rippe JM, Irwin RS, Alpert JS, Fink MP (eds): Intensive Care Medicine, pp 33–42. Boston: Little, Brown, 1985.
158. Crimm A, Severance HW Jr, Coffey K, et al: Prognostic significance of isolated sinus tachycardia during first three days of acute myocardial infarction. Am J Med 1984; 76:983–988.
159. Crenshaw BS, Ward SR, Stebbins AL, Granger CB, for the GUSTO Trial Investigators: Risk factors and outcomes in patients with atrial fibrillation following acute myocardial infarction [Abstract]. Circulation 1995; 92(suppl I):777.
160. Amsterdam EA: Efficacy of cardioselective beta-adrenergic blockade with intravenously administered metoprolol in the treatment of supraventricular tachyarrhythmias. J Clin Pharmacol 1991; 14:446–451.
161. Ellenbogen KA: A placebo-controlled trial of continuous intravenous diltiazem infusion for 24-hour heart rate control during atrial fibrillation and atrial flutter: a multicenter study. J Am Coll Cardiol 1991; 18:891–897.
162. Akiyama T, Pawitan Y, Greenberg H, et al: Increased risk of death and cardiac arrest from encainide and flecainide in patients after non–Q-wave acute myocardial infarction in the Cardiac Arrhythmia Suppression Trial: CAST investigators. Am J Cardiol 1991; 68:1551–1555.
163. Reimold SC, Chalmers TC, Berlin JA, Antman EM: Assessment of the efficacy and safety of antiarrhythmic therapy for chronic atrial fibrillation: observations on the role of trial design and implications of drug-related mortality. Am Heart J 1992; 24:924–932.
164. Mark DB, Dunham G: Therapeutic drug monitoring in the acutely ill patient. *In* Califf RM, Mark DB, Wagner GS (eds): Acute Coronary Care, 2nd ed, pp 481–488. St. Louis: Mosby–Year Book, 1995.
165. Podrid PJ: Amiodarone: reevaluation of an old drug. Ann Intern Med 1995; 122:689–700.
166. Lown B, Calvert AF, Armington R, Ryan M: Monitoring for serious arrhythmias and high risk of sudden death. Circulation 1975; 52:189–198.
167. MacMahon S, Collins R, Peto R: Effects of prophylactic lidocaine in suspected acute myocardial infarction. JAMA 1988; 260:1910–1916.
168. Cairns JA, Connolly SJ, Gent M, et al: Postmyocardial infarction mortality in patients with ventricular premature depolarizations. Canadian Amiodarone Myocardial Infarction Arrhythmia Trial pilot study. Circulation 1991; 84:550–557.
169. Ceremuzynski L, Kleczar E, Krezeminska-Pakula M, et al: Effect of amiodarone on mortality after myocardial infarction: a double-blind, placebo-controlled, pilot study. J Am Coll Cardiol 1992; 20:1056–1062.
170. Navarro-Lopez F, Cosin J, Marrugat J, et al: Comparison of the effects of amiodarone versus metoprolol on the frequency of ventricular arrhythmias and on mortality after acute myocardial infarction. Am J Cardiol 1995; 72:1243–1248.
171. Burkart F, Pfisterer M, Kiowski W, et al: Effect of antiarrhythmic therapy on mortality in survivors of myocardial infarction with asymptomatic complex ventricular arrhythmias: Basel Antiarrhythmic Study of Infarct Survival (BASIS). J Am Coll Cardiol 1995; 16:1711–1718.
172. Pfisterer M, Kiowski W, Burckhardt D, et al: Beneficial effect of amiodarone on cardiac mortality in patients with asymptomatic complex ventricular arrhythmias after acute myocardial infarction and preserved but not impaired left ventricular function. Am J Cardiol 1992; 69:1399–1402.
173. Windle JR, Easley AR Jr, Stratbucker RA: A multipurpose, self-adhesive patch electrode capable of external pacing, cardioversion defibrillation, and 12-lead electrocardiogram. Pacing Clin Electrophysiol 1993; 16:235–241.
174. Berger PB, Ruocco NA Jr, Ryan TJ, et al: Incidence and prognostic implications of heart block complicating inferior myocardial infarction treated with thrombolytic therapy: results from TIMI II. J Am Coll Cardiol 1992; 20:533–540.
175. Clemmensen P, Bates ER, Califf RM, et al: Complete atrioventricular block complicating inferior wall acute myocardial infarction treated with reperfusion therapy. TAMI Study Group. Am J Cardiol 1991; 67:225–230.
176. Lamas GA, Muller JE, Turi ZG, et al: A simplified method to predict occurrence of complete heart block during acute myocardial infarction. Am J Cardiol 1986; 57:1213–1219.
177. Zoll PM, Zoll RH, Falk RH, et al: External noninvasive temporary cardiac pacing: clinical trials. Circulation 1985; 71:937–944.
178. Barbagelata A, Granger CB, Topol EJ, et al: Isolated recurrent ischemia after thrombolytic therapy: incidence, importance, and cost. Am J Cardiol in press.
179. Betriu A, Califf RM, Granger C, for the GUSTO Investigators: Importance of clinical findings during post-infarction angina in determining prognosis: results from the GUSTO trial [Abstract]. J Am Coll Cardiol 1994; 23:27A.
180. White HD, Cross DB, Williams BF, Norris RM: Safety and efficacy of repeat thrombolytic treatment after acute myocardial infarction. Br Heart J 1990; 64:177–181.
181. Simoons ML, Arnout J, van den Brand M, et al: Retreatment with alteplase for early signs of reocclusion after thrombolysis. The European Cooperative Study Group. Am J Cardiol 1993; 71:524–528.
182. Purvis JA, McNeil AJ, Roberts MJD, et al: First-year follow-up after repeat thrombolytic therapy with recombinant-tissue plasminogen activator for myocardial reinfarction. Coron Artery Dis 1992; 3:713–720.
183. Barbash GI, Hod H, Roth A, et al: Repeat infusion of recombinant tissue-type plasminogen activator in patients with acute myocardial infarction and early recurrent myocardial ischemia. J Am Coll Cardiol 1990; 16:779–783.
184. Ellis SG, Debowey D, Bates ER, Topol EJ: Treatment of recurrent ischemia after thrombolysis and successful reperfusion for acute myocardial infarction: effect on in-hospital mortality and left ventricular function. J Am Coll Cardiol 1991; 17:752–757.
185. Califf RM, Harrell FE Jr, Lee KL, et al: The evolution of medical and surgical therapy for coronary artery disease. A 15-year perspective. JAMA 1989; 261:2077–2086.
186. deFeyter PJ, Serruys PW: Percutaneous transluminal coronary angioplasty for unstable angina. *In* Topol EJ (ed): Textbook of Interventional Cardiology, 2nd ed, vol 1, pp 274–291. Philadelphia: WB Saunders, 1994.
187. Ohman EM, Califf RM, Topol EJ, et al: Consequences of reocclusion after successful reperfusion therapy in acute myocardial infarction. TAMI Study Group. Circulation 1990; 82:781–791.
188. Ohman EM, Harrington RA, Granger CB: Recurrent ischemia and reinfarction after reperfusion. *In* Califf RM, Mark DB, Wagner GS (eds): Acute Coronary Care, 2nd ed, pp 584–598. St. Louis: Mosby–Year Book, 1995.
189. Hill JD, Stiles QR: Acute ischemic ventricular septal defect. Circulation 1989; 79(suppl I):112–115.
190. Tcheng JE, Jackman JD Jr, Nelson CL, et al: Outcome of patients sustaining acute ischemic mitral regurgitation during myocardial infarction. Ann Intern Med 1992; 117:18–24.
191. Hickey MS, Smith LR, Muhlbaier LH, et al: Current prognosis of ischemic mitral regurgitation. Implications for future management. Circulation 1988 (suppl I):51–59.
192. Yoran C, Yellin EL, Becker RM, et al: Mechanism of reduction of mitral regurgitation with vasodilator therapy. Am J Cardiol 1979; 43:773–777.
193. Harrington RA, Rippe JM: Acute mitral regurgitation. *In* Rippe JM, Irwin RS, Alpert JS, Fink MP (eds): Intensive Care Medicine, 2nd ed, pp 326–336. Boston: Little, Brown, 1991.
194. Wall TC, Califf RM, Harrelson-Woodlief L, et al: Usefulness of a pericardial friction rub after thrombolytic therapy during acute myocardial infarction in predicting amount of myocardial damage. The TAMI Study Group. Am J Cardiol 1990; 66:1418–1421.
195. Berman J, Haffajee CI, Alpert JS: Therapy of symptomatic pericarditis after myocardial infarction: retrospective and prospective studies of aspirin, indomethacin, prednisone, and spontaneous resolution. Am Heart J 1981; 101:750–753.
196. Jugdutt BI, Basualdo CA: Myocardial infarct expansion during indomethacin or ibuprofen therapy for symptomatic post infarction pericarditis: influence of other pharmacologic agents during early remodeling. Can J Cardiol 1989; 5:211–221.

197. Roberts R, de Mello V, Sobel BE: Deleterious effect of methyl-prednisone in patients with myocardial infarction. Circulation 1976; 53(suppl I):204–206.
198. Selker HP, Griffith JL, D'Agostino RB: A time-insensitive predictive instrument for acute myocardial infarction mortality: a multicenter study. Med Care 1991; 29:1196–1211.
199. Krucoff MW, Croll MA, Pope JE, et al: Continuous 12-lead ST segment recovery analysis in the TAMI 7 Study: performance of a noninvasive method for real time detection of failed myocardial reperfusion. Circulation 1993; 88:437–446.
200. Newby LK, Califf RM, for the GUSTO Investigators: Redefining uncomplicated myocardial infarction in the thrombolytic era [Abstract]. Circulation 1994; 90(suppl I):110.
201. Multicenter Post-Infarction Research Group: Risk stratification and survival after myocardial infarction. N Engl J Med 1983; 309:321–336.
202. Harris PJ, Harrell FE Jr, Lee KL, Rosati RA: Nonfatal myocardial infarction in medically treated patients with coronary artery disease. Am J Cardiol 1980; 46:937–942.
203. Morris KG: Use of radionuclide angiography following acute myocardial infarction. *In* Califf RM, Mark DB, Wagner GS (eds): Acute Coronary Care, 2nd ed, pp 797–813. St. Louis: Mosby–Year Book, 1995.
204. Yusuf S, Zucker D, Peduzzi P, et al: Effect of coronary artery bypass graft surgery on survival: overview of 10-year results from randomised trials by the coronary artery bypass graft surgery trialists collaboration. Lancet 1994; 344:563–570.
205. Garg R, Yusuf S: Overview of randomized trials of angiotensin-converting enzyme inhibitors on mortality and morbidity in patients with heart failure. JAMA 1995; 273:1450–1456.
206. Silver MT, Rose GA, Paul SD, et al: A clinical rule to predict preserved left ventricular ejection fraction in patients after myocardial infarction. Ann Intern Med 1994; 750–756.
207. Peterson ED, Shaw LJ, Kesler K, Califf RM: Is exercise treadmill testing useful for post infarction risk stratification in the thrombolytic era? A meta-analysis of the literature [Abstract]. Circulation 1995; 92(suppl I):272.
208. Beller GA, Gibson RS, Watson DD: Radionuclide methods of identifying patients who may require coronary artery bypass surgery. Circulation 1985; 72(suppl V):9–22.
209. Moss AJ, Goldstein RE, Hall WJ, et al: Detection and significance of myocardial ischemia in stable patients after recovery from an acute coronary event. JAMA 1993; 269:2379–2385.
210. Morris KG, Palmeri ST, Califf RM, et al: Value of radionuclide angiography for predicting specific cardiac events after acute myocardial infarction. Am J Cardiol 1985; 55:318–324.
211. Bigger JT Jr, Fleiss JL, Rolnitzky LM: Prevalence, characteristics and significance of ventricular tachycardia detected by 24-hour continuous electrocardiographic recordings in the late hospital phase of acute myocardial infarction. Am J Cardiol 1986; 58:1151–1160.
212. Denes P, el-Sherif N, Katz R, et al: Prognostic significance of signal-averaged electrocardiogram after thrombolytic therapy and/or angioplasty during acute myocardial infarction (CAST substudy). Am J Med 1994; 74:216–220.
213. Singh N, Mironov D, Armstrong PW, et al: Heart rate variability assessment early after acute myocardial infarction: pathophysiological and prognostic correlates. Circulation in press.
214. Gore JM, Goldberg RJ, Matsumoto AS, et al: Validity of serum total cholesterol level obtained within 24 hours of acute myocardial infarction. Am J Cardiol 1984; 54:722–725.
215. Krumholz HM, Cohen BJ, Tsevat J, et al: Cost-effectiveness of a smoking cessation program after myocardial infarction. J Am Coll Cardiol 1993; 22:1697–1702.
216. The Diabetes Control and Complications Trial (DCCT) Research Group: Effect of intensive diabetes management on macrovascular events and risk factors in the diabetes control and complications trial. Am J Cardiol 1995; 75:894–903.
217. Anticoagulants in the Secondary Prevention of Events in Coronary Thrombosis (ASPECT) Research Group: Effect of long-term oral anticoagulant treatment on mortality and cardiovascular morbidity after myocardial infarction. Lancet 1995; 343:499–503.
218. van Bergen PFMM, Jonker JJC, van Hout BA, et al: Costs and effects of long-term oral anticoagulant treatment after myocardial infarction. JAMA 1995; 273:925–928.
219. Cairns JA, Markham BA: Economics and efficacy in choosing oral anticoagulants or aspirin after myocardial infarction. JAMA 1995; 273:925–928.
220. O'Neill WW, Timmis GC, Bourdillon PD, et al: A prospective randomized clinical trial of intracoronary streptokinase versus coronary angioplasty for acute myocardial infarction. N Engl J Med 1986; 314:812–818.
221. DeWood MA, Fisher MJ, for the Spokane Heart Research Group: Direct PTCA versus intravenous rt-PA in acute myocardial infarction: preliminary results from a prospective randomized trial [Abstract]. Circulation 1989; 80(suppl II):418.
222. Zijlstra F, de Boer M, Hoorntje JCA, et al: A comparison of immediate coronary angioplasty with intravenous streptokinase in acute myocardial infarction. N Engl J Med 1993; 328:680–684.
223. Ribeiro EE, Silva LA, Carneiro R, et al: Randomized trial of direct coronary angioplasty versus intravenous streptokinase in acute myocardial infarction. J Am Coll Cardiol 1993; 22:376–380.
224. Elizaga J, Garcia EJ, Delcan JL, et al: Primary coronary angioplasty versus systemic thrombolysis in acute anterior myocardial infarction: in-hospital results from a prospective randomized trial [Abstract]. Circulation 1993; 88(suppl I):411.
225. Michels KB, Yusuf S: Does PTCA in acute myocardial infarction affect mortality and reinfarction rates? A quantitative overview (meta-analysis) of the randomized clinical trials. Circulation 1995; 91:476–485.
226. Hung J, Goris ML, Nash E, et al: Comparative value of maximal treadmill testing, exercise thallium myocardial perfusion scintigraphy and exercise radionuclide ventriculography for distinguishing high- and low-risk patients soon after acute myocardial infarction. Am J Cardiol 1984; 53:1221–1227.
227. Leppo JA, O'Brien J, Rothendler JA, et al: Dipyridamole–thallium-201 scintigraphy in the prediction of future cardiac events after myocardial infarction. N Engl J Med 1984; 310:1014–1018.
228. Gibson RS, Beller GA, Gheorghiade M, et al: The prevalence and clinical significance of residual myocardial ischemia 2 weeks after uncomplicated non–Q-wave infarction: a prospective natural history study. Circulation 1986; 73:1186–1198.
229. Abraham RD, Freedman SB, Dunn RF, et al: Prediction of multivessel coronary artery disease and prognosis early after acute myocardial infarction by exercise electrocardiography and thallium-201 myocardial perfusion scanning. Am J Cardiol 1986; 58:423–427.
230. Gimple LW, Hutter AM Jr, Guiney TE, Boucher CA: Prognostic utility of predischarge dipyridamole-thallium imaging compared to predischarge submaximal exercise electrocardiography and maximal exercise thallium imaging after uncomplicated acute myocardial infarction. Am J Cardiol 1989; 64:1243–1248.
231. Tilkemeier PL, Guiney TE, LaRaia PJ, Boucher CA: Prognostic value of predischarge low-level exercise thallium testing after thrombolytic treatment of acute myocardial infarction. Am J Cardiol 1990; 66:1203–1207.
232. Hendel RC, Gore JM, Alpert JS, Leppo JA: Prognosis following interventional therapy for acute myocardial infarction: utility of dipyridamole-thallium scintigraphy. Cardiology 1991; 79:73–80.
233. De Cock CC, Visser FC, van Eenige MJ, et al: Prognostic value of thallium-201 exercise scintigraphy in low-risk patients after Q-wave myocardial infarction: comparison with exercise testing and catheterization. Cardiology 1992; 81:342–350.
234. Nicod P, Corbett JR, Firth BG, et al: Prognostic value of resting and submaximal exercise radionuclide ventriculography after acute myocardial infarction in high-risk patients with single and multivessel disease. Am J Cardiol 1983; 52:30–36.
235. Dewhurst NG, Muir AL: Comparative prognostic value of radionuclide ventriculography at rest and during exercise in 100 patients after first myocardial infarction. Br Heart J 1983; 49:111–121.
236. Morris KG, Palmeri ST, Califf RM, et al: Value of radionuclide angiography for predicting specific cardiac events after acute myocardial infarction. Am J Cardiol 1985; 55:318–324.
237. Fioretti P, Brower RW, Simoons ML, et al: Relative value of clinical variables, bicycle ergometry, rest radionuclide ventriculography and 24-hour ambulatory electrocardiographic monitoring at discharge to predict 1-year survival after myocardial infarction. J Am Coll Cardiol 1986; 8:40–49.
238. Ryan T, Armstrong WF, O'Donnell JA, Feigenbaum H: Risk stratification after acute myocardial infarction by means of exercise two-dimensional echocardiography. Am Heart J 1987; 114:1305–1316.
239. Kuchar DL, Freund J, Yeates M, Sammel N: Enhanced prediction of major cardiac events after myocardial infarction using exercise radionuclide ventriculography. Aust N Z J Med 1987; 17:228–233.
240. Applegate RJ, Dell'Italia LJ, Crawford MH: Usefulness of two-dimen-

sional echocardiography during low-level exercise testing early after uncomplicated acute myocardial infarction. Am J Cardiol 1987; 60:10–14.

241. Abraham RD, Harris PJ, Roubin GS, et al: Usefulness of ejection fraction response to exercise one month after acute myocardial infarction in predicting coronary anatomy and prognosis. Am J Cardiol 1987; 60:225–230.

242. Bolognese L, Rossi L, Sarasso G, et al: Silent versus symptomatic dipyridamole-induced ischemia after myocardial infarction: clinical and prognostic significance. J Am Coll Cardiol 1992; 19:953–959.

243. Sclavo MG, Noussan P, Pallisco O, Presbitero P: Usefulness of dipyridamole-echocardiographic test to identify jeopardized myocardium after thrombolysis. Limited clinical predictivity of dipyridamole-echocardiographic test in convalescing acute myocardial infarction: correlation with coronary angiography. Eur Heart J 1992; 13:1348–1355.

244. Picano E, Landi P, Bolognese L, et al: Prognostic value of dipyridamole echocardiography early after uncomplicated myocardial infarction: a large-scale, multicenter trial. The EPIC Study Group. Am J Med 1993; 95:608–618.

SECTION TWO

Heart Failure

8 Pathophysiologic and Clinical Considerations in the Treatment of Heart Failure: An Overview

Wilson S. Colucci, MD

Heart failure (HF) can be defined as a clinical syndrome resulting from cardiac dysfunction and characterized by (1) signs and symptoms of intravascular and interstitial volume overload, including shortness of breath, rales, and edema, or (2) manifestations of inadequate tissue perfusion, such as fatigue or poor exercise tolerance.[1] HF is extremely common. In the United States there are an estimated 2–3 million patients with the diagnosis of HF, and about 400,000 new cases are diagnosed each year.[1] Despite a steady decrease in the incidence of cardiovascular disease in the United States, the prevalence of HF is increasing, in part because of the increasing age of the general population, and in part because patients with several types of cardiovascular disease, including HF, are surviving longer. HF is among the most common hospital discharge diagnoses in the United States and is the leading discharge diagnosis in patients older than 65 years. The economic impact of HF is enormous. Although many patients with mild HF are able to live relatively normal and productive lives, most patients with moderate or severe symptoms have a significant reduction in the quality of life, are unable to work, and are susceptible to episodes of decompensation that may require emergent treatment and/or admission to a hospital. It is estimated that the treatment costs for HF in the United States exceeded $10 billion in 1990.[1]

The last several years have brought meaningful advances in the therapy of HF. Whereas as recently as 1975 pharmacologic treatment of ambulatory patients with HF was largely limited to diuretics and digitalis, the options now include a choice of several vasodilators acting by a variety of mechanisms, numerous angiotensin converting enzyme (ACE) inhibitors, and potent loop diuretics as well as several types of investigational agents, which may act by novel mechanisms. Cardiac transplantation is an effective therapy for patients with end-stage disease, and mechanical assist devices are playing an increasingly important role in the support of patients awaiting a new heart.

GOALS OF THERAPY

The goals of therapy are context dependent. In the hospitalized patient with severe decompensated HF, the goal is to achieve hemodynamic stabilization, appropriate fluid balance, and acceptable metabolic parameters (see Chapter 10). Rapid and decisive intervention can be life-saving and often involves parenteral agents, mechanical support devices, and in some cases surgical intervention (e.g., coronary revascularization, valve replacement, transplantation). The results of therapy are rapid (minutes to hours) and readily measured in terms of hemodynamics, renal function, and metabolic status. Cardiac transplantation, although a mainstay in the treatment of end-stage disease, is severely restricted by the number of donor hearts (approximately 2500 per year in the United States) relative to the number of potential candidates (approximately 50,000 per year in the United States). However, advances in the development of xenografts and mechanical hearts may provide an alternative to transplantation in the future (see Chapter 15). After stabilization of the patient with acute decompensation, the goals of therapy should shift to longer term considerations as an oral regimen is introduced in preparation for discharge.

In the ambulatory patient with mild, moderate, or severe HF symptoms, the goals of therapy are to increase functional capacity, improve quality of life, reduce the need for hospitalization, and prolong survival (see Chapter 11). Although measurable, these goals are more difficult to quantify than for the hospitalized patient, and the temporal response to therapy may be long (weeks to months) and punctuated by numerous spontaneous fluctuations that can confound interpretation. It is difficult to prove the clinical value of therapy for such patients. Fortunately, recommendations for therapy in ambulatory patients with HF are increasingly supported by controlled trials.[1]

Still more difficult to quantify are the effects of therapy in patients with asymptomatic left ventricular dysfunction (see Chapter 12). In such patients, the goal of therapy is to delay the progression of the underlying myocardial process and thereby prevent the development of symptoms. Although an improvement in survival is difficult to prove in such patients, it is reasonable to expect that mortality will be reduced in concert with the slowing of disease progression. Observations with ACE inhibitors[2] and beta-adrenergic antagonists[3] suggest that the early use of these agents could have a major impact on the prevention of HF and raise as a challenge the early identification of asymptomatic patients who might benefit from early treatment with these or other newer agents.

The current approach to the treatment of HF involves the use of multiple agents that act by complementary mechanisms. The timing and choice of agents and approaches are constantly evolving as new therapies become available and information about established approaches is expanded. Although algorithms can be formulated, they rapidly become outdated. The following brief review of several key aspects of the pathophysiology and clinical manifestations of HF is intended to provide the outline of a conceptual basis on which to assess the value of currently available therapies and to evaluate the potential of new approaches as they become available for clinical use.

PATHOPHYSIOLOGY

Etiology

A large number of cardiovascular diseases may culminate in HF. It is convenient to distinguish HF caused by primary myocardial dysfunction from that caused by mechanical abnormalities (e.g., valvular lesions, shunts, and pericardial disease). In about 50% of the patients enrolled in contemporary therapeutic trials for HF, coronary artery disease was thought to be the underlying cause of HF; of the 50% attributed to nonischemic processes, about half were categorized as "idiopathic"[4] (Table 8–1). It is now apparent that many cases of idiopathic cardiomyopathy are hereditary or related to prior subclinical inflammatory or viral processes. The initial approach to the treatment of HF should include a careful search for remediable causes (e.g., coronary artery disease; valvular lesions; endocrine, metabolic, or rheumatologic causes).

Systolic vs. Diastolic Failure

HF may be caused by systolic or diastolic cardiac dysfunction, or a combination of both. In patients with predominantly systolic dysfunction, the left ventricular cavity is generally dilated and the ejection fraction is reduced (see Chapter 13). In patients with predominantly diastolic dysfunction, the left ventricular cavity may be normal or reduced in size and thick walled with a normal or increased ejection fraction.[5, 6] Systolic myocardial dysfunction is most common in patients with HF caused by chronic ischemic disease or any of the dilated cardiomyopathies. Diastolic dysfunction is most common in patients with hypertrophic or restrictive cardiomyopathies (infiltrative or idiopathic), in elderly patients, and in patients with a history of hypertension. Systolic and diastolic dysfunction coexist in many cases, and either may predominate at one time or another in a given patient.

Most clinical trials in HF have focused on patients with systolic dysfunction due to dilated cardiomyopathy. In contrast to the important role of digitalis, vasodilators, and ACE inhibitors in patients with systolic failure, these agents are not uniformly useful and can be deleterious in patients with predominant diastolic dysfunction, in whom the mainstays of therapy are careful management of intravascular volume and heart rate control. Because the treatments for systolic and diastolic dysfunction differ markedly, it is important that this distinction be made early in the design of a therapeutic plan. Systolic and diastolic dysfunction can often be distinguished by echocardiography to define chamber size and contractile function.

TABLE 8–1. ETIOLOGY OF HEART FAILURE IN CONTEMPORARY CLINICAL TRIALS

Etiology	Number of Patients (%)
Ischemic	936 (50.3)
Nonischemic	925 (49.7)
Etiology provided	678 (36.4)
Idiopathic	340 (18.2)
Valvular	75 (4.0)
Hypertensive	70 (3.8)
Ethanol	34 (1.8)
Viral	9 (0.4)
Postpartum	8 (0.4)
Amyloidosis	1 (0.1)
Other/unspecified	141 (7.6)
No etiology provided	247 (13.3)

Shown are the relative frequencies of various diagnoses in patients who were entered into heart failure treatment trials published in 1989–1990. Ischemic heart disease was the most common etiology, accounting for about half of the cases. Of the cases identified as nonischemic, about half were classified as idiopathic.

Adapted from Teerlink JR, Goldhaber SZ, Pfeffer MA: An overview of contemporary etiologies of congestive heart failure. Am J Cardiol 1991; 121:1852.

Compensatory Mechanisms

The fundamental cause of HF is usually a decrease in myocardial pump function. However, the resulting hemodynamic derangement provokes a complex and interrelated array of secondary neurohormonal and vascular adjustments that affect minute-to-minute cardiac function by altering preload, afterload, and heart rate (Fig. 8–1). In addition, the resulting changes in loading conditions, heart rate, and neurohormonal status may have important detrimental effects on myocardial and vascular remodeling and thereby contribute to the progression of myocardial failure.

Several of the current approaches to the therapy of HF involve the use of agents that counter vasoconstriction (e.g., vasodilators) and the effects of neurohormonal activation (ACE inhibitors, beta-adrenergic antagonists, digitalis by its antisympathetic and parasympathetic actions). It is likely that additional agents acting by these and other,

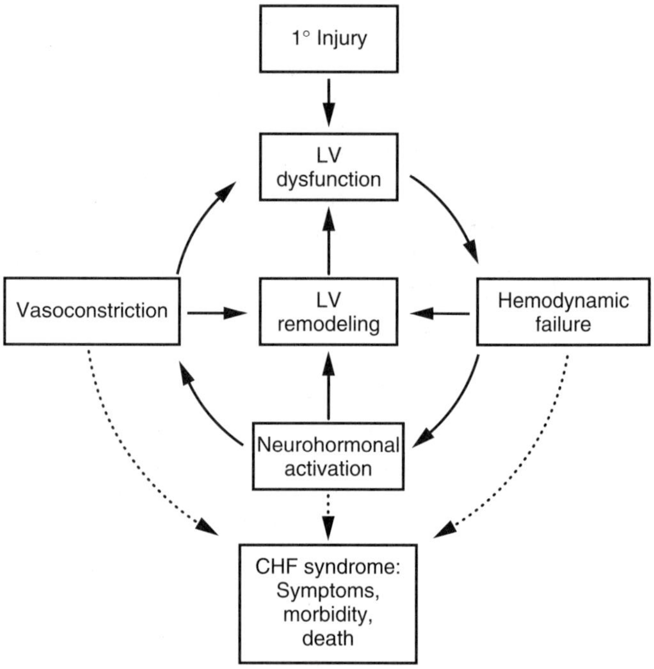

Figure 8–1. Schematic representation of the pathophysiologic process of heart failure. An injury to the myocardium resulting in left ventricular (LV) dysfunction initiates the cycle by causing hemodynamic impairment with reduced cardiac output and elevated ventricular filling pressures. Secondary neurohormonal activation ensues, involving the sympathetic nervous and renin-angiotensin systems, increased expression of endothelin by various cardiovascular tissues, and increased release of arginine vasopressin. These neurohormonal alterations, and possibly vascular remodeling and abnormal endothelium-dependent vasodilation, contribute to systemic and pulmonary vasoconstriction, vascular redistribution, and intravascular volume expansion as a result of salt and water retention. Systemic vasoconstriction and ventricular dilation result in an increase in the afterload against which the ventricle must work and thereby further depress systolic function. Increased ventricular loading conditions and chamber dilation act to augment systolic and diastolic myocardial wall stresses, which together with direct neurohormonal stimulation appear to be important stimuli for myocardial remodeling. As our understanding of the pathophysiologic events involved in heart failure improves, it may be possible to devise new pharmacologic and molecular approaches that will not only alleviate symptoms but also prevent disease progression and reverse existing myocardial dysfunction. *Abbreviation*: CHF, congestive heart failure.

newer mechanisms will be of further benefit in the treatment of HF in the future.

Systemic and Pulmonary Vasoconstriction

Generalized vasoconstriction and regional redistribution occur commonly in HF.[7] In addition to shunting blood away from the skin, gut, and kidneys, systemic vasoconstriction increases left ventricular afterload and thereby results in further depression of systolic function. Increased pulmonary vascular tone, together with passive elevation in pulmonary venous pressure, causes an increase in pulmonary arterial pressure and thereby contributes to right-sided heart failure and reduced exercise capacity. Increased vascular tone in HF appears to reflect the activation of neurohormonal systems, particularly the sympathetic nervous system and the renin-angiotensin system (RAS).[8, 9] Evidence that endothelium-dependent vasodilation is attenuated[10] and endothelin production is increased[11] in patients with HF suggests that these mechanisms may also contribute to systemic and pulmonary vasoconstriction.

Vasodilators that reduce arterial tone (e.g., nitroprusside, phentolamine, hydralazine) increase stroke volume and cardiac output in patients with HF, often without decreasing arterial pressure. Vasodilators with relative selectivity for the renal vasculature (e.g., ACE inhibitors) are particularly well suited to patients with HF who have reduced renal perfusion. No orally active vasodilators are specific for the pulmonary vasculature. The inhalation of nitric oxide causes selective pulmonary vasodilation in patients with HF but is accompanied by an elevation in left ventricular filling pressure that is apparently caused by increased venous return to a poorly compliant left ventricle.[12]

Neurohormonal Activation

Several neurohormone systems are activated in patients with HF.[8, 9] Elevated sympathetic nervous system activity is reflected by increased sympathetic nerve traffic and increased levels of urinary and plasma catecholamines.[13] A clinically relevant consequence of increased sympathetic nerve activity is that the contractile and chronotropic responses to beta-adrenergic receptor stimulation are attenuated[14, 15] and may limit the physiologic response to exercise and the effectiveness of agents such as dobutamine. Despite the fact that myocardial sympathetic nerve activity and catecholamine turnover are typically increased, myocardial stores of catecholamines are typically depleted, and consequently agents that act indirectly by a tyramine-like mechanism to increase neuronal norepinephrine release (e.g., dopamine) may be less effective than direct-acting beta-adrenergic agonists. The sympathetic nervous system appears to be activated even in patients with asymptomatic left ventricular dysfunction[16] and may thus contribute to early disease progression.

The RAS is activated in many patients with HF, as evidenced by increased plasma levels of renin, angiotensin, and aldosterone.[8, 9] In addition, there is evidence that tissue components of the RAS may be activated and could contribute to both vasoconstriction and remodeling of cardiovascular tissues.[17–19] Although ACE inhibitors have had a major impact on the clinical course of patients with HF, important questions remain regarding the role of the RAS and the mechanism of the beneficial effect of ACE inhibitors in HF. ACE inhibitors also inhibit the degradation of bradykinin, which may act by endothelium-dependent mechanisms to cause vasodilation and other beneficial tissue effects mediated by nitric oxide. Therefore, it is not clear to what extent ACE inhibitors reflect a reduction in angiotensin II levels, an increase in bradykinin levels, or both. Conversely, angiotensin may be generated by non–ACE-dependent pathways or by tissue ACE, which may not be fully inhibited by ACE inhibitors. Angiotensin receptor blocking agents that are now available for clinical use[20] should shed light on these issues and may prove to be of therapeutic value in HF.

Circulating levels of endothelin, arginine vasopressin (AVP), and atrial natriuretic factor (ANF) are often elevated in patients with HF. It is noteworthy that circulating endothelin levels correlate with the pulmonary vascular resistance.[11] AVP contributes to hyponatremia and possibly vasoconstriction in some patients with more severe decompensation. ANF is a vasodilator with relative renal specificity and probably acts as a counterregulatory factor to oppose the actions of vasoconstrictors. The contributions of endothelin and AVP to the pathophysiologic process of HF should be elucidated further by the imminent availability of antagonists for endothelin and AVP receptors. Conversely, the administration of natriuretic peptides such as ANF or brain natriuretic peptide, a closely related peptide made in the hypertrophied ventricle, or the inhibition of their degradation may be of value in the treatment of HF.

Inflammatory Cytokines

Increased levels of tumor necrosis factor-alpha have been observed in the plasma of patients with HF,[21] leading to the suggestion that inflammatory cytokines may be involved in the pathophysiology of the syndrome.[22] Inflammatory cytokines, acting in part through the increased production of nitric oxide, can attenuate beta-adrenergic responsiveness in the myocardium.[23] Inflammatory cytokines can also depress myocardial contractility independent of nitric oxide[24, 25] and affect the growth and phenotype of cardiac myocytes and fibroblasts.[26] The potential role of anticytokine agents in the treatment of HF remains to be explored. In this regard, it is intriguing that vesnarinone, an agent that may improve survival in patients with HF,[27] has been shown to suppress plasma levels of inflammatory cytokines in some patients.[28]

Myocardial Remodeling

Unless the underlying myocardial damage is corrected, myocardial dysfunction is generally a progressive condition marked by further ventricular dilation and reductions in systolic and/or diastolic function. This progressive change in the size and shape of the ventricular chamber is referred to as *remodeling*.[29] Although the initial pathophysiologic event may be limited in time and extent, remodeling of otherwise healthy tissue is a progressive process that can result in the onset of symptomatic disease months or years after the initial myocardial event (see Chapter 12).

At the molecular and cellular levels, HF is often accompanied by hypertrophy of cardiac myocytes with the addition of sarcomeres, proliferation of fibroblasts, alterations in the composition of the extracellular matrix, and altered expression of a variety of proteins involved in excitation/contraction coupling, the contractile apparatus, and signal transduction.[30] Increases in myocardial wall stress as a result of decreased systolic pump function and chamber dilation appear to play a central role in causing remodeling. In addition, a variety of neurohormones or paracrine-acting factors that are activated in patients with HF, including norepinephrine, angiotensin, and endothelin, are known to exert direct effects on cardiac myocytes and fibroblasts and may thus contribute to the remodeling process. There is evidence that peptide growth factors made by myocytes and nonmyocytes within the heart may be stimulated by mechanical and/or neurohormonal stimuli and thereby play a central role in orchestrating the remodeling process.[31] As the understanding of the signaling pathways involved in pathologic myocardial remodeling increases, it is possible that new pharmacologic agents (e.g., antagonists for growth factor receptors) and molecular approaches (e.g., overexpression or blocked expression of key molecules) that will allow manipulation of the remodeling process in a beneficial way will be devised.

TABLE 8–2. FRAMINGHAM CRITERIA FOR THE DIAGNOSIS OF HEART FAILURE

Major Criteria	*Minor Criteria*
Paroxysmal nocturnal dyspnea	Extremity edema
Neck vein distention	Night cough
Rales	Dyspnea on exertion
Cardiomegaly	Hepatomegaly
Acute pulmonary edema	Pleural effusion
S_3 gallop	Vital capacity reduced by one third from normal
Increased venous pressure (>16 cm H_2O)	Tachycardia (≥120 beats per minute)
Positive hepatojugular reflux	*Major or Minor*
	Weight loss ≥4.5 kg in a 5-day treatment period

The Framingham Heart Study used these symptoms and physical findings to establish the diagnosis of heart failure. The diagnosis of heart failure requires that at least one major and two minor criteria be present.

Adapted from Ho KKL, Anderson KM, Kannell WB, et al: Survival after the onset of congestive heart failure in Framingham Heart Study subjects. Circulation 1993; 88:107.

CLINICAL MANIFESTATIONS

Diagnostic Criteria

The hallmarks of HF are dyspnea and exercise intolerance.[32] Various diagnostic criteria, such as those used in the Framingham Heart Study[33] (Table 8–2), may be helpful in suggesting the diagnosis of HF and thereby prompt further evaluation of cardiac function.

Dyspnea

Dyspnea at rest or with exertion reflects an increase in pulmonary venous pressure secondary to an increase in left ventricular filling pressures. The ability to tolerate an increase in pulmonary venous pressure varies markedly from patient to patient. Patients with the new onset of increased left ventricular filling pressure may have pulmonary congestion or edema at relatively low pressures, whereas patients with gradually progressive chronic HF may tolerate much higher left ventricular filling pressures with only mild symptoms as a result of the development of increased pulmonary lymphatic capacity. Distinguishing between cardiac and pulmonary dyspnea may be difficult but is frequently possible on the basis of a careful history, physical examination, and appropriate cardiopulmonary testing.[34]

Exercise Intolerance

The ability to perform exercise is almost always decreased in patients with HF. Exercise may be limited by the development of dyspnea, as already discussed, or by leg weakness and fatigue, reflecting insufficient blood flow to the exercising skeletal muscles. Although the primary mechanism for reduced skeletal muscle blood flow is an insufficient increase in the cardiac output with exercise, other factors, including local changes in muscle metabolism and impaired vasodilation of the skeletal vasculature, may contribute.

Exercise capacity is most often quantified by means of a maximal exercise test during which the patient walks on a treadmill or pedals on an ergometer at progressively increasing workloads until further exercise is prevented by the development of dyspnea and/or leg weakness. Several exercise protocols may be used, and the testing may be quantified as to duration, maximal workload achieved, or oxygen consumed. The use of cardiopulmonary testing increases the objectivity of the evaluation by ascertaining whether a maximal anaerobic effort was achieved.[35] An alternative type of exercise test determines the ability to exercise at a submaximal workload by measuring either the duration of exercise at a given submaximal workload (chosen to be at or below the anaerobic threshold) or the distance walked in a fixed period (e.g., 6 mins).[36]

Quality of Life

HF can affect the quality of life in many ways, ranging from physical limitation to psychological depression. Although many instruments may be used to assess quality of life in patients with HF, one in particular, the Minnesota Living With Heart Failure Score, was designed specifically for patients with HF.[37] This self-administered questionnaire requires that the patient respond to 21 simple questions by grading each on a scale of 1–5. Although the Minnesota Living With Heart Failure Score has been used primarily in research settings to assess the response to therapy, it may be of value in the longitudinal assessment of individual patients.

Survival

Survival is reduced in patients with HF of all functional levels and also in patients with presymptomatic left ventricular dysfunction. Despite demonstrable improvements in prognosis with the use of ACE inhibitors, vasodilators, and possibly other newer agents, the survival of patients with HF is still severely limited. The 1-year mortality is in excess of 50%–60% in patients with severe HF; in the range of 15% to 30% in patients with mild to moderate HF; and in the range of 10% in patients with mild symptoms or asymptomatic left ventricular dysfunction (Fig. 8–2). The cause of death in patients with HF is generally refractory pump failure or arrhythmias, but the distinction may be difficult to make, particularly in previously ambulatory patients in whom death was not witnessed. Data from the Studies of Left Ventricular Dysfunction (SOLVD) treatment trial suggest that the ACE inhibitor enalapril reduced the rate of death

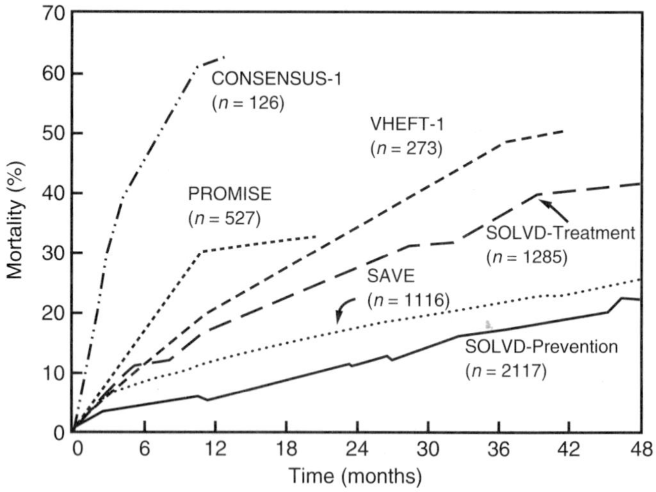

Figure 8–2. Mortality of patients with heart failure. Shown are the mortality curves from the placebo treatment arms of several controlled trials. The Cooperative North Scandinavian Enalapril Survival Study (CONSENSUS)–1 trial is representative of patients with predominantly New York Heart Association (NYHA) functional class IV heart failure. The Prospective Randomized Milrinone Survival Evaluation (PROMISE) trial enrolled patients who were in NYHA classes III and IV heart failure, whereas the Vasodilator Heart Failure Trial (VHEFT)–1 and Studies of Left Ventricular Dysfunction (SOLVD) treatment trials consisted predominantly of patients with NYHA classes II and III heart failure. The Survival and Ventricular Enlargement (SAVE) and SOLVD-prevention trials enrolled asymptomatic patients with left ventricular dysfunction. (Adapted from Young JB: Assessment of heart failure. *In* Colucci WS [ed]: Atlas of Heart Diseases, Volume IV: Heart Failure: Cardiac Function and Dysfunction, Chap. 7. St. Louis: CV Mosby, 1995.)

from pump failure but had little or no effect on the rate of sudden death.[38] Electrophysiologic testing, antiarrhythmic agents, (particularly amiodarone), and implantable defibrillators may have a role in selected patients, particularly those with symptomatic arrhythmias, but have not yet been shown to be of value in the majority of patients with HF who have a high level of asymptomatic arrhythmias.

Several clinical measures can be shown to predict survival in patients with HF, including left ventricular ejection fraction; maximal oxygen consumption; New York Heart Association functional class; hemodynamic parameters; ventricular ectopic activity; and neurohormones, including norepinephrine, angiotensin, and ANF[39] (see Chapter 11). Although any particular prognostic indicator may be of relatively little value in a given patient, the congruence of several indicators can provide a useful general sense of the prognosis.

REFERENCES

1. Konstam MA, Dracup K, Baker DW, et al: Heart failure: evaluation and care of patients with left-ventricular systolic dysfunction. *In* Clinical Practice Guideline, number 11. Agency for Health Care Policy and Research, June 1994. AHCPR publication 94–0612.
2. The SOLVD Investigators: Effect of enalapril on mortality and the development of heart failure in asymptomatic patients with reduced left ventricular ejection fractions. N Engl J Med 1992; 327:685.
3. Colucci WS, Packer M, Bristow MR, et al: Carvedilol inhibits clinical progression in patients with mild heart failure. Circulation 1995; 92(suppl I):395.
4. Teerlink JR, Goldhaber SZ, Pfeffer MA: An overview of contemporary etiologies of congestive heart failure. Am J Cardiol 1991; 121:1852.
5. Kessler KM: Heart failure with normal systolic function: update of prevalence, differential diagnosis, prognosis, and therapy [Editorial]. Arch Intern Med 1988; 148:2109.
6. Goldsmith SR, Dick C: Differentiating systolic from diastolic heart failure: pathophysiologic and therapeutic considerations. Am J Med 1993; 95:645.
7. Zelis R, Nellis S, Longhurst J, et al: Abnormalities in the regional circulations accompanying congestive heart failure. Prog Cardiovasc Dis 1975; 18:181.
8. Francis GS, Goldsmith SR, Levine BT, et al: The neurohumoral axis in congestive heart failure. Ann Intern Med 1984; 101:370.
9. Cusco JA, Creager MA: Neurohumoral, renal, and vascular adjustments in heart failure. *In* Colucci WS (ed): Atlas of Heart Diseases, Volume IV: Heart Failure: Cardiac Function and Dysfunction, Chap. 6. St. Louis: CV Mosby, 1995.
10. Kubo SH, Rector TS, Bank AJ, et al: Endothelium dependent vasodilation is attenuated in patients with heart failure. Circulation 1991; 84:1589.
11. Cody RJ, Haas GJ, Binkley PF, et al: Plasma endothelin correlates with the extent of the pulmonary hypertension in patients with chronic congestive heart failure. Circulation 1992; 67:719.
12. Loh E, Stamler JS, Hare JM, et al: Cardiovascular effects of inhaled nitric oxide in patients with left ventricular dysfunction. Circulation 1994; 90:2780.
13. Floras JS: Clinical aspects of sympathetic activation and parasympathetic withdrawal in heart failure. J Am Coll Cardiol 1993; 22:72A.
14. Colucci WS, Denniss AR, Leatherman GF, et al: Intracoronary infusion of dobutamine to patients with and without severe congestive heart failure. Dose-response relationships, correlation with circulating catecholamines, and effect of phosphodiesterase inhibition. J Clin Invest 1988; 81:1103.
15. Colucci WS, Ribeiro JP, Rocco MB, et al: Impaired chronotropic response to exercise in patients with congestive heart failure. Role of postsynaptic β-adrenergic desensitization. Circulation 1989; 80:314.
16. Francis GS, Benedict C, Johnstone DE, et al: Comparison of neuroendocrine activation in patients with left ventricular dysfunction with and without congestive heart failure. Circulation 1990; 82:1724.
17. Hirsch AT, Talsness CE, Schunkert H, et al: Tissue-specific activation of cardiac angiotensin converting enzyme in experimental heart failure. Circ Res 1991; 69:475.
18. Lindpaintner K, Lu W, Niedermajer N, et al: Selective activation of cardiac angiotensinogen gene expression in post-infarction ventricular remodeling in the rat. J Mol Cell Cardiol 1993; 25:133.
19. Meggs LG, Coupet J, Huang H, et al: Regulation of angiotensin II receptors on ventricular myocytes after myocardial infarction in rats. Circ Res 1993; 72:1149.
20. Gottlieb SS, Dickstein K, Fleck E, et al: Hemodynamic and neurohormonal effects of the angiotensin II antagonist losartan in patients with congestive heart failure. Circulation 1993; 88:1602.
21. Levine B, Kalman J, Mayer K, et al: Elevated circulating levels of tumor necrosis factor in severe chronic heart failure. N Engl J Med 1990; 223:236.
22. Mann DL, Young JB: Basic mechanisms in congestive heart failure. Recognizing the role of proinflammatory cytokines. Chest 1994; 105:897.
23. Balligand J-L, Ungureanu-Longrois D, Simmons WW, et al: Cytokine-inducible nitric oxide synthase (iNOS) expression in cardiac myocytes. Characterization and regulation of iNOS expression and detection of iNOS activity in single cardiac myocytes in vitro. J Biol Chem 1994; 269:27580.
24. Finkel MS, Oddis CV, Jacob TD, et al: Negative inotropic effects of cytokines on the heart mediated by nitric oxide. Science 1992; 257:387.
25. Yokoyama T, Vaca L, Rossen RD, et al: Cellular basis for the negative inotropic effects of tumor necrosis factor-alpha in the adult mammalian heart. J Clin Invest 1993; 92:2303.
26. Thaik CM, Calderone A, Takahashi N, Colucci WS: Interleukin-1β modulates the growth and phenotype of rat cardiac myocytes. J Clin Invest 1995; 96:1093–1099.
27. Feldman AM, Bristow MR, Parmley WW, et al: Effects of vesnarinone on morbidity and mortality in patients with heart failure. N Engl J Med 1993; 329:149.
28. Matsumori A, Shioi T, Yamada T, et al: Vesnarinone, a new inotropic agent, inhibits cytokine production by stimulated human blood from patients with heart failure. Circulation 1994; 89:955.
29. Pfeffer MA: Cardiac remodeling and its prevention. *In* Colucci WS (ed): Atlas of Heart Diseases, Volume IV: Heart Failure: Cardiac Function and Dysfunction, Chap. 5. St. Louis: CV Mosby, 1995.
30. Colucci WS: Treatment of stable heart failure: new approaches. *In* Colucci WS (ed): Atlas of Heart Diseases, Volume IV: Heart Failure: Cardiac Function and Dysfunction, Chap. 12. St. Louis: CV Mosby, 1995.
31. Takahashi N, Calderone A, Izzo NJ Jr, et al: Hypertrophic stimuli induce transforming growth factor-β_1 expression in rat ventricular myocytes. J Clin Invest 1994; 94:1470.
32. Young JB: Assessment of heart failure. *In* Colucci WS (ed): Atlas of Heart Diseases, Volume IV: Heart Failure: Cardiac Function and Dysfunction, Chap. 7. St. Louis: CV Mosby, 1995.
33. Ho KKL, Anderson KM, Kannell WB, et al: Survival after the onset of congestive heart failure in Framingham Heart Study subjects. Circulation 1993; 88:107.
34. Wassermann K: Dyspnea on exertion: is it the heart or the lungs? JAMA 1982; 248:2039.
35. Weber KT, Kinasewitz GT, Janicki JS, et al: Oxygen utilization during exercise in patients with chronic cardiac failure. Circulation 1982; 65:1213.
36. Lipkin DP, Bayliss J, Poole-Wilson PA: The ability of a submaximal exercise test to predict maximal exercise capacity in patients with heart failure. Eur Heart J 1985; 6:829.
37. Rector TS, Kubo SH, Cohn JN: Validity of the Minnesota Living With Heart Failure questionnaire as a measure of therapeutic response to enalapril or placebo. Am J Cardiol 1993; 71:1106.
38. The SOLVD Investigators: Effect of enalapril on survival in patients with reduced left ventricular ejection fractions and congestive heart failure. N Engl J Med 1991; 325:293.
39. Rector TS, Cohn JN: Prognosis, use of prognostic variables, and assessment of therapeutic responses. *In* Colucci WS (ed): Atlas of Heart Diseases, Volume IV: Heart Failure: Cardiac Function and Dysfunction, Chap. 8. St. Louis: CV Mosby, 1995.

9 The Pharmacology of Heart Failure Drugs

Ralph A. Kelly, MD
Thomas W. Smith, MD

This chapter focuses on drugs used in the management of heart failure caused by systolic and diastolic ventricular dysfunction. Treatment in all cases should be tailored to the underlying pathophysiologic process in the individual patient. In this chapter, the pharmacology of these agents is discussed only in the context of the treatment of heart failure. Vasodilators, particularly angiotensin converting enzyme (ACE) inhibitors, form the cornerstone of contemporary drug therapy for heart failure, and the rationale for their use is discussed in detail. Orally active formulations of several drugs that increase cyclic adenosine monophosphate (cAMP) levels in cardiac and vascular smooth muscle have not proved to be safe in long-term therapy of heart failure, whereas parenteral formulations remain essential for the short-term support of the circulation in patients with decompensated systolic ventricular dysfunction. The use of beta-adrenergic antagonists in heart failure patients, although still considered investigational, is also reviewed.

DIURETICS

The importance of diuretics in the treatment of heart failure is the result of the central role of the kidney as the target organ for many of the hemodynamic, hormonal, and autonomic nervous system changes that occur in response to a failing myocardium. The net effect of these physiologic responses is an increase in salt and water retention, resulting in expansion of the extracellular fluid volume.[1–4] This response sustains cardiac output and tissue perfusion by allowing the heart to operate higher on its ventricular function (i.e., Frank-Starling) curve (Fig. 9–1). However, these physiologic adaptations incur the cost of higher end-diastolic filling pressures, as well as increasing ventricular chamber dimensions and wall stress; these adverse effects eventually limit any further increase in cardiac output and also result in pulmonary venous congestion and peripheral edema.

Diuretics reduce intravascular and eventually extracellular fluid volume and ventricular filling pressures (i.e., preload). Except in the case of a natriuresis that results in a rapid decline in intravascular volume, diuretics do not usually cause a clinically important reduction in cardiac output, particularly in patients with advanced heart failure. This is because of the relative flatness of the ventricular function curve and increased chamber dimensions in most patients with advanced heart failure, in whom a decrease in high diastolic filling pressures will reduce congestive symptoms and ventricular wall stress but not stroke output. In patients with advanced heart failure, chronic diuretic therapy in conjunction with vasodilators tends to reduce the mitral regurgitation that often accompanies abnormally large left ventricular chamber dimensions. This effect helps to maintain forward cardiac output despite a decline in ventricular filling volume and pressure.

Diuretic Classes

NaK2Cl Symport Inhibitors (Loop Diuretics)

Of the loop diuretics available, only furosemide, bumetanide, or torasemide should be used in the treatment of most patients with heart failure. Ethacrynic acid should be reserved for patients who are allergic to sulfonamides or who have developed interstitial nephritis while taking alternative drugs because of the increased risk of ototoxicity in these patients. Loop diuretics inhibit a specific ion transport protein, the NaK2Cl symporter (cotransporter), a 115-kDa protein found on the apical membrane of renal epithelial cells in the ascending limb of the loop of Henle.[5–7] Several isoforms of a family of cation chloride cotransporters have been described in various cell types and tissues that share an overall 60% amino acid homology and a sensitivity to loop diuretics.[7] These drugs also decrease the absorption of calcium and magnesium, cations whose absorption is directly linked to NaCl uptake in this portion of the nephron. By preventing the resorption of solute in excess of water in the thick ascending limb of the loop of Henle and thereby reducing the tonicity of the medullary interstitium, loop diuretics also contribute to the development of hyponatremia in heart failure patients. The increased delivery of sodium and fluid to distal nephron segments also enhances potassium secretion. This tendency of loop diuretics to cause potassium wasting is exacerbated by the presence of elevated aldoste-

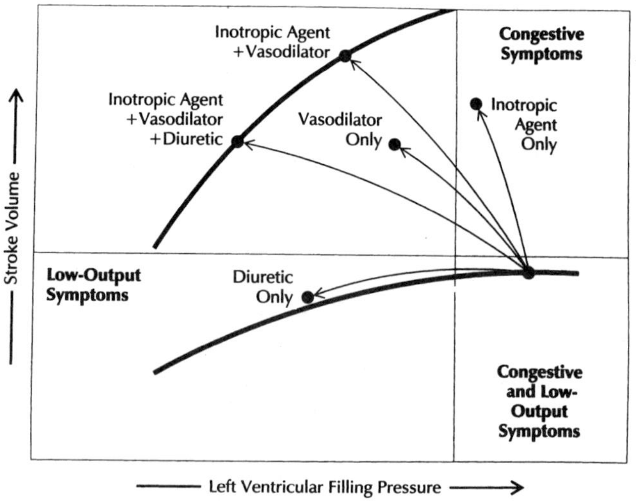

Figure 9–1. Physiologic response to pharmacologic interventions in heart failure. The relation between diastolic filling pressure (or preload) and cardiac output (or ventricular performance) is illustrated for a patient with heart failure caused by predominant systolic dysfunction before *(lower right)* and after *(upper left)* treatment as indicated. Notice that cardiac glycosides and other positively inotropic agents, such as sympathomimetic drugs, produce a higher ventricular function curve in these patients, indicating greater cardiac work for a given level of ventricular filling pressure. Vasodilators, such as angiotensin converting enzyme inhibitors, also produce improved ventricular function curves but reduce cardiac filling pressures. Diuretics improve symptoms of congestive heart failure by lowering cardiac filling pressures along the same ventricular function curve. Combinations of drugs often yield additive effects on hemodynamics.

rone levels, as is typically the case in heart failure patients. Hypokalemia can be minimized by concomitant use of drugs that inhibit aldosterone release (e.g., ACE inhibitors) or prevent receptor binding (e.g., spironolactone) or by diuretics that minimize distal nephron potassium wasting (e.g., amiloride).

Loop diuretics are often effective in advanced congestive heart failure as single diuretic agents because their oral bioavailability is unaffected by heart failure and because of the magnitude of the acute natriuresis that can be achieved over a short period.[5] Nevertheless, even in the absence of heart failure, compensatory changes may limit the patient's diuretic response to subsequent doses of diuretics. These changes are the result of diuretic-induced alterations in intrarenal hemodynamics as a result of tubuloglomerular feedback and increased sympathetic nervous system activity, among other mechanisms. This process is termed *diuretic adaptation*.[5, 8] In addition, because the elimination half-life is short for loop diuretics, multiple daily doses are often necessary. This is an acceptable strategy for managing ambulatory heart failure patients if there is adequate monitoring of daily body weight and blood electrolyte levels.

In hospitalized patients, an alternative strategy is to give the same total daily dose of a loop diuretic by continuous intravenous infusion.[9] This regimen results in a sustained natriuresis as a result of the constant presence of high diuretic drug levels within the renal tubular lumina. This approach also avoids the potential for ototoxicity that occurs with transient high blood levels of drug following intermittent intravenous loop diuretic dosing. A typical continuous furosemide infusion is initiated with a 20- to 40-mg loading dose as a bolus injection followed by a constant intravenous infusion of 5 mg/h, with repeated bolus injections that precede each additional upward titration of the infusion rate as necessary.

NaCl Symport Inhibitors (Thiazide Diuretics)

Although these agents have been in regular use for more than 40 years in the United States, the molecular target protein within the kidney for the thiazide diuretics has only recently been described. All thiazide diuretics exhibit weak carbonic anhydrase inhibitory activity, but their principal site of action is known to be the NaCl symporter (cotransporter) present in renal tubular epithelial cells in the distal convoluted tubule. This loop diuretic–insensitive 115-kDa protein exhibits 45% amino acid sequence homology with the absorptive NaK2Cl symporter isoform found in the loop of Henle, and is expressed in many tissues other than the kidney.[7, 10] This observation may shed light on the mechanisms of these drugs' less desirable metabolic side effects on lipid and glucose metabolism, as well as their possible effects on peripheral vascular resistance in the treatment of hypertension. The thiazide diuretics are generally useful as single drugs for the therapy of volume retention only in patients with relatively mild heart failure, because their site of action in the distal nephron permits rapid intrarenal adjustments of water and solute absorption to other more proximal nephron segments. Thiazide diuretics also are less effective in patients with moderate renal insufficiency (i.e., at glomerular filtration rates lower than 30 mL/min). However, thiazide diuretics exhibit a true synergism with loop diuretics, resulting in a natriuresis that is greater than the sum of either class of drugs given individually. This is useful in the treatment of diuretic resistance (discussed later).

Potassium-Sparing Diuretics

These drugs are not effective as single agents for the diuretic treatment of heart failure. However, they are useful in limiting potassium and magnesium wasting in combination with a loop diuretic. Potassium-sparing diuretics are divided into agents that inhibit apical membrane sodium conductance channels in epithelial cells of the collecting duct (e.g., amiloride, triamterene)[5, 11, 12] and aldosterone antagonists that also have their principal pharmacologic effect in the collecting duct (e.g., spironolactone, canrenone).[13, 14] Potassium-sparing diuretics should be administered cautiously to patients who are already receiving renin-angiotensin system (RAS) antagonists (e.g., ACE inhibitors), because these agents also increase the serum potassium concentration. Beta-adrenergic antagonists and nonsteroidal anti-inflammatory drugs (NSAIDs) can also induce hyperkalemia in patients receiving potassium-sparing diuretics.

Diuretic Resistance in Heart Failure Patients

The term *diuretic resistance* should not encompass the expected renal physiologic changes to repetitive doses of diuretic—that is, "diuretic adaptation" or "braking" that can be demonstrated in normal subjects as well as in heart failure patients, as noted previously, although this response may be exaggerated in heart failure patients.[5] With the administration of loop diuretics in heart failure patients, diuretic adaptation can be managed by more frequent intermittent or continuous intravenous dosing and more stringent dietary salt restriction.

The common causes of diuretic resistance are listed in Table 9–1. Pharmacokinetic causes of diuretic resistance (e.g., altered bioavailability, decreased drug access to the renal tubular lumen) are unusual in heart failure patients in the absence of renal insufficiency.[15–17] It is often difficult to distinguish clinically between intravascular volume depletion following aggressive diuretic and vasodilator therapy and a decrease in cardiac output and blood pressure as a result of primary cardiac failure, although a more marked decline in urea clearance than in creatinine clearance suggests intravascular volume depletion. Pulmonary arterial and venous or left atrial pressure monitoring may be required to make this distinction. In addition, all vasodilators commonly employed as afterload-reducing agents in heart failure patients dilate a number of central and peripheral vascular beds. Therefore, renal blood flow may be reduced despite an increase in cardiac output, resulting in a decline in diuretic effectiveness. Vasodilator therapy also may lower renal perfusion pressure below the level necessary to maintain normal autoregulation and glomerular filtration in patients with renal arterial stenoses as a result of atherosclerotic disease.

The unique role of angiotensin II as an intrarenal signaling autacoid means that RAS antagonists, unlike other vasodilators, can augment the effectiveness of diuretics by mechanisms that are independent of their ability to reduce systemic vascular resistance (discussed later).[18] However, these drugs can also diminish diuretic effectiveness by reducing the transglomerular perfusion pressure to the point that the glomerular filtration rate declines abruptly. This

TABLE 9–1. CAUSES OF DIURETIC RESISTANCE IN HEART FAILURE

Decreased Renal Perfusion and Glomerular Filtration Rate as a Result of
Excessive intravascular volume depletion as a result of aggressive diuretic therapy
Decline in cardiac output as a result of worsening heart failure, arrhythmias, or other primary cardiac causes
Decline in mean arterial pressure below that necessary to sustain renal autoregulation of glomerular perfusion pressure as a result of aggressive vasodilator therapy
Selective reduction in glomerular perfusion pressure following initiation or dose increase of renin-angiotensin system antagonists, including ACE inhibitor therapy
Nonsteroidal anti-inflammatory drugs
Primary Renal Pathology (e.g., Cholesterol Emboli, Renal Artery Stenosis, Drug-Induced Interstitial Nephritis, Obstructive Uropathy)
Noncompliance With Medical Regimen, Excess Dietary Sodium Intake, or Both

Abbreviation: ACE, angiotensin converting enzyme.

response is most commonly observed in patients with a decreased renal arterial perfusion pressure due to either renal artery stenosis or a limited cardiac output and for whom a high angiotensin II–mediated glomerular efferent arteriolar tone is necessary to maintain glomerular filtration. This cause of diuretic resistance is typically accompanied by a marked decline in the rate of creatinine clearance. This cause must be distinguished from the more common, limited increases in serum creatinine levels that often accompany initiation of ACE inhibitor therapy.

Decreased responsiveness to loop diuretics in patients otherwise receiving optimal medical management should initially be managed by increasing the frequency of loop diuretic doses. If this procedure is ineffective, then a thiazide diuretic administered with a loop diuretic will often result in a substantial natriuresis.[8, 15, 19, 20] Although effective, this diuretic combination can often result in profound intravascular volume depletion, hypotension, renal potassium wasting, hyponatremia, and a decrease in the glomerular filtration rate. Accordingly, this combination should be used cautiously, particularly in outpatients. Spironolactone combined with a loop diuretic may also be effective in these patients, although patients are at increased risk of hyperkalemia if they are concomitantly receiving a RAS antagonist. In hospitalized patients, dopamine administered at doses that cause selective dopaminergic receptor stimulation may increase renal blood flow and diuretic responsiveness (i.e., <2 μg/kg/min, based on estimated lean body weight). If diuretic resistance is the result of a decline in cardiac function, then this condition should be treated by optimizing vasodilator therapy and, in hospitalized patients, the short-term administration of sympathomimetic drugs or phosphodiesterase inhibitors and mechanical circulatory assist devices, if necessary. Other strategies under investigation include short-term infusions of recombinant atrial natriuretic peptide (ANP) or other natriuretic peptides or the administration of neutral endopeptidase inhibitors to enhance endogenous ANP levels and activity.[21–24]

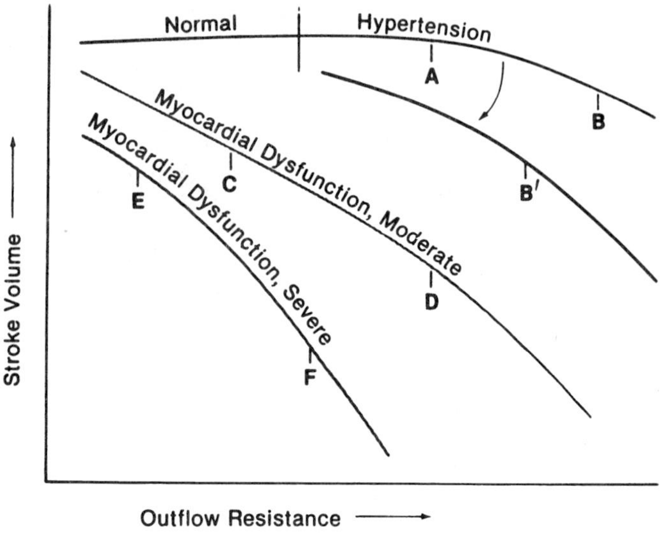

Figure 9–2. Relation of ventricular outflow resistance to stroke volume in patients with systolic ventricular dysfunction. Ventricular outflow resistance, a principal determinant of afterload, has little effect on stroke volume in normal hearts. In patients with systolic ventricular dysfunction, an increase in outflow resistance is often accompanied by a decline in ventricular stroke volume. Conversely, a reduction in systemic vascular resistance, one component of outflow resistance, after administration of an arterial vasodilator, may increase stroke volume in patients with severe myocardial dysfunction. This increase in stroke volume may prevent a decline in blood pressure despite arterial vasodilation in heart failure patients. (From Cohn JN, Franciosa JA: Vasodilator therapy of cardiac failure. N Engl J Med 1977; 297[1]:27–31.)

Metabolic Consequences of Diuretic Therapy

The most important adverse effect of diuretic therapy in heart failure patients is electrolyte abnormalities, including hyponatremia, hypokalemia, and hypochloremic metabolic alkalosis.[5, 25–27] The importance of significant magnesium deficiency with chronic use of diuretics remains controversial.[25, 28–30]

Both hypokalemia and renal magnesium wasting can be limited by concomitant administration of oral potassium chloride supplements or a potassium-sparing diuretic. Potassium-sparing drugs are probably safe, provided that renal function is not significantly impaired. Even moderate renal insufficiency tends to limit any natriuretic effect and promote hyperkalemia when potassium-sparing diuretics are administered. Routine monitoring of serum potassium levels is necessary, particularly when patients are also receiving other drugs that limit renal potassium losses (e.g., NSAIDs, beta-adrenergic antagonists, ACE inhibitors). Because primary cardiac arrhythmia is presumed to be the cause of sudden death in many patients with advanced heart failure, many of whom are also receiving a cardiac glycoside, routine monitoring of serum electrolytes is prudent and justified in any heart failure patient on chronic diuretic therapy.

VASODILATORS

The rationale for the use of vasodilators grew out of experience with parenteral sympatholytic agents and nitroprusside in patients with severe heart failure. Cohn and Franciosa,[31] in an influential 1977 article, reviewed the evidence and advocated the use of these drugs (Fig. 9–2). Studies of vasodilators in the following decade demonstrated that these agents are well tolerated and effective in improving symptoms in heart failure. The effectiveness of the isosorbide dinitrate–hydralazine combination[32] and of ACE inhibitors in reducing mortality in heart failure patients has been demonstrated in a number of prospective randomized controlled trials in the 1980s.[33] Additional trials have also supported an expansion of the indications for the use of vasodilator therapy (specifically, ACE inhibitors) to patients with ventricular dysfunction but without symptoms of overt heart failure and for the prevention of ventricular dilatation and the development of heart failure in patients following myocardial infarction. These trials are discussed in greater detail in Chapters 11 and 12. The vasodilator drugs commonly employed in heart failure patients are listed in Table 9–2.

Renin-Angiotensin System Antagonists

Renin-Angiotensin Systems

The importance of RAS in the pathophysiology of heart failure has been underscored by the effectiveness of RAS antagonists in improving symptoms and in reducing mortality in this syndrome. Classically, this system has been viewed as a renin-angiotensin-aldosterone axis, the activity of which is determined by the rate of renin released into the systemic circulation from the juxtaglomerular apparatus in the glomerular afferent arterioles.[34] Renin is released as a precursor peptide, prorenin, in response to a number of factors, including decreased renal perfusion pressure, increased sympathetic nervous system activity, and tubuloglomerular feedback mechanisms that sense the volume and composition of fluid in the lumen of the distal portion of the loop of Henle. Prorenin is activated within the circulation by unclear mechanisms to renin, a proteolytic enzyme that metabolizes renin substrate, angiotensinogen, to the decapeptide angiotensin I (Ang I). Most circulating angiotensinogen is produced in the liver, and its synthesis and release are markedly enhanced by other "acute phase reactants" following infection or administration of inflammatory cytokines. Angiotensin I is metabolized to angiotensin II (Ang II) by ACE, which is found circulating in plasma as well

TABLE 9–2. VASODILATOR DRUGS IN HEART FAILURE

Drug	Mechanism	Preload Reduction	Afterload Reduction	Usual Dose
Nitrovasodilators				
Nitroglycerin	Nitric oxide donors	+ + +	+	0.2–10 μg/kg/min IV
Isosorbide dinitrate		+ + +	+	5–6 mg transdermal
Nitroprusside		+ + +	+	10–60 mg q4h PO
		+ + +	+ + +	0.1–5 μg/kg/min IV
Renin-Angiotensin System Antagonists				
Captopril	Inhibition of renal systemic and tissue generation of angiotensin II by ACE; decreased metabolism of bradykinin	+ +	+ +	6.25–50 mg PO q8h
Enalapril		+ +	+ +	2.5–10 mg PO q12h
Enalaprilat		+ +	+ +	0.5–2.0 mg IV q12h
Quinapril		+ +	+ +	5–30 mg PO q24h
Lisinopril		+ +	+ +	2.5–20 mg PO q12h–q24h
Ramipril		+ +	+ +	1.25–5 mg PO q.d.
Losartan†	Blockade of angiotensin II (AT_1) receptors	+ +	+ +	25–50 mg q12h
Phosphodiesterase Inhibitors				
Amrinone	Inhibition of type III cAMP phosphodiesterase and other mechanisms	+ +	+ +	0.5 mg/kg, then 2–20 μg/kg/min IV
Milrinone		+ +	+ +	50 μg/kg, then 0.25–1 μg/kg/min IV
Vesnarinone*				60 mg PO q24h
Direct Vasodilators				
Hydralazine	Unclear	+	+ + +	10–100 mg PO q6h
Nicorandil*	Increased K^+ channel conductance and other mechanisms	+ +	+ + +	Not determined
Minoxidil		+	+ + +	5–30 mg/d
Diazoxide		+	+ + +	1–3 mg/kg q4h–q24h
Sympatholytics				
Prazosin (and other quinazoline derivatives)	α_1-Adrenergic receptor antagonist	+ + +	+ +	1–5 mg PO q8h
Phentolamine	Nonselective alpha-adrenergic blockade	+ +	+ +	0.5–1 mg/min IV
Lebetalol	Nonselective beta-	+	+ +	50–400 mg PO q12h
Carvedilol	adrenergic and α_1-			12.5–50 mg PO q12h
	adrenergic blockade	+	+ +	
Bucindolol	Additional mechanisms	+	+ +	6.25–100 mg PO q12h
Calcium Channel Blocking Drugs				
Nifedipine	Inhibition of L-type voltage-sensitive Ca^{2+} channels	+	+ + +	10–30 mg PO q8h
Amlodipine		+	+ + +	1.25–10 mg PO q24h
Sympathomimetics				
Dobutamine	Myocardial and vascular beta-adrenergic agonist	+	+ +	2–20 μg/kg/min IV
Dopamine	Selective renal arterial vasodilation			≤2 μg/kg/min IV

Abbreviation: ACE, angiotensin converting enzyme.
Many of these drugs have not been approved for the indication of heart failure by the U.S. Food and Drug Administration as of this writing.
*Investigational: Adapted from Kelly RA, Smith TW: The pharmacologic treatment of heart failure. In Hardman JG, Limbird LE (eds): Goodman and Gilman's The Pharmacologic Basis of Therapeutics, 9th ed. New York: McGraw-Hill, 1996.
†Not approved for heart failure indication.

as on the plasma membrane of endothelial cells and a number of other cell types. ACE is a relatively nonspecific zinc metalloprotease that also comprises the activity of kininase II, which is responsible for the metabolism of bradykinin. Among other actions, Ang II, acting at specific receptors (discussed later) found on many cell types in all organs, increases systemic vascular resistance and blood pressure and induces sodium retention through direct intrarenal actions and by inducing the synthesis and release of aldosterone by zona glomerulosa cells in the adrenal cortex.

With the advent of highly specific and highly sensitive technologies for the detection and cellular localization of components of RAS, it is now recognized that many local or tissue RASs exist throughout the vasculature and in parenchymal cells of most, if not all, organs.[34–37] Within the cellular components of blood vessels, for example, de novo synthesis and secretion of Ang II from aortic endothelial cells in vitro was described in 1987, and more recent evidence suggests that locally released Ang II acts within the vascular wall as a paracrine signaling peptide to promote the proliferation as well as the contraction of vascular smooth muscle cells.[38] Within the kidney, as well as within other organs classically associated with the renin-angiotensin-aldosterone axis (e.g., the adrenal), all components of the classic systemic RAS (i.e., renin, angiotensinogen, and ACE) can be found, suggesting that the activity of Ang II within each of these tissues is largely, if not exclusively, determined by its local synthesis, activation, and release. The relevance of the systemic renin-angiotensin-aldosterone axis to the pathophysiology of heart failure is unclear as a result of the rapidly expanding literature on the molecular pharmacology of Ang II as a locally acting autocrine/paracrine signaling peptide.

Angiotensin Receptors

Two classes of Ang II receptors have been described (AT1 and AT2), both of which bind Ang II with roughly equal affinities and are widely distributed on many tissues in a developmental and cell type–specific manner.[34] AT1 receptors are canonical GTP-binding protein–linked integral membrane proteins with seven transmembrane-spanning domains that bind the diphenylimidazole derivative losartan. The AT1 receptor subtypes are highly homologous and are linked to the activation of phospholipase C and release of inositol triphosphate (IP_3) and diacylglycerol (DAG), which, among other effects, increase intracellular calcium. The AT2 receptor is also a seven–transmembrane-spanning domain receptor with relatively low (≅33%) homology in its amino acid sequence with the AT1 receptor. The cellular signaling pathways initiated by Ang II binding at this receptor are not clear. Shortly after its identification, it was recognized that the AT2 receptor is abundantly expressed in a species- and tissue-specific manner during fetal development and early postnatal life but is subsequently downregulated.[39] Nevertheless, the AT2 receptor is expressed in many cell types in the adult heart. Both AT1 and AT2 receptors are expressed in normal human myocardium, although at relatively low levels (≅5–10 fmol/mg protein), and the AT2 receptor is the most abundant Ang II receptor found in adult human atrial and ventricular myocytes.[40, 41] The available literature on angiotensin receptors in mammalian, and particularly in human, cardiac muscle is limited.

Cardiovascular Actions of Angiotensins

The clinical trials that have documented the safety and efficacy of RAS antagonists are described in Chapters 11 and 12. Virtually all of these trials have used ACE inhibitors, which are not selective RAS antagonists, and the improved survival of patients following myocardial infarction or with symptomatic heart failure is not likely to be the result of the antihypertensive effects of these drugs, because earlier trials with other vasodilators that resulted in approximately equal declines in blood pressure had no effect on mortality in these patients. Several reviews and editorials have focused on possible direct and indirect effects of angiotensins on the vasculature and on myocardial remodeling and energetics, among other effects.[42, 43]

Vascular Actions of Angiotensin II. Angiotensins have direct vasoconstrictor activity in vascular smooth muscle. In addition, Ang II is known to enhance the activity of the sympathetic nervous system by several mechanisms, including blockade of norepinephrine reuptake and facilitation of norepinephrine release.[44, 45] Direct antiproliferative and antiatherogenic effects of ACE inhibitors have been demonstrated. A number of in vitro studies have documented that Ang II induces a sequence of biochemical signals within vascular smooth muscle cells that are associated with DNA replication and cellular proliferation. These actions are mediated at least in part by increased expression of peptide growth factors that, in turn, act as additional proliferative signals.[34, 46–49] ACE inhibitors have been shown to decrease the progression of atherosclerosis in rabbits with genetic hyperlipidemia and in cholesterol-fed monkeys.[50, 51] Antithrombotic effects of ACE inhibitors have also been demonstrated in vitro and in several animals models and may be the result of inhibition of both Ang II generation and bradykinin metabolism. Ang II directly increases synthesis and release of plasminogen activator inhibitor 1 (PAI-1), a prothrombolytic protein that is an inhibitor of endogenous fibrinolytic peptides such as tissue plasminogen activator (tPA).[52, 53] These prothrombotic, fibrolytic, and vasoactive actions of Ang II, in addition to possible direct atherogenic effects of this peptide, suggest that local vascular RAS may play a role in atherosclerotic plaque "activation" and subsequent rupture and thrombosis.

Myocardial Actions of Angiotensin II. Ang II has long been known to have a positively inotropic effect in isolated muscle strips from several animal species. However, it is unclear whether these effects of Ang II are relevant to human physiology, particularly because a negatively inotropic action of ACE inhibitors and AT1 receptor antagonists has not been described. Ang II released by an activated intracardiac RAS may play a role in mediating a decrease in ventricular compliance.[54] These observations have been extended to humans with aortic stenosis and left ventricular hypertrophy, in whom selective intracoronary infusion of the ACE inhibitor enalaprilat by Friedrich and colleagues[55] resulted in a downward, rightward shift of the late diastolic filling portion of the pressure volume relation. Although other explanations are possible (e.g., a coronary vasodilator response leading to decreased ischemia), these data suggest that ACE inhibitors have a direct, positively lusitropic action.

In vitro, Ang II is known to induce activation of signaling pathways that lead to cellular proliferation of fibroblasts isolated from cardiac muscle and that contribute to the increased fibrosis characteristic of some forms of cardiac hypertrophy and cardiomyopathy.[56–58] Ang II can cause proliferation of cardiac fibroblasts and induce hypertrophic growth of neonatal ventricular myocytes in vitro, and may do so in vivo as well, by potentiating the activity of the sympathetic nervous system and the release of norepinephrine, which is known to induce myocyte hypertrophy in vitro by acting through β_1-adrenergic receptors.[59] These actions of Ang II, in addition to its arterial and venous vasoconstrictor properties, probably contribute to the "remodeling" that occurs in surviving ventricular muscle following myocardial infarction. These data provide additional evidence that activation of an intracardiac RAS plays an important role in the initiation of compensatory change in ventricular growth or remodeling, changes that ultimately become deleterious and adversely affect survival.

In addition to inhibition of intracardiac RAS, renin-angiotensin antagonists, by virtue of their vasodilating activity, also reduce intracavity pressures and diminish wall stress, thereby decreasing myocardial oxygen demand. These agents also inhibit Ang II stimulation of aldosterone release, which reduces intravascular volume and preload and may have direct actions on the extent of interstitial collagen deposition in the heart.[60] ACE inhibitors have also been shown to decrease sympathetic nervous system activity and improve parasympathetic nervous system tone, which could result in reduced electrophysiologic instability in infarcted or cardiomyopathic muscle.[61, 62]

Renal Actions of Angiotensin II and RAS Antagonists. RAS antagonists also exhibit beneficial pharmacologic effects on sodium homeostasis in heart failure patients. These effects result from the important role of Ang II in the regulation of intrarenal hemodynamics, glomerular filtration, and tubular resorption of solute and water in the kidney (Fig. 9–3). Ang II also induces the release of aldosterone from the adrenal cortex, which facilitates sodium resorption in the distal nephron. Inhibitors of the RAS, therefore, have unique properties among the vasodilators in that they can potentiate the activity of diuretics in heart failure patients. This effect has been demonstrated in patients receiving chronic ACE inhibitor therapy for heart failure.[18] ACE inhibitors also may reduce potassium wasting and water resorption, particularly when combined with a loop diuretic, thus reducing the severity of both hyperkalemia and hypona-

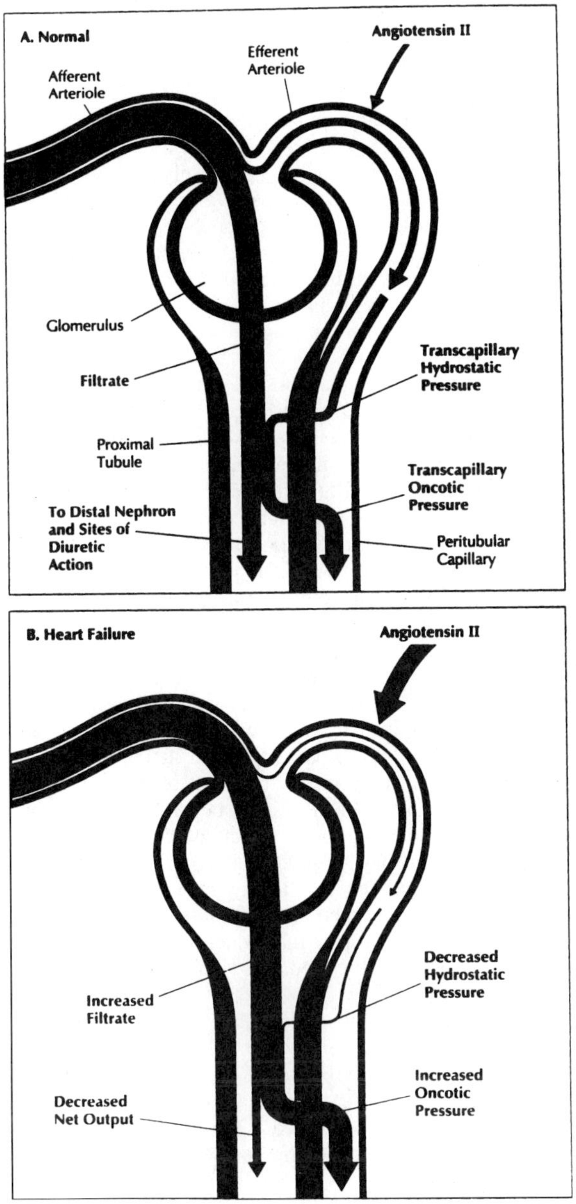

Figure 9–3. Role of intrarenal angiotensin II in the regulation of solute and water homeostasis in heart failure patients. Among other actions within the kidney, the intrarenal renin-angiotensin system is a physiologic regulator of the tone of glomerular efferent arterioles *(A)*, thereby determining in part the fraction of glomerular plasma that will be filtered at the glomerulus (i.e., the "filtration fraction"). In heart failure *(B)*, increased efferent arteriolar tone mediated by angiotensin II results in an increase in filtration fraction, which reduces transcapillary hydrostatic pressure and increases peritubular capillary oncotic pressure, thereby increasing sodium and water resorption in the proximal tubule. (Adapted from Humes HD, Gottlieb M, Brenner BM: The kidney in congestive heart failure. *In* Brenner BM [ed]: Contemporary Issues in Nephrology, vol 1, p 51. London: Churchill Livingstone, 1992.)

tremia, which are common in advanced heart failure. ACE inhibitors, by blocking the intrarenal metabolism of bradykinin, increase intrarenal bradykinin levels, which also facilitates renal salt and water loss.

Although RAS antagonists have several advantages over other classes of vasodilators, these drugs limit the kidneys' ability to autoregulate glomerular perfusion pressure and thereby maintain glomerular filtration. This may be particularly important in patients with a marginal cardiac output or blood pressure and can result in a decline in the glomerular filtration rate, resulting in an increase in serum creatinine levels. In the first Cooperative North Scandinavian Enalapril Survival Study (CONSENSUS I), in which the efficacy of enalapril was compared with that of a placebo in patients with severe (New York Heart Association [NYHA] classes III and IV) heart failure,[33] the serum creatinine increased by a factor of two or greater in only 11% of 123 patients, compared with 3% in the placebo group.[63] The maximal increase in serum creatinine correlated inversely with mean arterial pressure. Patients receiving high daily doses of loop diuretics were at a slightly higher risk for a significant elevation in serum creatinine.[64] The factors associated with a decline in renal function in heart failure in patients receiving an ACE inhibitor are listed in Table 9–3. Most patients in the CONSENSUS I trial tolerated enalapril well, and the serum creatinine in fact fell in 24% of patients. This has generally been the experience in most of the later trials involving ACE inhibitors (see Chapters 11 and 12), in which patients, on average, had less severe heart failure than those in the CONSENSUS I trial. In the arm of the Studies of Left Ventricular Dysfunction (SOLVD) trial that examined symptomatic patients with heart failure, approximately 11% of patients receiving enalapril had an increase in serum creatinine of more than 2 mg/dL compared with 8% receiving placebo.[65] In the Gruppo Italiano per lo Studio della Sopravvivenza nell-Infarto Miocardico (GISSI-3) trial, there was a small but significantly increased risk of renal dysfunction at 6 weeks after admission to the hospital in patients randomized to receive lisinopril who had normal renal function at the entry of study (0.6% for lisinopril vs. 0.3% among controls).[66]

An increase in serum creatinine need not require discontinuation of the RAS antagonist in the absence of uremic symptoms or a decline in sodium excretion. If the serum creatinine level more than doubles, the ACE inhibitor dose should be reduced or another class of vasodilator should be substituted. There is a growing role for RAS antagonists in the treatment of patients with renal failure. The rate of progression of renal insufficiency can be decreased by careful control of blood pressure (i.e., mean arterial pressure ≤ 90 mm Hg), and RAS antagonists, which invariably were ACE inhibitors in published clinical trials, appear to be superior to other classes of antihypertensive agents, with the possible exception of calcium channel antagonists.[67–69]

Angiotensin Converting Enzyme Inhibitors

The first orally bioavailable ACE inhibitor, captopril, was introduced in the late 1970s. A synthetic, nonpeptide ACE inhibitor,

TABLE 9–3. CONVERTING ENZYME INHIBITION IN CONGESTIVE HEART FAILURE

Factors Favoring Deterioration in Renal Function
Evidence of Na^+ depletion or poor renal perfusion
Large doses of diuretics
Increased urea-creatinine ratio
Mean arterial pressure < 80 mm Hg
Evidence of maximal neurohumoral activation
Presence of hyponatremia secondary to AVP activation
Interruption of counter-regulatory mechanisms
Coadministration of prostaglandin inhibitors
Presence of adrenergic dysfunction (e.g., diabetes mellitus)
Factors Favoring Improvement in Renal Function
Maintenance of Na^+ balance
Reduction in diuretic dosage
Increase in sodium intake
Mean arterial pressure > 80 mm Hg
Minimal neurohumoral activation
Intact counter-regulatory mechanisms

Abbreviations: AVP, arginine vasopressin. From Miller JA, Tobe SW, Skorecki KL: Control of extracellular fluid volume and the pathophysiology of edema. *In* Brenner BM (ed): Brenner & Rector's The Kidney, 5th ed, vol I, p 817. Philadelphia; WB Saunders, 1996.

teprotide, had been available for about a decade before captopril and had proved safe and effective in the treatment of hypertension and heart failure.[70] All orally active ACE inhibitors presently available fall into three general categories: (1) those with a sulfhydryl group that binds to the zinc moiety in ACE, including captopril and zofenopril; (2) those in which a carboxyl group was designed to bind the zinc moiety at the ACE catalytic site, which are the majority of ACE inhibitors, including enalapril, lisinopril, ramipril, cilazapril, quinopril, and others; and (3) proline derivatives, in which a phosphinic acid group is used to bind to the zinc moiety of which fosinopril is the prototype. Several of these drugs are inactive esters or prodrugs, such as zofenopril, enalapril and fosinopril, and must be de-esterified to the active drug in vivo.

Relatively tissue-specific effects have been described for some ACE inhibitors. These differences in ACE activity and physiologic responsiveness among members of the same class of RAS antagonists are probably the result of the accessibility to, or entrapment of, active drug within cellular sites of Ang II generation within a given tissue. Prodrug esters, which must be cleaved by plasma and tissue esterases to become active ACE inhibitors such as enalapril, trandolapril, ramipril, zofenopril, and quinapril, are more rapidly transported as prodrug esters into cells and accumulate following de-esterification, although fosinopril, interestingly, is more rapidly accumulated in myocardial tissue in its de-esterified form.[71–73] The clinical importance of these differences in the site and extent of accumulation of specific ACE inhibitors requires additional investigation.

ACE inhibitors are "balanced" vasodilators in that they induce venous as well as arterial vasodilation and therefore have direct effects on both preload and afterload. Mean arterial pressure tends to decline despite an increase in stroke volume and cardiac output, although this is often not accompanied by an increase in heart rate but probably is the result of their action to decrease sympathetic nervous system activity for the reasons noted previously. These effects are accompanied by a modest increase in ejection fraction and an improvement in myocardial energy metabolism as a result of a fall in ventricular end-diastolic pressure and volume. These early hemodynamic effects are sustained with the chronic use of these drugs (i.e., tolerance does not occur).

Initiating Therapy With ACE Inhibitors. It is advisable to begin therapy with an ACE inhibitor at low doses of a relatively short-acting drug (e.g., 6.25 mg captopril or 2.5 mg enalapril). An abrupt fall in blood pressure occasionally occurs after an initial dose of an ACE inhibitor, particularly in patients who are intravascularly volume depleted. This response is often unpredictable; therefore, caution is recommended when beginning these drugs in any patient who has significant left ventricular dysfunction or has received large doses of diuretics. Unacceptable hypotension can usually be reversed by intravascular volume expansion, although this is obviously not ideal in heart failure patients with an expanded extracellular fluid volume.

The maximal hypotensive response to an initial oral dose of captopril occurs 1–2 h after dosing, whereas the maximal response to oral enalapril occurs 4–6 h after dosing. In the SOLVD trials, of 7487 ambulatory patients undergoing a prerandomization drug challenge of open-label enalapril (2.5 mg/day), only 1.3% were unwilling to enter the trial because of unacceptable side effects.[65, 74, 75]

This benign experience with oral captopril and enalapril may not be directly transferable to other ACE inhibitor formulations because of differences in the rate of activation of prodrugs and other pharmacokinetic considerations. Infusion of intravenous enalaprilat leads to a much more rapid decline in arterial pressure than that seen with the oral formulation; this factor may have contributed to the high incidence in clinically significant hypotension in patients randomized to receive an ACE inhibitor in the CONSENSUS II trial.[76] These patients received an initial 1-mg dose of enalaprilat administered over a 2-h period, followed by a 2.5-mg oral dose of enalapril 6 h later. More recent trials of ACE inhibitors in acute myocardial infarction, including captopril in the Fourth International Study of Infarct Survival (ISIS-4),[77] zofenopril in the Survival of Myocardial Infarction Long-Term Evaluation (SMILE),[78] and lisinopril in GISSI-3,[66] showed a positive impact on survival. Initial doses of all these agents (6.25 mg captopril; 7.5 mg zofenopril; and 2.5 mg lisinopril) were well tolerated, although as patients approached the target doses in each trial, persistent hypotension requiring a reduction in dose or discontinuation of therapy was approximately two to three times more common in patients receiving active drug (about 8%–10% in ISIS-4,[77] GISI-3,[66] and SMILE[78]). Although it is reasonable to assume that other ACE inhibitors also confer a survival benefit in patients with acute myocardial infarction or chronic heart failure, determination of the extent and duration of first-dose effects on hemodynamics require dose-ranging studies of each drug in this patient population.

These data suggest that the initiation of ACE inhibitor therapy in patients with chronic left ventricular dysfunction or following myocardial infarction be limited to those drugs for which extensive pharmacokinetic data exist in this patient population (e.g., captopril, enalapril, lisinopril, ramipril). With careful observation of blood pressure, serum electrolytes, and serum creatinine levels, ACE inhibitor doses are customarily titrated upward over several days in hospitalized patients or over a few weeks in outpatients.

There is no precisely defined relation between dose and long-term clinical effectiveness of these drugs.[79, 80] The target doses of these drugs in several large prospective trials in which a positive effect of an ACE inhibitor was demonstrated on mortality as well as other endpoints were 50 mg of captopril two or three times per day[77, 81]; 10 mg of enalapril twice daily[82]; 10 mg of lisinopril once daily[66]; 5 mg of ramipril twice daily[83]; or 30 mg of zofenopril twice daily.[78] Higher doses are often used in the treatment of hypertension, but it is unclear whether increasing the dose beyond that used in these trials will result in additional hemodynamic or survival benefit.[79, 80] Upward dose titration may be prudent if a patient's blood pressure remains above a target level and may be of benefit in selected patients with significant functional mitral regurgitation (discussed later; see Chapter 10). Despite the evidence for a clear-cut effect with these drugs, Pitt[79] has argued that it may be unwise to assume that all ACE inhibitors are equal or that doses other than those shown to improve mortality in controlled clinical trials should be used in heart failure. Adding a second vasodilator (e.g., hydralazine, with or without nitrates) has been advocated by some investigators in patients with advanced heart failure. However, this approach has not yet been evaluated by controlled clinical survival trials.

Few consistent and clinically important pharmacokinetic drug interactions exist between the ACE inhibitors and most other classes of drugs that are commonly administered to patients with heart failure. There is no consistent evidence for an important interaction between any ACE inhibitor and digoxin. Because most ACE inhibitors are cleared primarily by the kidney, a reduction in dose, increase in dosing interval, or both may be necessary in patients with renal impairment. The most common pharmacodynamic interactions include an increased risk of hyperkalemia when ACE inhibitors are administered with renal epithelial Na^+ channel or aldosterone inhibitors (i.e., potassium-sparing diuretics), and a decrease in glomerular filtration rate when coadministered with NSAIDs.

ACE Inhibitors and Valvular Regurgitation. Many patients with advanced heart failure as a result of ventricular systolic dysfunction have functional mitral regurgitation because of left ventricular and mitral valve ring dilation. Treatment with sodium nitroprusside has been successful in the short term but is impractical as chronic therapy. In a monitored setting, intravenous enalaprilat (1.25 mg) reduced systemic vascular resistance and the volume of regurgitant flow and increased cardiac index significantly only in patients with severe functional mitral regurgitation.[84] In a prospective, randomized, double-blind study, captopril was compared with placebo in 23 patients with ischemic cardiomyopathies and functional mitral regurgitation in a trial design in which patients, after a test dose, received increasing doses of captopril (12.5 mg b.i.d., 25 mg b.i.d., and 50 mg b.i.d.) at 4-week intervals.[85] Importantly, significant improvements in stroke volume, systemic vascular resistance, left atrial size, and a daily activity status index were present only in patients receiving 100 mg/day of captopril. These data, when combined with results of the Survival and Ventricular Enlargement (SAVE) study[81] and SOLVD treatment trial,[74] demonstrate that progressive left ventricular dilation, which is associated with functional mitral regurgitation, can be prevented by ACE inhibitors, and that these drugs are effective in the chronic management of this complication of left ventricular dysfunction.

ACE Inhibitors and Cough. Cough is a relatively frequent and annoying side effect of long-term therapy with ACE inhibitors.[86–88] The prevalence of cough is probably between 5% and 20% of all patients receiving an ACE inhibitor and appears to be higher in patients with congestive heart failure. Patients with underlying structural lung disease or asthma are not at increased risk for this adverse effect. The frequency of cough in both the treatment and prevention arms of the SOLVD trials[65, 74] and the Veterans Heart Failure Trial–II (V-HeFT-II) study[82] was about 33%, but cough was also a frequent complaint in heart failure patients receiving either placebo or other classes of vasodilators (about 25%). Approximately 3% of patients in the SAVE study receiving active drug had to be withdrawn because of cough compared with 1% receiving placebo.[81] This symptom usually disappears within several days after discontinuing the drug but may take up to 2 weeks to disappear. Switching to a different ACE inhibitor is rarely effective in reducing this side effect.[87] Some patients respond to a reduction in dose. Angiotensin receptor antagonists (e.g., losartan) may be the best alternative for most patients with intractable cough. However, a clear survival benefit in patients with heart failure for this class of RAS antagonists has not yet been demonstrated. Inhaled sodium cromoglycate (40 mg/day in divided doses) has proved effective in reducing the frequency of cough in short-term trials.[88]

Angiotensin II Receptor Antagonists

The first Ang II receptor antagonist to undergo dose-ranging and safety trials in humans with heart failure was losartan. Despite its specificity for only one class of Ang II receptors (i.e., AT1) and the lack of bradykinin-potentiating activity that is characteristic of ACE inhibitors, losartan's spectrum of activity appears to be very similar to that of the ACE inhibitors,[89] although experience with patients in heart failure is limited. In patients with mild to moderate heart failure, losartan (25–50 mg/day given as a single daily dose) resulted in 10%–15% declines in mean arterial pressure, a fall in pulmonary capillary wedge pressure, and an increase in cardiac output.[90–92] As with ACE inhibitors, there was no reflex tachycardia associated with the decline in blood pressure and no evidence of tolerance to the drug's hemodynamic effects over a 12-week period.[91] In larger trials of losartan in the treatment of primary hypertension, there has been no increased frequency of cough associated with its use. Although losartan has a convenient pharmacokinetic profile, is well tolerated, and will probably prove to be an effective and safe drug for hypertension and heart failure patients, it does not appear to offer any important advantages over ACE inhibitors in the treatment of heart failure. Ang II receptor blockers may prove to be an acceptable alternative in patients who cannot tolerate ACE inhibitors.

Renin Inhibitors

The pharmaceutical industry has developed a number of agents that inhibit the enzymatic activity of renin, and new agents with high affinities for human renin are being generated that also have acceptable oral bioavailability. Intravenous infusion of remikiren (RO 42-5892) or enalkiren (A-64662) in patients with mild to moderate heart failure resulted in an immediate fall in mean arterial pressure that was similar in magnitude to that produced by intravenous enalaprilat.[93, 94] Administration of an ACE inhibitor to patients already receiving remikiren, or vice versa, resulted in no additional hemodynamic effect. Although it is likely that orally bioavailable and specific renin inhibitors will be developed in the near future, the available data do not suggest that these drugs will have a spectrum of activity in heart failure that is importantly different from those of the ACE inhibitors of AT1 receptor antagonists.

Nitrovasodilators

The specific cellular mechanisms responsible for the direct relaxation of vascular smooth muscle that is characteristic of the nitrovasodilators have become apparent only in the past decade despite the fact that these drugs are the oldest vasodilators in common clinical practice. It is now understood that these drugs mimic the activity of nitric oxide and its congeners, collectively termed nitrogen oxides (NO_x). These agents are autocrine and paracrine signaling autacoids that are formed in endothelial and smooth muscle cells throughout the vasculature, as well as in many other cell types, including cardiac muscle cells.[95–97] These autacoids subserve a number of cellular functions depending on the specific cell type and tissue in which they are synthesized, ranging from inhibition of platelet aggregation and bactericidal activity in macrophages to the regulation of memory formation in the brain, among numerous other functions.

Nitrogen oxides were originally identified as the bioactive factors responsible for endothelium-dependent relaxation of blood vessels.[98] Their activity is based on the ability of nitric oxide to bind to a heme moiety in soluble guanylate cyclase. Unlike nitroprusside, which is spontaneously converted to nitric oxide by endogenous intracellular reducing agents such as glutathione, nitroglycerin and other organic nitrates undergo a more complex enzymatic biotransformation to nitric oxide or bioactive S-nitrosothiols.[99] The activities of specific enzymes and cofactors required for this biotransformation, although not yet clearly identified, appear to differ within the vascular beds among organs and at different levels of the vasculature within an organ.

Nitroprusside

Nitroprusside is an effective venous and arterial vasodilator and acts to reduce both ventricular preload and afterload. Because it is quickly metabolized to cyanide and nitric oxide, its onset of action is rapid, and upward titration can usually be achieved expeditiously to achieve an optimal and predictable hemodynamic effect. For these reasons, nitroprusside is commonly used in intensive care settings for management of acutely decompensated heart failure when blood pressure is adequate to maintain cerebral, coronary, and renal perfusion. Ventricular filling pressures are rapidly reduced by an increase in venous compliance, resulting in a redistribution of blood volume from central to peripheral veins. This nitrovasodilator is among the most effective afterload-reducing agents because of its spectrum of vasodilating activity on different vascular beds.[100, 101] It reduces peripheral vascular resistance, increases aortic wall compliance, and, at optimal doses, improves ventricular-vascular coupling.[102] Nitroprusside also dilates pulmonary arterioles, thereby reducing right ventricular afterload.

This combination of preload- and afterload-reducing effects also improves myocardial energetics by reducing wall stress, which is of particular importance when oxygen delivery is limited, such as in an ischemic cardiomyopathy. However, care must be taken to ensure that blood pressure does not fall to the point of compromising diastolic coronary artery flow or activating a marked baroreflex-mediated increase in sympathetic nervous system tone. Nitroprusside is particularly effective in patients with congestive heart failure caused by or complicated by significant mitral regurgitation or left-to-right shunts through a ventricular septal defect.

As with most vasodilators, the commonest adverse effect of nitroprusside is hypotension. However, the redistribution of blood flow from central organs to peripheral vascular beds may limit or prevent any increase in renal blood flow in some patients, despite an increase in cardiac output. Nitroprusside-induced nonselective pulmonary arteriolar vasodilation may worsen ventilation-perfusion mismatches in patients with advanced chronic obstructive pulmonary disease or large pleural effusions. Arteriolar vasodilation throughout the coronary vascular bed may reduce perfusion pressure to muscle supplied by partially occluded vessels (i.e., coronary steal) in patients with heart failure and coronary atherosclerosis characterized by advanced fixed lesions of epicardial coronary arteries. This factor may account for an increase in the frequency of angina in occasional patients with an ischemic cardiomyopathy despite a favorable hemodynamic response to nitroprusside. An organic nitrate, in addition to hydralazine or an ACE inhibitor, should be substituted in these cases.

Hydrocyanic acid and cyanide are by-products of the biotransformation of nitroprusside. Cyanide toxicity is uncommon, however, because cyanide is rapidly metabolized by the liver to thiocyanate, which is cleared by the kidney. Thiocyanate toxicity, cyanide toxicity, or both may occur in the presence of hepatic or renal failure and following prolonged infusions of nitroprusside in patients with marginal cardiac output or passive congestion of the liver. Thiocyanate toxicity, which is more common in patients with renal insufficiency, should be suspected in any patient receiving nitroprusside who has unexplained abdominal pain, mental status changes, or convulsions. Clinical manifestations of cyanide toxicity are more subtle in onset than those of thiocyanate toxicity and are usually manifested by a decline in cardiac output accompanied by a metabolic acidosis as a result of accumulation of lactic acid. Assays for blood levels of both thiocyanate and cyanide are commonly available in clinical laboratories. Methemoglobinemia is another unusual complication of prolonged, high-dose nitroprusside infusion.

Organic Nitrates and Molsidomine

In acute as well as chronic congestive heart failure, isosorbide dinitrate; isosorbide mononitrate; nitroglycerin as an intravenous preparation, ointment, sublingual tablets, and lingual spray; and molsidomine are relatively safe and effective agents for reducing ventricular preload through an increase in peripheral venous capacitance. These drugs also decrease pulmonary and systemic vascular resistance, usually at doses higher than those required for an increase in venous capacitance. Tolerance does develop to these drugs (discussed later), but tolerance should be distinguished from a resistance to the initial vasodilating effects of nitroglycerin. Resistance is occasionally seen in some patients with advanced heart failure, elevated right and left heart filling pressures, and peripheral edema. These patients may respond to nitroglycerin only after intravascular volume and right atrial pressures have been decreased by diuretics.[103]

Because of their relatively selective vasodilating effects on the epicardial coronary vasculature, the organic nitrates may directly increase systolic and diastolic ventricular function by improving coronary flow in patients with an ischemic cardiomyopathy, in addition to their activity in reducing ventricular filling pressures, wall stress, and oxygen consumption.[104] In acute myocardial infarction, however, the effect of the routine use of nitrovasodilators on mortality remains controversial.[77, 105, 106] Recent trials of several nitrovasodilators (transdermal nitroglycerin in GISSI-3[66]; isosorbide mononitrate in ISIS-4[77]; and molsidomine in the European Study of Prevention of Infarct with Molsidomine [ESPRIM][105]) did not demonstrate any reduction in mortality with these drugs, although they were generally well tolerated by patients.

Despite its limited effects on systemic vascular resistance and the problem of pharmacologic tolerance (discussed below), isosorbide dinitrate has been shown to be more effective than placebo in improving exercise capacity and in reducing symptoms when administered chronically to heart failure patients, particularly when added to another class of vasodilator (e.g., hydralazine, captopril). The experience with newer nitrovasodilators, including isosorbide mononitrates and molsidomine, in the treatment of heart failure is limited compared with their use in the treatment of angina. Molsidomine, following formation of its active metabolite, linsidomine (SIN-1), in the liver, is effective in reducing systemic vascular resistance, pulmonary capillary wedge pressure, and right atrial pressure.[106] Tolerance to the arteriolar and venular vasodilating effects of this drug does develop, although its extent and time course may differ from tolerance associated with organic nitrates. The spectrum of activity of 5-isosorbide mononitrate would not be expected to differ from isosorbide dinitrate in heart failure. Although its greater bioavailability and longer elimination half-life may provide a convenient pharmacokinetic profile, among the nitrate formulations, only isosorbide dinitrate has been shown to increase exercise tolerance[107] and, with hydralazine, prolong survival in patients with heart failure.[32]

Nitrovasodilator Tolerance

The rapid development of tolerance to the venous and arteriolar vasodilating effects of the nitrovasodilators has been known for more than a century, and although well documented, the mechanisms responsible are not clearly understood.[108-110] It is likely that several mechanisms contribute to decreased responsiveness to nitrovasodilators with time, and that the importance of the relative contribution of each potential mechanism differs with the specific drug employed, the underlying disease (heart failure vs. angina), and the specific vascular bed.

There is good evidence that nitrovasodilators cause a shift in solute and water into the intravascular space within hours of their administration, presumably because of changes in the physical (Starling) forces across capillary beds. However, diuretics do not consistently blunt the development of nitrate tolerance. Although the activation of reflex neurohumoral and renal mechanisms would be expected to occur with any vasodilator that reduced mean arterial pressure, most of these pathways (e.g., the sympathetic nervous system, the intrarenal RAS) are chronically activated in advanced heart failure, and pressure may decrease as cardiac output improves and venous congestion diminishes. However, ACE inhibitors have been reported to blunt or to have no effect on the development of tolerance.[111-115] The remaining suggested mechanisms contributing to nitrovasodilator tolerance can be classified as "end-organ" tolerance, or decreased responsiveness of smooth muscle in the vasculature to the continuous presence of these drugs.[110] Much attention has focused on whether nitrate tolerance represents a decreased ability to form cyclic guanosine monophosphate (cGMP) or a deficit of cofactors and other intermediates necessary for the formation of nitrogen oxides from organic nitrates within smooth muscle cells, or an excess of superoxide anion produced by adjacent endothelial cells that could inactivate nitrogen oxides generated by nitrovasodilators.[109, 116] Treatment of nitrate tolerance in angina and heart failure has been attempted with excess sulfhydryl donors in vitro and in vivo, but the results are inconsistent.[109]

These apparently conflicting data probably reflect subtle but important differences in experimental design, differences in the clinical characteristics of each study population, the complex and poorly understood molecular pharmacology of these drugs at the cellular level, and perhaps most importantly, the need of many clinical investigations to provide a single unifying explanation for "end-organ" nitrate tolerance.

Hydralazine

Hydralazine is an effective antihypertensive drug, particularly when combined with other agents that blunt compensatory increases in sympathetic tone and salt and water retention, although its cellular mechanism of action remains poorly understood. In heart failure, hydralazine reduces right and left ventricular afterload by reducing systemic as well as pulmonary vascular resistance. Unlike its effects in hypertension, this is usually not accompanied by important reflex changes in sympathetic nervous system activity unless symptomatic hypotension occurs. These hemodynamic changes result in an augmentation of forward stroke volume and a reduction in ventricular systolic wall stress and the regurgitant fraction in mitral insufficiency. Hydralazine also appears to have "direct," modest, positively inotropic activity in cardiac muscle that is unrelated to afterload reduction. Haas and Leier[117] have argued that this property makes hydralazine an ideal agent with which to withdraw patients with decompensated end-stage congestive heart failure from intravenous inotropic agents such as dobutamine or milrinone. Hydralazine is effective in reducing renal vascular resistance and in increasing renal blood flow to a greater degree than most other vasodilators; therefore, it may be the vasodilator of choice in heart failure patients with renal dysfunction who cannot tolerate an ACE inhibitor.

Hydralazine has minimal effects on venous capacitance and therefore is most effective when combined with agents with venodilating activity (e.g., organic nitrates). The combination of hydralazine (300 mg/day) and isosorbide dinitrate was less effective than enalapril in reducing mortality in heart failure patients in the V-HeFT-II trial,[82] although this combination of agents did increase survival compared with placebo or the α_1-adrenergic antagonist prazosin in V-HeFT-I.[32] This is an important point because a number of promising vasodilator drugs, some of which also have direct effects on cardiac contractility (e.g., milrinone, flosequinan), have been shown to decrease survival in heart failure. Although not yet tested in clinical trials, hydralazine, administered with or without nitrates, may provide additional hemodynamic improvement for patients already being treated with conventional doses of an ACE inhibitor, digoxin, and diuretics in advanced heart failure.[118]

Adverse Effects

Side effects that may necessitate dose adjustment or withdrawal of hydralazine are common. For example, in the V-HeFT-I trial,[32] 20% of patients complained of symptoms that could have been related to hydralazine. The most common complaints—headache and dizziness—could also have been caused by the concomitantly administered nitrates, however. Often, the side effects diminish with time or respond to a reduction in dose.

Metabolism

Hydralazine metabolism is primarily mediated by hepatic acetylation.[119] Therefore, patients with a "slow acetylater" phenotype have a prolonged elimination half-life of the drug. At the usual doses and dosing intervals of hydralazine, these patients are at greater risk of developing arthritis or other components of a lupus-like syndrome. This complication is unusual in heart failure, however, perhaps because of the somewhat lower doses than typically are used for the treatment of hypertension. Hydralazine may induce a reflex increase in sympathetic tone sufficient to cause angina in some patients with ischemic cardiac disease, although this is less likely in heart failure patients because of the concomitant increase in cardiac output.

Drug Administration

Intravenous hydralazine is available but provides little practical advantage over oral formulations and is less predictable and more difficult to titrate than other intravenous vasodilators and inotropic agents (e.g., nitroprusside, dobutamine). The oral bioavailability and pharmacokinetics of elimination of hydralazine do not appear to be importantly affected by heart failure unless there is severe hepatic congestion or hypoperfusion. Intravenous hydralazine may be useful in heart failure during pregnancy, in which relative contraindications exist for most other vasodilators.

As with the ACE inhibitors, the most appropriate dose of hydralazine has not been determined in heart failure. A daily dose of 300 mg was employed in the V-HeFT trials[32, 82] and, in combination with isosorbide dinitrate, was documented to have a positive impact on survival. Although additional hemodynamic benefit may be demonstrable at doses higher than 300 mg/day, which were more commonly used before ACE inhibitors became available, this may not be translated into prolonged survival.

Calcium Channel Antagonists

Four classes of calcium channel antagonists are commonly available: phenylalkylamines (e.g., verapamil), benzothiazepenes (e.g., diltiazem), diarylaminopropylamines (e.g., bepridil), and dihydropyridines (e.g., nifedipine). All four of these are effective vasodilators; however, none has been shown to produce sustained improvement in symptoms in heart failure patients with predominant systolic ventricular dysfunction. These drugs appear to worsen symptoms and may increase mortality in patients with systolic dysfunction. This includes patients with heart failure as a result of ischemic disease.[120, 121] The reason for these adverse effects of calcium channel blockers in heart failure patients is unclear. It may be related to the known negative inotropic effects of these drugs or to reflex neurohumoral activation.

Second-generation calcium channel antagonists of the dihydropyridine class, particularly felodipine, appear to have fewer negatively inotropic effects than earlier drugs of this class and are being evaluated in randomized prospective trials to determine their effects on both symptoms and mortality in heart failure patients already receiving standard medical management.[121–124] Amlodipine has a prolonged elimination half-life (>36 h), resulting in more consistent vasodilation and less reflex tachycardia.[122–124] Whether these effects will translate into improved survival or improved hemodynamics and control of congestive symptoms is currently being evaluated in the Prospective Randomized Amlodipine Survival Evaluation (PRAISE) trial. Felodopine demonstrates a tenfold increase in selectivity for vascular smooth muscle over nifedipine, with little or no negative inotropic effect at clinically relevant doses.[121, 125] The combination of felodipine with an ACE inhibitor may result in additional hemodynamic benefit without significant sympathetic nervous system activation or adverse effects on survival. This possibility is being tested prospectively in the V-HeFT-III trial.[126]

It should be noted that calcium channel antagonists may be useful for the treatment of congestive heart failure symptoms caused by diastolic dysfunction, such as hypertensive or idiopathic hypertrophic cardiomyopathies. Both verapamil and diltiazem tend to facilitate diastolic relaxation and lower diastolic filling pressures, and both drugs also decrease heart rate, an important determinant of diastolic filling time. These agents can also be useful in the acute management of patients in heart failure caused by most supraventricular tachyarrhythmias in the absence of severe right or left ventricular systolic dysfunction. The exception are those patients with known or suspected extranodal atrioventricular accessory pathways.

Other Vasodilators

A number of additional classes of vasodilator drugs, including sympatholytic agents, are effective in reducing ventricular preload and afterload and improving symptoms in heart failure. None of these agents, however, has been shown to improve survival in heart failure patients, and their use should be restricted to the treatment of patients who are intolerant to or not adequately treated by the ACE inhibitors or hydralazine with a nitrovasodilator. Several new classes of drugs, including K^+ channel activators (e.g., nicorandil)[127] and "calcium sensitizers"[128, 129] that exhibit positive inotropic and vasodilating activity (e.g., levosimendan), are undergoing clinical testing. In addition, a mechanical aortic counterpulsation device (i.e., intra-aortic balloon pump) often provides the most effective short-term means to reduce left ventricular afterload and directly increase cardiac output for the treatment of acute or chronic decompensated heart failure that is refractory to treatment with standard drug regimens and is not complicated by significant aortic insufficiency.

INOTROPIC DRUGS

Cardiac Glycosides

The chemical structure of this venerable class of drugs includes a steroid nucleus containing an unsaturated lactone at the C_{17} position and one or more glycosidic residues at C_3. Examples are found in a large number of plants and several toad species, typically serving as a venom or toxin that alters the future behavior of predators.[130] William Withering's 1785 monograph contains the first comprehensive description of digitalis glycosides in the treatment of congestive heart failure.[131] This treatise describes the therapeutic efficacy and toxicities of the leaves of the common foxglove plant, *Digitalis purpurea*.[131] Other digitalis glycosides are derived from the leaves of *Digitalis lanata* (digitoxin and digoxin) and from the seeds of *Strophanthus gratus* (ouabain). The terms *digitalis glycoside* and *cardiac glycoside* are often used interchangeably, although cardiac glycoside is the more inclusive term, whereas digitalis glycoside should be reserved for compounds derived from *Digitalis* species. Digoxin is now the most commonly prescribed cardiac glycoside because of its convenient pharmacokinetics, alternative routes of administration, and widespread availability of serum drug level measurements.

Mechanisms of Action

Inhibition of Monovalent Cation Active Transport. All cardiac glycosides are potent and selective inhibitors of the active transport of Na^+ and K^+ across cell membranes. These drugs bind to a specific high-affinity site on the extracytoplasmic face of the alpha subunit of Na^+K^+-ATPase, the enzymatic equivalent of the cellular "sodium pump."[132] The affinity of the alpha subunit for cardiac glycosides varies among species and among the three known mammalian alpha subunit isoforms, each of which is encoded by a separate gene.

The presence of the ouabain binding site on the alpha subunit of Na^+K^+-ATPase has led to speculation that endogenous ouabain-like hormones or locally acting substances might exist that would serve as a regulatory ligand for the enzyme.[133, 134] The authors suggest the alternative possibility: that the evolutionary persistence of the ouabain binding site could be the result of a requirement for a specific amino acid sequence and conformation of the enzyme necessary for successful ion translocation but which has also provided a target for evolutionary selection favoring certain plants and toads by serving as a means of poisoning animal predators.

There is evidence from site-directed mutagenesis studies that the affinity of Na^+K^+-ATPase for cardiac glycosides is determined by the amino acid composition of the first transmembrane domain and the extracellular domain between the first and second (i.e., H_1 and H_2) transmembrane domains, and also the extracellular loop between the H_7 and H_8 transmembrane domains.[135] Cardiac glycoside binding to the alpha subunit of Na^+K^+-ATPase previously was thought to require the presence of an unsaturated lactone ring at C_{17}, a beta hydroxyl group at C_{14}, and *cis* stereochemical fusion of the A–B and C–D rings of the steroid nucleus, unlike the conformation of cholesterol and steroid hormones in which these ring junctions are *trans*. These structure-activity relations now appear to be unduly restrictive, because it has since been reported that certain derivatives of progesterone with a *trans* ring fusion characteristic of steroid hormones, such as 14-beta-hydroxy progesterone, bind to Na^+K^+-ATPase and inhibit Na^+K^+-ATPase activity.[136]

Cardiac glycoside binding to and inhibition of the Na^+K^+-ATPase sodium pump is reversible and entropically driven. Under physiologic conditions, these drugs bind preferentially to the enzyme following phosphorylation of a beta-aspartate on the cytoplasmic face of the alpha subunit, thus stabilizing this "E_2P" conformation.[132] Extracellular K^+ promotes dephosphorylation at this site as a step in this cation's active transport into the cytosol, which is accompanied by a decrease in the cardiac glycoside binding affinity of the enzyme. This presumably explains why increased extracellular K^+ tends to reverse some manifestations of digitalis toxicity.

Positive Inotropic Effect. Since about 1920, cardiac glycosides have been known to increase the velocity and extent of shortening of cardiac muscle, resulting in a shift upward and leftward of the ventricular function (Frank-Starling) curve relating stroke work to filling volume or pressure (see Fig. 9–1). This occurs in normal as well as failing myocardium and in atrial as well as ventricular muscle. The effect appears to be sustained for periods of weeks or months without evidence of desensitization or tolerance.[137, 138] This positive inotropic effect is the result of an increase in the availability of cytosolic Ca^{2+} during systole, thus increasing the velocity and extent of sarcomere shortening. This increase in intracellular Ca^{2+} is a consequence of cardiac glycoside–induced inhibition of the sarcolemmal Na^+K^+-ATPase.

Na^+ and Ca^{2+} ions enter the cardiac muscle cell during each cycle of depolarization, contraction, and repolarization (Fig. 9–4). After activation of the fast Na^+ channel and the consequent depolarization, Ca^{2+} enters the cell via the L-type Ca^{2+} channel and triggers the release of additional Ca^{2+} into the cytosol from the sarcoplasmic reticulum (SR). During repolarization and relaxation, Ca^{2+} is again sequestered in the SR by a Ca^{2+}-ATPase, and is also extruded from the cell by the Na^+-Ca^{2+} exchanger and by a sarcolemmal Ca^{2+}-ATPase. Because the capacity of the Na^+-Ca^{2+} exchanger to extrude Ca^{2+} from the cell depends on the intracellular Na^+ activity, binding of a cardiac glycoside to the sarcolemmal Na^+K^+-ATPase and inhibition of sodium pump activity reduces the rate of active Na^+ extrusion, and cytosolic Na^+ content rises. This reduces the transmembrane Na^+ gradient driving the extrusion of intracellular Ca^{2+}, and more Ca^{2+} is taken up by the SR and is available to activate contraction during the subsequent cell depolarization cycle. Evidence supporting this mechanism is available from studies in which radionuclide tracers, cation-selective microelectrodes, and intracellular aequorin or ion-sensitive fluorescent dyes were used. Widespread acceptance of this mechanism of action awaited demonstration that small changes in intracellular Na^+ activity are accompanied by substantial increases in developed tension.[132, 139] Excessive increases in intracellular Ca^{2+} are believed to contribute to cardiac glycoside toxicity when Ca^{2+} overload results in spontaneous cycles of Ca^{2+} release and reuptake. This may lead to Ca^{2+}-induced activation of inward Ca^{2+} current, resulting in transient late depolarizations (afterdepolarizations) that may be accompanied by aftercontractions (Fig. 9–5) and probably contribute to toxic electrophysiologic effects.

Other mechanisms that may contribute to the inotropic actions of cardiac glycosides include increased cytosolic Ca^{2+} acting as a positive feedback signal to increase Ca^{2+} entry through sarcolemmal L-type Ca^{2+} channels.[132] Cardiac glycosides have also been reported to increase Ca^{2+}-triggered Ca^{2+} release via cardiac (but not skeletal) muscle SR Ca^{2+} release channels in isolated SR vesicles as a result of the increased probability of channel openings (not increased single channel conductance) when cardiac glycosides in nanomolar concentrations were present at the cytosolic face of oriented SR vesicle preparations inserted into planar lipid membranes.[139]

Regulation of Sympathetic Nervous System Activity. Heart failure is well known to be accompanied by an increase in sympa-

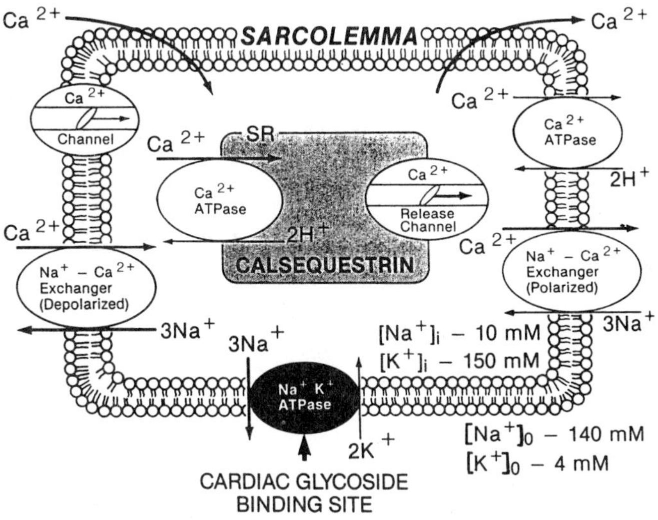

Figure 9–4. Sarcolemmal exchange of Na^+ and Ca^{2+} during cell depolarization and repolarization. Na^+ and Ca^{2+} ions enter mammalian cardiac muscle cells during each cycle of membrane depolarization. Ca^{2+} entry triggers the release through Ca^{2+} release channels of larger amounts of Ca^{2+} from internal stores in the sarcoplasmic reticulum (SR). The resulting increase in intracellular Ca^{2+} interacts with troponin C and is responsible for activating the cross-bridge interactions between actin filaments and myosin cross-bridges that result in sarcomere shortening. The electrochemical gradient for Na^+ across the sarcolemma is maintained by active (i.e., ATP-consuming) transport of Na^+ out of the cell by the sarcolemmal Na^+,K^+-ATPase. Na^+ is actively extruded by Na^+,K^+-ATPase, whereas the majority of cytosolic Ca^{2+} is pumped by a Ca^{2+}-ATPase back into the SR, where it is bound by the protein calsequestrin, and the remainder is removed from the cell by either a plasma membrane Ca^{2+}-ATPase or a high capacity Na^+-Ca^{2+} cation exchange protein. This sarcolemmal membrane protein exchanges three Na^+ ions for every Ca^{2+} ion, using the electrochemical potential of Na^+ to drive Ca^{2+} extrusion. Notice that the direction of cation transport may reverse briefly during depolarization, when the electrical gradient across the sarcolemma is transiently reversed. Beta-adrenergic agonists and phosphodiesterase inhibitors, by increasing intracellular cAMP levels, activate protein kinase A, which enhances the contractile state by phosphorylating target proteins including phospholamban and the subunit of the L-type Ca^{2+} channel. (Adapted from Smith TW, Braunwald E, Kelly RA: The management of heart failure. *In* Braunwald E [ed]: Heart Disease, 4th ed, p 480. Philadelphia: WB Saunders, 1992.)

thetic nervous system activity, in part as a result of a reduction in the sensitivity of the arterial baroreflex response to blood pressure. This reduction in sensitivity results in a decline in tonic baroreflex suppression of central nervous system–directed sympathetic activity. This loss of sensitivity of the normal baroreflex arc also appears to contribute to the sustained elevation in plasma norepinephrine, renin, and vasopressin levels characteristic of heart failure. This sustained activation of sympathetic nervous system activity, which initially serves to maintain blood pressure and cardiac output by increasing heart rate, contractility, and systemic vascular resistance, also contributes to decreasing excretion of salt and water by the kidneys. Despite the obvious evolutionary advantage of this adaptive response to stresses such as hypovolemia, the longer-term consequences in chronic heart failure may well be maladaptive.

Mason and colleagues[140] observed that intravenous ouabain increased mean arterial pressure, forearm vascular resistance, and venous tone in normal human subjects, probably as a result of direct effects on vascular smooth muscle. In contrast, patients with heart failure responded with a decline in heart rate and other effects that were consistent with enhanced baroreflex responsiveness. Direct effects of cardiac glycosides on carotid baroreflex responsiveness to changes in carotid sinus pressure have been reported in isolated baroreceptor preparations from animals with experimentally induced heart failure.[141] Ferguson and colleagues[142] demonstrated in patients with moderate to severe heart failure that infusion of deslanoside increased forearm blood flow and cardiac index and decreased heart rate, concomitant with a marked decrease in skeletal muscle sympathetic nerve activity measured as an indicator of centrally mediated sympathetic nervous system activity. In contrast, dobutamine, a sympathomimetic drug that increased cardiac output to a similar degree, did not affect muscle sympathetic nerve activity in these patients.[142, 143] Reduced neurohumoral activation may be an important mechanism contributing to the efficacy of cardiac glycosides in the treatment of patients with heart failure.

Electrophysiologic Actions. New classes of drugs (e.g., adenosine, L-type Ca^{2+} channel antagonists, beta-adrenergic blockers, amiodarone) have displaced digoxin as a first-line agent in the treatment of supraventricular cardiac arrhythmias, with the exception of atrial fibrillation, in which digoxin is often used alone or in combination with a beta-adrenergic blocking agent, verapamil, or diltiazem. Digoxin does, however, remain useful in the management of supraventricular arrhythmias in patients with systolic ventricular dysfunction.[144]

Atrial and ventricular muscle and specialized cardiac pacemaker and conduction fibers differ in their responses and sensitivity to cardiac glycosides. These responses represent the net of direct effects on cardiac cells added to indirect, neurally mediated effects. At usual therapeutic serum concentrations (1–1.5 ng/mL), digoxin usually decreases automaticity and increases maximal diastolic resting membrane potential in atrial and atrioventricular (AV) nodal cells as a result of augmented vagal tone and decreased sympathetic nervous system activity. These effects are accompanied by prolongation of effective refractory period and decreased AV nodal conduction velocity. At higher digoxin levels or in the presence of underlying disease, these effects may cause sinus bradycardia or arrest, prolongation of AV conduction, or heart block. At toxic levels, cardiac glycosides can increase sympathetic nervous system activity, potentially contributing to the generation of arrhythmias. Increased intracellular Ca^{2+} loading and increased sympathetic tone both contribute to an increased rate of spontaneous (phase 4) diastolic depolarization and also to delayed afterdepolarizations (see Fig. 9–5) that may reach threshold and generate propagated action potentials. The combination of increased automaticity and depressed conduction in the His-Purkinje network predisposes to arrhythmias, including ventricular tachycardia and fibrillation.

Pharmacokinetics and Dosing

Digoxin. The half-life for digoxin elimination of 36–48 h in patients with normal or near-normal renal function lies between those of ouabain and digitoxin and facilitates once-per-day dosing for these patients. In the absence of loading doses, near steady-state blood levels are achieved in four to five half-lives, or about 1 week following initiation of maintenance therapy if normal renal function is present. Digoxin is largely excreted unchanged, with a clearance rate proportional to the glomerular filtration rate, resulting in the excretion of approximately one third of body stores daily. In the presence of an elevated blood urea nitrogen-to-creatinine ratio (i.e., prerenal azotemia), digoxin clearance more closely parallels urea clearance, indicating that under these circumstances, some drug filtered at the glomerulus undergoes tubular reabsorption. In patients with heart failure and reduced cardiac reserve, increased cardiac output and renal blood flow in response to treatment with vasodilators or sympathomimetic agents may increase renal digoxin clearance, necessitating dosage adjustment. Digoxin is not removed effectively by peritoneal dialysis or hemodialysis because of its large (4–7 L/kg) volume of distribution. The principal body reservoir for digoxin is skeletal muscle rather than adipose tissue. Accordingly,

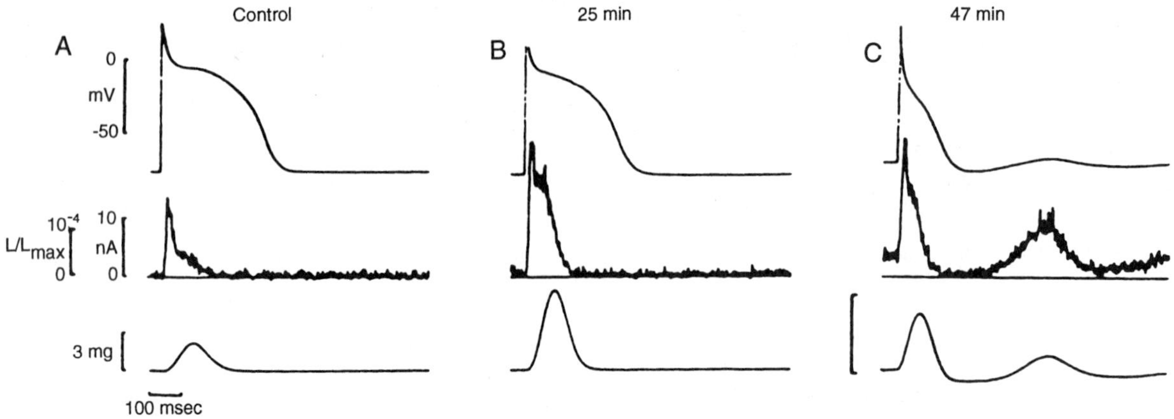

Figure 9–5. Role of intracellular calcium in mediating inotropic and toxic electrophysiologic effects of cardiac glycosides. Simultaneous recordings from an isolated Purkinje fiber of changes in membrane potential *(top trace)*, intracellular Ca^{2+} as reported by the Ca^{2+}-sensitive indicator aequorin *(center trace)*, and developed tension *(bottom trace)* at baseline (i.e., in the absence of a cardiac glycoside) *(A)*, after 25 min of exposure to ouabain *(B)*, and after 47 min exposure to ouabain *(C)*. Compared with the baseline tracing, there is a pronounced rise in the intracellular Ca^{2+} transient with an associated increase in developed tension at 25 min after exposure. However, as toxic effects of ouabain accumulate over time, a characteristic afterdepolarization and aftercontraction indicative of Ca^{2+} overload and cardiac glycoside toxicity become apparent at 47 min after exposure. These afterdepolarizations are a consequence of increasing intracellular Ca^{2+} content induced by the cardiac glycoside that results in spontaneous cycles of Ca^{2+} release and reuptake that are thought to contribute to digitalis-induced arrhythmias. (From Weir WG, Hess D: Excitation-contraction coupling in cardiac Purkinje fibers. Effects of cardiotonic steroids on the intracellular [Ca^{2+}] transient, membrane potential, and contraction. J Physiol 1984; 83:395.)

dosing should be based on estimated lean body mass. Neonates and infants tolerate and tend to require higher doses of digoxin for an equivalent therapeutic effect than older children or adults, although measured absorption and renal clearance rates are similar. Digoxin crosses the placenta, and drug levels in maternal and umbilical vein blood are similar to each other.

Current tablet preparations of digoxin average 70%–80% oral bioavailability; elixir and encapsulated gel preparations approach 90%–100% bioavailability. Parenteral digoxin is available for intravenous use. Loading or maintenance doses can be given by intravenous injection, which should be carried out over at least 15 min to avoid vasoconstrictor responses to more rapid injection. Intramuscu-

TABLE 9–4. DRUG INTERACTIONS WITH DIGOXIN

Drug	Mechanism	Direction and Magnitude of Change in Blood Level*	Suggested Clinical Management*
Cholestyramine, kaolin-pectin, neomycin, sulfasalazine	Decrease absorption	↓ 25%	Give digoxin 8 h before agent, or use solution or gel form
Antacids	Unclear	↓ 25%	Temporal dispersion of doses
Bran	Decreases absorption	↓ 25%	Temporal dispersion of doses
Propafenone, quinidine, verapamil, amiodarone	Decrease renal digoxin clearance, volume of distribution, or both	↑ 70%–100%	Decrease digoxin by 50% and monitor serum digoxin levels as necessary
Thyroxine	Increases volume of distribution and renal clearance	Variable decreases in digoxin blood levels	Monitor serum digoxin levels
Erythromycin, omeprazole, tetracycline	Increase digoxin absorption	↑ 40%–100%	Monitor serum dioxin levels
Albuterol	Increases volume of distribution	↓ 30%	Monitor serum digoxin levels
Captopril, diltiazem, nifedipine, nitrendipine	Variable moderate decrease in digoxin clearance, volume of distribution, or both	Variable increase in blood levels	Monitor serum digoxin levels
Cyclosporine	May decrease renal function	Variable increase in blood levels	Monitor serum digoxin levels frequently
Beta blockers, verapamil, diltiazem, flecainide, disopyramide, bepridil	↓ SA or AV junctional conduction of automaticity		Monitor ECG for evidence of SA or AV block
Kaliuretic diuretics	Decrease serum and tissue K^+, increases automaticity, and promotes inhibition of Na^+, K^+-ATPase by digoxin		Montior ECG for arrhythmias consistent with digoxin toxicity
Sympathomimetic drugs	Increase automaticity		Monitor ECG for arrhythmia
Verapamil, diltiazem, beta-adrenergic blocking agents	Diminish cardiac contractile state		Discontinue or lower dose of Ca^{2+} channel or beta-adrenergic blocker

Symbols and abbreviations: ↓, decreased; ↑, increased; AV, atrioventricular; ECG, electrocardiogram; SA, sinoatrial.
*Approximation only, to be monitored as clinically appropriate.

lar digoxin is absorbed unpredictably, causes local pain, and is not recommended.

Therapeutic Drug Monitoring. Nomograms are available for estimating loading and maintenance doses of digoxin but are not widely used because of variability in individual patient responsiveness to cardiac glycosides and the ready availability in most clinical settings of serum digoxin concentration assays. Various clinical conditions and drug interactions that can alter digoxin's pharmacokinetics (Tables 9–4, 9–5) are also reflected in the serum digoxin level. Reduced thyroid and renal function both decrease the volume of distribution of digoxin, necessitating downward adjustments in loading and maintenance doses. Table 9–5 lists disease states and alterations in plasma and tissue electrolytes that can change patient susceptibility to toxicity at any given dose or serum level of the drug.

Studies using noninvasive indices of ventricular function suggest that there is a nonlinear relation between the serum digoxin concentration and the observed inotropic effect, with the majority of the increase in contractility occurring by the time steady-state levels around 1.8 nmol/L (1.4 ng/mL) are reached (Fig. 9–6). The relation of serum digoxin level to therapeutic effect is less clear in the control of the ventricular rate among patients with atrial fibrillation. The effectiveness of cardiac glycosides given as single agents in controlling ventricular rate during exercise is limited at doses and serum levels in the usual therapeutic range. Overt toxicity tends to emerge at serum concentrations two to three times higher than the target 1.8 nmol/L, but it must always be remembered that a substantial overlap of serum levels exists among patients exhibiting symptoms and signs of toxicity and those with no clinical evidence of intoxication.[145] If ready access to serum digoxin assays is available, a reasonable approach to the initiation of therapy is to begin at 0.125–0.250 mg/day, depending on lean body mass and estimated creatinine clearance, and to measure a serum digoxin level 1 week later, with careful monitoring of the patient's clinical status in the interim. Patients with impaired renal function will not yet have reached steady state and will need to be monitored closely until four to five clearance half-lives have elapsed, which may be as long as 3 weeks. Oral or intravenous loading with digoxin, although generally safe, is rarely necessary, because other safer and more effective drugs exist for short-term inotropic support or for initial treatment of supraventricular arrhythmias (see Chapter 16).

Blood samples for serum digoxin level measurement should be taken 6–8 h following the last digoxin dose. Serum level monitoring is justified in patients with substantially altered drug clearance rates or volumes of distribution (e.g., very old, debilitated, or very obese patients). Adequacy of digoxin dosing and risk of toxicity in a given patient should never be based on a single isolated serum digoxin concentration measurement.

Digitoxin. Digitoxin is the principal native cardiac glycoside present in digitalis leaf. It is the least polar and most slowly excreted of all available cardiac glycosides. Oral bioavailability approaches 100% and is less affected by malabsorption syndromes than is digoxin. Unlike digoxin, digitoxin is about 97% bound to albumin in normal plasma and is extensively metabolized in the liver with minimal renal clearance of the native glycoside. Displacement of digitoxin from plasma protein by some drugs, including warfarin, can occur but rarely results in clinically important changes in serum levels at usual digitoxin doses. The elimination half-life is 4–6 days irrespective of renal function, resulting in a stable steady-state level of drug 3–4 weeks after initiation of a daily maintenance dose. Therapeutic serum or plasma concentrations are about ten times higher than those of digoxin as a result of serum protein binding.

TABLE 9–5. FACTORS THAT ALTER PATIENT SENSITIVITY TO CARDIAC GLYCOSIDES

Serum electrolyte abnormalities
Hypokalemia or hyperkalemia
Hypomagnesemia
Hypercalcemia
Acid-base imbalances
Thyroid status
Abnormal renal function
Autonomic nervous system tone
Respiratory disease
Concomitant drug therapy
Type and severity of underlying heart disease

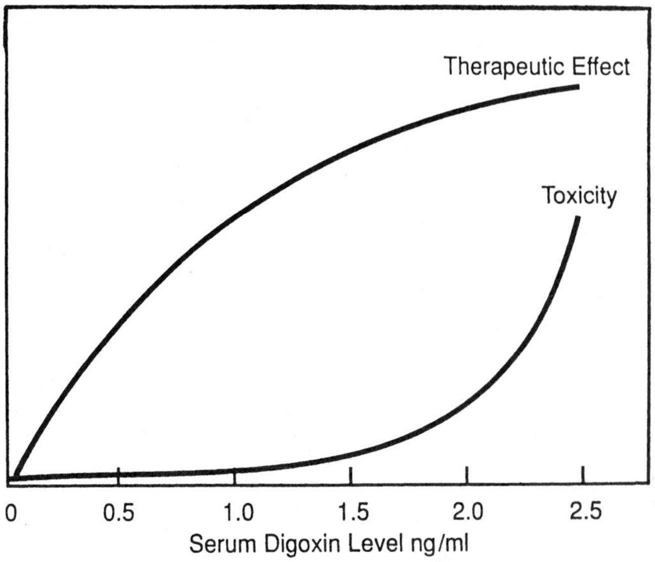

Figure 9–6. Conceptual relation between positive inotropic effect and risk of toxicity as a function of digoxin serum concentration. The expected rise in therapeutic effect with increasing serum levels of digoxin *(upper curve)* begins to flatten at serum levels higher than 1.5 ng/mL. The incidence of clinically important toxicity is low until approximately 2 ng/mL but rises more steeply thereafter. Despite a large body of clinical evidence that validates these observations for many patients with heart failure, individual persons differ in their response to "therapeutic" serum levels of digoxin. (Adapted from Leier CV [ed]: Cardiotonic Drugs: A Clinical Survey, p 85. New York: Marcel Dekker, 1987.)

Ouabain and Deslanoside. Before the development of other therapeutic approaches to the treatment of supraventricular arrhythmias, a number of relatively water-soluble and rapidly acting cardiac glycosides and cardioactive steroids such as ouabain and deslanoside were developed for parenteral administration. These agents are poorly absorbed by the gut and must be given intravenously. Ouabain and deslanoside undergo predominantly renal clearance, with an elimination half-life of 18–24 h in normal persons.

Drug Interactions With Digoxin

Drugs that have pharmacokinetic interactions with digoxin are listed in Table 9–4. Verapamil, quinidine, and amiodarone are commonly administered with digoxin, and dosing must be adjusted appropriately. Drugs that reduce digoxin's volume of distribution and renal clearance rate (e.g., quinidine) necessitate decreases in both loading and maintenance doses of the cardiac glycoside. Indirect pharmacokinetic interactions also occur. Cyclosporine, for example, often reduces renal function, and consequently digoxin clearance, in cardiac transplant patients. Pharmacodynamic interactions between digoxin and other drugs include those with sympathomimetic amines that can contribute to the genesis of arrhythmias at digoxin concentrations in the usual therapeutic range.

Digitalis Toxicity

The incidence and severity of digitalis toxicity have declined over the past two decades for several reasons. Safe and effective alternative drugs are available for the treatment of supraventricular arrhythmias; there is increased understanding of digoxin pharmacokinetics as well as recognition of important interactions between digoxin and a number of commonly used drugs; and there is widespread use of serum digoxin level monitoring.[146] Nevertheless, patients with heart failure—especially severe heart failure—are often at increased risk for adverse electrophysiologic effects of digitalis. The recognition of digitalis toxicity continues to be an important consideration in the assessment of arrhythmias and neurologic and gastrointestinal symptoms (Table 9–6) in patients receiving cardiac glycosides.[147]

Disturbances of cardiac impulse formation, conduction, or both are the hallmarks of digitalis toxicity. Among the common electrocardiographic manifestations are ectopic beats of AV junctional or ventricular origin, first-degree AV block, an excessively slow ventricular rate response to atrial fibrillation, and an accelerated AV junctional pacemaker. These manifestations may require only dosage adjustment and monitoring, as clinically appropriate. Sinus bradycardia, sinoatrial arrest or exit block, and second- or third-degree AV conduction delay often respond to atropine, but temporary ventricular pacing is sometimes necessary and should be available. Potassium administration is often useful for atrial, AV junctional, or ventricular ectopic rhythms, even when the serum potassium level is in the normal range, unless high-grade AV block is also present. Lidocaine and phenytoin, which in conventional doses have minimal effects on AV conduction, are useful in the management of worsening ventricular arrhythmias that threaten hemodynamic compromise. Electrical cardioversion can precipitate severe rhythm disturbances in patients with overt digitalis toxicity and should be used with particular caution. A more comprehensive discussion of the treatment of digitalis toxicity can be found elsewhere.[147]

Potentially life-threatening digoxin or digitoxin toxicity can be reversed by antidigoxin immunotherapy.[148] Purified Fab fragments from digoxin-specific antisera are available at most poison control centers and larger hospitals in North America and Europe. The smaller (molecular weight, 50,000) Fab fragments have a larger volume of distribution, more rapid onset of action, and more rapid clearance, as well as reduced immunogenicity compared with intact IgG. Clinical experience in adults and children has established the effectiveness and safety of antidigoxin Fab in treating life-threatening digoxin toxicity, including cases of massive ingestion with suicidal intent. Doses of Fab are calculated according to a simple formula based on either the estimated dose of drug ingested or the total body digoxin burden (Table 9–7) and are administered intravenously in saline over 30–60 min. Recrudescent digoxin toxicity is unusual, but can occur 24–48 h after Fab administration in patients with normal renal function or later in patients with renal impairment. Determination of the efficacy and cost effectiveness of less-than-complete neutralizing doses of digoxin-specific Fab fragments for suspected or moderate cases of digoxin toxicity requires further assessment.

TABLE 9–6. CENTRAL NERVOUS SYSTEM–MEDIATED TOXIC EFFECTS OF CARDIAC GLYCOSIDES

Psychiatric: Delirium, fatigue, malaise, confusion, dizziness, abnormal dreams
Visual: Disturbed color vision, halos
Gastrointestinal: Anorexia, nausea, vomiting, abdominal pain (may be a result of mesenteric arteriolar constriction)
Respiratory: Enhanced ventilatory response to hypoxia
Cardiac: Proarrhythmic effects (mediated by both direct and neurohormonal mechanisms)

ADRENERGIC SIGNALING IN HEART FAILURE

In this section, the changes in beta-adrenergic signaling in cardiac muscle that are relevant to the drug treatment of heart failure are briefly reviewed. For a more general overview of biogenic amine signaling, including the molecular pharmacology of GTP-binding protein-linked receptors, the reader is referred to several comprehensive overviews.[149–153] In the normal human myocardium, β_1 receptors predominate in cardiac myocytes, with a ratio of β_1 to β_2 receptors of approximately 3:1. Alpha-adrenergic receptors are present in human ventricular myocardium, and selective intracoronary infusion of an alpha agonist such as phenylephrine does increase myocardial contractility, but the amount of receptor protein is less than that of beta receptors.[154, 155] The importance of beta-adrenergic receptor-mediated signaling to physiologic abnormalities in human heart failure was not appreciated until the early 1980s. Bristow and colleagues[156] determined that isolated muscle fibers obtained from patients with end-stage heart disease had a markedly reduced responsiveness to isoproterenol and that this was the result of a reduced number of beta receptors when compared with muscle fibers from patients with normal cardiac function. These researchers later demonstrated that this "downregulation" of beta receptor number was the result of a selective decrease in β_1-adrenergic receptors, with little or no change in β_2 receptor number.[157] These data have been confirmed independently by a number of laboratories.[155, 158, 159] In addition to a decrease in β_1 receptor number, functional uncoupling or desensitization of beta receptors from downstream signaling pathways within cardiac myocytes also occurs. This is partly the result of an increase in total beta-adrenergic receptor kinase (βARK) activity, an enzyme responsible for posttranslational modifications of the receptor that uncouples receptor-initiated G-protein signaling. There is an increase in mRNA levels of a βARK isoform (βARK-1) in human heart failure.[160, 161]

In addition to a reduction in β_1 receptor number and evidence of desensitization, there are additional characteristic changes observed in beta-adrenergic signaling in heart failure patients.[155, 159, 162] There is a moderate decrease in β_2 receptor affinity that contributes to the reduced responsiveness to exogenous beta-adrenergic agonists.[155, 162, 163] In addition, accumulating evidence points to an increase in the activity of a G_i isoform in failing heart muscle.[162, 163] Although this isoform activity could contribute to the decreased responsiveness of failing myocardium to β_2-selective agonists, the increase in G_i appears to result in less important changes in cardiac function compared with the loss of β_1 receptors.[164]

The physiologic stimulus for β_1 receptor downregulation appears to be prolonged exposure to high, local concentrations of norepinephrine rather than high circulating levels of catecholamines. Bristow and colleagues[165] have compared adrenergic receptor densities and coupling to downstream effector proteins in right and left ventricular muscle between patients with heart failure as a result of biventricular idiopathic dilated cardiomyopathy and patients with heart failure as a result of primary pulmonary hypertension and chronic right ventricular failure. β_1 receptor density and tissue norepinephrine content were diminished in both ventricles in patients with idiopathic dilated cardiomyopathy, but despite high circulating levels of catecholamines, there was selective downregulation of β_1 receptors in the right ventricles of patients with primary pulmonary hypotension and heart failure.[165] Thus, although some inconsistencies remain unexplained, it appears that prolonged, high, local concentrations of norepinephrine, with its tenfold higher affinity for β_1-adrenergic receptors, are probably the proximate cause of β_1-adrenergic receptor downregulation in the failing heart.[166]

Although the amount of information on vascular responsiveness

TABLE 9–7. CALCULATION OF DOSE OF ANTICARDIAC GLYCOSIDE IMMUNOTHERAPY

The calculation of the amount of polyclonal antidigoxin Fab antibody fragments to be administered is based on a dose of Fab that is stoichiometrically equivalent to the total body burden of digoxin.

Estimation of total body digoxin burden (mg)

Total drug ingested following acute digoxin poisoning
(i.e., amount ingested × 0.80 [average oral bioavailability of tablet formulations])

OR

Known or suspected toxicity during chronic digoxin therapy:

$$\frac{\text{Serum digoxin concentration} \times \text{volume of distribution (5.6 L/kg)} \times \text{weight in kg}}{1000}$$

Calculation of Fab fragment dose, by either

$$\frac{\text{Molecular mass of Fab fragments} = 50{,}000 \times 64 \times \text{total body digoxin content in mg}}{\text{Molecular mass of digoxin} = 781}$$

$$= \text{dose of Fab fragments in mg}$$

OR, if using a standard formulation (e.g., Digibind [Burroughs Wellcome]),

$$\frac{\text{Estimated total body load of digoxin (mg)}}{0.6 \text{ (mg/vial)}}$$

$$= \text{Digibind dose in numbers of vials}$$

For reversal of digitoxin toxicity, substitute 1 for oral bioavailability and 0.56 L/kg for volume of distribution in the previous formulas.

to alpha- or beta-adrenergic agonists is much less than that on the characterization of these signaling pathways in cardiac muscle, the available evidence suggests that there is not an important difference between patients with heart failure and normal controls in this regard.[167, 168]

Beta-Adrenergic Receptor and Dopaminergic Receptor Agonists

Dopamine and dobutamine are sympathomimetic amines that constitute the positively inotropic agents of choice for short-term support of the circulation in advanced heart failure as well as in clinical settings of temporary myocardial dysfunction such as following cardiopulmonary bypass.[169] Despite short-term hemodynamic responses that would appear to favor the long-term use of beta-adrenergic agonists in heart failure accompanied by reduced systolic ventricular function, the rapid development of tolerance and unwanted side effects of orally active formulations that have been studied have discouraged the further development of such agents. Isoproterenol, epinephrine, and norepinephrine have little role in the treatment of most cases of severe heart failure but may on occasion be useful in the postcardiac surgery setting. Dobutamine and dopamine have comparable myocardial inotropic and lusitropic effects and also have a spectrum of vascular activities that is often preferable to that of other beta-adrenergic agonists. Dobutamine tends to cause less tachycardia and to be less arrhythmogenic than the endogenous catecholamines, isoproterenol, or dopamine.

Dobutamine

Dobutamine, as available clinically, is a racemic mixture that stimulates both β_1- and β_2-adrenergic receptor subtypes and either binds but does not activate alpha-adrenergic receptors ([+] enantiomer) or stimulates α_1 and α_2 receptor subtypes ([−] enantiomer). Lower doses resulting in a clear positive inotropic effect in humans exert a predominant β_1-adrenergic effect, whereas alpha-adrenergic agonist effects of the (−) enantiomer in the vasculature and myocardium are blocked by the alpha receptor antagonist effect of the (+) enantiomer. Dobutamine does not stimulate dopaminergic receptors and, unlike dopamine, does not selectively alter renal blood flow. Racemic dobutamine also acts as a vasodilator to reduce aortic impedance and systemic vascular resistance, thus reducing afterload and improving ventricular-vascular coupling.[170, 171] In contrast, dopamine may either have no effect or increase ventricular afterload, depending on the infusion rate. Therefore, dobutamine is preferable to dopamine for most patients with advanced heart failure who have not responded adequately to oral vasodilators, digoxin, and diuretics. Intravenous infusions of dobutamine of up to several days in duration are usually well tolerated, although pharmacologic tolerance generally limits long-term use. Dobutamine is typically initiated at 2–3 μg/kg/min without a loading dose and is titrated according to symptoms and diuretic responsiveness. Systemic arterial pressure may increase, not change, or decrease depending on the extent of vasodilation and change in cardiac output. Heart rate may decline after several hours if cardiac output is significantly increased and central sympathetic tone declines. Use of a flow-directed catheter to monitor pulmonary capillary wedge pressure and cardiac output allows more effective use of dobutamine alone or in conjunction with other vasodilators and diuretics.

Outpatient therapy with dobutamine, administered continuously by a portable infusion pump through a central venous catheter, has been evaluated in patients with advanced heart failure and symptoms that are refractory to other drugs.[172–174] Although this approach has been useful in maintaining compensation in some patients, it has not gained widespread clinical acceptance. Intermittent use of dobutamine ("dobutamine holiday") may be appropriate for selected patients. In a small, randomized, controlled trial of "pulsed inotropic therapy," with dobutamine given at a dose sufficient to raise the heart rate to 70%–80% of the predicted maximum in patients with moderate to severe heart failure for 30 min per day 4 days a week, patients treated with active drug had a higher maximal exercise tolerance, lower plasma norepinephrine levels, and improved symptoms at the end of 3 weeks, compared with control subjects matched for age and severity of heart failure.[175]

Patients who have become tolerant to dobutamine on continuous infusions may benefit from an intravenous class III cAMP phosphodiesterase inhibitor (e.g., milrinone) for several days, which may then allow dobutamine to be reinstituted. Weaning patients from intravenous sympathomimetics is often difficult and may require aggressive use of vasodilators (sometimes of more than one class) as well as digoxin and diuretics.

Dopamine

This endogenous catecholamine evokes vasodilatory responses by direct stimulation of dopaminergic postsynaptic type 1 and presynaptic type 2 receptors in the peripheral vasculature. Dopamine causes relatively selective vasodilation of splanchnic and renal arterial beds at doses less than or equal to 2 μg/kg/min.[176] This may be useful in promoting renal blood flow and maintaining glomerular filtration rate in patients who become refractory to diuretics, especially when this is the result of marginal renal perfusion, although the safety of this approach is controversial.[177, 178] Dopamine also has direct renal tubular effects that promote natriuresis. At intermediate (2–10 μg/kg/min) infusion rates, dopamine enhances norepinephrine release from vascular sympathetic neurons, resulting in increased beta-adrenergic receptor activation in the heart. At higher infusion rates (5–20 μg/kg/min), peripheral vasoconstriction occurs as a result of direct alpha-adrenergic receptor stimulation. Increases in systemic vascular resistance are common even at intermediate infusion rates. Tachycardia tends to be more pronounced with dopamine than with dobutamine and may worsen systolic and diastolic function in patients with ischemic cardiomyopathies. Dose ranges noted previously are based on estimated lean body weight rather than actual patient weight. Emergence of unexplained tachycardia or arrhythmias in a patient receiving "renal-range" dopamine should raise the suspicion of an inappropriately high dopamine infusion rate.

There is increasing debate regarding whether low-dose or "renal-range" dopamine improves renal function and diuretic effectiveness in patients with heart failure and a marginal cardiac output and prevents or attenuates acute renal failure in postoperative surgical patients with or without acute renal failure.[177, 178] In postoperative surgical patients, dopamine has been shown either to increase urine output without significantly affecting creatinine clearance or to have no effect on urine flow or urea or creatinine clearance.[179–181]

Dopexamine

Dopexamine is a synthetic sympathomimetic agent designed as a dopamine analog for intravenous use that has a sixtyfold higher affinity for β_2 receptors than dopamine.[182, 183] Dopexamine exhibits moderate dopaminergic receptor stimulation at clinically relevant infusion rates (0.25–1 μg/kg/min) and causes some selective vasodilation of hepatosplanchnic and renal vascular beds. At infusion rates higher than 1 μg/kg/min, patients may develop unacceptable ventricular ectopy or supraventricular tachycardias.[182, 183] Although dopexamine offers a hemodynamic profile that is intermediate between those of dobutamine and dopamine, there is no compelling evidence that dopexamine offers any important clinical advantages over the other two drugs.[184, 185]

Oral Dopamine Agonists

Orally active analogs of dopamine have been developed and include levodopa, ibopamine, and fenoldopam. These drugs have been shown to improve symptoms in some heart failure patients, but none has been subjected to rigorous examination in large, prospective randomized trials when added to standard therapy.[169] Levodopa causes unacceptable side effects in a majority of patients. Available evidence suggests that ibopamine may be effective in selected heart failure patients with marginal renal function or diuretic resistance, but its present status remains investigational. Digoxin proved superior to ibopamine in one randomized, placebo-controlled trial of patients who had mild to moderate heart failure symptoms receiving "background" therapy with diuretics alone.[186]

Phosphodiesterase Inhibitors

Agents such as theophylline, 3-isobutyl-1-methyl xanthine (IBMX), and caffeine have long been recognized as nonspecific cGMP and cAMP phosphodiesterase (PDE) inhibitors. The utility of this class of agents in heart failure was limited until the 1980s, when a number of PDE isoenzyme subclass-specific inhibitors became available. Table 9–8 summarizes the isoenzyme classification scheme of Beavo and Reifsnyder,[187] comprising five distinct but related gene families based largely on known complementary DNA sequences. Tissue and cellular PDE isoenzyme distribution, as well as subcellular localization and links to specific cGMP- and cAMP-dependent signaling pathways, are increasingly recognized.[188–190] Any specificity of "selective" inhibitors for most PDE isoenzymes exists only within a relatively narrow concentration range, with increasingly nonspecific inhibition at higher concentrations. Most PDE inhibitors have other known pharmacologic activities. For example, dipyridamole is an antagonist of adenosine uptake and metabolism. Of the types of PDE inhibitors, type III drugs have received the most attention for the treatment of heart failure.

Amrinone and Milrinone

Parenteral formulations of amrinone and milrinone have received U.S. Food and Drug Administration (FDA) approval for short-term support of the circulation in patients with advanced heart failure. Longer-term prospective trials of oral formulations of both drugs often caused intolerable side effects, exhibited minimal long-term efficacy, and in the doses used, caused increased mortality in heart failure patients.[191, 192] Both agents are bipyridine derivatives and relatively selective inhibitors of the cGMP-inhibited, cAMP PDE type III group. Both drugs cause vasodilation with a consequent fall in systemic vascular resistance, and increases in contractile force and in velocity of relaxation of cardiac muscle. Amrinone and milrinone are commonly used in combination with other oral or intravenous drugs for short-term treatment of patients with severe heart failure as a result of systolic right or left ventricular dysfunction. Both drugs are initiated by an intravenous loading dose followed by a continuous infusion, typically a 0.5 mg/kg bolus infusion followed by 2–20 μg/kg/min for amrinone. Milrinone is about 10 times more potent than amrinone, with a typical loading dose of 50 μg/kg and an infusion rate of 0.25–1 μg/kg/min. Half-lives of amrinone and milrinone clearance are 2–5 h and 0.5–2.0 h, respectively, and are approximately doubled in patients with advanced heart failure. Clinically significant thrombocytopenia is reported in about 10% of patients receiving amrinone but is rare with milrinone.

Because of its greater selectively for PDE III isoenzymes, shorter half-life, and fewer side effects, milrinone is the agent of choice among currently available PDE inhibitors for short-term parenteral inotropic support in patients with severe heart failure. Development of oral formulations of PDE inhibitors for treatment of chronic heart failure has been deterred by the premature termination of the Prospective Randomized Milrinone Survival Evaluation (PROMISE) trial,[191, 192] which documented a 53% increase in mortality in patients with NYHA class IV heart failure receiving milrinone. Unfavorable results were also evident in a smaller trial that compared oral milrinone to either digoxin or placebo.[193] Sustained hemodynamic im-

TABLE 9–8. CYCLIC NUCLEOTIDE PHOSPHODIESTERASE ISOENZYMES

Isoenzyme Family	Regulatory Characteristics	Selective Inhibitors	Known Functional Effects of Isoenzyme Inhibition
I	Ca^{2+}, calmodulin regulated with different K_m values for cGMP and cAMP hydrolysis	Vinpocetine	CNS modulation; vasorelaxation
II	cGMP-stimulated cAMP hydrolysis with high K_m for cAMP	None	
III	cGMP-inhibited cAMP hydrolysis; low K_m for cAMP and cGMP	Milrinone Amrinone Pimobendan Cilostamide Enoximone Peroximone Vesnarinone	Positive inotropism; vascular and airway dilation; inhibition of platelet aggregation; stimulation of lipolysis; inhibition of cytokine production*
IV	Low K_m for cAMP hydrolysis	Rolipram R020–1724	Airway smooth muscle relaxation; inhibition of inflammatory mediator release; CNS modulation; gastric acid secretion
V	High and low K_m isoforms for cGMP-specific hydrolysis	Zaprinast Dipyridamole	Platelet aggregation inhibition

Abbreviation: CNS, central nervous system.

*Reported only for vesnarinone; not proven to be related to phosphodiesterase inhibition.

Adapted from Nicholson CD, Challiss RAJ, Shadid M: Differential modulation of tissue function and therapeutic potential of selective inhibitors of cyclic nucleotide phosphodiesterase isoenzymes. Trends Pharmacol Sci 1991;12:19–27.

provement was lacking and the incidence of adverse events, particularly cardiac arrhythmias, was greater in the milrinone group.

Vesnarinone

This orally active, positively inotropic agent with vasodilator activity appears to act via multiple mechanisms. In addition to relatively selective inhibition of an isoform of cGMP-inhibited cAMP phosphodiesterase present in human myocardial and kidney tissue,[194] vesnarinone also affects sarcolemmal membrane voltage-activated sodium and potassium channels. This could contribute to the drug's positive inotropic action as well as exert electrophysiologic effects. The net effect at selected dose levels is a decrease in heart rate and prolongation of action potential duration, which is opposite to the result observed with other class III PDE inhibitors. Vesnarinone has also been reported to decrease production by lymphocytes of some inflammatory cytokines.[195]

Vesnarinone appeared to decrease mortality in one placebo-controlled trial.[196] Patients on standard therapy for moderate to moderately severe heart failure were randomized to placebo or vesnarinone at 60 mg or 120 mg/day. An apparent increase in mortality in patients receiving the larger dose of active drug caused the early termination of that arm of the trial. The lower dose of 60 mg/day of vesnarinone, however, was associated with a greater than 50% reduction in mortality at 12 weeks compared with placebo.[196] Symptoms of heart failure and quality of life improved in the 60-mg/day vesnarinone group, consistent with prior smaller trials. Results of additional clinical trials in progress are awaited.

BETA-ADRENERGIC ANTAGONISTS

The development of intravenous and oral formulations of beta-adrenergic *agonists* for the support of the circulation in heart failure caused by systolic ventricular dysfunction was based on the reasonable rationale that these drugs would improve contractile function and diastolic relaxation, much like endogenous catecholamines. By virtue of their β_2-adrenergic agonist activity, many of these agents were expected to also act as vasodilators, providing an additional useful pharmacologic effect in heart failure. This rationale seemed at first to be reinforced by evidence that cardiac muscle from heart failure patients and from animals with experimental heart failure exhibits a significant hyporesponsiveness to endogenous catecholamines. Indeed, there is a growing consensus that β_1-adrenergic receptor number is decreased in many patients with heart failure, whereas β_2 receptors appear to be functionally uncoupled from inducing postreceptor signaling.[155, 159, 164] However, despite this pathophysiologic substrate and these drugs' apparently favorable hemodynamic profile in short-term studies in patients with heart failure, beta-adrenergic agonists have not been found to be useful in the management of chronic heart failure and may be detrimental except for temporary circulatory support in hospitalized patients.

In contrast, beta-adrenergic *antagonists* may improve exercise tolerance and perhaps mortality in heart failure patients. Despite clinical and experimental animal data that these drugs had an initial negative inotropic effect and could worsen ventricular function, the introduction of beta-adrenergic antagonists in the treatment of heart failure was based largely on empirical evidence from small clinical trials. Beta-adrenergic antagonists are identified by their affinity for binding to beta-adrenergic receptors that is sufficiently high to antagonize the binding of endogenous agonists (i.e., norepinephrine and epinephrine) at blood and tissue concentrations that do not cause other, undesirable, effects. Historically, these agents have been classified based on their relative selectivity for the β_1- or β_2-adrenergic receptors, their ability to bind other adrenergic receptors (usually alpha receptors), and their ability to interact with other molecular targets at clinically relevant doses (e.g., the K^+ channel antagonist activity of the [+] enantiomer of sotalol). In addition, many beta-adrenergic antagonists are characterized by their ability not only to prevent the binding of endogenous catecholamines but also to act as weak agonists (i.e., intrinsic sympathomimetic activity [ISA]) or to bind to and inactivate beta receptors even in the absence of endogenous agonists (inverse agonism). Beta-adrenergic antagonists are also distinguished by the chemical characteristics of each compound (e.g., lipophilicity) that determine its tissue distribution and clearance mechanisms (Table 9–9).

In the 1970s, Waagstein and associates[197] in Sweden reported that beta-adrenergic blockers improved symptoms and several measures

TABLE 9–9. PHARMACODYNAMIC PROPERTIES OF BETA-ADRENERGIC ANTAGONISTS

Generic Name	Proprietary Names	Adrenergic Receptor Selectivity	Partial Agonism (ISA)	Inverse Agonism*	Lipid Solubility	Vasodilator Activity	Other Actions
Acebutolol	Sectral	$+\beta_1$	+		+	+	
Atenolol	Tenormin	$+\beta_1$	0		0	0	
Betaxolol	Kerlone	$+\beta_1$	0		0		
Bevantolol		$++\beta_1$	0		++	+	
Bisoprolol	Zebeta	$++\beta_1$	0		+	0	
Bucindolol		$0\beta_1\beta_2$	0		0	++	"Direct" vasodilator
Carteolol	Cartrol	$0\beta_1\beta_2$	++		0	0	
Carvedilol		$(+)\beta_1\alpha_1$	0	+	+	++	
Celiprolol		$+\beta_1$	$+\beta_2$		0	+	
Esmolol	Brevibloc	$+\beta_1$	0		0	0	
Labetalol	Trandate, Normodyne	$\beta_1,\beta_2\alpha_1$	0	++	++	++	
Metoprolol	Lopressor	$+\beta_1$	0		++	0	
Nadolol	Corgard	$\beta_1\beta_2$	0		0	0	
Nebivolol		$+\beta_1$	0		0	+	"Direct" vasodilator
Oxprenolol	Trasicor	$\beta_1\beta_2$	++		+	0	
Penbutolol	Levatol	$\beta_1\beta_2$	++		+++	0	
Pindolol	Visken	$\beta_1\beta_2$	+++	++	++	0	
Propranolol	Inderal	$\beta_1\beta_2$	0		+++	0	
Sotalol	Betapace	$\beta_1\beta_2$	0	+++	0	0	Class III antiarrhythmic
Timolol	Blocadren	$\beta_1\beta_2$	0		0	0	

Abbreviation: ISA, intrinsic sympathomimetic activity.

*Inverse agonism is the ability to bind and stabilize the inactive conformation of G-protein–linked receptors. It has not been well defined for most beta-adrenergic antagonists in the context of human cardiovascular pharmacology.

of ventricular function over a period of several months in patients with mild to severe heart failure as a result of idiopathic dilated cardiomyopathy.[198] Although several small clinical trials in the 1980s tended to support these observations, none was sufficiently large to provide definitive evidence regarding improvement in symptoms or exercise tolerance or to have the statistical power to detect a change in mortality.[199, 200] However, a meta-analysis of trials of beta-adrenergic antagonists administered to patients following myocardial infarction, as well as subgroup analyses of several of the larger secondary prevention trials, indicates that these drugs may decrease mortality in patients with heart failure.[201]

Since 1990, a number of additional trials have been reported, most of which have supported the hypothesis that beta-adrenergic antagonists improve symptoms and ventricular function in heart failure, although limited data on the survival benefits of these agents have only recently become available and there is no consensus as yet on either mechanism of action or which spectrum of pharmacologic characteristics of these agents is ideal.

The Metoprolol in Dilated Cardiomyopathy (MDC) trial[202] examined the efficacy of metoprolol in 383 patients with mild to moderate (classes II–III) heart failure as a result of an idiopathic dilated cardiomyopathy who were already receiving optimal medical management, including ACE inhibitors. Patients with clinically significant epicardial coronary artery disease were excluded. The average ejection fraction in patients randomized to receive either placebo or metoprolol was 0.22 in both groups. Metoprolol therapy was initiated as a test dose of 5 mg before randomization. Ninety-six percent of patients tolerated this dose and were randomized to placebo or active drug. The target dose was 100–150 mg/day achieved over 7 weeks, and the mean dose of those on active drug was 108 mg/day at 3 months. Although there was no difference in mortality after 12 months of follow-up, the number of patients requiring hospitalization for worsening heart failure or listing for cardiac transplantation was significantly less in the metoprolol group. Over 12 months, the ejection fraction improved significantly more in patients receiving metoprolol (.22–.34) than in patients receiving placebo (.22–.28).[202]

The results of the Cardiac Insufficiency Bisoprolol Study (CIBIS) trial,[203] which examined the effects of this β_1-selective antagonist in 641 heart failure patients with a NYHA class III functional status as a result of either an ischemic or a primary dilated cardiomyopathy, also did not show a significant reduction in mortality in patients already receiving a contemporary standard medical regimen including an ACE inhibitor. As in the MDC trial, however, functional status improved, and the incidence of clinical decompensation as a result of worsening heart failure declined. Despite the neutral results in the CIBIS trial[203] on the efficacy of β_1-selective adrenergic antagonists on mortality in patients with an ischemic cardiomyopathy, Fisher and colleagues[204] have confirmed that both functional status and the need for hospitalizations because of worsening heart failure were improved in 50 patients with known coronary artery disease and an ejection fraction below .40 who were randomized to receive metoprolol compared with placebo. Ejection fraction also improved significantly at 6 months compared with those receiving placebo. In a dose-ranging study of the efficacy of the nonselective beta-adrenergic agonist with vasodilating activity bucindolol in 139 heart failure patients with both idiopathic and ischemic cardiomyopathies, Bristow and colleagues[205] demonstrated improvement in functional status as well as ejection fraction, with the greatest improvement observed at the highest dose (200 mg/day) in patients with both ischemic and idiopathic cardiomyopathies. Although maximal exercise tolerance declined, there was a trend toward improvement in submaximal exercise tolerance, which may be a more reliable indicator of functional status for patients receiving drug therapy for heart failure.[206]

Other beta-adrenergic antagonists with vasodilating activity are being evaluated for use in heart failure patients. Drugs with partial β_2 agonist activity (ISA) include pindolol (nonselective) and celiprolol (β_1 selective) adrenergic antagonists.[206] Because of the negative survival data with the partial beta agonist xamoterol in one large randomized controlled trial,[207] it is unlikely that other beta-adrenergic antagonists with a significant degree of agonist activity will be widely tested in heart failure patients.

Labetalol, a nonselective β_1 and β_2 antagonist that also blocks α_1 receptors and is already licensed in the United States for the treatment of hypertension, has been evaluated in small trials of heart failure patients. In one placebo-controlled, randomized, crossover trial of 12 patients with idiopathic dilated cardiomyopathy, labetalol increased exercise tolerance, decreased systemic vascular resistance, and increased cardiac output over 3 months of follow-up.[208] Carvedilol, like labetalol, exhibits both α_1 and beta receptor antagonism, with no partial agonist (ISA) activity but modest, probably clinically irrelevant, β_1 selectivity and a longer elimination half-life (2–8 h) that permits once or twice daily dosing.[209] Carvedilol appears to be well tolerated in small trials of patients with both idiopathic and ischemic cardiomyopathies, and there are several preliminary reports of its efficacy in improving left ventricular ejection fraction, submaximal exercise tolerance, and symptoms.[209, 210] In a published report of 40 patients with idiopathic dilated cardiomyopathy randomized to receive either placebo or carvedilol (target dose, 25 mg b.i.d.) with background therapy of digoxin, diuretics, and an ACE inhibitor, carvedilol after 4 months improved symptoms, submaximal exercise capacity, and left ventricular ejection fraction (from .20–.30) and decreased pulmonary artery wedge pressure.[211]

The U.S. placebo-controlled dose-ranging efficacy and safety trials of carvedilol in heart failure patients have been discontinued prematurely by the Data and Safety Monitoring Board because of an unexpectedly strong positive effect of carvedilol on mortality.[212] If these results are confirmed by further analysis, carvedilol will be the first beta-adrenergic antagonist to show a benefit on survival in heart failure patients, in addition to improving resting hemodynamics, symptoms, and submaximal exercise tolerance when administered concurrently with contemporary medical therapy. Large survival trials involving bucindolol are also currently under way, including the β-Blocker Evaluation Survival Trial (BEST) that will help to further clarify this issue.

It remains unclear by what mechanisms beta-adrenergic antagonists may favorably affect ventricular function and clinical status in patients with heart failure as a result of predominant systolic dysfunction.[213] Nevertheless, available evidence supports a potential role for beta-adrenergic antagonists in the treatment of patients with idiopathic dilated cardiomyopathy, and probably ischemic cardiomyopathy as well. However, it should be emphasized that beta-adrenergic blocking drugs can be hazardous in patients with advanced heart failure. In all reported studies, the initial doses were low (e.g., 5-mg test doses for metoprolol, followed by 10 mg/day) and were slowly titrated upwards over 4–6 weeks. Although this approach appears promising, it is investigational and has not been approved by the FDA for the indication of heart failure.

REFERENCES

1. Awazu M, Ichikawa I: Alterations in renal function in experimental congestive heart failure. Semin Nephrol 1994; 14:401.
2. Rouse D, Suki WN: Effects of neural and humoral agents on the renal tubules in congestive heart failure. Semin Nephrol 1994; 14:412.
3. Miller JA, Tobe SW, Skorecki KL: Control of extracellular fluid volume and the pathophysiology of edema. *In* Brenner BM (ed): Brenner & Rector's The Kidney, 5th ed, vol I, p 817. Philadelphia: WB Saunders, 1996.
4. Young JB, Pratt CM: Hemodynamic and hormonal alterations in patients with heart failure: Toward a contemporary definition of heart failure. Semin Nephrol 1994; 14:427.
5. Section V: Management of the patient with renal failure. *In* Brenner BM (ed): Brenner & Rector's The Kidney, 5th ed, vol II, p 2297. Philadelphia: WB Saunders, 1996.
6. Jackson, EK: Diuretics and other agents employed in the mobilization of edema fluid. *In* Hardman JG, Limbird L (eds): Goodman & Gilman's The Pharmacological Basis of Therapeutics, 9th ed. New York: McGraw-Hill, 1996.
7. Haas M: The Na-K-Cl cotransporters. Am J Physiol 1994; 267:C869.
8. Ellison DH: The physiologic basis of diuretic synergism: Its role in treating diuretic resistance. Ann Intern Med 1991; 114:886.
9. Lahav M, Regev A, Ra'anani P, Theodor E: Intermittent administration of furosemide vs continuous infusion preceded by a loading dose for congestive heart failure. Chest 1992; 102:725.
10. Gamba G, Saltzberg SN, Lombardi M, et al: Primary structure and functional expression of a cDNA encoding the thiazide-sensitive, electroneutral sodium-chloride cotransporter. Proc Natl Acad Sci U S A 1993; 90:2749.
11. Palmer LG: Epithelial Na channels: Function and diversity. Annu Rev Physiol 1992; 54:51.
12. Canessa C, Schild L, Buell G, et al: Amiloride-sensitive epithelial Na^+ channel is made of three homologous subunits. Nature 1994; 367:463.
13. Weber KT, Villarreal D: Aldosterone and antialdosterone therapy in congestive heart failure. Am J Cardiol 1993; 71:3A.
14. Funder JW: Aldosterone action. Annu Rev Physiol 1993; 55:115.
15. Brater DC: Diuretic resistance: Mechanisms and therapeutic strategies. Cardiology 1994; 84:57.
16. Brater DC: Pharmacokinetics of loop diuretics in congestive heart failure. Br Heart J 1994; 72:S40.
17. Van Meyel JJM, Gerlag PGG, Smits P, et al: Absorption of high dose furosemide (frusemide) in congestive heart failure. Clin Pharmacokinet 1992; 22:308.
18. Good JM, Brady AJB, Noormohamed FH, et al: Effect of intense angiotensin II suppression on the diuretic response to furosemide during diuretic chronic ACE inhibition. Circulation 1994; 90:220.
19. Knauf H, Mutschler E: Functional state of the nephron and diuretic dose-response-rationale for low-dose combination therapy. Cardiology 1994; 84:18.
20. Kiyingi A, Field MJ, Pawsey CC, et al: Metolazone in treatment of severe refractory congestive cardiac failure. Lancet 1990; 335:29.
21. Tan AC, Russel FGM, Thien T, Benraad TJ: Atrial natriuretic peptide. An overview of clinical pharmacology and pharmacokinetics. Clin Pharmacokinet 1993; 24:28.
22. Deutsch A, Frishman WH, Sukenik D, et al: Atrial natriuretic peptide and its potential role in pharmacotherapy. J Clin Pharmacol 1994; 34:1133.
23. Connelly TP, Francis GS, Williams KJ, et al: Interaction of intravenous atrial natriuretic factor with furosemide in patients with heart failure. Am Heart J 1994; 127:392.
24. Semigran MJ, Aroney CN, Herrmann HC, et al: Effects of atrial natriuretic peptide on myocardial contractile and diastolic function in patients with heart failure. J Am Coll Cardiol 1992; 20:98.
25. Leier CV, Dei Cas L, Metra M: Clinical relevance and management of the major electrolyte abnormalities in congestive heart failure: Hyponatremia, hypokalemia, and hypomagnesemia. Am Heart J 1994; 128:564.
26. Cody RJ: Clinical trials of diuretic therapy in heart failure: Research directions and clinical considerations. J Am Coll Cardiol 1993; 22:165A.
27. Hampton JR: Results of clinical trials with diuretics in heart failure. Br Heart J 1994; 72:S68.
28. Woods KL, Fletcher S: Long-term outcome after intravenous magnesium sulphate in suspected acute myocardial infarction: The second Leicester Intravenous Magnesium Intervention Trial (LIMIT-2). Lancet 1994; 343:816.
29. Arsenian MA: Magnesium and cardiovascular disease. Prog Cardiovasc Dis 1993; 35:271, 1993.
30. Davies DL, Fraser R: Do diuretics cause magnesium deficiency? Br J Clin Pharmacol 1993; 36:1.
31. Cohn JN, Franciosa JA: Vasodilator therapy of cardiac failure. N Engl J Med 1977; 27:31:254.
32. Cohn JN, Archibald DG, Ziesche S, et al: Effect of vasodilator therapy on mortality in chronic congestive heart failure. Results of a Veterans Administration Cooperative Study. N Engl J Med 1986; 314:1547.
33. CONSENSUS Trial Study Group: Effects of enalapril on mortality in severe congestive heart failure. Results of the Cooperative North Scandinavian Enalapril Survival Group (CONSENSUS). N Engl J Med 1987; 316:1429.
34. Griendling KK, Murphy TJ, Alexander RW: Molecular biology of the renin-angiotensin system. Circulation 1993; 87:1816.
35. Paul M, Wagner J, Dzau VJ: Gene expression of the renin-angiotensin system in human tissues. Quantitative analysis by the polymerase chain reaction. J Clin Invest 1993; 91:2058.
36. Greenwald L, Becker RC: Expanding the paradigm of the renin-angiotensin system and angiotensin-converting enzyme inhibitors. Am Heart J 1994; 128:997.
37. Dzau VJ, Re R: Tissue angiotensin system in cardiovascular medicine: A paradigm shift? Circulation 1994; 89:493.
38. Kifor I, Dzau VJ: Endothelial renin-angiotensin pathways: Evidence for intracellular synthesis and secretion of angiotensins. Circ Res 1987; 60:422.
39. Sechi LA, Griffin CA, Grady EF, et al: Characterization of angiotensin II receptor in subtypes in rat heart. Circ Res 1992; 71:1482.

40. Regitz-Zagrosek V, Friedel N, Heymann A, et al: Regulation, chamber localization, and subtype distribution of angiotensin II receptors in human hearts. Circulation 1995; 91:1461.
41. Holubarsch C, Schmidt-Schweda S, Knorr A, et al: Functional significance of angiotensin receptors in human myocardium. Significant differences between atrial and ventricular myocardium. Eur Heart J 1994; 15:88.
42. Lonn EM, Yusuf S, Jha P, et al: Emerging role of angiotensin-converting enzyme inhibitors in cardiac and vascular protection. Circulation 1994; 90:2056.
43. Cody RJ: Comparing angiotensin-converting enzyme inhibitor trial results in patients with acute myocardial infarction. Arch Intern Med 1994; 154:2029.
44. Lyons D, Webster J, Benjamin N: Angiotensin II. Adrenergic sympathetic constrictor action in humans. Circulation 1995; 91:1457.
45. Goldsmith SR, Hasking GJ, Miller E: Angiotensin II and sympathetic activity in patients with congestive heart failure. J Am Coll Cardiol 1993; 21:1107.
46. Morishita R, Gibbons GH, Ellison KE, et al: Evidence for direct local effect of angiotensin in vascular hypertrophy. In vivo gene transfer of angiotensin converting enzyme. J Clin Invest 1994; 94:978.
47. Rakugi H, Jacob HJ, Krieger JE, et al: Vascular injury induces angiotensinogen gene expression in the media and neointima. Circulation 1993; 87:283.
48. Fishel RS, Thourani V, Eisenberg SJ, et al: Fibroblast growth factor stimulates angiotensin converting enzyme expression in vascular smooth muscle cells. Possible mediator of the response to vascular injury. J Clin Invest 1995; 95:377.
49. Daemen MJ, Lombardi DM, Bosman FT, Schwartz SM: Angiotensin II induces smooth muscle cell proliferation in the normal and injured rat arterial wall. Circ Res 1991; 68:450.
50. Aberg G, Ferrer P: Effects of captopril on atherosclerosis in cynomolgus monkeys. J Cardiovasc Pharmacol 1990; 15:S65.
51. Chobanian AV, Haudenschild CC, Nickerson C, Drago R: Anti-atherogenic effect of captopril in the Watanabe heritable hyperlipidemic rabbit. Hypertension 1990; 15:327.
52. Vaughn DE, Lazos SA, Tong K: Angiotensin II regulates the expression of plasminogen activator inhibitor-1 in cultured endothelial cells. A potential link between the renin-angiotensin system and thrombosis. J Clin Invest 1995; 95:995.
53. Olson JA, Jr, Shiverick KT, Ogilvie S, et al: Angiotensin II induces secretion of plasminogen activator inhibitor 1 and a tissue metalloprotease inhibitor-related protein from rat brain astrocytes. Neurobiology 1991; 88:1928.
54. Weinberg EO, Schoen FJ, George D, et al: Angiotensin-converting enzyme inhibition prolongs survival and modifies the transition to heart failure in rats with pressure overload hypertrophy due to ascending aortic stenosis. Circulation 1994; 90:1410.
55. Friedrich SP, Lorell BH, Rousseau MF, et al: Intracardiac angiotensin-converting enzyme inhibition improves diastolic function in patients with left ventricular hypertrophy due to aortic stenosis. Circulation 1994; 90:2761.
56. Matsubara H, Kanasaki M, Murasawa S, et al: Differential gene expression and regulation of angiotensin II receptor subtypes in rat cardiac fibroblasts and cardiomyocytes in culture. J Clin Invest 1994; 93:1592.
57. Schorb W, Peeler TC, Madigan NN, et al: Angiotensin II-induced protein tyrosine phosphorylation in neonatal rat cardiac fibroblasts. J Biol Chem 1994; 269:19626.
58. Crabos M, Roth M, Hahn AWA, Erne P: Characterization of angiotensin II receptors in cultured adult rat cardiac fibroblasts. Coupling to signaling systems and gene expression. J Clin Invest 1994; 93:2372.
59. Waspe LE, Ordahl CP, Simpson PC. The cardiac-myosin heavy chain isogene is induced selectively in α_1-adrenergic receptor-stimulated hypertrophy of cultured rat heart myocytes. J Clin Invest 1990; 85:1206.
60. Weber KT, Brilla CG: Pathological hypertrophy and cardiac interstitium. Circulation 1991; 83:1849.
61. Binkley PF, Haas GJ, Starling RC, et al: Sustained augmentation of parasympathetic tone with angiotensin converting enzyme inhibition in patients with congestive heart failure. J Am Coll Cardiol 1993; 21:655.
62. Cody RJ, Franklin KW, Kluger J, Laragh JH: Mechanisms governing the postural response, and baroreceptor abnormalities in chronic congestive heart failure: Effects of acute and long-term converting enzyme inhibition. Circulation 1982; 66:135.
63. Ljungman S, Kjekshus J, Swedberg K, for the CONSENSUS Group: Renal function in severe congestive heart failure during treatment with enalapril (the Cooperative North Scandinavian Enalapril Survival Study [CONSENSUS] Trial). Am J Cardiol 1992; 70:479.
64. Mandal AK, Markert RJ, Saklayen MG, et al: Diuretics potentiate angiotensin converting enzyme inhibitor-induced acute renal failure. Clin Nephrol 1994; 42:170.
65. SOLVD Investigators: Effect of enalapril on survival in patients with reduced left ventricular ejection fractions and congestive heart failure. N Engl J Med 1991; 325:293.
66. Gruppo Italiano per lo Studio della Sopravvivenza nell'Infarto Miocardico: GISSI-3 Investigators: Effects of lisinopril and transdermal glyceryl trinitrate singly and together on 6-week mortality and ventricular function after acute myocardial infarction. Lancet 1994; 343:1115.
67. Maschio G: Protecting the residual renal function: How do ACE inhibitors and calcium antagonists compare? Nephron 1994; 67:257.
68. Hannedouche T, Landais P, Goldfarb B, et al: Randomized controlled trial of enalapril and blockers in non-diabetic chronic renal failure. Br Med J 1994; 309:833.
69. Lewis EJ, Hunsicker LG, Bain RP, et al: The effect of angiotensin-converting-enzyme inhibition on diabetic nephropathy. N Engl J Med 1993; 2329:1456.
70. Ondetti MA: From peptides to peptidases: A chronicle of drug discovery. Annu Rev Pharmacol 1994; 34:1.
71. Wiseman LR, McTavish D: Trandolapril. A review of its pharmacodynamic and pharmacokinetic properties, and therapeutic use in essential hypertension. Drugs 1994; 48:71.
72. Plosker GL, Sorkin EM: Quinapril. A reappraisal of its pharmacology and therapeutic efficacy in cardiovascular disorders. Drugs 1994; 48:227.
73. Zusman RM: Angiotensin-converting enzyme inhibitors: More different than alike? Focus on cardiac performance. Am J Cardiol 1993; 72:25H.
74. SOLVD Investigators: Effect of enalapril on mortality and the development of heart failure in asymptomatic patients with reduced left ventricular ejection fractions. N Engl J Med 1992; 327:685.
75. Kostis JB, Shelton BJ, Yusuf S, et al: Tolerability of enalapril initiation by patients with left ventricular dysfunction: Results of the medication challenge phase of the studies of left ventricular dysfunction. Am Heart J 1994; 128:358.
76. Swedberg K, Held R, Kjekshus J, et al: Effects of the early administration of enalapril on mortality in patients with acute myocardial infarction. Results of the Cooperative New Scandinavian Enalapril Survival Study II (CONSENSUS II). N Engl J Med 1992; 327:678.
77. ISIS-4 (Fourth International Study of Infarct Survival) Collaborative Group: ISIS-4: A randomized factorial trial assessing early oral captopril, oral mononitrate, and intravenous magnesium sulphate in 58,050 patients with suspected acute myocardial infarction. Lancet 1995; 345:669.
78. Ambrosioni E, Borghi C, Magnani B, for the Survival of Myocardial Infarction Long-Term Evaluation (SMILE) Study Investigators: The effect of the angiotensin-converting-enzyme inhibitor zofenopril on mortality and morbidity after anterior myocardial infarction. N Engl J Med 1995; 332:80.
79. Pitt B: Use of "xapril" in patients with chronic heart failure. A paradigm or epitaph for our times? Circulation 1994; 90:1550.
80. Pfeffer MA: Ace inhibition in acute myocardial infarction. N Engl J Med 1995; 332:118.
81. Pfeffer MA, Braunwald E, Moye LA, et al: Effect of captopril on mortality and morbidity in patients with left ventricular dysfunction after myocardial infarction. N Engl J Med 1992; 327:669.
82. Cohn JN, Johnson G, Ziesche S, et al: A comparison of enalapril with hydralazine-isosorbide dinitrate in the treatment of chronic congestive heart failure. N Engl J Med 1991; 325:303.
83. Acute Infarction Ramipril Efficacy (AIRE) Study Investigators: Effect of ramipril on mortality and morbidity of survivors of acute myocardial infarction with clinical evidence of heart failure. Lancet 1993; 342:821.
84. Varriale P, David W, Chryssos BE: Hemodynamic response to intravenous enalaprilat in patients with severe congestive heart failure and mitral regurgitation. Clin Cardiol 1993; 16:235.
85. Seneviratne B, Moore GA, West PD: Effect of captopril on functional mitral regurgitation in dilated heart failure: A randomized double blind placebo controlled trial. Br Heart J 1994; 72:63.
86. Israili ZH, Hall WD: Cough and angioneurotic edema associated with angiotensin-converting enzyme inhibitor therapy. Ann Intern Med 1992; 117:234.
87. Ravid D, Lishner M, Lang R, Ravid M: Angiotensin-converting enzyme inhibitors and cough: A prospective evaluation in hypertension and in congestive heart failure. J Clin Pharmacol 1994; 34:1116.

88. Hargreaves MR, Benson MK: Inhaled sodium cromoglycate in angiotensin-converting enzyme inhibitor cough. Lancet 1995; 345:13.
89. Sweet CS, Rucinska EJ: Losartan in heart failure: Preclinical experiences and initial clinical outcomes. Eur Heart J 1994; 15:139.
90. Gottlieb SS, Dickstein K, Fleck E, et al: Hemodynamic and neurohormonal effects of the angiotensin II antagonist losartan in patients with congestive heart failure. Circulation 1993; 88:1602.
91. Crozier I, Ikram H, Awan N, et al: Losartan in heart failure. Hemodynamic effects and tolerability. Circulation 1995; 91:691.
92. Brunner HR, Nussberger J, Waeber B: Dose-response relationships of ACE inhibitors and angiotensin II blockers. Eur Heart J 1994; 15:123.
93. Frishman WH, Fozailoff A, Lin C, Dike C: Renin inhibition: A new approach to cardiovascular therapy. J Clin Pharmacol 1994; 34:873.
94. Kiowski W, Beerman J, Rickenbacher P, et al: Angiotensinergic versus nonangiotensinergic hemodynamic effects of converting enzyme inhibition in patients with chronic heart failure. Assessment by acute renin and converting enzyme inhibition. Circulation 1994; 90:2748.
95. Stamler JS: Redox signaling: Nitrosylation and related target interactions of nitric oxide. Cell 199478:931.
96. Nathan C, Xie Q-W: Nitric oxide synthases: Roles, tolls, and controls. Cell 1994; 78:915.
97. Schmidt HHHW, Walter U: NO at work. Cell 1994; 78:919.
98. Furchgott RF, Zawadzki JV: The obligatory role of endothelial cells in the relaxation of arterial smooth muscle by acetylcholine. Nature 1980; 288:373.
99. Harrison DG, Bates JN: The nitrovasodilators. New ideas about old drugs. Circulation 1993; 87:1461.
100. Risoe C, Simonsen S, Rootwelt K, et al: Nitroprusside and regional vascular capacitance in patients with severe congestive heart failure. Circulation 1992; 85:997.
101. Kussmaul WG, Altschuler JA, Matthai WH, Laskey WK: Right ventricular-vascular interaction in congestive heart failure. Importance of low-frequency impedance. Circulation 1993; 88:1010.
102. Heesch CM, Hatfield BA, Marcoux L, Eichhorn EJ: Predictors of pressure and stroke volume response to afterload reduction with nitroprusside in patients with congestive heart failure secondary to idiopathic dilated cardiomyopathy. Am J Cardiol 1994; 74:951.
103. Varriale P, David WJ, Chryssos BE: Hemodynamic resistance to intravenous nitroglycerin in severe congestive heart failure and restored response after diuresis. Am J Cardiol 1991; 68:1400.
104. Fallen EL, Nahmias C, Scheffel A, et al: Redistribution of myocardial blood flow with topical nitroglycerin in patients with coronary artery disease. Circulation 1995; 91:1381.
105. European Study of Prevention of Infarct with Molsidomine (ESPRIM) Group: The ESPRIM trial: Short-term treatment of acute myocardial infarction with molsidomine. Lancet 1994; 344:91.
106. Unger P, Vachiery J-L, de Canniere D, Staroukine M, Berkenboom G: Comparison of the hemodynamic responses to molsidomine and isosorbide dinitrate in congestive heart failure. Am Heart J 1994; 128:557.
107. Leier CV, Huss P, Magouin RD, Unverferth DV: Improved exercise capacity and differing arterial and venous tolerance during chronic isosorbide dinitrate therapy for congestive heart failure. Circulation 1983; 67:817.
108. Elkayam U: Tolerance to organic nitrates: Evidence, mechanisms, clinical relevance, and strategies for prevention. Ann Intern Med 1991; 114:667.
109. Mangione NJ, Glasser SP: Phenomenon of nitrate tolerance. Am Heart J 1994; 128:137.
110. Dupuis J: Nitrates in congestive heart failure. Cardiovasc Drugs Ther 1994; 8:501.
111. Dupuis J, Lalonde G, Bichet D, Rouleau JL: Captopril does not prevent nitroglycerin tolerance in heart failure. Can J Cardiol 1990; 6:281.
112. Katz RJ, Levy WS, Buff L, Wasserman AG: Prevention of nitrate tolerance with angiotensin converting enzyme inhibitors. Circulation 1991; 83:1271.
113. Dakak N, Makhoul N, Frugelman MY, et al: Failure of captopril to prevent nitrate tolerance in congestive heart failure secondary to coronary artery disease. Am J Cardiol 1990; 66:608.
114. Meredith IT, Alison JF, Zhang FM, et al: Captopril potentiates the effects of nitroglycerin in the coronary vascular bed. J Am Coll Cardiol 1993; 22:581.
115. Parker JD, Parker JO: Effect of therapy with an angiotensin-converting enzyme inhibitor on hemodynamic and counter-regulatory responses during continuous therapy with nitroglycerin. J Am Coll Cardiol 1993; 21:1445.
116. Munzel T, Sayegh H, Freeman BA, et al: Evidence for enhanced vascular superoxide anion production in nitrate tolerance. A novel mechanism underlying tolerance and cross-tolerance. J Clin Invest 1995; 95:187.
117. Haas GJ, Leier CV: Vasodilators in congestive heart failure. *In* Hosenpud JD, Greenberg BH (eds): Congestive Heart Failure, p 400. New York: Springer-Verlag, 1994.
118. Binkley PF, Starling RC, Hammer DF, Leier CV: Usefulness of hydralazine to withdraw from dobutamine in severe congestive heart failure. Am J Cardiol 1991; 68:1103.
119. Hofstra AH: Metabolism of hydralazine: Relevance to drug-induced lupus. Drug Metab Rev 1994; 26:485.
120. Elkayam U, Shotan A, Mehra A, Ostrzega E: Calcium channel blockers in the heart. J Am Coll Cardiol 1993; 22:139A.
121. Conti CR: Use of calcium antagonists to treat heart failure. Clin Cardiol 1994; 17:101.
122. van Zwieten PA, Pfaffendord, M: Similarities and differences between calcium antagonists: Pharmacological aspects. J Hypertens 1993; 11:S3.
123. Lehmann G, Reiniger G, Beyerle A, Rudolph W: Pharmacokinetics and additional anti-ischemic effectiveness of amlodipine, a once-daily calcium antagonist during acute and long-term therapy of stable angina pectoris in patients pretreated with a beta-blocker. Eur Heart J 1993; 14:1531.
124. Burges R, Moisey D: Unique pharmacologic properties of amlodipine. Am J Cardiol 1994; 73:2A.
125. Todd PA, Faulds D: Felodipine. A review of the pharmacology and therapeutic uses of the extended release formulation in cardiovascular disorders. Drugs 1992; 44:251.
126. Cohn JN: Vasodilators in heart failure. Conclusions from V-HeFT II and rationale for V-HeFT III. Drugs 1994; 47:47.
127. Escande D, Henry P: Potassium channels as pharmacological targets in cardiovascular medicine. Eur Heart J 1993; 14:2.
128. Lilleberg J, Antila S, Karlsson N, et al: Pharmacokinetics and pharmacodynamics of simendan, a novel calcium sensitizer, in healthy volunteers. Clin Pharmacol Ther 1994; 56:554.
129. Pollesello P, Ovaska M, Kaivola J, et al: Binding of a new Ca^{2+} sensitizer, levosimendan, to recombinant human cardiac troponin C. A molecular modelling, fluorescence probe, and protein nuclear magnetic resonance study. J Biol Chem 1994; 269:28584.
130. Guntert TW, Linde HHA: Chemistry and structure-activity relationships of cardioactive steroids. Handbook Exp Pharmacol 1981; 56/I:13.
131. Withering W: An account of the foxglove and some of its medical uses, with practical remarks on dropsy, and other diseases. *In* Willius FA, Keys TE (eds): Classics of Cardiology, vol 1 , p 231. Dover, NY: 1941.
132. Eisner DA, Smith TW: The Na-K pump and its effectors in cardiac muscle. *In* Fozzard HA, Haber E, Katz AM, Morgan HE (eds): The Heart and Cardiovascular System, p 863. New York: Raven Press, 1992.
133. Kelly RA, Smith TW: The search for the endogenous digitalis: An alternative hypothesis. Am J Physiol 1989; 256:C937.
134. Kelly RA, Smith TW: Endogenous cardiac glycosides. Adv Pharmacol 1994; 25:263.
135. Lingrel JB, Van Huysse J, O'Brien W, et al: Structure-function studies of the Na,K-ATPase. Kidney Int 1994; 45:S32.
136. Templeton JF, Ling Y, Sashi Kumar VP, et al: Synthesis and structure-activity relationships of 14-hydroxy-5-pregnanes:pregnanes that bind to the cardiac glycoside receptor. Steroids 1993; 58:518.
137. Schmidt TA, Holm-Nielsen P, Kjeldsen J: No upregulation of digitalis glycoside receptor (Na,K-ATPase) concentration in human heart left ventricle samples obtained at necropsy after long-term digitalization. Cardiovasc Res 1991; 25:684.
138. Schmidt TA, Allen PD, Colucci WS, et al: No adaptation to digitalization as evaluated by digitalis receptor (Na,K-ATPase) quantification in explanted hearts from donors without heart disease and from digitalized recipients with end-stage heart failure. Am J Cardiol 1992; 70:110.
139. Harrison SM, McCall E, Boyett MR: The relationship between contraction and intracellular sodium in rat and guinea-pig ventricular myocytes. J Physiol (Lond) 1992; 449:517.
140. Mason DT, Braunwald E, Karsh RB, et al: Studies on digitalis. X. Effects of oubain on forearm vascular resistance and venous tone in normal subjects and in patients in heart failure. J Clin Invest 1964; 43:532.
141. Wang W, Chen J-S, Zucker IH: Carotid sinus baroreceptor sensitivity in experimental heart failure. Circulation 1990; 81:1959.
142. Ferguson DW, Berg WJ, Sanders JS, et al: Sympathoinhibitory responses to digitalis glycosides in heart failure patients. Direct evidence from sympathetic neural recordings. Circulation 1989; 80:65.

143. Gheorghiade M, Ferguson D: Digoxin. A neurohormonal modulator in heart failure? Circulation 1991; 84:2181.
144. Sarter BH, Marchlinski FE: Redefining the role of digoxin in the treatment of atrial fibrillation. Am J Cardiol 1992; 69:71G.
145. Kelly RA, Smith TW: Use and misuse of digitalis blood levels. Heart Dis Stroke 1992; 1:117.
146. Mahdyoon H, Battilana G, Rosman H, et al: The evolving pattern of digoxin intoxication: observations at a large urban hospital from 1980–1988. Am Heart J 1990; 120:1189.
147. Kelly RA, Smith TW: Recognition and management of digitalis toxicity. Am J Cardiol 1992; 69:108G.
148. Kelly RA, Smith TW: Antibody therapies for drug overdose. *In* Austen KF, Burakoff SJ, Rosen FS, Strom TR (eds): Therapeutic Immunology. Cambridge, MA: Blackwell Scientific, 1996.
149. Neer EJ: Heterotrimeric G proteins: Organizers of transmembrane signals. Cell 1995; 80:249.
150. Civelli O, Bunzow JR, Grandy DK: Molecular diversity of the dopamine receptors. Annu Rev Pharmacol Toxicol 1993; 32:281.
151. Ostrowski J, Kjelsberg MA, Caron MG, Lefkowitz RJ: Mutagenesis of the β_2-adrenergic receptor: How structure elucidates function. Annu Rev Pharmacol Toxicol 1992; 32:167.
152. Ruffolo RR Jr, Nichols AJ, Stadel JM, Hieble JP: Pharmacologic and therapeutic applications of α_2-adrenoceptor subtypes. Annu Rev Pharmacol Toxicol 1993; 32:243.
153. Hoffman BB, Lefkowitz RJ: Catecholamines; sympathomimetic drugs; and adrenergic receptor antagonists. *In* Hardman JG, Limbird LE (eds): Goodman and Gilman's The Pharmacologic Basis of Therapeutics, Chap. 10. New York: McGraw-Hill, in press.
154. Landzberg JS, Parker JD, Gauthier DF, Colucci WS: Effects of myocardial α_1-adrenergic receptor stimulation and blockade on contractility in humans. Circulation 1991; 84:1608.
155. Bristow MR: Changes in myocardial and vascular receptors in heart failure. J Am Coll Cardiol 1993; 22:61A.
156. Bristow MR, Ginsburg R, Minobe W, et al: Decreased catecholamine sensitivity and -adrenergic-receptor density in failing human hearts. N Engl J Med 1982; 307:205.
157. Bristow MR, Ginsburg R, Umans V, et al: β_1- and β_2-adrenergic receptor subpopulations in non-failing and failing human ventricular myocardium: Coupling of both receptor subtypes to muscle contraction and selective β_1-receptor down regulation in heart failure. Circ Res 1986; 59:297.
158. Merlet P, Delforge J, Syrota A, et al: Positron emission tomography with ^{11}C CGP-12177 to assess β-adrenergic receptor concentration in idiopathic dilated cardiomyopathy. Circulation 1993; 87:1169.
159. Insel PA: β-Adrenergic receptors in heart failure. J Clin Invest 1993; 92:2563.
160. Ungerer M, Bohm M, Elce JS, et al: Altered expression of β-adrenergic receptor kinase and β_1-adrenergic receptors in the failing human heart. Circulation 1993; 87:454.
161. Ungerer M, Parruti G, Bohm M, et al: Expression of β-arrestins and β-adrenergic receptor kinases in the failing human heart. Circ Res 1994; 74:206.
162. Harding SE, Brown LA, Wynne DG, et al: Mechanisms of adrenoceptor desensitization in the failing human heart. Cardiovasc Res 1994; 28; 1451.
163. White M, Roden R, Minobe W, et al: Age-related changes in β-adrenergic neuroeffector systems in the human heart. Circulation 1994; 90:1225.
164. Hershberger RE: Beta-adrenergic receptor agonists and antagonists in heart failure. *In* Hosenpud JD, Greenberg BH (eds): Congestive Heart Failure, p 454. New York: Springer-Verlag, 1994.
165. Bristow MR, Minobe W, Rasmussen R, et al: β-Adrenergic neuroeffector abnormalities in the failing human heart are produced by local rather than systemic mechanisms. J Clin Invest 1992; 89:803.
166. Gilbert EM, Sandoval A, Larrabee P, et al: Lisinopril lowers cardiac adrenergic drive and increases β-receptor density in the failing human heart. Circulation 1993; 88:472.
167. Creager MA, Quigg RJ, Ren CJ, et al: Limb vascular responsiveness to β-adrenergic receptor stimulation in patients with congestive heart failure. Circulation 1991; 83:1873.
168. Kubo SH, Rector TS, Heifetz SM, Cohn JN: α_2-Receptor-mediated vasoconstriction in patients with congestive heart failure. Circulation 1989; 80:1660.
169. Leier CV: Current status of non-digitalis positive inotropic drugs. Am J Cardiol 1992; 69:120G.
170. Binkley PF, VanFossen DV, Nunziata E, et al: Influence of positive inotropic therapy on pulsatile hydraulic load and ventricular-vascular coupling in congestive heart failure. J Am Coll Cardiol 1990; 15:1127.
171. Binkley PF, Murray KD, Watson KM, et al: Dobutamine increases cardiac output of total artificial heart. Implications for vascular contribution of inotropic agents to augmented ventricular function. Circulation 1991; 84:1210.
172. Sacher HL, Sacher ML, Landau SW, et al: Outpatient dobutamine therapy: The rhyme and the riddle. J Clin Pharmacol 1992; 32:141.
173. Kataoka T, Keteyian SJ, Marks CC, et al: Exercise training in a patient with congestive heart failure on continuous dobutamine. Med Sci Sports Exer 1993; p 678.
174. Miller LW: Outpatient dobutamine for refractory congestive heart failure: Advantages, techniques, and results. J Heart Lung Transplant 1991; 10:482.
175. Adamopoulos S, Piepoli M, Qiang F, et al: Effects of pulsed β-stimulant therapy on β-adrenoceptors and chronotropic responsiveness in chronic heart failure. Lancet 1995; 345:344.
176. Good J, Frost G, Oakley CM, Cleland GF: The renal effects of dopamine and dobutamine in stable chronic heart failure. Postgrad Med J 1992; 68:S7.
177. Vendegna TR, Anderson RJ: Are dopamine and/or dobutamine renoprotective in intensive care unit patients? Crit Care Med 1994; 22:1893.
178. Thompson BT, Cockrill BA: Renal-dose dopamine: A siren song? Lancet 1994; 344:7.
179. Duke GJ, Briedis JH, Weaver RA: Renal support in critically ill patients: Low-dose dopamine or low-dose dobutamine? Crit Care Med 1994; 22:1919.
180. Flancbaum L, Choban PS, Dasta JF: Quantitative effects of low-dose dopamine on urine output in oliguric surgical intensive care unit patients. Crit Care Med 1994; 22:61.
181. Baldwin L, Henderson A, Hickman P: Effect of postoperative low-dose dopamine on renal function after elective major vascular surgery. Ann Intern Med 1994; 120:744.
182. van Veldhuisen DJ, Girbes ARJ, de Graeff PA, Lie KI: Effects of dopaminergic agents on cardiac and renal function in normal man and in patients with congestive heart failure. Int J Cardiol 1992; 37:293.
183. Leier CV, Binkley PF, Carpenter J, et al: Cardiovascular pharmacology of dopexamine in low output congestive heart failure. Am J Cardiol 1988; 62:94.
184. Baumann G, Felix SB, Filcek SAL: Usefulness of dopexamine hydrochloride versus dobutamine in chronic congestive heart failure and effects on hemodynamics and urine output. Am J Cardiol 1990; 65:748.
185. MacGregor DA, Butterworth JF IV, Zaloga GP, et al: Hemodynamic and renal effects of dopexamine and dobutamine in patients with reduced cardiac output following coronary artery bypass grafting. Chest 1994; 106:835.
186. van Veldhuisen DJ, Manin T, Veld AJ, et al.: Double-blind placebo-controlled study of ibopamine and digoxin in patients with mild to moderate heart failure: Results of the Dutch Ibopamine Multicenter Trial (DIMT). J Am Coll Cardiol 1993; 22:1564.
187. Beavo JA, Reifsnyder DH: Primary sequence of cyclic nucleotide phosphodiesterase isozymes and the design of selective inhibitors. Trends Pharmacol Sci 1990; 11:150.
188. Nicholson CD, Challiss RAJ, Shahid M: Differential modulation of tissue function and therapeutic potential of selective inhibitors of cyclic nucleotide phosphodiesterase isoenzymes. Trends Pharmacol Sci 1991; 12:19.
189. Bode DC, Kanter JR, Brunton LL: Cellular distribution of phosphodiesterase isoforms in rat cardiac tissue. Circ Res 1991; 68:1070.
190. Beavo JA: cGMP inhibition of heart phosphodiesterase: Is it clinically relevant? J Clin Invest 1995; 95:444.
191. Packer M, Carver JR, Rodeheffer RJ, et al: Effect of oral milrinone on mortality in severe chronic heart failure. N Engl J Med 1991; 325:1468.
192. Packer M: The development of positive inotropic agents for chronic heart failure: How have we gone astray? J Am Coll Cardiol 1993; 22:119A.
193. DiBianco R, Shabetai R, Kostik W, et al: A comparison of oral milrinone, digoxin, and their combination in the treatment of patients with chronic heart failure. N Engl J Med 1989; 320:677.
194. Meacci E, Taira M, Moos M Jr, et al: Molecular cloning and expression of human myocardial cGMP-inhibited cAMP phosphodiesterase. Proc Natl Acad Sci U S A 1992; 89:3721.
195. Matsui S, Matsumori A, Matoba Y, et al: Treatment of virus-induced myocardial injury with a novel immunomodulating agent, vesnarinone.

Suppression of natural killer cell activity and tumor necrosis factor-α production. J Clin Invest 1944; 94:1212.
196. Feldman AM, Bristow MR, Parmley WW, et al: Effects of vesnarinone on morbidity and mortality in patients with heart failure. N Engl J Med 1993; 329:149.
197. Waagstein F, Hjalmarson A, Varnauskas E, Wallentin F: Effect of chronic beta-adrenergic receptor blockade in congestive cardiomyopathy. Br Heart J 1975; 37:1022.
198. Swedberg K: Initial experience with beta blockers in dilated cardiomyopathy. Am J Cardiol 1993; 71:30C.
199. Fowler MB: Controlled trials with beta blockers in heart failure: Metoprolol as the prototype. Am J Cardiol 1993; 71:45C.
200. Doughty RN, MacMahon S, Sharpe N: Beta-blockers in heart failure: Promising or proved? J Am Coll Cardiol 1994; 23:814.
201. The Beta-Blocker Pooling Project Research Group: The Beta-Blocker Pooling Project (BPPP); Subgroup findings from randomized trials in post-infarction patients. Eur Heart J 1988; 9:8.
202. Waagstein F, Bristow MR, Swedberg K, et al: Beneficial effects of metoprolol in idiopathic dilated cardiomyopathy. Lancet 1993; 342:1441.
203. CIBIS Investigators and Committees: A randomized trial of β-blockade in heart failure. The Cardiac Insufficiency Bisoprolol Study (CIBIS). Circulation 1994; 90:1765.
204. Fisher ML, Gottlieb SS, Plotnick GD, et al: Beneficial effects of metoprolol in heart failure associated with coronary artery disease: A randomized trial. J Am Coll Cardiol 1994; 23:943.
205. Bristow MR, O'Connell JB, Gilbert EM, et al, for the Bucindolol Investigators: Dose-response of chronic -blocker treatment in heart failure from either idiopathic dilated or ischemic cardiomyopathy. Circulation 1994; 89:1632.
206. Bristow MR: Pathophysiologic and pharmacologic rationales for clinical management of chronic heart failure with beta-blocking agents. Am J Cardiol 1993; 21:12C.
207. The Xamoterol in Severe Heart Failure Study Group: Xamoterol in severe heart failure. Lancet 1990; 336:1.
208. Leung WH, Lau CP, Wong CK, et al: Improvement in exercise performance and hemodynamics by labetalol in patients with idiopathic dilated cardiomyopathy. Am Heart J 1990; 199:884.
209. Fowler MB: Beta-blockers in heart failure: Potential of carvedilol. J Hum Hypertens 1993; 7:S62.
210. Krum H, Sackner-Bernstein JD, Goldsmith RL, et al: Double-blind, placebo-controlled study of the long-term efficacy of carvedilol in patients with severe chronic heart failure. Circulation 1995; 92:1499.
211. Metra M, Nardi M, Giubbini R, Dei Cas L: Effects of short- and long-term carvedilol administration on rest and exercise hemodynamic variables, exercise capacity and clinical conditions in patients with idiopathic dilated cardiomyopathy. J Am Coll Cardiol 1994; 24:1678.
212. SmithKline Beecham Statement on Carvedilol. March 1995.
213. Ertl G, Neubauer S, Gaudron P, et al: Beta-blockers in cardiac failure. Eur Heart J 1994; 15:16.

10 Management of Patients Hospitalized With Heart Failure

Lynne Warner Stevenson, MD
Wilson S. Colucci, MD

INTRODUCTION

Patients may require treatment of heart failure during hospitalization in a variety of situations. The majority of patients hospitalized for heart failure have previously been diagnosed with heart failure but have subsequently developed progressive hemodynamic decompensation that leads to admission. In some cases, the rate or degree of decompensation is sufficiently alarming that urgent or semiurgent admission is indicated in order to avert impending collapse. In other cases, hospital admission may be scheduled more electively to initiate or modify therapy that might otherwise be difficult or dangerous in the outpatient setting. Patients admitted with another cardiac diagnosis such as angina, arrhythmia, or an embolic event may require initiation of therapy for heart failure that was not previously recognized. Less commonly, patients may undergo evaluation and therapy for heart failure after an initial diagnosis of a noncardiac problem such as chronic pulmonary disease or pneumonia.

The approach to therapy for all patients with heart failure should first include a careful search for potentially correctable factors (Table 10–1). The subsequent steps depend on multiple factors, including the acuity of onset, the level of hemodynamic compromise, the rate of deterioration, and the underlying etiology. In the patient with critical compromise, particularly with precipitous onset or rapid progression, the first goal of therapy is stabilization of the circulation and protection of the vital organs. This may necessitate rapid management decisions regarding the use of intravenous inotropic and direct-acting vasoactive agents (e.g., dobutamine, nitroprusside, dopamine) and, less often, mechanical support (e.g., intra-aortic balloon counterpulsation or a ventricular assist device). At the other end of the spectrum, in the patient admitted to the hospital with gradual progression of chronic heart failure, therapy is more likely to be directed at the initiation or modification of chronic oral medications

TABLE 10–1. POTENTIALLY REVERSIBLE FACTORS CONTRIBUTING TO DECOMPENSATION IN PATIENTS WITH HEART FAILURE

Myocardial ischemia amenable to revascularization
Recent viral illness
Heavy alcohol consumption
Tachyarrhythmias
Thyroid disease
Periodic hypoxia (e.g., sleep apnea)
Anemia
Noncompliance with medications and/or salt and fluid restriction
Nonsteroidal anti-inflammatory agents

with the goal of improving functional status, preventing the progression of the underlying myocardial dysfunction, and improving survival. In this chapter, both types of patients are discussed. The treatment of ambulatory patients who do not require admission to the hospital is discussed in Chapter 11.

EVALUATION OF THE PATIENT

Importance of Rapid Assessment

The potential availability of invasive hemodynamic measurement does not diminish the critical importance of rapid bedside estimation of circulatory status. Although patients are often admitted to the hospital "electively" for the treatment of heart failure, the admission in many cases is prompted by the premonition of imminent deterioration. Therefore, it is prudent to perform a brief clinical evaluation of newly admitted patients even before review of the medical records, which are often extensive. Severe elevation of intracardiac filling pressures and the adequacy or inadequacy of systemic perfusion can usually be ascertained within a few minutes.[1–7] It is sometimes necessary to initiate therapy on the basis of the clinical assessment, although subsequent hemodynamic monitoring may be necessary for optimal adjustment of therapy. As a first approximation, patients can be categorized on the basis of the presence or absence of clinical evidence for elevated filling pressures and critically reduced organ perfusion.

Intracardiac Filling Pressures and Volume Status

The presence of severely elevated filling pressures is often not appreciated in patients with chronic heart failure. Chronic extravasation of fluid as a result of high filling pressures in the pulmonary vascular bed can markedly increase the capacity for lymphatic drainage, in such a way that the pulmonary capillary wedge pressures of over 30 mm Hg may be tolerated. The presence of rales is therefore a relatively insensitive sign for elevated filling pressures in chronic heart failure.[1–3] On the other hand, the presence of diffuse rales or respiratory distress in the upright position is a relatively specific sign of a severe elevation of left-sided filling pressures. Such patients may require urgent intervention to avert respiratory failure (see Emergency Therapy section).

The absence, presence, or intensity of a left-sided third heart sound rarely indicates the level of left ventricular filling pressure, except in the occasional patient in whom the third heart sound is known by the examiner to have changed recently in the absence of a concomitant change in rhythm or rate. The chest radiograph can provide multiple clues to the presence of chronic heart failure, but is not a reliable guide to current hemodynamic status.[5] In addition, it should be recognized that changes in the "left-sided heart border" in chronic dilated heart failure are frequently caused by changes in right ventricular size.

Signs of elevated right ventricular filling pressures are relatively reliable indicators of elevated left ventricular filling pressures, although in the more acute setting they are less sensitive. On occasion, the presence of independent right ventricular pathology such as right ventricular infarction, primary right-sided valve lesions, right ventricular dysplasia, or intrinsic pulmonary hypertension may cause dissociation of right and left ventricular filling pressures. Right-sided filling pressures are best assessed by inspecting the jugular veins,[6] which should be assessed in all patients with heart failure. Either internal or external jugular veins may be used if venous pulsations confirm free flow to the right atrium. The patient should be raised or lowered until the height of the blood column becomes visible, and the vertical height of the jugular venous pressure above the sternal angle, which itself is about 5 cm above the right atrium, should be estimated.

In the absence of primary liver disease, ascites is a specific but very insensitive indicator of fluid status in the patient with heart failure, inasmuch as some patients do not develop ascites despite marked hepatic engorgement and abdominal discomfort. Peripheral edema is a more sensitive sign of volume overload than is ascites, but it is much less sensitive than an elevation of the jugular venous pressure. Obesity, previous vein graft harvesting, other venous disease, and lymphatic obstruction can cause peripheral edema out of proportion to central venous pressures. Before a decrease in peripheral edema is considered to reflect clinical improvement in a hospitalized patient, it is important to ascertain whether gravity has merely shifted the fluid to the dependent presacral area.

Examination of the peripheral pulse with a blood pressure cuff during a bedside Valsalva maneuver can help to clarify volume status in patients with heart failure.[1] Although this maneuver requires considerable physician practice and patient cooperation, it can provide valuable information. An automated noninvasive device that quantifies the fingertip blood pressure response to a Valsalva maneuver has been validated.[4]

Adequacy of Perfusion

It is important to distinguish patients with a chronically reduced cardiac output from those in whom the cardiac output is deteriorating rapidly. Obvious mental obtundation and anuria suggest acute hypoperfusion. It is often helpful to look for cold skin on the forearms and thighs, in addition to the hands and feet. Some patients may have frank cyanosis when cardiac output is critically reduced.

An important part of the noninvasive assessment of systemic perfusion is careful measurement of the blood pressure by the examiner. The cuff should be deflated slowly in order to determine the exact level at which Korotkoff sounds start and stop. The difference between the systolic and diastolic pressure, expressed as the proportional pulse pressure is calculated as follows, omitting beats that follow premature ventricular contractions:

$$\text{Proportional Pulse Pressure} = \frac{\text{Systolic Blood Pressure} - \text{Diastolic Blood Pressure}}{\text{Systolic Blood Pressure}}$$

Assessment of the pulse pressure is complicated by the presence of atrial fibrillation, unless the rate is fairly regular. The presence of pulsus alternans also complicates this assessment but is itself often an indication of very compromised stroke volume. When the pulse pressure is less than 25% of the systolic pressure, the cardiac index is generally below 2.2 L/min/m^2.[3] This level of hypoperfusion is alarming in a patient with new heart failure. Pulse pressures of less than 15% of the systolic pressure often indicate more severe compromise and a greater need for immediate intervention. Although many patients with critically reduced perfusion have a systolic blood pressure below 80 mm Hg, blood pressures of 110/100 mm Hg are also common and frequently are charted as 110/80 mm Hg if the cuff has been deflated too rapidly.

Invasive Assessment

The insertion of a pulmonary artery catheter is rarely necessary for initial hemodynamic classification of the patient with chronic heart failure. In most cases, the measured hemodynamic parameters are not necessary for the diagnosis of compromise, but they can allow more systematic adjustment of therapy, particularly the optimization of loading conditions and choice of agents. The initiation of urgent therapy for severely elevated filling pressures and/or critically reduced perfusion should not be delayed for the exact hemodynamic measurements.

The need for an invasive arterial pressure monitor is determined to a large extent by nursing practice in a given unit. Although inexact, the noninvasive blood pressure cuff frequently provides adequate blood pressure trends during adjustment of therapy, even in patients with systolic blood pressures in the vicinity of 80 mm Hg. Electrocardiographic monitoring is routine for most patients admitted for therapy of heart failure. The rapidity of changes in fluid and electrolyte status during diuresis may predispose to arrhythmias, which can be worsened by potentially arrhythmogenic drugs such as dopamine or dobutamine. In addition, the patient with decompensated heart failure has an increased risk of sudden death from multiple intrinsic mechanisms.[8]

A urinary catheter is important when hourly urine outputs are being observed as an indication of perfusion and may also be helpful for documenting the adequacy of the initial diuretic regimen and for avoiding very frequent urination during mobilization of a large excess volume, but in general it should be removed within 24–48 h to minimize the risk of infection.

Determining the Primary and Secondary Causes

The syndrome of heart failure is nonspecific and can result from a wide range of pathologic conditions that may dictate disparate types of therapy. This aspect of evaluation is particularly critical in heart failure of new onset, causes of which include acute myocardial infarction, valvular regurgitation, and myocarditis, as well as exacerbation of previously occult ventricular dysfunction. Urgent revascularization or valve replacement may in some cases avert progression to chronic heart failure.

The initial evaluation of all heart failure should include consideration of coronary artery disease, primary valvular lesions, pericardial disease, and extracardiac disease such as primary pulmonary hypertension or intrinsic pulmonary parenchymal disease. When myocardial failure appears primary, it should be characterized, usually by echocardiography, to determine whether it is predominantly caused by a dilated, hypertrophic, or restrictive cardiomyopathy. Distinguishing between patients with a low left ventricular ejection fraction (predominant systolic failure) and those with a relatively preserved ejection fraction (predominant diastolic failure) is important in selecting the appropriate form of therapy (see Chapter 13). Clues to the presence of primary diastolic dysfunction include advanced age and a history of diabetes mellitus or hypertension.

Multiple factors can cause decompensation in chronic heart failure or precipitate new symptoms of heart failure in a patient with previous asymptomatic left ventricular dysfunction (see Table 10–1). The most common cause is fluid retention related to excess salt intake or inadequate use of diuretics. Alcohol intake that is moderate by general standards (about two glasses of wine per day) may cause further myocardial depression in an impaired ventricle, although this amount has not been implicated as a primary cause of cardiomyopathy in an otherwise healthy person. It is worth addressing this issue explicitly because many patients extrapolate to their heart failure the publicized benefits of wine for coronary artery disease. Atrial arrhythmias, most often atrial fibrillation, commonly bring heart failure to attention and in some cases may be the underlying cause of heart failure which is potentially reversible with effective antiarrhythmic therapy.[9] Common viral infections frequently precipitate deterioration for several weeks in patients with chronic heart failure, who then may recover compensation if carefully managed.

STRATEGIES FOR INITIAL TREATMENT

General Principles

For both emergent and less urgent situations, initial therapeutic decisions reflect the estimated severity of pulmonary congestion and systemic hypoperfusion. Ongoing evaluation guides subsequent therapy, which may in some cases be facilitated by hemodynamic monitoring for more precise adjustment of medications to the desired endpoints (Table 10–2). Although the general approach is described for broad hemodynamic profiles, there are many unique situations that necessitate individualization of the strategy.

TABLE 10–2. SUGGESTED INDICATIONS FOR HEMODYNAMIC MONITORING DURING THERAPY FOR DECOMPENSATED HEART FAILURE

Presence of hypoperfusion suspected from:
Narrow pulse pressure
Mental obtundation
Declining renal function with high volume status
Intense neurohormonal activation suggested by:
Serum sodium below 133 mEq/L
Persistent systemic hypotension with low doses of ACE inhibitors
Symptoms of congestion at rest in the presence of:
Frequent angina or other evidence of ischemia
Frequent symptomatic ventricular arrhythmias
Baseline impairment of renal function
Severe intrinsic pulmonary disease
Persistent or recurrent symptoms of congestion at rest or minimal exertion despite:
Administration of high doses of loop diuretics
Addition of metolazone or hydrochlorothiazide
Salt and fluid restriction
Consideration of cardiac transplantation for primary indication of heart failure

Profile A: Clinical Compensation

When initial assessment fails to reveal evidence of resting congestion or hypoperfusion, despite presentation with symptoms of heart failure at rest or during minimal exertion, patients should be evaluated for intermittent conditions such as ischemia or arrhythmias (which could cause transient elevation of filling pressures), pulmonary disease, and other noncardiac causes of dyspnea. When there is doubt as to whether cardiac abnormalities are responsible for the symptoms, the number of repeated hospitalizations may be reduced by insertion of a pulmonary artery catheter to measure hemodynamics at rest. Hemodynamics should be assessed during exercise if resting hemodynamics do not explain exertional limitation. Many patients with ejection fractions of less than .25 are well compensated with few symptoms, and therefore it should not be assumed that all symptoms in a patient with a low ejection fraction are caused by heart failure.

Profile B: Congestion With Adequate Perfusion

In such patients, the majority of symptoms reflect the elevations in right- and left-sided intracardiac filling pressures that are transmitted to the pulmonary and systemic venous system. Typically, the systolic blood pressure is >85 mm Hg and the proportional pulse pressure is >25%. Both systemic volume expansion and vasoconstriction contribute to the elevated intracardiac filling pressures. The relative emphasis on diuretics vs. vasodilators is determined in part by the degree of apparent volume overload. Most patients admitted with symptoms of severe congestion have some fluid retention and benefit from 2–4 L of net fluid loss. Some patients with obvious extravascular volume reservoirs such as ascites and peripheral edema require extensive diuresis, often on the order of 10–20 L. Initial diuretic therapy generally requires an intravenous loop diuretic and may require a second agent such as metolazone or hydrochlorothiazide (see Diuretics section).

Initiation or adjustment of angiotensin converting enzyme (ACE) inhibitors should be pursued in most patients. Even in the patient without an apparent severe decrease in cardiac output, a reduction of systemic vascular resistance often facilitates reduction of intraventricular filling pressures, and inhibition of aldosterone production may limit diuretic requirements. If the patient is not receiving an

ACE inhibitor and has no contraindications, an agent should be started at low dosages and increased carefully. Use of a short-acting agent may be safest for initiation in the decompensated patient. For patients already receiving ACE inhibitors, either short- or long-acting, the dosages may be increased empirically to target doses (captopril: 50 mg t.i.d.;[10] enalapril: 10 mg b.i.d.;[11, 12] or their equivalents), as tolerated. Concomitant optimization of volume status and vascular tone is often necessary for restoring stabilization but can be difficult to achieve empirically. It has at times been recommended that diuretics be decreased or stopped before initiation of ACE inhibition in the outpatient setting. In hospitalized patients without obvious hypoperfusion, it is generally safe to initiate and adjust ACE inhibitors or other vasodilators empirically while a diuresis occurs.

The patient requires frequent evaluation as diuresis proceeds. Most patients should be rendered free of pulmonary congestion and peripheral edema. Orthopnea and dyspnea upon walking a short distance generally indicate that further diuresis is required. Most patients with chronic heart failure describe freedom from both orthopnea and dyspnea on light exertion when the pulmonary capillary wedge pressure is less than 25 mm Hg, and some patients are asymptomatic at a pulmonary capillary wedge pressure of 30 mm Hg. Reduction of filling pressures in most patients should ideally continue until the jugular venous pressure is less than 7–8 mm Hg. In most cases, the pulmonary capillary wedge pressure is usually not higher than 20 mm Hg at this time. The benefit of further reduction of filling pressures has not been established; however, reduction of the pulmonary capillary wedge pressure to 15–16 mm Hg may be associated with a small additional increase in stroke volume in some patients,[13, 14] and the ability to achieve this degree of lowering of left-sided filling pressure may be associated with a better prognosis.[14]

Patients in whom clinical evidence of congestion persists despite empiric adjustment of diuretics and vasodilators may be considered for further adjustment of therapy guided by invasive hemodynamic monitoring. Empiric therapy may be limited by hypotension, declining renal function, or inability to achieve an adequate diuresis. In patients with active angina, sudden changes in systemic vascular resistance and coronary perfusion pressures may aggravate ischemia, although more often the reduction in ventricular filling pressures reduces the number of ischemic episodes. Ventricular arrhythmias may be aggravated by reflex sympathetic stimulation resulting from sudden vasodilatation or diuresis, as well as by electrolyte shifts. In patients with a serum sodium level of less than 133 mEq/L, in whom the renin-angiotensin system is highly activated,[16] stabilization with oral ACE inhibitors may be more difficult without hemodynamic monitoring.

Profile C: Hypoperfusion Without Congestion

When the blood pressure, mental status, or peripheral signs indicate reduced systemic perfusion, the patient should be evaluated rapidly to determine the need for urgent intervention. Because, as discussed previously, signs of pulmonary congestion may be absent even in patients with elevated left-sided filling pressures, invasive monitoring is often helpful for guiding therapy. Even though systemic vascular resistance may be markedly elevated, the use of vasodilators in such patients is often accompanied by hypotension, and it may be necessary to cautiously increase the intravascular volume so that vasodilators can be tolerated. When such patients are critically compromised, therapy should include positive inotropic agents, which may in some cases be combined with vasodilator agents if the systemic vascular resistance is high.

Profile D: Congestion With Hypoperfusion

The combination of congestion and hypoperfusion is probably the most common profile in patients hospitalized with heart failure. In such patients, hemodynamic monitoring may allow the simultaneous optimization of filling pressures and systemic vascular resistance through the use of intravenous agents (e.g., nitroprusside, dobutamine, milrinone), which can often be titrated to approach hemodynamic goals within 24–48 h. When initial filling pressures and systemic vascular resistance are close to target levels, oral agents may be initiated and adjusted without the intermediate step of intravenous therapy.

Once hemodynamic monitoring is in place, there are often a number of reasonable approaches, and the optimal regimen may be arrived at only by therapeutic trial. However, in selecting the initial intravenous drug regimen, the physician should pay particular attention to the systemic vascular resistance, because this parameter is an important determinant of whether the patient will respond favorably to a vasodilator (Table 10–3). Patients with an elevated systemic vascular resistance are generally responsive to vasodilators such as nitroprusside. As discussed later, although the vasodilator of choice is most often nitroprusside, nitroglycerin can also be used for this purpose and may be the preferred agent if active ischemia is a concern. At the other end of the spectrum are patients in whom the systemic vascular resistance is at the low normal range or below normal. In these patients, the drug of choice is most often dobutamine, because further reduction in the systemic vascular resistance without inotropic support may result in an unacceptable fall in the arterial pressure. In patients with a systemic vascular resistance in the "normal" range, either vasodilators or positive inotropic agents are often effective and frequently may be used in combination to achieve an optimal result. When nitroprusside or nitroglycerin alone is ineffective as a vasodilator or not tolerated, these agents may be combined with dobutamine or dopamine or replaced by a phosphodiesterase inhibitor such as milrinone that exerts both effects.

In most patients admitted with decompensation resulting from chronic heart failure, the tailoring of intravenous followed by oral vasodilators can generally be achieved during 72–96 h of hemodynamic monitoring[17] (see Adjustment of Oral Medications section). Maintenance of an indwelling pulmonary artery line, however, requires that the patient remain close to the bed and does present a risk for infection, although this risk is minimized by careful attention to sterile insertion and the use of a catheter sleeve. For these reasons, insertion of the catheter may be postponed until the information can best guide therapy. In a stable patient with massive volume overload evidenced by ascites and anasarca, the need for diuresis is clear without quantitation of filling pressures and cardiac output. This diuresis can proceed empirically for several days until limited by hypotension or azotemia or until further and more precise adjustment of filling pressures and vasodilatation is required.

Emergency Therapy

For the patient who is first seen with critical compromise, rapid therapy may be needed to avert potentially fatal hemodynamic col-

TABLE 10–3. SELECTION OF DRUGS IN PATIENTS WITH BOTH ELEVATED FILLING PRESSURES AND A REDUCED CARDIAC OUTPUT

Cardiac Output	Low	Low	Low
PCW	High	High	High
Systemic vascular resistance	High	Normal	Low
Initial agent	Nitroprusside	Nitroprusside, milrinone, or dobutamine/ nitroprusside	Dobutamine or dopamine

lapse or prolonged organ dysfunction. The emergency therapy of respiratory distress approaching pulmonary edema includes *sublingual nitroglycerin* until an intravenous nitroglycerin drip can be initiated (one 1/150-grain sublingual tablet every 4 min is equivalent to approximately 100 μg/min intravenously), in addition to maintaining the patient in a *sitting position* with oxygen supplementation. Concomitant *intravenous diuretic* therapy may be given to patients with chronic heart failure but should be used cautiously in the setting of acute myocardial infarction, in which there is often maldistribution of fluid rather than total body fluid overload. Intravenous *morphine* (2- to 5-mg boluses) causes vasodilatation and sedation but should be carefully monitored because excessive sedation may precipitate the need for intubation in a patient with declining respiratory strength. *Intubation* may reduce work, sympathetic drive, and ischemia in a patient with pulmonary edema associated with an acute myocardial infarction. Intubation is rarely required in patients with an exacerbation of chronic heart failure without other problems; however, it may become necessary in a patient with chronic heart failure complicated by intrinsic lung disease or acute infection.

Pulmonary edema may occur in the setting of low, normal, or even high cardiac output. When the adequacy of perfusion is in doubt in the emergency setting, it may be necessary to progress to therapy with positive inotropic agents (e.g., dobutamine) or inotropic vasodilators (e.g., milrinone) before hemodynamic measurements have been made. As discussed in the next section, the use of these agents is strongly guided by the hemodynamic profile, and therefore their empiric use is suboptimal. Nevertheless, because the hemodynamic profile in patients with a critically reduced cardiac output in the setting of acute decompensation often includes elevated systemic vascular resistance and elevated filling pressures, these agents can frequently be administered before the initiation of invasive monitoring. Dobutamine is the most versatile drug for this setting. Occasionally, patients present in a low-output state with relative vasodilatation, such as sepsis or after spinal anesthesia, for which an agent such as dopamine or epinephrine may provide more support of the arterial pressure until hemodynamic information is available. The intravenous phosphodiesterase inhibitors have both inotropic and vasodilator effects. Because of the prolonged half-lives of these agents, they are best used after hemodynamic monitoring has been initiated. The use of vasodilators can potentially aggravate the situation if filling pressures or systemic vascular resistances are already low, and therefore they should be started at relatively low dosages and then carefully titrated upward as tolerated or until invasive monitoring is available.

Prolonged attempts to stabilize patients in an emergency situation with pharmacologic therapy should not delay consideration of further support with an intra-aortic balloon pump or mechanical ventricular assist devices (see Chapter 15). Such devices are most often indicated in the setting of an acute event such as myocardial infarction, valve rupture, or, in rare instances, acute viral myocarditis. For the patient in whom the situation is less urgent, initial therapy should be based on a more systematic analysis of the underlying hemodynamic status.

HEMODYNAMIC GOALS FOR GUIDING THERAPY

Effective therapy can often by guided by noninvasive clinical estimation of the hemodynamic profile discussed above. Insertion of a pulmonary artery catheter, however, whether for the indications in Table 10–2 or as part of an evaluation for cardiac transplantation, provides an opportunity for more precise adjustment to specific hemodynamic goals.

Intracardiac Filling Pressures

The goals of therapy should include a pulmonary capillary wedge pressure in the range of 15–18 mm Hg in patients with chronic heart failure.[13] Appropriate filling pressures for maximal cardiac output may be slightly higher in situations of decreased ventricular compliance without major dilation, such as in acute myocardial infarction.[18] A right atrial pressure of less than 7–8 mm Hg has been suggested as a general target but cannot always be achieved. The optimal right atrial pressures in the presence of right ventricular infarction may be higher, although the aggressive volume loading once recommended in this setting is now recognized to compromise left ventricular function. In practical terms, the right atrial pressure is most helpful as a guide to diuresis and venodilatation.

Cardiac Output

The normal cardiac index is at least 2.5 L/min/m^2. When the cardiac index falls below this level, particularly if the fall is acute, there may be hypoperfusion of vital organs resulting in reduced mentation, renal insufficiency, and hepatic and/or gut dysfunction. Becaues it is often important to improve organ perfusion in such patients, a major focus of therapy is to increase the cardiac output. A cardiac index of 2.0–2.2 L/min/m^2 is usually well tolerated, and even lower cardiac indices may cause relatively little organ dysfunction in some patients, particularly if the low output state has developed gradually. Therefore, the goal of therapy should be to achieve a cardiac output that is sufficient to maintain normal organ function. The cardiac index target may vary widely from patient to patient and from day to day in the same patient; however, as a first approximation, a cardiac index in the range of 2.2–2.5 L/min/m^2 is a reasonable goal for in-hospital therapy. Mixed venous oxygen saturation may also provide a measure of the adequacy of perfusion and may be used to calculate the cardiac output by the Fick equation on the basis of an assumed oxygen consumption.

Systemic Vascular Resistance

The normal systemic vascular resistance (SVR) is 1000–1300 dynes/sec/cm^{-5} and lower for very large persons. SVR is sometimes multiplied by body surface area to give an SVR index. It is generally useful to titrate vasodilator therapy to achieve an SVR in the range of 1000–1200 dynes/sec/cm^{-5}, and many patients may have a further increase in cardiac output when the SVR is lowered to the range of 800–900 dynes/sec/cm^{-5}. However, excessive vasodilatation can activate baroreflexes, leading to increased sympathetic tone and tachycardia. Also, a degree of vasodilatation that is tolerated in the supine position may predispose to postural hypotension when the patient becomes ambulatory.

USE OF SPECIFIC INTRAVENOUS AGENTS

Nitroprusside (Figs. 10–1, 10–2)

An initial dosage of 10 μg/min can be increased by 20 μg/min every 10–15 min while filling pressures and blood pressure are monitored. Goals of titration are often to reduce the systemic vascular resistance to the range of 1000–1200 dynes/sec/cm^{-5} while a systolic blood pressure of $\geq$80 mm Hg is maintained. Both arterial and venous dilation contribute to the decrease in pulmonary capillary wedge pressure, which is most marked in patients without major volume overload. Right atrial pressures are also reduced. Once an effect on filling pressure or arterial pressure becomes evident during the upward titration, cardiac output and systemic vascular resistance should be calculated and measured frequently during subsequent adjustments until the target hemodynamics are achieved.

Dosages over 300 μg/min are rarely required in order to achieve adequate vasodilatation, and they increase the chance of cyanide toxicity. Nitroprusside rapidly releases cyanide that is converted to thiocyanate in the liver and is excreted by the kidney. Liver dysfunction and prolonged infusion may predispose to the accumulation of cyanide, which inactivates the cytochrome oxidase system and causes

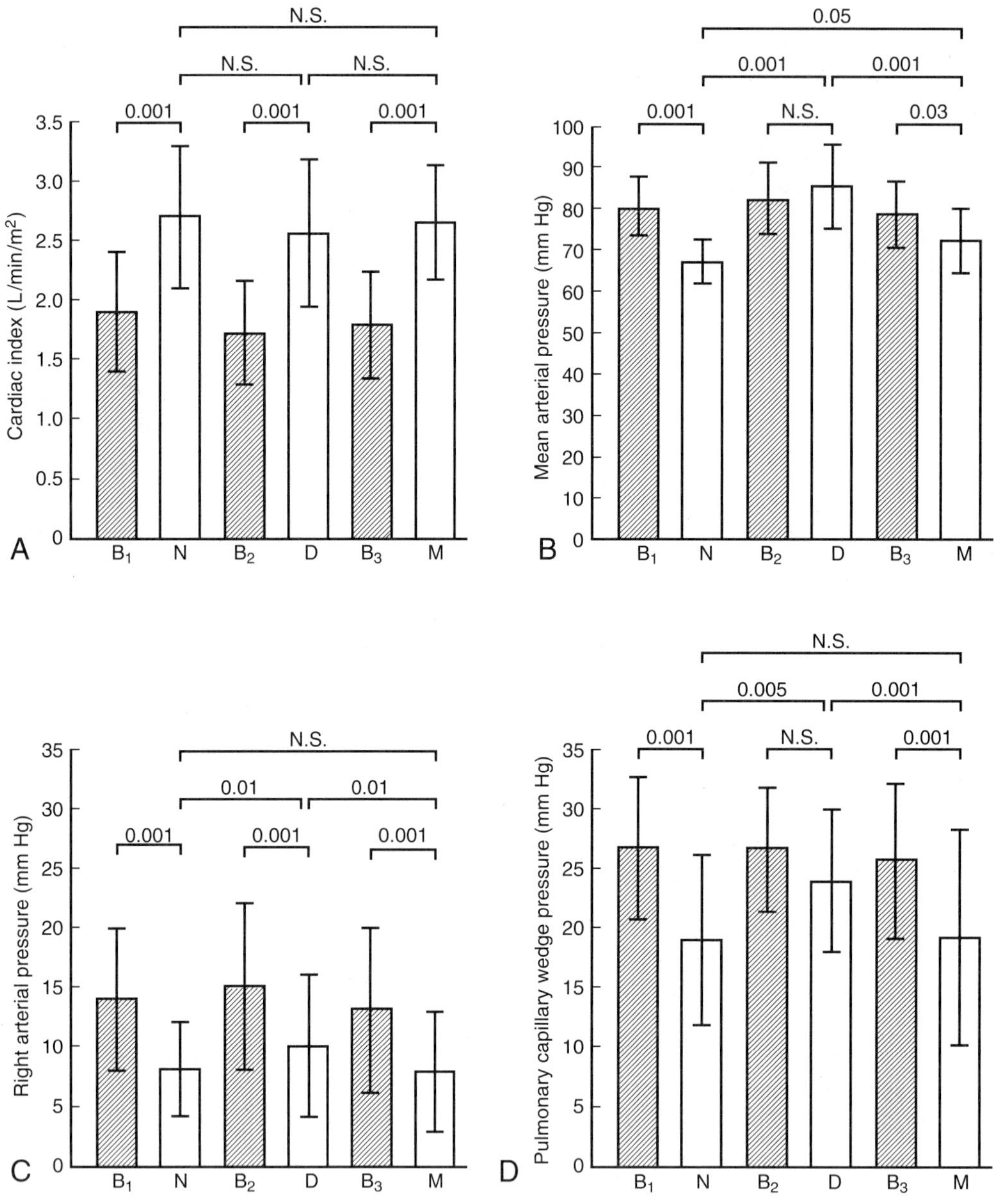

Figure 10–1. Shown are the comparative effects of nitroprusside (N), dobutamine (D), and milrinone (M) on cardiac index, mean arterial pressure, right atrial pressure, and pulmonary capillary wedge pressure in patients with severe heart failure (B_1, B_2, and B_3 = baseline measurements). The three agents were administered in doses that caused comparable increases in cardiac index (*A*). Under these conditions, nitroprusside and milrinone significantly reduced mean arterial pressure (*B*), but dobutamine had no effect. All three agents reduced right atrial pressure (*C*), although the effect of dobutamine was slightly less pronounced. Both nitroprusside and milrinone significantly reduced pulmonary capillary wedge pressure (*D*), and this effect was significantly more pronounced than the effect of dobutamine. (Adapted from Monrad ES, Baim DS, Smith HS, et al: Effects of milrinone on coronary hemodynamics and myocardial energetics in patients with congestive heart failure. Circulation 1985; 71:972–979.)

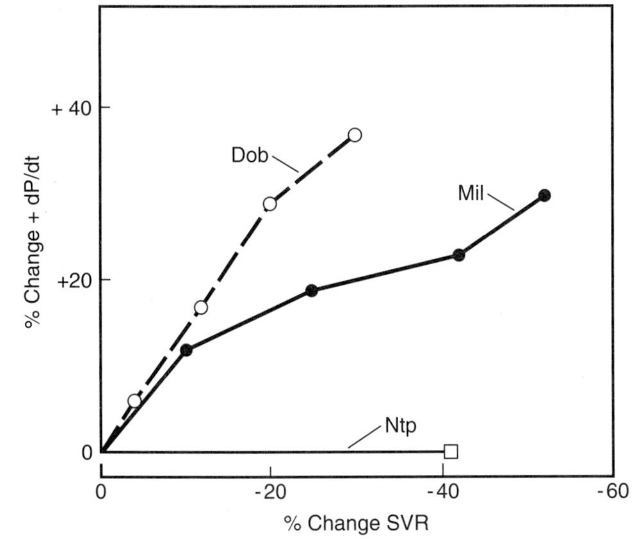

Figure 10–2. The relative effects of dobutamine (DOB), milrinone (MIL), and nitroprusside (NTP) on left ventricular contractility, as reflected by peak +dP/dt and systemic vascular resistance (SVR) in patients with severe heart failure. (From Colucci WS, Wright RF, Jaski BE, et al: Milrinone and dobutamine in severe heart failure: differing hemodynamic effects and individual patient responsiveness. Circulation 1986; 73:III-175–III-173.)

lactic acidosis. Patients may complain first of nausea, restlessness, and dysphoria. Cyanide toxicity from nitroprusside rarely requires specific therapy other than discontinuation of nitroprusside, but it can be treated with sodium nitrite, which reacts to form methemoglobin to bind cyanide; thiosulfate, which facilitates conversion of cyanide to thiocyanate; or hydroxycobalamin (vitamin B_{12}), which combines with cyanide to form cyanocobalamin. More gradual toxicity accompanied by fatigue, nausea, psychosis, and seizures can result over days from thiocyanate accumulation.

Intravenous Nitroglycerin

Intravenous nitroglycerin is generally used at dosages of 50–400 μg/min with titration guided by filling pressures and the systemic vascular resistance. Traditionally considered to be venodilators at low doses and arterial vasodilators at higher doses, nitrates, even in low doses, may decrease systemic vascular resistance in some patients. However, a given decrease in systemic vascular resistance is generally accompanied by a greater decrease in ventricular filling pressures with nitroglycerin than with nitroprusside. Although used less often than nitroprusside for the management of heart failure, intravenous nitroglycerin may be of particular value in patients with disproportionate right-sided failure or intolerance to nitroprusside. There is some evidence that nitroglycerin may cause less coronary steal than does nitroprusside, which theoretically could worsen myocardial perfusion in the setting of recent infarction or ischemia.

Dobutamine (see Figs. 10–1, 10–2; Figs. 10–3, 10–4)

The predominant effect of dobutamine is to increase the cardiac output by increasing myocardial contractility.[19, 20] In addition, there are modest decreases in the systemic vascular resistance and cardiac filling pressures as a result of a combination of the direct myocardial and vascular effects of the drug, and withdrawal of sympathetic tone secondary to the improvement in hemodynamic function. However, these effects are mild and seldom limit the ability to titrate the drug.

Dobutamine is commonly infused at rates ranging from 2–15 μg/kg/min, although higher infusion rates may occasionally be used.

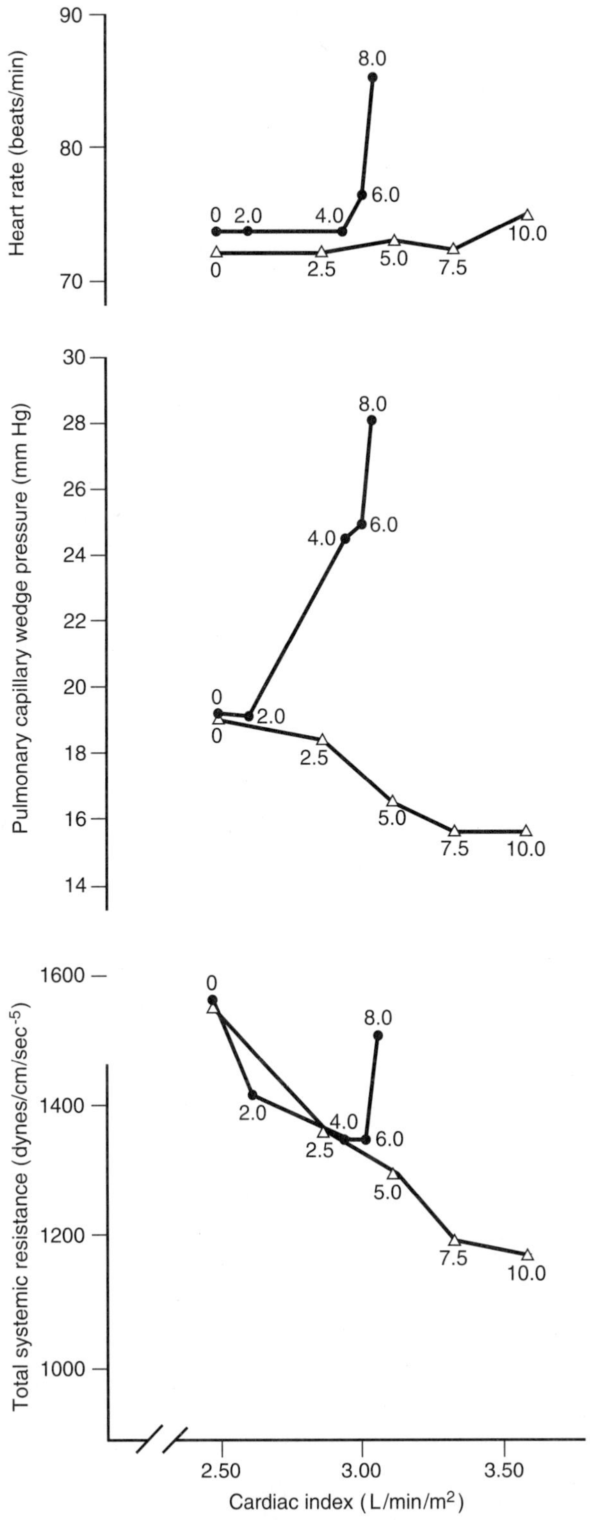

Figure 10–3. Comparative effects of dopamine (•) and dobutamine (Δ) on heart rate, pulmonary capillary wedge pressure, and total systemic resistance in patients with moderate to severe heart failure. Each agent was titrated over the doses shown. These data illustrate that dopamine, at infusion rates that exceed 2–4 μg/kg/min, exerts a constrictor effect, as evidenced by the increase in total systemic resistance. When given alone to patients with severe heart failure, dopamine in high doses increases pulmonary capillary wedge pressure, as a result of both the increase in arterial pressure and venoconstriction. (Adapted from Leier CV, Heban PT, Huss P, et al: Comparative systemic and regional hemodynamic effects of dopamine and dobutamine in patients with cardiomyopathic heart failure. Circulation 1978; 58:466–475.)

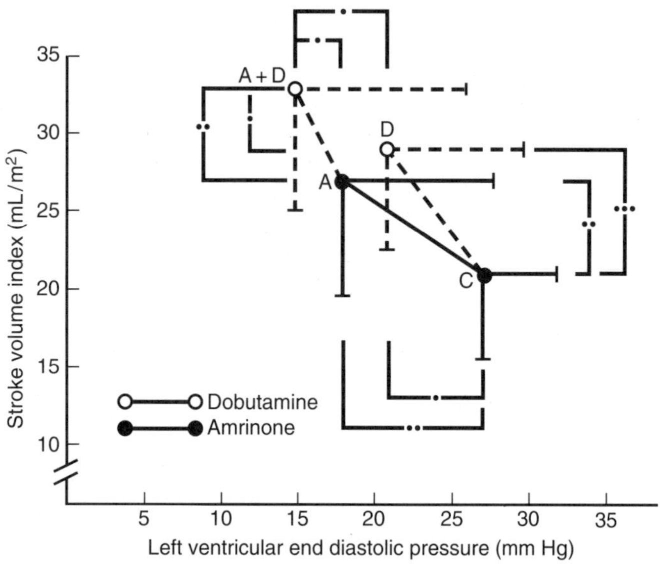

Figure 10–4. Hemodynamic effects of dobutamine (D), amrinone (A), and the combination (A + D) in patients with moderate to severe heart failure. As shown here, the additive effect of the two agents may exceed the effect of either agent alone. *Other abbreviation:* C, control measurements. (Adapted from Gage J, Rutman H, Lucido D, LeJemtel TH: Additive effects of dobutamine and amrinone on myocardial contractility and ventricular performance in patients with severe heart failure. Circulation 1986; 74:367–373.)

The responsiveness to dobutamine can vary greatly from patient to patient and from day to day in the same patient, partly because of differing levels of beta-adrenergic desensitization. In general, patients with long-standing heart failure and/or more severe decompensation are less responsive to dobutamine than are patients with mild failure and/or failure of recent onset. In most patients with clinically important decompensation and a reduced cardiac output, dobutamine can be started at a rate of 2.5 μg/kg/min with upward titration to rates of 5, 7.5, 10, 12.5, and 15 μg/kg/min at 15- to 30-min intervals. The upward titration should be guided by the hemodynamic goals of treatment or the development of a dose-limiting response, most often an unacceptable increase in heart rate or arrhythmias, which should lead to a reduction in dosage to the prior level. In rare instances, patients receiving dobutamine complain of nausea and tremulousness. The responsiveness to a given infusion rate of dobutamine may increase or decrease with time and is not entirely predictable. Therefore, the infusion rate should be reevaluated periodically.

If the maximally tolerated infusion rate of dobutamine does not yield an adequate therapeutic response, consideration should be given to the addition of a second drug. If the systemic vascular resistance is elevated, the addition of a vasodilator such as nitroprusside or nitroglycerin may be of value.[21] The combination of dobutamine with a phosphodiesterase inhibitor (e.g., milrinone or amrinone) may be helpful in potentiating the positive inotropic response and also by providing vasodilatation.[22, 23] In patients with severe hypotension who receive dobutamine, it may be necessary to add a pressor dosage of dopamine (i.e., >5 μg/kg/min) in order to support the arterial pressure. In patients with heart failure, the need for pressor support frequently presages the need for mechanical support such as intra-aortic balloon counterpulsation or the use of a left ventricular assist device (see Chapter 15).

Dopamine (see Fig. 10–3)

In patients with heart failure, a major role for dopamine is to improve renal function by increasing renal blood flow.[24] This effect occurs at low "renal" dosages of 1–4 μg/kg/min, with which mild systemic vasodilatation may also be observed in some patients. Higher infusion rates do not increase renal blood flow further unless there is severe hypotension, and they may actually decrease renal blood flow by causing alpha-adrenergic receptor–mediated constriction. At infusion rates greater than 5 μg/kg/min, dopamine also exerts a positive inotropic effect by stimulating beta-adrenergic receptors and a vasoconstrictor effect by stimulating alpha-adrenergic receptors.

It is unusual to use dopamine primarily as a positive inotropic agent in patients with heart failure. Although the vasoconstrictor action of dopamine may be important in maintaining arterial pressure in some patients with severe decompensation, this effect is not desirable for most patients with heart failure, in whom dosages over 5 μg/kg/min should be avoided. When higher pressor dosages are required, the drug should be titrated upward to achieve the minimal acceptable arterial pressure. As with dobutamine, the upward titration is generally limited by tachycardia and arrhythmias.

Milrinone and Amrinone (see Figs. 10–1, 10–2, 10–4)

The phosphodiesterase inhibitors (PDEI) amrinone and milrinone exert a direct positive inotropic effect on the myocardium[25] and a direct dilator effect on the vasculature.[26] The vasodilator action of these agents, like that of nitroprusside, is "balanced," with both arterial and venous dilatation, and these agents are therefore of most benefit when the cardiac output is reduced in the presence of elevations in systemic vascular resistance and left-sided filling pressure. Because of the dual mechanism of action, the PDEIs cause a greater increase in cardiac output than does nitroprusside, despite causing comparable decreases in systemic vascular resistance and left-sided filling pressure.[27] Likewise, for any given increase in cardiac index, the PDEIs cause greater decreases in systemic vascular resistance and filling pressures than does dobutamine.[28] However, because these agents are potent vasodilators, they may not be tolerated in patients with normal or reduced systemic vascular resistance and/or left-sided filling pressure.

Amrinone was the prototype PDEI for clinical use.[29] Although it is still available, its use has largely been supplanted by milrinone,[30] a second-generation agent. In contrast to dobutamine, which has a half-life of only a few minutes, milrinone has a half-life of 20–45 min in patients with heart failure. For this reason, milrinone therapy is initiated by giving a bolus of drug (50 μg/kg over 10 minutes), followed by a constant infusion at the rate of 0.375–0.75 μg/kg/min. As with dobutamine, the dose of the drug tolerated may be limited by cyclic adenosine monophosphate (cAMP)–mediated side effects, particularly tachycardia and arrhythmias. In addition, as noted earlier, the dose may be limited by hypotension in patients who cannot tolerate the arterial or venous dilatation.

Intravenous Diuretics (see also Chapter 9)

Hospitalizations for heart failure are often prolonged unnecessarily because of delays in establishing effective diuresis. The loop diuretics are the most effective agents generally used. As the diuretic acts from the tubular lumen, the high tubular concentrations required are most often achieved with intravenous administration. Furosemide is currently the most common loop diuretic used in the hospital. Bumetanide has a similar action with slightly higher cost and a significant incidence of myalgia. Ethacrynic acid has a higher incidence of ototoxicity and is less often used. An agent more recently approved by the U.S. Food and Drug Administration (FDA) is torsemide, which has more consistent bioavailability and longer action than the other loop diuretics; its role remains to be determined.

Frequent reevaluation is the key to effective diuresis. The diuretic response and the patient's condition should be reviewed frequently and diuretic orders revised. Intravenous furosemide is given initially in dosages of 20–100 mg, depending on previous diuretic history, and dosages of up to 240 mg may be necessary. The addition of a thiazide, such as chlorothiazide or metolazone, often markedly potentiates the diuresis. Acetazolamide is occasionally added as well. The aldosterone antagonists, which are useful in fluid retention associated with cirrhosis, can cause a modest increment in diuresis. A constant intravenous infusion of furosemide at 5–20 mg/h may be effective in treating refractory fluid retention but should be preceded by a trial of low-dosage dopamine (2–4 μg/kg/min) to enhance renal perfusion. In patients with massive fluid overload that cannot be mobilized with any pharmacologic combination, ultrafiltration may be effective.[31] Patients with massive ascites may also benefit from slow paracentesis to remove intra-abdominal fluid.

ADJUSTMENT OF ORAL MEDICATIONS

Angiotensin Converting Enzyme Inhibitors

A goal of hospitalization may be to initiate or adjust the dosage of an ACE inhibitor. For patients without evident hypoperfusion, ACE inhibitors can often be initiated or increased empirically. However, in patients with low serum sodium levels (in general, <134 mEq/L) or a resting systolic blood pressure less than 90 mm Hg, marked hypotension may develop with the initial dose of an ACE inhibitor. In such patients, therapy should be initiated with low dosages of captopril (e.g., 6.25 mg).

Patients stabilized on intravenous nitroprusside (or nitroglycerin) can usually be weaned to an ACE inhibitor, often in combination with nitrates. In such patients, the rate of nitroprusside infusion may be decreased slightly before the oral agent is given; the oral agent is then titrated upward gradually as the intravenous vasodilator is weaned. It is important to record hemodynamics at the time of hypotension, particularly if the hypotensive response persists. The dose of captopril is increased every 2–4 h until there is evidence of a vasodilator response. The titration is then continued with dosing every 6 h until the target level of vasodilatation is achieved.

Nitrates

When therapy is adjusted to the hemodynamic goals achieved on nitroprusside, the addition of isosorbide dinitrate to captopril frequently reduces systemic vascular resistance and ventricular filling pressures more effectively than does captopril alone. In some patients who cannot tolerate either captopril or hydralazine, isosorbide dinitrate alone can be an effective vasodilator.[32] Most experience has been with isosorbide dinitrate, which is begun in doses of 10 mg t.i.d. and increased as needed, sometimes up to 80 mg t.i.d. The development of nitrate tolerance varies greatly but may be minimized by use of a nitrate-free interval of 10–12 h.[33] This nitrate-free interval may be timed to the diurnal period of fewest symptoms, generally at night.

Hydralazine

For patients in whom weaning from intravenous agents has been particularly difficult, or in whom ACE inhibitors are not tolerated or do not adequately optimize resting hemodynamics, hydralazine may be of value, often in combination with oral nitrates.[12] The usual starting dose is 25 mg, and the usual maximal dose is 150–200 mg q.i.d. The most common side effect necessitating discontinuation of hydralazine is nausea, which occurs in approximately 25% of patients with heart failure. Hydralazine-induced lupus occurs only rarely in patients with heart failure.

Oral Diuretics

Once fluid balance has been restored, the selection of an oral diuretic dose for discharge is empiric, and further adjustment is almost always required both in the hospital and after discharge. It should be noted that patients have a different salt and fluid intake at home than in the hospital. As a first approximation, the dose of intravenous diuretic that was effective may be given as an oral dose twice per day.

Consolidation of the Medical Regimen Before Discharge

Patients who have undergone a major revision of vasodilator regimen should be observed on the new regimen for 24–48 h of ambulation before discharge. Most patients with heart failure tolerate systolic blood pressures of 80 mm Hg or higher. Final adjustment of vasodilator regimens can be delayed unnecessarily by withholding the medication on the basis of blood pressure parameters that are too strict for this population. In general, dosages should be decreased or delayed by 1 h for low blood pressures but should not be omitted. During this adjustment period, patients receiving two vasodilator agents may need to have the doses staggered.

As soon as optimal fluid status is achieved, diuretics should be given orally, as described earlier. Daily weight measurements and careful fluid intake/output records help track fluid status. This process should include patient education about the importance of daily weight measurements after discharge and a strategy of diuretic adjustment for weight gain. Creatinine and blood urea nitrogen levels should be measured until discharge. Modest elevations of these indices of renal function in the first few weeks after aggressive diuresis are common among patients with long-standing fluid retention and, in the absence of other signs of deterioration, usually do not indicate poor systemic perfusion. Patients should not be discharged, however, if the creatinine level continues to rise.

The design and communication of a clear plan before discharge may reduce readmissions for heart failure.[34] By the time of discharge, patients should be able to take their own medications according to schedule, understand sodium and fluid restriction and the diuretic regimen, and recognize symptoms of pulmonary congestion and postural hypotension. A specific activity prescription is very helpful for patients, many of whom have previously been told to "take it easy." This may be facilitated, before or soon after discharge, by an exercise test with gas exchange measurements, which allows identification of a target heart rate at which anaerobic metabolism is reached. A clear line of communication should be established for questions that arise early after discharge. An unsolicited phone call by the physician or nurse specialist after 3 days can identify early problems that might otherwise have progressed to necessitate readmission. Patients who are discharged after major redesign of their regimen should be seen within the next 7 days, at which time electrolytes and renal function should again be evaluated.

OTHER MANAGEMENT ISSUES

Electrolyte Replacement

Appropriate potassium replacement is determined less by the serum potassium level than by the adequacy of renal function, anticipated further urinary losses, concomitant therapy with ACE inhibitors or potassium-sparing diuretics, and conditions such as alkalosis or diabetes mellitus that impair movement of potassium into cells. Safe replacement requires recognition that 98% of potassium is intracellular. Although a reduction of the steady-state serum potassium level by 1 mEq/L indicates an approximately 300-mEq total deficit of potassium, potassium replacement goes initially into the extracellular volume, which is only about 15 L. Rapid replacement of 30 mEq can thus acutely raise potassium concentration by 2 mEq/L, although later redistribution occurs. Because the electrophysiologic consequences of hyperkalemia result from the altered gradient between the intracellular and extracellular concentrations, the risk of clinical hyperkalemic arrhythmias is highest during potassium replacement, when intracellular potassium concentrations are still low. Hyperkalemia is a common cause of iatrogenic morbidity, and occasionally, mortality, during hospitalization for heart failure.[34]

Magnesium is also depleted during diuretic therapy, and hypomagnesemia has been associated with increased ventricular arrhythmias, particularly torsades de pointes. Although replacement to a magnesium level of 1.8 mEq/L is recommended, more vigorous replacement has not been shown to have any clear benefit.

Severe muscle cramps may occur in patients undergoing a rapid diuresis but are usually not associated with detectable serum electrolyte abnormalities and rarely respond to electrolyte replacement. Pain from such cramps may be sufficiently intense to necessitate the use of narcotics, but usually resolves within 12 h.

Sodium and Fluid Restriction

The majority of patients with advanced heart failure should receive a restricted sodium diet (2 g/day) while in the hospital, except in rare cases in which oral nutritional intake is of overriding importance. Although effective use of diuretic combinations in the hospital renders sodium restriction less important for the initial correction of volume overload, strict restriction of sodium is critical for the stability of fluid balance after discharge. To allow a patient more liberal sodium intake in the hospital delivers the wrong message about the importance of this restriction. In addition, education regarding sodium content of food is often enhanced during an admission.

Patients with intense neurohumoral activation, usually indicated by a low plasma sodium concentration, may have marked thirst, which dominates all other issues. Diuresis may intensify thirst initially, although the patient should be assured that the thirst mechanism will soon "reset" after the lower volume status is maintained for 1–2 weeks. Restriction to a total fluid intake of 2000 mL/day is adequate for most hospitalized patients and is also a reasonable guideline after discharge.

Because hyponatremia generally progresses slowly in patients with heart failure, the risk of central nervous system effects is very small. Patients with a serum sodium level in the range of 125 mEq/L may improve when given a small amount of oral replacement (e.g., soup or potato chips) during continued diuresis. When the serum sodium level is less than 120 mEq/L, fluid should be restricted to 1000 mL/day, and it may be necessary to simultaneously administer normal saline and diuretics.

Oxygen Supplementation

In the absence of frank respiratory failure, concomitant pulmonary disease, or significant right-to-left shunting, patients with chronic heart failure rarely have arterial desaturation. In such patients, supplemental oxygen does not generally improve systemic oxygen delivery and has the drawback of causing airway irritation and limitation of movement. In the absence of arterial desaturation, the use of nasal oxygen is often empiric and may be based on whether the patient derives a subjective benefit. However, in some patients, oxygen may decrease elevated pulmonary vascular resistance and secondarily improve right-heart function.

Ventricular Arrhythmias

Premature ventricular contractions in pairs and triplets may occur in up to 80% of patients hospitalized with heart failure. Their appearance is correlated with the severity of heart failure and all-cause mortality, but there is no evidence that suppression with antiarrhythmic agents improves prognosis. Ventricular arrhythmias of sufficient frequency to compromise perfusion or cause symptoms should be treated. Prolonged runs of asymptomatic ventricular tachycardia at rapid rates may also merit treatment. Suppression with agents such as lidocaine is rarely necessary and is often complicated by decreased clearance, which can lead to toxicity. The oral antiarrhythmic agent of choice is generally amiodarone.

Anticoagulation

Although patients with a low ejection fraction and a dilated ventricle are at increased risk of embolic events, the indications for anticoagulation are best recognized for patients with additional risk factors such as atrial fibrillation,[35] a history of embolic events, and echocardiographic or angiographic evidence of a mobile ventricular thrombus. During hospitalization, such patients are often administered intravenous heparin, which can be discontinued for invasive procedures. The routine use of chronic anticoagulation in other patients with heart failure has not been established.[36]

MANAGEMENT OF ACUTE-ONSET HEART FAILURE

The principles described here have been developed primarily to treat decompensation of chronic heart failure. Similar principles apply, however, to acute heart failure, with some special considerations. Unlike the approach to exacerbations of chronic heart failure, therapy for acute heart failure is generally designed for temporary stabilization until definitive mechanical intervention or spontaneous recovery can occur. The design of an effective oral regimen for outpatient stabilization is not a major goal, at least initially.

Heart failure in the setting of acute myocardial infarction can develop and progress rapidly. Diagnosis is occasionally delayed when blood pressure is initially maintained in the setting of marked sinus tachycardia. Intravenous inotropic support in the compromised patient should not be postponed on account of concern about increasing myocardial oxygen demand, which is also raised by excessive ventricular filling pressures. Dobutamine can be initiated while a pulmonary artery catheter is inserted to monitor loading conditions, and it can be continued if stroke volume remains low. In contrast to the hemodynamic goals in the chronically dilated heart, low systemic blood pressures and low cardiac outputs may be less tolerated by patients with previously normal hemodynamics. Likewise, higher filling pressures, in the range of 18 mm Hg, may be required in order to maximize cardiac output.[18] Intravenous nitroglycerin is frequently used to decrease ischemia, and may also provide arterial vasodilatation when the systemic vascular resistance is high. Intravenous nitroprusside may potentially cause a "coronary steal" in the setting of acute ischemia and is generally reserved for patients with severe hypertension. Because total body volume status is usually normal, diuretics are rarely needed during acute infarction except as initial emergency therapy to avoid respiratory failure from pulmonary edema. Insertion of an intra-aortic balloon for counterpulsation should be considered if cardiac output is reduced, ventricular filling pressures are severely elevated, or evidence of ongoing ischemia persists. Evaluation for definitive intervention such as angioplasty, surgical revascularization, or valve replacement should not be delayed by prolonged attempts to stabilize a patient on pharmacologic therapy.

Patients with acute heart failure caused by new mitral or aortic valvular regurgitation are exquisitely sensitive to afterload. As in acute infarction, optimization of forward flow in these patients may best be guided by invasive hemodynamic monitoring. Arterial vasodilatation with intravenous nitroprusside, followed by oral vasodilators, often improves forward flow markedly and allows elective consideration of valve replacement.

MANAGEMENT OF PATIENTS WITH DIASTOLIC DYSFUNCTION

Diastolic dysfunction is discussed in detail in Chapter 13. Admission with this diagnosis is often precipitated by hypertension, ischemia, or fluid overload, all of which should be treated aggressively. Although cardiac output may be reduced, intravenous inotropic support is seldom necessary to preserve cardiac output. Low-dosage dopamine may aid diuresis in some cases. Elevated systemic blood pressure is often a target for vasodilator therapy, which can then be adjusted without invasive hemodynamic monitoring. ACE inhibitors and calcium channel blocking agents can lower blood pressure and improve ventricular compliance. Nitrate therapy may help to relieve elevated filling pressures, especially when used in anticipation of activity. Postural hypotension may be more common among these patients than among patients with predominant systolic ventricular failure.

REFERENCES

1. Zema MJ, Restivo B, Sos T, et al: Left ventricular dysfunction—bedside Valsalva maneuver. Br Heart J 1980; 44:560–569.
2. Ewy GA: The abdominojugular test: technique and hemodynamic correlates. Ann Intern Med 1988; 109:456–460.
3. Stevenson LW, Perloff JK: The limited reliability of physical signs for the estimation of hemodynamics in chronic heart failure. JAMA 1989; 261:884–888.
4. McIntyre KM, Vita JA, Lambrew CT, et al: A non-invasive method of predicting pulmonary-capillary wedge pressure. N Engl J Med 1992; 327:1715–1720.
5. Chakko S, Woska D, Martinez H, et al: Clinical, radiographic, and hemodynamic correlations in chronic congestive heart failure: conflicting results may lead to inappropriate care. Am J Med 1991; 90:353–359.
6. Perloff JK: Physical Examination of the Heart and Circulation, p 93. Philadelphia: WB Saunders, 1982.
7. Young JB: Assessment of heart failure. *In* Braunwald E (ed) (Colucci WS, vol ed.): Atlas of Heart Disease, vol 4, pp 7.2–8.1. St. Louis: CV Mosby, 1995.
8. Luu M, Stevenson WG, Stevenson LW, et al: Diverse mechanisms of unexpected cardiac arrest in advanced heart failure. Circulation 1989; 80:1675–1680.
9. Grogan M, Smith HC, Gersh BJ, Wood DW: Left ventricular dysfunction due to atrial fibrillation in patients initially believed to have idiopathic dilated cardiomyopathy. Am J Cardiol 1992; 69:1570–1573.
10. Pfeffer MA, Braunwald E, Moye LA, et al: Effect of captopril on mortality and morbidity in patients with left ventricular dysfunction after myocardial infarction: results of the survival and ventricular enlargement trial. N Engl J Med 1992; 327:669–677.
11. The SOLVD Investigators: Effect of enalapril on survival in patients with reduced left ventricular ejection fractions and congestive heart failure. N Engl J Med 1991; 325:293–302.
12. Cohn JN, Johnson G, Ziesche S, et al: A comparison of enalapril with hydralazine-isosorbide dinitrate in the treatment of chronic congestive heart failure. N Engl J Med 1991; 325:303–310.
13. Stevenson LW, Tillisch JH: Maintenance of cardiac output with normal filling pressures in dilated heart failure. Circulation 1986; 74:1303–1308.
14. Stevenson LW, Belil D, Grover McKay M, et al: Effects of afterload reduction on left ventricular volume and mitral regurgitation in severe congestive heart failure. Am J Cardiol 1987; 60:654–658.
15. Stevenson LW, Tillisch JH, Hamilton M, et al: Importance of hemodynamic response to therapy in predicting survival with ejection fraction <20% secondary to ischemic or non-ischemic dilated cardiomyopathy. Am J Cardiol 1990; 66:1348–1354.
16. Lee WH, Packer M: Prognostic importance of serum sodium concentration and its modification by converting enzyme inhibition in patients with severe chronic heart failure. Circulation 1986; 73:257–267.
17. Fonarow GC, Chelimsky-Fallick C, Stevenson LW, et al: Effect of direct vasodilation with hydralazine versus angiotensin-converting enzyme inhibition with captopril on mortality in advanced heart failure: the Hy-C trial. J Am Coll Cardiol 1992; 19:842–850.
18. Forrester JS, Diamond G, Chatterjee K, Swan HJC: Medical therapy of acute myocardial infarction by application of hemodynamic subsets. N Engl J Med 1976; 295:1356–1362; 1404–1412.
19. Tuttle RR, Mills J: Dobutamine: development of a new catecholamine to selectively increase cardiac contractility. Circ Res 1975; 36:185–196.
20. Leier CV, Webel J, Bush CA: The cardiovascular effects of dobutamine in patients with severe cardiac failure. Circulation 1977; 56:468–472.
21. Awan NA, Evenson MK, Needham KE, et al: Effect of combined nitroglycerin and dobutamine infusion in left ventricular dysfunction. Am Heart J 1983; 106:35–40.
22. Gage J, Rutman H, Lucido D, LeJemtel TH: Additive effects of dobutamine and amrinone on myocardial contractility and ventricular performance in patients with severe heart failure. Circulation 1986; 74:367–373.
23. Colucci WS, Denniss AR, Leatherman GF, et al: Intracoronary infusion of dobutamine to patients with and without severe congestive heart failure. Dose-response relationships, correlation with circulating catecholamines, and effect of phosphodiesterase inhibition. J Clin Invest 1988; 81:1103–1110.
24. Leier CV, Heban PT, Huss P, et al: Comparative systemic and regional hemodynamic effects of dopamine and dobutamine in patients with cardiomyopathic heart failure. Circulation 1978; 58:466–475.
25. Ludmer PL, Wright RF, Arnold MO, et al: Separation of the direct myocardial and vasodilator actions of milrinone administered by an intracoronary infusion technique. Circulation 1986; 73:130–137.
26. Cody RJ, Muller FB, Kubo SH, et al: Identification of the direct vasodilator effect of milrinone with an isolated limb preparation in patients with chronic congestive heart failure. Circulation 1986; 73:124–129.
27. Jaski BE, Fifer MA, Wright RF, et al: Positive inotropic and vasodilator actions of milrinone in patients with severe congestive heart failure. Dose-response relationships and comparison to nitroprusside. J Clin Invest 1985; 75:643–649.
28. Colucci WS, Wright RF, Jaski BE, et al: Milrinone and dobutamine in severe heart failure: differing hemodynamic effects and individual patient responsiveness. Circulation 1986; 73:III-175–III-183.
29. Benotti JR, Grossman W, Braunwald E, et al: Hemodynamic assessment of amrinone. A new inotropic agent. N Engl J Med 1978; 299:1373–1377.
30. Maskin CS, Sinoway L, Chadwick B, et al: Sustained hemodynamic and clinical effects of a new cardiotonic agent, WIN 47203, in patients with severe congestive heart failure. Circulation 1983; 67:1065–1070.
31. Agostoni PG, Marenzi GC, Pepi M, et al: Isolated ultrafiltration in moderate congestive heart failure. J Am Coll Cardiol 1993; 21:424–431.
32. Cohn JN: Nitrates are effective in the treatment of chronic congestive heart failure: the protagonist's view. Am J Cardiol 1990; 66:444.
33. Parker JO, Farrell B, Lahey KA, Moe G: Effect of intervals between doses on the development of tolerance to isosorbide dinitrate. N Engl J Med 1987; 316:1440–1444.
34. Ashton CM, Kuykendall DH, Johnson ML, et al: The association between the quality of inpatient care and early readmission. Ann Intern Med 1995; 122:415–421.
35. Chakko SC, Frutchey J, Gheorghiade M: Life-threatening hyperkalemia in severe heart failure. Am Heart J 1989; 117:1083–1091.
36. Flaker CG, Blackshear JL, McBride R, et al: Antiarrhythmic drug therapy and cardiac mortality in atrial fibrillation. The Stroke Prevention in Atrial Fibrillation Investigators. J Am Coll Cardiol 1992; 20:527–532.

11 Long-Term Treatment of the Ambulatory Patient With Heart Failure

Spencer H. Kubo, MD
Jay N. Cohn, MD

In addition to the accumulation of many statistics describing the public health problem of heart failure,[1–8] there has been considerable advancement in our understanding of basic pathophysiologic mechanisms contributing to the common signs and symptoms, the progressive nature of left ventricular dysfunction, and the high mortality rates. Furthermore, there has been an enormous effort in numerous clinical trials demonstrating that certain treatments, such as the angiotensin converting enzyme (ACE) inhibitors, reduce mortality and improve functional status. Nonetheless, the morbidity associated with heart failure remains excessive. On the basis of surveys and chart reviews that suggest ACE inhibitors are prescribed for only a small fraction of appropriate patients,[9, 10] it is the strong impression among specialists in heart failure that many patients may not be optimally treated. These observations have stimulated the formulation and publication of specific recommendations and guidelines for the treatment of patients with heart failure, such as the report from the Agency for Health Care Policy and Research.[11] Thus, a major emphasis for the 1990s will include not only the traditional search for more effective therapies but also a significant educational effort that will assist a wide range of health care providers to better use existing therapies.

This chapter reviews the current state-of-the-art treatment strategies for ambulatory patients with chronic heart failure. In each section, we provide some of the most pertinent information regarding pathophysiologic mechanisms as well as data from important clinical trials that provide the scientific rationale and justification for the treatment recommendation. For areas in which there are few data on mechanisms and treatment, the consensus opinion among heart failure specialists is presented. In addition, each section includes practical recommendations that can be used in everyday clinical encounters.

BACKGROUND PATHOPHYSIOLOGY

The basic pathophysiology of heart failure due to left ventricular systolic dysfunction including abnormalities in myocardial function, peripheral vasoconstriction, and neurohormonal activation is extensively discussed in E. Braunwald's *Heart Disease*, fifth edition (Philadelphia: WB Saunders, 1995), (Chapter 14) as well as other reviews.[12–14] It is instructive to review three important pathophysiologic concepts that have had a substantial impact on the overall treatment strategy. The first concept recognizes the systemic nature of the clinical syndrome of heart failure. Although the primary problem is related to an abnormality in the myocardium, many of the presenting signs and symptoms are related to dysfunction of different end organs. Thus, shortness of breath can be related to excess extracellular volume in the pleural and alveolar spaces, whereas liver dysfunction and early satiety may be due to a combination of splanchnic congestion and hypoperfusion. Exercise intolerance appears to be related to many different factors including but not limited to an inadequate chronotropic and inotropic response, peripheral vasoconstriction, ventilatory abnormalities, and abnormal muscle metabolism.[15] The fact that heart failure is a systemic process makes it unlikely that any single treatment will be capable of a complete treatment response. Indeed, one of the hallmarks of the current treatment strategy is *combination* drug therapy. Thus, most patients with heart failure are currently treated with multiple drugs, each with a different mechanism of action and different treatment endpoints.

A second important concept involves the interaction between myocardial dysfunction, peripheral vasoconstriction, and neurohormonal activation as summarized in Figure 11–1. This model emphasizes that the clinical syndrome of heart failure is related to a primary abnormality in myocardial function. However, further decreases in myocardial function as well as progressive hypertrophy and dilatation (remodeling) can occur in the absence of additional direct injury to the myocardium owing to the adverse effects of neurohormonal activation and peripheral vasoconstriction. Furthermore, because neurohormonal activation and peripheral vasoconstriction promote salt and water retention by the kidneys and restrict blood flow to vital organs, these factors are important in the pathogenesis of many signs and symptoms of heart failure. Therefore, this model can help explain the absence of signs and symptoms of "heart failure" in some patients who have significant ventricular dysfunction. It can be anticipated that these patients do not have activation of salt-retaining neurohormonal systems or the reduction in blood flow to exercising muscle and therefore may not manifest all of the characteristic signs of systemic end-organ dysfunction. However, despite the absence of signs and symptoms in these patients, treatment directed at their myocardial dysfunction is still appropriate and is reviewed in Chapter 12.

The model in Figure 11–1 also emphasizes the observation that treatments that do not have an intrinsic action on the primary myocardial abnormality can still have substantial benefit for patients with heart failure. Thus, ACE inhibitors and vasodilators reduce vasoconstrictor tone and/or neurohormonal activation and are associated with marked improvement in symptoms and survival. In contrast, it has been observed that the tendency to activate neurohormonal pathways[16] is a common characteristic of drugs that appear to have an adverse effect on long-term survival in heart failure.

A third concept that has evolved from the activity in clinical trials is that all therapeutic interventions must be critically examined with

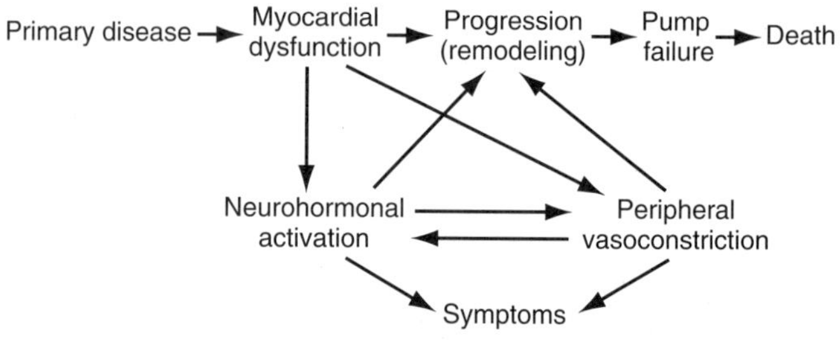

Figure 11–1. Interaction between myocardial dysfunction, peripheral vasoconstriction, and neurohormonal activation as a basic pathophysiologic mechanism in heart failure. For discussion, see text.

respect to two different but equally important endpoints—an improvement in symptoms or quality of life and an improvement in survival.[17, 18] Although it is obviously preferable that all interventions have a concordant effect on these endpoints, this is not always the case. For example, diuretics are effective in reducing clinical signs and symptoms in patients with an expanded extracellular volume, but their effects on survival are unknown. In contrast, there are convincing data that ACE inhibitors not only improve symptoms, reduce hospitalizations, and improve exercise tolerance but also prolong survival. The distinction between the two endpoints is also reflected in prioritization of treatment for different subgroups of patients. For example, patients with asymptomatic left ventricular dysfunction do not require therapy that will reduce symptoms, but a treatment regimen that prolongs life would be highly desirable. In contrast, a patient with advanced heart failure benefits from any treatment that relieves symptoms. Finally, the traditional paradigm for most clinicians emphasized symptom reduction as the most important treatment objective. Nonetheless, because of the high mortality rates associated with heart failure, it has become increasingly important to consider the impact of treatment on survival. Therefore, most current treatment strategies are considerably more aggressive than those of a decade ago[19] and include a major emphasis on the use of ACE inhibitors, which are the class of drugs shown repeatedly to improve survival.

DIETARY SODIUM RESTRICTION

Pathophysiologic Mechanisms

One of the most common abnormalities in patients with heart failure is an expanded extracellular volume that is manifested by pulmonary congestion, peripheral edema, ascites, and elevated jugular venous pulse; symptoms include ankle swelling, dyspnea on exertion, shortness of breath, and orthopnea. These abnormalities are related in part to avid sodium retention by the kidney, which is caused by a complex interaction between decreased cardiac output, decreased renal blood flow, redistribution of intrarenal blood flow to the sodium-conserving medulla, neurohormonal activation, and increased renal sympathetic nerve activity. The complex pathophysiologic process of the expansion of extracellular volume in heart failure and other edematous disorders has been reviewed in detail.[20–25]

Diuretics are the most commonly prescribed drugs for patients with signs and symptoms related to an expanded extracellular volume. Although restriction of dietary sodium intake is universally recommended for patients with heart failure who are given diuretics, it is the repeated experience of many heart failure specialists that this recommendation is inadequately implemented. The failure to correctly implement a sodium-restricted diet will diminish the effectiveness of diuretics, increase the dosage requirement, and aggravate potassium loss.

Few experimental data specifically assess the effect of dietary sodium intake in heart failure. Cody and associates[26] studied 10 patients with severe heart failure who were monitored in a clinical research center after all vasodilator and diuretic therapy was discontinued during a diet containing a very low sodium (approximately 200 mg/day) or a moderate sodium intake (approximately 2000 mg/day). The very low sodium diet was associated with a significant reduction in weight (76.5 $\pm$ 5.0 kg vs. 78.5 $\pm$ 4.9 kg; $p < .05$), mean pulmonary artery pressure (27 $\pm$ 4 mm Hg versus 36 $\pm$ 3 mm Hg; $p < .05$), and mean pulmonary wedge pressure (16 $\pm$ 3 mm Hg vs. 24 $\pm$ 1 mm Hg; $p < .03$). Volpe and coworkers[27] studied 12 patients with mild heart failure (New York Heart Association [NYHA] class I to II) and demonstrated that a high-salt diet resulted in a significant increase in left ventricular end-diastolic and end-systolic volumes, a failure of plasma levels of atrial natriuretic factor to increase, and a systematic reduction in the daily sodium excretion. Thus, even in patients with mild heart failure who do not have signs or symptoms of congestion, there is a reduced ability to excrete a sodium load. Other studies performed in patients with salt-sensitive hypertension[28] and classic experiments in animal models of heart failure[29, 30] clearly demonstrate that the level of sodium intake in the diet can have an important effect on hemodynamics and clinical status.

Our clinical observations with patients referred to the Heart Failure–Heart Transplantation Program are supportive of the importance of dietary sodium restriction. An important subset of patients who are referred for consideration of transplantation because of repeated hospitalizations or persistent edema despite large doses of diuretics commonly experience marked benefit when the pharmacologic regimen is coupled with an effective sodium-restricted diet.[31]

Practical Considerations

The decision to restrict dietary sodium intake and to what level is related in part to the severity of edema formation. In patients who have asymptomatic left ventricular dysfunction, a judicious restriction of sodium intake to no more than 3500 mg/day is probably useful, although there are no data on the long-term effects of such a recommendation. Patients with mild symptoms of an expanded extracellular volume typically require restriction to less than 2500 mg/day. Patients with more severe heart failure often obtain satisfactory results only when the intake is reduced to less than 2000 mg/day.

Thorough and repeated instruction is key. Many patients find a patient-oriented text to be useful.[32] Several general principles must be observed. Because a single teaspoon of salt contains 1938 mg of sodium, it is difficult to stay below the recommended minimum if there is a saltshaker in the house. Second, most foods contain sodium naturally, so that it is not possible (or recommended) to eliminate sodium entirely from the diet. Nonetheless, several common foods contain large amounts of sodium, such as 1 medium dill pickle (928 mg), 1 Big Mac (980 mg), and 1 oz of corn chips (231 mg), all of which should be avoided. Patients must also recognize that total sodium intake can accumulate when they take large quantities of foods with relatively low sodium content, such as 1 slice of bread (114 mg), 1 cup of low-fat yogurt (133 mg), and 1 cup of milk (122 mg).

Many patients are assisted by pocket-sized books that contain the sodium content of foods used at home or eaten in restaurants. Table 11–1 lists representative examples. Herbs and other spices are encouraged as salt substitutes. Compliance is improved by building in some flexibility and by encouraging patients to take responsibility for this aspect of their medical management. Commercial substitutes can often be helpful. However, one must be careful concerning the specific sodium and potassium content of each salt substitute.

DIURETICS

Adverse Effects

Diuretics are a cornerstone in the pharmacologic management of patients with heart failure.[33, 34] Diuretics inhibit sodium reabsorption in the kidney, leading to increased urinary sodium excretion. There are several available diuretics that are usually classified according to their site of action in the kidney.[35, 36] The pharmacology of diuretics is discussed in detail in Chapter 9.

Despite the wide acceptance of diuretics, they have a number of long-term adverse effects that are well known to clinicians, including hypokalemia, hyponatremia, hypocalcemia, hyperuricemia, hypomagnesemia, metabolic alkalosis, and carbohydrate intolerance. One adverse effect that may be particularly important in patients with heart failure is activation of neurohormonal pathways.[14, 37] Francis and colleagues[38] demonstrated that intravenous furosemide given to patients with heart failure was associated with significant increases in mean arterial pressure, systemic vascular resistance, plasma renin activity, and plasma norepinephrine. Neurohormonal activation has now been described even with standard doses of oral furosemide in

TABLE 11–1. SODIUM CONTENT OF EVERYDAY FOODS

Food	Portion	Sodium (mg)
Beer	12 fl oz	25
Cola, low-calorie	8 fl oz	21
Coffee	8 fl oz	1
American cheese	1 oz	406
Milk	1 cup	122
Ice cream	1 cup	75
Egg	1	57
Herring, smoked	3 oz	5234
Salmon, broiled	3 oz	99
Tuna, canned	3 oz	288
Beef, cooked	3 oz	55
Ham	3 oz	1114
Frankfurter	1	639
Pizza with pepperoni	½ pie	813
Spaghetti sauce, canned	7.5 oz	1054
Apple, raw	1	2
Bread, white	1 slice	114
Corn chips	1 oz	231
Chicken noodle soup	1 cup	1107
Soup beans, frozen	3 oz	3
Soup beans, canned	1 cup	326
Corn, frozen	1 cup	7
Corn, canned	1 cup	384
Barbeque sauce	1 tbsp	130
Soy sauce	1 tbsp	1029
Italian dressing	1 tbsp	116
Hamburger, Whopper	1	990
Big Mac	1	980

Source: U.S. Department of Agriculture.

patients with mild heart failure.[39, 40] The mechanisms by which diuretics stimulate renin and norepinephrine release have not been completely defined,[41] but there are three important pathophysiologic consequences. First, renin secretion results in increased secretion of aldosterone, which will promote sodium retention. Thus, activation of the renin-angiotensin system is a part of the natural counterregulatory system that will diminish the action of the diuretic. Second, increased vasoconstriction secondary to increased levels of angiotensin II and norepinephrine may have a positive feedback effect in which the increased impedance to ventricular emptying results in progressive ventricular dysfunction. Finally, it is well documented that neurohormonal activation manifested by increased plasma norepinephrine, increased plasma renin activity, and hyponatremia is a strong predictor of increased mortality.[5, 42, 43] Therefore, it is possible, although unproven, that diuretic-associated neurohormonal stimulation could be associated with an adverse effect on long-term mortality.

The association of diuretic therapy with neurohormonal activation has an important influence on the optimal use of diuretics for patients with heart failure. It is useful to reinforce dietary sodium restriction in patients who appear to require large doses of diuretics. Second, many of the adverse effects of neurohormonal stimulation by diuretics can be blocked by the concomitant administration of an ACE inhibitor. With this combination therapy, one may obtain the beneficial effect of diuretics but block the increase in angiotensin II and aldosterone. Several clinical trials reviewed in later sections have now strongly confirmed the clinical benefits of combining ACE inhibitors with diuretics over diuretic therapy alone.

It is also important to understand the effects of secondary processes, commonly termed diuretic adaptation, that can cause overall sodium balance to return to neutral despite continued diuretic administration. The response to a diuretic-induced reduction of extracellular volume is a further reduction in sodium and chloride excretion through stimulation of proximal tubule reabsorption, increased renal sympathetic nerve activity, and increased aldosterone.[44, 45] Furthermore, evidence suggests that long-term diuretic treatment induces a number of changes in the collecting duct and distal tubule, including an increase in mitochondrial volume, a proliferation of basement membrane, an increase in adenosine triphosphatase activity, and cellular hypertrophy, all of which increase distal tubule reabsorption.[46–48] Thus, increases in proximal and distal tubule sodium reabsorption result in a compensatory "braking action" that increases sodium and chloride retention and will clearly limit the effectiveness of diuretics when they are given as monotherapy.

The pharmacokinetics and pharmacodynamic effects of diuretics can be abnormal in patients with heart failure.[33, 49] In many patients with peripheral and bowel wall edema, the absorption of orally administered drugs can be reduced, thereby delaying the time to appearance and peak concentration of the diuretic in the urine. Unless the glomerular filtration rate is less than 30 mL/min, the pharmacokinetics of intravenous formulations is largely normal in heart failure, which explains why this route is typically more effective in the decompensated patient. Furthermore, the pharmacodynamic response is reduced in heart failure so that the rate of sodium excretion is reduced at any given renal tubule diuretic concentration.[49, 50] Thus, the ceiling dose, or that dose above which further sodium excretion is minimal, is typically double in patients with heart failure compared with that in normal subjects. It is for this reason that a larger dose is commonly more effective than increasing the frequency (e.g., b.i.d. or t.i.d.) of administration.

Practical Considerations

The decision to initiate diuretics in the management of patients with heart failure can be guided by the simplified treatment algorithm summarized in Figure 11–2. The first step is to identify patients with overt manifestations of congestion. Patients may have the common symptoms of orthopnea, paroxysmal nocturnal dyspnea, dyspnea on exertion, exercise intolerance, cough, shortness of breath, or fatigue in combination with rales, pleural effusions, elevated jugular venous pulse, peripheral edema, ascites, S_3 gallop, and a narrow pulse pressure. Other clinical characteristics include frequent outpatient visits and hospitalizations. Common diagnostic tests that are frequently performed in this population of patients include chest radiography, echocardiography, and cardiac catheterization. These tests typically reveal ventricular enlargement, reduced ejection fraction, reduced cardiac output, and elevated cardiac filling pressures.

Patients without any of these common signs or symptoms typically do not require initiation of treatment with diuretics. For patients with mild congestive symptoms, the first treatment should include instruction regarding a sodium-restricted diet. If signs and/or symptoms persist, the most commonly used drug will be a diuretic. Some physicians find that thiazide diuretics are often adequate in maintaining an acceptable intravascular volume in patients with mild heart failure. The primary site of action of the thiazide diuretics is the distal tubule, where approximately 5%–10% of the filtered load of sodium is reabsorbed. However, as cardiac function, renal perfusion, and renal function all decrease, proximal tubule sodium reabsorption increases from 67% to 80%–90% of the filtered load. Therefore, in heart failure, the filtered load delivered to the distal tubule is decreased, which makes the thiazide diuretics less effective. For these reasons, the most commonly prescribed diuretic for patients with overt manifestations of heart failure is a loop diuretic.

Although diuretics have traditionally been the first-line agent for patients with heart failure, the current treatment algorithm contains two additional recommendations for patients treated with a diuretic. The first is to reinforce a sodium-restricted diet, which will clearly enhance the effectiveness of a diuretic in normalizing volume status. The second is to add an ACE inhibitor at the onset to block diuretic-

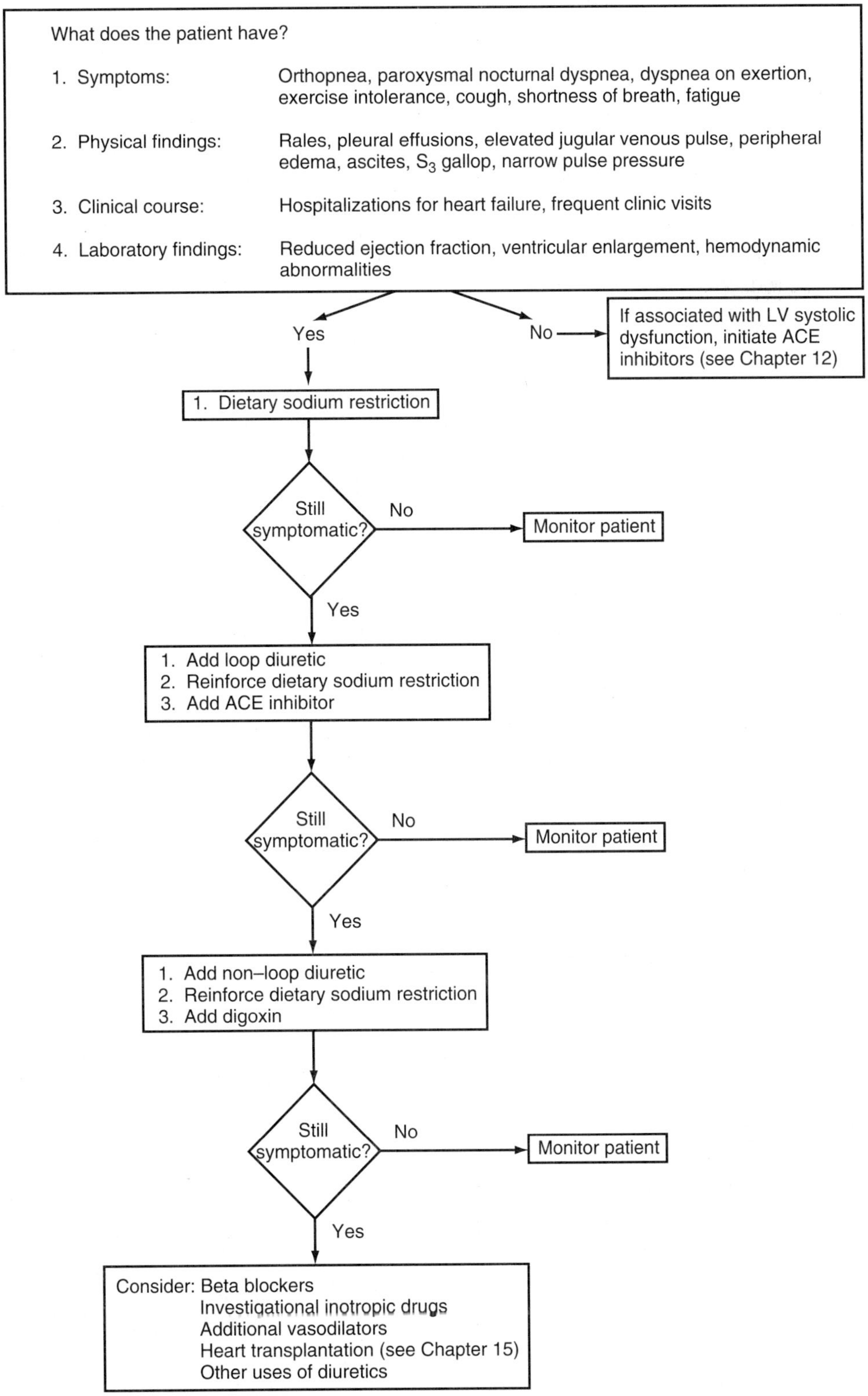
What does the patient have?
1. Symptoms:
Orthopnea, paroxysmal nocturnal dyspnea, dyspnea on exertion, exercise intolerance, cough, shortness of breath, fatigue
2. Physical findings:
Rales, pleural effusions, elevated jugular venous pulse, peripheral edema, ascites, S_3 gallop, narrow pulse pressure
3. Clinical course:
Hospitalizations for heart failure, frequent clinic visits
4. Laboratory findings:
Reduced ejection fraction, ventricular enlargement, hemodynamic abnormalities
Yes
No
If associated with LV systolic dysfunction, initiate ACE inhibitors (see Chapter 12)
1. Dietary sodium restriction
Still symptomatic?
No
Monitor patient
Yes
1. Add loop diuretic
2. Reinforce dietary sodium restriction
3. Add ACE inhibitor
Still symptomatic?
No
Monitor patient
Yes
1. Add non–loop diuretic
2. Reinforce dietary sodium restriction
3. Add digoxin
Still symptomatic?
No
Monitor patient
Yes
Consider: Beta blockers
Investigational inotropic drugs
Additional vasodilators
Heart transplantation (see Chapter 15)
Other uses of diuretics

Figure 11–2. Treatment algorithm for the ambulatory patient with heart failure. For discussion, see text.

induced neurohormonal activation and because of the important clinical benefits discussed in greater detail in the next section. Thus, the current standard practice differs from only a decade ago in that diuretics should not be used as monotherapy.

There are several endpoints to monitor in patients treated with diuretics. Because the main indication is symptom relief, one may reduce the dose of diuretics to maintenance levels once there is a satisfactory reduction in dyspnea, orthopnea, and edema. Selected patients do not require any maintenance doses of diuretics especially if they are effective in reducing dietary sodium intake.[51] An alternative strategy is to guide dosing by normalization of the jugular venous pulse, which is thought by some to be an important factor in preventing progression of left ventricular dysfunction.

Some patients have refractory signs and symptoms and are frequently labeled *diuretic resistant.* It is common to find that such patients may be noncompliant with their medication regimens or ineffective in limiting dietary sodium intake and that reinforcement of the management strategy is required. In patients with obvious peripheral edema, significant bowel wall edema may limit oral absorption, so that intravenous formulations (e.g., furosemide and/or chlorothiazide) may be effective in initiating a diuresis. In other patients, the problem is inadequate sodium delivery to the tubule lumen due to reduced renal perfusion and impaired tubule secretion of diuretics. Most patients respond to doubling the dose rather than giving the same dose twice daily.

In other patients, the combination of a loop diuretic with a thiazide diuretic, which facilitates the action of the loop diuretic, may be particularly effective.[52, 53] The mechanisms of diuretic synergism between a loop and a thiazide diuretic are not fully defined but are likely to be related to their inhibition of transport in different segments of the nephron.[44] As discussed previously, the adaptive response to long-term loop diuretic therapy is an increase in sodium and chloride transport in the distal tubule because of the increased concentration of sodium presented to the distal tubule as well as cellular hypertrophy. Distal tubule sodium absorption is thiazide sensitive. Thus, adding a thiazide diuretic inhibits the compensatory distal tubule adaptations and results in a diuresis much greater than that obtained by simply increasing the dose of the loop diuretic. The addition of a thiazide diuretic may also be used for transient episodes of fluid accumulation. This "booster pill" strategy allows one to keep the dose of the loop diuretic constant and minimize errors associated with frequent dose changes. Furthermore, by using the additional diuretic only on a temporary basis, one tends to reduce the amount of the diuretic that the patient will be exposed to long term. However, one must be cautious because this combination pill strategy can lead to overdiuresis.

During long-term treatment, and particularly during changes in diuretic regimens, it is important to monitor levels of potassium, given the marked kaliuretic effects of diuretic drugs. One should also observe renal function because this parameter may be sensitive to changes in blood volume and/or vasoconstrictor hormones. Excessive volume depletion should be avoided because it will have a major effect on hypotension and renal dysfunction.

In our clinical experience, we have found it extremely useful to have patients weigh themselves daily. This process helps to engage patients in their medical care, alert them to the effect of dietary indiscretions, and facilitate "fine tuning" of medications. For patients with a rapid weight gain of 2–3 lb, a temporary increase in diuretic dosage, or the addition of a thiazide diuretic for 1 to 3 days, is often sufficient to return the patient to "dry" weight.

Other techniques may be useful in highly refractory patients who are more commonly seen in the hospital setting. Bolus administration of large doses of furosemide (500 to 1000 mg)[54, 55] may be necessary to achieve adequate drug levels within the tubule lumen, especially in the presence of renal insufficiency, when accumulation of endogenous organic acids may reduce tubule secretion. Another technique is a constant infusion of a loop diuretic.[56, 57] The constant infusion limits the ability of the kidney to retain sodium and chloride once the tubule levels of the diuretic decrease to below threshold levels. Thus, there is a greater net sodium excretion despite comparable total drug excretion and lower serum drug concentrations. Finally, in extreme areas with refractory ascites, ultrafiltration or high-volume paracentesis has been used for symptomatic relief.[58]

ACE INHIBITORS AND VASODILATORS

Pathophysiologic Mechanisms

One of the most important advances in the treatment of heart failure was the recognition that pump function in heart failure was critically dependent on the outflow resistance against which the ventricle must empty.[59] It is now well established that vasodilator drugs that relax peripheral arterioles shift the ventricular function curve upward and to the left, resulting in an increase in cardiac output without a large change in blood pressure. Moreover, drugs that increase the capacitance of the venous circulation redistribute blood volume from the central to peripheral reservoirs and therefore decrease the signs and symptoms of elevated cardiac filling pressures. Since these original observations, there have been an extraordinary number of clinical studies reviewed elsewhere[60, 61] that have investigated the mechanisms of action as well as the systemic and regional hemodynamic effects of different vasodilators in patients with heart failure. These studies have characterized vasodilators that act predominantly on the arterioles, leading to a reduction in impedance (e.g., hydralazine); vasodilators that act predominantly on venous tone (e.g., nitrates); and vasodilators that have a balanced effect on arterioles and veins (e.g., ACE inhibitors).

The most widely used vasodilators are the ACE inhibitors. The traditional view is that the primary mechanism of action of ACE inhibitors is a reduction in angiotensin II–mediated vasoconstriction (Fig. 11–3). Evidence supporting this mechanism includes the observation that the magnitude of the acute reduction in blood pressure and systemic vascular resistance are strongly correlated with plasma renin activity.[62] The reduction of angiotensin II also results in a decrease in release of aldosterone from the adrenal gland and also of norepinephrine in the synaptic cleft.

More recent data, however, suggest that the ACE inhibitors have actions that are considerably more complex than a simple effect on circulating levels of angiotensin II. Because kininase is identical to converting enzyme, ACE inhibitors also reduce the metabolism of bradykinin. Bradykinin can stimulate the release of nitric oxide and other endothelium-dependent vasodilators, including prostaglan-

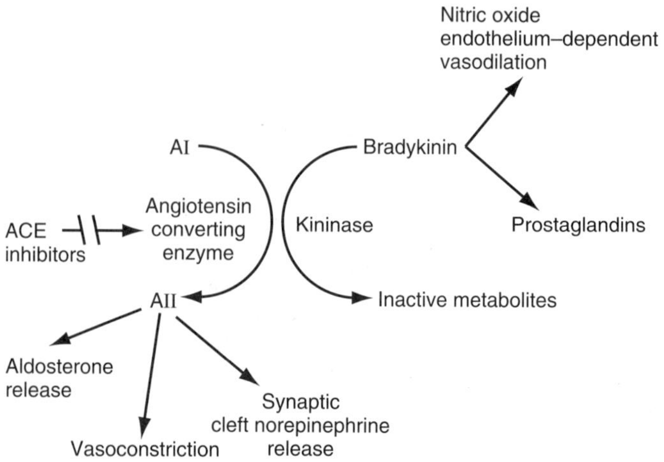

Figure 11–3. Mechanism of action of angiotensin converting enzyme (ACE) inhibitors. For discussion, see text. *Abbreviations*: AI, AII, angiotensin I and II; NE, norepinephrine.

dins.[63] Finally, there is now considerable evidence regarding tissue renin-angiotensin systems in blood vessels and the heart and that ACE inhibitors have an important effect on vascular and myocardial hypertrophy.[64] Any or all of these actions may have an important effect mediating the clinical efficacy of the ACE inhibitors.

Clinical Efficacy

Numerous prospective, placebo-controlled studies[65–79] have demonstrated the beneficial effects of ACE inhibitors and vasodilators on exercise tolerance, salt and water balance, clinical signs and symptoms, neurohormonal stimulation, quality of life, and survival in patients with chronic heart failure (Table 11–2). The concordance of findings in these multicenter trials has provided a strong scientific basis for the widespread use of ACE inhibitors in the management of heart failure. Several multicenter trials deserve comment.

Vasodilator Heart Failure Trial (VHEFT)

VHEFT was the first placebo-controlled trial to test the hypothesis that vasodilators could prolong survival in patients with heart failure.[65] The vasodilators tested were prazosin, an alpha-adrenergic blocker, and the combination of hydralazine and isosorbide dinitrate. Both drug regimens had been shown in previous studies to have similar acute hemodynamic benefit manifested by decreases in cardiac filling pressures and systemic vascular resistance and increases in cardiac output. The study included 642 men with reduced exercise capacity (peak oxygen consumption less than 25 mL/kg/min) and either a cardiothoracic ratio greater than .55, a left ventricular internal dimension greater than 2.7 cm/m^2, or a left ventricular ejection fraction less than .45. In a mean follow-up period of 2.3 years, the cumulative mortality rate was 25.6% in the hydralazine–isosorbide dinitrate group and 34.3% in the placebo group (risk reduction 34%; $p < .028$). In contrast, the mortality rate for the prazosin group was virtually identical to that for the placebo group.

Cooperative North Scandinavian Enalapril Survival Study (CONSENSUS)

The CONSENSUS trial randomized 253 hospitalized patients with class IV symptoms to either enalapril or placebo in addition to treatment with digoxin, diuretics, and non-ACE vasodilators.[66] On the basis of an interim analysis, enalapril was associated with a highly significant survival benefit compared with placebo (36% vs. 52%). Therefore, this trial was prematurely terminated, because it was deemed unethical to continue a trial in which half of the participants could have been randomized to placebo.

VHEFT-2

VHEFT-2 was designed to compare hydralazine–isosorbide dinitrate, which was the superior drug combination in VHEFT-1, with enalapril in the treatment of patients similar to those enrolled in VHEFT-1.[67] The enalapril group had a lower 2-year mortality rate compared with that of patients randomized to hydralazine–isosorbide dinitrate (18% vs. 25%, mortality reduction 28%, $p = .016$). Interestingly, exercise time and left ventricular function improved to a greater degree in the patients randomized to hydralazine–isosorbide dinitrate.

Studies of Left Ventricular Dysfunction (SOLVD)

SOLVD[68] was a randomized, double-blind, placebo-controlled trial in patients with an ejection fraction of .35 or less. The treatment trial of SOLVD enrolled 2567 patients who had signs and symptoms of heart failure and required treatment with digitalis and diuretics. After a mean follow-up of 41.4 months, there were significantly more deaths in the placebo group compared with the enalapril group (510 vs. 452; 16% mortality reduction). Furthermore, enalapril was associated with a significant 30% reduction in hospitalizations for heart failure. This mortality reduction probably underestimated the true effect of enalapril, because nearly 30% of the patients in the placebo group were taking open label converting enzyme inhibitors at the end of the trial.

SOLVD Prevention Trial

The SOLVD prevention trial[69] was run concurrently with the treatment trial and used the same experimental design except for the restriction to patients who had no signs or symptoms or any treatment for overt heart failure. After an average follow-up of 37.4 months, there were 334 deaths in the placebo group compared with 313 in the enalapril group. This 8% mortality reduction approached but did not achieve statistical significance. More impressive were the highly significant reductions in the first hospitalizations for heart failure (36%) and in the onset of heart failure requiring pharmacologic therapy (37%).

Assessment of Treatment With Lisinopril and Survival (ATLAS)

The ATLAS trial is currently in progress and expected to end in 1996. This trial will compare the effects of high- and low-dose lisinopril on mortality in 3000 patients with a left ventricular ejection fraction less than .30. Although this trial is not placebo controlled, it is hoped that it will provide important insight regarding the dependency on the dose of the ACE inhibitor.

Postinfarction Trials

Table 11–2 also contains the results of several trials that studied the effects of ACE inhibitors on mortality in the post–myocardial infarction population.[80] These trials, which are discussed in greater detail in Chapter 12, focused on a patient population that is not entirely comparable to the patients with left ventricular dysfunction and overt heart failure who were enrolled in the VHEFT, CONSENSUS, and SOLVD trials. Nonetheless, the results of the postinfarction trials have two important implications when treatment for patients with heart failure is considered.

First, the majority of these trials demonstrated that treatment with an ACE inhibitor initiated early after myocardial infarction had a small but significant benefit in reducing short-term mortality. This finding is significant because most of the patients enrolled in the postinfarction trials did not have overt heart failure. Both the treatment and prevention trials of SOLVD[68, 69] suggested that the benefit of enalapril was less in patients with mild heart failure. This finding has suggested to some that the strategy of treating patients without overt heart failure is not warranted. However, the experience in the postinfarction trials involving more than 50,000 patients suggests that there is indeed a small but significant benefit of early treatment.

The second and more compelling issue is that early intervention with an ACE inhibitor can prevent or at least delay the onset of overt heart failure. The Survival and Ventricular Enlargement (SAVE) trial demonstrated that captopril was associated with a 37% reduction in the development of heart failure and a 22% reduction in hospitalizations for heart failure. The CONSENSUS-2 trial demonstrated that enalapril reduced the need to change therapy for heart failure by 10%.[24] The Survival of Myocardial Infarction Long-term Evaluation (SMILE) trial demonstrated that the early use of zofenopril reduced the occurrence of severe congestive heart failure that developed within 6 weeks of the infarction.[77] These data are consistent with the

TABLE 11–2. KEY TRIALS IN HEART FAILURE: VASODILATORS AND ANGIOTENSIN CONVERTING ENZYME INHIBITORS

Trial	*N*	Agent	Entry Criteria	Follow-up Duration	Primary Endpoint	Findings/Status
VHEFT-1 (Vasodilator Heart Failure Trial)[65]	642	Prazosin vs. hydralazine–isosorbide dinitrate vs. placebo	CTR > .55 LVID > 2.7 cm/m^2 LVEF < .45 Decreased exercise tolerance	2.3 years	Mortality	2 years: Placebo 34.3% Prazosin 34.3% H/I 25.6% Reduction 34%
CONSENSUS (Cooperative North Scandinavian Enalapril Survival Study)[66]	253	Enalapril vs. placebo	NYHA IV	Average: 188 days	Mortality	1 year: P 52% E 36% Reduction 40%
VHEFT-2 (Vasodilator Heart Failure Trial)[67]	804	Hydralazine–isosorbide dinitrate vs. enalapril	CTR > .55 LVID > 2.7 cm/m^2 LVEF < .45 Decreased exercise tolerance	2.5 years	Mortality	2 years: H/I 25% E 18% Reduction 28%
SOLVD treatment trial (Studies of Left Ventricular Dysfunction)[68]	2567	Enalapril vs. placebo	LVEF ≤ .35 Signs/symptoms or drug therapy for HF	41.4 months	Mortality	P 39.7% E 35.2% Reduction 16%
SOLVD prevention trial (Studies of Left Ventricular Dysfunction)[69]	4228	Enalapril vs. placebo	LVEF ≤ .35 No signs/symptoms or drug therapy for HF	37.4 months	Mortality	P 15.8% E 14.8% Reduction 8%, p = .30
ATLAS (Assessment of Treatment with Lisinopril and Survival)	3000	High-dose lisinopril vs. low-dose lisinopril	LVEF < .30	2 years	Mortality	Expected end date 12/96
PROFILE (Prospective Randomized Flosequinan Longevity Evaluation)[70]	2304	Flosequinan vs. placebo	LVEF < .35 NYHA III-IV Digoxin, diuretic, ACE inhibitor	22 months	Mortality	F 20.6% P 15.4% Trial terminated 2° increased risk
Post-infarction Trials						
SAVE (Survival and Ventricular Enlargement)[71]	2231	Captopril vs. placebo	LVEF ≤ .40 3–16 days post MI	42 months	Mortality	P 25% C 20% Reduction 19%

AIRE (Acute Infarction Ramipril Efficacy)[72]	2006	Ramipril vs. placebo	3–10 days post MI Clinical evidence of HF	15 months	Mortality	P 23% R 17% Reduction 27%
ISIS-4 (International Study of Infarct Survival)[73]	29,022 (58,000 total)	Captopril vs. placebo	24 h post MI	6 months	Mortality	35-day mortality P 7.3% C 6.8% Risk reduction 5.2%, $p < .02$
CONSENSUS-2 (Cooperative North Scandinavian Enalapril Survival Study)[74]	6090	Enalapril IV/PO vs. placebo	24 h post MI	6 months	Mortality	P 10.2% E 11%
GISSI-3 (Gruppo Italiano per lo Studio della Sopravvivenza nell Infarto (Miocardio)[75]	19,394	Lisinopril vs. placebo	24 h post MI	6 weeks	Mortality	6-week mortality P 7.1% L 6.3% 11% risk reduction, $p = .03$
Chinese Captopril Trial[76]	12,629	Captopril vs. placebo	36 h post MI	1 month	Mortality	P 9.7% C 9.0%
SMILE (Survival of Myocardial Infarction Long-term Evaluation)[77]	1556	Zofenopril vs. placebo	24 h post MI	6 weeks	Mortality Heart failure	P 6.5% Z 4.9% Reduction 25%, $p = .19$ Heart failure P 4.1% Z 22%
PRACTICAL (Placebo-controlled Randomized, ACE Inhibitors, Comparative Trial in Cardiac Infarction and LV Function)[78]	225	Enalapril vs. captopril vs. placebo	24 h post MI	3 months	Left ventricular function Mortality	ACE increased LVEF Enalapril improved survival
TRACE (Trandolapril Cardiac Evaluation)[79]	1749	Trandolapril vs. placebo	Post MI LVEF ≤ .35	Minimum 24 months	Mortality	Expected end date 7/94

Abbreviations: ACE, angiotensin converting enzyme; CTR, cardiothoracic ratio; HF, heart failure; LVEF, left ventricular ejection fraction; LVID, left ventricular internal dimension; MI, myocardial infarction; NYHA, New York Heart Association class.

results of the prevention trial of SOLVD, which demonstrated a 20% reduction in hospitalizations for heart failure and a 29% reduction in the development of heart failure. These cumulative data suggest that ACE inhibitors will have a significant clinical benefit even in patients at relatively low risk.

Practical Considerations

ACE Inhibitors

Despite this overwhelming database from numerous clinical trials as well as the consensus among expert opinion leaders,[81–84] the application of ACE inhibitors to the large population of patients with heart failure appears to be much slower than anticipated. There may be several factors contributing to this slow trend. First, the use of ACE inhibitors appears to vary widely among different specialties; the percentage of cardiologists prescribing ACE inhibitors is larger than the percentage of primary care physicians.[9, 10] This difference may be related to a reliance on previous "step care" algorithms that reserved ACE inhibitors for patients with advanced heart failure. The perception that ACE inhibitors should be used primarily by cardiologists in patients with advanced heart failure may have even greater consequences under managed care initiatives where primary care physicians will manage the greatest number of patients with heart failure.

Second, it is a common perception that the ACE inhibitors are associated with a high frequency of significant adverse effects as listed in Table 11–3. However, the controlled experience from CONSENSUS and SOLVD in a large population of ambulatory patients suggests that the actual frequency of these complications is low and in the acceptable range when the potential benefit is considered.[68, 85, 86] Furthermore, management and avoidance of these complications can be facilitated by knowledge of certain predisposing factors and by institution of a few precautionary measures.

The most important problem to monitor during the initiation of ACE inhibitors is hypotension. Patients at highest risk for this complication are those who are volume depleted, receiving large doses of diuretics or concomitant vasodilator therapy, or older than 75 years. Patients who demonstrate activation of the renin-angiotensin system as manifested by increased plasma renin activity are those who have angiotensin II–mediated vasoconstriction and who are also at risk for hypotension (Fig. 11–4). As shown by Cody and Laragh,[62] the percentage decrease in systemic vascular resistance and pulmonary wedge pressure, as well as the percentage increase in cardiac index and stroke index, after a single oral dose of captopril, highly correlated with baseline plasma renin activity. Thus, patients with an activated renin-angiotensin system, as manifested by an elevated plasma renin activity, had more marked hemodynamic changes with captopril. In contrast, hemodynamic changes were minimal in patients with suppressed activity of the renin-angiotensin system. Because measurements of plasma renin activity are not readily available in most laboratories, most clinicians take advantage of the relatively tight inverse correlation between plasma renin activity and serum sodium concentration.[87, 88] Therefore, patients with a low serum sodium level (<130 mg/L) are more likely to have hypotension during the initiation of therapy. Useful strategies in all these groups of patients include temporary withholding of diuretics and the use of a test dose of a short-acting ACE inhibitor (e.g., 6.25 mg captopril) followed by gradual titration upward in a period of several weeks.

TABLE 11–3. ADVERSE EFFECTS OF ANGIOTENSIN CONVERTING ENZYME INHIBITORS

Hypotension	Cough
Renal insufficiency	Skin rash
Hyperkalemia	Dysgeusia

Although mild renal insufficiency may concern clinicians, there are many misperceptions.[89–92] Many patients with heart failure actually have an *improvement* in renal function with the initiation of ACE inhibitors probably mediated by an increase in cardiac output and renal perfusion.[93] Second, as discussed before, the frequency and magnitude of renal insufficiency in controlled trials are low, and only a small percentage of patients must be withdrawn from therapy. The mechanisms contributing to renal insufficiency are complex and are accentuated by concomitant drug therapy and hemodynamic abnormalities that are characteristic of heart failure.[89, 90] Patients at risk for renal insufficiency share many of the same features of patients at risk for hypotension. It is generally recommended that patients be reassessed approximately 1 week after initiation of an ACE inhibitor to monitor renal function and blood pressure. If there is an increase in serum creatinine greater than 1 mg/dL, the volume status and diuretic dose should be reassessed. In the majority of cases, renal function will return to baseline level once volume status has been returned to normal or if the diuretic dose is decreased. It is also advisable to check for concomitant medications that can aggravate renal insufficiency, such as the nonsteroidal anti-inflammatory drugs that reduce vasodilatory prostaglandins.

Hyperkalemia can occur in patients receiving ACE inhibitors because of the reduction in angiotensin II–mediated aldosterone secretion. Therefore, the dosage of potassium supplements and potassium levels should be monitored approximately 1 week after initiation of ACE inhibitors. Potassium-sparing diuretics should be used with caution.

The other side effects of ACE inhibitors, such as dysgeusia, skin rash, and cough, are commonly self-limited or reversible with discontinuation of the drug.[86, 94] Clinicians must be particularly cautious about stopping ACE inhibitors because of cough. Cough is a common manifestation of heart failure and will often respond to an increased dose of diuretics, ACE inhibitor, or both. If the cough is intolerable, a smaller dose or temporary discontinuation can be tried. Many patients tolerate a mild cough in exchange for the important improvements in survival and quality of life.

Tachyphylaxis or the attenuation of the beneficial effect is not a major problem during maintenance therapy with an ACE inhibitor. However, heart failure and the renin-angiotensin system are dynamic processes and are influenced by many factors, such as dietary sodium intake. Increased dietary sodium intake could exacerbate edema formation, suppress renin activity, and give the appearance of a "treatment failure."

Doses of ACE inhibitors should be titrated upward for 2 to 3 weeks until target doses are achieved (e.g., 25–50 mg three times daily for captopril, 10 mg twice daily for enalapril). The issue of the optimal dose is controversial because it is a common impression that many patients are being treated with substantially smaller doses.[95] It is possible that the same clinical benefit that was observed in clinical trials can be derived with a substantially smaller dose, but there are no clinical data to support this assumption. Therefore, it is generally recommended to use the same doses that were used in the large controlled clinical trials.

Another issue of considerable controversy is whether the beneficial effects of ACE inhibitors are class or drug specific.[96] This issue has become even more important because the number of ACE inhibitors that are available continues to increase and now includes captopril, enalapril, lisinopril, fosinopril, benazepril, ramipril, and quinapril. Currently, captopril, enalapril, lisinopril, and quinapril are indicated for the treatment of symptomatic heart failure. Captopril is the only ACE inhibitor indicated for post–myocardial infarction patients, and enalapril is the only ACE inhibitor indicated for the prevention of heart failure in asymptomatic patients. At present, there are insufficient scientific data that would conclusively prove whether the benefits demonstrated in clinical trials are applicable to all ACE inhibitors or only to the specific drug studied. There are some differences in structure, pharmacokinetics, and pharmacodynamics among the ACE inhibitors,[97–100] but it is not known whether these differences have a

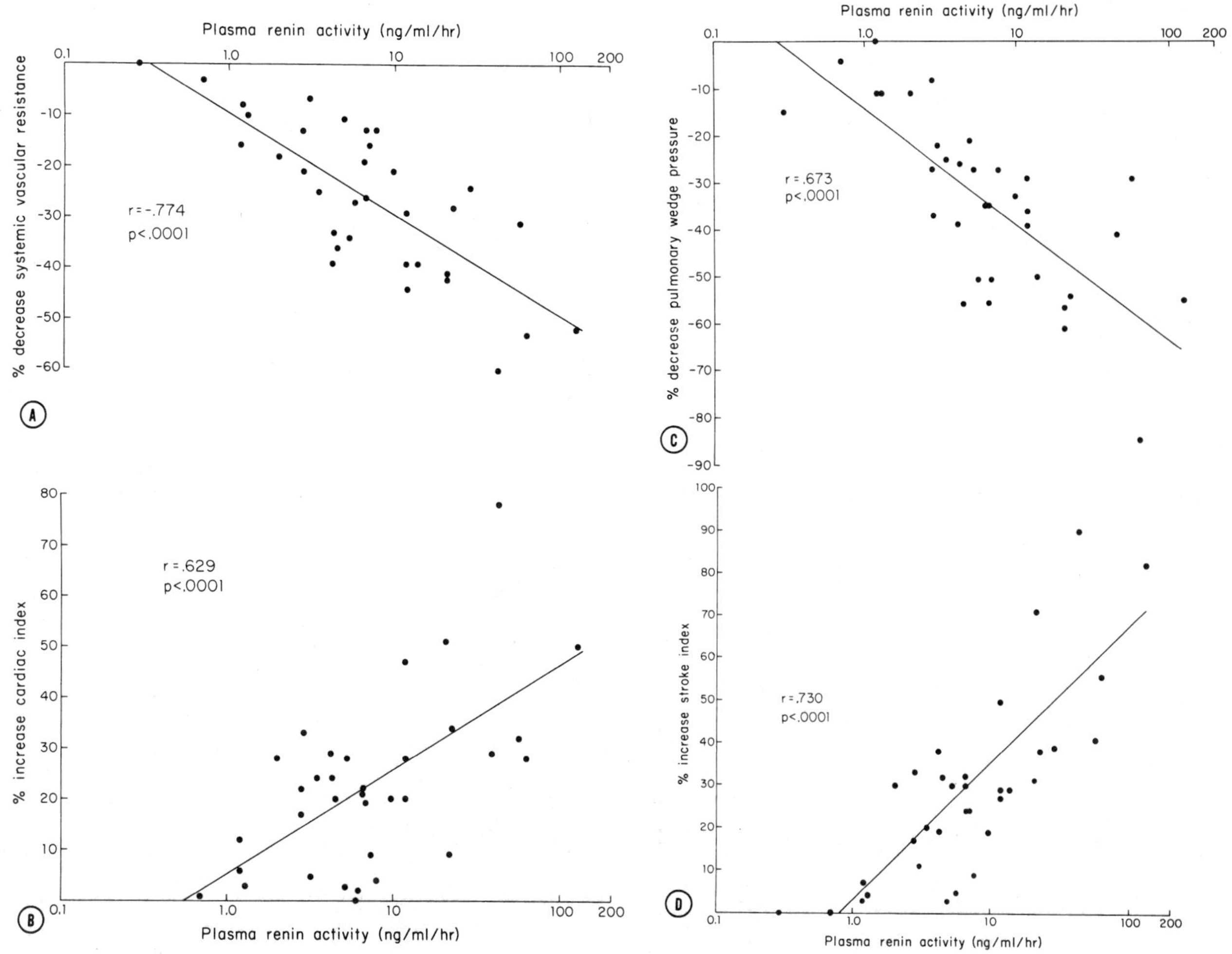

Figure 11–4. Correlation between baseline plasma renin activity and acute hemodynamic changes at time of peak response to an oral dose of captopril (25 mg). The percentage decrease in systemic vascular resistance *(A)*, the percentage increase in cardiac index *(B)*, the percentage decrease in pulmonary wedge pressure *(C)*, and the percentage increase in stroke index *(D)* were all highly correlated with activation of the renin-angiotensin system, as manifested by plasma renin activity. Thus, patients with activated renin-angiotensin systems, manifested by an elevated plasma renin activity, had more marked hemodynamic changes. (From Cody RJ, Laragh JH: Use of captopril to estimate renin-angiotensin-aldosterone activity in the pathophysiology of chronic heart failure. Am Heart J 1982; 104:1184–1189.)

significant impact on clinical outcomes. Furthermore, cost has become a dominant issue in many different situations. However, the precise mechanism of benefit of the ACE inhibitors is still not known, and many physicians choose to use the ACE inhibitors with the largest investigative experience.[95]

Hydralazine and Isosorbide Dinitrate

The combination of hydralazine and isosorbide dinitrate was shown in VHEFT-1 to be an efficacious combination in terms of an improvement in survival compared with placebo.[65] Moreover, in VHEFT-2, this combination tended to increase exercise capacity and ejection fraction more than enalapril did.[67] The experience from these two large trials clearly demonstrated the utility and benefits of this drug combination.

Nonetheless, a number of factors have limited the widespread application of this drug combination to patients with heart failure. First, in VHEFT-2, the ACE inhibitor enalapril resulted in a statistically significant improvement in survival compared with those patients treated with hydralazine and isosorbide dinitrate.[67] Second, this combination is considerably more cumbersome for patient compliance because the target doses used in the VHEFT trials were 160 mg of isosorbide dinitrate (40 mg four times daily) and 300 mg of hydralazine (75 mg four times daily). Third, this combination has a number of side effects, primarily related to the headaches associated with nitrate preparations. In the VHEFT trials, between 18% and 33% of patients discontinued one or both of the medications because of side effects.[65, 67]

In clinical practice, the combination of hydralazine and isosorbide dinitrate appears to be particularly useful in those patients who require vasodilator therapy but are unable to tolerate ACE inhibitors. Many physicians use nitrates in their patients with heart failure. On the basis of trial data, it would be prudent to administer nitrates in combination with hydralazine. A combination product is currently in development. The long-term experience is limited, but the drug combination is useful and well tolerated.[101] Some patients have symptoms that are refractory to an ACE inhibitor, diuretics, and digitalis and may derive hemodynamic and clinical benefit with these two additional vasodilators. Massie and coworkers[102] demonstrated the additive hemodynamic benefits of adding hydralazine to captopril.

The most important recommendation regarding this regimen is to initiate therapy with small doses followed by gradual dose titration for several weeks. We have found that initial doses greater than 10 mg of isosorbide dinitrate and 25 mg of hydralazine are generally not well tolerated. Prophylactic acetaminophen can reduce the problems associated with nitrate-induced headache, but nonsteroidal anti-inflammatory agents should be avoided. Several long-acting nitrate preparations are now available, but the clinical experience in patients with heart failure is limited.

Calcium Channel Blockers

Calcium channel blocking agents have been considered for patients with heart failure because these drugs have potent vasodilator actions and may also reduce ischemia in patients with left ventricular dysfunction due to coronary artery disease.[103] Several hemodynamic studies have demonstrated that the acute administration of calcium channel blockers is associated with a reduction in systemic vascular resistance and an increase in cardiac output.[104] However, the acute hemodynamic effects of nifedipine, verapamil, and diltiazem have not been uniform and have not been associated with consistent short- or long-term clinical benefit.

The deleterious responses in patients with heart failure may be related to the direct negative inotropic actions that may predominate when calcium channel blockers are given long term. In addition, calcium channel blockers can stimulate the release of neurohormones both directly and indirectly by a fall in blood pressure. Finally, a post hoc analysis of the Multicenter Diltiazem Postinfarction Trial demonstrated that diltiazem was associated with an increased frequency of new or worsening heart failure in patients with an ejection fraction less than .40.[105] On the basis of these cumulative data, it is generally recommended that calcium channel blockers be used only with great caution in patients with heart failure. The primary benefit may be mainly from a reduction of ischemia, rather than from the vasodilator action per se. Furthermore, it is generally recommended that these drugs certainly be used in conjunction with an ACE inhibitor.

Several newer calcium channel blockers with greater selectivity for vascular actions are being developed. The limited experience to date with nicardipine, nitrendipine, felodipine, and amlodipine[106, 107] suggests a potent hemodynamic action but with variable clinical efficacy. Felodipine and amlodipine are currently being investigated in VHEFT-3 and the Prospective Randomized Amlodipine Survival Evaluation (PRAISE) trials, respectively. These multicenter trials should provide important information on the long-term clinical efficacy of these agents in patients with heart failure.

Flosequinan

Flosequinan is an orally active quinolone derivative with vasodilator properties. Although flosequinan will not be available for use in patients with heart failure, the experience with this agent in clinical trials highlights several important points regarding vasodilator therapy.

Several hemodynamic studies demonstrated that flosequinan had a balanced vasodilator action characterized by a decrease in systemic vascular resistance, an increase in cardiac output, and a decrease in cardiac filling pressure.[108] In three clinical trials that included 31 patients maintained on digoxin and diuretics,[109] 322 patients maintained on digoxin, diuretics, and ACE inhibitors,[110] and 88 patients in whom digoxin and diuretics were continued after a 2-week withdrawal of ACE inhibitors,[111] flosequinan was associated with an improvement in exercise capacity and symptoms. However, shortly after the market release of flosequinan in March 1993, the interim results of a multicenter mortality trial suggested that patients receiving 100 mg/day of flosequinan had an increased risk of death compared with that of patients receiving placebo. The mechanisms of this increased mortality are not known but may be related to neurohormonal stimulation or to a mild positive inotropic effect.

These findings should be contrasted with the repeated demonstration that ACE inhibitors prolong life in this population of patients. This contrast clearly demonstrates that not all vasodilators are equivalent. Because the hemodynamic actions are similar, these data raise the possibility that the mechanism of survival benefit with an ACE inhibitor may not be solely dependent on hemodynamic changes.

DIGOXIN

Clinical Effects

The mechanisms of action and the pharmacology of digoxin are discussed in Chapters 9 and 17 as well as other references.[112, 118] Although digoxin has been commonly used in the management of heart failure, there was considerable controversy regarding the precise documentation of its clinical efficacy.[113–116] Early studies were conflicting, and interpretation was difficult because of small sample sizes and dependence on less precise clinical measures. It is therefore appropriate to review the more recent data from some of the larger and more conclusive randomized placebo-controlled trials[117–130] that have provided the firm scientific data to recommend the routine use of digoxin in patients with symptomatic heart failure (Table 11–4).

Many of the early trials that evaluated the efficacy of digoxin used a crossover design and sample sizes that are considered small in comparison with more recent multicenter trials. Fleg[117] and Taggart[118] and coworkers reported crossover trials in 30 and 22 patients, respectively, both observed for 3 months. There were no significant differences between placebo and digoxin in terms of exercise duration, frequency and severity of symptoms, or other clinical endpoints. In contrast, the trial by Lee and colleagues[119] received considerable attention for the use of a scoring system based on clinical assessments, physical findings, and radiographic and echocardiographic findings. Fourteen of 25 patients were considered digoxin responders with a marked improvement in the heart failure score. Of interest, it was commonly noted that this trial suggested that only patients with an S_3 gallop would respond to digoxin. However, the scoring system used in this study ranged from 0 to 14. Because the lowest score possible was 0, the ability for any intervention to improve the clinical status of patients with a low score, such as the clustering of patients without an S_3 gallop, was extremely limited. Because the finding of an S_3 gallop is not always reliable or reproducible, it is more appropriate to consider digoxin for all patients with heart failure irrespective of an S_3 gallop.

Subsequent trials have used a parallel design in which digoxin was compared with placebo and other agents including xamoterol, captopril, milrinone, and ibopamine. Whereas the primary intent of these trials was to demonstrate the efficacy of these newer agents, the trials nonetheless provided important information on the use of digoxin. The German and Austrian Xamoterol Study Group randomized 433 patients to placebo, digoxin, or xamoterol, a mixed beta agonist with some beta antagonist activity.[123] Both digoxin and xamoterol decreased symptoms of heart failure compared with placebo. The Captopril-Digoxin Multicenter Research group randomized 300 patients to placebo, digoxin, or captopril.[124] At 6 months, digoxin increased ejection fraction, whereas captopril improved exercise duration and NYHA functional class. Both digoxin and captopril reduced the need for additional diuretics as well as hospitalizations and emergency room visits for heart failure. DiBianco and coworkers[127] reported the results of a trial that randomized 230 patients to one of four groups including placebo, digoxin, milrinone (a phosphodiesterase inhibitor), and the combination of digoxin and milrinone. Digoxin improved ejection fraction and exercise tolerance and markedly decreased the frequency of clinical decompensation compared with placebo. Finally, the Dutch Ibopamine Multicenter Trial (DIMT) randomized 161 patients to placebo, digoxin, or ibopamine, a dopamine agonist.[128] Digoxin improved exercise time and decreased neurohormonal activation.

Two trials[129, 130] employed a withdrawal design in either patients who were treated with a diuretic only (Prospective Randomized Study of Ventricular Failure and the Efficacy of Digoxin [PROVED]) or patients who were treated with a diuretic and an ACE inhibitor (Randomized Assessment of Digoxin on Inhibitors of the Angiotensin Converting Enzyme [RADIANCE]). In both trials, the groups treated with digoxin for a 3-month period exhibited a higher ejection fraction, better exercise tolerance, and fewer episodes and symptoms of heart failure compared with the placebo group.

Although these studies demonstrated the beneficial effects of digoxin on clinical endpoints, the effects on mortality are not known. Virtually all of the clinical studies have been unable to assess an effect on survival because of inadequate sample size.[131] Some but not all studies in patients recovering from acute myocardial infarction have shown that patients treated with digoxin had increased mortality rates compared with patients who were not taking digoxin, even when corrected for the prevalence of symptomatic heart failure in digoxin-treated patients.[132–136] The specific effects of digitalis on mortality are currently being assessed in the Digitalis Investigation Group (DIG) trial, a randomized prospective study sponsored by the National Heart, Lung, and Blood Institute of the National Institutes of Health with an estimated enrollment of 8000 patients.[131] Data from the DIG trial and from the VHEFT-3 trial, which uses a 2 × 2 factorial design with digoxin and felodipine, are anticipated to be available in early 1996. It is hoped that these trials will provide firm evidence of whether the effects of digitalis on clinical parameters and survival are concordant.

The cumulative data from controlled trials would suggest that digitalis is associated with important clinical improvements and would support the addition of digoxin to a regimen of a diuretic and an ACE inhibitor for patients with left ventricular systolic dysfunction and significant heart failure. However, digoxin has not been shown to have efficacy in patients with heart failure primarily due to diastolic dysfunction and might have adverse effects in patients with ongoing myocardial ischemia. Furthermore, there are no data to support the use of digitalis in patients who have asymptomatic left ventricular dysfunction.

Practical Considerations

Previous practice typically involved the use of full digitalizing doses to more rapidly achieve therapeutic levels. However, this is usually not necessary for most patients who can be started on maintenance doses, ranging from 0.125 to 0.375 mg/day. Steady-state levels will be reached in approximately 1 week. The gelatin capsule increases oral bioavailability by up to 90%, so that there should be a 10% reduction in the total daily dose. Because drug elimination is primarily by the kidneys, digoxin doses must be adjusted in renal insufficiency. There are a number of drug interactions that can significantly influence the efficacy and toxicity of digoxin. Drugs known to increase digoxin levels include quinidine, verapamil, diltiazem, and amiodarone. It is common practice to empirically reduce digoxin doses on initiating therapy with these drugs with close follow-up of digoxin levels.

Measurement of serum digoxin levels can be helpful especially in identifying patients who are receiving subtherapeutic doses. The value of obtaining digoxin levels on a routine basis is unknown, but it is probably reasonable to check a level in follow-up to be certain that the dose has achieved a serum level between 0.7 and 1.5 mg/mL. Digoxin levels are important in the evaluation of toxic effects, such as evidence of nausea, arrhythmias, atrioventricular block, or confusion. Patients with advanced heart failure were once considered candidates for intensified digoxin therapy, and doses were occasionally pushed to the point of development of toxic effects. With the availability of other treatments, this is no longer appropriate.

For many years, digoxin has been used to control the ventricular response rate in atrial fibrillation. In many situations, however, digoxin may not provide adequate rate control, especially during exercise or in patients with high sympathetic tone. Many such patients respond to the judicious addition of a beta blocker or a calcium channel blocker such as diltiazem or verapamil for adjustment of rate control. In selected patients, atrioventricular nodal ablation followed by dual-chamber pacing may be necessary.

OPTIONS FOR PATIENTS WITH PERSISTENT SIGNS AND SYMPTOMS

Patients who have persistent signs and symptoms of heart failure despite intensive treatment with diuretics, dietary sodium restriction, ACE inhibitors, and digoxin present a difficult challenge for physicians dealing with patients with heart failure. As listed in Figure 11–2, several options can be considered individually or in combination for patients with refractory heart failure. Some patients will require multiple diuretics (e.g., loop and thiazide diuretics) or multiple vasodilators (e.g., combination of ACE inhibitors, hydralazine, and isosorbide dinitrate) as discussed in previous sections of this chapter. Many patients will be candidates for heart transplantations, which is discussed in Chapter 15. The remainder of this section summarizes the experience with and potential roles of two other pharmacologic options, beta blockers and inotropic agents, that are under intensive investigation.

Beta Blockers

Beta blockers have traditionally been contraindicated in patients with heart failure because of concerns that the negative inotropic action could result in clinically important deteriorations.[137] This dogma has been challenged by laboratory and clinical studies suggesting that beta blockers may have important short- and long-term benefits for this population of patients.[138, 139]

It is well established that sympathetic activation in heart failure is associated with beta receptor "downregulation," a complex sequence of biochemical and molecular events that results in a decreased number of surface beta receptors and uncoupling of the beta receptor complex.[140, 141] Several clinical trials have shown that carefully administered beta blockers can result in improved ventricular function, hemodynamics, functional class, and beta receptor density.[142–145] Furthermore, two small trials suggested that beta blocker therapy may also be associated with a significant improvement in survival.[146, 147]

The effects of beta blockade on survival have now been assessed in the Metoprolol in Dilated Cardiomyopathy (MDC) and the Cardiac Insufficiency Bisoprolol Study (CIBIS) trials[148, 149] (Table 11–5). The MDC trial randomized 380 patients to either metoprolol or placebo. In an 18-month follow-up period, metoprolol did not affect mortality but was associated with a 34% reduction in the need for cardiac transplantation. The CIBIS trial randomized 641 patients to either bisoprolol or placebo. In a 2-year follow-up, total mortality was slightly but not significantly reduced in the bisoprolol group (21 vs. 17; $p = .22$).

Why these trials did not demonstrate an improvement in mortality is not known, but the reason could be related to the small sample size. Therefore, the National Institutes of Health and the Veterans Administration Medical Centers are organizing a multicenter trial (Beta Blocker Evaluation of Survival [BEST]) anticipated to enroll 2800 patients to more definitively determine whether bucindolol has a beneficial effect in this population of patients.[150] This trial was initiated in 1995.

There is additional interest in the effects of carvedilol, a nonselective beta antagonist with vasodilator properties due to alpha-adrenergic antagonism, on clinical endpoints and survival, which are being evaluated by the Australian and New Zealand Heart Failure Research Collaborative Group (ANZ), the Multicenter Oral Carvedilol in Heart Failure Assessment (MOCHA), and the Prospective Randomized Evaluation of Carvedilol in Symptoms and Exercise (PRECISE) trials (see Table 11–5). It is hoped that these trials will add to the scientific database regarding the advisability of beta blocker therapy in patients with heart failure. Until these additional data are complete,

TABLE 11–4. RANDOMIZED PROSPECTIVE PLACEBO-CONTROLLED TRIALS WITH DIGOXIN

Reference	Year	Patients	NYHA	LVEF	Study Design	Duration	Findings	Comments
Fleg et al[117]	1982	30	II–III	.23	Crossover	3 months	No significant difference in exercise duration, frequency and severity of symptoms	Withdrawal produced a small increase in cardiac size
Taggart et al[118]	1983	22	I–III	NA	Crossover	3 months	No improvement in clinical endpoints	Digoxin decreased heart rate and improved systolic time intervals
Lee et al[119]	1982	25	I–III	.29	Crossover	5–80 days	14/25 patients were digoxin responders—improvement in clinical and radiographic heart failure score	
Guyatt et al[120]	1988	20	I–III	.17	Crossover	7 weeks	Digoxin group had small differences in dyspnea, clinical assessment, and walking test score	7 patients receiving placebo prematurely terminated from the study
Aronow et al[121]	1986	10	NA	.45	Withdrawal	4 months	No patient required reinstitution of digoxin after withdrawal	
Alicandri et al[122]	1987	16	II–III	NA	Crossover Digoxin Captopril	1 month	Both drugs increased exercise tolerance and cardiac function	
German and Austrian Xamoterol Study Group[123]	1988	433	I–III	NA	Parallel Digoxin (104) Xamoterol (220) Placebo (109)	3 months	Xamoterol increased exercise duration Both digoxin and Xamoterol decreased symptoms Digoxin reduced cardiothoracic ratio	Xamoterol subsequently found to increase mortality

Captopril-Digoxin Multicenter Research Group[124]	1988	300	I–III	.25	Parallel Digoxin Captopril Placebo	6 months	Digoxin improved ejection fraction Both digoxin and captopril reduced need for additional diuretics and hospitalizations and emergency department visits for heart failure	Captopril improved exercise duration and NYHA class
Davies et al[125]	1991	145	II–III	.30	Parallel Enalapril Digoxin	4 weeks	Clinical response to digoxin and captopril similar between 4 and 14 weeks	Enalapril patients had fewer adverse events and less fatigue during exercise
Drexler et al[126]	1992	196	II–III	.48–.55	Parallel Digoxin Captopril Placebo	1 year	Digoxin improved symptoms and NYHA class	Neither drug affected exercise capacity
DiBianco et al[127]	1989	230	II–IV	.21	Parallel Digoxin Milrinone Digoxin and milrinone Placebo	3 months	Digoxin improved ejection fraction and exercise tolerance and decreased clinical deteriorations	Milrinone later withdrawn
DIMT[128]	1993	161	II–III	.29	Parallel Digoxin, N = 55 Ibopamine, N = 53 Placebo, N = 53	6 months	Digoxin improved exercise time and decreased neurohormonal activation	
PROVED[129]	1993	88	II–III	.28	Parallel withdrawal Digoxin Placebo	3 months	Decreased episodes of HF Improved exercise tolerance Increased LVEF	No ACE inhibitor allowed
RADIANCE[130]	1993	173	II–III	$< .27$	Parallel withdrawal Digoxin Placebo	3 months	Decreased episodes of HF Increased exercise tolerance Increased LVEF	All patients received ACE inhibitors

Abbreviations: ACE, angiotensin converting enzyme; HF, heart failure; LVEF, left ventricular ejection fraction; NA, not available; NYHA, New York Heart Association class.

TABLE 11–5. KEY TRIALS IN HEART FAILURE: BETA BLOCKERS

Trial	*N*	Agent	Entry Criteria	Follow-up Duration	Primary Endpoint	Findings/Status
MDC (Metoprolol in Dilated Cardiomyopathy)[148]	380	Metoprolol vs. placebo	EF < .40	18 months	Mortality and cardiac transplant	No effect on mortality 34% reduction in need for cardiac transplant
CIBIS (Cardiac Insufficiency Bisoprolol Study)[149]	641	Bisoprolol vs. placebo	LVEF < .40 NYHA III–IV	1.9 years	Mortality	P 21% B 16.6%, $p = .22$ B improved functional status
ANZ (Australian and New Zealand Heart Failure Research Collaborative Group)[206]	415	Carvedilol vs. placebo	LVEF < .40	3 years	Mortality	Carvedilol improved ejection fraction 52%
MOCHA (Multicenter Oral Carvedilol in Heart Failure Assessment)[207]	345	Carvedilol vs. placebo (6.25, 12.5, 25 mg)	LVEF < .35	6 months	Clinical efficacy	Carvedilol caused dose-related increase in ejection fraction and survival
PRECISE (Prospective Randomized Evaluation of Carvedilol in Symptoms and Exercise)[208]	276	Carvedilol vs. placebo (25–50 mg)	LVEF < .35	6 months	Clinical efficacy	Carvedilol improved ejection fraction, quality of life, and symptoms
BEST (Beta Blocker Evaluation of Survival Trial)	2800	Bucindolol vs. placebo	LVEF < .35 NYHA III–IV	3 years	Mortality	Expected start date 3/95

Abbreviations: EF, ejection fraction; LVEF, left ventricular ejection fraction; NYHA, New York Heart Association class.

beta blockers are typically reserved for selected patients under highly monitored conditions.

Orally Administered Positive Inotropic Agents

Safe and clinically effective inotropic agents are sought for patients with heart failure because this clinical syndrome is the result of a primary defect in myocardial contractility and because many patients have symptoms that are refractory to intensive treatments with diuretics, dietary sodium restriction, ACE inhibitors, vasodilators, and digoxin. In the last 15 years, there has been an extraordinary effort to develop an orally administered inotropic agent.[151] The majority of the studies have focused on the phosphodiesterase inhibitors, which produce a marked acute hemodynamic benefit. However, enthusiasm for the potential therapeutic effects of this class of drugs decreased significantly when several multicenter trials failed to detect a significant improvement in exercise tolerance and when the Prospective Randomized Milrinone Survival Evaluation (PROMISE) trial demonstrated increased mortality rates in patients treated with milrinone.[152–156]

Data from these trials must be carefully interpreted, however, because these adverse features may not be applicable to all inotropic drugs.[157–159] It has been suggested that the adverse outcomes were specifically related to phosphodiesterase inhibition and increased levels of cyclic adenosine monophosphate (cAMP) so that inotropic agents with alternative mechanisms of action might have more favorable clinical effects. Furthermore, the use of fixed large doses, the criteria for selection of patients, and the extent of background drug therapy may have contributed to the adverse outcomes in these trials.[160, 161]

Although several drugs may have some potential as inotropic drugs, vesnarinone (OPC-8212) and pimobendan are the farthest along in development (Table 11–6). Vesnarinone is a quinolinone derivative with unique membrane actions that are not dependent on phosphodiesterase inhibition.[162, 163] Some but not all of the early clinical trials demonstrated clinical benefit.[164, 165] A subsequent large multicenter randomized placebo-controlled trial in 477 patients demonstrated a striking 62% reduction in mortality with 60 mg/day of vesnarinone.[166] The 120 mg/day dose was discontinued because of excess mortality, which suggests an unusual dose-response relationship. Study of the effects of a lower dosage of vesnarinone (30 mg/day and 60 mg/day vs. placebo) is currently under way in VEST (vesnarinone trial).

Pimobendan is a benzimidazole-pyridazinone derivative that appears to use calcium sensitization of the myofilament as its primary mechanism of action. A controlled trial in 198 patients demonstrated important improvements in exercise time, peak oxygen consumption, and quality of life.[167] Again, the effects appeared to favor the low dosage, because the efficacy of 5 mg/day was greater than that of 10 mg/day. The effects of pimobendan on mortality are not known.

Table 11–6 also lists two trials that are currently in progress. The DIG trial, which was discussed in the section on digoxin, will specifically assess the effects of digoxin on morbidity. The VHEFT-3 trial uses a 2 × 2 factorial design to assess the effects of digoxin and felodipine on exercise tolerance and survival.

One additional treatment that can be used in patients who have signs and symptoms of heart failure that are refractory to standard treatment regimens is intravenous dobutamine.[168] Anecdotal experience with use of central venous access and low-dose infusions (generally < 5 μg/kg/min) has been favorable, especially in patients waiting for heart transplantation.[169, 170] Because dobutamine can be given on an ambulatory basis with specially calibrated pocket-sized pumps, many patients enjoy an improvement in quality of life. The adverse effect profile is acceptable, especially if the dose adminis-

TABLE 11–6. KEY TRIALS IN HEART FAILURE: INOTROPIC AGENTS

Trial	*N*	Agent	Entry Criteria	Follow-up Duration	Primary Endpoint	Findings/Status
PROMISE (Prospective Randomized Milrinone Survival Evaluation)[155]	1088	Milrinone vs. placebo	NYHA III–IV LVEF ≤ .35 Digoxin, diuretic, ACE inhibitor	6.1 months	Mortality	P 24% M 30% Increase 28% Study terminated prematurely
Vesnarinone (OPC-8212)[166]	477	Vesnarinone vs. placebo	LVEF ≤ .30	6 months	Mortality Morbidity	V 5.4% P 13.9% Reduction 62% 120-mg dose discontinued because of excess mortality
Pimobendan[167]	198	Pimobendan vs. placebo	LVEF < .45 Digoxin, diuretic, single vasodilator	12 weeks	Exercise Quality of life	Pimobendan increased exercise time, peak oxygen consumption, and quality of life 5 mg/day superior to 10 mg/day
DIG (Digitalis Investigators Group)	8000	Digoxin vs. placebo	Clinical HF NSR Stratified LVEF	2 years	Mortality	Expected end date 12/95
VHEFT-3 (Vasodilator Heart Failure Trial)[209]	451	Felodipine, digoxin, placebo (2 × 2 factorial design)	LVEF < .45 CTR > .55	2 years	Exercise tolerance	Felodipine had no effect on mortality or on peak exercise capacity
VEST (Vesnarinone trial)	3618	Vesnarinone (30 or 60 mg) vs. placebo	LVEF ≤ .30 NYHA III–IV	18 months	Mortality	Expected end date 6/97

Abbreviations: ACE, angiotensin converting enzyme; CTR, cardiothoracic ratio; HF, heart failure; LVEF, left ventricular ejection fraction; NSR, normal sinus rhythm; NYHA, New York Heart Association class.

tered is not escalated. It is postulated that the adverse experience and increased mortality rates observed in the controlled trial with outpatient dobutamine infusions were related to the titration to higher than necessary dosages.

ADJUNCTIVE THERAPY

Anticoagulants

Many clinicians have recommended anticoagulants for patients with dilated cardiomyopathy and symptomatic heart failure in the absence of specific contraindications for prophylaxis against thromboembolic complications and stroke.[171, 172] This recommendation was based on the frequent presence of ventricular thrombus in up to 75% of cases of dilated cardiomyopathy[173] and the repeated observation of an extremely high frequency of embolic episodes in this population of patients.[172, 174–177] Finally, retrospective analyses appeared to suggest that the occurrence of emboli was reduced in patients who were taking anticoagulants.

However, these recommendations are being reconsidered in view of data from more recent multicenter trials. In VHEFT-2, there were only 46 embolic events in 804 patients observed an average of 2.56 years.[178] In SOLVD, only 5.3% of patients experienced an embolism during 39.2 months of follow-up.[179] Furthermore, the use of anticoagulants, as directed by individual physicians, was not associated with a reduced frequency of thromboembolic complications. Thus, because the risk of thromboembolism and the benefit of anticoagulant therapy may not be as large as once considered, in the absence of data from a controlled trial,[180] recommendations for anticoagulation for patients with heart failure should be made on an individual basis. An alternative regimen used by many clinicians is to use a single daily dose of aspirin, but there are few controlled data on the efficacy of this recommendation.

Antiarrhythmic Agents

The indications for and the efficacy of antiarrhythmic agents are some of the most controversial issues in the management of heart failure.[181, 182] The rationale for considering these agents as adjunctive therapy is based on the observation that as many as 30% to 50% of all deaths in patients with heart failure can be classified as sudden death.[183] Frequent ventricular premature contractions and nonsustained ventricular tachycardia on Holter recordings are almost universal in patients with heart failure[181, 184] and are frequent sources of concern in hospitalized patients who are on telemetry monitoring. These arrhythmias are probably related to a number of factors including fibrosis, wall stress, left ventricular dilatation, electrolyte imbalances, high levels of circulating catecholamines, and drug therapy such as digitalis. All of these factors have suggested that antiarrhythmic therapy and suppression of high-risk arrhythmias would be beneficial in this population of patients.

However, there are a number of significant problems with this therapeutic strategy. The association between ventricular arrhythmias and an increased risk of sudden death has not been uniform,[185] possibly because ventricular arrhythmias may be a nonspecific manifestation of poor left ventricular function rather than a specific arrhythmogenic substrate. Second, the mechanisms of sudden death in heart failure may also be related to ischemia or bradyarrhythmias.[186] Third, a number of adverse events are associated with the use of antiarrhythmic agents in patients with heart failure, including a proarrhythmic effect[187] as well as aggravation of heart failure.[188] Most important, the Cardiac Arrhythmia Suppression Trial[189] demonstrated that type I antiarrhythmic agents, although decreasing the frequency of ventricular ectopy, were associated with an *increase* in mortality in patients who had sustained a recent myocardial infarction. Therefore, it is prudent to avoid the routine use of conventional antiarrhythmic drug therapy in patients with heart failure.

More recent studies have suggested that amiodarone may substantially reduce the frequency and complexity of asymptomatic ventricular arrhythmias as well as total mortality in patients with chronic heart failure.[190, 191] There are now two multicenter trials that have prospectively addressed the beneficial effects of amiodarone. The Grupo de Estudio de la Sobrevida en la Insufficiencia Cardiaca en Argentina (GESICA) trial included 516 patients from 26 hospitals in Argentina. This unblinded trial demonstrated a 28% reduction in mortality.[192] In contrast, the Congestive Heart Failure Survival Trial of Antiarrhythmia Therapy (CHF-STAT) trial, which enrolled patients from Veterans Administration Medical Centers in the United States, did not demonstrate a significant benefit of amiodarone.[193]

It is difficult to reconcile the conflicting results of these two trials. It is possible that differences in etiology, severity of heart failure, dose of amiodarone, and prior drug exposure may all be important. There is currently insufficient evidence to recommend the routine use of amiodarone in patients with heart failure. Nonetheless, amiodarone is favored by many physicians in patients with a history of sudden death, ventricular tachycardia, or inducible ventricular arrhythmias during electrophysiologic testing.

There is increasing experience with the implantable cardioverter-defibrillators for patients with symptomatic ventricular tachycardia and ventricular fibrillation. These devices can reliably detect and terminate lethal rhythms and have dramatically changed the expected survival curves.[194, 195] Recent improvements include the ability to pace terminate arrhythmias and nonthoracotomy lead systems. At present, these devices are indicated only for patients with heart failure who have symptomatic ventricular arrhythmias.

Physical Training

Complete bed rest in the past was a common recommendation for patients with heart failure to reduce myocardial oxygen demand. However, it is now well established that skeletal muscle structure and function are abnormal in heart failure and that these abnormalities contribute to deconditioning and exercise intolerance.[196–198] Small clinical trials have suggested that regular physical exercise is associated with improvement in symptoms, clinical status, and exercise duration.[199, 200] On the basis of these findings, most physicians recommended a program of regular exercise for their patients. Such programs are often facilitated by initial supervision in a cardiac rehabilitation program and by restriction of aerobic exercise to levels that are below the anaerobic threshold.

SPECIAL CONSIDERATIONS

The majority of ambulatory patients with chronic heart failure have impairment of left ventricular systolic performance and can be treated according to the algorithms presented in this chapter. However, several subgroups of patients merit special consideration because other therapeutic options may provide important clinical benefit. Patients with atherosclerotic coronary artery disease and evidence of myocardial ischemia and patients with significant valvular heart disease are considered in this section. Patients with primary diastolic dysfunction and patients with active myocarditis are considered in Chapters 13 and 14, respectively.

Patients With Atherosclerotic Coronary Vascular Disease

There are several ways in which atherosclerotic coronary artery disease can complicate the treatment of patients with chronic heart failure. Symptoms of angina pectoris and myocardial ischemia are often difficult to distinguish from the exertional dyspnea and fatigue associated with heart failure. However, patients who have myocardial ischemia frequently require additional anti-ischemic medication to maximize clinical improvement. Thus, in addition to standard treatment with digoxin, diuretics, and ACE inhibitors, such patients may improve further with the addition of nitrates, beta blockers, and occasionally calcium channel blockers. Exercise testing with thallium scintigraphy may be able to detect important ischemia, but the specificity of electrocardiographic and imaging findings is clearly reduced in these patients. In many instances, the addition of anti-ischemic drugs to the regimen is simply based on the presence of significant obstructive lesions and presumed ischemia.

Other patients with atherosclerotic coronary artery disease may have periodic decompensations that are triggered by episodes of myocardial ischemia. One example is the patient with "flash pulmonary edema" with an abrupt presentation of heart failure. In addition to anti-ischemic pharmacologic interventions, these patients may benefit from coronary revascularization with either coronary artery bypass surgery or coronary angioplasty.

Another important therapeutic consideration in patients with underlying atherosclerotic coronary vascular disease is the issue of hibernating myocardium.[201, 202] It is a well-established clinical observation that many patients will experience striking improvement in left ventricular systolic function after bypass surgery.[203] The mechanisms of this improvement are not fully known but are probably related to the restoration of blood flow to viable myocardium. This improvement in ejection fraction can occur even in patients without symptoms of angina pectoris.

There is no widely accepted or reliable method that will consistently identify those patients who would be expected to derive benefit from anti-ischemic medications and/or revascularization. Some patients have symptoms of angina pectoris that occur out of proportion to symptoms of excess extracellular volume that are more typical of heart failure. Coronary angiography is important for demonstration of significant stenoses that would be amenable to revascularization. Physiologic tests for ischemia including exercise or dipyridamole-thallium scintigraphy, positron emission tomography, or exercise radionuclide or echocardiographic imaging are important in defining patients who would be expected to have the greatest likelihood of a favorable response to reperfusion.[202]

An increased survival with bypass surgery has clearly been demonstrated in the subset of patients with a reduced ejection fraction and three-vessel coronary artery disease.[204, 205] Frequently, however, the decision to pursue or defer consideration of revascularization is strongly influenced by negative factors or conditions that either preclude intervention or substantially reduce the potential benefit. Such factors include history of previous cardiac surgery; severe comorbid diseases, such as renal failure, chronic obstructive lung disease, and diabetes; and moderate to severe mitral regurgitation. In addition, patients with low ejection fractions below .20 are often considered to have an excessive risk of bypass surgery. In some patients, heart transplantation is the preferred option.

Patients With Valvular Heart Disease

Patients with significant regurgitant valvular heart disease represent another difficult subgroup. Many patients with significant left ventricular dilatation will have mitral regurgitation due to annular dilatation. Other patients will have concomitant disease of the mitral apparatus related to a prior history of rheumatic heart disease or due to ischemic heart disease and papillary muscle dysfunction. Frequently, the use of vasodilator therapy will adequately reduce the regurgitant volume to permit symptomatic improvement. In other cases, however, it must be considered that abnormalities in the mitral apparatus make a primary contribution to symptoms and left ventricular dysfunction and that repair and/or valve replacement may have important therapeutic benefit. However, no reliable method will consistently distinguish those patients who will benefit from mitral valve surgery from those who experience a progressive decline in ventricular function after mitral surgery.

REFERENCES

1. Smith MW: Epidemiology of congestive heart failure. Am J Cardiol 1985; 55:3A–8A.
2. Kannel WB, Belanger AJ: Epidemiology of heart failure. Am Heart J 1991; 121:851–957.
3. Schocken DD, Arieta MI, Leaverton PE, Ross EA: Prevalence and mortality rate of congestive heart failure in the United States. J Am Coll Cardiol 1992; 20:301–306.
4. Ho KKL, Anderson KM, Kannel WB, et al: Survival after the onset of congestive heart failure in Framingham Heart Study patients. Circulation 1993; 88:107–115.
5. Francis GS, Kubo SH: Prognostic factors affecting diagnosis and treatment of congestive heart failure. Curr Probl Cardiol 1989; 14:631–671.
6. Vinson J, Rich NW, Sperry JC, et al: Early readmission of elderly patients with congestive heart failure. J Am Geriatr Soc 1990; 38:1290–1295.
7. O'Connell JB, Bristow MR: Economic impact of heart failure in the United States: time for a different approach. J Heart Lung Transplant 1993; 13:S107–S112.
8. Ghali JK, Cooper R, Ford E: Trends in hospitalization rates for heart failure in the United States, 1973–1986: evidence for increasing population prevalence. Arch Intern Med 1990; 150:769–773.
9. Bourassa MG, Gurne O, Bangdiwala SI, et al, for The Studies of Left Ventricular Dysfunction (SOLVD) Investigators: Natural history and patterns of current practice in heart failure. J Am Coll Cardiol 1993; 22:14A–19A.
10. Rajfer SI: Perspective of the pharmaceutical industry on the development of new drugs for heart failure. J Am Coll Cardiol 1993; 22:198A–200A.
11. Baker DW, Konstam M, Bolterff M, Pitt B: Management of heart failure: I. Pharmacologic treatment JAMA 1994; 272:1361–1366.
12. Cohn JN: Heart failure. *In* Willerson JT, Cohn JN (eds): Cardiovascular Medicine, pp 947–978. New York: Churchill Livingstone, 1994.
13. Goldsmith SR, Kubo SH: Pathophysiology of heart failure: peripheral vascular factors and neurohormonal mechanisms. *In* Cohn JN (ed): Drug Treatment of Heart Failure, pp 49–78. Secaucus, NJ: Advanced Therapeutics Communications International, 1988.
14. Cody RS, Laragh JH: The renin-angiotensin-aldosterone system in chronic heart failure: pathophysiology and implications for treatment. *In* Cohn JN (ed): Drug Treatment of Heart Failure, pp 79–104. Secaucus, NJ: Advanced Therapeutics Communications International, 1988.
15. Myers J, Froehlicher VF: Hemodynamic determinants of exercise capacity in chronic heart failure. Ann Intern Med 1991; 115:377–386.
16. Packer M: How should physicians view heart failure? The philosophical and physiological evaluation of three conceptual models of the disease. Am J Cardiol 1993; 71:3C–11C.
17. Rector TS, Cohn JN: Assessment of therapeutic efficacy in patients with chronic heart failure. *In* Barnett DB, Pouleur H, Francis GS (eds): Congestive Cardiac Failure: Pathophysiology and Treatment, pp 93–102. New York: Marcel Dekker, Inc. 1993.
18. Cohn JN: Current therapy of the failing heart. Circulation 1988; 78:1099–1107.
19. Hlatky MA, Fleg JL, Hinton PC, et al: Physician practice in the management of congestive heart failure. J Am Coll Cardiol 1986; 8:966–970.
20. Schrier RW: Body fluid volume regulation in health and disease: a unifying hypothesis. Ann Intern Med 1990; 113:155–159.
21. Hollenberg NK: The role of the kidney in heart failure. *In* Cohn JN (ed): Drug Treatment of Heart Failure, pp 105–106. Secaucus, NJ: Advanced Therapeutics Communications International, 1988.
22. Anand IS, Ferrari R, Kalra GS, et al: Edema of cardiac origin. Studies of body water and sodium, renal function, hemodynamic indexes, and plasma hormones in untreated congestive cardiac failure. Circulation 1989; 80:299–305.
23. Chonko AM, Bay WH, Stein JH, Ferris TF: The role of renin and aldosterone in the salt retention of edema. Am J Med 1977; 63:881–889.
24. Cody RJ, Ljungman S, Covit AB, et al: Regulation of glomerular filtration rate in chronic congestive heart failure patients. Kidney Int 1988; 34:361–367.
25. Mettauer B, Rouleau JL, Bichet D, et al: Sodium and water excretion abnormalities in congestive heart failure: determinant factors and clinical implications. Ann Intern Med 1986; 105:161–167.
26. Cody RJ, Covit AB, Schaer BL, et al: Sodium and water balance in chronic congestive heart failure. J Clin Invest 1986; 77:1441–1452.
27. Volpe M, Tritto C, DeLuca N, et al: Abnormalities of sodium handling and of cardiovascular adaptations during high salt diet in patients with mild heart failure. Circulation 1993; 88:1620–1627.
28. Muntzel M, Drueke T: A comprehensive review of the salt and blood pressure relationship. Am J Hypertens 1992; 5:1S–42S.
29. Braunwald E, Plauth WH, Morrow AG: A method for the detection and quantification of impaired sodium excretion. Circulation 1965; 32:223–231.
30. Barger AC, Ross RS, Price HL: Reduced sodium excretion in dogs with mild valvular lesions of the heart and in dogs with congestive heart failure. Am J Physiol 1955; 180:249–260.
31. Kubo SH, Ormaza SM, Francis GS, et al: Trends in patient selection for heart transplant. J Am Coll Cardiol 1993; 21:975–981.
32. Silver MA: Success With Heart Failure: Help and Hope for Those With Congestive Heart Failure. New York: Plenum Press, 1994.
33. Cody RJ, Kubo SH, Pickworth KK: Diuretic utilization for the sodium retention of congestive heart failure. Arch Intern Med, in press.
34. Mokrzyeki MH: Diuretic treatment of heart failure. Heart Failure 1994; Oct/Nov:181–191.
35. Mudge GH, Weiner IM: Drugs affecting renal function and electrolyte metabolism. *In* Goodman LS, Gilman A, Gilman AG, Koelle GB (eds): The Pharmacologic Basis of Therapeutics, 7th ed, pp 879–907. New York: Macmillan, 1985.
36. Wilcox CS: Diuretics. *In* Brenner BM, Rector FC Jr: The Kidney, 4th ed, pp 2133–2147. Philadelphia: WB Saunders, 1991.
37. Ikram H, Chan W, Espiner EA, et al: Haemodynamic and hormone responses to acute and chronic furosemide therapy in congestive heart failure. Clin Sci 1980; 59:443–449.
38. Francis GS, Siegel RM, Goldsmith SR, et al: Acute vasoconstrictor response to intravenous furosemide in patients with chronic congestive heart failure. Ann Intern Med 1985; 103:1–6.
39. Kubo SH, Clark M, Laragh JH, et al: Identification of normal neurohormonal activity in mild congestive heart failure and stimulating effect of upright posture and diuretics. Am J Cardiol 1987; 60:1322–1328.
40. Bayliss J, Norell M, Canepa-Anson R, et al: Untreated heart failure: clinical and neuroendocrine effects of introducing diuretics. Br Heart J 1987; 57:17–22.
41. Chen M, Schnermann J, Malvin RL, et al: Time course of stimulation of renal renin messenger RNA by furosemide. Hypertension 1993; 21:36–41.
42. Lee WH, Packer M: Prognostic importance of serum sodium concentration and its modification by converting enzyme inhibition in patients with severe chronic heart failure. Circulation 1986; 73:257–267.
43. Swedberg K, Emeroth P, Kjekshus J, Wilhelmson L, for the CONSENSUS Trial Study Group: Hormones regulating cardiovascular function in patients with severe heart failure and their relation to mortality. Circulation 1990; 82:1730–1736.
44. Ellison DH: The physiologic basis of diuretic synergism: its role in treating diuretic resistance. Am Intern Med 1991; 114:886–894.
45. Wilcox CS, Mitch WE, Kelly RA, et al: Response of the kidney to furosemide I. Effects of salt intake and renal compensation. J Lab Clin Med 1983; 102:450–458.
46. Ellison DH, Velazquez H, Wright FS: Adaptation of the distal convoluted tubule of the rat: structural and functional effects of dietary salt intake and chronic diuretic infusion. J Clin Invest 1989; 83:113–126.
47. Kaissling B, Stanton BA: Adaptation of distal tubule and collecting duct to increased sodium delivery I. Ultrastructure. Am J Physiol 1988; 255:F1256–F1268.
48. Stanton BA, Kaissling B: Adaptation of distal tubule and collecting duct to increased sodium delivery II. Na and K transport. Am J Physiol 1988; 255:F1269–F1275.
49. Brater DC: Clinical pharmacology of loop diuretics. Drugs 1991; 42(suppl 3):14–22.
50. Brater DC: Resistance to loop diuretics: why it happens and what to do about it. Drugs 1985; 30:427–443.
51. Grinstead WC, Francis MJ, Marks GF, et al: Discontinuation of chronic diuretic therapy in stable congestive heart failure secondary to coronary artery disease or to idiopathic dilated cardiomyopathy. Am J Cardiol 1994; 73:881–886.
52. Wollam GL, Tarazi RC, Bravo EL, Dustan HP: Diuretic potency of combined hydrochlorothiazide and furosemide therapy in patients with angiotensin. Am J Med 1982; 72:929–938.
53. Gage JS, Mancini DM, Gumbardo DJ, et al: Efficacy of combined diuretic therapy with metolazone and furosemide in patients with refractory congestive heart failure. Cardiovasc Rev Rep 1986; 7:814–817.

54. Gerlag PG, Van Meijel JJM: High dose furosemide in the treatment of refractory congestive heart failure. Arch Intern Med 1988; 148:286–291.
55. Kuchar DL, O'Rourke MF: High dose furosemide in refractory cardiac failure. Eur Heart J 1985; 6:954–958.
56. Rudy DW, Voelker JR, Greene PK, et al: Loop diuretics for chronic renal insufficiency: a continuous infusion is more efficacious than bolus therapy. Ann Intern Med 1991; 115:360–366.
57. Lahav M, Regev A, Ra'anani P, et al: Intermittent administration of furosemide vs continuous infusion preceded by a loading dose for congestive heart failure. Chest 1992; 102:725–731.
58. Agostoni PG, Marenzi GC, Pepi M, et al: Isolated ultrafiltration in moderate congestive heart failure. J Am Coll Cardiol 1993; 21:424–431.
59. Cohn JN, Franciosa JA: Vasodilator therapy of cardiac failure. N Engl J Med 1977; 297:27–31, 254–258.
60. Packer M: Vasodilator and inotropic drugs in the treatment of chronic heart failure: distinguishing hype from hope. J Am Coll Cardiol 1988; 12:1299–1317.
61. Parmley WW: Angiotensin converting enzyme inhibitors in the treatment of heart failure. *In* Cohn JN (ed): Drug Treatment of Heart Failure, pp 227–250. Secaucus, NJ: Advanced Therapeutics Communications International, 1988.
62. Cody RJ, Laragh JH: Use of captopril to estimate renin-angiotensin-aldosterone activity in the pathophysiology of chronic heart failure. Am Heart J 1982; 104:1184–1189.
63. Vanhoutte PM: Endothelium and control of vascular function: state of the art lecture. Hypertension 1986; 12:797–806.
64. Dzau VJ: Circulating versus local renin angiotensin system in cardiovascular homeostasis. Circulation 1988; 77(suppl I):I-4–I-13.
65. Cohn JN, Archibald DG, Ziesche S, et al: Effect of vasodilator therapy on mortality in chronic congestive heart failure. Results of a Veterans Administration Cooperative Study. N Engl J Med 1986; 314:1547–1552.
66. The CONSENSUS Trial Study Group: Effects of enalapril on mortality in severe congestive heart failure. Results of the Cooperative North Scandinavian Enalapril Survival Study (CONSENSUS). N Engl J Med 1987; 316:1429–1435.
67. Cohn JN, Johnson G, Ziesche S, et al: A comparison of enalapril with hydralazine–isosorbide dinitrate in the treatment of chronic congestive heart failure. N Engl J Med 1991; 325:303–310.
68. The SOLVD Investigators: Effect of enalapril on survival in patients with reduced left ventricular ejection fractions and congestive heart failure. N Engl J Med 1991; 325:293–302.
69. The SOLVD Investigators: Effect of enalapril on mortality and the development of heart failure in asymptomatic patients with reduced left ventricular ejection fractions. N Engl J Med 1992; 327:685–691.
70. Packer M, Rouleau J, Swedberg K, et al, and the PROFILE Investigators: Effect of flosequinan on survival in chronic heart failure: preliminary results of the PROFILE Study [Abstract]. Circulation 1993; 88:I-301.
71. Pfeffer MA, Braunwald E, Moye LA, et al, on behalf of the SAVE Investigators: Effect of captopril on mortality and morbidity in patients with left ventricular dysfunction after myocardial infarction. Results of the survival and ventricular enlargement trial. N Engl J Med 1992; 327:669–677.
72. The Acute Infarction Ramipril Efficacy (AIRE) Study Investigators: Effect of ramipril on mortality and morbidity of survivors of acute myocardial infarction with clinical evidence of heart failure. Lancet 1993; 342:821–828.
73. ISIS Collaborative Group: ISIS-4: randomised study of oral captopril in over 50,000 patients with suspected acute myocardial infarction [Abstract]. Circulation 1993; 88(pt 2):I-394.
74. Swedberg K, Held P, Kjekshus J, et al, on behalf of the CONSENSUS II Study Group: Effects of the early administration of enalapril on mortality in patients with acute myocardial infarction. Results of the Cooperative New Scandinavian Enalapril Survival Study II (CONSENSUS II). N Engl J Med 1992; 327:678–684.
75. Gruppo Italiano per lo Studio della Sopravvivenza nell'Infarto Miocardio (GISSI): GISSI-3: effects of lisinopril and transdermal glyceryl trinitrate singly and together on 6 week mortality and ventricular function after acute myocardial infarction. Lancet 1994; 343:1115–1122.
76. The Chinese Captopril Trial: Oral presentation at the 66th Scientific Sessions of the American Heart Association, Atlanta, GA, November 1993.
77. Ambrosioni E, Borghi C, Magnani B, for the Survival of Myocardial Infarction Long-Term Evaluation (SMILE) Study Investigators: The effect of the angiotensin-converting enzyme inhibitor zofenopril on mortality and morbidity after anterior myocardial infarction. N Engl J Med 1995; 332:80–85.
78. Foy SG, Crozier IG, Turner JG, et al: Comparison of enalapril versus captopril on left ventricular function and survival three months after acute myocardial infarction. Am J Cardiol 1994; 73:1180–1186.
79. The Trace Study Group: The Trandopril Cardiac Evaluation (TRACE) Study: rationale, design, and baseline characteristics of the screened population. Am J Cardiol 1994; 73:44C–50C.
80. Lonn EM, Yusuf S, Ika P, et al: Emerging role of angiotensin-converting enzyme inhibitors in cardiac and vascular protection. Circulation 1994; 90:2056–2069.
81. Braunwald E: ACE inhibitors—a cornerstone of the treatment of heart failure. N Engl J Med 1991; 325:351–353.
82. Cohn JN: The prevention of heart failure: a new agenda. N Engl J Med 1992; 327:725–727.
83. Massie BM: All patients with left ventricular systolic dysfunction should be treated with an angiotensin-converting enzyme inhibitor: a protagonist's viewpoint. Am J Cardiol 1990; 66:439–443.
84. Poole-Wilson PA, Lindsay D: Advances in the treatment of heart failure. BMJ 1992; 304:1069–1070.
85. Ljungman S, Kjekshus J, Swedberg K, for the CONSENSUS Trial Group: Renal function in severe congestive heart failure during treatment with enalapril. Am J Cardiol 1992; 70:479–487.
86. Williams GH: Converting enzyme inhibitors in the treatment of hypertension. N Engl J Med 1988; 319:1517–1525.
87. Levine TB, Franciosa JA, Vrobel T, et al: Hyponatremia as a marker for high renin heart failure. Br Heart J 1982; 47:161–166.
88. Packer M, Medina N, Yushak M: Relation between serum sodium concentration and the hemodynamic and clinical responses to converting enzyme inhibition with captopril in severe heart failure. J Am Coll Cardiol 1984; 3:1035–1043.
89. Keane WF, Anderson S, Aurell M, et al: Angiotensin converting enzyme inhibitors and progressive renal insufficiency: current experience and future directions. Ann Intern Med 1989; 111:503–516.
90. Suki WN: Renal hemodynamic consequences of angiotensin-converting enzyme inhibition in congestive heart failure. Arch Intern Med 1989; 149:669–673.
91. Packer M: Identification of risk factors predisposing to the development of functional renal insufficiency during treatment with converting-enzyme inhibitors in chronic heart failure. Cardiology 1989; 76:50–55.
92. Packer M, Lee WH, Medina N, et al: Functional renal insufficiency during long term therapy with captopril and enalapril in severe chronic heart failure. Ann Intern Med 1987; 106:346–354.
93. Pierpont GL, Francis GS, Cohn JN: Effect of captopril on renal function in patients with congestive heart failure. Br Heart J 1981; 46:522–527.
94. Israili ZH, Hall WD: Cough and angioneurotic edema associated with angiotensin converting enzyme inhibitor therapy: a review of the literature and pathophysiology. Ann Intern Med 1992; 117:234–242.
95. Pitt B: Use of 'xapril' in patients with chronic heart failure: a paradigm or epitaph for our times? Circulation 1994; 90:1550–1551.
96. Pitt B: Angiotensin-converting enzyme inhibitors in patients with congestive heart failure: a class effect? Am J Cardiol 1991; 68:106–108.
97. Kubo SH, Cody RJ: Clinical and hemodynamic aspects of angiotensin converting enzyme inhibition for the management of congestive heart failure. *In* Ferguson RK, Vlasses PH (eds): The Clinical Applications of the Converting Enzyme Inhibitors, pp 87–136. Mt. Kisco, NY: Futura Publishing, 1987.
98. Herman AG: Differences in structure of angiotensin converting enzyme inhibitors might predict differences in action. Am J Cardiol 1992; 70:102C–108C.
99. Unger TH, Ganten D, Lang RE, Scholkens BA: Is tissue converting enzyme inhibition a determinant of the antihypertensive efficacy of converting enzyme inhibitors? Studies with the different compounds HOE 498 and MK421 in spontaneously hypertensive rats. J Cardiovasc Pharmacol 1984; 6:872–880.
100. Cushman DW, Wang FL, Fung WC, et al: Differentiation of angiotensin-converting enzyme (ACE) inhibitors by their selective inhibition of ACE in physiologically important target organs. Am J Hypertens 1989; 2:294–306.
101. Fonarow GC, Chelimsky-Fallick C, Stevenson LW, et al: Effect of direct vasodilation with hydralazine versus angiotensin-converting enzyme inhibition with captopril on mortality in advanced heart failure: the Hy-C trial. J Am Coll Cardiol 1992; 19:842–850.
102. Massie BM, Packer M, Hanlon JT, Combs DT: Hemodynamic responses to combined therapy with captopril and hydralazine in patients with severe heart failure. J Am Coll Cardiol 1983; 2:338–344.

103. Colucci WS: Usefulness of calcium antagonists for congestive heart failure. Am J Cardiol 1987; 59:52B–58B.
104. Packer M: Pathophysiological mechanisms underlying the adverse effects of calcium channel-blocking drugs in patients with chronic heart failure. Circulation 1989; 80(suppl IV):IV-59–IV-67.
105. Goldstein RE, Boccuzzi SJ, Cruess D, et al, the Adverse Experience Committee, and the Multicenter Diltiazem Postinfarction Research Group: Diltiazem increases late-onset congestive heart failure in postinfarction patients with early reduction in ejection fraction. Circulation 1991; 83:52–60.
106. Kubo SH, Olivari MT, Cohn JN: Calcium antagonists in heart failure. Ann N Y Acad Sci 1988; 522:553–564.
107. Ryman KS, Kubo SH, Lystash J, et al: The effect of nicardipine on rest and exercise hemodynamics in chronic congestive heart failure. Am J Cardiol 1986; 58:583–588.
108. Haas GJ, Binkley PF, Carpenter JA, et al: Central and regional hemodynamic effects of flosequinan for congestive heart failure. Am J Cardiol 1989; 63:1354–1359.
109. Pinsky DJ, Wilson PB, Ahem D, et al: Flosequinan improves symptoms and exercise tolerance in heart failure. Results of placebo controlled trial [Abstract]. Circulation 1990; 82:322.
110. Massie BM, Berk MR, Brozena S, et al, for the FACET Investigators: Can further benefit be achieved by adding a vasodilator to triple therapy in CHF: results of the flosequinan–ACE inhibitor trial (FACET) [Abstract]. Circulation 1992; 86:I-645.
111. Packer M, Pitt B, on behalf of the REFLECT I and REFLECT II Study Groups: Efficacy of flosequinan in patients with heart failure who are withdrawn from therapy with converting-enzyme inhibitors: a double-blind controlled study [Abstract]. Circulation 1992; 86:I-644.
112. Smith TW: Digitalis: mechanisms of action and clinical use. N Engl J Med 1988; 318:358–365.
113. Smith JR, Gheorghiade M, Goldstein S: The current role of digoxin in the treatment of heart failure. Coronary Artery Disease 1993; 4:16–26.
114. Kelly RA, Smith TW: Digoxin in heart failure: implications of recent trials. J Am Coll Cardiol 1993; 22:107A–112A.
115. Mulrow CD, Feusner JR, Valez R: Reevaluation of digitalis efficacy: new light on an old leaf. Ann Intern Med 1984; 101:113–117.
116. Jaeschke R, Oxman AD, Guyatt GH: To what extent do congestive heart failure patients in sinus rhythm benefit from digoxin therapy? A systematic overview and meta-analysis. Am J Med 1990; 88:279–286.
117. Fleg L, Gottlieb SH, Lakatta EG: Is digoxin really important in compensated heart failure? Am J Med 1982; 73:244–250.
118. Taggart AJ, Johnston GD, McDevitt DG: Digoxin withdrawal after cardiac failure in patients with sinus rhythm. J Cardiovasc Pharmacol 1983; 5:229–234.
119. Lee DC-S, Johnson RA, Bingham JB, et al: Heart failure in outpatients: a randomized trial of digoxin versus placebo. N Engl J Med 1982; 306:699–705.
120. Guyatt GH, Sullivan MJJ, Fallen EL, et al: A controlled trial of digoxin in congestive heart failure. Am J Cardiol 1988; 61:371–375.
121. Aronow WS, Starling L, Etienne F: Lack of efficacy of digoxin in treatment of compensated congestive heart failure with third heart sound and sinus rhythm in elderly patients receiving diuretic therapy. Am J Cardiol 1986; 58:168–169.
122. Alicandri C, Fariello R, Boni E, et al: Captopril versus digoxin in mild-moderate chronic heart failure: a crossover study. J Cardiovasc Pharmacol 1987; 9:S61–S67.
123. German and Austrian Xamoterol Study Group: Double-blind placebo-controlled comparison of digoxin and xamoterol in chronic heart failure. Lancet 1988; 1:489–493.
124. The Captopril-Digoxin Multicenter Research Group: Comparative effects of therapy with captopril and digoxin in patients with mild to moderate heart failure. JAMA 1988; 259:539–544.
125. Davies RF, Beanlands DS, Nadeau C, et al: Enalapril versus digoxin in patients with congestive heart failure: a multicenter study. J Am Coll Cardiol 1991; 18:1602–1609.
126. Drexler H, Schumacher M, Siegrist J, Just H, for the CADS Multicenter Study Group: Effect of captopril and digoxin on quality of life and clinical symptoms in patients with coronary artery disease and mild heart failure [Abstract]. J Am Coll Cardiol 1992; 19(suppl A):260A.
127. DiBianco R, Shabetai R, Kostuk WT, et al: A comparison of oral milrinone, digoxin, and their combination in the treatment of patients with chronic heart failure. N Engl J Med 1989; 320:677–683.
128. vanVeldhuisen DJ, Man In't Veld AJ, Dunselman PHJM, et al: Double-blind placebo-controlled study of ibopamine and digoxin in patients with mild to moderate heart failure: results of the Dutch Ibopamine Multicenter Trial (DIMT). J Am Coll Cardiol 1993; 22:1564–1573.
129. Uretsky BF, Young JB, Shahidi FE, et al: Randomized study assessing the effect of digoxin withdrawal in patients with mild to moderate chronic congestive heart failure: results of the PROVED trial [Prospective Randomized Study of Ventricular Failure and the Efficacy of Digoxin]. J Am Coll Cardiol 1993; 22:955–962.
130. Packer M, Gheorghiade M, Young JB, et al: Withdrawal of digoxin from patients with chronic heart failure treated with angiotensin-converting-enzyme inhibitors [RADIANCE (Randomized Assessment of Digoxin on Inhibitors of the Angiotensin Converting Enzyme)]. N Engl J Med 1993; 329:1–7.
131. Yusuf S, Garg R, Held P, Gorlin R: Need for a large randomized trial to evaluate the effects of digitalis on morbidity and mortality in congestive heart failure. Am J Cardiol 1992; 66:64G–70G.
132. Moss AJ, Davis HT, Conrad DL, et al: Digitalis associated cardiac mortality after myocardial infarction. Circulation 1981; 64:1150–1156.
133. Bigger JT, Fleiss JL, Rolnitsky LA, et al: Effect of digitalis treatment on survival after acute myocardial infarction. Am J Cardiol 1985; 55:623–630.
134. Muller JE, Turi ZG, Stone PH, et al, and the MILIS Study Group: Digoxin therapy and mortality following myocardial infarction: experience in the MILIS study. N Engl J Med 1986; 314:265–271.
135. Ryan TJ, Bailey KR, McCabe CH, et al: The effects of digitalis on survival in high risk patients with coronary artery disease: the Coronary Artery Surgery Study (CASS). Circulation 1983; 67:735–742.
136. Byrington R, Goldstein S, for the BHAT Research Group: Association of digitalis therapy with mortality in survivors of acute myocardial infarction: observations in the Beta-Blocker Heart Attack Trial. J Am Coll Cardiol 1985; 6:976–982.
137. Packer M: Role of the sympathetic nervous system in chronic heart failure: a historical and philosophical perspective. Circulation 1990; 82(suppl I):I-1–I-6.
138. Eichhorn EJ: The paradox of β-adrenergic blockade for the management of congestive heart failure. Am J Med 1992; 92:527–533.
139. Eichhorn EJ, Hjalmarson A: β-Blocker treatment for chronic heart failure: the frog prince. Circulation 1994; 90:2153–2156.
140. Bristow MR, Hershberger RE, Port JD, et al: β-Adrenergic pathways in nonfailing and failing human ventricular myocardium. Circulation 1990; 82(suppl I):I-12–I-25.
141. Colucci WS: In vivo studies of myocardial β-adrenergic receptor pharmacology in patients with congestive heart failure. Circulation 1990; 82(suppl I):I-47–I-51.
142. Waagstein F, Hjalmarson A, Varnauskas E, et al: Effect of chronic beta-adrenergic receptor blockade in congestive cardiomyopathy. Br Heart J 1975; 37:1022–1036.
143. Heilbrunn SM, Shah P, Bristow MR, et al: Increased β-receptor density and improved hemodynamic response to catecholamine stimulation during long-term metoprolol therapy in heart failure from dilated cardiomyopathy. Circulation 1989; 79:483–490.
144. Engelmeier RS, O'Connell JB, Walsh R, et al: Improvement in symptoms and exercise tolerance by metoprolol in patients with dilated cardiomyopathy: a double-blind, randomized placebo-controlled trial. Circulation 1985; 72:536–546.
145. Gilbert EM, Anderson JL, Deitchman D: Chronic β-blocker–vasodilator therapy improves cardiac function in idiopathic dilated cardiomyopathy: a double-blind, randomized study of bucindolol versus placebo. Am J Med 1990; 88:223–229.
146. Swedberg K, Waagstein F, Hjalmarson A, et al: Prolongation of survival in congestive cardiomyopathy by beta receptor blockade. Lancet 1979; 1:1374–1376.
147. Anderson JL, Lutz JR, Gilbert EM, et al: A randomized trial of low-dose beta-blockade therapy for idiopathic dilated cardiomyopathy. Am J Cardiol 1985; 55:471–475.
148. The MDC Trial Study Group: Metoprolol in dilated cardiomyopathy. Multicenter randomized placebo-controlled trial. Lancet 1993; 342:1441–1446.
149. CIBIS Investigators and Committees: A randomized trial of β-blockade in heart failure: the Cardiac Insufficiency Bisoprolol Study (CIBIS). Circulation 1994; 90:1765–1773.
150. Domanski MJ, Eichhorn EJ: Beta blockade in congestive heart failure—the need for a definitive study. Am J Cardiol 1994; 73:597–599.
151. Colucci WS, Wright RF, Braunwald E: New positive inotropic agents in the treatment of congestive heart failure. Mechanisms of action and recent clinical developments. N Engl J Med 1986; 314:290–299, 349–358.
152. Uretsky BF, Jessup M, Konstam MA, et al: Multicenter trial of oral enoximone in patients with moderate to moderately severe congestive heart failure: lack of benefit compared to placebo. Circulation 1990; 82:774–780.

153. Massie B, Bourassa M, DiBianco R, et al, for the Amrinone Multicenter Trial Group: Long-term oral administration of amrinone for congestive heart failure: lack of efficacy in a multicenter controlled trial. Circulation 1985; 71:963–971.
154. Hood WB: Controlled and uncontrolled studies of phosphodiesterase III inhibitors in contemporary cardiovascular medicine. Am J Cardiol 1989; 63:46A–53A.
155. Packer M, Carver JR, Rodeheffer RJ, et al, for the PROMISE Study Research Group: Effect of oral milrinone on mortality in severe chronic heart failure. N Engl J Med 1991; 325:1468–1475.
156. Packer M: Effect of phosphodiesterase inhibitors on survival of patients with chronic congestive heart failure. Am J Cardiol 1989; 63:41A–45A.
157. Packer M: Do positive inotropic agents adversely affect the survival of patients with chronic congestive heart failure? Protagonist's viewpoint. J Am Coll Cardiol 1988; 12:562–565.
158. Colucci WS: Do positive inotropic agents adversely affect the survival of patients with chronic congestive heart failure? Antagonist's viewpoint. J Am Coll Cardiol 1988; 12:566–569.
159. Sonnenblick EH, Demopoulos L, Le Jemtel TH: Aims of positive inotropic therapy in congestive heart failure. Heart Failure 1993; 9:148–155.
160. Bristow MR, Lowes BD: Low dose inotropic therapy for ambulatory heart failure. Coronary Artery Disease 1994; 5:112–118.
161. Kubo SH: Inotropic agents with calcium-sensitizing properties: clinical and hemodynamic effects of pimobendan. Coronary Artery Disease 1994; 5:119–126.
162. Feldman AM, Strobeck JE: Quinolinone derivatives in the management of congestive heart failure. Coronary Artery Disease 1994; 5:107–111.
163. Masuoka H, Ito M, Sugioka M, et al: Two isoforms of cGMP inhibited cyclic nucleotide phosphodiesterases in human tissue distinguished by their responses to vesnarinone, a new cardiotonic agent. Biochem Biophys Res Commun 1993; 190:412–417.
164. Feldman AM, Baughman KL, Lee WK, et al: Usefulness of OPC-8212, a quinolinone derivative, for chronic congestive heart failure in patients with ischemic heart disease or idiopathic dilated cardiomyopathy. Am J Cardiol 1991; 68:1203–1210.
165. Kubo SH, Rector TS, Strobeck JE, et al: OPC-8212 in the treatment of congestive heart failure: results of a pilot study. Cardiovasc Drugs Ther 1988; 2:653–660.
166. Feldman AM, Bristow MR, Parmley WW, et al, for the Vesnarinone Study Group: Effects of vesnarinone on morbidity and mortality in patients with heart failure. N Engl J Med 1993; 329:149–155.
167. Kubo SH, Gollub S, Bourge R, et al, for the Pimobendan Multicenter Research Group: Beneficial effects of pimobendan on exercise tolerance and quality of life in patients with heart failure. Results of a multicenter trial. Circulation 1992; 85:942–949.
168. Unverferth DV, Magorien RD, Lewis RP, Leier CV: Long-term benefit of dobutamine in patients with congestive cardiomyopathy. Am Heart J 1980; 100:622–630.
169. Appelfeld MM, Newman KA, Sutton FJ, et al: Outpatient dobutamine and dopamine infusions in the management of chronic heart failure: clinical experience in 21 patients. Am Heart J 1987; 114:589–595.
170. Miller LW: Outpatient dobutamine for refractory congestive heart failure: advantages, techniques, and results. J Heart Lung Transplant 1991; 10:482–487.
171. Meltzer RS, Visser CA, Fuster V: Intracardiac thrombi and systemic embolization. Ann Intern Med 1986; 104:689–698.
172. Fuster V, Gersh BJ, Giuliani ER, et al: The natural history of idiopathic dilated cardiomyopathy. Am J Cardiol 1981; 47:521–525.
173. Roberts WC, Siegel RJ, McManus BM: Idiopathic dilated cardiomyopathy: analysis of 152 necropsy patients. Am J Cardiol 1987; 60:1340–1355.
174. Kyrle PA, Korninger C, Gossinger H, et al: Prevention of arterial and pulmonary embolism by oral anticoagulants in patients with dilated cardiomyopathy. Thromb Haemost 1985; 54:521–523.
175. Lapeyre AC, Steele PM, Kazmise FJ, et al: Systemic embolization in chronic left ventricular aneurysm: incidence and the role of anticoagulation. J Am Coll Cardiol 1985; 6:524–538.
176. Gottdiener JS, Gay SA, VanVorhees L, et al: Frequency and embolic potential of left ventricular thrombus in dilated cardiomyopathy: assessment by 2-dimensional echocardiography. Am J Cardiol 1983; 52:1281–1285.
177. Stratton JR, Nemanich JW, Johannessen KA, Resnick AD: Fate of left ventricular thrombi in patients with remote myocardial infarction or idiopathic cardiomyopathy. Circulation 1988; 78:1388–1393.
178. Dunkman WB, Johnson GR, Carson PE, et al, and the VA Cooperative Study Group: Incidence of thromboembolic events in congestive heart failure [Abstract]. Circulation 1993; 87:VI-94–VI-101.
179. Cohn JN, Benedict CR, LeJemtel TH, et al, SOLVD Investigators: Risk of thromboembolism in left ventricular dysfunction: SOLVD [Abstract]. Circulation 1992; 86:I-252.
180. Falk RH: A plea for a clinical trial of anticoagulation in dilated cardiomyopathy. Am J Cardiol 1990; 65:914–915.
181. Francis GS: Should asymptomatic ventricular arrhythmias in patients with congestive heart failure be treated with antiarrhythmic drugs? J Am Coll Cardiol 1988; 12:274–283.
182. Podrid PJ, Fogel RI, Fuchs TT: Ventricular arrhythmia in congestive heart failure. Am J Cardiol 1992; 69:82G–98G.
183. Goldman S, Johnson G, Cohn JN, et al, for the VHEFT Cooperative Studies Group: Mechanism of death in heart failure and the Vasodilator Heart Failure Trials. Circulation 1993; 87:VI-24–VI-31.
184. Holmes J, Kubo SH, Cody RJ, et al: Arrhythmias in ischemic and nonischemic dilated cardiomyopathy: prediction of mortality by ambulatory electrocardiography. Am J Cardiol 1985; 55:146–151.
185. Packer M: Lack of relation between ventricular arrhythmias and sudden death in patients with chronic heart failure. Circulation 1992; 85(suppl I):I-50–I-56.
186. Luu M, Stevenson WG, Stevenson LW, et al: Diverse mechanisms of unexpected cardiac arrest in advanced heart failure. Circulation 1989; 80:1675–1680.
187. Velebit V, Podrid P, Lown B, et al: Aggravation and provocation of ventricular arrhythmias by antiarrhythmic drugs. Circulation 1982; 65:886–894.
188. Ravid S, Podrid PJ, Lampert S, et al: Congestive heart failure induced by six of the newer antiarrhythmic drugs. J Am Coll Cardiol 1989; 14:1326–1330.
189. Echt DS, Liebson PR, Mitchell LB, et al, and the CAST Investigators: Mortality and morbidity in patients receiving encainide, flecainide, or placebo. The Cardiac Arrhythmia Suppression Trial. N Engl J Med 1991; 324:781–788.
190. Cleland JGF, Dargie HJ, Findlay IN, et al: Clinical, haemodynamic and antiarrhythmic effects of long term treatment with amiodarone in patients in heart failure. Br Heart J 1987; 57:436–445.
191. Neri R, Mestroni L, Salvi A, et al: Ventricular arrhythmias in dilated cardiomyopathy: efficacy of amiodarone. Am Heart J 1987; 113:707–715.
192. Doval HC, Nul OR, Grancelli HO, et al, for the Grupo de Estudio de la Sobrevida en la Insufficiencia Cardiaca en Argentina (GESICA): Randomised trial of low dose amiodarone in severe congestive heart failure. Lancet 1994; 344:439–498.
193. Singh SN, Fletcher RD, Fisher SG, et al, and the CHF-STAT Investigators: Results of the Congestive Heart Failure Survival Trial of Antiarrhythmia Therapy (Veterans Affairs Cooperative Studies Program #320) [Abstract]. Circulation 1994; 90:I-546.
194. Winkle RA, Mead RH, Ruder MA, et al: Long-term outcome with the automatic implantable cardioverter-defibrillator. J Am Coll Cardiol 1989; 13:1353–1361.
195. Tchou PJ, Kadri N, Anderzin J, et al: Automatic implantable cardioverter defibrillators and survival of patients with left ventricular dysfunction and malignant ventricular arrhythmias. Ann Intern Med 1988; 109:529–534.
196. Sullivan MJ, Green HJ, Cobb FR: Skeletal muscle biochemistry and histology in ambulatory patients with long-term heart failure. Circulation 1990; 81:518–527.
197. Massie BM, Conway M, Yonge R, et al: ^{31}P Nuclear magnetic resonance evidence of abnormal skeletal muscle metabolism in patients with congestive heart failure. Am J Cardiol 1987; 60:309–315.
198. Drexler H, Riede U, Munzel T, et al: Alterations of skeletal muscle in chronic heart failure. Circulation 1992; 85:1751–1759.
199. Sullivan MJ, Higginbotham MB, Cobb FR: Exercise training in patients with chronic heart failure delays ventilatory anaerobic threshold and improves submaximal exercise performance. Circulation 1989; 79:324–329.
200. Adamopoulos S, Coats AJS, Brunotte F, et al: Physical training improves skeletal muscle metabolism in patients with chronic heart failure. J Am Coll Cardiol 1993; 21:1101–1106.
201. Bolli R: Mechanism of myocardial "stunning." Circulation 1990; 82:723–738.
202. Dilsizian V, Bonow RO: Current diagnostic techniques of assessing myocardial variability in patients with hibernating and stunned myocardium. Circulation 1993; 87:1–20.
203. Brundage BH, Massie BM, Botvinick EH: Improved regional ventricular function after successful surgical revascularization. J Am Coll Cardiol 1984; 3:902–908.
204. Alderman EL, Fisher LD, Litwin P, et al: Results of coronary artery surgery in patients with poor left ventricular function (CASS). Circulation 1983; 68:785–795.
205. Pigott JD, Kouchoukos NT, Oberman A, Cutter GR: Late results of

surgical and medical therapy for patients with coronary artery disease and depressed left ventricular function. J Am Coll Cardiol 1985; 5:1036–1045.
206. Sharpe N, MacMahon S, on behalf of the Australia-New Zealand Heart Failure Research Collaborative Group: Effects of 12 months treatment with carvedilol on left ventricular function and exercise performance in patients with heart failure of ischemic etiology. Circulation 1995; 92(suppl I):I-394.
207. Bristow MR, Gilbert EM, Abraham WT, et al: Multicenter oral carvedilol heart failure assessment (MOCHA): a six-month dose-response evaluation in Class II-IV patients. Circulation 1995; 92(suppl I):I-142.
208. Packer M, Colucci WS, Sackner-Berstein J, et al: Prospective randomized evaluation of carvedilol on symptoms and exercise tolerance in chronic heart failure: results of the PRECISE Trial. Circulation 1995; 92(suppl I):I-143.
209. Cohn JN, Ziesche SM, Loss LE, et al: Effect of Felodipine on short-term exercise and neurohormone and long-term mortality in heart failure: results of V-HeFT VIII: Circulation 1995; 92(suppl I):I-143.

12 Prevention of Heart Failure and Treatment of Asymptomatic Left Ventricular Dysfunction

Marc A. Pfeffer, MD, PhD

Heart failure is an all-encompassing term that describes an inability, as a result of any one of many etiologies, of the ventricular chambers to deliver an adequate volume of oxygenated blood to body tissues. Thus heart failure is considered a "final common pathway" for a myriad of diseases that lead to inadequate cardiac function. Despite the multitude of causes, the predominant pathophysiologic insults that result in the syndrome of congestive heart failure can be grossly categorized by three often overlapping mechanisms: (1) conditions that impose a sustained heightened extrinsic demand on cardiac function, such as congenital defects, valvular heart disease, and, most prominent, hypertension; (2) intrinsic abnormalities of contractile function, such as myopathies, either primary or secondary such as those produced by toxins (ethanol, doxorubicin [Adriamycin]); and (3) a large category of vascular insufficiency states wherein the fundamental insult is impairment of flow to otherwise viable myocytes. In clinical practice, various combinations of extrinsic demand, intrinsic dysfunction, and vascular insufficiency are common.

STRATEGIES FOR PRIMARY PREVENTION OF HEART FAILURE

The most effective treatment of congestive heart failure would, of course, be preventive measures to reduce the number of people who ever manifest the clinical syndrome. Because the etiologies of congestive heart failure are so diverse, multiple strategies of primary prevention are needed. In certain regions of the globe, environmental efforts to eliminate the hematophagous insect vector for *Trypanosoma cruzi* would be considered a highly desirable primary preventive measure for reducing the incidence of Chagas cardiomyopathy, a common cause of heart failure in South and now Central America.

In most other effective prevention strategies, population-based approaches entail broad screening to identify persons with a specific modifiable risk factor. In this approach, it is assumed that therapy effective in reducing the likelihood of the disease is available. Such therapy, however, should be directed only toward persons with the potential to benefit. Among the best-studied examples of population-based risk-factor modification are the efforts to identify and treat persons with hypertension.[1] By mass screening, the segment of the population at risk for morbidity and premature mortality from hypertension was identified and treated with antihypertensive therapy. By virtue of the numbers of people at risk, the treatment of hypertension is indeed one of the most effective population-based means of reducing the incidence of congestive heart failure. The adoption of such a preventive strategy implies both screening and the implementation of an effective intervention. Also implicit in this approach is that large numbers of otherwise healthy persons must be screened in order to identify a subpopulation in need of chronic antihypertensive therapy. Thus preventive therapy should be safe, efficacious, and cost effective in relation to other accepted interventions.

In addition to antihypertensive therapy, other primary prevention measures that reduce the incidence of atherosclerosis, such as favorable modification of lipid levels, discontinuation of or abstinence from cigarette smoking, avoidance of obesity, and adoption of a more active lifestyle, can lead to a reduction in congestive heart failure by limiting the incidence of myocardial infarction. These well-known primary preventive strategies are effective and are now entrenched as fundamental tenets of medical care. Because relatively large numbers of people must be treated to prevent few clinical events, health care economists frequently debate the precise operational definition of the point in the spectrum of risk at which a specific intervention becomes cost effective.

STRATEGIES FOR SECONDARY PREVENTION OF HEART FAILURE

At the other end of the spectrum is the treatment of the much smaller group of patients who already present with signs and symptoms of congestive heart failure. Because these persons seek medical attention, screening is much less of an issue. Because of the high rates of morbidity and mortality associated with congestive heart failure, effective therapies are more readily demonstrated and accepted (see Chapter 11). This chapter focuses on the rationale for identifying asymptomatic patients with ventricular dysfunction and treating them with an angiotensin converting enzyme (ACE) inhibitor. This new approach and the use of this therapy is a strategy

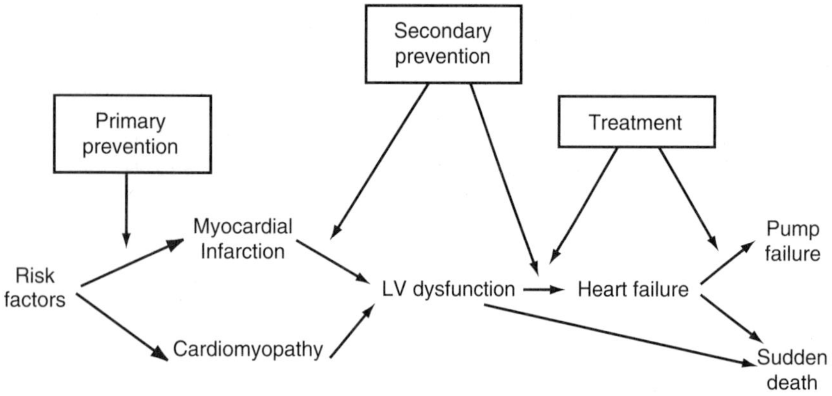

Figure 12–1. Conceptual framework for the points of intervention for heart failure prevention and treatment. In addition to primary prevention and symptomatic treatment, therapy directed to patients with impaired hearts who remain relatively asymptomatic provides yet another focus to limit the overall morbidity and mortality from this syndrome of heart failure. (From the National Heart Lung and Blood Institute Report of the Task Force on Research in Heart Failure, May 1994.)

intermediate between the broad primary prevention measures targeted to entire populations and the individualized treatment regimens for patients with existing symptomatic congestive heart failure. Therefore, the strategy of identifying and treating asymptomatic individuals with left ventricular (LV) dysfunction offers unique challenges as well as life-saving opportunities (Fig. 12–1).

The preventive use of ACE inhibitor therapy requires the identification of a patient population with asymptomatic LV dysfunction. Although noninvasive measures of cardiac function are reliable, they are expensive. Another issue of both clinical and ethical concern is the exposure of an asymptomatic person to the potential adverse effects and expense of pharmacologic therapy. However, recent data have provided sufficient justification for the identification of asymptomatic patients with LV dysfunction and for treating them with an ACE inhibitor not only to reduce the risk of developing symptomatic congestive heart failure but also to prolong survival. In this regard, this new use of ACE inhibition therapy in the appropriate patient population is preventive.

Secondary Prevention in Patients With Left Ventricular Dysfunction: The SOLVD Trial

One of the two arms of the Studies of Left Ventricular Dysfunction (SOLVD) was a direct test of the hypothesis that identifying patients with asymptomatic LV dysfunction and treating them with an ACE inhibitor (enalapril) would lead to a reduction in rates of cardiovascular morbidity and mortality.[2] Overall, the trial had two components: the prevention arm and the treatment arm. Eligibility for both required an objective determination of systolic dysfunction, as defined by a criterion of LV ejection fraction of .35 or less. No etiology of this ventricular dysfunction was specified, and the only major cardiovascular exclusions were recent myocardial infarction (within 30 days), unstable angina, uncontrolled hypertension, complex congenital heart disease, and cor pulmonale.

The determination as to whether the patient was randomized into the prevention arm or the treatment arm was purely clinical and relied totally on the physician's assessment. Patients assigned to the prevention arm were considered to have little or no limitations of exercise tolerance that were attributed to dyspnea or fatigue and did not require treatment with digitalis, diuretics, or vasodilators for heart failure before randomization. On the other hand, those allocated to the treatment arm of the trial were assessed as having "clear clinical evidence" of congestive heart failure and currently required treatment with diuretics, inotropic drugs or vasodilators, or a combination of these for symptomatic relief.[2] Of importance is that neither the LV ejection fraction nor other objective measures provided information that could be used to differentiate the symptomatic from the asymptomatic patients. However, on average the symptomatic patients had lower ejection fractions (symptomatic, .25; asymptomatic, .28) and greater activation of neurohormones such as norepinephrine, plasma renin activity, and atrial natriuretic factor (ANF) than did the asymptomatic patients.[3] Again, because there was marked overlap, these measurements could not be used to distinguish the asymptomatic from the symptomatic patients.

This clinical assessment of symptomatic status was extremely important because the prognostic implications of this clinical classification (i.e., symptomatic or asymptomatic) were profound. Of those assigned to the treatment trial (symptomatic patients), the mortality rate at 41 months among the patients receiving placebo was approximately 40%.[4] In contrast, despite the same requirement for depressed LV ejection fraction, the all-cause mortality rate among placebo recipients in the prevention arm (asymptomatic patients) was only 16% after 37 months of follow-up.[5] This striking difference in the mortality rates between the placebo groups in the prevention and treatment arms of SOLVD is an important direct illustration of the discriminatory capacity of the physician's clinical assessment of symptomatic status.

Of the 6794 patients randomized into the SOLVD studies, 4228 were clinically designated as having asymptomatic LV dysfunction and were entered into the prevention trial.[5] These patients were then randomized to receive either the ACE inhibitor enalapril (commencing at 2.5 mg b.i.d. and gradually increasing to the target dose of 10 mg b.i.d.) or matching placebo. The mean baseline age and mean blood pressure of patients in this group were 59 years and 125/78 mm Hg, respectively. Serum electrolytes and creatinine levels were normal, and two thirds of the patients were categorized in functional class I according to the criteria of the New York Heart Association. For most patients (83%) the etiology of the heart disease was considered to be ischemic heart disease. The diagnosis of idiopathic dilated cardiomyopathy was made in only about 10% of these asymptomatic patients. A history of hypertension or diabetes was present in 37% and 15%, respectively, in the SOLVD prevention trial. Almost three quarters of these patients were not currently receiving either digitalis or diuretics. In general, this population was perceived to be at low risk, except for the objective finding of an LV ejection fraction of .35 (average, .28).

The SOLVD investigators had successfully identified a new target population for their study of the effects of ACE inhibition. With 3.5 years of detailed follow-up experience on these 4228 patients, the group receiving enalapril demonstrated a strong trend for reduced cardiovascular mortality (14.1% vs. 12.6% of the placebo recipients; risk reduction, 12%; 95% confidence interval [CI], −3%–26%; p = .12). However, it must be recognized that this was an intent-to-treat analysis, in which the treating physician was free to initiate nonprotocol use of ACE inhibition therapy for any patient whose clinical status deteriorated to the point of becoming symptomatic. Indeed, a higher rate of clinical deterioration was observed in the placebo group, which was one of the most striking findings of the SOLVD prevention trial. Regardless of whether heart failure was defined by the study physician's assessment that overt signs and symptoms of failure had developed or by the criterion that hospital-

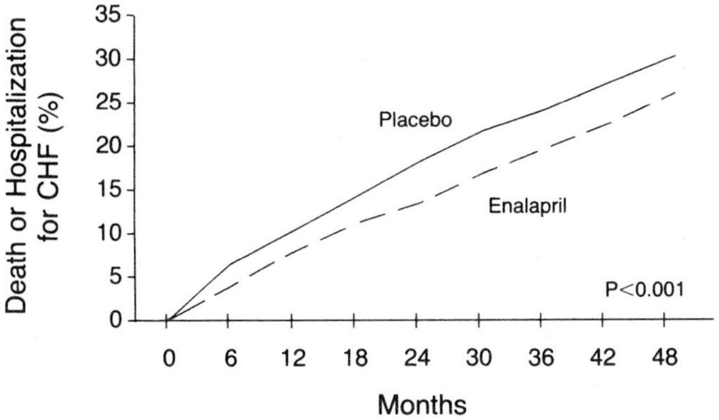

Figure 12–2. Death or hospitalization for congestive heart failure (CHF). (From the SOLVD Investigators: Effect of enalapril on mortality and the development of heart failure in asymptomatic patients with reduced left ventricular ejection fractions. N Engl J Med 1992; 327:685–691.)

ization was required for management of heart failure, patients randomized to receive the ACE inhibitor exhibited a striking reduction in the risk of developing either of these heart failure endpoints. Over 30% of the placebo recipients developed symptomatic congestive heart failure, and randomization to enalapril reduced the incidence to only 20.7% (risk reduction, 37%; 95% CI, 28%–44%; $p < .0001$). Similarly, the need for hospitalization for congestive heart failure also was significantly reduced, from 12.9% to 8.7% (risk reduction, 36%; 95% CI, 22%–46%; $p < .001$) (Fig. 12–2).

The relationship between clinical deterioration to symptomatic status and subsequent mortality in the SOLVD prevention study provides important mechanistic information. Regardless of therapy assignment, the chance of death among patients who eventually deteriorated to symptomatic status was twice as high as that among patients who remained asymptomatic. The effectiveness of ACE inhibitor therapy in the SOLVD prevention arm appeared to be attributable to a reduction in the incidence of becoming symptomatic, inasmuch as the risks of death among patients who developed symptoms or were hospitalized for heart failure were comparable in the two treatment arms.

This well-conducted study identified a previously unstudied population of patients with LV dysfunction (ejection fraction, .35) who were clinically classified as asymptomatic and among whom the overall mortality rate was less than half that among symptomatic patients. However, it could be demonstrated that a strategy of prophylactic use of an ACE inhibitor for patients with asymptomatic LV dysfunction did indeed lead to a reduction in the incidence of eventual symptomatic heart failure. Altering this progression from asymptomatic to symptomatic status resulted in a reduction in the risk for subsequent cardiovascular mortality. To achieve this benefit, enalapril was used at a target dose of 10 mg twice a day. With regard to adverse effects of treatment, it is important to note that an excess of dizziness, cough, and a small but statistically significant increase in serum potassium and creatinine levels were associated with this new use of an ACE inhibitor as preventive therapy.

Preventive Therapy After Myocardial Infarction

Survivors of myocardial infarction are logical subjects for studies aimed at preventing the development of congestive heart failure. The Framingham Heart Study[6] demonstrated that the risk of developing symptomatic congestive heart failure was increased by tenfold in a survivor of an infarct in comparison with the normal population and was even several times higher than the risk among persons with a clinical history of angina but no discrete myocardial infarction (Fig. 12–3). In the same well-characterized population, the actual clinical development of congestive heart failure was most often observed to occur years after the myocardial infarction rather than immediately[7] (Fig. 12–4).

Along with these epidemiologic data, clinical trials have consistently demonstrated a time-related risk of developing heart failure in survivors of myocardial infarction. In the Cardiac Arrhythmia Pilot Study (CAPS), 61 (12%) of the 502 patients developed heart failure that necessitated hospitalization during the first year after the infarct.[8] When stratified for ejection fraction, this risk ranged from 4% for those with an ejection fraction of more than .50 to 30% for those

Figure 12–3. Age-adjusted risk of developing congestive heart failure according to prior coronary heart disease status in the Framingham Study: Men and women 45–74; 18 year follow-up. (From Kannel WB, Savage D, Castelli WP: Cardiac failure in the Framingham Study: Twenty-year follow-up. *In* Braunwald E, Mock MB, Watson JT (eds): Congestive Heart Failure: Current Research and Clinical Applications, p 15. New York: Grune & Stratton, Inc., 1982.)

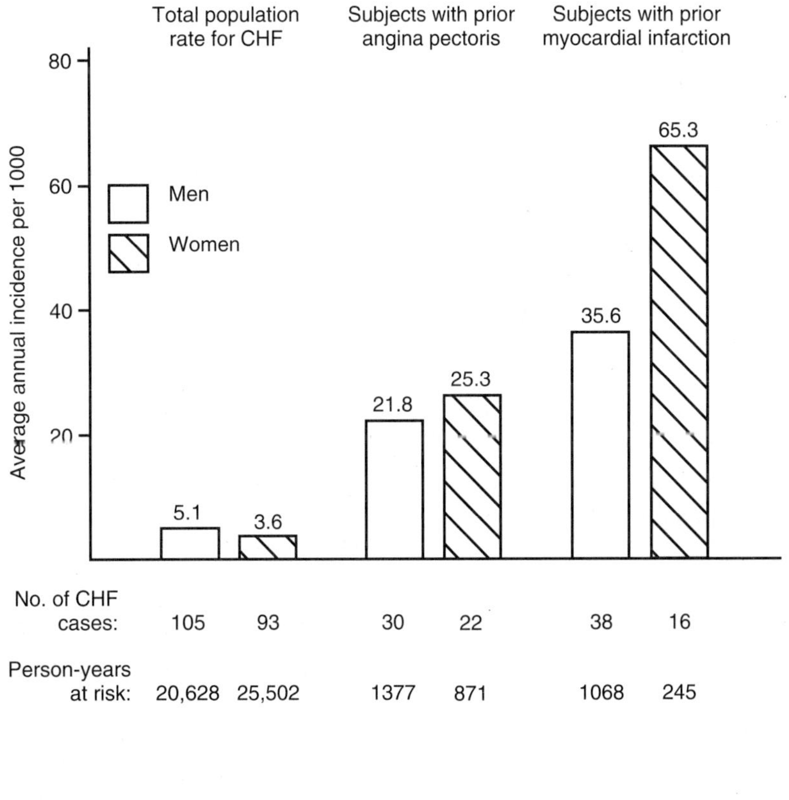

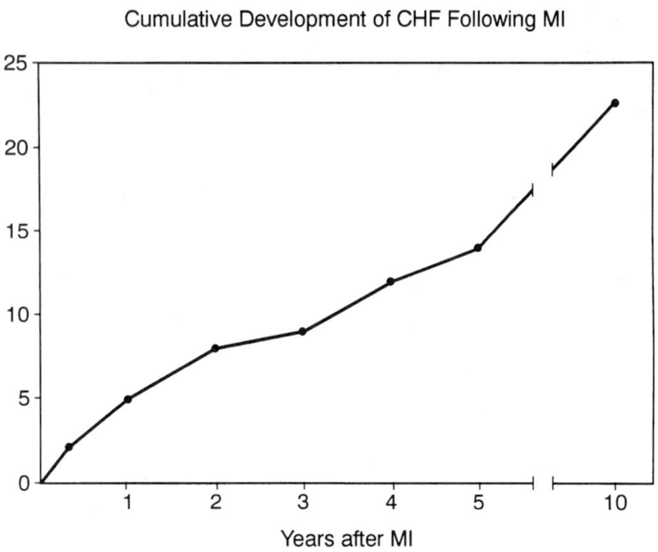

Figure 12–4. Cumulative development of symptomatic congestive heart failure following myocardial infarction. (Adapted from Kannell WB, Sorlie P, McNamara P: Prognosis after initial myocardial infarction: The Framingham Study. Am J Cardiol 1979; 44:53–59.)

with an ejection fraction of less than .21. During the 2.5 years of observation in the Multicenter Diltiazem Post Infarction Trial (MDPIT), 24% of the placebo-assigned patients were reported to require treatment for symptomatic congestive heart failure.[9] Assignment to the active treatment arm, in which the calcium channel blocker diltiazem was used, was associated with an increased mortality rate among patients with any of the following prerandomization indicators of a higher risk myocardial infarction: pulmonary congestion, anterior lateral Q wave, or ejection fraction of less than .40.[10] This important study demonstrated the fragility of patients with LV dysfunction and added a cautionary note to the use of a calcium channel blocker in this patient population. Again, however, this risk of developing symptomatic congestive heart failure after myocardial infarction was strongly related to the LV ejection fraction. Therefore, the selection of survivors of infarcts, especially those with depressed LV ejection fraction, results in the identification of a potentially large group of patients at risk for developing symptomatic congestive heart failure.

Understanding Pathogenesis Provides a Rationale for Treatment. By definition, a myocardial infarction is the end result of the necrosis of contractile tissue caused by abrupt interruption of coronary blood flow. Although the loss of contractile units is acute, as discussed previously, the clinical development of the syndrome of congestive heart failure often takes years to become evident. A major clue to the possible sequence of events during this clinically silent phase from the myocardial infarction to the appearance of symptoms came from studies in experimental animals. In the rat model of coronary artery ligation, the abrupt insult of a myocardial infarction was shown to initiate an insidious process of ventricular chamber enlargement (remodeling) that was associated with a time-dependent deterioration of ventricular function.[11] It has since become clear that such progressive enlargement of the ventricle is a prominent feature of ventricular dysfunction in several experimental models. Whether the impairment of cardiac function is produced by microsphere embolization of the coronary vasculature,[12] direct current shock myocardial damage,[13] or isoproterenol cardiotoxicity,[14] a time-dependent increase in ventricular volume ensues. The clinical importance of these observations has been established by a number of studies measuring the LV cavity volume in survivors of myocardial infarction; these measurements demonstrated that progressive LV dilatation occurs in a substantial proportion of these patients.[15–21]

Although the early ventricular dilatation may serve to restore stroke volume of the impaired ventricle, this structural change creates additional stimuli for further remodeling.[22] The change in the ventricular geometry increases myocardial wall stress, which in turn promotes a further increase in cavity volume, thereby creating an unrelenting stimulus for further dilatation. This progressive deterioration in cardiac function and structure may well explain the late appearance of congestive heart failure in certain survivors of infarcts even in the absence of further myocardial necrosis.

Both in animal studies and in humans, the extent of the myocardial infarction is the major determinant of the magnitude of ventricular enlargement. Treatments that reduce the infarct size (restoration of coronary flow) during the acute infarct period can be considered therapies preventive of both remodeling and congestive heart failure. However, once the damage has occurred and reperfusion can no longer salvage myocytes, ACE inhibition therapy provides another opportunity to reduce the risk of the development of heart failure. In an experimental model of myocardial infarction in rats, long-term ACE inhibition therapy attenuated enlargement and limited the time-dependent deterioration of ventricular function.[23] In this animal model, in which confounding factors are experimentally minimized and comparisons could be based on the degree of histologic damage, ACE inhibitor therapy was associated with preservation of ventricular function and geometry and, more important, with prolongation of survival.[24]

The relevance of these observations from animal studies was directly tested by several well-designed mechanistic clinical studies.[25–29] Patients with recent myocardial infarctions and asymptomatic LV dysfunction were randomized to receive either conventional therapy alone or conventional therapy plus an ACE inhibitor. A common theme of these studies was that quantitative measures of ventricular volume increased in the survivors of myocardial infarction and that ACE inhibitor therapy attenuated this time-dependent ventricular enlargement.[25–29] These clinical observations that a favorable modification of ventricular remodeling after infarction was associated with the use of ACE inhibitor therapy provided the initial rationale for treatment of asymptomatic patients with ventricular dysfunction. The concept was that interruption of the remodeling process would lower the risk of congestive heart failure (prevention) and prolong survival. This hypothesis has since been tested in clinical trials.

The SAVE Study. The Survival and Ventricular Enlargement (SAVE) study[30] was the first direct test of the hypothesis that treatment of an asymptomatic patient with LV dysfunction after myocardial infarction would lead to an improvement in clinical outcome and not just in ventricular volumes. Patients who had recently had a myocardial infarction but who were not considered, on clinical grounds, to have congestive heart failure were screened; those with an ejection fraction of .40 or less were identified as potential trial participants. On days 3–16 after the infarction, patients were randomized to receive either placebo or the ACE inhibitor captopril. This timing allowed for clinical assessment of the patient's stability as well as for decisions regarding catheterization and revascularization procedures. In keeping with the theme of prevention of heart failure, patients who already manifested symptomatic congestive heart failure were excluded from this trial; therefore, the study was a test of the new use of an ACE inhibitor for prevention of cardiovascular morbidity and mortality. Before actual randomization, captopril was started at the initial dose of 6.25 mg, which was tolerated by all but 19 of the 2250 patients who were otherwise eligible and gave informed consent. The remaining 2231 patients were entered into the trial. The target dose of captopril or matching placebo was 25 mg three times per day during the hospitalization; the dose was increased to 50 mg three times per day for the remainder of the ambulatory phase.

TABLE 12–1. RELATIVE RISK OF DEATH IN PATIENTS EXPERIENCING MANIFESTATIONS OF CHF

Event	Incidence	Relative Risk (95% CI)
Hospitalization	15%	6.4 (5.3 to 7.8)
ACE Inhibitor Therapy	13%	4.5 (3.6 to 5.6)
Initiate or Augment Digitalis/Diuretic for CHF	28%	4.7 (3.9 to 5.7)

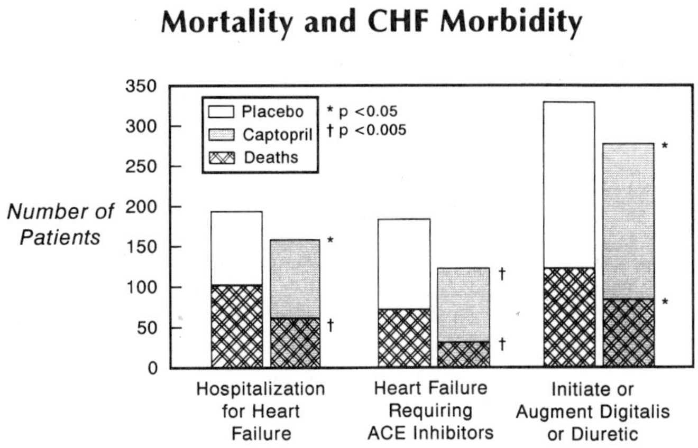

Figure 12–5. Development of symptomatic heart failure in the Survival and Ventricular Enlargement (SAVE) trial. Three prospective definitions of heart failure are shown and, for each, the difference between placebo and captopril assignment was demonstrated. Not only were less patients in the active therapy arm likely to experience each of the specific definitions of clinical deterioration from heart failure but in each case there were less subsequent fatal events (hatched portion of the bars). (From Pfeffer MA: Mechanistic lessons from the SAVE study. AJH 1994; 7:106s–111s.)

During the 3.5 years of follow-up, approximately 15% of the patients manifested heart failure that, by clinical criteria, necessitated the use of an ACE inhibitor or prompted a hospitalization for management. Regardless of therapy assignment, the patients who developed clinical manifestations of heart failure after randomization were three to six times more likely than other SAVE patients to suffer a fatal event (Table 12–1). Even though this population was selected for LV dysfunction, the majority of patients did not manifest symptomatic failure. As anticipated, the risk of developing heart failure was not uniform with older age; a lower ejection fraction, the presence of mitral regurgitation, and a history of hypertension, diabetes, or multiple infarctions all emerged as independent predictors of increased odds for heart failure.[31] In a subset of patients for whom neurohormonal sampling was done, a higher level of the N-terminal portion of pro-ANF in serum was an important additional independent measure of heightened cardiovascular risk, particularly the risk of developing congestive heart failure;[32] this measure is currently of investigative interest.

Randomization to the prophylactic use of an ACE inhibitor reduced the incidence of congestive heart failure by any of three prospectively defined criteria: (1) clinical deterioration necessitating ACE inhibition, (2) hospitalization for management of heart failure, or (3) clinical need to initiate or augment digitalis or diuretic therapy for symptoms of congestive failure (Fig. 12–5). As equally important as the reduction in incidence of congestive heart failure was the fact that the number of patients who exhibited these heart failure endpoints and subsequently died was also reduced by this prophylactic use of the ACE inhibitor (see Fig. 12–5). These observations of reduced appearance and subsequent death with the treatment of asymptomatic patients with LV dysfunction after myocardial infarction does indeed provide direct evidence for the preventive action of the ACE inhibitor in this patient population before the development of signs and symptoms of heart failure.

A prospective mechanistic echocardiographic study supports the initial hypothesis that attenuating ventricular enlargement would reduce the incidence of heart failure and subsequent death.[33] This quantitative echocardiographic study did indicate that patients who manifested enlargement were more likely to experience clinical cardiovascular events than were those who did not manifest enlargement. By reducing the incidence of further ventricular enlargement, ACE inhibitor therapy also reduced the risk for fatal and nonfatal cardiovascular events. Of particular interest was a group of patients who, despite randomization to active therapy (captopril), demonstrated progressive ventricular enlargement. In these patients, the risk of cardiovascular events was comparable to that of placebo-assigned patients with ventricular enlargement.[33] This quantitative echocardiographic study provided a link between the attenuation of LV enlargement and at least a component of the benefit of chronic ACE inhibitor therapy for asymptomatic LV dysfunction (Fig. 12–6).

FUTURE DIRECTIONS

An intriguing observation from both the SAVE and the SOLVD studies that has become the focus of continued investigative interest has been the reduction in myocardial infarctions that was observed

Figure 12–6. SAVE study quantitative echocardiographic data demonstrating greater increases in left ventricular area between baseline and 1 year in patients who experienced adverse cardiovascular (CV) events compared with those with an uncomplicated clinical course following myocardial infarction. (From St. John Sutton M, Pfeffer MA, Plappert T, et al: Quantitative two-dimensional echocardiographic measurements are major predictors of adverse cardiovascular events after acute myocardial infarction: the protective effects of captopril. Circulation 1994; 89:68–75.)

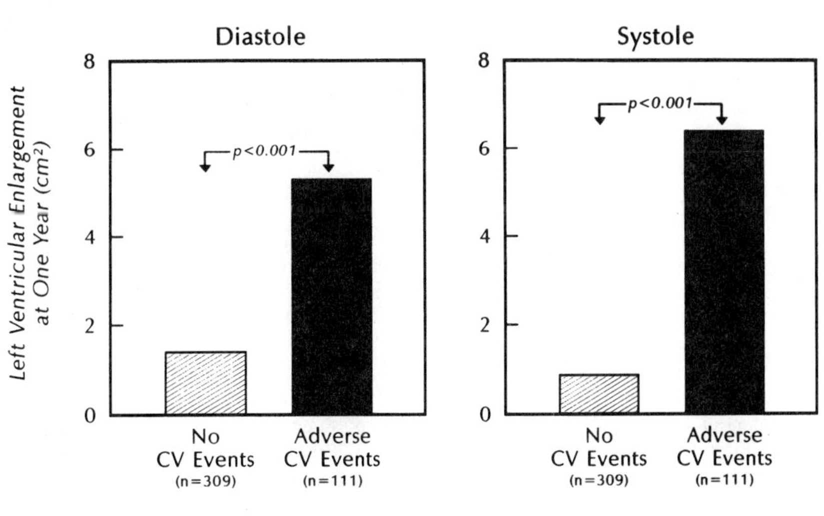

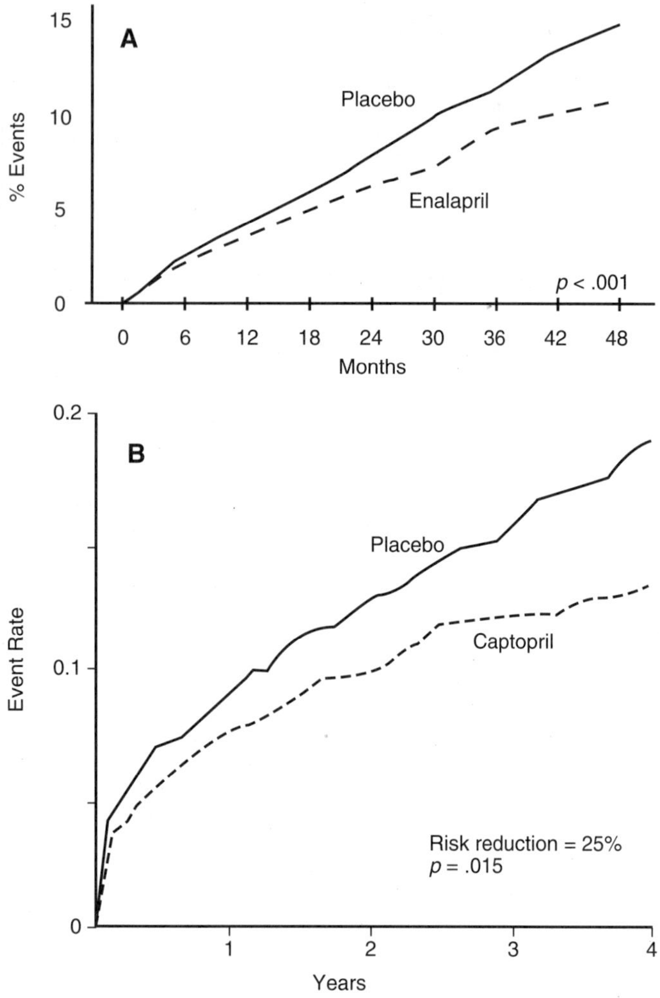

Figure 12–7. The number of patients experiencing a myocardial infarction following randomization in the SOLVD study *(A)* or the SAVE study *(B)*. Note the similar time course and magnitude of the reduction of risk of experiencing a myocardial infarction following randomization to either of the ACE inhibitors. (*A* from Yusuf S, Pepine CJ, Garces C, et al: Effects of enalapril on myocardial infarction and unstable angina in patients with low ejection fractions. Lancet 1992; 340:1173–1178. *B* from Pfeffer MA, Braunwald E, Moyé LA, et al: Effects of captopril on mortality and morbidity in patients with left ventricular dysfunction after myocardial infarction. Results of the Survival and Ventricular Enlargement Trial. N Engl J Med 1992; 327:669.)

in both populations (Fig. 12–7). In the SOLVD study, regardless of whether patients were selected for the treatment arm or the prevention arm (symptomatic or asymptomatic), there was a reduction in the reports of myocardial infarction from patients assigned to enalapril therapy.[34] Similarly in the SAVE study, patients randomized to the ACE inhibitor captopril were less likely to suffer a myocardial infarction during the follow-up period.[30]

The magnitude and time course of these reductions were similar in these trials with two different ACE inhibitors. Although reduced ejection fraction was an entry criterion for both studies, the level of ejection fraction was not a predictor of either the risk of myocardial infarction or the benefits of ACE inhibitor therapy in reducing myocardial infarction.[33, 35]

Although it is currently unknown whether these observations will extend to the broader population with more preserved LV function, the potential public health implications are important. Two major trials, Heart Outcomes Prevention Evaluation (HOPE) and Prevention of Events with ACE Inhibition (PEACE), will directly test this hypothesis that ACE inhibition therapy will reduce the rates of cardiovascular-related death and myocardial infarction even in the absence of LV dysfunction. A favorable outcome in these trials would expand the preventive aspect of ACE inhibitor therapy from the already demonstrated clinical benefits achieved in attenuating secondary ventricular remodeling to the primary preventive strategies of risk factor modification (see Fig. 12–1).

REFERENCES

1. Cutler JA, Psaty BM, MacMahon S, Furberg CD: Public health issues in hypertension control: what has been learned from clinical trials. *In* Laragh JH, Brenner BM (eds): Hypertension: Pathophysiology, Diagnosis and Management, 2nd ed, p 253. New York: Raven Press, 1995.
2. The SOLVD Investigators: Studies of left ventricular dysfunction (SOLVD)—rationale, design and methods: two trials that evaluate the effect of enalapril in patients with reduced ejection fraction. Am J Cardiol 1990; 66:315–322.
3. Francis GS, Benedict C, Johnstone DE, et al: Comparison of neuroendocrine activation in patients with left ventricular dysfunction with and without congestive heart failure. A substudy of the Studies of Left Ventricular Dysfunction (SOLVD). Circulation 1990; 82:1724–1729.
4. The SOLVD Investigators: Effect of enalapril on survival in patients with reduced left ventricular ejection fractions and congestive heart failure. N Engl J Med 1991; 325:293–302.
5. The SOLVD Investigators: Effect of enalapril on mortality and the development of heart failure in asymptomatic patients with reduced left ventricular ejection fractions. N Engl J Med 1992; 327:685–691.
6. Kannel WB, Savage D, Castelli WP: Cardiac failure in the Framingham Study: twenty-year follow-up. *In* Braunwald E, Mock MB, Watson JT (eds): Congestive Heart Failure: Current Research and Clinical Applications, p 15. New York: Grune & Stratton, 1982.
7. Kannel WB, Sorlie P, McNamara PM: Prognosis after initial myocardial infarction: the Framingham Study. Am J Cardiol 1979; 44:53–59.
8. Greene HL, Richardson DW, Hallstrom AP, et al: Congestive heart failure after acute myocardial infarction in patients receiving antiarrhythmic agents for ventricular premature complexes (Cardiac Arrhythmia Pilot Study). Am J Cardiol 1989; 63:393–398.
9. Lichstein E, Hager WD, Gregory JJ, et al: Relation between beta-adrenergic blocker use, various correlates of left ventricular function and the chance of developing congestive heart failure. J Am Coll Cardiol 1990; 16(6):1327–1332.
10. Moss AJ, Oakes D, Benhorin J, et al: The interaction between diltiazem and left ventricular function after myocardial infarction. Circulation 1989; 80(IV):102–106.
11. Pfeffer JM, Pfeffer MA, Fletcher PJ, Braunwald E: Progressive ventricular remodeling in rat with myocardial infarction. Am J Physiol 1991; 260(HCP 29):H1406–H1414.
12. Sabbah HN, Stein PD, Kono T, et al: A canine model of chronic heart failure produced by multiple sequential coronary microembolizations. Am J Physiol 1991; 260(HCP 29):H1379–H1384.
13. McDonald KM, Francis GS, Carlyle PF, et al: Hemodynamic, left ventricular structural and hormonal changes after discrete myocardial damage in the dog. J Am Coll Cardiol 1992; 19:460–467.
14. Teerlink JR, Pfeffer JM, Pfeffer MA: Progressive ventricular remodeling in response to diffuse isoproterenol-induced myocardial necrosis in rats. Circ Res 1994; 75:105–113.
15. Erlebacher JA, Weiss JL, Eaton LW, et al: Late effects of acute infarct dilation on heart size: a two dimensional echocardiographic study. Am J Cardiol 1982; 49:1120–1126.
16. Lamas GA, Pfeffer MA: Increased left ventricular volume following myocardial infarction in man. Am Heart J 1986; 111:30–35.
17. Gadsboll N, Hoilund-Carlsen PF, Badsberg JH, et al: Late ventricular dilatation in survivors of acute myocardial infarction. Am J Cardiol 1989; 64:961–966.
18. Jeremy RW, Allman KC, Bautovitch G, Harris PJ: Patterns of left ventricular dilation during the six months after myocardial infarction. J Am Coll Cardiol 1989; 13:304–310.
19. Kostuk WJ, Kazamias TM, Gander MP, et al: Left ventricular size after acute myocardial infarction: serial changes and their prognostic significance. Circulation 1973; 47:1174–1179.
20. Gaudron P, Eilles C, Kugler I, Ertl G: Progressive left ventricular dys-

function and remodeling after myocardial infarction: potential mechanisms and early predictors. Circulation 1993; 87:755–763.
21. Rumberger JA, Behrenbeck T, Breen JR, et al: Nonparallel changes in global left ventricular chamber volume and muscle mass during the first year after transmural myocardial infarction in humans. J Am Coll Cardiol 1993; 21:673–682.
22. Pfeffer MA, Pfeffer JM: Ventricular enlargement and reduced survival after myocardial infarction. Circulation 1987; 75(IV):93–97.
23. Pfeffer JM, Pfeffer MA, Braunwald E: Influence of chronic captopril therapy on the infarcted left ventricle of the rat. Circ Res 1985; 57:84–95.
24. Pfeffer MA, Pfeffer JM, Steinberg C, Finn P: Survival after an experimental myocardial infarction: beneficial effects of long-term therapy with captopril. Circulation 1985; 72:406–412.
25. Pfeffer MA, Lamas GA, Vaughan DE, et al: Effect of captopril on progressive ventricular dilatation after anterior myocardial infarction. N Engl J Med 1988; 319:80–86.
26. Sharpe N, Smith H, Murphy J, Hannan S: Treatment of patients with symptomless left ventricular dysfunction after myocardial infarction. Lancet 1988; 1:255–259.
27. Bonaduce D, Petretta M, Arrichiello P, et al: Effects of captopril treatment on left ventricular remodeling and function after anterior myocardial infarction: comparison with digitalis. J Am Coll Cardiol 1992; 19:858–863.
28. Ray SG, Pye M, Oldroyd KG, et al: Early treatment with captopril after acute myocardial infarction. Br Heart J 1993; 69:215–222.
29. Foy SG, Crozier IG, Turner JG, et al: Comparison of enalapril versus captopril on left ventricular function and survival three months after acute myocardial infarction (the "PRACTICAL" study). Am J Cardiol 1994; 73:1180–1186.
30. Pfeffer MA, Braunwald E, Moyé LA, et al: Effect of captopril on mortality and morbidity in patients with left ventricular dysfunction after myocardial infarction. Results of the Survival and Ventricular Enlargement Trial. N Engl J Med 1992; 327:669–677.
31. Arnold JMO, Rouleau JL, Geltman EM, et al: Predictors for the development of heart failure in patients with left ventricular dysfunction (LVEF ≤40%) after myocardial infarction [Abstract]. Circulation 1994; 90(I):380.
32. Hall C, Rouleau JL, Moyé L, et al: N-terminal proatrial natriuretic factor—an independent predictor of long-term prognosis after myocardial infarction. Circulation 1994; 89:1934–1942.
33. St. John Sutton M, Pfeffer MA, Plappert T, et al: Quantitative two-dimensional echocardiographic measurements are major predictors of adverse cardiovascular events after acute myocardial infarction: the protective effects of captopril. Circulation 1994; 89:68–75.
34. Yusuf S, Pepine CJ, Garces C, et al: Effect of enalapril on myocardial infarction and unstable angina in patients with low ejection fractions. Lancet 1992; 340:1173–1178.
35. Rutherford JD, Pfeffer MA, Moyé LA, et al: Effects of captopril on ischemic events after myocardial infarction. Results of the Survival and Ventricular Enlargement Trial. Circulation 1994; 90:1731–1738.

13 Management of Left Ventricular Diastolic Dysfunction

William H. Gaasch, MD
Edgar C. Schick, MD
Michael R. Zile, MD

Diastolic dysfunction of the left ventricle can be defined as a condition in which the ventricle exhibits an impaired relaxation and a limited ability to fill; in pure diastolic dysfunction, the left ventricular (LV) chamber is not enlarged and the ejection fraction is normal.[1–6] The most common causes are LV hypertrophy and ischemia. Mild forms of diastolic dysfunction may be manifested as a slow or delayed pattern of relaxation and filling with little or no elevation of LV diastolic pressure and no cardiac symptoms. In some patients, the ventricle exhibits a limited ability to use the Frank-Starling mechanism; despite an increased filling pressure, the ejection fraction and stroke volume fail to rise during exercise, and the patient experiences dyspnea and fatigue.[7–9] Slow or delayed myocardial relaxation can adversely affect coronary blood flow and flow reserve and contribute to the development of myocardial ischemia;[10, 11] thus, angina or silent ischemia may be part of the clinical syndrome, even if there is little or no epicardial coronary artery disease. In its most severe form, diastolic dysfunction presents as overt congestive heart failure (CHF).

As many as one third of patients presenting with CHF have a normal ejection fraction; most such patients have clinically significant diastolic dysfunction.[12–14] The prevalence of diastolic dysfunction, however, depends on age, gender, and the population under consideration. It is relatively uncommon in young or middle-aged patients who have been preselected for clinical research or other specialized care.[15] By contrast, the prevalence of CHF with a normal ejection fraction can exceed .50 in older patients, notably elderly women residing in nursing homes.[16–18]

The prognosis of patients with CHF due to diastolic dysfunction is less ominous than in those patients with systolic dysfunction.[15] The annual mortality of patients with CHF in the presence of a normal LV ejection fraction is approximately .07 to .08.[15, 19–21] Mortality may be substantially higher in patients with coronary disease and diastolic dysfunction;[20] it can be less than 2% per year in those without coronary disease.[20, 21] Despite a relatively low mortality, morbidity can be high; treatment failures are common, and hospital readmissions are frequent.

An evaluation of LV size and function is mandatory in all patients suspected of having LV systolic or diastolic dysfunction, especially those with overt CHF.[22] If there is clinical evidence of pulmonary venous hypertension and the chest film exhibits features of elevated pulmonary venous pressure in the presence of a normal heart size, diastolic dysfunction should be considered. The diagnosis is confirmed if an echocardiogram or angiogram reveals a normal or nearly normal LV ejection fraction. This clinical approach can be supplemented and refined by measuring or calculating indices of LV relaxation derived from the LV isovolumic relaxation period or the LV filling period. Such indices are, however, influenced by hemodynamic loads, chamber stiffness, and multiple other factors; these indices are used principally for clinical investigation.[1–6]

The standard echocardiogram can be used to further define the pathophysiologic process. For example, increased wall thickness, especially a high relative wall thickness, implicates LV hypertrophy or, less commonly, an infiltrative process.[23, 24] When the latter is a serious consideration, a myocardial biopsy should be performed.[25] Coronary artery disease should be considered, especially in patients with little or no LV hypertrophy. Depending on the results of noninvasive stress tests, a coronary angiogram may be necessary to confirm or exclude the diagnosis of coronary disease and to design an appropriate therapeutic plan.

GENERAL PRINCIPLES OF MANAGEMENT

Large randomized trials have confirmed survival and other benefits of treatment with vasodilators and angiotensin converting enzyme (ACE) inhibitors in patients with systolic dysfunction and an ejection fraction that is less than .35 to .40.[22] Unfortunately, there are no such trials in patients with diastolic dysfunction. As a result, therapy of LV diastolic dysfunction is based on the results of clinical investigations and observations in relatively small groups of patients[17, 26–28] and concepts based on an understanding of pathophysiology.[1–6]

Treatment of Presenting Symptoms

With few exceptions, the initial treatment of patients with LV diastolic dysfunction presenting with CHF, angina, or hypertension is similar to that of patients with systolic dysfunction of the left ventricle. Pulmonary edema, with or without signs of systemic venous congestion, can be treated with parenteral diuretics, morphine, intravenous or cutaneous nitroglycerin, and rotating tourniquets. The last two techniques are rapidly reversible and, therefore, advantageous in patients who become hypotensive. Hypotension can be a significant problem in diastolic dysfunction; in such patients, a steep LV diastolic pressure-volume curve can be responsible for large changes in filling pressure and cardiac output with only modest changes in volume. For this reason, diuretic therapy is initiated with a small dose of a loop diuretic (e.g., 10 to 20 mg furosemide intravenously). If a prompt diuresis is not achieved with the administration of a loop diuretic, the dose is increased and/or a second agent (e.g., hydrochlorothiazide or metolazone) is used in combination.

Beta agonists can have a salutary effect on splanchnic blood flow and facilitate diuresis; these agents can also promote myocardial relaxation and augment cardiac output, even in patients with a normal ejection fraction. Thus, it can be argued that dopamine (2 to 3 μg/kg/min) should be used in the initial treatment of patients with acute CHF and pulmonary edema caused by diastolic dysfunction, just as it is used in systolic dysfunction. Unfortunately, beta agonists may precipitate or promote myocardial ischemia;[29] therefore, it is advisable to administer such agents cautiously and only for limited periods.

Define Etiology and Plan Long-Term Therapy

Any attempt to develop a long-term therapeutic plan must be based on a careful consideration of the cause of the diastolic dysfunction and its potential response to treatment. For example, verapamil can be effective in symptomatic patients with hypertrophic cardiomyopathy,[27] but it is contraindicated in patients with clinically significant cardiac amyloidosis.[25] Coronary artery disease, hypertensive heart disease, chronic constrictive pericarditis, and aortic stenosis provide relatively specific therapeutic targets. However, the problem is commonly less specific. Indeed, the mechanisms underlying diastolic dysfunction in hypertensive hypertrophic cardiomyopathy of the elderly tend to preclude a single or specific therapeutic intervention. For this reason, emphasis is placed on control of arterial hypertension, prevention of myocardial ischemia, treatment of congestive symptoms, and maintenance of normal sinus rhythm.

Avoid Positive Inotropic Drugs

Most patients with congestive heart failure caused by LV systolic dysfunction (and those with mixed systolic-diastolic dysfunction) benefit from treatment with positive inotropic agents. Such therapy is generally not used in the long-term treatment of patients with pure diastolic dysfunction because the LV ejection fraction is preserved and there appears to be little potential for a beneficial effect.[17, 26] Moreover, positive inotropic agents have the potential to worsen the pathophysiologic processes that cause diastolic dysfunction.

Digitalis, by inhibiting the sodium-potassium-ATPase pump, augments intracellular calcium through a sodium-calcium exchange mechanism and thereby augments contractile state. In this manner, digitalis produces an increase in systolic energy demands while adding to a relative calcium overload in diastole. These effects may not be clinically apparent under many circumstances, but during hemodynamic stress or ischemia, digitalis may promote or contribute to diastolic dysfunction.[30] Therefore, with the possible exception of patients with chronic atrial fibrillation (who might benefit from a small dose of digitalis in combination with other drugs to slow atrioventricular conduction and ventricular rate), digitalis should not be used in the treatment of pure diastolic dysfunction.

Beta-adrenergic agonists, by increasing intracellular cyclic adenosine monophosphate (cAMP), enhance calcium sequestration by the sarcoplasmic reticulum and thereby promote a more rapid and complete myocardial relaxation between beats.[31, 32] Beta agonists can also increase venous capacitance, which leads to a reduction in ventricular filling pressures. Phosphodiesterase inhibitors can produce similar salutary effects on myocardial relaxation and venous capacitance.[33] Unfortunately, all cAMP-dependent agents promote calcium influx into the cell and augment myocardial energy demands. Thus, dopamine, amrinone, and similar agents can be useful in the short-term management of patients with CHF (see previous text), but their use can be complicated by myocardial ischemia and serious arrhythmias. They have not been shown to be effective in long-term therapy.

Conceptually, an ideal therapeutic agent should augment myocardial relaxation without promoting calcium overload. A combination of verapamil (which blocks calcium influx) and dopamine (which stimulates calcium uptake by the sarcoplasmic reticulum) might achieve this goal.[34] Similarly, zatebradine (a specific bradycardiac agent) and a beta agonist might also have potential therapeutic utility.[35] Xamoterol, or other partial beta-adrenergic agonists, might be useful in long-term therapy.[36] Unfortunately, the efficacy of such treatments has not been evaluated in human beings with LV diastolic dysfunction.

SINUS RHYTHM AND RATE CONTROL

Tachycardia is poorly tolerated by patients with most cardiac disorders. Atrial tachyarrhythmias and even sinus tachycardia have a negative impact on diastolic function for several reasons. First, rapid heart rates cause an increase in myocardial oxygen demands and a decrease in coronary perfusion time; thus, rapid rate can promote ischemic diastolic dysfunction, even in the absence of epicardial coronary disease. Second, there may be incomplete relaxation between beats, and as a result there is an increase in diastolic pressure relative to volume; thus, LV effective distensibility is reduced. Third, rapid rates reduce the diastolic filling time and ventricular filling. For these and other reasons, most clinicians use beta blockers or calcium channel blockers to prevent excessive tachycardias and produce a relative bradycardia in patients with diastolic dysfunction. However, excessive bradycardia can result in a fall in cardiac output despite an increase in LV filling.[29, 37] Such considerations underscore the need for individualizing therapeutic interventions that affect heart rate.

Benefits of Bradycardia

Biophysical considerations indicate that intrinsic heart rate is inversely related to heart weight.[38] Whereas the optimal rate of hypertrophic or large failing hearts is not known, it is likely that such hearts would function most efficiently at slow rates. A relative bradycardia has several potentially beneficial effects. Both the salutary effects on myocardial energetics and the prolonged diastolic interval that allows complete relaxation and more filling are important. Slow rate is also associated with an increased capillary density in hypertrophic hearts.[39] In addition, hypertrophied and failing hearts exhibit a flat or even negative force-frequency relation;[37, 40, 41] thus, in contrast to normal hearts, function may improve as the rate is slowed. The optimal heart rate may differ in systolic and diastolic dysfunction, so attempts to correct an excessive heart rate must be individualized. An initial goal might be a resting rate of approximately 60 beats per minute with a blunted exercise-induced increase in heart rate.

Most beta blockers and some calcium blockers exert a substantial negative chronotropic effect, but the use of such agents can be limited by hypotension and other disabling side effects. With the development of specific bradycardiac agents,[35] it might be possible to selectively lower the heart rate with little direct effect on the remainder of the cardiovascular system.

SPECIFIC THERAPEUTIC TARGETS

Venous Congestion

The renin-angiotensin-aldosterone system is activated in patients with chronic CHF, but the mechanisms that evoke its activation remain especially unclear in patients with LV diastolic dysfunction. Myocardial ischemia, uncontrolled hypertension, and excessive dietary sodium may contribute to the development of congestion. In some patients, limited distensibility of the atria may attenuate the secretion of atrial natriuretic factor and thereby reduce its diuretic effect.[42] In others, low systemic vascular resistance and/or low arterial pressure may contribute to salt and water retention.[43, 44] Elevated venous pressure may directly cause renal sodium retention.[45] Despite a limited understanding of the pathogenesis of salt and water retention in patients with diastolic dysfunction, diuretics remain the mainstay of therapy for venous congestion.

After the initial treatment of congestive failure caused by LV diastolic dysfunction, most patients require salt restriction and long-term administration of a diuretic. These agents effectively reduce the central blood volume, lower the ventricular diastolic pressures, and thus alleviate the symptoms of the congestive state. Lower LV diastolic pressures may promote subendocardial blood flow. With the exception of their antihypertensive effects, diuretics do not affect the primary disease processes that led to diastolic dysfunction.

Thiazide diuretics can occasionally suffice for management of mild CHF, but the carbohydrate intolerance and hyperuricemia induced by these agents can limit their use. Loop diuretics such as furosemide are more potent than the thiazides, especially when the glomerular filtration rate is reduced. The combination of furosemide and a thiazide can be especially useful when edema is refractory to either agent alone. The potassium-sparing diuretic spironolactone, used in combination with thiazides or loop diuretics, can be particularly effective in patients with hypokalemia or high aldosterone levels. Spironolactone also has the potential to retard the fibrosis that contributes to abnormal chamber stiffness (see subsequent text).

The reduction in blood volume that follows the use of diuretics triggers an increase in sympathetic tone and further activation of the renin-angiotensin system. Such neurohormonal activation can lead to vasoconstriction and a worsening of the congestive state. Some vasodilators, particularly nitrates and pure arteriolar vasodilators, evoke a similar response. By contrast, ACE inhibitors (and beta blockers) blunt the neurohormonal activation and decrease the salt and water retention that complicates the treatment of heart failure. The ACE inhibitors may also have salutary effects on the active and passive properties of the left ventricle (see subsequent text). If hypotension does not limit their use, ACE inhibitors can provide useful adjunctive therapy in patients with diastolic dysfunction.

Atrial Arrhythmias

Atrial fibrillation is poorly tolerated in patients with LV diastolic dysfunction. In hypertrophic cardiomyopathy, for example, atrial fibrillation is usually accompanied by a substantial increase in ventricular diastolic and atrial pressures, leading eventually to pulmonary edema and hypotension. Similar changes may be anticipated when atrial fibrillation develops in patients with acute or chronic coronary heart disease, hypertensive heart disease, or restrictive cardiomyopathy. Overt decompensation occurs partly because of inadequate time for complete ventricular relaxation (see previous text) and partly because of the loss of atrial mechanical function and its contribution to ventricular filling.

Restoration of sinus rhythm is mandatory. Direct-current cardioversion may be necessary on an emergency basis. In less urgent situations, electrical or chemical cardioversion can be performed after rate control with digitalis, beta blockers, or calcium channel blockers. In hypertrophic obstructive cardiomyopathy, atrial fibrillation can be an indication for surgical ventricular myectomy.

Myocardial Ischemia

An extensive clinical and experimental literature documents the substantial deleterious effect of ischemia on the diastolic properties of the left ventricle.[46, 47] Thus, a transient increase in LV stiffness and diastolic pressure develops during myocardial ischemia caused by coronary spasm, exercise, rapid atrial pacing, angioplasty balloon inflation, and spontaneous angina.[48] Ischemia can be treated (1) with nitrates, beta blockers, and calcium channel blockers; (2) with coronary angioplasty; or (3) with surgical bypass grafts. On occasion, the signs of ischemic diastolic dysfunction may be especially prominent; such circumstances can dictate an aggressive approach.[49]

Hypertension and Hypertrophy

Several factors contribute to the diastolic dysfunction seen in hypertensive heart disease.[50] First, the abnormal loading conditions imposed by arterial hypertension can reduce the LV relaxation and filling rates. Second, concentrically hypertrophied hearts exhibit an increased passive stiffness (caused by a low volume/mass and fibrosis) and an impaired relaxation that is independent of hemodynamic loads. Third, a limited coronary vascular reserve can be responsible for myocardial ischemia, even in the absence of epicardial coronary disease. Each of these factors should be considered in the treatment of patients with hypertensive heart disease and diastolic dysfunction.

Because abnormalities of diastolic function can be detected in asymptomatic hypertensive patients with or without a measurable increment in LV mass,[51, 52] it could be argued that early treatment directed at normalization of the diastolic disorder might be desirable. There are, however, no data that could be used to support such an early treatment of diastolic dysfunction. Treatment of such asymptomatic patients should be directed primarily at preventing the known complications of hypertension (e.g., stroke); a secondary goal can be the prevention of hypertrophy and fibrosis.

The short-term treatment of elevated systemic arterial pressure, especially in severely hypertensive patients, provides a beneficial clinical effect on LV diastolic function.[53] Such a salutary effect of load reduction is more difficult to demonstrate during long-term therapy. Indeed, there is considerable variation in the effects of different antihypertensive agents on myocardial relaxation.[50] For example, despite an equivalent decrease in arterial pressure, nifedipine augments LV filling rate and other relaxation indices, but propranolol does not.[54] Other studies of patients with hypertensive heart disease indicate that diastolic dysfunction improves as LV hypertrophy regresses.[55–57] Still others confirm an improved diastolic function, prolonged exercise duration, and better heart failure scores in verapamil-treated patients with hypertensive heart disease and clinically significant LV diastolic dysfunction;[28] these clinical benefits were not closely related to changes in blood pressure or heart rate. Differences in the effects of treatment on diastolic function probably depend on the amount of hypertrophy regression, the alterations in ventricular loading conditions, the direct myocardial effect of the antihypertensive agent, and possibly the changes in coronary reserve.

A progressive interstitial fibrosis accompanies the hypertrophic response to arterial hypertension; fibrosis can also be prominent in the LV hypertrophy seen with aortic stenosis and hypertrophic cardiomyopathy. Such abnormal accumulation of fibrillar collagen is a result of enhanced collagen synthesis by cardiac fibroblasts that is related in part to the activity of the renin-angiotensin-aldosterone system. Thus, nonmyocyte cells in the cardiac interstitium are stimulated to produce a progressive interstitial and perivascular fibrosis whose important functional consequences include increased myocardial stiffness and impaired coronary flow reserve. In experimental studies, ACE inhibitors or spironolactone appears to protect against the exaggerated fibrous tissue response.[58, 59] For these reasons, the imperative to treat arterial hypertension may include prevention of the deleterious effects of angiotensin II and aldosterone. These preventive and treatment strategies have not yet been tested in humans with diastolic dysfunction. ACE inhibitors, however, are widely used effective antihypertensive agents that can produce regression of LV hypertrophy; a salutary effect on cardiac fibrosis may constitute an unexpected bonus.

Hypertrophic Cardiomyopathy and Relaxation

Diastolic dysfunction is a most important component of the pathophysiologic process of hypertrophic cardiomyopathy. The dysfunction is caused by (1) an increase in passive stiffness of the ventricle and (2) abnormal myocardial relaxation. The first is caused by a low volume/mass ratio combined with fibrosis and possibly fiber disarray.[60, 61] The second is related to a combination of abnormal myocardial calcium metabolism, altered ventricular loading conditions, and nonuniformity. Thus, as a result of depressed calcium sequestration by the sarcoplasmic reticulum and perhaps an increase in membrane calcium channels, myocardial calcium overload contributes to a slow or delayed myocardial relaxation (a slow and prolonged dissociation of actin-myosin), which leads to increased diastolic tone or tension.[41, 62, 63] Such prolonged relaxation can persist throughout the entire diastolic interval, especially in the presence of tachycardia. Assuming that the alterations in passive stiffness are relatively fixed and irreversible, medical therapy is directed toward the relaxation abnormalities.

The calcium antagonists verapamil, diltiazem, and nifedipine can correct many of the abnormal indices of relaxation and provide symptomatic relief.[63, 64] Verapamil, the most widely used calcium antagonist in hypertrophic cardiomyopathy, has a beneficial effect on angina and dyspnea; it also produces an improved exercise capacity.[27] Therapy is initiated at a low dosage (120 to 240 mg/day) and gradually increased to 360 to 480 mg/day; the optimal dose is determined by the symptomatic response of the patient.

Unfortunately, the vasodilating effects of the calcium antagonists can lead unpredictably to intensification of an outflow obstruction or hypotension even in the absence of obstruction.

Although beta blockers do not directly stimulate ventricular relaxation, they are commonly used in patients with hypertrophic cardiomyopathy. Angina, dyspnea, and presyncopal symptoms tend to improve during treatment.[65] Angina seems to respond more favorably than dyspnea. If propranolol is used, therapy is initiated with 40 mg two or three times daily, and the dose is gradually increased to 240–320 mg/day. Some patients require larger doses to achieve a beneficial effect on exercise capacity and symptoms.

When symptoms prove refractory to medical therapy, surgical procedures such as myotomy-myectomy, mitral valve replacement, or atrioventricular sequential pacemakers may favorably influence the diastolic properties of the left ventricle and produce symptomatic relief in selected patients with hypertrophic obstructive cardiomyopathy.[66–70] These approaches are not useful in nonobstructive hypertrophic cardiomyopathy or other causes of diastolic dysfunction.

Exercise Intolerance

Patients with a history of CHF and a normal ejection fraction (even those with diastolic dysfunction and little or no congestion) exhibit an exercise intolerance that has two major causes. First, elevated LV diastolic, left atrial, and pulmonary venous pressures cause a reduction in lung compliance; this increases the work of breathing and evokes the symptom of dyspnea. Increased LV diastolic pressure during exercise may also limit subendocardial blood flow during a period of increased myocardial oxygen demands, further worsening diastolic function. Second, an inadequate cardiac output during exercise contributes to anaerobic metabolism of skeletal muscles, lactate accumulation, and consequently fatigue of the legs and the accessory muscles of respiration. Neither of these pathophysiologic mechanisms provides a complete explanation for exercise intolerance in patients with heart failure.[7–9, 71–73] With such limited understanding of the precise factors responsible for dyspnea and fatigue, it has been difficult to develop a standard treatment plan for patients with LV diastolic dysfunction. Certainly, hypertension, myocardial ischemia, and clinically apparent congestion must be treated, but caution must be exercised to avoid even mild volume depletion that can contribute to a reduced cardiac output.

Calcium blockers and beta blockers have a salutary effect on symptoms in many if not most patients with clinically significant LV diastolic dysfunction. However, the beneficial effect of these agents on exercise tolerance is not always paralleled by improved LV diastolic function or increased relaxation rate. For example, in symptomatic patients with hypertrophic cardiomyopathy, a placebo-controlled, double-blind comparison of the effects of verapamil and propranolol on exercise tolerance indicated that both agents produced an increase in exercise duration; however, relaxation rate increased with verapamil and decreased with propranolol.[74] The observation that such verapamil effects persist long term[27] and that it is effective in patients with other causes of diastolic dysfunction[28] makes this agent a treatment of choice.

Beta-adrenergic receptor blocking agents produce a decrease in exercise capacity in normal individuals, but these agents can produce an improvement in exercise tolerance in patients with hypertrophic cardiomyopathy.[74] This salutary effect of beta blockers on exercise tolerance, despite a direct depressant effect on myocardial relaxation, makes this class of agents an acceptable alternative to the calcium blockers in hypertrophic cardiomyopathy. It is well known that beta blockers (and revascularization procedures) promote exercise capacity in patients with coronary heart disease, but it is not known whether beta blockers are effective in older patients with other causes of LV diastolic dysfunction.[75]

SUMMARY

The treatment of LV diastolic dysfunction has two major objectives. The first is to eliminate or reduce the factors responsible for diastolic dysfunction; the second is to reverse the consequences of diastolic dysfunction, particularly venous congestion. In general, the former is a long-term goal, whereas the latter can usually be

TABLE 13–1. TREATMENT GOALS AND METHODS

Reduce the congestive state
Salt restriction, diuretics, angiotensin converting enzyme (ACE) inhibitors
Dialysis or plasmapheresis
Maintain atrial contraction
Direct-current or pharmacologic cardioversion
Sequential atrioventricular pacing
Prevent tachycardia and promote bradycardia
Beta blockers, calcium blockers
Radiofrequency ablation and pacing
Treat and prevent myocardial ischemia
Nitrates, beta blockers, calcium blockers
Bypass surgery, angioplasty
Control hypertension and promote regression of hypertrophy
Antihypertensive agents
Attenuate neurohormonal activation
Beta blockers, ACE inhibitors
Prevent fibrosis and promote regression of fibrosis
ACE inhibitors, spironolactone
Anti-ischemic agents
Improve ventricular relaxation
Beta-adrenergic agonists
Systolic unloading
Treat ischemia
Calcium blockers (in hypertrophic cardiomyopathy)

achieved promptly. Treatment goals and methods are summarized in Table 13–1.

In some patients with severe refractory diastolic dysfunction, dialysis or plasmapheresis may be required to relieve life-threatening elevations of venous pressure. Direct removal of pleural or ascitic fluid can produce symptomatic improvement; on occasion, such a mechanical approach can initiate a diuresis. The role of surgery to correct valvular disease or myocardial ischemia should always be considered. The ultimate therapeutic measure is cardiac transplantation.[76]

REFERENCES

1. Stauffer JC, Gaasch WH: Recognition and treatment of left ventricular diastolic dysfunction. Prog Cardiovasc Dis 1990; 32:319.
2. Lorell BH: Significance of diastolic dysfunction of the heart. Annu Rev Med 1991; 42:411.
3. Bonow RO, Udelson JE: Left ventricular diastolic dysfunction as a cause of congestive heart failure: mechanisms and management. Ann Intern Med 1992; 117:502.
4. Litwin SE, Grossman W: Diastolic dysfunction as a cause of heart failure. J Am Coll Cardiol 1993; 22:49.
5. Brutsaert DL, Sys SU, Gillebert TC: Diastolic failure: pathophysiology and therapeutic implications. J Am Coll Cardiol 1993; 22:318.
6. Gaasch WH, Blaustein AS, LeWinter MM: Heart failure and clinical disorders of left ventricular diastolic dysfunction. *In* Gaasch WH, Le Winter MM (eds): Left Ventricular Diastolic Dysfunction and Heart Failure, p 245. Philadelphia: Lea & Febiger, 1994.
7. Cuocolo A, Sax FL, Brush JE, et al: Left ventricular hypertrophy and impaired diastolic filling in essential hypertension: diastolic mechanisms for systolic dysfunction during exercise. Circulation 1990; 81:978.
8. Clyne CA, Arrighi JA, Maron BJ, et al: Systemic and left ventricular response to exercise stress in asymptomatic patients with valvular stenosis. Am J Cardiol 1991; 68:1469.
9. Kitzman DW, Higginbotham MB, Cobb FR, et al: Exercise intolerance in patients with heart failure and preserved left ventricular systolic function: failure of the Frank-Starling mechanism. J Am Coll Cardiol 1991; 17:1065.
10. Watanabe J, Levine MJ, Bellotto F, et al: Left ventricular diastolic chamber stiffness and intramyocardial coronary capacitance in isolated dog hearts. Circulation 1993; 88:2929.
11. Udelson JE, Bonow RO, O'Gara PT, et al: Verapamil prevents silent myocardial perfusion abnormalities during exercise in asymptomatic patients with hypertrophic cardiomyopathy. Circulation 1989; 79:1052.
12. Echeverria HH, Bilisker MS, Myerburg RJ, Kessler KM: Congestive heart failure: echocardiographic insights. Am J Med 1983; 75:750.
13. Dougherty AH, Naccarelli GV, Grey EL, et al: Congestive heart failure with normal systolic function. Am J Cardiol 1984; 54:778.
14. Soufer R, Wohlgelernter D, Vita NA, et al: Intact systolic left ventricular function in clinical congestive heart failure. Am J Cardiol 1985; 55:1032.
15. Cohn JN, Johnson G, and the Veterans Administration Cooperative Study Group: Heart failure with normal ejection fraction: the V-HeFT study. Circulation 1980; 81(suppl III):48.
16. Luchi RJ, Snow E, Luchi JM, et al: Left ventricular function in hospitalized geriatric patients. J Am Geriatr Soc 1982; 30:702.
17. Forman DE, Coletta D, Kenny D, et al: Clinical issues related to discontinuing digoxin therapy in elderly nursing home patients. Arch Intern Med 1991; 151:2194.
18. Wong WF, Gold S, Fukuyama O, Blanchette PL: Diastolic dysfunction in elderly patients with congestive heart failure. Am J Cardiol 1989; 63:1526.
19. Setaro JF, Soufer R, Remetz MS, et al: Long-term outcome in patients with congestive heart failure and intact systolic left ventricular performance. Am J Cardiol 1992; 69:1212.
20. Judge KW, Pawitan Y, Caldwell J, et al: Congestive heart failure in patients with preserved left ventricular systolic function: analysis of the CASS registry. J Am Coll Cardiol 1991; 18:377.
21. Brogen WC, Hillis LD, Flores ED, et al: The natural history of isolated left ventricular diastolic dysfunction. Am J Med 1992; 92:627.
22. Gaasch WH: Diagnosis and treatment of heart failure based on left ventricular systolic or diastolic dysfunction. JAMA 1994; 271:1276.
23. Gaasch WH: Left ventricular radius to wall thickness ratio. Am J Cardiol 1979; 43:1189.
24. Carroll JD, Gaasch WH, McAdam KPWJ: Amyloid cardiomyopathy: characterization by a distinctive voltage/mass relation. Am J Cardiol 1982; 49:9.
25. Pollak A, Falk RH: Left ventricular systolic dysfunction precipitated by verapamil in cardiac amyloidosis. Chest 1993; 104:618.
26. Topol EJ, Traill TA, Fortuin NJ: Hypertensive hypertrophic cardiomyopathy of the elderly. N Engl J Med 1985; 312:277.
27. Bonow RO, Dilsizian V, Rosing DR, et al: Verapamil-induced improvement in left ventricular filling and increased exercise tolerance in patients with hypertrophic cardiomyopathy: short and long term results. Circulation 1985; 72:853.
28. Setaro JF, Zaret BL, Schulman DS, et al: Usefulness of verapamil for congestive heart failure associated with abnormal left ventricular diastolic filling and normal left ventricular systolic performance. Am J Cardiol 1990; 66:981.
29. Udelson JE, Cannon RO, Bacharach SL, et al: Beta adrenergic stimulation with isoproterenol enhances left ventricular diastolic performance in hypertrophic cardiomyopathy despite potentiation of myocardial ischemia: comparison to rapid atrial pacing. Circulation 1989; 79:371.
30. Lorell BH, Isoyama S, Grice WN, et al: Effects of ouabain and isoproterenol on left ventricular diastolic function during low-flow ischemia in isolated, blood-perfused rabbit hearts. Circ Res 1988; 63:457.
31. Morad M, Rolett EL: Relaxing effect of catecholamines on mammalian heart. J Physiol (Lond) 1972; 244:537.
32. Lang RM, Carroll JD, Nakamura S, et al: Role of adrenoceptors and dopamine receptors in modulating left ventricular diastolic function. Circ Res 1988; 63:126.
33. Monrad ES, McKay R, Baim DS, et al: Improvement in indexes of diastolic performance in patients with congestive heart failure treated with milrinone. Circulation 1984; 70:1030.
34. Apstein CS, Morgan JP: Cellular mechanisms underlying left ventricular diastolic dysfunction. *In* Gaasch WH, LeWinter MM (eds): Left Ventricular Diastolic Dysfunction and Heart Failure, p 3. Philadelphia: Lea & Febiger, 1994.
35. Breall JA, Watanabe J, Grossman W: Effect of zatebradine on contractility, relaxation, and coronary blood flow. J Am Coll Cardiol 1993; 21:471.
36. Marlow HF: Review of clinical experience with xamoterol: effects on exercise capacity and symptoms of heart failure. Circulation 1990; 81(suppl III):93.
37. Liu CP, Ting CT, Lawrence W, et al: Diminished contractile response to increased heart rate in intact human left ventricular hypertrophy: systolic versus diastolic determinants. Circulation 1993; 88:1893.

38. Levine HJ: Optimum heart rate of large failing hearts. Am J Cardiol 1988; 61:633.
39. Wright AJA, Hudlicka O, Brown MD: Beneficial effect of chronic bradycardial pacing on capillary growth and heart performance in volume overload heart hypertrophy. Circ Res 1989; 64:1205.
40. Mulieri LA, Hasenfuss G, Leavitt B, et al: Altered myocardial force-frequency relation in human heart failure. Circulation 1992; 85:1743.
41. Gwathmey JK, Warren SE, Briggs M, et al: Diastolic dysfunction in hypertrophic cardiomyopathy: effect on active force generation during systole. J Clin Invest 1991; 87:1023.
42. Anand IS, Ferrari R, Kalra GS, et al: Pathogenesis of edema in constrictive pericarditis: studies of body water and sodium, renal function, hemodynamics, and plasma hormones before and after pericardiectomy. Circulation 1991; 83:1880.
43. Anand IS, Chandrashekhar Y, Ferrari R, et al: Pathogenesis of congestive state in chronic obstructive pulmonary disease: studies of body water and sodium, renal function, hemodynamics, and plasma hormones during edema and after recovery. Circulation 1992; 86:12.
44. Anand IS, Chandrashekhar Y, Ferrari R, et al: Pathogenesis of oedema in chronic severe anemia: studies of body water and sodium, renal function, hemodynamic variables, and plasma hormones. Br Heart J 1993; 70:357.
45. Firth JD, Raine AEG, Ledingham JGG: Raised venous pressure: a direct cause of renal sodium retention in oedema. Lancet 1988; 1:1033.
46. Grossman W: Why is left ventricular diastolic pressure increased during angina pectoris? J Am Coll Cardiol 1985; 5:607.
47. Gilbert J, Glantz S: Determinants of left ventricular filling and of the diastolic pressure-volume relation. Circ Res 1989; 64:827.
48. Paulus WJ, Bronzwaer JGF, de Bruyne B, Grossman W: Different effects of "supply" and "demand" ischemia on left ventricular diastolic function in humans. *In* Gaasch WH, LeWinter MM (eds): Left Ventricular Diastolic Dysfunction and Heart Failure, p 286. Philadelphia: Lea & Febiger, 1994.
49. Kunis R, Greenberg H, Yeoh CG, et al: Coronary revascularization for recurrent pulmonary edema in elderly patients with ischemic heart disease and preserved ventricular function. N Engl J Med 1985; 313:1207.
50. Hoit BD, Walsh RA: Diastolic function in hypertensive heart disease. *In* Gaasch WH, LeWinter MM (eds): Left Ventricular Diastolic Dysfunction and Heart Failure, p 354. Philadelphia: Lea & Febiger, 1994.
51. Inouye I, Massie B, Loge D, et al: Abnormal left ventricular filling: an early finding in mild to moderate systemic hypertension. Am J Cardiol 1984; 53:120.
52. Fouad-Tarazi FM: Ventricular diastolic function of the heart in systemic hypertension. Am J Cardiol 1990; 65:85G.
53. Given BD, Lee TH, Stone PH, et al: Nifedipine in severely hypertensive patients with congestive heart failure and preserved ventricular function. Arch Intern Med 1985; 145:281.
54. Zusman RM: Nifedipine but not propranolol improves left ventricular systolic and diastolic function in patients with hypertension. Am J Cardiol 1989; 64:51F.
55. Smith VE, White WB, Meeran MK, Karimeddini MK: Improved left ventricular filling accompanies reduced left ventricular mass during therapy of essential hypertension. J Am Coll Cardiol 1986; 8:1449.
56. Schulman SP, Weiss JL, Becker LC, et al: The effects of antihypertensive therapy on left ventricular mass in elderly patients. N Engl J Med 1990; 322:1350.
57. Betocchi S, Chiariello M: Effects of antihypertensive therapy on diastolic dysfunction in left ventricular hypertrophy. J Cardiovasc Pharmacol 1992; 19:S116.
58. Weber KT, Brilla CG: Pathological hypertrophy and cardiac interstitium: fibrosis and renin-angiotensin-aldosterone system. Circulation 1991; 83:1849.
59. Weber KT, Sun Y, Guarda E: Structural remodeling in hypertensive heart disease and the role of hormones. Hypertension 1994; 23:869.
60. Wigle ED, Sasson Z, Henderson MA, et al: Hypertrophic cardiomyopathy: the importance of the site and the extent of hypertrophy. Prog Cardiovasc Dis 1985; 28:1.
61. Wigle ED, Wilansky S: Diastolic dysfunction in hypertrophic cardiomyopathy. Heart Failure 1987; 3:82.
62. Wagner JA, Sax FL, Weisman HF, et al: Calcium-antagonist receptors in the atrial tissue of patients with hypertrophic cardiomyopathy. N Engl J Med 1989; 320:755.
63. Udelson JE, Bonow RO: Left ventricular diastolic function and calcium channel blockers in hypertrophic cardiomyopathy. *In* Gaasch WH, Le Winter MM (eds): Left Ventricular Diastolic Dysfunction and Heart Failure, p 465. Philadelphia: Lea & Febiger, 1994.
64. Chatterjee K: Calcium antagonist agents in hypertrophic cardiomyopathy. Am J Cardiol 1987; 59:146B.
65. Maron BJ, Bonow RO, Cannon RO, et al: Hypertrophic cardiomyopathy: interrelationships of clinical manifestations, pathophysiology, and therapy. N Engl J Med 1987; 316:780.
66. McIntosh CL, Maron BJ: Current operative treatment of obstructive hypertrophic cardiomyopathy. Circulation 1988; 78:487.
67. Leachman RD, Krajcer Z, Azic T, Cooley DA: Mitral valve replacement in hypertrophic cardiomyopathy: ten year follow up in 54 patients. Am J Cardiol 1987; 60:1416.
68. Fananapazir L, Cannon RO, Tripodi D, Panza JA: Impact of dual chamber permanent pacing in patients with obstructive hypertrophic cardiomyopathy with symptoms refractory to verapamil and beta adrenergic blocker therapy. Circulation 1992; 85:2149.
69. Cannon RO, Tripodi D, Dilsizian V, et al: Results of permanent dual chamber pacing in symptomatic nonobstructive hypertrophic cardiomyopathy. Am J Cardiol 1994; 73:571.
70. Fananapazir L, Epstein ND, Curiel RV, et al: Long-term results of dual chamber (DDD) pacing in obstructive hypertrophic cardiomyopathy. Circulation 1994; 90:2731.
71. Packer M: Abnormalities of diastolic function as a potential cause of exercise intolerance in chronic heart failure. Circulation 1990; 81(suppl III):78.
72. Chikamori T, Counihan PJ, Doi YL, et al: Mechanisms of exercise limitation in hypertrophic cardiomyopathy. J Am Coll Cardiol 1992; 19:507.
73. Bonow RO: Determinants of exercise capacity in hypertrophic cardiomyopathy. J Am Coll Cardiol 1992; 19:513.
74. Rosing DR, Kent KM, Maron BJ, Epstein SE: Verapamil therapy: a new approach to the pharmacologic treatment of hypertrophic cardiomyopathy. II. Effects on exercise capacity and symptomatic status. Circulation 1979; 60:1208.
75. Wei JY: Age and the cardiovascular system. N Engl J Med 1992; 327:1735.
76. Warren SE, Cohn LH, Schoen FJ, et al: Advanced diastolic heart failure in familial hypertrophic cardiomyopathy managed with cardiac transplantation. J Appl Cardiol 1988; 3:415.

14 Treatment of Myocarditis

Kenneth L. Baughman, MD
Ralph H. Hruban, MD

One of the most challenging areas of cardiology is the diagnosis and treatment of myocarditis. Myocarditis is rare, its pathophysiologic mechanism is not understood, there is no diagnostic "gold standard," and all currently available treatments are considered controversial. Nonetheless, myocarditis is an exceedingly important cause of heart muscle disease. Whereas many patients with myocarditis have a subclinical, benign course, the disease may cause supraventricular or ventricular arrhythmias, sudden death, or fulminant acute left ventricular dysfunction. Furthermore, progressive myocardial damage and myocarditis may account for up to 40% of patients in whom a dilated cardiomyopathy ultimately develops.

Myocarditis can be classified as either primary or secondary (Table 14–1). Primary myocarditis is believed to be the result of viral and postviral immunologic effects on the heart. Secondary myocarditis is myocardial inflammation caused by a known agent. For patients with secondary myocarditis, treatment of the causative agent frequently resolves the myocardial inflammation. This chapter concentrates on the treatment of *primary* myocarditis.

PATHOPHYSIOLOGY

The first link between viral infection and heart disease was reported in the late 1800s, when cardiac symptoms in patients with mumps were reported.[1] In 1929, Lucke described the postmortem findings of myocarditis in patients dying of epidemic influenza.[2] The first report of enterovirus and associated myocarditis was by Saphir,[3] who described the postmortem findings of myocarditis in patients dying with poliomyelitis. Enteroviruses were widely recognized in the 1950s and 1960s as the most frequent cause of myocarditis.[4] Approximately 70 serotypes of enterovirus have been associated with human heart disease. These have been confirmed by (1) isolation of the virus directly from cardiac tissue; (2) isolation of a virus during the acute illness (particularly in neonates) from the nasal passageways, oropharynx, or stool; or (3) demonstration of a fourfold increase in convalescent immunoglobulin titers to a specific viral agent in patients with documented myocardial inflammation. It is now believed that enteroviruses are responsible for more than 50% of the cases of documented myocarditis. Enteroviruses, single-stranded RNA viruses that lack an envelope, are capable of causing myocarditis and include the following, in descending order of frequency: coxsackie B, coxsackie A, echovirus, poliovirus, adenovirus, cytomegalovirus, influenza A and B, rubella, rubeola, mumps, hepatitis A and B, varicella zoster, rabies, and lymphocytic choriomeningitis. During endemic viral infections, cardiac disease develops in approximately 5% of patients with a systemic viral illness, and cardiac manifestations may develop in as many as 12% of viremic patients during epidemic intervals.

TABLE 14–1. PRIMARY AND SECONDARY CAUSES OF MYOCARDITIS

Cause of Myocarditis	Examples
Rickettsial	Rocky Mountain spotted fever
	Scrub typhus
Bacterial	Diphtheria
	Salmonellosis
	Tuberculosis
Spirochetal	Syphilis
Fungal	Aspergillosis
	Blastomycosis
	Candidiasis
	Histoplasmosis
Protozoal	Trypanosomiasis
	Toxoplasmosis
Drugs	Cocaine
	Lithium
	Catecholamines
	Doxorubicin hypersensitivity
Chemicals	Lead
	Arsenic
	Carbon monoxide
Physical agents	Radiation therapy
	Hyperthermia and hypothermia
Other	Systemic lupus erythematosus
	Connective tissue disease
	Sarcoidosis
	Kawasaki syndrome

Phases of Infection

Viral infection of the heart and subsequent immune damage progress through several distinct phases typical of any infection.[4–6]

Phase I. Phase I is characterized by a direct viral invasion of myocardial cells. The virus initially attaches to the myocyte by specific viral receptors on the cell surface and subsequently enters the myocyte. Viral replication proceeds within the myocardial cell, which diminishes the intrinsic DNA, RNA, and cell protein production, resulting in cell damage and loss of contractility within 1 to 2 days. During this early phase of viral infection, there may be destruction of myofibers and filaments as well as the appearance of viral vesicles within the cell. Thus, during the initial phase, there is viral infection of cardiac myocytes, subclinical injury to the myocytes, and release of a variety of previously sequestered myocyte antigens into the circulation.

Phase II. Phase II of postviral myocarditis is characterized by an inflammatory response to the viral cellular invasion. Depending on the cause of the myocarditis, the primary inflammatory cells may be lymphocytes, macrophages, polymorphonuclear leukocytes, or eosinophils. This acute cellular inflammation results in myocyte dysfunction.

Phase III. Phase III of the postviral response is the development of a specific T cell response.

Role of Antigen Presenting Cells

Some of the myocyte antigens shed during the acute infection of myocytes are taken up by antigen presenting cells (APCs), including macrophages and dendritic cells. These APCs then process the antigens as they would a foreign antigen and present peptide fragments derived from these antigens to $CD4^+$ T helper cells. These antigens are then presented on the surface of the APCs in conjunction with class II major histocompatibility complex (MHC) antigens; in some patients, $CD4^+$ T helper cells recognize this peptide–class II antigen complex as foreign, triggering an immune response. Thus, the release of previously sequestered myocardial antigens during the acute phase of viral infection can lead to the triggering of an immune reaction. Alternatively, in a process termed *molecular mimicry,* viral antigens expressed during the acute infection may share immune determinants with normal myocyte proteins, and the immune system, in mounting an immune response to the viral antigen, also mounts an immune response to cross-reacting myocyte protein.

Cytokine Response

Once antigen presented by APCs has activated T helper cells, the activated lymphocytes release a variety of cytokines, which in turn activate the effector mechanisms responsible for further myocyte injury. For example, T_H2 cells release interleukin (IL)–4 and IL-5, which stimulate B cell maturation into plasma cells, resulting in the development of a humoral (antibody-mediated) response. T_H1 T helper cells release IL-2, interferon-gamma, and tumor necrosis factor-beta (TNF-β), which activate $CD8^+$ cytotoxic T cells and macrophages.

Activated T Cell Response

Activated $CD8^+$ cytotoxic T cells can bind to peptide–class I MHC complexes on myocytes and injure the myocytes directly by a variety of processes, including granule exocytosis. In contrast, macrophages activated within the myocardium will locally release a variety of factors, such as tumor necrosis factor-alpha (TNF-α), acid hydrolases, and hydrogen peroxide, which will nonspecifically injure myocytes. Thus, regardless of which mechanism actually triggers the immune response in a given patient with myocarditis, the important points to remember are (1) that the injury to the myocardium can take place after most of the virus has been cleared from the heart, (2) that the primary injury to the heart is immunologic, and (3) that a variety of different immune mediators, including both cellular and humoral immunity, play a role in the development of myocarditis.

Vascular Reaction

A vascular reaction is also associated with phase III.[4] Enteroviruses infect endothelial as well as myocyte cells, and anti–endothelial cell and adhesion molecule (specifically intercellular adhesion molecule [ICAM]) antibodies can be identified in patients suffering from viral myocarditis. The initial vascular infection and subsequent immunologic response with its associated free radical generation and calcium overload may result in diffuse small-vessel vasculitis and vascular spasm. These abnormalities may result in focal coronary insufficiency contributing to the myocardial necrosis and fibrosis seen with ongoing myocarditis.

Viral Persistence

Whereas it was previously presumed that the immune response successfully cleared the myocardium of the offending viral agent and that the subsequent myocardial damage was due to the ongoing immune or autoimmune response to the initial viral infection, there is increasing evidence that not all of the virus may be cleared from the heart.[7–10] The virus may persist in small quantity, hidden in areas of fibrosis, necrosis, and mononuclear cell reaction. This viral persistence may result in continued antigen or neoantigen production, triggering some patients into a persistent immune response and ongoing myocardial damage.

Variability of Clinical Response to Viral Myocarditis

Although the pathophysiologic process seems clear-cut, descriptions of the human condition of myocarditis vary dramatically. Animal models of myocarditis have demonstrated that this variation is probably due to differences in the infecting virus and in the host immune response, which may be inferenced by variables such as gender, age, and pregnancy. In a mouse model, coxsackie B_3 causes a severe myocarditis with a high mortality rate. Coxsackie A_9 in the same animal model causes only a self-limited myocarditis with no residua.[11–13] Encephalomyocarditis in some mouse species results in a dilated cardiomyopathy with a chronic active myocardial inflammatory infiltrate.[14] Therefore, the differences in presentation seen in human patients may be due to differences in the viral agent infecting them. In addition, animal models indicate that males respond with somewhat greater T cell proliferation than females do, that very young and very old are more susceptible to infection, and that pregnancy enhances the capability for viral infection. These variations in viral etiology and host response probably account for the dramatic variation in the presentation of patients with myocarditis and in their response to treatment.

CLINICAL PRESENTATION

Symptoms

Most patients with myocarditis have a history of an acute viral illness. Symptoms include fever, chills, coryza, and constitutional symptoms. Patients with myalgias, palpitations, and symptoms of pericarditis as part of their initial illness are more likely to develop symptomatic myocarditis. In adults, there is usually a delay between the initial viral illness and the onset of symptoms of heart muscle disease. This delay is dependent on the viral etiology and host response variations noted before. In contrast, children often present with symptoms of severe myocardial dysfunction and acute viral illness simultaneously. Adults with fulminant acute myocarditis display the least delay between viral illness and myocarditis and have profound left ventricular dysfunction between 1 and 3 weeks after the initial viral illness. Patients with other clinicopathologic varieties of myocarditis have an insidious onset of myocardial infection and associated myocardial dysfunction occurring weeks to months after their initial illness. The apparent timing of the preceding viral illness is often confused owing to the patient's physician misinterpreting the symptoms of acute left ventricular dysfunction, such as a persistent nonproductive cough, as being caused by the viral illness itself. Pediatric and adult patients virtually always present with evidence of congestive heart failure including exertional weakness and fatigability, shortness of breath, orthopnea, paroxysmal nocturnal dyspnea, and occasionally right-sided congestive heart failure.

Rarely, patients may present with embolic phenomenon, and there is evidence to suggest that patients with acute myocarditis are predisposed to ventricular thrombosis. Patients with myocarditis may also present with sudden death. Burke and colleagues[15] evaluated sports-related and non–sports-related sudden deaths in subjects 14–40 years of age and found that 6% of the patients with sports-related deaths had myocarditis and 4.5% of the patients with non–sports-related deaths had myocardial inflammation. Myocarditis may also account for nonsustained ventricular tachycardia. A number of investigators[16–18] have documented that up to 50% of patients with no other cause of ventricular tachycardia after full cardiac evaluation may have myocarditis on endomyocardial biopsy, which presumably accounts for their arrhythmia.

Physical Examination

Physical examination may be normal or reveal jugular venous distention, hepatic engorgement, and edema if the inflammatory process involves both ventricles or if the left ventricular dysfunction is so severe as to cause right ventricular compromise. The patients may be in profound cardiogenic shock, but even less severely affected patients display some evidence of decreased forward cardiac output. The lungs may show evidence of congestion, depending on the degree of compromise of the heart and associated elevation of end-diastolic pressure. The first heart sound is usually diminished because of decreased myocardial contractility. The second heart sound is characterized by a narrowed split or, occasionally, a paradoxical splitting due to depressed left ventricular contraction. A loud pulmonic component of the second sound is present if there is pulmonary hypertension. S_3 gallop rhythms are common, as are murmurs of mitral and tricuspid regurgitation, if there is sufficient ventricular dilatation. A pericardial friction rub may be present but is unusual.

Laboratory Tests

The electrocardiogram may display supraventricular or ventricular arrhythmias. There are virtually always nonspecific ST-T wave abnormalities, and a pseudoinfarct pattern has been reported in some patients. Chest radiography shows variable heart size with or without congestive heart failure. Echocardiography usually demonstrates evidence of left ventricular compromise. The more acute the patient's presentation, the more likely it is that the left ventricle will be of normal or nearly normal size and that it will have thickened left ventricular walls, presumably because of associated myocardial edema. Patients farther in time from acute onset may have a pattern typical of a dilated cardiomyopathy with thin walls, enlarged chambers, and reduced activity.

CRITERIA FOR THE DIAGNOSIS OF MYOCARDITIS

Attempts should be made to isolate a viral pathogen in patients presenting with an acute viral myocarditis. This includes culturing the nasopharynx, oropharynx, stool, and blood. Acute and convalescent titers for viral pathogens have been used as an indication of the etiology of an acute viral illness. Although both culture and acute and convalescent titers may be of some assistance in determining the most likely cause of myocarditis, these tests do not establish the diagnosis of myocarditis but rather suggest an acute viral illness that may or may not be associated with myocardial inflammation.

Noninvasive Studies

Noninvasive nuclear scans have been evaluated in patients with presumed acute myocarditis. Gallium is a bone scan radioisotope that has an affinity for tumors and inflammation. O'Connell and coworkers[19] reported a sensitivity of only 36% with this technique but a specificity of 98% in a group of patients with preserved myocarditis. Patients with positive gallium scan responses treated with immunosuppressive agents and demonstrating decreased gallium uptake also had an improvement in ejection fraction and survival compared with those who failed to improve.[20] Antimyosin is a radiolabeled Fab fragment that attaches to exposed myosin in any condition that interrupts integrity of the cell membrane of the myocyte. Because myocarditis is associated with myocyte disruption that may expose myosin, this agent may be useful for the noninvasive detection of myocardial inflammation. Dec and colleagues[21] reported that this technique has a sensitivity of 83%, specificity of 53%, and predictive value of 92%. Scans may be of some benefit to select patients appropriate for endomyocardial biopsy; however, a relatively high false-negative rate with both gallium and antimyosin has been demonstrated compared with endomyocardial biopsy.[22]

Light Microscopic Studies

Myocarditis is a histologic diagnosis. Before 1986, even the histologic criteria for establishing this diagnosis were ill defined, resulting in dramatic variations in the incidence of "myocarditis" demonstrated in patients with new left ventricular dysfunction submitted to endomyocardial biopsy. A group of distinguished cardiac pathologists met in 1984 to resolve this issue and in 1986 published what have been termed the Dallas criteria (Table 14–2), so named for the site of their meeting.[23] The criteria for establishing the diagnosis of myocarditis and borderline myocarditis are stated later.

The inflammatory infiltrate should be subclassified as lymphocytic, eosinophilic, neutrophilic, giant cell, granulomatous, or mixed. The amount of inflammatory infiltrate and its distribution should be described as mild, moderate, or severe and focal, confluent, or diffuse, respectively. The amount and distribution of fibrosis, if present, can be described similarly and should also be characterized as endocardial, replacement, or interstitial.

The diagnosis of myocarditis requires evidence of myocyte damage associated with an inflammatory cell infiltrate not typical of that seen with the other causes of cell death, such as ischemia. Borderline myocarditis lacks the histologic changes of myocyte damage but does require a significant inflammatory cell infiltrate. Despite these criteria, there remains significant interobserver and intraobserver variability. The diagnosis of myocarditis is highly dependent on a qualified cardiac pathologist who has experience in reviewing cardiac tissue. The appearance of myocyte damage may appear artifactually, caused by crush, tear, or fixation changes. In addition, endothelial cells, fibrocytes, and tissue histiocytes can mimic inflammatory cells. Immunohistochemical staining of the tissue sections to characterize the cells that are present in the biopsy sample enhances the diagnostic sensitivity of the endomyocardial biopsy. Finally, Tazelaar and Billingham[24] reported that 87% of patients with end-stage dilated cardiomyopathy at the time of transplantation have an average of 6.2 lymphocytes per high-power field. This makes the distinction between myocarditis and cardiomyopathy even more of a problem in patients with advanced ventricular dysfunction.

Endomyocardial Biopsy: Sensitivity and Specificity

The tissue for establishing the histologic diagnosis is acquired by endomyocardial biopsy. This technique has evolved, and it can now be performed percutaneously on an outpatient basis. Performance of endomyocardial biopsy is associated with an approximately 6% risk of complications.[25] Of these complications, 45% are associated with the insertion of the venous cannula and encompass complications

TABLE 14–2. THE DALLAS CRITERIA FOR THE DIAGNOSIS OF MYOCARDITIS

Definition

An inflammatory infiltrate of the myocardium with necrosis and/or degeneration of adjacent myocytes not typical of the ischemic damage associated with coronary artery disease

Classification

Myocarditis, with or without fibrosis
Borderline myocarditis (repeated biopsy may be indicated)
No myocarditis

such as carotid artery or femoral artery puncture, vasovagal reaction, bleeding, pneumothorax, or neurovascular damage. The remaining 55% of complications occur during the biopsy itself, and of these, only myocardial perforation with pericardial tamponade is life-threatening. The authors have documented two deaths as a result of perforation in more than 6000 endomyocardial biopsies at their institution.

Although endomyocardial biopsy with histopathologic demonstration of myocarditis is the gold standard for establishing the diagnosis of myocarditis, the biopsy is relatively insensitive. Using autopsy specimens of patients dying of myocarditis from a number of primary and secondary causes, Chow[26] and Hauck[27] and coworkers evaluated the sensitivity of endomyocardial biopsies. Each independent endomyocardial sample had only a 17%–28% chance of demonstrating myocarditis. Overall, even with multiple biopsies, the diagnosis of myocarditis could be established in only 63%–64% of patients. This often required a large number of specimens, which is impractical. Hauck and colleagues[27] reported a false-negative biopsy rate of 83% with one specimen, 55% with five specimens, and 37% with ten specimens. Although including patients with borderline myocarditis would increase the odds of making a histologic diagnosis, it is evident from these postmortem studies that myocarditis often involves the epimyocardial and midmyocardial wall and is not accessible to the endomyocardial biopsy.

Tissue Immunologic Studies

Immunopathologic staining may assist in the diagnosis of myocarditis by confirming that mononuclear cells are lymphocytic in origin. Fresh-frozen tissue can be stained for the presence of immunoglobulin or complement, and the deposit of either of these or cardiac myocytes supports the diagnosis of immune injury to the heart. Similarly, fresh-frozen tissue can be stained for MHC antigens.[28] Myocarditis is often associated with the induction of MHC antigens on cardiac myocytes. Despite the use of immunopathologic analysis and determination of MHC expression, myocarditis is a focal process, and even endomyocardial biopsy is an imperfect gold standard for diagnosing this condition.

Electron Microscopy

Electron microscopy of endomyocardial biopsy specimens is of no benefit, because viral pathogens are frequently indistinguishable from the normally appearing ribosomes in their density and size. Viral isolation is also virtually impossible, except in the acute phases of illness.

Serum Antibodies

Enterovirus-specific immunoglobulin M (IgM) antibodies have been developed.[29] The presence of these antibodies, particularly in high titer, may imply a significant and/or ongoing exposure to enteroviruses. Seventeen percent of blood donors have been found to be antibody positive, whereas 36% of those with acute pericarditis and 48% of those with aseptic meningitis display the enterovirus IgM in high titer. Approximately one third of patients with dilated cardiomyopathy are antibody positive, whereas 64% of those with chronic relapsing pericarditis have high IgM antibody titers in a 1- to 10-year interval.

Molecular Approaches

Because it has been difficult to demonstrate myocardial inflammation and myocyte necrosis by endomyocardial biopsy, a multitude of investigators have attempted to identify the virus itself with molecular biologic techniques. In 1985, Zahringer first reported viral signal in mouse heart muscle after a neoviral infection by molecular hybridization.[6] Kandolf and associates[7] in 1987 isolated enteroviral genome in human tissue by in situ hybridization. Bowles and coworkers[8] reported coxsackie B virus–specific RNA sequences in approximately 41% of patients with healed myocarditis or dilated cardiomyopathy. They subsequently found a persistent virus in 6 of 21 patients with dilated cardiomyopathy, compared with 1 of 19 patients with ischemic cardiomyopathy, at the time of heart transplantation. More important, there was no correlation between the presence of virus and evidence of inflammatory heart disease. It was subsequently demonstrated that this technique had a high degree of cross-reactivity with normal myocardial cellular constituents, and the concept of viral persistence in the myocardium was called into question.

Subsequently, more sensitive and specific polymerase chain reaction (PCR)–based studies have been performed. These techniques allow a minute quantity of a specific nucleic acid sequence to be detected after extensive selective amplification. This technique is ideal for the analysis of endomyocardial biopsy specimens because low copy numbers of viral genes can be detected in small pieces of tissue. Whereas cDNA probe techniques reported a frequency of viral persistence of 29%–46% in patients with dilated cardiomyopathy and 47% in patients with myocarditis compared with 0%–5% in control subjects, PCR techniques report the frequency to be 0%–15% for dilated cardiomyopathy, 7% to 22% for myocarditis, and 0%–17% for control subjects.[9] Clearly, sample heterogeneity and the focal nature of this illness may limit the capability of the molecular as well as the histologic techniques noted before.

In situ hybridization is an attractive molecular method of detecting viral sequences because the tissue is intact and one can identify which cells hybridize to the probe.[10] These techniques have been used to demonstrate that persistent viral genome is present not only in the cardiac muscle cells but also in the adventitia of blood cells. Furthermore, work by Kandolf[10] has suggested that in some patients, the virus is capable of myocyte-to-myocyte transfer. Most investigators now agree that small quantities of viral genome may persist in some patients with or after myocarditis and that viral persistence is usually found in areas of fibrosis or inflammation.

The importance of diagnosing myocarditis histologically cannot be overstated, despite the problems noted, because the history, physical examination findings, and other laboratory data to suggest the condition are even less specific than the biopsy results.

CLINICAL CLASSIFICATION

Several attempts have been made to classify the histopathologic features and clinical course of patients with biopsy-proven myocarditis. Fenoglio and coworkers[30] retrospectively documented myocarditis in 34 of 135 patients submitted to endomyocardial biopsy. Only one endomyocardial biopsy sample was submitted to histologic examination, and this work was published before the Dallas criteria were established. Fenoglio described three categories of myocarditis: acute, rapidly progressive, and chronic myocarditis. Patients in the *acute* category had a short duration of illness of less than 2 months and had extensive cellular damage with little evidence of healing and limited fibrosis. Five of these seven patients were dead within 8 weeks, including four of five treated with immunosuppressive agents. The *rapidly progressive* group had an illness of approximately 2 years' duration and displayed limited acute inflammation but marked healing and fibrosis. Seventeen of these patients died within 2 years; none of the seven treated patients responded to immunosuppressive therapy. Nine patients with *chronic* symptoms of more than 3 years' duration and focal inflammation, healing, and fibrosis remained alive; four of the nine improved with immunosuppressives.

Dec and colleagues[31] found pre–Dallas criteria myocarditis in 27 of 179 patients evaluated with symptoms of heart failure of less than 6 months' duration. The frequency of myocarditis was 89% in the patients who had been ill for less than 4 weeks. Diffuse and focal areas of myocyte inflammation and necrosis were described; however, the histology correlated poorly with outcome. The rate of spontaneous improvement was approximately 40%, regardless of the presence of myocarditis, and the rate of improvement with immunosuppressive therapy was no different from the rate of spontaneous improvement (44% vs. 33%).

Lieberman and coworkers[32] reported Dallas criteria myocarditis in 35 of 348 consecutive patients (10%) undergoing endomyocardial biopsy at The Johns Hopkins Hospital for the new onset of heart failure. Patients with secondary myocarditis were excluded; there was a high proportion of follow-up biopsies; and patients, if treated with immunosuppressives, followed a standard regimen. Four clinicopathologic categories were established (Fig. 14–1). Four patients displayed fulminant myocarditis. Like Fenoglio's group, these patients had an abrupt onset of congestive heart failure shortly after a preceding viral illness, profound left ventricular dysfunction without dilatation, and dramatically positive biopsy results for myocyte necrosis and inflammatory cells, and they either died or improved spontaneously within 2 weeks. Twenty-six patients had acute myocarditis. These patients had a more insidious onset of left ventricular compromise weeks after a presumed viral illness. Patients had modest left ventricular dilatation and biopsy findings that were much less dramatic than those in the fulminant category. These patients improved mildly or progressed to a severe dilated cardiomyopathy. Chronic active myocarditis was found in three patients. These patients had an onset similar to that of patients with acute myocarditis. Unfortunately, these patients had recurrent episodes of symptomatic deterioration associated with increasing fibrosis and giant-cell formation on follow-up biopsy. This group went on to develop a mildly dilated restrictive cardiomyopathy in a period of several months. Two patients with chronic persistent myocarditis were described. These patients had normal ventricular function despite evidence on repeated biopsies of myocardial inflammation with or without myocyte necrosis. Despite normal ventricular function, these patients displayed cardiac symptoms, including palpitations and chest pain.

The marked variability in clinical presentation demonstrated in these series of biopsy-proven myocarditis may reflect alterations in viral pathogen, viral strain, or host response. Unfortunately, these important issues are not yet answerable.

EVALUATION OF THE PATIENT (Fig. 14–2)

As noted in the preceding section, patients with myocarditis may present with a variety of manifestations, the most common of which is cardiac dysfunction with the new onset of congestive heart failure. Patients may also, however, present with pericarditis, symptomatic arrhythmia, sudden death, or embolic events. Children and some adult patients with fulminant myocarditis may present with viral symptoms at the same time as their cardiac manifestations.

A complete history should be taken, not only as it relates to the current illness, but to investigate other potential causes of cardiac dysfunction, including preceding heart murmurs, toxin exposure, alcohol and/or drug use, or other medical conditions that cause cardiac muscle weakness. Risk factors for coronary atherosclerosis, including hypertension, diabetes, cholesterol abnormalities, family history of premature atherosclerosis or cardiomyopathy, and smoking, should be sought. It should be recalled that perhaps 10% of all patients with cardiomyopathy have a family history of familial-related cardiomyopathy. In addition, the duration of symptoms should be investigated. The biopsy will have the highest yield of identifying treatable heart dysfunction in patients with heart failure less than 6 months in duration. The true onset of the patient's illness can often be determined by inquiring as to whether the patient was ever told that he or she had a large heart and by investigating the onset of early symptoms of heart failure that may have been termed "bronchitis."

The physical examination should concentrate on signs of left and/or right ventricular heart failure. Patients should also be evaluated for ongoing evidence of viral infection, including examination of the eyes, nasopharynx, throat, skin, and lymph nodes. Finally, features of other causes of cardiomyopathy should be sought, including evidence of drug use, vitamin deficiency, or endocrinopathy.

An *electrocardiogram* should be obtained on all patients. This may display evidence of a clear-cut myocardial infarction. Often, patients with heart dysfunction and cardiomyopathies have "pseudoinfarct" patterns of poor R wave progression or nonspecific axis deviation and Q wave appearance. Evidence of left ventricular hypertrophy or left atrial abnormality may suggest that the illness has been longer standing and may imply hypertension as an etiologic factor. Supraventricular or ventricular arrhythmias may be diagnosed with a routine electrocardiogram. *Chest radiography* should be performed to determine heart size, the severity of pulmonary congestion, and other causes of heart failure suggested by aortic valve, mitral valve, or pericardial calcification. *Laboratory analysis* includes routine hematologic and chemistry studies. These rarely provide an indication of the cause of the patient's left ventricular compromise but help assess its severity in terms of renal and liver congestion and underperfusion. In patients with severe anemia, leukemia, or myeloma, these diagnoses may be "discovered" by such screening studies. The authors do not routinely obtain *viral titers* on patients, because the collection of acute and viral titers is costly, is time consuming, and rarely defines etiology in time to be of any benefit to the patient. They do obtain an *antinuclear antibody* on all patients to rule out connective tissue disorders. They also obtain *thyroid-stimulating hormone* levels and *urinary vanillylmandelic acid* levels to rule out endocrinopathy-related heart dysfunction.

Echocardiography should be done on all patients with suspected myocarditis. This allows physicians to determine cardiac chamber size and the degree of ventricular dysfunction. It also allows physicians to determine segmental and nonsegmental cardiac involvement, identifies patients with significant valvular abnormalities, and allows clinicians to absolutely quantitate the presence and severity of peri-

MYOCARDITIS

	Fulminant	Acute	Chronic Active	Chronic Persistent
Onset	Distinct	Indistinct	Indistinct	Indistinct
LV dysfunction	Severe	Moderate	Moderate	None
Biopsy	Multiple foci active	Active or borderline	Active or borderline	Active or borderline
Clinical history	Complete recovery or death	Incomplete recovery or dilated CM	Mildly dilated CM	Normal LV, non-CHF symptoms
Histologic history	Complete resolution	Complete resolution	Ongoing fibrosis giant cells	Ongoing

Figure 14–1. Pathophysiologic classification of myocarditis.

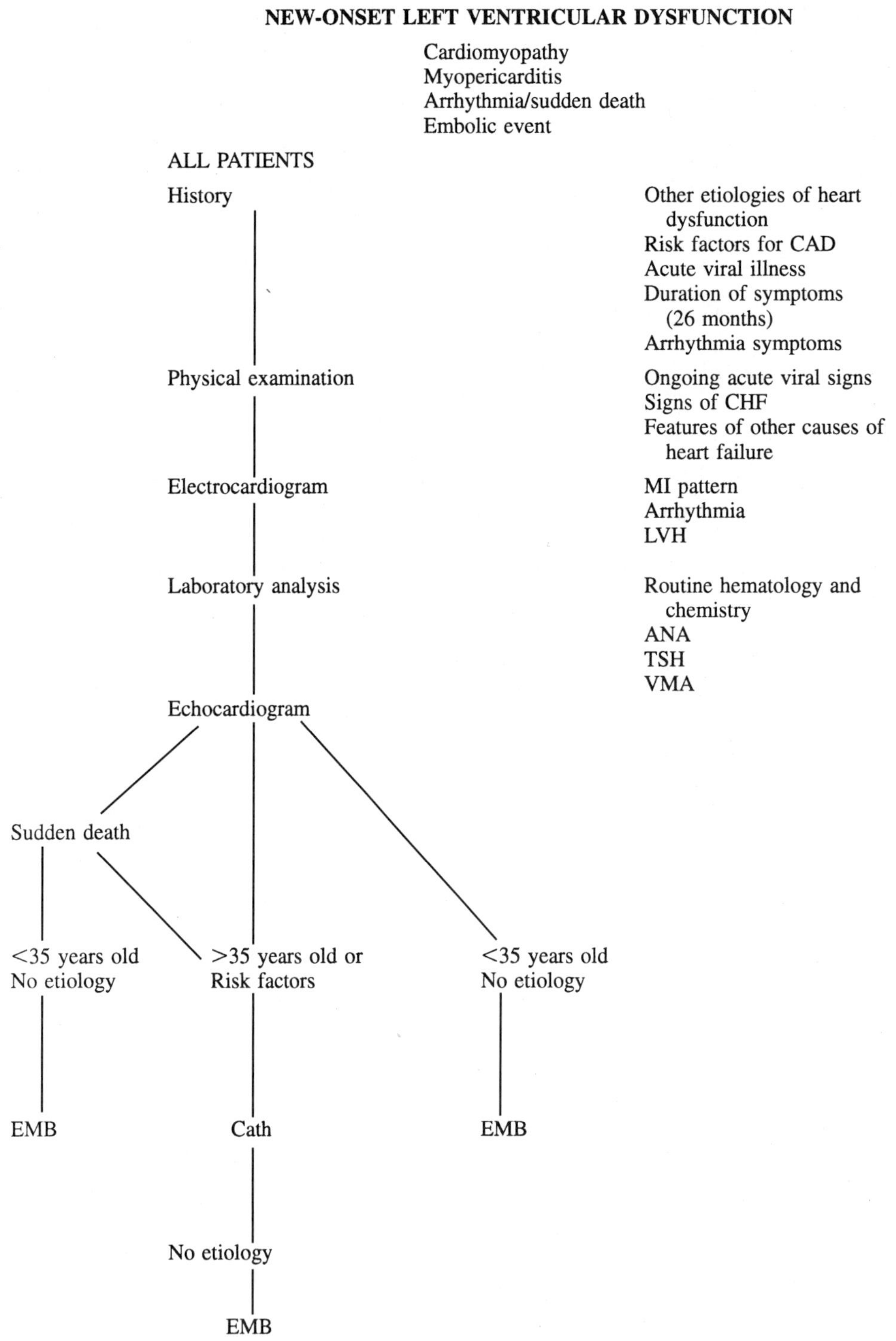

Figure 14–2. Approach to the evaluation of patients presenting with the onset of left ventricular dysfunction and suspected myocarditis.

cardial effusions. In our experience, patients with more acute forms of myocarditis have less dilated, more thickened, yet hypofunctional hearts. Patients should also be evaluated for valvular abnormalities including critical aortic stenosis and significant aortic and mitral regurgitation.

If patients present with sudden death or syncope, the authors routinely proceed with *electrophysiologic study.* The endocardial electrodes from electrophysiologic studies may result in some focal endocardial damage, making interpretation of a subsequent heart biopsy more difficult. Therefore, whenever possible, the endomyocardial biopsy should be performed before electrophysiologic study.

Coronary angiography should be performed in patients with evidence of infarction by electrocardiogram and who are older than 35 years or younger than 35 years but with multiple risk factors for coronary atherosclerosis. The authors prefer to perform endomyocardial biopsy before coronary angiography, particularly in patients who are at high risk for dye exposure, such as those with renal insufficiency, diabetes, or persistent left ventricular failure. These patients may have ischemic cardiomyopathy diagnosed by endomyocardial biopsy.

EXPERIMENTAL OBSERVATIONS ON TREATMENT
(Table 14–3)

Antiviral Agents

Currently, there are no clinically acceptable antiviral drugs for the enterovirus agents that cause most cases of primary myocarditis. Ribavirin is a broad-spectrum antiviral agent that inhibits RNA polymerase.[33] This agent has been effective in encephalomyocarditis models of myocarditis, even when it is given 4 days after infection. Unfortunately, the doses necessary to be effective in humans have thus far proved to be toxic. Disoxaril is another antiviral agent that prevents viral encoding.[34] This agent also is not currently available for clinical use. Unless there is evidence that the myocarditis is due to cytomegalovirus, ganciclovir or acyclovir would be ineffective. Similarly, immunization to prevent myocarditis is impossible because of the large number of potential etiologic agents.

Immunosuppressive Agents

Because most cases of myocarditis are believed to be caused by an immune reaction in the absence of significant numbers of viral particles, immunosuppressive agents have received the most attention in the quest to find an effective agent to treat myocarditis. Agents that have been investigated include prednisone (a diffuse suppressant of cytokines and inflammatory necrosis), cyclosporine (a depressor of IL-2 production and receptor expression), and azathioprine (alters purine metabolism). In general, immunosuppressive agents that decrease CD4 and CD8 cell populations tend to decrease the intensity of the myocarditis, whereas agents that diminish natural killer cells increase inflammation and viral production. Although there is some species and immunosuppressive agent variability, animal studies have failed to demonstrate significant changes in mortality, histopathology, or viral production when immunosuppressive agents are given before, coincident with, or after an infectious viral agent.[35] Immunosuppressive agents may acutely increase viral replication and/or allow a virus to persist longer in some animal models. There is evidence that nonspecific immunosuppressive agents like prednisone may benefit antigen (myosin)–induced myocarditis, which may imply some benefit for animals or humans with immune rather than infectious myocardial inflammation.[13, 36]

Immunosuppressive agents have been used in patients with myocarditis. The rationale for the use of these agents has been based primarily on the histopathologic similarities between myocarditis and cardiac rejection after transplantation. Clearly, there must be significant differences because myocarditis demonstrates patchy, limited myocardial necrosis and inflammation with profound ventricular compromise, whereas cardiac rejection often demonstrates severe lymphocytic infiltration and myocyte necrosis with nearly normal cardiac function. In 1984, Kereiakes and Parmley[37] reported the results of treating 82 cases of biopsy-proven (non–Dallas criteria) myocarditis with prednisone or a combination of prednisone and azathioprine. Overall, 49 of 82 patients (60%) demonstrated some improvement. Of note, however, only 1 of 21 patients (5%) improved if there was acute or rapidly progressive myocarditis by biopsy. This contrasts with 20 of 22 patients (91%) who improved with chronic myocarditis. More recent experience, including the authors', confirms that adult patients with fulminant myocarditis respond poorly to immunosuppressive therapy, whereas in most patients with fulminant myocarditis who receive heart failure support but not immunosuppressive therapy, a dramatic recovery may occur in a short time. However, these observations are anecdotal.

There are numerous case reports concerning the management of adult and pediatric patients with fulminant myocarditis.[38–47] All of these series have documented children or young adults with preceding or ongoing viral illnesses presenting abruptly with profound congestive heart failure and profound myocardial dysfunction with only minimal cardiac dilatation. These patients meet the criteria for fulminant myocarditis as proposed by Lieberman and coworkers.[32] Some of these reports attribute the dramatic improvements in their patients' ventricular function in a short period to corticosteroids or OKT-3 (a monoclonal antibody to CD3 surface antigens of T lymphocytes). In these reports, patients received standard medical therapy and, in most cases, pressor agents, such as dopamine, dobutamine, norepinephrine, or amrinone. A high proportion of these patients were also supported with extracorporeal membrane oxygenation or left ventricular assist device.[42–47] All reported patients had improvement, if not normalization, of ventricular function within 1 week of the institution of therapy. The rate of improvement in ventricular performance is much greater than one would anticipate from the use of immunosuppressive agents, and it is likely that these patients recovered spontaneously. These series support the use of aggressive management of left ventricular compromise and the use of afterload, preload, and assist device therapy to limit the mechanical strain on the inflamed myocardium to prevent distention during this period of "plasticity."

The prospective, randomized, immunosuppressive vs. placebo-controlled National Institutes of Health–supported trial of the treatment of myocarditis is complete.[48] More than 2000 patients with possible myocarditis were submitted for inclusion; however, only 200 patients had acceptable histopathology. Of these, only 111 were randomized, because others either had a return of ventricular function to nearly normal or refused to participate. One of the treatment arms (prednisone and azathioprine) was eliminated because of low enrollment, which ultimately resulted in a treatment cohort of 64 patients (prednisone and cyclosporine) and a control cohort of 47 subjects. It has generally been presumed that treatment demonstrated no significant improvement in ventricular performance or survival; however, no primary results have been published to this date.[48, 49]

Jones and colleagues[50] described 20 patients with Dallas criteria myocarditis (9 myocarditis and 11 borderline myocarditis). All patients with myocarditis or borderline myocarditis were treated with prednisone (1 mg/kg/day) and azathioprine (1.5 mg/kg/day) for 6 to 8 weeks, at which time repeated biopsy was performed followed by a tapering dose of prednisone for another 6- to 8-week interval. Patients with a borderline myocarditis had greater improvement as determined by left ventricular stroke work index/end-diastolic volume ratio, heart rate–corrected circumferential fiber shortening, left ventricular ejection fraction, and left ventricular size compared with patients with acute myocarditis. These data support previous observations suggesting that patients with chronic disease are more responsive to therapy than are those with an acute course.

Parillo and associates[51] randomized 102 patients with established dilated cardiomyopathy without myocarditis to prednisone or stan-

TABLE 14–3. POTENTIAL APPROACHES TO THE TREATMENT OF MYOCARDITIS

- Immune regulation
  - Immune suppression
  - Immune absorption
  - Immune stimulation
- Cytokine regulation
  - Interleukin-1
  - Interleukin-2
  - Tumor necrosis factor-alpha
- Interferon
- Immunoglobulin administration
- Antivirals
- Calcium channel blockade

dard therapy. At 3 months, there was a transient improvement in ejection fraction of .055 in the prednisone-treated group compared with an increase of .023 in the placebo group. In addition, 67% of patients with "reactive" features (increased erythrocyte sedimentation rate, positive gallium scan response, biopsy with immunoglobulin or inflammatory/fibroblastic biopsy) improved their ejection fraction by .05 compared with 28% of "nonreactive" control subjects. However, this improvement was not sustained, and the ejection fractions diminished by .066 in the treated group at the end of 9 months. This would imply that the long-term response of patients with chronic myocarditis to immunosuppressive therapy (if one exists at all) does not extend to the patient population with a well-developed chronic dilated cardiomyopathy.

Cytokines

Cytokines have been investigated as potential avenues for treating myocarditis.[52–55] Cytokines evaluated include IL-1, IL-2, anti–IL-2, tumor necrosis factor, anti–tumor necrosis factor, interferon-beta, and interferon-gamma. IL-1 may be cytotoxic and contribute to decreased myocyte contractility. IL-1 release locally may exacerbate release of myocyte antigens.[52] IL-1 blockade could potentially block the autoimmune phase of myocarditis. IL-2 is a T cell–derived cytokine that stimulates the growth of T cells, regulates natural killer cell activity, and stimulates cytotoxic T cell effects (see Fig. 14–1). If given early, IL-2 decreases evidence of myocarditis by enhancing natural killer cell activity.[52] After this interval, treatment with IL-2 worsens myocarditis as demonstrated by decreased survival and an increase in the inflammatory cell infiltrate, myocyte necrosis, and T cell infiltration.[53] Anti–IL-2 antibodies have been administered in vivo to animals and are capable of modulating these effects of IL-2.

TNF-α is released by macrophages and has a multitude of cytokine regulatory effects.[54, 55] TNF-α increases the expression of ICAM-1 and endothelial leukocyte adhesion molecules on endothelial cells, both of which result in increased binding of leukocytes to the endothelium and increased migration of inflammatory cells into the area of active myocarditis. TNF-α may also affect the expression of class I and II MHC antigens as well as ICAM expression. TNF-α levels increase in patients with myocarditis. In animal models, TNF-α may attenuate or exacerbate viral replication, depending on the concentration and viral pathogen.[54] Anti–TNF-α blocks IL-2–mediated growth and inhibits binding of IL-2 to cellular receptors. Anti–TNF-α has been demonstrated to be of benefit in limiting the severity of myocarditis only when it is administered 1 day before viral infection or induction of other myocarditis models.[55]

Interferon-gamma activates macrophages and monocytes, induces class I and II MHC antigen expression, inhibits CD4 cells, and increases ICAM expression.[56] Interferon-beta and interferon-gamma can independently diminish viral titers and numbers of infected cells in animal models of myocarditis. Much larger doses of either agent alone are required, whereas interferon-gamma and interferon-beta are synergistic and can be used in a smaller dose together. All cytokines are capable of producing independent systemic effects including myalgias, fever, anorexia, and myelosuppression if given in high enough dosage. Neither cytokine nor anticytokine therapy is available for patients to date.[56]

It has been noted for many years that activated immune cells produce soluble inhibitors of myocyte contractile function. This response has been traced to inhibition of signal transduction and G protein stimulation of adenylate cyclase.[57] This soluble mediator affecting the beta-adrenergic receptor appears to be, at least in part, nitric oxide.[58]

Immunoabsorptive Therapy

Immunoabsorptive therapy has been suggested.[59] In the course of immunologic reaction to myocarditis, a number of antibodies are created to specific autoantigens. These include antibodies to myosin, adenosine nucleotide translocator (ANT), and the beta-adrenergic receptor.[59, 60] Synthetic peptides to ANT and myosin immobilized on a thiopropyl-sepharose column have been used to remove autoantibodies from circulation. Although theoretically possible, this therapy may be of limited value because it would (1) require determination of the autoantigens targeted by each patient's immune reaction, (2) immunoabsorb only circulating antibodies, and (3) not decrease antibody production.

Immunostimulants

Immunostimulants have been used in animals.[61, 62] FK565 is a low-molecular-weight immunoactive compound that increases macrophage function, including attachment of substrate, free radical production, and lysosomal enzyme production. The agent may also increase natural killer cell activity but has no direct antiviral effect. FK565 has inhibited viral multiplication in isolated mouse cell lines and has inhibited viral replication and decreased cellular inflammation, myocyte necrosis, and calcification in mice infected with coxsackievirus B_3 and given FK565 simultaneously.[61] Survival has also been demonstrated to increase from 30% to 60% in FK565-treated animals.[62] This agent appears to "treat" myocarditis by an activation of host defense mechanisms.

Immunoglobulins

Immunoglobulins have received attention in the treatment of myocarditis. Immunoglobulins have been demonstrated, in coxsackievirus B_3–infected mice models, to diminish evidence of myocarditis and viral titers while improving survival in a dose-dependent manner.[63] Drucker and coworkers[64] reported the use of gammaglobulin in 21 children with presumed myocarditis compared with 25 historical control subjects. Although most patients underwent endomyocardial biopsy, not all biopsy specimens demonstrated myocarditis. Regardless, children with acute left ventricular compromise were treated with intravenous gammaglobulin at a dose of 2 g/kg in a period of 24 h. In this retrospective, uncontrolled trial, those treated with gammaglobulin had a decrease in left ventricular end-diastolic diameter and a higher fractional shortening rate by echocardiography at 3 to 6 and 6 to 12 months after treatment. In addition, survival in the treated population was 84%, compared with 60% in the historical control group. Kawasaki disease is an acute inflammatory condition of unknown etiology that acutely is associated with myopericarditis and, after 1–2 weeks, coronary arteritis.[65] Coronary aneurysms, which develop in 15%–25% of those infected, may cause myocardial infarction, chronic coronary artery disease, or sudden cardiac death. A randomized prospective trial of gammaglobulin (400 mg/kg/day × 4 days plus aspirin 100 mg/kg/day × 14 days, then 3–5 mg/kg/day) compared with aspirin treatment alone demonstrated a significant decline in coronary artery aneurysms at 2 and 7 weeks (8% vs. 23% at 2 weeks and 4% vs. 18% at 7 weeks) in the gammaglobulin group.[66] Gammaglobulin also diminished evidence of an inflammatory state and fever. The mechanism by which immunoglobulins might have an effect on myocarditis is unclear. It is presumed that the immunoglobulin preparation contains antibodies to the pathogen causing the myocarditis. Immunoglobulin may saturate antigen receptors and the reticuloendothelial system. Finally, immunoglobulin may decrease the CD4 lymphocyte population with its attendant change in CD4 cell immunologic function.

Calcium Channel Blockers

Another potential approach to the treatment of myocarditis is the use of calcium channel blocking agents, specifically verapamil. Verapamil, when given before or at peak viremic times after infection

(4 days) in animal models of myocarditis, has been shown to decrease inflammation, myonecrosis, and microvascular disease. These changes were associated with decreased fibrosis and calcification of the myocardium. The effect of verapamil is similar to that seen in other animal models of cardiomyopathy including the Syrian hamster model of spontaneously developing hypertrophic cardiomyopathy and the chagasic model of postinfectious cardiomyopathy. Both of these animal models are associated with significant coronary vasoconstriction.

Many of the processes that perpetuate myocarditis are calcium dependent.[4, 67] In phase I of viral myocarditis, calcium channel blockers may decrease viral replication by their effects on assembly and budding. These effects are controlled through the membrane and cytoskeletal activities of viruses that are calcium dependent. In phase II of myocarditis, T cell activation and proliferation may also affect calcium-dependent T cell function. Calcium blockade may, therefore, alter interleukin production. In addition, myocyte exposure to autoantibodies results in calcium overload and death. Calcium blockade may prevent or delay myocyte cell death. Finally, the vascular abnormalities associated with myocarditis may be decreased or eliminated by the use of calcium blocking agents to prevent vasospasm and eliminate exposure to free radical lipid peroxidation. There have been no trials using verapamil or other calcium channel blockers in patients with myocarditis.[67] Such trials would be potentially dangerous in view of the negative inotropic effects of verapamil. Other agents affecting microvascular tone, such as angiotensin converting enzyme inhibitors and prazosin, may prevent some microvascular vasoconstriction, but their benefits have not been demonstrated in animal models or humans.

CURRENT RECOMMENDATIONS FOR TREATMENT

There are no adequate data to recommend firmly a course of treatment for diagnosed myocarditis. The following reflects a synthesis of existing clinical knowledge and the authors' experience with this condition (Fig. 14–3).

Adults

Adult patients presenting with *fulminant* myocarditis should undergo endomyocardial biopsy on presentation to ensure that the diagnosis is correct. Immunosuppressive therapy should be specifically withheld in this group of patients for 2 weeks. If, after this time, the patient has failed to improve, these patients should be listed for cardiac transplantation. More important, patients with fulminant myocarditis should receive hemodynamic support to ensure their survival. This may include use of intravenous pressors, intra-aortic balloon counterpulsation, or a left ventricular assist device.

IMMUNOSUPPRESSIVE TREATMENT OF MYOCARDITIS IN ADULTS

Fulminant Myocarditis	Acute Myocarditis		Dilated Cardiomyopathy
Avoid treatment			Avoid treatment
	Infectious stage: avoid treatment	Immune stage: possible treatment benefit	

Figure 14–3. Approach to the treatment of patients with myocarditis. Patients with fulminant myocarditis should not receive immunosuppressive therapy, as there is evidence that this worsens myocardial function. Likewise, patients with acute myocarditis still in the infectious stage of inflammation should not be treated with agents to suppress the immune response, and in fact, immune stimulating agents may be of more benefit in such patients. Patients who have fixed dilated cardiomyopathies have been demonstrated not to improve with corticosteroid therapy. Therefore, only patients in the immune stage of an active myocarditis may benefit from immune suppression. The mechanism of identifying such patients, however, remains ill defined.

Patients with *acute* biopsy-proven myocarditis should be treated with standard heart failure therapy. If, after 2 weeks, the patient has shown no improvement in noninvasive measurements of ventricular function, treatment with immunosuppressive agents should be initiated. Immunosuppressive agents that may be used include prednisone, azathioprine, and/or cyclosporine. Patients are usually treated for 6 to 8 weeks with relatively high dosages. Repeated endomyocardial biopsy, right-sided heart catheterization, and noninvasive assessment of ventricular function is performed to assess efficacy. Patients with histologic resolution or resolving myocarditis who have responded hemodynamically or by echocardiogram to immunosuppressive therapy should continue immunosuppressive therapy in the tapering dose for an additional 8 weeks, whereupon prednisone and then azathioprine are discontinued. Patients not responding histologically or hemodynamically should have immunosuppressive agents tapered rapidly in a 4-week period. Patients successfully treated may display a rebound immune activation, which after histologic documentation requires reinstitution of immunosuppressive therapy and then gradual lowering of immunosuppressive agents to the least possible maintenance dose.

Patients with chronic active myocarditis at the time of initial biopsy or who have changes of chronic active myocarditis in follow-up of acute myocarditis are at high risk for progression to a mildly dilated restrictive cardiomyopathy. There has been no therapy demonstrated to alter their disease. It may be that immunosuppressive agents are ineffective, that the dose is inadequate, or that treatment should be directed to persistent viral stimulation.

Patients with chronic persistent myocarditis should not receive immunosuppressive therapy. There has been no demonstration of progression to left ventricular dysfunction in this condition.

For treated patients, the authors currently recommend prednisone in a dose of 1 mg/kg/day in two divided doses. We do not administer more than 60 mg of prednisone per day, regardless of the patient's weight. Azathioprine is given at 1.5 mg/kg/day in a single dose. Cyclosporine is usually administered at 2–3 mg/kg/day in two divided doses. Doses are tapered in patients with acute myocarditis after 8 weeks by decreasing prednisone by 10 mg/day each week until doses of 20 mg/day are reached, at which time the decrease is by 5 mg/day a week. The morning dose is always the larger of the two doses when they are unevenly split. Azathioprine or cyclosporine is usually continued for 2–3 weeks after discontinuation of prednisone.

Significant side effects may occur with any immunosuppressive agent used. The most devastating acute side effects for patients include alterations in their appearance with redistribution of fat, acne, and weight gain. The subacute effects of osteoporosis, gastric irritation, glucose intolerance, and skin fragility affect many patients. A few patients will have aseptic necrosis, even with short-term exposure to corticosteroids. Azathioprine may result in a significant decrease in white blood cell count because of either a dose effect or an idiosyncratic reaction. To ensure no dose-effect response, patients should have their white blood cell counts measured at least every other week during treatment with azathioprine, and the drug should be discontinued if the white blood cell count is below 5000 mm^3. Patients with an idiosyncratic decrease in granulocytes or excessive granulocyte lowering with standard treatment will complain of a flulike illness. Any patient complaining of such symptoms should be seen immediately and treated appropriately with hospitalization and prophylactic antibiotics if the total granulocyte count falls below 1000 mm^3. Cyclosporine results in hypertension and some hirsutism, even in short-term exposure. Moderate renal tubular dysfunction may also develop in some patients, and hypertension may be exacerbated in others. Cyclosporin A levels should be observed and kept in the low therapeutic range. Creatinine concentration should be monitored every other week to ensure its stability, and cyclosporine should be discontinued if there is more than a 1-mg/dL increase in the creatinine concentration without another explanation.

Children

Children presenting with acute fulminant myocarditis and evidence of an ongoing viral process should undergo endomyocardial biopsy and be treated with immunoglobulin or entered into the national trial of immunoglobulin treatment in this disorder. The currently recommended dose is 2 g/kg in a 24-h period. Some patients are treated with a similar dose at 3–5 days.

Supportive Therapy

Treatment should include limitation of oxygen demands to the myocardium by imposing rest and supplemental oxygen. Similarly, the arrhythmias and congestive heart failure associated with myocarditis should be treated appropriately regardless of the potential to treat the myocarditis itself. This includes diuretics, afterload reduction, and inotropic support, if necessary. Digoxin is usually withheld, unless it is necessary to control the ventricular response to atrial fibrillation, because of concern that this agent may exacerbate coronary artery and microvascular spasm.

The most clear therapeutic principle in patients with myocarditis, particularly fulminant myocarditis with significant inflammatory infiltrate and edema, is to provide maximal hemodynamic support and unloading of the heart. This support should include the use of a left ventricular assist device or intra-aortic balloon pump, if necessary. Patients with fulminant myocarditis and cardiogenic shock may require support with an intra-aortic balloon pump, extracorporeal membrane oxygenation, or a left ventricular assist device.

REFERENCES

1. Bergtsson E, Orndale G: Complications of mumps with special reference to the incidence of myocarditis. Acta Med Scand 1954; 149:381–388.
2. Lucke B, Wight T, Kiure E: Pathologic anatomy and bacteriology of influenza: epidemic of autumn. Arch Intern Med 1929; 24:154–237.
3. Saphir O, Wile SA: Myocarditis in poliomyelitis. Am J Med Sci 1942; 203:781–788.
4. See DM, Tilles JG: Viral myocarditis. Rev Infect Dis 1991; 13:951–956.
5. Sole MJ, Liu P: Viral myocarditis: a paradigm for understanding the pathogenesis and treatment of dilated cardiomyopathy. J Am Coll Cardiol 1993; 22(suppl A):99A–105A.
6. Martino TA, Liu P, Sole MJ: Viral infection and the pathogenesis of dilated cardiomyopathy. Circ Res 1994; 74:182–188.
7. Kandolf R, Ameis D, Kirschner P, et al: In situ detection of enteroviral genomes in myocardial cells by nucleic acid hybridization: an approach to the diagnosis of viral heart disease. Proc Natl Acad Sci U S A 1987; 84:6272–6276.
8. Bowles NE, Rose ML, Taylor P, et al: End-stage dilated cardiomyopathy. Circulation 1989; 80:1128–1136.
9. Keeling PJ, Jeffery S, Caforio AL, et al: Similar prevalence of enteroviral genome within the myocardium from patients with idiopathic dilated cardiomyopathy and controls by the polymerase chain reaction. Br Heart J 1992; 68:554–559.
10. Klingel K, Hohenadl C, Canu A, et al: Ongoing enterovirus-induced myocarditis is associated with persistent heart muscle infection: quantitative analysis of virus replication, tissue damage, and inflammation. Proc Natl Acad Sci U S A 1992; 89:314–318.
11. Rose NR, Herskowitz A, Neumann DA: Autoimmunity in myocarditis: models and mechanisms. Clin Immunol Immunopathol 1993; 68:95–99.
12. Neumann DA, Rose NR, Ansari AA, Herskowitz A: Induction of multiple heart autoantibodies in mice with coxsackievirus B_3- and cardiac myosin–induced autoimmune myocarditis. J Immunol 1994; 152:343–350.
13. Neumann D, Herskowitz A, Rose NR: Myosin: autoantigen in myocarditis. *In* Khaw B, Narula J, Strauss H (eds): Monoclonal Antibodies in Cardiovascular Diseases. Philadelphia: Lea & Febiger, 1994.
14. Neumann DA, Wulff SM, Leppo MK, et al: Pathologic changes in the cardiac interstitium of mice infected with encephalomyocarditis virus. Cardiovasc Pathol 1993; 2:117–126.
15. Burke AP, Farb A, Virmani R, et al: Sports-related and non–sports-related sudden cardiac death in young adults. Am Heart J 1991; 121:568–575.
16. Vignola PA, Aonuma K, Swaye PS, et al: Lymphocytic myocarditis presenting as unexplained ventricular arrhythmias: diagnosis with endomyocardial biopsy and response to immunosuppression. J Am Coll Cardiol 1984; 4:812–819.
17. Strain JE, Grose RM, Factor SM, Fisher JD: Results of endomyocardial biopsy in patients with spontaneous ventricular tachycardia but without apparent structural heart disease. Circulation 1983; 68:1171–1181.
18. Sugrue DD, Holmes DR, Gersh BJ, et al: Cardiac histologic findings in patients with life-threatening ventricular arrhythmias of unknown origin. J Am Coll Cardiol 1984; 4:952–957.
19. O'Connell JB, Henkin RE, Robinson JA, et al: Gallium-67 imaging in patients with dilated cardiomyopathy and biopsy-proven myocarditis. Circulation 1984; 70:58–62.
20. O'Connell JB, Robinson JA, Henkin RE, Gunnar RM: Immunosuppressive therapy in patients with congestive cardiomyopathy and myocardial uptake of gallium-67. Circulation 1981; 64:780–786.
21. Dec GW, Palacios I, Yasuda T, et al: Antimyosin antibody cardiac imaging: its role in the diagnosis of myocarditis. J Am Coll Cardiol 1990; 16:97–104.
22. Bouhour JB, Helias J, DeLaJartre AY, et al: Detection of myocarditis during the first year after discovery of a dilated cardiomyopathy by endomyocardial biopsy and gallium-67 myocardial scintigraphy: prospective multicentre French study of 91 patients. Eur Heart J 1988; 9:520–528.
23. Aretz HT, Billingham ME, Edwards WD, et al: Myocarditis: histopathologic definition and classification. Am J Cardiovasc Pathol 1986; 1:3–14.
24. Tazelaar HD, Billingham ME: Leukocytic infiltrates in idiopathic dilated cardiomyopathy: a source of confusion with active myocarditis. Am J Surg Pathol 1986; 10:405–412.
25. Deckers JW, Hare JM, Baughman KL: Complications of transvenous right ventricular endomyocardial biopsy in adult patients with cardiomyopathy: a seven-year survey of 546 consecutive diagnostic procedures in a tertiary referral center. J Am Coll Cardiol 1992; 19:43–47.
26. Chow LH, Radio SJ, Sears TD, McManus BM: Insensitivity of right ventricular endomyocardial biopsy in the diagnosis of myocarditis. J Am Coll Cardiol 1989; 14:915–920.
27. Hauck AJ, Kearney DL, Edwards WD: Evaluation of postmortem endomyocardial biopsy specimens from 38 patients with lymphocytic myocarditis: implications for role of sampling error. Mayo Clin Proc 1989; 64:1235–1245.
28. Ansari AA, Wang YC, Danner DJ, et al: Abnormal expression of histocompatibility and mitochondrial antigens by cardiac tissue from patients with myocarditis and dilated cardiomyopathy. Am J Pathol 1991; 139:337–354.
29. Muir P, Tizey AJ, English TAH, et al: Chronic relapsing pericarditis and dilated cardiomyopathy: serological evidence of persistent enterovirus infection. Lancet 1989; 1:804–807.
30. Fenoglio JJ, Ursell PC, Kellogg CF, et al: Diagnosis and classification of myocarditis by endomyocardial biopsy. N Engl J Med 1983; 308:12–18.
31. Dec GW, Palacios IF, Fallon JT, et al: Active myocarditis in the spectrum of acute dilated cardiomyopathies. N Engl J Med 1985; 312:885–890.
32. Lieberman EB, Hutchins GM, Herskowitz A, et al: Clinicopathologic description of myocarditis. J Am Coll Cardiol 1991; 18:1617–1626.
33. Matsumori A, Wang H, Abelmann WH, Crumpacker CS: Treatment of viral myocarditis with ribavirin in animal preparation. Circulation 1985; 71:834–839.
34. Jubelt B, Wilson AK, Ropka SL, et al: Clearance of a persistent enterovirus infection of the mouse central nervous system by the antiviral agent disoxaril. J Infect Dis 1989; 159:866–870.
35. Herzum M, Huber SA, Weller R, et al: Treatment of experimental murine coxsackie B_3 myocarditis. Eur Heart J 1991; 12:200–202.
36. Rose NR, Hill SL, Neumann DA: Experimental myocarditis. *In*: Autoimmune Disease Models: A Guidebook. New York: Academic Press, 1994.
37. Kereiakes DJ, Parmley WW: Myocarditis and cardiomyopathy. Am Heart J 1984; 8:1318–1326.
38. Chan KY, Iwahara M, Benson LN, et al: Immunosuppressive therapy in the management of acute myocarditis in children: a clinical trial. J Am Coll Cardiol 1991; 17:458–460.
39. Khoury Z, Keren A, Benhorin J, Stern S: Aborted sudden death in a young patient with isolated granulomatous myocarditis. Eur Heart J 1994; 15:397–399.

40. Cox DM: Complete heart block in the pediatric patient. J Emerg Nursing 1992; 18:497–500.
41. Gilbert EM, O'Connell JB, Hammond ME, et al: Treatment of myocarditis with OKT3 monoclonal antibody [Letter]. Lancet 1988; 1:759.
42. Jett GK, Miller A, Savino D, Gonwa T: Reversal of acute fulminant lymphocytic myocarditis with combined technology of OKT3 monoclonal antibody and mechanical circulatory support. J Heart Lung Transplant 1992; 11:733–738.
43. Moreno-Cabral CE, Moreno-Cabral RJ, McNamara JJ, et al: Prolonged extracorporeal circulation for acute myocarditis. Int J Artif Organs 1992; 15:475–480.
44. Stallion A, Rafferty JF, Warner BW, et al: Myocardial calcification: a predictor of poor outcome for myocarditis treated with extracorporeal life support. J Pediatr Surg 1994; 29:492–494.
45. Chang AC, Hanley FL, Weindling SN, et al: Left heart support with a ventricular assist device in an infant with acute myocarditis. Crit Care Med 1992; 20:712–715.
46. Grundl PD, Miller SA, Nido PJ, et al: Successful treatment of acute myocarditis using extracorporeal membrane oxygenation. Crit Care Med 1993; 21:302–304.
47. Rockman HA, Adamson RM, Dembitsky WP, et al: Acute fulminant myocarditis: long-term follow-up after circulatory support with left ventricular assist device. Am Heart J 1991; 121:922–926.
48. Davies MJ, Ward DE: How can myocarditis be diagnosed and should it be treated? Br Heart J 1992; 68:346–347.
49. Peters NS, Poole-Wilson PA: Myocarditis—continuing clinical and pathologic confusion. Am Heart J 1991; 121:942–946.
50. Jones SR, Herskowitz A, Hutchins GM, Baughman KL: Effects of immunosuppressive therapy in biopsy-proved myocarditis and borderline myocarditis on left ventricular function. Am J Cardiol 1991; 68:370–376.
51. Parrillo JE, Cunnion RE, Epstein SE, et al: A prospective, randomized, controlled trial of prednisone for dilated cardiomyopathy. N Engl J Med 1989; 321:1061–1068.
52. Kishimoto C, Kuroki Y, Hiraoka Y, et al: Cytokine and murine coxsackievirus B_3 myocarditis. Circulation 1994; 89:2836–2842.
53. Matsumori A, Yamada T, Kawai C: Immunomodulating therapy in viral myocarditis: effects of tumour necrosis factor, interleukin 2 and anti–interleukin-2 receptor antibody in an animal model. Eur Heart J 1991; 12:203–205.
54. Yamada T, Matsumori A, Sasayama S: Therapeutic effect of anti–tumor necrosis factor-alpha antibody on the murine model of viral myocarditis induced by encephalomyocarditis virus. Circulation 1994; 89:846–851.
55. Smith SC, Allen PM: Neutralization of endogenous tumor necrosis factor ameliorates the severity of myosin-induced myocarditis. Circ Res 1992; 70:856–863.
56. Heim A, Canu A, Kirschner P, et al: Synergistic interaction of interferon-β and interferon-γ in coxsackievirus B_3–infected carrier cultures of human myocardial fibroblasts. J Infect Dis 1992; 166:958–965.
57. Chung MK, Gulick TS, Rotondo RE, et al: Mechanism of cytokine inhibition of β-adrenergic agonist stimulation of cyclic AMP in rat cardiac myocytes. Circ Res 1990; 67:753–763.
58. Balligand JL, Ungureanu D, Kelly RA, et al: Abnormal contractile function due to induction of nitric oxide synthesis in rat cardiac myocytes follows exposure to activated macrophage-conditioned medium. J Clin Invest 1993; 91:2314–2319.
59. Schwimmbeck PL, Bland NK, Schultheiss HP, Strauer BE: The possible value of synthetic peptides in the diagnosis and therapy of myocarditis and dilated cardiomyopathy. Eur Heart J 1991; 12:76–80.
60. Limas CJ, Goldenberg IF, Limas C: Autoantibodies against β-adrenoceptors in human idiopathic dilated cardiomyopathy. Circ Res 1989; 64:97–103.
61. Sato Y, Maruyama S, Kawai C, Matsumori A: Effect of immunostimulant therapy on acute viral myocarditis in an animal model. Am Heart J 1992; 124:428–434.
62. Sato Y, Matsumori A: Treatment of coxsackievirus B_3 myocarditis by immunoactive peptide in an animal model. Clin Immunol Immunopathol 1992; 65:65–69.
63. Weller AH, Hall M, Huber SA: Polyclonal immunoglobulin therapy protects against cardiac damage in experimental coxsackievirus-induced myocarditis. Eur Heart J 1992; 13:115–119.
64. Drucker NA, Colan SD, Lewis AB, et al: γ-Globulin treatment of acute myocarditis in the pediatric population. Circulation 1994; 89:252–257.
65. Kao CH, Hsieh KS, Wang YL, et al: Tc-99m HMPAO WBC imaging to detect carditis and to evaluate the results of high-dose γ-globulin treatment in Kawasaki disease. Clin Nucl Med 1992; 17:623–626.
66. Newburger JW, Takahashi M, Burns JC, et al: The treatment of Kawasaki syndrome with intravenous γ-globulin. N Engl J Med 1986; 315:341–347.
67. Dong R, Liu P, Wee L, et al: Verapamil ameliorates the clinical and pathological course of murine myocarditis. J Clin Invest 1992; 90:2022–2030.

15 Cardiac Transplantation and Circulatory Assistance

Lynne Warner Stevenson, MD
Eric A. Rose, MD

The majority of patients with heart failure can maintain a good functional capacity and quality of life with medical therapy. For those patients who remain severely limited after optimal medical therapy and consideration of revascularization or valve replacement, newer surgical therapies may be considered. Cardiac transplantation has evolved to be considered standard "best therapy" for eligible candidates. The problems of rejection, infection, and graft vasculopathy detract from the success of the procedure, but substantial benefit in quality and length of life is experienced by most recipients. Unfortunately, the number of heart transplant recipients is limited by the scarcity of donor hearts—only 2500 yearly in the United States. Mechanical support devices can provide temporary support and increasingly serve as bridges to transplantation for hospitalized patients. Models of mechanical support devices are being developed which will be worn by outpatients for more permanent support. The potential roles for cardiomyoplasty and the total artificial heart remain to be defined.

CARDIAC TRANSPLANTATION

The number of potential candidates for cardiac transplantation has been estimated to be 30,000–40,000 annually in the United States.[1]

Because fewer than 10% of these patients can actually undergo heart transplantation, this section emphasizes the evaluation of the potential candidate for transplantation and outlines the general problems of the transplant recipient.

Indications

Selection for cardiac transplantation was once largely a matter of eliminating patients with contraindications. Growing waiting lists for transplantation and improving prognoses for patients with advanced heart failure with both medical therapy and transplantation mandate careful consideration of indications as well (Fig. 15–1). Heart failure is the primary reason for referral in more than 90% of adults considered for heart transplantation. The majority of these patients have systolic failure with left ventricular ejection fractions of less than .25, with almost equal incidence of coronary artery disease and nonischemic cardiomyopathy. Fewer than 10% have other diagnoses, such as valvular disease, restrictive cardiomyopathy, adult congenital heart disease, cardiac tumors, or trauma.[2] All heart failure patients must be evaluated for potentially reversible factors contributing to heart failure. Despite severe decompensation at the time of referral to the cardiologist, many patients can regain a good quality of life and functional capacity with optimization of medical therapy without transplantation.[3] In most medical centers, hospital admission is routine to effectively combine evaluation for transplantation with maximization of alternative therapy. Insertion of a pulmonary artery catheter to measure pulmonary pressures for candidacy also allows further monitoring to redesign the vasodilator and diuretic regimen in those patients with a pulmonary capillary wedge pressure higher than 20 mm Hg and/or cardiac index of less than 2.2 L/min/m^2. Increasing pressure to complete candidate evaluation without hospitalization is not ultimately cost effective because of the missed opportunity to supervise the optimization of medical management, which may render transplantation unnecessary.

Selection of patients for transplantation should distribute scarce donor hearts to maximize the difference between the expected outcome with transplantation and the expected outcome without transplantation in terms of both quality and length of life.[4] The current 1-year mortality after heart transplantation is 10%–15%,[2] compared with the mortality for transplant candidates without transplantation, which is assumed to be 40%–50% at 1 year after referral, better than the "negligible chance of 6-month survival" described for candidates a decade ago. Eligible patients who remain critically decompensated in the hospital can expect a major improvement from transplantation in both quality and length of life. Outpatients with persistent symptoms of congestion can also expect major improvement with transplantation. Patients who can achieve stability as outpatients may have similar 2-year survival and quality of life with and without transplantation. However, these patients face the continuing risks of sudden death and deterioration to the point at which they require transplantation more urgently. Considerable effort has been devoted to identifying outpatients at particularly high risk of poor outcome without transplantation.[5–7]

A history of previous New York Heart Association clinical class IV symptoms does not identify a group at uniformly high risk, because marked improvement can often result from redesigning medical therapy.[8] Once the left ventricular ejection fraction is below .30, the degree of reduction does not correlate well with symptoms or prognosis. The measurement of peak oxygen consumption has provided an objective measurement of functional capacity that is also helpful for identifying survivors. Early work demonstrated high mortality in the group with peak exercise oxygen consumption of less than 14 mL/kg/min,[7] whereas more recent analysis suggests that the biggest difference is in patients with peak oxygen consumption of less than 11 mL/kg/min (Table 15–1).[9] This measurement also allows comparison of current peak functional capacity for each heart failure patient with that predicted after transplantation, which is usually 50%–70% of the predicted normal for age, gender, and size.[3] Exercise testing is not necessary to document limitation in patients who are bedridden or have evidence of congestive symptoms at rest. Peak oxygen consumption should be measured after obvious decompensation has been treated and the patient has regained ambulatory status.

A small number of patients undergo transplantation primarily for reasons other than heart failure symptoms, although most do have underlying heart failure. The occasional development of refractory ventricular arrhythmias leading to frequent activation of an implantable defibrillator despite antiarrhythmic drug therapy can be an indication for transplantation. Patients with intractable symptoms of ischemia not amenable to revascularization may be considered for transplantation, although noncardiac chest pain and narcotic-seeking behavior must be considered. Transplantation may be considered for intractable endocarditis.[10] Patients with restrictive cardiomyopathies and "burned out" hypertrophic cardiomyopathy may become transplant candidates because of severe congestive symptoms despite ejection fractions higher than .30. It is important to recognize that a low ejection fraction is neither a necessary nor a sufficient indication for transplantation (Table 15–2).[9]

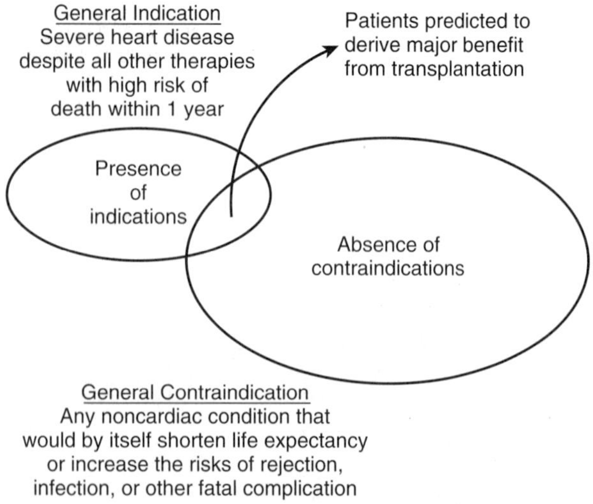

Figure 15–1. Venn diagram emphasizing the limited intersection between presence of indications and lack of contraindications in patients evaluated for cardiac transplantation.

Contraindications

In practice, evaluation of indications and contraindications generally proceeds simultaneously, because even the patients who show initial improvement may later decline to the point at which they need urgent consideration. In general, a contraindication is a condition that itself shortens life expectancy or increases the risk of death from rejection or from complications of immunosuppression, particularly infection (Table 15–3).[4, 9, 11, 12] Depending on the screening process before complete evaluation, approximately 30%–60% of potential candidates are accepted for transplantation (Fig. 15–2). Conditions that limit the potential for full rehabilitation are also relative contraindications, but using these conditions as contraindications for heart transplant raises issues regarding discrimination against the handicapped. The ideal candidate is sick enough to need a transplant but sufficiently well to expect a good result.

Age remains a controversial criterion. Although highly selected older patients may have good outcomes after transplantation,[12, 13] large series consistently demonstrate decreased long-term survival in older recipients.[14, 15] The longest reported single-center series of cyclosporine-treated recipients describes 82% vs. 76% survival at 1

TABLE 15–1. PEAK EXERCISE OXYGEN CONSUMPTION AND EXPECTED BENEFIT FROM TRANSPLANTATION

Peak VO_2 With Heart Failure	Expected Peak VO_2 After Transplant	Estimated 1-Y Survival With Heart Failure (%)	Estimated 1-Y Survival After Transplant (%)	Decision Regarding Transplant
<10	<14–18	<50	<80–90	Transplant (if eligible)
10–14	14–18	60–75	80–90	Toward transplant
14–18	14–18	75–85	80–90	Away from transplant
>18	>14–18	85–95	>80–90	No transplant (unless other indications)

Adapted from Mancini DM, Eisen H, Kussmaul W, et al: Value of peak exercise oxygen consumption for optimal timing of cardiac transplantation in ambulatory patients with heart failure. Circulation 1991; 83:778–786; and Stevenson LW, Sietsema K, Tillisch JH, et al: Exercise capacity for survivors of cardiac transplantation or sustained medical therapy for heart failure. Circulation 1990; 81:78–85.

year and 62% vs. 45% survival at 5 years for adults younger than and older than 50 years of age, respectively.[14] Potential candidates older than 60 years of age are generally evaluated more carefully for evidence of diseases that cause comorbidity in this age group.

Search for the cause of heart failure is important to exclude those patients with active diseases such as lupus erythematosus, rheumatoid arthritis, or scleroderma, which would continue after transplantation. Amyloidosis is a contraindication in most programs because of the tendency for systemic progression and recurrence in the allograft.[11] Patients undergoing transplantation for Chagas cardiomyopathy frequently demonstrate reactivation of disease following transplantation, but the ability to suppress this infection remains controversial.[16] Considerable emotional pressure is frequently generated in favor of patients with major systemic conditions that have the potential to persist or deteriorate during immunosuppression, particularly because some of these patients might do well after transplantation. Faced with a severe shortage of donor hearts, however, it is not feasible to collect systematic data about transplantation in all conditions. As described by Copeland and colleagues, selection must be based on "a combination of empirically derived contraindications with limited natural history data and considerable common sense."[17]

Diabetes mellitus is no longer an absolute contraindication to transplantation. Dependence on high doses of insulin is a relative contraindication, because glucose intolerance is increased by steroid therapy, and posttransplant hyperglycemia predisposes to severe infections. The evaluation of the diabetic patient includes a search for evidence of end-organ damage such as peripheral neuropathy, proteinuria indicative of diabetic nephropathy, retinopathy indicative of systemic arteriopathy, and small vessel peripheral vascular disease, any of which are usually criteria for exclusion. Patients with juvenile onset diabetes are generally excluded.

Pulmonary hypertension, which can develop after long-standing heart failure, presents a major immediate risk to the newly transplanted right ventricle, even if the pulmonary pressures subsequently decrease. The specific definitions for unacceptable pulmonary hypertension vary, but they generally include a consideration of pulmonary vascular resistance, which should usually be reducible to below 300 dynes/sec/cm^{-5}, and pulmonary artery systolic pressure, which should be reducible to levels below 60 mm Hg with pharmacologic ther-

TABLE 15–2. INDICATIONS FOR CARDIAC TRANSPLANTATION

Accepted Indications
- Peak VO_2 <10 mL/kg/min with achievement of anaerobic metabolism
- Severe ischemia severely limiting routine activity not amenable to bypass surgery or angioplasty
- Recurrent symptomatic ventricular arrhythmias refractory to all accepted therapeutic modalities

Probable Indications
- Peak VO_2 <14 mg/kg/min and major limitation of the patient's daily activities
- Recurrent severe unstable ischemia not amenable to bypass or angioplasty
- Instability of fluid balance or renal function not the result of patient noncompliance with regimen of weight monitoring, salt restriction, and flexible use of diuretic drugs

Inadequate Indication
- Ejection fraction ≤.20
- History of functional class III or IV symptoms of heart failure
- Previous ventricular arrhythmias
- Peak VO_2 >15 mL/kg/min without other indications

Adapted from Mudge GH, Goldstein S, Addonizio LJ, et al: Task Force 3: Recipient guidelines/prioritization. J Am Coll Cardiol 1993; 22(1):21–31.

TABLE 15–3. CONTRAINDICATIONS FOR CARDIAC TRANSPLANTATION

General Eligibility
- Absence of any noncardiac condition that would itself shorten life expectancy or increase the risk of death from rejection or from complications of immunosuppression, particularly infection

Relative Contraindications
- Over the upper age limit of 60–65 y (various programs)
- Active infection
- Active ulcer disease
- Active malignancy
- Severe diabetes mellitus with severe end-organ damage
- Severe peripheral vascular disease
- Pulmonary function (FEV_1, FVC) <50%–60%* or history of chronic bronchitis
- Serum creatinine >2–2.5 mg/dL; creatinine clearance <40–50 mL/min*
- Bilirubin >2.5 mg/dL, transaminases >2 times normal*
- Pulmonary artery systolic pressure >50–60 mm Hg*
- Mean transpulmonary gradient >12–15 mm Hg*
- High risk of life-threatening noncompliance
  - Inability to make strong consistent commitment to transplantation program
  - Cognitive impairment severe enough to limit comprehension of medical regimen
  - Psychiatric instability severe enough to jeopardize incentive for adherence to long-term medical regimen
  - Personality disorder compromising provision of necessary medical care
  - History of recurring alcohol or drug abuse
  - Failure to establish stable address or telephone number
  - Previous demonstration of repeated noncompliance with medication or follow-up

*May need to provide optimal hemodynamics with nitroprusside, dobutamine, or both for several days to assess reversibility of organ dysfunction caused by heart failure.

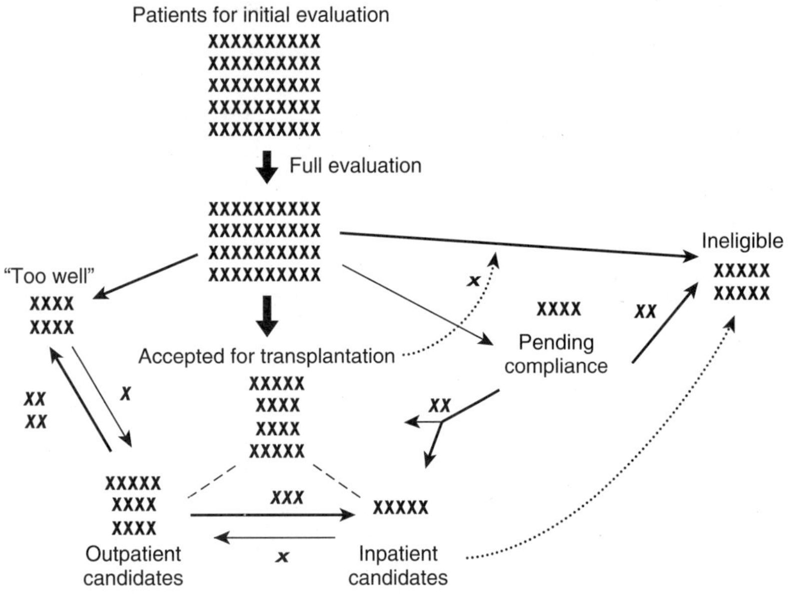

Figure 15–2. Algorithm of the evaluation process demonstrating the dynamic nature of eligibility for transplantation. The importance of an integrated program providing both transplantation and medical therapies for heart failure is apparent.

apy.[18] The transpulmonary gradient (mean pulmonary artery pressure minus mean pulmonary capillary wedge pressure) is the least influenced by the degree of hemodynamic compensation (Table 15–4) and in acceptable candidates is generally below 15 mm Hg.[19] Patients with initially high pulmonary pressures may undergo acute therapy with nitroprusside or other vasodilators in the catheterization suite to demonstrate reversibility. Patients with pulmonary capillary wedge pressures greater than or equal to 25 mm Hg, however, are more likely to demonstrate acceptable pulmonary pressures and resistances after sustained reduction in filling pressures over several days. Even if more acute reductions can be achieved, these patients are likely to benefit chronically from revision of their medical regimen under hemodynamic monitoring to maintain lower filling pressures after discharge. The rare patient whose pulmonary pressures are still borderline despite successful reduction of filling pressures may have significant perioperative risk. A brief trial of prostaglandin E1 or nitric oxide[20] may establish ultimate reversibility and assist in planning a strategy for early postoperative management. Patients with irreversible pulmonary hypertension are at unacceptably high risk for acute right heart failure and should not undergo orthotopic transplantation (replacement of old heart with new). Heterotopic transplantation, in which the new heart is "piggy-backed" onto the old, has occasionally been performed in patients with pulmonary hypertension, but reported survival has been lower than in most experiences of orthotopic transplantation.[21]

Pulmonary function is compromised by the congestive state.[22] Patients with severely elevated filling pressures should undergo pulmonary function testing after pulmonary capillary wedge pressure has been reduced for at least 5 days, and again later if pulmonary function is still unacceptable. The general criteria are at least 50% of predicted forced vital capacity and forced expired volume in 1 sec (see Table 15–3). In most centers, patients must not smoke for at least 3 months before transplantation. This prohibition reflects not only the risks of perioperative pulmonary complications but also the risk of postoperative resumption of smoking, which frequently happens and appears to increase the chance of accelerated graft arteriopathy.[23] Continued smoking also raises concerns about patient commitment to achieving and maintaining health. Patients who stop smoking at least 1 year before transplantation have been shown to have a better outcome than those who do not.[24] Regardless of pulmonary function results, a history of morning sputum production and "smoker's cough" is considered by some programs to be a relative contraindication because of the high risk for later pulmonary infection during immunosuppression. There is no organized data regarding outcome for patients with mild intrinsic asthma, which is generally not a contraindication.

Hemodynamic compromise also affects renal and hepatic function. Renal function is generally optimized by several days of inotropic infusions to improve cardiac output and renal perfusion. Creatinine clearance of at least 50 mL/min is preferred. Occasionally, lower

TABLE 15–4. PREOPERATIVE REVERSIBILITY OF PULMONARY HYPERTENSION DURING TAILORED THERAPY* IN 100 TRANSPLANT RECIPIENTS

	Initial PAS > 50 mm Hg	Initial PVR > 240 dynes/sec/cm^{-5}	Initial TPG > 15 mm Hg
No	35% (6%)	59% (9%)	86% (7%)
Yes	65% (8%)	41% (5%)	14% (7%)
If yes, reversible	41% (3%)	25% (11%)	8% (17%)
If yes, not reversible	24% (10%)	16% (0%)	6% (0%)

Numbers in parentheses indicate 30-day mortality after transplantation.

*Reversibility determined after 72 h of therapy tailored to reduced pulmonary capillary wedge pressure to 15 mm Hg, followed in 5% of patients by a trial of prostaglandin E1, if necessary.

Abbreviations: PAS, pulmonary artery systolic pressure; PVR, pulmonary vascular resistance; TPG = transpulmonary gradient (mean pulmonary artery pressure minus pulmonary capillary wedge pressure).

rates may be accepted if they are clearly related to acute decompensation and there is normal renal size on ultrasonography and an absence of significant proteinuria. Hepatic function, on the other hand, is optimized by the maintenance of low right-sided filling pressures with minimization of the retrograde flow from tricuspid regurgitation. Although elevated bilirubin and alkaline phosphatase may be the most common pattern, all patterns of abnormal liver function tests have been seen. The rare elevation of transaminases into the thousands generally reflects a recent period of critical hypoperfusion. In such cases, liver function should be allowed to recover during support with either drugs or devices before cardiac transplantation is performed.

The risk of developing malignancy is multiplied by immunosuppression, which is assumed to interfere with normal policing of early malignant clones.[25] Neoplasms within the previous 3–5 years, other than superficial skin lesions, are generally contraindications to cardiac transplantation. Particular concern is devoted to screening for recurrent disease in any patient with previous malignancy known for late recurrence, such as breast cancer. Many patients, however, have successfully undergone transplantation 5–10 years after successful therapy of lymphomas; these patients usually have heart failure resulting from doxorubicin (Adriamycin) cardiotoxicity.

Severe rejection episodes after transplantation often reflect noncompliance with medication or appointments. The heavy psychological toll of transplantation combined with mood swings related to glucocorticoid therapy can precipitate lethal episodes of overt suicidal behavior or passive suicide attempts through noncompliance with medication or clinic visits. Current alcohol or illicit drug use are contraindications. All psychiatric and social support factors are integrated into an assessment of the likelihood for maintained compliance.[26, 27] Relative weakness of either the patient's abilities or his or her family support can be counterbalanced by strength in the other component. One of the many benefits of the optimally integrated transplant and heart failure program[28] is the opportunity to establish better compliance profiles for patients who would have been rejected on the basis of previous history of noncompliance (see Fig. 15–2).

The emergency evaluation of a potential candidate in critical condition remains a challenge. When the patient's organ function and cognitive function are acutely impaired, decisions regarding both operative risk and patient commitment are based on experienced guesswork and emotional bias. Many of these patients must be refused transplant, with the initial cost of disappointment replacing the tragedy of prolonged postoperative misery and death. Dying patients who can be rescued by transplantation, however, may be the most rewarding examples of transplantation. Greater risks will continue to be taken, and occasional mistakes made, for such patients who ultimately have the most to gain from transplantation in terms of survival and quality of life. The increasing availability of mechanical support devices may allow some of these patients to be stabilized for both physiologic and psychologic candidacy, following which the chance of favorable posttransplant outcome can be enhanced (discussed later).

Management of the Transplant Candidate

The major principles regarding care before transplantation are elucidated in Chapters 10 and 11. It has been established by the Consensus Conference on Transplantation that outpatients should preferably be seen at least monthly, but certainly no less often than every 2 months, at the center where the transplant will be performed.[11] More frequent clinic visits with the patient's local cardiologist are necessary for monitoring electrolytes, renal function, and anticoagulation. Progressive right heart failure, renal dysfunction, or hepatic dysfunction are indications for hospitalization. Patients whose condition renders them bedridden need hospitalization or help to increase their activity level. Although the patients with the most severe compromise can expect the greatest improvement, preoperative condition is an important determinant of postoperative outcome. Patients with clinical volume overload before transplantation may be more likely to have perioperative problems with pulmonary hypertension, prolonged intubation, coagulopathy, and hepatic dysfunction complicating recovery.

During the long waiting periods for a donor heart, candidacy for transplantation is considered to be a dynamic state from which movement is possible (see Fig. 15–2). Patients may develop infections, new diabetic complications, noncompliance, or other contraindications for transplantation. The risk of becoming ineligible is particularly high for hospitalized patients who are critically ill, such as those on assist devices (discussed later). As many as 30% of these patients may become ineligible as a result of infection, multiorgan failure, coagulopathy, or other problems.[29, 30]

Other patients may improve without transplantation. The highest risk of death is in the early period after listing, after which time some of the factors which led to deterioration before referral may resolve spontaneously and the benefits of optimized medical therapy may be realized. Current policy dictates periodic reevaluation of candidates to identify those patients in whom functional capacity and prognosis may have improved sufficiently that transplantation can be deferred. This reevaluation is based on criteria of clinical stability and improvement of functional capacity confirmed by measurement of peak oxygen consumption (Table 15–5). After this reevaluation, candidates remaining on the list should still meet the indications described previously for initial candidacy (see Table 15–2). As many as 30% of ambulatory candidates may be able to leave the active waiting list with subsequent 2-year survival similar to that after transplantation.[31]

Patients awaiting transplantation generally carry long-range beepers. In general, candidates should be able to reach the transplant center within 3 h of notification. Almost one half of planned transplants are canceled because of deterioration of the donor or donor disease noted at the time of harvest. Patients need to be aware of the chance of "practice runs," which will be even more frequent for patients living at long distances from the transplant center who may need to begin their trip many hours before the anticipated time of harvesting.

Assessment of Potential Donor Hearts for Transplantation

Evaluation and management of the potential heart donor are evolving. In the presence of irreversible brain injury, the circulation is

TABLE 15–5. PROPOSED CRITERIA FOR STABILITY AND IMPROVEMENT DURING REEVALUATION OF CANDIDATES AWAITING TRANSPLANT

Clinical Criteria
- Stable fluid balance without orthopnea, elevated jugular venous pressures, or other evidence of congestion on flexible diuretic regimen
- Stable blood pressure with systolic pressure $\geq$ 80 mm Hg
- Stable serum sodium and renal function
- Absence of symptomatic ventricular arrhythmias
- Absence of frequent angina
- Absence of severe drug side effects
- Stable or improving activity level without dyspnea during self-care or 1-block exertion

Exercise Criteria (if initial peak VO_2 < 14 mL/kg/min)
- Improvement in peak oxygen consumption of $\geq$ 2 mL/kg/min
- Peak oxygen consumption $\geq$ 12 mL/kg/min

Adapted from Stevenson LW, Steimle AE, Fonarow W, et al: Improvement in exercise capacity of candidates awaiting heart transplantation. J Am Coll Cardiol 1995; 25:163–170.

often unstable because of severe volume depletion from diabetes insipidus and marked fluctuations in autonomic tone. Vigorous therapy with vasopressin and replacement of urine volumes often decrease the need for intravenous inotropic agents, which commonly include dopamine. Measurement of central venous pressure may help to optimize volume status.

Absolute contraindications to donation include evidence of infection with the human immunodeficiency virus, hepatitis B, and usually hepatitis C infection. History of major drug use, alcoholism, or known cardiac disease are also contraindications (Table 15–6). Echocardiography has become a vital tool for donor assessment. Age and risk factors for coronary artery disease may influence the decision regarding whether a potential donor should be further evaluated with coronary arteriography. Selection of donor hearts has evolved to encompass more "marginal" donors because of the increasing disparity between the number of patients on the waiting list and the limited donor supply.[32–34]

Distribution of Donor Hearts

Once patients have been accepted for transplantation in the United States, they are placed on a national computerized waiting list through the United Network of Organ Sharing (UNOS), a private organization under federal contract to distribute organs equitably. Priority for transplantation is generally classified as either regular status (UNOS 2) or high status (UNOS 1); high status is awarded to patients requiring inotropic infusions or mechanical support in intensive care units. Several regions have sanctioned "variances" by which patients are divided into more subcategories with intermediate levels of priority.

Patients are listed by blood type within a given donor weight range. When a donor heart becomes available for the next appropriate patient on the list, the transplant center is notified, and extensive communication begins. Some patients with significant numbers of antibodies detected on screening require a crossmatch between donor lymphocytes and recipient serum to prevent implantation of a donor heart to which the recipient has pre-existing antibodies. Many of the considerations described for general donor evaluation are particularly important in relation to a given recipient (see Table 15–5). Patients with higher pulmonary pressures may be at greater risk of early right heart failure if the donor is older, smaller than the recipient, or at a distance from the recipient that will require a longer ischemic time.

TABLE 15–6. CONSIDERATIONS IN DONOR EVALUATION

Time and Circumstances of Brain Death
Age of Donor
- May be considered in relation to recipient's age in conjunction with risk factors, including male gender, and availability of donor catheterization

Cardiac Function
- History of risk factors for coronary artery disease or cardiomyopathy
- Recent insult
  - Cause of death
  - Anoxia
  - Prolonged resuscitation
- Electrocardiographic evidence of chronic disease or acute injury
- Ventricular wall motion on echocardiography
- Ventricular hypertrophy on echocardiography
- Need for high-dose pressor support despite adequate volume

Potential Infection
- Active donor infection
- Risk factors or serology for human immunodeficiency virus
- Positive serology for hepatitis B or C
- Cytomegalovirus status when known prior to transplant

Compatibility With Recipient
- Blood type
- Body size and gender (smaller hearts in women)
- Recipient pulmonary artery pressures
- Recipient antibodies to potential donor

Anticipated Ischemic Time Between Harvesting and Reimplantation

Technique of Transplantation

The general sequence of the surgical transplantation procedure is described by Reitz.[35] The most common technique of anastomosis has been that originally performed by Lower and Shumway,[36] in which both atria of the recipient heart are opened behind their appendages and the posterior atrial segments anastomosed to the right and left atria of the donor heart, creating snowman-shaped atria. Atrial torsion and distortion may lead to mitral and tricuspid valvular incompetence and sinus node dysfunction. The asynchronous contraction of the donor and recipient atria may detract from effective ventricular filling.

An alternative method using bicaval anastomoses removes all of the recipient right atria and portions of the recipient venae cavae. The remaining recipient venae cavae are then anastomosed to the donor venae cavae, which enter the now-intact donor right atrium.[37, 38] With this approach, the left atrium is either partially excised, leaving the pulmonary vein entrances as in the Lower and Shumway technique, or the inflow portions of the pulmonary veins are transplanted with the donor heart (Fig. 15–3). Preliminary experience with the bicaval techniques suggests a reduction in valvular regurgitation[39] and in the need for postoperative pacing for bradycardia. Potential disadvantages of this modified technique include delayed stenosis of the caval anastomoses, bleeding from the inaccessible medial aspects of the pulmonary venous anastomoses, and longer operative time.

Care of the Transplant Recipient

Because transplant cardiology has become a recognized subspecialty area, care of the cardiac transplant recipient is guided in almost all cases either by a local transplant cardiologist or a regional transplant cardiologist in close collaboration with a community physician. The aspects emphasized in this chapter are those relating to hospitalizations and the general principles that determine the clinical success of the procedure.

Early Postoperative Period

The primary concern in the immediate postoperative period is the function of the newly transplanted heart. Donor heart dysfunction can result from problems with preservation and ischemia, unrecognized primary cardiac pathology, right heart decompensation, or, more rarely, pericardial tamponade in the recipient. Monitoring of pulmonary pressures, left-sided filling pressures, and cardiac output is critical to allow specific hemodynamic intervention. Prolonged difficulty during initial weaning from cardiopulmonary bypass may predict instability during the next 24 h.

Low-dose dobutamine, or less often, isoproterenol, and dopamine are routinely employed by most surgeons. In addition to providing inotropic support, these agents stimulate the newly denervated sinus node, which is frequently exquisitely sensitive to changes in circulating catecholamines. Right heart failure is a dreaded early complication, occurring in 10%–20% of recipients.[40] Relative right heart dysfunction is suggested by right atrial pressures that are higher than or equal to left-sided filling pressures and can be confirmed by echocardiography. Reduction of pulmonary pressures is crucial in the setting of right heart dysfunction, even if these levels are only modestly elevated. Dobutamine and isoproterenol are useful in reducing pulmonary pressures, and vasoconstrictor agents like high-dose dopamine and norepinephrine should be avoided or minimized. Ni-

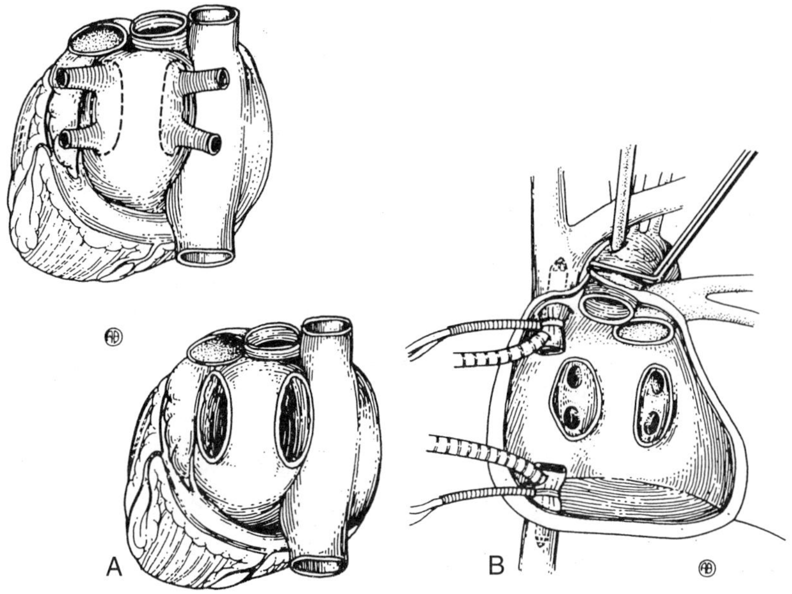

Figure 15–3. *A,* Donor heart harvesting for total replacement involves the pulmonary veins and long cuffs of the recipient superior and inferior venae cavae for bicaval anastomoses. *B,* In recipient heart explantation and cannulation, the posterior aspects of the left and right atria are resected, leaving two cuffs with the origin of the right and left pulmonary veins. The venae cavae are transected completely.

troglycerin and nitroprusside are frequently helpful in reducing pulmonary pressures. Prostaglandin E1 can be very effective in dilating the pulmonary bed, particularly if infused directly into the right atrium.[41] As seen in postoperative congenital heart surgery, the use of inhaled nitric oxide can provide short-term benefit.[20] Refractory right heart dysfunction may rarely require use of a mechanical right ventricular assist device (VAD).

Atrial arrhythmias are common early after transplantation, as with other open-heart procedures. Although usually well tolerated and transient, atrial arrhythmias can precipitate collapse in a patient with marginal hemodynamic function. It is important to recognize that digitalis will not slow atrioventricular conduction in the denervated heart, which is, however, very sensitive to calcium channel blocking agents. Isolated premature ventricular contractions are common, but sustained ventricular arrhythmias are rare and usually indicate ischemic injury. In the early postoperative period, the electrocardiogram often shows bizarre ST and T wave segment abnormalities with prolonged QT interval, all presumably reflecting changes after denervation (Fig. 15–4). These abnormalities usually resolve after a few months. Occasional anterior or inferior Q waves suggestive of a myocardial infarction without corresponding wall motion abnormalities may appear. If the recipient sinus node remains, the recipient P

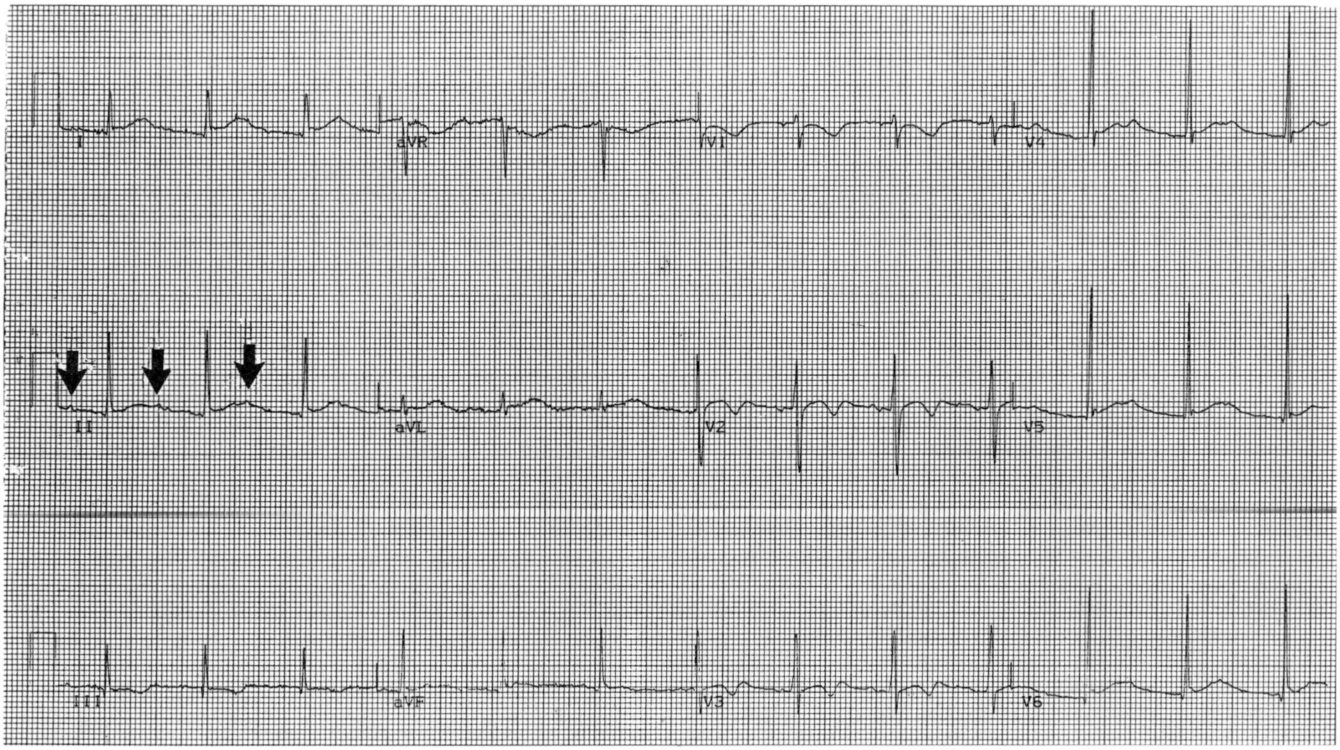

Figure 15–4. An electrocardiogram from a transplant recipient 12 hours after transplantation demonstrates typical QT prolongation and T wave abnormalities and dissociation of the recipient P wave *(arrows)* from the donor P-QRS complexes.

wave may be seen as an "extra" P wave dissociated from the P-QRS complex of the transplanted heart. The recipient sinus node is generally removed during the bicaval anastomotic technique. Right bundle branch block and right ventricular conduction commonly occur and persist after transplantation, possibly as a result of septal torsion or other factors during harvesting.

Renal function often becomes a major concern at 12–24 h after transplantation. Renal function in the cardiac transplant candidate is often compromised by chronically decreased renal perfusion and occasionally by unappreciated vascular disease and diabetic involvement. Transplantation further insults the kidneys through cardiopulmonary bypass, rapid fluctuations in renal perfusion, and the administration of cyclosporine, which is both acutely and chronically nephrotoxic.[42] Some cardiac transplant programs avoid the use of cyclosporine in the first 72 h after transplant in patients with risk factors for postoperative renal failure,[43] which include preoperative dependence on inotropic agents, blood urea nitrogen levels higher than 50 mg/dL, or creatinine levels higher than 1.5 mg/dL. For these high-risk patients, or for other patients demonstrating unexpected renal compromise, therapy with the monoclonal preparation OKT3 is often used without cyclosporine until renal function becomes adequate. Many patients demonstrate a period of relative postoperative oliguria for 24 h after surgery which requires careful monitoring of fluid balance and potassium.

The majority of early transplant recipients have total-body volume overload. Patients with obvious major hypervolemia at the time of transplantation should be considered for intraoperative ultrafiltration. Even without pretransplant peripheral edema, volume overload usually does not resolve spontaneously after transplantation and requires intravenous diuretics. Pulmonary and hepatic function may be unnecessarily compromised by postoperative congestion.

Other issues become important after the first 48 h posttransplant. Some patients develop significant hypertension, which requires vigorous therapy. Nitroprusside is occasionally necessary. An added effect of calcium channel blockers such as diltiazem is a decrease of hepatic cyclosporine metabolism, which necessitates close monitoring of cyclosporine levels and decreasing cyclosporine doses. Sublingual nifedipine may help to decrease high pressures quickly. Angiotensin converting enzyme (ACE) inhibitors are effective for hypertension, but they occasionally cause hyperkalemia in patients who are also receiving cyclosporine. Uncontrolled hypertension may be associated with seizures, particularly in younger patients receiving cyclosporine.

Malnutrition commonly accompanies severe chronic heart failure. In the postoperative period, high doses of glucocorticoids increase catabolism. Appetite, however, is often exuberant. Careful attention must be paid to caloric requirements and replacement of electrolytes such as magnesium and phosphate. Magnesium depletion is particularly to be avoided, because magnesium excretion is enhanced by cyclosporine, and low magnesium levels have been associated with an increased incidence of cyclosporine-induced seizures. Hyperglycemia is exacerbated by glucocorticoid administration and may necessitate insulin use in patients previously controlled through diet or the use of oral hypoglycemic agents.

The rate of general recovery after transplantation reflects the patient's functional state before transplantation. Extubation is generally achieved within 24–48 h after transplant. Often, patients can be sitting up by the second day and walking slowly by the fourth day after transplantation. Bedside bicycling is encouraged within the first week. The usual length of stay required for resolution of postoperative issues and establishment of the initial immunosuppressive regimen is usually 2 weeks, but earlier discharges are planned when appropriately skilled outpatient support services are available.

Patient teaching is a critical component of the initial hospitalization. Patients must understand the importance of limiting lipid intake and total caloric intake. An exercise program not only aids peripheral reconditioning but strengthens bones at risk for osteoporosis. Patients must learn to be vigilant for early signs of infection or rejection, for which they should seek immediate attention. The average individual must increase his or her compliance from about 60% to more than 90%, particularly with immunosuppressive medications. A representative discharge regimen is shown in Table 15–7. The immunosuppressive medications and prophylaxis against infection are discussed later. Histamine-2 antagonists are often used to prevent peptic ulcers and gastritis during periods of high corticosteroid dosing.

General Considerations for Rehospitalization After Transplantation

The majority of rehospitalizations are triggered by infection or rejection. All patients are instructed to take their temperature daily and to call their transplant physician whenever their temperature rises above 38°C (100°F). Except in occasional cases of classic familial upper respiratory syndromes, patients with fever must undergo evaluation with careful examination, chest radiographs, and blood and urine cultures. Particular vigilance is necessary during the 6 weeks following therapy for rejection and in patients developing severe neutropenia as a result of azathioprine, methotrexate, or cytomegalovirus (CMV) infection.

In addition to the usual focus on lungs, blood, urine, and gastrointestinal tract, areas of potential infection in the transplant recipient include the sinuses and the central nervous system. Gastrointestinal complications are common, the clinical evidence of which may be blunted by the use of glucocorticoids.[44, 45] Peptic ulcer disease and gastritis may develop during high-dose prednisone administration. Toxic megacolon can occur rapidly, particularly in a patient with constipation. The incidence of cholecystitis may be increased, because cyclosporine decreases bile salt secretion, promoting cholestasis.[46]

Although most episodes of rejection are treated with oral or intravenous corticosteroids without hospitalization, patients are admitted for rejection associated with hemodynamic compromise or refractory rejection necessitating therapy with antilymphocyte sera. Despite the frequency of surveillance biopsies, rejection episodes occasionally present first with clinical symptoms. In addition to symptoms of infection, any complaint of unusual fatigue, shortness of breath, presyncope, or syncope merits immediate evaluation in the closest emergency department. Evidence of hemodynamic compromise necessitates transfer to the transplant center. Echocardiography is a frequent emergency-department procedure to estimate left ventricular function in a patient with vague complaints or in a patient with hypotension that could be the result of either rejection or sepsis. In patients with frank circulatory collapse, the distinction between primary rejection and myocardial depression as a result of sepsis can be difficult. In cases of circulatory compromise in the absence of apparent sepsis, intravenous glucocorticoids should be given immediately for presumed rejection without waiting for the results of endomyocardial biopsy.

Hospitalization can be required for apparently minor gastrointestinal syndromes that impair the patient's ability to take oral immuno-

TABLE 15–7. SAMPLE DISCHARGE REGIMEN

Cyclosporin A
Prednisone
Azathioprine
Furosemide
Diltiazem
H_2 blocker
(Consider HMG-CoA reductase inhibitor)
Trimethoprim-sulfamethoxazole
Nystatin or clotrimazole
(Consider antiviral prophylaxis)

suppressive medications. To change to intravenous administration of the regular oral regimen, 80% of the daily prednisone dose is given as methylprednisolone, approximately 30% of the daily cyclosporine dose is given intravenously over 12–24 h or in 1-h infusions twice daily, and the oral azathioprine dose is unchanged. Other newer immunosuppressive agents are generally withheld until resolution of the gastrointestinal syndrome. Guidelines for intravenous immunosuppression are similar to those for general surgical procedures except that patients undergoing surgery who have been on low-dose or no maintenance corticosteroid therapy should receive "stress" doses of glucocorticoids (the equivalent of at least 100 mg of hydrocortisone) which should rapidly be tapered as the situation stabilizes. Cyclosporine levels should be monitored frequently during changes in clinical condition and other therapies because of the potential alterations in metabolism. It is important to recognize that infections and other events may trigger immune responses and rejection.

The degree of vigilance regarding protective isolation of transplant patients varies among centers. Gowns, masks, and gloves have not been shown to decrease infection rates[45] but do effectively decrease casual traffic. Patients are at greatest risk of acquiring infection within the first few months after transplant or after recent therapy for rejection. Patients with infected surgical wounds or active pulmonary infections are not appropriate roommates for transplant recipients. Careful handwashing and masks for staff and visitors with viral infections are essential. Universal precautions should be observed by hospital staff. Wearing of a mask is often recommended for patients exposed to family members with an infection, crowded hospital clinics, and open excavation sites.

Immunosuppression and Rejection

Rejection. Rejection remains the central challenge of transplantation. Immune injury can be caused by cytotoxic T lymphocytes, natural killer cells, monocyte-macrophages, cytokine effects, and multiple antibody-mediated mechanisms. Hyperacute rejection occurring within minutes after recipient blood flow to the transplanted heart indicates the presence of preformed antibodies specific for the donor, whereas most other clinical syndromes of rejection probably reflect a concert of immunologic mechanisms (Table 15–8), although considerable confusion has arisen from attempts to characterize vascular/"humoral" rejection. The majority of patients develop at least one episode of rejection within the first year after transplantation. The cumulative rate in the Cardiac Transplant Research Database from 25 institutions was 0.8 episodes by the third month, 1.1 episodes by 6 months, and 1.3 by 12 months after transplantation, although 37% of patients had no rejection during that time.[47] The risk of rejection declines dramatically over the first year, but of patients who did have rejection during the first year, 17% had later episodes of rejection. Risk factors for rejection include younger recipient age, female recipient, and female donor heart.[47]

True hyperacute rejection is rare and generally fatal, although initial graft dysfunction from other causes such as prolonged ischemic time may improve. Because it is also attributed to circulating antibodies, rejection occurring within the first 72 h after transplantation may in some cases be treated with plasmapheresis and intensive glucocorticoid therapy.

The majority of rejection episodes are diagnosed by review of the results of surveillance endomyocardial biopsy, routinely performed weekly for the first 4 postoperative weeks and monthly after 6 months. Biopsies are generally repeated within 2–3 weeks after therapy for a rejection episode. Controversy exists regarding the timing of surveillance biopsies after the first year. In attempts to decrease the required frequency of these uncomfortable and resource-intensive biopsies, a battalion of other noninvasive techniques has been introduced, but none has shown sufficient sensitivity to replace biopsy in the outpatient setting. Multiple different grading scales exist, but the best standardization has been provided by the scale of the International Society of Heart and Lung Transplantation (Table 15–9).[48] Severe rejection as defined on this scale is rarely seen in patients on cyclosporine therapy, even in those with life-threatening hemodynamic compromise. The distribution of biopsy grades in 4400 biopsies from a representative institution is shown in Figure 15–5.

Biopsy-revealed grade I rejection generally does not require treatment. Patients with grade II biopsy results are treated in some institutions, but the rejection frequently resolves without therapy. Patients with grade III biopsy results are usually treated, and the rare patient with a grade IV result should be treated aggressively (Fig. 15–6). The terms "vascular" or "humoral" rejection originally referred to the presence of endothelial swelling and inflammation or positive immunofluorescence staining for immunoglobulin and complement in vessels captured on biopsy[49] but have been loosely employed to describe clinical syndromes.

More than 80% of episodes considered on the basis of biopsy results to need specific augmentation of immunosuppression are clinically silent.[47] Atrial arrhythmias are occasionally associated with rejection. Syncope occasionally occurs as an indication of a major rejection episode. In the era of transplantation before cyclosporine, decreases in electrocardiographic voltage reflected intramyocardial edema from rejection. This edema is usually less marked during cyclosporine therapy, but an obvious decrease in QRS amplitude should raise concern about rejection or transplant coronary artery disease (TCAD). Low-grade fever has been described as an indicator of rejection but is a rare concomitant in current experience and usually results from infection. One of the most common signs of rejection is the new apparent control of previously refractory hypertension. Vague shortness of breath and fatigue can herald rejection

TABLE 15–8. PRESENTATIONS OF REJECTION

- Hyperacute rejection causing graft failure at implantation
- Acute cellular rejection diagnosed on routine surveillance biopsy
- Acute cellular rejection with hemodynamic compromise
- Vascular rejection diagnosed on biopsy, with or without accompanying cellular infiltrate
- Reversible graft dysfunction without cellular infiltrate
- Chronic irreversible graft dysfunction without cellular infiltrate
- Transplant coronary artery disease detected by angiography or autopsy

TABLE 15–9. BIOPSY GRADING SCALE

Grade	New Nomenclature	Old Nomenclature
0	No rejection	No rejection
1A	Focal perivascular or interstitial infiltrate without necrosis	Mild rejection
1B	Diffuse but sparse infiltrate without necrosis	
2	One focus only with aggressive infiltration and/or focal myocyte damage	Focal moderate rejection
3A	Multifocal aggressive infiltrates and/or myocyte damage	Low moderate rejection
3B	Diffuse inflammatory process with necrosis	Borderline severe rejection
4	Diffuse aggressive polymorphous infiltrate with or without edema, hemorrhage, and vasculitis; with necrosis	Severe acute rejection

Adapted from Billingham ME, Cary NR, Hammond ME, et al: A working formulation for the standardization of nomenclature in the diagnosis of heart and lung rejection: Heart Rejection Study Group. J Heart Trans 1990; 9:587–593.

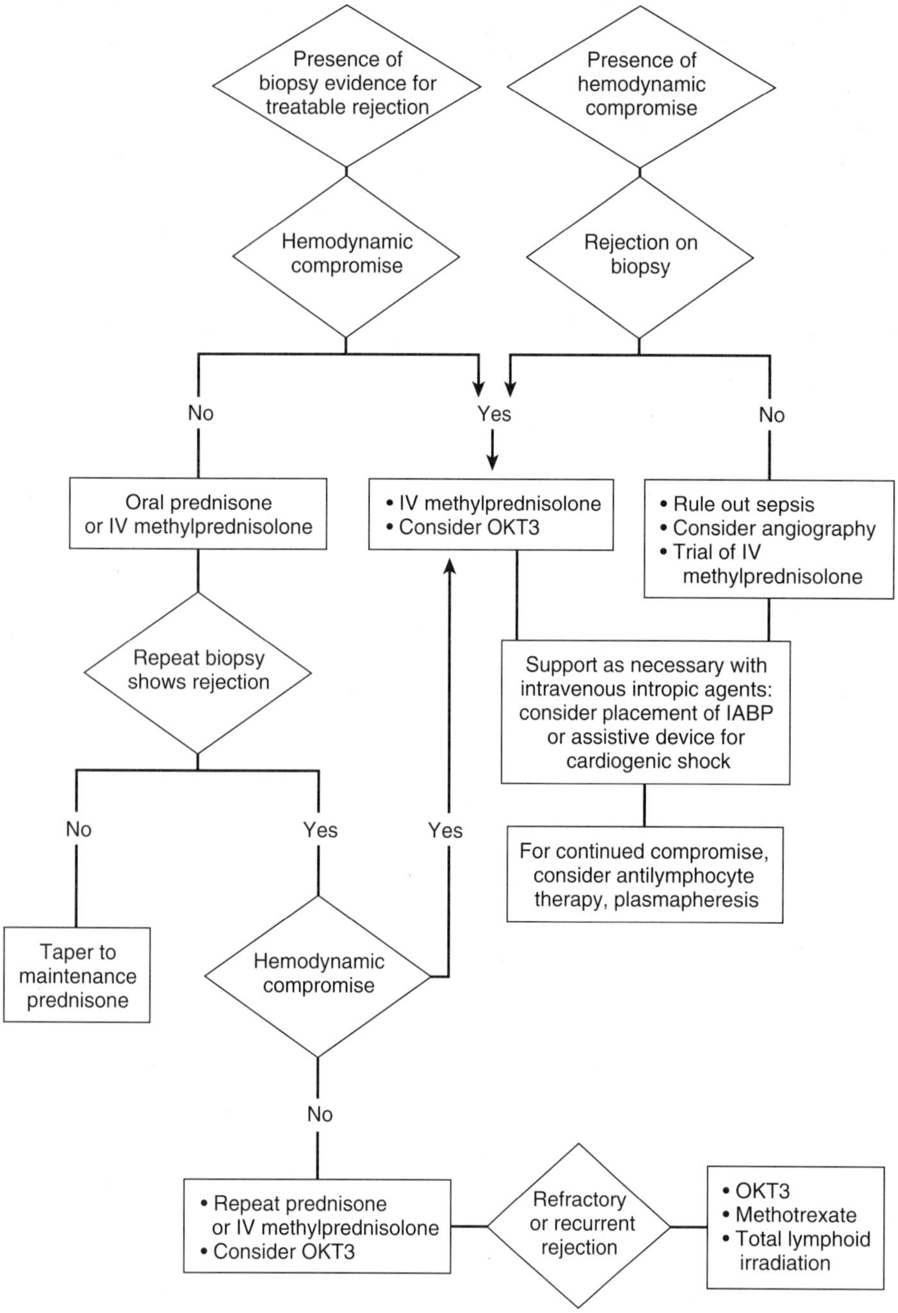

Figure 15–5. Distribution of biopsy grades among 4400 biopsy specimens from 250 transplant recipients. (Figure courtesy of Gayle Winters.)

with hemodynamic compromise. Peripheral edema can also occur but more often results from poor compliance with salt restriction, use of nifedipine for hypertension, and the chronically blunted response to fluid retention (discussed later). Patients who have developed an apparent decrease in left ventricular function without cellular rejection on biopsy specimens are sometimes considered to have humoral or vascular rejection attributed to antibody-mediated injury, even in the absence of biopsy evidence. The presumptive diagnosis of rejection in these cases without cellular infiltrate is often supported retrospectively by improvement in ventricular function after intensification of immunosuppression. Some patients with new left ventricular dysfunction that does not reverse are found to have previously unsuspected coronary artery disease.

Of 918 episodes of rejection in the multicenter series, 16% were associated with hemodynamic compromise. Almost one third of these clinical episodes occurred without major cellular rejection on biopsy.[47] Hemodynamic compromise from rejection can progress to circulatory collapse in hours and may require rapid escalation of therapy (see Fig. 15–6). Any patient presenting with unexplained weakness, shortness of breath, syncope, or hypotension should undergo immediate echocardiography to evaluate left ventricular function. In the absence of evidence of sepsis, patients with new hypotension and decreased left ventricular function are generally treated immediately with intravenous methylprednisolone for presumed rejection, even before a biopsy specimen is obtained. In patients with hemodynamic compromise, intense cytokine activation may be a major mediator of depressed left ventricular function, which can improve dramatically within hours of glucocorticoid therapy. Plasmapheresis is occasionally employed in these patients.

There are a small number of patients who develop gradual reduction in systolic function during the first year or later after transplantation; this often occurs in patients who received relatively small

TABLE 15–10. CARDIAC TRANSPLANT IMMUNOSUPPRESSION

	Cyclosporine	Methylprednisolone	Prednisone	Azathioprine
Preoperative	None or 2–6 mg/kg PO	None	None	0–2 mg/kg
Intraoperative	None	500–1000 mg for 1–2 doses	None	None
Immediate postoperative	IV or oral twice/d titrating to slightly higher level than that used for chronic dosing	125 mg IV every 12 h for 3 doses	After methylprednisolone, start at 0.5–1 mg/kg/d, gradually taper to 0.2–0.3 mg/kg/d by 2–4 wk	1.5–3 mg/kg/d
Long-term therapy	Titrate 3–8 mg/kg/d to blood levels, may decrease slightly in progressive renal dysfunction	None	Target for 0.1 mg/kg/d by 3–6 mo; selected patients may be "weaned" from prednisone	2 mg/kg/d or less as needed to maintain white blood cell count >4000/mm^3

hearts. Restrictive physiology may be apparent. Exercise tolerance and fluid balance are markedly impaired. A previous history of major rejection episodes may be more common in these patients. A trial of enhanced immunosuppression is appropriate if there is any evidence of rejection in biopsy specimens. Cardiac catheterization may be indicated to identify the early onset of accelerated TCAD, which can lead to impaired coronary vascular reserve and diastolic dysfunction.

Standard Therapy for Prevention and Treatment of Rejection. Current immunosuppression therapy includes a chronic regimen of drugs adjusted to blunt the ongoing immune response to the transplanted heart (Table 15–10) and acute supplementation with those or other therapies if rejection occurs (see Fig. 15–6). Cyclosporine and the newer drug FK506 both block production of interleukin-2 by activated lymphocytes.[50] Although hypertension is less of a problem with FK506, nephrotoxicity is similar to that with cyclosporine and neurotoxicity is more severe; therefore, cyclosporine remains the major immunosuppressive agent used for heart transplantation.[51]

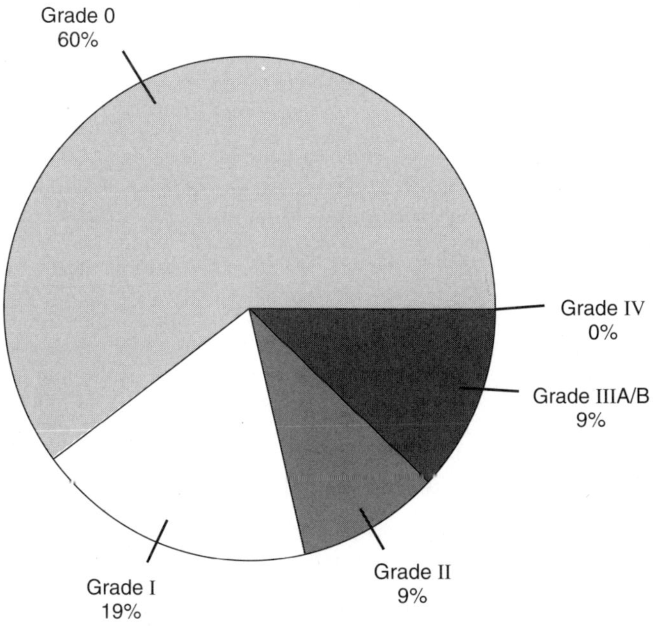

Figure 15–6. Algorithm for therapy for biopsy-proven rejection episodes, with or without hemodynamic compromise, and for acute hemodynamic compromise, with or without biopsy evidence of rejection. *Abbreviations:* IABP, intra-aortic balloon counterpulsation; IV, intravenous; MP, methylprednisolone.

The method of initiation of cyclosporine in the perioperative period varies according to renal function, as described previously. Some programs employ an oral preoperative cyclosporine loading dose (see Table 15–9). Postoperative administration may be either intravenous or oral, with intravenous infusion totaling approximately 30% of the oral dose. Maintenance oral doses range from 3 to 8 mg/kg/day. Dosing may be increased when modest grades of rejection are being observed without intensification of other therapy. Previous use of cyclosporine was characterized by much higher doses and greater toxicity than those currently observed during blood level monitoring. Blood levels, assayed by various methods, are generally checked daily during the initial hospitalization and frequently during major changes in therapy. Many medications affect the metabolism of cyclosporine (Table 15–11). Management of seizure disorders is particularly troublesome, because most anticonvulsant medications accelerate cyclosporine metabolism and decrease blood levels markedly. Cyclosporine levels should be observed during any gastrointestinal illness that might affect cyclosporine absorption, and intravenous cyclosporine therapy should be instituted if necessary.

Nephrotoxicity and hypertension occur in most patients taking cyclosporine (Table 15–12).[52] Occasionally, patients must discontinue cyclosporine late after heart transplantation to prevent the need for dialysis or renal transplantation. Symptoms of cyclosporine neurotoxicity include headaches, tremors, and dysesthesias, which generally improve within the first few months after initiation of therapy.[53] Hirsutism is common, and many female patients use depilatories to remove excess hair growth.

Azathioprine, which inhibits purine biosynthesis, is part of the current standard "triple-therapy" approach to immunosuppression. The addition of azathioprine to cyclosporine allows reduced maintenance doses of glucocorticoids. Administration of azathioprine is begun intravenously or orally in doses of 1.5–2 mg/kg/day early after surgery. This drug is generally adjusted to maintain white blood cell counts of at least 4000/mm^3. Unlike other maintenance

TABLE 15–11. COMMON DRUG INTERACTIONS WITH CYCLOSPORINE

Increased Cyclosporine Levels	Decreased Cyclosporine Levels
Diltiazem	Ethanol
Cimetidine	Cholestyramine
Ranitidine	Phenobarbital
Metoclopramide	Phenytoin
Ciprofloxacin	Ethambutol
Erythromycin	Nafcillin
Ketoconazole	Isoniazid
	Sulfamethoxazole

TABLE 15–12. POTENTIAL ADVERSE EFFECTS OF TRIPLE-DRUG IMMUNOSUPPRESSION

Cyclosporine	Diabetes exacerbation
Hypertension	Obesity
Renal dysfunction	Labile emotions
Hyperkalemia	Sodium retention
Hypomagnesemia	Hyperlipidemia
Hyperuricemia	Easy bruisability
Hepatic dysfunction	Peptic ulcers
CNS	Cataracts
Seizures	Insomnia
Tremor	Avascular bone necrosis
Paresthesia	Corticosteroid myopathy
Anxiety	Growth retardation in children
Insomnia	*Azathioprine*
Hirsutism	Leukopenia
Rhinorrhea	Thrombocytopenia
Gingival hyperplasia	Macrocytic anemia
Malignancy	Pancreatitis
Corticosteroids	Cholestatic jaundice
Cushingoid habitus	Hepatitis
Osteoporosis	Interstitial pneumonitis

Adapted from Kobashigawa JA, Stevenson LW: Post-operative treatment of heart transplant recipients. J Crit Illness 1993; 8:607–615.

immunosuppressive agents, azathioprine is not part of the acute therapy for rejection episodes, although the chronic dose may be increased, when allowed by the white blood cell count, to provide additional baseline immunosuppression to prevent future recurrence. Azathioprine is metabolized by the xanthine oxidase pathway, and the dose must be decreased by approximately 75% if allopurinol is taken concomitantly, as may be necessary for some patients with gout.

Glucocorticoids are given in high doses in the perioperative period, initially as intravenous methylprednisolone, and later as oral prednisone (see Table 15–10). Subsequent reduction yields an average dose of 20 mg/day by 30 days in most centers. Rejection is treated with increased doses of glucocorticoids, which may be given as intravenous boluses of 250–1000 mg of methylprednisolone for 3 days or in oral pulses of 50–100 mg daily, tapering to maintenance doses over the next 7–14 days.[54] Some centers initiate steroid-free maintenance after the first month, with reinstitution of chronic maintenance glucocorticoid therapy only in the 20%–40% of patients who demonstrate multiple episodes of rejection.[55] Mild levels of rejection seen in biopsy specimens are treated more aggressively in patients who are not receiving chronic glucocorticoid therapy. Withdrawal of glucocorticoid therapy after the first 6 months can be successful in as many as 85% of patients.[56] There is some concern that these patients are more vulnerable to hemodynamic compromise should late rejection occur. The anticipated benefits of "steroid-free maintenance" for plasma lipid levels, diabetes, obesity, and osteoporosis have not been uniformly demonstrated. Greater genetic homogeneity between recipients and donors in some regions may influence the likelihood of rejection and the strategies used at different centers.

Lymphocyte antibody preparations include locally prepared rabbit antithymocyte globulins (ATG) and antilymphocyte globulins (ALG) and commercial equine ATGs, all of which are polyclonal. The mouse monoclonal preparation OKT3 is directed against the CD3 complex on the lymphocyte surface. These preparations were given for the first 5–14 days after transplantation in an attempt to induce partial graft tolerance, termed "induction therapy." Once used routinely by approximately 50% of transplant programs, induction therapy may delay but probably does not decrease the incidence of rejection[47] and may increase the appearance of vascular rejection, which has been associated with poorer prognosis.[49] Use of induction therapy has also been implicated in higher rates of CMV infection and posttransplant lymphoproliferative disease (PTLD).[57] These preparations may be used in shorter courses to allow delay of initial cyclosporine therapy in patients with precarious renal function.[42]

The major role of the antilymphocyte preparations is for the "rescue" therapy of refractory rejection, which is usually treated with 5 mg of intravenous OKT3 daily for 10–14 days.[58] The first dose of OKT3, and less commonly, the second or third doses, may be associated with fever, respiratory distress, and occasionally, circulatory collapse attributed to intense cytokine release from activation of lymphocytes. These symptoms are minimized by the prior administration of corticosteroids, diphenhydramine, acetaminophen, and in some cases, nonsteroidal anti-inflammatory agents. The chance of acute respiratory failure is higher in the setting of marked elevation in fluid volume and pulmonary pressures. When given in the perioperative period, the apparent first-dose reaction is decreased by giving the first dose while the patient is still anesthetized in the operating room. For treatment of rejection, administration of the first two or three doses should be done under close supervision with epinephrine and intubation available. Aseptic meningitis, characterized by pleocytosis in sterile cerebrospinal fluid and variable neurologic symptoms, can occur at any time during the course of OKT3 administration. Although the last doses of OKT3 can occasionally be administered in an outpatient setting, concern regarding the severity of rejection and potential OKT3 side effects often mandate continued hospitalization. To avoid "rebound" rejection during recovery of the lymphocyte population 1–2 weeks after OKT3 therapy, high prednisone doses are usually maintained during this time.

Human antibodies develop to the mouse antibody in 20%–80% of patients and are detected by flow cytometry or enzyme-linked immunosorbent assays or inferred by an unexpected rise in peripheral blood CD3-positive lymphocytes, which are monitored frequently during therapy. In some cases, administration of the higher dose of 10 mg is effective as therapy for rejection in the presence of antibodies. The presence of antibodies may be associated with a higher incidence of vascular rejection.[49]

There is a theoretical rationale for the use of broader antilymphocyte therapy, such as polyclonal ATG or locally manufactured preparations of ALG, when a major component of antibody-mediated response is suspected. There is currently no controlled data demonstrating clinical differences between polyclonal and monoclonal preparations in suppression of antibody-mediated responses during hemodynamic compromise. Polyclonal preparations may occasionally be contaminated with antibodies to other blood components, such as platelets.

Therapies Used for Recurrent or Refractory Rejection. Patients with many episodes of recurrent rejection, particularly those in high-risk groups such as multiparous women, may require additional immunosuppressive therapy. Methotrexate is a folic acid analog that inhibits DNA synthesis by binding competitively to dihydrofolic reductase. It is generally given orally, 5 mg one to three times weekly.[59] Methotrexate should be markedly reduced or avoided in the presence of significant renal dysfunction. Azathioprine may or may not be reduced simultaneously, depending on the white blood cell count, which should be checked at least weekly during methotrexate administration. Adverse effects of methotrexate include nausea, mucositis, fatigue, leukopenia, and leukemoid reactions, in addition to the expected increase in risk of infection. The duration of therapy is generally about 8 weeks and has led to reversal of rejection in the majority of cases. More prolonged courses of methotrexate may be employed to reduce maintenance corticosteroid requirement.

Total lymphoid irradiation (TLI), developed as therapy for Hodgkin disease, leads to prolonged suppression of cell-mediated immunity and appears to induce some level of specific tolerance.[60] Radiation is delivered to a thoracic "mantle" and inverted Y abdominal field, 80 cGy twice weekly or less frequently as tolerated by the white blood cell and platelet counts, to a planned total of 800 cGy.

Because of the time required (minimum 5 weeks) and the frequent need to discontinue azathioprine, TLI does not constitute therapy for severe acute rejection but can lead to dramatic improvement in some patients with smoldering or recurrent rejection.

Plasmapheresis is occasionally employed before transplantation in patients with high levels of sensitization to random panel antigens. Acute rejection with severe hemodynamic compromise in the first weeks after transplantation and possibly later may involve intense antibody reactions. Although the rationale for plasmapheresis is the removal of these antibodies, circulating cytokines and soluble antigens may also be depleted and other components of the immune response modulated.[50]

Newer agents under investigation include cyclosporine analogs and FK506, both of which inhibit interleukin-2 production; rapamycin (or sirolimus), which inhibits interleukin-2 receptor binding; mycophenolate mofetil, which inhibits purine biosynthesis and may suppress antibody formation related to TCAD; brequinar, which inhibits pyrimidine synthesis; and 15-deoxyspergualin, which inhibits generation of cytotoxic T lymphocytes and maturation of B lymphocytes.[50] Many new targets have been identified for monoclonal antibodies, including the T-cell receptor complex, interleukin-2 receptors, tumor necrosis factor-alpha, and intracellular adhesion molecules. Another therapy under investigation is photopheresis, in which the peripheral blood mononuclear cells of patients given 8-methoxypsoralen are exposed ex vivo to ultraviolet light. The proposed mechanism involves cell surface alteration that incites suppressor activity from other effector cells in vivo.

Transplant Coronary Artery Disease

Diffuse disease of the coronary arteries is evident on angiography in 50% of transplant recipients by 5 years but can appear within the first few months after the procedure.[11, 61] TCAD is a common cause of death late after transplantation (Fig. 15–7). Intracoronary ultrasonography frequently detects abnormalities of the intima before compromise of the lumina is seen on angiograms. Because the pathologic specimens show less lipid and calcium infiltration than in native atherosclerosis, the term arteriopathy has been suggested for this condition. In addition, concomitant involvement of veins and venules has given rise to the term "graft vasculopathy." This major cause of late death after transplantation appears to result from the interaction of circulating and local immune responses, endothelial activation and infiltration,[62] and other factors such as obesity, hyperlipidemia, and smoking.[23, 61] TCAD occurs with and without cyclosporine administration and with and without glucocorticoid maintenance, and it occurs in similar frequencies even in geographic regions with lower incidences of acute rejection. Risk may be increased by CMV infection, which causes increased expression of surface antigens in infected cells.

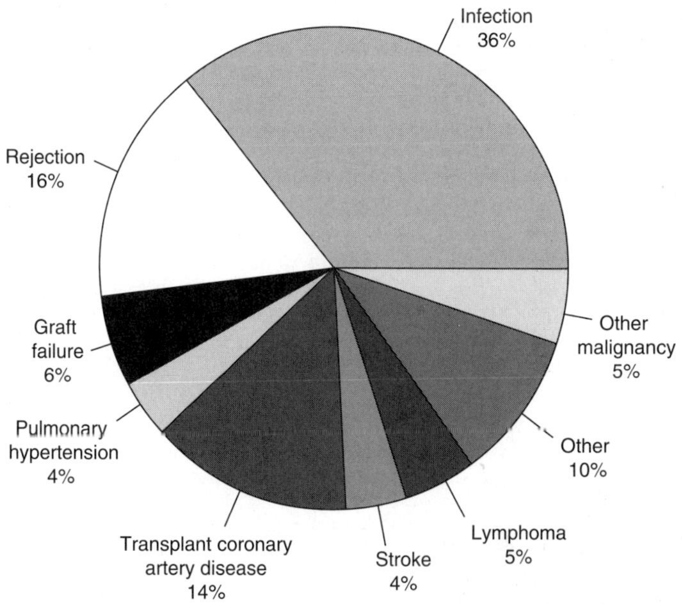

Figure 15–7. Causes of mortality after transplantation in the extended Stanford experience of 310 patients who underwent transplantation with cyclosporine therapy after 1980. *Abbreviations:* HTN, hypertension; TCAD, transplant coronary artery disease.

Coronary artery disease in the denervated heart is usually asymptomatic until left ventricular dysfunction has developed. Rare patients demonstrate a typical or atypical chest pain pattern that suggests partial re-enervation. Worsening exercise tolerance or syncope may be the presenting symptom. It seems reasonable to treat patients with TCAD with nitrates and beta blockers, if tolerated, but there is no good evidence that anti-ischemic agents impact on either ischemia or survival in this population.

There are no known interventions that slow progression or cause regression of TCAD after it has been diagnosed. The calcium channel antagonist diltiazem has been suggested to decrease the development of TCAD.[63] Aggressive use of hydroxy-3-methylglutaryl coenzyme A (HMG-CoA) reductase inhibitors beginning on the day of transplantation may decrease the incidences of both rejection and vasculopathy, perhaps from direct effects on membrane function of immune effector cells, as well as effects on circulating lipids. Cyclosporine reduces the metabolism of reductase inhibitors, which can accumulate and cause rhabdomyolysis in transplant recipients if creatine phosphokinase levels are not closely monitored.[64] Once the disease is evident angiographically, the number of vessels involved and the level of left ventricular function are important prognostic factors. Patients with three-vessel disease and a left ventricular ejection fraction of less than .40 have less than 50% survival during the year following diagnosis, and most deaths occur suddenly.

Angioplasty has been performed with technical success in areas of relatively discrete stenoses with demonstrable distal ischemia.[65] The rate of restenosis is high, but the major problem after angioplasty is rapid progression of the disease in other areas. Coronary artery bypass has been undertaken in rare cases; its use is limited primarily by poor downstream flow in diseased resistance vessels. Retransplantation is the therapy of choice in patients who remain eligible for transplantation but is often excluded because of the presence of renal disease and other conditions. Even in optimal candidates, retransplantation has been associated with a 1-year survival rate of only 60%, compared with a survival rate of 80%–85% with first-time transplantation.[15] Calculation of survival after transplantation may overestimate the success of transplantation per heart transplanted unless retransplantation is considered as an endpoint (Fig. 15–8). Sudden death is the most common endpoint for patients with TCAD, presumably as a result of ventricular arrhythmias in the setting of ischemia.

Infection

Suppression of the immune system provides opportunity for infection after heart transplantation, but these patients are much more robust than patients who are granulocytopenic after cancer chemotherapy or bone marrow transplantation. The widespread use of cyclosporine has led to a decrease in the severity of infection and mortality from infection, but infection remains the leading cause of death after transplantation. Review of a recent 25-center experience showed the incidence of serious infection, defined primarily as episodes severe enough to require intravenous therapy, to be 0.62 infections per patient during the first year following transplantation, with the majority of episodes occurring during the first 3 months.[66] Multiple infections often occur in the same patient, whereas 67% of

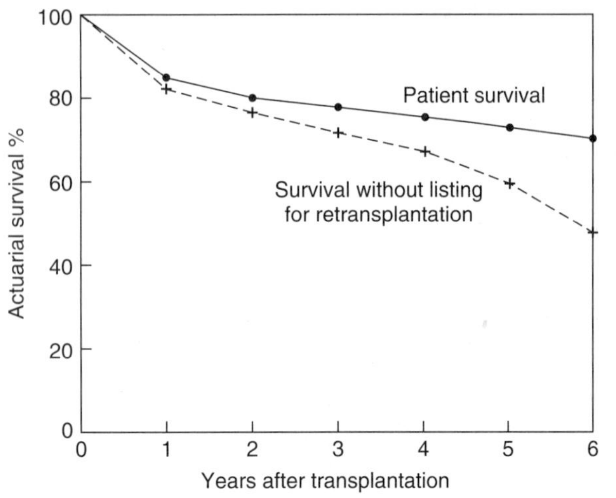

Figure 15–8. Actuarial survival curve in 400 transplant recipients demonstrates good survival at 6 years after transplant but a progressive increase in the number of patients with sufficient graft compromise to warrant retransplantation. (Data obtained with the collaboration of Jon A. Kobashigawa.)

patients are free of major infection during the first year. Death occurred in 17% of overall episodes and in 36% of fungal infections.

Bacteria are the most common causes of infection during the first month after transplantation, particularly *Staphylococcus* species and gram-negative organisms (Fig. 15–9). Opportunistic infections with CMV, *Pneumocystis* species, and fungi dominate from the second month after transplantation. Herpes simplex, however, often causes superficial infection early after transplantation or rejection therapy and may appear at sites of skin trauma. Toxoplasmosis can occur in the first few months after transplantation and possibly may be transmitted from the donor. After the first 6 months, there may be an increasing incidence of more common community-acquired bacterial infections.

The most common single infection is CMV. Clinical syndromes of CMV infection occur in 10%–30% of heart transplant recipients, and antilymphocyte therapy is associated with increased risk. Most patients are seropositive for CMV by the first year after transplantation. To diagnose active infection, CMV may be cultured from the urine or buffy coat of blood or identified by polymerase chain reaction. For the 25-center study, even the approximately two thirds of recipients who are seropositive before transplantation showed a 9% incidence of clinical reactivation. The group at greatest risk, however, are patients who are seronegative for CMV who then receive a heart from a seropositive donor. This group, which constitutes about 15% of all heart transplant recipients, is the focus of numerous prophylactic regimens with ganciclovir or hyperimmune globulin, which are anticipated to reduce the severity of subsequent CMV infection.[67] Many patients who develop positive CMV serology demonstrate none of the clinical syndromes of vague fevers, upper or lower gastrointestinal pain or bleeding, pulmonary infection, or possible CMV myocarditis demonstrated by polymerase chain reaction on endomyocardial biopsy specimens. In addition to these concerns, CMV infection appears to predispose to coinfection with other organisms such as *Pneumocystis carinii* and to the development of accelerated graft vasculopathy. At one time, therapy of CMV was restricted to cases with pathologic evidence of tissue invasion, but ganciclovir is now instituted for most clinical CMV syndromes.

The lung is the most common site of infection in heart transplant patients (see Fig. 15–9). Blood, urine, and the gastrointestinal tract are also frequent sites of infection. Sternal wound infection occurs rarely, but can be fatal. In the search for a source of infection, the sinuses and central nervous system should always be suspected. In the absence of a toxic appearance or an obvious source of infection, fever should generally not be treated initially with empiric broad-spectrum antibiotics, which will confound subsequent diagnosis and may predispose to subsequent infection with resistant organisms or fungi.

Community-acquired viral upper respiratory syndromes are generally well tolerated by heart transplant patients, who may be at slightly higher risk for secondary bacterial pulmonary infections. Exposure to chickenpox is a major concern, however, and should be avoided whenever possible. Prophylactic treatment with hyperimmune globulin may decrease the severity of infection if administered soon after known contact in a nonimmune transplant recipient. When given after the first 6 months after transplantation, vaccination against influenza appears to produce appropriate titer responses without stimulating rejection. Live-virus vaccines should be avoided.

In many centers, trimethoprim-sulfamethoxazole is administered twice weekly for prevention of *Pneumocystis* infection in cardiac transplant patients. Nystatin or clotrimazole preparations are used to prevent oral candidiasis (i.e., thrush). The optimal prophylactic regimen for prevention of CMV in the CMV-negative recipient of a CMV-positive donor organ has not yet been established but may include ganciclovir or hyperimmune globulin. CMV titers are routinely observed after transplantation, but broad "surveillance" cultures are no longer routine in most transplant centers. Protective isolation procedures do not appear to reduce the incidence of overall or specific infections but do tend to decrease traffic into the transplant patients' rooms. When overall vigilance is high, good handwashing procedures and wearing of masks by staff and family with viral syndromes may be sufficient. Considering the exposure to multiple

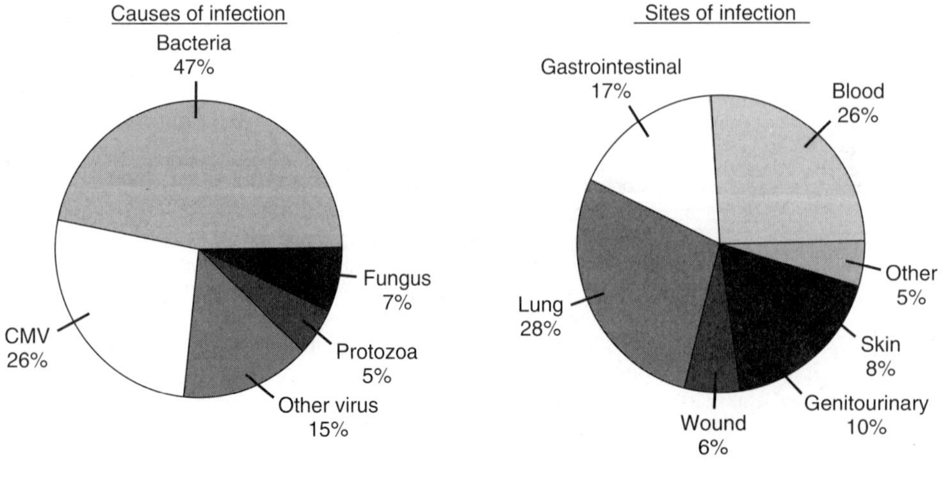

Figure 15–9. Pie chart demonstrating the sites and organisms implicated in 409 infectious episodes from the Cardiac Transplant Research Database, which includes patients from 25 major transplant centers. Episodes were defined as infections severe enough to require intravenous therapy or life-saving oral therapy. *Abbreviation:* CMV, cytomegalovirus. (Adapted from Miller LW, Naftel DC, Bourge RC: Infection after heart transplantation: A multi-institutional study. J Heart Lung Trans 1994; 13:381–393.)

hospital organisms, some programs suggest that transplant recipients wear masks when they return for clinic visits and biopsies. Every center is plagued by occasional outbreaks of specific infections which can at times be traced to environmental factors, such as aspergillosis from construction sites or *Serratia* infections from contaminated water pipes, but more often, these outbreaks subside spontaneously without changes in infection management strategy.

Malignancy

The risk of developing malignancy after transplantation is estimated at 1%–4% yearly.[25] This increased incidence is attributed to general suppression of the immune policing of early malignant clones. There is no detectable increase in lung, breast, and colon malignancies.

Cutaneous malignancies are particularly associated with the use of azathioprine, which may relate to its metabolite nitromidazole, which enhances photosensitivity. Generous use of sunscreens and protective clothing are advised in cardiac transplant patients. Posttransplant lymphoproliferative disease (PTLD) is a unique form of lymphoma that is usually of B-cell origin. The Epstein-Barr virus has been repeatedly implicated in PTLD.[68] Previous use of antilymphocyte preparations may increase the incidence of PTLD.[57] This lymphoma is more likely than other lymphomas to present in extranodal locations such as the central nervous system and the gastrointestinal tract. Drastic reduction of immunosuppression has led to regression of PTLD, which is otherwise treated with chemotherapy, in as many as 40% of cases. Although most cases of PTLD occur after the first year after transplantation, this disease can appear earlier, in which case the prognosis is usually very poor.

Function After Transplantation

Cardiac Function and Exercise. The systolic function of the transplanted heart is usually normal, except in the setting of rejection or TCAD, but diastolic function is slightly impaired, perhaps as a result of denervation, fibrosis from rejection, or cyclosporine.[69, 70] The product of the higher heart rate and slightly lower stroke volume is a cardiac output that is normal or slightly reduced at rest. Multiple factors can compromise function of the transplanted hearts during exercise (Table 15–13).[69] The peak oxygen consumption, peak workload, and exercise time are generally about 50%–70% of that predicted for gender, age, and body size.[3] This impairment represents both the limited cardiac reserve and peripheral muscle factors, which include prior deconditioning and the effects of glucocorticoid therapy. Some patients are limited by bone pain related to osteoporosis or aseptic necrosis. Exercise training has been shown to increase peak capacity by about 20%.[71] However, patients are generally advised to avoid vigorous exercise after therapy for rejection, until a biopsy specimen demonstrating improvement is obtained.

TABLE 15–13. FACTORS AFFECTING CARDIAC PERFORMANCE AFTER TRANSPLANTATION

Before Implantation
Donor
Donor size and cardiac function
Adequacy of preservation
Ischemic time
Recipient
Irreversible pulmonary hypertension causing right heart failure
Obesity
Diabetes
Denervation
Afferent denervation
Impaired reflex response of peripheral circulation
Impaired neural regulation of fluid balance and renal function
Absence of anginal symptoms during ischemia
Efferent denervation
Absent vagal tone
Elevated resting heart rate
Delayed heart rate response to increased demand
Limited maximal heart rate response
Possible impairment of relaxation
Hypersensitivity to catecholamines, adenosine
Atrial Anastomoses
Atrial distortion and asynchronous contraction
Mitral and tricuspid regurgitation
Increased baseline atrial natriuretic factor
Effects of Rejection
Acute myocardial depression from cytokines
Chronic fibrosis
Nonspecific graft dysfunction
Decreased coronary vascular reserve
Epicardial coronary artery disease
Complications of Hypertension
Left ventricular hypertrophy
Increased peripheral afterload
Cardiodepressant effects of calcium channel blockers, beta blockers
Obesity

Denervation and Dysrhythmias. Harvesting of the donor heart creates both afferent and efferent denervation.[69] Afferent interruption impairs the rapid vasoregulatory and slower sympathorenal responses to volume changes. Afferent denervation eliminates the sensation of angina except in rare patients with partial sympathetic reinnervation. Lack of efferent innervation eliminates the balancing effects of vagal and sympathetic outflow on heart rate and contractility in response to demand. The use of beta-blocking agents, which are sometimes employed to treat hypertension, has been shown to decrease contractility and exercise capacity but is clinically tolerated in some patients.

The sinus rate is generally elevated as a result of the loss of tonic vagal input. Approximately 10% of posttransplant patients demonstrate persistent sinus node dysfunction, which sometimes responds to oral theophylline or terbutaline. Even though persistent sinus node dysfunction often resolves by 6 months postoperatively, early implantation of a pacemaker allows rehabilitation and discharge to proceed as scheduled. Atrioventricular node function is usually normal. Atrial arrhythmias are common in the early postoperative period and can also occur during rejection episodes. Absence of direct sympathetic innervation leads to exaggerated responses to calcium channel blockers and beta blockers. Bradyarrhythmias can develop during rejection or for unexplained reasons later after transplantation. Rarely, coronary artery spasm is diagnosed in patients with bradyarrhythmias. Ventricular arrhythmias are rare except in the setting of coronary disease.

The effects of antiarrhythmic therapy are influenced by denervation. Digoxin does not slow atrioventricular conduction in the absence of direct vagal innervation except at high and potentially toxic doses. Drugs with vagolytic activity in the native heart, such as quinidine and disopyramide, can decrease heart rate and atrioventricular conduction in the transplanted heart.[69] The denervated heart appears to have increased sensitivity to acetylcholine and adenosine, which can produce marked bradyarrhythmias.

Hypertension. Hypertension occurs in 50%–90% of heart transplant recipients on cyclosporine and typically develops within the first few months after transplantation.[72] Disproportionate diastolic hypertension is common, and the normal diurnal variation in blood pressure is lost. Hypertension in patients on cyclosporine may reflect the combined effects of increased sympathetic tone, increased endothelin levels, stimulation of the renin-angiotensin system, and nephrotoxicity. Considerations in the choice of therapy for hypertension include the cyclosporine-sparing effect of diltiazem and its possible role in reducing TCAD and potential worsening of exercise capacity on beta-receptor antagonists. ACE inhibitors are also effective but occasionally cause hyperkalemia when administered in combination with cyclosporine; therefore, potassium levels should be monitored during initiation of ACE inhibitor therapy. Calcium channel blocking agents are effective in reducing hypertension but can cause peripheral edema and predispose to postural symptoms in some patients. Many transplant recipients need more than one antihypertensive agent to maintain blood pressures below 140/100 mm Hg.

Fluid Status and Renal Function. Cardiac transplant patients tend to retain fluid as a result of glucocorticoid therapy and impaired neural volume regulation despite the cardiac production of atrial natriuretic peptides, which is not only preserved but often enhanced. Diuretics are often necessary to maintain fluid balance, but hypovolemia, particularly when assuming a standing position, is also difficult for a circulatory system with a denervated heart to buffer. Slightly elevated filling pressures may be necessary in some patients to achieve adequate filling in the setting of decreased ventricular compliance. In patients with significant impairment of renal function by cyclosporine, maintenance of higher volume status may be necessary to prevent further deterioration. As in heart failure patients, the use of prostaglandin inhibitors can cause worsening of renal function, although it is usually tolerated for brief periods of musculoskeletal problems or gout. Potassium replacement is rarely necessary because of the potassium-retaining effects of cyclosporine.

Osteoporosis. Osteoporosis eventually occurs in at least 10% of transplant recipients. Postmenopausal women are at highest risk, but osteoporosis is a concern in all transplant patients.[73] Both glucocorticoids and cyclosporine compromise bone mass, which is frequently reduced before transplantation. Reduction or elimination of glucocorticoids is ideal but frequently is not feasible. Oral calcium supplementation, vitamin D, fluoride, biphosphonates, hydrochlorothiazide, intramuscular calcitonin injections, and periodic supplementation with estrogen or testosterone are frequently employed.

Success of Rehabilitation. The most important lesson for the candidate for heart transplantation is that the procedure exchanges one burden of problems, those associated with heart failure, for another burden of problems, those associated with rejection and the complications of immunosuppression. Because transplantation does not restore normal quality of life or life expectancy, it can improve them only when they are otherwise severely limited.

Restoration of normal hemodynamics does not translate immediately into increased activity. In patients with previous chronic debility, the pretransplant peripheral muscle deconditioning reverses slowly after transplantation, particularly in the presence of corticosteroid therapy. Formal exercise training within the first weeks after discharge accelerates improvement in peak oxygen consumption and ventilatory efficiency.[74]

Much of the information regarding quality of life after transplantation is derived from the National Cooperative Transplantation Study of 85% of transplant programs in the United States based on patients undergoing transplantation before 1990.[75] Based on global measures of activity, 85% of survivors are "physically active," although 66% perceived themselves as limited in some way from doing something they desired. This limitation was in activities of daily living in only 1%. Health problems restricted 7% of patients to home most of the time. Physical concerns caused 34% of patients problems walking several blocks or climbing stairs, 43% of patients had trouble bending or lifting, and 47% considered themselves physically limited in workload at work or home. Although at least 50% of patients could theoretically be employed, fewer than 33% returned to work. The low reemployment rate reflects not only physical limitations but many nonmedical problems, such as dependence on disability income and employer liability.

Despite the numerous physiologic limitations experienced after heart transplantation, it remains the best therapy for selected patients with end-stage heart failure. The National Cooperative Transplantation Study reported that heart transplant recipients rated their level of well-being as similar to that of the healthy population,[75] results that were equivalent to those in the kidney and pancreas transplant populations. This may in some measure reflect the contrast from previous illness and also the intensity of the transplant experience. Beyond the potential physiologic benefits, many patients describe a rejuvenation after transplantation. Receipt of a heart harvested from tragedy restores to many recipients a gratitude and energy which is not diminished by the knowledge that their future health remains uncertain.

CIRCULATORY SUPPORT DEVICES

As heart transplant waiting lists become longer, mechanical circulatory assistance offers extended support for patients who deteriorate hemodynamically and are otherwise unlikely to survive to receive a heart.[29, 30] These devices also serve effectively as bridges to spontaneous improvement from acute myocarditis, myocardial infarction, and postcardiotomy shock. The spectrum of potential devices includes the intra-aortic balloon counterpulsation pump (IABP), extracorporeal membrane oxygenation (ECMO), univentricular and biventricular nonpulsatile and pulsatile devices, and the total artificial heart.

The indications for emergency mechanical support, which differ depending on the cause of ventricular failure, remain controversial and are often best recognized in retrospect. Decisions may need to be made very rapidly in settings of acute deterioration from which spontaneous recovery is possible. Patients with a long history of heart failure usually deteriorate more slowly than those with recent onset unless an acute insult is added. Exacerbation of chronic heart failure frequently reverses without mechanical support after vigorous diuresis, readjustment of medications, and resolution of any concurrent problems such as infection.

Obvious indications for escalating support are evidence of critical hypoperfusion, such as mental obtundation or anuria without other cause, and accumulation of lactate. Conversely, respiratory failure as a result of heart failure is usually a consequence of severely elevated filling pressures rather than low output and can in most cases be treated pharmacologically, except when caused by intermittent severe ischemia without baseline congestion. Most hepatic dysfunction reflects severely elevated venous pressures rather than low output, except when severe prolonged hypoperfusion causes "shock liver," which is characterized by transaminase levels in the thousands.

The impact of hemodynamic parameters differs widely among patients, but at the most severe end of the spectrum, mechanical support is generally indicated in patients who have an inability to maintain systolic blood pressure greater than or equal to 75–80 mm Hg, cardiac index of more than 1.5–1.8 L/min/m^2, and pulmonary venous saturation of more than 50% on maximal pharmacologic support. As long as ventricular filling pressures exclude hypovolemia, the degree of filling pressure elevation is not often a factor in the decision of whether or not to provide mechanical support. Pharmacologic reduction of left ventricular filling pressures higher than 30 mm Hg frequently leads to improved cardiac output through reduction of mitral regurgitation.[76] Right atrial pressures that remain higher than 20 mm Hg when pulmonary capillary wedge pressures are equivalent identify patients who have a poor likelihood of long-term stabilization but may also be at risk for right heart failure after device placement. Patients with systemic vascular resistances higher than 1800 dynes-sec-cm^{-5} often improve with vasodilatation. On maximal therapy, more subtle trends of declining cardiac index and renal function are difficult to interpret, but intervention should not be delayed when a trend of progressive deterioration is obvious.[77]

The choice of circulatory support device depends on the situation (Fig. 15–10). Patients with potentially reversible conditions may be supported with short-term devices such as the IABP or external assistance of one or both ventricles. Patients in whom improvement is unlikely may or may not receive IABP support before undergoing

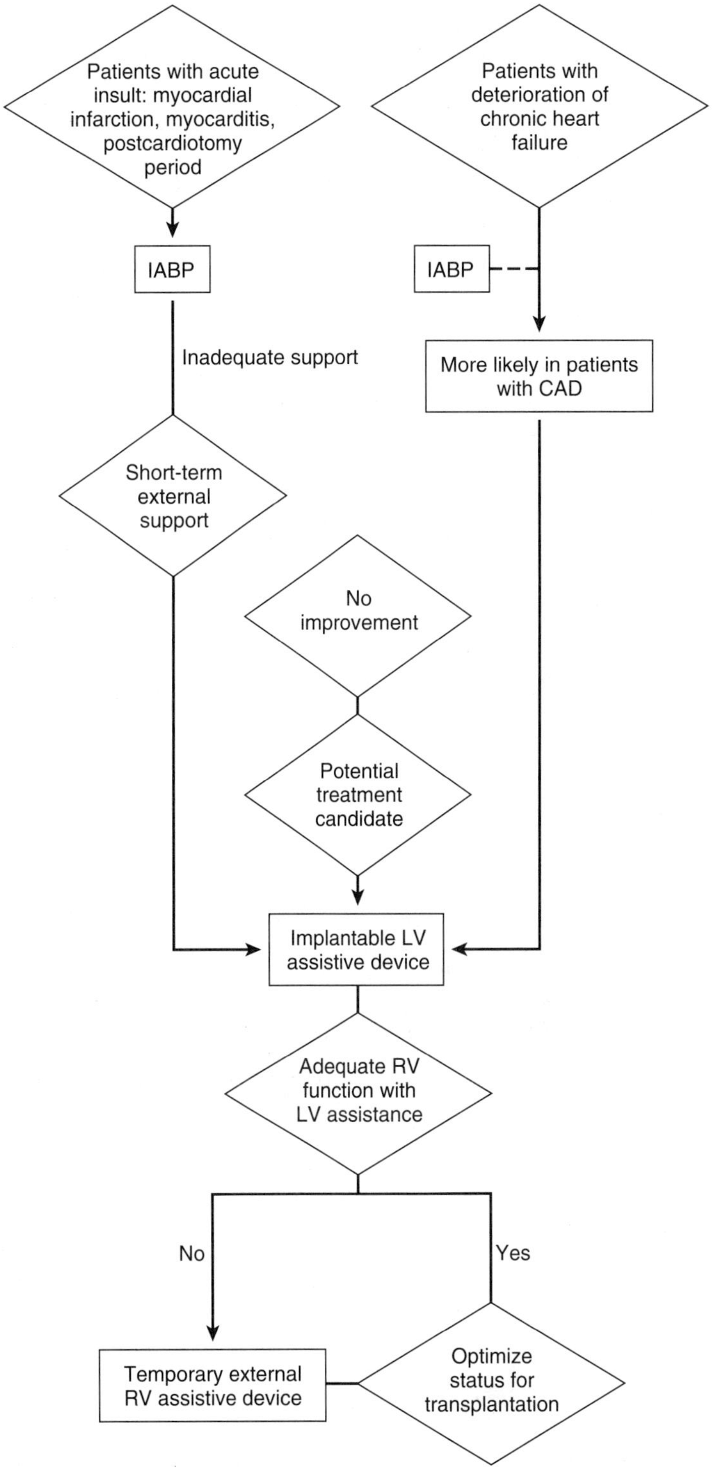

Figure 15–10. Algorithm for the use of mechanical assist devices for circulatory failure despite maximal pharmacologic therapy. Patients with an acute insult are more likely to recover sufficient intrinsic ventricular function to allow device removal. Patients with deterioration of chronic heart failure may be considered for an implantable assist device, with or without a trial of intra-aortic balloon support. *Abbreviations:* CAD, coronary artery disease; IABP, intra-aortic balloon counterpulsation; LV, left ventricle; RV, right ventricle.

placement of an implantable left ventricular assist device (LVAD) for extended stabilization and ambulation. Approximately 10%–30% of patients receiving LVADs require temporary right ventricular assistance with a separate device, which can usually be subsequently removed.

In the critically ill patient, early mortality or ineligibility for transplantation after device placement is in the range of 25%–35%;[30] therefore, this risk should be exceeded by the anticipated risk without support. The early posttransplant mortality for severely compromised patients may be reduced by implantable LVADs from 15%–20% to 10%, and this factor should also be considered. As the devices progress to provide long-term support for the ambulatory patient with less immediate risk after device insertion or medical therapy, the criteria for insertion will be based less on acute decompensation and more on the extended prognosis.

Intra-Aortic Balloon Counterpulsation

The largest experience with any mechanical circulatory support device is that with the IABP, which can provide a brief period of respite until more definitive intervention for a failing ventricle or for recovery of left ventricular "stunning" after infarction, cardiac arrest, or postcardiotomy shock can be attempted.[78] The cardiac output of a supported ventricle may increase by 10%–20% depending on the intrinsic contractility and the extent of myocardial injury.

The IABP has successfully bridged patients to transplantation,[78] but as the waiting periods grow longer even for hospitalized patients, this device cannot provide adequate sustained support. A major disadvantage of the IABP is the requirement for the patient to be recumbent in an intensive care unit, which precludes pretransplantation rehabilitation from heart failure. The IABP may be of greatest use in providing immediate support until stabilization and semielective insertion of a more permanent device as an extended bridge to transplantation can be undertaken.

Centrifugal Pumps

Centrifugal pumps have been used commonly for postcardiotomy support.[79] The Biomedicus bio-pump is one example (Fig. 15–11). Introduced in the late 1970s and early 1980s, these devices have gained acceptance as a result of their efficacy, simplicity, and reasonable cost.[80] Although they have been used as a short-term bridge to transplantation, they are not approved for long-term use as bridging devices. The duration of feasible support without major complications is measured only in days. In general, centrifugal pumps can maintain patient candidacy for transplant for a short period but rarely improve organ function or preoperative status from the time of implantation.

All centrifugal pumps require venous and arterial cannulation, through which they provide continuous nonpulsatile flow. Left ventricular support is accomplished by placing a large (36-Fr or larger) cannula in the right superior pulmonary vein at its junction with the left atrium while blood is returned to the aorta or femoral artery. Right ventricular assistance is provided by large cannulae positioned in the right atrium and inferior vena cava. Blood is returned to the pulmonary artery. All patients supported with these devices require continuous anticoagulation.

Complications associated with centrifugal pumps include bleeding, coagulopathy, thromboembolism, renal dysfunction, and sepsis. As of December 1992, the combined registry of the American Society of Artificial Internal Organs and the International Society for Heart and Lung Transplantation (ASAIO-ISHLT) included 853 patients supported by centrifugal pumps.[80] Bleeding occurred in as many as 55% of patients and device failure in as many as 15%.[80] Management requires continuous attendance of perfusionists in the intensive care unit setting, where patients remain bedridden without potential for rehabilitation. These devices have pivotal roles in salvaging some postcardiotomy patients but are not feasible for extended support before transplantation.

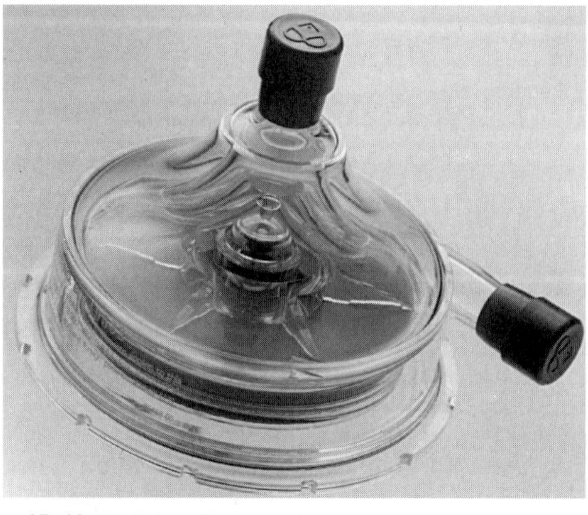

Figure 15–11. The Biomedicus centrifugal pump. (Courtesy of Medronic Bio-Medicus, Inc., Eden Prairie, MN.)

TABLE 15–14. VENTRICULAR ASSIST DEVICES

Extracorporeal Nonpulsatile
Centrifugal pumps
Extracorporeal membrane oxygenator (ECMO)
Extracorporeal Pulsatile
Thoratec (Pierce-Donachy)
Abiomed BVS 5000
*Intracorporeal Pulsatile**
Novacor
HeartMate
Total Artificial Heart (early trials)
CardioWest 70 and 100
Penn State Pneumatic

*The intra-aortic balloon pump is intracorporeal and pulsatile but is not included here because it does not produce its own stroke volume.

Extracorporeal Membrane Oxygenation

An ECMO unit is similar to a centrifugal pump, except that an oxygenator, usually of a membrane type similar to that used during cardiopulmonary bypass for open-heart procedures, is spliced into the circuit. Some circuits use a roller rather than a centrifugal pump. Groin cannulation is the most common technique, either via a cutdown method or percutaneously. Bleeding is a common complication associated with an ECMO circuit, because, like the centrifugal pump, ECMO requires continuous heparin anticoagulation and also causes hemolysis. ECMO has an undisputed role in neonatal respiratory failure. Experience is accumulating from support of postcardiotomy and posttransplant ventricular dysfunction in children,[81, 82] but the results in adults have been largely unfavorable. The limited length of time until development of organ failure and diffuse coagulopathy renders ECMO a very limited option during an unpredictable waiting period.

Ventricular Assist Devices

VADs currently provide the best alternatives for extended support of patients awaiting transplantation. In addition to the longer period of possible support, these devices allow ambulation and rehabilitation. Several VADs are available for clinical use, including extracorporeal pulsatile pumps and intracorporeal (implantable) pulsatile devices with an external power and control console (Table 15–14).

External Ventricular Assist Devices

The Thoratec device is a pneumatic device with a stroke volume of 65 mL which can be used for left-sided, right-sided, or bilateral ventricular support. Inflow cannulation is via the respective atria or ventricles, and outflow cannulation is via either the pulmonary artery or the aorta, depending on the ventricle being supported. Insertion requires a median sternotomy and cardiopulmonary bypass. Because the pump housing is external, it can be placed in patients of any body habitus.[83] Anticoagulation with warfarin or heparin is required.

The Abiomed BVS 5000 is a pneumatically driven vertical blood pump that also is capable of either right or left ventricular assistance. Its maximal stroke volume is 80 mL, determined by the venous return pulled by gravity from cannulae placed in the right or left atrium. Outflow cannulae are inserted in the main pulmonary artery or aorta. This device is suitable only for short-term postcardiotomy support, because its cannulae exit through the sternum to a bedside housing and impair patient mobility. Continuous anticoagulation is also required with the use of this device.

Implantable Ventricular Assist Devices

Implantable VADs are attached to the left ventricle and aorta. Right ventricular support is not provided. External connections provide venting and access to the power source and controls (Table 15–15). Confusion has arisen from the terminology. In general, an "implantable" device refers to a device with an internalized pumping mechanism (i.e., prosthetic ventricle). The control unit, pump actuator, and venting or compliance chamber are located outside the patient (Fig. 15–12). The power/control console can sit at the bedside like the console for an IABP, or the "wearable" model has been miniaturized to be carried by the patient. A "fully implantable" VAD with no extracorporeal components has yet to be implanted clinically. This reflects both the engineering challenges of a responsive compliance chamber and concerns regarding backup mechanisms for device reliability. All of the implantable VADs share five general components (see Table 15–15).

Clinical experience with the Novacor and HeartMate devices is increasing (Table 15–16). The wearable systems allow independent patient function. The Novacor LVAD is a double–pusher-plate, electrically powered pump. The blood pump and electromechanical energy converter are implanted, whereas the control unit is external.[84] The pump stroke volume of the Novacor LVAD is 70 mL. In the United States, more than 100 patients have undergone implantation of the Novacor LVAD, primarily as a bridge to transplantation. Patients receive full anticoagulation while supported with this device.

The HeartMate 1000IP LVAD, which is pneumatically driven, and the HeartMate 1205 VE, which is electrically driven, are pusher-plate blood pumps with stroke volumes of 85 mL. The titanium housing, which contacts the blood, promotes the formation and adherence of a pseudoneointima.[85] As a result, anticoagulation requirements are reduced if not eliminated.[86]

Patient Selection for Implantable Ventricular Assist Devices

Indications. As with many new therapies, success with the implantable LVAD as a bridge to transplant hinges on correct patient

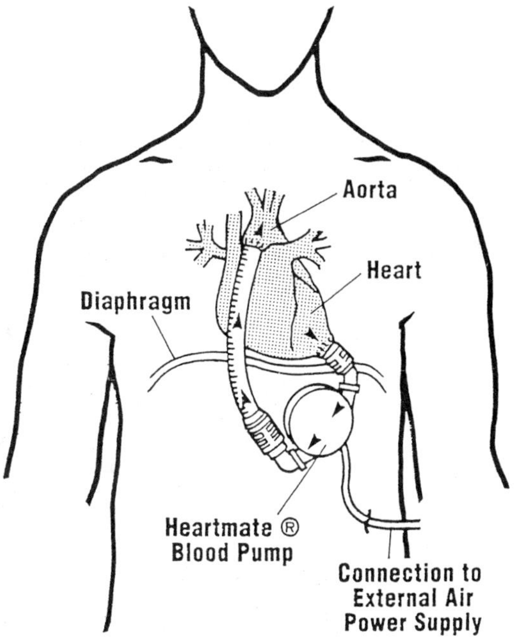

Figure 15–12. A "wearable" vented electrical ventricular assist device with inflow cannula in the ventricular apex and outflow graft to the ascending aorta. The pump is positioned in the left upper quadrant, either intra-abdominally or preperitoneally. Exiting through a fascial tunnel is the drive line with electrical connections to the device and an air vent which may be used as an emergency backup with a mechanical hand-powered pump. The power supply can be carried on a holster.

selection. Initially, VADs were used in extremely ill patients, with predictably poor results. General hemodynamic considerations with VADs are described earlier in this section. Hemodynamic criteria previously in frequent use for VADs were adapted from those originally suggested by Norman and colleagues[87] for IABP insertion, including a cardiac index of less than 2 L/min/m^2, pulmonary capillary wedge pressure higher than 20 mm Hg, systolic blood pressure lower than 90 mm Hg, and systemic vascular resistance higher than 2100 dynes/sec/cm^{-5}. These criteria are present initially in many potential transplant candidates who can later be rendered ambulatory on oral vasodilators and diuretics without mechanical assistance. Specific hemodynamic criteria are neither necessary nor sufficient indications for insertion of a VAD, compared with the assessment of an experienced heart failure team of surgeons and cardiologists that all other therapies have been exhausted and irreversible circulatory collapse and organ failure are imminent without mechanical support.

Timing of device insertion postcardiotomy depends on many fac-

TABLE 15–15. COMPONENTS AND CONFIGURATIONS OF IMPLANTABLE VENTRICULAR ASSIST DEVICES

Components
- Prosthetic ventricle
  - Inflow and outflow valves
  - Pumping chamber
  - Lining surface
- Control unit
- Pump actuator (driver)
  - Pneumatic or electric
- Power supply for driver
  - Alternating current, battery pack, or both
- Air displacement system
  - Venting line or compliance chamber

Configurations
- External console at bedside (currently approved for qualified centers)
- "Wearable": miniaturized control and power systems that can be carried by patient (continuing clinical investigation)
- Fully implantable: all components internalized except transcutaneous energy transmission system (yet to be implanted clinically)

TABLE 15–16. USE OF IMPLANTABLE LEFT VENTRICULAR ASSIST DEVICES AS BRIDGES TO HEART TRANSPLANTATION

Patient Outcome	Novacor (n = 180)	HeartMate (n = 157)
Died before transplant	68 (38%)	44 (28%)
Currently supported on device	10	25
Survived to undergo transplant	102	88
Discharged from hospital after transplant	93 (91% of transplant recipients)	74 (84% of transplant recipients)

tors and varies widely. Patients who cannot be weaned from cardiopulmonary bypass in the operating room or those likely to recover from postcardiotomy cardiogenic shock should have "short-term" left ventricular assistance with an IABP or extracorporeal pulsatile support in addition to maximal inotropic support. Over the next few days, either patient improvement or insertion of an implantable LVAD should occur (see Fig. 15–10). Use of assist devices as bridges to transplantation for patients in chronic heart failure is currently based on the assessment of imminent circulatory collapse but may increasingly be extended to avert progressive organ system dysfunction, which compromises posttransplant outcome.[77]

Contraindications. A number of major contraindications to long-term implantable LVAD placement have been established. Concerns specific to device implantation include a body surface area less than 1.5 m^2, which causes technical difficulties. Structural heart disease should be carefully sought and, if found, is a contraindication. Significant aortic valve insufficiency may become severe enough after device insertion to detract from net forward flow, and tricuspid regurgitation should be corrected to optimize right ventricular performance. Septal defects should also be repaired at the time of device insertion to avoid right-to-left shunting caused by sudden reduction in left-sided filling pressures. Atrial arrhythmias may decrease right ventricular function and device filling in the crucial 48 h after device insertion but are not absolute contraindications. Evaluation of right heart function remains controversial but critical, because right heart failure causes death in up to 20% of LVAD recipients. The dependence of right heart function on left heart pressures renders evaluation difficult. Preoperative right ventricular stroke work index may be a useful predictor.[88] Because most experience has been with these devices used as a prelude to transplantation, other contraindications are those for heart transplantation. Diabetes mellitus is not itself a contraindication, but it predisposes to other organ failure and to infection, which may compromise the chance of subsequent transplantation.

There are several reports of risk factors for recipients of LVADs.[89–91] A risk factor summation scale (RFSS) has been devised to predict patients who are unlikely to survive device insertion and for whom intervention is not likely to be successful.[91] Liver, kidney, and lung dysfunction; fever; and technical obstacles are included in the RFSS; this allows stratification into high-, medium-, and low-risk groups. Prospective testing of the RFSS system may allow elimination of high-risk patients from consideration because expected early survival is too low, whereas patients currently too compromised for heart transplantation may have an acceptably low risk for device implantation, which may lead to improvement and transplant candidacy.

Complications of Left Ventricular Assist Device Placement

Bleeding, right heart failure, air embolism, and progressive multiorgan system failure can occur early after implantation of an LVAD. Thromboembolism, infection, and device failure are later complications. The pathophysiology of these complications is discussed in detail elsewhere.[92]

The incidence of severe bleeding with LVADs has decreased with experience. Coagulopathy before device insertion results from congested liver dysfunction and thrombocytopenia. Cardiopulmonary bypass and previous sternotomies contribute to perioperative bleeding. In the implantable VAD experience, 50% of patients required reoperation for bleeding.[30] The use of aprotinin appears to decrease the incidence of bleeding but may also alter vascular resistance through effects on thromboxane A_2.[93]

Right Heart Failure. A central focus of debate remains the potential for LVAD to treat what appears to be biventricular failure. The frequent improvement of right heart function after lung transplantation suggests that the right ventricle has greater plasticity than the left ventricle. The clinical experience with LVADs indicates that the majority of patients can derive major benefit from left ventricular assistance, with subsequent improvement of right heart performance.

Right heart failure of sufficient severity to warrant use of a right VAD occurs in at least 20% of recipients.[86] Preoperative pulmonary vascular resistance is a less powerful predictor for right-sided heart failure with an LVAD than for right heart failure with a new heart posttransplant, because ability to meet high pressures may indicate some reserve in the current right ventricle.[88] The close association between ongoing blood loss and right heart dysfunction reflects not only the coagulopathy of congestion but also the pulmonary vascular effects of cytokine production and thromboxane A_2 release from blood product infusions.[93] Improved recognition of and response to early compromise have reduced the frequency of right heart failure from 40% to 20% in experienced centers. Reduction of excess fluid and judicious use of inotropic agents and pulmonary vasodilators can help to optimize right heart function.

Thromboembolism. Thromboemboli have been reported in 10%–35% of patients receiving the Novacor device[94] and warfarin anticoagulation. Device modification of the inflow conduit–valve mechanism and addition of other anticoagulation agents may decrease this risk further. The HeartMate device has a unique textured surface that leads to the formation of pseudoneointima, with lower risk of thromboembolic events.[85] The reported incidence of embolic events with the HeartMate device in 57 patients was two episodes, one from a fungal vegetation on the device and the other apparently from a native mechanical aortic valve, for an incidence of 0.2 episodes per patient year. These patients did not receive heparin or warfarin after the first 2 weeks after surgery. Intraoperative air embolism occurs rarely because the devices are de-aired and the left ventricle filled before device activation.

Infection. Most infections in LVAD recipients are nosocomial pneumonias or incidences of sepsis from central venous catheters. Early removal of indwelling central lines and appropriate, aggressive use of intravenous antibiotics help avoid pump infection. Device-related infections occur in 25% of patients secondary to drive-line infection.[86] Such infections generally do not preclude these patients from transplantation. The continuous administration of antibiotics in the absence of documented infectious sources is not advocated, because it does not prevent infection and may lead to superinfection.

Multiorgan Failure. The most common cause of death after LVAD placement is progressive multiorgan failure secondary to sepsis.[86, 30] In the absence of sepsis or pre-existing multiorgan failure, multiorgan failure rarely develops, because of the adequacy of hemodynamic support from the implantable devices.

Hemolysis. Hemolysis is more commonly associated with patients on centrifugal pump support than those with VADs.[80] The potential for erythrocyte damage is recognized with implantable devices but has rarely been detected.

Treatment of Arrhythmias. Although not a complication of device placement, native arrhythmias require careful management, particularly early after insertion. During the initial days required for the reversal of pulmonary hypertension, atrial arrhythmias can impair right and left heart function and device filling. Ventricular arrhythmias can also compromise right heart function and ventricular interdependence during this time. Intracardiac thrombi can result from sustained atrial arrhythmias. Vigorous attempts should be made to restore and maintain sinus rhythm. After initial stabilization, however, later appearance of atrial and even ventricular fibrillation are usually well tolerated.[95]

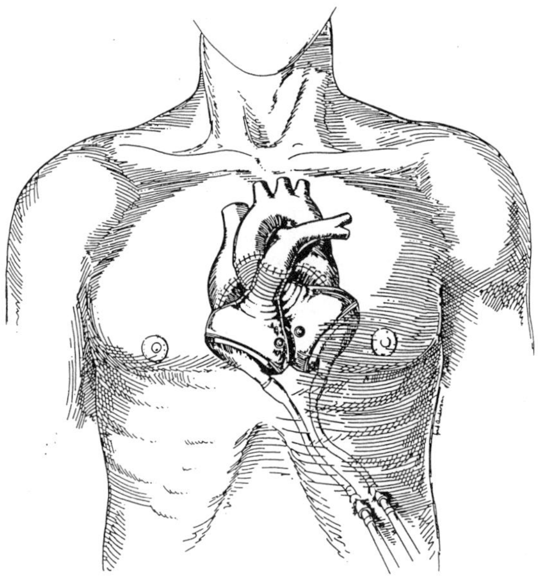

Figure 15–13. The CardioWest C-70 total artificial heart. (Courtesy of CardioWest Technologies, Inc., Tucson, AZ.)

Outcome After Mechanical Circulatory Support

Since the first successful bridge to transplant with an IABP in 1978,[78] univentricular and biventricular devices and ECMO have been used. Implantable LVADs have become the primary bridge because of the lengthening waiting time for donor hearts. As of November 1993, 180 Novacor and 157 HeartMate devices had been implanted in the United States.[30] The measured endpoints of perioperative survival to transplantation and survival following transplantation are similar with the two devices (see Table 15–16), with 33% of patients dying before transplantation. Of the patients who survived and then underwent transplantation, 88% were discharged from the hospital.

Intermediate outcomes of stabilization and rehabilitation have also been positive.[96] Cardiac output is increased by approximately 30%, and hepatic, renal, and neurohormonal functions are normalized.[86] Exercise capacity is also improved. The devices have occasionally been used for longer than 500 days before transplantation. Patients with Novacor devices and patients with HeartMate devices have been supervised as outpatients.[97, 98] It should be recognized that both devices in clinical use require transcutaneous energy cables that remain potential entry points for infection and mechanical misadventures, which can hopefully be minimized by future advances in design. Increasing experience may eventually allow a dramatic reduction in the hospitalization cost for these transplant candidates and set the precedent for long-term support without transplantation. This might address the problem of refractory heart failure to a much greater degree than will be possible for cardiac transplantation, which is limited to approximately 2500 patients yearly.

TOTAL ARTIFICIAL HEART

The need for a total artificial heart persists for patients who require both right and left ventricular support. After the first permanent artificial heart implantation in 1982, problems with hemodynamic, thromboembolic, and hemostatic complications hindered further development.[99–102] The CardioWest (Fig. 15–13) and Penn State pneumatic hearts are currently approved by the U.S. Food and Drug Administration for investigation as bridges to transplantation. Potential advantages include not only the biventricular support but also the orthotopic location, which eliminates the need to use the abdominal body cavity, and a smaller intrathoracic compliance chamber. Thromboembolic complications have been reduced but remain a focus of concern. The largest experience is with the CardioWest total artificial heart (derived from the Jarvik heart), used in four North American centers in a total of 33 recipients. Considerable additional experience is needed to determine the role of these devices.[102]

CARDIOMYOPLASTY

Dynamic cardiomyoplasty is a procedure in which skeletal muscle is used as a graft wrapped around the myocardium and stimulated by a pacemaker to contract in synchrony with the heart. Use of the patient's own latissimus dorsi muscle renders this an attractive approach for cardiac assistance (Fig. 15–14). The procedure involves

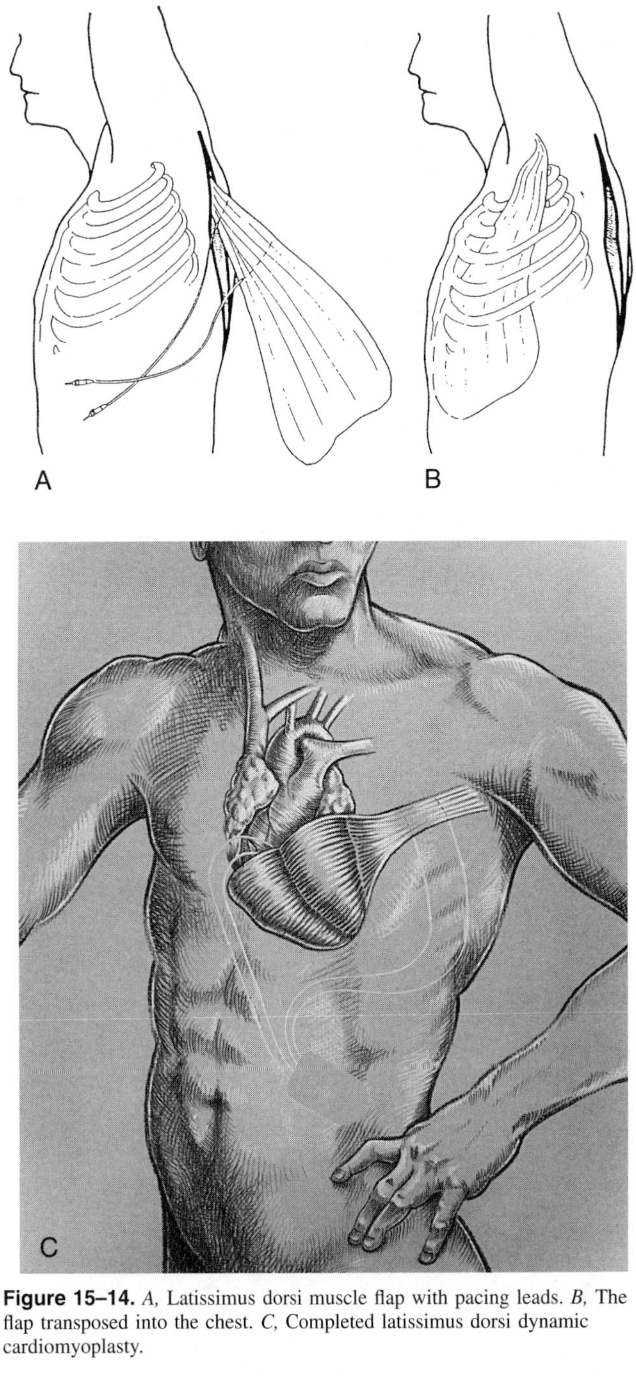

Figure 15–14. *A,* Latissimus dorsi muscle flap with pacing leads. *B,* The flap transposed into the chest. *C,* Completed latissimus dorsi dynamic cardiomyoplasty.

dissection of the latissimus dorsi (usually the left) with preservation of the neurovascular pedicle. Through a median sternotomy, the free end of the muscle is sutured to surround the lateral and anterior walls of both ventricles.[103] An intramyocardial sensing electrode is placed into the ventricular wall to sense depolarization and, together with a muscle pacing electrode, is connected to a cardiomyostimulator.

After 2 weeks of postoperative recovery, muscle stimulation is gradually increased over 6 weeks to an impulse train. During this time, the muscle transforms from the fast-twitch type IIB fibers to fatigue-resistant type I fibers. This transformation leads to some loss of muscle mass, power, and speed of contraction and relaxation,[104] although the remaining function is estimated to be adequate for cardiac support.[105] Alternative stimulation techniques in animals suggest the eventual possibility of sustained intermediate transformation to type IIA fibers.

Clinical Experience

Before 1990, initial experience with cardiomyoplasty demonstrated 33% perioperative mortality in patients considered to have New York Heart Association class IV symptoms, with approximately 30% additional mortality during the year after the procedure. In more recent experience, primarily in patients with class III symptoms, operative mortality was 12% and 1-year survival 68%,[106] which does not exceed the expected survival for class III patients without cardiomyoplasty. Modest improvements in hemodynamic parameters and ejection fraction have been significant in some populations.[107] Peak exercise capacity measured by gas exchange analysis may be more likely to improve in patients with the lowest initial capacity. Reported improvements in quality of life assessments and estimated clinical class have exceeded improvement in more objective measurements.[105] Some animal models and anecdotal clinical experience suggest that a major benefit may be the "girdling" to prevent progressive ventricular dilatation. A randomized trial is currently in progress at several United States centers.

Indications for Cardiomyoplasty

Although available only as an investigational procedure, cardiomyoplasty has stimulated sufficient interest to lead many patients to seek this option. Contraindications frequently cited include class IV symptoms, previous cardiac surgery, severe mitral regurgitation, right ventricular ejection fraction of less than .30, dysrhythmias necessitating pacemaker or implantable cardioverter-defibrillator, peak oxygen consumption below 10 or greater than 22 mL/kg/min, and major dysfunction of other organ systems.

DEVELOPMENT OF SURGICAL THERAPIES FOR HEART FAILURE

The vast majority of patients with heart failure can maintain good quality of life with currently available medical therapies, which, with wider use, may decrease the rate of progression to heart failure requiring surgical intervention. For patients with refractory symptoms of heart failure with optimal medical therapy, cardiac transplantation currently offers the best chance of improved quality of life and prolonged survival. The 10- to 20-fold disparity between the number of these patients and the number of suitable donor hearts limits the impact of transplantation on the problem of heart failure. In addition, the problem of TCAD limits the lifespan of transplanted hearts.

Developments in mechanical assist devices and techniques for skeletal muscle assistance offer hope for therapies that can be distributed more widely to those in need. The initial challenge is to select patients who will demonstrate success of the investigational therapies, as in the early days of cardiac transplantation, when many contraindications were absolute. As multiple new approaches become available, however, the challenge for the physician treating heart failure patients is not to identify the best patient for each new therapy, but to choose from all available therapies the best therapy for each patient.

Acknowledgment

Sharon A. Hunt and the following chairs of the Cardiology Task Forces from the 24th Bethesda Conference on Cardiac Transplantation are gratefully acknowledged for their suggestions regarding the Transplantation section of this chapter: John B. O'Connell, Gilbert H. Mudge, James B. Young, Leslie W. Miller, and Maria Rosa Constanzo.

REFERENCES

1. O'Connell JB, Gunnar RM, Evans RW, Fricker FJ, et al: Task Force 1: organization of heart transplantation in the U.S. J Am Coll Cardiol 1993; 22(1):8–14.
2. Hosenpud JD, Novick RJ, Breen TJ, Daily OP: The registry of the International Society for Heart and Lung Transplantation: eleventh official report—1994. J Heart Lung Transplant 1994; 13:561–570.
3. Stevenson LW, Sietsema K, Tillisch JH, et al: Exercise capacity for survivors of cardiac transplantation or sustained medical therapy for heart failure. Circulation 1990; 81:78–85.
4. Stevenson LW, Miller L: Cardiac transplantation as therapy for heart failure. Curr Prob Cardiol 1991; 16(4):219–305.
5. Francis GS: Determinants of prognosis in patients with heart failure. J Heart Lung Transplant 1994; 13:S113–S116.
6. Stevenson WG, Stevenson LW, Middlekauff HR, Saxon LA: Sudden death prevention in patients with advanced left ventricular dysfunction. Circulation 1993; 88:2953–2961.
7. Mancini DM, Eisen H, Kussmaul W, et al: Value of peak exercise oxygen consumption for optimal timing of cardiac transplantation in ambulatory patients with heart failure. Circulation 1991; 83:778–786.
8. Stevenson LW: Tailored therapy before transplantation for treatment of advanced heart failure: effective use of vasodilators and diuretics. J Heart Lung Transplant 1991; 10:468–476.
9. Mudge GH, Goldstein S, Addonizio LJ, et al: Task Force 3: recipient guidelines/prioritization. J Am Coll Cardiol 1993; 22(1):21–31.
10. DiSesa VJ, Sloss LJ, Cohn JH: Cardiac transplantation for intractable prosthetic valve endocarditis. J Heart Lung Transplant 1990; 9:142–143.
11. Miller LW, Kubo SH, Young JB, et al: Report of the Consensus Conference on candidate selection for cardiac transplantation. J Heart Lung Trans 1995, 14:562–571.
12. O'Connell JB, Bourge RC, Costanzo-Nordin MR, et al: Cardiac transplantation: recipient selection, donor procurement, and medical follow-up. AHA position statement. Circulation 1992; 86:1061–1079.
13. Olivari MT, Antolick A, Kaye MP, et al: Heart transplantation in elderly patients. J Heart Lung Transplant 1988; 7:258–264.
14. Grattan MT, Moreno-Cabral CE, Starnes VA, et al: Eight-year results of cyclosporine-treated patients with cardiac transplants. J Thorac Cardiovasc Surg 1990; 99:500–509.
15. Kaye MP: Registry of the International Society for Heart and Lung Transplantation: tenth official report—1993. J Heart Lung Transplant 1993; 12:541–548.
16. Stolf NAG, Higushi L, Bocchi E, et al: Heart transplantation in patients with Chagas' disease cardiomyopathy. J Heart Lung Transplant 1987; 5:307–312.
17. Copeland JG, Emery RW, Levinson MM, et al: Selection of patients for cardiac transplantation. Circulation 1987; 75:2–9.
18. Costard-Jackle A, Fowler MB: Influence of preoperative pulmonary artery pressure on mortality after heart transplantation: testing of potential reversibility of pulmonary hypertension with nitroprusside is useful in defining a high risk group. J Am Coll Cardiol 1992; 19:48–54.
19. Erickson KW, Costanzo-Nordin MR, O'Sullivan EJ, et al: Influence of preoperative transpulmonary gradient on late mortality after orthotopic heart transplantation. J Heart Lung Trans 1990; 9:526–537.
20. Loh E, Stamler JS, Hare JM, et al: Cardiovascular effects of inhaled nitric oxide in patients with left ventricular dysfunction. Circulation 1994; 90:2780–2785.
21. Desruennes M, Muneretto C, Gandjbakhch I, et al: Heterotopic heart

transplantation: current status in 1988. J Heart Lung Transplant 1989; 8:479–485.
22. Wright RS, Levine MS, Bellamy PE, et al: Ventilatory and diffusion abnormalities in potential heart-transplant recipients. Chest 1990; 98:816–820.
23. Radovancevic B, Poindexter S, Birovljev S, et al: Risk factors for development of accelerated coronary artery disease in cardiac transplant recipients. Eur J Cardiothorac Surg 1990; 4:309–312.
24. Bussieres LM, Cardella CJ, Daly PA, et al: Relationship between preoperative pulmonary status and outcome after heart transplantation. J Heart Lung Trans 1990; 9:124–128.
25. Penn I: Cancers after cyclosporine therapy. Transplant Proc 1988; 20:276–279.
26. Olbrisch ME, Levenson JL: Psychological evaluation of heart transplantation candidates: an international survey of process, criteria and outcomes. J Heart Lung Transplant 1991; 10:948–955.
27. Rodriguez MD, Colon A, Santiago-Delphin EA: Psychosocial profile of noncompliant patients. Transplant Proc 1991; 23:1807–1809.
28. Herrick CM, Mealey PC, Tischner LL, Holland CS: Combined heart failure-transplant program: Advantages in assessing medical compliance. J Heart Lung Trans 1987; 6:141–145.
29. Levin HR, Chen JM, Oz MC, et al: Potential of left ventricular assist devices as outpatient therapy while awaiting transplantation. Ann Thorac Surg 1994; 58:1515.
30. McCarthy PM, Sabik JF: Implantable circulatory support devices as a bridge to heart transplantation. Semin Thorac Cardiovasc Surg 1994; 6(3):174.
31. Stevenson LW, Steimle AE, Fonarow G, et al: Improvement in exercise capacity of candidates awaiting heart transplantation. J Am Coll Cardiol 1995; 25:163–170.
32. Sweeney MS, Lammermeier DE, Frazier OH, et al: Extension of donor criteria in cardiac transplantation: Surgical risk versus supply-side economics. Ann Thorac Surg 1990; 50:7.
33. Ott GY, Herschberger RE, Ratkovec RR, et al: Cardiac allograft from high-risk donors: excellent clinical results. Ann Thorac Surg 1994; 57:76.
34. Blackbourne LH, Tribble CG, Langenburg SE, et al: Successful use of undersized donors for orthotopic heart transplantation—with a caveat. Ann Thorac Surg 1994; 57:1472.
35. Reitz B: Heart and heart-lung transplantation. *In* Braunwald E (ed): Heart Disease: A Textbook of Cardiovascular Medicine, pp 520–534. Philadelphia: WB Saunders, 1992.
36. Lower RR, Shumway NE: Studies in orthotopic homotransplantation of the canine heart. Surg Forum 1960; 11:18.
37. Dreyfus G, Jebara V, Mihaileanu S, et al: Total orthotopic heart transplantation: an alternative to the standard technique. Ann Thorac Surg 1991; 52:1181.
38. Blanche C, Czer LSC, Valenza M, et al: Alternative technique for orthotopic heart transplantation. Ann Thorac Surg 1994; 57:765.
39. Sievers HH, Leyh R, Jahnke A, et al: Bicaval versus atrial anastomoses in cardiac transplantation: Right atrial dimension and tricuspid valve function at rest and during exercise up to thirty-six months after transplantation. J Thorac Cardiovasc Surg 1994; 108:780.
40. Hosenpud JD, Norman DF, Cobanoglu MA, et al: Serial echocardiographic findings early after heart transplantation: Evidence for reversible right ventricular dysfunction and myocardial edema. J Heart Trans 1987; 6:343–347.
41. Pascual JMS, Fiorelli AI, Bellotti GM: Prostacyclin in the management of pulmonary hypertension after heart transplantation. J Heart Lung Transplant 1990; 9:664–651.
42. Myer BD, Ross J, Newton L, et al: Cyclosporine associated with chronic nephropathy. New Engl J Med 1984; 311:699.
43. Macris MP, Van Buren CG, Sweeney MS, et al: Selective use of OKT3 in heart transplantation with the use of risk factor analysis. J Heart Lung Transplant 1989, 8.296–302.
44. Merrell SW, Ames SA, Nelson EW, et al: Major abdominal complications following cardiac transplantation. Arch Surg 1989; 124:889–894.
45. Miller LW, Schlant RC, Kobashigawa JA, et al: Bethesda Conference on Transplantation. Task Force 5: complications of transplantation. J Am Coll Cardiol 1993; 22:41–54.
46. Spes CH, Angermann CE, Beyer RW, et al: Increased evidence for cholelithiasis in heart transplant recipients receiving cyclosporine therapy. J Heart Lung Transplant 1990; 9:404–407.
47. Kobashigawa JA, Kirklin JK, Naftel DC, et al: Pretransplantation risk factors for acute rejection after heart transplantation: a multi-institutional study. J Heart Lung Trans 1993; 12: 255–366.
48. Billingham ME, Cary NR, Hammond ME, et al: A working formulation for the standardization of nomenclature in the diagnosis of heart and lung rejection: Heart Rejection Study Group. J Heart Lung Transplant 1990; 9:587–593.
49. Hammond EH, Wittwer CT, Greenwood J, et al: Relationship of OKT3 sensitization and vascular rejection in cardiac transplant patients receiving OKT3 rejection prophylaxis. Transplantation 1990; 50:776–782.
50. Costanzo-Nordin MR, Cooper DKC, Jessup M, et al: Bethesda Conference on Transplantation. Task Force 6: future developments. J Am Coll Cardiol 1993; 22:54–64.
51. Armitage JM, Fricker FJ, Del Nido P, et al: The clinical trial of FK506 as primary and rescue immunosuppression in adult cardiac transplantation. Transplant Proc 1991; 23:3058–3060.
52. Kahan BD: Cyclosporine. N Engl J Med 1989; 321:1725–1738.
53. Kobashigawa JA, Stevenson LW: Post-operative treatment of heart transplant recipients. J Crit Illness 1993; 8:607–615.
54. Kobashigawa JA, Stevenson LW, Moriguchi JD, et al: Is intravenous glucocorticoid therapy better than an oral regimen for asymptomatic cardiac rejection? A randomized trial. J Am Coll Cardiol 1993; 21:1142–1144.
55. Renlund DG, Bristow MR, Crandall BG, et al: Hypercholesterolemia after heart transplantation: amelioration by corticosteroid-free maintenance immunosuppression. J Heart Lung Transplant 1989; 8:214–220.
56. Kobashigawa JA, Stevenson LW, Brownfield ED, et al: Initial success of steroid weaning late after heart transplantation. J Heart Lung Transplant 1992; 11:428–430.
57. Costanzo-Nordin MR, O'Sullivan EJ, Johnson MR, et al: Prospective randomized trial of OKT3 vs. horse antithymocyte globulin–based immunosuppressive prophylaxis in heart transplantation. J Heart Lung Transplant 1990; 9:306–315.
58. O'Connell JB, Renlund DG, Gay WA, et al: Efficacy of OKT3 retreatment for refractory cardiac allograft rejection. Transplantation 1989; 47:788–792.
59. Costanzo-Nordin MR, Grusk DB, Silver MA, et al: Reversal of recalcitrant cardiac allograft rejection with methotrexate. Circulation 1988; 78(suppl III):47–57.
60. Salter MM, Kirklin JK, Bourge RC: Total lymphoid irradiation in the treatment of early or recurrent heart rejection. J Heart Lung Transplant 1992; 11:902–912.
61. Uretsky BF, Murali S, Reddy PS, et al: Development of coronary artery disease in cardiac transplant patients receiving immunosuppressive therapy with cyclosporine and prednisone. Circulation 1987; 76:827–834.
62. Salomon RN, Hughes CCW, Schoen FJ, et al: Human coronary transplantation-associated arteriosclerosis: evidence for a chronic immune reaction to activated graft endothelial cells. Am J Pathol 1991; 138:791–798.
63. Schroeder JS, Gao SZ, Alderman EA, et al: A preliminary study of diltiazem in the prevention of coronary artery disease in heart transplant recipients. N Engl J Med 1993; l328:164–170.
64. Kobashigawa JA, Murphy FL, Stevenson LW, et al: Low-dose lovastatin safely lowers cholesterol after cardiac transplantation. Circulation 1990; 82(suppl IV):281–283.
65. Halle AA, Wilson RF, Vetrovec GW, for the Cardiac Transplant Angioplasty Study Group: Multicenter evaluation of percutaneous transluminal coronary angioplasty in heart transplant recipients. J Heart Lung Transplant 1992; 11:S138–S141.
66. Miller LW, Naftel DC, Bourge RC: Infection after heart transplantation: a multi-institutional study. J Heart Lung Transplant 1994; 13:381–393.
67. Merigan TC, Renlung DG, Keay S, et al: A controlled trial of ganciclovir to prevent cytomegalovirus disease after heart transplantation. N Engl J Med 1992; 326:1182–1186.
68. Randhawa PS, Youosem SA, Paradis IL, et al: The clinical spectrum, pathology, and clonal analysis of Epstein-Barr virus associated lymphoproliferative disorders in heart-lung transplant recipients. Am J Clin Pathol 1989; 92:177–185.
69. Young JB, Winters WL, Bourge R, Uretsky BF: Task Force 4: function of the heart transplant recipient. J Am Coll Cardiol 1993; 22(1):31–41.
70. Uretsky BF: Physiology of the transplanted heart. *In* Brest AN (ed): Cardiovascular Clinics, pp 23–40. Philadelphia: FA Davis, 1990.
71. Kavanagh T, Yacoub MH, Mertner DJ, et al: Cardiorespiratory responses to exercise training after orthotopic cardiac transplantation. Circulation 1988; 77:162–171.
72. Luke RG: Mechanisms of cyclosporine-induced hypertension. Am J Hypertens 1991; 4:468–471.
73. Rich GM, Mudge GH, Laffel GL, et al: Cyclosporin A and prednisone-

associated osteoporosis in heart transplant recipients. J Heart Lung Transplant 1992; 11:940–948.
74. Kobashigawa JA, Leaf DA, Gleeson MP, et al: Benefit of cardiac rehabilitation in heart transplant patients: A randomized trial. J Heart Lung Transplant 1994; 90(1, part II):S77.
75. Evans RW: Executive Summary: The National Cooperative Transplantation Study. Report BHARC-100-91-020. Seattle: Battelle Seattle Research Center, 1991.
76. Stevenson LW, Belil D, Grover-McKay M, et al: Effects of afterload reduction on left ventricular volume and mitral regurgitation in severe congestive heart failure. Am J Cardiol 1987; 60:654–658.
77. Loisance DY, Deleuze PH, Houel R, et al: Pharmacologic bridge to cardiac transplantation: current limitations. Ann Thorac Surg 1993; 55:310–313.
78. Reemstma K, Drusin R, Edie R, et al: Cardiac transplantation for patients requiring mechanical circulatory support. N Engl J Med 1978; 298:670.
79. Pae WE Jr, Miller CA, Mathews Y: Ventricular assist devices for postcardiotomy shock. J Thorac Cardiovasc Surg 1992; 104:541.
80. Curtis JJ: Centrifugal mechanical assist for postcardiotomy ventricular failure. Semin Thorac Cardiovasc Surg 1994; 6(3):140.
81. Karl TR: Extracorporeal circulatory support in infants and children. Semin Thorac Cardiovasc Surg 1994; 6(3):154.
82. Galantowicz ME, Stolar CJ: Extracorporeal membrane oxygenation for perioperative support in pediatric heart transplantation. J Thorac Cardiovasc Surg 1991; 102:148.
83. Votapka TV, Pennington DG: Circulatory assist devices in congestive heart failure. Cardiol Clin 1994; 12:143.
84. Rowles JR, Mortimer BJ, Olsen DB: Ventricular assist and total artificial heart devices for clinical use in 1993. ASAIO J 1993; 39:840.
85. Rose EA, Levin HR, Oz MC, et al: Artificial circulatory support with textured interior surfaces: a counterintuitive approach to minimizing thromboembolism. Circulation 1994; 90(suppl II):87.
86. Frazier OH, Rose EA, Macmanus Q, et al: Multicenter clinical evaluation of the HeartMate 1000IP left ventricular assist device. Ann Thorac Surg 1992; 53:1080.
87. Norman JC, Colley DA, Igo SR, et al: Prognostic indices for survival during postcardiotomy intra-aortic balloon pumping. J Thorac Cardiovasc Surg 1977; 74:709.
88. Levin HR, Burkoff D, Oz MC, et al: Pre-operative right ventricular stroke work is a major determinant of right heart failure in patients after LVAD implantation. J Heart Lung Transplant 1994; 13(1):S73.
89. Farrar DJ, Thoratec Investigators: Preoperative predictors of survival in patients with Thoratec ventricular asist devices as a bridge to heart transplantation. J Heart Lung Transplant 1994; 13:93.
90. Reedy JE, Swartz MT, Termuhlen DF, et al: Bridge to heart transplantation: Importance of patient selection. J Heart Lung Transplant 1990; 9:473.
91. Oz MC, Pepino P, Goldstein D, et al: Selection scale predicts patients successfully receiving long-term, implantable left ventricular assist devices [Abstract]. Circulation 1994; 90(4, suppl I):I-308.
92. Pennington G, Swartz MC: Assisted circulation and the mechanical heart. *In* Braunwald E (ed): Heart Disease: A Textbook of Cardiovascular Medicine, pp 535–550. Philadelphia: WB Saunders, 1992.
93. Goldstein DJ, Seldomridge JA, Chen JM, et al: Use of aprotinin in LVAD recipients reduces blood loss, blood use, and perioperative mortality. Ann Thorac Surg 1995; 59:1063.
94. McCarthy PM, Portner PM, Tobler HG, et al: Clinical experience with the Novacor ventricular assist system. J Thorac Cardiovasc Surg 1991; 102:578.
95. Oz MC, Rose EA, Levin HR: Selection criteria for ventricular assist device placement. Am Heart J 1995; 129:173.
96. Estrada-Quintero T, Uretsky BF, Murali S, et al: Amelioration of the heart failure state with left ventricular assist system support. J Am Coll Cardiol 1992; 19(3):254A.
97. Levin HR, Chen JM, Oz MC, et al: Potential of left ventricular assist devices as outpatient therapy while awaiting transplantation. Ann Thorac Surg 1994; 58:1515.
98. Dew MA, Kormos RL, Roth LH, et al: Life quality in the era of bridging to cardiac transplantation: Bridge patients in an out of hospital setting. ASAIO J 1993; 39:145.
99. Griffith BP: Interim use of the Jarvik-7 artificial heart: lessons learned at Presbyterian-University Hospital of Pittsburgh. Ann Thorac Surg 1989; 47:158.
100. Muneretto C, Solis E, Pavie A, et al: Total artificial heart: survival and complications. Ann Thorac Surg 1989; 47:151.
101. Johnson KE, Prieto M, Joyce L, et al: Summary of the clinical use of the Symbion total artificial heart: a registry report. J Heart Lung Transplant 1992; 11:103.
102. Sapirstein JS, Pae WE Jr, Rosenberg G, et al: The development of permanent circulatory support systems. Semin Thorac Cardiovasc Surg 1994; 6(3):188.
103. Carpentier A, Chachques JC: Clinical dynamic cardiomyoplasty: method and outcome. Semin Thorac Cardiovasc Surg 1991; 3:136.
104. Lucas CM, Van der Veen FH, Cheriex EC, et al: Long-term follow-up (12 to 35 weeks) after dynamic cardiomyoplasty. J Am Coll Cardiol 1993; 22(3):758–767.
105. El Oakley RM, Jarvis JC: Cardiomyoplasty: a critical review of experimental and clinical results. Circulation 1994; 90:2085–2090.
106. Furnary AP, Moreira LFP, Jessup M, et al: Dynamic cardiomyoplasty improves systolic ventricular function [Abstract]. Circulation 1994; 90(suppl I):I–309.
107. Moreira LFP, Bocchi EA, Stolf NA, et al: Current expectations in dynamic cardiomyoplasty. Ann Thorac Surg 1993; 55:299.

SECTION THREE

Arrhythmias/Conduction Disturbances

16 Drug Treatment of Supraventricular Tachycardias

John P. DiMarco, MD, PhD

Drug therapy remains an important component of the management of patients with supraventricular arrhythmias. Appropriate use of drugs in these patients requires an understanding of the electrophysiologic mechanisms and pathways responsible for each particular arrhythmia, the pharmacology of the tissue or tissues involved, and the properties of the antiarrhythmic drugs available. It is also important to define the goal of any therapeutic intervention. When a patient presents with the new onset of a tachycardia, rapid control of symptoms is the immediate goal. This may involve measures either to control rate or to restore sinus rhythm. When control of rate is the goal, treatment is often directed at the atrioventricular (AV) node rather than the tissue responsible for the arrhythmia itself, because rate control at the level of the node is facilitated by the potential for concealed conduction of impulses as they pass through that structure. In arrhythmias involving reentry over a single circuit, a single block in conduction is sufficient to terminate the arrhythmia. When multiple circuits of reentry are involved, simultaneous blocks in most or all of these circuits must occur. Termination of reentrant arrhythmias may require only an instantaneous drug effect. In contrast, arrhythmias caused by enhanced, abnormal, or triggered automaticity require more sustained effects to suppress the focus or foci involved.

Prophylaxis of recurrent arrhythmias may require a different strategy than does termination. In reentrant arrhythmias, complete and permanent conduction block in the circuits involved is only rarely achievable, and if the structure involved is required during normal conduction, complete, permanent block may not be desirable. Effective approaches may include facilitation of early termination, drug-induced changes in conduction times, or production of block only in abnormal, nonvital conduction pathways. Chronic suppression of automatic arrhythmias often requires approaches to eliminate or modify precipitating stimuli or to suppress or selectively eliminate the responsible tissues. In some cases, the arrhythmia cannot be terminated or chronically prevented, and strategies to modify its effects, usually by modifying AV conduction to decrease ventricular rate, must be employed. When the arrhythmia is allowed to persist and, because of stasis as a result of loss of atrial contraction, is associated with an increased embolic risk, anticoagulation is also an important part of comprehensive drug therapy.

PHARMACOLOGY OF SUPRAVENTRICULAR ARRHYTHMIAS

Drug therapy of supraventricular arrhythmias is often based on the concept of a "vulnerable parameter" that is the primary target of drug action.[1] The sinus node and the AV node have calcium-mediated action potentials and are therefore sensitive to direct effects of calcium channel blockers and adenosine and indirect (autonomically mediated) effects of beta-adrenergic blockers or cardiac glycosides. Conduction in atrial and ventricular muscles is depressed by sodium channel blockers, and refractory periods are prolonged by potassium channel blockers. Enhanced or abnormal automaticity in atrial and ventricular muscle may be the result of many causes; therefore, muscarinic agonists, beta-adrenergic antagonists, calcium channel blockers, and sodium channel blockers may also be effective in selected cases. Most accessory pathways behave like atrial or ventricular muscle. Conduction and refractory periods of accessory pathways are most susceptible to sodium and potassium channel blockers, but a few pathways that are sensitive to adenosine have been described. Although there are limitations to the Vaughan-Williams classification of antiarrhythmic drugs,[2] it is still useful as a general guide for selecting drug therapy (Tables 16–1 and 16–2).

EVALUATION OF THERAPY

Several types of studies have been used to establish the effectiveness of drug therapy in supraventricular arrhythmias. The most useful studies are randomized comparisons of the drug being studied to either a placebo control or some other agent. The range of doses studied during the course of drug evaluation should include both minimally and maximally effective doses. When two agents are compared, it is important that each drug be tested at doses expected to produce a clinically relevant response.

The efficacy of a drug for acute termination of an episode of tachycardia is relatively easy to evaluate. Patients presenting with an appropriate arrhythmia are entered into the trial. Both spontaneous and stimulation-induced episodes of arrhythmia may be included. After an observation period to establish stability of the tachycardia, the patient is given one or more doses of the drug under study or

TABLE 16–1. DRUG ACTIONS IN SUPRAVENTRICULAR ARRHYTHMIAS

	ECG				Electrophysiology		
Class	**PR/VR**	**QRS**	**QTc**	**JTc**	**A/V**	**AP**	**AVN**
I. Na^+ channel blockers							
Ia	NC	(↑)	↑	↑	ERP-↑ COND-↓	ERP-↑ COND-↓	ERP-NC COND-NC
Ic	↑	↑↑	(↑)	NC	ERP-↑ COND-↓↓	ERP-↑ COND-↓↓	ERP-↑ COND-↓
II. Beta-adrenergic blockers	↑	NC	NC	NC	ERP-NC COND-NC	ERP-NC COND-NC	ERP-↑ COND-↓
III. K^+ channel blockers*	↑	NC	↑↑	↑ ↑	ERP-(↑) COND-↑	ERP-↑ COND-↑	ERP-↑ COND-↓
IV. Ca^{2+} channel blockers	↑	NC	NC	NC	ERP-NC COND-NC	ERP-NC ERP-NC	ERP-↑↑ COND-↑↑
Adenosine	↑	NC	NC	NC	ERP (A)-↓ ERP (V)-NC COND-NC	ERP-↓ COND-↑	ERP-↑↑ COND-↓↓
Digoxin	↑	NC	NC	NC	ERP (A)-↓ ERP (V)-NC COND-NC	ERP-↓ or NC COND-↑ or NC	ERP-↑ COND-↑

*Clinically available agents, sotalol and amiodarone, have other actions not related to K^+ channel blockade.
Abbreviations: ↓, decreased; ↑, increased; A, atrium; AP, accessory pathway; AVN, atrioventricular node; COND, conduction velocity or capability; ECG, electrocardiogram; ERP, effective refractory period; NC, no change; V, ventricle; VR, ventricular rate. Parentheses indicate slight effect.

the active or inactive control. Total response is determined by the fraction of episodes converted within a specified period of time. This study design is most commonly used for evaluation of intravenous drugs, because absorption of orally administered agents during a rapid tachycardia is usually delayed in an unpredictable fashion. However, in patients with arrhythmias that have few hemodynamic consequences (e.g., atrial fibrillation with well-controlled ventricular rates), oral drug therapy can be studied through the use of a similar protocol with a longer period of observation. In any protocol studying acute termination, it is important to have some estimate of the probability for spontaneous termination. For some arrhythmias, the spontaneous conversion rate for new onset arrhythmias is quite high, and uncontrolled anecdotal reports of drug efficacy can be highly misleading (Fig. 16–1).[3]

Supraventricular arrhythmias are rarely immediately life-threatening. Therefore, the most relevant clinical endpoint for a study of drug efficacy may not be complete prevention of all arrhythmias. Pritchett and coworkers[4] and others[5] have established elegant designs for studying the effects of drugs on paroxysmal arrhythmias. The patient is entered into the study, and arrhythmia frequency is established during a drug-free control period. Double-blind treatment is

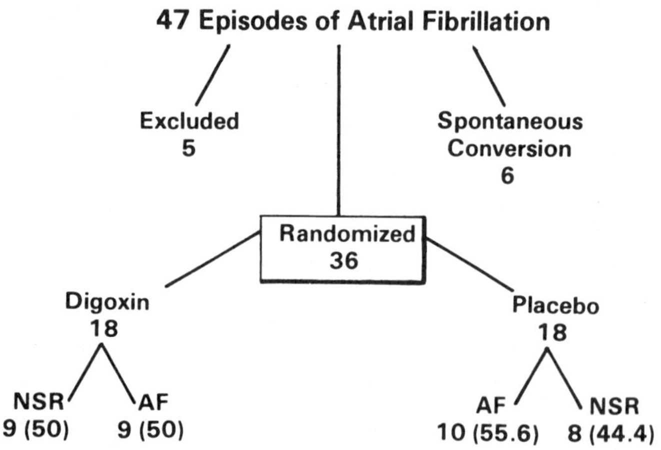

Figure 16–1. Digoxin in new-onset atrial fibrillation. Patients presenting with new-onset atrial fibrillation were randomized to receive either digoxin or placebo. The conversion rate was not different between the two groups. Conversion was observed in 13% before drug therapy, in 44% who received placebo, and in 50% of those treated with digoxin. Numbers in parentheses are percentages. *Abbreviations:* AF, atrial fibrillation; NSR, normal sinus rhythm. (From Falk RH, Knowlton AA, Bernard SA, et al: Digoxin for converting recent-onset atrial fibrillation to sinus rhythm. Ann Intern Med 1987; 106:503.)

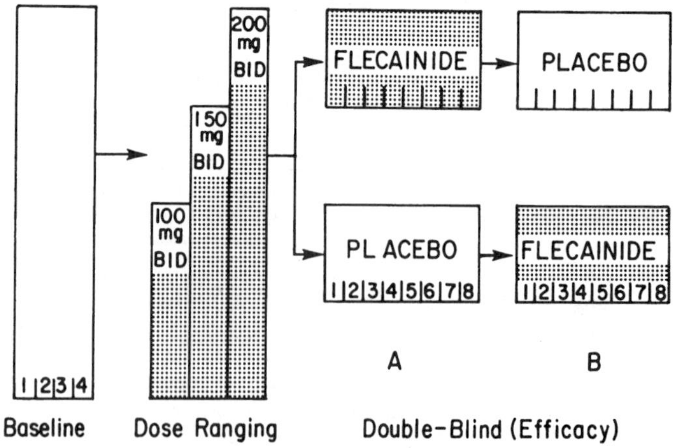

Figure 16–2. Design for drug studies in paroxysmal arrhythmias. Patients undergo a baseline observation period (4 weeks) during which one or more arrhythmia episodes are documented. A dose-titration phase is then used to establish tolerability of the drug to be studied. Patients then enter a double-blind, placebo-controlled treatment phase on the highest tolerated dose. Crossover is permitted after two or more recurrences in each block. Possible endpoints are time to first recurrence, interval between attacks, and fraction free of recurrence. (From Anderson JL, Gilbert EM, Alpert BL, et al: Prevention of symptomatic recurrences of paroxysmal atrial fibrillation in patients initially tolerating antiarrhythmic therapy. A multicenter, double-blind, crossover study of flecainide and placebo with transtelephonic monitoring. Circulation 1989; 80: 1557.)

TABLE 16–2. ANTIARRHYTHMIC DRUGS USED IN TREATING SUPRAVENTRICULAR ARRHYTHMIAS

Class	Indications	Agent(s)	Proarrhythmia	IV Dose	Oral Dose* (mg/d)	Common Adverse Effects
Ia	Conversion/ prophylaxis of AFib, AFlut	Quinidine SO_4†	↑ QTc, ↑ QRS, torsades de pointes, AFib → AFlut	NR	600–1200	GI, blood, rash, fever
		Procainamide	As above	15 mg/kg load, 2–4 mg/min	3000–6000	Lupus-like syndrome, agranulocytosis, GI
		Disopyramide	As above	NA	450–900	Constipation, anticholinergic effects, ↓ LV function
Ic	Conversion/ prophylaxis of AFib, ATach; prophylaxis of PSVT	Flecainide	↑ QRS, ↑ pacing threshold, AFib → AFlut, incessant VT	NA	150–400	CNS, ↓ LV function
		Propafenone	As above	NA	450–900	Dysgeusia, CNS, ↓ LV function
		Moricizine‡	As above	NA	600–900	CNS
II	Rate control—AFib, MAT, ATach; prophylaxis of PSVT, ?ATach, ?AFib	Many preparations	Sinus bradycardia, AV block			↓ LV function, bronchospasm, CNS
III	Prophylaxis/ conversion of AFib, AFlut, PSVT, ATach	Sotalol	↑ QTc, polymorphic VT, bradycardia	NA	160–320	Bronchospasm, ↓ LV function
		Amiodarone	As above, less polymorphic VT	NA	100–300‖	GI, ocular, pulmonary, thyroid, neurologic
IV	Conversion/ prophylaxis of PSVT; rate control AFib, ?MAT	Verapamil	Bradycardia, sinus arrest, ↑ AFib duration	5–15 mg§	240–480	Constipation, ↓ LV function, hypotension
		Diltiazem	As above	15–50 mg§	180–360	↓ LV function, hypotension
Other agents	Conversion of PSVT	Adenosine	Bradycardia, atrial and ventricular ectopy, secondary ↑ heart rate, AFib	3–12 mg	NA	Flushing, chest pain, dyspnea
	Rate control AFib	Digoxin	Bradycardia, ATach, ventricular ectopy	0.5–1.0 mg§	0.125–0.5	GI, visual

*Total daily dose range. Dosage schedule may depend on preparation used.
†Other quinidine salts are available. Dosage adjustment is required.
‡Classification based on profile during clinical use.
‖Loading period is required.
§Divided doses.
Abbreviations: ↑, increased; ↓, decreased; AFib, atrial fibrillation; AFlut, atrial flutter; ATach, atrial tachycardia; CNS, central nervous system reactions; GI, gastrointestinal; LV, left ventricular; MAT, multifocal atrial tachycardia; NA, not available; NR, not recommended for supraventricular arrhythmias; PSVT, paroxysmal supraventricular tachycardia.

then begun, and the endpoints evaluated are time to first occurrence and intervals between recurrent episodes (Fig. 16–2). Quality of life during chronic therapy should also be routinely assessed. In this type of study, either fixed doses or maximally tolerated doses of the agent under study can be used. This study design provides the most reliable statistical data but is not appropriate for patients who have infrequent episodes or for patients in whom severe symptoms during tachycardia or a need for electrical cardioversion makes multiple recurrent episodes of tachycardia undesirable. Therefore, most studies in the literature that deal with recurrence of atrial fibrillation after cardioversion use life-table analyses of the first recurrent episode of sustained atrial fibrillation as their measure of effect.

In patients with ventricular arrhythmias, prevention of arrhythmia induction in an electrophysiologic study during drug therapy has been widely used to predict future efficacy of a drug. This approach has been less widely used clinically in patients with supraventricular arrhythmias for several reasons. There has been no pressing need to establish absolute drug efficacy, because recurrences are only rarely life-threatening or fatal. Additionally, the role of autonomic nervous system influences on arrhythmia initiation and maintenance can be profound, and in many cases, changes in autonomic tone can override drug effects.[6] Finally, protocols for initiation of supraventricular arrhythmias and the correlations between changes in response to stimulation and clinical efficacy are not well established.

ATRIAL FIBRILLATION

Atrial fibrillation is the most common sustained cardiac arrhythmia. Its prevalence increases with age, and in the very elderly, as much as 15% of the population may have atrial fibrillation. Atrial fibrillation is not usually thought of as a life-threatening arrhythmia, but it is associated with significant patient morbidity. Atrial fibrillation results in a loss of atrial transport, and the ventricular rate becomes irregular. This causes a reduction in cardiac output that can be large and unpredictable. Even when the average ventricular rate is within an acceptable range, many patients, particularly those with noncompliant ventricles or with reduced ejection fractions, are hemodynamically compromised while they are in atrial fibrillation. In addition, with loss of atrial contractility, abnormal patterns of blood flow within the atria exist, and an increased risk for thromboembolism is present. Anticoagulation, therefore, is a major consideration in drug therapy in patients with chronic or recurrent atrial fibrillation.

Termination of Atrial Fibrillation

Atrial fibrillation presents in some patients as a paroxysmal, highly symptomatic arrhythmia with an abrupt and clearly identifiable onset. In other patients, atrial fibrillation presents insidiously, with the patient either being totally free of symptoms or having only mild, nonspecific symptoms of fatigue or dyspnea which he or she does not associate with any changes in rhythm.

When a patient with atrial fibrillation first presents, several questions should immediately be asked. Does the arrhythmia require either urgent electrical cardioversion or intravenous drugs to slow ventricular rates for the control of serious symptoms? Is an attempt at conversion of atrial fibrillation and maintenance of sinus rhythm likely to be successful? Is anticoagulation required before the conversion attempt?

An assessment of both the possible reversible causes and the immediate consequences of atrial fibrillation should be made before a course of treatment is selected. Indications for emergency cardioversion might include life-threatening ischemia, loss of consciousness, severe hypotension, or congestive failure. Patients with extremely rapid ventricular rates that are unlikely to be controlled easily (e.g., patients with Wolff-Parkinson-White syndrome) also are candidates for urgent electrical cardioversion. In most other patients, the first step in therapy should be an attempt to control excessive ventricular rate with drugs that block or delay AV nodal conduction. Depending on the acuity of presentation, this can be accomplished with either intravenous or oral agents, as discussed later.

After the ventricular rate has been reduced sufficiently to relieve major symptoms, the possibility of a reversible cause should be considered. Uncontrolled conditions such as untreated hyperthyroidism, active pericarditis, or drug or substance toxicity or withdrawal make an attempt at early conversion unwise, because the possibility of recurrence is unacceptably high until the basic problem is addressed. Other conditions that might make attempts at cardioversion unwise include greatly enlarged atrial dimensions and known or suspected sinus node dysfunction without appropriate protection with a pacemaker. Duration of atrial fibrillation appears to be an important factor influencing cardioversion strategy for several reasons. Atrial electrophysiology becomes progressively abnormal as atrial fibrillation persists[7]; therefore, it is preferable to attempt conversion as soon as possible after the arrhythmia develops. Duration of atrial fibrillation is also a determinant of the risk of stroke or embolism after cardioversion. It is recommended that all patients with atrial fibrillation of longer than 2 days in duration undergo 3–4 weeks of anticoagulation before an elective cardioversion attempt.[8] For these reasons, it is prudent to attempt conversion within 48 h of arrhythmia onset whenever possible. If the patient presents within 48 h of onset but cardioversion is delayed until several days have passed to allow drug loading, diagnostic studies, or correction of concomitant problems, interim anticoagulation with heparin should be considered.

It is important to recognize that many, if not most, cases of new onset atrial fibrillation convert spontaneously. This fact was highlighted in a study by Falk and colleagues[3] that examined the efficacy of intravenous digoxin for conversion of new-onset atrial fibrillation. Patients were randomly assigned to either intravenous digoxin or a placebo control. Nine of 18 patients who received digoxin converted to sinus rhythm, as did 8 of 18 patients who received only placebo (see Fig. 16–1). The difference between digoxin and placebo was obviously not significant. Studies involving oral or intravenous doses of standard antiarrhythmic drugs have often included patients with varying durations of atrial fibrillation; this makes comparisons between studies difficult. Conversion rates after oral or intravenous administration of sodium or potassium channel blocking drugs such as flecainide, propafenone, quinidine, procainamide, disopyramide, sotalol, and amiodarone range between 60% and 90% if atrial fibrillation is of less than 48 h duration but are only 15%–30% if the arrhythmia has been present longer.[9–19] More recently developed agents such as dofetilide, bidisomide, and ibutilide may be somewhat more effective, but only limited data are available.[20-22]

The possibility of an adverse reaction must be expected whenever an attempt at pharmacologic conversion of atrial fibrillation is made. Intravenous quinidine, and to a lesser extent, procainamide, are vasodilators. Their use can result in a lowering of blood pressure, which will then increase sympathetic tone on the AV node and result in faster ventricular rates while the patient is still in atrial fibrillation. It is also common for an antiarrhythmic drug to organize atrial fibrillation into atrial flutter. Because the drugs also prolong the typical atrial cycle in flutter length, 1:1 AV conduction can occur, with potentially catastrophic consequences.[23] This is most commonly seen with agents such as flecainide or propafenone but can also been observed with other agents, including quinidine and procainamide. Conversion of atrial fibrillation commonly unmasks sinus node dysfunction in elderly patients, and syncope as a result of unexpected sinus arrest or bradycardia-induced tachyarrhythmia can occur. QT prolongation and torsades de pointes may occur with agents that prolong repolarization, including sotalol, quinidine, procainamide, and many of the newer potassium channel blocking antiarrhythmic drugs.

Rate Control During Atrial Fibrillation

During atrial fibrillation, atrial activity is ongoing at rates of 400 beats per minute or higher, with patterns of both regular and irregular activity.[24] Langendorf and associates[25] developed the concept of "concealed conduction" to describe how the AV node controls and modulates ventricular rates during atrial fibrillation. Atrial impulses arriving at the AV node have a variety of fates. Some arrive when the node has fully recovered and conduct to the His-Purkinje system and ventricles. Other impulses arrive when the node is fully refractory and are blocked without influencing the properties of the node. Some impulses, however, enter the AV node and reset the refractory period without conducting to the ventricle. These "concealed" impulses thus affect subsequent impulses by "delaying it, blocking it or causing repetitive concealed conduction."[25] Thus, the net ventricular rate during atrial fibrillation is primarily determined by the effective and functional refractory periods of the AV node, which are strongly influenced by both the sympathetic and parasympathetic branches of the autonomic nervous system. A secondary influence on ventricular rate is the rate and regularity of atrial activity.[26] When atrial cycle lengths are short or irregular, there is a greater opportunity for concealed conduction, and net rates will slow. This phenomenon may explain some of the changes in ventricular rate after administration of antiarrhythmic drugs that are thought to have little direct effect on the AV node.

The goal of therapy to control ventricular rate in atrial fibrillation may be difficult to define with precision. In the symptomatic patient with new-onset atrial fibrillation, the immediate goal is usually to lower the rate sufficiently to relieve symptoms. In patients with sinus rhythm, however, there is an essentially linear relation between heart rate and metabolic demand.[27] A similar relation should be the goal of rate-control therapy during atrial fibrillation, but this is difficult to achieve. An accurate assessment requires documentation of adequate rate control at rest, during exercise, and during daily activities appropriate to the patient's condition. Cardiac glycosides, calcium channel blockers, and beta-adrenergic blockers are the primary agents used for rate control. Each agent or class of drugs has advantages and disadvantages.

Cardiac Glycosides

Digoxin and other cardiac glycosides have been used to control rates in patients with atrial fibrillation for many years. Although these agents have some direct effects on the AV node, their primary action is an augmentation of parasympathetic tone.[28] Digoxin often produces acceptable heart rates in the resting state, but unless the patient is sedentary, optimal rate control throughout a full range of daily activities is only rarely achieved. Other limitations to monotherapy with a cardiac glycoside have also been noted. In new-onset arrhythmia, the onset of rate slowing is usually delayed 4–8 h after initiation of therapy.[29] During exercise, digoxin has little effect on heart rate at a standard oxygen consumption.[28] In patients with paroxysmal atrial fibrillation, digoxin has little effect on heart rate at initiation of the episode.[30, 31] Although digoxin therapy offers significant advantages in terms of dosage schedule and cost of therapy, careful evaluation of its effects is necessary when it is used as the only agent for rate control. In many cases, overreliance on digoxin alone leads to delays in achieving rate control and inconsistent maintenance of satisfactory rates.[32]

Failure to achieve satisfactory rate control with digoxin therapy is often an indicator of increased sympathetic drive. Further attempts to control rates by increasing digoxin doses are likely to be ineffective and may produce toxicity. Digoxin plasma levels should not be allowed to rise above 2 ng/mL.

Calcium Channel Blockers

The calcium channel blockers verapamil and diltiazem are effective drugs for rate control in atrial fibrillation. They produce frequency-dependent effects on the AV node to delay conduction and prolong its effective and functional refractory periods.[33] Both verapamil and diltiazem are available in intravenous formulations which permit rapid, titratable administration for rapid control of ventricular rates. In many patients with chronic atrial fibrillation, oral therapy with both verapamil and diltiazem controls ventricular rates, improves exercise tolerance, and decreases symptoms.

Calcium channel blockers are also effective antihypertensive and antianginal agents, and there may be additional reasons for selecting them in patients with atrial fibrillation who might also benefit from these actions. In patients with clinical signs of congestive heart failure, calcium channel blockers may be associated with an increased mortality and should be used with caution.

Several possible forms of proarrhythmia are possible during the use of calcium channel blockers. Sinus node suppression may appear, particularly in patients with bradycardia-tachycardia syndromes. Two reports have suggested that calcium blockers may not be the drugs of choice in patients with paroxysmal atrial fibrillation. Shenasa and associates[34] evaluated the effects of oral and intravenous verapamil and diltiazem on the duration of induced atrial fibrillation in patients undergoing electrophysiologic studies. Calcium channel blockers, both oral and intravenous, prolonged the duration of atrial fibrillation episodes, with the most dramatic effects seen among patients with a history of prior atrial fibrillation. In another study, Kumagai and colleagues[35] reported that verapamil prolonged intra-atrial conduction times and increased fragmentation of atrial electrograms in patients with paroxysmal atrial fibrillation. These laboratory observations have not been confirmed by parallel observations during chronic therapy in patients with paroxysmal arrhythmias, but they do raise questions for further study.

Beta-Adrenergic Blocking Drugs

Sympathetic stimulation shortens refractory periods and increases conduction velocity in the AV node. Beta-adrenergic blockers are therefore often helpful for controlling rates during atrial fibrillation. All beta blockers decrease maximal heart rates during exercise or stress. The choice of a particular beta blocker can be made based on desired duration of action, optimal route of administration, and the agent's cardioselectivity. In patients with resting bradycardia while in atrial fibrillation or in those with sinus bradycardia and paroxysmal episodes of tachycardia, agents with intrinsic sympathomimetic activity (e.g., pindolol or xamoterol) can be used. Although beta blockers are generally effective in reducing symptoms caused by poor rate control during atrial fibrillation, studies during maximal exercise in patients with chronic atrial fibrillation have not shown consistent improvements in exercise capacity. One study showed marked improvement in patients with atrial fibrillation and mitral stenosis,[36] but patients with other diagnoses may manifest either no change or a decrease in maximal exercise capacity.[37]

Nonpharmacologic Therapy

Alternative approaches to controlling rate in atrial fibrillation have been developed. Catheter techniques for radiofrequency ablation of AV conduction are very reliable and relatively safe. Adaptive-rate pacemakers have sophisticated sensors that permit highly accurate physiologic control of ventricular rate both at rest and during daily activities. A number of studies have documented improvements in left ventricular function, exercise tolerance, general health, and psychological symptom scores in patients with poorly controlled paroxysmal or chronic atrial fibrillation who have undergone this procedure.[38–41] As more sophisticated physiologic sensors for pacemakers are introduced, the ability of the implanted pacemaker to respond optimally to demands should further improve. This approach should be considered in patients in whom pharmacologic control of rate proves difficult.

Another catheter technique for modulating AV nodal conduction has been described.[42, 43] This approach attempts to limit conduction through the AV node by interrupting atrial inputs to the node via its posterior and midseptal approaches. In selected patients, this technique has been effective during short-term follow-up, and permanent pacing has not been required.

Clinical Considerations

Any strategy for rate control must account for special clinical circumstances that may limit or enhance the effectiveness of the various therapeutic options available. Atrial fibrillation is a common complication of chronic lung disease. These patients have high adrenergic tone or are chronically exposed to sympathomimetic agents and will therefore respond poorly to digoxin. Beta blockers, even if cardioselective, may not be tolerated if bronchospasm is present. Calcium channel blockers are the agents of choice, but AV junctional ablation is often necessary. Patients with hyperthyroidism respond best to beta-adrenergic blockers. Beta blockers are preferred when atrial fibrillation occurs after cardiac surgery. In this situation, digoxin alone is of little benefit because of high adrenergic tone, and the possibility that episodes could be prolonged by a calcium channel blocker should be considered.

Patients with paroxysmal atrial fibrillation are often particularly difficult to manage. Most of the time they are in sinus rhythm, and under this condition, it is difficult to judge the effects of a rate control strategy for atrial fibrillation. Paroxysms can occur during periods of either high sympathetic or high parasympathetic tone, and it is often the abrupt change in rate that is most disturbing for the patient. In elderly patients and in those with associated abnormalities of sinus node function, AV junctional ablation with pacemaker insertion is often the most efficient method for controlling the patient's symptoms. Patients with Wolff-Parkinson-White syndrome who present with atrial fibrillation require a different management approach. In these patients, AV conduction may occur exclusively or preferentially over the accessory pathway rather than the AV node. Almost all accessory pathways capable of conducting at rapid rates are insensitive to the agents usually used to block AV nodal conduction. Paradoxical accelerations of rate may be seen after administration of cardiac glycosides,[44] calcium channel blockers,[45] and adenosine.[46] If immediate cardioversion is not required, intravenous procainamide is the usual drug of choice (Fig. 16–3).

Anticoagulation

Atrial fibrillation is an important risk factor for stroke and other forms of thromboembolism. This is true in patients with rheumatic valvular heart disease, those with other forms of heart disease, the elderly, and with some qualifications, in those without structural heart disease. It has been estimated that about 15% of all ischemic strokes are the result of atrial fibrillation. Between 1989 and 1992, five randomized clinical trials[47–51] were reported describing the effects of warfarin anticoagulation on the incidence of stroke in patients with nonvalvular atrial fibrillation (Table 16–3). Two of these trials also included groups treated with aspirin.[47, 49] The results of these trials have recently been subjected to a meta-analysis.[52] If an intention-to-treat analysis is used, warfarin is shown to reduce the risk of stroke by 68% (95% confidence limit, 50%–79%). Four independent risk factors for stroke were identified in this meta-analysis: (1) history of prior stroke or transient ischemic attack, (2) increasing age, (3) hypertension, and (4) diabetes. In all groups analyzed, except those younger than age 65 with *no* other risk factors, warfarin dramatically reduced the risk of stroke. Warfarin was also shown to produce approximately the same degree of risk reduction in a secondary prevention trial, the European Atrial Fibrillation Trial (EAFT).[53]

The effects of aspirin on stroke risk in atrial fibrillation remain

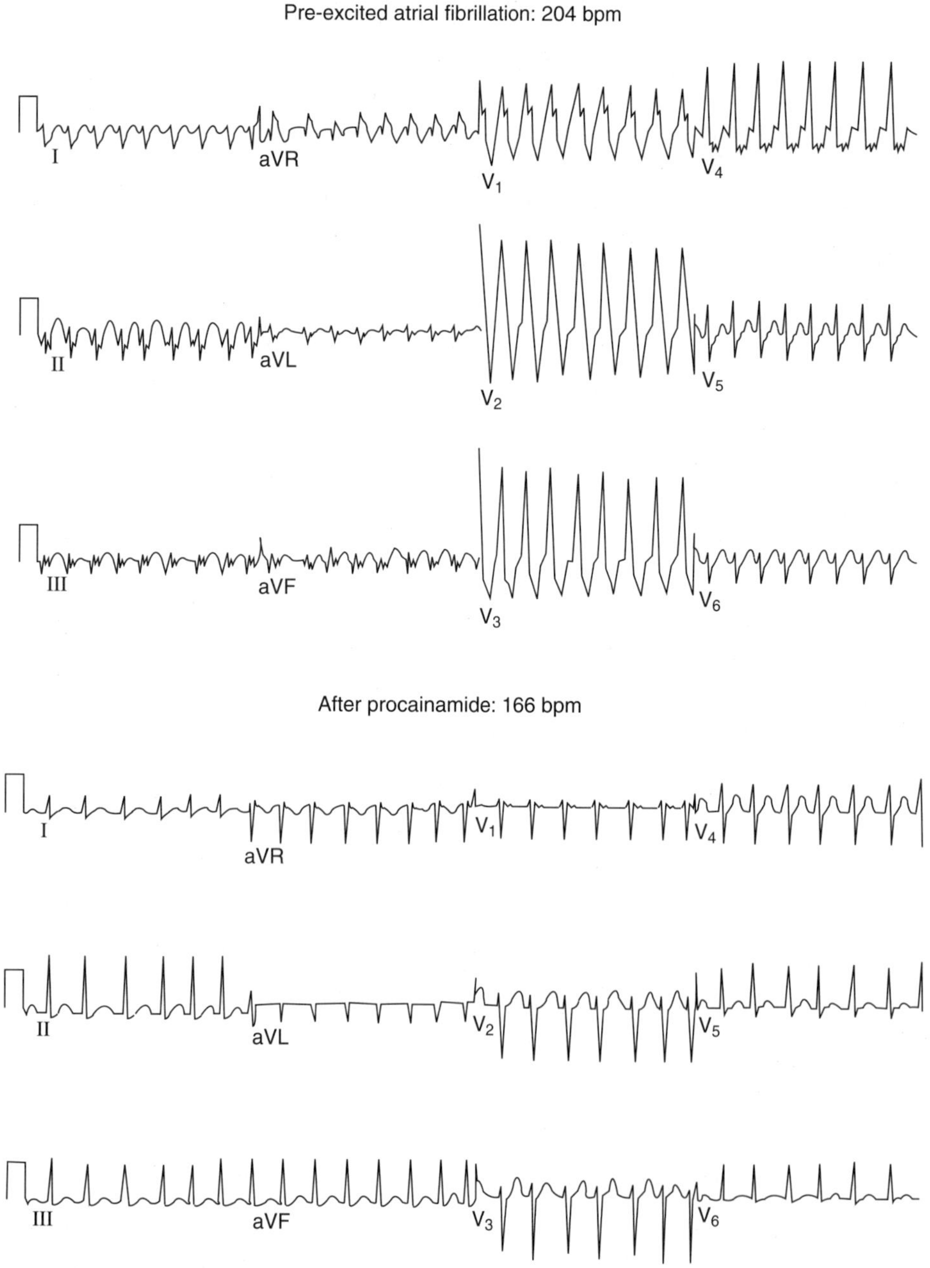

Figure 16–3. Atrial fibrillation in Wolff-Parkinson-White syndrome. This patient with a left free wall accessory pathway presented with palpitations and pre-excited atrial fibrillation (top). He was given procainamide. Accessory pathway conduction disappeared, and atrial fibrillation then continued over the normal conduction system at a reduced rate (bottom). Shortly thereafter, he converted to normal sinus rhythm.

TABLE 16–3. ANTICOAGULATION TRIALS IN NONRHEUMATIC ATRIAL FIBRILLATION

Trial	No. of Patients	Anticoagulation Target	Annual Rate of Primary Events* (%)
AFASAK[47]			
Control	335		5.5
Aspirin (80 mg)	336		5.5
Warfarin	335	INR: 2.8–4.2	2.0
SPAF I[49]			
Group 1			
Control	211		8.3
Warfarin	210	PTR: 1.3–1.8	2.3
Groups 1 and 2			
Control	528		6.3
Aspirin (325 mg)	517		3.2
BAATAF[48]			
Control	208		3.0
Warfarin	212	PTR: 1.2–1.5	0.4
SPINAF[51]			
Control	265		4.3
Warfarin	260	PTR: 1.2–1.5	0.9
CAFA[50]			
Control	191		5.2
Warfarin	187	INR: 2.0–3.0	3.5
SPAF II[55]			
Age ≤75 y			
Aspirin (325 mg)	357		1.9
Warfarin	358	PTR: 1.3–1.8	1.3
Age >75 y			
Aspirin (325 mg)	188		4.8
Warfarin	197	PTR: 1.3–1.8	3.6
EAFT[53]			
Control	378		19
Aspirin (325 mg)	404		15
Control	214		17
Warfarin	255	INR: 2.5–4.0	8

*Primary events included ischemic stroke in all studies. Inclusion of other embolic events was variable.

Abbreviations: INR, international normalized ratio; PTR, prothrombin time ratio.

controversial. In the Atrial Fibrillation Aspirin Anticoagulation Trial (AFASAK) study,[47] aspirin produced a nonsignificant decrease in risk. However, in one of the subgroups in a Stroke Prevention in Atrial Fibrillation trial (SPAF I), a significant 42% reduction in risk was observed. The risk reduction with aspirin in EAFT was 14% (95% confidence interval, −15%–36%).[53] In a retrospective analysis of nonrandomized aspirin use in the Boston area trial,[54] no benefit was observed.

There remain numerous questions concerning the optimal anticoagulation strategy for patients with atrial fibrillation. The optimal degree of anticoagulation has yet to be established. Most authors currently recommend an International Normalized Ratio (INR) of 1.5–3 or 2–3.[52] The influence of frequency and duration of episodes in patients with paroxysmal atrial fibrillation on stroke risk has not been examined, and it is uncertain at what point anticoagulation should be required. The role of therapy in low-risk patients (i.e., those younger than age 65 without risk factors) is also uncertain, and many physicians prefer aspirin over warfarin in these patients. As shown in the SPAF II trial,[55] chronic anticoagulation is not without potential hazards, and better methods for selecting patients for this therapy are needed.

Prevention of Recurrent Atrial Fibrillation

Previously, quinidine and other class Ia sodium channel blockers were the agents usually selected for prevention of recurrent atrial fibrillation after conversion of an initial episode. This approach has been challenged. In a meta-analysis of six randomized, placebo-controlled trials of quinidine for maintenance of sinus rhythm after cardioversion, Coplen and colleagues[56] showed that quinidine was associated with a lower recurrence rate than that seen during placebo therapy (Fig. 16–4). The analysis also showed that mortality was higher among the quinidine-treated patients. Many of the studies included in this analysis were conducted before many of the possible proarrhythmic effects and drug interactions of quinidine were recognized, and some deaths were not cardiac in nature. However, the threefold excess mortality should not be completely ignored. In a retrospective analysis of mortality in the SPAF I trial, Flaker and associates[57] reported that antiarrhythmic drug therapy increased risk for death in patients with a history of congestive heart failure. These observations should not be surprising in view of the known potential for proarrhythmia observed with these agents. Unfortunately, even though the newer agents have fewer extracardiac side effects and may be better tolerated during chronic therapy, proarrhythmia can be seen with all active antiarrhythmic drugs. Therefore, the risks and benefits of chronic suppressive drug therapy must always be a consideration when a physician considers initiating therapy. It is also important to remember that a single recurrence of atrial fibrillation should not always be considered a drug failure and a reason to change therapy. For patients with arrhythmias that are not life-threatening, intervals between episodes and symptoms during recurrence are often more important considerations.

Flecainide and propafenone are attractive alternatives to class Ia agents in patients without ischemic heart disease who have normal ventricular function.[58–60] In many patients with paroxysmal episodes of atrial fibrillation, these drugs increase the time to first recurrence and the average interval between episodes (Fig. 16–5). Although not yet well studied, moricizine is likely to produce similar results. Because these drugs also tend to slow AV nodal conduction, recurrent episodes may be better tolerated than before drug administration. Experience with these agents in patients with atrial fibrillation in the setting of some form of structural heart disease is limited. In view of the excess mortality among drug-treated patients reported in the

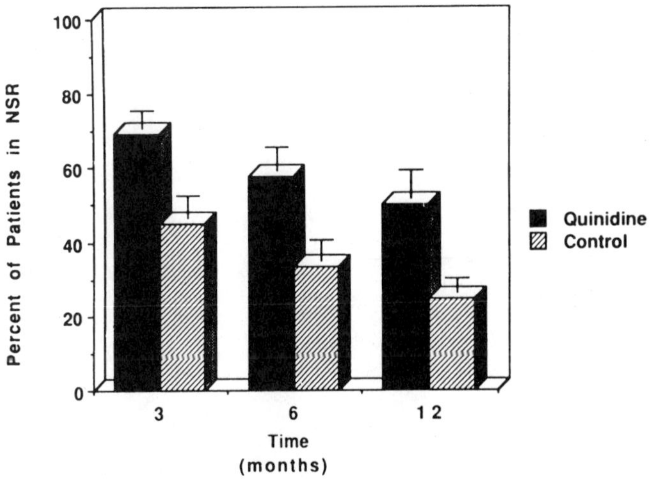

Figure 16–4. Efficacy of quinidine for maintaining sinus rhythm after cardioversion of atrial fibrillation. The data represent a meta-analysis of six studies involving 808 patients. *Abbreviation:* NSR, normal sinus rhythm. (From Coplen SE, Antman EM, Berlin JA, et al: Efficacy and safety of quinidine therapy for maintenance of sinus rhythm after cardioversion: A meta-analysis of randomized controlled trials. Circulation 1990; 82:1106.)

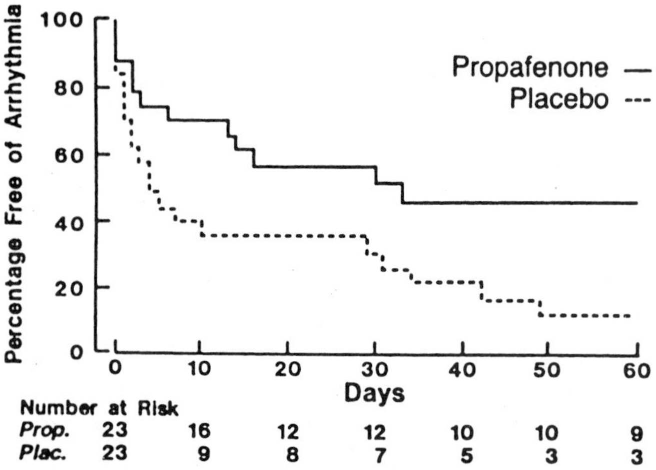

Figure 16–5. Propafenone for paroxysmal atrial fibrillation. A life table analysis of first arrhythmia recurrence is illustrated. *Abbreviations:* Prop, propafenone; Plac, placebo. (From Pritchett EL, McCarthy EA, Wilkinson WE: Propafenone treatment of symptomatic paroxysmal supraventricular arrhythmias: a randomized, placebo-controlled, crossover trial in patients tolerating oral therapy. Ann Intern Med 1991; 114:539.)

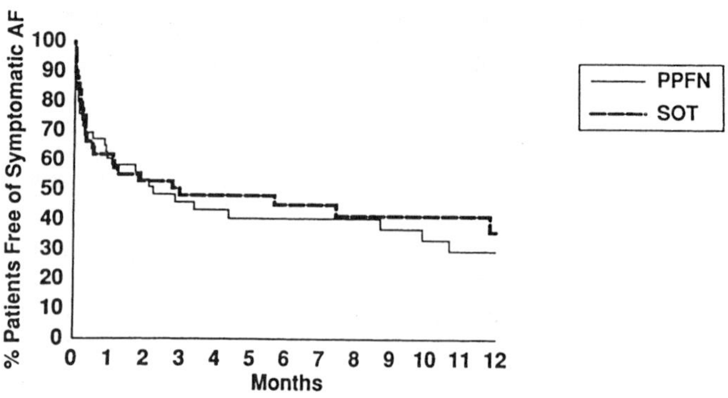

Figure 16–7. Randomized comparison of propafenone and sotalol. Patients were randomized between the two drugs after failure of a class IA agent. No difference in recurrence rate was noted. *Abbreviations:* AF, atrial fibrillation; PPFN, propafenone; SOT, sotalol. (From Reimold SC, Cantillon CO, Friedman PL, et al: Propafenone versus sotalol for suppression of recurrent symptomatic atrial fibrillation. Am J Cardiol 1993; 71:558.)

Cardiac Arrhythmia Suppression Trials,[61, 62] these agents should not be used in patients with known ischemic heart disease.

Sotalol is a class III antiarrhythmic drug that also produces beta-adrenergic blockade. Although currently marketed in the United States only for treatment of life-threatening ventricular arrhythmias, it is widely used in patients with atrial fibrillation. Juul-Möller and associates[63] compared sotalol to quinidine in 183 patients after conversion from atrial fibrillation to normal sinus rhythm. The two drugs were associated with similar recurrence rates (Fig. 16–6), but sotalol was better tolerated because of fewer extracardiac adverse reactions. Reimold and colleagues[64] compared propafenone and sotalol in a randomized trial of 100 patients with recurrent atrial fibrillation. Similar recurrence rates were noted with the two agents (Fig. 16–7). The major toxicities associated with sotalol are QTc prolongation, bradycardia, and torsades de pointes. Patients with electrolyte imbalance, bradycardia-tachycardia syndromes, ventricular hypertrophy, and female gender are at highest risk for the latter, which is a potentially life-threatening complication of sotalol.

Amiodarone has been reported to be effective both for paroxysmal atrial fibrillation and for maintenance of sinus rhythm after cardioversion.[64–67] Amiodarone produces toxicity in many organ systems, but at chronic doses of 200 mg per day or less, therapy is usually well tolerated. In contrast to most other antiarrhythmic agents, excess mortality has not been associated with amiodarone use in postmyocardial infarction populations or in patients with congestive heart failure, and some studies have indicated benefit.[68, 69] This record of safety and the long period of time required for peak drug effect allow outpatient initiation of therapy in patients with tolerated atrial fibrillation. The most common doses used are 400–600 mg daily for 2–4 weeks, followed by 200 mg per day.

In view of the limited efficacy of all available antiarrhythmic drugs in patients with atrial fibrillation, some authors have proposed a stepwise approach to therapy beginning with a class Ia or Ic agent followed by class III agents (i.e., sotalol followed by amiodarone; Fig. 16–8).[70, 71] Although this approach seems reasonable, it should be remembered that a single recurrence does not necessarily indicate drug failure. If episodes are well tolerated and of acceptable frequency, there is no need to change therapy with every recurrence. Few patients will remain totally arrhythmia-free during long-term follow-up, and palliation of symptom frequency and severity, rather than total abolition of arrhythmia, is a more practical therapeutic goal.

Atrial Fibrillation After Cardiac Surgery

Atrial fibrillation and atrial flutter are common problems after cardiac surgery. In patients without heart failure and without a history

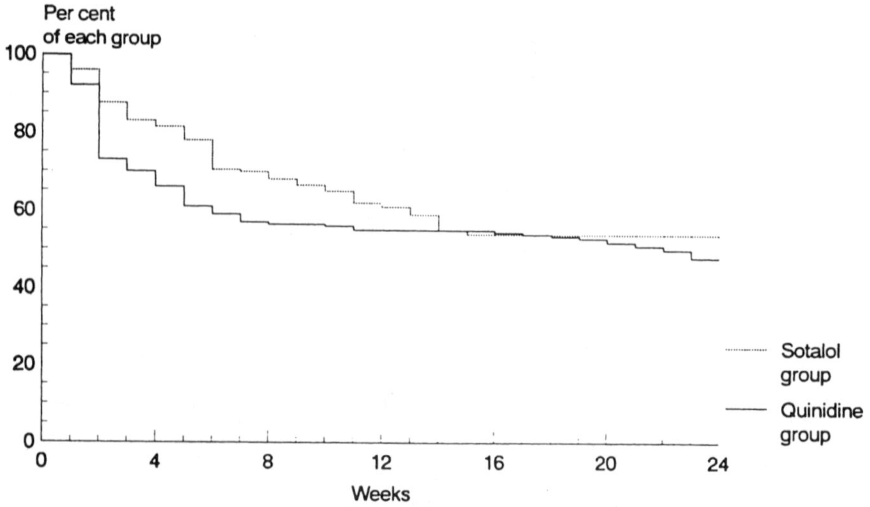

Figure 16–6. Sotalol versus quinidine for maintaining sinus rhythm after conversion of atrial fibrillation. Patients were randomized to either sotalol or quinidine after a successful cardioversion. There was no significant difference in rate of recurrence, but sotalol was better tolerated because it produced fewer adverse effects. (From Juul-Möller S, Edvardsson N, Rehnqvist-Ahlberg N: Sotalol versus quinidine for the maintenance of sinus rhythm after direct current conversion of atrial fibrillation. Circulation 1990; 82:1932.)

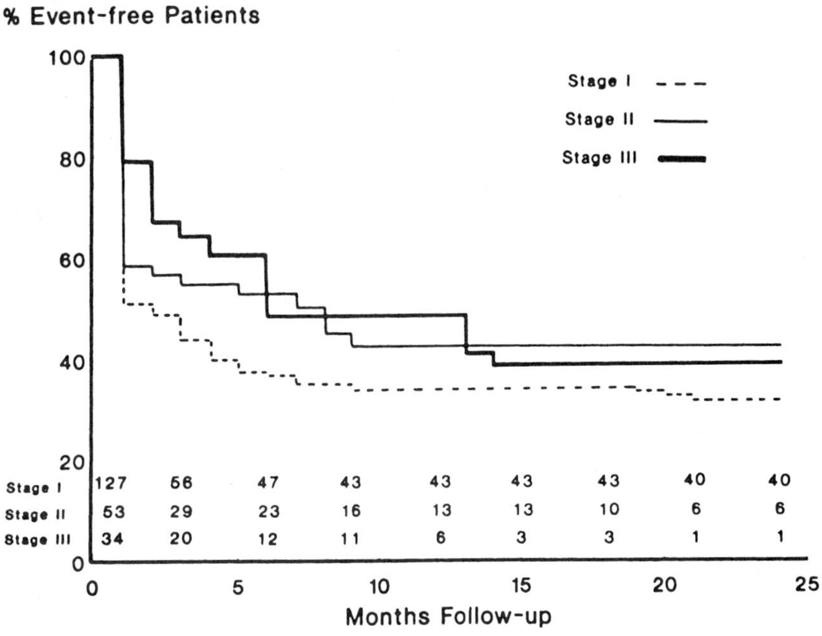

Figure 16–8. Staged-care management of atrial fibrillation. Patients were treated with flecainide in stage I, sotalol or quinidine in stage II, and amiodarone in stage III. About 40% of patients responded during each stage. Most failures were noted to occur early during therapy. If failures occur after 3 to 6 months of treatment, it would be reasonable to cardiovert and continue the same agent. (From Crijns HJ, Van Gelder IC, Van Gilst WH, et al: Serial antiarrhythmic drug treatment to maintain sinus rhythm after electrical cardioversion for chronic atrial fibrillation or atrial flutter. Am J Cardiol 1991; 68:335.)

of prior atrial fibrillation, postoperative atrial fibrillation usually develops in the interval between 2 and 10 days after operation and then will spontaneously resolve. Advanced age, prior beta blocker therapy, and, possibly, right coronary artery disease have been identified as potential risk factors for developing postoperative atrial arrhythmias after cardiac surgery.[72] Because adrenergic tone is high during this period, stable rate control is often difficult, and in patients with frequent paroxysms, hospital stay may be greatly prolonged. A number of trials have evaluated the effects of prophylactic drug therapy for preventing atrial fibrillation and atrial flutter after coronary artery surgery. Two meta-analyses of data from these trials have been published (Table 16–4). Kowey and associates[73] analyzed data from seven beta blocker trials, five digoxin trials, and two trials that combined the two drugs. Andrews and colleagues,[74] using somewhat different criteria for study selection, evaluated 18 beta blocker trials, three verapamil trials, and five digoxin trials. Prophylactic administration of either verapamil or digoxin had no effect on the incidence of atrial fibrillation after surgery. In contrast, beta-adrenergic blockers were shown to reduce atrial fibrillation incidence in both meta-analyses, from 34% to 8.4% in the Andrews study and from 20.2% to 9.8% in the Kowey report. The beta blocker chosen did not appear to be important. Combination therapy with digoxin and a beta blocker was also effective, but only two trials which enrolled a total of 292 patients studied this question. On the basis of these data, it appears reasonable to recommend prophylactic beta blockade after coronary artery bypass surgery, particularly in those with the risk factors mentioned previously. Prophylactic therapy need be continued for only 7–10 days after operation. Once atrial fibrillation has developed, management of the acute episodes is similar to that for other forms of atrial fibrillation.

ATRIAL FLUTTER

Although atrial flutter and atrial fibrillation share many common causes and some patients will manifest both arrhythmias, management of atrial flutter episodes requires a significantly different approach from that of atrial fibrillation. Atrial flutter is most commonly caused by a single macroreentrant circuit with a counterclockwise rotation in the right atrium. The atrial cycle is 200 ± 40 msec (250–350 per minute) but may be slower when atrial flutter develops during drug therapy. Because the cycle length is regular, alternate impulses arriving at the AV node are either conducted or completely blocked, and there is little opportunity to control ventricular rate via enhancement of concealed conduction. Ventricular rates lower than 150 beats per minute (>2:1 AV conduction ratio) tend to be unstable, with sudden accelerations or decelerations with changes in autonomic tone. Therefore, in the absence of significant intrinsic AV conduction

TABLE 16–4. PREVENTION OF ATRIAL FIBRILLATION* AFTER CARDIAC SURGERY—META-ANALYSIS RESULTS

Author	Drug	Number of Studies Reviewed	Number of Patients	AF (%)	
				Control	Treated
Kowey[73]	Beta blocker	7	1418	20.2	9.8
	Digoxin	5	875	19.1	15.4
	Digoxin plus beta blocker	2	292	29.4	2.2
Andrews[74]	Verapamil	3	432	18.2	18.2
	Digoxin	5	507	17.6	14.2
	Beta blockers	18	1549	34	8.7

*Most studies included all atrial tachyarrhythmias without specifying types.
Abbreviation: AF, atrial fibrillation.

disease that limits changes in rate, patients with atrial flutter should not be allowed to remain in the arrhythmia chronically.

Termination of Atrial Flutter

Studies in animal models have shown that drugs may terminate atrial flutter either by producing a large increase in the wavelength of the impulse within the circuit or by disrupting the lateral boundaries of the circuit, thus encouraging major cycle length oscillations and termination.[75, 76] As in atrial fibrillation, class Ia, class Ic, and class III antiarrhythmic agents may all be effective, but the anticipated response rates (20%–30%) are disappointing. In most cases, drugs that block AV nodal conduction must simultaneously be administered to guard against 1:1 conduction as the atrial cycle length slows. If drug administration alone fails to terminate atrial flutter, cardioversion, with the use of either direct current shock or rapid atrial pacing, should be performed. Drug therapy may facilitate termination of atrial flutter with rapid pacing.[77]

Few data concerning the need for anticoagulation before termination of an episode of atrial flutter are available. Most patients with atrial flutter have unstable rates and present soon after arrhythmia onset. Several weeks of anticoagulation are often not feasible; therefore, termination is usually attempted soon after onset without prior anticoagulation. However, when atrial flutter presents in a chronic setting and adequate rate control can be effectively maintained, anticoagulation before attempted cardioversion is reasonable.

Chronic Management of Atrial Flutter

Atrial flutter is much less common than atrial fibrillation, and in many patients, the presence of both atrial flutter and atrial fibrillation may be documented. Few data are available that specifically focus on the long-term efficacy of drug therapy of atrial flutter. Chronic rate control may be an option in selected patients who have intrinsic conduction system disease, but because concealed conduction is not prominent as a result of the regularity of the atrial cycle length, effective long-term rate control is difficult. The approach to prophylactic drug therapy is similar to that used in patients with atrial fibrillation, as outlined previously. AV nodal blocking agents are usually also prescribed to protect against 1:1 conduction should atrial flutter recur with a cycle length prolonged by the drug. Several approaches for catheter ablation of atrial flutter in selected patients have recently been described, and the initial results appear highly promising.[78, 79] Additional long-term follow-up data and more experience in patients with a variety of cardiac disorders are necessary before the role of catheter ablation is fully defined.

PAROXYSMAL SUPRAVENTRICULAR TACHYCARDIA

Several electrophysiologic mechanisms may be responsible for episodes of paroxysmal supraventricular tachycardia (PSVT). Reentry within the AV nodal region is the most common form. In this arrhythmia, two or more functionally distinct conduction pathways may be identified in the perinodal area.[80] These pathways are characterized by their relative conduction times as either "fast" or "slow." In the common or typical form of AV node reentry, anterograde conduction occurs over a slow pathway and retrograde conduction occurs over a fast pathway. Electrocardiography (ECG) shows a narrow QRS complex tachycardia, and P waves are usually obscured by the QRS. Other patterns, including "fast-slow" and "slow-slow" tachycardias, may be observed but are less common. Mapping and ablation studies indicate that fast pathways are likely to be located in the anterior approaches to the compact AV node, whereas slow pathways tend to be posterior in location. AV reentry is the second most common form of PSVT. The usual reentry circuit involves anterograde conduction over the AV node and retrograde conduction over an accessory pathway; this pattern is described as orthodromic reentry. Other patterns, including use of the accessory pathway for anterograde conduction (i.e., antidromic reentry) and reentry through multiple accessory pathways, are also possible but are clinically much less common than orthodromic reentry. Sinus node reentry and atrial tachycardias are other forms of PSVT that require different approaches to acute therapy, because the AV node is not actively involved in the arrhythmia circuit. These forms of PSVT are discussed separately.

Termination of PSVT

Some patients with PSVT can terminate their tachycardias with vagal maneuvers, particularly when they are employed at the initiation of an episode, before reflex sympathetic tone increases. The Valsalva maneuver appears to be the most effective technique in adults,[81] whereas in infants, facial immersion is easier to use and is more effective.[82] Patients can be instructed to lie down and try a vagal maneuver as soon as possible after tachycardia onset. When an episode has lasted sufficiently long for the patient to seek medical assistance, drug therapy is often required to terminate the arrhythmia. Various agents, including digitalis, beta blockers, edrophonium, and phenylephrine, were used in the past in patients with PSVT. Intravenous doses of more recently introduced agents such as flecainide,[83, 84] propafenone,[83, 85, 86] and sotalol[87, 88] are effective for terminating acute episodes. However, because of their relative safety, ease of administration, and high response rates, adenosine and calcium channel blockers are now the agents of choice.

Adenosine

Adenosine is an endogenous purine nucleoside that produces electrophysiologic effects in several cardiac tissues.[89–91] These actions are produced by an interaction with a specific cell surface receptor known as the A_1 receptor. Other adenosine receptors are present in the body but do not mediate electrophysiologic effects. Using G-proteins as mediators, adenosine directly increases outward potassium conductance in supraventricular tissues and indirectly blocks catecholamine-mediated inward calcium currents throughout the heart. This results in decreased automaticity in the sinus node and some atrial pacemakers, and decreased conduction and increased refractoriness in the AV node. Atrial refractory periods shorten, and atrial fibrillation may be precipitated by atrial extrastimuli.[92] Most accessory pathways are not directly affected by adenosine.[93] A few accessory pathways may show conduction block after adenosine, and many pathways will indirectly shorten their refractory periods during the sympathetic discharge that follows adenosine's direct effects. Exogenously administered adenosine is rapidly cleared from the circulation by cellular uptake and metabolism, with an estimated eliminated half-time of 1–5 sec. As a result, direct effects of adenosine after bolus injection are of very brief duration, with onset of action during the first pass through the circulation and a duration of action of less than 15 sec. Adenosine also produces a secondary sympathetic reflex response that may cause a sinus tachycardia after the direct effects have resolved. During constant intravenous infusions, the direct negative chronotropic and dromotropic effects are usually not observed, and only increased sympathetic activity is seen.[94]

These unusual pharmacodynamic and pharmacokinetic properties led to studies of the clinical utility of adenosine in patients with PSVT.[95–99] In both AV nodal reentry and AV reentry, conduction through the AV node is a required portion of the arrhythmia circuit. A single block in impulse conduction breaks the circuit and terminates the episode. The ultrashort duration of adenosine's actions after intravenous infusion allows AV nodal conduction to be safely interrupted to break the tachycardia during the brief period of drug effect.

The onset of adenosine's action in patients with PSVT typically occurs 15–30 sec after peripheral infusion. More rapid effects and lower dose requirements are observed with central administration, because less time is available for metabolism.[100] Because the drug is so rapidly metabolized, other factors, including mixing volumes, circulation time, and dead space at injection ports, may influence dose response. Interindividual differences in drug sensitivity are also possible. Because adenosine does not accumulate between doses, most authors recommend the use of gradually increasing doses until termination occurs. In adult patients, the reported effective dose range is 2.5–25 mg, with termination occurring in essentially all patients if no upper limit on dosage is imposed. One controlled study used sequential doses of 3, 6, 9, and 12 mg at 2-min intervals in patients with PSVT.[97] Conversion rates were 35%, 62%, 80%, and 91% for the these four doses, respectively, compared with a total conversion rate of 16% with placebo (Fig. 16–9). In the same study, 93% of patients with PSVT responded to a 6-mg dose of adenosine, followed, if necessary, by a 12-mg dose. Adenosine can be used safely in pediatric populations.[101–103] The dose range in pediatric patients has been reported to be 50–250 μg/kg.

Block during anterograde or retrograde AV nodal conduction is the most common pattern of arrhythmia termination. Block during accessory pathway conduction is possible in certain arrhythmias if the pathway is sensitive to adenosine (e.g., the permanent form of junctional reciprocating tachycardia).[104] Adenosine-induced atrial or ventricular premature beats may also terminate some episodes.

A number of arrhythmias have been reported to occur after termination of PSVT by adenosine. These may occur both during the early phase of adenosine's direct action as well as during the reflex-mediated period of increased sympathetic tone. A few seconds of sinus arrest, AV block, or both are commonly seen but are usually of no consequence unless inappropriately large doses of adenosine are administered. Atrial and ventricular ectopy occur around the time of arrhythmia termination in as many as one third of patients.[97] Isolated cases of polymorphic ventricular tachycardia have been described in patients with prolonged QT intervals as a result of either drug effects or excessive bradycardia.[105–106] Adenosine shortens atrial action potential duration and can facilitate induction of atrial fibrillation if appropriately timed atrial premature beats occur or are introduced.[92] Reinitiation of PSVT can occur after the period of adenosine-induced AV nodal block has passed. In one series, this occurred in 9% of patients.[97] Reinitiation can be managed either by a repeat of the same dose of adenosine or by substitution of a calcium channel blocker. Acceleration of ventricular rates during atrial arrhythmias that are not terminated by adenosine is possible as a result of shortened refractory periods in accessory pathways and secondary sympathetic effects on the AV node.

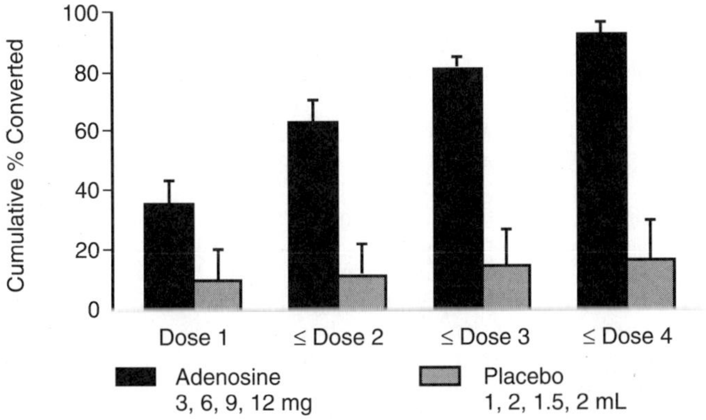

Figure 16–9. Adenosine dose ranging. Patients with paroxysmal supraventricular tachycardia were given increasing doses of adenosine (3, 6, 9, and 12 mg) or placebo at 2-min intervals. Higher doses may be required in some patients but were not permitted in this trial. (From DiMarco JP, Miles W, Akhtar M, et al: Adenosine for paroxysmal supraventricular tachycardia: dose ranging and comparison with verapamil in placebo-controlled, multicenter trials. Ann Intern Med 1990; 113:104.)

Transient side effects are reported by most patients who receive adenosine. The most commonly reported sensations are chest pain, flushing, and dyspnea. These side effects are dose related in both severity and duration and usually subside within 30–60 sec after injection. Therapy is not required. Aerosolized adenosine produces bronchoconstriction. Although a bronchospastic response is probably quite rare after intravenous administration, adenosine should probably be avoided in patients with active symptoms of asthma. Hypotension after arrhythmia termination does not occur, because the drug is metabolized before it reaches the peripheral arterioles (Fig. 16–10).

Adenosine metabolism or action is affected by several commonly prescribed medications. Dipyridamole blocks uptake of adenosine and greatly enhances and prolongs the effects of adenosine. Theophylline and other methylxanthines are competitive antagonists of adenosine at the A_1 receptor, and adenosine use in patients with therapeutic plasma theophylline concentrations is ineffective. Adenosine should be used in caution in patients with drug-induced or spontaneous long QT intervals because of the potential risk of inducing polymorphic ventricular tachycardia during the pause after arrhythmia termination.[106] Because adenosine clears from the circulation so rapidly, other drugs can be administered after its use without fear of interaction.

Calcium Channel Blockers

The calcium channel blockers verapamil and diltiazem also prolong AV nodal refractoriness and facilitate development of second-degree AV nodal block. This action is not shared with the dihydropyridine-type calcium channel blockers. Both verapamil[107, 108] and diltiazem[108–110] are highly effective for terminating acute episodes of PSVT by either AV nodal reentry or AV reentry. The recommended dose of verapamil in adults is 5 mg intravenously over 2 min, followed in 5–10 min by a second dose of 5–7.5 mg, if necessary. For diltiazem, the usual initial dose is 20 mg (0.25 mg/kg), followed, if necessary, by a second dose of 25–30 mg (0.35 mg/kg). Termination of PSVT occurs within 5 min after infusion of the effective dose of either agent. Among hemodynamically stable patients, more than 90% of episodes of PSVT are terminated by these dosages.

Arrhythmias can occur after the administration of calcium channel blockers. Atrial and ventricular premature beats are commonly seen around the time of arrhythmia termination. Induction of atrial fibrillation has been observed in a small number of patients.[111] Intravenous calcium channel blockers shorten the anterograde refractory period of many accessory pathways and may cause hypotension and collapse if mistakenly given to patients with pre-excited atrial arrhythmias.[112]

Adverse reactions to calcium channel blockers are rare in adult patients who are normotensive and free of heart failure during tachycardia. Calcium channel blockers are also vasodilators; therefore, they must be used with caution if hypotension is present. Use of doses lower than those recommended in hypotensive patients may decrease conversion rates without improving safety. Some authors recommend pre-treatment with intravenous calcium to moderate verapamil-induced hypotension,[113, 114] but this is not usually required. Sinus node suppression with symptomatic bradycardias can occur in patients with sinus node dysfunction or in those who have previously received intravenous beta-adrenergic blockers. Cardiovascular collapse has been reported in infants and neonates who received verapamil for PSVT.[115–117] Although similar data for diltiazem are lacking, both drugs should be avoided in patients younger than 1 year of age.

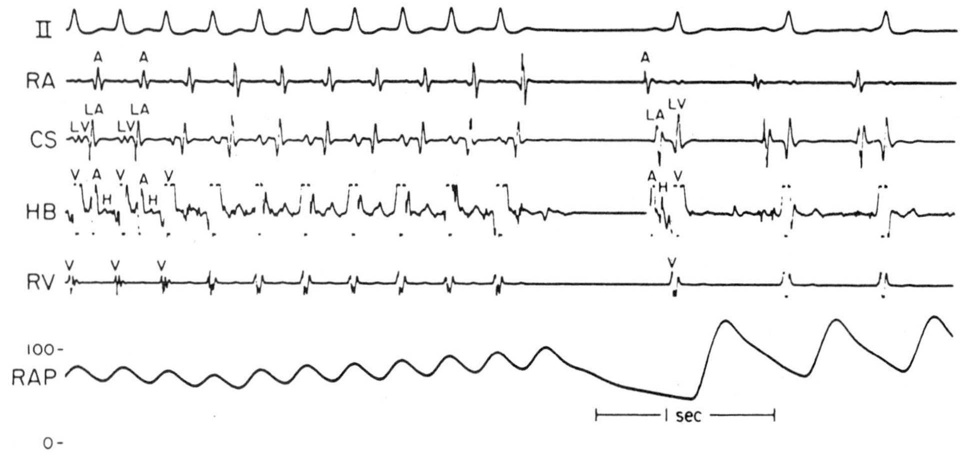

Figure 16–10. Adenosine in AV reentrant tachycardia. The tracings represent surface electrocardiographic lead II; intracardiac recordings from the right atrium (RA), coronary sinus (CS), bundle of His (HB), and right ventricle (RV); and a radial artery pressure (RAP). Twenty-two seconds after infusion of adenosine, anterograde block in the AV node terminates the tachycardia, and sinus rhythm is restored. Arterial pressure improved with resumption of sinus rhythm. *Other abbreviations:* A, atrium; H, His potential; LA, left atrium; LV, left ventricle; V, ventricle. (From DiMarco JP, Sellers TD, Lerman BB, et al: Diagnostic and therapeutic use of adenosine in patients with supraventricular tachyarrhythmias. J Am Coll Cardiol 1985; 6:417.)

Choice of Agent

Adenosine and verapamil have been compared in several randomized, controlled trials.[97, 118–121] In these studies, there has been no difference in efficacy between the two compounds. Although a similar direct comparison is not available between adenosine and diltiazem, the same results would be expected. The vast majority of patients with acute episodes of PSVT can be managed safely with either adenosine or a calcium channel blocker. Adenosine is the drug of choice in patients with hypotension or heart failure, in infants and neonates, and in patients who have recently received intravenous beta blockers. Verapamil or diltiazem should be selected in patients with active bronchospasm, in those receiving dipyridamole or theophylline, and whenever poor venous access does not allow administration of a rapid bolus. Patients who fail on either adenosine or a calcium channel blocker may safely be switched to the other. However, the response rate to appropriate administration of recommended doses of either agent among patients with PSVT as a result of either AV node reentry or AV reentry is so high that failure should make the physician question the accuracy of his or her original diagnosis.

In certain situations, the diagnosis of a narrow complex tachycardia may be uncertain, and as in atrial tachycardias, the arrhythmia may not depend on the AV node for continuation. In these situations, calcium channel blockers may cause excess hypotension if the tachycardia is not terminated, and adenosine may be a safer agent. In wide-complex tachycardias, caution must be exercised with both calcium channel blockers and adenosine unless the mechanism responsible for the arrhythmia is known. In pre-excited rhythms or in the most common types of ventricular tachycardia, hypotension, chest pain, and accelerated conduction over accessory pathways are potential complications of adenosine or calcium blocker administration. A careful assessment of the probable mechanism for the wide-complex tachycardia based on clinical and ECG findings is necessary before the use of test doses of adenosine or calcium channel blockers. Unless there are strong reasons to suspect AV node reentry or AV reentry with aberration, it is advisable to use drugs that are known to be efficacious and safe in pre-excited or ventricular tachycardias.

Prevention of Recurrent PSVT

When episodes of PSVT are well tolerated, can always be self-terminated, and occur infrequently, chronic prophylactic drug therapy is unnecessary. When chronic therapy is indicated, either a nonpharmacologic approach with catheter ablation or a pharmacologic approach may be most appropriate in individual patients. Catheter ablation has the advantage of offering an opportunity for "cure" of the arrhythmia by elimination of the anatomic substrate required. However, the immediate financial cost of catheter ablation may be significant, and although the serious complication rate for catheter ablation is low, it is not zero. Drug therapy has a lower short-term cost, and most drug toxicity is reversible if the drug is discontinued. However, the cost of the drugs, the need for acute and routine medical care, and deleterious effects of arrhythmia episodes and continuous drug therapy on quality of life make catheter ablation an option preferred by many patients.

Because the common forms of PSVT require AV nodal conduction, agents that block the AV node are often the first steps in chronic therapy. Calcium channel blockers and beta-adrenergic blockers have been shown to be chronically effective in 60%–80% of patients with well-tolerated PSVT.[107, 108, 122–126] When AV nodal blocking agents are ineffective or cannot be tolerated, sodium channel blockers may be effective. Class Ia drugs have only modest effects on accessory pathways and on fast AV nodal pathways, but these agents may be useful in some patients.[127, 128] Flecainide[129–135] and propafenone[60, 136–138] have been extensively studied in patients with PSVT. These agents have clinically significant effects on both accessory pathways and the AV node and are highly efficacious in delaying PSVT recurrence. Class Ic agents should be considered as the drugs of choice in patients without structural heart disease. Pritchett and Wilkinson have reported that the risk for ventricular proarrhythmia is low in these patients.[139] In this study, one death was observed among 236 patients treated with flecainide with a mean follow-up of 311 days. Nine deaths occurred among encainide-treated patients followed for a mean of 609 days. Comparison to a control group of arrhythmia patients from Duke University showed no significant difference in survival. In contrast, these drugs should be avoided in patients with structural heart disease, particularly those with prior myocardial infarction or congestive heart failure. Sotalol is effective for preventing PSVT because of both its beta blocker and its class III antiarrhythmic activities.[140] Amiodarone is highly effective in preventing PSVT recurrence, but the frequent toxicity observed during long-term therapy indicates that this drug should be used only in carefully selected patients in whom other drug or nonpharmacologic approaches are unsuccessful or inadvisable.[141] Combination therapy of a class I antiarrhythmic drug with a beta blocker may prove successful when single-agent therapy fails. Catecholamine stimulation can reverse effects of many drugs on accessory pathways or AV nodal conduction (Fig. 16–11).[6] Some authors have advocated isoproterenol challenge to help predict those patients in whom combination therapy will be necessary.[142]

ATRIAL TACHYCARDIAS

Atrial tachycardias other than atrial flutter and atrial fibrillation are much less common than AV nodal reentry and AV reentry through an accessory pathway. Therefore, data from controlled trials

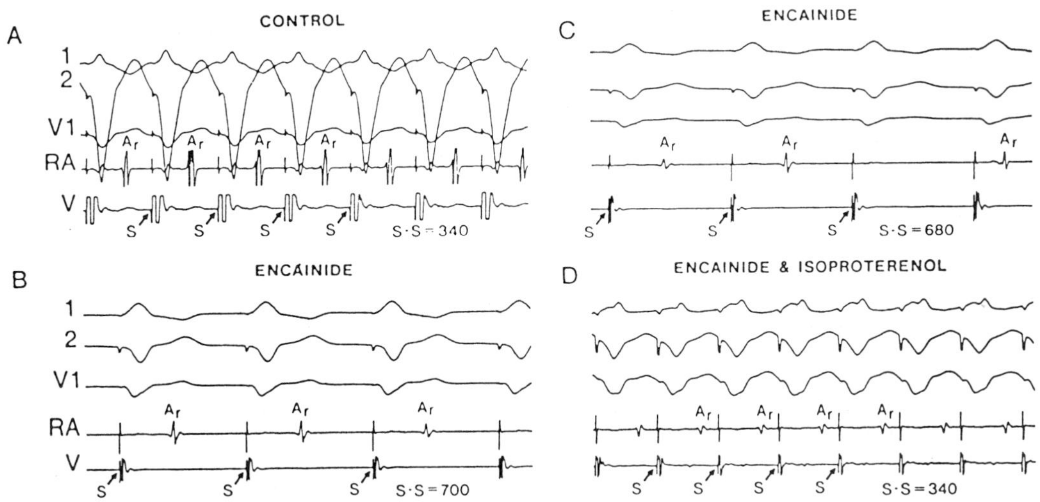

Figure 16–11. Reversal of drug effect by isoproterenol. The tracings show electrophysiologic recording in a patient with retrograde conduction over an accessory pathway. At baseline *(A)*, 1:1 VA conduction is maintained to a cycle length of 340 msec. During encainide (*B* and *C*), conduction is present at 700 msec, but block occurs at 680 msec. When isoproterenol is infused *(D)*, 1:1 conduction at 340 msec is restored. *Abbreviations:* A_r, retrograde atrial electrogram; RA, right atrium; S, stimulus; V, ventricular electrogram. (Akhtar M, Niazi I, Naccarelli GV, et al: Role of adrenergic stimulation by isoproterenol in reversal of effects of encainide in supraventricular tachycardia. Am J Cardiol 1988; 62:45L.)

concerning the treatment of these arrhythmias are usually unavailable, and the therapies described in the following sections are based primarily on anecdotal observations from clinical reports, each of which included relatively small numbers of patients. The electrophysiologic mechanisms responsible for these arrhythmias are poorly characterized.[143] ECG patterns in atrial tachycardia provide information concerning the site of origin in the atrium but not concerning the mechanism of the arrhythmia. Pharmacologic responses may not be specific for determining electrophysiologic mechanisms.[144, 145]

Tachycardias Originating in the Sinus Node

Inappropriate sinus tachycardia is a relatively common clinical finding that is believed to be caused by a disturbance of autonomic nervous system control of the sinus node.[146, 147] The prevalence of this condition is illustrated by the fact that as many as 50% of patients who present with a complaint of palpitations have sinus rhythm or sinus tachycardia during symptoms.[148] Patterns of both persistent tachycardia and unexplained alternations between a relatively slow sinus arrhythmia and sinus tachycardia can be observed. Although psychologic causes (e.g., panic attacks) can sometimes be identified, in many patients, no physical or psychologic abnormalities are discovered. Inappropriate sinus tachycardia has also been reported to occur with increased frequency after radiofrequency modulation of the AV node in patients with AV nodal reentry; the mechanism responsible for this phenomenon remains uncertain.[147] Patients with inappropriate sinus tachycardia require a careful evaluation for reversible causes of the syndrome. Excess circulating catecholamines, hyperthyroidism, hypotension, anemia, fever, psychiatric disorders, and drug effects must be excluded. If no reversible cause can be identified, reassurance should be the first approach. If symptoms persist, beta-adrenergic blockers can be prescribed. In those patients in whom alternating sinus bradycardias and tachycardias are documented, a beta blocker with intrinsic sympathomimetic activity, such as pindolol, may prove most effective.

Sinus node reentry has been described in both animals and humans.[149] It can be distinguished from inappropriate sinus tachycardia by its paroxysmal nature with abrupt onset and termination. Short episodes of sinus node reentry are fairly common, particularly in elderly patients, but sustained episodes are rare.[149, 150] Adenosine, verapamil, and vagal maneuvers all appear to be effective measures for terminating sinus node reentry.[150] Data concerning long-term therapy in these patients are lacking, but calcium channel blockers, beta blockers, and class I and class III antiarrhythmic drugs have been described as effective.

Atrial Tachycardias

Atrial tachycardias may be caused by enhanced automaticity, triggered activity, and reentry.[144] Each of these mechanisms may be catecholamine-sensitive or -dependent. Clinical presentations range from paroxysmal episodes of sustained or nonsustained tachycardia to incessant patterns of repetitive short bursts or continuous tachycardia. When the tachycardia is incessant, a tachycardia-induced myopathy may occur, and atrial tachycardia should be considered in the differential diagnosis of unexplained heart failure, particularly in children, adolescents, and young adults. Digoxin toxicity has been associated with atrial tachycardia with second- or third-degree AV block but is responsible for only a minority of patients presenting with this ECG pattern.

The pharmacologic management of atrial tachycardias is largely empiric. The acute response to standard doses of verapamil, adenosine, or a combination of these may be either tachycardia termination or the production of transient AV block.[96, 144, 145, 151] Many atrial tachycardias become intermittent in response to beta-adrenergic blockers. Few data concerning long-term drug suppression of atrial tachycardia are available. Flecainide,[152, 153] propafenone,[154] moricizine,[155] and amiodarone[151, 156, 157] have all been described as effective in small numbers of patients. Atrial mapping and catheter ablation can also be used in these patients and may be preferred to drugs in many situations.[158–161]

Multifocal Atrial Tachycardia

Multifocal atrial tachycardia (MAT) is a tachycardia characterized by three or more discrete P-wave morphologies occurring irregularly, with a total atrial rate between 120 and 180 beats per minute.[162, 163] One-to-one AV conduction is usually observed, but occasional early atrial beats may be blocked. MAT is most frequently seen in critically ill patients, particularly those with respiratory decompensation or failure. Theophylline toxicity is an important factor in the pathogenesis of this condition, leading some researchers to speculate that MAT is caused by triggered activity in multiple atrial sites.[164] MAT must be distinguished from atrial fibrillation, the other irregular narrow-complex tachycardia, because MAT is not responsive to cardioversion and may be exacerbated by digoxin. In children, a multifocal tachycardia, often called *chaotic atrial tachycardia*, that is not associated with acute illness or methylxanthine toxicity has been reported.

Because MAT is usually seen only in the setting of acute illness, the first steps at therapy should be directed at correction of the underlying disease process. Electrolyte disorders should be corrected, and the necessity for continued use of methylxanthines or catecholamines reviewed. Some authors recommend pharmacologic doses of magnesium.[165] Therapy with class I antiarrhythmic drugs has been generally ineffective. Beta blockers and calcium channel blockers have been of some value in scattered reports.[164, 166, 167] In a small controlled study comparing verapamil, metoprolol, and placebo, metoprolol was the most effective therapy.[168] Eight of nine patients responded to metoprolol, with response defined as either reversion to sinus rhythm or a 15% decrease in ventricular rate. Two of nine and four of nine patients had similar responses to placebo and verapamil, respectively. Unfortunately, many patients with MAT cannot tolerate even a cardioselective beta blocker, and therapy must be administered cautiously.

MAT usually resolves if the underlying illness is effectively treated. If MAT recurs frequently or persists despite best medical therapy, consideration of either a trial of amiodarone[169] or AV junctional ablation with permanent ventricular pacemaker insertion is indicated.

Junctional Ectopic Tachycardia

Junctional ectopic tachycardia has been seen primarily in infants and children. Both congenital and postoperative forms have been described.[170, 171] The congenital form usually presents with congestive heart failure in infancy. The postoperative form is seen after surgery to repair tetralogy of Fallot, transposition of the great vessels, and other forms of complex congenital heart disease. The mechanism for both arrhythmias is thought to be enhanced automaticity in the AV junction somewhere above the region that gives rise to the His potential. Because of the incessant nature of the tachycardia and its resistance to cardioversion and most forms of drug therapy, mortality is high.[163] Limited experience with sotalol,[172] propafenone,[173] and amiodarone[164] suggests that trials with these drugs are warranted. Catheter ablation and permanent pacing may be required in patients who fail to respond to drugs.

REFERENCES

1. Task Force of the Working Group on Arrhythmias of the European Society of Cardiology: The Sicilian gambit: a new approach to the classification of antiarrhythmic drugs based on their actions on arrhythmogenic mechanisms. Circulation 1991; 84:1831.
2. Vaughan-Williams EM: A classification of antiarrhythmic actions reassessed after a decade of new drugs. J Clin Pharmacol 1984; 24:129.
3. Falk RH, Knowlton AA, Bernard SA, et al: Digoxin for converting recent-onset atrial fibrillation to sinus rhythm. Ann Intern Med 1987; 106:503.
4. Pritchett ELC, Lee KL: Designing clinical trials for paroxysmal atrial tachycardia and other paroxysmal arrhythmias. J Clin Epidemiol 1988; 41:851.
5. Anderson JL, Gilbert EM, Alpert BL, et al: Prevention of symptomatic recurrences of paroxysmal atrial fibrillation in patients initially tolerating antiarrhythmic therapy. A multicenter, double-blind, crossover study of flecainide and placebo with transtelephonic monitoring. Circulation 1989; 80:1557.
6. Akhtar M, Niazi I, Naccarelli GV, et al: Role of adrenergic stimulation by isoproterenol in reversal of effects of encainide in supraventricular tachycardia. Am J Cardiol 1988; 62:45L.
7. Allessie M, Konings K, Wijffels M: Electrophysiological mechanisms of atrial fibrillation. *In* DiMarco JP, Prystowsky EN (eds): Atrial Arrhythmias: State of the Art, pp 155–161. Armonk, NY: Futura, 1994.
8. Laupacis A, Albers G, Dunn M, et al: Antithrombotic therapy in atrial fibrillation. Chest 1992; 102(suppl 4):426S.
9. Borgeat A, Goy JJ, Maendly R, et al: Flecainide versus quinidine for conversion of atrial fibrillation to sinus rhythm. Am J Cardiol 1986; 58:496.
10. Hellestrand KJ: Intravenous flecainide acetate for supraventricular tachycardias. Am J Cardiol 1988; 62:16D.
11. Goy JJ, Kaufmann U, Kappenberger LJ, et al: Restoration of sinus rhythm with flecainide in patients with atrial fibrillation. Am J Cardiol 1988; 62:38D.
12. Bianconi L, Boccadamo R, Pappalardo A, et al: Effectiveness of intravenous propafenone for conversion of atrial fibrillation and flutter of recent onset. Am J Cardiol 1989; 64:335.
13. Suttorp MJ, Kingma JH, Lie AH, et al: Intravenous flecainide versus verapamil for acute conversion of paroxysmal atrial fibrillation or flutter to sinus rhythm. Am J Cardiol 1989; 63:693.
14. Crijns HJ, Van Wijk LM, Van Gilst WH, et al: Acute conversion of atrial fibrillation to sinus rhythm: clinical efficacy of flecainide acetate: comparison of two regimens. Eur Heart J 1988; 9:634.
15. Suttorp MJ, Kingma JH, Jessurun ER, et al: The value of class IC antiarrhythmic drugs for acute conversion of paroxysmal atrial fibrillation or flutter to sinus rhythm. J Am Coll Cardiol 1990; 16:1722.
16. Murdock CJ, Davis MJE: A double-blind, controlled study of sotalol compared to propranolol and placebo in the treatment of acute atrial fibrillation. Aust N Z J Med 1988; 18:364.
17. Strasberg B, Arditti A, Sclarovsky S, et al: Efficacy of intravenous amiodarone in the management of a paroxysmal or new atrial fibrillation with fast ventricular response. Int J Cardiol 1985; 7:47.
18. Mostow ND, Vrobel TR, Noon D, et al: Rapid control of refractory atrial tachyarrhythmias with high-dose oral amiodarone. Am Heart J 1990; 120:1356.
19. Faniel R, Schoenfeld P: Efficacy of i.v. amiodarone in converting rapid atrial fibrillation and flutter to sinus rhythm in intensive care patients. Eur Heart J 1983; 4:180.
20. Suttorp MJ, Polak PE, van't Hof A, et al: Efficacy and safety of a new selective class III antiarrhythmic agent dofetilide in paroxysmal atrial fibrillation or atrial flutter. Am J Cardiol 1992; 69:417.
21. Gibson JK, Buchanan LV, Kabell G, et al: Ibutilide, a class III antiarrhythmic agent, rapidly terminates atrial flutter in a canine mode. Pharmacologist 1992; 34:165.
22. Ellenbogen KA, Wood MA, Stambler BS, et al: Conversion of atrial fibrillation and flutter by intravenous ibutilide [Abstract]. J Am Coll Cardiol 1994; 23:227A.
23. Falk RH: Proarrhythmia in patients treated for atrial fibrillation or flutter. Ann Intern Med 1992; 117:141.
24. Konings KT, Kirchof CJ, Smeets JR, et al: High-density mapping of electrically-induced atrial fibrillation in humans. Circulation 1994; 89:1665.
25. Langendorf R, Pick A, Katz LN: Ventricular response in atrial fibrillation: role of concealed conduction in the AV junction. Circulation 1965; 32:69.
26. Chorro FJ, Kirchhof CJHJ, Brugada J, et al: Ventricular response during irregular atrial pacing and atrial fibrillation. Am J Physiol 1990; 259(Heart Circ Physiol 28):H1015.
27. Corbelli R, Masterson M, Wilkoff BL: Chronotropic response to exercise in patients with atrial fibrillation. PACE Pacing Clin Electrophysiol 1990; 13:179.
28. Beasley R, Smith DA, McHaffie DJ: Exercise heart rates at different serum digoxin concentrations in patients with atrial fibrillation. Br Med J 1985; 290:9.
29. Weiner P, Bassan MM, Jarchovsky J, et al: Clinical course of acute atrial fibrillation treated with rapid digitalization. Am Heart J 1983; 105:223.
30. Rawles JM, Metcalfe MJ, Jennings K: Time of occurrence, duration, and ventricular rate of paroxysmal atrial fibrillation: the effect of digoxin. Br Heart J 1990; 63:225.
31. Murgatroyd FD, O'Nunain S, Gibson SM, et al: The results of CRAFT-1: a multicenter, double-blind, placebo-controlled crossover study of digoxin in symptomatic paroxysmal atrial fibrillation [Abstract]. J Am Coll Cardiol 1993; 21:478A.
32. Roberts SA, Diaz C, Nolan PE, et al: Effectiveness and costs of digoxin treatment for atrial fibrillation and flutter. Am J Cardiol 1993; 72:567.
33. Ellenbogen KA, German LD, O'Callaghan WG, et al: Frequency-dependent effects of verapamil on atrioventricular nodal conduction in man. Circulation 1985; 72:344.

34. Shenasa M, Kus T, Fromer M, et al: Effect of intravenous and oral calcium antagonists (diltiazem and verapamil) on sustenance of atrial fibrillation. Am J Cardiol 1988; 62:403.
35. Kumagai K, Matsuo K, Ono M, et al: Effects of verapamil on electrophysiological properties in paroxysmal atrial fibrillation. PACE Pacing Clin Electrophysiol 1993; 16:309.
36. Ahuja RC, Sinha N, Saran RK, et al: Digoxin or verapamil or metoprolol for heart rate control in patients with mitral stenosis: a randomised cross-over study. Int J Cardiol 1989; 25:325.
37. Matsuda M, Matsuda Y, Yamagishi T, et al: Effects of digoxin, propranolol, and verapamil on exercise in patients with chronic isolated atrial fibrillation. Cardiovasc Res 1991; 25:453.
38. Heinz G, Siostrzonek P, Kreiner G, et al: Improvement in left ventricular systolic function after successful radiofrequency His bundle ablation for drug refractory, chronic atrial fibrillation and recurrent atrial flutter. Am J Cardiol 1992; 69:489.
39. Twidale N, Sutton K, Bartlett L, et al: Effects on cardiac performance of atrioventricular node catheter ablation using radiofrequency energy for drug-refractory atrial arrhythmias. PACE Pacing Clin Electrophysiol 1993; 16:1275.
40. Rodriguez LM, Smeets JL, Xie B, et al: Improvement in left ventricular function by ablation of atrioventricular nodal conduction in selected patients with lone atrial fibrillation. Am J Cardiol 1993; 72:1137.
41. Kay GN, Bubien RS, Epstein AE, et al: Effect of catheter ablation of the atrioventricular junction on quality of life and exercise tolerance in paroxysmal atrial fibrillation. Am J Cardiol 1988; 62:741.
42. Williamson BD, Man KC, Daoud E, et al: Radiofrequency catheter modification of atrioventricular conduction to control the ventricular rate during atrial fibrillation. N Engl J Med 1994; 331:910.
43. Della Bella P, Carbucicchio C, Tondo C, et al: Modulation of atrioventricular conduction by ablation of the "slow" atrioventricular node pathway in patients with drug-refractory atrial fibrillation or flutter. J Am Coll Cardiol 1995; 25:39.
44. Sellers TD Jr, Bashore TM, Gallagher JJ: Digitalis in the pre-excitation syndrome. Analysis during atrial fibrillation. Circulation 1977; 56:260.
45. Gulamhusein S, Ko P, Klein GJ: Ventricular fibrillation following verapamil in the Wolff-Parkinson-White syndrome. Am Heart J 1983; 106:145.
46. Garratt CJ, Griffith MJ, O'Nunain S, et al: Effects of intravenous adenosine on antegrade refractoriness of accessory connections. Circulation 1991; 84:1962.
47. Petersen P, Godtfredsen J, Boysen G, et al: Placebo-controlled, randomised trial of warfarin and aspirin for prevention of thromboembolic complications in chronic atrial fibrillation: the Copenhagen AFASAK study. Lancet 1989; 1:175.
48. The Boston Area Anticoagulation Trial for Atrial Fibrillation Investigators: The effect of low-dose warfarin on the risk of stroke in patients with nonrheumatic atrial fibrillation. N Engl J Med 1990; 323:1505.
49. Stroke Prevention in Atrial Fibrillation Investigators: Stroke Prevention in Atrial Fibrillation Study: final result. Circulation 1991; 84:527.
50. Connolly SJ, Laupacis A, Gent M, et al: Canadian Atrial Fibrillation Anticoagulation (CAFA) Study. J Am Coll Cardiol 1991; 18:349.
51. Ezekowitz MD, Bridgers SI, James KE, et al: Warfarin in the prevention of stroke associated with nonrheumatic atrial fibrillation. N Engl J Med 1992; 327:1406.
52. Atrial Fibrillation Investigators: Risk factors for stroke and efficacy of antithrombotic therapy in atrial fibrillation. Arch Intern Med 1994; 154:1449.
53. European Atrial Fibrillation Study Group: Secondary prevention in nonrheumatic atrial fibrillation after transient ischaemic attack or minor stroke. Lancet 1993; 342:1255.
54. Singer DE, Hughes RA, Gress DR, et al: The effect of aspirin on the risk of stroke in patients with nonrheumatic atrial fibrillation: the BAATAF Study. Am Heart J 1992; 124:1567.
55. Stroke Prevention in Atrial Fibrillation Investigators: Warfarin versus aspirin for prevention of thromboembolism in atrial fibrillation: Stroke Prevention in Atrial Fibrillation II Study. Lancet 1994; 343:687.
56. Coplen SE, Antman EM, Berlin JA, et al: Efficacy and safety of quinidine therapy for maintenance of sinus rhythm after cardioversion: a meta-analysis of randomized controlled trials. Circulation 1990; 82:1106.
57. Flaker GC, Blackshear JL, McBride R, et al: Antiarrhythmic drug therapy and cardiac mortality in atrial fibrillation. J Am Coll Cardiol 1992; 20:527.
58. Pietersen AH, Hellemann H: Usefulness of flecainide for prevention of paroxysmal atrial fibrillation and flutter: Danish-Norwegian Flecainide Multicenter Study Group. Am J Cardiol 1991; 67:713.
59. Clementy J, Dulhoste MN, Laiter C, et al: Flecainide acetate in the prevention of paroxysmal atrial fibrillation: a nine-month follow-up of more than 500 patients. Am J Cardiol 1992; 70:44A.
60. Pritchett EL, McCarthy EA, Wilkinson WE: Propafenone treatment of symptomatic paroxysmal supraventricular arrhythmias: a randomized, placebo-controlled, crossover trial in patients tolerating oral therapy. Ann Intern Med 1991; 114:539.
61. The Cardiac Arrhythmia Suppression Trial (CAST) Investigators: Preliminary report: effect of encainide and flecainide on mortality in a randomized trial of arrhythmia suppression after myocardial infarction. N Engl J Med 1989; 321:406.
62. Cardiac Arrhythmia Suppression Trial II Investigators: Ethmozine exerts an adverse effect on mortality in survivors of acute myocardial infarction. N Engl J Med 1992; 1327:227.
63. Juul-Möller S, Edvardsson N, Rehnqvist-Ahlberg N: Sotalol versus quinidine for the maintenance of sinus rhythm after direct current conversion of atrial fibrillation. Circulation 1990; 82:1932.
64. Reimold SC, Cantillon CO, Friedman PL, et al: Propafenone versus sotalol for suppression of recurrent symptomatic atrial fibrillation. Am J Cardiol 1993; 71:558.
65. Gosselink AT, Crijns HJ, Van Gelder IC, et al: Low-dose amiodarone for maintenance of sinus rhythm after cardioversion of atrial fibrillation or flutter. JAMA 1992; 267:3289.
66. Horowitz LN, Spielman SR, Greenspan AM, et al: Use of amiodarone in the treatment of persistent and paroxysmal atrial fibrillation. J Am Coll Cardiol 1985; 6:1402.
67. Disch DL, Greenberg ML, Holzberger PT, et al: Managing chronic atrial fibrillation: a Markov decision analysis comparing warfarin, quinidine, and low-dose amiodarone. Ann Intern Med 1994; 120:449.
68. Ceremuzynski L, Kleczar E, Krezeminska-Pakula M, et al: Effect of amiodarone on mortality after myocardial infarction: a double-blind, placebo-controlled pilot study. J Am Coll Cardiol 1992; 20:1056.
69. Burkart F, Pfisterer M, Kiowski W, et al: Effect of antiarrhythmic therapy on mortality in survivors of myocardial infarction with asymptomatic complex ventricular arrhythmias: Basel Antiarrhythmic Study of Infarct Survival (BASIS). J Am Coll Cardiol 1990; 16:1711.
70. Antman EM, Beamer AD, Cantillon C, et al: Therapy of refractory symptomatic atrial fibrillation and atrial flutter: a staged care approach with new antiarrhythmic drugs. J Am Coll Cardiol 1990; 15:698.
71. Crijns HJ, Van Gelder IC, Van Gilst WH, et al: Serial antiarrhythmic drug treatment to maintain sinus rhythm after electrical cardioversion for chronic atrial fibrillation or atrial flutter. Am J Cardiol 1991; 68:335.
72. Laver MS, Eagle KA, Buckley MF, et al: Atrial fibrillation following coronary artery bypass surgery. Prog Cardiovasc Dis 1989; 31:367.
73. Kowey PR, Taylor JE, Rials SJ, et al: Meta-analysis of the effectiveness of prophylactic drug therapy in preventing supraventricular arrhythmia early after coronary artery bypass grafting. Am J Cardiol 1992; 69:963.
74. Andrews TC, Reimold SC, Berlin JA, et al: Prevention of supraventricular arrhythmias after coronary artery bypass surgery. A meta-analysis of randomized control trials. Circulation 1991; 84(suppl):III-236.
75. Spinelli W, Hoffman BF: Mechanisms of termination of reentrant atrial arrhythmias by class I and class III antiarrhythmic agents. Circ Res 1989; 65:1565.
76. Pinto JM, Graziano JN, Boyden PA: Endocardial mapping of reentry around an anatomical barrier in the canine right atrium: observations during the action of the class Ic agent flecainide. J Cardiovasc Electrophysiol 1993; 4:672.
77. Olshansky B, Okumura K, Hess PG, et al: Use of procainamide with rapid atrial pacing for successful conversion of atrial flutter to sinus rhythm. J Am Coll Cardiol 1988; 11:359.
78. Cosio FG, Lopez-Gil M, Goicolea A, et al: Radiofrequency ablation of the inferior vena cava–tricuspid valve isthmus in common atrial flutter. Am J Cardiol 1993; 71:705.
79. Feld GK, Fleck RP, Chen PS, et al: Radiofrequency catheter ablation for the treatment of human type 1 atrial flutter. Identification of a critical zone in the reentrant circuit by endocardial mapping techniques. Circulation 1992; 86:1233.
80. Jazayeri MR, Sra JS, Akhtar M: Atrioventricular nodal reentrant tachycardia: electrophysiologic characteristics, therapeutic interventions, and specific reference to anatomic boundary of the reentrant circuit. Cardiovasc Clin 1993; 11:151.
81. Mehta D, Wafa S, Ward DE, et al: Relative efficacy of various physical manoeuvres in the termination of junctional tachycardia. Lancet 1988; 1:1181.

82. Sreeram N, Wren C: Supraventricular tachycardia in infants: response to treatment. Arch Dis Child 1990; 65:127.
83. O'Nunain S, Garratt CJ, Linker NJ, et al: A comparison of intravenous propafenone and flecainide in the treatment of tachycardias associated with the Wolff-Parkinson-White syndrome. PACE Pacing Clin Electrophysiol 1991; 14:2028.
84. Hellestrand KJ: Intravenous flecainide acetate for supraventricular tachycardias. Am J Cardiol 1988; 62:16D.
85. Hammill SC, McLaren CJ, Wood DL, et al: Double-blind study of intravenous propafenone for paroxysmal supraventricular reentrant tachycardia. J Am Coll Cardiol 1987; 9:1364.
86. Vignati G, Mauri L, Figini A: The use of propafenone in the treatment of tachyarrhythmias in children. Eur Heart J 1993; 14:546.
87. Teo KK, Harte M, Morgan JH: Sotalol infusion in the treatment of supraventricular tachyarrhythmias. Chest 1985; 87:113.
88. Jordaens L, Gorgels A, Stroobandt R, et al: Efficacy and safety of intravenous sotalol for termination of paroxysmal supraventricular tachycardia. The Sotalol Versus Placebo Multicenter Study Group. Am J Cardiol 1991; 68:35.
89. Camm AJ, Garratt CJ: Adenosine and supraventricular tachycardia. N Engl J Med 1991; 325:1621.
90. DiMarco JP: Adenosine: diagnostic and therapeutic uses in cardiac arrhythmias. Cardiol Rev 1994; 2:33.
91. Faulds D, Chrisp P, Buckley MM-T: Adenosine: an evaluation of its use in cardiac diagnostic procedures, and in the treatment of paroxysmal supraventricular tachycardia. Drugs 1991; 41:596.
92. O'Nunain S, Garratt C, Paul V, et al: Effect of intravenous adenosine on human atrial and ventricular repolarization. Cardiovasc Res 1992; 26:939.
93. Garratt CJ, Griffith MJ, O'Nunain S, et al: Effects of intravenous adenosine on antegrade refractoriness of accessory connections. Circulation 1991; 84:1962.
94. Biaggioni I, Olafsson B, Robertson RM, et al: Cardiovascular and respiratory effects of adenosine in conscious man. Evidence for chemoreceptor activation. Circ Res 1987; 61:779.
95. DiMarco JP, Sellers TD, Berne RM, et al: Adenosine: electrophysiologic effects and therapeutic use for terminating paroxysmal supraventricular tachycardia. Circulation 1983; 68:1254.
96. DiMarco JP, Sellers TD, Lerman BB, et al: Diagnostic and therapeutic use of adenosine in patients with supraventricular tachyarrhythmias. J Am Coll Cardiol 1985; 6:417.
97. DiMarco JP, Miles W, Akhtar M, et al: Adenosine for paroxysmal supraventricular tachycardia: dose ranging and comparison with verapamil in placebo-controlled, multicenter trials. Ann Intern Med 1990; 113:104.
98. Marco CA, Cardinale JF: Adenosine for the treatment of supraventricular tachycardia in the ED. Am J Emerg Med 1994; 12:485.
99. Gausche M, Persse DE, Sugarman T, et al: Adenosine for the prehospital treatment of paroxysmal supraventricular tachycardia. Ann Emerg Med 1994; 24:183.
100. McIntosh-Yellin NL, Drew BJ, Scheinman MM: Safety and efficacy of central intravenous bolus administration of adenosine for termination of supraventricular tachycardia. J Am Coll Cardiol 1993; 22:741.
101. Overholt ED, Rheuban KS, Gutgesell HP, et al: Usefulness of adenosine for arrhythmias in infants and children. Am J Cardiol 1988; 61:336.
102. Till J, Shinebourne EA, Rigby ML: Efficacy and safety of adenosine in the treatment of supraventricular tachycardia in infants and children. Br Heart J 1989; 62:204.
103. Ralston MA, Knilans TK, Hannon DW, et al: Use of adenosine for diagnosis and treatment of tachyarrhythmias in pediatric patients. J Pediatr 1994; 124:139.
104. Lerman BB, Greenberg M, Overholt ED, et al: Differential electrophysiologic properties of decremental retrograde pathways in long RP′ tachycardia. Circulation 1987; 76:21.
105. Ben-Sorek ES, Wiesel J: Ventricular fibrillation following adenosine administration. A case report. Arch Intern Med 1993; 153:2701.
106. Wesley RC Jr, Turnquest P: Torsades de pointes after intravenous adenosine in the presence of prolonged QT syndrome. Am Heart J 1992; 123:794.
107. Wellens HJJ, Tan SL, Bär FWH, et al: Effect of verapamil studied by electrical stimulation of the heart in patients with paroxysmal reentrant supraventricular tachycardia. Br Heart J 1977; 39:1058.
108. Akhtar M, Tchou P, Jazayeri M: Use of calcium channel entry blockers in the treatment of cardiac arrhythmias. Circulation 1989; 80(suppl):IV-31.
109. Dougherty AH, Jackman WM, Naccarelli GV, et al: Acute conversion of paroxysmal supraventricular tachycardia with intravenous diltiazem. IV Diltiazem Study Group. Am J Cardiol 1992; 70:587.
110. Frabetti L, Capucci A, Gerometta PS, et al: Intravenous diltiazem in patients with paroxysmal re-entrant supraventricular tachycardia. Int J Cardiol 1989; 23:215.
111. Belhassen B, Viskin S, Laniado S: Sustained atrial fibrillation after conversion of paroxysmal reciprocating junctional tachycardia by intravenous verapamil. Am J Cardiol 1988; 62:835.
112. McGovern B, Garan H, Ruskin JN: Precipitation of cardiac arrest by verapamil in patients with Wolff-Parkinson-White syndrome. Ann Intern Med 1986; 104:791.
113. Barnett JC, Touchon RC: Short-term control of supraventricular tachycardia with verapamil infusion and calcium pretreatment. Chest 1990; 97:1106.
114. Salerno DM, Anderson B, Sharkey PJ, et al: Intravenous verapamil for treatment of multifocal atrial tachycardia with and without calcium pretreatment. Ann Intern Med 1987; 107:623.
115. Radford D: Side effects of verapamil in infants. Arch Dis Child 1983; 58:465.
116. Epstein ML, Kiel EA, Victoria BE: Cardiac decompensation following verapamil therapy in infants with supraventricular tachycardia. Pediatrics 1985; 75:737.
117. Garland JS, Berens RJ, Losek JD, et al: An infant fatality following verapamil therapy for supraventricular tachycardia: cardiovascular collapse following intravenous verapamil. Pediatr Emerg Care 1985; 1:198.
118. Rankin AC, Rae AP, Oldroyd KG, et al: Verapamil or adenosine for the immediate treatment of supraventricular tachycardia. Q J Med 1990; 74:203.
119. Belhassen B, Glick A, Laniado S: Comparative clinical and electrophysiologic effects of adenosine triphosphate and verapamil on paroxysmal reciprocating junctional tachycardia. Circulation 1988; 77:795.
120. Garratt C, Linker N, Griffith M, et al: Comparison of adenosine and verapamil for termination of paroxysmal junctional tachycardia. Am J Cardiol 1989; 64:1310.
121. Hood MA, Smith WM: Adenosine versus verapamil in the treatment of supraventricular tachycardia. Am Heart J 1992; 123:1543.
122. Mauritson DR, Winniford MD, Walker WS, et al: Oral verapamil for paroxysmal supraventricular tachycardia. Ann Intern Med 1982; 96:409.
123. Lai WT, Voon WC, Yen HW, et al: Comparison of the electrophysiologic effects of oral sustained-release and intravenous verapamil in patients with paroxysmal supraventricular tachycardia. Am J Cardiol 1993; 71:405.
124. Clair WK, Wilkinson WE, McCarthy EA, et al: Treatment of paroxysmal supraventricular tachycardia with oral diltiazem. Clin Pharmacol Ther 1992; 51:562.
125. Mehta AV, Chidambaram B: Efficacy and safety of intravenous and oral nadolol for supraventricular tachycardia in children. J Am Coll Cardiol 1992; 19:630.
126. Moller B, Ringquist C: Metoprolol in the treatment of supraventricular tachyarrhythmias. Ann Clin Res 1979; 11:34.
127. Bauernfeind RA, Wyndham CR, Dhingra RC, et al: Serial electrophysiologic testing of multiple drugs in patients with atrioventricular nodal reentrant paroxysmal tachycardia. Circulation 1980; 62:1341.
128. Wellens HJJ, Bär FW, Dassen WRM, et al: Effect of drugs in the Wolff-Parkinson-White syndrome. Am J Cardiol 1980; 46:665.
129. Henthorn RW, Waldo AL, Anderson JL, et al: Flecainide acetate prevents recurrence of symptomatic paroxysmal supraventricular tachycardia. The Flecainide Supraventricular Tachycardia Study Group. Circulation 1991; 83:119.
130. Neuss H, Schlepper M: Long-term efficacy and safety of flecainide for supraventricular tachycardia. Am J Cardiol 1988; 62:56D.
131. Hoff PI, Tronstad A, Oie B, et al: Electrophysiologic and clinical effects of flecainide for recurrent paroxysmal supraventricular tachycardia. Am J Cardiol 1988; 62:585.
132. Hohnloser SH, Zabel M: Short- and long-term efficacy and safety of flecainide acetate for supraventricular tachycardia. Am J Cardiol 1992; 70:3A.
133. Till JA, Rowland E, Shinebourne EA, et al: Treatment of refractory supraventricular arrhythmias with flecainide acetate. Arch Dis Child 1987; 62:247.
134. Priestley KA, Ladusans EJ, Rosenthal E, et al: Experience with flecainide for the treatment of cardiac arrhythmias in children. Eur Heart J 1988; 9:1284.
135. Cockrell JL, Scheinman MM, Titus C, et al: Safety and efficacy of oral

flecainide therapy in patients with atrioventricular re-entrant tachycardia. Ann Intern Med 1991; 114:189.
136. Breithardt G, Borggrefe M, Wiebringhaus E, et al: Effect of propafenone in Wolff-Parkinson-White syndrome: electrophysiologic findings and long-term follow-up. Am J Cardiol 1984; 54:29D
137. Manz M, Steinbeck G, Lüderitz B: Usefulness of programmed stimulation in predicting efficacy of propafenone in long-term antiarrhythmic therapy for paroxysmal supraventricular tachycardia. Am J Cardiol 1985; 56:593.
138. Musto B, D'Onofrio A, Cavallaro C, et al: Electrophysiological effects and clinical efficacy of propafenone in children with recurrent paroxysmal supraventricular tachycardia. Circulation 1988; 78:863.
139. Pritchett ELC, Wilkinson WE: Mortality in patients treated with flecainide and encainide for supraventricular arrhythmias. Am J Cardiol 1991; 67:976.
140. Knuze KP, Schluter M, Kuck KH: Sotalol in patients with Wolff-Parkinson-White syndrome. Circulation 1987; 75:1050.
141. Kopelman HA, Horowitz LN: Efficacy and toxicity of amiodarone for the treatment of supraventricular tachyarrhythmias. Prog Cardiovasc Dis 1989; 31:355.
142. Niazi I, Naccarelli G, Dougherty A, et al: Treatment of atrioventricular node reentrant tachycardia with encainide: reversal of drug effect with isoproterenol. J Am Coll Cardiol 1989; 13:904.
143. Dhala AA, Case CL, Gillette PC: Evolving treatment strategies for managing atrial ectopic tachycardia in children. Am J Cardiol 1994; 74:283.
144. Engelstein ED, Lippman N, Stein KM, et al: Mechanism-specific effects of adenosine on atrial tachycardia. Circulation 1994; 89:2645.
145. Chen S-A, Chiang C-E, Yang C-J, et al: Sustained atrial tachycardia in adult patients. Electrophysiological characteristics, pharmacological response, possible mechanisms, and effects of radiofrequency ablation. Circulation 1994; 90:1262.
146. Morillo CA, Klein GJ, Thakur RK, et al: Mechanism of "inappropriate" sinus tachycardia. Role of sympathovagal balance. Circulation 1994; 90:873.
147. Skeberis V, Simonis F, Tsakonas K, et al: Inappropriate sinus tachycardia following radiofrequency ablation of AV nodal tachycardia: incidence and clinical significance. PACE Pacing Clin Electrophysiol 1994; 17:924.
148. DiMarco JP, Philbrick JT: Use of ambulatory electrocardiographic (Holter) monitoring. Ann Intern Med 1990; 113:53.
149. Reiffel JA: Normal sinus rhythm and its variants (sinus arrhythmia, sinus tachycardia, sinus bradycardia), sinus node reentry and sinus node dysfunction (sick sinus syndrome): mechanisms, recognition and management. *In* Podrid PJ, Kowey PR (eds): Cardiac Arrhythmias, pp 750–767. Baltimore: Williams & Wilkins, 1994.
150. Gomes JA, Hariman RJ, Kang PS, et al: Sustained symptomatic sinus node reentrant tachycardia: incidence, clinical significance, electrophysiologic observations and the effects of antiarrhythmic agents. J Am Coll Cardiol 1985; 5:45.
151. Haines DE, DiMarco JP: Sustained intraatrial reentrant tachycardia: clinical, electrocardiographic and electrophysiologic characteristics and long-term follow-up. J Am Coll Cardiol 1990; 15:1345.
152. Priestley KA, Ladusans EJ, Rosenthal E, et al: Experience with flecainide for the treatment of cardiac arrhythmias in children. Eur Heart J 1988; 9:1284.
153. Kunze KP, Kuck KH, Schluter M, et al: Effect of encainide and flecainide on chronic ectopic atrial tachycardia. J Am Coll Cardiol 1986; 7:1121.
154. Reimer A, Paul T, Kallfelz HC: Efficacy and safety of intravenous and oral propafenone in pediatric cardiac dysrhythmias. Am J Cardiol 1991; 68:741.
155. Evans VL, Garson A Jr, Smith RT, et al: Ethmozine (moricizine HCl): a promising drug for "automatic" atrial ectopic tachycardia. Am J Cardiol 1987; 60:83F.
156. Haines DE, Lerman BB, DiMarco JP: Repetitive supraventricular tachycardia: clinical manifestations and response to therapy with amiodarone. PACE Pacing Clin Electrophysiol 1985; 9:130.
157. Mehta AV, Sanchez GR, Sacks EJ, et al: Ectopic automatic atrial tachycardia in children: clinical characteristics, management and follow-up. J Am Coll Cardiol 1988; 11:379.
158. Chen SA, Chiang CE, Yang CJ, et al: Radiofrequency catheter ablation of sustained intra-atrial reentrant tachycardia in adult patients. Identification of electrophysiological characteristics and endocardial mapping techniques. Circulation 1993; 88:578.
159. Kay GN, Chong F, Epstein AE, et al: Radiofrequency ablation for treatment of primary atrial tachycardias. J Am Coll Cardiol 1993; 21:901.
160. Goldberger J, Kall J, Ehlert F, et al: Effectiveness of radiofrequency catheter ablation for treatment of atrial tachycardia. Am J Cardiol 1993; 72:787.
161. Lesh MD, Van Hare GF, Epstein LM, et al: Radiofrequency catheter ablation of atrial arrhythmias. Results and mechanisms. Circulation 1994; 89:1074.
162. Kastor JA: Multifocal atrial tachycardia. N Engl J Med 1990; 322:1713.
163. Scher DL, Asura EL: Multifocal atrial tachycardia: mechanisms, clinical correlates and treatment. Am Heart J 1989; 118:574.
164. Levine JH, Michael JR, Guarnieri T: Treatment of multifocal atrial tachycardia with verapamil. N Engl J Med 1985; 312:21.
165. Iseri LT, Fairshter RD, Hardemann JL, Brodsky MA: Magnesium and potassium therapy in multifocal atrial tachycardia. Am Heart J 1985; 110:789.
166. Hanau SP, Solar M, Arsura EL: Metoprolol in the treatment of multifocal atrial tachycardia. Cardiovasc Rev Rep 1984; 5:1182.
167. Hill GA, Owens SD: Esmolol in the treatment of multifocal atrial tachycardia. Chest 1992; 101:1726.
168. Arsura E, Lefkin AS, Scher DL, et al: A randomized, double-blind, placebo-controlled study of verapamil and metoprolol in treatment of multifocal atrial tachycardia. Am J Med 1988; 85:519.
169. Kouvaras G, Calkins DV, Halal G, et al: The effective treatment of multifocal atrial tachycardia with amiodarone. Am Heart J 1989; 120:301.
170. Villain E, Vetter VL, Garcia JM, et al: Evolving concepts in the management of congenital junctional ectopic tachycardia. A multicenter study. Circulation 1990; 81:1544.
171. Case CL, Gillette PC: Automatic atrial and junctional tachycardias in the pediatric patient: strategies for diagnosis and management. PACE Pacing Clin Electrophysiol 1993; 16:1323.
172. Maragnes P, Fournier A, Davignon A: Usefulness of oral sotalol for the treatment of junctional ectopic tachycardia. Int J Cardiol 1992; 35:165.
173. Paul T, Reimer A, Janousek J, et al: Efficacy and safety of propafenone in congenital junctional ectopic tachycardia. J Am Coll Cardiol 1992; 20:911.

17 Nonpharmacologic Treatment of Supraventricular Tachycardias

William M. Miles, MD
Lawrence S. Klein, MD
Raul D. Mitrani, MD
David P. Rardon, MD
Douglas P. Zipes, MD

The purpose of this chapter is to review nonpharmacologic techniques for the management of various supraventricular tachyarrhythmias. These arrhythmias include atrioventricular (AV) nodal reentrant tachycardia, tachycardias using accessory pathways, atrial tachycardias, atrial flutter, and atrial fibrillation. Although antitachycardia pacing and surgical techniques are considered briefly, the most important nonpharmacologic therapeutic modality is catheter ablation. Catheter ablation techniques are potential first-line therapies for elimination of AV nodal reentrant tachycardia and tachycardias using accessory pathways (Table 17–1). On the other hand, catheter ablation is not appropriate for all patients with atrial tachycardia or atrial flutter, although selected patients with these arrhythmias may enjoy a high success rate. Catheter ablation for atrial fibrillation is commonly used to effect control of the ventricular response without eliminating the atrial fibrillation; however, surgical procedures to eliminate atrial fibrillation have been successful in highly selected patients, and catheter ablation techniques for elimination of atrial fibrillation are being actively investigated.

MECHANISMS OF SUPRAVENTRICULAR TACHYCARDIAS

Understanding the mechanisms of the various supraventricular tachycardias is essential for designing a therapeutic approach.[1] Supraventricular tachycardias are defined as those that do not arise solely from the ventricles or the bundle branches. Most supraventricular tachycardias involve only "supraventricular" cardiac tissue, specifically the sinus node, the atria, and/or the AV node. However, AV reciprocating (or reentrant) tachycardia (employing an accessory pathway in the tachycardia circuit, see later) is also considered a supraventricular tachycardia, even though the ventricles are a necessary part of the tachycardia circuit.

Although supraventricular tachycardias usually have narrow QRS complexes, they can be associated with wide QRS complexes if there is a pre-existing bundle branch block or if functional bundle branch block occurs on initiation of the arrhythmia. Atrial fibrillation and atrial flutter are the most common of the supraventricular tachyarrhythmias and usually occur in patients with underlying structural heart disease. The term paroxysmal supraventricular tachycardia refers to regular tachycardias with sudden onset and sudden termination; they occur most often in younger patients without evidence of structural heart disease. Of these paroxysmal supraventricular tachycardias, approximately two thirds represent AV nodal reentrant tachycardia. Approximately 30% represent AV reentrant tachycardia; the normal AV node/His-Purkinje system is used for anterograde conduction and either a manifest or a concealed (retrogradely conducting only) accessory pathway for retrograde conduction. The remainder are atrial tachycardias, arising exclusively from atrial tissue. A special form of atrial tachycardia is sinoatrial nodal reentrant tachycardia, in which a portion of the sinus node is believed to participate in the tachycardia reentrant circuit.

AV Nodal Reentrant Tachycardia

Although it was previously thought that the reentrant circuit responsible for AV nodal reentrant tachycardia was confined within the AV node itself,[2] it has become apparent from surgical[3–8] and subsequent catheter ablation[9–16] data that the reentrant circuit uses both AV nodal tissue and perinodal atrial tissue. The anterosuperior atrial inputs to the AV node represent the "fast pathway," and the more posteroinferior approaches to the AV node (near the coronary sinus ostium in the posterior aspect of Koch's triangle) represent the "slow pathway." Dual AV nodal physiology is common even in the absence of AV nodal reentrant tachycardia, and multiple slow path-

Sponsored in part by the Herman C. Krannert Fund; by grants HL–42370 and HL–01782 from the National Heart, Lung, and Blood Institute of the National Institutes of Health, US Public Health Service; and by the American Heart Association, Indiana Affiliate, Inc.

TABLE 17–1. CATHETER ABLATION OF SUPRAVENTRICULAR ARRHYTHMIAS

Arrhythmia	Ablation Potentially "Curative"	Acceptable First-Line Therapy for All Patients With This Arrhythmia	Patient Selection Necessary	Estimated Success Rate
Atrioventricular nodal reentrant tachycardia	Yes	Yes	No	95%
Accessory pathway	Yes	Yes	No	90%–95%
Atrial tachycardia	Yes	No	Yes	90%†
Atrial flutter	Yes	No	Yes	90%†
Atrial fibrillation	No*	—	—	—

*Except for investigational catheter "maze" procedure.
†Optimal candidates selected.

ways may exist.[17–19] In the *typical* variety of AV nodal reentrant tachycardia, the circuit consists of anterograde conduction via a slow AV nodal pathway and retrograde conduction via a fast AV nodal pathway. This usually results in atrial and ventricular activation being simultaneous during tachycardia.

Atypical varieties of AV nodal reentrant tachycardia occur less frequently (approximately 10% of cases).[1, 13] One atypical form represents reversal of the circuit described before for typical AV nodal reentrant tachycardia (e.g., anterograde conduction occurs via the fast AV nodal pathway, and retrograde conduction occurs via the slow AV nodal pathway). This is manifested by a longer RP than PR interval during tachycardia with inverted P waves in leads II, III, and aVF. In addition, retrograde atrial activation during tachycardia is earliest posteriorly in Koch's triangle near the coronary sinus ostium rather than more anterosuperiorly as in typical AV nodal reentry. A third variety of AV nodal reentry has been termed "slow-slow" AV nodal reentrant tachycardia. The RP interval is shorter than the PR interval during tachycardia, and the P wave is inscribed in the ST segment. Earliest retrograde atrial activation is also located posteriorly in this variety, and therefore it has been postulated that anterograde conduction is via one slow AV nodal pathway and retrograde conduction is via a second slow AV nodal pathway.

Arrhythmias Occurring Via Accessory Pathways

Accessory pathways, also referred to as accessory AV connections, are composed of atrial muscle tissue that can bridge the AV groove anywhere along the tricuspid or mitral annulus except in the region where the aorta and mitral annulus are contiguous.[20] Most of these pathways are capable of both anterograde and retrograde conduction, although pathways that conduct only retrogradely or (less commonly) only anterogradely[21] occur. Pathways that conduct anterogradely result in ventricular pre-excitation during sinus rhythm; that is, the QRS complex represents a fusion between ventricular activation using the accessory pathway and ventricular activation via the normal AV node/His-Purkinje system. When an accessory pathway conducts retrogradely only, there is no evidence of pre-excitation during sinus rhythm, and the pathway is termed *concealed.* A concealed accessory pathway may still participate in AV reentrant tachycardia as described later but is not associated with a risk of excessively rapid ventricular response should atrial fibrillation occur.

In patients with accessory pathways, reentrant tachycardia includes both the atria and the ventricles and is termed AV reentrant tachycardia.[22] If the direction of conduction through the AV node/His-Purkinje system during AV reciprocating tachycardia is in the normal anterograde direction, the tachycardia is termed *orthodromic* AV reciprocating tachycardia; anterograde conduction is via the normal AV node/His-Purkinje system, and retrograde conduction is via the accessory pathway. This results in a tachycardia with narrow QRS complexes (unless functional bundle branch block occurs) without pre-excitation. In an unusual form of reciprocating tachycardia termed *antidromic,* anterograde conduction is via the accessory pathway and retrograde conduction via the His-Purkinje/AV node.[23–25] This tachycardia is termed *maximally pre-excited* because the QRS complexes are wide and represent activation of the ventricles entirely via the accessory pathway.

The most common arrhythmia in patients with accessory pathways is orthodromic AV reciprocating tachycardia. The second most common arrhythmia is atrial fibrillation or flutter, often with a rapid ventricular response via the accessory pathway, which does not delay conduction like the normal AV node. The least common arrhythmia in patients with accessory pathways is antidromic AV reciprocating tachycardia (< 5% of tachycardias). On rare occasions, an antidromic tachycardia can result from anterograde conduction via one accessory pathway and retrograde conduction via a second accessory pathway. In the unusual situation in which an accessory pathway conducts anterograde only, atrial fibrillation with a rapid ventricular response and antidromic AV reciprocating tachycardia can occur, but orthodromic AV reciprocating tachycardia with narrow QRS complexes cannot occur.

Atrial Tachycardias

Atrial tachycardias are tachycardias that arise exclusively from atrial tissue. They typically have rates between 110 and 250 per minute. These arrhythmias can be due to abnormal automaticity, triggered activity, or intra-atrial reentry, although these mechanisms are often difficult to distinguish clinically. From an ablation standpoint, the atrial tachycardias can be divided into either *focal* or *macroreentrant* varieties. Focal atrial tachycardias can be due to either automatic or microreentrant mechanisms; in either case, the arrhythmia originates from a relatively small area, and the origin of the tachycardia can be mapped by searching for the earliest site of atrial activation during tachycardia. In macroreentrant varieties, the tachycardia uses a reentrant circuit that travels around an anatomic barrier. In this situation, atrial activation can be recorded over large areas throughout systole and diastole, and interruption of either a narrow isthmus of tissue critical to the tachycardia circuit or a region of critical slow conduction may be required for elimination of the tachycardia.

Sinoatrial reentrant tachycardia is thought to include the sinus node as a portion of the reentrant circuit, with perinodal atrial tissue composing the remainder of the circuit.[26] This tachycardia can be induced and terminated with programmed atrial stimulation and terminated with maneuvers that increase vagal tone, such as carotid sinus massage. However, some atrial tachycardias arising from areas distant from the sinus node can also be terminated by vagal maneuvers, verapamil, or adenosine.[27, 28]

Atrial Flutter

In atrial flutter, atrial activation is regular with rates of approximately 300 per minute (in the absence of drug therapy). Atrial flutter consists of typical and atypical varieties. Typical atrial flutter demonstrates negative "sawtooth" flutter waves in the inferior electrocardiographic leads. Typical atrial flutter is generated by an atrial macroreentrant circuit where the impulse travels superiorly up the atrial septum and back down inferiorly via the right atrial free wall.[29, 30] An anatomic isthmus in the region of the inferior vena cava, coronary sinus, and tricupsid annulus is necessary for completion of the tachycardia circuit. Typical atrial flutter is particularly amenable to ablation techniques. This intra-atrial macroreentrant circuit of typical atrial flutter can be reversed, resulting in atrial flutter with a similar rate but with flutter waves that are upright in the inferior leads. This pattern is less common than the typical pattern but is also amenable to ablation. However, other varieties of atypical atrial flutter that tend to be more rapid and less organized are more difficult to eliminate successfully with ablation.

Atrial Fibrillation

Atrial fibrillation is a disorganized atrial rhythm that is thought to be due to multiple intra-atrial reentrant wavelets.[31, 32] A critical mass of atrial tissue is necessary to perpetuate these multiple wavelets. Therefore, therapy for directly eliminating atrial fibrillation is based on the premise that multiple surgical lesions[33] (or possibly linear catheter ablation lesions[34]) placed within the right and left atria can eliminate atrial fibrillation by dividing the atrial muscle into portions that are too small to maintain fibrillation.

In addition, symptoms from atrial fibrillation can be palliated by slowing the ventricular response with use of catheter ablation or modification of the AV node.

PRINCIPLES OF ABLATION

Catheter ablation in humans was first reported for elimination of AV conduction to prevent the rapid ventricular response to atrial tachyarrhythmias.[35, 36] Ablation was originally accomplished by use of a defibrillator to deliver a direct-current shock between a catheter placed adjacent to the cardiac structure to be targeted and a large surface area adhesive electrode applied to the skin. However, because of complications related to intracardiac direct-current shocks,[37] ablation did not become commonplace for arrhythmia therapy until the advent of radiofrequency catheter ablation.[12, 38] Typically, up to 50 watts of 500-kHz radiofrequency energy are delivered between a 4-mm distal catheter electrode and a large surface area adhesive skin patch for up to 60 sec.[39–41] Tissue that is heated above 50°C by the radiofrequency energy is irreversibly damaged[42–45] (Fig. 17–1). Currently available energy delivery systems result in lesions that are approximately 5 mm in diameter and 3 mm deep, although the size of lesions varies significantly with catheter tip contact and the cooling effect of the blood flow.

Radiofrequency energy produces lesions that are homogeneous and well demarcated from the surrounding tissue. The delivery of radiofrequency current is not associated with barotrauma (pressure shock wave due to release of gases) as is direct-current shock ablation. Damage to valve tissue or the fibrous skeleton of the heart, as well as cardiac perforation, is unusual with the currently approved systems. Although the small lesion size is a potential advantage of radiofrequency ablation, in situations in which a larger lesion would be preferable because of a deeper location of an arrhythmia focus or difficulty stabilizing the catheter close to the site of arrhythmia origin, the small lesion size may represent a disadvantage.

The size of lesions produced by radiofrequency energy is limited by the fact that when tissue at the catheter tip is heated to 100°C, a tissue coagulum forms on the catheter that prevents further energy delivery (so-called impedance rise). Radiofrequency ablation has been aided by catheters that allow monitoring of the temperature at the tip (to ensure good catheter-tissue contact and signal an impending impedance rise)[46, 47] and by monitoring the system impedance, which normally decreases by 5–10 ohms during the first few seconds of energy delivery if good catheter-tissue contact is present.[48] Newer developments include guidance of catheter location with intracardiac echocardiography;[49] larger electrodes with higher radiofrequency power delivery;[50] catheters designed to produce linear lesions; irrigation techniques to cool the ablation catheter;[51] new energy sources, such as laser, microwave, or ultrasound energy; and multielectrode mapping catheters.[52]

Complications of catheter ablation can occur during the diagnostic/mapping portion of the electrophysiology procedure or be related to delivery of the radiofrequency energy itself; the former is much more common than the latter. Potential complications include femoral vein thrombosis; pulmonary thromboembolism; damage to the femoral artery, including pseudoaneurysm formation, pneumothorax, or hemothorax if subclavian or internal jugular venous access is obtained; cardiac perforation with or without cardiac tamponade; systemic or cerebral embolism if left ventricular catheterization is necessary; or damage to the aortic valve due to catheter trauma. Although its necessity is not clearly proven, many investigators recommend an antiplatelet agent such as aspirin for approximately 6 weeks after ablation to prevent formation of thrombus at the endocardial site of energy delivery. Damage to the normal AV conduction system is a hazard if energy is delivered close to the AV node or His bundle.

Elderly patients can undergo catheter ablation safely in most cases, but the risk of cardiac perforation appears to be higher in this population of patients.[53, 54] Although catheter ablation can be performed safely in young children,[55–57] animal data suggest that the lesion produced by the ablation procedure in immature sheep myocardium can enlarge as the animal grows; therefore, catheter ablation should be performed in infants and small children only if the arrhythmias are drug refractory and highly symptomatic.[58, 59] There is a small increase in risk for development of a malignant neoplasm or genetic defect as a result of radiation exposure from fluoroscopy;[60, 61] this risk may be accentuated in children. Radiation exposure can be minimized by the operator's experience and the use of pulse fluoroscopy.

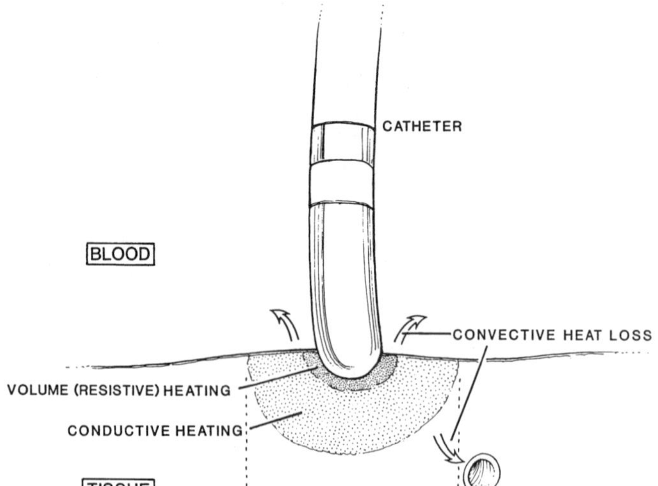

Figure 17–1. Schematic of myocardial lesion formation during radiofrequency energy delivery. A catheter with a large distal electrode is positioned at the interface of the blood and the endocardium. A small rim of tissue around the tip of the catheter is directly heated by the passage of radiofrequency current through the tissue; this is termed volume or resistive heating. The larger portion of the lesion is created by heat transfer from the region of resistive heating, termed conductive heating. There is cooling of the catheter tip by blood flowing past the catheter and cooling of deeper tissues by blood flow in intramyocardial blood vessels. The resultant lesion with use of current methods is approximately 5 mm in diameter.

ANTITACHYCARDIA PACING FOR SUPRAVENTRICULAR TACHYCARDIAS

Antitachycardia pacing techniques such as burst or ramp atrial pacing can terminate supraventricular tachycardias such as atrial flutter, AV nodal reentrant tachycardia, atrial tachycardia, and AV reentrant tachycardias in selected patients.[62] However, there are several disadvantages of using permanent implantable antitachycardia pacing devices to treat supraventricular tachycardias:

1. Antitachycardia pacing does not prevent but rather terminates tachycardia once it occurs, thus not totally eliminating symptoms.
2. Antitachycardia pacing is not effective for many patients with supraventricular tachycardias, and efficacy in any given patient is frequently inconsistent because of changes in autonomic tone, body position, and activity level.
3. Antitachycardia pacing may be proarrhythmic, especially by inducing atrial fibrillation that does not respond to pacing techniques. This may be particularly dangerous in patients who have an anterogradely conducting accessory pathway.
4. Antitachycardia pacing requires implantation of a permanent device.

With the advent of ablation, most tachycardias that are amenable to antitachycardia pacing can be permanently eliminated with ablation. Therefore, although antitachycardia pacing is an important therapy for ventricular tachycardia when it is incorporated into an implantable device with defibrillation capabilities, it is now infrequently used for supraventricular tachycardias.

NONPHARMACOLOGIC THERAPY FOR SPECIFIC SUPRAVENTRICULAR TACHYCARDIAS

AV Nodal Reentrant Tachycardia

Techniques

Although of historical interest, surgical and antitachycardia pacing therapies for AV nodal reentrant tachycardia have been almost completely abandoned in favor of radiofrequency ablation.[11, 12] Ablation for elimination of AV nodal reentrant tachycardia is performed by delivering energy to either the anterosuperior (fast pathway)[12, 63] or posteroinferior (slow pathway) inputs into the AV node.[11, 64–70] The earliest investigators targeted the fast pathway, but this has largely been abandoned in favor of a selective slow pathway ablation because of the decreased risk of inadvertent AV block with use of this technique.

If the diagnosis of AV nodal reentrant tachycardia has not been established before electrophysiologic study, both diagnostic and ablation procedures can be performed at the same time. Slow pathway elimination is accomplished by ablation in the posterior aspect of Koch's triangle along the tricuspid annulus at the level of the coronary sinus ostium, or occasionally at the ostium of the coronary sinus (Fig. 17–2). The location of energy delivery is guided by anatomic localization of the catheter with fluoroscopy,[65, 67, 69, 70] by the relative size of atrial and ventricular electrograms (usually a small atrial and large ventricular deflection), and by fractionation of the atrial electrogram that may or may not represent recording of a slow pathway potential[11, 71–73] (Fig. 17–3). Ablation success is assessed by attempting to reinduce AV nodal reentrant tachycardia after energy delivery, assuming it was reproducibly induced before energy delivery. If necessary, isoproterenol is infused to facilitate tachycardia induction. Characteristic junctional extrasystoles usually (but not necessarily) occur during energy delivery at an appropriate anatomic site,[74] indicating good catheter position and tissue heating. The PR interval should not increase after selective slow pathway ablation.

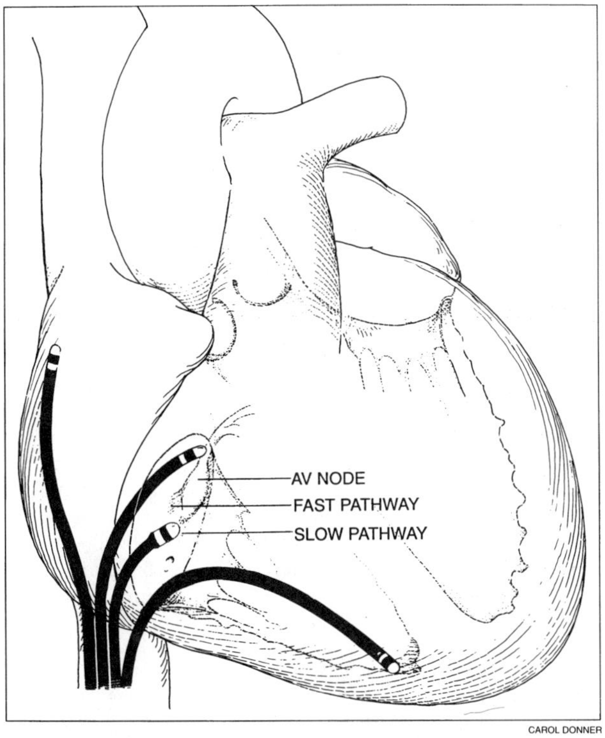

Figure 17–2. Schematic of catheter position for ablation of the slow pathway in atrioventricular (AV) nodal reentrant tachycardia. Diagnostic electrode catheters in the high right atrium and right ventricular apex as well as a catheter at the tricuspid annulus anterosuperiorly adjacent to the proximal His bundle are shown. The ablation catheter is located along the posteroinferior aspect of the tricuspid annulus in the region of the posterior (slow pathway) inputs to the AV node. If one were to deliver energy through the catheter recording the His bundle potential, complete AV block would result. If this catheter were withdrawn approximately 0.5 cm, it would be in an appropriate location to effect selective fast pathway ablation. (From Klein LS, Miles WM: Radiofrequency ablation of cardiac arrhythmias. Scient Am Science Med 1994; 1:48–57.)

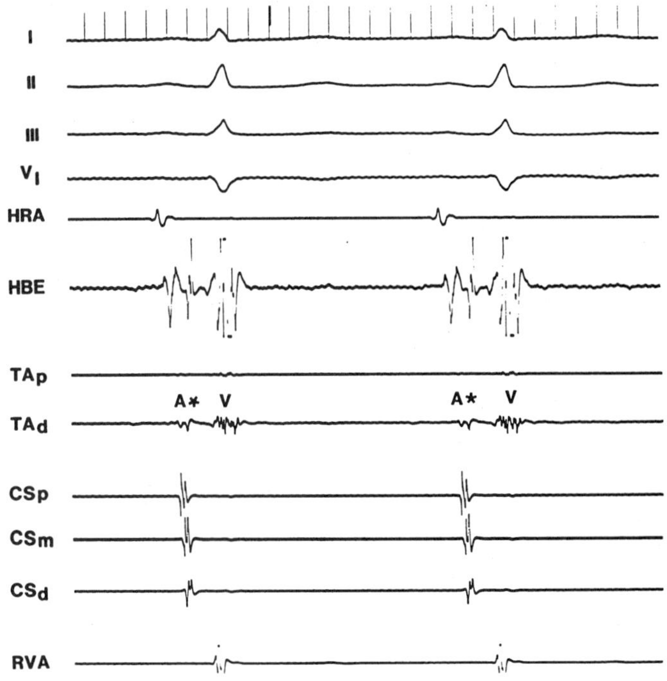

Figure 17–3. Possible slow pathway potentials recorded from the tricuspid annulus at the site of successful selective slow pathway ablation for elimination of AV nodal reentrant tachycardia. Surface leads I, II, III, and V_1 are displayed along with intracardiac high right atrial (HRA), His bundle (HBE), proximal (TAp) and distal (TAd) tricuspid annulus, proximal coronary sinus (CSp), middle coronary sinus (CSm), distal (CSd) coronary sinus, and right ventricular apical (RVA) electrograms. On the distal electrode positioned at the tricuspid annulus (TAd), a fractionated atrial potential (A*) and a larger ventricular potential (V) are recorded. The last sharp component of the atrial potential (asterisk) may represent a slow pathway potential. However, whether this electrogram represents a true slow pathway potential or merely a fractionated atrial potential, the electrogram is characteristic of a successful site for selective slow pathway ablation.

Indications

Either radiofrequency catheter ablation or pharmacologic agents can be considered first-line therapy for AV nodal reentrant tachycardia, depending on the patient's preference. Because of the small risk (<1%) of heart block with slow pathway ablation techniques and the fact that many patients may respond to pharmacologic agents that slow conduction in the AV node (e.g., digitalis, beta blockers, verapamil, or diltiazem), some patients may prefer a trial of these drugs before considering ablation. However, therapy with type I or type III drugs (sodium or potassium channel blockers, respectively, such as quinidine, flecainide, sotalol, amiodarone, and others) is not preferred to ablation except in patients whose overall general medical condition prohibits performance of an invasive procedure or in patients with a strong preference in favor of drug therapy. Ablation is preferred in patients with severe symptoms due to AV nodal reentrant tachycardia (e.g., syncope or near-syncope), patients in whom AV nodal blocking drugs fail to prevent symptomatic episodes or produce side effects, patients who are particularly active or participate in competitive athletics, female patients who wish to discontinue drug therapy in anticipation of pregnancy, and patients who wish to avoid lifelong drug therapy.

Efficacy

Acute success at eliminating AV nodal reentrant tachycardia by use of selective slow pathway ablation techniques is approximately 95%.[11, 12, 63–70] In half of these patients, single AV nodal reentrant echocardiographic beats are still inducible after ablation; these are probably not predictive of arrhythmia recurrence, although this is controversial.[66, 75–77] The fact that single AV nodal reentrant echoes may be inducible after apparently successful ablations implies that it is not necessary to destroy all the posterior inputs to the AV node, and the "slow pathway" may consist of multiple fibers. Ablation is effective in patients with either typical or atypical varieties of AV nodal reentry,[78] although in the slow-slow variety of AV nodal reentrant tachycardia, the fast pathway approach may not be applicable. In an occasional patient, a fast pathway ablation may be purposely or inadvertently performed if there is difficulty obtaining an adequate result from ablation energy delivered posteriorly to the slow pathway regions. Approximately 10% of patients having an initially successful ablation experience recurrent tachycardia and require a second ablation procedure; ablation of recurrences is successful in more than 90% of patients.

Routine follow-up electrophysiologic studies are not necessary. However, patients with recurrent palpitations after ablation, patients with severe hemodynamic symptoms from tachycardia before ablation, and selected patients with occupations involving public safety (e.g., airline pilots) should undergo follow-up electrophysiologic study several weeks after the procedure to document ablation success.

Complications

The frequency of heart block with the posterior approach is less than 1% but is not zero. It is difficult to predict who will have heart block from the procedure; it is related to inadvertent catheter movement during energy delivery in some cases, and there can be posterior displacement of the AV node in others. Rare patients with AV nodal reentrant tachycardia may have no anterograde fast pathway conduction as manifested by first-degree AV block during sinus rhythm; these patients may have a higher frequency of AV block after ablation.[79, 80] The late development of AV block (days to weeks) after an ablation procedure occurs occasionally with selective fast, but not slow, pathway ablation.

A phenomenon peculiar to the ablation for AV nodal reentrant tachycardia is the occurrence of sinus tachycardia after ablation that can be symptomatic in some patients. It is not clear whether patients with AV nodal reentry are susceptible to sinus tachycardia before ablation or whether sinus tachycardia is caused by the ablation procedure. One study suggests that radiofrequency ablation in the posteroseptal area alters vagal innervation to the heart as demonstrated by a decrease in heart rate variability after ablation.[81] In addition, this phenomenon may be exacerbated in some patients by withdrawal of beta blocker therapy. Measures generally consist of reassurance, ruling out of recurrent AV nodal reentrant tachycardia, and treatment with beta blockers. In addition, palpitations due to premature atrial or ventricular extrasystoles are also common after ablation.

Other potential complications include those of the catheterization procedure itself and are not peculiar to AV nodal reentrant tachycardia ablation; these include venous thrombosis, pulmonary thromboembolism, and cardiac perforation from diagnostic catheters. Cerebrovascular events and myocardial infarction are rare because the arterial system is not entered.

Tachyarrhythmias Associated With Accessory Pathways

Techniques

Accessory AV connections located anywhere along the mitral or tricuspid annuli can be ablated with radiofrequency catheter techniques[12, 38, 55, 82–85] (Fig. 17–4). Left-sided accessory pathways can be approached by use of a retrograde transaortic technique in which the catheter is passed from the femoral artery across the aortic valve and stabilized on the AV groove just underneath the mitral valve on its ventricular aspect, or superior to the mitral valve on its atrial aspect[86] (Figs. 17–5, 17–6). Some operators prefer a transseptal technique, approaching the left atrium from the right atrium and delivering the ablation energy along the atrial aspect of the mitral annulus.[87, 88] Left-sided accessory pathways that are more epicardial in location can be approached via the coronary sinus.[89–93] Right-sided accessory pathways can be ablated by introducing catheters into either the femoral vein–inferior vena caval or the subclavian or internal jugular vein–superior vena caval systems. The catheters are stabilized on the atrial or, less frequently, the ventricular aspect of the tricuspid annulus.[94] Right anteroseptal and midseptal accessory pathways can be close to the normal AV conduction system but can be ablated with a low risk (<1%) of AV block by careful mapping to avoid the AV node or His bundle or by delivering the ablation energy on the ventricular aspect of the tricuspid annulus where the His bundle is deep in the septum.[95, 96] The posteroseptal region is a complex triangular space,[97] bounded on the right by the region of the coronary sinus os, anteriorly by the midseptal locations, and extending to the left approximately 1 cm into the coronary sinus. Posteroseptal pathways can be approached from the venous system via the tricuspid annulus, from the arterial system via the mitral annulus, or from within the coronary sinus or its branches such as the middle cardiac vein.[91, 98] Posteroseptal accessory pathways may occasionally be asso-

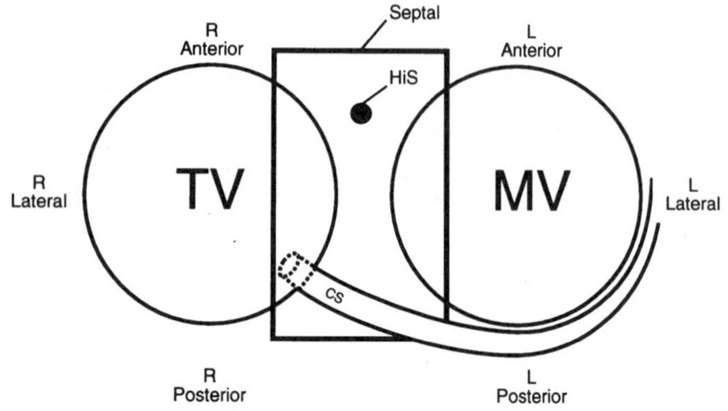

Figure 17–4. Schematic for terminology of accessory pathway locations. The mitral and tricuspid annuli are illustrated as viewed from the left anterior oblique fluoroscopic view (TV, tricuspid valve; MV, mitral valve). The septal region is complex and is greatly simplified in this schematic. The His bundle occupies the anteroseptal region. The coronary sinus passes through the posteroseptal region. (From Miles WM, Zipes DP, Klein LS: Ablation of free wall accessory pathways. *In* Zipes DP [ed]: Catheter Ablation of Arrhythmias, pp 211–230. Armonk, NY: Futura Publishing, 1994.)

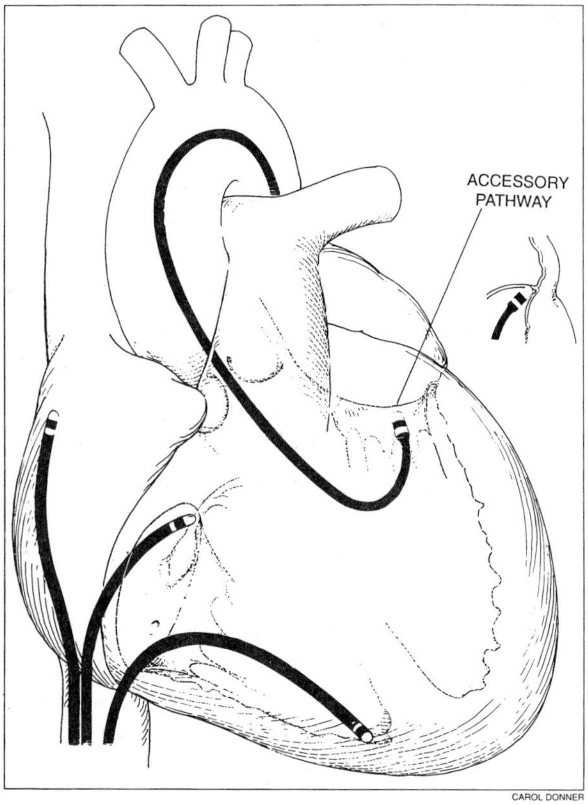

Figure 17–5. Schematic of the retrograde transaortic approach for ablation of left free wall accessory pathways. Diagnostic catheters are illustrated in the high right atrium, across the tricuspid valve in the region of His bundle, and in the right ventricular apex. An ablation catheter is advanced retrogradely via the aorta across the aortic valve and stabilized underneath the mitral valve annulus along the left ventricular free wall. The inset on the right of the illustration shows positioning of the ablation catheter underneath the mitral valve leaflet. (From Klein LS, Miles WM: Radiofrequency ablation of cardiac arrhythmias. Scient Am Science Med 1994; 1:48–57.)

ciated with abnormalities of the coronary sinus, such as coronary sinus diverticula.[99]

The delta wave axis on a pre-excited surface electrocardiogram helps localize an accessory pathway before ablation.[100, 101] Positive delta waves in lead V_1 suggest a left-sided accessory pathway, and isoelectric or negative delta waves in V_1 suggest a right-sided accessory pathway. Positive delta waves in the inferior leads suggest an anterior location, and negative delta waves suggest a posterior location. The presence of multiple accessory pathways or associated anomalies such as Ebstein anomaly may make the procedure more difficult, but high success rates can still be obtained. Patients with anteroseptal or midseptal accessory pathways should be warned of the slightly increased risk of AV block.

When the ablation catheter is stabilized on the mitral or tricuspid annulus, both atrial and ventricular electrograms are recorded simultaneously on the distal electrode;[102, 103] large atrial and small ventricular potentials are recorded if the catheter is located on the atrial aspect of the AV groove, and large ventricular and small atrial potentials are recorded if the catheter is located on the ventricular aspect of the AV groove. If pre-excitation is present during sinus rhythm or atrial pacing, local ventricular activation at the successful ablation site should precede the onset of the delta wave on the surface electrocardiogram. During ventricular pacing with retrograde conduction via the accessory pathway or during orthodromic AV reciprocating tachycardia, the site of earliest atrial activation along the atrial aspect of the annulus represents a favorable ablation site. Recording of a potential arising from the accessory pathway (Figs. 17–7 to 17–9) identifies a favorable ablation site.[38, 104, 105] Local atrial and ventricular potentials recorded from the successful site are usually close to one another (within 40 msec), but this does not always occur if the accessory pathway has a prolonged conduction time.

Indications

Orthodromic AV reentrant tachycardia is the most common arrhythmia in patients with accessory pathways. The degree of symp-

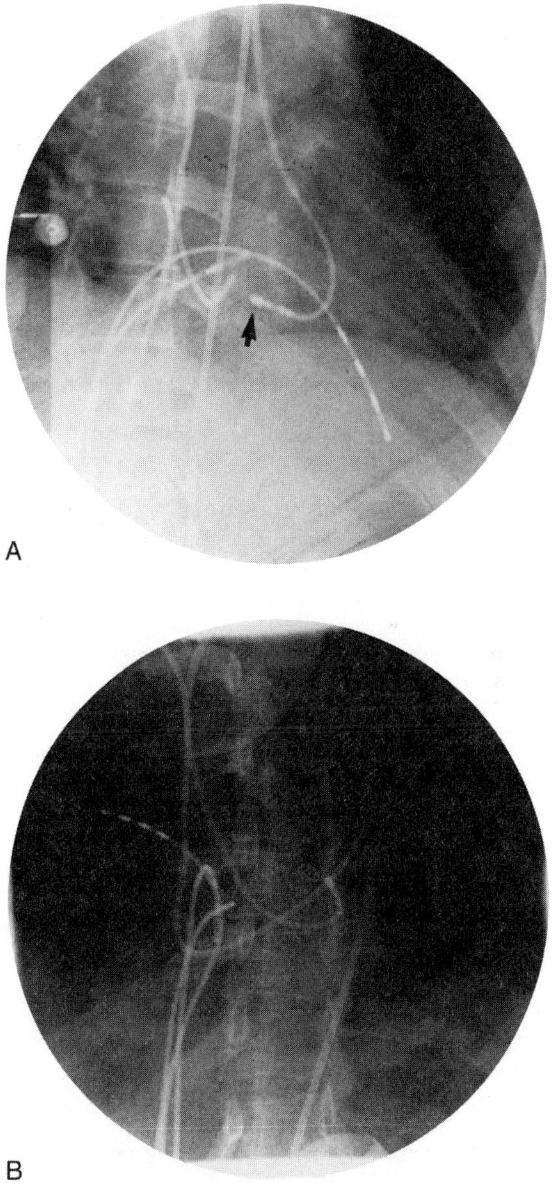

A

B

Figure 17–6. Fluoroscopic appearance of a typical ablation catheter location *(arrow)* for ablation of a left free wall accessory pathway by the retrograde transaortic approach. Both right anterior oblique *(A)* and left anterior oblique *(B)* projections are shown. The ablation catheter enters the left ventricle through the aortic valve and turns back on itself underneath the mitral valve apparatus at the AV groove, using the coronary sinus catheter as a target. High right atrial, His bundle, right ventricular, and coronary sinus catheters are in place. (From Miles WM, Zipes DP, Klein LS: Ablation of free wall accessory pathways. *In* Zipes DP [ed]: Catheter Ablation of Arrhythmias, pp 211–230. Armonk, NY: Futura Publishing, 1994.)

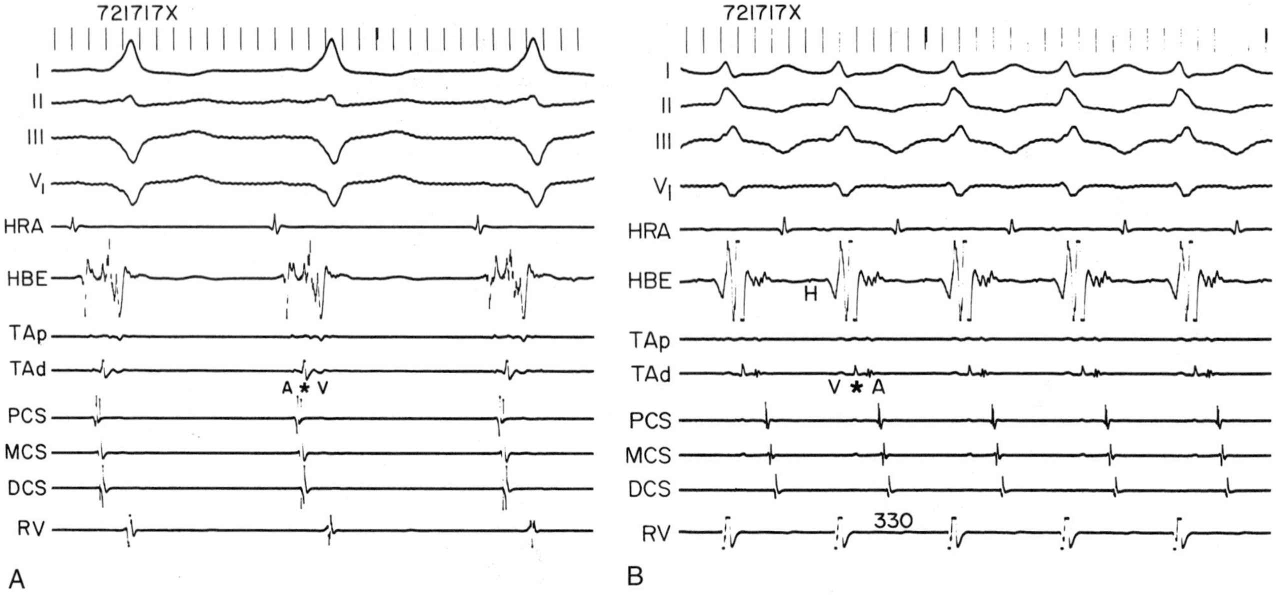

Figure 17–7. Localization of a right posteroseptal accessory pathway before ablation by recording accessory pathway potentials (Figs. 17–7 to 17–9 are from the same patient). TAp and TAd represent proximal and distal electrograms recorded from an ablation catheter positioned along the posteroseptal tricuspid annulus. Surface leads I, II, III, and V_1 are illustrated along with high right atrial (HRA), His bundle (HBE), proximal coronary sinus (PCS), middle coronary sinus (MCS), distal coronary sinus (DCS), and right ventricular (RV) electrograms. *A*, Sinus rhythm with a delta wave consistent with a right posteroseptal accessory pathway. On the distal tricuspid annulus electrodes, an accessory pathway potential (*) is recorded between the atrial potential (A) and the ventricular potential (V). *B*, Orthodromic AV reciprocating tachycardia using the right posteroseptal accessory pathway as the retrograde limb. An accessory pathway potential (*) is now recorded between ventricular activation (V) and atrial activation (A). *Other abbreviation:* H, His bundle activation. (From Miles WM, Klein LS, Rardon DP, et al: Atrioventricular reentry and variants: mechanisms, clinical features and management. *In* Zipes DP, Jalife J [eds]: Cardiac Electrophysiology: From Cell to Bedside, 2nd ed, pp 638–655. Philadelphia: WB Saunders, 1995.)

toms from this arrhythmia varies, but it is often associated with hemodynamic compromise with presyncope and occasionally syncope. In patients with rapid anterograde accessory pathway conduction, atrial fibrillation poses a risk. In patients without underlying structural heart disease, atrial fibrillation frequently arises after the initiation of rapid AV reciprocating tachycardia; therefore, ablation of the accessory pathway that eliminates AV reentrant tachycardia in this group of patients usually eliminates episodes of atrial fibrillation.[106, 107] However, in older patients with underlying structural heart disease, atrial fibrillation without pre-excitation may recur after successful accessory pathway ablation. There is a small risk of sudden cardiac death (approximately 1 sudden death per 1000 patient-years of follow-up) in patients with Wolff-Parkinson-White syndrome, presumably due to atrial fibrillation with rapid ventricular response leading to ventricular fibrillation.[108–110] Most experts currently recommend that patients with delta waves found incidentally on their electrocardiogram but without symptoms of tachyarrhythmias *not* undergo evaluation by electrophysiologic study and not receive therapy, including ablation of the accessory pathway. A possible exception is in patients with potentially hazardous occupations such as airline pilots, in whom the first occurrence of an arrhythmia could result in danger to themselves or others.

In patients with accessory pathways who have symptomatic tachycardia necessitating therapy, radiofrequency ablation of the accessory pathway should be offered as a possible initial therapy. If atrial fibrillation with rapid anterograde accessory pathway conduction is

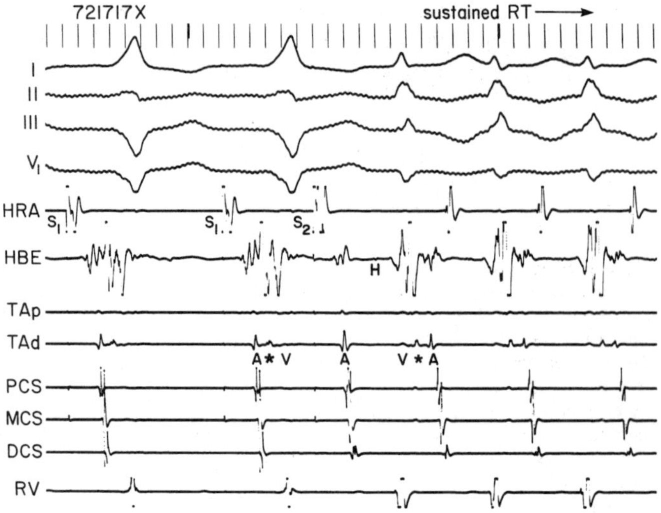

Figure 17–8. Induction of orthodromic AV reciprocating tachycardia (RT) in the same patient as in Figure 17–7. Surface leads I, II, III, and V_1 are illustrated along with high right atrial (HRA), His bundle (HBE), proximal (TAp) and distal (TAd) tricuspid annulus, proximal coronary sinus (PCS), middle coronary sinus (MCS), distal coronary sinus (DCS), and right ventricular (RV) electrograms. During atrial pacing (S_1), the right posteroseptal tricuspid annulus electrodes (TAd) record an accessory pathway potential (*) between atrial activation (A) and ventricular activation (V). After introduction of an atrial extrastimulus (S_2), there is anterograde block in the accessory pathway, and the accessory pathway potential is not recorded after atrial activation. The impulse reaches the ventricle via the normal AV node/His-Purkinje system (H), and AV reciprocating tachycardia is induced. The TAd electrodes now record a reversal of activation with a ventricular electrogram followed by the accessory pathway and then atrial activation. The accessory pathway potential could be dissociated from the atrial potential with atrial pacing techniques, proving that it was not part of the atrial potential. (From Miles WM, Klein LS, Rardon DP, et al: Atrioventricular reentry and variants: mechanisms, clinical features and management. *In* Zipes DP, Jalife J [eds]: Cardiac Electrophysiology: From Cell to Bedside, 2nd ed, pp 638–655. Philadelphia: WB Saunders, 1995.)

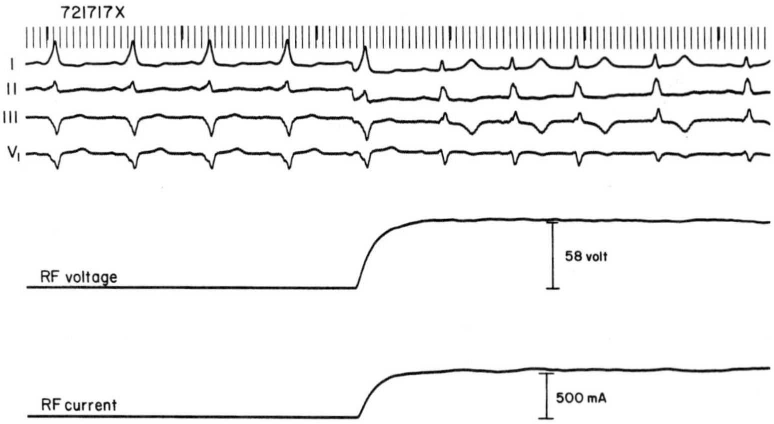

Figure 17–9. Ablation of the accessory pathway illustrated in Figures 17–7 and 17–8. Surface electrocardiographic leads are displayed along with radiofrequency (RF) voltage and current. When radiofrequency energy is delivered through the electrode labeled TAd in the previous figures, the delta wave disappears almost immediately. (From Miles WM, et al: Atrioventricular reentry and variants: mechanisms, clinical features and management. *In* Zipes DP, Jalife J [eds]: Cardiac Electrophysiology: From Cell to Bedside, 2nd ed, pp 638–655. Philadelphia: WB Saunders, 1995.)

not a possibility, other potential first-line therapies include drugs that slow AV nodal conduction, such as beta blockers, verapamil, or diltiazem. Digitalis can be used in patients with concealed accessory pathways, but because it may decrease anterograde refractoriness of accessory pathways, it should not be used in patients with manifest accessory pathways unless the anterograde characteristics of the pathway are known. Type I and type III antiarrhythmic drugs prolong accessory pathway conduction and refractoriness and may protect against a rapid ventricular response in atrial fibrillation, but the risks involved with the use of these drugs[111] must be weighed against the small risk of complications from an ablation procedure. Because any pharmacologic therapy has potential drawbacks of noncompliance, incomplete efficacy, and side effects (including risks to the fetus), patients with moderate to severe symptoms during tachycardia, patients with rapid anterograde accessory pathway conduction, and young patients who will be participating in vigorous activity may benefit from ablation rather than from pharmacologic therapy. Catheter ablation is the therapy of choice for patients who have had rapid AV reciprocating tachycardia or atrial fibrillation leading to cardiac arrest.

On occasion, surgical ablation[112–114] of accessory pathways is warranted. This includes patients with highly symptomatic arrhythmias in whom one or more attempts at catheter ablation have failed, or patients who are undergoing cardiac surgery for another indication (e.g., coronary artery bypass grafting).

Efficacy

Catheter ablation of accessory pathways is successful in 90%–95% of patients;[12, 38, 81–96, 98] the success rate for posteroseptal accessory pathways may be slightly lower. In 5%–10% of patients, accessory pathway conduction can recur, usually within days to weeks of the ablation procedure.[115, 116] The majority (more than 90%) of patients with recurrent pathway conduction can undergo successful reablation at a second procedure. As in patients after AV nodal reentry ablation, follow-up electrophysiologic studies are not necessary in most patients unless recurrent symptoms occur.

Complications

Minor complications occur in approximately 5% of patients, and major complications occur in fewer than 1% of patients. Major complications from ablation of left-sided accessory pathways include cerebral thromboembolism, myocardial infarction from inadvertent catheter manipulation or energy delivery in the coronary arteries, or damage to the aortic valve. There is a small risk of complete AV block from energy delivered in the right anteroseptal, left anteroseptal, or right midseptal regions. Complications common to all pathway locations include cardiac perforation and venous thromboembolism. The risk of venous perforation when energy is delivered into a small vessel such as the middle cardiac vein can be minimized by temperature monitoring and appropriate decrease in power output. Arterial complications such as pseudoaneurysms can occur. Transseptal punctures can be complicated by arterial thromboembolism, air embolism, aortic puncture, or cardiac perforation; these are rare in skilled hands.[87, 88]

Pre-Excitation Variants

Two variants of the pre-excitation syndrome deserve special mention. The first is the so-called Mahaim tachycardia.[117] This is an unusual antidromic AV reentrant tachycardia with anterograde conduction via an atriofascicular fiber (connecting the right atrial free wall near the AV groove to the distal right bundle branch) and retrograde conduction via the His-Purkinje system and AV node.[118–125] Tachycardia has a left bundle branch block QRS morphology. Manifest pre-excitation is usually noted only during rapid atrial pacing or tachycardia. The atriofascicular fibers conduct only anterogradely and have decremental (AV node–like) conduction properties. They are thought possibly to represent a congenital duplication of the AV node/His-Purkinje system. Indications for ablation in these patients are similar to those in patients with more typical AV connections; sudden death is not recognized as a common outcome.

The permanent form of junctional reciprocating tachycardia is an incessant supraventricular tachycardia often presenting in childhood. The tachycardia mechanism is orthodromic AV reciprocating tachycardia; the AV node/His-Purkinje system is used for anterograde conduction, and retrograde conduction is via a slowly conducting accessory pathway with decremental conduction properties, usually located in the posteroseptal region.[126–129] A tachycardia-induced cardiomyopathy may develop from the incessant tachycardia. These tachycardias are often drug refractory or can be exacerbated by drugs that prolong the conduction properties of the circuit. Catheter ablation is highly effective for these tachycardias and is the therapy of choice in most patients.

Atrial Tachycardias

Atrial tachycardias can arise in either the right or the left atrium. Many focal atrial tachycardias arise from the right atrium along the crista terminalis[130] or in the left atrium at the insertion of the pulmonary veins. The right atrium is approached from either the inferior or superior vena cava. The left atrium is usually approached by use of a transseptal puncture or through a patent foramen ovale.

Localization of an ablation site to eliminate the atrial tachycardia differs, depending on the tachycardia mechanisms. Focal atrial tachycardias arise from one relatively small location. The site for ablation is localized by identifying the earliest atrial activation during tachycardia (activation mapping) (Fig. 17–10) or the catheter location

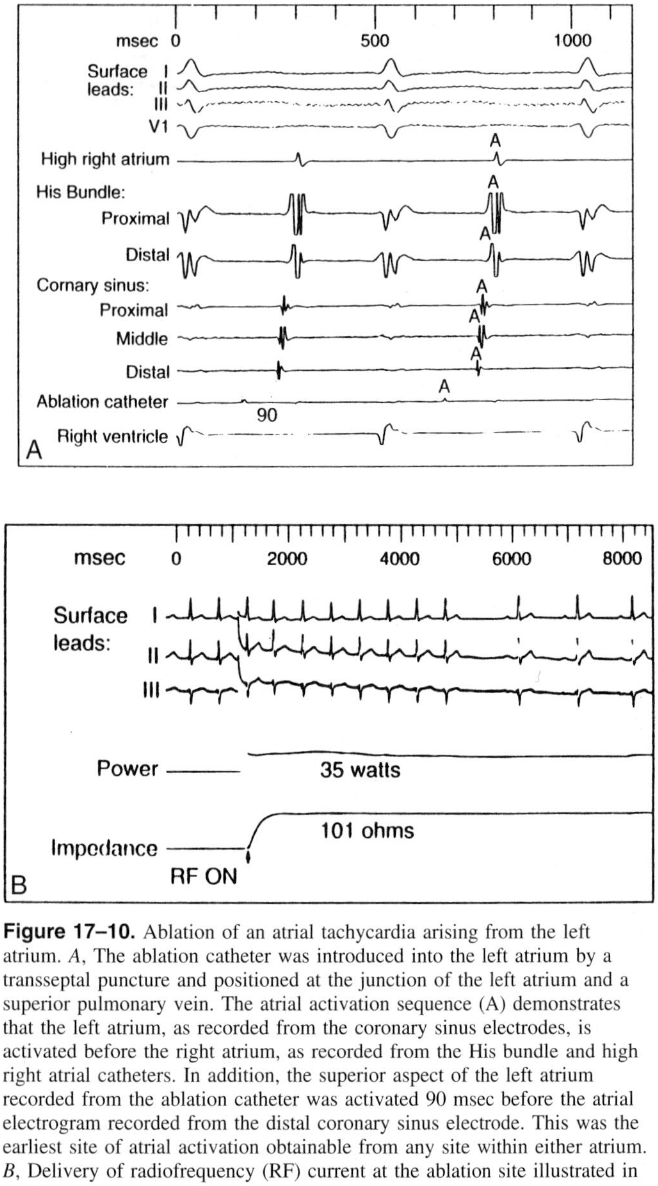

Figure 17–10. Ablation of an atrial tachycardia arising from the left atrium. *A*, The ablation catheter was introduced into the left atrium by a transseptal puncture and positioned at the junction of the left atrium and a superior pulmonary vein. The atrial activation sequence (A) demonstrates that the left atrium, as recorded from the coronary sinus electrodes, is activated before the right atrium, as recorded from the His bundle and high right atrial catheters. In addition, the superior aspect of the left atrium recorded from the ablation catheter was activated 90 msec before the atrial electrogram recorded from the distal coronary sinus electrode. This was the earliest site of atrial activation obtainable from any site within either atrium. *B*, Delivery of radiofrequency (RF) current at the ablation site illustrated in *A*. The patient was in atrial tachycardia at the beginning of radiofrequency energy delivery. The atrial tachycardia suddenly terminated 4 sec after the onset of radiofrequency energy delivery, and sinus rhythm ensued. (From Klein LS, Miles WM: Radiofrequency ablation of cardiac arrhythmias. Scient Am Science Med 1994; 1:48–57.)

where paced P waves or intracardiac activation sequences match those during tachycardia (pace mapping).[131] On the other hand, patients with macroreentrant atrial tachycardias require more sophisticated mapping techniques and are often more difficult to ablate successfully. These include patients who have had previous cardiac surgery for congenital defects (e.g., a Mustard or Fontan procedure), in whom the success rate is reduced because of the difficulty localizing the macroreentrant circuit and because of the markedly dilated atria.[132] It is thought that the macroreentrant circuit encircles the surgical scar. In these patients, a zone of slow conduction can be identified by tachycardia entrainment techniques, or anatomic linear lesions can be created in regions thought to represent a narrow isthmus critical for tachycardia maintenance.

Indications

In contrast with patients with AV nodal reentrant tachycardia and tachycardias in whom accessory pathways are used, catheter ablation is first-line therapy in only selected patients with atrial tachycardias. Some atrial tachycardias (probably those due to abnormal automaticity or triggered activity) are responsive to verapamil or beta blockers.[27, 28] In many patients, drugs with type I or type III actions are necessary. In younger patients or in patients who have failed drug therapy, nonpharmacologic therapy may be considered. Good candidates for catheter ablation include patients who have a single monomorphic P wave morphology during tachycardia and in whom tachycardia is either frequent or readily inducible in the laboratory (using either pacing techniques or isoproterenol infusion). Ablation in patients with multiple atrial tachycardia foci is associated with decreased success rates because of the difficulty in approaching multiple locations and because the existence of multiple atrial tachycardias implies the presence of underlying myocardial disease. The success rate in patients who have episodes of atrial fibrillation as well as atrial tachycardia is also lower; however, if atrial tachycardia is the predominant rhythm, or if atrial tachycardia apparently leads to atrial fibrillation, then ablation of the atrial tachycardia may be a reasonable option.

Efficacy

Success rates for atrial tachycardia ablation depend on the population of patients studied. Patients with frequent uniform single atrial tachycardias tend to be selected; in many studies, patients with significant structural heart disease, congenital defects with surgical correction, or markedly dilated atria have been excluded. Most published studies report an acute success rate approaching 90%.[28, 131, 133–138] Follow-up in most series has been brief, but there appears to be a 10% to 20% recurrence rate. Repeated ablation procedures are often successful. Although successes have been reported in patients with multiple atrial tachycardias and in patients with atrial tachycardias associated with surgically corrected congenital heart lesions, the overall success rate is lower. In these situations, ablation should be reserved for highly symptomatic patients whose conditions are refractory to drug treatment. Long-term effectiveness of surgical treatment of atrial tachycardia has been reported.[139]

Complications

Complications from ablation in patients with atrial tachycardias that can be approached from the right atrium are infrequent, but reported series are small. Although the atria are thin-walled structures, perforation of the atria during radiofrequency energy delivery is rare as long as excessive power is not delivered. If energy must be delivered to the high lateral right atrium near the superior vena caval–right atrial junction, pacing should be performed at high outputs from the catheter before energy delivery to detect proximity of the catheter to the phrenic nerve; damage to the phrenic nerve from radiofrequency energy can cause paralysis of the hemidiaphragm. Ablation of left atrial tachycardia may require transseptal catheterization with its attendant risks.

Sinoatrial Nodal Reentrant Tachycardia

Sinoatrial nodal reentrant tachycardia is an atrial tachycardia in which a portion of the sinus node is included in the tachycardia circuit.[26] These tachycardias are usually relatively slow (110 to 150 per minute), although they can cause symptoms, especially during adrenergic stimulation. In patients in whom digitalis, beta blockers, verapamil, or diltiazem does not eliminate the tachycardia or cause side effects, ablation of the sinus nodal area is a reasonable option to eliminate the tachycardia. Energy is delivered to the site of earliest atrial activation during sinus nodal reentrant tachycardia. The atrial electrogram at the successful site is usually fractionated and precedes the onset of the P wave in the surface electrocardiogram.[140] Reported series are small, and true success rates are unknown. Potential unique complications include damage to the phrenic nerve with hemidiaphragmatic paralysis and excessive damage to the sinus node with resultant slow junctional rhythm requiring pacemaker implantation. However, the sinus node is a large structure, and discrete radiofrequency burns usually do not interfere with its pacemaker function.

Inappropriate Sinus Tachycardia

In the syndrome of inappropriate sinus tachycardia, patients have a persistent sinus tachycardia inappropriate for the metabolic needs of the body.[141] It is associated with palpitations that can be highly symptomatic in some patients. The initial therapy for this entity is beta blockade, although beta blockers are either ineffective or not tolerated in many patients. Other causes of sinus tachycardia (such as hyperthyroidism, pheochromocytoma, occult infection, anemia) should be excluded. In rare patients with highly symptomatic inappropriate sinus tachycardia, destruction of the sinus nodal region with catheter ablation may relieve symptoms. The pacemaker focus shifts from the high right atrium to the lower right atrium when success is achieved, and the maximal heart rate obtainable during sympathetic stimulation decreases (Fig. 17–11). Series are small, but improvement in symptoms has been reported. A pacemaker can be required acutely or late after the procedure if subsidiary atrial pacemaker rates are inadequate.

Atrial Flutter

Techniques

Atrial flutter represents a macroreentrant intra-atrial arrhythmia (Fig. 17–12). The typical variety uses the atrial septum for low to high conduction and the right atrial free wall for high to low conduction.[29, 30] A narrow region of slow conduction bounded by the inferior vena cava, tricuspid annulus, and coronary sinus appears to be critical for tachycardia maintenance. Catheter ablation for typical atrial flutter is effected by creating linear lesions between the tricuspid annulus and the inferior vena cava, between the tricuspid annulus and the coronary sinus, and between the coronary sinus and the inferior vena cava. Success rates appear to be better with this anatomic-based procedure than with electrical mapping techniques such as entrainment or activation mapping.[142–144] Atrial flutter in which a circuit reversed from that described before is used can also be amenable to these techniques. Other atypical flutters are difficult to ablate adequately.

Atrial flutter can be approached surgically by producing lesions similar to those described for catheter ablation. However, indications for a surgical approach are rare.

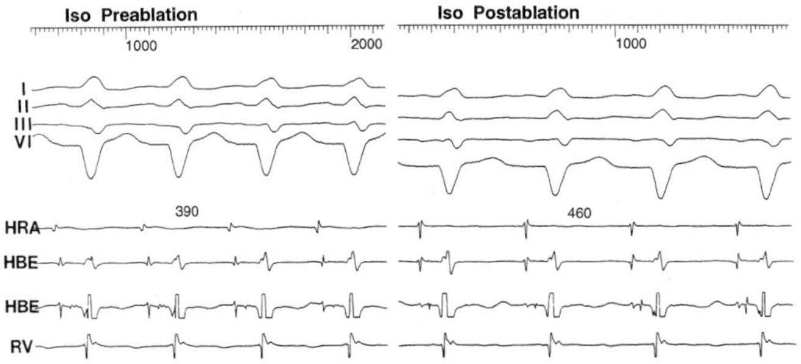

Figure 17–11. Catheter ablation of the sinus nodal region in a patient with inappropriate sinus tachycardia. Surface leads I, II, III, and V_1 are illustrated along with high right atrial (HRA), proximal (upper) and distal (lower) His bundle (HBE), and right ventricular (RV) electrograms. The patient had a pre-existing fixed left bundle branch block. Isoproterenol was infused at the same dose throughout the procedure. *Left panel*, Preablation, the atrial cycle length during isoproterenol infusion was 390 msec. The P waves were positive in leads II and III, and the right atrial activation was high to low; that is, the atrial electrogram recorded from the high right atrium preceded that from the low right atrium as recorded from the His bundle electrogram. *Right panel*, During continued isoproterenol infusion after ablation of the sinus nodal regions, the sinus cycle length was 460 msec. The P waves were flat in lead II and negative in lead III, and there was simultaneous atrial activation recorded from the high right atrial and His bundle catheters; therefore, the intrinsic cardiac pacemaker has shifted from the sinus nodal to a low atrial origin region. This patient has experienced relief from symptoms of inappropriate tachycardia in a 6-month follow-up period.

Indications

Favorable candidates for ablation of atrial flutter are patients with typical atrial flutter and no associated atrial fibrillation. In these patients, ablation may be offered as a potential first-line therapy, although drug therapy to maintain sinus rhythm is also a first-line option according to the patient's preferences. Ablation can also be first-line therapy in patients with the reversed circuit variant of atrial flutter described before. Patients with predominantly typical atrial flutter but occasional episodes of atrial fibrillation may benefit from an atrial flutter ablation to diminish the total amount of arrhythmia; the possibility that ablation of atrial flutter can also eliminate associated atrial fibrillation is speculative. In patients with large left atria, marked structural cardiac disease, atypical atrial flutters, or associated atrial fibrillation, ablation should not be considered primary therapy.

Efficacy

As with atrial tachycardias, the success rate of atrial flutter ablation depends on the patients selected. In patients with typical atrial flutter or reversed circuit atrial flutter, the acute success rate is approximately 90% in most series using the anatomic procedure described.[142–144] However, the recurrence rate is approximately 20%. In patients with recurrent atrial flutter after ablation, a repeated ablation procedure is commonly successful. In distinction to AV nodal reentry and AV reentry, a progressive frequency of arrhythmia recurrence over time may not be unexpected because of the common presence of underlying structural heart disease.

Complications

Complications from atrial flutter ablation are infrequent. The chances of cardiac perforation or AV block are low when energy is delivered to the posterior aspects of Koch's triangle. Because several linear ablation lesions are required, there is a small risk of atrial thrombus formation.

Atrial Fibrillation

Procedures for Control of Ventricular Response During Atrial Fibrillation

AV Junctional Ablation. Catheter ablation techniques can be used to either totally ablate or modify AV conduction, blunting the rapid ventricular response to atrial fibrillation.[35, 36, 145–151] Ablation is not employed as initial therapy for ventricular rate control but can be useful in patients in whom drug therapy to control the ventricular response has been ineffective or not tolerated, and in whom atrial fibrillation cannot be prevented by drug therapy.[152] When complete junctional ablation is employed, implantation of a permanent pacemaker is required. In patients with chronic atrial fibrillation, this pacemaker should be a VVIR model; that is, it paces only the ventricle but can increase its rate when metabolic demand is increased. In patients with intermittent atrial fibrillation, a dual-cham-

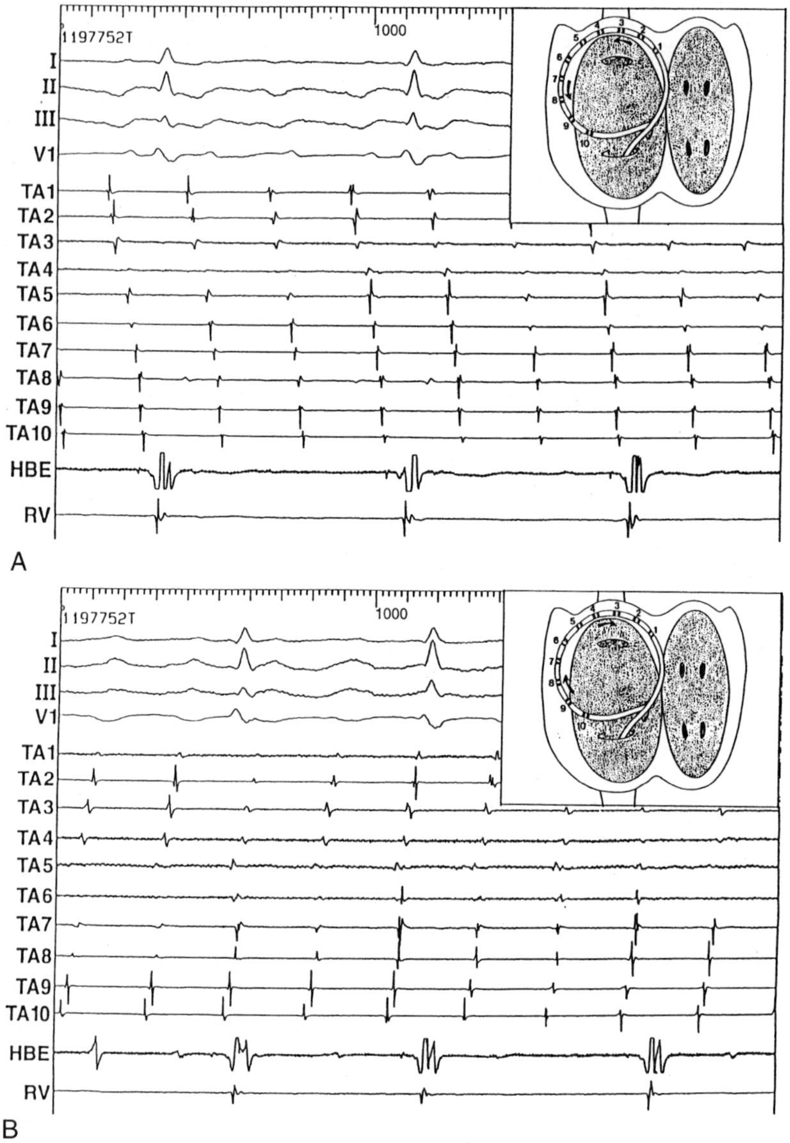

Figure 17–12. Mapping of typical (counterclockwise) and reverse-circuit (clockwise) atrial flutter in the same patient. Surface electrocardiograms I, II, III, and V_1 are illustrated along with His bundle (HBE), right ventricle (RV), and 10 electrograms (TA1–TA10) recorded from a "halo" catheter positioned in the right atrium as illustrated in the schematic at the upper right of each panel. *A*, The patient has typical atrial flutter as illustrated by the negative flutter waves in leads II and III. Atrial mapping revealed earliest activation in electrode pair TA1 and latest in TA10, demonstrating that atrial activation was low to high along the septum and high to low along the right atrial free wall (i.e., counterclockwise rotation of the flutter circuit). *B*, Subsequently in the study, atrial flutter having positive flutter waves in leads II and III was induced. Intracardiac mapping revealed that earliest atrial activation was recorded in TA10 and traveled around the atrium to TA1 in a clockwise fashion. This represents the same tachycardia circuit as in *A* but with reversal of direction as illustrated by the arrows. Both atrial flutters were eliminated with linear radiofrequency lesions created from the tricuspid annulus to the inferior vena cava.

ber pacemaker with "mode switching" should be employed; that is, the pacemaker employs the DDDR mode when the patient is in sinus rhythm but switches automatically to the VVIR mode when atrial tachyarrhythmias are sensed.

Advantages of complete AV junctional ablation with pacemaker implantation in patients with atrial fibrillation who are drug refractory or drug intolerant include (Table 17–2) (1) avoidance of excessively rapid rates during atrial fibrillation, (2) regularization of the ventricular rate (in some patients, symptoms can be caused by the irregularity of the ventricular rate), and (3) avoidance of side effects from pharmacologic agents. The physiologic increase in ventricular rate during exercise can be preserved by implanting a rate-adaptive pacemaker. The major disadvantage of the procedure is that the atria may continue to fibrillate; therefore, there is loss of sinus control of the ventricular rate, loss of AV synchrony, and continued risk of arterial thromboembolism requiring anticoagulation.

The AV junction can be ablated in most patients by delivering energy to the anterosuperior aspect of the tricuspid annulus near the septal leaflet where low atrial, His bundle, and ventricular potentials are recorded. In unusual cases, ablation of the AV junction requires delivering energy to the left septum.[153] The most common complications from the procedure are those incurred by permanent pacing, including pacemaker infection and lead dislodgment. Most patients have reasonable junctional escape intervals (rates of 40 to 50 per minute), and therefore sudden pacemaker failure is unlikely to cause death.

In series using both direct-current shock and radiofrequency energy to ablate the AV junction, investigators have reported an approximately 2% per year incidence of sudden death on follow-up.[150, 154, 155] One possible explanation is that this population of patients has significant pre-existing structural heart disease, and the sudden death is not related to the ablation procedure. However, there is anecdotal evidence that polymorphic ventricular tachyarrhythmias can occur in patients who had rapid ventricular rates before ablation and who were paced at relatively slow rates after ablation, possibly related to QT prolongation exacerbated by electrolyte abnormalities. Therefore, many investigators recommend pacing patients at a relatively rapid rate (greater than 80 per minute) for the first few weeks after ablation.

AV Junctional Modification. Techniques for modifying AV nodal conduction rather than total ablation have been developed, obviating the need in selected patients for implantation of a pacemaker.[156–159] This technique is based on the theory that the "slow" posterior

TABLE 17–2. NONPHARMACOLOGIC THERAPY FOR ATRIAL FIBRILLATION

	Likelihood of Long-Term Efficacy	Prevention of Rapid Ventricular Rate	Sinus Control of Rate	Atrioventricular Synchrony	Atrial Transport	Regularization of Rate	↓ Rate of Thromboembolism	Major Drawbacks
Drugs	±	+	+	+	+	+	+	Incomplete efficacy; side effects
Atrioventricular junctional ablation (modification)	+(±)	+	0	0	−	+(0)	0	Pacemaker complications
Surgical maze (catheter maze)	+(?)	+	+	+	+	+	+	Major surgery; catheter techniques investigational
Atrial defibrillator	±	+	+	+	+	+	+	Discomfort from shocks; risk of ventricular fibrillation induction

inputs to the AV node usually have shorter refractory periods than the more anterior "fast" AV nodal inputs (even in patients without AV nodal reentry). Therefore, if the posterior inputs of the AV node were ablated, the overall AV nodal refractoriness would increase, and therefore the ventricular response to atrial fibrillation would decrease. This technique has the advantage of avoiding implantation of a pacemaker with its resultant complications. Disadvantages include unknown long-term efficacy and the fact that only approximately 75% of patients can be adequately treated with this technique (the remainder require total AV junctional ablation). In addition, the atria continue to fibrillate, and the resultant ventricular rate is still not regular. It may be reasonable initially to attempt AV nodal modification in patients referred for AV junctional ablation and, if that is not successful, then perform complete AV junctional ablation; a second procedure may be required if the decrease in the ventricular response from AV nodal modification is not maintained on follow-up.

AV junctional ablation and modification should be carried out in patients in whom the rapid ventricular response is thought to be responsible for symptoms. Symptoms related to loss of AV synchrony or sinus control of the heart rate will not be improved by these techniques.

Techniques for Elimination of Atrial Fibrillation

Surgical[160–163] and, more recently, catheter ablation data[34] have demonstrated that atrial fibrillation can be eliminated by producing multiple atrial incisions or linear ablation lesions. Catheter ablation procedures for elimination of atrial fibrillation are in early stages of development, although clinical data have been reported.[164–166]

The most successful surgical technique for elimination of atrial fibrillation is the maze procedure.[160, 161, 163] It can be performed in patients with either paroxysmal or chronic atrial fibrillation. Theoretic advantages of the maze procedure over AV junctional ablation or modification procedures include preservation of sinus control of the ventricular rate, maintenance of AV synchrony, prevention of thromboembolism, and preservation of atrial transport function. The major disadvantage is that it is a major surgical procedure with sternotomy. Postoperatively, approximately 40% of patients still require permanent pacing because of atrial chronotropic incompetence due to underlying sick sinus syndrome possibly exacerbated by the operation. In skilled hands, the success rate of surgery alone is 90%; another 9% of patients have recurrent atrial flutter amenable to drug therapy or possibly catheter ablation.

Dual-Chamber Pacing for Prevention of Atrial Fibrillation

Small nonrandomized studies suggest that paroxysmal atrial fibrillation can be prevented in some patients by preventing bradycardia with dual-chamber pacing, or by employing dual-chamber rather than ventricular demand pacing in patients requiring pacemakers. Presumably, the mechanism is by improving hemodynamics, lessening atrial stretch, and/or preventing atrial ectopy during bradycardia. Until further data are available, prevention of paroxysms of atrial fibrillation is not sufficient in itself to justify pacemaker implantation.

Implantable Atrial Defibrillator

Clinical trials are currently under way to validate the feasibility, safety, and efficacy of an implantable atrial defibrillator.[167–171] Potential candidates for such a device would be patients with intermittent atrial fibrillation. There is a theoretic possibility that avoidance of prolonged episodes of atrial fibrillation can prevent the eventual development of chronic atrial fibrillation. In addition, the patient would be spared the risk of thromboembolism and anticoagulation as well as potential risks and side effects of antiarrhythmic drugs used to prevent atrial fibrillation or to slow the ventricular response during atrial fibrillation.

Potential limitations of this technology include the discomfort from the shock delivered to terminate atrial fibrillation in the awake patient. Preliminary research with catheter-based systems involving the use of biphasic waveforms shows that shocks of less than 2 joules can often defibrillate the atria, although these shocks may not be universally tolerated by patients. A second major limitation of the technology is that an atrial shock that is mistimed, is delivered by a lead that has migrated to the ventricle, or occurs during the ventricular vulnerable period after a short preceding RR interval may precipitate ventricular fibrillation. Preliminary data show that this is likely to be a rare event.

Acknowledgment

The authors appreciate the expert secretarial assistance of Sue Mills.

REFERENCES

1. Ganz LI, Friedman PL: Supraventricular tachycardia. N Engl J Med 1995; 332:162–173.
2. Miller JM, Rosenthal ME, Vassallo JA, et al: Atrioventricular nodal reentrant tachycardia: studies on upper and lower "common pathways." Circulation 1987; 75:930–940.
3. Ross DL, Johnson DC, Denniss AR, et al: Curative surgery for atrioventricular junctional ("AV nodal") reentrant tachycardia. J Am Coll Cardiol 1985; 6:1383–1392.
4. Cox JL, Holman WL, Gain ME: Cryosurgical treatment of atrioventricular node reentrant tachycardia. Circulation 1987; 76:1329–1336.

5. Holman WL, Hackel DB, Lease JG, et al: Cryosurgical ablation of atrioventricular nodal reentry: histologic localization of the proximal common pathway. Circulation 1988; 77:1356–1362.
6. Keim S, Werner P, Jazayeri M, et al: Localization of the fast and slow pathways in atrioventricular nodal reentrant tachycardia by intraoperative ice mapping. Circulation 1992; 86:919–925.
7. McGuire MA, Roboton M, Yip ASB, et al: Electrophysiologic and histologic effects of dissection of the connection between the atrium and posterior part of the atrioventricular node. J Am Coll Cardiol 1994; 23:693–701.
8. McGuire MA, Yip ASB, Robotin M, et al: Surgical procedure for the cure of atrioventricular junctional ("AV node") reentrant tachycardia: anatomic and electrophysiologic effects of dissection of the anterior atrionodal connections in a canine model. J Am Coll Cardiol 1994; 24:784–794.
9. Haissaguerre M, Warin JF, Lemetayer P, et al: Closed-chest ablation of retrograde conduction in patients with atrioventricular nodal reentrant tachycardia. N Engl J Med 1989; 320:426–433.
10. Epstein LM, Scheinman MM, Langberg JJ, et al: Percutaneous catheter modification of the atrioventricular node. A potential cure for atrioventricular nodal reentrant tachycardia. Circulation 1989; 80:757–768.
11. Jackman WM, Beckman KJ, McClelland JH, et al: Treatment of supraventricular tachycardia due to atrioventricular nodal reentry by radiofrequency catheter ablation of slow-pathway conduction. N Engl J Med 1992; 327:313–318.
12. Calkins H, Sousa J, El-Atassi, et al: Diagnosis and cure of the Wolff-Parkinson-White syndrome or paroxysmal supraventricular tachycardias during a single electrophysiologic test. N Engl J Med 1991; 324:1612–1618.
13. Akhtar M, Jazayeri MR, Sra J, et al: Atrioventricular nodal reentry. Clinical, electrophysiological, and therapeutic considerations. Circulation 1993; 88:282–295.
14. Janse MJ, Anderson RH, McGuire MA, et al: "AV nodal" reentry: Part I: "AV nodal" reentry revisited. J Cardiovasc Electrophysiol 1993; 4:561–572.
15. McGuire MA, Janse MJ, Ross DL: "AV nodal" reentry: Part II: AV nodal, AV junctional, or atrionodal reentry? J Cardiovasc Electrophysiol 1993; 4:573–586.
16. Miles WM, Hubbard JE, Zipes DP, et al: Elimination of AV nodal reentrant tachycardia with 2:1 VA block by posteroseptal ablation. J Cardiovasc Electrophysiol 1994; 5:510–516.
17. Ho SY, McComb JM, Scott CD, et al: Morphology of the cardiac conduction system in patients with electrophysiologically proven dual atrioventricular nodal pathways. J Cardiovasc Electrophysiol 1993; 4:504–512.
18. Racker DK: Transmission and reentrant activity in the sinoventricular conducting system and in the circumferential lamina of the tricuspid valve. J Cardiovasc Electrophysiol 1993; 4:513–525.
19. Ward DE, Garratt CJ: The substrate for atrioventricular "nodal" reentrant tachycardia: is there a "third pathway"? J Cardiovasc Electrophysiol 1993; 4:62–67.
20. Gallagher JJ, Pritchett ELC, Sealy WC, et al: The preexcitation syndromes. Prog Cardiovasc Dis 1978; 20:285–327.
21. Hammill SC, Pritchett ELC, Klein GJ, et al: Accessory atrioventricular pathways that conduct only in the antegrade direction. Circulation 1980; 62:1335–1340.
22. Miles WM, Klein LS, Rardon DP, et al: Atrioventricular reentry and variants: mechanisms, clinical features and management. *In* Zipes DP, Jalife J (eds): Cardiac Electrophysiology: From Cell to Bedside, 2nd ed, pp 638–655. Philadelphia: WB Saunders, 1995.
23. Bardy GH, Packer DL, German LD, et al: Preexcited reciprocating tachycardia in patients with Wolff-Parkinson-White syndrome: incidence and mechanisms. Circulation 1984; 70:377–391.
24. Packer DL, Gallagher JJ, Prystowsky EN: Physiological substrate for antidromic reciprocating tachycardia. Prerequisite characteristics of the accessory pathway and atrioventricular conduction system. Circulation 1992; 85:574–588.
25. Lehmann MH, Tchou P, Mahmud R, et al: Electrophysiological determinants of antidromic reentry induced during atrial extrastimulation. Insights from a pacing model of Wolff-Parkinson-White syndrome. Circ Res 1989; 65:295–306.
26. Gomes JA, Hariman RJ, Kang PS, et al: Sustained symptomatic sinus node reentrant tachycardia: incidence, clinical significance, electrophysiologic observations and the effects of antiarrhythmic agents. J Am Coll Cardiol 1985; 5:45–57.
27. Engelstein ED, Lippman N, Stein KM, et al: Mechanism-specific effects of adenosine on atrial tachycardia. Circulation 1994; 89:2645–2654.
28. Chen SA, Chiang CE, Yang CJ, et al: Sustained atrial tachycardia in adult patients. Electrophysiological characteristics, pharmacological response, possible mechanisms, and effects of radiofrequency ablation. Circulation 1994; 90:1262–1278.
29. Olshansky B, Okumura K, Hess PG, et al: Demonstration of an area of slow conduction in human atrial flutter. J Am Coll Cardiol 1990; 16:1639–1648.
30. Isber N, Restivo M, Gough WB, et al: Circus movement atrial flutter in the canine sterile pericarditis model. Cryothermal termination from the epicardial site of the slow zone of the reentrant circuit. Circulation 1993; 87:1649–1660.
31. Allessie MA: Reentrant mechanisms underlying atrial fibrillation. *In* Zipes DP, Jalife J (eds): Cardiac Electrophysiology: From Cell to Bedside, 2nd ed, pp 562–566. Philadelphia: WB Saunders, 1995.
32. Cox JL, Canavan TE, Schuessler RB, et al: The surgical treatment of atrial fibrillation. II. Intraoperative electrophysiologic mapping and description of the electrophysiologic basis of atrial flutter and fibrillation. J Thorac Cardiovasc Surg 1991; 101:406–426.
33. Cox JL, Schuessler RD, D'Agostino HJ, et al: The surgical treatment of atrial fibrillation. III. Development of a definitive surgical procedure. J Thorac Cardiovasc Surg 1991; 101:569–583.
34. Elvan A, Pride HR, Eble JN, et al: Radiofrequency catheter ablation of the atria reduces the inducibility and duration of atrial fibrillation in dogs. Circulation 1995; 91:2235–2244.
35. Gallagher JJ, Svenson RH, Kasell JH, et al: Catheter technique for closed-chest ablation of the atrioventricular conduction system. N Engl J Med 1982; 306:194–200.
36. Scheinman MM, Morady F, Hess DS, et al: Catheter-induced ablation of the atrioventricular function to control refractory supraventricular arrhythmia. JAMA 1982; 248:851–855.
37. Bardy GH, Ivey TD, Coltorti F, et al: Developments, complications and limitations of catheter-mediated electrical ablation of posterior accessory atrioventricular pathways. Am J Cardiol 1988; 61:309–316.
38. Jackman WM, Wang X, Friday KJ, et al: Catheter ablation of accessory atrioventricular pathways (Wolff-Parkinson-White syndrome) by radiofrequency current. N Engl J Med 1991; 324:1605–1611.
39. Kalbfleisch SJ, Langberg JJ: Catheter ablation with radiofrequency energy: biophysical aspects and clinical applications. J Cardiovasc Electrophysiol 1992; 3:173–186.
40. Avitall B, Khan M, Krum D, et al: Physics and engineering of transcatheter cardiac tissue ablation. J Am Coll Cardiol 1993; 22:921–932.
41. Nath S, DiMarco JP, Haines DE: Basic aspects of radiofrequency catheter ablation. J Cardiovasc Electrophysiol 1994; 5:863–876.
42. Haverkamp W, Hindricks G, Gulker H, et al: Coagulation of ventricular myocardium using radiofrequency alternating current: Bio-physical aspects and experimental findings. PACE 1989; 12:187–195.
43. Haines DE, Watson DD: Tissue heating during radiofrequency catheter ablation: a thermodynamic model and observations in isolated perfused and superfused canine right ventricular free wall. PACE 1989; 12:962–976.
44. Haines DE, Verow AF: Observations on electrode-tissue interface temperature and effect on electrical impedance during radiofrequency ablation of ventricular myocardium. Circulation 1990; 82:1034–1038.
45. Wittkampf FHM: Temperature response in radiofrequency catheter ablation. Circulation 1992; 86:1648–1650.
46. Langberg JJ, Calkins H, El-Atassi R, et al: Temperature monitoring during radiofrequency catheter ablation of accessory pathways. Circulation 1992; 86:1469–1474.
47. Calkins H, Prystowsky E, Carlson M, et al: Temperature monitoring during radiofrequency catheter ablation procedures using closed loop control. Circulation 1994; 90:1279–1286.
48. Harvey M, Kim YN, Sousa J, et al: Impedance monitoring during radiofrequency catheter ablation in humans. PACE 1992; 15:22–27.
49. Chu E, Kalman JM, Kwasman MA, et al: Intracardiac echocardiography during radiofrequency catheter ablation of cardiac arrhythmias in humans. J Am Coll Cardiol 1994; 24:1351–1357.
50. Langberg JJ, Gallagher M, Strickberger SA, et al: Temperature-guided radiofrequency catheter ablation with very large distal electrodes. Circulation 1993; 88:245–249.
51. Nakagawa H, Yamanashi WS, Pitha JV, et al: Comparison of in vivo tissue temperature profile and lesion geometry for radiofrequency ablation with a saline-irrigated electrode versus temperature control in a canine thigh muscle preparation. Circulation 1995; 91:2264–2273.

52. Jenkins KJ, Walsh EP, Colan SD, et al: Multipolar endocardial mapping of the right atrium during cardiac catheterization: description of a new technique. J Am Coll Cardiol 1993; 22:1105–1110.
53. Epstein LM, Chiesa N, Wong MN, et al: Radiofrequency catheter ablation in the treatment of supraventricular tachycardia in the elderly. J Am Coll Cardiol 1994; 23:1356–1362.
54. Mitrani R, Klein L, Rardon D, et al: Major complications during radiofrequency ablation occur more frequently in elderly patients [Abstract]. PACE 1994; 17:418.
55. Dick M, O'Connor BK, Serwer GA, et al: Use of radiofrequency current to ablate accessory pathway connections in children. Circulation 1991; 84:2318–2324.
56. Van Hare GF, Witherell CL, Lesh MD: Follow-up of radiofrequency catheter ablation in children: results in 100 consecutive patients. J Am Coll Cardiol 1994; 23:1651–1659.
57. Saul JP, Hulse JE, De W, et al: Catheter manipulation for ablation of accessory atrioventricular pathways in young patients: use of long vascular sheath, the transseptal approach and a retrograde left posterior parallel approach. J Am Coll Cardiol 1993; 21:571–583.
58. Saul JP, Hulse JE, Papagiannis J, et al: Late enlargement of radiofrequency lesions in infant lambs. Implications for ablation procedures in small children. Circulation 1994; 90:492–499.
59. Kugler JD: Radiofrequency catheter ablation for supraventricular tachycardia. Should it be used in infants and small children? Circulation 1994; 90:639–641.
60. Calkins H, Niklason L, Sousa J, et al: Radiation exposure during radiofrequency catheter ablation of accessory atrioventricular connections. Circulation 1991; 84:2376–2382.
61. Lindsay BD, Eichling JO, Ambos HD, et al: Radiation exposure to patients and medical personnel during radiofrequency catheter ablation for supraventricular tachycardia. Am J Cardiol 1992; 70:218–233.
62. den Dulk K, Brugada P, Smeets JLRM, et al: Pacing for supraventricular tachycardias. *In* Zipes DP, Jalife J (eds): Cardiac Electrophysiology: From Cell to Bedside, pp 934–942. Philadelphia: WB Saunders, 1990.
63. Langberg JJ, Harvey M, Calkins H, et al: Titration of power output during radiofrequency catheter ablation of atrioventricular nodal reentrant tachycardia. J Am Coll Cardiol 1994; 23:716–723.
64. Kay GN, Epstein AE, Dailey SM, et al: Selective radiofrequency ablation of the slow pathway for the treatment of atrioventricular nodal reentrant tachycardia: evidence for involvement of perinodal myocardium within the reentrant circuit. Circulation 1992; 85:1675–1688.
65. Jazayeri MR, Hempe SL, Sra JS, et al: Selective transcatheter ablation of the fast and slow pathways using radiofrequency energy in patients with atrioventricular nodal reentrant tachycardia. Circulation 1992; 85:1318–1328.
66. Mitrani RD, Klein LS, Hackett FK, et al: Radiofrequency ablation for atrioventricular node reentrant tachycardia: comparison between fast (anterior) and slow (posterior) pathway ablation. J Am Coll Cardiol 1993; 21:432–441.
67. Wu D, Yeh SJ, Wang CC, et al: A simple technique for selective radiofrequency ablation of the slow pathway in atrioventricular node reentrant tachycardia. J Am Coll Cardiol 1993; 21:1612–1621.
68. Langberg JJ, Leon A, Borganelli M, et al: A randomized, prospective comparison of anterior and posterior approaches to radiofrequency catheter ablation of atrioventricular nodal reentry tachycardia. Circulation 1993; 87:1551–1556.
69. Moulton K, Miller B, Scott J, et al: Radiofrequency catheter ablation for AV nodal reentry: a technique for rapid transection of the slow AV nodal pathway. PACE 1993; 16:760–768.
70. Kalbfleisch SJ, Strickberger SA, Williamson B, et al: Randomized comparison of anatomic and electrogram mapping approaches to ablation of the slow pathway of atrioventricular node reentrant tachycardia. J Am Coll Cardiol 1994; 23:716–723.
71. Haissaguerre M, Gaita F, Fischer B, et al: Elimination of atrioventricular nodal reentrant tachycardia using discrete slow potentials to guide application of radiofrequency energy. Circulation 1992; 85:2162–2175.
72. de Bakker JMT, Coronel R, McGuire MA, et al: Slow potentials in the atrioventricular junctional area of patients operated on for atrioventricular node tachycardias and in isolated porcine hearts. J Am Coll Cardiol 1994; 23:709–715.
73. McGuire MA, de Bakker JMT, Vermeulen JT, et al: Origin and significance of double potentials near the atrioventricular node. Correlation of extracellular potentials, intracellular potentials, and histology. Circulation 1994; 89:2351–2360.
74. Jentzer JH, Goyal R, Williamson BD, et al: Analysis of junctional ectopy during radiofrequency ablation of the slow pathway in patients with atrioventricular nodal reentrant tachycardia. Circulation 1994; 90:2820–2826.
75. Lindsay BD, Chung MK, Gamache C, et al: Therapeutic end points for the treatment of atrioventricular node reentrant tachycardia by catheter-guided radiofrequency current. J Am Coll Cardiol 1993; 22:733–740.
76. Li HG, Klein GJ, Stites HW, et al: Elimination of slow pathway conduction: an accurate indicator of clinical success after radiofrequency atrioventricular node modification. J Am Coll Cardiol 1993; 22:1849–1853.
77. Manolis AS, Wang PJ, Estes NAM: Radiofrequency ablation of slow pathway in patients with atrioventricular nodal reentrant tachycardia. Do arrhythmia recurrences correlate with persistent slow pathway conduction or site of successful ablation? Circulation 1994; 90:2815–2819.
78. Strickberger SA, Kalbfleisch SJ, Williamson B, et al: Radiofrequency catheter ablation of atypical atrioventricular nodal reentrant tachycardia. J Cardiovasc Electrophysiol 1993; 22:526–532.
79. Sra JS, Jazayeri MR, Blanck Z, et al: Slow pathway ablation in patients with atrioventricular node reentrant tachycardia and a prolonged PR interval. J Am Coll Cardiol 1994; 24:1064–1068.
80. Rigden LB, Klein LS, Mitrani RD, et al: Increased risk of heart block following slow pathway ablation for AV nodal reentrant tachycardia in patients with marked PR interval prolongation during sinus rhythm [Abstract]. PACE 1995; 18:918.
81. Kocovic DZ, Harada T, Shea JB, et al: Alterations of heart rate and of heart rate variability after radiofrequency catheter ablation of supraventricular tachycardia. Delineation of parasympathetic pathways in the human heart. Circulation 1993; 88(pt 1):1671–1681.
82. Lesh MD, VanHare GF, Schamp DJ, et al: Curative percutaneous catheter ablation using radiofrequency energy for accessory pathways in all locations: results in 100 consecutive patients. J Am Coll Cardiol 1992; 19:1303–1309.
83. Kay GN, Epstein AE, Dailey SM, et al: Role of radiofrequency ablation in the management of supraventricular arrhythmias. Experience in 760 consecutive patients. J Cardiovasc Electrophysiol 1993; 4:371–389.
84. Kuck KH, Schlüter M: Single-catheter approach to radiofrequency current ablation of left-sided accessory pathways in patients with Wolff-Parkinson-White syndrome. Circulation 1991; 84:2366–2375.
85. Calkins H, Langberg J, Sousa J, et al: Radiofrequency catheter ablation of accessory atrioventricular connections in 250 patients. Circulation 1992; 85:1337–1346.
86. Jackman WM, Kuck KH, Naccarelli GV, et al: Radiofrequency current directed across the mitral anulus with a bipolar epicardial-endocardial catheter electrode configuration in dogs. Circulation 1988; 78:1288–1298.
87. Swartz JF, Tracy CM, Fletcher RD: Radiofrequency endocardial catheter ablation of accessory atrioventricular pathway atrial insertion sites. Circulation 1993; 87:487–499.
88. Lesh MD, Van Hare GF, Scheinman MM, et al: Comparison of the retrograde and transseptal methods for ablation of left free wall accessory pathways. J Am Coll Cardiol 1993; 22:542–549.
89. Cappato R, Schlüter M, Mont L, et al: Anatomic, electrical, and mechanical factors affecting bipolar endocardial electrograms. Impact on catheter ablation of manifest left free-wall accessory pathways. Circulation 1994; 90:884–894.
90. Langberg J, Griffin JC, Herre JM, et al: Catheter ablation of accessory pathways using radiofrequency energy in the canine coronary sinus. J Am Coll Cardiol 1989; 13:491–496.
91. Dhala AA, Deshpande SS, Bremmer S, et al: Transcatheter ablation of posteroseptal accessory pathways using a venous approach and radiofrequency energy. Circulation 1994; 90:1799–1810.
92. Haissaguerre M, Gaita F, Fischer B, et al: Radiofrequency catheter ablation of left lateral accessory pathways via the coronary sinus. Circulation 1992; 86:1464–1468.
93. Langberg JJ, Man KC, Vorperian VR, et al: Recognition and catheter ablation of subepicardial accessory pathways. J Am Coll Cardiol 1993; 22:1100–1104.
94. Miles WM, Zipes DP, Klein LS: Ablation of free wall accessory pathways. *In* Zipes DP (ed): Catheter Ablation of Arrhythmias, pp 211–230. Armonk, NY: Futura Publishing, 1994.
95. Kuck KH, Schlüter M, Gürsoy S: Preservation of atrioventricular nodal conduction during radiofrequency current catheter ablation of midseptal accessory pathways. Circulation 1992; 86:1743–1752.
96. Haissaguerre M, Marcus F, Poquet F, et al: Electrocardiographic characteristics and catheter ablation of parahissian accessory pathways. Circulation 1994; 90:1124–1128.

97. Dean JW, Ho SY, Rowland E, et al: Clinical anatomy of the atrioventricular junctions. J Am Coll Cardiol 1994; 24:1725–1731.
98. Bashir Y, Heald SC, O'Nunain S, et al: Radiofrequency current delivery by way of a bipolar tricuspid annulus–mitral annulus electrode configuration for ablation of posteroseptal accessory pathways. J Am Coll Cardiol 1993; 22:550–556.
99. Guiraudon GM, Guiraudon CM, Klein GJ, et al: The coronary sinus diverticulum: a pathological entity associated with the Wolff-Parkinson-White syndrome. Am J Cardiol 1988; 62:733–735.
100. Milstein S, Sharma AD, Guiraudon GM, et al: An algorithm for the electrocardiographic localization of accessory pathways in the Wolff-Parkinson-White syndrome. PACE 1987; 10:555–563.
101. Fitzpatrick AP, Gonzales RP, Lesh MD, et al: New algorithm for the localization of accessory atrioventricular connections using a baseline electrocardiogram. J Am Coll Cardiol 1994; 23:107–116.
102. Calkins H, Kim YN, Schmaltz S, et al: Electrogram criteria for identification of appropriate target sites for radiofrequency catheter ablation of accessory atrioventricular connections. Circulation 1992; 85:565–573.
103. Chen X, Borggrefe M, Shenasa M, et al: Characteristics of local electrogram predicting successful transcatheter radiofrequency ablation of left-sided accessory pathways. J Am Coll Cardiol 1992; 20:656–665.
104. Prystowsky EN, Browne KF, Zipes DP: Intracardiac recording by catheter electrode of accessory pathway depolarization. J Am Coll Cardiol 1983; 1:468–470.
105. Jackman WM, Friday KJ, Yeung-Lai-Wah JA, et al: New catheter technique for recording left free-wall accessory atrioventricular pathway activation. Identification of pathway fiber orientation. Circulation 1988; 78:598–610.
106. Sharma AD, Klein GJ, Guiraudon GM, et al: Atrial fibrillation in patients with Wolff-Parkinson-White syndrome: incidence after surgical ablation of the accessory pathway. Circulation 1985; 72:161–169.
107. Waspe LE, Brodman R, Kim SG, et al: Susceptibility to atrial fibrillation and ventricular tachyarrhythmia in the Wolff-Parkinson-White syndrome: role of the accessory pathway. Am Heart J 1986; 112:1141–1152.
108. Klein GJ, Bashore TM, Sellers TD, et al: Ventricular fibrillation in the Wolff-Parkinson-White syndrome. N Engl J Med 1979; 301:1080–1085.
109. Klein GJ, Prystowsky EN, Yee R, et al: Asymptomatic Wolff-Parkinson-White. Should we intervene? Circulation 1989; 80:1902–1905.
110. Munger TM, Packer DL, Hammill SC, et al: A population study of the natural history of Wolff-Parkinson-White syndrome in Olmsted County, Minnesota, 1953–1989. Circulation 1993; 87:866–873.
111. Roden DM: Risks and benefits of antiarrhythmic therapy. N Engl J Med 1994; 331:785–791.
112. Cox JL, Gallagher JJ, Cain ME: Experience with 118 consecutive patients undergoing operation for Wolff-Parkinson-White syndrome. J Thorac Cardiovasc Surg 1985; 90:490–501.
113. Guiraudon GM, Klein GL, Sharma AD, et al: Surgery for Wolff-Parkinson-White syndrome: further experience with an epicardial approach. Circulation 1986; 74:525–529.
114. Mahomed Y, King RD, Zipes DP, et al: Surgical division of Wolff-Parkinson-White pathways utilizing the closed-heart technique: a 2-year experience in 47 patients. Ann Thorac Surg 1988; 45:495–504.
115. Langberg JJ, Calkins H, Kim YN, et al: Recurrence of conduction in accessory atrioventricular connections after initially successful radiofrequency catheter ablation. J Am Coll Cardiol 1992; 19:1588–1592.
116. Chen X, Kottkamp H, Hindricks G, et al: Recurrence and late block of accessory pathway conduction following radiofrequency catheter ablation. J Cardiovasc Electrophysiol 1994; 5:650–658.
117. Gallagher JJ, Smith WM, Kasell JH, et al: Role of Mahaim fibers in cardiac arrhythmias in man. Circulation 1981; 64:176–189.
118. Klein GJ, Guiraudon GM, Kerr CR, et al: "Nodoventricular" accessory pathway: evidence for a distinct accessory atrioventricular pathway with atrioventricular node-like properties. J Am Coll Cardiol 1988; 11:1035–1040.
119. Tchou P, Lehmann MH, Jazayeri M, et al: Atriofascicular connection or a nodoventricular Mahaim fiber? Electrophysiologic elucidation of the pathway and associated reentrant circuit. Circulation 1988; 77:837–848.
120. Haissaguerre M, Warin J-F, Metayer P, et al: Catheter ablation of Mahaim fibers with preservation of atrioventricular nodal conduction. Circulation 1990; 82:418–427.
121. Okishige K, Strickberger SA, Walsh EP, et al: Catheter ablation of the atrial origin of a detrimentally conducting atriofascicular accessory pathway by radiofrequency current. J Cardiovasc Electrophysiol 1991; 2:465–475.
122. Klein LS, Hackett FK, Zipes DP, et al: Radiofrequency catheter ablation of Mahaim fibers at the tricuspid annulus. Circulation 1993; 87:738–747.
123. Leitch J, Klein GJ, Yee R, et al: New concepts on nodoventricular accessory pathways. J Cardiovasc Electrophysiol 1990; 1:220–230.
124. Benditt DG, Milstein S: Nodoventricular accessory connections: a misnomer or a structural functional spectrum. J Cardiovasc Electrophysiol 1990; 1:231–237.
125. McClelland JH, Xunzhang W, Beckman KJ, et al: Radiofrequency catheter ablation of right atriofascicular (Mahaim) accessory pathways guided by accessory pathway activation potentials. Circulation 1994; 89:2655–2666.
126. Critelli G, Gallagher JJ, Monda V, et al: Anatomic and electrophysiologic substrate of the permanent form of junctional reciprocating tachycardia. J Am Coll Cardiol 1984; 4:601–610.
127. Shih H, Miles W, Klein L, et al: Multiple accessory pathways in the permanent form of junctional reciprocating tachycardia. Am J Cardiol 1994; 73:361–367.
128. Chien WW, Cohen TJ, Lee MA, et al: Electrophysiological findings and long-term follow-up of patients with the permanent form of junctional reciprocating tachycardia treated by catheter ablation. Circulation 1992; 85:1329–1336.
129. Gaita F, Haissaguerre M, Giustetto C, et al: Catheter ablation of permanent junctional reciprocating tachycardia with radiofrequency current. J Am Coll Cardiol 1995; 25:648–654.
130. Shenasa H, Merrill JJ, Hamer ME, et al: Distribution of ectopic atrial tachycardias along the crista terminalis: an atrial ring of fire? [Abstract] Circulation 1993; 88:I-29.
131. Tracy CM, Swartz JF, Fletcher RD, et al: Radiofrequency catheter ablation of ectopic atrial tachycardia using paced activation sequence mapping. J Am Coll Cardiol 1993; 21:910–917.
132. Triedman JK, Saul JP, Weindling SN, et al: Radiofrequency ablation of intra-atrial reentrant tachycardia after surgical palliation of congenital heart disease. Circulation 1995; 91:707–714.
133. Walsh EP, Saul JP, Hulse JE, et al: Transcatheter ablation of ectopic atrial tachycardia in young patients using radiofrequency current. Circulation 1992; 86:1138–1146.
134. Gillette PC: Successful transcatheter ablation of ectopic atrial tachycardia in young patients using radiofrequency current. Circulation 1992; 86:1339–1340.
135. Kay GN, Chong F, Epstein AE, et al: Radiofrequency ablation for treatment of primary atrial tachycardias. J Am Coll Cardiol 1993; 21:901–909.
136. Chen SA, Chiang CE, Yang CJ, et al: Radiofrequency catheter ablation of sustained intra-atrial reentrant tachycardia in adult patients. Identification of electrophysiological characteristics and endocardial mapping techniques. Circulation 1993; 88:578–587.
137. Lesh MD, Van Hare GF, Epstein LM, et al: Radiofrequency catheter ablation of atrial arrhythmias. Results and mechanisms. Circulation 1994; 89:1074–1089.
138. Van Hare GF, Lesh MD, Stranger P: Radiofrequency catheter ablation of supraventricular arrhythmias in patients with congenital heart disease: results and technical considerations. J Am Coll Cardiol 1993; 22:883–890.
139. Prager NA, Cox JL, Lindsay BD, et al: Long-term effectiveness of surgical treatment of ectopic atrial tachycardia. J Am Coll Cardiol 1993; 22:85–92.
140. Sanders WE, Sorrentino RA, Greenfield RA, et al: Catheter ablation of sinoatrial node reentrant tachycardia. J Am Coll Cardiol 1994; 23:926–934.
141. Morillo CA, Klein GJ, Thakur RK, et al: Mechanism of "inappropriate" sinus tachycardia. Role of sympathovagal balance. Circulation 1994; 90:873–877.
142. Feld GK, Fleck RP, Chen PS, et al: Radiofrequency catheter ablation for the treatment of human type I atrial flutter. Identification of a critical zone in the reentrant circuit by endocardial mapping techniques. Circulation 1992; 86:1233–1240.
143. Cosio FG, López-Gil M, Goicolea A, et al: Radiofrequency ablation of the inferior vena cava–tricuspid valve isthmus in common atrial flutter. Am J Cardiol 1993; 71:705–709.
144. Kirkorian G, Moncada E, Chevalier P, et al: Radiofrequency ablation of atrial flutter. Efficacy of an anatomically guided approach. Circulation 1994; 90:2804–2814.
145. Huang SK, Bharati S, Graham AR, et al: Closed chest catheter desiccation of the atrioventricular junction using radiofrequency energy—a new method of catheter ablation. J Am Coll Cardiol 1987; 9:349–358.
146. Langberg JJ, Chin MC, Rosenqvist M, et al: Catheter ablation of the atrioventricular junction with radiofrequency energy. Circulation 1989; 80:1527–1535.

147. Jackman WM, Wang X, Friday KJ, et al: Catheter ablation of atrioventricular junction using radiofrequency current in 17 patients: comparison of standard and large-tip catheter electronics. Circulation 1991; 83:1562–1576.
148. Yeung-Lai-Wah JA, Alison JF, Lonergan L, et al: High success rate of atrioventricular node ablation with radiofrequency energy. J Am Coll Cardiol 1991; 18:1753–1758.
149. Morady F, Calkins H, Langberg JJ, et al: A prospective randomized comparison of direct current and radiofrequency ablation of the atrioventricular junction. J Am Coll Cardiol 1993; 21:102–109.
150. Olgin JE, Scheinman MM: Comparison of high energy direct current and radiofrequency catheter ablation of the atrioventricular junction. J Am Coll Cardiol 1993; 21:557–564.
151. Fisher JD: Direct current and radiofrequency catheter ablation: so far and yet so near. J Am Coll Cardiol 1993; 21:565–566.
152. Pritchett ELC: Management of atrial fibrillation. N Engl J Med 1992; 326:1264–1271.
153. Sousa J, El-Atassi R, Rosenheck S, et al: Radiofrequency catheter ablation of the atrioventricular junction from the left ventricle. Circulation 1991; 84:567–571.
154. Evans GT, Scheinman MM, Zipes DP, et al: The Percutaneous Cardiac Mapping and Ablation Registry: final summary of results. PACE 1988; 11:1621–1626.
155. Evans GT, Scheinman MM, Bardy G, et al: Predictors of in-hospital mortality after DC catheter ablation of atrioventricular junction. Results of a prospective, international, multicenter study. Circulation 1991; 84:1924–1937.
156. Williamson BD, Man KC, Daoud E, et al: Radiofrequency catheter modification of atrioventricular conduction to control the ventricular rate during atrial fibrillation. N Engl J Med 1994; 331:910–917.
157. Wellens HJJ: Atrial fibrillation—the last big hurdle in treating supraventricular tachycardia. N Engl J Med 1994; 331:944–945.
158. Feld GK, Fleck P, Fujimura O, et al: Control of rapid ventricular response by radiofrequency catheter modification of the atrioventricular node in patients with medically refractory atrial fibrillation. Circulation 1994; 90:2299–2307.
159. Della Bella P, Carbucicchio C, Tondo C, et al: Modulation of atrioventricular conduction by ablation of the "slow" atrioventricular node pathway in patients with drug-refractory atrial fibrillation or flutter. J Am Coll Cardiol 1995; 25:39–46.
160. Cox JL, Boineau JP, Schuessler RB, et al: Five-year experience with the maze procedure for atrial fibrillation. Ann Thorac Surg 1993; 56:814–824.
161. Cox JL, Boineau JP, Schuessler RB, et al: A review of surgery for atrial fibrillation. J Cardiovasc Electrophysiol 1991; 2:541–561.
162. Feinberg MS, Waggoner AD, Kater KM, et al: Restoration of atrial function after the maze procedure for patients with atrial fibrillation. Assessment by Doppler echocardiography. Circulation 1994; 90(pt 2):II-285–II-292.
163. Ferguson TB: The future of arrhythmia surgery. J Cardiovasc Electrophysiol 1994; 5:621–634.
164. Haissaguerre M, Marcus FI, Fischer B, et al: Radiofrequency catheter ablation in unusual mechanisms of atrial fibrillation: report of three cases. J Cardiovasc Electrophysiol 1994; 5:743–751.
165. Haissaguerre M, Gencel L, Fischer B, et al: Successful catheter ablation of atrial fibrillation. J Cardiovasc Electrophysiol 1994; 5:1045–1052.
166. Swartz JF, Pellersels G, Silvers J, et al: A catheter-based curative approach to atrial fibrillation in humans [Abstract]. Circulation 1994; 90(pt 2):I-335.
167. Powell AC, Garan H, McGovern BA, et al: Low energy cardioversion of atrial fibrillation in the sheep. J Am Coll Cardiol 1992; 20:707–711.
168. Cooper RAS, Alferness CA, Smith WM, et al: Internal cardioversion of atrial fibrillation in sheep. Circulation 1993; 87:1673–1686.
169. Levy S, Camm J: An implantable atrial defibrillator. An impossible dream? Circulation 1993; 87:1769–1772.
170. Ayers GM, Alferness CA, Ilina M, et al: Ventricular proarrhythmic effects of ventricular cycle length and shock strength in a sheep mode of transvenous atrial defibrillation. Circulation 1994; 89:413–422.
171. Lévy S, Richard P: Is there any indication for an intracardiac defibrillator for the treatment of atrial fibrillation? J Cardiovasc Electrophysiol 1994; 5:982–985.

18 Drug Treatment of Ventricular Tachycardias

William G. Stevenson, MD
Peter L. Friedman, MD, PhD

Ventricular tachycardia results from reentry, triggered activity, or automaticity in ventricular myocardium or the His-Purkinje system below the His bundle, producing a tachycardia with a wide QRS duration that typically exceeds 0.12 sec.[1,2] Management is guided by the clinical presentation and associated heart disease. Tachycardia is considered to be sustained if it requires an intervention for termination, such as cardioversion or drug administration, if it produces severe symptoms, such as syncope, or if it persists for 30 sec or longer. Self-terminating ventricular tachycardias three or more consecutive beats in duration but lasting less than 30 sec are designated nonsustained. The QRS morphologic characteristics of ventricular tachycardia are an important clue to its cause (Table 18–1). Monomorphic ventricular tachycardias have similar QRS complexes from beat to beat (Fig. 18–1*A*). Polymorphic ventricular tachycardias have different beat-to-beat QRS morphologic features (see Fig. 18–1*B*). Polymorphic ventricular tachycardia should also be distinguished from two or more distinct monomorphic ventricular tachycardias occurring in the same patient. Sinusoidal ventricular tachycardias have a sine wave configuration, making it difficult to distinguish the T wave from the QRS complex (see Fig. 18–1*C*). This occurs in very rapid monomorphic ventricular tachycardia, also known as ventricular flutter, which may have the same mechanisms as slower monomorphic ventricular tachycardias. Slow sinusoidal ventricular tachycardia results from marked slowing of ventricular conduction, most commonly due to hyperkalemia or an antiarrhythmic drug. Ventricular fibrillation is characterized by chaotic electrical activity without discernable QRS complexes (see Fig. 18–1*D*). Ventricular fibrillation can be caused by deterioration of ventricular tachycardia and may also occur as a primary arrhythmia. Detailed discussions of pathophysiology and clinical presentation of ventricu-

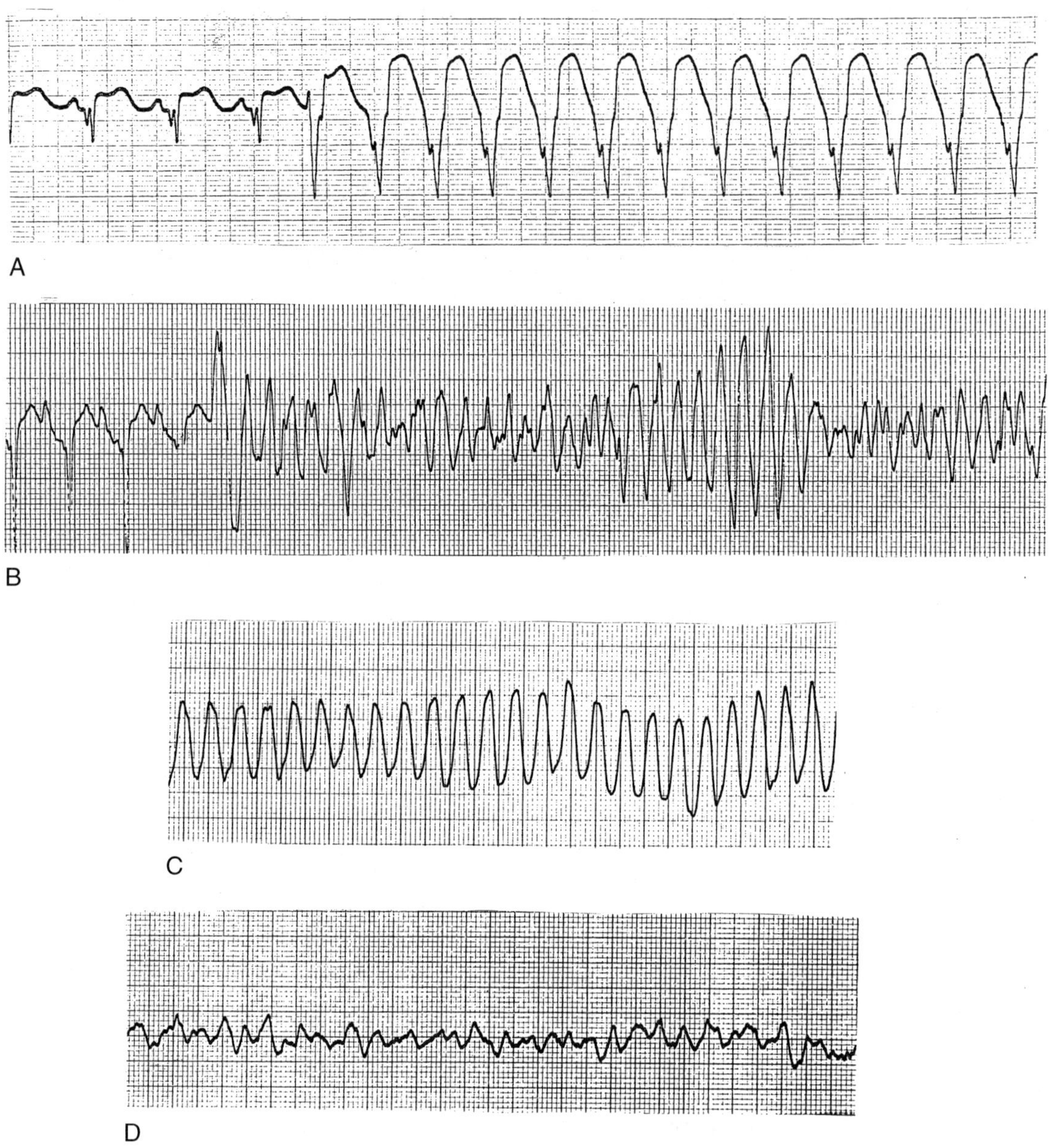

Figure 18–1. Four different sustained ventricular arrhythmias are shown. *A,* Spontaneous initiation of sustained monomorphic ventricular tachycardia. *B,* Spontaneous initiation of polymorphic ventricular tachycardia during acute myocardial infarction. *C,* Sinusoidal ventricular tachycardia also known as ventricular flutter. *D,* Ventricular fibrillation.

lar tachycardias may be found in Zipes[1] and Akhtar.[2] This chapter focuses primarily on management considerations.

MANAGEMENT OF THE ACUTE EPISODE

Initial Approach to the Patient

When first assessing a patient with a sustained ventricular tachyarrhythmia, the hemodynamic impact of the arrhythmia is the most important consideration. Arrhythmias that produce hemodynamic collapse, such as ventricular fibrillation or rapid ventricular tachycardia, should be treated with prompt direct current (DC) cardioversion. Slower sustained monomorphic ventricular tachycardias may have less severe hemodynamic consequences, allowing consideration of acute drug therapy or further diagnostic steps before resorting to cardioversion. Immediate DC cardioversion should be performed if ventricular tachycardia causes hypotension, with evidence of shock, severe angina, or pulmonary edema.

Cardioversion and Defibrillation

The method of DC cardioversion depends on the nature and the rate of the ventricular arrhythmia. Cardioversion of ventricular fibrillation or sustained polymorphic ventricular tachycardia is performed without attempting to synchronize the shock to a QRS complex because the rapid, disorganized, electrical activity of these arrhythmias results in unreliable sensing. Attempts to deliver a shock synchronized to a QRS complex during such arrhythmias causes unnecessary delays. An initial shock of 200 joule is recommended and is usually effective, particularly if the arrhythmia has been of brief duration, as might occur in an intensive care unit.[3, 4] Polymorphic ventricular tachycardia is almost always interrupted by a single

TABLE 18–1. CAUSES OF SUSTAINED VENTRICULAR TACHYCARDIA

Sustained Monomorphic VT
Associated With Abnormal Ventricular Wall Motion
Healed myocardial infarct
Dilated cardiomyopathy
Chagas disease
Sarcoidosis
Right ventricular dysplasia
Cardiac tumors
Scleroderma
After repair of tetralogy of Fallot
Bundle branch reentry
Normal Ventricular Function
Idiopathic
Bundle branch reentry
Digitalis toxicity
Polymorphic VT/VF
Torsades de Pointes Associated With QT Prolongation
Congenital
Acquired
QT Prolongation May Be Present But Is Not Required
Evolving or Transient Electrophysiologic Abnormalities
Acute myocardial ischemia
Digitalis toxicity
Acute myocarditis
Cocaine ingestion
Degeneration from sustained monomorphic VT
Myocardial Hypertrophy
Hypertrophic cardiomyopathy
Aortic stenosis
Dilated cardiomyopathy
Sinusoidal VT
Rapid Monomorphic VT
Associated With Globally Slow Ventricular Conduction
Hyperkalemia
Antiarrhythmics
Phenothiazines
Antidepressants
Severe global ischemia

Abbreviation: VT, ventricular tachycardia.

200-joule DC shock. Ventricular fibrillation may persist after a 200-joule shock, particularly when the fibrillatory waves are of low amplitude or the arrhythmia has been present for an indeterminate time. Additional high-energy shocks of 300 and 360 joule, respectively, should then be delivered immediately (Fig. 18–2). If ventricular fibrillation is still present, epinephrine, 1:10,000 dilution, is given as a 1-mg bolus intravenously, followed by up to three additional 360-joule shocks if necessary.

In patients with sustained monomorphic ventricular tachycardia who require immediate DC cardioversion, the rate and QRS morphologic characteristics should be considered. When the tachycardia rate is relatively slow, that is, less than 200 beats per minute, and the QRS amplitude is much greater than the T wave amplitude, most cardioversion devices sense the QRS complex reliably, and the shock should be synchronized to the QRS complex. Monomorphic ventricular tachycardia can often be terminated by relatively low-energy shocks of 10–50 joule. If a low-energy shock is ineffective, higher energy shocks of up to 360 joule should be applied. Reliable QRS sensing may not be possible when the rate of ventricular tachycardia is much faster than 200 beats per minute or for sinusoidal ventricular tachycardias. A nonsynchronized shock, usually beginning with a shock energy of 200 joules, should be delivered. Attempts to synchronize the shock to a QRS complex can result in the shock's being delivered during the T wave at a time when there are marked regional disparities in repolarization. This often precipitates ventricular fibrillation. Sustained monomorphic ventricular tachycardia is almost always interrupted by a high-energy DC shock. When it persists, one should be alert to the possibility that other factors, such as hyperkalemia, drug toxicity, or proarrhythmia (see later discussion) may be involved.

Acute Antiarrhythmic Drug Therapy

If DC cardioversion of ventricular tachycardia or ventricular fibrillation has been unsuccessful or if the arrhythmia recurs immediately after a successful cardioversion, intravenous antiarrhythmic drug therapy is required (see Fig. 18–2). Table 18–2 lists drugs that are available for acute intravenous administration. Lidocaine is usually the drug of first choice, although its value during cardiopulmonary resuscitation has not been conclusively demonstrated. The use of lidocaine in patients with persistent ventricular fibrillation despite repeated cardioversion may not improve outcome and may actually increase the likelihood of converting the rhythm to asystole.[5] Lidocaine may be of more value in patients who have repeated recurrences of ventricular tachycardia or fibrillation after initial successful cardioversion. If lidocaine is ineffective, procainamide or bretylium tosylate should be considered (see Table 18–2). A superiority of one of these agents over the other has not been demonstrated. Procainamide causes vasodilation, which can cause severe hypotension during rapid intravenous administration. The onset of electrophysiologic effects is rapid. Administration of bretylium causes an initial release of norepinephrine from sympathetic nerve terminals, which increases myocardial contractility but at the risk of aggravating the ventricular arrhythmia.[6] During chronic intravenous therapy, blockade of sympathetic neural function occurs, which may increase responsiveness to circulating catecholamines and could theoretically aggravate arrhythmias. The full antiarrhythmic effect of bretylium may not be seen for 20–30 min or more after its intravenous administration.

Amiodarone is available as an intravenous formulation approved by the U.S. Food and Drug Administration (FDA) for emergency use in patients with hemodynamically compromising ventricular tachyarrhythmias that are unresponsive to DC shock or are not suppressed by other intravenous antiarrhythmic drugs. Intravenous administration of amiodarone can be efficacious in patients with intractable ventricular fibrillation and sustained monomorphic ventricular tachycardia[7–11] as well as refractory polymorphic ventricular tachycardia.[12] Its role in the emergency management of intractable ventricular fibrillation or ventricular tachycardia is still being defined. Its efficacy in these situations appears to be similar to that of bretylium, and it may be better tolerated hemodynamically.[10] Amiodarone should be considered when lidocaine, procainamide, and bretylium are ineffective. It may also be a reasonable alternative to bretylium. In one study, during prolonged cardiac arrests in which repeated cardioversions were unsuccessful, an organized rhythm was restored in nearly 80% of patients after administration of intravenous amiodarone.[7] Frequent recurrences of sustained monomorphic ventricular tachycardia that do not respond to other antiarrhythmic drugs are markedly reduced or eliminated in 50%–80% of patients.[8, 11] In an emergency situation, amiodarone is administered intravenously in an initial loading dose of 150 mg as a bolus (15 mg/min), followed by a constant infusion of 1 mg/min for 6 h and then a maintenance infusion of 0.5 mg/min. The acute antiarrhythmic effects of the drug are not seen if the initial bolus is omitted. Supplemental intravenous bolus infusions of 150 mg may be given for arrhythmias that recur during the constant infusion. The total dose should not exceed 2100 mg in 24 h. Continuous infusion into a peripheral vein often causes phlebitis; a large central vein is the preferred route of administration. Hypotension occurs in 20%–40% of patients, likely because of the vehicles polysorbate 80 and benzyl alcohol, which are necessary to render amiodarone soluble in aqueous solution.[9–11, 13] The hypotension may result in part from release of histamine from mast cells triggered by polysorbate 80.[14] Supplemental intravenous fluids and

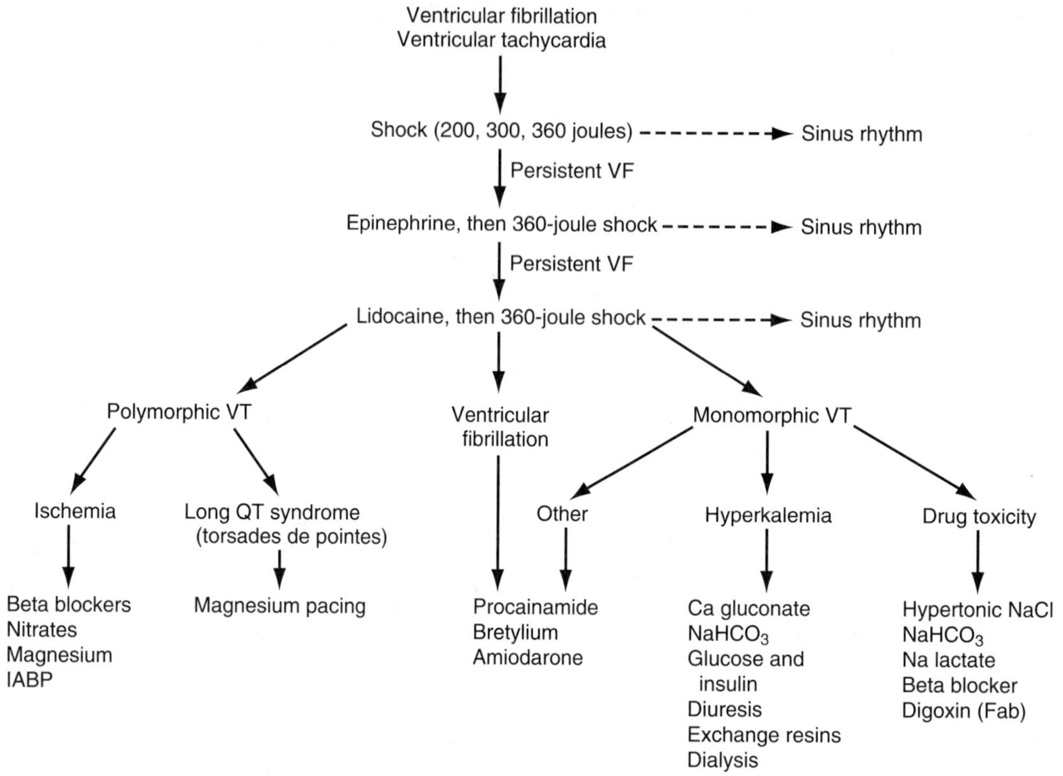

Figure 18–2. Flow diagram for the emergency treatment of ventricular fibrillation or sustained ventricular tachycardia with hemodynamic collapse. *Abbreviation:* IABP, intra-aortic balloon counterpulsation.

vasopressors may be needed to counteract these effects. Intravenous amiodarone can cause bradycardia because of sinus node dysfunction or atrioventricular (AV) block; temporary pacing is occasionally necessary.[8, 11] Provocation of polymorphic ventricular tachycardia as a proarrhythmic response (see further on) has been reported but is rare.

When ventricular tachycardia does not respond to DC cardioversion and antiarrhythmic drug administration, underlying, potentially correctable causes should be particularly considered. Refractory polymorphic ventricular tachycardia suggests that acute myocardial ischemia or a form of the long QT syndrome may be present (see discussion of polymorphic ventricular tachycardia further on). Magnesium sulfate, 1–2 g, administered as an intravenous bolus may be effective for either cause. Intravenous amiodarone has also been effective in selected patients in this setting.[12] If ischemia is likely, intravenous administration of beta-adrenergic blockers and nitrates, and intra-aortic balloon counterpulsation should be considered. Emergent coronary angiography followed by angioplasty or surgical revascularization may be required.

Incessant monomorphic ventricular tachycardia can be the consequence of drug toxicity, most commonly from agents that depress myocardial conduction, such as the class IA and IC antiarrhythmic drugs or tricyclic antidepressants.[6, 15–19] Administration of other antiarrhythmic drugs that depress conduction may exacerbate the arrhythmia and should be avoided. Administration of intravenous beta blockers, hypertonic sodium bicarbonate, or sodium lactate is sometimes helpful.[16–19] Sodium loading reduces drug-induced slowing of conduction velocity.[20] In patients with tricyclic antidepressant overdosage, hypertonic saline and neostigmine or pyridostigmine may be useful to reverse the anticholinergic effects of the tricyclics.

Digitalis intoxication can cause incessant ventricular tachycardia. It deserves special consideration because cardioversion can cause deterioration to ventricular fibrillation. Sustained monomorphic ventricular tachycardia resulting from moderate degrees of digitalis excess is thought to be caused by triggered activity in cells located high in the His-Purkinje system.[21] Such ventricular tachycardias are referred to as fascicular tachycardias and are characterized by relatively narrow QRS complexes, usually with a right bundle branch block configuration indicating a focus of origin in the left bundle branch (Fig. 18–3). Some patients also have a pattern of alternating left and right axis deviation in the frontal plane, causing bidirectional ventricular tachycardia.[21] Incessant ventricular fibrillation due to digitalis toxicity is rare and usually results from a massive overdose. Although phenytoin or lidocaine may be effective in some patients with ventricular tachycardia or ventricular fibrillation caused by digitalis toxicity,[22] the treatment of choice is the administration of intravenous digoxin-specific antigen-binding fragments (Fab).[23]

Electrolyte derangements, particularly hyper- or hypokalemia, can contribute to or cause incessant ventricular tachycardia. Wide QRS tachycardia caused by hyperkalemia typically has a relatively slow rate, that is, less than 160 beats per minute, and extremely wide QRS complexes (Fig. 18–4). Acute administration of calcium gluconate or sodium bicarbonate rapidly reverses the electrophysiologic effects of hyperkalemia and produces immediate narrowing of the QRS complex. This allows time for the administration of hypertonic glucose and insulin, which has a delayed effect, and the use of forced diuresis, administration of cationic exchange resins via a nasogastric tube or rectal enema and, if necessary, peritoneal or hemodialysis to remove potassium.

Wide QRS Tachycardia Without Hemodynamic Compromise

In some patients, sustained monomorphic ventricular tachycardia does not cause hemodynamic compromise. The clinical presentation depends on the tachycardia rate, the nature of the underlying heart disease, left ventricular function, and the sequence of ventricular

TABLE 18–2. DOSAGE AND PHARMACOKINETICS OF INTRAVENOUS ANTIARRHYTHMIC DRUGS

	Intravenous Loading Dose	Maintenance Infusion (mg/min)	Therapeutic Plasma Concentration (μg/mL)	Major Route of Elimination	Acute Toxicity
Lidocaine	1–2 mg/kg at 20–50 mg/min; repeat 1 mg/kg bolus q5 min × 1 or 2 *or* 0.5 mg/kg bolus q8 min 1–4 times as needed; total dose not to exceed 3 mg/kg	1–4	1–5	Hepatic	Bradycardia, CNS symptoms, nausea
Procainamide	6–17 mg/kg at 25 to 30 mg/min *or* 100 mg q5 min × 5–10 doses; total dose not to exceed 2000 mg	2–6	4–10	Renal-hepatic	Hypotension, CNS, nausea, bradycardia, AV block, incessant VT, torsades de pointes
Bretylium	5 mg/kg IV push; repeat doses after 5 min of 10 mg/kg q15 min × 2 as needed *or* 5–10 mg/kg at 1–2 mg/kg/min; total dose not to exceed 25 mg/kg	0.5–2	0.04–0.9	Renal	Hypotension, proarrhythmia, nausea
Amiodarone	150-mg bolus (15 mg/min × 10 min), then 1 mg/min × 6 h, then 0.5 mg/min maintenance; repeat bolus of 150 mg for arrhythmia recurrence	0.4–1	1–3.5	Hepatic	Bradycardia, AV block, hypotension, torsades de pointes, thrombophlebitis, acute hepatitis
Adenosine	6 mg, rapid push; if no effect, repeat 12-mg dose	—	—	Metabolized in endothelium	Hypotension, AV block, cutaneous flushing, headache
Magnesium sulfate	1–2 g over 1–2 min	1–4 g/h	—	Renal	Neuromuscular depression
Propranolol	1–3 mg at 1 mg/min; repeat dose × 1 after 2 min as needed	—	1–2.5	Hepatic	Hypotension, heart failure, bronchospasm, bradycardia, AV block

Abbreviations: CNS, central nervous system; AV, atrioventricular; VT, ventricular tachycardia; IV, intravenous.

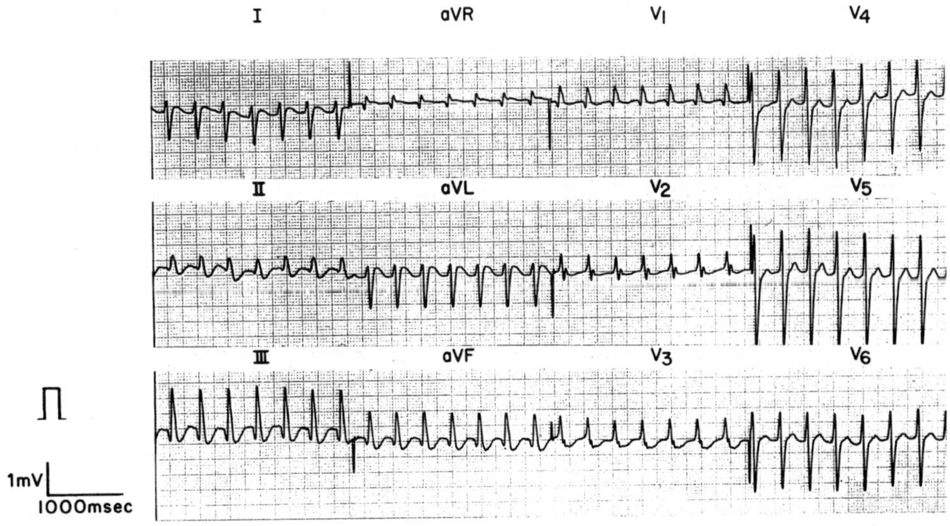

Figure 18–3. Fascicular ventricular tachycardia due to digitalis intoxication. *Abbreviations:* aVR, augmented unipolar lead, right arm; aVL, augmented unipolar lead, left arm; aVF, augmented unipolar lead, left leg. (From Friedman PL, Antman EM: Electrocardiographic manifestations of digitalis toxicity. *In* Smith TW [ed]: Digitalis Glycosides, p 268. Orlando, FL: Grune & Stratton, 1985.)

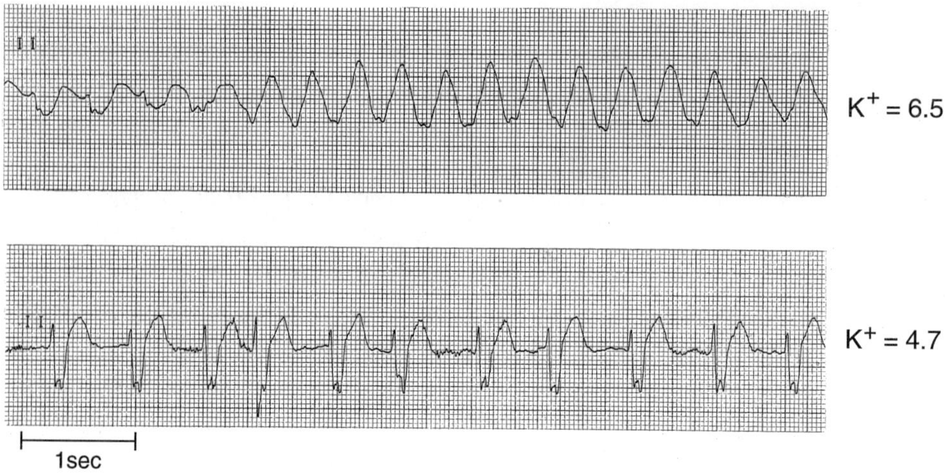

Figure 18–4. *Top,* Sinusoidal ventricular tachycardia resulting from hyperkalemia. *Bottom,* Atrial fibrillation and bundle branch block in the presence of a normal serum potassium level.

activation during tachycardia. When the tachycardia is well tolerated, emergency cardioversion is not required as the first treatment. One should first attempt to establish the diagnosis and institute a therapy that is likely to restore sinus rhythm, while minimizing the chance of transforming a hemodynamically stable rhythm into one that is unstable. Distinguishing supraventricular tachycardia with aberrant intraventricular conduction from ventricular tachycardia is the first step. The clinical history is the single most useful tool. When there is a history of prior myocardial infarction, ventricular tachycardia is the correct diagnosis in 90% or more of patients.[24] A 12-lead electrocardiogram should be recorded. The presence of AV dissociation, fusion, or capture beats establishes ventricular tachycardia as the diagnosis. In the absence of these factors, analysis of the QRS morphology is often helpful.[25] If the diagnosis is still in doubt, administration of intravenous adenosine can be used as a diagnostic maneuver.[26, 29] Administered into a peripheral vein as a rapid bolus of 6 mg, followed if necessary by a second bolus dose of 12 mg, adenosine terminates most paroxysmal supraventricular tachycardias due to AV nodal reentry or to AV reentry over the AV node and an accessory AV pathway. When it is administered into a central vein, the effects are more pronounced; the initial dose should be 3 mg. If atrial tachycardia or atrial flutter with aberrant conduction over the AV node and His-Purkinje system is present, the diagnosis becomes apparent during the transient high-grade AV block that is produced by the drug. If atrial tachycardia or atrial flutter with conduction to the ventricle over an accessory AV pathway is present, adenosine usually has no effect. Degeneration to atrial fibrillation is possible, however, and could precipitate ventricular fibrillation.[6] If this diagnosis is possible, intravenous procainamide should be administered. Termination of ventricular tachycardia by adenosine is rare, but it can occur, particularly when the tachycardia originates in the right ventricular outflow tract. In ventricular tachycardia with 1:1 ventriculoatrial conduction, adenosine administration usually causes transient ventriculoatrial dissociation, a finding that confirms ventricular tachycardia as the diagnosis. Adenosine has been administered to patients with documented ventricular tachycardia induced in the electrophysiology laboratory, and it is safe in such patients. Although it can cause peripheral vasodilation and arterial hypotension, its extremely brief duration of action ensures that these effects are fleeting. Verapamil and other calcium antagonists, in contrast, have more profound and long-lasting hypotensive effects as well as significant negative inotropic effects. When administered during ventricular tachycardia, these agents frequently cause hemodynamic collapse with potentially catastrophic consequences.[30, 31] They should never be administered to patients with a sustained wide QRS complex tachycardia of uncertain origin.

Once the diagnosis of ventricular tachycardia has been confirmed in a patient with a hemodynamically well-tolerated wide QRS tachycardia, and the possibility that the tachycardia represents a proarrhythmic effect of an antiarrhythmic drug has been excluded, an antiarrhythmic drug should be administered in an effort to restore sinus rhythm. Although oral administration of quinidine, disopyramide, flecainide, propafenone, or sotalol has been used in carefully selected patients, intravenous administration is preferred in most circumstances (see Table 18–2). Lidocaine is the drug of first choice in most situations because of its favorable hemodynamic profile and low risk of ventricular proarrhythmia, but it terminates sustained ventricular tachycardia in only 30% of patients.[29] Lidocaine has a rapid rate of redistribution after an intravenous bolus; plasma concentrations quickly fall to less than therapeutic levels. If lidocaine boluses are ineffective, a second agent can be administered safely. Procainamide is often effective. It should be administered at a rate of 30 mg/min or slower, with careful monitoring for hypotension. If ventricular tachycardia persists, or significant symptoms develop, DC cardioversion should be performed. Administration of a third or a fourth drug to terminate tachycardia is not advisable because the risk of ventricular proarrhythmia and hemodynamic compromise is likely to increase with multidrug combinations. Patients who experience hemodynamically stable sustained monomorphic ventricular tachycardia during chronic oral therapy with the class IC drugs flecainide or propafenone, which prominently slow ventricular conduction velocity, are best treated by DC cardioversion without administration of additional antiarrhythmic agents. The additional conduction slowing caused by lidocaine or procainamide may increase the risk of proarrhythmia and may even cause the tachycardia to become incessant.[6, 15]

EVALUATION AFTER THE ACUTE EVENT

After conversion of the ventricular arrhythmia and stabilization, the presence and severity of underlying heart disease should be assessed. In most cases, coronary angiography is warranted. If coronary artery disease is absent, a careful search for other structural heart disease should be performed. Echocardiography is useful to assess right and left ventricular function, ventricular wall motion abnormalities, and the presence of valvular heart disease. The risk of arrhythmia recurrence depends on the type of ventricular tachycardia and severity of heart disease.

Sustained Monomorphic Ventricular Tachycardia

Distinguishing ventricular tachycardia from supraventricular tachycardia with aberrancy is of paramount importance for selecting therapy and assessing prognosis. If there is any doubt, invasive electrophysiologic studies should be performed.[1] Programmed electrical stimulation initiates sustained monomorphic ventricular tachycardia in more than 90% of patients who have this arrhythmia as a consequence of structural heart disease.[32] Electrophysiologic study also detects most supraventricular tachycardias. If ventricular tachycardia is provokable, evaluation in the electrophysiology laboratory is often helpful in establishing the site or origin and mechanism of the arrhythmia.[2, 25] Electrophysiologic study is a safe procedure in experienced hands, with a 0.06% risk of death.[33] The major complications of cardiac perforation, significant hemorrhage, and venous thrombosis occur in 0.2%, 0.05%, and 0.2% of patients, respectively.

Polymorphic Ventricular Tachycardia and Ventricular Fibrillation

The differential diagnosis and approach to the patient resuscitated from sustained polymorphic ventricular tachycardia or ventricular fibrillation is presented in Figure 18–5.[34] Acute reversible causes should be excluded (see Table 18–1). A 12-lead electrocardiogram and serum markers of acute myocardial infarction should be evaluated. Serum electrolyte levels should be obtained. If the corrected QT (QT_c) interval is prolonged to longer than 0.46 sec and precipitating factors for torsades de pointes are present, this must be considered the likely diagnosis (see further on); electrophysiology testing is not required. If acute myocardial infarction is present with ST elevation and unequivocal serum enzyme markers, polymorphic ventricular tachycradia or ventricular fibrillation can be attributed to the acute infarct (see further on). Other potential causes are transient myocardial ischemia and reentry in a region of scar. In rare instances, ventricular fibrillation is precipitated by a supraventricular arrhythmia, usually in a patient with severe underlying heart disease, or by atrial fibrillation in a patient with the Wolff-Parkinson-White syndrome.[25, 35] Other causes are much less common (see Table 18–1).

CONSIDERATIONS IN SELECTING CHRONIC ANTIARRHYTHMIC THERAPY

In patients at risk for recurrent episodes of sustained arrhythmias, antiarrhythmic drug therapy, implantable cardioverter-defibrillators, and surgical or catheter ablation are therapeutic options (see Chapter 19). A number of antiarrhythmic drugs are approved for chronic oral therapy of life-threatening ventricular arrhythmias (Table 18–3).[6] The class III drugs amiodarone and sotalol prolong action potential duration and refractoriness and in addition possess other actions. The class I drugs block the fast sodium current, slowing conduction velocity; several also have additional effects, such as action potential prolongation. Side effects are common with antiarrhythmic drugs and are often a major determinant of the therapy selected (Table 18–4). The potential for proarrhythmia necessitates initiation of drug therapy in a hospital setting with electrocardiographic monitoring. A loading dose shortens the time to an electrophysiologic effect but may increase the risk of proarrhythmia and is not generally used for sotalol and class IC drugs. The initial maintenance dose of medication should be low and gradually increased in a manner appropriate for the pharmacokinetics of the drug to a dose that achieves the desired effect (see Table 18–3). Many patients with ventricular arrhythmias have depressed ventricular function and impaired renal or hepatic function, which increases the risk of drug accumulation to toxic levels. The route of drug elimination, negative inotropic effects, and drug interactions (Table 18–5) are also important considerations.

Proarrhythmia

Proarrhythmia is the emergence of a new arrhythmia, such as torsades de pointes (see further on) or severe bradycardia, or aggravation of an existing arrhythmia by an antiarrhythmic drug.[15, 19, 36–39] The incidence and type of proarrhythmia varies with the drug, the

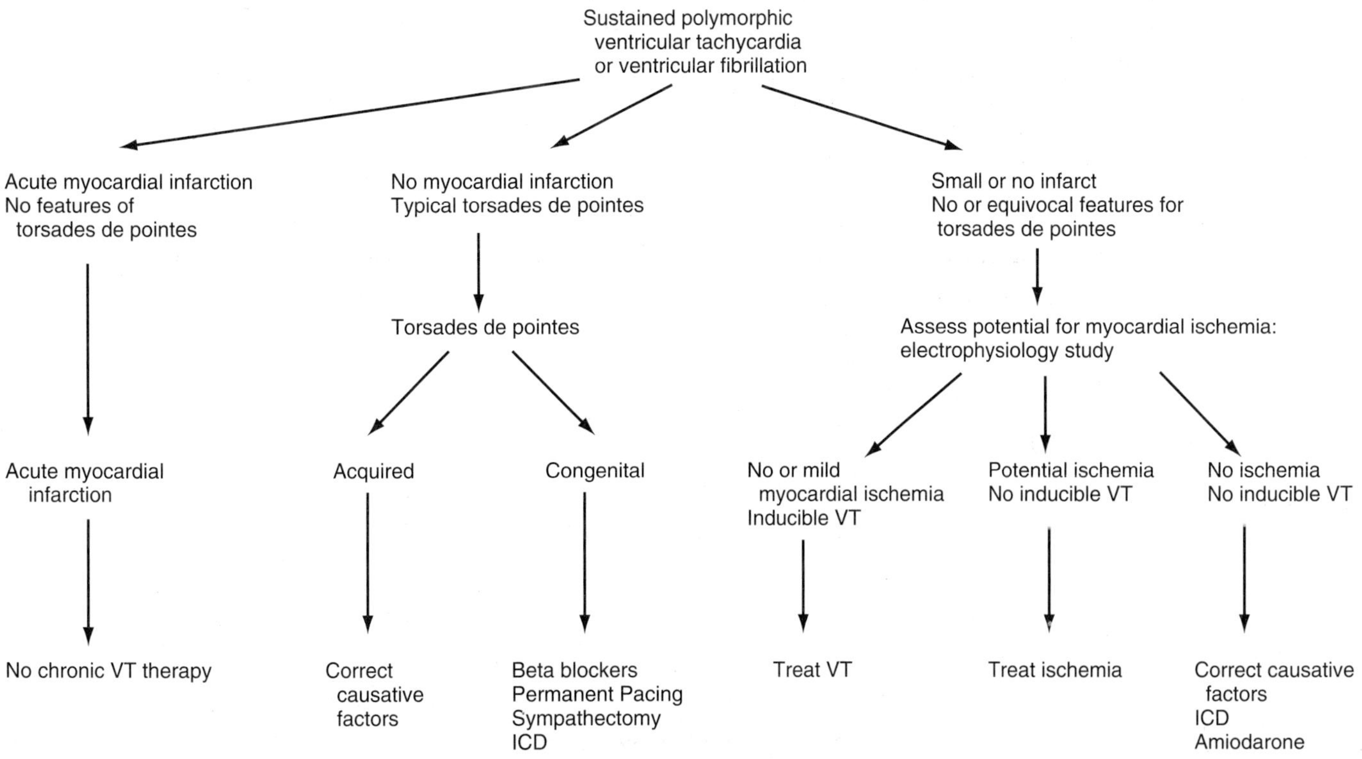

Figure 18–5. Flow diagram for selecting chronic therapy for patients resuscitated from polymorphic ventricular tachycardia or ventricular fibrillation. *Abbreviations:* ICD, implantable cardioverter-defibrillator; VT, ventricular tachycardia.

TABLE 18–3. DOSAGE AND PHARMACOKINETICS OF ORAL ANTIARRHYTHMIC AGENTS

	Loading (mg)	Maintenance (mg)	Time to Peak Plasma Concentration (h)	Effective Serum or Plasma Concentration (μg/mL)	Elimination Half-Life (h)	Bio-availability (%)	Active Metabolite	Major Route of Elimination
Class IA*								
Quinidine	200–300 q2 h × 2–4	300–600 q6–8 h	1.5–3	3–6	5–9	60–80	No	Hepatic
Procainamide	500–1000	350–1000 q3–6 h	1	4–10	3–5	70–85	*N*-acetyl procainamide	Renal/hepatic
Disopyramide	200–400	100–400 q6–8 h	1–2	2–5	4–10	80–90	Yes	Renal/hepatic
Class IB*								
Mexiletine	400–600	150–300 q6–8 h	2–4	0.75–2	10–17	90	No	Hepatic
Tocainide	400–600	400–600 q8–12 h	0.5–2	4–10	11	90	No	Renal/hepatic
Class IC*								
Moricizine	300	100–400 q8 h	0.5–2	0.1	1–3	40	Yes	Hepatic
Flecainide		50–200 q12 h	1–6	0.2–1.0	20	95	No	Renal/hepatic
Propafenone		150–300 q8–12 h	1–3	0.2–3	5–8	25–75	Yes	Hepatic
Class III*								
Amiodarone	800–1600 daily for 1–3 wk	200–400 daily	3–7	1–2.5	50 days	35–65	Yes	Hepatic
Sotalol		80–320 q12 h	2–4	>1.2	12	90–100	No	Renal

*Vaughn Williams-Singh Classification:[6] class I sodium channel blockade with fast onset and offset kinetics (IB), slow onset and offset kinetics (IC), or intermediate onset and offset kinetics (IA). Class II blockade of beta-adrenergic receptors, class III blockade of potassium channels with prolongation action of repolarization. Class IV blockade of the slow calcium channel.

From Zipes DP: Management of cardiac arrhythmias: Pharmacological, electrical, and surgical techniques. *In* Braunwald E (ed): Heart Disease, A Textbook of Cardiovascular Medicine, 4th ed, p 628. Philadelphia: WB Saunders, 1992; *and* Hohnloser SH, Woosley RL: Sotalol. N Engl J Med 1994; 331(1):31–38.

arrhythmia being treated, and the severity of heart disease (see Table 18–4). Patients with a history of sustained ventricular tachycardia and depressed ventricular function are at greater risk for proarrhythmia.

Life-threatening ventricular tachycardia develops during the initiation of drug therapy in 7% of patients who have previously suffered sustained ventricular tachycardia.[37] A single arrhythmia recurrence is likely to indicate failure to suppress the arrhythmia being treated rather than proarrhythmia. Proarrhythmia is likely, however, when a patient who was previously subject to rare attacks suffers repeated episodes of ventricular tachycardia after antiarrhythmic drug therapy is begun. Occasionally, tachycardia becomes incessant. This is most frequent with drugs that markedly slow conduction, such as flecainide and propafenone, but it can occur with any drug.[19] This type of proarrhythmia usually occurs within 4 days of initiating drug therapy. Treatment involves withdrawing the drug and supporting the patient hemodynamically.

Proarrhythmia is less frequent in patients who have not previously suffered a sustained arrhythmia. In one study, during initiation of flecainide, encainide, or moricizine therapy in myocardial infarction survivors, 0.7% suffered nonfatal sustained ventricular tachycardia and 1.6% suffered a fatal arrhythmia.[39] Distinguishing an arrhythmia caused by medication from one that is the consequence of associated heart disease can be difficult. The antiarrhythmic drug should be withdrawn. Invasive electrophysiologic study may be useful.[38, 40] The presence of an inducible, sustained monomorphic ventricular tachycardia in the absence of the drug may identify patients who are

TABLE 18–4. ADVERSE CARDIAC EFFECTS OF ANTIARRHYTHMIC AGENTS

	Proarrhythmia			
	Torsades de Pointes	Sustained Ventricular Tachycardia/Ventricular Fibrillation in High-Risk Patients*	Bradyarrhythmias	Negative Inotropic Effects
Quinidine	2%	1%	+	0
Procainamide	1–2%	1%	+	+
Disopyramide	1–2%	1%	+	+ + +
Moricizine		5–45%	+	+ +
Mexiletine		1%	+	+ +
Tocainide		1%	+	+ +
Flecainide		4–16%	+ +	+ +
Propafenone		5%	+ +	+ + +
Amiodarone	0.7%	2–4%	+ + +	0
Sotalol	2–4%	8%	+ + +	+ + +
Beta blocker	—	0	+ + +	+ + +

Symbols: +, mild; + +, moderate; + + +, pronounced.
*Patients with a history of sustained ventricular tachycardia and ventricular dysfunction.
Data from references 15, 37, 80, 82, 89, 90, and 91.

TABLE 18–5. DRUG INTERACTIONS

Antiarrhythmic Drugs	Effects
Amiodarone	Reduces clearance of warfarin phenytoin digoxin quinidine procainamide
Quinidine	Reduces clearance of propranolol Reduces volume of distribution digoxin
Moricizine	Reduces clearance of warfarin? Increases clearance of theophylline
Mexiletine	Reduces clearance of theophylline
Other Drugs	**Effects on Antiarrhythmic Drugs**
Phenytoin Phenobarbital Rifampin	Increase clearance of quinidine disopyramide mexiletine
Cimetidine	Reduces clearance of quinidine lidocaine procainamide flecainide moricizine
Propranolol	Reduces clearance of lidocaine
Acetazolamide	Reduces clearance of quinidine

at risk for arrhythmia recurrences even if the drug is withheld. Patients without structural heart disease who do not have inducible ventricular tachycardia have a low risk of subsequent severe arrhythmias if antiarrhythmic drugs are withheld.

Proarrhythmia may also be manifested by an increase in nonsustained ventricular tachycardia and ambient ventricular ectopic activity. The latter varies markedly over time, however, and spontaneous fluctuations can mimic a drug's antiarrhythmic or proarrhythmic effect. A marked increase in ventricular ectopy has been observed during initiation of antiarrhythmic therapy in 3%–5% of patients with prior myocardial infarction.[39] These patients often had a similar response to therapy with a second antiarrhythmic drug and an increased mortality rate even though they were not treated chronically with the drug.

Antiarrhythmic drugs may promote an arrhythmia in concert with another factor such as myocardial ischemia. Therapy with flecainide in myocardial infarct survivors continues to increase mortality, even months after initiation of therapy, an effect that has been attributed to "late proarrhythmia."[41] One suggested mechanism is an increase in fatal arrhythmias during episodes of myocardial ischemia.

Negative Inotropic Effects

The hemodynamic and inotropic effects of antiarrhythmic drugs are often due to a complex interplay of actions. Blockade of the fast sodium channel, slow calcium channel, and beta-adrenergic receptors diminishes contractility. Action potential prolongation, which allows more time for calcium transit during systole, and vasodilation tend to offset direct negative inotropic effects. With the exception of quinidine and amiodarone given during chronic oral therapy, all antiarrhythmic drugs have negative inotropic effects,[42–44] which are usually mild and not clinically evident in patients with normal ventricular function. In patients with depressed ventricular function, symptomatic heart failure can occur. Of 167 patients with stable, compensated heart failure, 10% suffered an exacerbation of heart failure when treated with an antiarrhythmic drug.[42] Patients who had severely depressed ventricular function, usually with a left ventricular ejection fraction of less than 0.25 were most susceptible. Even if the drug does not precipitate overt heart failure, negative inotropic effects are a concern during long-term therapy. This may not apply to beta-adrenergic blocking drugs, which improve mortality and reduce sudden death in myocardial infarction survivors who are able to tolerate these drugs.[45, 46]

Interactions with Implantable Defibrillators

Even when a drug does not prevent an arrhythmia, it may be useful for decreasing arrhythmia recurrences and shocks in patients with implanted cardioverter-defibrillators. A variety of potential interactions with the device are possible.[47] Amiodarone can increase the current required for defibrillation. In animal models, other antiarrhythmic drugs may increase, decrease, or have no effect on defibrillation thresholds. Drugs often slow the rate of ventricular tachycardia. Recurrences of ventricular tachycardia may be slower than the detection rate of the device and escape detection. Drugs can alter the pacing threshold and the effectiveness of pacing algorithms for arrhythmia termination. Bradycardia that follows a shock may theoretically be more severe during therapy with drugs that suppress automaticity in the sinus and AV nodes. After a change in antiarrhythmic drug therapy, reevaluation of defibrillator function should be considered, particularly if defibrillation thresholds at implantation were marginal.

Predicting Antiarrhythmic Drug Efficacy

In most patients, recurrences of ventricular tachycardia are infrequent and unpredictable. Absence of ventricular tachycardia during observation for a few days in the hospital does not ensure long-term freedom from attacks. For patients with arrhythmias that are not life-threatening, or if an antiarrhythmic drug has high efficacy, empirical drug therapy is an option. The medication is administered to achieve a desired serum level, electrocardiographic effect, or dose. This approach is often used with amiodarone. For patients with potentially life-threatening arrhythmias, a means of predicting drug efficacy is desirable. The most useful clinical predictor is ventricular function. The risk of arrhythmia recurrences and sudden death increases with decreasing ventricular function.

Invasive Electrophysiologic Testing

In patients with sustained ventricular tachycardia that can be initiated by pacing, antiarrhythmic drug effects can be assessed during electrophysiologic study.[48–53] The exact pacing protocol and criteria for drug efficacy vary from laboratory to laboratory.[32] The patient is first studied in the absence of medication to define the inducible arrhythmia. The antiarrhythmic drug is then administered until the desired serum level and/or electrocardiographic effect is achieved, and the study is repeated. If the ventricular tachycardia is still provokable, a period for drug washout is allowed, followed by a second drug test, a process referred to as serial testing. A drug that suppresses initiation of ventricular tachycardia can be identified in 20%–50% of patients. An effective drug is identified in fewer than 25% of patients who have had prior myocardial infarction and have a left ventricular ejection fraction less than 0.25, but a drug that is efficacious is identified in more than 40% of patients who have a left ventricular ejection fraction greater than 0.40. Patients who have a favorable response to one drug, or to intravenous procainamide, are more likely to respond to other drugs as well.

The accuracy of electrophysiologic study for predicting long-term prevention of arrhythmia recurrences is controversial and probably modest. Patients in whom a drug suppresses ventricular tachycardia have a lower risk of sudden death than do patients in whom a drug does not suppress ventricular tachycardia.[50–52] During therapy with drugs predicted to be effective by electrophysiologic study in the Electrophysiologic Study Versus Electrocardiographic Monitoring (ESVEM) trial (Table 18–6), the probability of death from arrhythmia was 10% at 1 year and 24% at 4 years.[48] The probability of an arrhythmia recurrence was 32% at 1 year and 64% at 4 years. It is possible that more aggressive stimulation protocols than were used in this trial could have identified patients with lower arrhythmia recurrence rates at the expense of identifying fewer acute drug responders. The prognostic significance of inducible ventricular tachycardia during therapy with amiodarone, which was not assessed in the ESVEM trial, is even less clear (see discussion further on).

Antiarrhythmic drugs often slow ventricular tachycardia, improving hemodynamic tolerance. This can also be assessed during electrophysiologic study, but the prognostic significance is controversial.[49]

Suppression of Ventricular Ectopy

Assessing suppression of ambient ventricular ectopic activity on electrocardiographic monitoring has also been used to predict drug efficacy.[48, 52] This requires the presence of frequent ventricular ectopy at baseline because spontaneous ventricular ectopic activity varies markedly from day to day. In the ESVEM trial, a minimum of 10 premature ventricular ectopic beats hourly during a 48-h recording period were required.[48] This severity of ectopy was present in 84% of patients who had suffered a sustained arrhythmia. Arrhythmia suppression by a drug was defined as suppression of 70% of total premature ventricular contractions, 80% of couplets, and 90% of ventricular tachycardia runs, with no runs longer than 15 beats. Arrhythmia suppression was achieved in 77% of patients and varied among drugs (see Table 18–6). Despite suppression of ambient ventricular ectopy, the probability of arrhythmia recurrence was 41% at 1 year and 67% by 4 years. Death resulting from an arrhythmia occurred in 9% of patients at 1 year and 17% at 4 years.

Exercise Testing

Some ventricular tachycardias are reliably provoked by exercise so that exercise testing can be used to assess drug effects. Circulating and myocardial catecholamines and the increase in heart rate are major factors in initiating these arrhythmias. Beta-adrenergic stimulation reduces the electrophysiologic effects of antiarrhythmic drugs.[54, 55] An increase in heart rate during activity or emotional upset can also alter drug effects.[56] During therapy with quinidine and sotalol, the drug-induced prolongation of action potential duration decreases as heart rate increases. This phenomenon is refered to as reverse use dependence.[56] Exercise may thereby reverse drug effects and precipitate an arrhythmia recurrence. Exercise testing is also useful for exposing proarrhythmic effects with some drugs.[57] The class IC drugs flecainide and propafenone have marked use-dependent conduction slowing effects.[6] Rapid heart rates can precipitate marked QRS widening with hemodynamic deterioration and occasionally ventricular fibrillation.

Specific Antiarrhythmic Drugs

Amiodarone

Amiodarone is a potent class III antiarrhythmic drug with important toxicities and drug interactions (see Table 18–5).[6, 58–61] In contrast to quinidine and sotalol, its effect on repolarization does not display reverse use dependency. It also blunts the chronotropic response to beta-adrenergic stimulation. It has a large volume of distribution and a slow elimination half-life that exceeds 25 days. During oral administration, the onset of action requires 2–3 days, and electrophysiologic effects may continue to increase over weeks. For patients with sustained ventricular tachycardia, a loading dose of 800–1600 mg/day is administered in divided doses for 1–2 weeks. The daily dose may then be reduced to 600–800 mg for 1–2 weeks or reduced to 400 mg. If a rapid onset of action is desired for life-threatening, frequent ventricular tachycardia, intravenous amiodarone can be administered (see preceding discussion). Alternatively, if gastrointestinal absorption is intact, 50 mg/kg/day administered orally can achieve an effect within 24–48 h.[60] After 3 days, the dose can be reduced for the remainder of the loading period. The electrophysiologic effects are manifested as slowing of the heart rate, QT interval prolongation, and suppression of ventricular ectopic beats.[61] To reduce side effects during chronic maintenance therapy, the dose should be tapered to the minimum required. In patients treated for sustained ventricular tachycardia, the usual maintenance dose is 300–400 mg/day. For less severe arrhythmias, doses of 200 mg/day and occasionally lower are often used. The long half-life allows administration of maintenance doses once daily and in some cases less frequently. During long-term therapy, plasma concentrations exceeding 0.5–1 μg/dL have been associated with suppression of ventricular ectopy.[59] Concentrations exceeding 2.5 μg/dL have been associated with increased toxicity.

Amiodarone alters the metabolism of a number of drugs (see Table 18–5). The effect of warfarin is potentiated and serum digoxin levels are increased. The doses of these medications should be reduced by one third to one half when amiodarone therapy is initiated. Further dose adjustments are often required.

TABLE 18–6. EFFICACY AND ADVERSE EVENTS OF ANTIARRHYTHMIC AGENTS IN THE ELECTROPHYSIOLOGIC STUDY VERSUS ELECTROCARDIOGRAPHIC MONITORING (ESVEM) TRIAL

	Suppression of Ventricular Ectopy (%)	Suppression of Inducible Ventricular Tachycardia (%)	Discontinued Because of Adverse Event* (%)	1-Year Recurrence of Ventricular Tachycardia During Chronic Therapy (%)
Sotalol	56	35	23	20
Quinidine	59	16	56	45
Procainamide	50	26	55	46
Mexiletine	67	12	46	50
Propafenone	48	14	39	38

*Adverse event includes cardiac and noncardiac side effects and arrhythmias during initial dose titration and follow-up.

From Mason JW for the Electrophysiologic Study Versus Electrocardiographic Monitoring Investigators: A comparison of seven antiarrhythmic drugs in patients with ventricular tachyarrhythmia. N Engl J Med 1993; 329:452–458.

Amiodarone has often been used as a last-resort antiarrhythmic drug when other agents are ineffective.[62-64] In patients who had life-threatening ventricular arrhythmias, the risk of an arrhythmia recurrence during amiodarone therapy was 15%–19% at 1 year and 38%–43% at 5 years. Death attributed to an arrhythmia occurred in 9% of patients at 1 year and 21%–22% of patients at 5 years. As with other drugs, the risk of arrhythmia recurrences and sudden death is higher in patients with severely depressed ventricular function. Predicting outcome with invasive electrophysiologic study or ambulatory electrocardiographic recordings is difficult.[65, 66] The optimal time for evaluation is not clear because of the long half-life of the drug. The majority of patients do not suffer arrhythmia recurrences despite the persistence of inducible ventricular tachycardia. An analysis of several trials found that inducible ventricular tachycardia was suppressed in only 31% of patients.[65] The probability of an arrhythmia recurrence was 14% in patients whose tachycardia was rendered noninducible and 37% for patients with persistently inducible ventricular tachycardia. Suppression of ventricular ectopy has been of variable utility for predicting efficacy.[65, 66]

The risk of proarrhythmia during amiodarone therapy is relatively low.[67] Amiodarone can cause torsades de pointes, but this is rare when it is administered as the sole antiarrhythmic agent. Proarrhythmia occasionally becomes manifested as frequent or incessant ventricular tachycardia. Amiodarone is relatively safe in patients with coronary artery disease.[58, 68] It does not increase arrhythmia-related mortality in myocardial infarction survivors. Amiodarone reduces angina, probably by coronary vasodilation and heart rate slowing.[69] It can, however, increase serum lipid levels.[70] It increases the current required for defibrillation by implantable defibrillators but is more effective in reducing defibrillator discharges than are class I drugs.[47, 71]

During long-term therapy, the majority of patients experience some side effect.[62, 63, 71] Therapy is discontinued because of an adverse effect in 10%–29% of patients by 2 years and in 18%–37% of patients by 5 years. Most side effects are dose- and time-related. Only 5% of myocardial infarction survivors receiving 200 mg of amiodarone daily discontinued the drug because of side effects during therapy for a median of 2.9 years.[68]

Amiodarone potently suppresses sinus node automaticity and AV node conduction. It should not be administered to patients who have symptomatic bradyarrhythmias in the absence of a permanent pacemaker. Monitoring for bradyarrhythmias during the first 4–7 days of therapy is prudent in patients with conduction system disease. Bradyarrhythmias can be exacerbated by combining amiodarone with beta-adrenergic blockers, calcium channel blockers, and digoxin. When bradyarrhythmias develop during long-term therapy, hypothyroidism caused by the drug should be considered (see later discussion).

In patients with severely depressed ventricular function, heart rate slowing during oral loading can cause a fall in cardiac output and increase cardiac filling pressures, although stroke volume is preserved.[72] During chronic oral therapy, amiodarone is well tolerated in patients with depressed ventricular function; left ventricular ejection fraction and exercise capacity often improve during chronic therapy.[73, 74] Intravenous amiodarone has negative inotropic and vasodilatory effects, which can precipitate cardiogenic shock when administered rapidly in patients with heart failure (see earlier discussion).

Noncardiac toxicities are a major concern. Patients should be followed closely for pulmonary, hepatic, and thyroid toxicities. Pulmonary toxicity occurs in 1.8% of patients yearly and has a mortality rate of 9.1%.[75, 76] Older patients and those with reduced pulmonary diffusing capacity are most susceptible. Pulmonary toxicity occurs most frequently after 3–12 months of therapy and is uncommon at maintenance doses of 300 mg/day or less. The clinical presentation is variable and can be difficult to distinguish from heart failure. During chronic therapy, chest radiographs should be obtained every 3–6 months in patients receiving more than 300 mg/day. The value of serial pulmonary function testing is controversial. If pulmonary toxicity develops, the drug should be discontinued immediately.

Amiodarone has been associated with an increased risk of postoperative adult respiratory distress syndrome in patients undergoing heart surgery.[77, 78] It has been suggested that oxygen free radicals generated during exposure to high oxygen concentrations are involved. In some cases, unrecognized pulmonary toxicity may have been present preoperatively. A careful evaluation for pulmonary toxicity is warranted when surgery is anticipated. The drug should be discontinued before heart surgery when possible. In patients undergoing heart transplantation, prior amiodarone therapy increases postoperative bradyarrhythmias but has not been associated with increased pulmonary toxicity.[79] Amiodarone may increase the need for inotropic agents after surgery.[77]

Amiodarone accumulates in the liver during chronic therapy. Elevation of hepatic transaminases is common. Persistent elevation greater than twice normal warrants a decrease in dose or discontinuation of the drug. Cirrhosis can occur but is rare.[6]

Amiodarone has some structural similarities to thyroid hormone.[80] Each molecule contains two iodine atoms. Amiodarone diminishes conversion of thyroxine (T_4) to triiodothyronine (T_3). During chronic therapy, T_4 levels are usually elevated, whereas serum T_3 and thyroid-stimulating hormone (TSH) remain in the normal range. Hyper- or hypothyroidism develops in 5%–10% of patients. In regions where dietary iodine intake is low, hyperthyroidism predominates. In other regions, hypothyroidism is more common. A TSH level should be obtained before initiating therapy and every 6 months during chronic therapy. Asymptomatic, subclinical hypothyroidism indicated by a mild elevation of TSH does not necessitate replacement therapy. More severe hypothyroidism can be managed by careful titration of supplemental thyroxine to suppress TSH into the normal range. Hyperthyroidism is confirmed by reduced serum TSH and is more difficult to control. Treatment with propylthiouracil or methimazole and withdrawal of amiodarone may be required.

Amiodarone often causes cutaneous photosensitivity, increasing susceptibility to sunburn in patients with fair complexions. Susceptible patients should use sunblock and protective clothing during prolonged sun exposure.

Sotalol

Sotalol is a potent class III drug that prolongs action potential duration and refractoriness in Purkinje fibers and ventricular muscle.[56, 81] It possesses noncardioselective beta-adrenergic blocking activity similar in potency to that of propranolol. Sotalol is available as a racemic mixture of *d*- and *l*- isomers. The *d*-isomer possesses 1/50 of the beta-blocking activity of the *l*-isomer.

Sotalol was compared with several class I agents in patients with sustained ventricular arrhythmias in the ESVEM trial (see Table 18–6).[53] Sotalol suppressed inducible ventricular tachycardia in 35% of patients. Tachycardia that remaind inducible was slowed in approximately half of patients.[81] Ambient ventricular ectopy was markedly suppressed in 56% of patients. In patients with sustained ventricular tachycardia in whom ambient ventricular ectopy or inducible ventricular tachycardia was suppressed, the probability of an arrhythmia recurrence during the next year was 20%.

During therapy for ventricular tachycardia, proarrhythmic events occur in up to 8% of patients.[81] Torsades de pointes (see later discussion) occurs in 2%–4% of patients. The incidence is dose-related and exceeds 4% at doses of 480 mg/day or more. Torsades de pointes occurs in fewer than 2% of patients when the QT_C interval during therapy is less than 0.5 $sec^{-1/2}$ and occurs in more than 5% of patients when the QT_C interval exceeds 0.55 $sec^{-1/2}$. Episodes usually occur within 7 days of initiating therapy. Later episodes may be precipitated by hypokalemia or bradycardia. Particular caution should be used in patients who are receiving potassium-wasting diuretic drugs.

Side effects prevent long-term therapy in approximately 16% of patients and are often related to the drug's beta-adrenergic blocking activity.[53] Sotalol is generally avoided in patients with severely depressed ventricular function. Aggravation of heart failure has been observed in 3% of patients.[81] Because of the risk of bradyarrhythmias, sotalol should not be administered to patients with sick sinus syndrome or AV block in the absence of a pacemaker. Hypotension, bronchospasm, and fatigue also occur.

Quinidine

Quinidine is a class IA drug that also prolongs action potential duration.[6] Quinidine suppresses inducible ventricular tachycardia on electrophysiologic study in 16% of patients and ventricular ectopy and nonsustained ventricular tachycardia on electrocardiographic monitoring in 59% of patients (see Table 18–6).[53] Ventricular tachycardia that remains inducible is often slowed. In patients in whom the drug suppresses inducible ventricular tachycardia or ambient ventricular ectopy, the risk of arrhythmia recurrence during the following year is as high as 45%. In contrast to other sodium channel blocking drugs and sotalol, it does not have negative inotropic effects in vivo.[44] Torsades de pointes occurs in up to 2% of patients, most commonly during the first 3 days of therapy.[82] Episodes that occur late during chronic therapy are often precipitated by an additional factor that prolongs repolarization, such as hypokalemia. Side effects, most frequently nausea and diarrhea, prevent long-term therapy in 30%–40% of patients.[53] In some cases, diarrhea can be ameliorated by a psyllium preparation such as Metamucil.

Procainamide

Procainamide is a class IA drug that also prolongs the duration of the action potential.[83] It is metabolized in the liver to *N*-acetylprocainamide, which is excreted through the kidney. Two phenotypes for acetylation are present. Rapid acetylation, observed in 50% of the U.S. population and in 80% of Asians, generally produces an *N*-acetylprocainamide level equal to or exceeding that of procainamide during chronic therapy. *N*-acetylprocainamide prolongs action potential duration but does not block the fast sodium current. Sustained-release procainamide preparations allow dosing at 6- to 8-h intervals.

Procainamide suppresses inducible ventricular tachycardia on electrophysiologic study in 26% of patients and markedly suppresses ambient ventricular ectopy in 50% of patients.[53] Ventricular tachycardia that remains inducible is often slowed. The effects of intravenous procainamide on inducible ventricular tachycardia do not necessarily predict the response to oral procainamide.

Proarrhythmic effects are infrequent.[37] In patients with renal insufficiency, *N*-acetylprocainamide can accumulate to high levels and cause torsades de pointes. Procainamide possesses mild negative inotropic effects, which can be clinically significant in patients with severely depressed ventricular function.[43, 44] Noncardiac side effects, including rash and nausea, and neurologic side effects are common. During long- term therapy, 60%–70% of patients acquire antinuclear antibodies and 20%–30% experience symptomatic systemic lupus erythematosus, which resolves over weeks to months after discontinuation of the drug. Agranulocytosis can also occur.

Disopyramide

Disopyramide is a class IA drug that also prolongs repolarization.[6] It has prominent negative inotropic effects and can precipitate hemodynamic collapse in patients with severe ventricular dysfunction. Anticholinergic side effects frequently cause xerostomia and blurred vision. Acute urinary retention can occur in susceptible patients. The drug is therefore avoided in men older than 50 years of age who are likely to have prostatic hypertrophy. Disopyramide prolongs the QT interval and can produce torsades de pointes.

Mexiletine

Mexiletine is a class IB drug with electrophysiologic effects similar to those of lidocaine. Mexiletine suppresses inducible ventricular tachycardia on electrophysiologic study in only 12% of patients and markedly suppresses ambient ventricular ectopy in 67% of patients (see Table 18–6).[53] Proarrhythmic effects are infrequent and are observed in 1.2% of patients.[37] The drug does not prolong the QT interval and does not appear to cause torsades de pointes. Mexiletine has often been given in combination with quinidine, disopyramide, procainamide, amiodarone, or flecainide.[84, 85] The combination is occasionally effective when neither drug individually suppresses ventricular tachycardia. Mexiletine has mild negative inotropic effects that can exacerbate heart failure in patients with impaired ventricular function.[42, 44] It can precipitate bradyarrhythmias in patients with sinus node or conduction system disease. Its major limitations are neurologic toxicity, most commonly tremor, and nausea.

Tocainide

Tocainide is a class IB drug with electrophysiologic actions similar to those of mexiletine.[6] It does not prolong the QT interval. Proarrhythmic effects are infrequent. Its use has been restricted to serious ventricular arrhythmias that have not responded to other drugs because of a 0.2% incidence of agranulocytosis. It has negative inotropic effects that can exacerbate heart failure in patients with impaired ventricular function.[43] Neurologic side effects are frequent.

Flecainide

Flecainide is a class IC drug that blocks the fast sodium current in a use-dependent manner with slow onset and offset kinetics.[6, 57] At rapid rates, ventricular conduction can be markedly slowed. Flecainide suppresses inducible ventricular tachycardia in 14% of patients who have suffered spontaneous ventricular tachycardia.[15] Proarrhythmia is a major concern. Frequent or incessant ventricular tachycardia is observed in up to 30% of patients treated for sustained ventricular arrhythmias who have depressed ventricular function.[6, 15, 37] Because of the marked use-dependent effects, rapid heart rates during exercise or supraventricular arrhythmias occasionally precipitate sustained, wide QRS sinusoidal ventricular tachycardia.[57, 86] This usually occurs in patients with underlying heart disease. Exercise testing has been recommended before hospital discharge to screen for proarrhythmia.

Flecainide suppresses ventricular ectopy and nonsustained ventricular tachycardia in more than 80% of patients with these arrhythmias after myocardial infarction, but mortality is increased despite arrhythmia suppression.[87, 88] The cause of the excess deaths is not established, but proarrhythmia has been suggested. Flecainide does not prolong repolarization; torsades de pointes, if it occurs, is rare.

Flecainide can exacerbate bradyarrhythmias and should not be administered to patients with sick sinus syndrome or AV block in the absence of a pacemaker. Negative inotropic effects can exacerbate heart failure. Mild neurologic side effects occur in up to 30% of patients.[88]

Propafenone

Propafenone is a class IC drug that blocks the fast sodium current in a use-dependent manner with slow onset and offset kinetics.[6] It is hepatically metabolized to 5-hydroxy-propafenone and *N*-dealkylpropafenone, both of which have sodium channel blocking activity.[89] The parent compound also has beta-adrenergic blocking properties. Approximately 7% of the U.S. population is deficient in the enzyme producing the 5-hydroxy metabolite, which has little beta-adrenergic blocking activity. These patients have higher levels of the parent drug, with consequent greater beta-adrenergic blocking effects.

Propafenone suppresses inducible ventricular tachycardia on electrophysiologic study in 14% of patients and markedly suppresses spontaneous ventricular ectopy in 48% of patients (see Table 18–6).[53] Ventricular tachycardia that remains inducible is often slowed. During therapy of ventricular arrhythmias, life-threatening proarrhythmia has been observed in up to 5% of patients.[37, 90] Because of prominent use-dependent conduction slowing, proarrhythmia precipitated by rapid heart rates can occur, as with flecainide. Propafenone rarely prolongs action potential duration, and torsades de pointes, if it occurs, is rare. It suppresses sinus and AV node function and can cause severe bradyarrhythmias in susceptible patients. Noncardiac adverse effects are generally minor and result in drug discontinuation in 6% of patients.

Moricizine

Moricizine is a class I drug. It suppresses inducible ventricular tachycardia in 10%–30% of patients and often slows the rate of inducible ventricular tachycardia.[91] Frequent ventricular ectopy and spontaneous nonsustained ventricular tachycardia are suppressed in 60%–80% of patients.[88, 91] The risk of proarrhythmic effects ranges from 3.2% to as high as 38% in patients with depressed ventricular function who have a history of sustained ventricular arrhythmias.[91, 92] In the Cardiac Arrhythmia Suppression Trial (CAST),[93] survivors of myocardial infarction who had a left ventricular ejection fraction of less than 0.40 and frequent ventricular ectopy had an increased risk of death or cardiac arrest during the first 14 days of moricizine therapy (2.5% as compared with 0.5% for the placebo group). After this early period, deaths were not increased during long-term therapy. Moricizine does not prolong repolarization, but possible cases of torsades de pointes have been reported.[92] Moricizine has negative inotropic effects; aggravation of heart failure is observed in 5%–15% of patients who have a prior history of heart failure.[42, 91] Bradyarrhythmias and conduction defects have been observed in 2% of patients.

Beta-Adrenergic Blockers

Many ventricular arrhythmias are exacerbated by increased sympathetic nervous system activity such as occurs with exertion or emotional upset. Beta-adrenergic blockers can blunt the adverse effects of sympathetic activation. These agents alone rarely achieve complete arrhythmia supression. In patients with inducible sustained ventricular tachycardia, treatment with only a beta blocker is associated with a high risk of arrhythmia recurrence.[50, 85] Steinbeck and coworkers randomized patients resuscitated from sustained ventricular tachycardia or ventricular fibrillation to empirical therapy with metoprolol or an antiarrhythmic drug selected by electrophysiologic testing.[50] During a mean follow-up of 23 months, sudden death occurred in 15% of patients treated with metoprolol alone, compared with 10% of patients treated with an antiarrhythmic drug that suppressed inducible ventricular tachycardia. Ventricular tachycardia recurred but was not fatal in 37% of the metoprolol-treated patients as compared with 10% of patients whose ventricular tachycardia was rendered noninducible during electrophysiologic study. Beta-adrenergic blockers are often useful when administered in combination with an antiarrhythmic drug.[54, 55, 94–96] Sympathetic stimulation can markedly reduce the electrophysiologic effects of antiarrhythmic drugs. The addition of a beta-adrenergic blocker can potentially preserve drug effects during increases in sympathetic tone. Therapy with beta-adrenergic blockers is limited by negative inotropic effects, hypotension, and aggravation of bradyarrhythmias, particularly when given in combination with antiarrhythmic drugs that cause similar adverse effects.

VENTRICULAR ARRHYTHMIAS RESULTING FROM CORONARY ARTERY DISEASE

Ventricular Arrhythmias During Acute Myocardial Infarction

Ventricular fibrillation or polymorphic ventricular tachycardia (see Fig. 18–1*B*) degenerating to ventricular fibrillation occurs in 1%–5% of patients during the first day in the hospital.[97, 98] The risk of ventricular fibrillation during acute myocardial infarction is greatest in the first hour and then diminishes rapidly. After defibrillation, the risk of recurrent ventricular fibrillation is relatively low. The risk of ventricular fibrillation during the first 2 weeks in the hospital is 15%. Patients with ventricular fibrillation preceded by heart failure or hypotension, referred to as secondary ventricular fibrillation, have an in-hospital mortality rate of up to 56%, probably resulting from associated large myocardial infarctions.[99] After resuscitation, attention should focus on management of the infarction. Many centers initiate therapy with intravenous lidocaine for 24 h. Recurrent episodes of polymorphic ventricular tachycardia or ventricular fibrillation suggest ongoing myocardial ischemia or a terminal event occurring during cardiogenic shock. Patients who survive to hospital discharge do not have an increased risk of sudden death during long-term follow-up and, in the absence of late recurrences, do not generally require long-term antiarrhythmic therapy.

During acute myocardial infarction, ventricular premature beats occur in virtually all patients, and nonsustained ventricular tachycardia or accelerated idioventricular rhythms occur in more than 50% of patients.[100] Although ventricular ectopy, and particularly idioventricular rhythms, are common during acute reperfusion, the incidence of ventricular fibrillation is not increased and may be reduced by thrombolytic therapy.[97, 100] Routine administration of prophylactic lidocaine decreases the risk of ventricular fibrillation but may increase the risk of death from asystole and is therefore not warranted.[97, 98] Beta-adrenergic blockers decreased the incidence of ventricular fibrillation during acute infarction in trials that did not administer thrombolytic therapy.[100] Intravenous magnesium sulfate reduces the incidence of ventricular fibrillation when administered before thrombolytic therapy.[101]

Long runs of ventricular tachycardia, lasting several seconds or minutes, occur in 2% of patients during acute myocardial infarction.[100] They are often relatively slow, 120–150 beats per minute, and frequently terminate spontaneously without producing hemodynamic compromise. The mechanism may be automaticity, and this arrhythmia does not indicate an increased risk for future arrhythmic events.

Sustained Monomorphic Ventricular Tachycardia After Myocardial Infarction

Sustained monomorphic ventricular tachycardia (see Fig. 18–1*A*) later than 48 h after myocardial infarction is due to reentry in the region of the infarct.[1] Tachycardia usually occurs in the absence of apparent myocardial ischemia and indicates a chronic substrate. Patients are subject to recurrent episodes, often over several years.

Sustained monomorphic ventricular tachycardia may present as hemodynamically tolerated wide complex tachycardia, syncope, or out-of-hospital cardiac arrest (also discussed further on). In the latter case, ventricular tachycardia has usually degenerated to ventricular fibrillation by the time paramedics arrive. Serum enzyme evidence of acute myocardial infarction is usually absent but occasionally occurs as a consequence of the hypotension and diminished myocardial perfusion produced by ventricular tachycardia.[102] Recurrences are likely if therapy is directed only to correcting ischemia.

The severity of coronary artery disease should be assessed. In most cases, coronary angiography should be performed and left ventricular ejection fraction and segmental wall motion abnormalities should be defined. In the vast majority of cases, a discrete region of akinesis or dyskinesis on ventriculography or echocardiography indicates a prior myocardial infarction that is the source of the arrhythmia. If ventricular wall motion is entirely normal, other possibilities must be considered, including supraventricular tachycardia with aberrancy, bundle branch reentry, and idiopathic ventricular tachycardia (see later discussion).

If the diagnosis is in question, an electrophysiologic study should be performed. In more than 90% of patients who have had spontaneous sustained monomorphic ventricular tachycardia, programmed electrical stimulation initiates this arrhythmia.[32] Most patients have the potential for more than one QRS morphologic characteristic of ventricular tachycardia.[103]

Patients who have suffered an episode of sustained monomorphic ventricular tachycardia late after myocardial infarction are subject to recurrences. Of 390 patients who survived sustained ventricular tachycardia or ventricular fibrillation late after myocardial infarction, 49% suffered a nonfatal arrhythmia recurrence and 19% died suddenly during the following 2 years despite therapy with antiarrhythmic drugs or surgery.[104] The majority of arrhythmia recurrences do not cause sudden death.[48, 104] Factors associated with an increased risk of death are ventricular tachycardia within 6–8 weeks of myocardial infarction, cardiac arrest at presentation, and severe ventricular dysfunction as indicated by multiple prior myocardial infarctions, heart failure during the acute infarction, a left ventricular ejection fraction less than 0.30, and New York Heart Association functional class III or worse because of dyspnea.[104–108]

Therapeutic options include antiarrhythmic drugs, implantable cardioverter-defibrillators (see Chapter 21), and ablative therapy (see Chapter 19). Selection of therapy should be based on prognostic factors, the severity of coronary artery disease, functional status, and the patient's concerns and preferences (Fig. 18–6). If coronary artery disease warrants coronary artery bypass grafting, concomitant ablative ventricular tachycardia surgery or implantation of a cardioverter-defibrillator should be considered (see Chapters 19 and 21). If episodes of tachycardia are frequent, ablative therapy or antiarrhythmic drugs are required to control symptoms. The likelihood that a drug will suppress ventricular tachycardia diminishes and the risk of proarrhythmia increases with the severity of left ventricular dysfunction.[48, 62] The drugs with the highest efficacy are amiodarone and sotalol.[53, 62, 63] The beta-adrenergic blocking properties of sotalol are beneficial in coronary artery disease, but associated side effects limit its use in many patients. Amiodarone is hemodynamically well tolerated and has desirable anti-ischemic effects and a low potential for proarrhythmia, but long-term side effects are a major problem. Amiodarone also has the potential to increase the current required for defibrillation by implantable defibrillators.[47] If cardiac surgery is an option, the possible increased perioperative risk of pulmonary complications should be considered before initiating therapy with amiodarone.[77, 78] Class I antiarrhythmic drugs are less effective but are useful in some patients. Because flecainide and moricizine increase mortality in myocardial infarct survivors, these drugs should be avoided.[93] In the preliminary analysis of one trial, propafenone was less effective in preventing death than was an implantable cardioverter-defibrillator.[109]

One approach to selecting the initial therapy is shown in Figure 18–6. Patients who have hemodynamically well-tolerated ventricular tachycardia and a left ventricular ejection fraction greater than 0.40 have a low risk of sudden death and often respond to an antiarrhythmic drug.[52, 108] Therapy with sotalol is initiated in the hospital, and the patient is monitored for proarrhythmic effects before discharge. If sotalol is not tolerated, empirical therapy with amiodarone or a class I drug guided by electrophysiologic testing or suppression of ambient ventricular ectopy is considered. Exercise testing is prudent before hospital discharge if the initial arrhythmia was provoked by exertion or excitement. If ventricular tachycardia is well tolerated but symptomatic heart failure is present or left ventricular function is severely depressed with a left ventricular ejection fraction of less than 0.25, amiodarone is chosen as the initial agent.

Patients with monomorphic ventricular tachycardia presenting with cardiac arrest have a 15%–21% risk of sudden death over the following 2 years, and the risk is even higher in those with severely depressed ventricular function.[52, 64, 105, 107] Even if inducible ventricular tachycardia is suppressed by a class I drug on electrophysiologic testing, patients with a left ventricular ejection fraction of less than 0.30 have a 2-year mortality rate exceeding 30%. An implantable cardioverter-defibrillator or therapy with amiodarone or sotalol should be considered.

Amiodarone is initiated in the hospital, with monitoring for 7–10

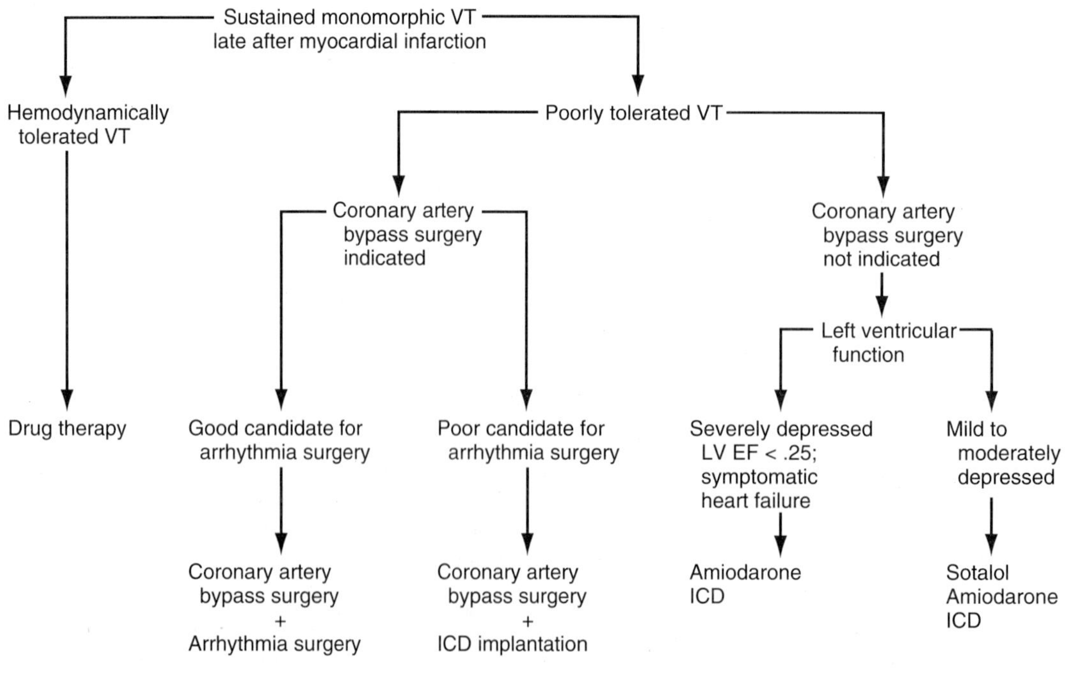

Figure 18–6. Flow diagram for selecting initial therapy for sustained monomorphic ventricular tachycardia caused by previous myocardial infarction. *Abbreviations:* LV EF, left ventricular ejection fraction; ICD, implantable cardioverter-defibrillator; VT, ventricular tachycardia.

days to ensure that an electrophysiologic effect is present before discharge. Patients with preserved ventricular function and a left ventricular ejection fraction greater than 0.30 are more likely to have a favorable drug response. Because of the high risk of arrhythmia recurrences during therapy with a class I drug or sotalol, an electrophysiologic study is often considered to assess the presence of inducible ventricular tachycardia and the hemodynamic response to the induced tachycardia.[49, 52] If ventricular tachycardia remains inducible and is poorly tolerated, nonpharmacologic therapy or amiodarone is considered.

As discussed previously, beta-adrenergic blockers can be useful adjuncts to amiodarone or class I drugs.[94–96] Drug combinations must be used cautiously to avoid bradyarrhythmias and aggravation of heart failure.

The Out-of-Hospital Ventricular Fibrillation Survivor

In patients with coronary artery disease, ventricular fibrillation most commonly results from one of three causes: acute myocardial infarction, transient myocardial ischemia, or ventricular tachycardia that degenerates to ventricular fibrillation.[34, 106, 110] When paramedics arrive, the cause of the ventricular fibrillation is usually unclear. After resuscitation, evidence for acute myocardial infarction should be sought and the severity of coronary artery disease defined (see Fig. 18–5). In the absence of a new thrombotic myocardial infarction, reentrant ventricular tachycardia must be strongly considered, particularly in patients with an old infarct. Electrophysiologic testing induces sustained monomorphic ventricular tachycardia in 32% of patients, almost all of whom have a healed myocardial infarction.[107] Induced ventricular tachycardia is usually faster than 200 beats per minute and often produces syncope, suggesting that ventricular tachycardia degenerating to ventricular fibrillation caused the cardiac arrest.[32, 106] The risk of recurrent ventricular tachycardia is high; these patients should be managed as discussed earlier.

If severe coronary artery disease is present but no ventricular tachycardia is inducible on electrophysiologic study, the most likely mechanism of the arrest was ventricular fibrillation related to a transient episode of ischemia. Absence of a prior myocardial infarct scar to serve as the potential cause of a reentrant ventricular tachycardia further supports this diagnosis. If coronary artery disease is present but does not appear to be severe, an assessment of provokable myocardial ischemia with exercise testing and perfusion imaging may be helpful in assessing likely ischemia. Coronary artery spasm should also be considered.[34] Therapy focuses on treatment of ischemia. In appropriate candidates, coronary artery bypass surgery is associated with a risk of recurrent cardiac arrest of less than 5% over 3 years and should be strongly considered.[111, 112]

In 16% of patients resuscitated from ventricular fibrillation in the absence of myocardial infarction, programmed stimulation induces polymorphic ventricular tachycardia or ventricular fibrillation.[32, 49, 107] Although this arrhythmia can be a nonspecific response to programmed stimulation, in this subgroup of patients it may also indicate the cause of the arrest. If myocardial ischemia is not the likely cause of the arrest, an implantable cardioverter-defibrillator or antiarrhythmic drug therapy, as for sustained monomorphic ventricular tachycardia, should be considered.

In some cases, ventricular tachycardia or ischemia, or a combination of the two, remain as potential causes after evaluation. Therapy should be directed at both. Occasionally, postoperative electrophysiologic testing is useful. Polymorphic ventricular tachycardia inducible before coronary artery revascularization but absent postoperatively suggests a role for transient ischemia in causing cardiac arrest.[112]

Syncope

Ventricular tachycardia may cause syncope before terminating spontaneously.[113] Of 41 patients with prior myocardial infarction referred for electrophysiologic study to evaluate syncope, 37% had inducible sustained monomorphic ventricular tachycardia, suggesting this as the cause.[114] Management is as discussed previously for poorly tolerated ventricular tachycardia (see Fig. 18–6).

Nonsustained Ventricular Tachycardia and Ventricular Ectopy

Nonsustained ventricular tachycardia is observed on 24-h electrocardiogram recordings in 7%–8% of myocardial infarction survivors.[115, 116] These tachycardias are usually slower than 200 beats per minute and shorter than 10 beats in duration. Frequent ventricular ectopic activity and nonsustained ventricular tachycardia are more common in patients with depressed ventricular function but are independent predictors of mortality and sudden death. Antiarrhythmic drug therapy with flecainide, encainide, or moricizine increases mortality despite suppression of nonsustained ventricular tachycardia.[87, 93] Meta-analysis of trials including other class I antiarrhythmic drugs suggest no benefit and also support the possibility that mortality could be increased.[117] Routine treatment of ventricular ectopy and nonsustained ventricular tachycardia in patients with coronary artery disease is not warranted.

Beta-adrenergic blocking drugs reduce ventricular ectopy in some patients and reduce sudden death in survivors of myocardial infarction, although this may not be related to an effect on ambient arrhythmias.[46, 117] Beta-adrenergic blockers should be administered to those patients able to tolerate them. In patients with symptomatic ventricular ectopy, beta-adrenergic blockers may alleviate symptoms and are safe, although they do not potently suppress ventricular ectopy.

In patients who are unable to tolerate beta-adrenergic blockers but in whom ventricular ectopy produces intolerable symptoms, therapy with amiodarone can be considered, but it must be balanced against the risk of long-term toxicities.[58, 118] Meta-analysis of trials involving 1140 patients after myocardial infarction found that amiodarone therapy (200–400 mg/day) reduced sudden death from 6.9% to 3.1% and total mortality from 11.2% to 6.1%.[118] For this purpose, a loading dose of 600–800 mg/day for 1–2 weeks followed by a maintenance dose of 200 mg/day is often administered. In some patients, the dose can be reduced even further. Amiodarone can also be considered for patients with severely depressed ventricular function and frequent ventricular ectopy.[73, 74, 79] In two large trials of patients with heart failure that included patients with coronary artery disease, amiodarone reduced mortality in patients with severe heart failure in one trial and had no effect on survival, either adverse or beneficial, in the other.[73, 74]

Additional testing can be performed to identify high- and low-risk subgroups of patients after myocardial infarction, but the clinical benefit is not established.[119–122] It is not known if antiarrhythmic therapy is beneficial or harmful in the high-risk group. In patients evaluated within a few weeks of myocardial infarction, a left ventricular ejection fraction of less than 0.40, depressed heart rate variability, an abnormal signal-averaged electrocardiogram, and inducible ventricular tachycardia during electrophysiologic study are associated with an increased risk of sudden death or sustained ventricular tachycardia during the next 1–2 years. Invasive electrophysiologic study within several weeks of the acute infarction induces sustained ventricular tachycardia in 6% of patients.[122] Inducible ventricular tachycardia is more frequent in patients with large, non-reperfused infarctions, a left ventricular ejection fraction of less than 0.40, and an abnormal signal-averaged electrocardiogram.[1] Inducible ventricular tachycardia predicts a 20% risk of spontaneous ventricular tachycardia or sudden death during the next year. Arrhythmic events occur in fewer than 3% of patients who do not have inducible ventricular tachycardia, but the incidence may be higher in patients with myocardial infarction complicated by heart failure. Late after myocardial infarction, sustained ventricular tachycardia is initiated in up to 37%

of patients who have a left ventricular ejection fraction of less than 0.40 and nonsustained ventricular tachycardia on ambulatory electrocardiogram recordings.[120] In one study, patients with a left ventricular ejection fraction of less than 0.40 but no inducible ventricular tachycardia had a 6% probability of sudden death within 2 years.[120] Sudden death or cardiac arrest occurred in 11 of 43 (26%) patients with inducible ventricular tachycardia who were treated with antiarrhythmic drugs. In three patients, cardiac arrest occurred in the hospital shortly after drug therapy was initiated, suggesting a proarrhythmic effect.

VENTRICULAR TACHYCARDIAS UNRELATED TO CORONARY ARTERY DISEASE

Nonischemic Dilated Cardiomyopathy

Sustained Monomorphic Ventricular Tachycardia

Sustained monomorphic ventricular tachycardia is infrequent in patients with nonischemic dilated cardiomyopathy.[79, 123] Of patients referred for possible cardiac transplantation, only 0.5% have a history of sustained monomorphic ventricular tachycardia. The mechanisms of these tachycardias are less well defined than those in coronary artery disease. Programmed ventricular stimulation initiates ventricular tachycardia in 43%–80% of patients, suggesting reentry or triggered automaticity as the tachycardia mechanism. Macroreentry involving the bundle branches causes up to 36% of inducible tachycardias as compared with fewer than 6% of monomorphic ventricular tachycardias in patients with ischemic heart disease.[2] Recognition of bundle branch reentry is important because it can be cured by catheter ablation (see Chapter 19).

Sustained monomorphic ventricular tachycardia is associated with a high risk of recurrent arrhythmias; 20%–25% of patients die suddenly during the following 3 years.[79, 123] Evaluation and therapy are as for sustained monomorphic ventricular tachycardia associated with coronary artery disease. These patients often have severely depressed ventricular function. Negative inotropic effects of antiarrhythmic drugs and proarrhythmia are important considerations.

Ventricular Fibrillation

Causes of ventricular fibrillation in patients with heart failure resulting from dilated cardiomyopathy include torsades de pointes, hyperkalemia, myocardial ischemia from coronary artery emboli, and ventricular tachycardia.[79] In many cases a cause cannot be established. In the absence of a clear cause, electrophysiologic testing should be performed. Sustained monomorphic ventricular tachycardia is inducible in 20%–36% of patients; bundle branch reentry should be excluded.[2] Even if the cause of the cardiac arrest cannot be determined, the risk of recurrence is high. In one study, the 3-year probability of sudden death was 29% for patients resuscitated from sustained ventricular tachycardia or ventricular fibrillation.[123] If the cause cannot be corrected, amiodarone or an implantable cardioverter-defibrillator should be considered.

Nonsustained Ventricular Tachycardia

Nonsustained ventricular tachycardia is observed in 20%–80% of patients with dilated, nonischemic cardiomyopathy.[79] The relation of nonsustained ventricular tachycardia and frequent ventricular ectopy to sudden death is less clear than in myocardial infarction survivors. In the multicenter Vasodilator Heart Failure Trial, 47% of patients had heart failure without coronary artery disease.[124] Nonsustained ventricular tachycardia or ventricular couplets during a 4- to 8-h electrocardiogram recording were associated with a lower left ventricular ejection fraction, poorer exercise capacity, and higher rates of mortality, but not increased rates of sudden death. Electrophysiologic testing is not useful for risk stratification because fewer than 5% of patients have inducible ventricular tachycardia, and the risk of sudden death is high regardless of the results of programmed stimulation when ventricular function is severely depressed. An abnormal signal-averaged electrocardiogram predicted an increased risk in one study, but not in others.[125]

Class I antiarrhythmic drugs generally should be avoided. There is no evidence that suppression of ventricular ectopic activity with these agents is beneficial, and proarrhythmic and negative inotropic effects could conceivably increase mortality. Low-dose amiodarone can be considered for patients with symptomatic ventricular ectopy or severely depressed ventricular function and ventricular ectopy.[73, 74, 79] The benefit must be weighed against the long-term side effects. A loading dose of 600–800 mg/day followed by 200–300 mg/day has been used. It has been suggested that the heart rate slowing effect of amiodarone may be particularly beneficial in patients with inappropriate tachycardia. Bradyarrhythmias, however, are a potentially important cause of sudden death in heart failure. Amiodarone should be avoided in patients with sick sinus syndrome or first-degree or greater AV block unless a pacemaker is present. Two large randomized trials of amiodarone therapy in patients with heart failure resulting from ischemic and nonischemic causes have shown conflicting results. The Grupo de Estudio de la Sobrevida en la Insuficiencia Cardiaca en Argentina (GESICA) trial randomized 516 patients who had an average left ventricular ejection fraction of 0.19–0.20.[74] A third of patients had nonsustained ventricular tachycardia. Amiodarone (maintenance dose 300 mg/day) reduced mortality from 41.4% to 33.5% at 2 years. Functional capacity improved in patients treated with amiodarone. The drug was discontinued because of side effects in 4.6% of patients. In the Veterans Affairs Cooperative Study Program Trial, 674 patients with a left ventricular ejection fraction of less than 0.40 and 10 or more ventricular ectopic beats per hour were randomized to amiodarone, 400–300 mg/day, or placebo.[73] The mortality rate was 28% at 2 years and was similar in the amiodarone- and placebo-treated patients.

Hypertrophic Cardiomyopathy

The risk of sudden death for patients with hypertrophic cardiomyopathy is 1%–6% per year.[126–129] Sustained monomorphic ventricular tachycardia is rare; the majority of cardiac arrests are due to polymorphic ventricular tachycardia or ventricular fibrillation. The latter can occasionally be provoked by rapid supraventricular arrhythmias.[130] Patients resuscitated from ventricular fibrillation should undergo evaluation to exclude other precipitating factors. The severity of left ventricular outflow obstruction and the presence of coronary artery disease in patients with risk factors should be defined. An electrophysiologic study is warranted. In one series of 30 patients who had been resuscitated from cardiac arrest, a supraventricular tachycardia that produced hypotension was identified in 4 patients.[130] Programmed stimulation induced sustained polymorphic ventricular tachycardia or ventricular fibrillation in two thirds of patients and monomorphic ventricular tachycardia in two patients. Five patients were treated with antiarrhythmic drugs, and three patients died suddenly, including two who had been treated with amiodarone. Eighteen patients received implantable defibrillators, none of whom died suddenly, and four subsequently received a spontaneous shock from the device, suggesting an arrhythmia recurrence. Although there are no controlled trials of this therapy, an implantable defibrillator should be considered.

Nonsustained ventricular tachycardia is present in a quarter of patients. Although it has been associated with an increased risk of sudden death in some studies, the predictive value is poor.[127, 129] Young age at diagnosis, a history of syncope, and a family history of hypertrophic cardiomyopathy are associated with an increased risk of sudden death. Therapy with beta-adrenergic blockers or calcium channel blockers should be considered, although the effect on survival is unknown.[131] Disopyramide has been used for its negative inotropic effects, which may produce hemodynamic benefits. If a history of syncope or presyncope is present, exercise testing and electrophysiologic study should be considered to exclude exercise-induced or other arrhythmias as the mechanism. Inducible polymorphic ventricular tachycardia or ventricular fibrillation on electrophysiologic study may identify high-risk patients.[129] The optimal therapeutic approach to high-risk patients has not been defined. Suppression of nonsustained ventricular tachycardia with amiodarone was associated with a favorable prognosis when compared with historical controls in one study; however, in a higher risk population of patients with a history of syncope or presyncope, the 2-year probability of sudden death during amiodarone therapy was 20%.[132]

Right Ventricular Dysplasia

Right ventricular dysplasia is a rare disease characterized by replacement of variable portions of the right ventricular myocardium by fatty and fibrous tissue.[1, 2, 133–135] Many, but not all, patients suffer from episodes of sustained monomorphic ventricular tachycardia due to reentry in regions of the involved ventricle. Ventricular tachycardia has a left bundle branch block configuration in the precordial leads. The major differential diagnosis is idiopathic right ventricular outflow tract tachycardia (see further on). In the vast majority of cases, a region of abnormal right ventricular wall motion is present on the echocardiogram. When right ventricular function appears normal on echocardiography, contrast ventriculography or magnetic resonance imaging may show subtle focal right ventricular abnormalities.[133, 134] Right ventricular dysplasia is favored by abnormal right ventricular wall motion, complete or incomplete right bundle branch block during sinus rhythm, inverted T waves in the precordial electrocardiographic leads, and an abnormal signal-averaged electrocardiogram. Right ventricular biopsy results are often abnormal, but biopsy is usually not required for the diagnosis.[133] Programmed electrical stimulation initiates sustained monomorphic ventricular tachycardia in 83% of patients who have had this arrhythmia spontaneously.[135]

Sudden death can be the initial presentation. Sudden death is relatively uncommon once the patient is under medical care, although 10% of patients suffer nonfatal arrhythmia recurrences.[135, 136] In one study, the probability of sudden death was 3% at 5 years.[136] In a series of 81 patients, sotalol was the most effective antiarrhythmic drug, but class I antiarrhythmic drugs and amiodarone can also be effective.[135] Beta-adrenergic blockers are useful in some patients. Patients should refrain from strenuous exercise. Nonpharmacologic therapies are considered for patients with frequent arrhythmia recurrences.

Other Structural Heart Disease

Sustained monomorphic ventricular tachycardia also occurs with diseases that produce focal areas of myocardial scarring (see Table 18–1). These include Chagas disease,[137] sarcoidosis,[138] and progressive systemic sclerosis. Prognosis is determined largely by the progression of cardiac disease. The arrhythmia is managed in the same manner as for ventricular tachycardia associated with an old myocardial infarction.

Idiopathic Ventricular Tachycardia

By definition, idiopathic ventricular tachycardia occurs in the absence of structural heart disease.[2] Idiopathic sustained monomorphic ventricular tachycardia is uncommon, accounting for 10% or fewer of patients who are referred for treatment of ventricular tachycardia.[139, 140] It may arise in either the left or the right ventricle. The site of origin of ventricular tachycardia is suggested by the morphology of the QRS complexes during tachycardia. Ventricular tachycardia with a predominantly negative QRS complex in lead V_1, resembling a left bundle branch block pattern, usually originates from the right ventricle. In contrast, tachycardia with a QRS complex in lead V_1 that is predominantly positive, resembling right bundle branch block, likely originates from the left ventricle. These arrhythmias can also be categorized based on other features, including whether they are provoked by exercise, whether they are sustained or nonsustained, their response to programmed electrical stimulation, and their response to drugs.[2, 142–146] Although certain patterns emerge, the mechanisms are diverse, and the response to antiarrhythmic drug therapy can be difficult to predict.

Idiopathic Right Ventricular Tachycardia

The most common electrocardiographic pattern of idiopathic right ventricular tachycardia is that of a left bundle branch block type of QRS complex with an inferior or rightward axis (+90 degrees or greater) deviation in the frontal plane (Fig. 18–7).[139, 142] These tachycardias arise from the right ventricular outflow tract. They frequently are exercise-induced and can be induced in a majority of patients by rapid pacing or programmed electrical stimulation, particularly during infusion of isoproterenol. The major diagnostic concern is to exclude right ventricular dysplasia (see earlier discussion).

Unlike sustained monomorphic ventricular tachycardia in patients with a previous infarct or dilated cardiomyopathy, some idiopathic ventricular tachycardias arising from the right ventricular outflow tract are terminated by intravenous administration of verapamil or

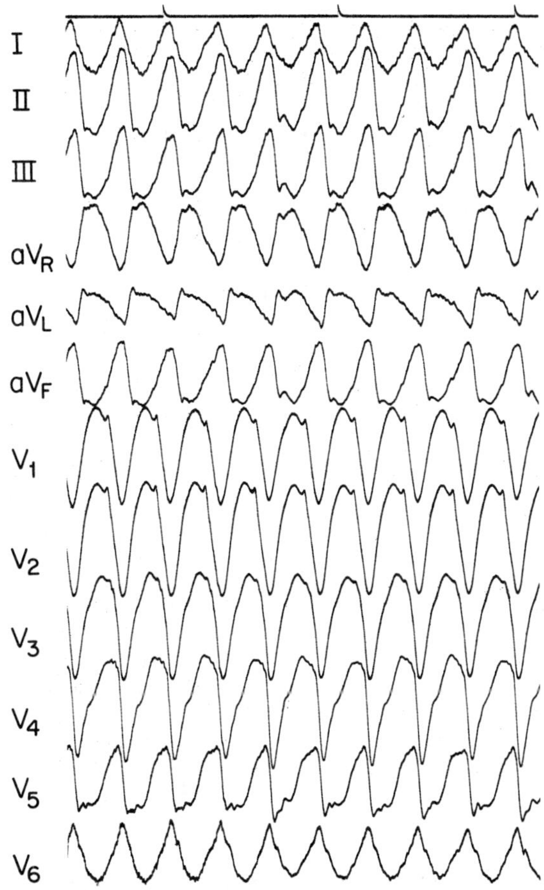

Figure 18–7. Idiopathic right ventricular outflow tract ventricular tachycardia. *Abbreviations:* aV_R, augmented unipolar lead, right arm; aV_L, augmented unipolar lead, left arm; aV_F, augmented unipolar lead, left leg.

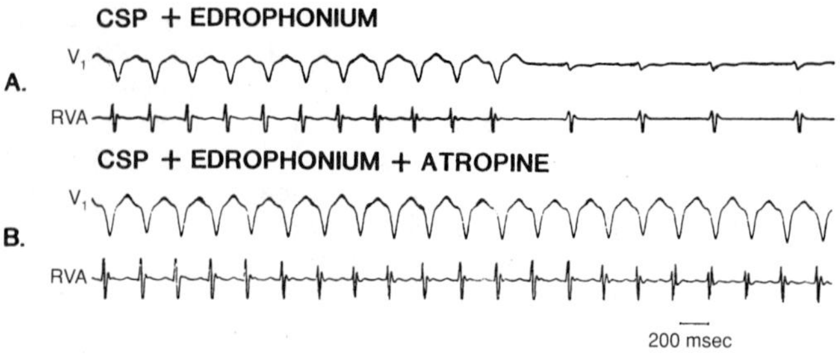

Figure 18–8. A, Termination of idiopathic right ventricular outflow tract tachycardia by carotid sinus pressure (CSP) and edrophonium. *B,* In the presence of a muscarinic cholinergic receptor blocker, CSP and edrophonium have no effect. *Abbreviation:* RVA = right ventricular apex bipolar electrogram. (From Lerman BB: Response of nonreentrant ventricular tachycardia to endogenous adenosine and acetylcholine. Evidence for myocardial receptor-mediated effects. Circulation 1993; 87:382–390.)

adenosine or by vagotonic maneuvers (Fig. 18–8).[141, 143, 145] Catecholamine-induced, cyclic adenosine monophosphate–mediated, triggered activity has been suggested as the underlying mechanism of these tachycardias. Some idiopathic right ventricular tachycardias may be due to catecholamine-induced enhanced automaticity rather than triggered activity and are suppressed by beta-adrenergic blocking agents but not by calcium antagonists.[146] Others may result from reentry and are not responsive to either beta blockers or calcium antagonists.[143] Tachycardias with a left bundle branch block–like configuration in lead V_1 but with a left axis deviation in the frontal plane typically originate from the inferior or inflow portion of the right ventricle and are usually not responsive to verapamil.[147]

Patients with idiopathic right ventricular tachycardia have an excellent prognosis with or without therapy, although there are rare reported instances of cardiac arrest.[148] Some patients experience long arrhythmia-free intervals without treatment. Patients with frequent episodes should be considered for long-term drug therapy or catheter ablation (see Chapter 19), particularly if ventricular tachycardia is rapid or causes severe symptoms. It is difficult to predict which drugs will be effective. Choosing a drug with as few nuisance side effects as possible and with a pharmacokinetic profile that allows for once- daily dosing helps to ensure patient compliance. Drugs with a low likelihood of proarrhythmia should be selected first. Since many idiopathic right ventricular tachycardias are provoked by exercise, one might think that beta-adrenergic blockers would be effective.[2, 149, 150] These drugs are safe but provide adequate control in only 25% of patients. Oral verapamil, 120 mg three times per day, or an equivalent dose of a long-acting verapamil preparation, effectively suppresses recurrences of ventricular tachycardia in approximately two thirds of patients.[147] Approximately 5% of patients treated with verapamil experience more frequent or longer lasting episodes of ventricular tachycardia or more hemodynamic compromise during the arrhythmia. In patients who do not respond to verapamil, the combination of verapamil plus a beta blocker can be tried (Fig. 18–9). Beta blockers in combination with a class IA antiarrhythmic drug have been effective in up to 90% of patients.[149] Class IC drugs have been used with moderate success[151, 152] and may be preferable to the class IA drugs because they are less likely to cause torsades de pointes. The class III drugs sotalol and amiodarone may also be effective. Except in resistent cases, these agents should be avoided because of the long-term side effects of amiodarone and the risk of torsades de pointes with sotalol.

Idiopathic Left Ventricular Tachycardia

The most common electrocardiographic pattern of idiopathic left ventricular tachycardia is that of a right bundle branch block type of QRS complex with a superior or leftward axis (−30 degrees or less) in the frontal plane (Fig. 18–10).[2, 140, 146, 153–155] In rare patients, right axis deviation in the frontal plane is seen. Idiopathic left ventricular tachycardia is often provoked with exercise, is more commonly seen in males, and is readily inducible during electrophysiologic study. In general, the tachycardia is well tolerated hemodynamically and is often incorrectly diagnosed as supraventricular tachycardia with aberrant intraventricular conduction. The arrhythmia can also be incessant and can lead to the development of tachycardia-related cardiomyopathy.[140] Idiopathic left ventricular tachycardia with a right bundle branch block and left axis deviation QRS configuration appears to originate from reentry in cells generating calcium-dependent slow responses in or near the distal ramifications of the His-Purkinje system in the posteroapical portion of the left ventricular septum.[140, 153, 155, 156] This tachycardia is interrupted by intravenous verapamil (Fig. 18–11) but does not usually respond to adenosine or vagal maneuvers. Intravenous lidocaine or procainamide usually does not terminate the tachycardia but may slow the tachycardia rate (Fig. 18–12). Idiopathic left ventricular tachycardia with a right bundle branch block–type QRS complex and right axis deviation can also be interrupted with intravenous verapamil and may also be terminated by intravenous adenosine, suggesting cyclic adenosine monophosphate–mediated triggered activity as the mechanism akin to that seen in patients with idiopathic right ventricular outflow tract tachycardia.[144]

Although a high proportion of idiopathic ventricular tachycardias are terminated by administration of intravenous verapamil, extreme caution should be exercised when calcium channel blockers are used in patients with a wide QRS complex tachycardia of uncertain cause. The vast majority of sustained ventricular tachycardias are *not* idiopathic but rather the consequence of serious underlying structural heart disease. Intravenous verapamil is likely to cause hemodynamic collapse with persistence rather than termination of the arrhythmia.[30, 31] When the patient is young, has no prior history of heart disease other than palpitations, is known to have a completely normal electrocardiogram in sinus rhythm, and is known to have a completely normal echocardiogram, it is reasonable to try intravenous verapamil if adenosine has not been successful in terminating the tachycardia. If any of these essential components of the patient's evaluation are missing, however, it is more prudent *not* to give verapamil and to give a drug such as lidocaine or procainamide instead. Although idiopathic left ventricular tachycardia can be exquisitely sensitive to intravenous verapamil, long-term oral therapy with verapamil often fails to prevent arrhythmia recurrences. Beta blocker therapy is also usually disappointing in these patients. There is limited experience with the use of class I or class III drugs for chronic therapy. Catheter ablation can be effective (see Chapter 19).

POLYMORPHIC VENTRICULAR TACHYCARDIA

Polymorphic ventricular tachycardia associated with QT interval prolongation is referred to as torsades de pointes ventricular tachy-

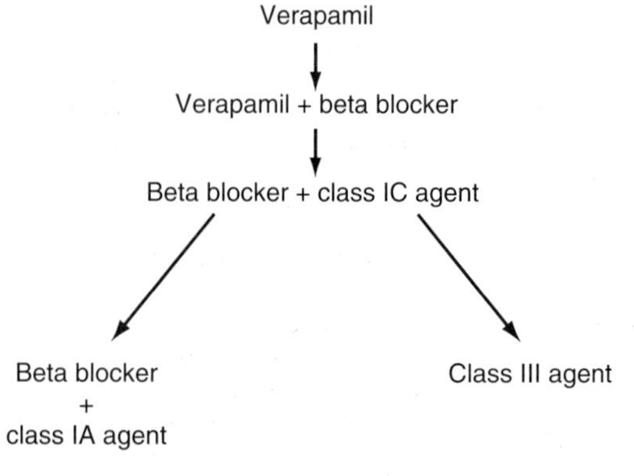

Figure 18–9. Flow diagram for chronic treatment of idiopathic right ventricular tachycardia.

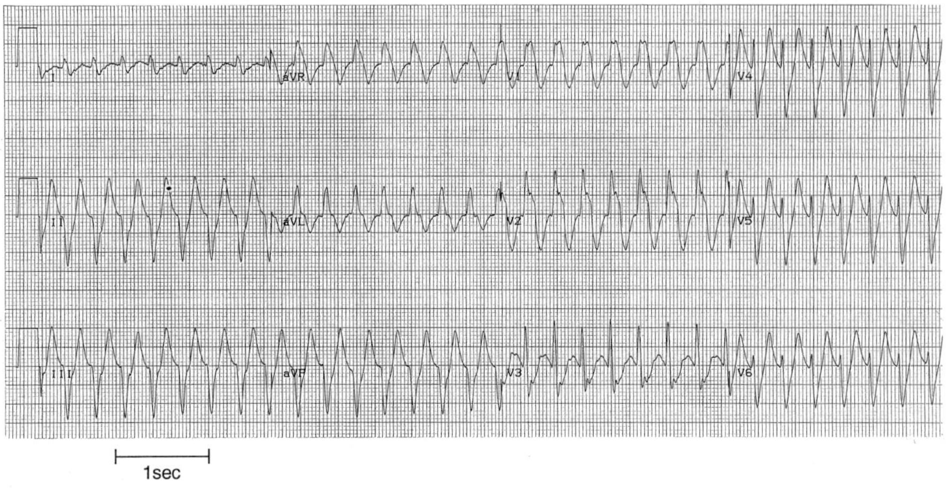

Figure 18–10. Twelve-lead ECG of idiopathic left ventricular tachycardia.

cardia.[157–159] QT interval prolongation may be acquired (resulting from an electrolyte abnormality or drug) or congenital. Polymorphic ventricular tachycardia can also be caused by a transient or evolving abnormality or severe underlying heart disease without marked QT interval prolongation (see Table 18–1). Acute myocardial ischemia is the most common cause (see previous discussion). The manner of tachycardia initiation is useful in suggesting the cause. Polymorphic ventricular tachycardia that occurs after a sudden deceleration in heart rate, such as might occur after a sinus pause, a nonconducted P wave, a long RR interval during atrial fibrillation, a pause after a ventricular premature depolarization, or during severe bradycardia, is designated as pause-dependent (Fig. 18–13). This pattern of initiation is commonly observed with many polymorphic ventricular tachycardias, but especially with torsades de pointes.[159] Polymorphic ventricular tachycardia that occurs without a preceding pause (see Fig. 18–1*B*) is more likely to be due to another cause. Polymorphic ventricular tachycardia may last only a few seconds, terminating spontaneously without causing any symptoms. Longer episodes usually cause syncope and may terminate after a minute or more (Fig. 18–14) or degenerate to ventricular fibrillation.

Torsades de Pointes

Acquired Long QT Syndrome

The mechanism of torsades de pointes is not established but may be triggered activity or reentry over continuously changing circuits.[1, 25, 157] Any drug or electrolyte abnormality that prolongs the action potential duration can be a culprit (Table 18–7). With some drugs, such as quinidine or procainamide, torsades de pointes may be an idiosyncratic reaction and can occur at low plasma drug concentrations.[158] With sotalol, torsades de pointes appears to be dose-related. Amiodarone often causes striking prolongation of the QT interval, but provocation of torsades de pointes is rare.[67] Increased heterogeneity of myocardial repolarization caused by a drug, which may be reflected in QT interval dispersion among different leads in the surface electrocardiogram, may be a more important factor predisposing to the development of torsades de pointes than the magnitude of QT prolongation caused by the drug.[160] Acquired torsades de pointes can occasionally occur in the absence of striking QT prolongation in the surface electrocardiogram, but evidence for pause dependence is present if the initiation of the arrhythmia is observed.[158, 159] Onset of the arrhythmia after a long RR interval (see Fig. 18–13) or in the setting of bradycardia should immediately trigger a search for possible underlying causes (see Table 18–7).

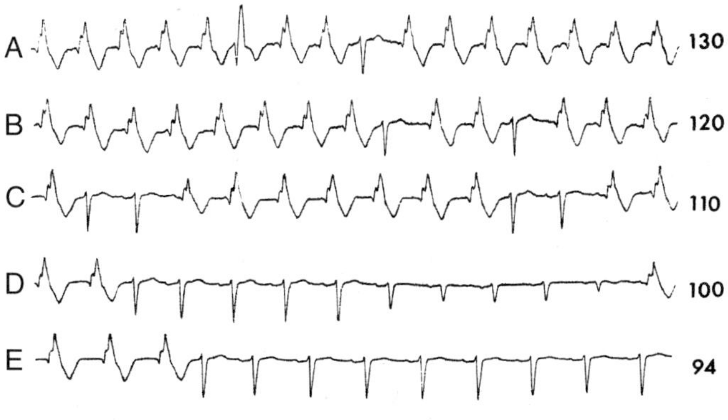

Figure 18–11. Slowing and then termination of idiopathic left ventricular tachycardia after intravenous administration of verapamil. (From Belhassen B, Shapira I, Pelleg A, et al: Idiopathic recurrent sustained ventricular tachycardia responsive to verapamil: an ECG-electrophysiologic entity. Am Heart J 1984; 108:1034–1037.)

Therapy should first concentrate on termination of the arrhythmia and prevention of immediate recurrences (see Fig. 18–2). After defibrillation, the initial treatment is magnesium sulfate administered as a 1- to 2-g bolus intravenously. This can be followed by a constant infusion if necessary to prevent short-term recurrences (see Table 18–2). If magnesium is ineffective or marked bradycardia is present, measures to increase the heart rate should be employed. The most direct method is temporary atrial or ventricular pacing. The heart rate should be increased sufficiently to prevent ventricular ectopy, usually to a rate between 90 and 120 beats per minute. An intravenous infusion of isoproterenol at doses of 1–5 μg/min or intravenous atropine given as a single bolus injection of 0.5 or 1 mg can be used if temporary pacing is not possible. Antiarrhythmic drugs that decrease action potential duration and shorten the QT interval theoretically may be of benefit. Lidocaine, however, is effective in fewer than 50% of patients.[158] Experience with phenytoin is extremely limited. Drugs that lengthen the QT interval should be scrupulously avoided because they are ineffective and may aggravate the arrhythmia. Verapamil has been reported to be effective in rare cases, consistent with a proposed mechanism involving early after-depolarizations, but experience is limited.[161]

Once the acute episodes have been brought under control, attention should focus on correction of underlying metabolic and electrolyte abnormalities and elimination of drugs that may have been causative (see Table 18–7). If an antiarrhythmic drug was the cause, the indication for antiarrhythmic drug therapy should be reconsidered. Treatment with another drug that prolongs the QT interval, with the exception of amiodarone, is associated with a high risk of recurrence exceeding 20%.[159] If antiarrhythmic drug therapy is deemed to be essential, propafenone, flecainide, mexiletine, or tocainide, which do

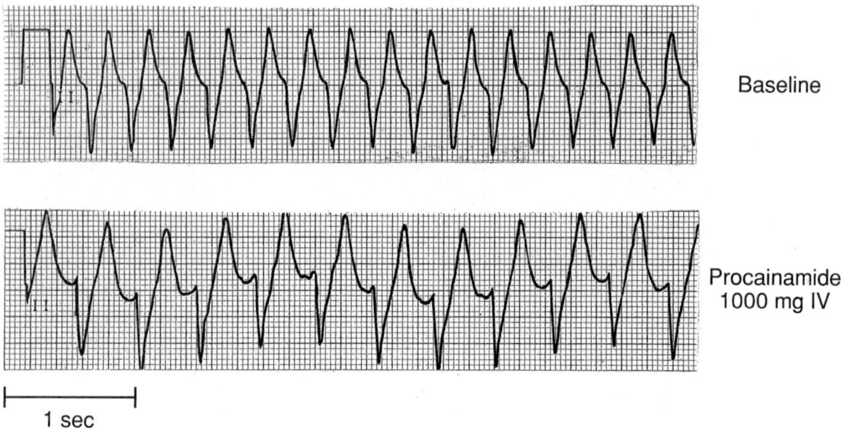

Figure 18–12. Slowing of the rate of idiopathic left ventricular tachycardia without termination after procainamide. Same patient as illustrated in Figure 18–10.

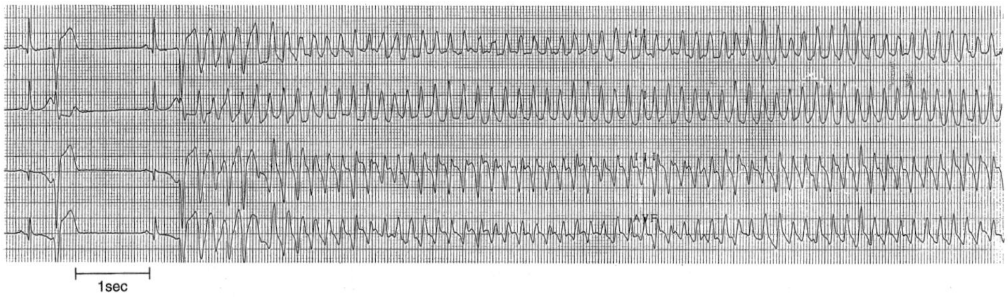

Figure 18–13. Pause-dependent polymorphic ventricular tachycardia.

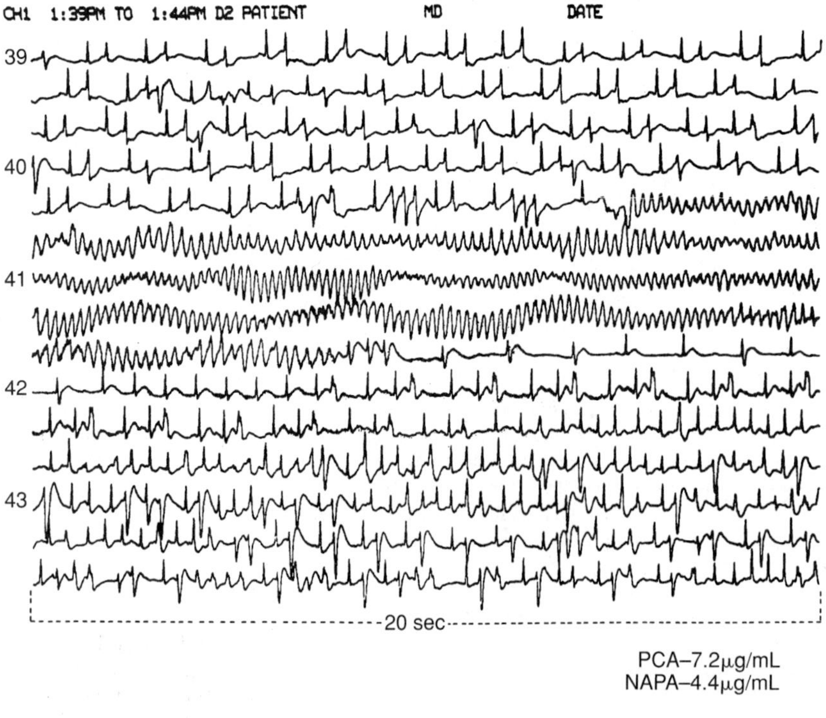

Figure 18–14. A long-lasting episode of torsades de pointes resulting from the acquired long QT syndrome. Note pause dependence of this arrhythmia. Frequent premature ventricular contractions are followed by three-beat runs of ventricular tachycardia (fifth row) followed by a 70-sec run of polymorphic ventricular tachycardia, which terminates spontaneously (ninth row). *Abbreviations:* PCA, procainamide; NAPA, *N*-acetyl procainamide.

TABLE 18–7. CAUSES OF THE ACQUIRED LONG QT SYNDROME

Drugs	Antidepressants
Antiarrhythmics	Tricyclics
Quinidine	Tetracyclics
Procainamide	Phenothiazines
N-acetyl procainamide	Organophosphates
Disopyramide	**Bradycardia**
Aprindine	
Moricizine	**Metabolic Causes**
Sotalol	Hypokalemia
Amiodarone	Hypomagnesemia
Antibiotics	Hypothermia
Ampicillin	Myocardial ischemia-infarction
Erythromycin	Liquid protein diets
Pentamidine	Starvation
Trimethoprim-sulfamethoxazole	Anorexia nervosa
Tetracycline	**Neurologic Causes**
Nonsedating antihistamines	Stroke
Astemizole	Encephalitis
Terfenadine	Subarachnoid hemorrhage
Calcium antagonists	Intracranial trauma
Lidoflazine	Radical neck dissection
Bepridil	Carotid endarterectomy

not prolong ventricular repolarization, or amiodarone, which has a very low likelihood of provoking torsades de pointes, can be considered.[67, 160, 161] Patients with severe heart failure who suffer torsades de pointes have a high risk of sudden death, even when the offending drug is replaced by amiodarone.[162]

Congenital Long QT Syndrome

The congenital long QT syndrome is either inherited or the result of a spontaneous genetic mutation in individuals without a clear family history of the condition. QT prolongation in the absence of an acquired cause is the hallmark of this syndrome. Some patients have minimal prolongation of the QT interval on the resting electrocardiogram but have abnormal T waves or experience abnormal ventricular repolarization during exercise.[163] Torsades de pointes is often provoked by stress, anxiety, fear, or physical exertion, pointing to the sympathetic nervous system as a key promoting factor. For this reason, torsades de pointes in the congenital long QT syndrome is considered to be adrenergic-dependent, in contrast to pause-dependent.[159] The distinction between adrenergic-dependent and pause-dependent torsades de pointes is not universally applicable, however, because many patients with congenital long QT syndrome have abnormally slow resting heart rates, a blunted chronotropic response to exercise, and torsades de pointes that may occur during periods of excessive bradycardia or after a sinus pause.[157, 164]

Drugs that prolong the QT interval are contraindicated (see Table 18–7). Beta-adrenergic blockade is the cornerstone of drug therapy. An agent that lacks intrinsic sympathomimetic activity should be used. The dose should be adequate to blunt the chronotropic response to exercise. One approach is to keep the peak exercise heart rate at less than 120 beats per minute. In some individuals, the dose of beta blocker required causes excessive sinus bradycardia at rest. Implantation of a permanent pacemaker is then required for continuation of beta blocker administration at an appropriate dose. This offers a greater degree of protection than withholding the pacemaker and using an inadequate dose of beta blocker. Despite beta-adrenergic blockade, nearly 20% of patients who have experienced symptoms continue to have syncope or suffer sudden death from torsades de pointes.[164] Unfortunately, these high-risk patients cannot be identified from resting QT intervals or the heart rate response to exercise. In one study, patients in whom beta blocker therapy failed had a greater degree of QT interval dispersion than did both patients who responded to beta blockers and healthy control subjects.[165] Further evaluation is warranted to determine whether QT interval dispersion is useful in identifying those individuals at high risk who therefore are candidates for alternative therapy.

Patients who fail to respond to beta blocker therapy with or without cardiac pacing are candidates for either left-sided cardiac sympathectomy or an implantable cardioverter-defibrillator.[164] The observation that some patients in whom beta blocker therapy fails respond to left-sided cardiac sympathectomy suggests that alpha-adrenergic stimulation may contribute to the genesis of torsades de pointes in congenital long QT syndrome.[166] The utility of alpha-adrenergic blocking agents is unknown.[167] There is also interest in a novel group of drugs that shorten action potential duration by increasing K^+ conductance through ATP-sensitive potassium channels.[168, 169] These drugs abolish early after-depolarizations and torsades de pointes in experimental preparations but have not yet been evaluated in patients with either idiopathic or acquired long QT syndrome.

Polymorphic Ventricular Tachycardia Without QT Prolongation

Polymorphic ventricular tachycardia occasionally occurs in the absence of prolongation of the QT interval or known causes of QT prolongation and without clinical features or a family history suggesting the congenital form of long QT syndrome. The tachycardia in these patients often, but not always, lacks the pause dependence seen in acquired long QT syndrome (see Fig. 18–1*B*). Significant underlying structural heart disease is usually present. Acute myocardial ischemia or infarction (see earlier) is the most common cause (see Table 18–1). In rare instances, the arrhythmia occurs because of acute myocarditis or drug toxicity or early after cardiac surgery. In these settings, it is often transient if the underlying disease process can be stabilized. It is particularly important to distinguish polymorphic ventricular tachycardia caused by ischemia from that resulting from the acquired long QT syndrome because the arrhythmia in the former group will be aggravated by rapid pacing and catecholamines, treatment modalities that are beneficial in the latter group.

Idiopathic Ventricular Fibrillation

In rare patients, ventricular fibrillation occurs in the absence of structural heart disease or the long QT syndrome. Patients are typically less than 40 years of age and most commonly male.[170–172] Ventricular fibrillation often begins with polymorphic ventricular tachycardia. Unlike torsades de pointes, the polymorphic ventricular tachycardia usually starts with a closely coupled ventricular premature depolarization not preceded by a pause. The majority of cases are not related to stress or exertion. A careful evaluation to exclude underlying heart disease should be performed, including echocardiography and coronary angiography. Exercise testing occasionally reveals rapid polymorphic nonsustained ventricular tachycardia. Electrocardiographic abnormalities are present in some patients.[171] Endomyocardial biopsy to detect acute myocarditis and evaluation for coronary artery spasm should be considered if the cause remains obscure. On electrophysiologic study, sustained polymorphic ventricular tachycardia or ventricular fibrillation is induced in approximately a third of patients. In rare instances, sustained monomorphic ventricular tachycardia is inducible.

Of 37 patients in two series, 11 suffered recurrent cardiac arrests or experienced an implantable defibrillator shock preceded by symptoms suggesting an arrhythmia recurrence during the initial 3 years after evaluation.[170, 172] Beta blockers, class IA antiarrhythmics, and amiodarone have been used in selected patients, but their efficacy is difficult to predict. An implantable cardioverter-defibrillator device should be considered for initial therapy.

REFERENCES

1. Zipes DP: Genesis of cardiac arrhythmias: electrophysiological considerations. *In* Braunwald E (ed): Heart Disease, A Textbook of Cardiovascular Medicine, 4th ed, p 588. Philadelphia: WB Saunders, 1992.
2. Akhtar M: Clinical spectrum of ventricular tachycardia. Circulation 1990; 82:1561–1573.
3. Gascho JA, Crampton RS, Cherwek ML, et al: Determinants of ventricular defibrillation in adults. Circulation 1979; 60:231–240.
4. Winkle RA, Mead RH, Ruder MA, et al: Effect of duration of ventricular fibrillation on defibrillation efficacy in humans. Circulation 1990; 81:1477–1481.
5. Weaver WD, Fahrenbruch CE, Johnson DD, et al: Effect of epinephrine and lidocaine therapy on outcome after cardiac arrest due to ventricular fibrillation. Circulation 1990; 82:2027–2034.
6. Zipes DP: Management of cardiac arrhythmias: pharmacological, electrical, and surgical techniques. *In* Braunwald E (ed): Heart Disease, A Textbook of Cardiovascular Medicine, 4th ed, p 628. Philadelphia: WB Saunders, 1992.
7. Williams ML, Woelfel A, Cascio WE, et al: Intravenous amiodarone during prolonged resuscitation from cardiac arrest. Ann Intern Med 1989; 110:839–842.
8. Moss AN, Mohiuddin SM, Hee TT, et al: Efficacy and tolerance of high-dose intravenous amiodarone for recurrent, refractory ventricular tachycardia. Am J Cardiol 1990; 65:609–614.
9. Scheinman MM for the IV Amiodarone Study Group: Multicenter study of the dose response to intravenous amiodarone in patients with refractory ventricular tachycardia/fibrillation. Circulation 1993; 88:I-396.
10. Kowey PR for the IV Amiodarone Investigators, Lankenau Hospital and Medical Research Center, Wynnewood, PA: A multicenter randomized double-blind comparison of intravenous beryllium with amiodarone in patients with frequent malignant ventricular arrhythmia. Circulation 1993; 88:I-396.
11. Nalos PC, Ismail Y, Pappas JM, et al: Intravenous amiodarone for short-term treatment of refractory ventricular tachycardia or fibrillation. Am Heart J 1991; 122:1629–1632.
12. Wolfe CL, Nibley C, Bhandari A, et al: Polymorphous ventricular tachycardia associated with acute myocardial infarction. Circulation 1991; 84:1543–1551.
13. Path GJ, Dai XZ, Schwartz JS, et al: Effects of amiodarone with and without polysorbate 80 on myocardial oxygen consumption and coronary blood flow during treadmill exercise in the dog. J Cardiovasc Pharm 1991; 18:11–16.
14. Massini E, Plachenault J, Pezziardi F, et al: Histamine-releasing properties of polysorbate 80 in vitro and in vivo: correlation with its hypotensive action in the dog. Agents Actions 1985; 16:470–477.
15. Herre JM, Titus C, Oeff M, et al: Inefficacy and proarrhythmic effects of flecainide and encainide for sustained ventricular tachycardia and ventricular fibrillation. Ann Intern Med 1990; 113:671–676.
16. Wasserman F, Brodsky L, Dick MM, et al: Successful treatment of quinidine and procainamide intoxication. Report of three cases. N Engl J Med 1958; 259:797–802.
17. Pentel PR, Goldsmith SR, Salerno DM, et al: Effect of hypertonic sodium bicarbonate on encainide overdose. Am J Cardiol 1986; 57:878–880.
18. Windelmann BR, Leinberger H: Life-threatening flecainide toxicity. A pharmacologic approach. Ann Intern Med 1987; 106:807–814.
19. Myerburg RJ, Kessler KM, Cox MM, et al: Reversal of proarrhythmic effects of flecainide acetate and encainide hydrochloride by propranolol. Circulation 1989; 80:1571–1579.
20. Bajaj AK, Woosley RL, Roden DM: Acute electrophysiologic effects of sodium administration in dogs treated with *O*-desmethyl encainide. Circulation 1989; 80:994–1002.
21. Friedman PL, Antman EM: Electrocardiographic manifestations of digitalis toxicity. *In* Smith TW (ed): Digitalis Glycosides. Orlando, FL: Grune & Stratton, 1985.
22. Friedman PL, Antman EM, Smith TW: Clinical management of digitalis toxicity. *In* Smith TW (ed): Digitalis Glycosides. Orlando, FL: Grune & Stratton, 1985.
23. Wenger TL, Butler VP, Haver E, et al: Treatment of 63 severely digitalis-toxic patients with digoxin-specific antibody fragments. J Am Coll Cardiol 1985; 5:118A–123A.
24. Aktar M, Shasa M, Jazayeri M, et al: Wide QRS complex tachycardia. Reappraisal of a common clinical problem. Ann Intern Med 1988; 105:905–912.
25. Zipes DP: Specific arrhythmias: diagnosis and treatment. *In* Braunwald E (ed): Heart Disease, A Textbook of Cardiovascular Medicine, 4th ed, p 667. Philadelphia: WB Saunders, 1992.
26. Griffith MJ, Linker NJ, Ward DE, Camm AJ: Adenosine in the diagnosis of broad complex tachycardia. Lancet 1988; 1:672–675.
27. Rankin AC, Oldroyd KG, Chong E, et al: Value and limitations of adenosine in the diagnosis and treatment of narrow and broad complex tachycardias. Br Heart J 1989; 62:195–203.
28. Sharma AD, Klein GJ, Yee R: Intravenous adenosine triphosphate during wide QRS complex tachycardia: safety, therapeutic efficacy, and diagnostic utility. Am J Med 1990; 88:337–343.
29. Giffith MJ, Linker NJ, Garratt CJ, et al: Relative efficacy and safety of intravenous drugs for termination of sustained ventricular tachycardia. Lancet 1990; 336:670–673.
30. Buxton AE, Marchlinski FE, Doherty JU, et al: Hazards of intravenous verapamil for sustained ventricular tachycardia. Am J Cardiol 1987; 59:1107–1110.
31. Stewart RB, Bardy GH, Greene HL: Wide complex tachycardia: misdiagnosis and outcome after emergent therapy. Ann Intern Med 1986; 104:766–771.
32. Wellens HJJ, Brugada P, Stevenson WG: Programmed electrical stimulation: its role in the management of ventricular arrhythmias in coronary heart disease. Prog Cardiovasc Dis 1986; 29:165–180.
33. Horowitz LN: Safety of electrophysiologic studies. Circulation 1986; 73(suppl II):28–31.
34. Myerburg RJ, Castellanos A: Cardiac arrest and sudden cardiac death. *In* Braunwald E (ed): Heart Disease, A Textbook of Cardiovascular Medicine, 4th ed, p 756. Philadelphia: WB Saunders, 1992.
35. Hays LJ, Lerman BB, DiMarco JP: Nonventricular arrhythmias as precursors of ventricular fibrillation in patients with out-of-hospital cardiac arrest. Am Heart J 1989; 118:53–57.
36. Roden DM: Risks and benefits of antiarrhythmic therapy. N Engl J Med 1994; 331(12):785–792.
37. Stanton MS, Prystowsky EN, Fineberg NS, et al: Arrhythmogenic effects of antiarrhythmic drugs: a study of 506 patients treated for ventricular tachycardia or fibrillation. J Am Coll Cardiol 1989; 14:209–215.
38. Ruskin JN, McGovern B, Garan H, et al: Antiarrhythmic drugs: a possible cause of out-of-hospital cardiac arrest. N Engl J Med 1983; 309(21):1303–1306.
39. Wyse DG, Morganroth J, Ledingham R, et al: New insights into the definition and meaning of proarrhythmia during initiation of antiarrhythmic drug therapy from the Cardiac Arrhythmia Suppression Trial and its pilot study. J Am Coll Cardiol 1994; 23:1130–1140.
40. Kudenchuk PJ, Kron J, Walance C, et al: Spontaneous sustained ventricular tachyarrhythmias during treatment with type IA antiarrhythmic agents. Am J Cardiol 1990; 65:446–452.
41. Task Force of the Working Group of Arrhythmias of the European Society of Cardiology: CAST and beyond, implications of the Cardiac Arrhythmia Suppression Trial. Circulation 1990; 81(3):1123–1127.
42. Ravid S, Podrid PJ, Lampert S, et al: Congestive heart failure induced by six of the newer antiarrhythmic drugs. J Am Coll Cardiol 1989; 14:1326–1330.
43. Gottlieb SS, Kukin ML, Medina N, et al: Comparative hemodynamic effects of procainamide, tocainide, and encainide in severe chronic heart failure. Circulation 1990; 81:860–864.
44. Packer M: Hemodynamic consequences of antiarrhythmic drug therapy in patients with chronic congestive heart failure. J Cardiovasc Electrophysiol 1991; 25:240–247.
45. Viscoli CM, Horowitz RI, Singer BH: Beta-blockers after myocardial infarction: influence of first-year clinical course on long-term effectiveness. Ann Intern Med 1993; 118:99–105.
46. Friedman CM, Byington RP, Capone RJ, et al: Effect of propranolol in patients with myocardial infarction and ventricular arrhythmia. J Am Coll Cardiol 1986; 7:1–8.
47. Manz M, Jung W, Lüderitz B: Interactions between drugs and devices: experimental and clinical studies. Am Heart J 1994; 127:978–984.
48. Mason JW for the Electrophysiologic Study versus Electrocardiographic Monitoring Investigators: A comparison of electrophysiologic testing with Holter monitoring to predict antiarrhythmic-drug efficacy for ventricular tachyarrhythmia. N Engl J Med 1993; 329:445–451.
49. Wood M, Stambler B, Ellenbogen K: Recent insights in programmed electrical stimulation for the management of sustained ventricular arrhythmias. Curr Opin Cardiol 1994; 9:3–11.

50. Steinbeck G, Andresen D, Bagh P, et al: A comparison of electrophysiologically guided antiarrhythmic drug therapy with beta-blocker therapy in patients with symptomatic, sustained ventricular tachyarrhythmias. N Engl J Med 1992; 327:987–992.
51. Kavanagh KM, Wyse DG, Duff HJ, et al: Drug therapy for ventricular tachyarrhythmias: how many electropharmacologic trials are appropriate? J Am Coll Cardiol 1991; 17:391–396.
52. Stevenson WG, Middlekauff HR: Antiarrhythmic drug response in patients at risk for sustained ventricular arrhythmias: can we identify successful long-term responders? J Cardiovasc Electrophysiol 1991; 2:S212–S220.
53. Mason JW for the Electrophysiologic Study versus Electrocardiographic Monitoring Investigators: A comparison of seven antiarrhythmic drugs in patients with ventricular tachyarrhythmia. N Engl J Med 1993; 329:452–458.
54. Calkins H, El-Atassi R, Schmaltz S, et al: Reversal of antiarrhythmic drug effects by epinephrine: quinidine versus amiodarone. J Am Coll Cardiol 1991; 19:347–352.
55. Markel ML, Miles MM, Luck JC, et al: Differential effects of isoproterenol on sustained ventricular tachycardia before and during procainamide and quinidine antiarrhythmic drug therapy. Circulation 1993; 87:783–792.
56. Singh BN: Electrophysiologic basis for the antiarrhythmic actions of sotalol and comparison with other agents. Am J Cardiol 1993; 72:8A–18A.
57. Ranger S, Talajic M, Lemery R, et al: Amplification of flecainide-induced ventricular conduction slowing by exercise, a potentially significant clinical consequence of use-dependent sodium channel blockade. Circulation 1989; 79:1000–1006.
58. Nademanee K, Singh BN, Stevenson WG, et al: Amiodarone and post-MI patients. Circulation 1993; 88(2):764–774.
59. Roden DM: Pharmacokinetics of amiodarone: implications for drug therapy. Am J Cardiol 1993; 72:45F–50F.
60. Evans SJL, Myers M, Zaher C, et al: High dose oral amiodarone loading: electrophysiologic effects and clinical tolerance. J Am Coll Cardiol 1992; 19:169–173.
61. Kim SG, Mannino MM, Chou R, et al: Rapid suppression of spontaneous ventricular arrhythmias during oral amiodarone loading. Ann Intern Med 1992; 117(3):197–201.
62. Herre JM, Sauve MJ, Malone P, et al: Long-term results of amiodarone therapy in patients with recurrent sustained ventricular tachycardia or ventricular fibrillation. J Am Coll Cardiol 1989; 13:442–449.
63. Weinberg BA, Miles WM, Klein LS, et al: Five-year follow-up of 589 patients treated with amiodarone. Am Heart J 1993; 125:109–120.
64. Olson PJ, Woelfel A, Simpson RJ, et al: Stratification of sudden death risk in patients receiving long-term amiodarone treatment for sustained ventricular tachycardia or ventricular fibrillation. Am J Cardiol 1993; 71:823–826.
65. Roberts SA, Viana MA, Nazari J, et al: Invasive and noninvasive methods to predict the long-term efficacy of amiodarone: a compilation of clinical observations using meta-analysis. PACE 1994; 17:1590–1602.
66. Nasir N, Doyle TK, Wheeler SH, et al: Usefulness of Holter monitoring in predicting efficacy of amiodarone therapy for sustained ventricular tachycardia associated with coronary artery disease. Am J Cardiol 1994; 73:554–558.
67. Hohnloser SH, Klingenheben T, Singh BN: Amiodarone-associated proarrhythmic effects, a review with special reference to torsades de pointes tachycardia. Ann Intern Med 1994; 121:529–535.
68. Navarro-Lopez F, Cosin J, Marrugat J, et al: Comparison of the effects of amiodarone versus metoprolol on the frequency of ventricular arrhythmias and on mortality after acute myocardial infarction. Am J Cardiol 1993; 72:1243–1248.
69. Meyer BJ, Amann FW: Additional antianginal efficacy of amiodarone in patients with limiting angina pectoris. Am Heart J 1993; 125(4):996–1001.
70. Wiersinga WM, Trip MK, van Beeren MH, et al: An increase in plasma cholesterol independent of thyroid function during long-term amiodarone therapy. Ann Intern Med 1991; 114:128–132.
71. Greene HL for the CASCADE Investigators: The CASCADE Study: randomized antiarrhythmic drug therapy in survivors of cardiac arrest in Seattle. Am J Cardiol 1993; 72:70F–74F.
72. Gottlieb SS, Riggio DW, Lauria S, et al: High dose oral amiodarone loading exerts important hemodynamic actions in patients with congestive heart failure. J Am Coll Cardiol 1994; 23:560–564.
73. Singh SN, Fletcher RD, Fisher SG, et al: Amiodarone in patients with congestive heart failure and asymptomatic ventricular arrhythmia. N Engl J Med 1995; 333:77–82.
74. Doval HC, Nul DR, Grancelli HO, et al: Randomized trial of low-dose amiodarone in severe congestive heart failure. Lancet 1994; 344:493–498.
75. Dusman RE, Stanton MS, Miles WM, et al: Clinical features of amiodarone-induced pulmonary toxicity. Circulation 1990; 82:51–59.
76. Fraire AE, Guntupalli KK, Greenberg SD, et al: Amiodarone pulmonary toxicity: a multidisciplinary review of current status. South Med J 1993; 86(1):67–77.
77. Gallagher JD: Class III antiarrhythmic agents: bretylium, sotalol, amiodarone. *In* Lynch C III (ed): Clinical Cardiac Electrophysiology, Perioperative Considerations, pp 113–156. Philadelphia: JB Lippincott, 1994.
78. Greenspon AJ, Kidwell GA, Hurley W, et al: Amiodarone-related postoperative adult respiratory distress syndrome. Circulation 1991; 84(suppl III):III-407–III-415.
79. Stevenson WG, Stevenson LW, Middlekauff HR, et al: Sudden death prevention in patients with advanced ventricular dysfunction. Circulation 1993; 88(6):2953–2961.
80. Figge HL, Figge J: The effects of amiodarone on thyroid hormone function: a review of the physiology and clinical manifestations. J Clin Pharmacol 1990; 30:588–595.
81. Hohnloser SH, Woosley RL: Sotalol. N Engl J Med 1994; 331(1):31–38.
82. Oberg KC, O'Toole MF, Gallastegui JL, et al: "Late" proarrhythmia due to quinidine. Am J Cardiol 1994; 74:192–194.
83. Ellenbogen KA, Wood MA, Stambler BS: Procainamide: a perspective on its value and danger. Heart Dis Stroke 1993; 2:473–476.
84. Jung W, Mletzko R, Manz M, et al: Efficacy and safety of combination therapy with amiodarone and type I agents for treatment of inducible ventricular tachycardia. PACE 1993; 16(I):778–788.
85. Whitford EG, McGovern B, Schoenfeld MH, et al: Long-term efficacy of mexiletine alone and in combination with class Ia antiarrhythmic drugs for refractory ventricular arrhythmias. Am Heart J 1988; 115:360–366.
86. Falk RH: Flecainide-induced ventricular tachycardia and fibrillation in patients treated for atrial fibrillation. Ann Intern Med 1989; 111:107–111.
87. The Cardiac Arrhythmia Suppression Trial (CAST) Investigators: CAST mortality and morbidity. Treatment versus placebo. N Engl J Med 1991; 324:781–788.
88. The Cardiac Arrhythmia Pilot Study (CAPS) Investigators: Effects of encainide, flecainide, imipramine and moricizine on ventricular arrhythmias during the year after acute myocardial infarction: the CAPS. Am J Cardiol 1988; 61:501–509.
89. Lee JT, Kroemer HK, Silberstein DJ, et al: The role of genetically determined polymorphic drug metabolism in the beta-blockade produced by propafenone. N Engl J Med 1990; 322:1764–1768.
90. Hernandez M, Reder RF, Marinchak RA, et al: Propafenone for malignant ventricular arrhythmia: an analysis of the literature. Am Heart J 1991; 121(4[1]):1178–1184.
91. Clyne CA, Estes NAM, Wang PJ: Moricizine. N Engl J Med 1992; 327(4):255–260.
92. Pratt CM: Proarrhythmic potential of moricizine: strengths and limitations of a data base analysis. Am J Cardiol 1990; 65:51D–55D.
93. The Cardiac Arrhythmia Suppression Trial II Investigators: Effect of the antiarrhythmic agent moricizine on survival after myocardial infarction. N Engl J Med 1992; 327:227–233.
94. Leclercq J-F, Leenhardt A, Lemarec H, et al: Predictive value of electrophysiologic studies during treatment of ventricular tachycardia with the beta-blocking agent nadolol. J Am Coll Cardiol 1990; 16:413–417.
95. Friehling TD, Lipshutz H, Marinchak RA, et al: Effectiveness of propranolol added to a type I antiarrhythmic agent for sustained ventricular tachycardia secondary to coronary artery disease. Am J Cardiol 1990; 65:1328–1333.
96. Bashir Y, Paul VE, Griffith MJ, et al: A prospective study of the efficacy and safety of adjuvant metoprolol and xamoterol in combination with amiodarone for resistant ventricular tachycardia associated with impaired left ventricular function. Am Heart J 1992; 124:1233–1240.
97. Solomon SD, Ridker PM, Antman EM: Ventricular arrhythmias in trials of thrombolytic therapy for acute myocardial infarction. A meta-analysis. Circulation 1993; 88(6):2575–2581.
98. Antman EM, Berlin JA: Declining incidence of ventricular fibrillation in myocardial infarction. Implications for the prophylactic use of lidocaine. Circulation 1992; 86(3):764–773.

99. Behar S, Reicher-Reiss H, Shechter M, et al: Frequency and prognostic significance of secondary ventricular fibrillation complicating acute myocardial infarction. Am J Cardiol 1993; 71:152–156.
100. Heidbüchel H, Tack J, Vanneste L, et al: Significance of arrhythmias during the first 24 hours of acute myocardial infarction treated with alteplase and effect of early administration of a β-blocker or a bradycardiac agent on their incidence. Circulation 1994; 89:1051–1059.
101. Horner SM: Efficacy of intravenous magnesium in acute myocardial infarction in reducing arrhythmias and mortality. Meta-analysis of magnesium in acute myocardial infarction. Circulation 1992; 86(3):774–779.
102. Woelfel A, Wohns DHW, Foster JR: Implications of sustained monomorphic ventricular tachycardia associated with myocardial injury. Ann Intern Med 1990; 112:141–143.
103. Mitrani RD, Biblo LA, Carlson MD, et al: Multiple monomorphic ventricular tachycardia configurations predict failure of antiarrhythmic drug therapy guided by electrophysiologic study. J Am Coll Cardiol 1993; 22:1117–1122.
104. Willems AR, Tijussen JG, Van Capelle FJL, et al: Determinants of prognosis in symptomatic ventricular tachycardia or ventricular fibrillation late after myocardial infarction. J Am Coll Cardiol 1990; 16:521–530.
105. Wilber DJ, Garan H, Finkelstein D, et al: Out-of-hospital cardiac arrest: use of electrophysiologic testing in the prediction of long-term outcome. N Engl J Med 1988; 318:19–24.
106. Adhar GC, Larson LW, Bardy GH, et al: Sustained ventricular arrhythmia: differences between survivors of cardiac arrest and patients with recurrent sustained ventricular tachycardia. J Am Coll Cardiol 1988; 12:159–165.
107. Poole JE, Mathisen TL, Kudenchuk PJ, et al: Long-term outcome in patients who survive out of hospital ventricular fibrillation and undergo electrophysiologic studies: evaluation by electrophysiologic subgroups. J Am Coll Cardiol 1990; 16:657–665.
108. Brugada P, Talajic M, Milleneers R, et al: The value of the clinical history to assess prognosis of patients with ventricular tachycardia or ventricular fibrillation after myocardial infarction. Eur Heart J 1989; 10:747–752.
109. Siebels J, Cappato R, Ruppel R, et al: Preliminary results of the Cardiac Arrest Study Hamburg (CASH). Am J Cardiol 1993; 72:109F–113F.
110. Greene HL: Sudden arrhythmic cardiac death—mechanisms, resuscitation and classification: the Seattle perspective. Am J Cardiol 1990; 65:4B–12B.
111. Every NR, Fahrenbruch CE, Hallstrom AP, et al: Influence of coronary bypass surgery on subsequent outcome of patients resuscitated from out of hospital cardiac arrest. J Am Coll Cardiol 1992; 19:1435–1439.
112. Kelly P, Ruskin JN, Vlahakes GJ, et al: Surgical coronary revascularization in survivors of prehospital cardiac arrest: its effect on inducible ventricular arrhythmias and long-term survival. J Am Coll Cardiol 1990; 15:267–273.
113. Kapoor W: Hypotension and syncope. *In* Braunwald E (ed): Heart Disease, A Textbook of Cardiovascular Medicine, 4th ed, p 875. Philadelphia: WB Saunders, 1992.
114. Moazez F, Peter T, Simonson J, et al: Syncope of unknown origin: clinical, noninvasive, and electrophysiologic determinants of arrhythmia induction and symptom recurrence during long-term follow-up. Am Heart J 1991; 121:81–88.
115. Maggioni AP, Zuanetti G, Franzosi MG, et al: Prevalence and prognostic significance of ventricular arrhythmias after acute myocardial infarction in the fibrinolytic era. GISSI-2 results. Circulation 1993; 87:312–322.
116. Connolly SJ, Cairns JA, the CAMIAT Pilot Study Group: Comparison of one-, six- and 24-hour ambulatory electrocardiographic monitoring for ventricular arrhythmia as a predictor of mortality in survivors of acute myocardial infarction. Am J Cardiol 1992; 69:308–313.
117. Teo KK, Yusuf S, Furberg CD: Effects of prophylactic antiarrhythmic drug therapy in acute myocardial infarction. An overview of results from randomized controlled trials. JAMA 1993; 270(13):1589–1595.
118. Zarembski DG, Nolan PE, Slack MK, et al: Empiric long-term amiodarone prophylaxis following myocardial infarction. Arch Intern Med 1993; 153:2661–2667.
119. Pedretti R, Etro MD, Laporta A, et al: Prediction of late arrhythmic events after acute myocardial infarction from combined use of noninvasive prognostic variables and inducibility of sustained monomorphic ventricular tachycardia. Am J Cardiol 1993; 71:1131–1141.
120. Wilber DJ, Olshansky B, Moran JF, et al: Electrophysiological testing and nonsustained ventricular tachycardia: use and limitations in patients with coronary artery disease and impaired ventricular function. Circulation 1990; 82:350–358.
121. Farrell TG, Bashir Y, Cripps T, et al: Risk stratification for arrhythmic events in postinfarction patients based on heart rate variability, ambulatory electrocardiographic variables and the signal-averaged electrocardiogram. J Am Coll Cardiol 1991; 18:687–697.
122. Bourke JP, Richards DAB, Ross DL, et al: Routine programmed electrical stimulation in survivors of acute myocardial infarction for prediction of spontaneous ventricular tachyarrhythmias during follow-up results, optimal stimulation protocol and cost-effective screening. J Am Coll Cardiol 1991; 18:780–788.
123. Chen X, Shenasa M, Borggrefe M, et al: Role of programmed ventricular stimulation in patients with idiopathic dilated cardiomyopathy and documented sustained ventricular tachyarrhythmias: inducibility and prognostic value in 102 patients. Eur Heart J 1994; 15:76–82.
124. Cohn JN, Johnson GR, Shabetai R, et al: Ejection fraction, peak exercise oxygen consumption, cardiothoracic ratio, ventricular arrhythmias, and plasma norepinephrine as determinants of prognosis in heart failure. Circulation 1993; 87(VI):VI-5–VI-16.
125. Mancini DM, Wong KL, Simson MB: Prognostic value of an abnormal signal-averaged electrocardiogram in patients with nonischemic congestive cardiomyopathy. Circulation 1993; 87:1083–1092.
126. Almendral JM, Ormaetxe J, Martinez-Alday JD, et al: Treatment of ventricular arrhythmias in patients with hypertrophic cardiomyopathy. Eur Heart J Soc 1993; 14(suppl J):71–72.
127. McKenna WJ: Sudden death in hypertrophic cardiomyopathy: assessment of patients at high risk. Circulation 1989; 80:1489–1482.
128. Kofflard MJ, Waldstein DJ, Vos J, et al: Prognosis in hypertrophic cardiomyopathy observed in a large clinic population. Am J Cardiol 1993; 72:939–943.
129. Fananapazir L, Chang AC, Epstein SE, et al: Prognostic determinants in hypertrophic cardiomyopathy. Prospective evaluation of a therapeutic strategy based on clinical, Holter, hemodynamic, and electrophysiological findings. Circulation 1992; 86:730–740.
130. Fananapazir L, Epstein SE: Hemodynamic and electrophysiologic evaluation of patients with hypertrophic cardiomyopathy surviving cardiac arrest. Am J Cardiol 1991; 67:280–287.
131. Hess OM, Krayenbuehl HP: Management of hypertrophic cardiomyopathy. Curr Opin Cardiol 1993; 8:434–440.
132. Fananapazir L, Leon MB, Bonow RO, et al: Sudden death during empiric amiodarone therapy in symptomatic hypertrophic cardiomyopathy. Am J Cardiol 1991; 67:169–174.
133. Mehta D, Davies MJ, Ward DE, et al: Ventricular tachycardias of right ventricular origin: markers of subclinical right ventricular disease. Am Heart J 1994; 127:360–366.
134. Carlson MD, White RD, Trohman RG, et al: Right ventricular outflow tract ventricular tachycardia: detection of previously unrecognized anatomic abnormalities using cine magnetic resonance imaging. J Am Coll Cardiol 1994; 24:720–727.
135. Wichter T, Borggrefe M, Haverkamp W, et al: Efficacy of antiarrhythmic drugs in patients with arrhythmogenic right ventricular disease. Results in patients with inducible and noninducible ventricular tachycardia. Circulation 1992; 86:29–37.
136. Leclercq J-F, Coumel F, Denjoy I, et al: Long-term follow-up after sustained monomorphic ventricular tachycardia: causes, pump failure, and empiric antiarrhythmic therapy that modify survival. Am Heart J 1991; 6(1):1685–1692.
137. Filho MM, Sosa E, Nishioka S, et al: Clinical and electrophysiologic features of syncope in chronic chagasic heart disease. J Cardiovasc Electrophysiol 1994; 5:563–570.
138. Winters SL, Cohen M, Greenberg S, et al: Sustained ventricular tachycardia associated with sarcoidosis: assessment of the underlying cardiac anatomy and the prospective utility of programmed ventricular stimulation, drug therapy and an implantable antitachycardia device. J Am Coll Cardiol 1991; 18(4):937–943.
139. Brooks R, Burgess JH: Idiopathic ventricular tachycardia. A review. Medicine 1988; 67:271–294.
140. Belhassen B, Viskin S: Idiopathic ventricular tachycardia and fibrillation. J Cardiovasc Electrophysiol 1993; 4:356–368.
141. Lerman BB, Belardinelli L, West GA, et al: Adenosine-sensitive ventricular tachycardia: evidence suggesting cyclic AMP–mediated triggered activity. Circulation 1986; 74:270–280.
142. Mont L, Seixas T, Brugada P, et al: The electrocardiographic, clinical, and electrophysiologic spectrum of idiopathic monomorphic ventricular tachycardia. Am Heart J 1992; 124:746–753.
143. Sung RJ, Shaprio WA, Shen EN, et al: Effects of verapamil on ventricular tachycardias possibly caused by reentry, automaticity, and triggered activity. J Clin Invest 1983; 72:250–360.

144. Lerman BB: Response of nonreentrant catecholamine-mediated ventricular tachycardia to endogenous adenosine and acetylcholine. Evidence for myocardial receptor-mediated effects. Circulation 1993; 87:382–390.
145. Wilber DJ, Baerman J, Olshansky B, et al: Adenosine-sensitive ventricular tachycardia. Clinical characteristics and response to catheter ablation. Circulation 1993; 87:126–134.
146. Sung RJ, Keung EC, Nguyen NX, et al: Effects of β-adrenergic blockade on verapamil-responsive and verapamil-irresponsive sustained ventricular tachycardias. J Clin Invest 1988; 81:688–699.
147. Gill JS, Blaszyk K, Ward DE, et al: Verapamil for the suppression of idiopathic ventricular tachycardia of left bundle branch–like morphology. Am Heart J 1993; 126:1126–1133.
148. Wesley RC Jr, Taylor R, Nadamanee K: Catecholamine-sensitive right ventricular tachycardia in the absence of structural heart disease: a mechanism of exercise-induced cardiac arrest. Cardiology 1991; 79:237–243.
149. Ritchie AH, Kerr CR, Qi A, et al: Nonsustained ventricular tachycardia arising from the right ventricular outflow tract. Am J Cardiol 1989; 64:594–598.
150. Mont L, Seixas T, Brugada P, et al: Clinical and electrophysiologic characteristics of exercise-related idiopathic ventricular tachycardia. Am J Cardiol 1991; 68:897–900.
151. Rahilly GT, Prystowsky EN, Zipes DP, et al: Clinical and electrophysiologic findings in patients with repetitive monomorphic ventricular tachycardia and otherwise normal electrocardiogram. Am J Cardiol 1982; 50:459–468.
152. Proclemer A, Ciani R, Feruglio GA: Right ventricular tachycardia with left bundle branch block and inferior axis morphology: clinical and arrhythmological characteristics in 15 patients. PACE 1989; 12:977–989.
153. Ohe T, Shimomura K, Aihara N, et al: Idiopathic sustained left ventricular tachycardia: clinical and electrophysiologic characteristics. Circulation 1988; 77:560–568.
154. Sethi KK, Manoharan S, Mohan JC, et al: Verapamil in idiopathic ventricular tachycardia of right bundle branch block morphology: observations during electrophysiologic and exercise testing. PACE 1986; 9:8–16.
155. Belhassen B, Shapira I, Pelleg A, et al: Idiopathic recurrent sustained ventricular tachycardia responsive to verapamil: an ECG-electrophysiologic entity. Am Heart J 1984; 108:1034–1037.
156. Okumura K, Matsuyama K, Miyagi H, et al: Entrainment of idiopathic ventricular tachycardia of left ventricular origin with evidence for reentry with an area of slow conduction and effect of verapamil. Am J Cardiol 1988; 62:727–732.
157. Leenhardt A, Coumel P, Slama R: Torsades de pointes. J Cardiovasc Electrophysiol 1992; 3:281–292.
158. Nguyen PT, Scheinman MM, Seger J: Polymorphous ventricular tachycardia: clinical characterization, therapy, and the QT interval. Circulation 1986; 74:340–349.
159. Jackman WM, Friday KJ, Anderson JL, et al: The long QT syndromes: a critical review, new clinical observations and a unifying hypothesis. Prog Cardiovasc Dis 1988; 31:115–172.
160. Hii JTY, Wyse DG, Gillis AM, et al: Precordial QT interval dispersion as a marker of torsades de pointes: disparate effects of class Ia antiarrhythmic drugs and amiodarone. Circulation 1992; 86:1376–1382.
161. Cosio FG, Goicolea A, Lopez Gil M, et al: Suppression of torsades de pointes with verapamil in patients with atrio-ventricular block. Eur Heart J 1991; 12:635–638.
162. Stevenson WG, Middlekauff HM, Stevenson LW, et al: Significance of aborted cardiac arrest and sustained ventricular tachycardia in patients referred for therapy of advanced heart failure. Am Heart J 1992; 124:123–130.
163. Schwartz PJ, Moss AJ, Vincent GM, et al: Diagnostic criteria for the long QT syndrome. An update. Circulation 1993; 88:782–784.
164. Schwartz PJ, Bonazzi O, Locati E, et al: Pathogenesis and therapy of the idiopathic long QT syndrome. Ann NY Acad Sci 1992; 644:112–141.
165. Priori SG, Napolitano C, Diehl L, et al: Dispersion of the QT interval. A marker of therapeutic efficacy in the idiopathic long QT syndrome. Circulation 1994; 89:1681–1689.
166. Schwartz PJ, Locati EH, Moss AJ, et al: Left cardiac sympathetic denervation in the therapy of congenital long QT syndrome. A worldwide report. Circulation 1991; 84:503–511.
167. Grubb BP: The use of oral labetalol in the treatment of arrhythmias associated to the long QT syndrome. Chest 1991; 100:1724–1725.
168. Wilde AAM, Janse MJ: Electrophysiological effects of ATP sensitive potassium channel modulation: implications for arrhythmogenesis. Cardiovasc Res 1994; 28:16–24.
169. Vos MA, Gorgels APM, Lipcsei GC, et al: Mechanism-specific antiarrhythmic effects of the potassium channel activator levcromakalim against repolarization-dependent tachycardias. J Cardiovasc Electrophysiol 1994; 5:731–742.
170. Meissner MD, Lehmann MH, Steinman RT, et al: Ventricular fibrillation in patients without significant structural heart disease: a multicenter experience with implantable cardioverter-defibrillator therapy. J Am Coll Cardiol 1993; 21:1406–1412.
171. Brugada P, Brugada J: Right bundle branch block, persistent ST segment elevation and sudden cardiac death: a distinct clinical and electrocardiographic syndrome. A multicenter report. J Am Coll Cardiol 1992; 20:1391–1396.
172. Wever EFD, Hauer RNW, Oomen A, et al: Unfavorable outcome in patients with primary electrical disease who survived an episode of ventricular fibrillation. Circulation 1993; 88:1021–1029.

19 Catheter Ablation of Ventricular Tachycardia

Lawrence S. Klein, MD
William M. Miles, MD
Raul D. Mitrani, MD
Douglas P. Zipes, MD

Although pharmacologic therapy of ventricular arrhythmias remains the mainstay of therapy for most patients with ventricular arrhythmias, nonpharmacologic approaches have been increasingly employed for several reasons.[1, 2] These include an improvement in the understanding of the mechanisms of ventricular arrhythmias, important technological advances, and an increasing desire among patients and physicians to eliminate tachycardia rather than suppressing the arrhythmia by using antiarrhythmic drugs. The risk of proarrhythmia, side effects, and long-term expense of antiarrhythmic drugs have also contributed to the allure of nonpharmacologic approaches (Table 19–1).

Implantable cardioverter defibrillators (ICDs) are most appropriate in patients who have had sudden cardiac death as a result of ventricular fibrillation or in patients with symptomatic sustained ventricular tachycardia (VT), especially when VT is associated with hemodynamic instability.[2] However, catheter ablation of VT is being increasingly utilized in patients with VT amenable to elimination by this technique.[3–16] Appropriate target arrhythmias include VT in patients without structural heart disease (idiopathic VT), left posterior fascicular VT (sometimes referred to as verapamil-sensitive VT), bundle branch reentrant VT, and stable monomorphic VTs in patients with coronary artery disease (CAD), usually patients with only one morphology of VT. Each of these applications are discussed in this chapter. Patients with hypotensive sustained VT, polymorphic VT, or ventricular fibrillation are not candidates for catheter ablation because of either the inability to map the arrhythmia (hemodynamic instability) or the inability to eliminate the arrhythmia (i.e., multiple foci or complex mechanisms as in ventricular fibrillation). Nonpharmacologic techniques to ablate VT include direct current (DC) shocks, intracoronary ethanol infusion, and radiofrequency (RF) energy. Although the latter technique is most common today, the other two techniques are important for historical reasons and are discussed briefly.

ABLATION OF VENTRICULAR TACHYCARDIA WITH THE USE OF DIRECT-CURRENT SHOCKS

DC capacitor discharge (other than for transthoracic electrical cardioversion) was initially applied to ablate the atrioventricular (AV) junction and control rapid ventricular rates associated with atrial tachyarrhythmias, most commonly atrial fibrillation.[17, 18] An early report[19] in 1983 demonstrated successful ablation of VT in three patients with the use of DC shocks administered through a catheter. In this report, one patient had idiopathic VT arising from the right ventricular outflow tract (RVOT), and two patients had VT because of CAD. Although there were no complications in this report, DC energy to ablate VT, especially in candidates for surgical elimination of VT or for implantable defibrillators, poses significant risks. These risks are, in part, because the procedure is cumbersome and complicated by the unavailability of catheters with a deflectable tip, making precise localization of the origin of VT and stable catheter contact with endocardium difficult and tedious. Other problems include the need for general anesthesia because of the pain associated with a capacitor discharge shock in the chest and damage to the electrode. If a second shock is necessary, the catheter has to be removed and replaced with a new catheter. This necessitates repeating the mapping procedure and adds to the length of the procedure and, possibly, to the risk of complications.[20, 21] In addition, DC ablation causes a pressure wave (barotrauma) that poses risk to cardiac structures, resulting in cardiac perforation in some instances.[20] Other disadvantages include a less homogeneous lesion whose size or location was less predictable because it depended on the impedance of the tissues being ablated and the catheter orientation, factors that are not always predictable through the use of fluoroscopic localization techniques. These inhomogeneous lesions have the potential for proarrhythmia. DC energy cannot be titrated, because it is delivered over only a few milliseconds.

In contrast, RF energy can be delivered in a more controlled fashion over a longer duration of time, typically 30 to 60 sec, thus giving the operator the ability to terminate energy delivery at any time if the desired effect is achieved (or not achieved) or if an adverse effect occurs. For these reasons, the role of DC ablation for VT has been limited, especially in recent years, as RF techniques have been refined and demonstrated to be safe. However, there are some advantages of DC ablation over RF. With available catheter designs and power availability with RF systems, only 50 W of power are available, resulting in a small lesion, generally 4–5 mm in diameter. Because a DC shock creates a larger and deeper lesion, an intramyocardial or epicardial focus could potentially be more easily approached with a DC shock. For practical purposes, however, such foci may be better treated with some of the newer enhancements of RF energy delivery, such as larger-tipped electrode catheters with higher current delivery, with other metals such as gold that produce a more efficient heat transfer, or possibly with a water-cooled electrode tip to allow for longer RF delivery time and therefore larger lesion size.

Some of the pros and cons of early attempts to ablate VT with the use of DC energy were demonstrated in the percutaneous mapping and ablation registry for VT[22] reported in 1988. This was a voluntary registry of patients undergoing ablation of the AV junction or VT with the use of DC techniques. Importantly, these ablations were performed early in the experience of most investigators and before the availability of RF energy or deflectable catheters. Also,

TABLE 19–1. BENEFITS OF RADIOFREQUENCY ABLATION VERSUS ANTIARRHYTHMIC DRUGS

Cure versus suppression
No proarrhythmia
No long-term side effects
Lower long-term expense
No noncompliance problems
No drug interaction problems

TABLE 19–2. ADVANTAGES AND DISADVANTAGES OF DIRECT CURRENT AND RADIOFREQUENCY ABLATION

Direct Current Ablation		Radiofrequency Ablation	
Advantages	**Disadvantages**	**Advantages**	**Disadvantages**
Larger lesion	Barotrauma	Deep anesthesia not needed	Smaller lesion
?Better penetration of scar/clot	Catheter damage	No barotrauma	Coagulum
Catheter-endocardium contact less essential	Need general anesthesia	Can titrate energy delivery	Limited scar/clot penetration
	Inhomogeneous lesion	No catheter damage	Catheter-endocardium contact essential
		No proarrhythmia	
		No valve/coronary artery damage	
		Homogeneous lesion	

these patients were ill, and the procedure was done as a "last resort." Patients in the registry had significant structural heart disease and had failed drug therapy. They were also thought not to be candidates for surgical arrhythmia management, which emphasizes the extent of structural heart disease in this patient cohort. In all, 164 patients followed for 12 ± 11 months were entered into the registry. Eighteen percent of the patients had no recurrent VT and were believed to have been cured of their arrhythmias. Another 41% also had no VT, but they required an antiarrhythmic drug to achieve this endpoint. Therefore, the total "success" rate was 59%, assuming that a previously ineffective antiarrhythmic drug becoming effective after ablation qualifies as a "success." The remaining 41% of patients had recurrent VT or procedure-related death (11 patients). Thus, although the success of catheter ablation of VT with DC energy was encouraging, the risks of the procedure combined with the failure rate left the door open for future developments that would provide safer and more effective techniques to ablate VT.[23]

USE OF RADIOFREQUENCY ENERGY IN ABLATION PROCEDURES

Because RF ablation techniques are described in several chapters in this text, the technique of RF ablation is only briefly described in this chapter. It is clear that RF ablation has revolutionized therapy for Wolff-Parkinson-White syndrome[24] and AV nodal reentry,[25] as well as for atrial tachyarrhythmias in selected patients.[26] RF ablation has also offered a new therapeutic alternative for many patients with VT. When used for the treatment of VT and other arrhythmia ablations, RF energy is delivered as alternating current with a frequency between 30 kHz and 300 MHz. RF energy is typically delivered as a continuous, unmodulated sine wave with a frequency of 500 kHz.[27] Although the same energy form is used for surgical electrocautery, the voltage used for ablation is about 20 times lower and is continuous rather than intermittent. Therefore, the energy waveform used for ablation procedures heats tissue without cutting it.[27, 28] In ablation procedures, RF energy is typically delivered between a 4-mm-long catheter electrode and a large skin electrode, although the ideal size and shape of the catheter electrode is a subject of continuous investigation and refinement. The cardiac lesion caused by RF ablation is typically 4 to 5 mm in diameter and about 3 mm in depth and is caused by heating. Advantages of RF energy over DC energy (Table 19–2) include the lack of the need for general anesthesia (although sedation is frequently used during most RF ablation procedures), absence of barotrauma, and a more controlled energy delivery, giving the operator the ability to titrate power. Furthermore, there is no catheter damage from RF energy delivery; therefore, energy can be delivered multiple times to a region of the heart without removing the catheter from the body. The lesion produced by RF energy is limited, homogeneous, and discrete, thus potentially minimizing the risk of proarrhythmia. These advantages of RF energy can also be considered a disadvantage in that the lesion is limited in size.

Additionally, because RF techniques use heat to destroy targeted cardiac tissue, if the temperature approaches or exceeds 100°C, a coagulum forms on the tip of the catheter, thus limiting current delivery to tissue and limiting lesion size.[28] This is referred to as an "impedance rise." When an impedance rise occurs, the catheter must be removed from the body and the coagulum wiped from the electrode. Impedance rises can usually be prevented by monitoring tip temperature of the electrode catheter with the use of a thermistor or thermocouple embedded in the tip or middle of the electrode. This may prevent the temperature from reaching or exceeding 100°C.[29] Other important aspects of RF energy delivery are that the catheter must be in good contact with tissue for a successful ablation (adequate lesion) to occur. Catheter-tip temperature monitoring may also help verify good catheter tip–tissue contact and may aid the operator in titrating power delivery.[29] An important limitation of RF energy is its inability to penetrate scar or clot. This is particularly important in patients with VT as a result of CAD. Of importance is that RF energy does not appear to damage cardiac valve structures.

CATHETER ABLATION OF VENTRICULAR TACHYCARDIA

Feasibility and Limitations

Certain VTs are readily amenable to catheter ablation, particularly by RF techniques. One such example is bundle branch reentry, in which conduction in the right bundle branch (RBB), or occasionally the left bundle branch (LBB), is typically eliminated, thereby interrupting the arrhythmia circuit.[30–34] This is a relatively simple procedure with a well-defined endpoint (i.e., creation of right bundle branch block). Several potential factors may limit the efficacy of catheter ablation for other types of VT (Table 19–3). As noted previously, these factors include the presence of endocardial scar or clot, limiting energy delivery to the desired site. An intramyocardial or epicardial VT focus, or perhaps multiple morphologies of VT or polymorphic VT, may limit the ability of catheter ablation techniques to eliminate the targeted substrate. Other patients have VT that cannot be induced in the electrophysiology (EP) laboratory, or if VT is induced, it is hemodynamically unstable and therefore unsafe for

TABLE 19–3. LIMITATIONS OF RADIOFREQUENCY ABLATION FOR VENTRICULAR TACHYCARDIA

Endocardial scar or clot
Intramyocardial or epicardial focus
Multiple ventricular tachycardia morphologies
Noninducible ventricular tachycardia
Polymorphic ventricular tachycardia
Hemodynamically unstable (rapid) ventricular tachycardia

TABLE 19–4. RADIOFREQUENCY ABLATION OF VENTRICULAR TACHYCARDIA

Selection of Patients	Reasons
Better Candidates	
Bundle branch reentry	Right or left bundle branch easily localized
Idiopathic (especially outflow tract) VT	High success rate, especially if RV outflow tract
VT in patients with coronary artery disease	If one morphology and hemodynamically stable
Worse Candidates	
RV dysplasia or dilated cardiomyopathy	New VTs may appear
Polymorphic VT	Mapping complexity
Rapid VT	Unsafe hypotension during mapping

Abbreviations: RV, right ventricular; VT, ventricular tachycardia.

mapping. In all of these instances, catheter ablation is not currently feasible. There is hope that these limitations ultimately can be overcome, at least to some extent, with multielectrode mapping catheters or perhaps computer mapping techniques.

Catheter stability and tissue contact are extremely important, especially with RF techniques as noted previously, but catheter tip–tissue contact is sometimes difficult to obtain in certain areas of the ventricle, at least with currently available deflectable catheters. VT in patients with CAD presents difficulties in mapping, because the relatively easier techniques of endocardial activation and pace mapping are frequently inaccurate in localizing the critical zone of slow conduction that needs to be eliminated to ablate a VT. Furthermore, new VTs can appear after an ablation procedure in patients who have progressive underlying structural heart disease, such as another myocardial infarction or worsening of a congestive dilated cardiomyopathy.

Given these limitations, catheter ablation of VT may not always be first-line therapy. However, in patients with bundle branch reentry or idiopathic VT, VT ablation may be the initial therapeutic choice (Table 19–4).

Intracoronary Ethanol Ablation

Although mostly limited to historical interest, some laboratories still perform intracoronary ethanol catheter ablation.[35–38] Because it is infrequently performed, this technique is only briefly described.

Transcoronary chemical ablation has two primary goals: to bypass the thickened and scarred endocardium that might impede the ability of an endocardial catheter to reach the VT focus, and to target arrhythmia therapy to a specific arrhythmogenic region. This technique was initially shown to effectively ablate aconitine-induced VT in dogs[38] and has been subsequently used in a limited fashion in humans.[35–37] Intracoronary ethanol ablation involves identifying the arrhythmogenic focus through intracardiac catheter mapping. Subsequently, the coronary branch supplying this area is identified angiographically, and when found, is selectively cannulated and injected with either iced saline or an antiarrhythmic agent such as lidocaine or procainamide during sustained VT (Figs. 19–1 to 19–3). Termination of the arrhythmia by such an injection is strong evidence that the targeted and cannulated coronary branch is providing the blood supply to the arrhythmogenic region. If such an arterial branch is identified, blood flow through the artery is permanently interrupted by injection of 1 or 2 mL of 95% ethanol. Although some successes with this technique have been reported, intracoronary ethanol ablation is cumbersome, and the tachycardia-specific artery may either not be identified or not be found in many patients. Furthermore, the size of the lesion is very difficult to control, and inadvertent reflux of ethanol into other arterial branches may create a larger-than-desired infarct.[35]

Catheter Ablation of Bundle Branch Reentrant Ventricular Tachycardia

His-Purkinje system reentry has been recognized for more than two decades, although elucidation of the mechanism of sustained bundle branch reentry in humans has occurred more recently. Now that the tachycardia circuit is well understood, catheter ablation to eliminate this arrhythmia is readily achieved.[30–34]

A diagnostic electrophysiologic study is essential to confirm the diagnosis of bundle branch reentry. Typically, bundle branch reentrant tachycardia results in AV dissociation during VT, probably as a result of the rapid rates and relatively poor ventriculoatrial conduction in these patients. A His potential or RBB potential usually precedes each QRS complex. The duration of the His-ventricular (H-V) or RBB-ventricular (RBB-V) interval during tachycardia is usually the same or longer than the H-V or RBB-V interval of supraventricular complexes. Furthermore, the spontaneous H-H or RBB-RBB cycle length variations precede a change in VT cycle length (Fig. 19–4). Finally, the His-to-RBB conduction time during tachycardia is identical to or shorter than the His-to-RBB conduction time during sinus rhythm. Typical bundle branch reentrant VT has the QRS morphology of a left bundle branch block (LBBB), because the circuit is anterograde down the RBB. LBBB is usually associated with left axis deviation. Bundle branch reentry is usually seen in patients with a dilated cardiomyopathy but can occur in patients with CAD or, rarely, in patients without known structural heart disease but in whom His-Purkinje conduction delay has been demonstrated.[34] The key factor underlying the presence of bundle branch reentry is His-Purkinje conduction delay. It is important to differentiate bundle branch reentrant VT from supraventricular tachycardia with aberration or intraventricular reentrant VT. Other arrhythmias that must be differentiated include fascicular tachycardia and antidromic AV reentry through an atriofascicular (Mahaim) fiber. The change in H-H intervals preceding changes in ventricular cycle length is important, because intramyocardial VT with retrograde activation of the bundle branches results in H-H cycle length changes *after* changes in the tachycardia cycle length. Bundle branch reentry accounted for 6% of all VTs in an active referral EP laboratory and for 40% of sustained VTs having an LBBB morphology in patients with an idiopathic dilated cardiomyopathy.[30] Bundle branch reentrant VT frequently is rapid and is associated with syncope and hemodynamic collapse. In an occasional patient, the direction of the tachycardia circuit may be reversed (i.e., retrograde up the RBB), giving rise to a tachycardia with a RBB block (RBBB) QRS morphology. Rarely, there may be reentry within the left anterior and left posterior fascicles (i.e., interfascicular reentry).[34]

After the diagnosis of bundle branch reentry has been confirmed, ablation of the RBB eliminates tachycardia. If it fails to do so, it may be because the tachycardia is interfascicular (i.e., utilizing the left posterior and left anterior fascicles) and the RBB is a bystander. To ablate the RBB, the ablation electrode must be positioned across

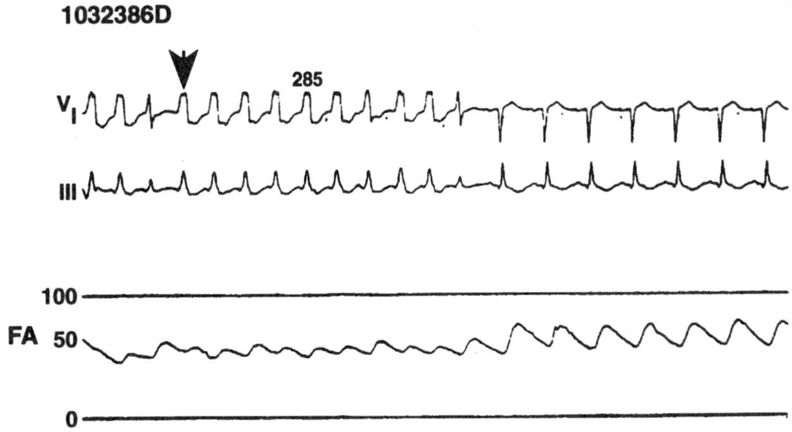

Figure 19–1. Sustained ventricular tachycardia (VT) was terminated with an intracoronary injection of iced saline. This recording is from a patient whose VT was refractory to all antiarrhythmic medications, including amiodarone. The tachycardia-specific coronary artery was cannulated, and VT was reproducibly terminated with iced saline. This procedure identified the blood supply to the arrhythmogenic region. *Abbreviation:* FA, femoral artery pressure recording. (From Nora MO, Miles WM, Klein LS, et al: Alcohol ablation of ventricular tachycardia. J Cardiovasc Electrophysiol 1991; 2:456.)

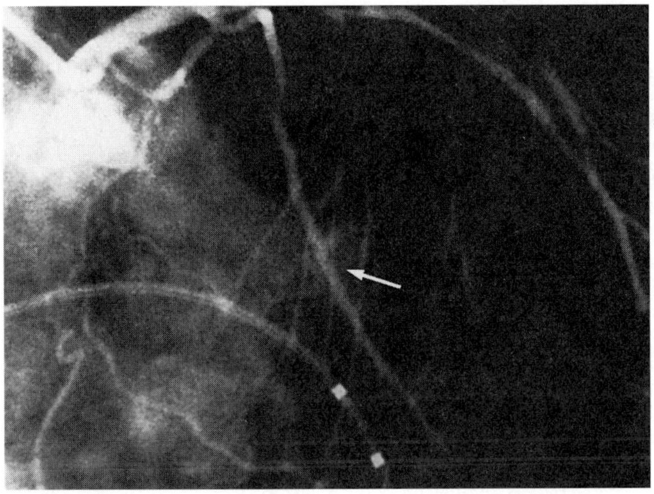

Figure 19–2. Radiograph of the coronary arterial tree from the patient in Figure 19–1, in whom iced saline terminated ventricular tachycardia. A marginal branch was the tachycardia-specific artery *(arrow)*. (From Nora MO, Miles WM, Klein LS, et al: Alcohol ablation of ventricular tachycardia. J Cardiovasc Electrophysiol 1991; 2:456.)

Figure 19–3. Radiograph from the patient in Figures 19–1 and 19–2. The marginal branch has become occluded *(arrow)* after injection of intracoronary ethanol. This permanently eliminated ventricular tachycardia in this patient. (From Nora MO, Miles WM, Klein LS, et al: Alcohol ablation of ventricular tachycardia. J Cardiovasc Electrophysiol 1991; 2:456.)

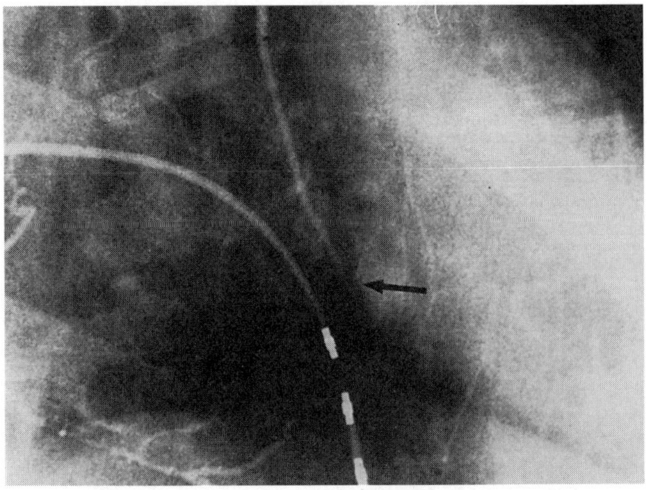

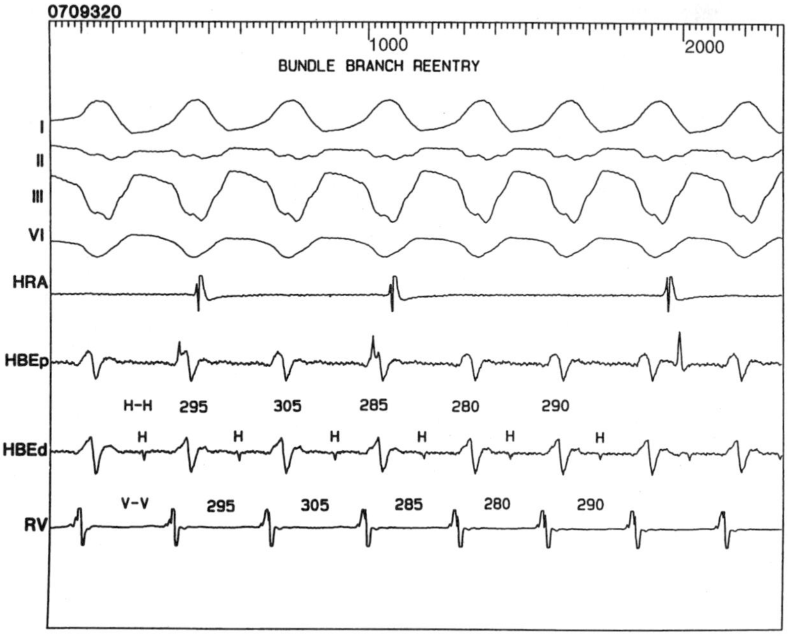

Figure 19–4. Sustained bundle branch reentry tachycardia. There is atrioventricular dissociation during ventricular tachycardia (VT), and VT has the morphology of a left bundle branch block with a leftward axis, typical for bundle branch reentry. The His-His (H-H) intervals during cycle length changes precede the ventricular-ventricular (V-V) interval changes. This is characteristic of bundle branch reentry and argues strongly against intramyocardial reentrant VT with retrograde penetration of the His-Purkinje system. *Abbreviations:* HBEd, distal His bundle lead; HBEp, proximal His bundle lead; HRA, high right atrium; RV, right ventricle.

the anterior leaflet of the tricuspid valve. A His potential may be recorded in this location. The catheter is then advanced farther across the valve until a large ventricular and an RBB potential are recorded and little or no atrial potential is seen. The interval between the RBB potential and ventricular activation is usually 20 msec shorter than the H-V interval. RF energy is then delivered to this region, and complete RBBB occurs (Fig. 19–5). When this procedure is successful, the tachycardia can no longer be induced.

Although ablation of the RBB eliminates bundle branch reentrant VT, many of the patients who have bundle branch reentry have severe underlying structural heart disease and may have VTs as a result of other mechanisms. Therefore, these patients frequently require antiarrhythmic drugs or ICDs in addition to ablation. Because these patients originally have long H-V intervals in sinus rhythm, and the RBB becomes eliminated as a target of ablation, a permanent pacemaker may be needed in some patients because of the risk of complete heart block. The indications for permanent pacing in these cases is not well defined, although many investigators implant a pacemaker if the final H-V interval exceeds 100 msec, and certainly if His-Purkinje block can be demonstrated with atrial pacing. Ablation of the LBB in patients with underlying LBBB as a result of delay in the left bundle may prevent the need for a permanent pacemaker in some patients.[33]

IDIOPATHIC VENTRICULAR TACHYCARDIA

Diagnosis

Because this chapter is focused on therapy, diagnostic information is not stressed. However, when considering the use of ablation for idiopathic VT, the diagnosis must be secure. Idiopathic VT may account for as much as 10% of patients with VT referred for EP study.

Classification of idiopathic VT is complex, in large part because the mechanisms of this form of VT is still relatively poorly understood, and many of the syndromes overlap. Most commonly, these arrhythmias are grouped into three classes: (1) Repetitive monomorphic VT; (2) Paroxysmal sustained VT; and (3) Idiopathic left ventricu-

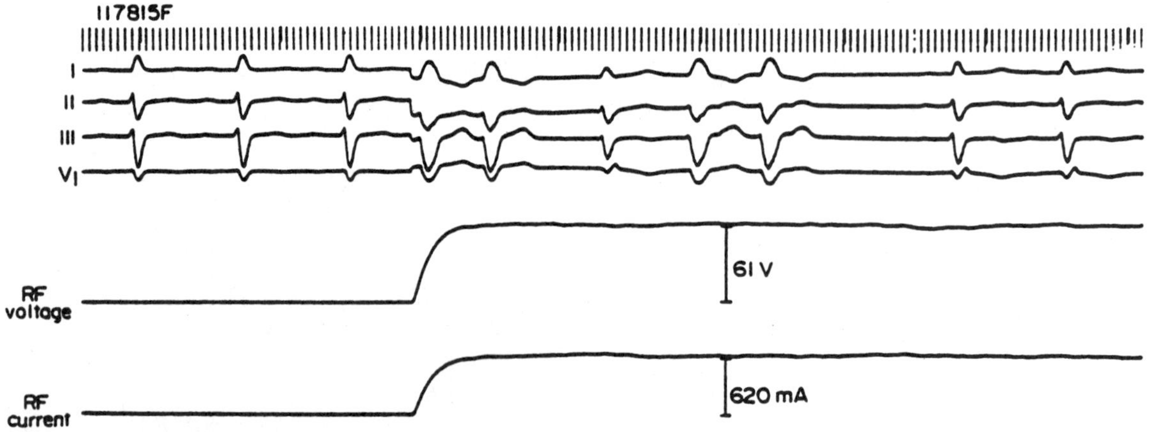

Figure 19–5. Ablation of the right bundle branch in a patient with bundle branch reentry. The rhythm in this tracing is sinus. Radiofrequency (RF) current is delivered, and within a couple of seconds, right bundle branch block occurs, indicating successful ablation of the right bundle branch. This therapy is curative for sustained bundle branch reentry tachycardia but does not eliminate other intramyocardial reentrant ventricular tachycardias that may also be present in these patients.

TABLE 19–5. IDIOPATHIC VENTRICULAR TACHYCARDIA

Ventricular Tachycardia Type	Characteristics
Repetitive monomorphic	Nonsustained Often adenosine-sensitive Good long-term prognosis; syncope rare Mechanism: ? triggered activity
Paroxysmal sustained	Sustained Often catecholamine-sensitive May terminate with adenosine May cause syncope Mechanisms: ? triggered activity
Idiopathic left	Usually verapamil-sensitive Occasionally adenosine-sensitive Usually sustained May cause syncope Origin: Usually left posterior fascicle region Mechanism: ? reentry

lar (LV) tachycardia. Many investigators refer to paroxysmal sustained VT as catecholamine-sensitive or exercise-induced VT if such is the case. Another term for idiopathic left ventricular VT is verapamil-sensitive VT, if the VT is suppressed by verapamil. These VTs frequently arise from or near the left posterior fascicle (Table 19–5).

The mechanisms of idiopathic VT are not discussed in detail here. Briefly, idiopathic LV VT is thought to be caused by reentry. Repetitive monomorphic VT and paroxysmal sustained VT are thought to be the result of triggered activity, possibly due to either early or delayed afterdepolarizations.

Catheter Ablation of Idiopathic VT

Attempts to ablate idiopathic VT initially used DC shocks guided by pace mapping and, occasionally, endocardial activation mapping.[38] More recently, attempts to ablate idiopathic VT have used RF energy sources. Our initial experience[3] included 16 patients; VT was eliminated in 15 of these patients by using RF energy delivered through a catheter. In this series, one patient had VT arising from the left ventricle. The remainder of the patients had VT arising from the right ventricle, the majority of whom had RVOT VT. However, three VTs arose from the right ventricular (RV) inflow tract and one VT from the free wall of the RV. There were no complications in this early series. Subsequent to that, Calkins and colleagues[5] reported similar success rates, but found that VTs arising from sites other than the RVOT were less likely to be successfully ablated with current technology. Our more recent experience confirms their findings.

Our experience with idiopathic VT ablation with the use of RF energy includes 58 patients (24 women) with a mean age of 37 years. The mean follow-up was 24 months. Symptoms before ablation included presyncope (28 patients), palpitations (21 patients), syncope (8 patients), and chest pain (1 patient). The mean duration of symptomatic VT before ablation was 4.2 years. A mean of 2.3 drug trials failed to control VT. VT was mapped to the RVOT in 36 of the 58 patients. Fourteen of 22 non-RVOT VTs mapped to the left ventricle, and eight mapped to the right ventricle (six, RV inflow; two, RV free wall). Eight of the 14 LV VTs were left posterior fascicular. RF ablation targeting nonfascicular VTs was guided by localization of the earliest local ventricular activation time and by pace mapping. Fascicular VT ablation was guided by early Purkinje potentials. RF ablation eliminated VT in 49 of 58 patients (85% success rate). In patients with RVOT VT, RF ablation eliminated VT in 35 of the 36 patients (97% success rate). Non-RVOT VT was successfully ablated in 14 of 22 patients (63% success rate). Three patients required two RF ablation sessions to successfully eliminate VT. Two patients were treated for postprocedure pericardial effusions, and one developed a transient segmental wall motion abnormality seen by echocardiography. During follow-up, no patient had spontaneous or inducible VT. We conclude from these results that RF ablation for idiopathic VT is feasible and safe. The acute success rate for RVOT VT approaches 100%. Neither late recurrence nor proarrhythmia has been observed in our experience.

When pace mapping is used to identify the site of origin of an idiopathic VT, the pacing-induced QRS complex must be morphologically identical to the spontaneous VT in at least 11 of 12 electrocardiography (ECG) leads, and usually, a 12-of-12 match is necessary (Figs. 19–6, 19–7). In our series, the mean endocardial activation time from successful ablation sites was 38 msec before the onset of the QRS complex during VT (Figs. 19–8 to 19–12). In patients who presented with sustained VT, the majority (about 90%) had inducible sustained VT at EP study. Of patients presenting with nonsustained VT, all had nonsustained VT induced at EP study, although most required isoproterenol infusion for induction. Isoproterenol is required to induce sustained VT in the EP laboratory in most patients with nonsustained VT. In a few patients presenting with sustained VT in whom sustained VT cannot be induced either at control or during isoproterenol infusion, epinephrine infusion (0.1–0.3 μg/kg/min) has been used to facilitate VT induction. Overall, the mean number of RF pulses was six, and the median number of RF pulses was three. Twelve patients required only one RF pulse. Of the six patients who had a failed ablation, one (a patient with spontaneous, hypotensive sustained VT) received an implantable antitachycardia device, two received sotalol, one received flecainide, one received verapamil, and one received a beta blocker.

Although we no longer obtain signal-averaged ECGs in these patients, our early experience suggested that the majority of these patients had a normal signal-averaged ECG both before and after the ablation session.

Verapamil-sensitive LV tachycardias appear to be a special case in which VT can arise from or adjacent to the Purkinje system, usually the left posterior fascicle.[4, 9] This fact helps with the mapping procedure for these tachycardias, in that a fascicular potential can frequently be recorded from the site at which RF energy delivery eliminates VT (see Fig. 19–12; Figs. 19–13, 19–14). Because these tachycardias can often be entrained, the mechanism is thought to be reentry. Importantly, when attempting to ablate this form of VT, the fascicular potential, if recorded, is usually earliest at the successful ablation site. Nakagawa and associates[4] reported a series of these patients in whom they used Purkinje potentials to guide ablation. These investigators found that activation and pace mapping were generally not useful for predicting ablation success. Other investigators have found the Purkinje potential to be less useful and a nonspecific marker.[9] We have found that a combined approach of an early Purkinje potential and pace mapping is frequently a reasonable method for approaching these VTs.

ABLATION OF VENTRICULAR TACHYCARDIA IN PATIENTS WITH STRUCTURAL HEART DISEASE

Structural heart disease contributes to the genesis of VT in most patients who present with this arrhythmia. Most investigations of ablation techniques for VT in patients with structural heart disease have been in patients with CAD.[10–16] It is thought that VT in patients with CAD results from a combination of a region of slow conduction and a region of anatomic or functional block, allowing reentry to occur, often around a border zone adjacent to an area of myocardial infarction.

Mapping the VT location and then ablating the VT in these patients is confounded by the structural cardiac abnormalities that are often present in patients with CAD (Table 19–3). Often, a large, deep lesion is required to eliminate a tachycardia substrate, and this

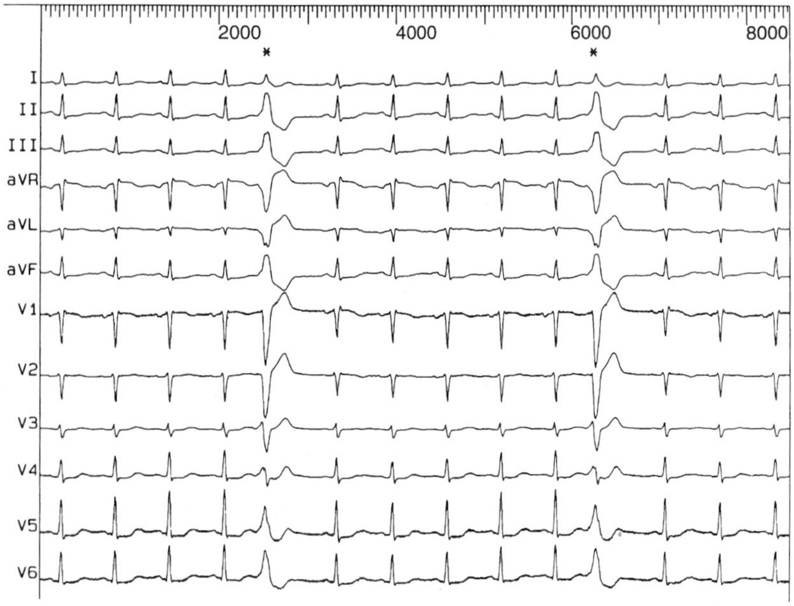

Figure 19–6. Premature ventricular complexes (PVCs) in a patient with idiopathic ventricular tachycardia (VT). Occasionally, in these patients, VT cannot be induced in the electrophysiology laboratory. PVCs having the same morphology as VT can be used for mapping. *Abbreviations:* aVF, augmented unipolar lead, left leg; aVL, augmented unipolar lead, left arm; aVR, augmented unipolar lead, right arm.

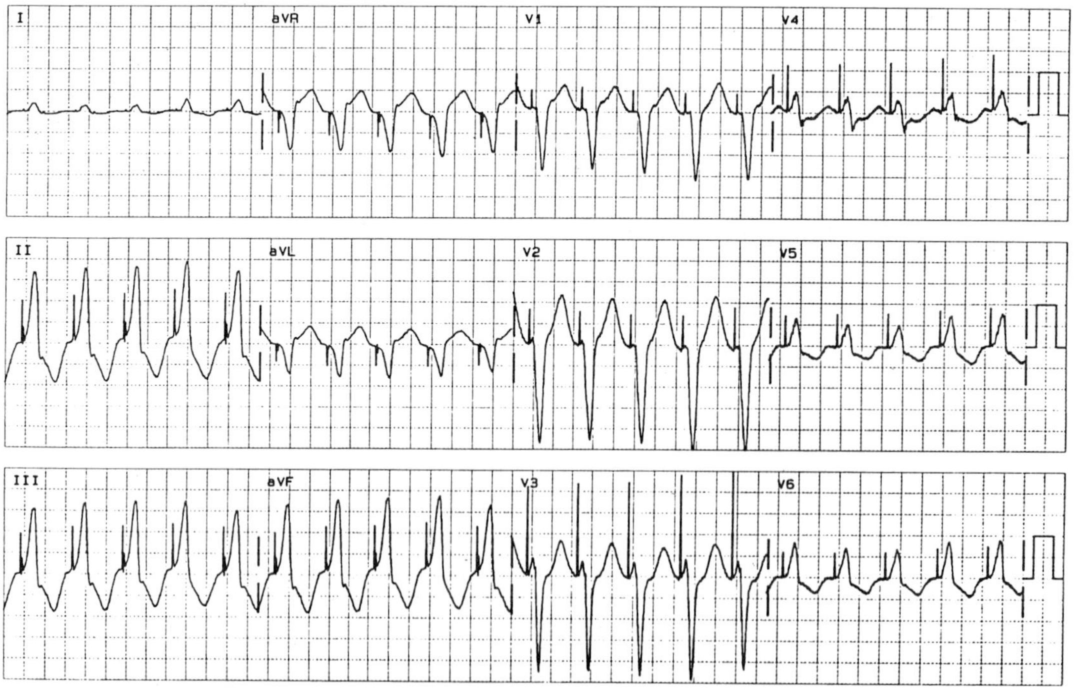

Figure 19–7. In the patient in Figure 19–6, pace mapping was used in an attempt to mimic the QRS morphology of the spontaneous premature ventricular complexes (PVCs). This is an example of a 12-of-12 pace-mapping match. Ablation from the site from which this pace map was obtained eliminated both the PVCs and ventricular tachycardia in this patient. *Abbreviations:* aVF, augmented unipolar lead, left leg; aVL, augmented unipolar lead, left arm; aVR, augmented unipolar lead, right arm.

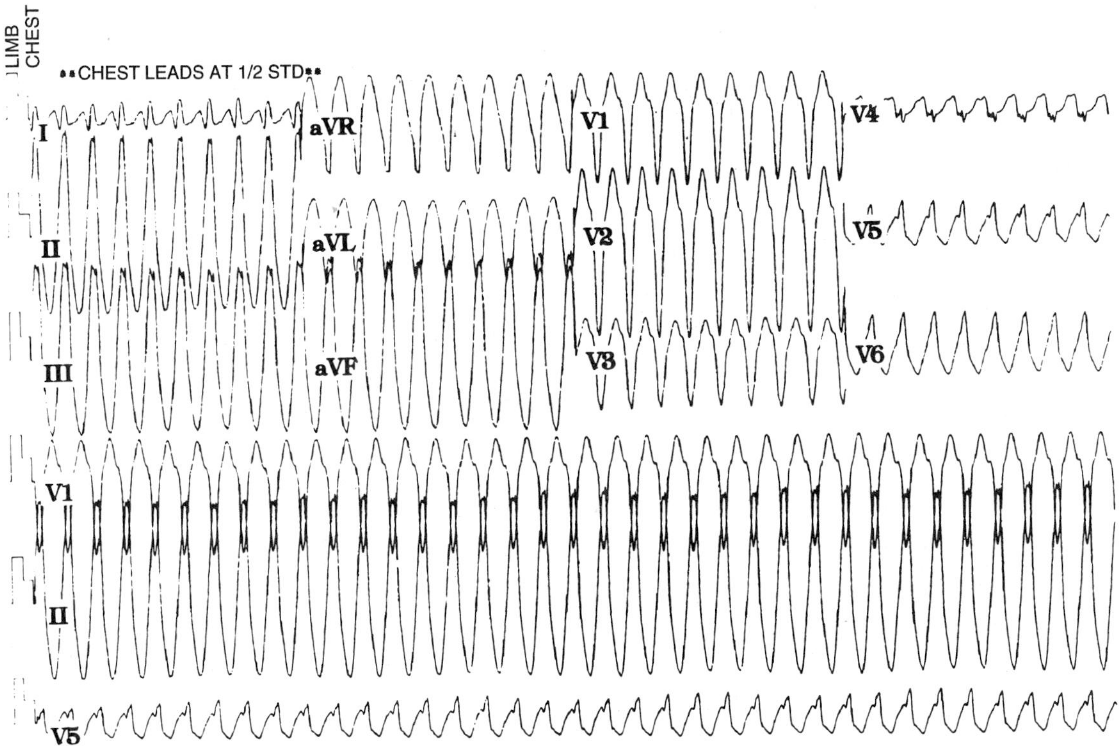

Figure 19–8. Scalar 12-lead electrocardiogram of ventricular tachycardia (VT) in a patient without structural heart disease who had paroxysmal sustained VT. *Abbreviations:* aVF, augmented unipolar lead, left leg; aVL, augmented unipolar lead, left arm; aVR, augmented unipolar lead, right arm.

Figure 19–9. Intracardiac recordings from the site from which delivery of radiofrequency energy eliminated ventricular tachycardia (VT). Note that the endocardial ventricular electrogram from the successful ablation site precedes the onset of the QRS complex on the surface electrocardiogram by 35 msec. The first complex in this tracing is a fusion beat, and the next three complexes are VT. Surface leads I, II, III, and V1 and intracardiac recordings from the ablation catheter, high right atrium (HRA), proximal and distal His bundle leads (HBEP and HBED, respectively), and the right ventricle (RV) are shown.

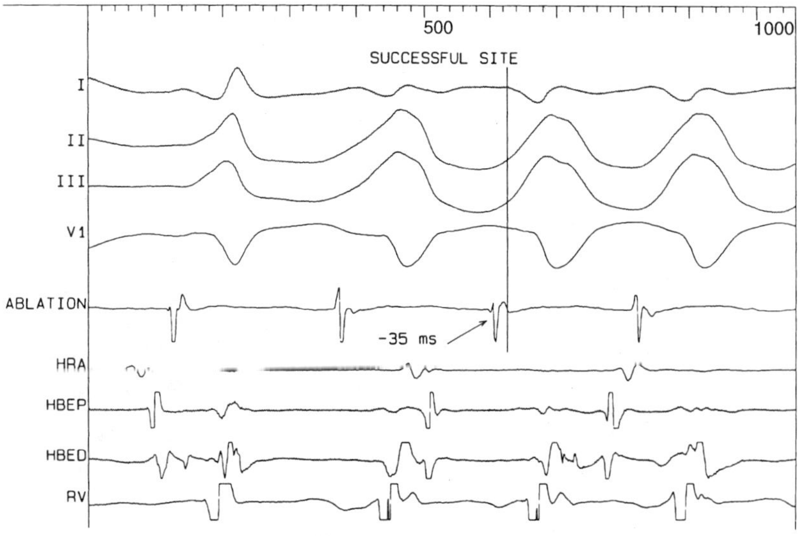

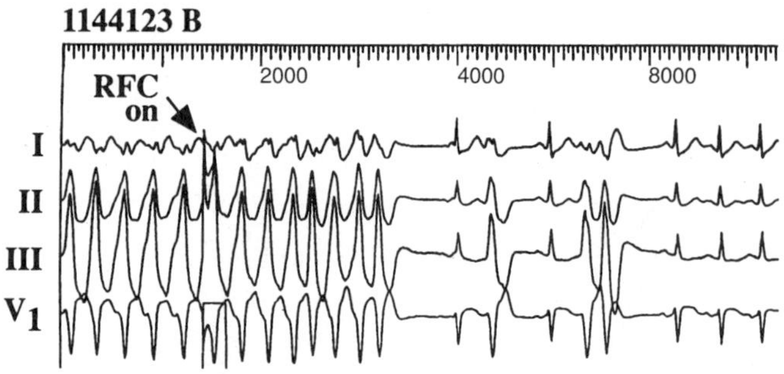

Figure 19–10. Idiopathic ventricular tachycardia (VT) arising from the right ventricular outflow tract. Illustrated is the successful radiofrequency pulse delivery. Note that within 2 sec of the onset of radiofrequency current (RFC), VT terminates. VT was no longer inducible in this patient after delivery of this RF pulse. Premature ventricular complexes (PVCs) having the morphology of VT early during the burn are common. These are thought to be caused by enhanced automaticity as a result of surrounding regions of hyperthermia.

may not be possible with RF energy through a 4-mm tip and with current technology. Additionally, pace mapping and endocardial activation are not as reliable in these patients as they are in patients with idiopathic VT, probably because of myocardial fibrosis altering myocardial activation patterns and different mechanisms of VT in the two patient populations.

Five techniques (Table 19–6) have been proposed for mapping VT in patients with structural heart disease (predominantly those with CAD): (1) early endocardial activation during VT (the local ventricular electrogram precedes the onset of the QRS complex on the surface ECG during VT); (2) isolated middiastolic potentials, probably representing activation of a critical region of slow conduction in the VT circuit during diastole (Figs. 19–15, 19–16); (3) pace mapping, as in patients with idiopathic VT; (4) local subthreshold burst pacing to terminate VT; and (5) concealed entrainment. Concealed entrainment refers to a technique in which pacing from the ablation or mapping catheter is performed in the region of slow conduction, thereby avoiding fusion with VT. The goal of this technique is to accelerate the tachycardia to the pacing rate (i.e., entrain it) without changing the QRS morphology during rapid or different pacing rates. If the QRS morphology changes at different pacing rates from a region from which VT can be entrained, "classic entrainment" has occurred and is probably caused by pacing from an entrance site to

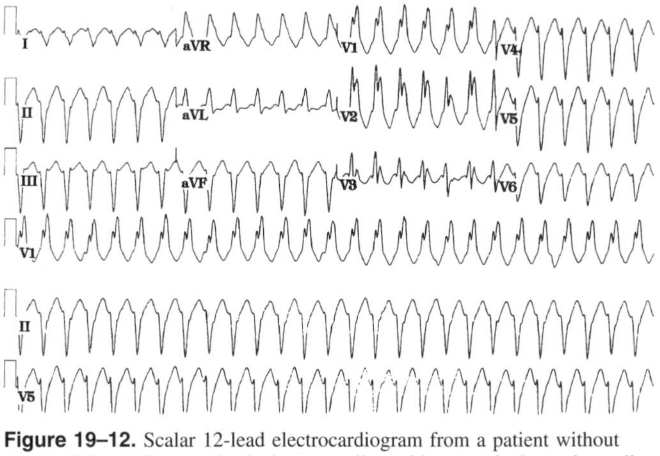

Figure 19–12. Scalar 12-lead electrocardiogram from a patient without structural heart disease who had verapamil-sensitive ventricular tachycardia (VT). The morphology of the QRS complexes is that of a right bundle branch block with an extreme leftward axis, typical for a VT arising from or near the left posterior fascicle. *Abbreviations:* aVF, augmented unipolar lead, left leg; aVL, augmented unipolar lead, left arm; aVR, augmented unipolar lead, right arm.

the region of slow conduction. No single criterion has been found to be universally successful in predicting a successful site for VT ablation. However, Morady and colleagues[12] reported using all of the criteria noted previously (except subthreshold stimulation) in combination and achieved success rates of up to 80% to eliminate a targeted VT. It should be noted that patients in this study remained on antiarrhythmic drugs, and other VTs were inducible in many of these patients. Patients participating in this and similar studies have been highly selected for being appropriate for catheter ablation, and these patients probably represent less than 10% of patients with CAD referred for management of VT. Although ablation in patients with multiple VT morphologies is often extraordinarily difficult, in some instances, VT with different morphologies may use the same area of slow conduction and be eliminated with a single RF pulse.

Stevenson and associates[11] used stimulus to QRS intervals and electrogram to QRS intervals in patients in whom concealed entrainment was demonstrated to differentiate slow conduction zones from bystander areas adjacent to the circuit during catheter mapping based on a computer simulation model. When this model was tested in 31 monomorphic VTs in 15 patients, RF current terminated VT in 24

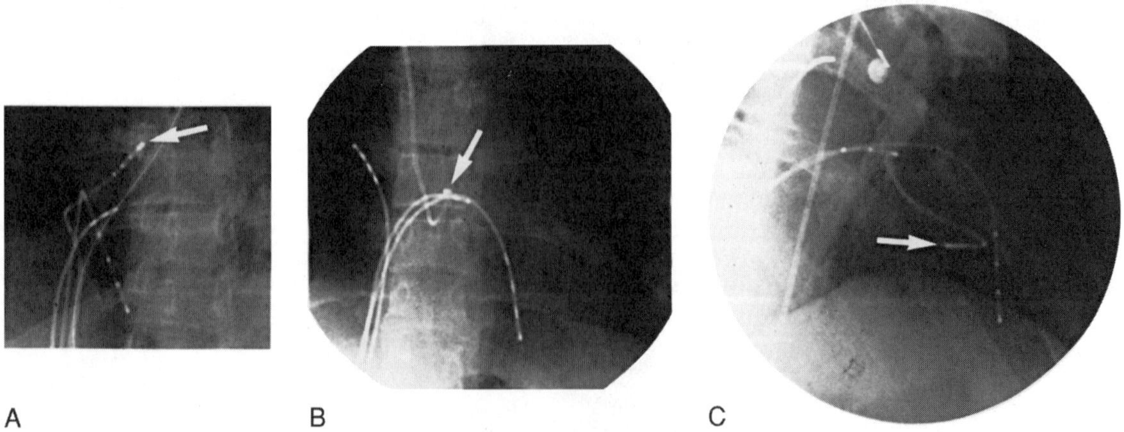

A B C

Figure 19–11. Three radiographs of typical catheter positions from which idiopathic ventricular tachycardia (VT) can be ablated. These three positions do not account for all successful ablation sites but represent three of the more common ones. In each instance, the catheter with the large distal tip is indicated. This is the distal ablating electrode *(arrow)*. *A,* A right ventricular outflow tract location. *B,* A right ventricular inflow tract location. Note the proximity of the ablation catheter tip to the catheter recording the His potential. *C,* A left posterior fascicular VT is being ablated. (From Klein LS, Shih HT, Hackett FK, et al: Radiofrequency catheter ablation of ventricular tachycardia in patients without structural heart disease. Circulation 1992; 85:1666–1674.)

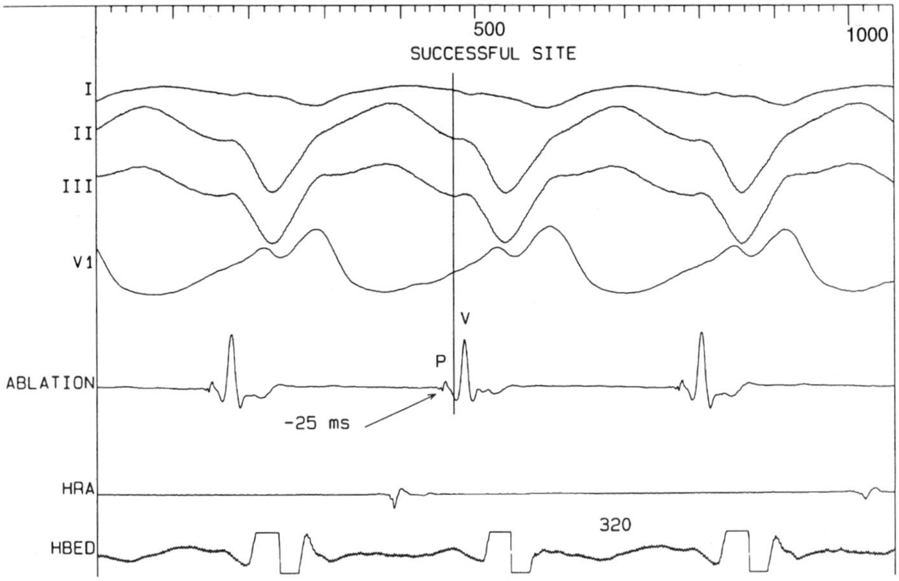

Figure 19–13. Intracardiac recording from the distal poles of the ablation catheter in the left ventricle at a site where delivery of radiofrequency current eliminated ventricular tachycardia in the patient in Figure 19–12. Note that from the successful ablation site, an early potential ("Purkinje" potential) precedes the onset of the ventricular (V) electrogram. *Abbreviations:* HBED, distal His bundle leads; HRA, high right atrium; P, Purkinje potential.

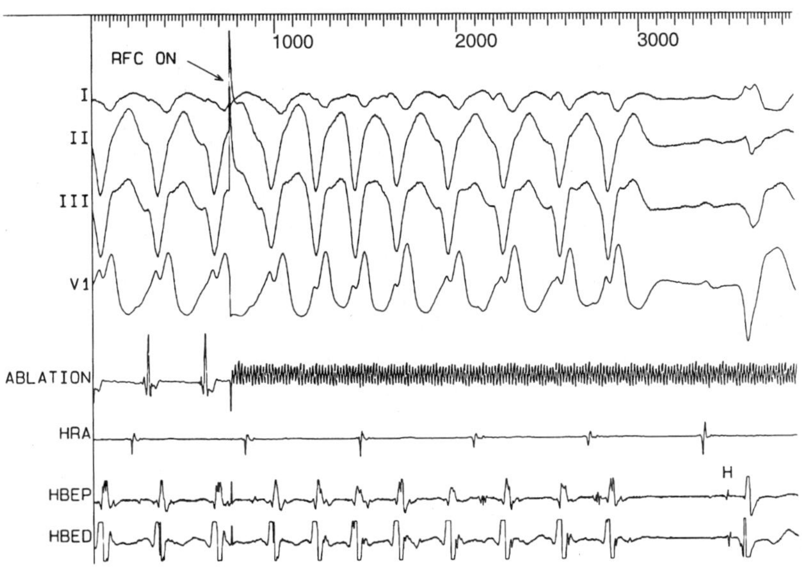

Figure 19–14. Delivery of radiofrequency current (RFC) in the patient in Figures 19–12 and 19–13. RFC promptly terminated ventricular tachycardia (VT) within 2 sec, and VT was no longer inducible after delivery of this RF pulse. This was, therefore, a successful ablation of an idiopathic left VT (left posterior fascicular VT). *Other abbreviations:* HBED, distal His bundle leads; HBEP, proximal His bundle leads; HRA, high right atrium.

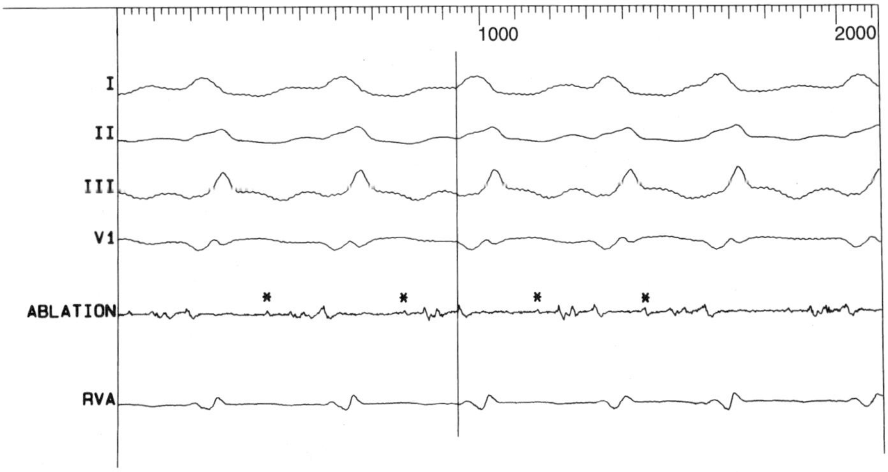

Figure 19–15. An isolated mid-diastolic potential *(asterisks).* These potentials are thought to be the result of recording at or near the region of slow conduction responsible for maintenance of ventricular tachycardia (VT). Delivery of radiofrequency energy to a site recording such a potential is frequently successful in eliminating VT, as it was in this case (see Fig. 19–16.) *Other abbreviation:* RVA, right ventricular apex.

(10%) of 241 sites in 12 (80%) of 15 patients. VT termination occurred more frequently at sites with concealed entrainment, a postpacing interval approximating the VT cycle length, and S-QRS interval during entrainment of more than 60 msec and less than 70% of the VT cycle length. VT termination was also predicted by the presence of isolated middiastolic potentials or continuous electrical activity, but these electrograms were infrequent (8% of all sites). Combinations of entrainment with concealed fusion, postpacing interval, S-QRS intervals and isolated middiastolic potentials or continuous electrical activity predicted a more than 35% VT termination rate during RF current application versus a 4% termination rate when none of these features were present. At restudy 1 week later, six patients had no inducible VT, and four patients had "modified" VT.

In another study, Kim and colleagues[13] used similar criteria and demonstrated that during follow-up after RF ablation of VT in patients with CAD, nine of 20 (45%) had recurrent VT. They concluded that RF ablation was feasible, but felt their success was only "moderately high" and it occurred in a very small and selected group of patients.

In general, patients with structural heart disease who may be candidates for RF ablation of VT include patients with incessant VT and those in whom implantation of an ICD is contraindicated. Ideally, a candidate for ICD should have one type of monomorphic VT that is inducible. Furthermore, induced VT must be hemodynamically stable to allow the time required for a potentially lengthy mapping procedure. Also, some patients may have VT that occurs frequently and terminates spontaneously. Such a patient is not a good candidate for an ICD and may be an appropriate candidate for an RF ablation procedure. In many instances, VT ablation is a useful adjunct to an ICD implant in a patient who may be receiving frequent therapies from the device. The ablation may either eliminate or reduce the number of therapies, especially if these therapies are painful shocks.

There is comparatively little experience with ablation of VT associated with other forms of structural heart disease. In patients with dilated cardiomyopathy, ablation of a monomorphic VT may be attempted, but because of the known progression of cardiomyopathy in most of these patients, the risk of development of new VTs in such patients makes ablation of VT unlikely to result in long-term cure of the arrhythmia. However, one must be careful to exclude bundle branch reentry as a mechanism of tachycardia in these patients, especially if a long HV interval is present. If such is the case, the arrhythmia may be easily treatable by RF ablation, assuming no other VTs are present.

Ablation with RF energy has occasionally been useful in patients with VT caused by arrhythmogenic RV dysplasia.[39] However, these patients tend to have multiple morphologies of VT and also generally have progression of the underlying structural abnormality (RV dilation and thinning). Furthermore, the risk of ventricular perforation may be increased because of the thin RV free wall. However, in patients with RV dysplasia who have one predominant tachycardia morphology that is inducible and hemodynamically stable, ablation may be a useful option, but it is often adjunctive therapy to an ICD. These patients are more likely to require antiarrhythmic medication after the ablation procedure, as well as the ICD. In one report,[40] the acute success rate of VT ablation in 11 patients was high (10 of 11 patients), but in a follow-up of 8 to 20 months, five of the ten patients had recurrent VT of a different morphology.

TABLE 19–6. TECHNIQUES TO MAP VENTRICULAR TACHYCARDIA

Endocardial activation
Isolated mid-diastolic potentials
QRS morphology by pace mapping
Termination by subthreshold burst pacing
Demonstration of concealed entrainment

FUTURE DIRECTIONS

Ablation of VT, particularly in patients with structural heart disease, is one of the most active areas of investigation in the field of catheter ablation. A high level of interest is directed toward finding ways to improve targeting of tachycardia by improved mapping techniques. New catheters are being developed to improve their ease of manipulation in the ventricle. Catheters with multiple electrodes or electrode arrays are in development in hopes of mapping multiple sites simultaneously, particularly through computerized mapping methods. Intracardiac echocardiography may also aid in catheter placement and lesion formation. There are attempts to increase lesion size with larger tipped catheter electrodes through the use of higher levels of RF power to maintain current density on the larger tip.[41] There are new types of electrodes that may allow for more efficient heating of tissue (i.e., gold and porous catheter tips), and additional energy sources are also under development (e.g., microwave, laser, ultrasound). In addition, a water-cooled catheter tip appears promising in increasing lesion diameter and depth. It is hoped that these and other advances will allow for larger and deeper lesions or lesions with varying contours that may help with certain ablation procedures. Also, these newer energy sources and electrode types may allow penetration of fibrous (scar) tissue or clots. Furthermore, although the efficacy of other energy sources and larger lesions is being

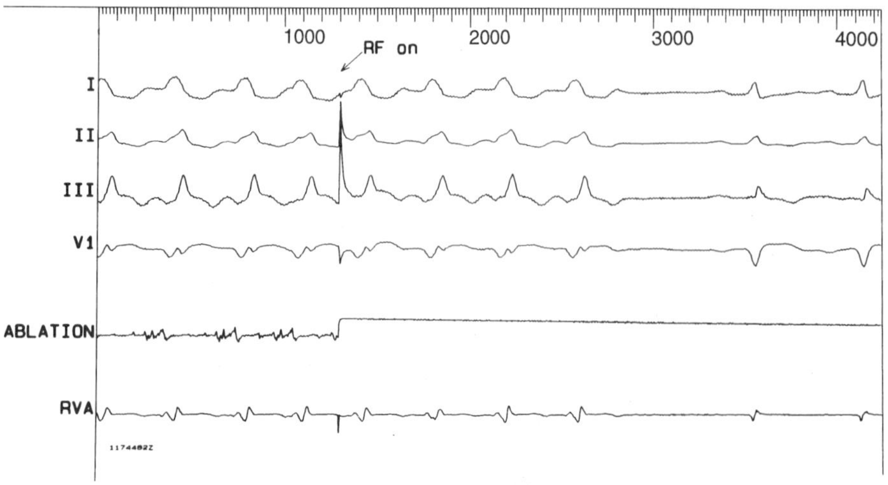

Figure 19–16. Termination of ventricular tachycardia by radiofrequency (RF) current delivery in the same patient as in Figure 19–15. Termination in such a fashion frequently signifies a successful ablation. *Other abbreviation:* RVA, right ventricular apex.

investigated, the safety of these techniques also requires investigation, because RF ablation, at least as currently employed, has enjoyed a considerable degree of safety along with a growing degree of efficacy. Therefore, future developments hopefully will allow for a greater percentage of patients with VT to be candidates for curative therapy through ablative techniques.

Acknowledgments

Supported in part by the Herman C. Krannert Fund; by grants HL-42370 and HL-07182 from the National Heart, Lung and Blood Institute of the National Institutes of Health, U.S. Public Health Service; and by the American Heart Association, Indiana Affiliate, Inc.

REFERENCES

1. Zipes DP, Klein LS, Miles WM: Nonpharmacologic therapy: can it replace antiarrhythmic drug therapy? J Cardiovasc Electrophysiol 1991; 2:255.
2. Klein LS, Miles WM, Zipes DP: Antitachycardia devices: realities and promises. J Am Coll Cardiol 1991; 18:1349–1362.
3. Klein LS, Shih HT, Hackett FK, et al: Radiofrequency catheter ablation of ventricular tachycardia in patients without structural heart disease. Circulation 1992; 85:1666–1674.
4. Nakagawa H, Beckman KJ, McClelland JH, et al: Radiofrequency catheter ablation of idiopathic left ventricular tachycardia guided by a Purkinje potential. Circulation 1993; 88:2607–2617.
5. Calkins H, Kalbfleisch SJ, El-Atassi R, et al: Relation between efficacy of radiofrequency catheter ablation and site of origin of idiopathic ventricular tachycardia. Am J Cardiol 1993; 71:827–833.
6. Wilber DJ, Baerman J, Olshansky B, et al: Adenosine-sensitive ventricular tachycardia. Circulation 1993:87:126–134.
7. Page RL, Shenasa H, Evans JJ, et al: Radiofrequency catheter ablation of idiopathic recurrent ventricular tachycardia with right bundle branch block, left axis morphology. PACE Pacing Clin Electrophysiol 1993; 16:327–336.
8. Kottkamp H, Chen X, Hindricks G, et al: Radiofrequency catheter ablation of idiopathic left ventricular tachycardia: further evidence for microreentry as the underlying mechanism. J Cardiovasc Electrophysiol 1994; 5:268–273.
9. Wen MS, Yeh SJ, Wang CC, et al: Radiofrequency ablation therapy in idiopathic left ventricular tachycardia with no obvious structural heart disease. Circulation 1994; 89:1690–1696.
10. Fitzgerald DM, Friday KJ, Yeung-Lai-Wah JA, et al: Myocardial regions of slow conduction participating in the reentrant circuit of multiple ventricular tachycardias: report on then patients. J Cardiovasc Electrophysiol 1991; 2:193–206.
11. Stevenson WG, Khan H, Sager P, et al: Identification of reentry circuit sites during catheter mapping and radiofrequency ablation of ventricular tachycardia late after myocardial infarction. Circulation 1993; 88:1647–1670.
12. Morady F, Harvey M, Kalbfleisch SJ, et al: Radiofrequency catheter ablation of ventricular tachycardia in patients with coronary artery disease. Circulation 1993; 87:363–372.
13. Kim YH, Sosa-Suarez G, Trouton TG, et al: Treatment of ventricular tachycardia by transcatheter radiofrequency ablation in patients with ischemic heart disease. Circulation 1994; 89:1094–1102.
14. Morady F: Further insight into mechanisms of ventricular tachycardia from the clinical electrophysiology laboratory. J Cardiovasc Electrophysiol 1991; 2:207–214.
15. Kuck KH, Schluter M, Geiger M, et al: Successful catheter ablation of human ventricular tachycardia with radiofrequency current guided by an endocardial map of the area of slow conduction. PACE Pacing Clin Electrophysiol 1991; 14:1060–1071.
16. Davis MJE, Murdock C: Radiofrequency catheter ablation of refractory ventricular tachycardia. PACE Pacing Clin Electrophysiol 1988; 11:725–729.
17. Gallagher JJ, Svenson RH, Kasell JH, et al: Catheter technique for closed-chest ablation of the atrioventricular conduction system. A therapeutic alternative for the treatment of refractory supraventricular tachycardia. N Engl J Med 1982; 306:194.
18. Scheinman MM, Morady F, Hess DS, et al: Catheter induced ablation of the atrioventricular junction to control refractory supraventricular arrhythmias. JAMA 1982; 248:851.
19. Hartzler GO: Electrode catheter ablation of refractory focal ventricular tachycardia. J Am Coll Cardiol 1983; 2:1107.
20. Bardy GH, Ivey TD, Coltori F, et al: Developments, complications, and limitations of catheter-mediated electrical ablation of posterior accessory atrioventricular pathways. Am J Cardiol 1988; 61:309.
21. Morady F, Scheinman MM, Di Carlo La, et al: Catheter ablation of ventricular tachycardia with intracardiac shocks: results in 33 patients. Circulation 1987; 75:1037.
22. Evans GT Jr, Scheinman MM, Zipes DP, et al: The Percutaneous Cardiac Mapping and Ablation Registry: final summary of results. PACE 1988; 11:1621.
23. Scheinman MM: Patterns of catheter ablation practice in the United States: results of the 1992 NASPE survey. PACE Pacing Clin Electrophysiol 1994; 17:873–875.
24. Jackman WM, Wang X, Friday KJ, et al: Catheter ablation of accessory atrioventricular pathways (Wolff-Parkinson-White syndrome) by radiofrequency current. N Engl J Med 1991; 324:1605.
25. Mitrani R, Klein L, Hackett F, et al: Radiofrequency catheter ablation for atrioventricular nodal reentrant tachycardia: comparison between fast (anterior) and slow (posterior) pathway ablation. J Am Coll Cardiol 1993; 21:432–441.
26. Lesh MD, Van Hare GF, Epstein LM, et al: Radiofrequency catheter ablation of atrial arrhythmias. Circulation 1994; 89:1074–1089.
27. Kalbfleisch SJ, Langberg JJ: Catheter ablation with radiofrequency energy: biophysical aspects and clinical applications. J Cardiovasc Electrophysiol 1992; 3:173.
28. Haines DE, Watson DD: Tissue heating during radiofrequency catheter ablation: a thermodynamic model and observations in isolated perfused and superfused canine right ventricular free wall. PACE Pacing Clin Electrophysiol 1989; 12:962–976.
29. Langberg JJ, Calkins H, El-Atassi R, et al: Temperature monitoring during radiofrequency catheter ablation of accessory pathways. Circulation 1992; 86:1469.
30. Tchou P, Jazayeri M, Denker S, et al: Transcatheter electrical ablation of right bundle branch. Circulation 1988; 78:246–257.
31. Langberg JJ, Desai J, Dullet N, et al: Treatment of macroreentrant ventricular tachycardia with radiofrequency ablation of the right bundle branch. Am J Cardiol 1989; 63:1010–1013.
32. Cohen TJ, Chien WW, Lurie KG, et al: Radiofrequency catheter ablation for treatment of bundle branch reentrant ventricular tachycardia: results and long-term follow-up. J Am Coll Cardiol 1991; 18:1767–1773.
33. Chien WW, Scheinman MM, Cohen TJ, et al: Importance of recording the right bundle branch deflection in the diagnosis of His-Purkinje reentrant tachycardia. PACE Pacing Clin Electrophysiol 1992; 15:1015–1024.
34. Blanck Z, Dhala A, Deshpande S, et al: Bundle branch reentrant ventricular tachycardia: cumulative experience in 48 patients. J Cardiovasc Electrophysiol 1993; 4:253–262.
35. Brugada P, de Swart H, Smeets J, et al: Transcoronary chemical ablation of ventricular tachycardia. Circulation 1989; 79:475.
36. Nora MO, Miles WM, Klein LS, et al: Alcohol ablation of ventricular tachycardia. J Cardiovasc Electrophysiol 1991; 2:456.
37. Okishige K, Friedman PL: Alcohol ablation for tachycardia therapy. J Cardiovasc Electrophysiol 1992; 3:354.
38. Inoue H, Waller B, Zipes DP: Intracoronary ethyl alcohol or phenol injection ablates aconitine-induced ventricular tachycardia in dogs. J Am Coll Cardiol 1987; 10:1342.
39. Morady F, Kadish AH, Di Carlo LA, et al: Long-term results of catheter ablation of idiopathic right ventricular tachycardia. Circulation 1990; 82.2093.
40. Shoda M, Kasanuki H, Ohnishi S, et al: Recurrence of new ventricular tachycardia after successful catheter ablation in patients with arrhythmogenic right ventricular dysplasia [Abstract]. Circulation 1992; 86:(suppl 1):580.
41. Langberg JJ, Gallagher M, Strickberger SA, et al: Temperature-guided radiofrequency catheter ablation with very large distal electrodes. Circulation 1993; 88:245–249.

20 Management of Bradyarrhythmias

David P. Rardon, MD
Raul D. Mitrani, MD
Lawrence S. Klein, MD
William M. Miles, MD
Douglas P. Zipes, MD

The normal cardiac impulse originates in the sinus node and traverses the atrium, antrioventricular (AV) node, and His-Purkinje system before activating the ventricle. Bradyarrhythmias may occur secondary to either intrinsic or extrinsic conduction system disorders.

Altered anatomy or loss of functional integrity of the sinus node, surrounding atrium, AV node, or His-Purkinje system can produce bradyarrhythmias that are intrinsic in origin. Examples include sinus arrest, which occurs when sinus node automaticity fails, or complete AV block, which occurs secondary to fibrotic changes in the His-Purkinje system. Disturbances of autonomic neural control[1, 2] or effects of cardioactive drugs (e.g., sympatholytic agents or antiarrhythmic drugs)[3] produce bradyarrhythmias that are extrinsic in origin.

Most bradyarrhythmias are encompassed within two broad general categories of sinus node dysfunction, or "sick sinus syndrome," and AV block. Manifestations of sinus node dysfunction include (1) severe sinus bradycardia, (2) sinus pauses or sinus arrest, (3) sinoatrial exit block, (4) chronic atrial tachyarrhythmias (especially atrial fibrillation associated with a slow ventricular response), (5) alternating bradyarrhythmias and tachyarrhythmias, and (6) inappropriate heart rate responses during physical activity or emotional stress (chronotropic incompetence).[4] AV block is classified as first-degree when all P waves conduct, but with delay; second-degree when some P waves conduct and others block; and third-degree when no P waves conduct.

Many patients with sinus node dysfunction or AV block can be asymptomatic. In asymptomatic individuals, no specific therapy may be required. On the other hand, many patients with bradyarrhythmias secondary to either sinus node dysfunction or AV block can exhibit a broad range of symptoms, including syncope, presyncope, shortness of breath, palpitations, fatigue, and lethargy.[5, 6] Bradyarrhythmias can exacerbate congestive heart failure and preclude effective treatment of coronary artery disease or associated tachyarrhythmias. Patients with symptomatic bradyarrhythmias require treatment aimed at removal of extrinsic causes when possible or correction with a pacemaker designed to maintain a cardiac rhythm that mimics normal cardiac function when possible. Specific recommendations for therapy of sinus node dysfunction and AV block are summarized in the following sections.

PACEMAKER THERAPY: GENERAL CONSIDERATIONS

Many patients with symptomatic bradyarrhythmias secondary to sinus node dysfunction or AV block require therapy with a pacemaker. This section provides general information about cardiac pacemakers that is applicable to management of all patients with bradyarrhythmias.

Pacing systems can be classified as single-lead ventricular or atrial demand pacemakers or dual-chamber DDD pacemakers, which sense and pace from both the atrial and ventricular chambers. These pacing modalities may or may not be rate adaptive or sensor driven. The North American Society of Pacing and Electrophysiology (NASPE) generic pacemaker code is summarized in Table 20–1. The first three or four letters of the code are used most frequently. The first three positions of the code define the chamber paced, the chamber sensed, and the response to pacing, respectively. The fourth position is used most frequently to define a rate-modulated unit.[7] For example, a VVIR pacemaker paces the ventricle, senses in the ventricle, responds to sensing by inhibition, and functions as a rate-responsive ventricular demand pacemaker.

In choosing a pacemaker for an individual patient, the following three questions need to be addressed:

1. Can the atrium be paced and/or sensed?
2. Is there latent or overt AV block?
3. Is there atrial chronotropic competence?

These questions dictate the need for an atrial lead, a ventricular lead, and a rate-responsive pulse generator, respectively. An algorithm for determining the optimal pacemaker mode that uses the information from these questions is given in Figure 20–1.[8]

TABLE 20–1. GENERIC PACEMAKER CODE

I Chamber Paced	II Chamber Sensed	III Response to Sensing	IV Programmability, Rate Modulation	V Antitachyarrhythmia Function
O, none	O, none	O, none	O, none	O, none
A, atrium	A, atrium	T, triggered	P, simple programmable	P, pacing
V, ventricle	V, ventricle	I, inhibited	M, multiprogrammable	S, shock
D, dual (A and V)	D, dual (A and V)	D, dual (T and I)	R, rate modulation	D, dual (P and S)

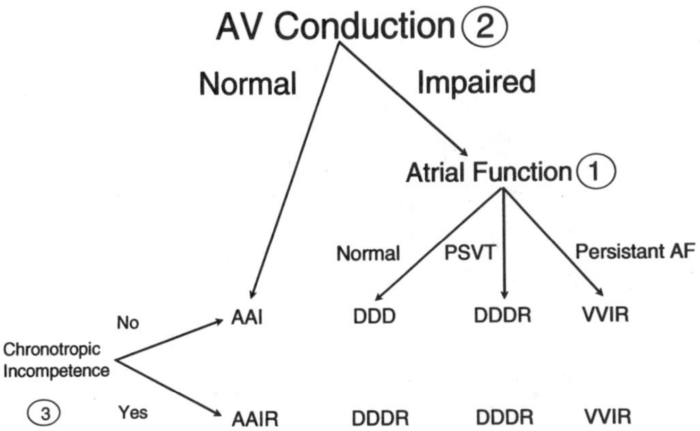

Figure 20–1. Algorithm for determining the optimal pacemaker mode. Numbers 1, 2, and 3 refer to questions to be addressed in choosing a pacemaker. See text for more details. *Abbreviations*: AF, atrial fibrillation; AV, atrioventricular; PSVT, paroxysmal supraventricular tachycardia.

SINUS NODE DYSFUNCTION

Sinus Pause or Arrest

Sinus pause or arrest implies failure of normal pacemaker discharge. This is characterized by lack of an expected sinus P wave on the surface electrocardiogram. Asymptomatic sinus pauses longer than 2 sec in duration are not uncommon and occur frequently in healthy young subjects and in trained athletes.[9] In patients with symptomatic sinus pauses, efforts should be made to discontinue cardiac glycosides, beta adrenoceptor blockers, calcium channel blockers, membrane-active antiarrhythmic agents, and other medications including lithium carbonate, cimetidine, amitriptyline, and the phenothiazines that may cause or potentiate the duration of pauses. Pacing therapy is indicated in patients with symptomatic sinus pauses without a correctable cause.

Sinus Exit Block

Sinoatrial exit block implies failure of a normal sinus impulse to exit the sinus nodal region and excite the atrium. This is characterized by lack of an expected sinus P wave on the surface electrocardiogram (Fig. 20–2). Sinoatrial exit blocks are classified in a manner analogous to AV blocks. First-degree sinoatrial exit block implies conduction delay from the sinus node to the atrium. This is not apparent on the surface electrocardiogram. Second-degree Mobitz type I sinoatrial exit block is characterized by progressive PP interval shortening before the unexpected lack of a P wave on the surface electrocardiogram. Second-degree Mobitz type II sinoatrial exit block is characterized by failure of one or more expected sinus P waves on the electrocardiogram. The duration of the pause should be an exact multiple of the preceding PP interval (see Fig. 20–2).[10]

The management of patients with sinoatrial exit block is similar to the management of patients with sinus pauses. Cardiac pacing is indicated in patients with symptomatic sinoatrial exit block without an identifiable reversible cause.

Bradycardia-Tachycardia Syndrome

Bradycardia-tachycardia syndrome is characterized by periods of tachyarrhythmia, such as atrial fibrillation or flutter or AV node reentry, that are followed by prolonged pauses when the tachyarrhythmia spontaneously terminates (Fig. 20–3). The bradyarrhythmia may be sinus, junctional, or rarely ventricular in origin. Medications required to treat the tachyarrhythmia may exacerbate symptoms from the pauses and bradycardia. Bradycardia pacing therapy is indicated for patients with symptoms related to pauses or excessive bradycardia not eliminated by discontinuation of drugs known to exacerbate the pauses. Pacing therapy is also indicated for patients in whom medications required to treat the tachyarrhythmia cannot be discontinued. The normal heart rate in adults is usually considered to be 60 to 100 beats per minute. Many healthy resting individuals have heart rates as slow as 35 to 40 beats per minute; in addition, well-trained athletes can have extremely low resting heart rates not associated with symptoms. Patients with sinus bradycardia (usually with rates less than 40 beats per minute) associated with symptoms related to the bradycardia that occurs as a consequence of long-term (essential) drug therapy of a type and dose for which there are no acceptable alternatives are candidates for bradycardia pacing therapy.

In addition, patients with atrial fibrillation in association with a slow ventricular response (not related to drugs) or prolonged pauses with symptoms (Fig. 20–4) are candidates for pacing therapy.

ATRIOVENTRICULAR BLOCK

First-Degree AV Block

First-degree AV block is present when the PR interval exceeds 200 msec. All P waves conduct to the ventricle with a constant but

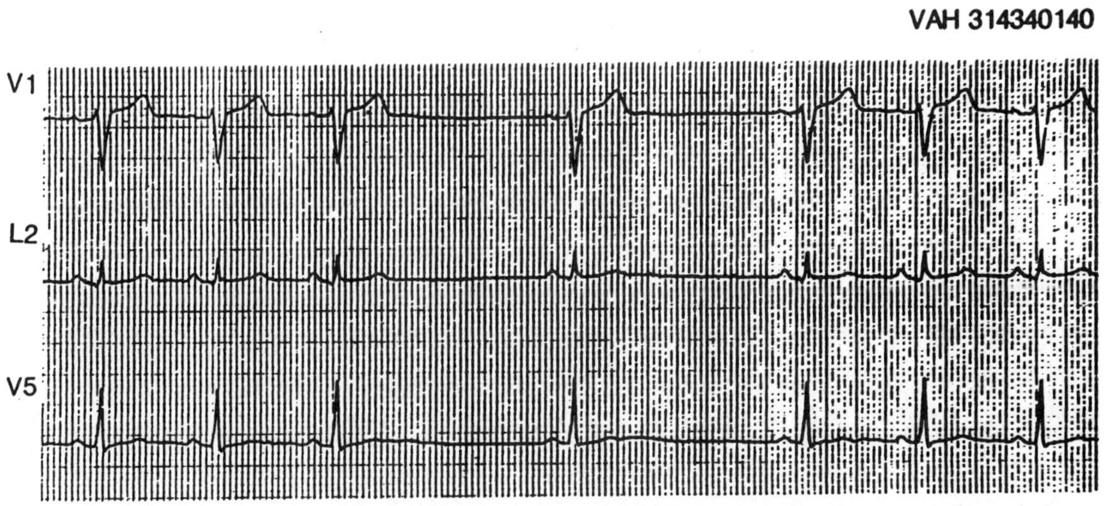

Figure 20–2. Recording of sinoatrial exit block. The rhythm is sinus with a rate of 75 per minute (800 msec). The pauses are twice the sinus cycle length (1600 msec) with absence of an expected P wave. This suggests that the sinus discharges on time but the impulse intermittently fails to conduct to the atrium.

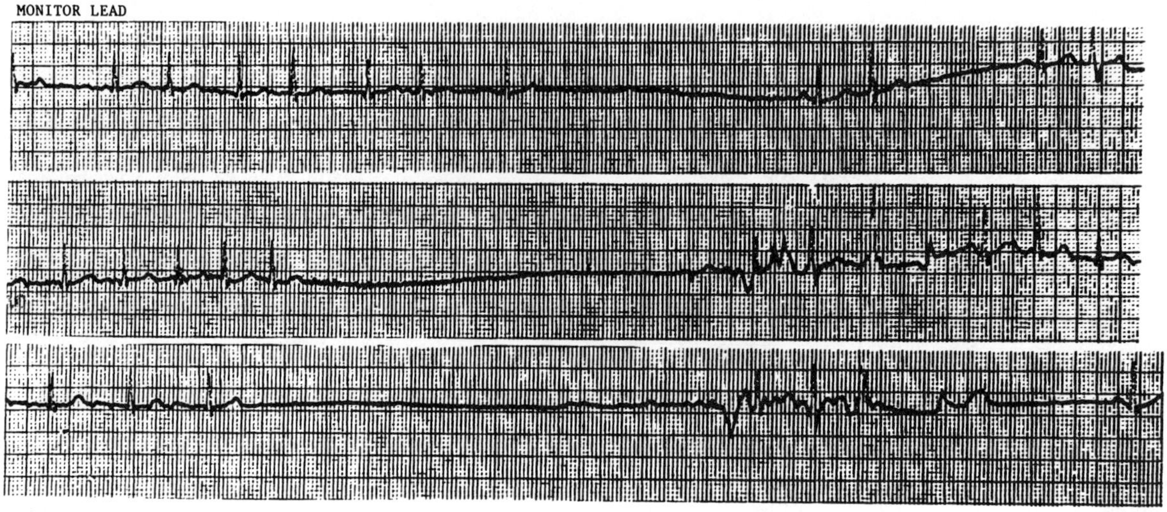

Figure 20–3. Bradycardia-tachycardia syndrome. The three strips are a continuous record of a monitor lead. The initial rhythm is atrial fibrillation, which terminates with a prolonged pause in each strip. The escape complexes are most likely sinus in origin. The frequent pauses were associated with presyncope, and the patient required a pacemaker and pharmacologic therapy to control the atrial fibrillation.

prolonged PR interval. The prognosis for patients with first-degree AV block is excellent, and no specific therapy is indicated. Even when first-degree AV block is associated with chronic bifascicular block, the rate of progression to third-degree AV block is low, and prophylactic pacing is not indicated in the asymptomatic patient.

Second-Degree AV Block

Type I second-degree AV nodal Wenckebach block is characterized by four features: (1) progressive prolongation of the PR intervals; (2) PR interval prolongation of progressively decreasing increments; (3) progressive shortening of the RR intervals; and (4) the pause encompassing the blocked P wave is less than the sum of two PP cycles (Figs. 20–5, 20–6). When type I second-degree AV block occurs with a QRS of normal duration, the block is almost always within the AV node proximal to the His bundle. In rare instances type I AV block occurs within the distal His bundle (intra-Hisian block). If the QRS duration is prolonged, the block may be within the AV node, within the His bundle, or below the His bundle in the bundle branches. Long PR intervals are more consistent with AV nodal block.

The prognosis and management of patients with type I second-degree AV block depend on the clinical setting and the presence of associated structural heart disease. Type I second-degree AV block occurs in a small percentage of normal persons during sleep and with some increased frequency in well-trained athletes.[11, 12] For asymptomatic individuals without structural heart disease, type I second-degree AV block has an excellent prognosis, and no therapy is required. When type I second-degree AV block occurs in patients with significant structural heart disease, the clinical course is usually determined by the extent and severity of the structural heart disease and is not secondary to the AV block. Routine prophylactic permanent pacing is not recommended in patients with AV nodal Wenckebach block and structural heart disease, unless they are symptomatic with recurrence of syncope, presyncope, or bradycardia that exacerbates congestive heart failure or angina. Permanent ventricular or AV sequential pacing is indicated for patients with type I second-degree AV block with syncope.

Type II second-degree AV block is characterized by three features:

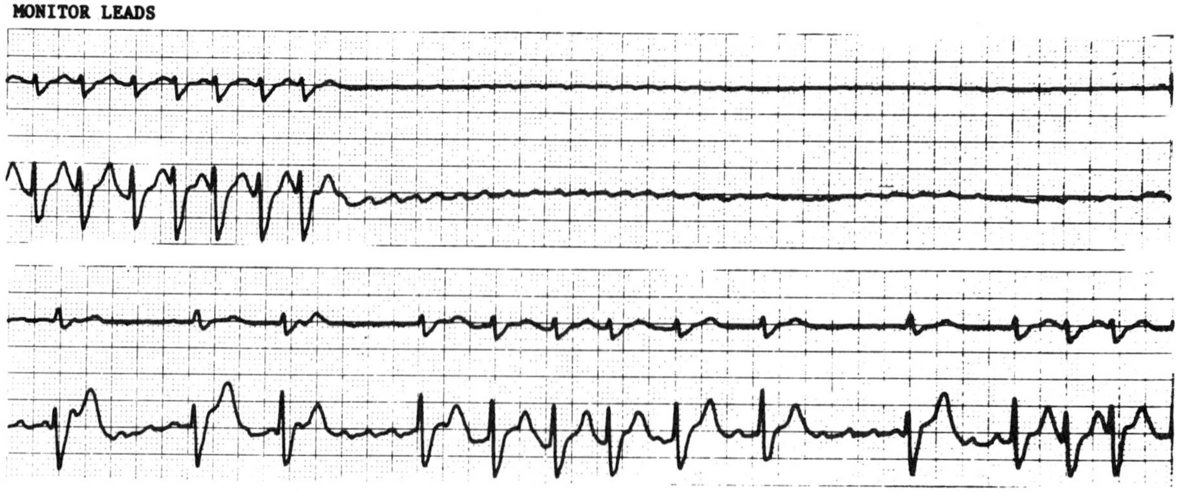

Figure 20–4. Atrial fibrillation with a prolonged pause. The record is continuous with two simultaneous monitor leads. The initial rhythm is atrial fibrillation with a rapid ventricular response.

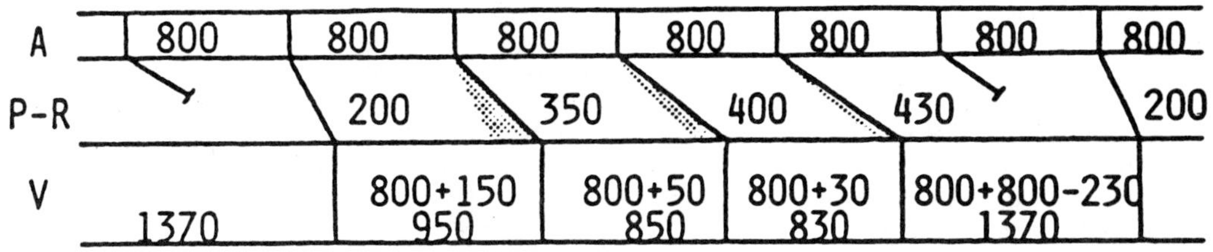

Figure 20–5. The structure of a "typical" AV nodal Wenckebach cycle. All intervals are in milliseconds. The PP interval is constant at 800 msec. The PR interval progressively lengthens (200–350–400–430 msec); the greatest increment in PR interval occurs between the first and second conducted P waves. Therefore, the RR intervals progressively shorten (950–850–830 msec). The pause encompassing the blocked P wave is less than the sum of two basic cycles by an amount equal to the total delay at the AV node (800 + 800 − 150 − 50 − 30 = 1370 msec).

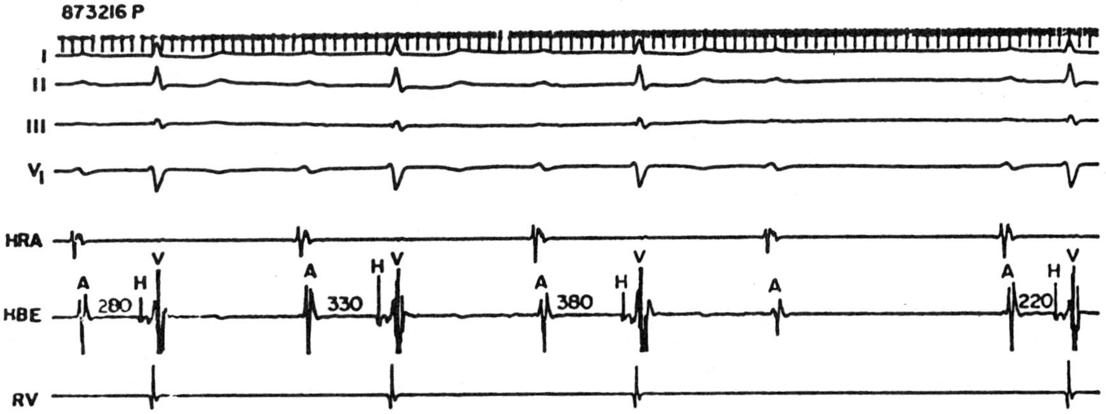

Figure 20–6. Second-degree AV block type I. The depicted leads are surface electrocardiograms leads I, II, III, and V_1 with intracardiac recordings from the high right atrium (HRA), the His bundle (HBS), and the right ventricle (RV). The rhythm is sinus. The AH interval gradually prolongs from 280 to 380 msec before the failure of the fourth atrial depolarization to conduct to the ventricle. The nonconducted atrial complex is not followed by a His potential, which demonstrates that the site of AV block is within the AV node. (Modified from Miles WM, Klein LS: Sinus nodal dysfunction and atrioventricular conduction disturbances. *In* Naccarelli GV [ed]: Cardiac Arrhythmias: A Practical Approach, pp 243–282. Mount Kisco, NY: Futura, 1991.)

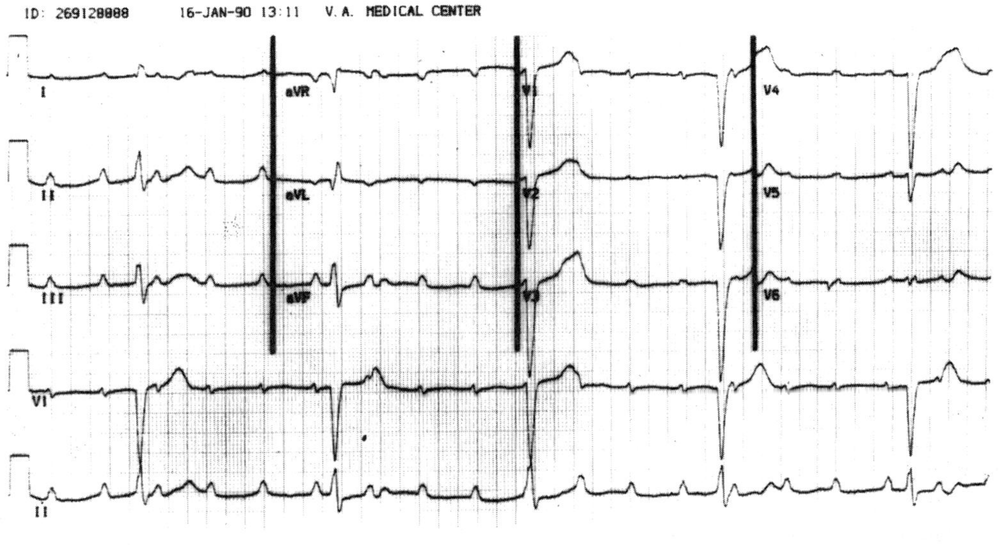

Figure 20–7. Acquired third-degree AV block. The rhythm is sinus tachycardia at 105 beats per minute. The ventricular rate is 33 beats per minute with left bundle branch block morphology. (From Rardon DP, Miles WM, Mitrani RD, et al: Atrioventricular block and dissociation. *In* Zipes DP, Jalife J [eds]: Cardiac Electrophysiology: From Cell to Bedside, p 939. Philadelphia: WB Saunders, 1995.)

(1) constant PP intervals and RR intervals; (2) constant PR intervals before the unexpected failure of a P wave to conduct the ventricle; and (3) a pause encompassing the blocked P wave that equals two PP cycles. Type II AV block occurs almost exclusively in association with a bundle branch block, and the anatomic site of block is virtually always within or below the His bundle.

Type II AV block often progresses to complete AV block, producing Adams-Stokes syncopal attacks. Therefore, prophylatic ventricular or AV sequential pacing is indicated in most patients, even those who initially present without symptoms.

A 2:1 AV block can be a form of either type I or type II AV block. A 2:1 block with a normal QRS duration supports block within the AV node (type I block), and a prolonged QRS favors but is not diagnostic of block below the His bundle (type II block). In general, the treatment of patients with 2:1 AV block does not substantially differ from that outlined earlier for those with type I or type II AV block.

Third-Degree AV Block

Third-degree AV block can be acquired or congenital and is characterized by failure of all P waves to conduct to the ventricle, which results in the complete dissociation of P waves and QRS complexes. The rate of the subsidiary pacemaker is slow, approximately 40 to 60 beats per minute in the presence of a junctional pacemaker (producing a narrow QRS complex in the absence of a pre-existing bundle branch block) and approximately 20–40 beats per minute if the impulse originates in the ventricles (wide QRS complex) (Fig. 20–7).

In patients with acquired complete AV block, permanent pacing is indicated, particularly if bradycardia is responsible for the symptoms, such as transient dizziness, lightheadedness, near-syncope, syncope, or more generalized symptoms of marked exercise intolerance or congestive heart failure. Even in asymptomatic patients with acquired complete AV block in the His-Purkinje system, the natural history suggests progression to the point of development of symptoms, and prophylactic pacing is recommended.

Treatment of the newborn with congenital complete heart block should be directed at correction of the low cardiac output and prevention of sudden death.[13] Treatment is not required for the asymptomatic child. Patients usually remain asymptomatic during childhood and adolescence; some patients have symptoms later in life. Pacing is indicated for patients with congenital second- or third-degree AV block with symptomatic bradycardia. Pacing has been recommended for patients with congenital AV block and a wide QRS escape rhythm (suggesting block distal to the His bundle) or for asymptomatic patients with an average ventricular rate of less than 50 beats per minute. Pacing is recommended for patients with documented infra-Hisian block, but it is not recommended for patients with asymptomatic congenital heart block without symptom-producing bradycardia (defined in terms of normal age-adjusted heart rate).[14]

Paroxysmal AV Block

Paroxysmal AV block is characterized by abrupt and persistent AV block in the presence of otherwise normal AV conduction (Fig. 20–8). Patients with paroxysmal AV block usually require permanent AV sequential pacemakers.

AV Block Associated With Acute Myocardial Infarction

Second- and third-degree AV heart block occur in 4% to 30% of patients admitted to the coronary unit with acute myocardial infarction.[15] Type I AV block occurs more commonly in association with acute inferior than anterior myocardial infarctions. The definitive cause of block has not been established. Inferior or posterior myocardial infarctions are associated with an increase in vagal tone accounting for sinus bradycardia, first-degree AV block, and possibly type I or advanced AV block. Type I AV block occurring in the course of an acute inferior myocardial infarction is usually transient and commonly resolves in the first 48–72 h after the infarction. Most patients are asymptomatic, and rarely does type I AV block progress to second- or third-degree block. Therefore, no specific therapy is warranted. Rarely, therapy may be required because of symptomatic bradycardia associated with hypotension, ventricular arrhythmias, or myocardial ischemia. Atropine therapy may be beneficial. Temporary transvenous ventricular pacing is occasionally required for persistent symptomatic bradycardia or hypotension that fails to respond to atropine.

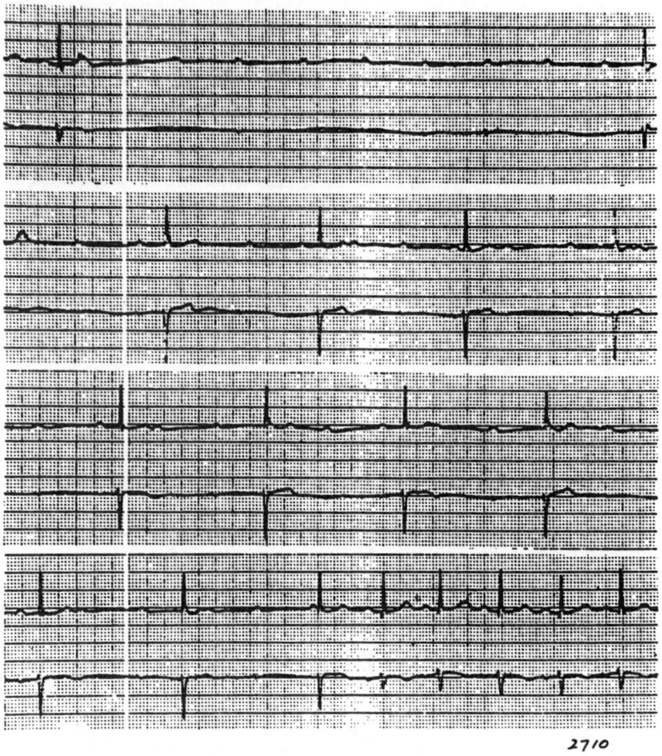

Figure 20–8. Paroxysmal AV block. The rhythm is sinus with a PP interval of 700 msec and normal QRS morphology. In the top strip, the rhythm is interrupted by a single atrial premature complex with a sinus return cycle of 1100 msec. AV conduction fails until the bottom panel. The ventricular escape complexes in the second and third panels are presumably junctional in origin. (From Rardon DP, Miles WM, Mitrani RD, et al: Atrioventricular block and dissociation. *In* Zipes DP, Jalife J [eds]: Cardiac Electrophysiology: From Cell to Bedside, p 940. Philadelphia: WB Saunders, 1995.)

Type II second-degree AV block occurs in approximately 1% of patients with acute myocardial infarction. Type II second-degree AV block occurs more commonly in patients with anterior as opposed to inferior myocardial infarctions. Because of the potential for progression to complete heart block, patients with type II second-degree AV block should be treated with temporary transvenous ventricular demand pacemakers.

Complete heart block occurs in 5% to 8% of patients with acute myocardial infarction. Complete heart block can occur with either inferior or anterior myocardial infarctions. It is generally agreed that temporary ventricular demand pacing is indicated for most patients with acute inferior myocardial infarction and complete AV block, particularly if the ventricular rate is slow (less than 45 beats per minute) or there is associated hypotension. Atropine may be used in this setting but is rarely of value. In patients with anterior myocardial infarction, complete AV block is often preceded by fascicular block, bundle branch block, or type II AV block. The escape rhythm is generally ventricular in origin, with rates less than 40 beats per minute. The block is usually distal to the His bundle. Temporary transvenous ventricular demand pacing is indicated in all patients with acute anterior infarctions and newly acquired complete AV block. This population of patients has a high mortality owing to the large size of infarction and resultant left ventricular dysfunction.

REFERENCES

1. Jordan JL, Yamaguchi I, Mandel WL: Studies on the mechanisms of sinus node dysfunction in the sick sinus syndrome. Circulation 1978; 57:217–223.
2. Desai JM, Scheinman MM, Strauss HC, et al: Electrophysiologic effects of combined autonomic blockade in patients with sinus node disease. Circulation 1981; 63:953–960.
3. Scheinman MM, Strauss HC, Evans GT, et al: Adverse effects of sympatholytic agents in patients with hypertension and sinus node dysfunction. Am J Med 1978; 64:1013–1020.
4. Benditt DG, Sakoguichi S, Goldstein MA, et al: Sinus node dysfunction: pathophysiology, clinical features, evaluation, and treatment. *In* Zipes DP, Jalife J (eds): Cardiac Electrophysiology: From Cell to Bedside, pp 1215–1247. Philadelphia: WB Saunders, 1995.
5. Ferrer MI: The sick sinus syndrome. Circulation 1973; 47:635–641.
6. Strauss HC, Prystowsky EN, Scheinman MM: Sino-atrial and atrial electrogenesis. Prog Cardiovasc Dis 1977; 19:385–404.
7. Bernstein AD, Camm AJ, Fletcher RD, et al: The NAPSE/BPEG generic pacemaker code for antibradyarrhythmia and adaptive-rate pacing and antitachyarrhythmia devices. PACE 1987; 10:794–799.
8. Griffin J: The optimal pacing mode for the individual patient. The rule of DDDR. *In* Barold SS, Mugica J (eds): New Perspectives in Cardiac Pacing 2, pp 325–338. Mount Kisco, NY: Futura Publishing, 1991.
9. Viitasalo MT, Kala R, Eisalo A: Ambulatory electrocardiographic recording in endurance athletes. Br Heart J 1982; 47:213–220.
10. Wu D, Yeh S-J, Lin F-C, et al: Sinus automaticity and sinoatrial conduction in severe symptomatic sick sinus syndrome. J Am Coll Cardiol 1992; 19:355–364.
11. Strasberg B, Amat-Y-Leon F, Dhingra RC, et al: Natural history of chronic second-degree atrioventricular nodal block. Circulation 1981; 63:1043–1049.
12. Meytes I, Kaplinsky E, Yahini JH, et al: Wenckebach A-V block, a frequent feature following heavy physical training. Am Heart J 1975; 90:426–430.
13. Pinsky WW, Gillette PC, Garson T: Diagnosis, management, and long term results of patients with complete atrioventricular block. Pediatrics 1982; 69:728–733.
14. Sholler GF, Walsch EP: Congenital complete heart block in patients without anatomic cardiac defects. Am Heart J 1989; 118:1193–1198.
15. Tans AC, Lie KI, Durrer D: Clinical setting and prognostic significance of high grade atrioventricular block in acute inferior myocardial infarction: a study of 144 patients. Am Heart J 1980; 99:4–8.

21 Use of the Implantable Cardioverter-Defibrillator for Ventricular Arrhythmias

Raul D. Mitrani, MD
Lawrence S. Klein, MD
Douglas P. Zipes, MD
William M. Miles, MD

The implantable cardioverter-defibrillator (ICD) has become standard therapy for patients with sustained or life-threatening ventricular arrhythmias. To date, the ICD has not been demonstrated to prolong survival in a controlled prospective trial.[1–4] However, several retrospective studies have suggested improved survival with the ICD.[5–12] Nevertheless, the ability of an ICD to terminate ventricular arrhythmias and prevent sudden cardiac death is unquestioned (Fig. 21–1).

The first ICD approved by the U.S. Food and Drug Administration was the Automatic Implantable Cardiac Defibrillator (AICD) by Cardiac Pacemakers, Incorporated (CPI) in 1985. This early defibrillator was capable only of delivering high-energy shocks for tachycardias that exceeded a predetermined or programmed rate. Today, many ICDs are available with both epicardial and endocardial lead systems. Most current ICDs offer bradycardia pacing support, antitachycardia pacing, low-energy cardioversion, and high-energy defibrillation. Multiple detection zones and multiple detection algorithms can be programmed to enable the ICD to treat slower ventricular tachycardias (VTs) with antitachycardia pacing and faster ventricular arrhythmias with cardioversion or defibrillation. VT detection is no longer limited to simple rate cut-off. Detection algorithms are available to differentiate atrial fibrillation, sinus tachycardia, and supraventricular tachycardia from VT.

Despite the increased complexities of ICD programming, some patients still receive inappropriate therapies and ICD shocks for non-VT rhythms. Overprogramming an ICD to prevent inappropriate therapies can cause nondetection of VT.[13]

This chapter reviews the use of ICDs as a therapeutic tool to treat ventricular tachyarrhythmias and prevent sudden cardiac death. Experience with the different ICD detection and treatment features is reviewed, and interactions of ICDs with pacemakers and drugs are discussed.

HISTORICAL PERSPECTIVES

The concept of ICDs originated in the late 1960s. Initially, there was much controversy regarding their development and applicability.[14, 15] The first human implant of an ICD occurred in 1980.[16]

Early ICDs lacked capabilities for antitachycardia pacing, low-energy cardioversions, or bradycardia pacing, which limited their usefulness in many patient populations. Nevertheless, the CPI AICD Ventak P became a popular defibrillator, and more than 30,000 implants were performed by 1994. Earlier experience with an implantable transvenous cardioverter demonstrated the efficacy of low-energy cardioversion for VT but also showed the need for backup

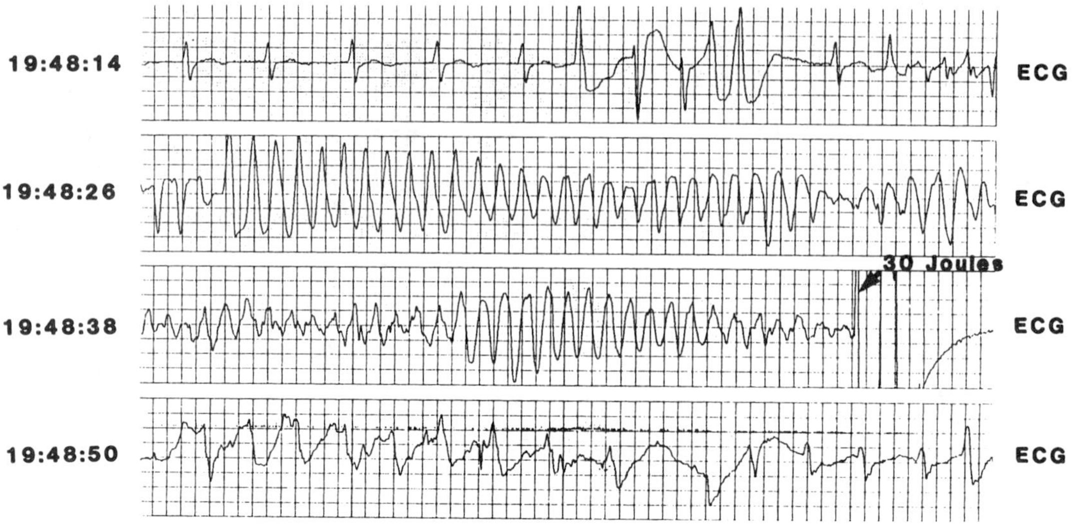

Figure 21–1. This electrocardiogram (ECG) is from a patient with an implantable defibrillator who had a spontaneous episode of ventricular fibrillation. The implantable cardioverter-defibrillator appropriately defibrillated the heart, restoring sinus rhythm.

defibrillation in any unit with automatic detection and treatment of ventricular arrhythmias.[17] Therefore, it became apparent that devices capable of delivering tiered therapy were required.

Rapid evolution of technology has led to improved ICD design and function, reducing their size and facilitating transvenous implantation. Implantation of transvenous ICDs has become standard therapy. The concept of the "ideal" defibrillator was conceived many years ago (Table 21–1); today, many devices are approaching this ideal. However, not all devices require all of the features listed in Table 21–1. A device that is too complex may be inappropriately programmed.[13] A patient with a history of sudden cardiac death without any clinical or inducible VT probably needs only a device that can effectively defibrillate ventricular fibrillation (VF) and perhaps also have backup bradycardia pacing. ICD features need to be programmed for specific patient needs.

TABLE 21–1. THE "IDEAL" ANTITACHYCARDIA DEVICE

Sensing
Distinguish ventricular from supraventricular tachycardias
Differentiate among two or more pathologic tachycardias
Noncommitted therapy for nonsustained tachycardias
Automatic sensitivity gain for different rhythms (sinus versus ventricular tachycardia or ventricular fibrillation)
Dual-chamber–sensing algorithms to be able to precisely differentiate atrial fibrillation and other supraventricular tachycardias from ventricular tachycardias
Hemodynamic or other physiologic monitoring that is incorporated into the sensing and/or therapy algorithms

Pacing
Bradycardia pacing (single and dual-chamber, rate-responsive with physiologic sensors, high output after shock)
Antitachycardia pacing (burst, adaptive) for ventricular and atrial tachycardias
Different antitachycardia therapies for different recognized pathologic tachycardias
Noninvasive electrophysiologic study capabilities

Cardioversion Defibrillation
Low-energy synchronized cardioversion
High-energy cardioversion or defibrillation
Biphasic shocks

Device Features
Small size
Single lead with transvenous approach and subpectoral implant
Memory (tachycardia rate, therapy delivered, number of successful therapies), extensive electrogram storage capabilities
Long battery life
Automatic capacitor reformation
Ability to interrogate and reprogram by telephone

PATIENT SELECTION AND INDICATIONS FOR ICD THERAPY

Guidelines for ICD implantation have been proposed by the American College of Cardiology/American Heart Association Joint Task Force[18] and the North American Society of Pacing and Electrophysiology (NASPE) Policy Statement.[19] In general, ICDs should be reserved for patients who have arrhythmias that are life-threatening, produce hemodynamic compromise or syncope, and are not secondary to reversible causes such as myocardial infarction, ischemia, or proarrhythmia caused by drugs or electrolyte disturbances. These guidelines are summarized in Table 21–2.

Prevention of Sudden Cardiac Death

The ability of an ICD to prevent sudden cardiac death depends on the patient population. Patients with left ventricular (LV) systolic dysfunction who have survived an episode of sudden cardiac death are at increased risk for recurrent cardiac arrest.[20] The risk for recurrent sudden cardiac death is between 15% and 50% within 2–3 years.[20–23] Patients with good LV function, well-tolerated VT, or both have better prognoses than those with poor LV function.[20, 24, 25]

The ICD is extremely effective at terminating episodes of VF or VT. In Figure 21–1, an episode of VF was terminated just as the patient was experiencing symptoms of lightheadedness. Had this arrhythmia occurred outside the hospital setting in a patient without a defibrillator, the patient probably would have died.

Many studies have demonstrated that ICD therapy reduces the occurrence of sudden cardiac death to less than 2% per year.[5, 12, 26–30] Total mortality remains at 30%–40% at 5 years postimplant,[30, 31] and it is unclear whether ICD therapy reduces total mortality or changes the mode of death so that patients expire from progressive pump failure rather than from VF. Even with an implantable ICD, long-term survival depends to a great extent on the LV ejection fraction.[7, 11, 31–33]

TABLE 21–2. INDICATIONS FOR ICD IMPLANTATIONS

Class I: Conditions for Which There Is General Agreement That an ICD Should Be Implanted
One or more documented episodes of hemodynamically significant ventricular tachycardia or ventricular fibrillation in a patient in whom electrophysiologic testing and ambulatory monitoring cannot be used to accurately predict efficacy of therapy
One or more documented episodes of hemodynamically significant ventricular tachycardia or ventricular fibrillation in a patient in whom no drug was found to be effective or no available and appropriate drug was tolerated
Continued inducibility at electrophysiologic study of hemodynamically significant ventricular tachycardia or ventricular fibrillation despite the best available drug therapy or despite surgery or catheter ablation if drug therapy has failed
Class II: Conditions for Which ICDs Are Frequently Used but There Is Divergence of Opinion with Respect to Need of Implantation
One or more documented episodes of hemodynamically significant ventricular tachycardia or ventricular fibrillation in a patient in whom drug efficacy testing is possible
Recurrent syncope of undetermined origin in a patient with hemodynamically significant ventricular tachycardia or ventricular fibrillation induced at electrophysiologic study in whom no effective or no tolerated drug is available or appropriate
Class III: Conditions for Which There Is General Agreement That ICDs Are Unnecessary
Recurrent syncope of undetermined cause in a patient without inducible tachyarrhythmias
Arrhythmias not the result of hemodynamically significant ventricular tachycardia or ventricular fibrillation
Incessant ventricular tachycardia or fibrillation

Adapted from Dreifus LS, Fisch C, Griffin JC, et al: Guidelines for implantation of cardiac pacemakers and antiarrhythmic devices. J Am Coll Cardiol 1991; 18:1–13.
Abbreviation: ICD, implantable cardioverter-defibrillator.

Although the ICD has not been proven to reduce total mortality in a randomized prospective trial, survival curve comparisons with historical controls or with projected patient deaths have shown better patient outcomes with an ICD than without one. Typical of these studies is one performed by Powell and colleagues[7] (Fig. 21–2) in

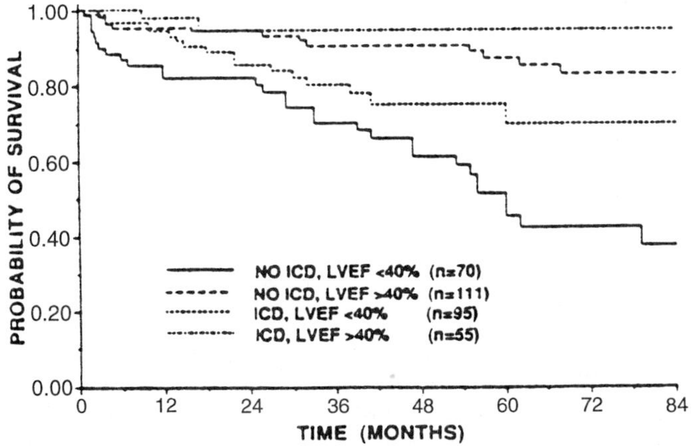

Figure 21–2. Plot of cardiac mortality in patients with and without an implantable cardioverter-defibrillator (ICD), stratified by left ventricular ejection fraction (LVEF). In this retrospective study, patients with ICDs had better survival rates, stratified for LVEF. (From Powell AC, Fuchs T, Finkelstein DM, et al: Influence of implantable cardioverter-defibrillators on the long-term prognosis of survivors of out-of-hospital cardiac arrest. Circulation 1993; 88:1083–1092.)

which patients with malignant ventricular arrhythmias treated with ICD had decreased cardiac mortality compared with patients treated with medications. In contrast, other investigators feel that these comparisons are flawed and that anything other than a randomized cohort for comparison is inappropriate.[34]

Many studies attempt to determine ICD efficacy by the number of "appropriate" shocks that patients experience over time. Depending on the device and its data storage capability, the ability to accurately stratify shocks as appropriate versus inappropriate can be difficult or impossible. Traditionally, it has been assumed that the presence of symptoms before an ICD discharge signifies that an appropriate shock for VT occurred. However, such symptoms can occur with supraventricular tachycardia and nonsustained VT. Furthermore, a device discharge for VT does not necessarily mean that the VT would have led to sudden cardiac death. Conversely, it has been assumed that a device discharge to an asymptomatic patient may be inappropriate; recent studies have shown that lack of symptoms before ICD shock can occur with both appropriate and inappropriate discharges.[35] Therefore, many retrospective studies detailing ICD experience are flawed by the inability to precisely determine the frequency of appropriate shocks.

Despite these limitations, the frequency of appropriate ICD shocks over a 2- to 5-year period is approximately 33%–70%.[10–12, 30, 32, 36] In some studies, "appropriate" ICD use[31] or sudden cardiac death[32] did not differ between patients with moderately depressed LV function and those with severely depressed LV function. Total and cardiac mortality was higher in patients with lower ejection fractions (EFs). Therefore, it can be concluded that ICD reduces arrhythmic mortality in patients in the highest risk group[11]; conversely, it can be concluded that ICDs overstate survival benefit because some high-risk patients expire from other causes.

ICD benefit could also be evaluated by examining the expected or actual survival for patients receiving appropriate ICD shocks. The mean survival after an appropriate ICD discharge is approximately 2 years,[12] which suggests a survival benefit in patients with ICDs who receive an appropriate discharge. In another study, 51 of 105 patients had appropriate shocks, and 26 of these patients received therapies for fast VT.[10] Figure 21–3 shows the expected benefit from an ICD by comparing any arrhythmia-related death with episodes of fast VT or VF. The assumption in this report[10] is that any detected episodes of fast VT or VF would have led to sudden cardiac death. Therefore, based on these and other reports, it appears that there are patients who receive appropriate ICD discharges and derive a subsequent survival benefit.

Although many retrospective studies on patients with ICDs have shown impressive reductions in sudden cardiac death, it remains unclear whether total mortality is reduced. One confounding variable is that many clinical series include heterogeneous patient populations. The spectrum of diseases (e.g., coronary artery disease, cardiomyopathies, structurally normal hearts), degrees of ventricular function, and modes of presentation differ among studies. The following sections describe ICD outcomes in better-defined patient populations.

Survivors of Out-of-Hospital Sudden Cardiac Death

Patients who survive an episode of cardiac arrest remain at high risk for recurrence. A multicenter retrospective series on 300 patients receiving ICDs who presented with VF and coronary artery disease reported that total mortality was not different between patients who did or did not receive ICD shocks.[37] These authors concluded that ICDs improved survival in patients who received shocks to a level observed in comparable patients who did not have recurrent VT or VF.

Retrospective studies comparing survivors of aborted sudden cardiac death who did or did not receive an ICD have produced conflicting results.[7, 9] Although the ICD decreased deaths from arrhythmias in both studies, overall survival was not different in one study[9]

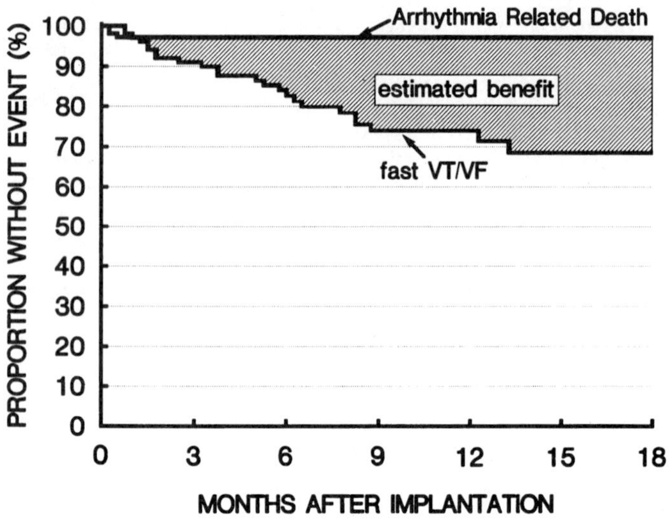

Figure 21–3. This graph estimates the survival benefit conferred by implantable cardiac defibrillators. The estimated benefit is obtained by comparing arrhythmia-related death versus any episode of fast ventricular tachycardia (VT) or ventricular fibrillation (VF) that presumably would have been life-threatening. (From Bocker K, Block M, Isbruch F, et al: Do patients with an implantable defibrillator live longer? J Am Coll Cardiol 1993; 124:1608–1614.)

and was improved by the ICD in another.[7] Even in the study by Powell and colleagues,[7] which demonstrated a reduction in total and cardiac mortality (see Fig. 21–2), other factors such as LV function and patient age were more powerful predictors of total cardiac mortality. This and other retrospective studies tend to be biased, because the assignment of ICD versus medical therapy is nonrandom, and "sicker" patients often receive medical therapy.[34] Therefore, it appears that ICD therapy is appropriate for patients who survive an episode of sudden cardiac death, although it is unclear whether overall survival is affected.

Patients with nonischemic cardiomyopathy have similar outcomes with ICD compared with patients with coronary artery disease[36]; therefore, treatment of these groups of patients should be similar.

Patients With Structurally Normal Hearts

Patients resuscitated from a cardiac arrest who are subsequently found to have no significant heart disease make up 5% of sudden cardiac death survivors.[21, 38] In the largest multicenter series on 28 such patients who received ICDs with a mean 2.5-year follow-up, it was concluded that these patients have an excellent three-year survival rate.[39] Most of these patients (61%) had no inducible ventricular arrhythmias. There were no cardiac deaths and two noncardiac deaths in this 28 patient cohort. Of note, only four patients received "appropriate" shocks, and a total of 31 shock episodes were termed "indeterminate." Because there were no control patients in this study, and because the classification of shocks into appropriate versus indeterminate was speculative, it is unclear to what extent mortality was reduced by defibrillators in this highly defined patient subgroup.

Other studies[2, 40, 41] confirmed that in patients with no identifiable heart disease who receive an ICD, 30%–75% of the patients received "appropriate" shocks. It has been suggested that ICD therapy is superior to other therapies if the clinical arrhythmia is not clinically reproducible in the electrophysiology laboratory.[40] Thus, it appears that in patients with idiopathic VF and in those who survived cardiac arrest, the use of ICD therapy is reasonable and is possibly life-saving.

Long QT Syndrome

There are little published data on ICD therapy in patients with the long QT syndrome. In the registry by Schwartz and associates,[42] there was a 1.3% annual incidence of sudden death. Clearly, therapies such as beta blockade, bradycardia pacing, and left stellectomy have been used and can alleviate symptoms such as syncope and possibly prevent some episodes of sudden cardiac death.[40, 42, 43] However, these therapies, used either individually or in combination, are imperfect. Because these patients are young and have otherwise structurally normal hearts, there is a dilemma as to whom should receive an ICD.

In a pediatric series of 14 patients with the long QT syndrome who received an ICD, 11 patients received an "appropriate" defibrillator discharge.[44] In our practice, one of three patients, all of whom were women aged 22–33 years, with the long QT syndrome who received an ICD following an episode of aborted sudden cardiac death received appropriate shocks for recurrent VT.

Because of the limited data available, no definitive recommendations can be made as to which patients with the long QT syndrome should receive an ICD. For patients with VF or those who survive an episode of sudden cardiac death, we strongly consider an ICD as primary therapy, along with beta blockade or other concomitant therapy. In patients with the long QT syndrome and markers that place them at risk for sudden cardiac death, the decision to implant an ICD must be individualized, probably after an attempt at medical therapy.

Pediatric Patients

Patients younger than 20 years of age who have received an ICD tend to be survivors of sudden cardiac death.[44] The spectrum of associated diseases is different in the pediatric population than in adults. Pediatric patients have more hypertrophic and dilated cardiomyopathies (54%), primary electrical diseases (26%), and congenital heart defects (18%). A multicenter cooperative study on pediatric patients receiving an ICD reported that 59% of patients received an "appropriate" shock, and 20% of patients received a "spurious" shock. Overall sudden death–free survival was comparable with that seen in adults—97%, 95%, and 90% at 1, 2, and 5 years after ICD implantation, respectively. Furthermore, abnormal ventricular function was the only significant predictor of mortality.[44]

High-Risk Patients Without Documented Sustained Ventricular Arrhythmias

There are no published data to support the use of a prophylactic ICD in high-risk patients who have not had documented sustained ventricular arrhythmias, nor is prophylactic ICD use recommended by the American College of Cardiology/American Heart Association Joint Task Force[18] or NASPE[19] in this patient group. In theory, potential survival benefit from an ICD in high-risk patients may exceed risks of implantation, especially with the newer transvenous defibrillators with biphasic shock capabilities. Before the use of the prophylactic ICD can become routine, other issues, such as cost effectiveness and quality of life, must be addressed, preferably in well-designed prospective trials.[45, 46]

There are a variety of noninvasive and invasive tests available to the clinician to identify patients, particularly postinfarction patients, who are at increased risk for sudden cardiac death.[26, 47] Three prospective studies are underway that evaluate the prophylactic use of ICDs for such high-risk patients with coronary artery disease.[26, 45, 47–50] The Multicenter Automatic Defibrillator Implantation Trial (MADIT)[50] enrolls patients with coronary artery disease, depressed LV function, nonsustained VT, and inducible VT. The hypothesis in MADIT is that implantation of an ICD in these high-risk patients improves overall survival compared with conventional therapy. In the Multicenter Unsustained Tachycardia Trial (MUSTT),[47] similar high-risk patients are enrolled to receive either no therapy or electrophysiology study–guided therapy. ICDs are implanted in patients randomized to electrophysiology study–guided therapy in whom no drug is found to be effective. In the Coronary Artery Bypass Grafting-Patch (CABG-Patch)[49] trial, patients with high-risk markers (i.e., decreased LV function and an abnormal signal-averaged electrocardiogram) who are undergoing coronary artery bypass grafting are randomized to receive an ICD at the time of grafting. Because these studies are ongoing, no recommendations can be made about the prophylactic use of an ICD in a high-risk patient who has not had a sustained ventricular arrhythmia.

USE OF ICD SYSTEMS

Hardware

Over the last decade, the actual hardware required to implant a defibrillator has been simplified. Epicardial defibrillators generally consist of a generator, two epicardial patches, and two rate-sensing epicardial screw-in leads. Current nonthoracotomy ICD systems consist of a pulse generator, one or two transvenous leads, and possibly, a subcutaneous patch or lead array system. With the use of biphasic waveforms, a nonthoracotomy lead system defibrillator can be implanted in 95%–99% of patients who require an ICD. Furthermore, most patients can have a totally transvenous ICD system, avoiding the use of a subcutaneous patch.[51]

The pulse generators weigh approximately 125–140 g (Table 21–3). The external encasement is made of titanium. The defibrillators commonly use 3.2 or 2 lithium silver vanadium oxide batteries to provide 6.4 V, which provides energy for pacing and defibrillation. The epicardial patches vary in size and material, but in general, larger patches are associated with lower defibrillation thresholds (DFTs). The headers vary according to the manufacturer and model of the defibrillator. Pacing and sensing leads attach to the header with a standard IS1 pacing configuration or bifurcated leads. There is a new industry standard for high-voltage defibrillating leads known as DF1, which uses a 3.2-mm lead. However, many older and currently used defibrillating leads or patches use a 5- to 6-mm lead. Adapters are used to connect leads to headers when there is a mismatch between lead sizes and defibrillator header sizes.

Nonthoracotomy Lead Systems

The CPI Endotak lead system was the first nonthoracotomy lead system available in the United States. It consists of the Endotak C lead, which is a 70- or 100-cm-long tined endocardial lead that combines bipolar sensing, pacing, and defibrillation in a single lead. The distal tip serves as the rate-sensing and pacing cathode. A distal right ventricular spring electrode serves as the sensing and pacing anode and defibrillation cathode (Fig. 21–4). A right atrial spring electrode typically serves as the defibrillation anode; therefore, pacing and sensing is between a distal pacing electrode and the distal high-voltage spring electrode. A subcutaneous patch can be added to this system to facilitate defibrillation in patients with elevated thresholds with a lead-alone system.

The Medtronic Transvene lead system was the second endocardial lead system to become available. The Transvene tripolar lead consists of two distal pacing electrodes for true bipolar sensing and pacing, as well as a distal high-voltage spring electrode. Defibrillation can be accomplished with a shock delivered between the distal high-voltage electrode and an "active" can of the defibrillator (Fig. 21–5*A*) implanted in a subpectoral position. Alternatively, an additional defibrillator lead can be implanted in a subclavian position (Fig. 21–5*B*). With the latter system (through two defibrillator leads), a subcutaneous patch can also be implanted in a subclavicular or axillary position when necessary to decrease DFTs.

Implantation of ICDs—General Principles

Implantation of an epicardial lead system ICD is associated with 1.5%–10% perioperative mortality. Factors such as low ejection

TABLE 21–3. CHARACTERISTICS OF DIFFERENT IMPLANTABLE CARDIOVERTER-DEFIBRILLATORS

	CPI				Medtronic					
Characteristic	Ventak P	P3	PRx	PRx3/Mini	PCD 7217	PCD 7219	Ventritex 110/115	Intermedics Res Q	Siemens Siecure	Telectronics Guardian—4215
Weight (g)	240	179	220	179/125	197	136	195/129	240	220	169
Displacement (mL)	145	97	130	97/68	130	83	130/73	150	120	102
Zones of VT detection	1	2	3	3	2	3	3	3	3	3
Algorithm for VT defect	PDF	PDF	Onset, stability, turning point morphology, SRD	Onset, stability, SRD	Onset, stability	Onset, stability	Onset	Onset, stability, sustained high rate	Onset, stability, duration	Onset, HRD
Real-time telemetry	No	Yes	No	Yes	Yes	Yes	Yes	Yes	Yes	Yes
NIPS	No	Yes	Yes	Yes	Yes	Yes	Yes	Yes	Yes	Yes
Stored electrogram/min	No	Yes/2.5 min	No	2.5/5 min	No	Yes/10 sec	2/8 min	No	No	Yes/"snapshot"
Bradycardia pacing	No	VVI	VVI	VVI	VVI	VVI	VVI	VVI	VVI	VVI
ATP	No	No	Yes	Yes	Yes	Yes	Yes	Yes	Yes	Yes
Maximum energy	30 joules	34 joules	34 joules	34/29 joules	34 joules	34 joules	750 volts	40 joules	40 joules	700 volts
Energy waveform	m	m, bi	m	m, bi	m, seq	m, bi	m, bi	bi	m	m, bi
Automatic capacitor reform	No	Yes	No	Yes	No	Yes	Yes	No	Yes	Yes
Committed therapy	Yes	Programmable	Programmable	Programmable	VT-no, VF-yes	Programmable	No	Yes	Yes	Programmable

Abbreviations: ATP, antitachycardia pacing; bi, biphasic; HRD, high rate duration; m, monophasic; NIPS, noninvasive programmed stimulation; PDF, probability density function; SRD, sustained rated duration; seq, sequential; VT, ventricular tachycardia; VF, ventricular fibrillation.

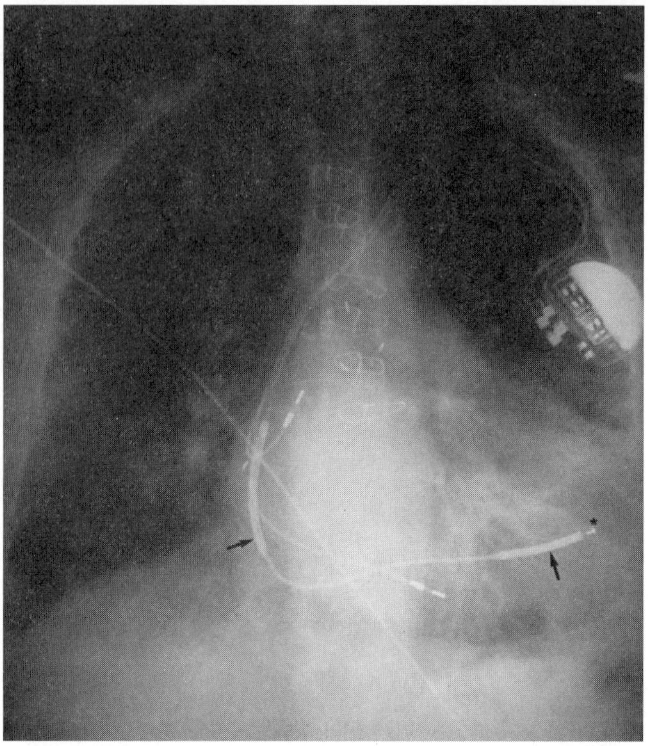

Figure 21–4. Chest roentgenogram of a patient with a transvenous implantable cardioverter-defibrillator (ICD) with which a CPI Endotak lead (Cardiac Pacemakers, Inc., St. Paul, MN) was used. The high-voltage spring electrodes *(arrows)* and distal pace-sensing electrode *(asterisk)* are demonstrated. This patient also has a dual-chamber bipolar pacemaker. Patients with ICDs and concomitant pacemakers need to have wide separation of the ICD sensing electrodes and the pacemaker leads. The ICD generator, which is implanted in the abdomen, is not shown.

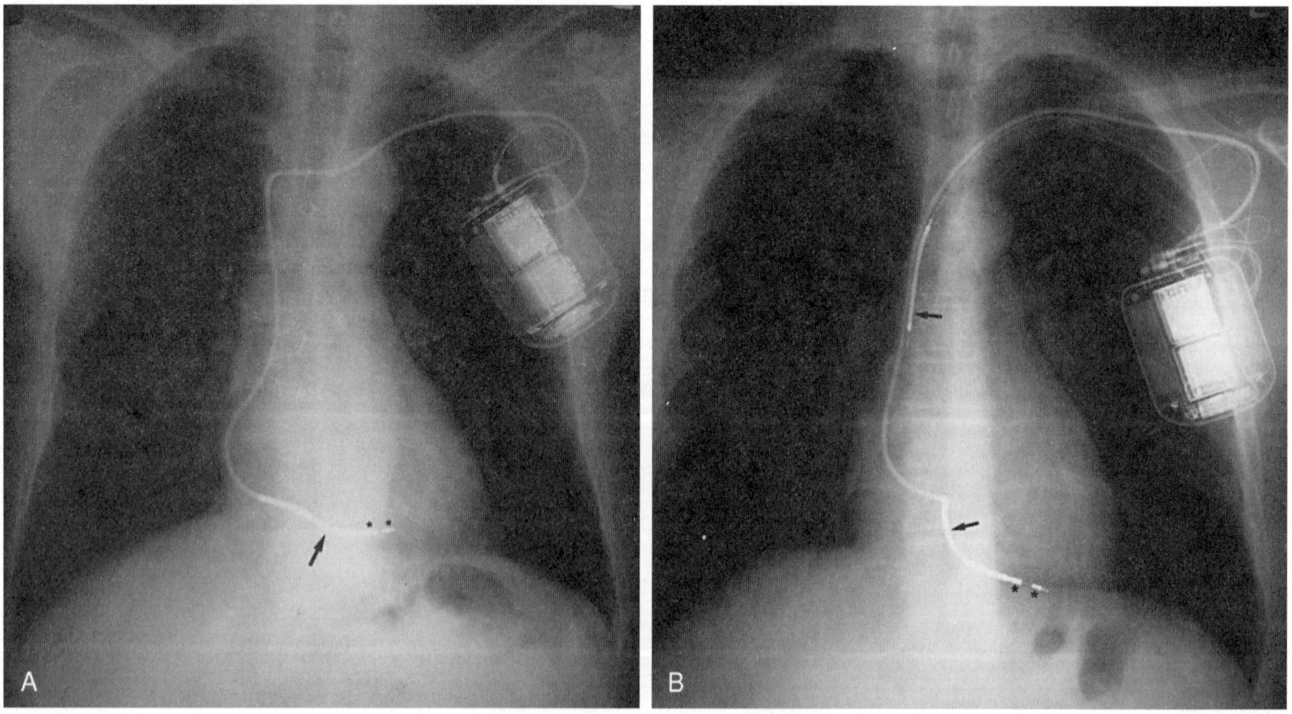

Figure 21–5. *A*, Chest roentgenogram of a patient with a Medtronic Jewel 7219C "hot can" (Medtronic, Inc., Minneapolis, MN). (There is only one high-voltage electrode *(arrow),* because defibrillation is accomplished between the high-voltage electrode and the shell of the defibrillator, which serves as a cathode or anode. Separate electrodes *(asterisks)* allow for true bipolar sensing and pacing. *B*, Chest roentgenogram of a patient with a Medtronic Jewel 7219D, which has two separate leads with high-voltage electrodes *(arrows).*

fraction and concomitant surgery[12, 33] increase the perioperative mortality.

Implantation of a nonthoracotomy lead system ICD can be performed with less morbidity and mortality than a system in which epicardial patches are used.[12, 29, 37, 52] Perioperative mortality in patients who receive nonthoracotomy ICDs is between 0% and 3.4%.[8, 10, 52, 53] The morbidity as expressed by length of hospital stay is reduced.[8, 53] The total 1-year mortality in patients receiving nonthoracotomy ICDs may be reduced compared with that in patients receiving epicardial ICDs because of the reduction in the perioperative mortality observed with the newer nonthoracotomy ICDs.[8] Other studies have shown equivalent long-term total survival between patients receiving thoracotomy and nonthoracotomy ICDs,[52] demonstrating at least equivalent efficacy for these newer defibrillator systems.

Three percent to 27% of patients receiving ICD implants experience lead-related problems.[52–54] Long-term lead complications were observed in 12.5% of 255 patients, most of whom had epicardial patches.[55] Lead fracture was the cause of the complication in one half of these patients. In another large series involving epicardial patch system ICDs, 21% of 241 patients experienced a complication requiring an operative procedure for correction.[56] Lead-related problems occurred in 8% of these patients, and infections requiring device explantation occurred in 5% of these patients. Lead dislodgment has occurred in up to 6% of patients with transvenous leads.[53, 54]

Infections occur in approximately 2.2%–13.1% of epicardial lead system ICD implants.[53, 54, 56, 57] In general, this complication is treated by explantation of the entire defibrillator system, although these patients may be managed by prolonged antibiotic therapy or other nonsurgical means.[58] Initial reports have shown comparable infection rates between thoracotomy and nonthoracotomy ICD systems.[53] Other reports demonstrate an infection rate of 0.6%–3.8% for nonthoracotomy ICDs.[52, 54, 59] Nonthoracotomy lead system defibrillators would be expected to have a lower infection rate because of the reduced amount of implanted hardware, shorter operative time, and smaller incision and wound size, especially with the subpectoral implants. However, most of the reports on nonthoracotomy ICD implants were with ICD systems that delivered monophasic shocks; therefore, a subcutaneous patch or crossover to an epicardial lead system ICD occurred in a significant number of patients. Thus, the expected infection and complication rates may be decreased further with the use of ICDs that deliver biphasic waveform defibrillation, because these systems are expected to have greater successful implantation rates as a totally transvenous system.

Because nonthoracotomy lead system defibrillators generally result in decreased operative morbidity and mortality, it is recommended that, in general, all patients receiving a new ICD have a transvenous ICD implanted. An exception to this recommendation is in patients undergoing concomitant cardiac surgery. In these patients, depending on the complexity of the surgery and experience of the surgeon with epicardial lead systems, it is reasonable to either implant an epicardial lead system defibrillator at the time of surgery or to implant a nonthoracotomy lead system ICD in the postoperative period. It is no longer advisable to implant only epicardial patches during a cardiac surgical procedure because of the high success rate of nonthoracotomy lead system ICDs.

In Table 21–4, we describe a strategy used to implant nonthoracotomy lead system defibrillators. In general, we prefer to implant the simplest system possible with the least amount of hardware to facilitate implantation and minimize complications. The DFT is acceptable when defibrillation is accomplished on three successive occasions with the use of defibrillation energy at least 10 joules less than the maximal energy output. We always start DFT testing by using biphasic waveforms (discussed later). It is preferable to attempt defibrillation at progressively lower energy outputs to obtain the "lowest energy of defibrillation." Clinical factors that can result in elevated DFTs include decreased LV systolic function and the use of antiarrhythmic drugs such as amiodarone.[60] DFT may increase over time[61] or with the addition of antiarrhythmic drugs[62]; therefore, patients with marginally acceptable DFTs may not have reliable defibrillation of rapid ventricular tachyarrhythmias on long-term follow-up.

When defibrillation is not accomplished with a totally transvenous system, lead repositioning or addition of another defibrillation lead or subcutaneous patch can facilitate implantation of a nonthoracotomy defibrillator. It should be noted that with progressive DFT testing, the actual DFT may rise. Potentially, there are transient and acute deleterious effects on cardiac function,[63] cardiac sympathetic responsiveness,[64] and postoperative neurologic function[65] associated with performing multiple DFT testing. Therefore, as outlined in Table 21–4, after multiple DFT tests are performed, it may be clinically prudent to discontinue DFT testing. If DFTs are marginal, implantation of leads and the ICD may be acceptable, provided follow-up DFT testing performed in the electrophysiology laboratory demonstrates an adequate DFT safety margin.

Defibrillation

Many methods are available to produce defibrillation. Historically, defibrillation was initially accomplished by truncated monophasic waveforms and was quite effective when defibrillators used epicardial patches. In the rare instances when epicardial DFTs were unacceptably elevated, use of a third epicardial patch or an endocardial defibrillation lead decreased DFTs by incorporating either simultaneous or sequential monophasic defibrillation shocks.[66–69]

Many patients fail to have adequate DFTs with the use of monophasic single-pathway shocks in totally transvenous defibrillator sys-

TABLE 21–4. IMPLANTATION OF A NONTHORACOTOMY DEFIBRILLATOR

1. Choose biphasic defibrillator systems according to operator preference and availability
   a. Single-lead system with one spring electrode and unipolar defibrillation
   b. Single-lead system with two spring high-voltage electrodes (e.g., CPI Endotak)
   c. Two-lead system (e.g., Medtronic Transvene)
2. Test biphasic defibrillation thresholds using a totally transvenous system
   a. If three of three defibrillations are accomplished with a minimal safety margin of ≥10 joules, implant defibrillator
   b. If there is inadequate defibrillation threshold, consider:
      repositioning lead or leads
      reversing polarity
   c. If defibrillation thresholds are still inadequate, then add a third endocardial electrode or a subcutaneous patch in a subpectoral or subaxillary position
3. If defibrillation thresholds remain elevated after trying mulitple configurations with leads, patches, or both, then consider the following
   a. If defibrillation thresholds are marginal and patient has undergone multiple defibrillation threshold tests, then consider implantation of the defibrillator with the "best" configuration; retest defibrillation threshold in the electrophysiology laboratory in a few days
   b. Terminate defibrillation threshold testing; return to the surgical suite in a few days to again try "best" lead configuration for nonthoracotomy defibrillation, followed by epicardial patch placement, if necessary
   c. Immediate implantation of one or two epicardial patches if the patient's clinical status is stable after multiple defibrillation threshold tests

TABLE 21–5. COMPARISON OF DEFIBRILLATION THRESHOLD USING BIPHASIC VERSUS MONOPHASIC WAVEFORMS IN NONTHORACOTOMY ICD SYSTEMS

Study	Defibrillation Pathway	DFT Monophasic (joules)	DFT Biphasic (joules)	*P* Value
Bardy et al.[75]*	Single	34.3	23.4	=.004
Jung et al.[76]	Dual	21.9	14.9	<.001
	Single	22.1	15	<.001
Saksena et al.[70]	Dual	15	9	<.02
Marks et al.[77]	Dual	28	14	<.0001
Neuzner et al.[78]	Single	22.2	12.5	<.0001
Wyse et al.[72]	Single	21.1	12.3	<.001

Abbreviations: DFT, defibrillation threshold; ICD, implantable cardioverter-defibrillator.

*Included data only from right ventricular electrode to chest wall patch.

TABLE 21–6. FACTORS TO CONSIDER WHEN PROGRAMMING AN ICD

Clinical Presentation of Patient
Cardiac arrest
Syncope
Blood pressure and symptoms during VT
Nonsustained VT

Electrophysiologic Properties of VTs
Spontaneous versus EPS-induced VTs
Rates of VTs
Number of different VTs
Presence of nonsustained or sponaneously terminating VT
Response to antitachycardia pacing (number of pacing stimuli, fixed burst, ramp)
Response to low-energy cardioversion (<2 joules with the ICD)

Possible Interaction with Supraventricular Rhythms
History of atrial fibrillation or atrial flutter
History of any supraventricular tachycardia
Maximal sinus rate and possible overlap with VT rate

Other Factors
Concurrent antiarrhythmic medication
  Possible elevation of defibrillation threshold
  Possible change in VT rate
Pacemaker-ICD interaction

Abbreviations: EPS, electrophysiology study; ICD, implantable cardioverter-defibrillator; VT, ventricular tachycardia.

tems. In general, with monophasic waveforms, successful implantation of such systems can be accomplished in 30%–70% of patients with the use of a totally transvenous system[52] and in 65%–90% of patients receiving a three-electrode configuration.[52, 59, 70] Multiple lead configurations, including a defibrillator lead in the coronary sinus, the use of a subcutaneous patch, reversal of defibrillation polarity, and simultaneous or sequential pulses, have been tried to reduce DFTs.[67–69, 71]

Biphasic waveform defibrillation is a superior method of defibrillation, especially when nonthoracotomy lead system defibrillators are used. Biphasic waveform defibrillation can be used in a two-lead, single-pathway defibrillation system or in a three-lead, simultaneous-pathway system. As seen in Table 21–5, biphasic waveform defibrillation resulted in a 32%–50% decrease in DFTs compared with monophasic waveform defibrillation[70, 72–78] and has led to decreased length of hospital stay compared with monophasic waveforms.[79] These data provide compelling evidence that patients should receive defibrillators with biphasic waveforms. However, it should be noted that in individual patients, depending on the electrode configuration, biphasic waveform DFT may be equal to or, rarely, in excess of monophasic DFT.[75]

The use of unipolar biphasic defibrillation between a right ventricular electrode and an active shell (can) of the defibrillator generator unit implanted in a subclavicular position may further reduce transvenous DFTs (see Fig. 21–5*A*).[76, 80, 81] The mean DFT with such a simplified system has been reported to be between 7 and 10 joules.[76, 81] Based on these preliminary data and our own experience, it is expected that this simplified unipolar defibrillating system will achieve sufficiently low DFTs to allow for implantation in almost anyone who can accommodate a subclavicular (subcutaneous or subpectoralis) implant.

Sensing: Detection Algorithms and Zones

The principle mode for tachycardia detection is the ventricular rate. Tachycardia is detected when the heart rate exceeds a preselected rate cut-off. Most defibrillators use autoadjusting sensitivity or automatic gain control, which varies the sensitivity on a beat-by-beat basis according to the amplitude of the detected R wave or to whether the patient is being paced. The maximal attainable sensitivity

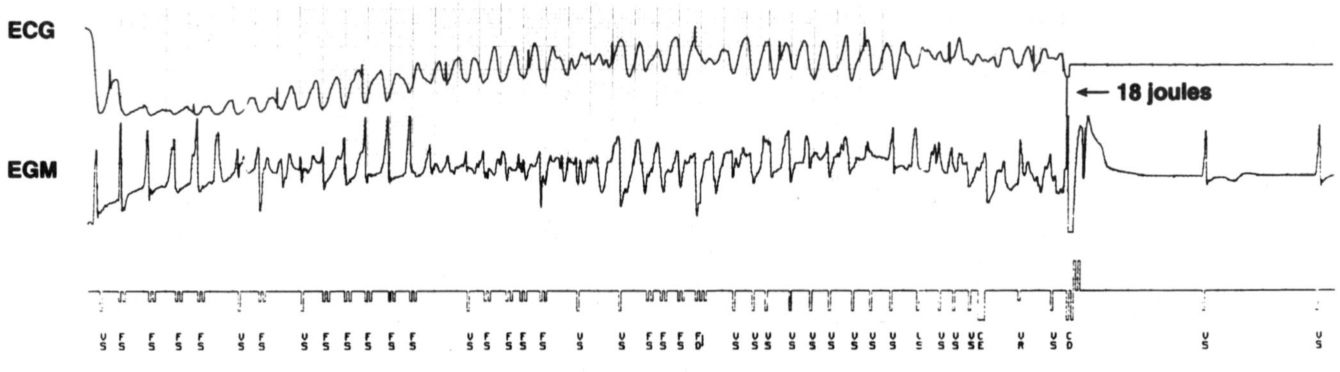

Figure 21–6. A surface electrocardiogram (ECG), intracardiac electrogram (EGM), and marker channel during an induced episode of ventricular fibrillation (VF). Note the EGM dropout, manifested by dropout of fibrillation sense (FS) markers, and the presence of normal ventricular sense (VS) markers during VF. Because the algorithm for VF detection allows for 18 of 24 complexes to be detected below the VF detection interval, there was only minimal delay before VF was detected (FD) and an 18-joule shock was delivered (CD). After VF is detected (FD), the marker channel normally records the rhythm with ventricular sense markers (VS) as the capacitors charge (CE) and the charge is delivered (CD). *Other abbreviation:* VR, ventricular refractor, which corresponds to a sensed event within 400 msec after capacitors have charged.

is generally in the level of 0.15–0.5 mV. There have been reports of undersensing of VT and VF in devices that rely on fixed-gain sensitivity[82, 83]; therefore, most current ICDs rely on autogain sensitivity.

Even with adequate sensing, ventricular electrogram amplitude may vary in rapid ventricular tachyarrhythmias or VF (Fig. 21–6). For this reason, most sensing algorithms require only a percentage of detected electrograms (e.g., 18 of 24) to fall within the tachycardia detection zone before initiating therapy. As shown in Figure 21–6, there was some dropout of ventricular electrograms, but VF was still detected without delay. Therefore, rate cut-off is very sensitive for detection of ventricular tachyarrhythmias, especially when an algorithm that allows for less than 100% detection is used. However, this algorithm lacks specificity, and any supraventricular arrhythmia that exceeds the rate cut-off (e.g., atrial fibrillation, supraventricular tachycardia, sinus tachycardia) will also be detected as a ventricular tachyarrhythmia and trigger a therapy (Fig. 21–7). Despite limitations of using rate cut-off alone for VT or VF detection, rate cut-off is the only criteria used for tachyarrhythmia detection in the majority of patients. In a report from Medtronic PCD with epicardial patches used in 1475 patients, 88% of patients' PCDs were programmed so that only rate cut-off for detection of VT or VF was used.[84]

Most ICDs currently offer more than one zone for detection of ventricular tachyarrhythmias. This allows for separate detection of VT and VF, which allows for specific and tiered therapy for one arrhythmia versus the other. The main feature that distinguishes these zones is ventricular rate, or RR intervals. A "VF" zone is programmed for arrhythmias with rapid ventricular rates (>185–240 bpm). Because detected arrhythmias at these rates are more likely to cause hemodynamic compromise, it is preferable that this zone be sensitive at the expense of specificity.

Some devices have multiple VT detection zones, and the algorithm can be altered to increase specificity for VT detection by requiring that other criteria be satisfied in addition to rate cut-off. These additional criteria can be programmed when the patient has the potential to have supraventricular arrhythmias (e.g., sinus tachycardia, atrial fibrillation) with ventricular rates that would otherwise fall within a VT detection zone. These features are outlined later in this chapter, and the decision to program these features is based on various clinical and electrophysiologic factors, as outlined in Table 21–6.

In general, patients with slower VTs are more likely to have overlap with inappropriate detection of supraventricular arrhythmias. Therefore, it is appropriate to attempt to differentiate these rhythms from VT. However, programming these features may decrease the sensitivity in detection of VT. Therefore, caution must be used, especially when patients have VT that causes hemodynamic compromise. Judicious use of specificity-enhancing features infrequently causes underdetection of VT; such underdetection can be corrected by reprogramming the ICD.[13]

In Figure 21–8, we propose an algorithm in programming VT and VF detection zones. In general, patients who present with cardiac arrest or rapid VT causing hemodynamic compromise have only one detection zone programmed (VF) unless there is also inducible VT that is terminated by antitachycardia pacing, low-energy cardioversion, or both. Patients with syncope and inducible VT may have a VT detection zone programmed if the VT is terminated by antitachycardia pacing and/or low-energy cardioversion. If a patient presents

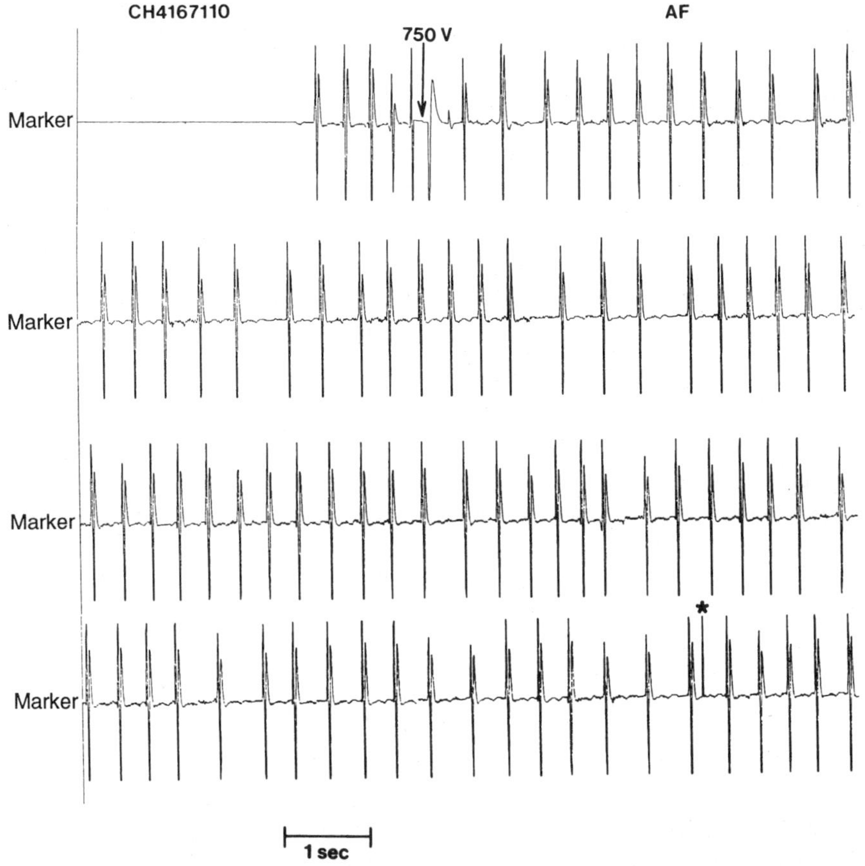

Figure 21–7. Stored electrograms from a patient who experienced an implantable cardioverter-defibrillator (ICD) discharge for atrial fibrillation. Note that the electrograms before and after delivery of a 750-V shock are identical, and the rhythm is irregularly irregular, consistent with atrial fibrillation. Because of the irregularity and because the ventricular response was near the tachycardia detection rate, the ICD took several seconds before declaring the rhythm to be below the tachycardia rate cut-off *(asterisk).*

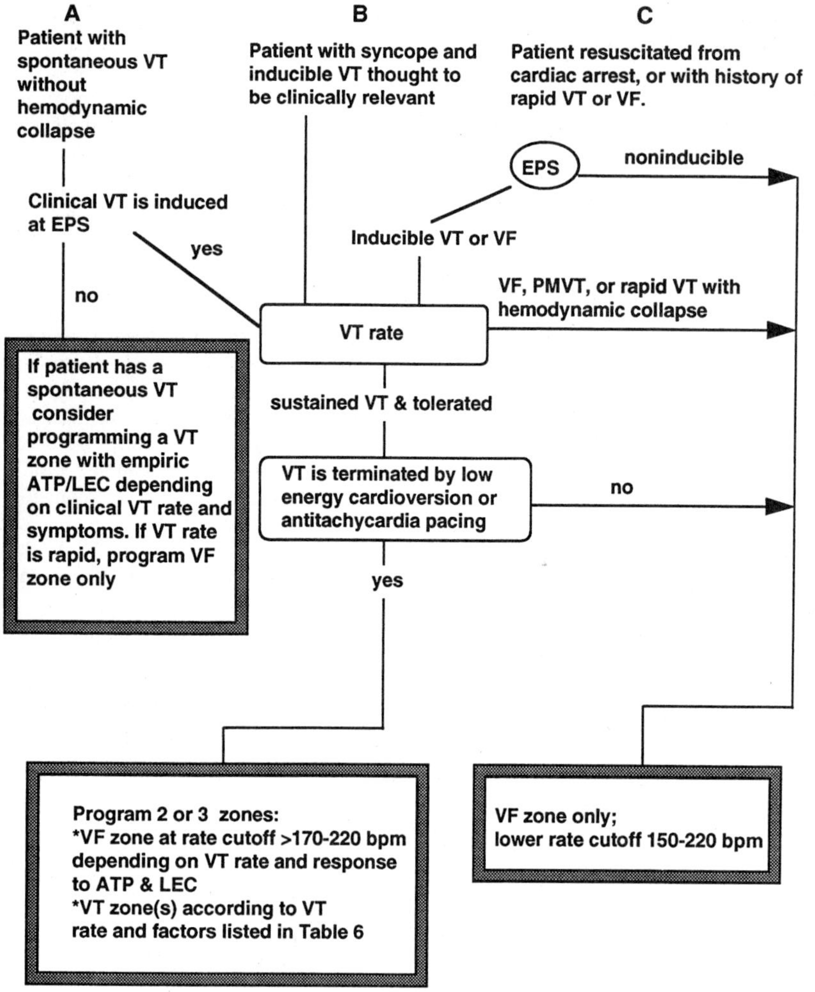

Figure 21–8. Algorithm for programming ventricular tachycardia (VT) and ventricular fibrillation (VF) detection zones. *Abbreviations:* ATP, antitachycardia pacing; bpm, beats per minute; EPS, electrophysiology study; LEC, low-energy cardioversion; PMVT, polymorphic ventricular tachycardia.

with a spontaneous VT that is well tolerated, then a VT detection zone is programmed unless that VT cannot be induced in the electrophysiology laboratory or terminated by antitachycardia pacing and low-energy cardioversion. In this situation, some clinicians program empiric antitachycardia pacing, low-energy cardioversion, or both.

The programming factors outlined in Table 21–6 must be considered, and ICD programming must be individualized. When it is necessary to enhance VT detection specificity, the features described in the following sections can be used, according to the type and model of the defibrillator. The following criteria and features can reduce the number of inappropriate shocks without compromising patient safety and VT detection.[85]

Onset Criteria

Patients with slow VTs that overlap in rate with sinus tachycardia may have inappropriate detection of sinus tachycardia (Fig. 21–9); this occurs in as many as 9% of patients.[85–87] To differentiate sinus tachycardia from VT, the onset criterion used by various manufacturers (see Table 21–3) examines the RR intervals before onset of tachycardia. A sinus tachycardia would be expected to have a gradually increasing rate before exceeding the tachycardia detection interval. A VT would be expected to have an abrupt change in the RR intervals before exceeding the tachycardia detection interval. Thus, the onset criterion would be satisfied if the rate of the tachycardia exceeds the tachycardia detection rate and there is change in the RR intervals before and after tachycardia that exceed a programmed value. The limitations of this feature include possible nondetection of an exercise-induced VT. In one study, a programmed onset ratio of 87% caused appropriate nondetection in 98% of episodes of sinus tachycardia while causing VT underdetection in only 0.5% of episodes.[86]

Rate Stability

Atrial fibrillation is a common arrhythmia in patients with ICDs and causes inappropriate tachycardia detections and therapies in as many as 12% of patients[85–87] (see Fig. 21–7). One algorithm to distinguish atrial fibrillation from VT is to examine the regularity of successive RR intervals (i.e., rate stability). If the differences in RR cycle lengths exceed a programmed value, then tachycardia detection would not be fulfilled, despite fulfillment of the rate criteria. Generally, a programmed stability value of 40 msec decreases detection of atrial fibrillation in more than 95% of patients with atrial fibrillation without compromising VT detection.[86] A lower stability value increases the specificity while decreasing sensitivity for VT detection. A greater stability value enhances VT sensitivity but decreases specificity. Obviously, this feature cannot be used for differentiating atrial fibrillation from VF. As with other specificity enhancement features, we recommend the use of this feature only in the VT detection zone.

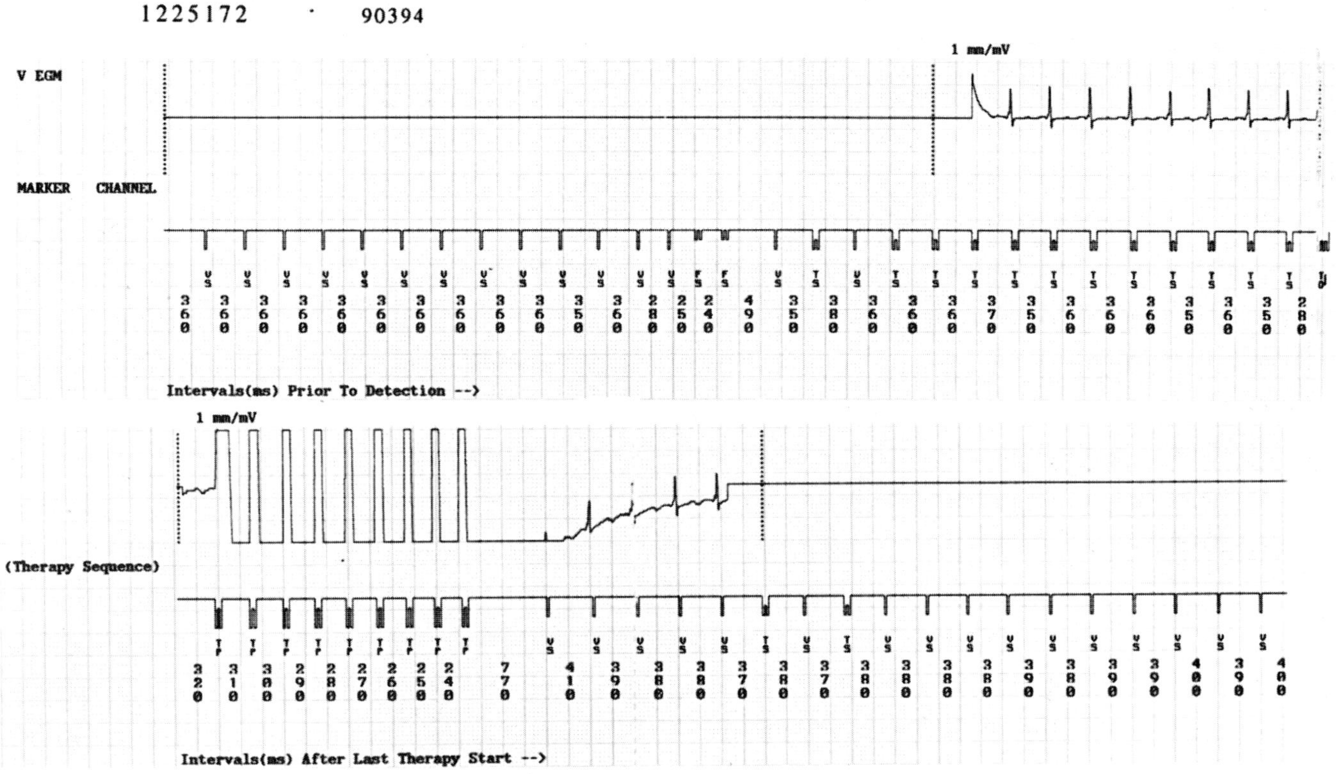

Figure 21–9. Intracardiac electrograms (V EGM) and marker channels of an episode of sinus tachycardia detected as a ventricular tachycardia (TD) before and after antitachycardia pacing (TP). The intervals demonstrated by the marker channel are in milliseconds. The onset feature was on, and the tachycardia detection interval was 380 msec. Initially, the sinus tachycardia was appropriately not detected as a ventricular tachycardia when the cycle length was below the tachycardia detection interval (360 msec; VS). However, a ventricular triplet at coupling interval 280–250–240 msec (VS-FS-FS) offset the detection algorithm such that the ensuing sinus tachycardia was detected as ventricular tachycardia (TS and TD). The intracardiac electrograms before and after therapy were identical, confirming inappropriate detection of sinus tachycardia. *Other abbreviation:* FS, fibrillation sense.

Noncommitted Therapy

After a tachycardia was detected, early ICDs were committed to delivering therapy despite spontaneous termination of the tachycardia (Fig. 21–10). Many newer devices offer "noncommitted" therapy, so that after initial detection of tachycardia and charging of the capacitors, the ICD reexamines the tachycardia just before delivering therapy and aborts therapy if tachycardia is no longer present. In one report, therapy was aborted in 2% of 4670 detected episodes of ventricular tachyarrhythmia.[88] These data demonstrate the benefits of noncommitted therapy in preventing inappropriate shocks or therapies and is a feature that we routinely use when programming all

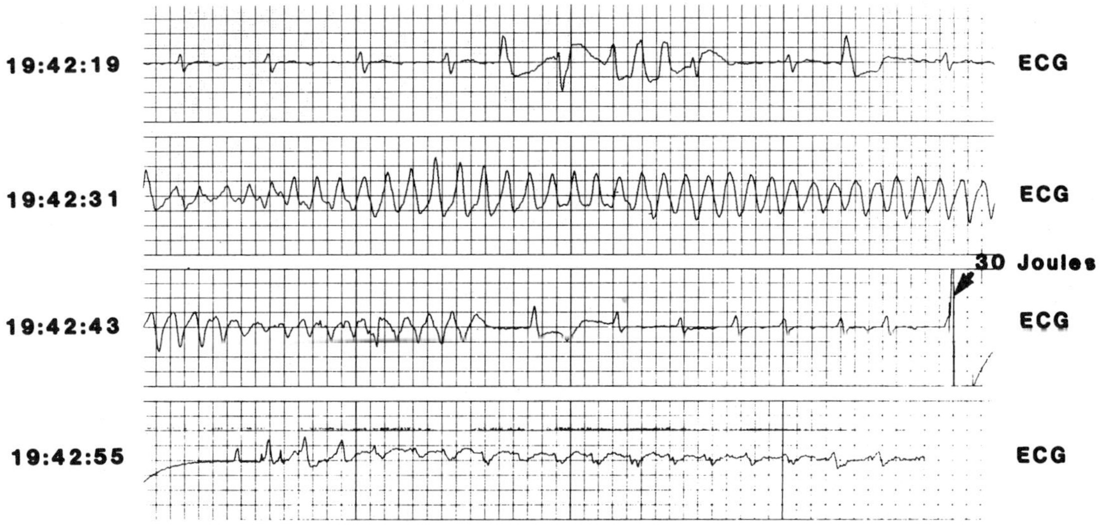

Figure 21–10. Electrocardiogram (ECG) from a patient with spontaneous nonsustained polymorphic ventricular tachycardia. This patient had a CPI AICD 1600 (Cardiac Pacemakers, Inc., Minneapolis, MN), which has noncommitted therapy; therefore, after the ventricular tachycardia was detected, a 30-joule shock was delivered, even though the ventricular tachycardia had terminated.

tachycardia detection zones, including the VF zone. The exception to this recommendation is in patients with "fine" VF, or poor sensing thresholds. In these patients, we program noncommitted therapy for VF, because the detected electrogram could deteriorate sufficiently during the capacitor charge time that VF is no longer detectable.

Extended High Rate

The extended high rate feature limits antitachycardia therapy after VT is detected. A programmable timer starts when a VT is detected, and if tachycardia is not terminated by the elapsed time, then the ICD automatically delivers the therapy programmed for VF.

Sustained Rate Detection

Sustained rate detection is a sensitivity-enhancing feature involving a programmable timer that begins when rate cut-off criteria is satisfied but VT is not detected because another feature, such as rate stability, is not satisfied. When the timer expires, VT detection is based on rate alone.

Other Sensing Issues

In general, oversensing of T waves, oversensing of electrical interference, and failure to sense electrograms during widely varying electrogram amplitude have been described and can cause underdetection, overdetection, or ineffective therapies for ventricular tachyarrhythmias.[89, 90]

Postshock Sensing

The amplitude of electrograms following ICD shocks is substantially reduced.[91] In the event of an unsuccessful shock for VF, redetection of VF may not be reliable.[91] Such underdetection of postshock VF electrograms is a greater problem in transvenous defibrillators that use integrated bipolar sensing (i.e., dedicated pace-sense electrode coupled to a shock electrode) than in systems that have true bipolar sensing.[83]

Bradycardia Pacing

Bradycardia pacing is available in most ICDs in the VVI mode. The advantage of having concomitant VVI pacing as part of an ICD is to avoid ICD-pacemaker interaction if a second device (e.g., a VVI pacemaker) is necessary. In general, antitachycardia pacing must be programmed at high outputs to ensure reliable ventricular capture during VT. Therefore, programming separate outputs for bradycardia and antitachycardia pacing minimizes current drain during bradycardia pacing while maintaining a safety threshold during antitachycardia pacing.

Antitachycardia Pacing

The ability to pace-terminate VT is based on the ability of a pacing impulse to capture excitable tissue within a reentrant circuit (Fig. 21–11). There is no universally acceptable antitachycardia pacing protocol.[92–98] Antitachycardia pacing protocols include fixed-burst pacing, when the pacing cycle length is determined by a programmed percentage of the tachycardia cycle length, and a programmed number of stimuli (4–15) are delivered at that cycle length. With autodecremental or ramp pacing, the first stimulus is determined by a programmed percentage of the tachycardia cycle length, and all subsequent stimuli are shortened by a programmed value (5–20 msec) or percentage.[92–99] These pacing modes can automatically increase the number of stimuli with multiple iterations of the antitachycardia pacing sequences. With either method, there is a risk of accelerating VT to a faster VT or to VF.

In the electrophysiology laboratory, antitachycardia pacing successfully terminates VT in 65%–90% of VTs and accelerates VT in up to 24%[92–99] of attempts. Eight-five percent to 99% of spontaneous VTs are successfully treated by antitachycardia pacing with acceleration rates of less than 5%.[93–100]

The greater efficacy of antitachycardia pacing for spontaneous VT compared with VT induced in the electrophysiology laboratory is probably partly the result of electrophysiologic-guided testing done for VT termination before programming such algorithms in the ICD. Therefore, algorithms known to be successful are programmed to treat spontaneous VTs, whereas algorithms that lead to acceleration are avoided. Antitachycardia pacing may be tested in the electrophysiology laboratory to establish the most effective antitachycardia pacing protocol and eliminate those protocols that accelerate VT to VF. However, algorithms that produce one result in the electrophysiology laboratory may have unexpected results outside the laboratory. Ambulatory patients probably have changes in autonomic tone that may alter conduction times and refractory periods within the reentrant loop, rendering antitachycardia pacing more difficult.[101] Additionally, the induced VT may be different than the spontaneously occurring VT. Therefore, it is unknown whether electrophysiologic-guided programming of antitachycardia pacing sequences is better than empiric programming of such algorithms; however, it is our practice to test pacing algorithms in the electrophysiology laboratory.

Antitachycardia pacing has been highly effective in terminating VT (see Fig. 21–11). In many patients, VT is terminated rapidly so that the patient remains free of symptoms. For the Ventritex Cadence, 94% of antitachycardia pacing protocols for spontaneous VT were successful; 5% of these resulted in unsuccessful therapy; and only 1% accelerated VT to a faster VT or VF.[88] Similar data were reported by Medtronic during their clinical trials with the PCD epicardial system, in which 90.7% of 15,646 ramp antitachycardia pacing attempts and 84.5% of 9704 burst antitachycardia pacing attempts successfully terminated VT.[84] Because of the small risk of acceleration as a result of antitachycardia pacing, ICDs are capable of identifying rapid VTs and advancing the therapy to cardioversion or defibrillation when such acceleration occurs.

Cardioversion

The ability to achieve low-energy cardioversion of VT through an endocardial catheter has been demonstrated.[102–104] Low-energy cardioversion (0.5–2 joules) for VT causes less patient discomfort[103–105] and preserves battery life compared with high-energy dis-

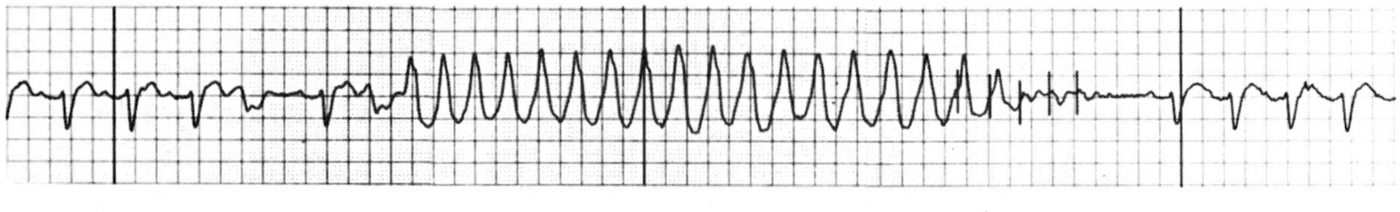

Figure 21–11. An example of spontaneous ventricular tachycardia at a cycle length of 320 msec. The implantable cardioverter-defibrillator delivered antitachycardia pacing consisting of five pulses, which quickly restored sinus rhythm. Sinus rhythm was restored within 7 sec of the start of ventricular tachycardia, preventing any symptoms from occurring in this patient.

charges. Studies have shown that the efficacy for VT termination is similar to that of antitachycardia pacing,[92, 93, 104, 105] as is the risk of arrhythmia acceleration (Fig. 21–12).

In data from clinical trials with the Ventritex Cadence,[88] 90% of 580 episodes of spontaneous VT were successfully treated with the first programmed cardioversion. Similar efficacy was obtained through the use of the Medtronic PCD epicardial system (89% of 3243 episodes) and the Transvene system (85% of 1685 episodes).[84] Caution must be used in interpreting these data, because it is likely that some episodes of "spontaneous ventricular tachycardia" reported in this study were in fact supraventricular rhythms or artifact. Nevertheless, these data demonstrate the high efficacy of low-energy cardioversion in terminating VT.

Data History and Stored Electrograms

The ability to differentiate appropriate from inappropriate shocks has improved greatly over the past several years. Initial ICDs were capable of providing information about the number of shocks delivered. Current ICDs provide more extensive data log histories or stored intracardiac electrograms preceding and following delivery of therapy. Interpretation of the events leading to antitachycardia therapy or a device shock has great implications for management of patients with ICDs. For instance, management of patients with "appropriate" shocks may include addition of or changes in antiarrhythmic drug therapy, changes in antitachycardia pacing protocols, changes in detection algorithms, or no change in medical or ICD programmed parameters. In contrast, management of patients who are thought to have received inappropriate ICD therapies may include medical therapy to control nonventricular tachyarrhythmias, changes in detection algorithms, or diagnosis of lead problems (Fig. 21–13).

A patient's clinical history is necessary to help determine whether or not device therapies were appropriate. In particular, it should be known whether a patient has a history of supraventricular tachyarrhythmias, nonsustained VT, or a concurrent bradycardia pacemaker. In addition, the patient's maximal sinus rate should be noted.

Symptoms preceding a device therapy may be helpful. Severe prodromal symptoms such as dizziness or syncope before a shock are suggestive of an appropriate ICD therapy.[35] With rapid detection and treatment of ventricular arrhythmias, patients often receive shocks for VT before onset of symptoms; therefore, lack of symptoms before ICD shock is not helpful in determining the cause of the shock.[35]

Analysis of RR intervals before and after ICD therapy helps to define the rhythm triggering ICD therapies. For instance, in Figure 21–9 the RR intervals are shown for a detected "VT." The detected tachycardia had RR intervals that were minimally shorter than the tachycardia detection interval, and the posttherapy rhythm had RR intervals that were minimally greater than the detection interval. Furthermore, the tachycardia detection interval was at an interval that corresponds to a relatively low rate cut-off. Therefore, based on the RR intervals, this detected "VT" was most likely a sinus tachycardia.

There are limitations involved to relying only on RR intervals to assess appropriateness of ICD therapy. Because only the rate and regularity of the rhythm are displayed, it is not possible to differentiate supraventricular tachycardia from VT. Furthermore, differentiation of atrial fibrillation from a somewhat irregular VT can be difficult. In an early report on the Medtronic PCD,[99] 19 of 144 episodes of detected VF were thought to be inappropriate (atrial fibrillation, 10; lead fracture, 7; oversensing, 2). Correction of these "inappropriate" shocks was made by changing tachycardia detection protocols, antiarrhythmic drugs, or leads.

Stored electrograms may provide a more accurate depiction of a patient's rhythm before receiving ICD therapy. Stored electrograms allow for analysis of the rate and electrogram morphology before detection and therapy. Figure 21–9 shows an example of the electrograms of a detected tachycardia that matched the electrograms during sinus rhythm, thereby confirming that sinus tachycardia, not VT, had occurred.

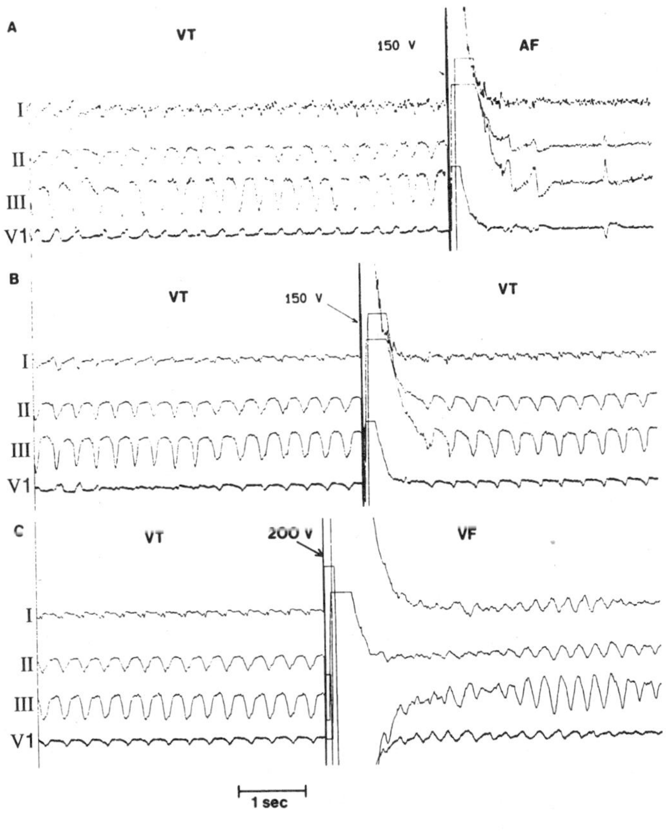

Figure 21–12. The three panels shown represent the variable response to low-energy cardioversion (150–200 V) to induced monomorphic ventricular tachycardia (VT) in one patient. The low-energy cardioversion either terminated the VT *(A),* did not affect the VT *(B),* or accelerated the VT to ventricular fibrillation *(C). Other abbreviations:* AF, atrial fibrillation; VF, ventricular fibrillation.

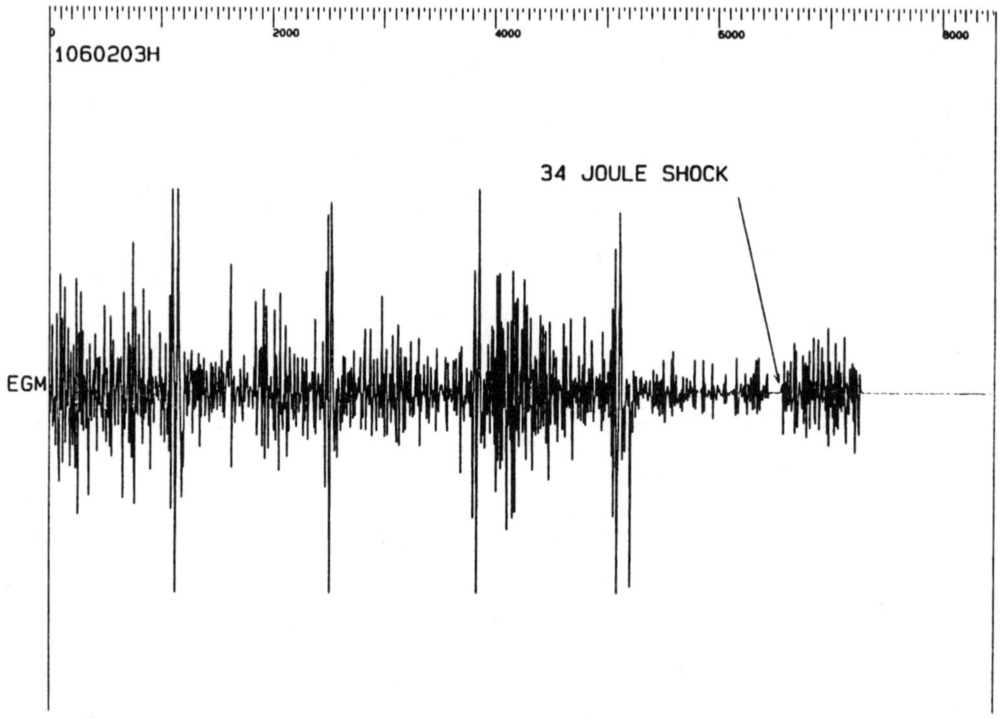

Figure 21–13. Stored electrogram (EGM) from a patient who received an inappropriate shock. Before receiving a 34-joule shock, the patient's spontaneous heart rate was 48 beats per minute. Electrical noise, apparent on the stored EGM, was detected as ventricular fibrillation.

Stored electrograms have aided in patient management. In one study, 60% of patients received antitachycardia therapies or device shocks.[106] Of 101 stored electrograms available for analysis, 74 were classified as VT, 13 as atrial fibrillation, 6 as supraventricular tachycardia, 4 as artifact, 1 as T wave oversensing, and 3 as indeterminate. Analysis of rate, mode of onset, and morphology of the tachycardia helped differentiate the VT from the non-VT rhythms. As a result of these diagnostic methods, changes made to the parameters of tachycardia detection or addition of antiarrhythmic drugs greatly reduced the number of "inappropriate" therapies for non-VT rhythms. Figure 21–13 is an example of electrical noise being detected as VF and being treated with a high-energy shock. This episode resulted in the detection and replacement of a defective transvenous endocardial pace-sense lead.

Stored electrograms are also of value for detected tachycardias that spontaneously terminate without device therapies. It has been reported that as many as 37% of patients with the Ventritex Cadence have such episodes of aborted therapies.[107] In that study, the causes for tachycardia detection with aborted therapies included nonsustained VT (12 patients), atrial fibrillation (5), supraventricular tachycardia (2), and artifact (13). These recorded events led to changes in defibrillator therapies, drug therapies, or lead adapters in many of these patients.

Thus, an effective data-recall system with stored electrograms can greatly aid in patient management and reduce the number of inappropriate therapies or shocks.

Special Features

There are many other features available in ICDs. Noninvasive programmed stimulation is available in many of the newer ICDs. As shown in Figure 21–14, various techniques can be used to induce VF to test defibrillation efficacy in the electrophysiology laboratory. In general, VF can be induced by burst ventricular pacing, high-frequency ventricular burst pacing, and low-energy shocks into the T wave. Programmed ventricular stimulation with introduction of ventricular extrastimuli can also be performed to induce VT.

Many of the ICDs have algorithms available to check pacing threshold and sinus rhythm R wave electrograms. Telemetry functions are available to check battery voltage and pacing and high-voltage lead impedances. Capacitor reformation can be performed manually or automatically at 2- to 3-month intervals.

PACEMAKER AND DRUG INTERACTIONS

As many as 70% of patients with ICDs receive antiarrhythmic medications to suppress recurrent VT or VF, slow down the rate of a VT to avoid syncope or to render it pace terminable, or to suppress supraventricular tachyarrhythmias to prevent inappropriate ICD discharges.[5, 62, 99] It is unknown whether antiarrhythmic drugs reduce the amount of ICD discharges.[108] However, data from the CASCADE trial[109] suggests that amiodarone reduces ICD discharges as compared with conventional antiarrhythmic medication, suggesting a beneficial role for amiodarone in treating patients with frequent recurrences of ICD shocks.

The effects of various antiarrhythmic drugs on DFTs have been reviewed.[62] Chronic amiodarone therapy appears to cause a significant increase in DFTs; in one study, the DFT increased from 10.9 to 20.0 joules,[110] and in another study, the DFT increased from 14.1 to 20.9 joules.[111] Thus, in patients with marginal DFT safety margins, repeat DFT testing after chronic amiodarone therapy is initiated should be considered. Other antiarrhythmic medications (e.g., quinidine, procainamide, propafenone, flecainide) either do not significantly affect DFT or may minimally increase DFT.[62] Sotalol may decrease DFT.[62] Based on animal studies, lidocaine may increase DFT in a dose-dependent manner.[62]

PACEMAKER AND ICD INTERACTIONS

Interactions between bradycardia pacemakers and ICDs were discovered during early concomitant use of both devices.[112–114] These interactions can lead to both inappropriate shocks and inappropriate nondetection of lethal ventricular tachyarrhythmias.

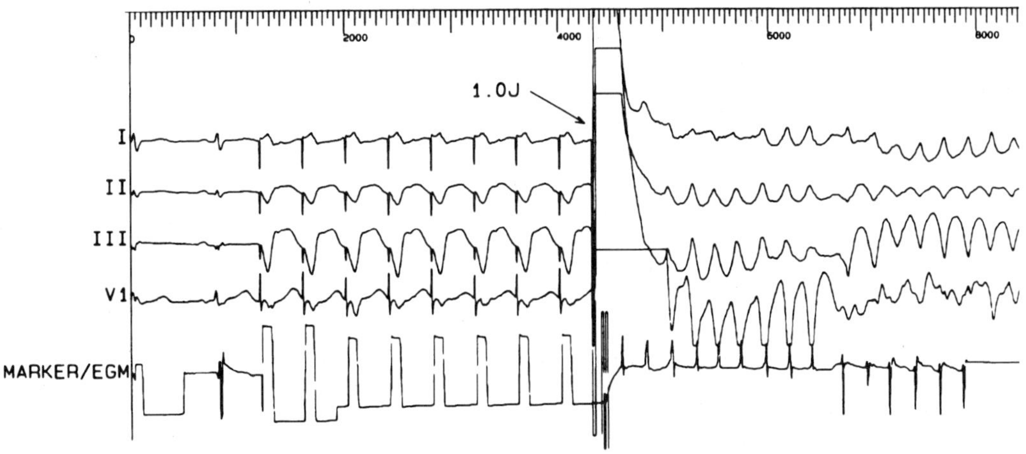

Figure 21–14. After delivering a drive train of eight stimuli at a cycle length of 400 msec, a 1-joule shock is delivered into the T wave, causing ventricular fibrillation. *Abbreviation:* EGM, electrogram.

The use of unipolar pacing is probably contraindicated in patients with ICDs. The unipolar pacemaker stimulus is more likely to be detected and sensed as a ventricular event than a bipolar stimulus. This can lead to double counting of a paced complex. In such a case, a paced rhythm greater than 50% of the tachycardia rate detection interval would be detected as VT.

Similarly, detection of a pacemaker stimulus may lead to ICD inhibition during VF. If VF fails to inhibit the pacemaker, the pacemaker output (for presumed asystole) may potentially inhibit the ICD. This problem is lessened with the use of a bipolar rather than a unipolar pacemaker. Nevertheless, any patient with an ICD and a pacemaker should have the ICD sensing checked during an episode of VF with the pacemaker programmed at maximal pacing output in the asynchronous mode. Care must be taken to place the ICD sensing electrodes far from the pacemaker electrodes (see Fig. 21–4).

A defibrillator discharge can alter pacemaker function. There can be a transient failure of the pacemaker to sense or capture after a defibrillator discharge. The ICD discharge can also reprogram a pacemaker to nominal settings, which can include changing polarity to unipolar. It therefore is recommended that committed bipolar pacemakers be used with ICDs.

MEDICOLEGAL ISSUES

Driving

There are no data as to the liability and risks involved in permitting patients with ICDs to drive private vehicles.[115, 116] Laws vary among states in the United States. Recommendations vary from allowing patients to drive after discharge from the hospital to restricting them from driving for life. A policy conference on driving in patients with arrhythmias took place in May 1994, and recommendations will probably be published by 1996. It appears that early after implantation patients are at increased risk for syncope, ICD discharge, or other arrhythmic events that may impair the ability to operate a motor vehicle.[115, 116] It is our policy to restrict patients from driving for as long as 6 months following ICD placement. At that time, the restriction is reevaluated, depending on the frequency and results of any ICD discharges and whether any instances of syncope have occurred.

Use of Nonapproved Device Combinations

Caution must be used when hybrid ICD systems (i.e., leads from one ICD company and a generator from another ICD company) are used, because a particular defibrillator's sensing circuits are designed for a particular lead and involve factors such as integrated bipolar versus true bipolar and spacing between the bipoles. It is possible that any hybrid system could lead to errors in sensing, as has been shown with approved systems.[89] Controversy surrounding the use of such systems has been noted, and there are no easy solutions to this problem.[117, 118] We recommend that clinicians generally follow guidelines established by the manufacturers of these products and by the U.S. Food and Drug Administration to insure that patients receive ICD systems that have been tested and have an adequate safety record. However, individual patient needs may necessitate the use of hybrid systems.

Acknowledgments

This chapter was sponsored in part by the Herman C. Krannert Fund; by grants HL-42370 and HL-07182 from the National Heart, Lung and Blood Institute of the National Institutes of Health, U.S. Public Health Service; and by the American Heart Association, Indiana Affiliate, Inc.

REFERENCES

1. Connolly SJ, Gent M, Roberts, et al (CIDS Co-Investigators): Canadian Implantable Defibrillator Study (CIDS). Study design and organization. Am J Cardiol 1993; 72:103F–108F.
2. Siebels J, Cappato R, Ruppel R, et al: Preliminary results of the Cardiac Arrest Study Hamburg (CASH). Am J Cardiol 1993; 72:108F–113F.
3. Epstein A: AVID necessity. PACE Pacing Clin Electrophysiol 1993; 16:1773–1775.
4. Sweeney MO, Ruskin JN: Mortality benefits and the implantable cardioverter-defibrillator. Circulation 1994; 89:1851–1858.
5. Winkle RA, Mead RH, Ruder MA, et al: Long-term outcome with the automatic implantable cardioverter-defibrillator. J Am Coll Cardiol 1989; 13:1353–1361.
6. Fogoros RN, Elson JJ, Bonnet CA, et al: Long-term outcome of survivors of cardiac arrest whose therapy is guided by electrophysiologic testing. J Am Coll Cardiol 1992; 19:780–788.
7. Powell AC, Fuchs T, Finkelstein DM, et al: Influence of implantable cardioverter-defibrillators on the long-term prognosis of survivors of out-of-hospital cardiac arrest. Circulation 1993; 88:1083–1092.
8. Block M, Breithardt G: Long term follow-up and clinical results of implantable cardioverter-defibrillators. *In* Zipes DP, Jalife J (eds): Cardiac Electrophysiology: From Cell to Bedside, 2nd ed, pp 1412–1425. Philadelphia: WB Saunders, 1995.
9. Crandall BG, Morris CD, Cutler JE, et al: Implantable cardioverter-defibrillator therapy in survivors of out-of-hospital sudden cardiac death without inducible arrhythmias. J Am Coll Cardiol 1993; 21:1186–1192.
10. Bocker K, Block M, Isbruch F, et al: Do patients with an implantable defibrillator live longer? J Am Coll Cardiol 1993; 21:1638–1644.

11. Mehta D, Saksena S, Krol RB: Survival of implantable cardioverter-defibrillator recipients: role of left ventricular function and its relationship to device use. Am Heart J 1992; 124:1608–1614.
12. Levine JH, Mellits D, Baumgardner RA, et al: Predictors of first discharge and subsequent survival in patients with automatic implantable cardioverter-defibrillators. Circulation 1991; 84:558-566.
13. Swedlow CD, Ahern T, Chen PS, et al: Underdetection of ventricular tachycardia by algorithms to enhance specificity in a tiered-therapy cardioverter-defibrillator. J Am Coll Cardiol 1994; 24:416-424.
14. Mirowski M, Mower MM, Gott VL, et al: Feasibility and effectiveness of low-energy catheter defibrillation in man. Circulation 1973; 48:79–85.
15. Lown B, Axelrod P: Editorial: implanted standby defibrillators. Circulation 1972; 46:637–639.
16. Mirowski M, Reid PR, Mower M, et al: Termination of malignant ventricular arrhythmias with an implanted automatic defibrillator in human beings. N Engl J Med 1980; 303:322–324.
17. Zipes DP, Heger JJ, Miles WM, et al: Early experience with an implantable cardioverter. N Engl J Med 1984; 311:485–490.
18. Dreifus LS, Fisch C, Griffin JC, et al: Guidelines for implantation of cardiac pacemakers and antiarrhythmia devices. J Am Coll Cardiol 1991; 18:1–13.
19. Lehmann MH, Saksena S: NASPE policy statement: implantable cardioverter defibrillators in cardiovascular practice. Report of the policy conference of the North American Society of Pacing and Electrophysiology. PACE Pacing Clin Electrophysiol 1991; 14:969–979.
20. Stevenson WG, Stevenson LW, Middlekauf HR, et al: Sudden death prevention in patients with advanced ventricular dysfunction. Circulation 1993; 88:2953–2961.
21. Wilbur D, Garan H, Finkelstein D, et al: Out-of-hospital cardiac arrest: use of electrophysiologic testing in the prediction of long-term outcome. N Engl J Med 1988; 318:19–24.
22. Weinberg BA, Miles WM, Klein LS, et al: Five-year follow-up of 589 patients treated with amiodarone. Am Heart J 1993; 125:109–120.
23. Sager PT, Choudhary R, Leon C, et al: The long-term prognosis of patients with out-of-hospital cardiac arrest but no inducible ventricular tachycardia. Am Heart J 1990; 120:1334–1342.
24. Poole JE, Mathisen TL, Kudenchuk PJ, et al: Long-term outcome in patients who survive out of hospital ventricular fibrillation and undergo electrophysiologic studies: evaluation by electrophysiologic subgroups. J Am Coll Cardiol 1990; 16:657–665.
25. Trappe HJ, Brugada P, Talajic M, et al: Prognosis of patients with ventricular tachycardia and ventricular fibrillation: role of the underlying etiology. J Am Coll Cardiol 1988; 12:166–174.
26. Wilbur DJ, Kopp D, Olshansky B, et al: Nonsustained ventricular tachycardia and other high risk predictors following myocardial infarction: implications for prophylactic AICD use. Prog Cardiovasc Dis 1993; 35:179–194.
27. Newman D, Sauve MJ, Herre J, et al: Survival after implantation of the cardioverter defibrillator. Am J Cardiol 1992; 69:899–903.
28. Forgoros RN, Elson JJ, Bonnet CA, et al: Efficacy of the implantable cardioverter defibrillator in prolonging survival in patients with severe underlying cardiac disease. J Am Coll Cardiol 1990; 16:381–386.
29. Mosteller RD, Lehman MH, Thomas AC, et al: Operative mortality with implantation of the automatic cardioverter-defibrillator. Am J Cardiol 1991; 68:1340–1345.
30. Gross JN, Song SL, Buckingham T, Furman S, Bilitch Registry Group. Influence of clinical characteristics and shock occurrence on ICD patient outcome: a multicenter report. PACE Pacing Clin Electrophysiol 1991; 14:1881–1886.
31. Kim SG, Maloney JD, Pinski SL, et al: Influence of left ventricular function on survival and mode of death after implantable defibrillator therapy (Cleveland Clinic Foundation and Montefiore Medical Center Experience). Am J Cardiol 1993; 72:1263–1267.
32. Kim SG, Fisher JD, Choue CW, et al: Influence of left ventricular function on outcome of patients treated with implantable defibrillators. Circulation 1992; 85:1304–1310.
33. Edel TB, Maloney JD, Moore SL, et al: Analysis of deaths in patients with an implantable cardioverter defibrillator. PACE Pacing Clin Electrophysiol 1992; 15:60–70.
34. Zipes, DP. Implantable cardioverter-defibrillator. Lifesaver or a device looking for a disease? Circulation 1994; 89:2943–2946.
35. Grimm W, Flores BF, Marchlinski FE: Symptoms and electrocardiographically documented rhythm preceding spontaneous shocks in patients with implantable cardioverter-defibrillator. Am J Cardiol 1993; 71:1415–1418.
36. Lessmeier TJ, Lehmann MH, Steinman RT, et al: Outcome with implantable cardioverter-defibrillator therapy for survivors of ventricular fibrillation secondary to idiopathic dilated cardiomyopathy or coronary artery disease without myocardial infarction. Am J Cardiol 1993; 72:911–915.
37. Lessmeier TJ, Lehmann MH, Steinman RT, et al: Implantable cardioverter-defibrillator therapy in 300 patients with coronary artery disease presenting exclusively with ventricular fibrillation. Am Heart J 1994; 128:211–218.
38. Myerburg RJ, Kessler KM, Estes D, et al: Long-term survival after prehospital cardiac arrest: analysis of outcome during an 8 year study. Circulation 1984; 70:538–546.
39. Meissner MD, Lehmann MH, Steinman RT, et al: Ventricular fibrillation in patients without significant structural heart disease: a multicenter experience with implantable cardioverter-defibrillator therapy. J Am Coll Cardiol 1993; 21:1406–1412.
40. Breithardt G, Wichter T, Haverkamp W, et al: Implantable cardioverter defibrillator therapy in patients with arrhythmogenic right ventricular cardiomyopathy, long QT syndrome, or no structural heart disease. Am Heart J 1994:127:1151–1158.
41. Wever EFD, Hauer RNW, Oomen A, et al: Unfavorable outcome in patients with primary electrical disease who survived an episode of ventricular fibrillation. Circulation 1993; 88:1021–1029.
42. Schwartz PJ, Locati EH, Moss AJ, et al: Left cardiac sympathetic denervation in the therapy of congenital long QT syndrome: a worldwide report. Circulation 1991; 84:503–511.
43. Schwartz PJ, Locati EH, Napolitano C, et al: The long QT syndrome. *In* Zipes DP, Jalife J (eds): Cardiac Electrophysiology: From Cell to Bedside, 2nd ed, pp 788–811. Philadelphia: WB Saunders, 1995.
44. Silka MJ, Kron J, Dunnigan A, et al: Sudden cardiac death and the use of implantable cardioverter-defibrillators in pediatric patients. Circulation 1993; 87:800–807.
45. Klein H, Trappe HJ, Fieguth G, et al: Prospective studies evaluating prophylactic ICD therapy for high risk patients with coronary artery disease. PACE Pacing Clin Electrophysiol 1993; 16:564–570.
46. Kuck KH: Value of prophylactic implantable cardioverter defibrillator therapy. PACE Pacing Clin Electrophysiol 1994; 17:514–516.
47. Kolettis TM, Saksena S: Prophylactic implantable cardioverter defibrillator therapy in high-risk patients with coronary artery disease. Am Heart J 1994; 127:1164–1170.
48. Brugada P, Andries E: The rationale for prophylactic implantation of a defibrillator in "high risk" patients. PACE Pacing Clin Electrophysiol 1993; 16:547–551.
49. Brachmann J, Freigang K, Sagau W: Coronary artery bypass graft patch trial. PACE Pacing Clin Electrophysiol 1993; 16:571–575.
50. MADIT Executive Committee. Multicenter Automatic Defibrillator Implantation Trial (MADIT): design and clinical protocol. PACE Pacing Clin Electrophysiol 1991; 14:920–927.
51. Manolis AS, Rastegar H, Wang PJ, et al: Fully transvenous cardioverter defibrillators: rare need for subcutaneous patch with two newer-generation systems. Am Heart J 1994; 128:808–815.
52. Brooks R, Garan H, Torchiana D, et al: Three-year outcome of a nonthoracotomy approach to cardoverter-defibrillator implantation in 189 consecutive patients. Am J Cardiol 1994; 74:1011–1015.
53. Kleman JM, Castle LW, Kidwell GA, et al: Nonthoracotomy- versus thoracotomy-implantable defibrillators. Intention-to-treat comparison of clinical outcomes. Circulation 1994; 90:2833–2842.
54. Pfeiffer D, Jung W, Fehske W, et al: Complications of pacemaker-defibrillator devices: diagnosis and management. Am Heart J 1994; 127:1073–1080.
55. Almassi GH, Olinger GN, Wetherbee JN, et al: Long-term complications of implantable cardioverter defibrillator lead systems. Ann Thorac Surg 1993; 55:888–892.
56. Grimm W, Flores BF, Marchlinski FE: Complications of implantable cardioverter defibrillator therapy: follow-up of 241 patients. PACE Pacing Clin Electrophysiol 1993; 16:218–222.
57. Bakker PFA, Hauer RNW, Wever EFD: Infections involving implanted cardioverter defibrillator devices. PACE Pacing Clin Electrophysiol 1992:15; 654–658.
58. Taylor RL, Cohen DJ, Widman LE, et al: Infection of an implantable cardioverter-defibrillator: management without removal of the device in selected cases. PACE Pacing Clin Electrophysiol 1990; 13:1352–1355.
59. Bardy GH, Hofer B, Johnson G, et al: Implantable transvenous cardioverter-defibrillators. Circulation 1993; 87:1152–1168.
60. Yee R, Klein GJ, Thakur RK: Clinical predictors of successful im-

plantable cardioverter defibrillator implantation. Am Heart J 1994; 127:1068–1072.
61. Venditti FJ, Martin DT, Vassolas G, et al: Rise in chronic defibrillation thresholds in nonthoracotomy implantable defibrillator. Circulation 1994; 89:216–223.
62. Manz M, Jung W, Luderitz B: Interactions between drugs and devices: experimental and clinical studies. Am Heart J 1994; 127:978–984.
63. Avitall B, Port S, Gal R, et al: Automatic implantable cardioverter/defibrillator discharges and acute myocardial injury. Circulation 1990; 81:1482–1487.
64. Ito M, Pride H, Zipes DP: Defibrillating shocks delivered to the heart impair efferent sympathetic responsivenss. Circulation 1993; 88:2661–2673.
65. Singer I, van der Laken J, Edmonds HL, et al: Is defibrillation testing safe? PACE Pacing Clin Electrophysiol 1991; 14:1899–1904.
66. Brooks R, Torchiana D, Vlahakes GJ, et al: Successful implantation of cardioverter-defibrillator systems in patients with elevated defibrillation thresholds. J Am Coll Cardiol 1993; 22:569–574.
67. Bardy GH, Stewart RB, Ivey TD, et al: Intraoperative comparison of sequential-pulse and single-pulse defibrillation in candidates for automatic implantable defibrillators. Am J Cardiol 1987; 60:618–624.
68. Jones DL, Klein GJ, Guiraudon GM, et al: Sequential pulse defibrillation in humans: orthogonal sequential pulse defibrillation with epicardial electrodes. J Am Coll Cardiol 1988; 11:590–596.
69. Bardy GH, Ivey TD, Allen MD, et al: Prospective comparison of sequential pulse and single pulse defibrillation with use of two different clinically available systems. J Am Coll Cardiol 1989; 14:165–171.
70. Saksena S, An H, Mehra R, et al: Prospective comparison of biphasic and monophasic shocks for implantable cardioverter-defibrillators using endocardial leads. Am J Cardiol 1992; 70:304–310.
71. Strickberger SA, Hummel JD, Horwood LE, et al: Effect of shock polarity on ventricular defibrillation threshold using a transvenous lead system. J Am Coll Cardiol 1994; 24:1069–1072.
72. Wyse DG, Kavanagh KM, Gillis AM, et al: Comparison of biphasic and monophasic shocks for defibrillation using a nonthoracotomy system. Am J Cardiol 1993; 71:197–202.
73. Winkle RA, Mead RH, Ruder MA, et al: Improved low energy defibrillation efficacy in man with the use of a biphasic truncated exponential waveform. Am Heart J 1989; 117:122–127.
74. Bardy GH, Ivey TD, Allen MD, et al: A prospective randomized evaluation of biphasic versus monophasic waveform pulses on defibrillation efficacy in humans. J Am Coll Cardiol 1989; 14:728–733.
75. Bardy GH, Troutman C, Johnson G, et al: Electrode system influence on biphasic waveform defibrillation efficacy in humans. Circulation 1991; 84:665–671.
76. Jung W, Manz M, Moosdorf R, et al: Clinical efficacy of shock waveforms and lead configurations for defibrillation. Am Heart J 1994; 127:985–993.
77. Marks ML, Johnson G, Hofer BO, et al: Biphasic waveform defibrillation using a three-electrode transvenous lead system in humans. J Cardiovasc Electrophysiol 1994; 5:103–108.
78. Neuzner J, Pitschner HF, Huth C, et al: Effect of biphasic waveform pulse on endocardial defibrillation efficacy in humans. PACE Pacing Clin Electrophysiol 1994; 17:207–212.
79. Natale A, Sra J, Axtell K, et al: Preliminary experience with a hybrid nonthoracotomy defibrillating system that includes a biphasic device: comparison with a standard monophasic device using the same lead system. J Am Coll Cardiol 1994; 24:406–412.
80. Bardy GH, Johnson G, Poole JE, et al: A simplified, single-lead unipolar transvenous cardioversion-defibrillation system. Circulation 1993; 88:543–547.
81. Bardy GH, Dolack L, Kudenchuck PJ, et al: Prospective, randomized comparison in humans of a unipolar defibrillation system with that using an additional superior vena cava electrode. Circulation 1994; 89:1090–1093.
82. Sperry RE, Ellenbogen KA, Wood MA, et al: Failure of a second and third generation implantable cardioverter defibrillator to sense ventricular tachycardia: implications for fixed-gain sensing devices. PACE Pacing Clin Electrophysiol 1992; 15:749–755.
83. Jones GK, Bardy GH: Considerations for ventricular fibrillation detection by implantable cardioverter defibrillators. Am Heart J 1994; 127:1107–1110.
84. PCD Epicardial System. Summary of Clinical Experience 1993. Minneapolis: Medtronic, Inc.
85. Grimm W, Flores BF, Marchlinski FE: Electrocardiographically documented unnecessary, spontaneous shocks in 241 patients with implantable cardioverter defibrillators. PACE Pacing Clin Electrophysiol 1992; 15:1667–1673.
86. Swerdlow CD, Chen PS, Kass RM, et al: Discrimination of ventricular tachycardia from sinus tachycardia and atrial fibrillation in a tiered therapy cardioverter-defibrillator. J Am Coll Cardiol 1994; 23:1342–1355.
87. Schmitt C, Montero M, Melichercik J: Significance of supraventricular tachyarrhythmias in patients with implanted pacing cardioverter defibrillators. PACE Pacing Clin Electrophysiol 1994; 17:295–302.
88. Fain ES, Winkle RA: Implantable cardioverter defibrillator: ventritex cadence. J Cardiovasc Electrophsiol 1993; 4:211–223.
89. Callans DJ, Hook BG, Kleiman RB, et al: Unique sensing errors in third-generation implantable cardioverter-defibrillators. J Am Coll Cardiol 1993; 22:1135–1140.
90. Kelly PA, Mann DE, Damle RS, et al: Oversensing during ventricular pacing in patients with a third-generation implantable cardioverter-defibrillator. J Am Coll Cardiol 1994; 23:1531–1534.
91. Jung W, Manz M, Moosdorf R, et al: Failure of an implantable cardioverter-defibrillator to redetect ventricular fibrillation in patients with a nonthoracotomy lead system. Circulation 1992; 86:1217–1222.
92. Bardy GH, Poole JE, Kudenchuk PJ, et al: A prospective randomized repeat-crossover comparison of antitachycardia pacing with low-energy cardioversion. Circulation 1993; 87:1889–1896.
93. Estes NAM, Haugh CJ, Wang PJ, et al: Antitachycardia pacing and low-energy cardioversion for ventricular tachycardia termination: a clinical perspective. Am Heart J 1994; 127:1038–1046.
94. Trappe HJ, Klein H, Kielblock B: Role of antitachycardia pacing in patients with third generation cardioverter defibrillators. PACE Pacing Clin Electrophysiol 1994; 17:506–513.
95. Gillis AM, Leitch JW, Sheldon RS, et al: A prospective randomized comparison of autodecremental pacing to burst pacing in device therapy for chronic ventricular tachycardia secondary to coronary artery disease. Am J Cardiol 1993; 72:1146–1151.
96. Cook JR, Kirchhoffer JB, Fitzgerald TF, et al: Comparison of decremental and burst overdrive pacing as treatment for ventricular tachycardia associated with coronary artery disease. Am J Cardiol 1992; 70:311–315.
97. Porterfield JG, Porterfield LM, Smith BA, et al: Conversion rates of induced versus spontaneous ventricular tachycardia by a third generation cardioverter defibrillator. PACE Pacing Clin Electrophysiol 1993; 16:170–173.
98. Newman D, Dorian P, Hardy J: Randomized controlled comparison of antitachycardia pacing algorithms for termination of ventricular tachycardia. J Am Coll Cardiol 1993; 21:1413–1418.
99. Bardy GH, Troutman C, Poole JE, et al: Clinical experience with a tiered-therapy, multiprogrammable antiarrhythmia device. Circulation 1992; 85:1689–1698.
100. Wietholt D, Block M, Isbruch F, et al: Clinical experience with antitachycadia pacing and improved detection algorithms in a new implantable cardioverter-defibrillator. J Am Coll Cardiol 1993; 21:885–894.
101. Schmidinger H, Sowton E: Physiological variation in the termination window of re-entry tachycardia studied by non-invasive programmed stimulation. Eur Heart J 1988; 9:997–1002.
102. Zipes DP, Jackman WM, Heger JJ: Clinical transvenous cardioversion of recurrent life-threatening ventricular tachyarrhythmias: low energy synchronized cardioversion of ventricular tachycardia and termination of ventricular fibrillation in patients using a catheter electrode. Am Heart J 1982; 103:789–794.
103. Yee R, Zipes DP, Gulamhusein S, et al: Low energy countershock using an intravascular catheter in an acute cardiac care setting. Am J Cardiol 1982; 50:1124–1129.
104. Waspe LE, Kim S, Matos JA: Role of a catheter lead system for transvenous countershock and pacing during electrophysiologic tests: an assessment of the usefulness of catheter shocks for terminating ventricular tachyarrhythmias. Am J Cardiol 1983; 52:477–484.
105. Saksena S, Chandran P, Shah Y, et al: Comparative efficacy of transvenous cardioversion and pacing in patients with sustained ventricular tachycardia: a prospective, randomized, crossover study. Circulation 1985; 72:153–160.
106. Hook BG, Callans DJ, Kleiman RB, et al: Implantable cardioverter-defibrillator therapy in the absence of significant symptoms. Circulation 1993; 87:1897–1906.
107. Hurwitz JL, Hook BG, Flores BT, Marchlinski FE: Importance of abortive shock capability with electrogram storage in cardioverter-defibrillator devices. J Am Coll Cardiol 1993; 21:895–900.
108. Kou WH, Kirsh MM, Boling SF, et al: Effect of antiarrhythmic drug

therapy on the incidence of shocks in patients who receive an implantable cardioverter-defibrillator after a single episode of ventricular tachycardia/fibrillation. PACE Pacing Clin Electrophysiol 1991; 14:1586–1592.
109. Dolack GL for the CASCADE Investigators: Clinical predictors of implantable cardioverter-defibrillator shocks (results of the CASCADE trial). Am J Cardiol 1994; 73:237–241.
110. Guarneiri T, Levine JH, Veltri EP, et al: Success of chronic defibrillation and the role of antiarrhythmic drugs with the automatic implantable cardioverter/defibrillator. Am J Cardiol 1987; 60:1061–1064.
111. Jung W, Manz M, Pizzulli L, et al: Effects of chronic amiodarone therapy on defibrillation threshold. Am J Cardiol 1992; 70:1023–1027.
112. Cohen AI, Wish MH, Fletcher RD, et al: The use and interaction of permanent pacemakers and the Automatic Implantable Cardioverter Defibrillator. PACE Pacing Clin Electrophysiol 1988; 11:704–711.
113. Epstein AE, Kay GN, Plumb VJ, et al: Combined automatic implantable cardioverter-defibrillator and pacemaker systems: implantation techniques and follow-up. J Am Coll Cardiol 1989; 13:121–131.
114. Furman S, Hayes DL, Holmes DR: A Practice of Cardiac Pacing, 3rd ed, pp 503–506. Mount Kisco, NY: Futura Publishing, 1993.
115. Larsen GC, Stupey MR, Walance CG, et al: Recurrent cardiac events in survivors of ventricular fibrillation or tachycardia. Implications for driving restrictions. JAMA 1994; 271:1335–1339.
116. Anderson MH, Camm AJ: Legal and ethical aspects of driving and working in patients with an implantable cardioverter defibrillator. Am Heart J 1994; 127:1185–1193.
117. Maloney JD, Khoury DS, Zhu W, et al: The art and science of mixing and matching. J Am Coll Cardiol 1994; 24:414–415.
118. Jones JD, Calahan TJ, Alpert S, et al: A Food and Drug Administration request for cooperation. J Am Coll Cardiol 1994; 24:413.

22 Treatment of Neurally Mediated Syncopal Syndromes

David G. Benditt, MD
Keith G. Lurie, MD

The neurally mediated syncopal syndromes constitute a group of conditions of which carotid sinus syndrome and the vasovagal faint are the best known (Table 22–1).[1–4] In general, the various neurally mediated syncopal syndromes are characterized by transient disturbances of reflex cardiovascular control, which usually lead to both inappropriate bradycardia and vasodilatation. Ultimately, if the bradycardia and vasodilatation are sufficiently severe, systemic hypotension with dizziness and syncope may occur.[1, 2] In addition, a number of concomitant symptoms (e.g., nausea, diaphoresis, loss of peripheral vision, and diminished hearing) are commonly associated with neurally mediated syncopal spells and often serve as warnings of an impending episode. Physical injury may occur if these warning symptoms either are not present (a relatively common circumstance in older persons) or are unheeded. Finally, it has been suggested that death may be an outcome in rare instances.[5]

In general, the principal factors differentiating the various forms of neurally mediated syncope are the specific initiating events. Thus, afferent neural signals triggering the episode may arise from within the central nervous system (e.g., syncope associated with fear, anxiety, unpleasant experiences) or from any of a variety of peripheral sites (receptors) subjected to mechanical stimuli (e.g., carotid sinus stimulation, cough, micturition), chemical stimuli, or pain. In the case of vasovagal syncope, the mechanisms remain poorly understood, but it seems that the initiating afferent neural signals may originate from any of several sites, including the cerebral cortex, as well as mechanically and chemically sensitive receptors within several organ systems (e.g., the ventricular myocardium, great vessels, gastrointestinal tract, bladder).

TABLE 22–1. NEURALLY MEDIATED SYNCOPAL SYNDROMES

Emotional syncope (common or "vasovagal" faint)
Carotid sinus syncope
Post-micturition syncope
Exercise-associated variant
Gastrointestinal stimulation
  swallow syncope, defecation syncope
Cough syncope
Sneeze syncope
Syncope associated with glossopharyngeal neuralgia
Airway stimulation
Raised intrathoracic pressure
  trumpet-playing, weight-lifting

Under normal circumstances, physiologic responses to "trigger" signals such as those just described initiate effective cardiovascular adaptation to the imposed stress. Thus, appropriate tachycardia and redistribution of blood flow to skeletal muscle beds are anticipated outcomes. However, when the efferent response is inappropriate (i.e., slowing of heart rate and peripheral vasodilatation), the ability of the cardiovascular system to maintain adequate cerebral blood flow is compromised, and loss of consciousness may occur. In some persons, the hypotension appears to be principally the result of bradycardia (asystole or, on occasion, paroxysmal atrioventricular [AV] block). These are termed predominantly *cardioinhibitory* in nature. In other persons, although much less frequently, hypotension is almost exclusively caused by vasodilatation, but heart rate appears to be normal (in fact, even in these cases the rate is usually inappropriately slow in view of the hypotension: i.e., "relative" bradycardia). These latter instances are termed primarily *vasodepressor.* Most cases manifest both cardioinhibitory and vasodepressor responses (i.e., they are a *mixed* form); the magnitude of the cardioinhibitory and vasodepressor responses usually differs among patients and possibly even within a given patient at various times.[1–3, 6, 7]

PRINCIPLES OF TREATMENT

Most cases of neurally mediated syncope are isolated events. Consequently, except for certain persons considered to be at high risk because of their occupations (e.g., commercial truck drivers, airplane pilots, sign painters, professional athletes), because of frailty (elderly persons prone to serious injury), or because they have already exhibited a dramatic presentation (e.g., worrisome physical injury, motor vehicle accident), little thought is usually given to long-term prophylactic treatment after a single syncopal event. Furthermore, in many other patients, syncopal episodes appear to cluster within a relatively brief period of time and seem to be causally related to unique, nonrecurring events (e.g., emotional upset occasioned by relationship difficulties, loss of a job, death in the family, altered health state as a result of concurrent illness). In such situations, attempts at chronic prophylaxis similarly do not appear to be warranted. However, a certain subset of patients appears to be particularly susceptible to recurring syncopal episodes over an extended period of time. Thus, although neurally mediated syncope may be expected to recur at least once in approximately 30% of patients over a several-year period after the first syncopal episode,[8–10] the apparently highly susceptible patient has multiple episodes over many years. These patients, along with the so-called high-risk patients described earlier, are the ones in whom attempts to achieve effective prophylaxis become an important concern (Figure 22–1).

The efficacy of current treatment strategies for most forms of neurally mediated syncope remains unproven. Nonetheless, certain principles of prophylaxis warrant attention (Figure 22–2). First, when appropriate, attention should be directed toward behavioral and situational modification, such as avoidance of emotional upset or uncomfortable environments or modification of individual responses to imposed stresses in patients particularly susceptible to vasovagal syncope. Second, medical treatment of associated conditions that may trigger syncopal episodes should be considered. For example, ameliorating pulmonary disease in patients with cough-induced syncope, ameliorating esophageal abnormalities in patients experiencing swallow-induced syncope, and warning of the potential relationship of alcohol intake to recurrences in persons with recurrent postmicturition syncope are desirable even if not easily accomplished.[1–2, 11–13] Similarly, in certain patients with carotid sinus syndrome, pathologic changes in the neck, such as tumors or the consequences of previous therapeutic irradiation, may necessitate surgical intervention in order to reduce recurrence risk. Third, attempts may be made to reduce individual susceptibility to neurally mediated fainting episodes by modifying responses within the neural reflex itself. Currently, these efforts focus on pharmacologic interventions, and although overall efficacy remains controversial, there is reason to believe that progress is being made. Finally, in certain settings it may be necessary to try to override the effects of the neural reflex. The best example is the use of cardiac pacemakers in selected cases (particularly carotid sinus–induced syncope) to prevent bradycardia. However, administration of vasoconstrictors to block vasodilatation also belongs to this category.

EVALUATION OF TREATMENT EFFICACY

The evaluation of candidate therapies for neurally mediated syncopal syndromes is not straightforward, particularly in vasovagal syncope. First, it is probably unrealistic to expect any treatment to be entirely effective. Therefore syncope recurrence alone is an inadequate endpoint. Techniques comparable with those proposed for evaluation of drug treatment in supraventricular tachycardias should be considered.[14–16] Thus the number of episodes and the duration of symptom-free intervals should be reported. Second, the effectiveness of a treatment measured solely from the results of follow-up tilt-table testing is similarly inadequate. In this regard, despite the fact that the conversion of a positive tilt to a negative tilt has been thought to indicate an effective treatment, the accuracy of such testing for predicting treatment benefit (or inadequacy) is unknown. Finally, placebo-controlled trials of relatively long duration are essential in view of the sporadic nature of syncopal episodes and the potentially powerful placebo effect of any proposed treatment.

PHARMACOLOGIC TREATMENT

Of the various neurally mediated syncopal syndromes, only in vasovagal syncope (as modeled by tilt-table testing) has there been a serious interest in developing pharmacologic interventions. Beta-adrenergic blocking drugs,[3, 6, 17–24] disopyramide,[3, 6, 18, 19, 22, 24, 25] and certain vasoconstrictor agents,[26, 27] have been the subject of the most intense study. Other options, such as serotonin reuptake blockers,[28, 29] are at an earlier stage of evaluation, and still others, such as theophylline and belladonna alkaloids (e.g., scopolamine),[30, 31] are currently of less interest. Finally, the role of volume expanders (e.g., fludrocortisone, salt tablets) has tended to diminish, but they are still used as adjuvants to other drugs.[32–34]

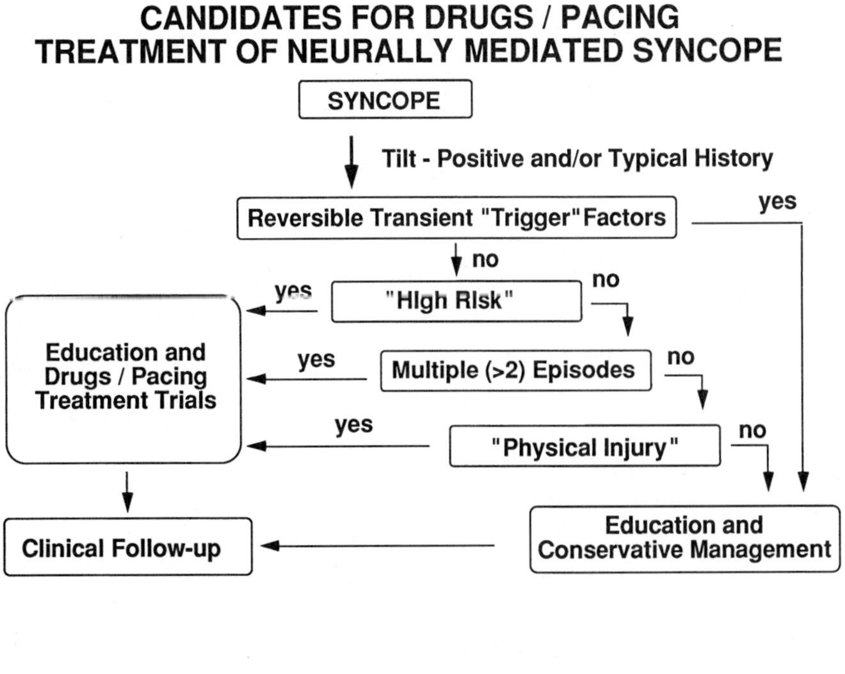

Figure 22–1. Schema depicting a decision process for determining which patients warrant initiation of treatment designed to prevent recurrences of neurally mediated syncope. "High risk" refers to occupation or avocation as described in the text. "Physical injury" also incorporates the concept of vehicular accidents even if actual injury did not occur.

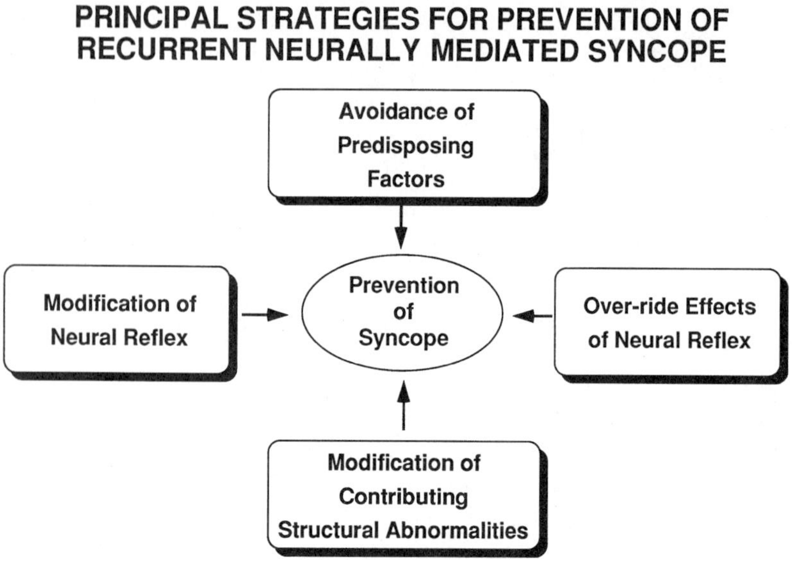

Figure 22–2. Diagram summarizing the principal current treatment strategies available for patients with recurrent neurally mediated syncope. It may be necessary to employ several strategies simultaneously in order to achieve adequate control.

In an attempt to assess the status of current pharmacologic approaches to prophylaxis (Fig. 22–3), this review focuses primarily on those studies in which treatment for vasovagal syncope was selected on the basis of tilt-table testing studies, but subsequent effectiveness was determined by clinical response during follow-up (usually categorized solely by syncope recurrence). A total of 11 reports encompassing findings in 169 patients observed for 18 ± 4.6 months were identified. In view of all therapeutic options chosen by the individual investigators, 152 (90%) of 169 patients remained without syncope recurrence during this period of time (Table 22–2). However, interpretation of this apparently favorable outcome must be tempered by the failure of the few available placebo-controlled studies to find benefit with current therapies.[10, 21, 27] For example, Brignole and colleagues[27] followed outcomes in 30 patients, 15 of whom were given placebo and 15 of whom were treated on the basis of outcome of tilt-table testing. During 10 ± 7 months follow-up, the number of syncope recurrences did not differ in the two experimental groups (20% of the treatment group, 27% of the placebo group).

Beta-Adrenergic Blocking Drugs

Beta-adrenergic blocking drugs were first proposed for prevention of syncope recurrences in a group of patients with tilt-table–proven vasovagal syncope in 1989.[6] Since then, these drugs have been the subject of considerable attention in this context. This popularity may be a result, in large part, of their being relatively safe and generally well tolerated over extended periods of time. However, they are also a seemingly logical choice from the perspective of the current understanding of the pathophysiologic process of vasovagal fainting. With regard to the latter, both spontaneous and induced fainting episodes in younger patients have been closely associated with very high circulating catecholamine concentrations, especially epinephrine.[35–37] These elevated catecholamine levels may act in multiple ways to increase susceptibility to fainting. First, catecholamines are believed to increase the sensitivity of the various participating peripheral receptors (including cardiac mechanoreceptors, as well as those in other organ systems) directly. Second, catecholamines enhance tissue responsiveness to the transiently increased vagal surge that is associated with these syndromes (so-called accentuated antagonism).[38] Finally, to the extent that increased myocardial contractility triggers afferent neural signals from ventricular mechanoreceptors, this too would be enhanced by catecholamines.

Of the drugs used for prevention of neurally mediated syncope, the beta-adrenergic blocking drugs are the most amenable to testing by acute intravenous administration. For example, Asso and associates[39] observed that in a cohort of 21 consecutive patients observed for at

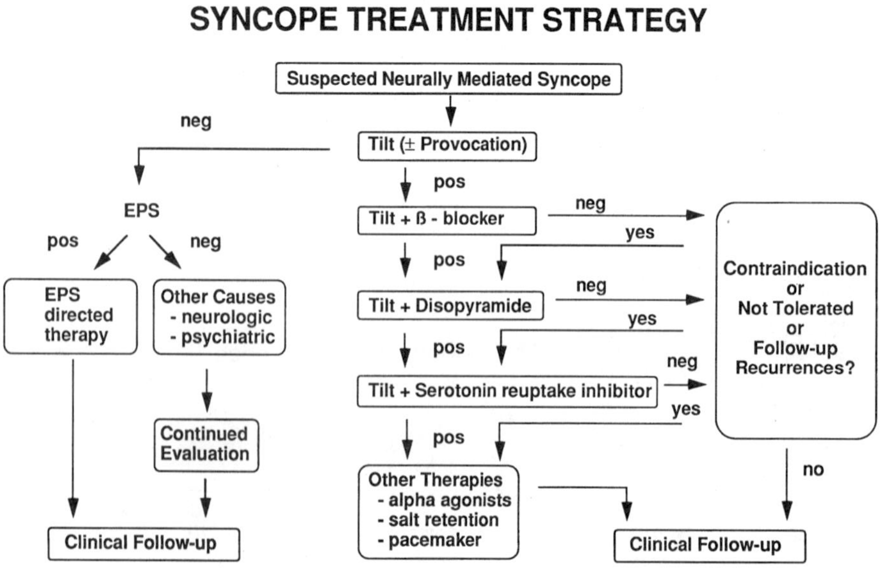

Figure 22–3. Diagram illustrating an approach to treatment selection in patients in whom it is desired to attempt prophylactic therapy for neurally mediated syncope. The efficacy of most of these treatment options remains unproven, and completion of definitive placebo-controlled trials is awaited.

TABLE 22–2. TILT-TABLE TESTING FOR PREDICTING EFFECTIVENESS OF THERAPY

Reference	Tilt-Neg on Proposed Treatment	Follow-up (months)	No Syncope During Follow-up	Therapies
Grubb et al[18]	15	16	14 (93%)	B-blk, Scop, Diso, Flcr
Sra et al[19]	34	18	32 (94%)	B-blk, Diso
Grubb et al[20]	10	21 ± 2	10 (100%)	B-blk, Scop, Diso, Pacer
Sra et al[24]	19	16	18 (94%)	B-blk, Diso, Theo
Milstein et al[25]	10	20 ± 5	9 (90%)	Diso
Raviele et al[26]	7	12 (9–16)	6 (86%)	Etileph, Scop
Brignole et al[27]	15	11 ± 7	7 (46%)	B-blk, Ergot, others
Asso et al[39]	11	13 (1–36)	9 (82%)	B-blk
Lurie et al[40]	17	19 ± 0.9	16 (94%)	B-blk
Grubb et al[77]	14	24 ± 11	14 (100%)	B-blk, Scop, Diso, B-blk + Flcr
Grubb et al[78]	17	23 ± 7	17 (100%)	Flcr, B-blk, Diso
Total	169	18 ± 4.6	152 (90%)	

Abbreviations: B-blk, beta-adrenergic blockade; Diso, disopyramide; Ergot, ergotamine; Etileph, etilephrine; Flcr, fludrocortisone; Pacer, pacemaker; Scop, scopolamine; Theo, theophylline.

least 3 years, 11 exhibited conversion of a positive tilt-table response to a negative response after careful parenteral administration of metoprolol (10 mg). During follow-up, only 1 of these 11 had a clear-cut syncopal episode. Patients who did not respond to metoprolol were treated with alternative agents; consequently, the value of a tilt test "failure" for predicting ineffectiveness of therapy could not be evaluated. Sra and colleagues[23] reported a similar experience: parenteral esmolol was evaluated after a positive tilt-table response in 27 syncope patients. Esmolol appeared to eliminate susceptibility to tilt-induced syncope in 16 of these 27. Ten of these patients had required isoproterenol infusion in order to induce syncope in the baseline state, whereas 6 had exhibited a positive tilt test result in the absence of pharmacologic provocation. In all 16 cases, subsequent oral beta-adrenergic blockade therapy was associated with apparent benefit.

Metoprolol, pindolol, and atenolol have been the most widely used beta-adrenergic blockers in published reports. Metoprolol and pindolol seem to be the currently preferred agents. Metoprolol was the first beta blocker used, on the basis of both its availability for parenteral testing in the United States and its relative cardioselectivity.[6] Cardioselectivity was thought to be important to help support the argument that cardiac receptor sites were the principal sources of afferent impulses that trigger vasovagal episodes. Pindolol has gained favor primarily because of its intrinsic sympathomimetic activity, which diminishes the severity of resting bradycardia in treated patients (Figure 22–4).[40]

Table 22–3 is a compilation of outcomes from published studies in which the apparent efficacy of beta-adrenergic blockade therapy was based on clinical outcomes during relatively long-term follow-up. Of 64 patients observed for 17 ± 4.9 months, 56 (88%) were reported to have experienced no syncope recurrence. Although not placebo controlled, these reports from a wide variety of centers suggest the potential utility of beta-blocker therapy in this setting.

Disopyramide Phosphate

Disopyramide phosphate, a class I antiarrhythmic agent with marked vagolytic properties, was first proposed for use in vasovagal syncope by the University of Minnesota group.[25] In this case it was thought that the well-known negative inotropic effect of the drug[41] (already used in hypertrophic cardiomyopathy[42]) might be helpful by reducing stretch on central cardiovascular receptors and thereby diminishing afferent neural traffic. In addition, the prominent vagolytic action of disopyramide was considered useful for maintaining heart rate and possibly alleviating many of the ancillary vagally mediated symptoms associated with vasovagal episodes (e.g., gastrointestinal distress). However, potential adverse consequences of disopyramide therapy (particularly torsades de pointes ventricular tachycardia secondary to QT interval prolongation) are a concern with this approach, particularly in patients with structural heart disease and those with prolonged QT intervals.[43] Similarly, care must be taken to avoid such treatment in patients with a predisposition to

TABLE 22–3. TILT-TABLE TESTING FOR PREDICTING EFFECTIVENESS OF THERAPY: BETA-ADRENERGIC BLOCKERS

Reference	Tilt-Neg on Proposed Treatment	Follow-up (months)	No Syncope During Follow-up	Therapies
Grubb et al[18]	9	16	8 (88%)	beta-blocker
Sra et al[24]	10	16	8 (80%)	Metoprolol
Brignole et al[27]	7	11 ± 7	5 (71%)	Atenolol
Asso et al[39]	11	13 (1–36)	9 (82%)	Metoprolol
Lurie et al[40]	17	19 ± 0.9	16 (94%)	Pindolol
Grubb et al[77]	5	24 ± 11	5 (100%)	beta-blocker
Grubb et al[78]	5	23 ± 7	5 (100%)	beta-blocker
Total	64	17 ± 4.9	56 (88%)	

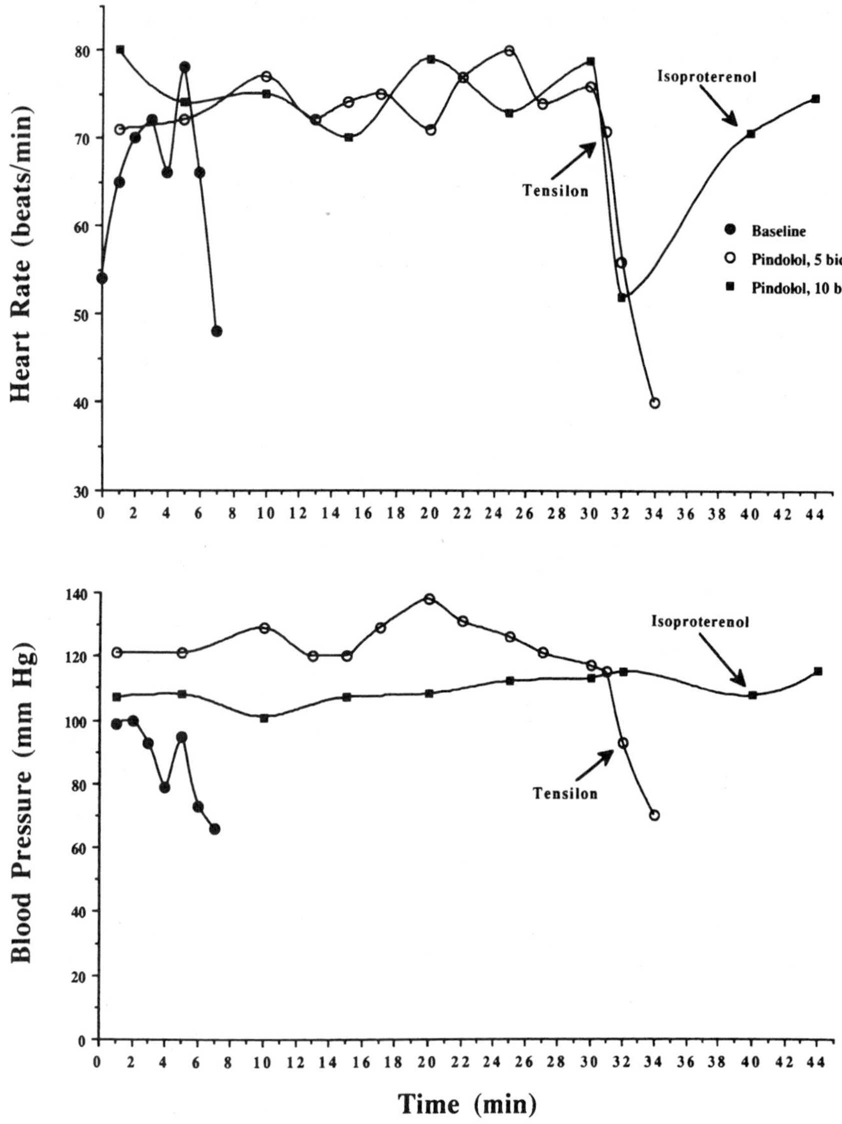

Figure 22–4. Graphs depicting heart rate *(upper panel)* and blood pressure *(lower panel)* changes (ordinate) in a patient who underwent a series of head-up tilt-table tests (test duration indicated in minutes on the abscissa). Each treatment status is depicted by a specific line. The untreated state was associated with an early and abrupt fall of heart rate and blood pressure (solid line, solid circles) accompanied by syncope. Treatment with pindolol resulted in increased tolerance to upright tilt even in the face of exposure to provocative agents such as isoproterenol and edrophonium (Tensilon).

urinary tract obstruction. Conversely, disopyramide may be better tolerated in young, active patients with fainting episodes (especially the athletically inclined) than is beta-adrenergic blockade.

The efficacy of disopyramide therapy remains uncertain and, indeed, has been brought into question as a result of observations by Morillo and associates[10] in a placebo-controlled study. In that report, among 21 patients followed for 29 ± 8 months, syncope recurrence was comparable in the disopyramide- and placebo-treated groups (27% and 30%). However, in three other noncontrolled published studies,[24, 25, 77] long-term clinical response to treatment with disopyramide phosphate seemed to be quite impressive (Table 22–4). The mean follow-up period in all four studies (including that of Morillo and associates[10]) was 21 ± 4.1 months. Of 29 patients treated with disopyramide, 25 (86%) remained free of syncope. It is clear that additional placebo-controlled experience is needed before clinicians can feel confident of the role of disopyramide in this patient population.

Serotonin Reuptake Blockers

Several lines of evidence suggest that within the central nervous system, serotonin participates in inhibiting sympathetic nervous system activity and thereby in facilitating hypotension.[29, 44] Selective serotonin reuptake blockers are believed to work reversibly in the synaptic cleft and thereby ultimately reduce serotonin effects on sympathetic neural activity. Using this insight, investigators from the Medical College of Ohio proposed the use of such agents in patients with neurally mediated syncope. An early uncontrolled report examined the effects of fluoxetine hydrochloride in 16 patients in whom conventional pharmacologic approaches (scopolamine, disopyramide, etc.) had failed.[28] Of these 16 patients, 13 (81%) tolerated long-term therapy, and 7 (44%) remained free of syncope during 19 ± 9 months' follow-up. Subsequently, the same group assessed the effects of the serotonin inhibitor sertraline hydrochloride in 17 patients.[29] Three patients (18%) were intolerant of therapy, and 5 (29%) continued to exhibit positive results on the tilt-table test. Of the remaining patients with negative tilt-table results, all were reported to have remained asymptomatic during 12 ± 5 months' follow-up.

Serotonin reuptake inhibitors also may have some applicability to forms of neurally mediated syncope other than vasovagal syncope. In carotid sinus syndrome, Grubb and colleagues[45] observed apparently beneficial effects of sertraline in one case and of fluoxetine in another. These observations, if confirmed, may prove quite valuable because other agents commonly used in neurally mediated syncope (particularly beta-adrenergic blockers) do not appear to be very useful other than in vasovagal syncope.[46]

TABLE 22–4. TILT-TABLE TESTING FOR PREDICTING EFFECTIVENESS OF THERAPY: DISOPYRAMIDE

Reference	Tilt-Neg on Proposed Treatment	Follow-up (months)	No Syncope During Follow-up
Sra et al[24]	6	16	6 (100%)
Milstein et al[25]	10	20±5	9 (90%)
Morillo et al[10]	? (n = 11)	25±8	8 (73%)
Grubb et al[77]	2	24±11	2 (100%)
Total	? (29)	21±4.1	25 (86%)

Other Pharmacologic Avenues

Theophylline has been proposed as a suitable agent for certain young patients with neurally mediated symptomatic bradyarrhythmias[47] and has been occasionally used in the treatment of vasovagal syncope.[31] As a rule, however, very few patients with vasovagal syncope appear to respond to theophylline alone. Consequently, theophylline is probably at best a third-line agent or possibly should be reserved for use as an adjuvant. Similarly, scopolamine is best considered an adjuvant. Although conveniently administered transcutaneously by application of a skin patch, scopolamine therapy tends to be associated with frequent troublesome side effects and also is accompanied by considerable tachyphylaxis.

Volume expanders such as fludrocortisone and salt supplements continue to be commonly considered options for pediatric patients with neurally mediated syncope. In adults, use of these agents has become less common because of concern regarding induction of hypertension and perhaps because of more willingness to employ some of the pharmacologic agents discussed earlier.

CARDIAC PACING

The utility of cardiac pacing has been a subject of particular interest in the treatment of carotid sinus syndrome and vasovagal syncope. For the former, cardiac pacing is accepted as an essential element of treatment in most cases and has been accorded a class 1 indication by the American Heart Association/American College of Cardiology Task Force on Cardiac Pacing.[48] In vasovagal syncope, the role of cardiac pacing is less certain, although the same Task Force accorded it a class 2 indication.

Pacing in Carotid Sinus Syndrome

The utility of cardiac pacing in carotid sinus syndrome appears to be well established despite the fact that pacing deals with only the cardioinhibitory element of the syndrome.[49–62] In one of the earliest examinations of this issue, Sugrue and associates[49] retrospectively assessed treatment and follow-up findings in 56 carotid sinus syndrome patients, of whom 47 (84%) were described as exhibiting primarily a cardioinhibitory response (asystolic pause of 3 sec or more), whereas 3 (5%) demonstrated predominantly vasodepressor findings (vasodepressor response of greater than 50 mmHg) and 6 (11%) demonstrated the mixed type. Thirteen patients (group 1) received no treatment, 20 received anticholinergic drug therapy (group 2), and 23 received pacemakers (group 3). Follow-up data (mean period, 40 months) were available in 53 cases and revealed that paced patients (group 3) tended to do well; 80% remained asymptomatic (vs. 54% of untreated group 1 patients). Although patients treated with anticholinergic therapy also fared well (group 2, 75% asymptomatic), this form of therapy has since lost favor because of the frequency with which undesirable side effects occur.

In a more detailed study of the utility of pacing in carotid sinus syndrome, Morley and colleagues[51] reported outcomes (mean follow-up period, 18 months) in 70 patients for whom selection of pacing therapy was based on symptom suppression during carotid sinus massage in the presence of temporary ventricular pacing. In this setting, long-term pacing rendered 62 (89%) asymptomatic, although several patients required pacing mode or device changes in order to achieve this result. Blanc and associates[54] also noted the effectiveness of cardiac pacing during follow-up in 54 patients with carotid sinus syndrome. Thirty-three patients were initially untreated, whereas 21 patients were treated with cardiac pacemakers. During follow-up, 19 (58%) of untreated patients experienced recurrences of syncope by 5 years, in comparison with only 1 (5%) of the patients who received pacemakers.

The most effective pacing mode for patients with carotid sinus syndrome has been the subject of a number of studies. Morley and colleagues[51, 52] were among the first to point out that because of the propensity for paroxysmal AV block to occur in carotid sinus syndrome, single-chamber atrial pacing (AAI or AAIR modes) is contraindicated in affected patients. Furthermore, although differences between single-chamber ventricular pacing and dual-chamber pacing were not striking in their study, Morley and colleagues[51] observed that there was a trend in favor of dual-chamber pacing, and that careful hemodynamic assessment during different pacing modes could be useful for optimal device selection.

Other investigators have also assessed the utility of hemodynamic evaluation before selection of pacing mode for patients with carotid sinus syndrome.[53–57, 59–62] Brignole and colleagues[57] evaluated pacing therapy prospectively in 60 consecutive patients presenting with syncope or presyncope. Dual-chamber pacing was selected for 26 patients on the basis of the presence of (1) cardioinhibitory carotid sinus syndrome with symptomatic "pacemaker effect" (i.e., hypotension induced by ventricular pacing alone), (2) mixed-type carotid sinus syndrome with intact ventriculoatrial conduction or orthostatic hypotension, or (3) severe sinus bradycardia. Single-chamber ventricular pacing (ventricular demand inhibited [VVI] mode) was selected in the remaining 34 patients. During follow-up (average period, 1 year), only two patients (one in each group) experienced a recurrence of syncope or presyncope; the overall rate of symptom suppression was 97%. Consequently, selection of pacing mode on the basis of hemodynamic findings identified patients who would most benefit from dual-chamber pacing and enabled the effective use of single-chamber ventricular pacing in the remaining 57% of patients. Other investigators have subsequently confirmed the utility of this approach.[56, 61] Nevertheless, the trend in North America is to favor use of dual-chamber pacing for all patients with carotid sinus syndrome.

Several reports emphasize the utility of selecting dual-chamber pacing modes for patients with carotid sinus syndrome. For example, Madigan and associates[53] examined hemodynamic responses in both supine and upright positions during dual-chamber (atrioventricular sequential [DVI] mode) and single-chamber ventricular (VVI mode) pacing. Eleven patients with a history of dizziness or syncope and who demonstrated evidence during carotid sinus massage of a pause of 3 sec or longer were included in the study. All patients had undergone implantation of dual-chamber pacemakers that could be programmed to VVI mode. An AV interval of 150 msec was chosen for testing in the dual-chamber mode, and pacing rate was set to just above the patients' baseline heart rate. Eight patients exhibited predominantly a cardioinhibitory form of carotid sinus syndrome (CSS) (vasodepressor response < 30 mmHg), whereas the remaining three patients had a mixed form. Findings revealed a clear-cut hemodynamic advantage for the dual-chamber mode during carotid sinus massage in terms of both diminishing the magnitude and rate of blood pressure fall, as well as the extent of symptoms induced. The latter findings were especially evident when testing was conducted with patients in the upright position.

Morley and colleagues[52] similarly examined long-term efficacy of dual-chamber and single-chamber pacing modes in 21 CSS patients, using a double-blind crossover method (6 weeks in each pacing mode). Daily symptoms were recorded by each patient during follow-up. Six patients could not tolerate the change from dual-chamber to single-chamber pacing and were removed from the study (all six exhibited pacemaker syndrome associated with 1:1 ventriculoatrial conduction). Among the remaining 15 patients, there was no apparent difference in terms of symptom frequency between the two pacing modes. However, almost two thirds of the patients indicated a preference for the dual-chamber mode. The only factor that was correlated with patient preference was the presence of ventriculoatrial conduction in all 13 (100%) patients who preferred dual-chamber pacing, in contrast to 3 of 8 (38%) of patients with no preference.

In summary, cardiac pacing is a key element in the treatment of patients with carotid sinus syndrome. In this regard, single-chamber ventricular pacing has proved effective in selected cases. Typically, these patients have a predominant cardioinhibitory mechanism with minimal ventricular pacing effect. However, dual-chamber pacing appears to be more effective than ventricular pacing in the more common mixed form of carotid sinus syndrome (in which there are clinically significant cardioinhibitory and vasodepressor components) and in patients with more severe ventricular pacing effect.

Pacing in Vasovagal Syncope

Only since 1990 has the potential utility of cardiac pacing for treatment of patients with recurrent vasovagal syncope become a subject of clinical interest.[24, 63–68] In a prospective evaluation of the effects of dual-chamber pacing in vasovagal syncope, Fitzpatrick and associates[66] reported hemodynamic and symptom status in 7 patients with recurrent syncope who underwent tilt-table testing and in whom vasovagal reactions were inducible on 2 successive days. The pacing protocol in this study involved the use of a hysteresis feature in which the base rate was 50 bpm and the subsequent pacing rate was 90 bpm. Pacing significantly improved cardiac index (1.0 ± 0.2 L/min/m^2 baseline vs. 1.6 ± 0.3 L/min/m^2 paced), mean arterial blood pressure (30 ± 11 mm Hg baseline vs. 48 ± 12 mm Hg paced), and the duration of tolerated upright posture (0.9 ± 1.2 min baseline vs. 3.2 ± 1.6 min paced) during induced vasovagal reactions. In five cases, syncope was prevented despite evident onset of a vasovagal reaction.

A comparable outcome was reported by Samoil and colleagues.[67] Six patients with reproducible positive tilt-table responses were studied in the unpaced state, during ventricular pacing, and again during dual-chamber cardiac pacing (pacing involved the use of rate hysteresis with a detection rate of <60 bpm, and the pacing rate was set to 20 bpm above resting rate). Findings indicated that ventricular pacing was ineffective, but dual-chamber pacing significantly ($p < .001$) improved upright tilt tolerance (25 ± 6 min dual-chamber pacing vs. 12 ± 6 min unpaced). Furthermore, dual-chamber pacing prevented syncope during tilt-table testing in three of the six patients tested.

In a controversial report, Sra and colleagues[24] concluded somewhat surprisingly that pacing offered little in the way of a practical therapeutic alternative in patients with vasovagal syncope. In coming to their conclusion, the authors examined the effect of temporary pacing for prevention of tilt-induced hypotension and bradycardia in 22 syncope patients with a positive outcome on an initial tilt-test in which bradycardia was thought to be of sufficient severity (heart rate nadir < 60 bpm) to trigger a pacing system. In a subsequent tilt-table test, pacing at a rate approximately 20% higher than the supine resting heart rate was initiated while the patients were supine and was continued throughout the period of upright posture. The actual pacing rates used were not reported. Most patients were evaluated during dual-chamber pacing, except for two with atrial fibrillation who were tested in a single-chamber ventricular pacing mode. During pacing, 1 patient remained asymptomatic, 15 patients reportedly experienced presyncope, and 5 developed syncope once again. The outcome in one additional patient was indeterminate. Subsequently, all patients underwent the tilt test again during pharmacologic therapy. During these later follow-up tilt-test observations, metoprolol prevented symptoms in 10 of 22 patients, theophylline in 3 of 12, and disopyramide in 6 of 9. Consequently, despite the authors' negative interpretation of the efficacy of pacing in these patients, the findings are in fact quite encouraging in terms of the potential utility of cardiac pacing in vasovagal syncope. Symptoms were clearly less severe than had been the case in the absence of pacing (syncope in 22).

Additional evidence in support of the potential utility of pacing in vasovagal syncope was provided by Petersen and associates.[68] This study reviewed experience with atrioventricular sequential (DDI) mode pacing (i.e., dual-chamber pacing and sensing, but with atrial-tracking capability disabled) in 37 patients with vasovagal syncope in whom apparent cardioinhibitory predominance was identified during tilt-table testing. Patients were observed for 39 ± 19 months, and symptomatic improvement was noted in 84%; 35% were asymptomatic.

Several factors account for the limited acceptance of cardiac pacing in vasovagal syncope. First, the almost universal presence of a clinically significant vasodepressor response is an important concern because it would not be expected to be altered by pacing. Second, vasovagal syncope is generally considered to have a benign prognosis, and consequently there is reasonable reluctance to implant a pacemaker. Third, unlike patients with carotid sinus syndrome, a substantial percentage of patients with vasovagal fainting episodes are relatively young and less inclined to accept pacemaker therapy. Finally, the benefits of pacing in vasovagal syncope have been the subject of investigative attention only since the early 1990s, and the published reports still only incorporate a relatively small number of patients.

ROLE OF TILT-TABLE TESTING IN TREATMENT SELECTION

There is general agreement that head-up tilt-table test plays a valuable diagnostic role in the evaluation of patients with recurrent syncope. Specifically, tilt-table testing has proved highly effective for distinguishing patients with marked susceptibility to neurally mediated syncope from the large population of patients presenting with recurrent syncope of unknown origin.[6, 18, 19, 69–71] However, the value of tilt-table testing for predicting treatment efficacy in individual patients remains less certain (Table 22–5).

Crucial to understanding the potential role of tilt-table testing for assessing treatment interventions is knowledge of test reproducibility. This has been the subject of a number of studies, and in general there has been a relatively high concordance (approximately 80%–85%) of outcomes in terms of syncope or no syncope within patients for two tests carried out either on the same day or even many days apart.[72–76] However, apart from whether syncope is or is not reproducible, treatment selection very much depends on reproducibility of electrophysiologic and hemodynamic characteristics during induced vasovagal spells. From the authors' own laboratory, Chen and associates[72] reported outcomes of two sequential 80° head-up tilt tests in 23 patients undergoing evaluation for recurrent syncope. Overall, 15 (65%) of the 23 individuals developed syncope in either the first or the second tilt procedure; 8 patients remained asymptomatic. Findings in the two tests were concordant in 20 (87%) of the 23 cases. Furthermore, there was a strong correlation between heart rate and hemodynamic findings in each of the two tests, which suggests that the characteristics of the induced episodes were very similar within a given patient.

The findings presented by Grubb and colleagues[73] similarly revealed that repeat tilts 3–7 days apart tended to exhibit strong intrapatient concordance for heart rate and blood pressure. However, Fish and associates[74] came to a somewhat different conclusion. In

TABLE 22–5. TILT-TABLE TESTING FOR PREDICTING EFFECTIVENESS OF THERAPY: PACING

Reference	Tilt-Neg on Proposed Treatment	Follow-up (months)	Improved During Follow-up	No Syncope During Follow-up
Sra et al[24]	3	16	3* (100%)	0 0%)
Petersen et al[68]	? (n = 37)	50 ± 24	23 (62%)	10 (27%)
Grubb et al[78]	4	21	2* (50%)	2 (50%)
Total	uncertain	29	63%	27%

* in conjunction with drug treatment.

their study, a series of 90° tilts for 15 min each were undertaken in the baseline state, followed if necessary by isoproterenol provocation. Findings revealed that syncope or presyncope was reproduced in 14 (67%) of 21 cases; an additional 4 patients (19%) exhibited milder symptoms in the second test. However, in this report, the patterns of physiologic response (i.e., cardioinhibitory, vasodepressor, mixed) often differed in the two tests. Thus despite a 67% reproducibility rate, these investigators were less convinced of the utility of head-up tilt as a useful method for assessing therapeutic interventions.

In view of the fact that a positive outcome on an initial tilt test may not be reproducible in approximately 20% of cases, it is uncertain whether tilt-table testing will prove as useful for predicting treatment as it appears to be as a diagnostic tool. Until this question is resolved, a reasonable approach is to interpret an apparently effective therapeutic outcome with caution. The latter is particularly important in view of the notoriously unpredictable nature of the condition and the propensity for many patients to experience long periods between syncopal episodes. Similarly, it is also premature to conclude that failure of therapy on the basis of tilt-table testing predicts subsequent spontaneous clinical failure. Studies employing careful correlation of long-term clinical follow-up with results of tilt-table studies are needed to address these issues.

CONCLUSION

Apart perhaps from the relatively well-defined role of cardiac pacing in carotid sinus syndrome, treatment strategies for most of the neurally mediated syncopal syndromes remain as yet incompletely defined. In particular, there is considerable uncertainty regarding the efficacy of any of the proposed pharmacologic treatment approaches for patients with recurrent vasovagal syncope. Large, carefully designed placebo-controlled studies (perhaps making use of important new epidemiologic observations described by Sheldon and colleagues[79]) are now needed. Continued study of the pathophysiologic processes of these conditions is essential if effective prophylaxis is to be provided for patients troubled by recurrent neurally mediated syncopal episodes.

Acknowledgment

The authors thank Barry L. S. Detloff and Wendy Markuson for assistance in preparation of this chapter.

REFERENCES

1. Benditt DG, Goldstein MA, Adler S, Sakaguchi S, Lurie K: Neurally mediated syncopal syndromes: Pathophysiology and clinical evaluation. *In* Mandel WJ (ed): Cardiac Arrhythmias, 3rd ed, pp 879–906. Philadelphia: JB Lippincott, 1995.
2. Ross RT: Syncope. London: WB Saunders, 1988.
3. Benditt DG, Sakaguchi S, Schultz JJ, et al: Syncope. Diagnostic considerations and the role of tilt table testing. Cardiol Rev 1993; 1:146–156.
4. Kapoor W: Evaluation and outcome of patients with syncope. Medicine 1990; 69:160–175.
5. Milstein S, Buetikofer J, Lesser J, et al: Cardiac asystole: a manifestation of neurally mediated hypotension-bradycardia. J Am Coll Cardiol 1989; 14:1626–1632.
6. Almquist A, Goldenberg IF, Milstein S, et al: Provocation of bradycardia and hypotension by isoproterenol and upright posture in patients with unexplained syncope. New Engl J Med 1989; 320:346–351.
7. Sutton R, Petersen M, Brignole M, et al: Proposed classification for tilt induced vasovagal syncope. Eur J Cardiac Pacing Electrophysiol 1992; 2:180–183.
8. Savage DD, Corwin L, McGee DL, et al: Epidemiologic features of isolated syncope: the Framingham study. Stroke 1985; 16:626–629.
9. Blanc JJ, Genet L, Mansourati J, et al: Interet du test d'inclinaison dans le diagnostic etiologique des pertes de connaissance. Presse Med 1990; 19:857–859.
10. Morillo C, Leitch JW, Yee R, Klein GJ: A placebo-controlled trial of intravenous and oral disopyramide for prevention of neurally mediated syncope induced by head-up tilt. J Am Coll Cardiol 1993; 22:1843–1848.
11. Lyle CB, Monroe JT, Flinn DE, Lamb LE: Micturition syncope. Report of 24 cases. N Engl J Med 1961; 265:982–986.
12. Lukash WM, Sawyer GT, Davies JE: Micturition syncope produced by orthostasis and bladder distention. N Engl J Med 1964; 270:341–344.
13. Kapoor WN, Peterson JR, Karpf M: Micturition syncope: a reappraisal. JAMA 1985; 253:796–798.
14. Pritchett EL, Smith MS, McCarthy EA, Lee K: The spontaneous occurrence of paroxysmal supraventricular tachycardia. Circulation 1984; 70:1–6.
15. Greer GS, Wilkinson WE, McCarthy EA, Pritchett EL: Random and nonrandom behaviour of symptomatic paroxysmal atrial fibrillation. Am J Cardiol 1989; 64:339–342.
16. Clair WK, Wilkinson WE, McCarthy EA, et al: Spontaneous occurrence of symptomatic paroxysmal atrial fibrillation and paroxysmal supraventricular tachycardia in untreated patients. Circulation 1993; 87:1114–1122.
17. Kus T, La Londe G, de Champlain J, Shenasa M: Vasovagal syncope: management with atrioventricular sequential pacing and beta-blockade. Can J Cardiol 1989; 5:375–378.
18. Grubb BP, Temesy-Aromos P, Hahn H, Elliott L: Utility of upright tilt-table testing in the evaluation and management of syncope of unknown origin. Am J Med 1991; 90:6–10.
19. Sra JS, Anderson AF, Sheikh SH, et al: Unexplained syncope evaluated by electrophysiologic studies and head-up tilt testing. Ann Intern Med 1991, 114.1013–1019.
20. Grubb BP, Gerard G, Roush K, et al: Differentiation of convulsive syncope and epilepsy with head-up tilt testing. Ann Intern Med 1991; 115:871–876.
21. Fitzpatrick AP, Ahmed R, Williams S, Sutton R: A randomised trial of medical therapy in "malignant vasovagal syndrome" or "neurally-mediated bradycardia hypotension syndrome." Eur J Cardiac Pacing Electrophysiol 1991; 2:99–102.
22. Grubb BP, Temesy-Armos P, Moore J, et al: Head-upright tilt-table testing in evaluation and management of the malignant vasovagal syndrome. Am J Cardiol 1992; 69:904–908.
23. Sra JS, Murthy VS, Jazayeri MR, et al: Use of intravenous esmolol

to predict efficacy of oral adrenergic blocker therapy in patients with neurocardiogenic syncope. J Am Coll Cardiol 1993; 19:402–408.
24. Sra J, Jazayeri MR, Avitall B, et al: Comparison of cardiac pacing with drug therapy in the treatment of neurocardiogenic (vasovagal) syncope with bradycardia or asystole. N Engl J Med 1993; 328:1085–1090.
25. Milstein S, Buetikofer J, Dunnigan A, et al: Usefulness of disopyramide for prevention of upright tilt-induced hypotension-bradycardia. Am J Cardiol 1990; 65:1339–1344.
26. Raviele A, Gasparini G, Di Pede F, et al: Usefulness of head-up tilt test in evaluating patients with syncope of unknown origin and negative electrophysiologic study. Am J Cardiol 1990; 65:1322–1327.
27. Brignole M, Menozzi C, Gianfranchi L, et al: A controlled trial of acute and long-term medical therapy in tilt-induced neurally-mediated syncope. Am J Cardiol 1992; 70:339–342.
28. Grubb BP, Wolfe D, Samoil D, et al: Usefulness of fluoxetine hydrochloride for prevention of resistent upright tilt induced syncope. PACE Pacing Clin Electrophysiol 1993; 16:458–464.
29. Kosinski DJ, Grubb BP, Temesy-Armos PN: The use of serotonin reuptake inhibitors in the treatment of neurally mediated cardiovascular disorders. J Serotonin Res 1994; 1:85–90.
30. Abi-Samra F, Maloney JD, Fouad-Tarazi FM, Castle L: The usefulness of head-up tilt testing and hemodynamic investigations in the workup of syncope of unknown origin. PACE Pacing Clin Electrophysiol 11:1202–1214, 1988.
31. Nelson S, Stanley M, Love C, Schaal SF: Autonomic and hemodynamic effects of oral theophylline in patients with vasodepressor syncope. Arch Intern Med 1991; 90:2425–2429.
32. Pongiglione G, Fish FA, Strasburger JF, Benson DW Jr: Heart rate and blood pressure response to upright tilt in young patients with unexplained syncope. Am J Cardiol 1990; 64:165–170.
33. Perry JC, Garson A Jr: The child with recurrent syncope: autonomic function testing and beta-adrenergic hypersensitivity. J Am Coll Cardiol 1991; 17:1168–1171.
34. Perry J, Friedman RA, Moak JP, Garson A Jr: Bradycardia and syncope in children not controlled by pacing: beta-adrenergic hypersensitivity. PACE Pacing Clin Electrophysiol 1991; 14:391–394.
35. Chosy JJ, Graham DT: Catecholamines in vasovagal fainting. J Psychosom Res 1965; 9:189–194.
36. Vingerhoets AJJM: Biochemical changes in two subjects succumbing to syncope. Psychosom Med 1984; 46:95–103.
37. Fitzpatrick A, Williams T, Ahmed R, Sutton R: Echocardiographic and endocrine changes during vasovagal syncope induced by prolonged head-up tilt. Eur J Cardiac Pacing Electrophysiol 1992; 2:121–128.
38. Levy MN, Martin P: Parasympathetic control of the heart. *In* Randall WC (ed): Nervous Control of Cardiovascular Function, pp 68–94. New York: Oxford University Press, 1984.
39. Asso A, Milstein S, Dunnigan A, et al: Prognostic significance of parenteral metoprolol during head-up tilt testing [Abstract]. Circulation 1991; 84(suppl II):409.
40. Lurie KG, Dutton J, Mangat R, Scheinman MM: Pindolol is effective in patients with vasovagal syncope [Abstract]. PACE Pacing Clin Electrophysiol 1992; 15:592.
41. Gottdiener JS, Dibianco R, Bates R, et al: Effects of disopyramide on left ventricular function: assessment by radionuclide cineangiography. Am J Cardiol 1983; 51:1554–1558.
42. Pollick C: Muscular subaortic stenosis: hemodynamic and clinical improvement after disopyramide. N Engl J Med 1982; 307:997–999.
43. Benditt DG, Benson DW Jr, Dunnigan A, et al: Drug therapy in sinus node dysfunction. *In* Rapaport E (ed): Cardiology Update, pp 79–102. New York: Elsevier, 1984.
44. Gonzalez-Heydrich J, Peroutka SJ: Serotonin receptor and reuptake sites: pharmacologic significance. J Clin Psychiatry 1990; 51(suppl 4):5–12.
45. Grubb BP, Samoil D, Kosinski D, et al: The use of serotonin reuptake inhibitors for the treatment of carotid sinus hypersensitivity syndrome unresponsive to dual chamber pacing. PACE Pacing Clin Electrophysiol 1994; 17:1434–1436.
46. Almquist A, Gornick C, Benson DW Jr, et al: Carotid sinus hypersensitivity: evaluation of the vasodepressor component. Circulation 1985; 71:927–936.
47. Benditt DG, Benson DW Jr, Kriett JM, et al: Electrophysiologic effects of theophylline in young patients with recurrent symptomatic bradyarrhythmias. Am J Cardiol 1983; 52:1223–1229.
48. Dreifus LS, Fisch C, Griffin JC, et al: Guidelines for implantation of cardiac pacemakers and antiarrhythmic devices. ACC/AHA Task Force report. J Am Coll Cardiol 1991; 18:1–13.
49. Sugrue DD, Gersh BJ, Holmes DR, et al: Symptomatic "isolated" carotid sinus hypersensitivity: natural history and results of treatment with anticholinergic drugs or pacemaker. J Am Coll Cardiol 1986; 7:158–162.
50. Strasberg B, Sagie A, Erdman S, et al: Carotid sinus hypersensitivity and carotid sinus syndrome. Prog Cardiovasc Dis 1989; 31:379–391.
51. Morley CA, Perrins EJ, Grant P, et al: Carotid sinus syncope treated by pacing. Analysis of persistent symptoms and role of atrioventricular sequential pacing. Br Heart J 1982; 47:411–418.
52. Morley CA, Perrins EJ, Chan SL, Sutton R: Long-term comparison of DVI and VVI pacing in carotid sinus syndrome. *In* Steinbach K (ed): Cardiac Pacing: Proceedings of the VIIth World Symposium on Cardiac Pacing, pp. 929–935. Steinkopff Verlag Darmstadt, 1983.
53. Madigan NP, Flaker GC, Curtis JJ, et al: Carotid sinus hypersensitivity: beneficial effects of dual-chamber pacing. Am J Cardiol 1984; 53:1034–1040.
54. Blanc JJ, Boschat J, Penther P: Hypersensibilité sino-carotidienne. Evolution à moyen terme en fonction du traitement et des symptômes. Arch Mal Coeur 1984; 77:330–336.
55. Peretz DI, Abdulla A: Management of cardioinhibitory hypersensitive carotid sinus syncope with permanent cardiac pacing—a seventeen year prospective study. Can J Cardiol 1985; 2:86–91.
56. Stryjer D, Friedensohn A, Schlesinger Z: Ventricular pacing as the preferable mode for long-term pacing in patients with carotid sinus syncope of the cardioinhibitory type. PACE Pacing Clin Electrophysiol 1986; 9:705–709.
57. Brignole M, Sartore B, Barra M, et al: Is DDD superior to VVI pacing in mixed carotid sinus syndrome? An acute and medium-term study. PACE Pacing Clin Electrophysiol 1988; 11:1902–1910.
58. Brignole M, Menozzi C, Lolli G, et al: Natural and unnatural history of patients with severe carotid sinus hypersensitivity: a preliminary study. PACE Pacing Clin Electrophysiol 1988; 11:1628–1635.
59. Brignole M, Sartore B, Barra M, et al: Ventricular and dual chamber pacing for treatment of carotid sinus syndrome. PACE Pacing Clin Electrophysiol 1989; 12:582–590.
60. Brignole M, Menozzi C, Lolli G, et al: Pacing for carotid sinus syndrome and sick sinus syndrome. PACE Pacing Clin Electrophysiol 1990; 13:2071–2075.
61. Deschamps D, Richard A, Citron B, et al: Hypersensibilité sino-carotidienne. Evolution à moyen et à long terme des patients traités par stimulation ventriculaire. Arch Mal Coeur 1990; 83:63–67.
62. Brignole M, Menozzi C, Lolli G, et al: Validation of a method for choice of pacing mode in carotid sinus syndrome with or without sinus bradycardia. PACE Pacing Clin Electrophysiol 1991; 14:196–203.
63. Benditt DG, Petersen M, Lurie KG, et al: Cardiac pacing for prevention of recurrent vasovagal syncope. Ann Intern Med 1995; 122:204–209.
64. Sapire DW, Casta A, Safley W, et al: Vasovagal syncope in children requiring pacemaker implantation. Am Heart J 1983; 106:1406–1411.
65. Fitzpatrick AP, Travill CM, Vardas PE, et al: Recurrent symptoms after ventricular pacing in unexplained syncope. PACE Pacing Clin Electrophysiol 1990; 13:619–624.
66. Fitzpatrick AP, Theodorakis G, Ahmed R, et al: Dual chamber pacing aborts vasovagal syncope induced by head-up 60° tilt. PACE Pacing Clin Electrophysiol 1991; 14:13–19.
67. Samoil D, Grubb BP, Brewster P, et al: Comparison of single and dual chamber pacing techniques in prevention of upright tilt induced vasovagal syncope. Eur J Cardiac Pacing Electrophysiol 1993; 1:36–41.
68. Petersen MEV, Chamberlain-Webber R, Fizpatrick AP, et al: Permanent pacing for cardio-inhibitory malignant vasovagal syndrome. Br Heart J 1994; 71:274–281.
69. Raviele A, Proclemer A, Gasparini G, et al: Long-term follow-up of patients with unexplained syncope and negative electrophysiologic study. Eur Heart J 1989; 10:127–132.
70. Benditt DG, Remole S, Bailin S, et al: Tilt-table testing for evaluation of neurally-mediated (cardioneurogenic) syncope: rationale and proposed protocols. PACE Pacing Clin Electrophysiol 1991; 14:1–10.
71. Fitzpatrick A, Theodorakis G, Vardas P, et al: The incidence of malignant vasovagal syndrome in patients with recurrent syncope. Eur Heart J 1991; 12:389–394.
72. Chen XC, Chen M-Y, Remole S, et al: Reproducibility of head-up tilt-table testing for eliciting susceptibility to neurally mediated syncope in patients without structural heart disease. Am J Cardiol 1992; 69:755–760.
73. Grubb BP, Wolfe D, Temesy-Armos P, et al: Reproducibility of head-upright test results in patients with syncope. PACE Pacing Clin Electrophysiol 1992; 15:1477–1481.

74. Fish FA, Strasburger JF, Benson DW Jr: Reproducibility of a symptomatic response to upright tilt in young patients with unexplained syncope. Am J Cardiol 1992; 70:605–609.
75. Buitleir M, Grogan EW Jr, Picone MF, Casteen JA: Immediate reproducibility of the tilt-table test in adults with unexplained syncope. Am J Cardiol 1993; 71:304–307.
76. Brooks R, Ruskin JN, Powell AC, et al: Prospective evaluation of day-to-day reproducibility of tilt-table testing in unexplained syncope. Am J Cardiol 1993; 71:1289–1292.
77. Grubb BP, Wolfe D, Samoil D, et al: Recurrent unexplained syncope in the elderly: the use of head-upright tilt-table testing in evaluation and management. J Am Geriatr Soc 1992; 40:1123–1128.
78. Grubb BP, Temesy-Armos P, Moore J, et al: Head upright tilt testing in the evaluation and management of the malignant vasovagal syndrome. Am J Cardiol 1992; 69:904–908.
79. Sheldon RS, Rose S, Flanagan P, et al: Multivariate predictors of syncope recurrence in drug-free patients following a positive tilt table test [Abstract]. Circulation 1994; 90:55.

SECTION

FOUR Dyslipoproteinemias/Atherosclerosis

23 Dyslipoproteinemias/Atherosclerosis: Introduction

Antonio M. Gotto, Jr., MD, DPhil
John A. Farmer, MD

Despite the accumulation of evidence linking dyslipidemia with coronary heart disease (CHD), the detection and treatment of dyslipidemia remain an underutilized means of reducing CHD risk. For example, a report from the Atherosclerosis Risk in Communities (ARIC) study showed that 42% of hypercholesterolemic subjects were aware of their condition, compared with 84% of hypertensive subjects, and only 4% of hypercholesterolemic subjects had their condition treated with medication and controlled, compared with 50% of hypertensive subjects.[1] According to the same report, awareness of hypercholesterolemia in hypercholesterolemic subjects increased from 31% in 1987 to 50% in 1989; concurrently, prevalence of hypercholesterolemia in study subjects decreased from 30% to 25%. During this time, the Adult Treatment Panel of the U.S. National Cholesterol Education Program issued guidelines for detecting and treating hypercholesterolemia.

In 1993, revised guidelines were issued by the Adult Treatment Panel II (ATP II).[2] The ATP II guidelines continue to emphasize lowering elevated low-density lipoprotein (LDL) cholesterol levels and place new emphasis on high-density lipoprotein (HDL) cholesterol as an important CHD risk factor. Increased attention is also given to the presence or absence of CHD in determining need for and intensity of lipid-regulating intervention.

LIPID METABOLISM

In order for lipids, which are insoluble in water, to be transported through the plasma, they are packaged into lipoproteins, spherical particles composed of a core of nonpolar lipids—cholesteryl ester and triglyceride—surrounded by a surface monolayer of polar lipids—phospholipid and cholesterol—and apolipoproteins. Lipoproteins are distinguished by composition, density, size, electrophoretic mobility, and the apolipoproteins on their surface (Table 23–1). It is the apolipoproteins that largely determine the metabolic fate of the lipoproteins to which they are attached. These proteins regulate enzyme activity, thereby affecting lipoprotein metabolism and core lipid composition, and, through recognition by membrane receptors, enable the lipoproteins to be removed from the circulation.

Exogenous and Endogenous Lipolytic Cascades

The transport of exogenous lipids begins with the packaging of dietary triglyceride and cholesterol into chylomicrons. The intestinal origin of these particles is reflected by the apolipoprotein (apo) B-48 on their surface. Very low density lipoprotein (VLDL), which is secreted by the liver, contains apo B-100, as do the other lipoproteins in the endogenous lipid cascade. Chylomicrons and VLDL, known collectively as triglyceride-rich lipoproteins, also contain apo C-II, which activates lipoprotein lipase.

Through the action of lipoprotein lipase, triglyceride is hydrolyzed from the triglyceride-rich lipoproteins, and the resulting free fatty acids are used as energy by muscle tissue or stored in adipose tissue for future energy needs. As the lipoprotein core shrinks, the excess surface components, including the A and C apolipoproteins, transfer to HDL.

Chylomicron remnants are quickly removed by the liver, apparently through receptor-mediated recognition and binding of the apo E on their surface. In the liver, cholesterol from these particles is converted into bile acids, excreted into the bile, or secreted in VLDL. Remnants of hydrolyzed VLDL—intermediate-density lipoprotein (IDL)—may be removed from the circulation by the B/E, or LDL, receptor, which recognizes and binds the apo E on the IDL surface. Alternatively, IDL may remain in the circulation, where, through the action of hepatic lipase, it is further hydrolyzed to become LDL. Approximately 70% of plasma cholesterol is transported in LDL, which delivers cholesterol to peripheral cells, where it is used to form cell membranes and steroid hormones. Removal of LDL by the B/E receptor is through recognition and binding of apo B-100, its sole major apolipoprotein.

B/E receptor activity decreases as intracellular cholesterol increases; conversely, B/E receptor activity is upregulated in response to decreased intracellular cholesterol concentration. Both B/E receptor activity and cholesterol synthesis by the liver are suppressed by excess dietary cholesterol. If B/E receptor activity is chronically suppressed, plasma LDL cholesterol level may become elevated. In general, the body derives 20%–40% of its cholesterol from the diet but is capable of synthesizing enough cholesterol for its needs.

LDL particles not removed by the B/E receptor may be removed through alternative receptor-mediated and non–receptor-mediated pathways, including the scavenger receptor on macrophages. Chemical modification of LDL, such as oxidation or acetylation, is thought to be necessary for removal of LDL by the scavenger receptor. Scavenger receptor activity is not downregulated as intracellular cholesterol accumulates, and continued uptake of cholesterol can convert the macrophage into a lipid-laden foam cell. Foam cells are the primary components of the fatty streak, which is thought to be the initial atherosclerotic lesion.

Through the action of cholesteryl ester transfer protein (CETP),

TABLE 23–1. PLASMA LIPOPROTEINS

Lipoprotein Class	Major Lipids	Density (g/mL)	Diameter (Å)	Electrophoretic Mobility	Apolipoproteins
Chylomicrons	Dietary triglyceride, cholesteryl ester	<0.95	800–5000	Origin	A-I, A-II, A-IV, B-48, C-I, C-II, C-III, E
Chylomicron remnants	Dietary cholesteryl ester	<1.006	>300	Origin	B-48, E
VLDL	Endogenous triglyceride	<1.006	300–800	Pre-beta	B-100, C-I, C-II, C-III, E
IDL	Cholesteryl ester, triglyceride	1.006–1.019	250–350	Broad-beta	B-100, E
LDL	Cholesteryl ester	1.019–1.063	180–280	Beta	B-100
HDL_2	Cholesteryl ester	1.063–1.125	90–120	Alpha	A-I, A-II, C-I, C-II, C-III, E
HDL_3	Cholesteryl ester	1.125–1.210	50–90	Alpha	A-I, A-II, C-I, C-II, C-III, E

Abbreviations: HDL, high-density lipoprotein; IDL, intermediate-density lipoprotein; LDL, low-density lipoprotein; VLDL, very low density lipoprotein.

triglyceride from the triglyceride-rich lipoproteins can be transferred to LDL in exchange for cholesteryl ester. The transferred triglyceride is hydrolyzed by hepatic lipase, resulting in LDL particles that are smaller and denser than normal LDL. A preponderance of small, dense LDL particles, which is more common in individuals with increased plasma triglyceride, has been associated with a threefold increased risk for myocardial infarction (MI).[3] Some studies have found that lowering triglyceride can convert small, dense LDL to normal, buoyant LDL.[4]

High-Density Lipoprotein and Reverse Cholesterol Transport

HDL is secreted by the liver and intestine as a discoidal precursor particle that acquires phospholipid and cholesterol from cell membranes and from surface components made redundant by the hydrolysis of the triglyceride-rich lipoproteins. Through the action of lecithin–cholesterol acyltransferase (LCAT) on the phospholipid and cholesterol in these particles, a core of cholesteryl ester is generated, and the disk is transformed into mature, spherical HDL. As HDL continues to acquire phospholipid and cholesterol, which serve as substrates for additional esterification by LCAT, the smaller HDL_3 particle is converted to the larger HDL_2, thereby increasing the amount of cholesterol carried in HDL.

HDL is thought to be the vehicle of reverse cholesterol transport, the putative process whereby cholesterol is returned from peripheral tissues to the liver for excretion. An increased number of HDL_2 particles would therefore enhance the efficiency of this process because of the increased cholesterol-carrying capacity. Conversely, this process may be compromised by the CETP-mediated exchange of triglyceride from chylomicrons and VLDL for cholesteryl ester in HDL. The transferred triglyceride then becomes a substrate for hydrolysis by hepatic lipase, and HDL_2 reverts to HDL_3, decreasing the volume of cholesterol carried in HDL. The cholesteryl ester transferred to chylomicrons and VLDL is removed from the plasma with chylomicron remnants, IDL, and LDL. The inverse relation between CHD incidence and HDL cholesterol level may be due to the increased capacity of reverse cholesterol transport when plasma HDL cholesterol is elevated, or high HDL cholesterol may reflect the efficient metabolism of triglyceride-rich lipoproteins, which are cleared from the plasma before their triglyceride is transferred to HDL and hydrolyzed.[5]

CHOLESTEROL LEVEL AND CORONARY HEART DISEASE

Blood cholesterol—in particular, cholesterol carried in LDL—has been linked with increased risk for CHD in observational epidemiologic, genetic, experimental, and clinical studies.

Observational Epidemiologic Evidence

Total cholesterol level has been directly associated with CHD risk in a number of observational epidemiologic studies. For example, in the Seven Countries Study, countries with higher mean serum cholesterol levels had higher coronary mortality rates than did countries with lower mean serum cholesterol levels.[6]

In the Ni-Hon-San Study, conducted in men of Japanese descent, there was a higher prevalence of elevated serum cholesterol in subjects living in California than in subjects living in Hawaii and a higher prevalence in subjects living in Hawaii than in subjects living in Japan.[7] Age-adjusted incidence of MI and CHD death was 50% higher in California than in Hawaii and twice as high in Hawaii as in Japan.[8]

In 356,222 men screened for the Multiple Risk Factor Intervention Trial, a continuous, graded relation was established between serum cholesterol and CHD mortality rate.[9] CHD mortality in men with serum cholesterol levels in the highest decile (≥264 mg/dL) was four times greater than in men with serum cholesterol levels in the lowest decile (≤167 mg/dL), and CHD mortality increased with each successive decile.

In the ongoing Framingham Heart Study, a direct relation was found between total serum cholesterol level and both cardiovascular mortality and total mortality in men and women younger than 50 years.[10] Each 10 mg/dL increase in total cholesterol increased cardiovascular mortality 9% and increased total mortality 5%.

Genetic Evidence

Evidence for the direct association between cholesterol level and CHD risk has also been provided by genetic disorders in which plasma cholesterol is elevated. CHD can develop in patients with these disorders who do not have any other CHD risk factors.

In patients with familial hypercholesterolemia (FH), a lack of competent B/E receptors causes plasma cholesterol—particularly LDL cholesterol—to increase because of impaired lipoprotein removal.[11] Patients with heterozygous FH have half the normal number of competent B/E receptors and twice the LDL cholesterol level of normal individuals. Symptomatic CHD typically develops by the age of 50 years in men with heterozygous FH and by the age of 60 years in women with heterozygous FH. Patients with homozygous FH, in whom competent B/E receptors are absent, have LDL cholesterol levels of 500 to 1000 mg/dL and often have symptomatic CHD before the age of 20 years.

Another genetic disorder characterized by increased plasma cholesterol and increased risk for CHD is familial defective apo B-100. In this disorder, a mutation in the gene for apo B-100 prevents its recognition and binding by the B/E receptor, resulting in an accumulation of LDL particles in the plasma. Most heterozygotes have total cholesterol and LDL cholesterol levels above the 95th percentile for age and sex, and by age 50 years, 40% of men and 20% of women with heterozygous familial defective apo B-100 have evidence of CHD.[12]

Experimental Evidence

Elevated cholesterol level has been found to cause atherosclerosis in many different animal species.[13] Atherosclerotic lesions have been induced by diets high in saturated fat and cholesterol[14] and have regressed with diets low in saturated fat and cholesterol.[15] The Watanabe heritable hyperlipidemic rabbit, which has no B/E receptors, serves as an animal model for FH.

Clinical Trial Evidence

In a number of interventional trials, cholesterol lowering by diet, drugs, and/or surgery has been associated with a reduction in CHD-related events. For example, in the Lipid Research Clinics Coronary Primary Prevention Trial, cholestyramine treatment significantly decreased total plasma cholesterol level 8% and significantly decreased LDL cholesterol level 12% compared with placebo. Combined incidence of CHD-related death and nonfatal MI was significantly reduced 19%.

In the Program on the Surgical Control of the Hyperlipidemias, partial ileal bypass surgery in subjects with one previous MI significantly decreased total cholesterol level 23% and significantly decreased LDL cholesterol level 38%, compared with control subjects assigned to usual care. Combined incidence of CHD-related death and nonfatal MI was significantly reduced 35% in the surgery group.[16]

A meta-analysis of seven lipid-lowering trials conducted in subjects with CHD determined that a 10% reduction in total cholesterol level, obtained with dietary and/or pharmacologic interventions, reduced MI incidence 15%.[17] In the same report, a meta-analysis of four lipid-lowering trials conducted in subjects without CHD at baseline evaluation showed that a 10% reduction in total cholesterol level, obtained with diet and/or drugs, reduced MI incidence 22%.

HIGH-DENSITY LIPOPROTEIN CHOLESTEROL LEVEL AND CORONARY HEART DISEASE

A strong, inverse relation between HDL cholesterol level and risk for CHD has been demonstrated in numerous epidemiologic studies. In the Framingham Heart Study, among subjects aged 50–79 years, risk for MI was 60%–70% greater in men with HDL cholesterol levels in the lower three quartiles (12–52 mg/dL) than in men with HDL cholesterol levels in the highest quartile (53–129 mg/dL), and risk for coronary events was six times greater in women with HDL cholesterol levels in the lowest quartile (23–46 mg/dL) than in women with HDL cholesterol levels in the highest quartile (67–139 mg/dL).[18] In women, HDL cholesterol level was inversely related to MI in every quartile. These differences were significant in women; the only significant difference in men was between the lowest and highest quartile of HDL cholesterol level. In another report from the Framingham Heart Study, each 10 mg/dL increase in HDL cholesterol significantly reduced CHD-related mortality 19% in men and 28% in women.[19]

In an analysis of four prospective U.S. studies, each 1 mg/dL increase in HDL cholesterol was associated with a significant 2% decrease in CHD risk in men and a significant 3% decrease in CHD risk in women.[20] Clinical trials specifically designed to determine whether increasing HDL cholesterol levels will decrease CHD-related morbidity and mortality are in progress.

TRIGLYCERIDE LEVEL AND CORONARY HEART DISEASE

Univariate analyses of data in many prospective observational studies have shown a direct relation between plasma triglyceride level and CHD incidence,[21] but this relation tends to diminish in multivariate analyses controlling for other CHD risk factors such as hypertension, physical inactivity, and obesity and may disappear when studies control for HDL cholesterol level, coagulation factors, or markers of abnormalities of glucose metabolism. Including HDL in the statistical analysis may cause the association between triglyceride level and CHD to be underestimated because of the close metabolic interrelation between HDL and the triglyceride-rich lipoproteins. In addition, plasma triglyceride measurements are highly variable within an individual and among individuals, potentially leading to the misclassification of subjects in epidemiologic and clinical trials.[22] Also, CHD risk at a given triglyceride level may vary depending on how much triglyceride is carried in each lipoprotein fraction. The triglyceride-rich lipoproteins are thought to differ in their atherogenicity: chylomicrons and normal, buoyant VLDL do not appear to confer increased atherosclerotic risk, but their remnants and small, dense VLDL (β-VLDL) are believed to be atherogenic.

In many studies, plasma triglyceride has been measured in a fasting sample; however, some researchers have suggested that assessment of postprandial lipemia may prove to be a more accurate predictor of CHD risk. Studies have found that indicators of the postprandial metabolism of triglyceride-rich lipoproteins are as accurate as HDL cholesterol in identifying CHD patients and control subjects.[23]

Although the association between plasma triglyceride level and CHD incidence remains controversial, increasing evidence from observational and interventional studies suggests that triglyceride plays an important role as part of a constellation of risk factors that together may allow a more refined assessment of CHD risk. In the observational Prospective Cardiovascular Münster (PROCAM) study, triglyceride levels of 200 mg/dL or greater were found in 39% of subjects who had an MI or died of CHD, compared with 21% of surviving subjects who did not have an MI or a stroke.[24] A significant association was found between triglyceride level and incidence of CHD events in univariate analysis but disappeared when total cholesterol or HDL cholesterol level was included in multivariate analysis. However, the group identified as having the highest risk for CHD events was characterized by a combination of a triglyceride level of 200 mg/dL or greater and an LDL cholesterol/HDL cholesterol ratio of 5 or greater. Although this subgroup represented less than 4% of subjects in this analysis, it accounted for almost 25% of CHD events reported.

A similar high-risk subgroup was identified in the Helsinki Heart Study, in which the effect on CHD events of gemfibrozil-induced changes in the lipid profile was evaluated.[25] Subjects at highest risk for a fatal or nonfatal MI or cardiac death were characterized by a combination of serum triglyceride level greater than 200 mg/dL and an LDL cholesterol/HDL cholesterol ratio greater than 5. Compared with subjects with a triglyceride level of 200 mg/dL or less and an LDL cholesterol/HDL cholesterol ratio of 5 or less, the relative risk for a CHD event in the high-risk subgroup was 3.8. In this high-risk subgroup, which accounted for approximately 10% of study subjects, CHD risk was reduced 71% with gemfibrozil treatment, compared with a 34% reduction in CHD risk in the entire group assigned to gemfibrozil.

GUIDELINES FOR DIAGNOSIS AND TREATMENT OF DYSLIPIDEMIA

The revised treatment guidelines of the ATP II provide a framework, to be applied with clinical judgment, for identifying and treating individuals whose lipid profile increases their risk for CHD.

The intensity of treatment is guided by the individual's overall risk status, which is influenced most strongly by the presence or absence of CHD or other atherosclerotic disease, such as peripheral arterial disease or symptomatic carotid artery disease. In individuals without atherosclerotic disease, CHD risk is stratified by cholesterol level combined with the number of other risk factors present. Positive risk factors included in the ATP II's algorithm are age (45 years or older in men; 55 years or older, or premature menopause without estrogen-replacement therapy, in women), family history of premature CHD (definite MI or sudden death before age 55 years in the father or other first-degree male relative, or before age 65 years in the mother or other first-degree female relative), current cigarette smoking, hypertension (140/90 mm Hg or greater confirmed on several occasions or the use of antihypertensive medication), low HDL cholesterol level (less than 35 mg/dL confirmed on several occasions), and diabetes mellitus; high HDL cholesterol level (60 mg/dL or greater confirmed on several occasions) is considered a negative risk factor to be subtracted from the number of positive risk factors in primary prevention. CHD risk factors not included for use in the ATP II's algorithm are obesity, which is usually found in conjunction with risk factors that are listed (hypertension, hyperlipidemia, low HDL cholesterol level, and diabetes mellitus), and physical inactivity. All modifiable risk factors are targets for intervention.

Assessment for Dyslipidemia

In individuals without CHD, the ATP II recommends the measurement of total blood cholesterol at least once every 5 years in all adults aged 20 years or older. HDL cholesterol should also be measured if accurate results are available and is used as an integral determinant of CHD risk. Nonfasting samples are adequate for these measurements. In individuals with CHD, a full fasting lipoprotein analysis is the initial assessment. The physician may prefer to perform a full fasting analysis initially in any patient.

In individuals without CHD, the ATP II classifies total cholesterol level less than 200 mg/dL as desirable, 200–239 mg/dL as borderline high, and 240 mg/dL or greater as high. However, because of the continuous and graded relation between cholesterol level and CHD risk, these categories should be regarded not as absolute cut points but as guides for clinical assessment.

In individuals without CHD, if total cholesterol level is desirable and HDL cholesterol level is 35 mg/dL or greater, no intervention is necessary. These individuals should be instructed in dietary recommendations for the general population and in risk factor reduction and should be retested in 5 years. Similar advice should be provided to individuals without CHD who have borderline-high total cholesterol level, HDL cholesterol level of 35 mg/dL or greater, and fewer than two other risk factors; lipid measurements and dietary information should be repeated in 1 to 2 years.

In patients with low HDL cholesterol levels, patients with borderline-high total cholesterol levels and two or more other risk factors, patients with high total cholesterol levels, and patients with CHD, a full fasting lipoprotein analysis is required to determine LDL cholesterol level. In patients recovering from an acute coronary event, LDL cholesterol level may be decreased for several weeks after the event, so LDL cholesterol measurements based on analyses performed during this time may not accurately reflect baseline values.

In a full fasting lipoprotein analysis, total cholesterol, HDL cholesterol, and total triglyceride levels are measured after a 12-hour fast, to allow the removal of chylomicrons from the circulation, and LDL cholesterol level is calculated by using the Friedewald formula, here given for lipid values in milligrams per deciliter:

$$\text{LDL cholesterol} = \text{total cholesterol} - \text{HDL cholesterol} - (\text{triglyceride}/5)$$

This formula is not accurate in patients with triglyceride level greater than 400 mg/dL or in patients with type III hyperlipidemia or apo $E_{2/2}$ phenotype.

Risk Status by Low-Density Lipoprotein Cholesterol Level

In patients without CHD, the ATP II classifies LDL cholesterol level less than 130 mg/dL as desirable, 130–159 mg/dL as borderline high, and 160 mg/dL or greater as high. Patients with desirable LDL cholesterol levels should be instructed in the dietary recommendations for the general population and in risk factor reduction and should be retested in 5 years. HDL cholesterol level less than 35 mg/dL and triglyceride level greater than 200 mg/dL should be treated as necessary.

In patients with borderline-high LDL cholesterol levels, the determination of risk status is guided by the consideration of other risk factors. If fewer than two other risk factors are present, the patient should be instructed in dietary modification and physical activity recommendations and should be retested by lipoprotein analysis in 1 year. If two or more other risk factors are present, or if LDL cholesterol level is high, lipoprotein analysis should be repeated within 1–8 weeks and the average LDL cholesterol value used to decide on treatment. If the LDL cholesterol values differ by more than 30 mg/dL, a third test is required, and treatment decisions should be based on the average of all three. If borderline-high or high LDL cholesterol level is confirmed, a clinical evaluation and lipid-regulating intervention are required. HDL cholesterol level less than 35 mg/dL and triglyceride level greater than 200 mg/dL should also be treated as necessary.

Because of the particularly high risk for a CHD-related event in patients with CHD or other atherosclerotic disease, LDL cholesterol level of 100 mg/dL or less is considered optimal by the ATP II. Patients with optimal LDL cholesterol level should receive individualized instruction on diet and physical activity and should be retested by lipoprotein analysis annually. HDL cholesterol level less than 35 mg/dL and triglyceride level greater than 200 mg/dL should also be treated as necessary. Patients whose LDL cholesterol level is higher than optimal require clinical evaluation and lipid-regulating intervention. Treatment decisions should be based on more than one assessment of LDL cholesterol.

Clinical Evaluation

A thorough clinical evaluation should be performed in patients without CHD who have high LDL cholesterol level or who have borderline-high LDL cholesterol level and two or more other risk factors and in patients with CHD whose LDL cholesterol level is higher than optimal. The clinical evaluation should include a history, physical examination, and basic laboratory tests. The physician should search for manifestations of atherosclerosis (e.g., peripheral pulses, vascular bruits) or dyslipidemia (e.g., corneal arcus, xanthelasmas/xanthomas, hepatosplenomegaly). The purpose of the evaluation is to determine whether the dyslipidemia is secondary to another condition or to diet or drugs, to assess for an underlying genetic disorder, and to refine estimation of the patient's risk status.

Important secondary causes of dyslipidemia include diabetes mellitus; hypothyroidism; nephrotic syndrome; obstructive liver disease; and the use of certain drugs, including progestins, anabolic steroids, corticosteroids, and certain antihypertensive agents. The underlying condition should be treated and, if possible, the responsible drug discontinued. LDL cholesterol level should then be re-evaluated.

The most common familial hyperlipidemias are familial combined hyperlipidemia, polygenic hypercholesterolemia, FH, and type III hyperlipidemia. If a genetic disorder is diagnosed, a family history should be obtained and cholesterol levels measured in family members, thereby potentially identifying other individuals who require lipid-regulating intervention to reduce CHD risk.

Consideration of CHD risk factors besides elevated LDL cholesterol level provides important information for assessing the patient's CHD risk. Modifiable risk factors provide additional targets for intervention, and both modifiable and nonmodifiable risk factors influence treatment decisions by better defining the patient's absolute risk.

Treatment of Hypercholesterolemia

Dietary Therapy

Primary treatment of elevated LDL cholesterol is dietary (see Chapter 24) and includes weight reduction in overweight patients and increased physical activity in sedentary patients. In patients without CHD who have fewer than two other risk factors, dietary therapy should be initiated if LDL cholesterol level is 160 mg/dL or greater; the treatment goal in these patients is LDL cholesterol level less than 160 mg/dL. In patients without CHD who have two or more other risk factors, dietary therapy should be initiated if LDL cholesterol level is 130 mg/dL or greater; the treatment goal in these patients is LDL cholesterol level less than 130 mg/dL. In patients with CHD, dietary therapy should be initiated if LDL cholesterol level is greater than 100 mg/dL; the treatment goal in these patients is LDL cholesterol level of 100 mg/dL or less.

The initial diet in patients without CHD is the Step I Diet, which is recommended for the general population aged 2 years and older. The Step I Diet consists of 30% or less of total calories from fat, 8%–10% of total calories from saturated fat, 10% or less of total calories from polyunsaturated fat, 15% or less of total calories from monounsaturated fat, 55% or more of total calories from carbohydrate, approximately 15% of total calories from protein, less than 300 mg/day of cholesterol, and total calories sufficient to achieve and maintain desirable weight. If, after 3 months' adherence to the Step I Diet, LDL cholesterol level remains elevated, the patient should proceed to the Step II Diet, which further reduces saturated fat to less than 7% of total calories and restricts cholesterol to less than 200 mg/day. In patients already following the Step I Diet at the time of assessment, the Step II Diet should be the initial therapy. The Step II Diet is the initial therapy in patients with CHD. On average, the institution of the Step I Diet in patients following a typical American diet decreases total cholesterol 5%–7%, and a Step II Diet decreases total cholesterol 10%–20%.[26]

Drug Therapy

In patients whose LDL cholesterol level remains elevated despite adherence to maximal dietary therapy, lipid-regulating drugs should be considered in addition to diet (Table 23–2). A 6-month trial is usually required to evaluate response to diet, although a shorter trial of dietary therapy may be preferable in patients with severe hypercholesterolemia that is not expected to be treated satisfactorily by diet and in patients with established atherosclerotic disease. Available lipid-regulating drugs are bile-acid sequestrants, nicotinic acid, 3-hydroxy-3-methylglutaryl coenzyme A (HMG-CoA) reductase inhibitors, fibric acid derivatives, and probucol (see Chapter 25). In postmenopausal women, estrogen-replacement therapy may provide an alternative to drug therapy.

In patients without CHD who have fewer than two other risk factors, drug therapy should be considered if LDL cholesterol level remains 190 mg/dL or greater on maximal dietary therapy; the treatment goal in these patients is LDL cholesterol level less than 160 mg/dL. In patients without CHD who have two or more other risk factors, drug therapy should be considered if LDL cholesterol level remains 160 mg/dL or greater; the treatment goal in these patients is LDL cholesterol level less than 130 mg/dL. In patients with CHD, drug therapy should be considered if LDL cholesterol level remains 130 mg/dL or greater; the treatment goal in these patients is LDL cholesterol level of 100 mg/dL or less. In all patients, drug therapy does not replace dietary therapy but should be used in conjunction with diet.

The ATP II recommends delaying drug therapy in younger patients without CHD (men younger than 35 years and women before menopause) unless LDL cholesterol level is 220 mg/dL or greater, except in patients with additional risk. However, clinical judgment is required to evaluate the patient's overall risk status. Similarly, clinical judgment is required to determine whether to initiate drug therapy in patients with CHD whose LDL cholesterol level is 100 to 129 mg/dL on maximal dietary therapy.

If a 3-month trial of lipid-lowering monotherapy does not adequately reduce LDL cholesterol level, combination drug therapy may be considered. Combination drug therapy may reduce side effects and cost and may increase compliance. Combining drugs with different mechanisms of action is particularly useful in patients with CHD and in patients with severe genetic dyslipidemias, because of the magnitude of lipid lowering required in these patients. Clinical judgment should be used in deciding whether to initiate combination drug therapy in patients with CHD whose LDL cholesterol level remains 100 to 129 mg/dL with a single lipid-regulating drug.

Other Therapies

In a few patients, primarily those with a severe hypercholesterolemia such as FH, LDL cholesterol level may not be adequately lowered even with combination drug therapy. These patients require referral to a lipid specialist, who can recommend specialized treatment such as partial ileal bypass surgery, plasmapheresis, LDL apheresis, plasma exchange, portacaval shunt, or liver transplantation (see Chapter 26).

TABLE 23–2. DRUG SELECTION RECOMMENDATIONS OF THE NATIONAL CHOLESTEROL EDUCATION PROGRAM ADULT TREATMENT PANEL II

Hyperlipidemia	Single Drug	Combination Drug
Elevated LDL cholesterol and triglyceride <200 mg/dL	Bile acid sequestrant HMG-CoA reductase inhibitor Nicotinic acid	Bile acid sequestrant + HMG-CoA reductase inhibitor Bile acid sequestrant + nicotinic acid HMG-CoA reductase inhibitor + nicotinic acid*
Elevated LDL cholesterol and triglyceride 200–400 mg/dL	Nicotinic acid HMG-CoA reductase inhibitor Gemfibrozil	Nicotinic acid + HMG-CoA reductase inhibitor* HMG-CoA reductase inhibitor + gemfibrozil† Nicotinic acid + bile acid sequestrant Nicotinic acid + gemfibrozil

Abbreviations: HMG-CoA, 3-hydroxy-3-methylglutaryl coenzyme A; LDL, low-density lipoprotein.
*Possible increased risk for myopathy or liver dysfunction.
†Increased risk for myopathy; must be used with caution.
From National Cholesterol Education Program: Second report of the Expert Panel on Detection, Evaluation, and Treatment of High Blood Cholesterol in Adults (Adult Treatment Panel II). Circulation 1994; 89:1329.

Treatment of Hypertriglyceridemia

In the ATP II guidelines, total triglyceride level less than 200 mg/dL is considered normal, 200–400 mg/dL is borderline high, 400–1000 mg/dL is high, and greater than 1000 mg/dL is very high. The primary therapy is dietary and should include weight reduction in overweight patients, reduction in dietary intake of saturated fat and cholesterol, institution of a regular program of physical activity, smoking cessation in patients who smoke, and, in certain patients, restricted intake of alcohol.

In hypertriglyceridemic patients with CHD, a family history of CHD, combined high total cholesterol (>240 mg/dL) and low HDL cholesterol (<35 mg/dL) levels, or a genetic hypertriglyceridemia associated with increased CHD risk, drug therapy may be considered to reduce CHD risk. Drug therapy may also be warranted in patients with high or very high triglyceride levels because of the increased risk for pancreatitis.

Treatment of Low Level of High-Density Lipoprotein Cholesterol

In patients with low HDL cholesterol level, the primary therapy is dietary therapy and includes weight reduction in overweight patients, smoking cessation in patients who smoke, and increased physical activity in sedentary patients. Low HDL cholesterol level may be secondary to hypertension, diabetes mellitus, and the use of certain drugs. As possible, these underlying causes should be corrected. In patients requiring drug therapy to lower LDL cholesterol level, drug selection should be guided by the effect on HDL cholesterol.

REFERENCES

1. Nieto FJ, Alonso J, Chambless LE, et al: Population awareness and control of hypertension and hypercholesterolemia: the Atherosclerosis Risk in Communities Study. Arch Intern Med 1995; 155:677.
2. National Cholesterol Education Program: Second report of the Expert Panel on Detection, Evaluation, and Treatment of High Blood Cholesterol in Adults (Adult Treatment Panel II). Circulation 1994; 89:1329.
3. Austin MA, Breslow JL, Hennekens CH, et al: Low-density lipoprotein subclass patterns and risk of myocardial infarction. JAMA 1988; 260:1917.
4. Eisenberg S, Gavish D, Oschry Y, et al: Abnormalities in very low, low, and high density lipoproteins in hypertriglyceridemia: reversal toward normal with bezafibrate treatment. J Clin Invest 1984; 74:470.
5. Patsch JR: Triglyceride-rich lipoproteins and atherosclerosis. Atherosclerosis 1994; 110:S23.
6. Keys A (ed): Coronary heart disease in seven countries [American Heart Association Monograph 29]. Circulation 1970; 41(suppl 1):1.
7. Marmot MG, Syme SL, Kagan A, et al: Epidemiologic studies of coronary heart disease and stroke in Japanese men living in Japan, Hawaii and California: prevalence of coronary and hypertensive heart disease and associated risk factors. Am J Epidemiol 1975; 102:514.
8. Robertson TL, Kato H, Rhoads GG, et al: Epidemiologic studies of coronary heart disease and stroke in Japanese men living in Japan, Hawaii and California: incidence of myocardial infarction and death from coronary heart disease. Am J Cardiol 1977; 39:239.
9. Stamler J, Wentworth D, Neaton JD, for the MRFIT Research Group: Is relationship between serum cholesterol and risk of premature death from coronary heart disease continuous and graded? Findings in 356,222 primary screenees of the Multiple Risk Factor Intervention Trial (MRFIT). JAMA 1986; 256:2823.
10. Anderson KM, Castelli WP, Levy D: Cholesterol and mortality: 30 years of follow-up from the Framingham Study. JAMA 1987; 257:2176.
11. Brown MS, Goldstein JL: A receptor-mediated pathway for cholesterol homeostasis. Science 1986; 232:34.
12. Tybjaerg-Hansen A, Humphries SE: Familial defective apolipoprotein B-100: a single mutation that causes hypercholesterolemia and premature coronary artery disease. Atherosclerosis 1992; 96:91.
13. Jokinen MP, Clarkson TB, Prichard RW: Animal models in atherosclerosis research. Exp Mol Pathol 1985; 42:1.
14. Reiser R, Sorrels MF, Williams MC: Influence of high levels of dietary fats and cholesterol on atherosclerosis and lipid distribution in swine. Circ Res 1959; 7:833.
15. Armstrong ML, Warner ED, Connor WE: Regression of coronary atheromatosis in rhesus monkeys. Circ Res 1970; 27:59.
16. Buchwald H, Varco RL, Matts JP, et al: Effect of partial ileal bypass surgery on mortality and morbidity from coronary heart disease in patients with hypercholesterolemia: report of the Program on the Surgical Control of the Hyperlipidemias (POSCH). N Engl J Med 1990; 323:946.
17. Rossouw JE, Lewis B, Rifkind BM: The value of lowering cholesterol after myocardial infarction. N Engl J Med 1990; 323:1112.
18. Abbott RD, Wilson PWF, Kannel WB, et al: High density lipoprotein cholesterol, total cholesterol screening, and myocardial infarction: the Framingham Study. Arteriosclerosis 1988; 8:207.
19. Wilson PWF, Abbott RD, Castelli WP: High density lipoprotein cholesterol and mortality: the Framingham Heart Study. Arteriosclerosis 1988; 8:737.
20. Gordon DJ, Probstfield JL, Garrison RJ, et al: High-density lipoprotein cholesterol and cardiovascular disease: four prospective American studies. Circulation 1989; 79:8.
21. Austin MA: Plasma triglyceride and coronary heart disease. Arterioscler Thromb 1991; 11:2.
22. Austin MA: Plasma triglyceride as a risk factor for coronary heart disease: the epidemiologic evidence and beyond. Am J Epidemiol 1989; 129:249.
23. Patsch JR, Miesenböck G, Hopferwieser T, et al: Relation of triglyceride metabolism and coronary artery disease: studies in the postprandial state. Arterioscler Thromb 1992; 12:1336.
24. Assmann G, Schulte H: Role of triglycerides in coronary artery disease: lessons from the Prospective Cardiovascular Münster study. Am J Cardiol 1992; 70:10H.
25. Manninen V, Tenkanen L, Koskinen P, et al: Joint effects of serum triglyceride and LDL cholesterol and HDL cholesterol concentrations on coronary heart disease risk in the Helsinki Heart Study: implications for treatment. Circulation 1992; 85:37.
26. Kris-Etherton PM, Krummel D, Russell ME, et al: The effect of diet on plasma lipids, lipoproteins, and coronary heart disease. J Am Diet Assoc 1988; 88:1373.

24 Dyslipoproteinemias/Atherosclerosis: Dietary Therapy

Margo A. Denke, MD
Scott M. Grundy, MD, PhD

The clinical management of patients with lipid disorders begins with dietary therapy. Despite the prominent role for diet, physicians may be hesitant to employ dietary therapy because of doubts about its feasibility and efficacy. This chapter examines, from a physician's perspective, the clinical use of therapeutic diets for lipid disorders. To achieve this goal, the chapter is divided into six sections: (1) the definition of a therapeutic diet, (2) the link between diet and lipoprotein metabolism, (3) the quantitative relationships between nutrient intake and lipoprotein levels, (4) the feasibility and implementation of a therapeutic diet, (5) the efficacy of a cholesterol-lowering diet, and (6) a stepwise approach for the dietary management of patients with specific lipid and lipoprotein patterns.

DEFINITION OF A THERAPEUTIC DIET

The current dietary recommendations of the National Cholesterol Education Program (NCEP)[1] and the American Heart Association[2] are based on the cause-effect relationship between the intake of specific macronutrients and risk factors for coronary heart disease (CHD). These recommendations are prescribed in two steps (Table 24–1) according to the level of CHD risk. CHD risk factors identified by the NCEP are age (45 years or older in men; 55 years or older, or premature menopause without estrogen-replacement therapy, in women), family history of premature CHD (myocardial infarction or sudden death before 55 years of age in father or other first-degree male relative or before 65 years of age in mother or other female first-degree relative), current cigarette smoking, hypertension (≥140/90 mm Hg or taking antihypertensive medication), high-density lipoprotein (HDL) cholesterol less than 35 mg/dL, and diabetes mellitus. The NCEP also includes a negative risk factor: if HDL cholesterol is 60 mg/dL or greater, one risk factor is to be subtracted from the total.

In patients without CHD who have fewer than two CHD risk factors, the Step I Diet is recommended if the low-density lipoprotein (LDL) cholesterol level is 160 mg/dL or greater. The treatment goal for this group is an LDL cholesterol level less than 160 mg/dL. In patients without CHD who have two or more risk factors, the Step I Diet should be initiated if LDL cholesterol level is 130 mg/dL or greater. The treatment goal for this group is an LDL cholesterol level less than 130 mg/dL. If the goal is not reached after 3 months of adherence to the diet, the patient should proceed to the Step II Diet. In patients already following a Step I Diet and in patients with CHD, the Step II Diet is the initial therapy. Educational materials concerning these diets are available from the American Heart Association, the NCEP, the American Dietetic Association, and other groups. To further assist their implementation, a dietitian can be invaluable in providing personalized counseling to the patient and his or her family. Nurses, physician assistants, and other qualified health care professionals can aid the physician in monitoring and reinforcing the diet.[3]

Unfortunately in practice, cholesterol-lowering diets are often perceived as a draconian restriction of the intake of good-tasting foods. Popular jokes support this common misperception: "If I eat any more chicken I am going to grow feathers and start clucking," "If it tastes good—spit it out," and "This diet doesn't make you live longer, it only *seems* longer."

Dietary therapy does not restrict the selection of foods per se. Because the dietary recommendations are defined by the macronutrient content of foods and not the foods themselves, a wide variety can be included in a therapeutic diet as long as the average daily intake meets the guidelines. For example, although the therapeutic diet calls for successive reductions in saturated fat and dietary cholesterol, implementation does not require the elimination of red meat from the diet. The recommendations instead require control of por-

TABLE 24–1. DIETARY THERAPY FOR CORONARY HEART DISEASE PREVENTION

	Recommended Daily Intake	
Nutrient	**Step I Diet**	**Step II Diet**
Total calories	To achieve and maintain desirable weight	To achieve and maintain desirable weight
Total fatty acids	<30% of total calories	<30% of total calories
Saturated	<10% of total calories	<7% of total calories
Polyunsaturated	Up to 10% of total calories	Up to 10% of total calories
Monounsaturated	10%–15% of total calories	10%–15% of total calories
Carbohydrates	50%–60% of total calories	50%–60% of total calories
Protein	10%–20% of total calories	10%–20% of total calories
Cholesterol	<300 mg	<200 mg
Sodium	1650–2400 mg	1650–2400 mg
Alcohol*	<30 g	<30 g

*Twelve ounces of beer, 5 oz of wine, or 1.5 oz of spirits contains 13.6 g of ethanol.

tion sizes of all meats including chicken (6–7 oz cooked meat per day) and selection of meats that are leaner. An example of how easily these diets can be implemented is shown in Table 24–2. Even the Step II Diet can be accomplished with the use of commonly consumed foods, often with only small adjustments in the overall eating plan.

The physician's role in dietary therapy is to prioritize the goals of dietary modification; this prioritizing should be based on the specific lipid goals of dietary therapy and an educated estimate of what can be expected, in quantitative terms, from the implementation of a therapeutic diet. This chapter uses two different frameworks to describe the complex interrelationships among dietary intake, lipoprotein metabolism, and CHD: the first is to consider each lipoprotein class (chylomicrons, very low density lipoprotein [VLDL], LDL, and HDL) and examine how diet may qualitatively influence the lipoprotein's metabolism and atherogenesis. The second is to review how a change in nutrient intake quantitatively effects a change in a patient's lipoprotein levels.

DIET AND LIPOPROTEIN METABOLISM

The function of lipoproteins is to transport the two major blood lipids, cholesterol and triglycerides, from one site to another. In humans, lipoproteins can be divided into four major classes that vary in origin, lipid content, half-life, and fate. Dietary intake can influence each of the four classes of lipoproteins by changing the composition of the lipoprotein particle or by changing its rate of production

TABLE 24–2. SAMPLE ONE-DAY MENUS REFLECTING THE AVERAGE AMERICAN INTAKE AND CHANGES NEEDED TO IMPLEMENT A STEP I DIET AND A STEP II DIET

Average American Intake	Step I Diet	Step II Diet
Breakfast	*Breakfast*	*Breakfast*
Bagel, plain (1 medium)	Bagel, plain (1 medium)	Bagel, plain (1 medium)
Cream cheese, regular (1 tbsp)	**Cream cheese, low-fat (2 tsp)**	**Margarine (2 tsp)**
Cereal, shredded wheat **(1 cup)**	Cereal, shredded wheat **(1½ cups)**	Cereal, shredded wheat **(1½ cups)**
Banana (1 small)	Banana (1 small)	Banana (1 small)
Milk, 2% (1 cup)	**Milk, 1% (1 cup)**	**Milk, skim (1 cup)**
Orange juice (¾ cup)	Orange juice (¾ cup)	Orange juice (¾ cup)
Coffee (1 cup)	Coffee (1 cup)	Coffee (1 cup)
Cream, half and half (1 tbsp)	**Milk, 1% (1 oz)**	**Milk, skim (1 oz)**
Lunch	*Lunch*	*Lunch*
Minestrone soup **(1 cup)**	Minestrone soup **(1 cup)**	Minestrone soup **(1½ cups)**
Roast beef sandwich	Roast beef sandwich	Roast beef sandwich
Whole wheat bread (2 slices)	Whole wheat bread (2 slices)	Whole wheat bread (2 slices)
Lean roast beef (3 oz)	Lean roast beef (3 oz)	Lean roast beef (3 oz)
American cheese, regular (¾ oz)	**American cheese, low-fat (¾ oz)**	**American cheese, low-fat (¾ oz)**
Lettuce (1 leaf)	Lettuce (1 leaf)	Lettuce (1 leaf)
Tomato (3 slices)	Tomato (3 slices)	Tomato (3 slices)
Mayonnaise, regular (1 tbsp)	**Mayonnaise, low-fat (2 tsp)**	**Margarine (2 tsp)**
Fruit and cottage cheese salad	Fruit and cottage cheese salad	Fruit and cottage cheese salad
Cottage cheese, regular (4% fat) (½ cup)	**Cottage cheese, 2% (½ cup)**	**Cottage cheese, 1% (½ cup)**
Peaches, canned in juice (½ cup)	Peaches, canned in juice (½ cup)	Peaches, canned in juice (½ cup)
Apple juice, unsweetened **(6 oz)**	Apple juice, unsweetened **(1 cup)**	Apple juice, unsweetened **(1 cup)**
Dinner	*Dinner*	*Dinner*
Salmon (3 oz)	**Salmon (3 oz)**	**Flounder (3 oz)**
Vegetable oil (1 tsp)	Vegetable oil (1 tsp)	Vegetable oil (1 tsp)
Baked potato (1 medium)	Baked potato (1 medium)	Baked potato (1 medium)
Margarine (2 tsp)	Margarine (2 tsp)	Margarine (2 tsp)
Green beans (½ cup), seasoned with margarine (½ tsp)	Green beans (½ cup), seasoned with margarine (½ tsp)	Green beans (½ cup), seasoned with margarine (½ tsp)
Carrots (½ cup), seasoned with margarine (½ tsp)	Carrots (½ cup), seasoned with margarine (½ tsp)	Carrots (½ cup), seasoned with margarine (½ tsp)
White dinner roll (1 medium)	White dinner roll (1 medium)	White dinner roll (1 medium)
Margarine (1 tsp)	Margarine (1 tsp)	Margarine (1 tsp)
Ice cream, regular (½ cup)	**Ice milk (1 cup)**	**Frozen yogurt (1 cup)**
Iced tea, unsweetened (1 cup)	Iced tea, unsweetened (1 cup)	Iced tea, unsweetened (1 cup)
Snack	*Snack*	*Snack*
Popcorn (3 cups)	Popcorn (3 cups)	Popcorn (3 cups)
Margarine (1 tbsp)	Margarine (1 tbsp)	Margarine (1 tbsp)

Nutritional Analysis

	Average American Intake	Step I Diet	Step II Diet
Calories	2546	2518	2533
Total fat, % kcal	37	29	28
SFA, % kcal	13	8.6	6.6
Cholesterol, mg	241	150	150
Dietary fiber, g	28	32	31

Abbreviation: SFA; saturated fatty acid.

From Kris-Etherton PM, Peterson S, Jaax S, et al: Implementing dietary change. *In* Rifkind BM (ed): Contemporary Issues in Cholesterol Lowering: Clinical and Population Aspects. New York: Marcel Dekker, 1995.

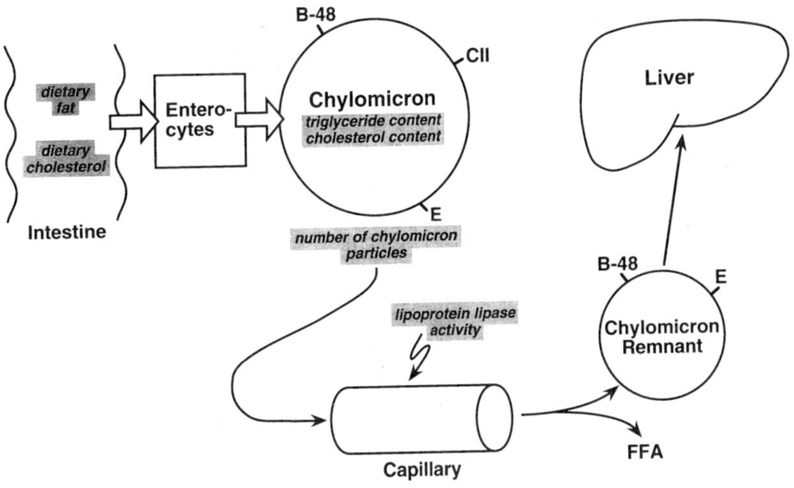

Figure 24–1. The interaction between chylomicron metabolism and diet. Chylomicrons are formed in enterocytes from dietary fat, dietary cholesterol, and endogenous triglycerides. Chylomicrons are secreted into the lymph and join the circulation at the thoracic duct; once they find their way to capillaries, they are acted on by lipoprotein lipase, which removes part of the triglyceride core, creating a chylomicron remnant. The number of chylomicron particles, their cholesterol and triglyceride content, and the activity of lipoprotein lipase are all influenced by dietary intake. *Abbreviations:* FFA, free fatty acid; B-48, apo B-48; CII, apo C-II; E, apo E.

or removal.[4] This section considers each lipoprotein class separately, reviewing its metabolism and its association with atherogenesis and how diet can alter these parameters.

Chylomicrons

Metabolism

Almost all our dietary fat is in the form of triglycerides. Once ingested, triglycerides undergo hydrolysis to fatty acids and monoglycerides under the catalytic action of pancreatic lipase in the small intestine. These fatty acids and monoglycerides, aided by biliary micelles, enter the intestinal mucosa, where they are resynthesized into triglycerides that are then incorporated into chylomicrons for transport.

Chylomicrons are large, spherical lipoproteins having a core of triglycerides and small amounts of cholesteryl esters; the surface coat of chylomicrons consists of unesterified cholesterol, phospholipids, and apolipoproteins. The predominant apolipoprotein is apolipoprotein (apo) B-48. Chylomicrons are generated by intestinal cells, are secreted into the intestinal lymph, and enter the systemic circulation through the thoracic duct (Fig. 24–1). As chylomicrons pass through the circulation, they come into contact with lipoprotein lipase (LPL), an enzyme found on capillary surfaces. LPL hydrolyzes and removes most of the chylomicron's core triglycerides. These triglycerides are, in turn, split into fatty acids and monoglycerides, both of which are taken up by adipose tissue. Adipocytes will reformulate the fatty acids and monoglycerides into triglycerides, storing them for future use. In the plasma, the triglyceride-depleted chylomicron particles, called chylomicron remnants, find their way to the liver, where they are removed.

Hepatic uptake of chylomicron remnants is believed to be mediated through the interaction of the particles' surface components with proteoglycans on the liver cell. Another apolipoprotein, apo E, appears to be involved in this interaction. The half-life of a chylomicron particle is only 20 minutes. However, since fat absorption in the small intestine occurs over a 4- to 6-hour period after ingestion, chylomicrons are often present in nonfasting serum.

Atherogenicity

Chylomicrons theoretically could increase coronary risk in several ways.[5] The most likely link is that chylomicron remnants are directly atherogenic. Another possibility is that chylomicrons, like any triglyceride-rich lipoprotein, raise triglyceride levels, even if only transiently. These triglycerides may enhance the thrombogenic tendency of the plasma and predispose the patient to coronary thrombosis. There is a limited amount of evidence to support each of these mechanisms, and the role that chylomicrons play in atherogenesis is still under investigation.

Diet's Effect on Chylomicron Content

Since all newly absorbed dietary cholesterol enters the body through chylomicrons, increasing the intake of dietary cholesterol will increase the cholesterol content of chylomicrons and chylomicron remnants. If chylomicrons are intrinsically atherogenic, these cholesterol-enriched chylomicron remnants would be particularly atherogenic.

Diet's Effect on Chylomicron Metabolism

Some patients, particularly those with fasting hypertriglyceridemia, have a prolonged duration of the normal 4- to 6-hour postprandial lipemia. A diet high in fat could prolong this period further. Specifically, high-fat diets provide more triglyceride-rich chylomicrons, which compete for clearance with existing triglyceride-containing particles, slowing down all triglyceride clearance.[6] Several studies claim that the duration of postprandial lipemia is increased in patients with premature CHD, suggesting that prolonged postprandial lipemia increases CHD risk.[5] This hypothesis, while attractive, has yet to be substantiated.

An indirect hypothesis linking diet with chylomicron metabolism and CHD is that high-fat diets promote coronary thrombosis.[7] The mechanism remains hypothetical and again is related to the ability of dietary fat to enhance postprandial hypertriglyceridemia, which, in turn, is speculated to promote thrombosis.[8] Some investigators believe that saturated fatty acids are more thrombogenic than are unsaturated fatty acids; stearic acid has been implicated as the most thrombogenic fatty acid.[9] These hypotheses are based on limited research, and whether dietary fat can promote thrombosis has yet to be proved.

Very Low Density Lipoproteins

Metabolism

VLDL is a triglyceride-rich lipoprotein that is formed in the liver. The triglycerides in VLDL are produced endogenously. VLDL particles are smaller than chylomicrons and contain less triglyceride in their lipid cores. The major apolipoprotein of VLDL is apo B-100, but VLDL also contains apo E and the C apolipoproteins, particularly apo C-II and apo C-III. The C apolipoproteins appear to be acquired after VLDL is secreted into the circulation. Apo C-II is required for the activation of LPL.

Like chylomicrons, VLDL particles pass into the peripheral circulation, where the particles interact with LPL and lose triglycerides by hydrolysis (Fig. 24–2). In the process, VLDL particles are transformed into smaller particles called VLDL remnants. Some of these remnants remain in the VLDL density range, whereas others fall into the intermediate-density lipoprotein (IDL) density range. VLDL remnants have one of two fates: they can be taken up by the liver or they can be converted to LDL. The half-life of a VLDL particle is 4–6 hours. Normally, about two thirds of VLDL remnants are removed by the liver. Hepatic uptake is mediated in part through proteoglycan interaction, similar to chylomicron remnant removal. Some VLDL remnants appear to be taken up by LDL receptors located on the surface of liver cells.

Atherogenicity

VLDL particles appear to have more atherogenic potential than do chylomicrons. This may be caused in part by (1) the smaller size of VLDL, which allows the lipoprotein particle to penetrate the arterial wall more readily, (2) the higher content of cholesteryl esters in VLDL, and (3) the presence of apo B-100 instead of apo B-48, the former having a tendency to become trapped within the artery wall. Some investigators believe that VLDL remnants are even more atherogenic than LDL, but not all workers are in agreement.[10]

Many epidemiologic studies indicate that triglyceride levels are positively correlated with the risk for CHD.[11] Since an excess of atherogenic VLDL remnants is present in patients with elevated triglyceride levels, the findings are consistent with the theory that VLDL is atherogenic.[12] High triglyceride levels may, however, induce other changes that additionally promote atherogenesis. For example, in the presence of high triglyceride levels, LDL particles become small and dense, and several reports suggest that small, dense LDL particles are unusually atherogenic.[11] In addition, elevated triglyceride levels are associated with low HDL cholesterol levels, and low HDL cholesterol levels also promote CHD. Finally, as reviewed previously, high triglyceride levels may induce a procoagulant state.[8] Thus, the association between high triglyceride levels and increased CHD risk may have several explanations, and VLDL may be only part of the explanation.

Diet's Effect on Very Low Density Lipoprotein Content

As with chylomicrons, higher intake of dietary cholesterol increases the cholesteryl ester content of VLDL particles. These cholesteryl ester–enriched particles may be particularly atherogenic in themselves or may, in turn, be converted to LDL particles that are similarly cholesterol-enriched.

Diet's Effect on Very Low Density Lipoprotein Metabolism

Although it might be expected that high-fat diets would raise VLDL levels and low-fat diets would lower them, just the opposite occurs. Low-fat, high-carbohydrate diets tend to raise fasting triglyceride levels, and high-fat diets tend to lower them.[13] This association between the fat content of the diet and fasting VLDL levels results from several factors: (1) fatty acids released from chylomicrons generated during a high-fat meal largely enter adipose tissue and are not directly available to the liver for resynthesis and incorporation into VLDL triglycerides; (2) by an unknown mechanism, low-fat, high-carbohydrate diets increase hepatic synthesis of triglycerides; and (3) low-fat diets may also reduce the synthesis of LPL, which, in turn, would reduce hydrolysis rates of VLDL triglycerides, prolonging their time in the circulation. High-carbohydrate diets generate VLDL particles that are larger but not increased in number. Thus, although these diets raise VLDL levels, they do not raise LDL levels because high-carbohydrate diets do not increase the output of apo B-100.

An interesting question is whether the different classes of fatty acids (saturated, monounsaturated, and polyunsaturated) have different effects on VLDL triglyceride levels.[14] Several reports suggest that saturated fatty acids lead to slightly higher VLDL levels than do unsaturated fatty acids, particularly polyunsaturated fatty acids. Polyunsaturated fatty acids can be further subclassified into two forms. The most abundant form of polyunsaturated fatty acids in the diet is the omega-6 type, of which linoleic acid is the major representative. Linoleic acid is derived mainly from vegetable oils. Compared with saturated and monounsaturated fatty acids, linoleic acid may have a VLDL-lowering action. In most individuals, the effect is relatively small, but in those with hypertriglyceridemia, it can be substantial. However, omega-3 fatty acids, which occur

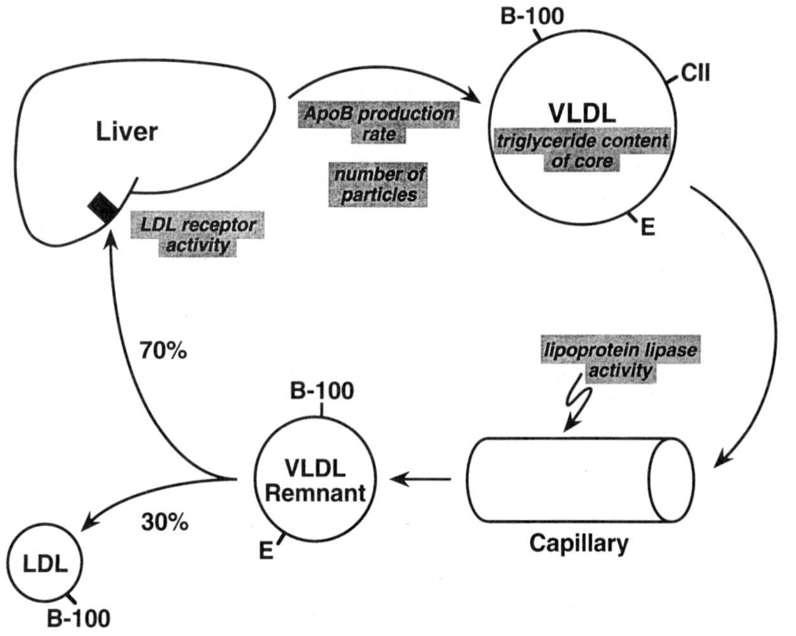

Figure 24–2. The interaction between VLDL metabolism and diet. Very low density lipoprotein (VLDL) particles are formed in the liver and secreted directly into the circulation. Apo B-100 is the major apoprotein of VLDL. Similar to chylomicrons, VLDL particles undergo catabolism by lipoprotein lipase, creating VLDL remnants. These remnants have two fates: one is to be taken up by hepatic low-density lipoprotein (LDL) receptors, and the other is to undergo further loss of core triglycerides and enrichment of core esterified cholesterol to become LDL. The production rate of apo B, the number of VLDL particles, the triglyceride content of the VLDL particle, and the activity of lipoprotein lipase are all influenced by dietary intake. *Abbreviations:* LDL, low-density lipoprotein; B-100, apo B-100; CII, apo C-II; E, apo E.

predominantly in fish oils, have a much greater triglyceride-lowering action.[15] They interfere with the formation of VLDL triglycerides in the liver and, as a result, the newly secreted VLDL particles are relatively depleted in triglycerides. It is of interest that the number of particles is not reduced, only their triglyceride content. Most of these lipoproteins are rapidly converted to LDL. Thus, although omega-3 fatty acids lower VLDL levels, they do not reduce total apo B-100 levels, and they often increase LDL cholesterol concentrations.

Another nutritional factor that raises VLDL levels is obesity. Obese patients have an increased synthesis of VLDL triglycerides.[16] Indeed, the total number of VLDL particles secreted by the liver appears to be increased in obese individuals. This response gives rise to an increase in both VLDL triglyceride and VLDL cholesterol levels and, since excess VLDL can be converted to LDL, to an increase in LDL levels.

A final dietary factor affecting VLDL triglycerides is alcohol. High intake of alcohol increases the synthesis of triglycerides in the liver and raises serum triglyceride levels.[17] Alcohol appears to increase the amount of triglycerides carried in each VLDL particle but not the total number of VLDL particles secreted by the liver. Hence, alcohol does not raise LDL levels, and it is doubtful that alcohol-induced hypertriglyceridemia is an atherogenic dyslipidemia.

Low-Density Lipoproteins

Metabolism

LDL particles contain mostly cholesteryl ester in their lipid cores. The only apoprotein of LDL is apo B-100. LDL is derived from the catabolism of VLDL remnants (Fig. 24–3). The removal of LDL from the circulation is relatively slow and occurs over a 2- to 3-day period in normal subjects. As a result, relatively large quantities of LDL accumulate in serum. Normally about two thirds of serum total cholesterol is contained in the LDL fraction. LDL is cleared from the circulation mainly by the liver; specific receptors residing on the surface of hepatic cells recognize the apo B-100 portion of the LDL surface.

Since LDL receptors are responsible for the removal of most serum LDL, the activity of LDL receptors is an important factor that controls serum concentrations of LDL. The expression of LDL receptors—that is, LDL receptor activity—depends on two factors: (1) genetic control of receptor synthesis and (2) metabolic control of receptor synthesis. Some individuals (about 1 in 500) inherit a defect in the gene encoding for LDL receptors. Normally, two alleles for the LDL receptor gene, one from each parent, are physiologically active and together define LDL receptor synthesis. When one gene is defective, LDL receptor synthesis falls by half, and serum LDL levels therefore double. The resulting condition is called heterozygous familial hypercholesterolemia. Absence of both genes results in homozygous familial hypercholesterolemia, characterized by marked elevations of LDL and severe early disease manifestations, including atherosclerotic cardiovascular disease. Other genetic factors appear to affect LDL receptor synthesis, and current research is directed toward elucidating other genetically determined control points. This research promises to shed new light on the causes of hypercholesterolemia. Beyond genetic control, however, LDL receptor synthesis depends on metabolic factors[18] such as the concentration of unesterified cholesterol within liver cells. A high content of cholesterol within the liver leads to suppression of LDL receptor synthesis, resulting in an increase in circulating LDL levels. Conversely, a reduced hepatic cholesterol content derepresses receptor synthesis, resulting in a reduction in serum LDL levels.

Two other regulating factors determine the LDL cholesterol level: (1) the rate of conversion of VLDL to LDL and (2) the amount of cholesterol carried in each LDL particle. A high input of LDL occurs in obese patients, in whom the secretion of VLDL is raised, and in some conditions such as familial combined hyperlipidemia, in which secretion of VLDL particles may be increased because of genetic factors. Finally, some individuals have an increased cholesterol level because of an abnormally high content of cholesterol in LDL particles. Reasons for this latter defect remain to be determined.

Atherogenicity

There is strong evidence that LDL is an atherogenic lipoprotein.[19] First, epidemiologic observations indicate that individuals with higher levels of LDL are at increased risk for CHD. Second, in genetic forms of elevated LDL cholesterol—for example, familial hypercholesterolemia—premature CHD is common. Third, in experimental animals, induction of high levels of LDL cholesterol results in rapid development of atherosclerosis. Fourth, in studies using model systems that simulate the arterial wall, LDL behaves in an atherogenic manner. Fifth, in clinical trials in which LDL cholesterol levels are lowered, rates of CHD are significantly reduced. Thus, there is little question that high levels of LDL increase the risk for CHD.

A new theory linking LDL particles with atherosclerosis involves the mechanism by which LDL is deposited in the arterial wall.[20] LDL is not normally taken up by macrophages in the arterial wall because macrophages have low LDL receptor activity. If LDL is modified, however, it is avidly taken up by macrophages. One type of modification of LDL occurs when the particle is exposed to oxygen free radicals that alter apo B-100 and fatty acid esters; even minimally oxidized LDL takes on highly atherogenic properties.

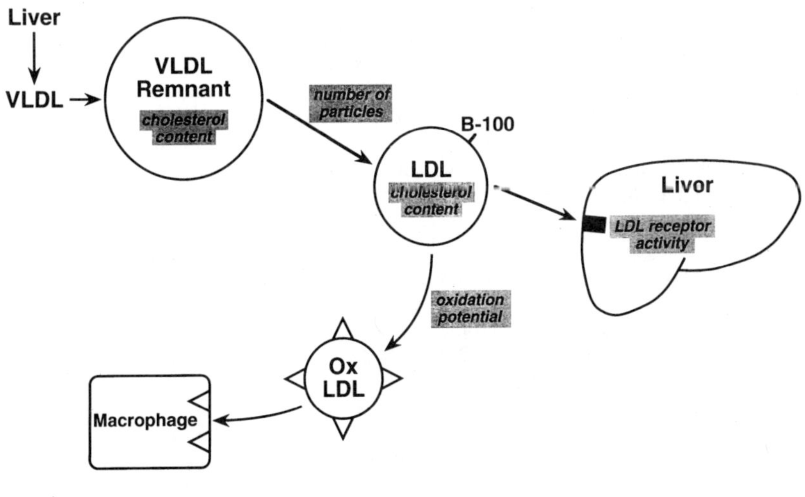

Figure 24–3. The interaction between LDL metabolism and diet. Low-density lipoprotein (LDL) particles are formed from very low density lipoprotein (VLDL) remnants. LDL is removed from the circulation by specific cellular receptors in the liver. If LDL becomes oxidized (Ox LDL), it is recognized by the macrophage scavenger receptor. The cholesterol content of LDL, the number of LDL particles, the LDL receptor activity, and the oxidation potential of LDL are all influenced by dietary intake. *Other abbreviation:* B 100, apo B-100.

Diet's Effect on Low-Density Lipoprotein Composition

The fatty acid content of LDL in part reflects dietary intake. For example, when LDL particles become enriched in polyunsaturated fatty acids, they are more susceptible to oxidation than when they are enriched with monounsaturated or saturated fatty acids.[21]

Vegetables and fruits contain vitamins, phenols, and other non-nutritive compounds that have antioxidant properties and may protect LDL from oxidation.[22] The substances that have been best characterized to date are the antioxidant vitamins. Vitamin E and beta carotene can be incorporated into LDL particles, and supplementation with these vitamins produces LDL particles that are less susceptible to oxidation. Diets high in vitamin C raise plasma levels of vitamin C and also may protect LDL against oxidation.

Diet's Effect on Low-Density Lipoprotein Metabolism

Many studies indicate that LDL levels respond to changes in dietary cholesterol and saturated fat intake; most of this change is mediated by changes in LDL receptor activity.[23] High intake of dietary cholesterol raises hepatic cholesterol content and suppresses LDL receptor synthesis. Serum LDL cholesterol concentrations consequently increase. Three common saturated fatty acids have been shown to raise LDL cholesterol levels: palmitic acid, myristic acid, and lauric acid. These saturated fatty acids raise LDL cholesterol levels by repressing LDL receptor activity. Recently, another type of fatty acid, trans-monounsaturated fatty acids, have also been shown to increase LDL levels.[24] The mechanism by which trans-fatty acids increase LDL cholesterol levels is unknown.

High-Density Lipoproteins

Metabolism

The final major system for lipid transport consists of HDL. The HDL system is made up of a variety of small lipoproteins that are smaller than LDL, but like LDL contain predominantly cholesteryl ester in their cores. Almost all HDL particles contain apo A-I as their major apolipoprotein. The HDL system can be further described by several classifications. One grouping divides HDL into smaller and larger particles, the most common small particle called HDL_3 and the larger particle called HDL_2. All HDL_2 and HDL_3 particles contain apo A-I. In addition, some particles in each subgroup contain apo A-II. This observation leads to another classification of HDL into HDL having only apo A-I (HDL A-I only) and HDL having both apo A-I and apo A-II (HDL A-I:A-II). It is likely that other subspecies of HDL will be characterized as having functional significance, but such properties have not been as well characterized.

The complexity of the preceding description of HDL is mirrored by the complexity of what is known about HDL metabolism. Many steps in HDL metabolism are not fully understood, but it seems that it is best described as a cycle. Figure 24–4 illustrates the metabolism of HDL A-I only, but presumably that for HDL A-I:A-II is similar. The cycle begins with HDL_3. The generation of HDL_3 begins with apo A-I, which is synthesized in both liver and gut and is secreted into the circulation. This free apo A-I serves as the scaffolding on which the HDL_3 particle is built, and the apo A-I becomes associated with phospholipids and unesterified cholesterol, which form the elements of the surface coat. At first, the HDL particle may contain only the components of the surface coat; this rudimentary lipoprotein has been called nascent HDL.[25] When nascent HDL comes into contact with the enzyme lecithin–cholesterol acyltransferase (LCAT), some of the surface coat cholesterol is esterified and becomes incorporated into the core. Additional unesterified cholesterol can be transferred from the surface of cells or from other lipoproteins on contact with nascent HDL. Through interaction with LCAT, this cholesterol is also esterified and added to the core. The final result is HDL_3.

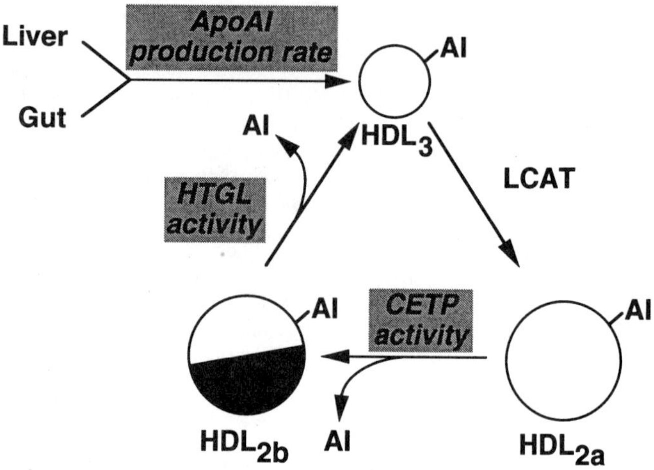

Figure 24–4. The interaction between HDL metabolism and diet. The metabolism of high-density lipoprotein (HDL) is best described as a cycle. The cycle is initiated by apo A-I synthesis, which occurs in both the liver and gut. Once this apo A-I becomes associated with phospholipids, cholesterol, and cholesteryl esters, it forms a small HDL_3 particle. Through the action of lecithin–cholesterol acyltransferase (LCAT), this small HDL_3 becomes further enriched with esterified cholesterol in its core, forming HDL_{2a}. Facilitated by cholesteryl ester transfer protein (CETP), HDL_3 interacts with triglyceride-rich lipoproteins. The core esterified cholesterol from HDL_{2a} is exchanged for the core triglycerides from very low density lipoprotein (VLDL) and chylomicrons. The resultant particle is called HDL_{2b}. Through the action of hepatic triglyceride lipase (HTGL), these triglycerides *(depicted in black)* are removed from HDL_{2b}, forming the smaller HDL_3. The cycle continues, and with each turn a small amount of apo A-I is lost. The production rate of apo A-I, the activity of CETP, and the activity of HTGL are all influenced by dietary intake.

Further accumulation of core cholesteryl ester leads to expansion of HDL_3 into a larger lipoprotein, HDL_{2a}. The latter undergoes further transformation by interaction with cholesteryl ester transfer protein (CETP). This protein aids the transfer of cholesteryl ester from HDL_{2a} to VLDL and chylomicrons. In addition, CETP transfers triglycerides from both VLDL and chylomicrons to HDL_{2a}. The result of this exchange is a triglyceride-enriched form of HDL_2 called HDL_{2b}. The latter then interacts with hepatic triglyceride lipase (HTGL), which degrades HDL_{2b} back to HDL_3, thus completing the HDL cycle. It appears that at each turn of the HDL cycle, some apo A-I is lost from the system. The average half-life of apo A-I is 5 days. If the cycle turns at a high rate, which may result from high levels of CETP or HTGL, the total pool size of HDL will be diminished. This is detected clinically as a low HDL cholesterol level.

Atherogenicity

Many epidemiologic studies reveal an inverse relationship between HDL cholesterol levels and risk for CHD.[26] Thus, a low HDL cholesterol level has been designated as a major risk factor for CHD. Just why a low level of HDL cholesterol would predispose an individual to CHD is not clear. Some investigators believe that HDL promotes "reverse cholesterol transport," that is, the removal of cholesterol from tissues so that it can be transported to the liver and excreted. Presumably this mechanism would extend to the arterial wall, where HDL might remove unesterified cholesterol found in atherosclerotic plaque. Alternatively, HDL may protect LDL against potentially atherogenic changes (e.g., oxidation and aggregation). Some changes in HDL levels appear to be associated particularly with CHD risk; for instance, the strongest inverse correlations between CHD and HDL are found for the HDL_2 and HDL A-I only subfractions. Generally these changes are manifested clinically by a low HDL cholesterol level.

In general, factors that lead to a decrease in HDL cholesterol levels should increase the risk for CHD. Various analyses suggest that about half the variation in HDL levels in the general population is explained by genetic factors.[27] The genes controlling the synthesis of apo A-I and HTGL appear to have the greatest effect on HDL levels. However, other nongenetic factors also affect HDL levels. Three of the most important are obesity, cigarette smoking, and lack of exercise. A favorable change in these factors provides one means to increase HDL cholesterol levels. Besides obesity, other dietary factors affect HDL concentrations,[28] and these can be reviewed briefly.

Diet's Effect on High-Density Lipoprotein Composition

Because of the complexity of the metabolism of HDL and its varying states, it has yet to be established if dietary intake alters HDL composition.

Diet's Effect on High-Density Lipoprotein Metabolism

The different dietary fatty acids appear to have a mild effect on HDL cholesterol levels.[28] The highest levels of HDL cholesterol have been observed in countries where large amounts of cholesterol-raising saturated fatty acids are consumed. In Finland, where the intake of saturated fatty acids is very high, average levels of HDL cholesterol are the highest in the world. Monounsaturated fatty acids also sustain a relatively high concentration of HDL cholesterol, almost as high as occurs with the dietary saturates. In contrast, a high intake of polyunsaturated fatty acids often produces a reduction in HDL cholesterol levels. The latter effect usually is demonstrable only when the intake of polyunsaturated fatty acids is more than 10% of energy; over the usual ranges of consumption of polyunsaturates, HDL cholesterol levels change little. Another category, the trans–fatty acids, also appears to produce a modest reduction in HDL cholesterol concentrations.

In contrast to the modest effect of different types of fatty acids on HDL cholesterol levels, the total fat content of the diet exerts a major effect on HDL cholesterol levels.[28] Diets that are low in fat (and high in carbohydrate) produce a much more pronounced reduction in HDL cholesterol levels. This effect appears to be the result of a decrease in synthesis of apo A-I. Whether the HDL-lowering action of high-carbohydrate diets raises the risk for CHD is a matter of dispute.

Finally, alcohol has been shown to raise HDL levels.[29] The mechanism for this action is unknown, but high intake of alcohol may inhibit the activities of both CETP and HTGL and, if so, HDL levels should rise. Epidemiologic surveys suggest that moderate intake of alcohol exerts a protective effect against CHD.[30] If true, some of this protective action might be mediated through an increase in HDL levels.

THE QUANTITATIVE RELATIONSHIP BETWEEN NUTRIENT INTAKE AND LIPID LEVELS

To complement the preceding review of the effects of diet on lipoprotein metabolism, we shift our frame of reference from lipoproteins to nutrients and discuss the effects of specific nutrients on lipid and lipoprotein levels. Because of the large number of studies evaluating this relationship, we can estimate in a quantitative fashion the expected effect of a change in nutrient intake.

Body Weight/Energy Balance

Perhaps the most important factor influencing serum lipid levels is an imbalance between energy intake and energy expenditure. The latest census-based national survey shows that Americans are becoming more obese.[31] This rise in the prevalence of obesity likely results from both an abundance in the food supply and a reduction in leisure time activities that involve physical activity.[32]

The Lipid Consequences of Excess Body Weight

Multiple cross-sectional population studies have shown that total cholesterol and LDL cholesterol levels correlate positively with body weight.[33, 34] Several large, prospective studies have observed that when participants gain weight, their total cholesterol levels rise. Conversely, when participants lose weight, serum cholesterol levels fall. These same associations have been observed in small, metabolic-ward studies and in meta-analyses of studies on exercise-induced weight loss[35] and diet-induced weight loss.[36] The Framingham Study has estimated that for every 10-lb weight gain, the total cholesterol level increases 7 mg/dL in men and 5 mg/dL in women.[37]

More striking is the association between body weight and HDL cholesterol levels. HDL cholesterol levels are inversely associated with body weight, and triglyceride levels are positively associated. To estimate the relative weight of a patient, the body mass index (BMI) (kg/m^2) can be calculated. For women, a BMI of 24–30 is considered overweight, and a BMI greater than 30 is obese (Table 24–3). For men, a BMI of 25–30 is overweight, and a BMI greater than 30 is considered obese (Table 24–4). In general, obese individuals—both men and women—have HDL cholesterol levels that are 5–10 mg/dL lower and triglyceride levels that are 35–110 mg/dL higher than those of their lean counterparts.

The Lipid Benefits of Weight Reduction

When weight loss occurs during cholesterol-lowering dietary modification, as in the Diet-Heart Feasibility Study,[38] the Multiple Risk Factor Intervention Trial (MRFIT),[39] and the Lipid Research Clinics Coronary Primary Prevention Trial,[40] greater cholesterol lowering is achieved. Specifically, in the MRFIT study, the Step I Diet produced on average a 9-mg/dL fall in LDL cholesterol, whereas dietary modification plus a 10-lb weight loss produced an average 14-mg/dL fall in LDL cholesterol levels.

Weight reduction through either caloric restriction or caloric expenditure has also been shown to lower triglyceride levels and raise HDL cholesterol levels. The time course of these changes should be noted.[41] Triglyceride levels change within a few days after changing caloric intake, but HDL cholesterol levels measured during a hypocaloric diet may be even lower than before the diet was initiated. After weight loss has been achieved and a steady state in weight is reestablished, HDL cholesterol levels typically rise over a 3- to 6-month period to a higher concentration.

Promoting Physical Activity: Weight Maintenance Plus Additional Lipid Benefits

Physical activity improves energy balance and can promote weight loss. The addition of exercise to the weight loss program will enhance the increase in HDL cholesterol levels above that of weight reduction alone.[42] Even if a patient does not lose weight, an increase in physical activity will increase HDL cholesterol levels. The effects of exercise on increasing HDL cholesterol vary with the intensity of exercise. Modest programs may result in a 2- to 3-mg/dL increase, and a vigorous aerobic program can produce an 8- to 10-mg/dL increase.[43]

Macronutrients

The macronutrient sources of energy—protein, fat, and carbohydrate—account for a substantial proportion of the effects of diet

TABLE 24–3. TRANSLATING BODY MASS INDEX CATEGORIES INTO SPECIFIC BODY WEIGHT (IN POUNDS) FOR COMMON MEN'S HEIGHTS (IN FEET AND INCHES)* WITH 1959 METROPOLITAN WEIGHT FOR MEDIUM FRAME FOR COMPARISON†

Height (ft/in)	Metropolitan Life	Body Mass Index Category					
		≤21.0	21.1–23	23.1–25	25.1–27	27.1–30	>30
5′4″	130	122	123–134	135–145	146–157	158–174	>174
5′5″	133	126	127–138	139–150	151–162	163–180	>180
5′6″	136	130	131–142	143–155	156–167	168–186	>188
5′7″	140	134	135–147	148–159	160–172	173–191	>191
5′8″	145	138	139–151	152–164	165–177	178–197	>197
5′9″	149	142	143–155	156–169	170–183	184–203	>203
5′10″	153	146	147–160	161–174	175–188	189–209	>209
5′11″	158	150	151–165	166–179	180–193	194–215	>215
6′0″	162	155	156–169	170–184	185–199	200–221	>221
6′1″	166	159	160–174	175–189	190–204	205–227	>227
6′2″	171	163	164–179	180–194	195–210	211–233	>233
6′3″	176	168	169–184	185–200	201–216	217–240	>240

*Adapted from Bray GA, Gray DS: Obesity Part I: Pathogenesis. *West J Med* 1988; 149:429–441.
†The Steering Committee of the American Heart Association: Cardiovascular and risk factor evaluation of healthy American adults. Circulation 1986; 75(6):1356A.

on serum lipids and lipoproteins. The quantitative effects of each nutrient group can be reviewed.

Protein

In certain animal species, dietary protein of animal origin can raise serum cholesterol levels. Studies in humans, however, have failed to demonstrate a consistent lipid-raising effect of animal protein or a lipid-lowering effect of vegetable protein. In the United States, the intake of dietary protein typically falls within a narrow range of 10%–20% of energy. Since protein appears to have a neutral effect on serum lipids, protein theoretically could be used as a substitute source of energy for macronutrients known to raise serum cholesterol levels. However, dietary protein is expensive, and an excess of dietary protein may have deleterious effects such as hastening the development of chronic renal insufficiency. For these reasons, the macronutrient emphasis in a cholesterol-lowering diet has focused on the balance between energy from carbohydrate and energy from fat.

Dietary Fat Versus Dietary Carbohydrate

Current recommendations call for a reduction of energy from total fat and an increase in energy from carbohydrate. These recommendations are made on the assumption that the major effect of diet on serum lipids is mediated by both the quantity and quality of dietary fat. However, data clearly indicate that the total fat content per se of the diet has little effect on total and LDL cholesterol levels if the fat is low in saturated fatty acids. Nonetheless, since all naturally occurring fats are a mixture of saturated, monounsaturated, and polyunsaturated fatty acids, strategies to reduce the total fat content of the diet in general also reduce the saturated fatty acid content of the diet. Hence, a simplistic approach in implementing a cholesterol-lowering diet is to eliminate as much fat as possible.

Unfortunately, if fat intake is severely restricted and carbohydrate intake is increased, in addition to a decrease in LDL cholesterol levels, an increase in triglyceride levels and a decrease in HDL cholesterol levels will occur.[44] Carbohydrates tend to raise triglyceride levels and lower HDL cholesterol levels, with clinically signifi-

TABLE 24–4. TRANSLATING BODY MASS INDEX CATEGORIES INTO SPECIFIC BODY WEIGHT (IN POUNDS) FOR COMMON WOMEN'S HEIGHTS (IN FEET AND INCHES)* WITH 1959 METROPOLITAN WEIGHT FOR MEDIUM FRAME FOR COMPARISON†

Height (ft/in)	Metropolitan Life	Body Mass Index Category					
		≤21.0	21.1–23	23.1–25	25.1–27	27.1–30	>30
4′10″	102	100	101–110	111–119	120–129	130–143	>143
4′11″	104	104	105–114	115–124	125–133	134–148	>148
5′0″	107	107	108–118	119–128	129–138	139–153	>153
5′1″	110	111	112–122	123–132	133–143	144–158	>158
5′2″	113	115	116–126	127–136	137–147	148–164	>164
5′3″	116	118	119–130	131–141	142–152	153–169	>169
5′4″	120	122	123–134	135–145	146–157	158–174	>174
5′5″	123	126	127–138	139–150	151–162	163–180	>180
5′6″	128	130	131–142	143–155	156–167	168–186	>186
5′7″	132	134	135–147	148–159	160–172	173–191	>191
5′8″	136	138	139–151	152–164	165–177	178–197	>197
5′9″	140	142	143–155	156–169	170–183	184–203	>203
5′10″	144	146	147–160	161–174	175–188	189–209	>209

*Adapted from Bray GA, Gray DS: Obesity Part I: Pathogenesis. *West J Med* 1988; 149:429–441.
†The Steering Committee of the American Heart Association: Cardiovascular and risk factor evaluation of healthy American adults. Circulation 1986; 75(6):1356A.

cant reductions seen when very low fat diets are consumed (i.e., less than 25% of calories from fat or more than 60% of calories from carbohydrate).[45] In normolipidemic subjects, the magnitude of the increase in triglyceride level resulting from very low fat diets is typically 30–100 mg/dL, with a concomitant reduction in HDL cholesterol of 3–8 mg/dL. Although some have argued that these lipid changes with high-carbohydrate, very low fat diets are transient,[46] an international sampling of lipid levels in young boys consuming diverse diets indicates that the relationship between carbohydrate/fat intake and HDL cholesterol levels is chronic and graded.[47] Since the recommended diets suggest a modest restriction in total fat to 30% of calories, the appearance of diet-induced high triglyceride levels and low HDL cholesterol levels may be limited to those individuals who have self-imposed, extreme restrictions in dietary fat intake.

Type of Fat

Fat is a mixture of saponifiable and unsaponifiable fractions. The saponifiable fraction represents 95% of the fat and is composed of triglycerides: three fatty acids attached by ester linkage to a glycerol backbone. There are three major classes of fatty acids, characterized by the presence of double bonds in the fatty acid carbon chain: saturated, monounsaturated, and polyunsaturated fatty acids. Although fat is typically characterized by its predominant fatty acid (e.g., a "saturated fat"), every fat contains a mixture of the three fatty acids (Table 24–5).

Saturated Fatty Acids. On the basis of results from metabolic-ward diet studies, a change in saturated fatty acid intake explains 60%–80% of the change observed in total cholesterol levels caused by isocaloric dietary modifications. For this reason, the primary focus of a cholesterol-lowering diet should be a reduction in saturated fatty acids.[48] Animal fats are rich in saturated fatty acids, but a few vegetable oils, notably palm kernel oil, coconut oil, palm oil, cocoa butter, and cottonseed oil, have a high content of saturated fatty acids as well (see Table 24–5).[49] The estimated intake of saturated fatty acid in the American diet is 20–60 g/day. Four saturated fatty acids account for 90% of the saturated fatty acids in the American diet: lauric acid (C12:0), myristic acid (C14:0), palmitic acid (C16:0), and stearic acid (C18:0). Only three of the four common saturated fatty acids raise serum cholesterol levels (denoted as S′ in Table 24–5). Stearic acid does not raise total or LDL cholesterol levels.

Although one can select specific fats for their saturated fat content (see Table 24–5), most saturated fat is consumed not as fat but as part of food: fatty meats, whole-fat dairy products, and fat hidden in products such as baked goods or casseroles. In general, ingestion of 10 g of saturated fatty acids daily for several weeks will raise total and LDL cholesterol levels 8–10 mg/dL.[50, 51] The effects of intermittent ingestion depend on the average intake of saturated fat for a several-week period.[52]

TABLE 24–5. FATTY ACID COMPOSITION OF COMMON FATS AND OILS RANKED BY CHOLESTEROL-RAISING SATURATED FATTY ACID CONTENT

Fat or Oil	S	S′	M	P	P/S Ratio
Palm kernel	81	72	11	2	0.0
Coconut	87	70	6	2	0.0
Palm	49	45	37	9	0.2
Butter oil	62	39	29	4	0.1
Beef tallow	50	30	42	4	0.1
Cocoa butter	60	26	33	3	0.1
Lard	39	25	45	11	0.3
Cottonseed	26	24	18	52	2.0
Chicken fat	30	23	50	21	0.7
Olive	14	11	74	8	0.6
Corn	13	11	24	59	4.6
Soybean	14	10	23	58	4.0
Peanut	17	10	46	32	1.9
Safflower	9	6	12	75	8.2
Canola	7	5	56	33	4.9
Safflower, high-oleic	6	5	75	14	2.3

Abbreviations: S, total saturated fatty acids, according to the definition currently used by the Food and Drug Administration; S′, cholesterol-raising saturated fatty acids (C12:0, C14:0, C16:0); M, monounsaturated fatty acids; P, polyunsaturated fatty acids.

From Denke MA: Diet and lifestyle modification and its relationship to atherosclerosis. Med Clin North Am 1994; 78:197–223.

Monounsaturated Fatty Acids. Monounsaturated fatty acids can be subcategorized by the positional isomer of the double bond: cis monounsaturated and trans monounsaturated.

Cis–Monounsaturated Fatty Acids. The most common cis–monounsaturated fatty acid is oleic acid (C18:1). Cis–monounsaturated fats are ubiquitous in both animal and vegetable fats. Although animal fats are high in oleic acid, they are also rich in saturated fatty acids. Low–saturated fat vegetable oils with more than 50% of their fatty acids as oleic acid include olive oil, canola oil, high-oleic safflower oil, and high-oleic sunflower oil (see Table 24–5).

The average intake of oleic acid is 20–50 g/day, with half coming from animal and half from vegetable sources. Oleic acid is neutral in that it neither raises nor lowers total and LDL cholesterol levels.[53] Diets high in oleic acid and low in saturated fatty acids, as consumed during the 1950s in the Mediterranean region, have been associated with low rates of CHD.[54]

Trans–Monounsaturated Fatty Acids. Although most monounsaturated fatty acids are of the cis configuration, trans-configured monounsaturates can be found in hydrogenated vegetable oils as well as in certain meat fats. Hydrogenation occurs naturally by action of bacterial degradation of fatty acids in ruminant animals; hence, small amounts of trans–fatty acids are present in milk fat, beef fat, and mutton fat. Hydrogenation is also a fat-processing technique by which vegetable oils with undesirable characteristics (melting point, tendency to become rancid, etc.) are altered to form hydrogenated fats with more desirable characteristics.[55] Hydrogenation converts polyunsaturated fatty acids into cis–monounsaturated fatty acids and trans–monounsaturated fatty acids; lesser quantities of stearic acid and trans–polyunsaturated fatty acids are also formed.

The estimated American intake of trans–fatty acids is 6–8 g/day. One third of the dietary trans–fatty acids comes from animal fats, whereas two thirds comes from hydrogenated vegetable oils. The trans–fatty acid content of a particular product containing hydrogenated oil depends on its manufacturing characteristics.[56] To remove easily oxidized polyunsaturated fatty acids, only minimal hydrogenation is required. For example, snack foods such as potato chips may contain 3%–10% of total fatty acids as trans–fatty acids. To change the melting point of a fat, more extensive hydrogenation is required. For example, tub margarines contain 13%–20% of total fat as trans–fatty acid, whereas stick margarines contain 25%–35% of total fat as trans–fatty acid. To change the properties of the fat to mimic the shortening quality of lard, even more extensive hydrogenation is required.

Several studies suggest that a specific trans–monounsaturated fatty acid, elaidic acid (C18:1), raises total and LDL cholesterol levels compared with oleic acid.[24] However, the overall effect of hydrogenated fats depends on what they are substituted for. Metabolic diet studies have clearly shown that hydrogenated fats, when substituted for more-saturated fats such as butter and lard, lower cholesterol levels. When substituted for less-saturated fats such as corn oil and safflower oil, however, hydrogenated fats raise cholesterol levels.

Trans–fatty acids may be one-third less potent than saturated fatty acids in raising total and LDL cholesterol levels. Ingestion of 8 g of elaidic acid can raise total and LDL cholesterol levels 5–7 mg/dL.

High doses (34 g/day) of trans–monounsaturated fatty acids have been shown to lower HDL cholesterol levels by about 6 mg/dL.[57] Whether typical intake of trans–fatty acids also produces lowering of HDL cholesterol has yet to be determined. If a linear relationship is confirmed, intake of 6–8 g/day of trans–fatty acids could produce a 1 mg/dL lowering of HDL cholesterol.

Polyunsaturated Fatty Acids. There are two types of polyunsaturated fatty acids: omega-6 and omega-3. These fatty acids are named by the location of the first double bond. Omega-6 fatty acids are primarily found in vegetable oils. Omega-3 fatty acids are primarily found in fish oils.

Omega-6 Fatty Acids. The most common omega-6 polyunsaturated fatty acid in the diet is linoleic acid (C18:2). Polyunsaturated fatty acids are found in high concentrations exclusively in vegetable oils. Common vegetable oils in which more than 50% of the fatty acids are polyunsaturated are safflower oil, corn oil, and soybean oil (see Table 24–5).

The average polyunsaturated fatty acid intake is 10–30 g/day. Polyunsaturated fatty acids were once thought to have a unique cholesterol-lowering property that could counterbalance the cholesterol-raising effects of saturated fatty acids. The desirability of a dietary fat was expressed in the popular press by the ratio of polyunsaturated to saturated fat, or P:S ratio. However, this ratio reflects neither the cholesterol-raising potential of a fat nor its effect on the risk for coronary disease. For example, olive oil (see Table 24–5) has an undesirable P:S ratio. Nonetheless, olive oil lowers serum cholesterol levels when substituted for butter, and geographic areas where people consume large amounts of olive oil have low rates of coronary disease. A better guide to the desirability of a fat is its content of cholesterol-raising saturated fatty acids.

More recent metabolic diet studies have shown that polyunsaturated fatty acids are roughly equivalent to monounsaturated fatty acids in their effects on total and LDL cholesterol levels; that is, both types are relatively neutral: neither type raises or lowers total and LDL cholesterol levels. No population has consumed a high–polyunsaturated fat diet for a prolonged enough period to establish the relationship between dietary intake and CHD rates.

Omega-3 Fatty Acids. The most common long-chain omega-3 fatty acids are eicosapentaenoic (EPA) (C20:4) and docosahexaenoic (DHA) (C22:6). Omega-3 fatty acids are found predominantly in fish oils; some vegetable oils (notably canola oil and soybean oil) have a shorter chain omega-3 fatty acid, linolenic acid (C18:3). The average omega-3 fatty acid intake in the United States is 0–5 g/day. Although initial reports suggested a unique cholesterol-lowering property for omega-3 fatty acids,[58] follow-up studies confirmed that omega-3 fatty acids are neutral in their effects on total and LDL cholesterol levels.[59] Nevertheless, countries with high dietary intakes of long-chain omega-3 fatty acids have low rates of CHD,[60] perhaps because of the beneficial effects of omega-3 on thromboxane metabolism.

The major lipid effect of long-chain omega-3 polyunsaturated fatty acids is on serum triglyceride levels. In normal subjects fed 3–7 g of fish oil concentrate, omega-3 fatty acids lower triglyceride levels 30–50 mg/dL, with little effect on HDL cholesterol levels. Since large quantities of fatty cold-water fish (salmon, mackerel) must be consumed to achieve this intake, from a practical standpoint small changes in dietary omega-3 consumption will have little effect on triglyceride levels in normal individuals.[61] In patients with hypertriglyceridemia, however, fish oil supplements have been shown to reduce fasting triglyceride levels 100–1200 mg/dL.[62]

Other Dietary Factors Known to Alter Lipids

Dietary Cholesterol

Dietary cholesterol is found in the unsaponifiable fraction of animal fats and in animal cell membranes. Dietary cholesterol is present in all animal products, including meats, poultry, and fish at 15–30 mg/oz and dairy fat. Egg yolks (213 mg/yolk) and organ meats (liver, 110 mg/oz; brain, 580 mg/oz) are also rich in dietary cholesterol.

The dietary intake of cholesterol in the United States typically ranges from 300–500 mg/day. Unlike fatty acids, of which greater than 95% is absorbed, only 40%–60% of dietary cholesterol is absorbed.[63] Even after correction for variable absorption, the effects of dietary cholesterol on total and LDL cholesterol levels remain variable. Some patients exhibit a marked increase in LDL cholesterol levels with chronic ingestion, whereas others show little response.[64] This variability in response remains unexplained. Theoretical explanations include variation in the chemical structure of apo E or inherent differences in the ability to downregulate endogenous cholesterol synthesis. For populations, the typical response in serum total and LDL cholesterol to 25 mg of dietary cholesterol is a 1-mg/dL increase in total and LDL cholesterol levels. The connection between dietary cholesterol and CHD is more impressive than the effects on lipid levels: multivariate analysis of several prospective studies has shown significant positive relationships between dietary cholesterol intake and subsequent CHD.[65]

Fiber

Dietary fiber can be characterized in several ways: digestible/nondigestible, soluble/insoluble, and crude/dietary. Water solubility appears to confer the cholesterol-lowering effect of fiber. Soluble fiber in the diet modestly lowers total and LDL cholesterol levels, but insoluble fiber does not. Daily intake of 2 oz of oat bran (11 g total fiber; 6 g soluble fiber) or oatmeal (5 g total fiber; 3 g soluble fiber) can lower total and LDL cholesterol levels by about 5 mg/dL.[66] The average intake of dietary fiber in the United States is 5–20 g/day.

Alcohol

Alcohol intake does not affect total cholesterol and LDL cholesterol levels in populations. Anecdotally, hypercholesterolemia in an alcoholic can remit with cessation of drinking, although controlled studies show consistent effects only on triglyceride levels. Alcohol intake is a strong predictor of triglyceride levels in population studies.[67] The effect of alcohol to raise triglyceride levels is only transient in metabolic-ward studies of young, lean, healthy subjects.[68] This could mean that alcohol ingestion by the population is intermittent; alternatively, it may indicate that the effect of alcohol observed in populations reflects the effects of alcohol only in older, fatter subjects who show a more chronic response. This latter hypothesis is supported by studies documenting the graded effects of alcohol on triglyceride and HDL cholesterol levels in older subjects.[17] The actions of alcohol on triglyceride levels appear to be both dose-dependent and dependent on the baseline triglyceride level: subjects with triglyceride levels less than 150 mg/dL typically have little increase in these levels with alcohol, whereas subjects with higher baseline triglyceride levels have greater increases, that is, 50–100 mg/dL.[69] Since overweight individuals already have an overproduction of triglyceride-rich lipoproteins,[16] alcohol is more likely to accentuate elevations of triglyceride levels in overweight individuals than in lean individuals. If hypertriglyceridemic individuals consume more than 7% of energy as alcohol, it will enhance their hypertriglyceridemia.[70]

In subjects with normal triglyceride levels, the predominant effect of alcohol on serum lipids is to raise HDL cholesterol levels.[71] This action is dose-dependent, and at a daily dose of 63 g of ethanol (four to five drinks; see Table 24–1), HDL cholesterol levels may increase by 5–12 mg/dL. Whether or not this increase in HDL cholesterol levels explains the reduced total mortality observed among light drinkers is unknown.[72] Current dietary recommendations do not advocate alcohol ingestion for the purpose of reducing CHD risk.

Coffee

Isolated reports have claimed that drinking caffeinated and decaffeinated coffee is associated with higher total and LDL cholesterol levels, but just as many reports have shown no association. Carefully performed metabolic studies suggest that the fat released during coffee bean boiling has an unsaponifiable fraction that can raise total and LDL cholesterol levels.[73] This fat is captured by paper filters; since Americans typically drink filtered coffee, it is unlikely that coffee consumption, either caffeinated or decaffeinated, will play a major role in altering lipid levels.

Vitamins

New evidence suggests that modification (particularly oxidation) of LDL is a necessary step for LDL to be recognized and taken up by macrophages, which, in turn, become foam cells—the progenitor of the arterial wall fatty streak. In vitro tests have been established to evaluate the susceptibility of LDL to oxidation.[74] LDL particles containing polyunsaturated fatty acids are more likely to undergo oxidation than are those containing either monounsaturated or saturated fatty acids. In addition to LDL fatty acid content, a high content of plasma vitamin C or a high LDL content of vitamin E or beta carotene appears to retard the oxidative process. Further research is needed regarding the benefit and need of antioxidant vitamin supplements for prevention of atherosclerosis. In the meantime, a CHD-prevention diet enriched with a variety of fruits, vegetables, and grains will provide these antioxidants, albeit in lower doses than can be achieved with supplementation.

EFFICACY OF A CHOLESTEROL-LOWERING DIET

Despite the extensive research that has quantitated the relationship between changes in dietary intake and changes in cholesterol levels, the efficacy of a cholesterol-lowering diet is still a concern for many physicians. Understanding the history of research documenting the efficacy of these diets may help the clinician make realistic expectations of what can be achieved by dietary therapy in the clinical setting.

In the 1950s and 1960s, several independent investigators conducted dietary experiments in men hospitalized in research wards, patients in nursing homes, and men in prisons. This choice of subjects and environments allowed maximal control of nutrient intake. Based on multiple experiments, changes in types of dietary fat were found to produce changes in total serum cholesterol levels. During the initial investigations, fat was characterized by its origin: animal species or vegetable species. In general, animal fats raised serum cholesterol levels, whereas vegetable oils lowered them. However, some vegetable oils—for example, coconut oil—behaved like animal fat and raised serum cholesterol levels. To improve characterization of dietary fat, techniques such as determining the iodine value of the fat were employed to estimate degree of unsaturation, which permitted a measurable trait of the fat to be correlated with its cholesterol-raising potential. With the introduction of gas-liquid chromatography, a more refined characterization of fat into its subcomponents of unsaponifiables (cholesterol, phytosterols, vitamins) and saponifiables (glycerol, saturated fatty acids, monounsaturated fatty acids, and polyunsaturated fatty acids) provided a more precise method of correlating the composition of a fat with its cholesterol-raising potential. Keys and colleagues[50] and Hegsted and coworkers[51] brought this initial phase of investigation to its logical conclusion by constructing equations to quantitate the changes in serum total cholesterol produced by specific dietary changes:

$$\text{Keys: change in serum cholesterol} = 2.7S - 1.35P + 1.5Z$$

and

$$\text{Hegsted: change in serum cholesterol} = 2.16S - 1.65P + 6.77C,$$

where S = percent calories from saturated fatty acids, P = percent calories from polyunsaturated fatty acids, Z = change in the square root of dietary cholesterol, expressed in mg/1000 calories, that is, $(\text{cholesterol content initial diet})^{1/2} - (\text{cholesterol content final diet})^{1/2}$, and C = change in dietary cholesterol in mg/2600 calories.

In general, saturated fatty acids raised cholesterol levels twice as much as polyunsaturated fatty acids lowered them. Monounsaturated fatty acids were found to be equivalent to carbohydrates in their effect on total cholesterol levels, and hence both carbohydrates and monounsaturated fatty acids were termed *neutral* in their effect. Dietary cholesterol was an additional nutrient that increased serum cholesterol levels. More recent investigations that have directly compared the effects of monounsaturated versus polyunsaturated fatty acids suggest that both equations may have overestimated the cholesterol-lowering effects of polyunsaturated fatty acids.[75] However, because large increases in dietary polyunsaturated fatty acids are no longer recommended[76] and because reductions in saturated fatty acids account for most of the response to a cholesterol-lowering diet,[50, 51] the equations remain generally applicable to populations today.

There are no data to suggest that the efficacy of a cholesterol-lowering diet is reduced in free-living individuals. In fact, clinical trials that employ intensive counseling and follow-up in outpatients have achieved the cholesterol lowering predicted from metabolic-ward studies.[77] Two trials of dietary therapy with intensive individualized counseling in individuals at usual risk for coronary disease achieved 75%–80% of the cholesterol lowering predicted by metabolic-ward studies and produced a 5%–14% reduction in total cholesterol levels.[38, 78] Studies in high-risk individuals have exceeded predictions and achieved a 4%–17% reduction in cholesterol levels.[77] Similar efficacy has been observed in six of seven published trials of dietary therapy for secondary prevention.[77] Studies of institutionalized individuals receiving dietary therapy show that the initial cholesterol lowering achieved by diet is maintained over time; this lack of tachyphylaxis to diet is also observed in free-living populations when dietary counseling continues throughout the duration of the study.[39, 40, 79, 80] In fact, the World Health Organization European Collaborative Trial[81] observed that greater cholesterol reductions were achieved during the years when more intensive dietary counseling occurred, and cholesterol levels reverted to baseline when counseling was discontinued. Therefore, the available evidence suggests that a cholesterol-lowering diet will maintain its initial effectiveness as long as dietary modification is maintained.

Strategies for Implementing the Step I and Step II Diets

Registered dietitians and other qualified nutrition professionals can be invaluable in identifying acceptable ways for a patient to implement the Step I and Step II Diets. Dietitians often employ three strategies to implement the Step I and Step II Diets[82]: (1) applying fat reduction strategies to food choices and food preparations, (2) counting grams of fat and saturated fat, and (3) using the American Heart Association Food Exchange Lists. These approaches can be applied singly or in combination and are outlined in the following sections.

Strategy No. 1: Apply One or More Fat Reduction Techniques to Meal Planning

Several food selection/preparation techniques can be used to reduce total fat, saturated fat, and cholesterol in the diet: (1) substituting low-fat foods for higher fat counterparts (e.g., skim milk in place of whole milk), (2) decreasing the quantity of high-fat foods, (3) replacing high-fat foods with foods that are lower in fat (e.g., flank steak for spare ribs), and (4) changing preparation techniques (e.g., broiling instead of frying).

Using the fat reduction strategy, lean cuts of red meat can be selected so that a 3-oz portion offers no more fat or saturated fat than do common cuts of poultry (Table 24–6). It has been estimated that implementing these fat reduction techniques will allow most patients to follow the Step I Diet.[83] If the dietary goal is a Step II Diet, however, the patient will likely need additional dietary advice.

Strategy No. 2: Count Grams of Fat and Saturated Fat

To use the second strategy, the caloric needs of the patient must be estimated; once estimated, the patient is given a target intake of fat in grams. Table 24–7 lists the maximum daily gram intake of fat and saturated fat allowable in diets that provide 1600–3000 calories. Since food labels now uniformly list grams of total fat and saturated fat on the label, patients can be instructed to add up their daily intake. (Supplemental booklets are available that list the fat content of meats and common restaurant foods.) Comparing the fat gram content of similar products may even guide the patient in selecting lower fat foods.

The drawback of this technique is its simplicity. Neither the total calorie intake nor the inclusion of food groups such as fruits, grains, or vegetables is addressed. This oversimplification of the dietary guidelines can lead to mistranslations of the dietary message. For example, some patients mistakenly view "no-fat" foods as foods that can be eaten as desired, and we have had patients gain weight when only fat grams were counted.

Strategy No. 3: Use the Exchange Lists from the American Heart Association

Some patients are already familiar with diet exchange lists and easily accept this approach. The American Heart Association Cookbook is a good reference book for this strategy; the cookbook defines each food group and gives examples of daily menus to help implement dietary change.[84] As with strategy no. 2, the caloric needs of the patient must be estimated. Table 24–8 lists the number of servings per day from the American Heart Association food groups for Step I and Step II Diets for different calorie levels. When using this approach, standard portion sizes must be emphasized, since the control of the intake of saturated fat is critically linked to portion size. The benefit of this approach is that it addresses issues of overall balance in the diet (e.g., adequacy of fruit and vegetable intake). The disadvantage is that implementation requires more instruction and menu planning than do other strategies.

TABLE 24–6. COMPARISON OF THE TOTAL FAT AND SATURATED FAT CONTENT OF LEAN AND HIGHER FAT BEEF, PORK, POULTRY, AND FISH

Type of Meat, Poultry, Fish (3 oz, cooked)	Total Fat (g)	Saturated Fat (g)
*Lean beef (choice grade, 0-in fat trim, broiled or braised**		
Top round	5.0	1.7
Top sirloin	6.7	2.6
Bottom round	7.5	2.5
Chuck arm pot roast	7.5	2.7
Higher fat beef		
Chuck blade roast (choice, 0-in fat trim)	12.6	4.9
Extra-lean ground beef	13.5	5.3
Regular ground beef	16.7	6.6
Prime rib (¼-in fat trim)	17.9	7.6
Lean pork (roasted)		
Lean ham, cured	4.7	1.5
Arm picnic, cured	6.0	2.1
Regular ham, cured	7.7	2.7
Higher fat pork		
Sirloin	11.3	3.9
Center rib	11.8	4.1
Loin	11.9	4.1
Boston blade	14.4	5.0
Lean poultry		
Turkey without skin, light meat roasted	2.7	1.0
Chicken without skin, light meat roasted	3.9	1.1
Turkey without skin, dark meat roasted	6.2	2.1
Turkey with skin, light meat roasted	7.1	2.0
Chicken without skin, dark meat roasted	8.3	2.3
Lean ground turkey	8.4	2.5
Chicken with skin, light meat roasted	9.3	2.7
Higher fat poultry		
Chicken without skin, dark meat fried	9.9	2.7
Turkey with skin, dark meat roasted	9.9	3.0
Chicken with skin, light meat fried	10.4	2.8
Ground turkey	11.4	3.1
Chicken with skin, dark meat roasted	13.5	3.8
Lean fish		
Lobster, boiled	0.5	0.09
Baked cod	0.7	0.09
Baked haddock	0.8	0.09
Shrimp, boiled	0.9	0.2
Crab, boiled	1.3	0.09
Tuna, packed in water	1.5	0.3
Swordfish, baked	4.4	1.2
Canned salmon	5.1	1.3
Higher fat fish		
Shrimp, fried	10.4	1.8
Mackerel, baked	15.0	3.3
Tuna, packed in oil	19.4	1.5

*Note: The value listed on the nutrition label is separable lean, 1/8-in fat trim.

From Kris-Etherton PM, Peterson S, Jaax S, et al: Implementing dietary change. *In* Rifkind BM (ed): Contemporary Issues in Cholesterol Lowering: Clinical and Population Aspects. New York: Marcel Dekker, 1995.

Promoting Adherence

In general, there are four areas in which patients have problems with adherence to a diet. First, patients may find it difficult to change their diet. Second, patients may have difficulty deciding how to make changes in food intake; the changes made may not always achieve the desired reduction of dietary saturated fatty acids and dietary cholesterol. Third, the assessment of the dietary change relies on self-reported dietary intakes that may not accurately reflect true intake. Fourth, patients may not receive adequate incentives to adhere to their diet after the initial counseling is completed. The physician can be instrumental in promoting long-term compliance by addressing each of these four areas.

Regarding the first area, the failure of a patient to adhere to the diet could be a failure to educate and motivate the patient. It is clear that to effect a substantial change in dietary intake, participants must receive both education and motivation to change.[85] We have found that if a patient understands his or her risk for coronary disease, and if family members are involved in supportive roles, the chances of dietary modification improve.

Second, the failure to achieve a change in nutrient intake may be due to a mistranslation of how the desired intake can be achieved

TABLE 24–7. MAXIMUM DAILY INTAKE OF FAT AND SATURATED FATTY ACIDS TO ACHIEVE THE STEP I AND STEP II DIETS*

	Total Calorie Level							
	1600	**1800**	**2000**	**2200**	**2400**	**2600**	**2800**	**3000**
Total fat, g†	53	60	767	73	80	87	93	100
Saturated fat—Step I, g‡	18	20	22	24	27	29	31	33
Saturated fat—Step II, g‡	12	14	16	17	19	20	22	23

*The average daily energy intake for women is 1800 calories; for men, it is 2500 calories.
†Total fat of both diets = 30% of calories (estimated by multiplying calorie level of the diet by 0.3 and dividing the product by 9 calories/g).
‡The recommended intake of saturated fat should be 8%–10% of total calories for the Step I Diet and less than 7% for the Step II Diet.
From National Cholesterol Education Program: Second report of the Expert Panel on Detection, Evaluation, and Treatment of High Blood Cholesterol in Adults (Adult Treatment Panel II). Circulation 1994; 89:1329–1445.

with food selections. We have found that effective dietary counseling must target the unique habits of each patient. Our initial dietary assessment always includes an evaluation of current detrimental habits, and counseling explores possible substitutions that are both acceptable to the patient and effective in achieving target dietary intakes. Besides bad habits, the counseling should explore the frequency and regularity of meals and snacks. The time, location, and flexibility of meals must be addressed—some patients have structured lunches in which no choice of menu is possible; solutions such as eating before the lunch, eating only part of the lunch, and so on must be discussed with the patient to help him or her realize that alternative eating strategies exist. Patients must be educated about how all possible permutations in food selections influence target nutrient intake. For example, excess saturated fatty acid could be consumed either by eating a few foods rich in saturated fatty acids or by eating many foods containing modest amounts of saturated fatty acids that added together exceed target intake. The physician can begin to explore these areas in a patient interview; a registered dietitian can provide reinforcement by defining specific and quantitative goals for the patient.

The third area of difficulty in assessing adherence is that changes in dietary intake may not be measured accurately. It must be acknowledged that self-reported intake does not have the accuracy that can be obtained in clinical studies in which intake can be directly measured. Self-reported intake, however, is the best available measure of dietary intake in free-living subjects. Several methods can be used to document intake: food frequency questionnaires, 24-hour dietary recall, and food records. A dietitian can use these techniques to assess and monitor intake. We have found that compliance is enhanced when patients are asked to report their dietary intake. This self-reported intake can identify problem areas that preclude adherence to the diet and can effectively and efficiently help target additional counseling.

The fourth, and perhaps least apparent, area is the need for persistent and consistent follow-up. Evaluating a patient's response to a cholesterol-lowering diet is more than simply measuring cholesterol levels. We have had several apparent "dietary failure" episodes in which patients have come in for blood testing only, the results of which revealed that their cholesterol levels had returned to baseline. What testing alone did not reveal is that the patient gained weight, ignored the diet or, in some cases, developed other conditions that needed medical attention (e.g., new-onset diabetes). Patients respond best to continued reinforcement of adherence when follow-up includes monitoring body weight, asking for a dietary history, and discussing problems with adherence (parties, holiday eating, and so on) on follow-up visits.

Nonresponse or Paradoxical Response to Diet

Although a cholesterol-lowering diet on average produces the desired effect, some individuals have almost no response or even a

TABLE 24–8. NUMBER OF SERVINGS PER DAY OF THE AMERICAN HEART ASSOCIATION FOOD EXCHANGE GROUPS TO IMPLEMENT THE STEP I OR STEP II DIET AT FOUR DIFFERENT CALORIC LEVELS

	Calorie Levels							
	1200		**1600**		**2000**		**2500**	
Food Groups	*Step I*	*Step II*	*Step I*	*Step II*	*Step I*	*Step II*	*Step I*	*Step II*
Meat, poultry, and seafood	6 oz	5 oz	6 oz	5 oz	6 oz	5 oz	6 oz	5 oz
Eggs (per week)	3	1	3	1	3	1	3	1
Dairy products	1	1	2	1	2	1	4	2
Fat	3	3	4	5	6	7	8	8
Bread, cereal, pasta, and starchy vegetables	3	4	4	5	7	8	10	10
Vegetables	4	4	4	4	4	4	4	5
Fruit	3	3	3	3	3	4	5	7
Optional foods*	0	0	2	2	2	2	2	2

*Optional foods include fat-modified desserts, fat-free or low-fat sweets, and alcoholic beverages. Each exchange from the "optional foods" group is equivalent to two exchanges of the "bread, cereal, pasta, and starchy vegetables" group plus one exchange of the "fat" group.
Source: Grundy SM, Winston M (eds): The American Heart Association Low-Fat, Low-Cholesterol Cookbook. New York: New York Times Books, 1989.

paradoxical response to dietary modification: their cholesterol levels increase on a cholesterol-lowering diet. This failure to achieve expected results could be due to the lack of adherence to dietary modification but could also result from individual differences in responsiveness. Both of these possibilities must be entertained for each patient, and the physician must "walk a fine line" between assuming the patient is not complying with the diet and excusing away noncompliance by assuming the patient has a biologically based resistance to diet.

The phenomenon of nonresponsiveness was clearly observed in the Diet-Heart Feasibility Study both in free-living men who were counseled to consume the test diet at home and in institutionalized men who were fed the test diet in a controlled manner.[38] Of the free-living men in the Diet-Heart Feasibility Study, 27.2% had either less than a 5% decrease in total cholesterol levels or a paradoxical increase. It is likely that more than half of this nonresponse to diet was due to noncompliance, since only 11.5% of the institutionalized men had a minimal response to dietary modification. Available data suggest that perhaps 10% of the general population will not achieve lipid lowering on a cholesterol-lowering diet;[79, 80] this percentage may be higher among patients in a tertiary clinic.

Why some patients do not respond to a cholesterol-lowering diet is still unclear. Certain genetic factors could account for some of the individual differences in the magnitude of response, and several candidate factors (variations in apo E, apo A-IV) are under active clinical investigation.[86] In the meantime, the clinician is still faced with the goal of lipid lowering.

Besides nonadherence, one clinical factor that should be modified is the presence of excess body weight. Several investigators have found that individuals who are overweight have a smaller magnitude of response to diet than do lean individuals.[87] This observation is consistent with the mechanisms of action of obesity and dietary intake on lipoprotein metabolism. Since obese patients with hypercholesterolemia have an overproduction of VLDL, increasing the clearance of LDL by reducing saturated fatty acid intake may not be sufficiently targeted at the metabolic defect to restore lipid levels to the normal range. Thus, for the overweight patient, a combination of modest weight reduction to reduce VLDL overproduction plus dietary modification may be more effective in accomplishing lipid lowering than dietary modification alone.

The nonresponse to dietary therapy, although clinically important for deciding when to advance to drug therapy, does not imply that the therapeutic diet has been ineffective at reducing the long-term risk for CHD. A therapeutic diet will be rich in fruits, grains, and vegetables and by this mechanism may provide other means to lower CHD risk than simply by lowering LDL cholesterol levels.

A STEPWISE APPROACH TO THE DIETARY MANAGEMENT OF PATIENTS WITH SPECIFIC LIPID AND LIPOPROTEIN PATTERNS

Since the actual prescription of diet depends on the individual's lipoprotein pattern, we have outlined our dietary approach for patients with five common lipid and lipoprotein patterns. It should be mentioned that the serum lipids are subject to random day-to-day variation and are influenced by medications and illness such as a recent myocardial infarction.[88] The mean of several measurements should be used to establish the patient's pattern, and the mean of several treatment measurements or trends in measurement should be used to evaluate the effectiveness of treatment.

Isolated Hypercholesterolemia (Type IIa)

Definition. Isolated hypercholesterolemia is defined by total cholesterol levels greater than 240 mg/dL. This increase is due to LDL cholesterol levels greater than 160 mg/dL. HDL cholesterol levels may or may not be low.

Etiology. Isolated elevations in total and LDL cholesterol levels are common in the United States and can be due to several metabolic disturbances. As discussed earlier, familial hypercholesterolemia is a well-characterized autosomal dominant disorder present in 1 of 500 individuals in the population.[89] Patients present with LDL cholesterol levels that are often greater than 220 mg/dL and may have clinical signs of tendon thickening, corneal arcus, and xanthelasma. Polygenic hypercholesterolemia is more common. Patients with polygenic hypercholesterolemia present with more moderate increases in the LDL cholesterol level, which is typically 160–200 mg/dL, and they account for the majority of patients one may encounter in clinical practice. Polygenic hypercholesterolemia is due to several causes and has been characterized by several metabolic defects[90]: some patients have suppressed LDL receptor activity, some have an overproduction of LDL that exceeds the capacity of LDL receptors, and others have abnormalities in the LDL particle itself. Age and excess body weight are environmental factors that may further enhance the expression of the hypercholesterolemia.[91] For this reason, cholesterol screening is recommended every 5 years even if initial levels are normal.[1]

Goals of Dietary Therapy

1. Since saturated fatty acids depress LDL receptor activity,[23] the primary focus of dietary therapy is a reduction in saturated fatty acid intake. The physician can begin the clinical instruction to the patient by reviewing the frequency and portion size of common sources of saturated fatty acids (full-fat dairy products, butter, cheese, ice cream, bacon, sausage, ribs, fatty meats, donuts). A registered dietitian can be invaluable in helping the patient make these important changes. The dietitian can work with the patient and recommend specific changes that are acceptable to the patient.
2. Dietary cholesterol also depresses LDL receptor activity and can contribute to elevated blood cholesterol levels. Dietary cholesterol comes from a few cholesterol-rich foods (organ meats, egg yolk) and from animal products. Every ounce of meat has approximately 25 mg of dietary cholesterol. Since many patients consume more than the recommended 6–7 oz of meat a day, the portion size of meat is a key way to reduce dietary cholesterol consumption. Physicians can be effective in counseling the patient about the portion size of meat intake; a piece of meat the size of a deck of cards is 3 oz, and only two portions are recommended each day.
3. Individuals who are overweight have an additional metabolic abnormality that is amenable to dietary therapy: obesity leads to an increased production of VLDL by the liver.[16] Reduction of body weight will reduce the production rate of these LDL precursors.
4. Isolated hypercholesterolemia can be secondary to another silent disorder, for example, undiagnosed diabetes, hypothyroidism, or primary liver disease such as biliary cirrhosis.[92] Treatment of the primary disorder will improve the hypercholesterolemia.

Expected Effect. The magnitude of reduction depends on the patient's initial diet, the initial body weight, and the patient's ability to alter his or her diet and weight. In general, LDL cholesterol reductions of 5%–11% can be achieved. Greater LDL cholesterol reductions are expected from individuals who have an initial diet rich in saturated fatty acids and dietary cholesterol. Greater LDL cholesterol reductions are expected from individuals who are able to achieve even modest reductions in body weight.

Isolated Borderline–High Hypertriglyceridemia (Type IV)

Definition. Isolated borderline–high hypertriglyceridemia is defined by fasting triglyceride levels of 200–400 mg/dL, with total cholesterol levels less than 240 mg/dL. HDL cholesterol levels may or may not be low.

Etiology. Hypertriglyceridemia may be genetic, and familial forms of hypertriglyceridemia have been characterized.[93] However, isolated hypertriglyceridemia in middle-aged adults is often influenced by environmental factors. Excess body weight, either by inducing overproduction of triglycerides by the liver or by inducing insulin resistance, can raise triglyceride levels.[33] Excess alcohol consumption, particularly when consumed in excess of 7% of calories, can contribute to increases in triglyceride levels.[70] Physical inactivity, resulting either in obesity or in reduced catabolism of triglycerides by muscle, is an additional factor that can raise fasting triglyceride levels.[43]

Goals of Dietary Therapy

1. Determine alcohol intake as percent of calories. Patients who make their own drinks need to use a jigger to measure alcohol and a measuring cup to measure wine intake. Limit hard liquor intake to no more than 1½ oz/day, beer intake to one 12-oz beer, and wine intake to 5 oz (2/3 cup).
2. Evaluate body weight by calculating the BMI and also by measuring excess fat at the waistline. Hypocaloric diets, even without significant weight loss (e.g., restricting caloric intake by only 200 calories/day), will improve fasting triglyceride levels.
3. Evaluate fasting blood glucose levels. Individuals with mild elevations of fasting glucose (e.g., glucose greater than 110 mg/dL) may have glucose intolerance, which can raise triglyceride levels. Dietary therapy aimed at improving glucose intolerance is appropriate for these patients. To improve glucose intolerance, weight reduction and spacing out calories with three meals and two snacks can improve lipid levels by reducing hepatic production of triglycerides and reducing input of dietary triglycerides to the liver.
4. Evaluate the percent calories from fat versus carbohydrate. Individuals with stringent very low fat diets (e.g., Pritikin or Ornish diet) may simply have a carbohydrate-induced mild hypertriglyceridemia, and adding back fats that are low in saturated and trans–fatty acids (e.g., vegetable oils, nuts, avocados) can reduce the triglyceride level and raise the HDL cholesterol level.
5. A regular exercise program can reduce triglyceride level by stimulating triglyceride uptake by metabolically active muscle.
6. Consider the use of omega-3 fatty acid supplementation with fish oil capsules to improve triglyceride level. A high dose of fish oil (6–12 g/day) can be effective therapy for hypertriglyceridemia. An unpleasant side effect is occasional belching with a fishy aftertaste, but this is uncommon. Of note, fish oil supplementation can worsen glucose intolerance;[94] the use of fish oil supplementation should be cautiously approached in patients with glucose intolerance or diabetes.

Expected Effect. Many patients with excess body weight can normalize their triglyceride levels when they lose weight. Similarly, those who consume excess calories from alcohol can improve triglyceride levels with alcohol restriction. Patients who are lean, do not drink, and do not have glucose intolerance are unlikely to respond to dietary maneuvers unless the cause of their high triglyceride level is a very low fat diet. A regular exercise program will reduce fasting triglyceride levels, but it is unlikely that exercise alone will normalize levels unless significant weight loss occurs.

Combined Elevations in Triglyceride and Cholesterol Levels (Combined Hyperlipidemia [Type IIb and Type III])

Definition. Combined elevations in triglyceride and cholesterol levels are defined by total cholesterol levels of 240–500 mg/dL and fasting triglyceride levels of 200–800 mg/dL. HDL cholesterol levels may be low or normal.

Etiology. Combined hyperlipidemia may be predominantly influenced by genetics (e.g., familial combined hyperlipidemia) or may be influenced by both environment and genetics (e.g., obesity plus polygenic hypercholesterolemia). It is important not to dismiss the value of dietary therapy for converting combined hyperlipidemia into simple hypercholesterolemia; such treatment, often accomplished with weight reduction, increases the number of classes of drugs that can be employed to treat this difficult lipid disorder.

A rare form of combined dyslipidemia is type III hyperlipidemia. Individuals with this disorder may be identified by clinical signs of tendon xanthoma and tuberoeruptive xanthoma. Clinically, these patients are exquisitely sensitive to body weight. When patients with type III hyperlipidemia gain weight, the lipoprotein disorder worsens; normalizing weight can make the disorder clinically inapparent.

Goals of Dietary Therapy

1. Evaluate body weight and BMI as well as excess fat at the waistline. As in disorders of simple hypertriglyceridemia, weight reduction can be effective in lowering triglyceride levels in combined hyperlipidemia. If triglyceride levels can be reduced to less than 250 mg/dL, drug therapy may be much more effective in normalizing the lipid levels.
2. Evaluate and quantitate the intake of alcohol. As with disorders of simple hypertriglyceridemia, alcohol will contribute to the hypertriglyceridemia in certain patients.
3. Evaluate other secondary causes of dyslipidemia, notably hypothyroidism, nephrotic syndrome, and diabetes mellitus or glucose intolerance.
4. As in simple hypercholesterolemia, reductions in saturated fatty acids and dietary cholesterol have also been shown to be effective in producing LDL cholesterol reductions in these patients.

Expected Effect. Dietary therapy will be most effective in patients with type III hyperlipidemia and in patients who are overweight.

Isolated Low High-Density Lipoprotein Cholesterol

Definition. Isolated low HDL cholesterol is defined by total cholesterol levels less than 240 mg/dL, triglyceride levels less than 200 mg/dL, and HDL cholesterol levels less than 35 mg/dL. LDL cholesterol values are variable.

Etiology. Low HDL cholesterol levels are frequently encountered in patients with CHD; these low levels are also encountered in individuals with very low total cholesterol levels (<160 mg/dL), in individuals with rare genetic disorders of HDL metabolism, in smokers, in obese individuals, and in individuals following a diet that is extremely restricted in total dietary fat. A given patient may have one or more of these influences.

Goals of Dietary Therapy

1. Since the most common cause of low HDL cholesterol levels is excess body weight, calculation of a patient's BMI and excess body weight is an important initial assessment. As in disorders of simple hypertriglyceridemia, weight reduction can be effective in raising HDL cholesterol levels.
2. Cessation of smoking will be beneficial for increasing HDL cholesterol levels and for reducing the risk for coronary disease in other ways.[95] When the clinician discusses smoking cessation, he or she should also explain that the patient may gain weight in the process. By openly discussing weight gain, the physician will help prioritize the relative risk of these two factors. Although both may lower HDL cholesterol levels, smoking is a much more powerful cardiovascular risk factor than is obesity. The small increase in cardiovascular risk that may occur from weight gain will be more than offset by the immediate risk reduction from cessation of smoking.

3. In patients who are deriving less than 25% of calories from total fat, an increase in dietary fat intake may raise HDL cholesterol levels. Because increases in saturated fat intake will also raise LDL cholesterol levels, the extra dietary fat should be low in saturated fat. Since fat is more calorically dense than carbohydrate, when recommending high fat intake it is important to caution the patient that concomitant reductions in intake of other foodstuffs must take place. An easy way to add fat back to a diet that is otherwise healthy is to add oil as salad dressing or to add 1/4 cup of nuts to the diet. Any type of nuts will do—all are low in saturated fatty acids. Raw or roasted nuts can be used; even if nuts are roasted in coconut oil, little of the roasting fat ends up on the roasted nut.

Expected Effect. The magnitude of increase in HDL cholesterol resulting from the preceding measures depends on how much of the patient's HDL cholesterol level is genetically determined and how much is modifiable by environment. We have seen individuals whose HDL cholesterol level rose from 23 mg/dL to 48 mg/dL by changing the fat content of the diet or as a result of smoking cessation, but these patients are clearly the exception rather than the rule. On average, a change of 4–6 mg/dL in HDL cholesterol can be expected from weight loss, smoking cessation, or changes in dietary consumption.

Moderate or Severe Hypertriglyceridemia (Type I and Type V)

Definition. Moderate hypertriglyceridemia is defined by fasting triglyceride levels of 400–800 mg/dL, and severe hypertriglyceridemia is defined by fasting triglyceride levels greater than 800 mg/dL; cholesterol levels are typically greater than 240 mg/dL. HDL cholesterol levels are typically low.

Etiology. This disorder is most commonly seen in patients with poorly controlled diabetes. The treatment of individuals with glucose intolerance should focus on improving glucose levels.

There are some patients with this disorder who do not have diabetes. Environmental influences such as excess alcohol intake and excess body weight should be evaluated. Drugs, particularly corticosteroids (e.g., prednisone taken for asthma or arthritis) can contribute to this disorder. Hypothyroidism can occasionally cause this disorder.

Goals of Dietary Therapy

1. Determine alcohol intake as percent of calories. Patients who make their own drinks need to use a jigger to measure alcohol and a measuring cup to measure wine intake. Limit hard liquor intake to no more than 1½ oz/day, beer intake to one 12-oz beer, and wine intake to 5 oz (2/3 cup).

2. Evaluate body weight by calculating the BMI and also by measuring excess fat at the waistline. Hypocaloric diets, even without significant weight loss (e.g., dietary restriction of caloric intake of only 200 calories/day) will improve fasting triglyceride levels.

3. Evaluate fasting blood glucose levels. In individuals with even mild elevations of fasting glucose (>110 mg/dL), glucose intolerance may contribute to this disorder. Dietary therapy aimed at improving glucose intolerance is appropriate for these patients. To improve glucose intolerance, weight reduction and spacing out calories by recommending three meals and two snacks each day can improve lipid levels by reducing hepatic production of triglycerides and by reducing the magnitude of a meal's input of dietary triglycerides to the liver.

4. Consider the use of omega-3 fatty acid supplementation with fish oil capsules to improve triglyceride levels. Fish oil supplementation can worsen glucose intolerance; therefore, the use of fish oil supplementation should be cautiously approached in patients with glucose intolerance or diabetes.

Expected Effect. The dyslipidemia of diabetes can markedly improve when blood glucose control is achieved. However, some diabetic patients will still have a lipid disorder despite optimal dietary management. Type V hyperlipidemia is unlikely to normalize with dietary therapy alone but will often convert to simple hypertriglyceridemia, which is more easily treated with drug therapy.

REFERENCES

1. The Expert Panel: Summary of the second report of the National Cholesterol Education Program (NCEP) Expert Panel on Detection, Evaluation, and Treatment of High Blood Cholesterol in Adults (Adult Treatment Panel II). JAMA 1993; 269:3015–3023.
2. Chait A, Brunzell JD, Denke MA, et al: AHA Medical/Scientific Statement: special report, rationale of the diet-heart statement of the American Heart Association: report of the Nutrition Committee. Circulation 1993; 88:3008–3029.
3. Hadley SA, Saarmann L: Lipid physiology and nutritional considerations in coronary heart disease. Crit Care Nurse 1991; 11:28–39.
4. Grundy SM, Denke MA: Dietary influences on serum lipids and lipoproteins. J Lipid Res 1990; 31:1149–1172.
5. Havel RJ: Postprandial hyperlipidemia and remnant lipoproteins. Curr Opin Lipidol 1994; 5:102–109.
6. Schneeman BO, Kotite L, Todd KM, Havel RJ: Relationships between the responses of triglyceride-rich lipoproteins in blood plasma containing apolipoproteins B-48 and B-100 to a fat-containing meal in normolipidemic humans. Proc Natl Acad Sci USA 1993; 90:2069–2073.
7. Nordoy A, Goodnight S: Dietary lipids and thrombosis. Arteriosclerosis 1990; 10:149–163.
8. Mammen EF, Gianturco SH, Wassef MK (eds): Hypertriglyceridemia, atherosclerosis, and thrombosis. Semin Thromb Hemost 1988; 14:137–292.
9. Hoak JC: Stearic acid, clotting, and thrombosis. Am J Clin Nutr 1994; 60(suppl):1050S–1053S.
10. Havel RJ: Role of triglyceride-rich lipoproteins in progression of atherosclerosis. Circulation 1990; 81:694–696.
11. Austin MA, Hokanson JE: Epidemiology of triglycerides, small dense low-density lipoprotein, and lipoprotein(a) as risk factors for coronary heart disease. Med Clin North Am 1994; 78:99–115.
12. Havel RJ: McCollum award lecture, 1993: Triglyceride-rich lipoproteins and atherosclerosis—new perspectives. Am J Clin Nutr 1994; 59:795-799.
13. Mensink RP, Katan MB: Effect of dietary fatty acids on serum lipids and lipoproteins: a meta-analysis of 27 trials. Arterioscler Thromb 1992; 12:911-919.
14. Chait A, Onitiri A, Nicoll A, et al: Reduction of serum triglyceride levels by polyunsaturated fat. Studies on the mode of action and on very low density lipoprotein composition. Atherosclerosis 1974; 20:347-364.
15. Harris WS, Connor WE, Inkeles SB, Illingworth DR: Dietary omega-3 acids prevent carbohydrate-induced hypertriglyceridemia. Metabolism 1984; 33:1016–1019.
16. Kesaniemi YA, Grundy SM: Increased low density lipoprotein production associated with obesity. Arteriosclerosis 1983; 3:170–177.
17. Seppä K, Sillanaukee P, Pitkäjärvi T, et al: Moderate and heavy alcohol consumption have no favorable effect on lipid values. Arch Intern Med 1992; 152:297–300.
18. Woollett LA, Dietschy JM: Effect of long-chain fatty acids on low-density-lipoprotein-cholesterol metabolism. Am J Clin Nutr 1994; 60(suppl):991S–996S.
19. Ginsberg HN: Lipoprotein metabolism and its relationship to atherosclerosis. Med Clin North Am 1994; 78:1–20.
20. O'Brien KD, Chait A: The biology of the artery wall in atherogenesis. Med Clin North Am 1994; 78:41–67.
21. Jialal I, Freeman DA, Grundy SM: Varying susceptibility of different low density lipoproteins to oxidative modification. Arterioscler Thromb 1991; 11:482–488.
22. Gaziano JM, Manson JE, Buring JE, Hennekens CH: Dietary antioxidants and cardiovascular disease. Ann N Y Acad Sci 1992; 669:249–259.
23. Spady DK, Dietschy JM: Dietary saturated triglycerides suppress hepatic low density lipoprotein receptors in the hamster. Proc Natl Acad Sci USA 1985; 82:4526–4530.

24. Mensink RP, Katan MB: Trans monounsaturated fatty acids in nutrition and their impact on serum lipoprotein levels in man. Progr Lipid Res 1993; 32:111–122.
25. Dashti N: Synthesis and secretion of nascent lipoprotein particles. Progr Lipid Res 1991; 30:219–230.
26. Gordon DJ, Rifkind BM: High-density lipoprotein—the clinical implication of recent studies. N Engl J Med 1989; 321:1311–1316.
27. Cohen JC, Wang Z, Grundy SM, et al: Variation at the hepatic lipase and apolipoprotein AI/CIII/AIV loci is a major cause of genetically determined variation in plasma HDL cholesterol levels. J Clin Invest 1994; 94:2377–2384.
28. Pietinen P, Huttunen JK: Dietary determinants of plasma high-density lipoprotein cholesterol. Am Heart J 1987; 113:620–625.
29. Belfrage P, Berg B, Hagerstrand I, et al: Alterations of lipid metabolism in healthy volunteers during long-term ethanol intake. Eur J Clin Invest 1977; 7:127–131.
30. Poikolainen K: Epidemiologic assessment of population risks and benefits of alcohol use. Alcohol Alcoholism 1991; 1:27–34.
31. Kuczmarski RJ, Flegal KM, Campbell SM, Johnson CL: Increasing prevalence of overweight among US adults. JAMA 1994; 272:205–211.
32. Stamler J: Epidemic obesity in the United States. Arch Intern Med 1993; 153:1040–1044.
33. Denke MA, Sempos CT, Grundy SM: Excess body weight: an under recognized contributor to high blood cholesterol in caucasian American men. Arch Intern Med 1993; 153:1093–1103.
34. Denke MA, Sempos CT, Grundy SM: Excess body weight: an underrecognized contributor to dyslipidemia in white American women. Arch Intern Med 1994; 154:401–410.
35. Tran AV, Weltman A: Differential effects of exercise on serum lipid and lipoprotein levels seen with changes in body weight: a meta analysis. JAMA 1985; 254:919–924.
36. Dattilo AM, Kris-Etherton PM: Effects of weight reduction on blood lipids and lipoproteins: a meta-analysis. Am J Clin Nutr 1992; 56:320–328.
37. Ashley FW, Kannel WB: Relation of weight change to changes in atherogenic traits. The Framingham Study. J Chronic Dis 1974; 27:103–114.
38. National Diet-Heart Study Research Group: The National Diet-Heart Study final report. Circulation 1968; 37(suppl 1):1–428.
39. Caggiula AQ, Christakis G, Farrant M, et al: The Multiple Risk Factor Intervention Trial (MRFIT) IV. Intervention on blood lipids. Prev Med 1981; 265:997–1001.
40. Gordon DJ, Salz KM, Roggenkamp KJ, Franklin FA: Dietary determinants of plasma cholesterol change in the recruitment phase of the Lipid Research Clinics Coronary Primary Prevention Trial. Arteriosclerosis 1982; 2:537–548.
41. Rössner S, Björvell H: Early and late effects of weight loss on lipoprotein metabolism in severe obesity. Atherosclerosis 1987; 64:125–130.
42. Wood PD, Stefanick ML, Williams PT, Haskell WL: The effects on plasma lipoproteins of a prudent weight-reducing diet, with or without exercise, in overweight men and women. N Engl J Med 1991; 325:461–466.
43. Bouchard C, Shephard RJ, Stephens T (eds): Physical Activity, Fitness and Health. Champaign, IL: Human Kinetics, 1994.
44. Sacks FM, Willett WW: More on chewing the fat. The good fat and the good cholesterol. N Engl J Med 1991; 325:1740–1742.
45. Nestel P, Hirsch E: Triglyceride turnover after diets rich in carbohydrate or animal fat. Asian Ann Med 1965; 14:265–269.
46. Ullmann D, Connor WE, Hatcher LF, et al: Will a high-carbohydrate, low-fat diet lower plasma lipids and lipoproteins without producing hypertriglyceridemia? Arterioscler Thromb 1994; 11:1059–1067.
47. West CE, Sullivan DR, Katan MB, et al: Boys from populations with high-carbohydrate intake have higher fasting triglyceride levels than boys from populations with high-fat intake. Am J Epidemiol 1990; 13:271–282.
48. Stone NJ: Diet, lipids, and coronary heart disease. Endocrinol Metab Clin North Am 1990; 19:321–344.
49. U.S. Department of Agriculture: Composition of Foods, "Fats and Oils." Agriculture Handbook No. 8-4. Washington, DC: U.S. Government Printing Office, 1979.
50. Keys A, Anderson JT, Grande F: Prediction of serum-cholesterol responses of man to changes in fats in the diet. Lancet 1957; 2:955–966.
51. Hegsted DM, McGandy RB, Myers ML, Stare FJ: Quantitative effects of dietary fat on serum cholesterol in man. Am J Clin Nutr 1965; 7:281–295.
52. Denke MA, Breslow JL: The effects of a low-fat diet with and without intermittent saturated fat and cholesterol ingestion on lipid, lipoprotein and apolipoprotein levels in normal volunteers. J Lipid Res 1988; 29:963–969.
53. Mattson FH, Grundy SM: Comparison of effects of dietary saturated, monounsaturated, and polyunsaturated fatty acids on plasma lipids and lipoproteins in man. J Lipid Res 1985; 26:194–202.
54. Keys A: Seven Countries: A Multivariate Analysis of Death and Coronary Heart Disease. Cambridge, MA: Harvard University Press, 1980.
55. Meyer WH, Anderson S, Applewhite TH, et al: The Technical Committee. Food Fats and Oils. Washington, DC: The Institute of Shortening and Edible Oils, 1988.
56. Hunter JE, Applewhite TH: Reassessment of trans fatty acid availability in the US diet. Am J Clin Nutr 1991; 54:363–369.
57. Mensink RP, Katan MB: Effect of dietary trans fatty acids on high-density and low-density lipoprotein cholesterol levels in healthy subjects. N Engl J Med 1990; 323:439–445.
58. Illingworth DR, Harris WS, Connor WE: Inhibition of low density lipoprotein synthesis by dietary omega-3 fatty acids in man. Arteriosclerosis 1984; 4:270–275.
59. Wilt TJ, Lofgren RP, Nichol KL, et al: Fish oil supplementation does not lower plasma cholesterol in men with hypercholesterolemia. Ann Intern Med 1989; 111:900–905.
60. Dyerberg J, Bang JO, Stofferson E, et al: Eicosapentaenoic acid and prevention of thrombosis and atherosclerosis. Lancet 1978; 2:117–119.
61. Singer P, Berger I, Lück K, et al: Long-term effect of mackerel diet on blood pressure, serum lipids and thromboxane formation in patients with mild essential hypertension. Atherosclerosis 1986; 62:259–265.
62. Harris WS, Dujovne CA, Zucker M, Johnson B: Effects of a low saturated fat, low cholesterol fish oil supplement in hypertriglyceridemic patients. Ann Intern Med 1988; 109:465–470.
63. Conner WE, Lin DS: The intestinal absorption of dietary cholesterol by hypercholesterolemic (type II) and normocholesterolemic humans. J Clin Invest 1974; 53:1062–1071.
64. The Relationship Between Dietary Cholesterol and Blood Cholesterol and Human Health and Nutrition. A Report to the Congress Pursuant to the Food Security Act of 1985, P.L. 99-198, Subtitle 5, Section 1453. Washington DC: U.S. Department of Agriculture, Department of Health and Human Services, 1985.
65. Stamler J, Shekelle R: Dietary cholesterol and human coronary heart disease. The epidemiologic evidence. Arch Pathol Lab Med 1988; 112:1032–1040.
66. Ripsin CM, Keenan JM, Jacobs DR, et al: Oat products and lipid lowering. A meta-analysis. JAMA 1992; 267:3317–3325.
67. Heiss G, Johnson NJ, Reiland S, et al: The epidemiology of plasma high-density lipoprotein cholesterol levels. The Lipid Research Clinics Program Prevalence Study. Summary. Circulation 1980; 62(suppl IV): 116-136.
68. Belfrage P, Berg B, Hagerstrand I, et al: Alterations of lipid metabolism in healthy volunteers during long-term ethanol intake. Eur J Clin Invest 1977; 7:127–131.
69. Ginsberg H, Olefsky J, Farquhar JW, Reaven GM: Moderate ethanol ingestion and plasma triglyceride levels. A study in normal and hypertriglyceridemic persons. Ann Intern Med 1974; 80:143–149.
70. Witztum JL, Dillingham MA, Giese W, et al: Normalization of triglycerides in type IV hyperlipoproteinemia fails to correct low levels of high-density-lipoprotein cholesterol. N Engl J Med 1980; 303:907–914.
71. Haskell WL, Camargo C, Williams PT, et al: The effect of cessation and resumption of moderate alcohol intake on serum high-density-lipoprotein subfractions. N Engl J Med 1984; 310:805–810.
72. Steinberg D, Pearson TA, Kuller LH: The Davis Conference, alcohol and atherosclerosis. Ann Intern Med 1991; 114:967–976.
73. Zock PL, Katan MB, Merkus MP, et al: Effect of a lipid-rich fraction from boiled coffee on serum cholesterol. Lancet 1990; 335:1235–1237.
74. Steinberg D, Berliner JA, Burton GW, et al: Antioxidants in the prevention of human atherosclerosis. Summary of the proceedings of a National Heart, Lung, and Blood Institute Workshop: September 5-6, 1991, Bethesda, MD. Circulation 1992; 85:2338–2345.
75. Dreon DM, Vranizan KM, Krauss RM, et al: The effects of polyunsaturated fat vs monounsaturated fat on plasma lipoproteins. JAMA 1990; 263:2462–2466.
76. Committee on Diet and Health, Food and Nutrition Board, Commission on Life Sciences, National Research Council, 1989. Diet and Health: Implication For Reducing Chronic Disease Risk. Washington, DC: National Academy Press, 1989.

77. Denke MA: Cholesterol lowering diets: a review of the evidence. Arch Intern Med 1995; 155:17–26.
78. Henderson MM, Kushi LH, Thompson DJ, et al: Feasibility of a randomized trial of a low-fat diet for the prevention of breast cancer: dietary compliance in the Women's Health Trial Vanguard Study. Prev Med 1990; 19:115–133.
79. Hjermann I, Velve BK, Holme I, Leren P: Effect of diet and smoking intervention on the incidence of coronary heart disease: report from the Oslo Study Group of a randomized trial in healthy men. Lancet 1981; 2:1303–1310.
80. Hjermann I: Smoking and diet intervention in healthy coronary high risk men: methods and 5-year follow-up of risk factors in a randomized trial: the Oslo Study. J Oslo City Hosp 1980; 30:3–17.
81. World Health Organization European Collaborative Group: European Collaborative Trial of Multifactorial Prevention of Coronary Heart Disease: final report on the 6-year results. Lancet 1986; 2:869–872.
82. Kris-Etherton PM, Wozniak-Wowk C, Scott LW, Jaax S: Implementation of blood cholesterol lowering diets using nutrition labels. Top Clin Nutr 1994; 10:14–26.
83. Smith-Schneider LM, Sigman-Grant MJ, Kris-Etherton PM: Dietary fat reduction strategies. J Am Diet Assoc 1992; 92:34–38.
84. Grundy SM, Winston M (eds): The American Heart Association Low-Fat, Low-Cholesterol Cookbook. New York: Random House, 1989.
85. Grundy SM: Adherence to cholesterol-lowering diets. Arch Intern Med 1992; 152:1139.
86. Denke MA: Review of human studies evaluating individual dietary responsiveness in patients with hypercholesterolemia. Am J Clin Nutr 1995; 62:471S–477S.
87. Cole TG, Bowen PE, Schmeisser D, et al: Differential reduction of plasma cholesterol by the American Heart Association Phase 3 Diet in moderately hypercholesterolemic, premenopausal women with different body mass indexes. Am J Clin Nutr 1992; 55:385–394.
88. Durrington PN: Biological variation in serum lipid concentrations. Scand J Clin Lab Invest Suppl. 1990; 198:86–91.
89. Brown MS, Goldstein JL: A receptor-mediated pathway for cholesterol homeostasis. Science 1986; 232:34–47.
90. Vega GL, Denke MA, Grundy SM: Metabolic basis of primary hypercholesterolemia. Circulation 1991; 84:118–128.
91. Miller NE, Nanjee MN: Hyperlipidemia in the elderly: metabolic changes underlying the increases in plasma cholesterol and triglycerides during aging. Cardiovasc Risk Factors 1992; 2:158–169.
92. Stone NJ: Secondary causes of hyperlipidemia. Med Clin North Am 1994; 78:117–142.
93. Brunzell JD, Schrott HG, Motulsky AG, et al: Myocardial infarction in the familial forms of hypertriglyceridemia. Metabolism 1976; 25:313–320.
94. Malasanos TH, Stacpoole PW: Biological effect of ω-3 fatty acids in diabetes mellitus. Diabetes Care 1991; 14:1160–1179.
95. Lakier JB: Smoking and cardiovascular disease. Am J Med 1992; 93(suppl 1A):8S–17S.

25 Dyslipoproteinemias/Atherosclerosis: Pharmacologic Therapy

John A. Farmer, MD
Antonio M. Gotto, Jr., MD, DPhil

Age-adjusted morbidity and mortality rates for coronary heart disease (CHD) have dropped dramatically during the past several decades. Contributing to this decline are increased recognition of CHD risk factors and the availability of pharmacologic agents to control modifiable risk factors such as dyslipidemia, hypertension, and diabetes. A variety of lipid-regulating pharmacologic agents have been demonstrated in clinical trials not only to improve circulating lipid levels but also to alter the clinical and anatomic course of atherosclerosis. This chapter focuses on the available lipid-regulating agents (Table 25–1) and their indications for use, mechanisms of action, side effects and drug interactions (Table 25–2), and validation in clinical trials. Special considerations for drug therapy of dyslipidemia in population subgroups are also addressed.

CLINICAL GUIDELINES

Determination of the need for pharmacologic therapy should be individualized according to the patient's risk factor profile, potential benefit of treatment, and potential adverse effects from drug therapy (which may be lifelong). The clinical guidelines established by the Adult Treatment Panel of the National Cholesterol Education Program (NCEP)[1] are based on the patient's overall risk, as defined by plasma level of low-density lipoprotein (LDL) cholesterol and presence of CHD or other atherosclerotic disease, as well as the following additional risk factors:

1. Age (45 years or older in men; 55 years or older, or premature menopause without estrogen-replacement therapy, in women).
2. Family history of CHD (definite myocardial infarction [MI] or sudden death before 55 years of age in the father or other first-degree male relative, or before 65 years of age in the mother or other first-degree female relative).
3. Current cigarette smoking.
4. Hypertension (140/90 mm Hg or greater confirmed on several occasions, or the use of antihypertensive medication).
5. Low level of high-density lipoprotein (HDL) cholesterol (less than 35 mg/dL confirmed on several occasions).
6. Diabetes mellitus.

The NCEP also defines one negative risk factor, high HDL cholesterol level (60 mg/dL or greater confirmed on several occasions), to be subtracted from the number of additional positive risk factors.

Treatment of Elevated Low-Density Lipoprotein Cholesterol Level

In patients without CHD and with fewer than two other risk factors, pharmacologic therapy should be considered if, after an

TABLE 25–1. APPROVED LIPID-REGULATING DRUGS

Agents	Mechanism of Action	Efficacy
Bile acid sequestrants Cholestyramine Colestipol	Decreased intrahepatic cholesterol due to nonspecific binding of bile acids; upregulation of LDL receptors	LDL-C decreases 15%–30% HDL-C increases 3%–5% TG usually unaffected; may increase
HMG-CoA reductase inhibitors Fluvastatin Lovastatin Pravastatin Simvastatin	Decreased cholesterol synthesis due to partial inhibition of HMG-CoA reductase; upregulation of LDL receptors	LDL-C decreases 20%–40% HDL-C increases 5%–15% TG decreases 10%–20%
Probucol	Increased fractional catabolic rate of LDL; decreased oxidation of LDL	LDL-C decreases 5%–15% HDL-C decreases 20%–30% TG usually unaffected
Nicotinic acid	Decreased production of VLDL; decreased release of free fatty acids into the circulation	LDL-C decreases 10%–25% HDL-C increases 15%–35% TG decreases 20%–50%
Fibric acid derivatives Gemfibrozil Clofibrate	Increased activity of lipoprotein lipase; decreased VLDL synthesis	LDL-C decreases 10%–15% with high LDL-C; may increase with high TG (variable) HDL-C increases 10%–15% TG decreases 20%–50%

Abbreviations: HDL-C, high-density lipoprotein cholesterol; HMG-CoA, 3-hydroxy-3-methylglutaryl coenzyme A; LDL, low-density lipoprotein; LDL-C, LDL cholesterol; TG, triglyceride; VLDL, very low density lipoprotein.

adequate trial of dietary therapy, LDL cholesterol level remains 190 mg/dL or greater; the LDL cholesterol goal for these patients is less than 160 mg/dL. However, because of questions raised concerning the risk/benefit ratio of long-term pharmacologic therapy in primary prevention, drug therapy should be delayed in men younger than 35 years of age and in premenopausal women whose LDL cholesterol levels are 190 to 220 mg/dL and who are without other risk. In patients without CHD and with two or more other risk factors, pharmacologic therapy should be considered if, after an adequate trial of dietary therapy, LDL cholesterol level remains 160 mg/dL or greater; the LDL cholesterol goal for these patients is less than 130 mg/dL. In secondary prevention, that is, in patients with existing CHD or other atherosclerotic disease, a more aggressive approach is warranted because these patients are at the highest risk for subsequent CHD events. In these patients, pharmacologic therapy should be considered if, after an adequate trial of dietary therapy, LDL cholesterol level remains 130 mg/dL or greater; the LDL cholesterol goal for this high-risk group is 100 mg/dL or less. The physician should exercise clinical judgment in deciding whether to initiate drug treatment in patients with CHD and LDL cholesterol level of 100 to 129 mg/dL. Because LDL cholesterol level is typically decreased during the first few weeks after an MI, risk factor reduction and dietary therapy should be implemented immediately and follow-up lipid measurements scheduled for 6 to 8 weeks after the acute event to determine the need for any additional therapy.

The NCEP recommends the use of bile acid sequestrants, nicotinic acid, 3-hydroxy-3-methylglutaryl coenzyme A (HMG-CoA) reductase inhibitors, fibric acid derivatives, and probucol to lower LDL cholesterol level. Because nicotinic acid and fibric acid derivatives also exert a strong triglyceride-lowering effect, they are so classified in the following sections.

Treatment of Elevated Triglyceride Level

Serum triglyceride levels are classified by the NCEP as normal (<200 mg/dL), borderline high (200 to 400 mg/dL), high (400 to 1000 mg/dL), and very high (>1000 mg/dL). As for hypercholesterolemia, the primary therapy for hypertriglyceridemia consists of lifestyle modifications: weight reduction if overweight, adherence to a diet low in saturated fat and cholesterol, adherence to a regular exercise program, smoking cessation, and, in some patients, restriction of alcohol consumption.

Drug therapy may be considered in patients with primary borderline-high triglyceride levels who have CHD, a family history of premature CHD, high total cholesterol (>240 mg/dL) combined with low HDL cholesterol (<35 mg/dL) levels, or a genetic hypertriglyceridemia associated with increased CHD risk, such as type III hyperlipidemia or familial combined hyperlipidemia. The pharmacologic agent selected should also decrease LDL cholesterol and increase HDL cholesterol. In some patients, some triglyceride-lowering agents may increase LDL cholesterol, but this increase may reflect a higher content of cholesteryl ester in larger, lipid-rich LDL particles, which are thought to be less atherogenic than small, dense LDL.

In patients with high triglyceride levels, possible causes of secondary hypertriglyceridemia, most commonly obesity, should be treated. Drug therapy may be required in order to prevent triglyceride from increasing to very high levels that may cause pancreatitis, especially in patients with a history of acute pancreatitis. In patients with very high triglyceride levels, vigorous efforts should be made to lower the triglyceride level because of the immediate risk for pancreatitis. Treatment of secondary causes of triglyceride elevation in these patients should include discontinuation of drugs that increase triglyceride, control of diabetes mellitus, restriction of alcohol consumption, and restriction of dietary fat to 10%–20% of total calories. If triglyceride level remains 1000 mg/dL or greater despite adherence to nonpharmacologic measures, drug therapy may be considered but can rarely reduce the triglyceride level to below 500 mg/dL in these patients. There is no effective drug therapy for chylomicronemia.

Treatment of Low High-Density Lipoprotein Cholesterol Level

The association of low HDL cholesterol level with increased CHD risk warrants the inclusion of interventions to raise HDL cholesterol level if necessary. The primary therapy is lifestyle modification, namely, dietary therapy and, as appropriate, weight reduction, smoking cessation, and increased physical activity. Hypertension and diabetes mellitus should be treated as necessary. Consideration should

TABLE 25–2. LIPID-REGULATING DRUG INTERACTIONS

Lipid-Regulating Agents	Clinical Manifestations of Drug Interactions	Interactive Agents
Bile acid sequestrants Cholestyramine Colestipol	Binding and decreased absorption of interactive agents	Thiazide diuretics Digitalis glycosides Beta blockers Coumarin anticoagulants (warfarin) Thyroid hormones Gemfibrozil (modest interaction with colestipol; with cholestyramine, may decrease lithogenicity of gemfibrozil) Oral hypoglycemic agents (sulfonylureas)
HMG-CoA reductase inhibitors Fluvastatin Lovastatin Pravastatin Simvastatin	Myopathy, rhabdomyolysis	Cyclosporine Prednisone Fibric acid derivatives Erythromycin
	Elevations in liver enzymes; possible muscle necrosis	Nicotinic acid
	Prolongation of prothrombin time	Coumarin
Probucol	Possible amplification of HDL cholesterol reduction	Androgens Progestins Beta blockers Other HDL-lowering agents
	Possible amplification of corrected QT interval prolongation	Group Ia antiarrhythmic agents (quinidine, procainamide, disopyramide) Tricyclic antidepressants Phenothiazines
Nicotinic acid	Increased level of nicotinic acid in the circulation	Aspirin (high dosage)
	Decreased efficacy of interactive agents	Uricosuric agents (sulfinpyrazone)
	Hepatocellular necrosis	Drugs that adversely affect hepatic structure or function
	Elevations in liver enzymes; possible muscle necrosis	HMG-CoA reductase inhibitors
	Possible potentiation of antihypertensive effects	Antihypertensive agents
Fibric acid derivatives Bezafibrate Ciprofibrate Clofibrate Fenofibrate Gemfibrozil	Binding and decreased absorption of gemfibrozil (modest)	Colestipol (with gemfibrozil)
	Rhabdomyolysis	HMG-CoA reductase inhibitors
	Increased anticoagulant activity	Warfarin
	Potentiation of hypoglycemic action	Glyburide (with gemfibrozil)

Abbreviations: HDL, high-density lipoprotein; HMG-CoA, 3-hydroxy-3-methylglutaryl coenzyme A.
Adapted from Farmer JA, Gotto AM Jr: Antihyperlipidaemic agents: drug interactions of clinical significance. Drug Safety 1994; 11:301. As amended in International Lipid Information Bureau: The ILIB Lipid Handbook for Clinical Practice: Blood Lipids and Coronary Heart Disease. Houston: International Lipid Information Bureau, 1995.

also be given to discontinuing drugs that decrease HDL cholesterol level. If drug therapy is required to lower LDL cholesterol level, an agent that also increases HDL cholesterol level should be preferred.

AGENTS WHOSE MAIN EFFECT IS TO LOWER CHOLESTEROL LEVEL

Bile Acid Sequestrants

Bile acid sequestrants have been used for more than 30 years in the treatment of patients with dyslipidemia. The mechanisms of action and efficacy and side effect profiles of resins are well established. Cholestyramine and colestipol, the resins currently available in the United States, are essentially pure LDL-lowering agents, although they have modest effects on other lipid fractions.

Mechanisms of Action

Both cholestyramine and colestipol are highly charged polycationic compounds that interrupt the enterohepatic circulation of bile acids by binding with the cholesterol-rich bile acid pool and decreasing its reabsorption.[2] Normally, only 3% of the bile acid pool is excreted by the fecal route, and the remainder is reabsorbed and undergoes enterohepatic recirculation. The bile acid sequestrants cause an increased conversion of cholesterol into bile acids by stimulating the rate-limiting enzyme 7α-hydroxylase. This enhanced conversion results in a decrease in intrahepatic levels of cholesterol, which in turn stimulates the number or function of the B/E (LDL) receptor and so increases the clearance of lipoproteins containing apolipoprotein (apo) B or apo E from the circulation. This secondary mechanism exerts an additive effect on the decrease in plasma cholesterol levels caused by the primary mechanism of enhanced fecal loss. However, the decrease in intrahepatic cholesterol also stimulates cholesterol biosynthesis through activation of HMG-CoA reductase, the rate-limiting enzyme of cholesterol biosynthesis, therefore increasing plasma cholesterol toward pretreatment levels.[3] Hence, there is frequently a more marked initial decline in plasma cholesterol level with bile acid sequestrant use followed by a diminution of efficacy because of increased production of cholesterol.

Efficacy

Cholestyramine is usually administered at 4–16 g/day (up to a maximum of 24 g/day) in divided doses. Colestipol is usually administered at 5–20 g/day (up to a maximum of 30 g/day) in divided doses. In patients receiving these agents, LDL cholesterol level may be expected to decrease an average of 15%–30%. HDL cholesterol level may increase 3%–5%, although the mechanism involved has not been fully established. Bile acid sequestrant therapy generally does not have a significant impact on triglyceride or very low density lipoprotein (VLDL) levels. However, plasma triglyceride levels may increase, particularly in patients with hypertriglyceridemia before therapy. The mechanism by which the bile acid sequestrants exacerbate hypertriglyceridemia may relate to an increased production or decreased degradation of triglyceride-rich lipoproteins.

Side Effects and Drug Interactions

Side effects are frequently the limiting factor in the clinical utility of the bile acid sequestrants. Because these agents are not absorbed into the circulation, their major side effects are gastrointestinal. Constipation is a common side effect with both of the bile acid sequestrants but can be improved by increasing intake of fluid and soluble fiber and by the use of stool softeners. The use of natural fibers containing guar gum may have an additive effect on cholesterol lowering. The usefulness of the resins, which are administered as powders, is also plagued by poor palatability and difficulty of ingestion. In an attempt to improve ease of administration, several modifications have been introduced, such as caplets and confectionery bars. Mixing the powders with juice or pulpy food may improve palatability and alter the consistency of these compounds.

Concern has been raised about possible carcinogenicity of these agents, because it has been suggested that prolonging the transit time of bile acids and consequently the exposure of the gastrointestinal endothelium may increase risk for malignant neoplasms. Cholestyramine has been reported to increase the frequency of 1,2-dimethylhydrazine–induced intestinal tumors in rats.[4] However, in the long-term clinical trials performed in human subjects, no increased risk for gastrointestinal malignant neoplasms with bile acid sequestrant therapy has been documented.

Because the bile acid sequestrants are nonspecific binders, they may decrease the absorption and clinical effects of concomitantly administered drugs. In patients receiving anticoagulants such as warfarin, anticoagulation efficiency may be decreased[5]; in patients receiving thiazide diuretics or digitalis preparations for congestive heart failure, volume overload and reduced inotropism may result from nonspecific binding of these agents by bile acid sequestrants. Other potentially affected agents are thyroxine, fat-soluble vitamins, and folic acid. Agents that may be bound by bile acid sequestrants should be administered 1 h before or at least 4 h after the resin to prevent decreased absorption.

Clinical Trials

Large-scale clinical trials have supported the use of bile acid sequestrants either as pharmacologic monotherapy or in combination with other agents. The Lipid Research Clinics Coronary Primary Prevention Trial (LRC-CPPT) was a landmark study demonstrating that clinical cardiac events could be decreased by the administration of cholestyramine. In this trial, 3806 men aged 35–59 years with total cholesterol level of 265 mg/dL or greater, LDL cholesterol level of 190 mg/dL or greater, triglyceride level of 300 mg/dL or less, and no known evidence of coronary disease were randomized to receive dietary therapy alone or in addition to cholestyramine 24 g/day in divided doses.[6] Average time on trial was 7.4 years. Dietary therapy alone decreased total cholesterol level by almost 5% and LDL cholesterol level by almost 8%. Respective decreases in the cholestyramine group were 13% and 20%, despite problems with compliance that reduced the power of the study, which had been designed with a goal of a 28% decrease in total cholesterol level with drug treatment. Nevertheless, the primary endpoint of definite CHD-related death combined with definite nonfatal MI was significantly decreased 19% in the cholestyramine group.

Additional cardiovascular endpoints that improved significantly with cholestyramine treatment in the LRC-CPPT included the development of angina, which was 20% lower in the cholestyramine group, and the development of new positive exercise test results, which decreased 25% in the cholestyramine group. Incidence of coronary bypass surgery was 21% lower in the cholestyramine group, but this difference was not significant. The LRC-CPPT was not able to demonstrate a decrease in total mortality because of an increase in accidents and violent deaths in the cholestyramine-treated group, although this difference was not significant. Cholestyramine therapy was not associated with an increase in malignant neoplasms. On the basis of the relation between the decrease in cholesterol level and the reduction in cardiac events seen in the LRC-CPPT, the rule of thumb developed that a 1% decrease in total cholesterol level is associated with a 2% reduction in CHD-related events. Subjects able to achieve the expected decrease in LDL cholesterol level of greater than 25%, who represented one third of the subjects randomized to receive cholestyramine therapy, had a 64% reduction in CHD risk.[7]

Bile acid sequestrants have been used as pharmacologic monotherapy or combination therapy in angiographically monitored trials that studied clinical and anatomic endpoints. The National Heart, Lung, and Blood Institute (NHLBI) Type II Coronary Intervention Study randomized 143 men and women aged 21 to 55 years with LDL cholesterol levels above the 90th percentile of the general population after diet to receive diet plus cholestyramine at a projected dose of 24 g/day or diet plus placebo.[8] The primary endpoint was change in severity of CHD as evaluated by coronary angiography at 5-year follow-up. Visual assessment of the angiograms revealed regression in a small proportion of both treated (6.8%) and control (7.1%) subjects. However, cholestyramine-treated subjects did demonstrate stabilization of lesions as indicated by significantly less progression (32%) than in the control subjects (49%). Total cholesterol level decreased 17% in the cholestyramine group, compared with 1% in the control group, and LDL cholesterol level decreased 26% and 5% in the respective groups. This trial was the first to demonstrate that anatomic progression of coronary lesions can be altered with pharmacologic lipid-lowering therapy.

Cholestyramine was also used as pharmacologic monotherapy in the St Thomas' Atherosclerosis Regression Study (STARS).[9] This trial assessed the effect of diet (fat limited to 27% of total calories, saturated fat limited to 8%–10% of total calories, omega-6 and omega-3 polyunsaturated fatty acids increased to 8% of total calories, and soluble fiber increased to 3.6 g per 1000 kcal), diet plus cholestyramine, and usual care on quantitatively analyzed angiographic endpoints in 90 men younger than 66 years with documented CHD and mean total cholesterol level of 280 mg/dL. Coronary angiography was repeated after an average of 39 months, and the mean absolute width of coronary artery segments was determined. Compared with the usual-care group, the two active-treatment groups showed significant improvement in coronary artery luminal diameter, which increased 0.103 mm in the diet-plus-cholestyramine group and 0.003 mm in the diet-only group but decreased 0.201 mm in the usual-care group. Respective decreases in total cholesterol level were 25%, 14%, and 2%, and respective decreases in LDL cholesterol level were 36%, 16%, and 3%. The diet-plus-cholestyramine group also experienced a dramatic improvement in total cardiac events. Only 4% of subjects randomized to this therapy experienced a cardiac event, compared with 11% of the diet-only group and 36% of the usual-care group. The usual-care group had significantly more events than did the two active-treatment groups.

Bile acid sequestrant therapy has also been studied in combination with other lipid-regulating agents. In the Cholesterol Lowering Atherosclerosis Study (CLAS), 162 nonsmoking men younger than 66 years with progressive coronary atherosclerosis, previous coronary bypass surgery, and entry fasting blood cholesterol levels of 185–350 mg/dL were randomized to a lipid-lowering diet alone or a more restrictive diet plus the combination of colestipol, 30 g/day, and nicotinic acid, 3–12 g/day.[10] The participants underwent a 6-week drug run-in period to establish that they could tolerate and respond to study doses of colestipol and nicotinic acid. Combination drug therapy resulted in significant improvement: in the group randomized to pharmacologic intervention, total cholesterol level decreased 22%, LDL cholesterol level decreased 39%, and HDL cholesterol level increased 35% compared with levels in the placebo group. At the end of the original 2-year trial period, repeat angiography demonstrated that 16% of subjects randomized to pharmacologic intervention had undergone definite regression of atherosclerosis in their native coronary arteries, compared with 4% of placebo subjects, which was a statistically significant difference. In addition, 45% of subjects who received aggressive therapy demonstrated stabilization of atherosclerotic lesions, compared with 37% of the placebo group. Benefit was seen in both native coronary vessels and saphenous vein bypass grafts. In the 103 subjects who continued on the study an additional 2 years, improvement of lipid parameters and angiographic endpoints persisted at 4-year follow-up.[11]

CLAS evaluated the potential role of triglyceride-rich lipoproteins in atherosclerosis. One of the major predictors of progression in drug-treated subjects was the concentration of apo C-III in the HDL fraction.[12] Apo C-III inhibits the metabolism of triglyceride-rich lipoproteins and their subsequent uptake by the liver, as opposed to apo C-II, which stimulates lipoprotein lipase activity. Sequestration of apo C-III in the HDL fraction removes this inhibitory effect and may facilitate the catabolism of triglyceride-rich lipoproteins and decrease the exposure time of the vessel wall to potentially atherogenic, partially hydrolyzed remnant particles.

In the Familial Atherosclerosis Treatment Study (FATS), 120 men aged 62 years or younger with apo B levels greater than 125 mg/dL, anatomically demonstrable coronary disease, and a family history of CHD received dietary therapy alone or in conjunction with combination drug therapy.[13] Colestipol, 30 g/day, was used in all three arms of the trial, including subjects randomized to conventional therapy whose baseline LDL cholesterol level was greater than the 90th percentile for age (43% of the group). In the two active-treatment groups, colestipol was combined with either lovastatin, 40–80 mg/day, or nicotinic acid, 4–6 g/day. The subjects were treated for 2.5 years and then underwent repeat angiography, which documented regression as the only change in 32% of subjects who received lovastatin plus colestipol, 39% of subjects who received nicotinic acid plus colestipol, and 11% of subjects who received conventional therapy; regression was reported in significantly more subjects in the active-treatment groups than in the conventional-therapy group. Progression as the only change was seen in 21%, 25%, and 46% of the respective groups. Total cholesterol level decreased 34% in the group receiving lovastatin plus colestipol and 23% in the group receiving nicotinic acid plus colestipol, compared with a 3% decrease in the conventional-therapy group. LDL cholesterol level decreased 46%, 32%, and 7% in the respective groups, and HDL cholesterol level increased 15%, 43%, and 5%. Despite modest but statistically significant decreases in mean percent stenosis of 0.7 percentage points with lovastatin plus colestipol and 0.9 percentage points with nicotinic acid plus colestipol compared with an increase of 2.1 percentage points with conventional therapy, combination therapy reduced by 73% the incidence of clinical events compared with conventional therapy, which was a statistically significant reduction. Clinical cardiovascular events (death, MI, or need for peripheral or coronary bypass or angioplasty) were reported in 3 of the 46 subjects randomized to lovastatin plus colestipol, 2 of the 48 subjects randomized to nicotinic acid plus colestipol, and 10 of the 52 subjects randomized to conventional therapy.

HMG-CoA Reductase Inhibitors

The advent of HMG-CoA reductase inhibitors marked a major advance in the pharmacologic treatment of dyslipidemia. The first reductase inhibitor to be used in human subjects was compactin (mevastatin), which was derived from extracts of the fungus *Penicillium citrinum.*[14] The initial studies using this agent demonstrated effective reductions of both total cholesterol and LDL cholesterol levels. Compactin was never released for clinical use for reasons that have not been clearly delineated but were apparently related to adverse effects in animals.

There are currently four HMG-CoA reductase inhibitors available in the United States: fluvastatin, lovastatin, pravastatin, and simvastatin. Fluvastatin is a synthetic, racemic mixture of active and inactive forms. Lovastatin and simvastatin, which are lactone derivatives, are lipophilic; fluvastatin and pravastatin are open-acid, hydrophilic compounds. The relative benefits of lipophilic and hydrophilic agents have not been demonstrated clinically. Hydrophilic agents may have decreased concentration in peripheral tissues such as muscle and so may have decreased potential for complications such as rhabdomyolysis. Conversely, lipophilic agents may be more completely extracted by the liver through a first-pass effect, localizing the drug-induced reduction in cholesterol synthesis to hepatic tissues, where this reduction may be of more therapeutic benefit than in peripheral tissues.

Mechanisms of Action

The major mechanism of action of all four reductase inhibitors is the partial competitive inhibition of HMG-CoA reductase. In addition to the decrease in cholesterol synthesis induced by these agents, the B/E receptor is upregulated in response to the decrease in intracellular cholesterol. This increase in receptor activity explains not only the decrease in circulating LDL levels but also the potential efficacy of these agents in decreasing levels of VLDL and intermediate-density lipoprotein (IDL), which carry apo E and apo B-100 on their surfaces. HMG-CoA reductase inhibitors may also decrease the hepatic secretion of apo B–containing lipoproteins,[15] although the lack of efficacy in homozygous familial hypercholesterolemia (FH), in which competent B/E receptors are lacking, is evidence against this potential mechanism.[16]

In addition to the effects on LDL and VLDL, a modest but significant rise in HDL level is usually induced by administration of a reductase inhibitor. The mechanism involved in this increase has not been completely elucidated but does not appear to be a direct effect on apo A synthesis.[17] Evidence has accumulated that cholesteryl ester may be transferred from HDL into apo B–containing particles; if the concentrations of apo B–containing particles are lowered, there may be a concomitant rise in HDL cholesterol.[18]

Efficacy

Fluvastatin administered at a dosage of 20–40 mg/day, lovastatin administered at a dosage of 10–80 mg/day, pravastatin administered at a dosage of 10–40 mg/day, or simvastatin administered at a dosage of 5–40 mg/day may be expected to decrease LDL cholesterol level 20%–40%. The reductase inhibitors are most effective in lowering LDL cholesterol level at lower dosages; as the dosage increases, LDL cholesterol level continues to decrease, but in smaller increments. Because the peak activity of HMG-CoA reductase occurs approximately at midnight, it is recommended that these agents be given in the evening. In particular, lovastatin should be administered with the evening meal, and pravastatin should be given at bedtime.

The effect of the reductase inhibitors on HDL cholesterol level is less predictable but is typically 3%–15%. Triglyceride level may decrease 10%–20%.

Side Effects and Drug Interactions

A major concern in the early use of HMG-CoA reductase inhibitors was the potential for formation of lens opacities or cataracts, based on prior experience with agents that blocked cholesterol synthesis after the steroid nucleus had been generated. For example, experimental animals treated with triparanol (MER-29) demonstrated an increase in lens opacities.[19] However, a large body of evidence accumulated from more than a decade of clinical use has not shown an increase in prevalence of lens opacities or cataract formation with administration of reductase inhibitors.

Problems associated with use of these agents include myopathy and hepatotoxicity. Initially, creatine kinase levels were monitored on a routine basis in an attempt to identify subclinical myopathy before the development of rhabdomyolysis. However, this enzyme is highly sensitive to a variety of other conditions as well, and the routine use of creatine kinase level as a screening test is not recommended. Approximately 0.1% of subjects who receive a reductase inhibitor as monotherapy may have clinically evident rhabdomyolysis characterized by marked elevations of creatine kinase, myoglobinuria, and muscle pain.[20] It is unclear whether this complication is a result of alteration of membrane stability caused by reduced cholesterol production or by reduced levels of ubiquinone, which is used for electron transport by the mitochondria. Although the mechanism responsible has not been established, the clinical event appears to be self-limited, and cessation of the drug generally results in reversal of the myopathic process. However, the incidence of muscle toxicity may be increased in combination therapy. Rhabdomyolysis is more common when a reductase inhibitor is combined with a fibric acid derivative,[21] erythromycin,[22] cyclosporine,[23] or nicotinic acid[24] or when patients have coexistent underlying renal insufficiency.[25]

Although the risk for rhabdomyolysis increases when a reductase inhibitor is combined with a fibric acid derivative, two studies of lovastatin and pravastatin indicate that this combination may be effective and relatively safe in selected patients. The combination of lovastatin and gemfibrozil was evaluated in a retrospective analysis of 80 men and women with primary mixed dyslipidemia that had not been corrected with either drug as monotherapy.[26] Subjects received both drugs in combination for an average of 21 months. Of the 714 creatine kinase measurements taken during the study, 9% were higher than the upper limit of normal, and only one (0.1%) was three times the upper limit of normal or higher. Myositis that could be attributed to the drug combination and that required discontinuation of the drugs occurred in 3% of patients and in 1% of patients with concurrent creatine kinase elevation. However, no subject had definite rhabdomyolysis or myoglobinuria.

Adverse events were also monitored in a prospective study in which 290 men and women with hypercholesterolemia were randomized to receive pravastatin, gemfibrozil, a combination, or placebo for 12 weeks.[27] Severe myopathy was not demonstrated during this trial, although study drugs were withdrawn from two subjects who had asymptomatic elevations of creatine kinase. Creatine kinase levels greater than four times the pretreatment level occurred in four subjects (5.4%) receiving combination therapy, two subjects (2.9%) receiving gemfibrozil alone, one subject (1.4%) receiving pravastatin alone, and one subject (1.4%) receiving placebo. The combination of pravastatin and gemfibrozil decreased LDL cholesterol level 37% and decreased VLDL cholesterol level 49%. There was a significant rise in HDL cholesterol of 17% with combination therapy. This study indicates that this drug combination is effective in lipid lowering but must be used only in carefully selected patients and then only with close observation for potential myositis.

In the Expanded Clinical Evaluation of Lovastatin (EXCEL) study, 977 of the 8245 men and women with moderate primary hypercholesterolemia (total cholesterol level 240–300 mg/dL, LDL cholesterol level 160 mg/dL or greater, and triglyceride level less than 350 mg/dL) originally randomized to lovastatin at various dosages or placebo for 1 year continued in the study for a second year.[28] During the 2-year period, rhabdomyolysis was not observed in any subject, and myopathy, defined as creatine kinase levels greater than 10 times the upper limit of normal, was seen in two subjects receiving lovastatin, 40 mg/day, and in four subjects receiving lovastatin, 80 mg/day. Creatine kinase elevation above the upper limit of normal occurred in 54% of placebo subjects during the 2-year period, emphasizing the nonspecificity of creatine kinase level as a marker for underlying reductase inhibitor toxicity. No subject in this study was diagnosed with clinical hepatitis, and there was no evidence of progressive liver disease. During the first year of the study, successive elevations of transaminase more than three times the upper limit of normal occurred in 45 of the 6582 subjects randomized to lovastatin treatment, and 87% of these cases occurred between 4 and 12 months of therapy. Only one lovastatin subject sustained transaminase elevations greater than three times the upper limit of normal during the second year of the trial. The mechanism whereby reductase inhibitors may induce hepatotoxicity is unknown, but it is recommended that patients have periodic determinations of circulating liver enzymes. Liver disease does not appear to be a clinical consequence of reductase inhibitor use.

There have been rare reports of adverse effects such as thrombocytopenia and arthralgias with reductase inhibitor use, but the mechanism remains unclear, and a causal relation has not been established.[29] Lovastatin, which is tightly protein bound, has been reported to increase the prothrombin time in patients also taking warfarin.[30] Because simvastatin is also tightly protein bound, it may have a similar effect when administered with oral anticoagulants.

Clinical Trials

Despite the relatively recent availability of the HMG-CoA reductase inhibitors for the pharmacologic management of coronary atherosclerosis, a large body of evidence supports their safety and efficacy in primary and secondary prevention. These agents have been used in trials that monitored not only anatomic and lipid parameters but also clinical endpoints such as coronary morbidity and mortality.

Lovastatin was studied as monotherapy in the Monitored Atherosclerosis Regression Study (MARS), in which 270 men and women, aged 37–67 years, with angiographically documented CHD and total cholesterol levels of 190–295 mg/dL were randomized to receive either a low-fat diet or the same diet plus high-dose lovastatin (80 mg/day) in divided doses for 2 years.[31] As reflected by the range of cholesterol levels included in this trial, subjects were not limited to patients with dyslipidemia. Lovastatin therapy decreased total cholesterol level 32%, LDL cholesterol level 45%, and triglyceride level 22% and increased HDL cholesterol level 8.5%, all of which were significantly different from changes of 2%–3% in the placebo group. On assessment by quantitative coronary angiography, lesions causing less than 50% stenosis at baseline evaluation showed no benefit with treatment. However, among lesions causing 50% or greater stenosis at baseline evaluation, those in lovastatin subjects showed a mean 4% decrease in percentage of diameter stenosis, compared with a 1% increase in placebo subjects. The primary endpoint of mean per-patient change in percent diameter stenosis as assessed by quantitative coronary angiography was not significantly different between the treatment groups, but the panel-assessed secondary endpoint of global change score showed significant improvement with lovastatin. By this visual assessment, subjects who received placebo were more likely to exhibit anatomic progression of atherosclerosis and less likely to exhibit anatomic regression than were subjects who received lovastatin. MARS did not demonstrate a difference between treatment groups in clinical coronary events.

Lovastatin was also used as monotherapy in the Canadian Coronary Atherosclerosis Intervention Trial (CCAIT), which randomized 331 dyslipidemic men and women (fasting total serum cholesterol levels 220–300 mg/dL) aged 21–70 years to placebo or lovastatin administered at a dosage titrated as necessary to reduce LDL cholesterol level to 90 to 130 mg/dL (mean lovastatin dosage 36 mg/day).[32] All subjects received dietary instruction. In the lovastatin group, total cholesterol level decreased 21% and LDL cholesterol level decreased 29%, compared with decreases of less than 2% in the placebo group. A coronary change score, defined as the per-patient mean of the minimal lumen diameter changes for all lesions measured, was determined on the basis of quantitative coronary angiography performed at baseline assessment and repeated after 2 years of treatment. The angiographic changes induced by lovastatin were small but statistically significant. Although both groups showed progression, that in the lovastatin group was less severe. In addition, new lesions were formed in significantly fewer subjects in the lovastatin group (16%) than in the placebo group (32%). Unlike MARS, CCAIT demonstrated greater benefit to lesions causing less than 50% stenosis at baseline assessment. Clinical events were also monitored in CCAIT and showed a small, insignificant trend in favor of lovastatin treatment.

Pravastatin monotherapy was studied in the Pravastatin Limitation of Atherosclerosis in the Coronary Arteries (PLAC I) study, a 3-year, randomized, multicenter trial conducted in 408 men and women with LDL cholesterol levels of 130–190 mg/dL and documented CHD including at least one lesion causing at least 50% stenosis.[33] The primary endpoint, change in mean diameter of 10 predefined coronary artery segments as assessed by quantitative coronary angiography, was not significantly different between treatment groups. However, events (MI, nonfatal MI plus death, nonfatal MI plus CHD-related death) occurring at least 90 days after the institution of therapy has been reported, implying lesion stabilization and decreased risk of plaque rupture with pravastatin treatment.

The West of Scotland Coronary Prevention Study (WOSCOPS) randomized 6595 men aged 45–64 with no previous myocardial infarction to receive pravastatin, 40 mg/day, or placebo; mean follow-up was 4.9 years.[33a] Relative risk for the primary endpoint, either nonfatal myocardial infarction or CHD death as a first event, was significantly reduced 31% with pravastatin.

Simvastatin monotherapy was studied in the Multicenter Anti-Atheroma Study (MAAS), which randomized 381 subjects aged 30–67 years with CHD to receive either simvastatin 20 mg/day or placebo for 4 years.[34] Dietary instruction was provided to all subjects according to the usual practice of each center. Compared with placebo, simvastatin decreased total cholesterol level 23%, LDL cholesterol level 31%, and triglyceride level 18% and increased HDL cholesterol level 9%. Coronary anatomy was evaluated by quantitative angiography performed at baseline assessment and repeated after 2 and 4 years of therapy. Although progression was the overall outcome in both groups, the per-patient average of mean lumen diameter of all coronary segments was 0.06 mm greater with simvastatin treatment, and the per-patient average of minimal lumen diameter of all coronary segments diseased at baseline assessment was 0.08 mm greater with simvastatin treatment. Both of these differences were statistically significant. Although MAAS was not powered to study the effects of therapy on mortality, cardiac death or MI was reported in 15 simvastatin subjects and 11 placebo subjects, but the difference was not significant. Percutaneous transluminal coronary angioplasty or coronary artery bypass surgery was performed in 23 simvastatin subjects, compared with 34 placebo subjects, but the difference was not statistically significant.

The effect of simvastatin monotherapy on mortality was evaluated in the Scandinavian Simvastatin Survival Study (4S), a double-blind, multicenter trial that randomized 4444 men and women aged 35–70 years with a history of angina or MI and with total cholesterol levels of 210–310 mg/dL and triglyceride levels of 220 mg/dL or less after diet to receive placebo or simvastatin administered at a dosage titrated as necessary to reduce total cholesterol level to 115–200 mg/dL.[35] Simvastatin dosage was increased from the initial 20 mg/day to 40 mg/day in 37% of simvastatin subjects and decreased to 10 mg/day in two subjects. After a median of 5.4 years of treatment, total mortality decreased 30% in the simvastatin group, which was highly significant. Cardiovascular mortality decreased 42%. The simvastatin group also obtained lipid benefits: total cholesterol level decreased 25%, LDL cholesterol level decreased 35%, HDL cholesterol level increased 8%, and triglyceride level decreased 10%, compared with respective increases of 1%, 1%, 1%, and 7% in the placebo group.

Probucol

Probucol is a bisphenol derivative with structural similarities to the antioxidant butylated hydroxytoluene.[36] Despite its long history of clinical use, its mechanism of action and effect on clinical cardiovascular endpoints remain obscure.

Mechanisms of Action

As opposed to other lipid-regulating drugs, probucol does not appear to require the presence of functioning B/E receptors to exert its cholesterol-lowering effect, because it has been shown to lower LDL cholesterol levels in patients with homozygous FH.[37] The decrease in LDL cholesterol level with probucol administration seems to be secondary to an increase in the fractional catabolic rate of LDL.[38] Other potential mechanisms of action attributed to probucol include reduction of hepatic cholesterol production, decreased secretion of lipoproteins from hepatocytes, and increased bile salt secretion.

There is increasing evidence that probucol may confer clinical benefits independent of lipid lowering. Dyslipidemic states are frequently associated with altered vascular reactivity, and increased vasoconstriction has been demonstrated in patients with hyperlipidemia.[39] Vasoconstriction induced in experimental animals by short-term cholesterol feeding and thought to be caused by LDL oxidized in vivo is improved by the administration of probucol.[40] In addition, antioxidant properties of probucol may slow progression of atherosclerosis. It appears that LDL must be oxidatively or otherwise modified to be recognized and internalized by the scavenger receptor on monocyte/macrophage cells. Oxidized LDL may have chemoattractant and cytotoxic properties that increase the migration of monocytes into areas with high concentrations of oxidized LDL and lead to further endothelial damage. Probucol may also exert a beneficial effect on naturally occurring antioxidants such as vitamin E.[41] In addition, studies performed in vitro have documented that probucol inhibits the uptake of acetylated LDL by macrophages and increases the release of cholesterol from macrophages.[42]

Efficacy

Probucol decreases LDL cholesterol levels 5%–15% and decreases HDL cholesterol levels 20%–30% but has essentially no effect on plasma triglyceride levels. The impact on HDL cholesterol appears to be related to pretreatment levels: patients whose pretreatment level of HDL cholesterol is normal to low appear to have a less dramatic decrease with probucol treatment.[43]

The probucol-induced decrease in HDL cholesterol is of uncertain mechanism and clinical significance. In a number of epidemiologic studies, high levels of HDL cholesterol have been associated with protection from coronary atherosclerosis, and the utility of probucol as a lipid-regulating agent has been questioned because of its effect on HDL cholesterol. Experimental studies have supported the premise that HDL is involved in reverse cholesterol transport, the putative process by which cholesterol is returned from the periphery to the liver for excretion or, through the action of cholesteryl ester transfer protein (CETP), transferred to apo B–containing particles. In vivo, however, it is difficult to monitor and measure this process. The impact of probucol on HDL level and metabolism is complicated and may be due to alteration of enzymes that remodel lipoproteins within the circulation, changes in apolipoprotein synthesis, or potential altering of the interaction of HDL with cholesterol-rich cells.[44]

In addition to decreasing plasma HDL cholesterol levels, probucol has been demonstrated to decrease the particle size of HDL, which may compromise reverse cholesterol transport. Experiments in hypercholesterolemic animals treated with probucol have demonstrated that apo A-I, a major apolipoprotein of HDL, was decreased secondary to an increase in fractional catabolic rate and a decrease in synthetic rate of apo A-I; the decreased synthetic rate continued 1 month after the discontinuation of probucol.[45] Probucol also increases circulating levels of CETP, resulting in an increased transfer of cholesteryl esters from HDL to lower density lipoproteins.[46]

The effect of these changes in circulating lipoproteins has been studied extensively in experimental animals, including the Watanabe heritable hyperlipidemic rabbit, which serves as a model for FH. These rabbits lack the B/E receptor and are susceptible to the development of severe, extensive atherosclerosis. The administration of probucol resulted in a marked decrease in the rate of progression of atherosclerosis in these animals despite the fact that HDL cholesterol level was decreased.[47]

In addition, probucol has been studied in human subjects with FH and associated tendinous xanthomas. In these patients, increased xanthoma regression after long-term administration of probucol was associated with greater decreases in HDL cholesterol.[48] The effect of probucol on circulating lipids in patients with FH may depend at least partially on the presence of apo E_4. Probucol administration produced significantly greater decreases in total cholesterol and in LDL cholesterol levels in patients with heterozygous FH who were homozygous for apo E_4 than in patients with heterozygous FH who did not have apo E_4; changes in triglyceride and VLDL cholesterol levels were also significantly different between the groups, decreasing in patients with apo E_4 and increasing slightly in patients without apo E_4.[49]

Side Effects and Drug Interactions

Probucol appears to be a safe lipid-regulating agent at the usual dosage of 500 mg twice a day. In general, side effects are mild clinical irritations such as increased prevalence of gastrointestinal dysfunction manifested by diarrhea, bloating, or heartburn. Less than 5% of patients discontinue probucol because of intolerable side effects.

However, probucol has been associated with prolongation of the QT interval and a possibility of increased susceptibility to polymorphic ventricular tachycardia (torsades de pointes). Early studies performed in several experimental animal species revealed an increased incidence of sudden cardiac death that was presumably due to induced ventricular arrhythmias.[50] Prolongation of the QT interval appears to be correlated with increased circulating probucol levels. Because probucol is highly lipophilic, its absorption is enhanced by a fatty meal; consequently, increased plasma levels of the drug may be seen in the postprandial state secondary to facilitated absorption. The potential risk may be minimized by giving probucol independently of meals or by more rigid adherence to a low-fat diet.

Although clinical trials have not established a definite correlation between probucol use and sudden cardiac death, QT prolongation has been documented in as many as 50% of patients who receive this drug.[51] Hence, in patients with underlying coronary disease or patients receiving concomitant medication known to be associated with QT prolongation, such as group Ia antiarrhythmic agents, tricyclic antidepressants, and phenothiazines, QT interval should be monitored. In addition, electrolyte status should be maintained in the normal range because hypokalemia, hypomagnesemia, and hypocalcemia can cause prolongation of repolarization.

Probucol has not been implicated in major drug interactions. Warfarin compounds may be safely coadministered without significant alteration of the prothrombin time.

Clinical Trials

The Probucol Quantitative Regression Swedish Trial (PQRST) was conducted in 274 men and women with femoral atherosclerosis, total cholesterol level greater than 265 mg/dL, LDL cholesterol level greater than 175 mg/dL, and triglyceride level of 350 mg/dL or less who received diet and cholestyramine as well as either probucol or placebo for 3 years.[52] Probucol was found to protect LDL from oxidation.[53] However, despite a 17% decrease in total cholesterol level and a 12% decrease in LDL cholesterol level with probucol treatment, the probucol-plus-cholestyramine group did not experience more atherosclerotic regression than the placebo-plus-cholestyramine group did. Lumen volume increased 0.6% in the group treated with probucol plus cholestyramine, which was not a significant increase from baseline values; lumen volume increased 4.2% in the group treated with cholestyramine alone, which was a significant improvement.

AGENTS WHOSE MAIN EFFECT IS TO LOWER TRIGLYCERIDE LEVEL

Nicotinic Acid

Nicotinic acid, a B complex vitamin, is a component of the nicotinamide adenine dinucleotide and the nicotinamide adenine dinucleotide phosphate coenzyme systems, which are involved in a variety of oxidation-reduction reactions. Deficiency of nicotinic acid results in pellagra, a chronic wasting disease typically associated with dementia, dermatitis, and diarrhea; adequate levels of dietary tryptophan may compensate for niacin deficiencies and mitigate pellagra. Pharmacologic doses of nicotinic acid exert beneficial effects on the endogenous lipid cascade, resulting in decreased triglyceride and LDL cholesterol levels and increased HDL cholesterol level.

Mechanisms of Action

The mechanisms by which nicotinic acid affects lipids are complex. The major activity is a reduction in hepatic synthesis and release of VLDL, which leads to a reduction in IDL and LDL because of the decrease in precursor particles.[54] Nicotinic acid also exerts a peripheral effect of decreased release of free fatty acids into the circulation. Free fatty acids are substrates for triglyceride synthesis, so this peripheral effect decreases hepatic production of triglyceride. However, the peripheral action of nicotinic acid appears to be transient, and its quantitative impact on the lipid profile remains controversial.

Plasma levels of the major apolipoproteins associated with VLDL, IDL, and LDL—especially apo B-100—are also decreased with nicotinic acid therapy. HDL levels rise as the result of decreased HDL catabolism, particularly in patients with hypertriglyceridemia before therapy.[55] Although Lp(a) levels are generally refractory to lipid-regulating drug therapy, nicotinic acid has been demonstrated to decrease Lp(a) levels.[56] The mechanism involved in Lp(a) lowering is unknown; although it is presumably beneficial, because of the association between Lp(a) and increased CHD risk found in many studies, the clinical impact of decreasing levels of this lipoprotein has not yet been addressed in clinical trials.

Efficacy

In general, nicotinic acid at doses of 2–6 g/day decreases LDL cholesterol level 10%–25% and increases HDL cholesterol level 15%–35%. Triglyceride level decreases 20%–50%. Nicotinic acid is beneficial in all dyslipidemias except those characterized by chylomicronemia. Familial defective apo B-100, a genetic disorder in which abnormal apo B-100 prevents the recognition of LDL by the B/E receptor, may be effectively treated with nicotinic acid.[57] This disorder cannot be managed effectively with agents whose primary hypolipidemic mechanism involves upregulation of the B/E receptor; therefore, reduction in LDL production is a more rational therapeutic approach.

Because of its broad spectrum of action, nicotinic acid may be used in the majority of genetic dyslipidemias. The amount of lipid lowering achieved with this agent is related at least in part to the underlying genetic abnormality, so that the individual response rate varies considerably.

Side Effects and Drug Interactions

Although most side effects of nicotinic acid are modest clinical irritations not associated with serious sequelae, their occurrence has limited widespread use of the agent. Flushing that may be diffuse and profound is virtually universal with nicotinic acid therapy and relates to prostaglandin-mediated vasodilatation that may be severe enough to cause systemic hypotension. The underlying mechanism may be blocked by the concomitant administration of prostaglandin inhibitors, such as aspirin. The flushing is frequently accompanied by pruritus. Another dermatologic complication, although a rare one, is acanthosis nigricans, which may be seen with long-term use of nicotinic acid.

Nicotinic acid has been associated with gastric irritation and should be used with extreme caution in patients with known peptic ulcer disease or with an underlying predisposition to the development of this condition. Hepatic function may be altered, and alanine transaminase and aspartate transaminase levels may be elevated. Mild transaminase elevation is not an absolute indication for halting drug administration, but if the enzyme levels remain in excess of three times normal, the agent should be discontinued. Fulminant hepatic necrosis has been associated with administration of nicotinic acid and is more frequently seen with sustained-release formulations.[58] Because of the increased incidence of hepatotoxicity reported with sustained-release nicotinic acid, the NCEP recommends that these preparations be used only in patients unable to tolerate the crystalline formulations (sustained-release preparations may minimize flushing) and unable to be treated adequately with other drugs.

Adverse metabolic effects that may be caused by nicotinic acid include hyperuricemia, and acute gouty arthritis may be precipitated by long-term therapy. Glucose tolerance may be decreased, and the unmasking of latent diabetes mellitus has been reported. If the decrease in glucose tolerance is mild, the diabetic regimen can be intensified and the drug continued. However, caution should be used in administering nicotinic acid to patients known to be diabetic or predisposed to diabetes. Acipimox, a nicotinic acid derivative, has been successfully administered to patients with diabetes. In 46 patients with non–insulin-dependent diabetes, 24 weeks of treatment with acipimox decreased total cholesterol level 9% and LDL cholesterol level 8% and increased HDL cholesterol level 30% compared with placebo; glycated hemoglobin values were significantly reduced in the acipimox group.[59] In addition, acipimox has been shown to improve glucose tolerance after an oral glucose load[60] and is apparently associated with fewer dermatologic problems.[61]

Another adverse effect of nicotinic acid is myositis, although the risk for rhabdomyolysis appears to be low in patients receiving nicotinic acid monotherapy but is increased when nicotinic acid is administered in combination with an HMG-CoA reductase inhibitor. Ophthalmologic problems such as toxic amblyopia and worsening glaucoma have been reported but are uncommon.

Clinical Trials

Nicotinic acid has been used as monotherapy and in combination with other agents in a number of large clinical trials. In the Coronary Drug Project, 1119 men with previous MI received nicotinic acid, 3 g/day for 5 years, and experienced decreases in total cholesterol level of 10% and in triglyceride level of 26% after correction for lipid changes in the placebo group.[62] This group also demonstrated a statistically significant 27% reduction in risk for nonfatal MI. Expected side effects were reflected in a higher frequency of dermal abnormalities, gastrointestinal problems, acute gouty arthritis, and increased plasma glucose levels than in the other treatment groups. Ten years after the termination of the trial, the group that had been randomized to receive nicotinic acid had an 11% reduction in total mortality compared with the placebo group, which was highly statistically significant and indicates that early reduction in CHD may result in long-term improvement in total mortality.[63]

In the Stockholm Ischaemic Heart Disease Secondary Prevention Study, 555 men and women with prior MI were randomized to a control group or to a treatment group receiving nicotinic acid, 3 g/day, plus clofibrate, 2 g/day.[64] After 5 years of nonblinded treatment, the combination of nicotinic acid and clofibrate decreased total cholesterol level 13% and decreased triglyceride level 19% compared with the control group. The drug-treated group also experienced a 36% reduction in CHD-related mortality and a 26% reduction in total mortality compared with the control group. In retrospective subset analysis, the decrease in CHD-related mortality appeared to be greatest in subjects who had the largest decrease in triglyceride levels but was unrelated to the decrease in cholesterol.

Fibric Acid Derivatives

Clofibrate was the initial fibrate used clinically. Currently, clofibrate and gemfibrozil are available in the United States; fenofibrate is approved but not yet available. Bezafibrate, ciprofibrate, and fenofibrate are available in other countries.

Mechanisms of Action

Although different in structure, the fibric acid derivatives appear to be similar in mode of action, but the precise underlying hypolipidemic mechanisms are complex and not completely understood. The primary effect of the fibrates is to enhance the catabolism of triglyceride-rich lipoproteins by increasing the activity of lipoprotein lipase. The increased catabolism increases the transfer of surface lipid components into the HDL fraction and results in increased HDL cholesterol levels.[65] In addition, there appears to be a hepatic action that results in decreased VLDL synthesis. Although the fibrates were initially thought to decrease cholesterol synthesis modestly, studies have shown no rise in urinary excretion of mevalonic acid with fibrate administration, which indicates that there is no alteration in the biosynthetic capacity of cholesterol.[66] LDL cholesterol appears to be decreased because of increased affinity of the B/E receptor for circulating LDL, in response to decreased intracellular cholesterol in hepatocytes.[67]

Efficacy

The predominant effects of fibric acid derivatives are to lower plasma triglyceride and raise HDL cholesterol levels; effects on total and LDL cholesterol levels are modest and vary according to the underlying hyperlipidemia. Clofibrate administered at a dosage of 2000 mg/day or gemfibrozil administered at a dosage of 1200 mg/day typically decreases triglyceride levels 20%–50% and increases HDL cholesterol levels approximately 10%–15%. LDL cholesterol level may be expected to decrease 10%–15%, but in patients with hypertriglyceridemia, LDL cholesterol level may increase. The variable effect on LDL cholesterol level may be a function of the efficiency of the B/E receptor in clearing the increased LDL generated by increased VLDL catabolism.

In addition to the changes in plasma lipid levels, fibrates have been found to alter the composition of lipoproteins. The small, dense LDL particles associated with hypertriglyceridemia are thought to be more atherogenic than normal LDL, and reduction of plasma triglyceride levels with fibrates has resulted in alteration in LDL composition to a potentially less atherogenic phenotype. Gemfibrozil administered to patients with primary hypercholesterolemia decreases circulating levels of small, dense LDL but not of more buoyant LDL and increases the amount of cholesteryl ester in the LDL particles, so that the atherogenicity of LDL may be decreased without a decrease in LDL cholesterol level.[68] Although the clinical benefit of altering LDL subclass has not been proved, it is theoretically attractive.

Some of the benefit of fibrate therapy may be achieved by alteration of coagulation variables and platelet function. Fibrates have been shown to reduce platelet aggregability and reactivity in response to epinephrine.[69] Fibrinogen, which has been linked to increased CHD risk in epidemiologic studies, is also decreased by fibric acid derivatives.[70] Gemfibrozil has been shown to decrease clotting factor VII–phospholipid complex level,[71] which is correlated with plasma triglyceride level.[72]

Side Effects and Drug Interactions

Fibrates are generally well tolerated, and the side effects encountered are often clinically mild but may occur in up to 5% of patients receiving these agents. The majority of side effects reported are gastrointestinal. Increased cholelithiasis has been reported with clofibrate use[62] but has not been definitely associated with the other fibrates. Liver function may occasionally be affected, but this alteration is usually limited to mild, reversible elevations of circulating alanine transaminase and aspartate transaminase. Myositis may occur with fibrate use, especially when a fibrate is combined with an HMG-CoA reductase inhibitor. However, rhabdomyolysis is extremely rare with fibrate monotherapy.

Other drug interactions involving fibric acid derivatives include increased anticoagulant activity of warfarin; therefore, prothrombin time should be monitored for potential changes when these agents are combined. Fibrate absorption, and consequently efficacy, may be decreased if the fibrate is coadministered with a bile acid sequestrant. The combination of nicotinic acid, which decreases VLDL production, and a fibric acid derivative, which increases VLDL catabolism, may be of benefit in patients with marked hypertriglyceridemia that cannot be controlled by either agent alone.

Clinical Trials

The World Health Organization (WHO) Cooperative Trial, begun in 1965, was a large primary-prevention study that randomized more than 10,000 men aged 30–59 years with hypercholesterolemia to receive clofibrate, 1600 mg/day, or placebo.[73] Average time on trial was 5.3 years. The reduction in total cholesterol level induced by clofibrate was a modest 9%, but this mild improvement was accompanied by a statistically significant 20% reduction in incidence of major ischemic heart disease. The WHO data were not originally analyzed on an intent-to-treat basis. The initial 47% excess in total mortality reported during the trial in the patients who received clofibrate was reduced to 11% during a 13-year follow-up period that included almost 8 years after the trial was completed.[74]

Clofibrate, 1600 mg/day, was administered to 1103 men with prior MI in the Coronary Drug Project.[62] After 5 years, total cholesterol level decreased 6% and triglyceride level decreased 22% compared with placebo. Small, nonsignificant improvements in cardiovascular mortality were reported, but no effect on total mortality was demonstrated. At 15-year follow-up, the group randomized to clofibrate had no increased mortality.[63]

The Helsinki Heart Study randomized 4081 men with non-HDL cholesterol level greater than 200 mg/dL and no evidence of CHD to receive gemfibrozil, 1200 mg/day, or placebo for 5 years.[75] Compared with placebo, gemfibrozil decreased total cholesterol level 10%, LDL cholesterol level 11%, and triglyceride level 35% and increased HDL cholesterol level 11%. However, despite these modest changes in total cholesterol and LDL cholesterol levels, CHD events, defined as fatal and nonfatal MI and cardiac death, were significantly reduced 34%. In a subgroup characterized by LDL cholesterol/HDL cholesterol ratio greater than 5 and triglyceride level greater than 200 mg/dL, which accounted for only 10% of the study population, CHD risk was reduced 70%. The investigators suggested that this subgroup may also have in common small, dense LDL, although the effect of gemfibrozil on this lipoprotein subclass was beyond the scope of the study.

OTHER PHARMACOLOGIC AGENTS

Estrogen

Observational epidemiologic studies have shown a high level of agreement that postmenopausal women are at increased risk for CHD. In the Framingham Heart Study, risk for a CHD event in postmenopausal women was more than twice that in premenopausal women; risk was increased whether menopause was natural or surgical.[76] CHD remains the leading cause of death in women in the United States, as it does for men, and the increase in CHD events that occurs in the postmenopausal years may be at least partly explained by the loss of estrogen. At 10-year follow-up of 48,470 postmenopausal women in the Nurses' Health Study, overall relative risk for major CHD events in subjects taking estrogen was 0.56 compared with subjects not taking estrogen.[77] This risk was reduced in subjects with natural and surgical menopause. Relative risk was 0.89 for total mortality and 0.72 for cardiovascular mortality in subjects currently or formerly taking estrogen. These and other observational studies suggest that estrogen may be used as a cardioprotective agent in postmenopausal women; its benefit is thought to be related to improvements in the lipid profile.

The Atherosclerosis Risk in Communities (ARIC) study included 4958 postmenopausal women classified according to hormone use.[78] Current users of estrogen or of estrogen plus progestin had significantly higher HDL cholesterol and significantly lower LDL cholesterol and Lp(a) levels than did nonusers. In addition to these benefits to the lipid profile, estrogen use produced lower levels of plasma fibrinogen and higher levels of factor VII. Fasting glucose levels were also lowered with estrogen use.

The Lipid Research Clinics Program Follow-up Study included evaluation of mortality in 2770 women, aged 40 to 69 years, during an average 8.5-year follow-up period.[79] Age-adjusted relative risk for cardiovascular death was 0.34 in estrogen users compared with nonusers. Although the mechanism by which estrogen decreased cardiovascular mortality could not be determined from this study, it was thought to be secondary to an estrogen-induced increase in HDL cholesterol.

A controversial exception to the body of clinical evidence supporting CHD risk reduction with estrogen use is a substudy of the Framingham Heart Study that evaluated the effect of estrogen on CHD incidence in 1234 postmenopausal women aged 50–83 years.[80] Relative risk for CHD was found to be 1.90 with estrogen use, although the risk for MI, eliminating the subjective reporting of angina, was not significantly increased.

Mechanisms of Action

The mechanisms by which estrogen confers its beneficial effects on CHD risk are unclear but may include improvement of coronary tone and alteration of platelet aggregation and other clotting factors. However, the bulk of evidence supports an improved lipid profile as a major source of clinical benefit with estrogen use. In addition to moderately increasing HDL cholesterol and moderately decreasing

LDL cholesterol levels in the circulation, as shown in numerous clinical studies,[81] estrogen has been shown in animal studies to reduce accumulation of LDL in the arterial wall.[82] Lp(a) levels may also be reduced[83]: a 50% reduction with a combination of estrogen and progesterone has been reported.[84] Although the medical implications of estrogen-induced Lp(a) reduction have not been elucidated, and the mechanism is unclear, increased Lp(a) level has been associated with increased risk for CHD in many studies, so it is theoretically attractive to normalize elevated levels of this atherogenic particle.

Efficacy

In postmenopausal women, orally administered estrogen may be expected to reduce LDL cholesterol levels by approximately 15% and increase HDL cholesterol levels by up to 15%. Triglyceride levels may increase, particularly in women with hypertriglyceridemia. Estrogen preparations commonly used are conjugated estrogen, at a dosage of 0.625 mg/day, and micronized estradiol, at a dosage of 2 mg/day. Transcutaneously or percutaneously administered estrogen appears to have less effect on lipoprotein levels than does orally administered estrogen. Exogenous estrogen has not yet received a U.S. Food and Drug Administration indication for lipid regulation or for reduction of CHD risk.

Side Effects

Postmenopausal estrogen use is not without risk, and the potential benefits must be weighed against the possibility of increased risk for endometrial cancer and other malignant neoplasms. The potential role of estrogen in breast cancer risk is unclear and highly controversial, although there may be a slight increase in risk with long-term use. Estrogen has been clearly associated with decreased risk for osteoporotic hip fracture but does not appear to affect risk for cerebrovascular disease.

Clinical Trials

In the multicenter, double-blind Postmenopausal Estrogen/Progestin Interventions (PEPI) trial, 875 healthy postmenopausal women aged 45 to 64 years were randomized to receive placebo; estrogen, 0.625 mg/day, alone; estrogen plus cyclic medroxyprogesterone acetate (MPA), 10 mg/day for 12 days/month; estrogen plus consecutive MPA, 2.5 mg/day; or estrogen plus cyclic micronized progesterone, 200 mg/day for 12 days/month.[85] The 3-year trial was powered to evaluate the effect of hormone-replacement therapy not on CHD directly but on selected factors thought to be associated with CHD risk: HDL cholesterol, blood pressure, insulin, and fibrinogen. HDL cholesterol differed significantly between the group receiving placebo, which had a slight decrease, and the groups receiving active treatment. Among the active-treatment groups, the slight increases in the groups receiving estrogen plus MPA were significantly less than the increases in the groups receiving estrogen alone or with micronized progesterone. Total cholesterol level was significantly lower in the groups receiving estrogen plus MPA than in the placebo group, and decreases in LDL cholesterol level were similar in all active-treatment groups and significantly different from placebo. Increases in triglyceride level were similar for all active-treatment groups and were significantly different from triglyceride level in the placebo group, which decreased slightly. Of the nonlipid primary endpoints, neither blood pressure nor 2-h insulin was significantly different between groups, although 2-h glucose, another measure of carbohydrate metabolism, increased significantly more with active treatment than with placebo. Fibrinogen increased significantly more in the placebo group than in the active-treatment groups; differences between active-treatment groups were not significant. The PEPI trial suggests that beneficial effects of estrogen on the CHD risk profile are not nullified by coadministration with progesterone, although MPA does significantly decrease the benefit to HDL cholesterol level. Estrogen alone was found to cause the greatest increase in HDL cholesterol level, but this regimen was also associated with increased endometrial hyperplasia. Micronized progesterone appears to preserve most of the benefit of estrogen administration without increasing risk for endometrial hyperplasia.

Among secondary-prevention trials, the Coronary Drug Project originally included two estrogen regimens, but both were discontinued because of adverse effects in the all-male study population.[62] Compared with placebo, conjugated estrogen at a dosage of 5.0 mg/day was associated with excess nonfatal cardiovascular events and lack of efficacy on total mortality, and conjugated estrogen at a dosage of 2.5 mg/day produced excess thromboembolism, cancer mortality, and total mortality.

Most published secondary-prevention studies with estrogen replacement have been retrospective studies instead of placebo-controlled, randomized trials. A retrospective study of 2268 women 55 years of age or older or with previous bilateral oophorectomy who were undergoing coronary angiography compared survival in patients who were currently using or had ever used estrogen with those who had never used estrogen.[86] In patients without angiographic evidence of CHD, there was no difference in 10-year survival between patients who had and patients who had not used estrogen. In subjects with coronary lesions causing less than 70% stenosis, 10-year survival was 85% in those who had never used estrogen and 96% in subjects who currently or formerly used estrogen, which was a statistically significant difference. In patients with coronary lesions causing 70% or greater stenosis, 10-year survival was 60% in those who had never used estrogen and 97% in those who currently or formerly used estrogen, which was a highly significant difference.

In 933 women aged 50–75 years who were undergoing coronary angiography, Gruchow and colleagues[87] assessed occlusion of coronary arteries by current use (within the 3 months before angiography) versus nonuse of estrogen-replacement therapy. Estrogen users were found to have less occlusion, and occlusion did not increase with age in this group as it did among nonusers. This protective effect of estrogen was not independent of HDL cholesterol, which suggests that estrogen confers cardioprotection by increasing HDL cholesterol level.

The NCEP recommends that oral estrogen be considered for LDL cholesterol lowering in postmenopausal women who require drug therapy. Estrogen-replacement therapy provides an alternative to the other pharmacologic agents in patients for whom the risk/benefit ratio appears favorable.

Fish Oil

Observational epidemiologic studies have documented that populations that consume increased quantities of omega-3 polyunsaturated fatty acids—predominantly eicosapentaenoic acid and docosahexaenoic acid—have decreased prevalence of atherosclerosis.[88] Autopsy studies of Alaskan natives have revealed less extensive coronary and peripheral artery disease.[89] In the Multiple Risk Factor Intervention Trial, CHD mortality was inversely related to the estimated dietary intake of omega-3 polyunsaturated fatty acids.[90] Although the mechanism by which increased consumption of cold-water fish and other marine animals with a high content of these polyunsaturates lowers lipids in humans remains controversial, in vitro studies have demonstrated a decrease in synthesis and secretion of apo B in cells incubated with eicosapentaenoic acid.[91] These studies have not been duplicated in humans, and their applicability to other species is not known.

In addition to their beneficial effects on the lipid profile, including decreasing plasma triglyceride and increasing apo A-I and HDL cholesterol levels, these agents have been documented to have nonlipid effects that may enhance their clinical benefit. Fish oils have been shown to prolong bleeding time, although more recent studies have demonstrated that the effects of these fatty acids on platelet function and hemostasis may be more limited than previously reported.[92] The role of neutrophil adhesion in acute ischemic syndromes is thought to be an important manifestation of MI. Fish oils decrease binding of leukocytes to the endothelium and displace the precursor of leukotriene B_4, an adhesion promoter.[93] In addition, dietary intake of fish oil has been shown in some studies to reduce coronary restenosis after angioplasty.[94] Until the role of omega-3 fatty acids has been clarified, however, the NCEP does not recommend supplemental dietary intake.

Antioxidant Therapy

LDL appears to require modification for recognition and binding by the scavenger receptor of monocyte/macrophages. After modification of LDL by, for example, acetylation or oxidation, cellular uptake is enhanced and foam cell generation is increased. Hence, agents that prevent the oxidative modification of LDL may confer clinical benefit by preventing this essential step in atherogenesis and so decreasing lipid accumulation in foam cells.

Antioxidant defense systems have been identified and may be membranous, intracellular, or extracellular in location. Alpha-tocopherol and beta-carotene are localized to the cell membrane. Intracellular antioxidants include superoxide dismutase, catalase, peroxidase, reduced glutathione, and ascorbic acid; extracellular antioxidants include ceruloplasmin, haptoglobin, ascorbic acid, and alpha-tocopherol. Within LDL, the major antioxidant appears to be alpha-tocopherol, although other antioxidants are also present.[95]

Although there is a large body of evidence from in vitro studies, the clinical implications of these studies are controversial. A European multicenter epidemiologic study demonstrated an inverse correlation between plasma levels of alpha-tocopherol and CHD-related mortality.[96] Supplementation of diet with large doses of vitamin E or C has been shown to increase plasma levels of these compounds.[97] Vitamin C supplementation decreases the susceptibility of LDL to oxidation in vitro, even though ascorbic acid is hydrophilic.

Dietary intake of certain fatty acids may increase the susceptibility of LDL to oxidative stress. Ingestion of large quantities of fish oil increases levels of thiobarbituric acid–reacting substances,[98] which provide a nonspecific measurement of oxidation. Diets rich in linoleic acid may also increase oxidative stress and so increase the susceptibility of LDL to oxidation.[99] Although evidence from observational epidemiologic studies supports the intake of naturally occurring antioxidants as protection against atherosclerosis, there are currently no prospective trials that demonstrate clinical benefit.

SPECIAL CONSIDERATIONS

Children and Adolescents

Children and adolescents in the United States have higher mean total cholesterol levels than do young people in many other countries, presumably because of higher intake of saturated fat and cholesterol. Pathologic examination of coronary arteries in the Bogalusa Heart Study,[100] which included subjects aged 7–24 years at time of death, and the Pathobiological Determinants of Atherosclerosis in Youth study,[101] which included subjects aged 15–34 years at time of death, indicates that coronary atherosclerosis begins in childhood and is associated with LDL cholesterol levels.

The NCEP convened an expert panel to establish evaluation and treatment guidelines for children and adolescents aged 2–19 years.[102] Although universal screening is not recommended in young people, children and adolescents from families with premature cardiovascular disease or dyslipidemia should be screened. However, a report from the Bogalusa Heart Study suggests that selective screening may not detect children at risk whose parents are too young for disease to have been diagnosed.[103]

As in adults, initial therapy for dyslipidemia in children at least 2 years of age is dietary. If 6 months to 1 year of adherence to dietary therapy does not achieve treatment goals, drug therapy should be considered in addition to dietary therapy for patients 10 years of age or older if LDL cholesterol level remains 190 mg/dL or greater or if LDL cholesterol level remains 160 mg/dL or greater in conjunction with either a positive family history of cardiovascular disease before the age of 55 or at least two other risk factors that have not been controlled despite vigorous efforts. The NCEP recommends that the choice of drugs be carefully considered and that LDL cholesterol, height, weight, and potential adverse effects of the drug selected be closely monitored in these patients.

The bile acid sequestrants appear to be safe when used in children. In this age group, the dosage of the resin should be determined not by body weight but by the levels of total cholesterol and LDL cholesterol. The child should begin with the lowest possible dosage, and then the dosage should be gradually titrated upward to achieve goals for total cholesterol and LDL cholesterol.

Nicotinic acid has been studied in children with FH, who did not suffer serious short-term effects.[104] However, this drug should be used with caution in children. Its use in this age group requires referral to a lipid specialist and should be considered only if diet and bile acid sequestrant therapy have proved inadequate for the attainment of treatment goals. As in adults, the normal safety measures required with nicotinic acid, including monitoring of blood uric acid, blood glucose, and liver enzyme levels, are necessary in children.

HMG-CoA reductase inhibitors, fibric acid derivatives, and probucol are currently not recommended in children and adolescents because of inadequate clinical experience in this age group.

The Elderly

Treatment of dyslipidemia in elderly patients has been controversial because of conflicting observational epidemiologic evidence and a lack of interventional trials that target this population. In the Kaiser Permanente Coronary Heart Disease in the Elderly Study, an observational epidemiologic study conducted in 2746 men aged 60–79 years without self-reported history of CHD, the excess risk for CHD-related mortality associated with elevated total cholesterol level increased more than fivefold with age.[105] A study of 997 men and women aged 65 years or older (mean age 79 years) reported that hypercholesterolemia is no longer a risk factor for CHD in individuals older than 70 years, but cholesterol values were based on nonfasting samples in 88% of subjects and were divided into fairly broad categories (<200 mg/dL, 200–240 mg/dL, and ≥240 mg/dL).[106] More clinical trial data are needed in this population.

Early studies used risk ratios that compared the prevalence of CHD in subjects whose cholesterol was in the highest quintile with that in subjects whose cholesterol was in the lowest quintile. As age increases, these risk ratios decrease, which has been interpreted to suggest that elderly subjects may not benefit from cholesterol reduction. However, the absolute number of individuals with coronary disease is increased in the elderly population, implying that more patients may benefit. In addition, chronologic and physiologic age may not be identical.

The current life expectancy after age 65 is 19 years in the United States. In a number of clinical trials, benefits of cholesterol lowering have not been seen during the first 2 or 3 years of the trial. Thus, if a patient's life expectancy is less than 5 years, cholesterol lowering may not be clinically indicated or cost effective.

There have been no data presented to establish that the process of atherosclerosis is different in the elderly population. Instead, evidence is accumulating that older individuals do benefit from interventions that reduce the risk for cardiovascular events. Risk factors for cardiac morbidity and mortality that apply to the general population have been shown to apply to the elderly as well. Although elderly patients with hypertension have frequently not been treated because of the widely accepted premise that irreversible vascular damage had already occurred and so lowering blood pressure would not be of benefit, trials such as the Systolic Hypertension in the Elderly Program (SHEP)[107] and Swedish Trial in Old Patients with Hypertension (STOP-Hypertension)[108] have shown a reduction in cardiovascular events in older patients treated for hypertension.

Clinical trials specifically designed to test the premise that lipid lowering in the elderly is of benefit have not been reported. However, in a subgroup analysis of 4S subjects, subjects aged 60 years or older had significant reductions in total mortality and in major coronary events.[35]

Drug therapy in the elderly should not be undertaken without careful evaluation of the patient's long-term prognosis, overall risk profile, existing CHD, and other medical conditions. In addition, elderly patients may be particularly susceptible to adverse drug effects, in part because of decreasing body size and cardiac output as well as the frequent coadministration of multiple medications, which increases the potential for drug interactions. Clinical judgment is essential in determining the need for aggressive therapy.

Bile acid sequestrants may be poorly tolerated in the elderly because of frequent gastrointestinal toxicity and may interfere with the absorption of coadministered drugs. Nicotinic acid may produce exaggerated side effects in this population, including flushing and dryness of the mouth and eyes. Diabetes mellitus increases in prevalence in the elderly, and in patients with glucose intolerance, diabetes may be unmasked by nicotinic acid administration. Hyperuricemia and increased risk for gout associated with nicotinic acid are also potential problems. Although the HMG-CoA reductase inhibitors are free from these side effects, extensive clinical experience in the elderly is lacking with these drugs. There is concern about possible increased risk for myopathy because most of the severe cases have been reported in older patients, particularly those with renal insufficiency. The use of fibric acid derivatives in the elderly is controversial because of their possible role in cholelithiasis, particularly with clofibrate use. In general, however, HMG-CoA reductase inhibitors and fibric acid derivatives are well tolerated in the elderly.

Drug therapy in primary prevention in the elderly should thus be undertaken only after thorough patient evaluation and with selection criteria clearly in mind. Secondary prevention, however, becomes more important because of the high prevalence of coronary disease in this age group. Patients older than 60 years who have known atherosclerosis should not be excluded a priori from aggressive therapy, because of the high rate of recurrence of vascular events in subjects with existing atherosclerosis.

Women

Coronary atherosclerotic events are fairly uncommon in women before menopause; however, the number of women who die of atherosclerosis-related events is roughly the same as the number of men because of the marked increase in CHD after menopause. The gender-mediated relative cardioprotection in women decreases after menopause and virtually disappears after the age of 70 years. LDL cholesterol increases sharply at menopause, and HDL cholesterol may decrease somewhat.

There is less clinical trial evidence of the effect of cholesterol lowering in women than in men because the majority of early trials excluded women, and in those that did enroll women, the number was generally too small to make definite conclusions about events. However, the decline in CHD during the past several decades has included decreased morbidity and mortality in women, and there are no data to suggest that the process of atherosclerosis in men is different from that in women. Lipid-regulating therapy with simvastatin was found to decrease incidence of major coronary events 35% in women, which was statistically significant.[35] Nevertheless, dyslipidemia in women remains a complicated issue. Hypertriglyceridemia was found to be an independent CHD risk factor in women but not in men in an analysis of Framingham Heart Study data.[109] HDL cholesterol may also be a stronger risk predictor in women than in men.

The NCEP recommends delaying drug therapy in premenopausal women without additional risk. Estrogen-replacement therapy may be used instead of lipid-regulating drugs in some postmenopausal women. As in men, drug therapy should be considered in postmenopausal women with very high LDL cholesterol levels or with multiple other risk factors.

Patients With Diabetes Mellitus

CHD, cerebrovascular disease, or peripheral vascular disease is the cause of death in 75% to 80% of adult patients with diabetes mellitus.[110] Premenopausal women with diabetes do not have the relative protection against CHD of premenopausal women without diabetes. In patients with diabetes, the typical dyslipidemia is increased plasma triglyceride and decreased HDL cholesterol levels. Patients with diabetes frequently have multiple CHD risk factors, but the associated risk factors do not explain all the excess risk in these patients.[111]

The American Diabetes Association Consensus Development Conference on the Detection and Management of Lipid Disorders in Diabetes[110] recommended that adult patients with diabetes receive a full fasting lipoprotein analysis annually. As in the NCEP guidelines, the aggressiveness of intervention is determined by the presence or absence of atherosclerotic disease. In patients without macrovascular disease, risk is further stratified by the presence of major cardiovascular risk factors, defined as HDL cholesterol level of 35 mg/dL or less, cigarette smoking, hypertension, and a family history of premature CHD.

In diabetic patients without macrovascular disease, if, after a 6-month trial of nonpharmacologic measures (low-fat diet, increased physical activity, and reduction of weight if overweight) and improved glycemic control, LDL cholesterol level remains 160 mg/dL or greater, or 130 mg/dL or greater in the presence of at least one other major risk factor, or if triglyceride level remains 400 mg/dL or greater, or 200 mg/dL or greater in the presence of at least one other major risk factor, drug therapy should be considered. In diabetic patients with macrovascular disease, if, after an adequate trial of nonpharmacologic measures and improved glycemic control (typically 3–6 months, although clinical judgment is especially required in these high-risk patients), LDL cholesterol level remains greater than 100 mg/dL or triglyceride level remains greater than 150 mg/dL, drug therapy should be considered. Patients whose triglyceride level is 1000 mg/dL or greater require special, immediate attention because of the increased risk for pancreatitis.

The fibric acid derivatives are useful in the diabetic patient because of their triglyceride-lowering and HDL cholesterol–raising effects. If LDL cholesterol becomes elevated with fibric acid derivative monotherapy, a bile acid sequestrant may be added at a low dosage. Fibrates do not appear to affect carbohydrate tolerance, but they may increase the risk for cholelithiasis, which is already increased in diabetes.

The HMG-CoA reductase inhibitors are useful for lowering LDL cholesterol level in diabetic patients. Triglyceride and HDL cholesterol levels may be improved, but these improvements are marginal if the triglyceride level is elevated and the HDL cholesterol level is low. The HMG-CoA reductase inhibitors have no effect on glucose control, but their effect on insulin resistance is not known. In familial forms of hypercholesterolemia, these agents may be used as monotherapy or in combination with a bile acid sequestrant.

Nicotinic acid is not recommended as first-line therapy in patients with diabetes because it increases insulin resistance, hyperglycemia, and hyperinsulinemia. Nicotinic acid should be used only in patients with refractory dyslipidemia and then only with careful monitoring; if glycemic control cannot be maintained, this agent must be discontinued. Nicotinic acid is relatively contraindicated in patients with insulin resistance because it may accelerate the development of clinical diabetes.

The bile acid sequestrants are not usually used as monotherapy in patients with diabetes because they can increase the triglyceride level, particularly if it is already elevated as is common in diabetes, and because their primary effect is to lower LDL cholesterol, which is not typically the sole dyslipidemia in diabetes. However, a low-dosage bile acid sequestrant may be added to a fibric acid derivative in patients with elevations in both VLDL and LDL, or to an HMG-CoA reductase inhibitor in patients with severe or familial forms of hypercholesterolemia; the latter combination is generally more effective and less toxic than HMG-CoA reductase inhibitor monotherapy. Bile acid sequestrants must be used with great care in diabetic patients with gastrointestinal autonomic neuropathy because of the increased risk for constipation or even fecal impaction. These agents have no adverse effect on glucose control.

TOTAL MORTALITY

The effect of cholesterol lowering on total mortality rates has been controversial.[112] Although secondary-prevention trials have generally documented decreased mortality with lipid lowering, primary-prevention trials such as the LRC-CPPT and the Helsinki Heart Study did not demonstrate decreased total mortality because of an increase in noncardiovascular deaths. However, in WOSCOPS, total mortality was decreased and noncardiovascular mortality was not increased.

Some observational studies have indicated increased mortality at lower cholesterol levels, but a causal relation has not been established. Low cholesterol can be a marker for decreased cholesterol production caused by serious illness, such as malignant neoplasm or cirrhosis of the liver, and these studies included individuals with these illnesses, as well as chronic obstructive pulmonary disease and hemorrhagic stroke.

Until recently, trials were not sufficiently powered to evaluate total mortality. However, with the publication of the results of 4S, which was designed specifically to measure total mortality, many of the questions concerning cholesterol lowering and mortality have been answered. In addition to the highly significant decrease in total mortality in the group treated with simvastatin, this study found no increase in noncardiovascular deaths with drug treatment.[35]

REFERENCES

1. National Cholesterol Education Program: Second report of the Expert Panel on Detection, Evaluation, and Treatment of High Blood Cholesterol in Adults (Adult Treatment Panel II). Circulation 1994; 89:1329.
2. Moore RB, Crane CA, Frantz ID Jr: Effect of cholestyramine on the fecal excretion of intravenously administered cholesterol-4-^{14}C and its degradation products in a hypercholesterolemic patient. J Clin Invest 1968; 47:1664.
3. Grundy SM, Ahrens EH Jr, Salen G: Interruption of the enterohepatic circulation of bile acids in man: comparative effects of cholestyramine and ileal exclusion on cholesterol metabolism. J Lab Clin Med 1971; 78:94.
4. Asano T, Pollard M, Madsen DC: Effect of cholestyramine on 1,2-dimethylhydrazine-induced enteric carcinoma in germfree rats. Proc Soc Exp Biol Med 1975; 150:780.
5. Gallo DG, Bailey KR, Sheffner AL: The interaction between cholestyramine and drugs. Proc Soc Exp Biol Med 1965; 120:60.
6. Lipid Research Clinics Program: The Lipid Research Clinics Coronary Primary Prevention Trial results. I. Reduction in incidence of coronary heart disease. JAMA 1984; 251:351.
7. Lipid Research Clinics Program: The Lipid Research Clinics Coronary Primary Prevention Trial results. II. The relationship of reduction in incidence of coronary heart disease to cholesterol lowering. JAMA 1984; 251:365.
8. Brensike JF, Levy RI, Kelsey SF, et al: Effects of therapy with cholestyramine on progression of coronary arteriosclerosis: results of the NHLBI Type II Coronary Intervention Study. Circulation 1984; 69:313.
9. Watts GF, Lewis B, Brunt JNH, et al: Effects on coronary artery disease of lipid-lowering diet, or diet plus cholestyramine, in the St Thomas' Atherosclerosis Regression Study (STARS). Lancet 1992; 339:563.
10. Blankenhorn DH, Nessim SA, Johnson RL, et al: Beneficial effects of combined colestipol-niacin therapy on coronary atherosclerosis and coronary venous bypass grafts. JAMA 1987; 257:3233.
11. Cashin-Hemphill L, Mack WJ, Pogoda JM, et al: Beneficial effects of colestipol-niacin on coronary atherosclerosis: a 4-year follow-up. JAMA 1990; 264:3013.
12. Blankenhorn DH, Alaupovic P, Wickham E, et al: Prediction of angiographic change in native human coronary arteries and aortocoronary bypass grafts: lipid and nonlipid factors. Circulation 1990; 81:470.
13. Brown G, Albers JJ, Fisher LD, et al: Regression of coronary artery disease as a result of intensive lipid-lowering therapy in men with high levels of apolipoprotein B. N Engl J Med 1990; 323:1289.
14. Endo A, Kuroda M, Tsujita Y: ML-236A, ML-236B, and ML-236C, new inhibitors of cholesterogenesis produced by *Penicillium citrinum.* J Antibiot (Tokyo) 1976; 29:1346.
15. Arad Y, Ramakrishnan R, Ginsberg HN: Lovastatin therapy reduces low density lipoprotein apoB levels in subjects with combined hyperlipidemia by reducing the production of apoB-containing lipoproteins: implications for the pathophysiology of apoB production. J Lipid Res 1990; 31:567.
16. Uauy R, Vega GL, Grundy SM, et al: Lovastatin therapy in receptor-negative homozygous familial hypercholesterolemia: lack of effect on low-density lipoprotein concentrations or turnover. J Pediatr 1988; 113:387.
17. Hunninghake DB: HMG CoA reductase inhibitors. Curr Opin Lipidol 1992; 3:22.
18. Grundy SM, Vega GL: Influence of mevinolin on the metabolism of low density lipoproteins in primary moderate hypercholesterolemia. J Lipid Res 1985; 26:1464.
19. Kirby TJ: Cataracts produced by triparanol. Trans Am Ophthalmol Soc 1967; 65:493.
20. Tobert JA, Shear CL, Chremos AN, et al: Clinical experience with lovastatin. Am J Cardiol 1990; 65:23F.
21. Pierce LR, Wysowski DK, Gross TP: Myopathy and rhabdomyolysis associated with lovastatin-gemfibrozil combination therapy. JAMA 1990; 264:71.
22. Spach DH, Bauwens JE, Clark CD, et al: Rhabdomyolysis associated with lovastatin and erythromycin use. West J Med 1991; 154:213.
23. Corpier CL, Jones PH, Suki WN, et al: Rhabdomyolysis and renal injury with lovastatin use. Report of two cases in cardiac transplant recipients. JAMA 1988; 260:239.
24. Tobert JA: Efficacy and long-term adverse effect pattern of lovastatin. Am J Cardiol 1988; 62:28J.
25. Grundy SM: HMG CoA reductase inhibitors: clinical applications and therapeutic potential. *In* Rifkind BM (ed): Drug Treatment of Hyperlipidemia, p 139. New York: Marcel Dekker, 1991.
26. Glueck CJ, Oakes N, Speirs J, et al: Gemfibrozil-lovastatin therapy for primary hyperlipoproteinemias. Am J Cardiol 1992; 70:1.
27. Wiklund O, Angelin B, Bergman M, et al: Pravastatin and gemfibrozil alone and in combination for the treatment of hypercholesterolemia. Am J Med 1993; 94:13.
28. Bradford RH, Shear CL, Chremos AN, et al: Expanded Clinical Evaluation of Lovastatin (EXCEL) study results: two-year efficacy and safety follow-up. Am J Cardiol 1994; 74:667.
29. Mantell G, Burke T, Staggers J: Extended clinical safety profile of lovastatin. Am J Cardiol 1990; 66:11B.
30. Ahmad S: Lovastatin: warfarin interaction. Arch Intern Med 1990; 150:2407.
31. Blankenhorn DH, Azen SP, Kramsch DM, et al: Coronary angiographic changes with lovastatin therapy: the Monitored Atherosclerosis Regression Study (MARS). Ann Intern Med 1993; 119:969.
32. Waters D, Higginson L, Gladstone P, et al: Effects of monotherapy with an HMG-CoA reductase inhibitor on the progression of coronary atherosclerosis as assessed by serial quantitative arteriography: the Canadian Coronary Atherosclerosis Intervention Trial. Circulation 1994; 89:959.

33. Pitt B, Mancini GBJ, Ellis SG, et al: Pravastatin Limitation of Atherosclerosis in the Coronary Arteries (PLAC I) [Abstract]. J Am Coll Cardiol 1995; 26:1133.
33a. Shephard J, Cobbe SM, Ford I, et al: Prevention of coronary heart disease with pravastatin in men with hypercholesterolemia. N Engl J Med 1995; 333:1301.
34. MAAS Investigators: Effect of simvastatin on coronary atheroma: the Multicentre Anti-Atheroma Study (MAAS). Lancet 1994; 344:633.
35. Scandinavian Simvastatin Survival Study Group: Randomised trial of cholesterol lowering in 4444 patients with coronary heart disease: the Scandinavian Simvastatin Survival Study (4S). Lancet 1994; 344:1383.
36. Steinberg D, Witztum JL: Probucol. *In* Rifkind BM (ed): Drug Treatment of Hyperlipidemia, p 169. New York: Marcel Dekker, 1991.
37. Baker SG, Joffe BI, Mendelsohn D, et al: Treatment of homozygous familial hypercholesterolemia with probucol. S Afr Med J 1982; 62:7.
38. Kesäniemi YA, Grundy SM: Influence of probucol on cholesterol and lipoprotein metabolism in man. J Lipid Res 1984; 25:780.
39. Gilligan DM, Guetta V, Panza JA, et al: Selective loss of microvascular endothelial function in human hypercholesterolemia. Circulation 1994; 90:35.
40. Kaplan R, Aynedjian HS, Schlondorff D, et al: Renal vasoconstriction caused by short-term cholesterol feeding is corrected by thromboxane antagonist or probucol. J Clin Invest 1990; 86:1707.
41. Finckh B, Niendorf A, Rath M, et al: Antiatherosclerotic effect of probucol in WHHL rabbits: are there plasma parameters to evaluate this effect? Eur J Clin Pharmacol 1991; 40(suppl 1):S77.
42. Yamamoto A, Hara H, Takaichi S, et al: Effect of probucol on macrophages, leading to regression of xanthomas and atheromatous vascular lesions. Am J Cardiol 1988; 62:31B.
43. Mellies MJ, Gartside PS, Glatfelder L, et al: Effects of probucol on plasma cholesterol, high and low density lipoprotein cholesterol, and apolipoproteins A1 and A2 in adults with primary familial hypercholesterolemia. Metabolism 1980; 29:956.
44. Berg A, Frey I, Baumstark M, et al: Influence of probucol administration on lipoprotein cholesterol and apolipoproteins in normolipemic males. Atherosclerosis 1988; 72:49.
45. Ying H, Saku K, Harada R, et al: Putative mechanisms of action of probucol on high-density lipoprotein apolipoprotein A-I and its isoproteins: kinetics in rabbits. Biochim Biophys Acta 1990; 1047:247.
46. Franceschini G, Sirtori M, Vaccarino V, et al: Mechanisms of HDL reduction after probucol. Changes in HDL subfractions and increased reverse cholesteryl ester transfer. Arteriosclerosis 1989; 9:462.
47. Carew TE, Schwenke DC, Steinberg D: Antiatherogenic effect of probucol unrelated to its hypocholesterolemic effect: evidence that antioxidants *in vivo* can selectively inhibit low density lipoprotein degradation in macrophage-rich fatty streaks and slow the progression of atherosclerosis in the Watanabe heritable hyperlipidemic rabbit. Proc Natl Acad Sci USA 1987; 84:7725.
48. Yamamoto A, Matsuzawa Y, Yokoyama S, et al: Effects of probucol on xanthomata regression in familial hypercholesterolemia. Am J Cardiol 1986; 57:29H.
49. Eto M, Sato T, Watanabe K, et al: Effects of probucol on plasma lipids and lipoproteins in familial hypercholesterolemic patients with and without apolipoprotein E4. Atherosclerosis 1990; 84:49.
50. Buckley MM-T, Goa KL, Price AH, et al: Probucol: a reappraisal of its pharmacological properties and therapeutic use in hypercholesterolaemia. Drugs 1989; 37:761.
51. Dujovne CA, Atkins F, Wong B, et al: Electrocardiographic effects of probucol. A controlled prospective clinical trial. Eur J Clin Pharmacol 1984; 26:735.
52. Walldius G, Erikson U, Olsson AG, et al: The effect of probucol on femoral atherosclerosis: the Probucol Quantitative Regression Swedish Trial (PQRST). Am J Cardiol 1994; 74:875.
53. Walldius G, Regnström J, Nilsson J, et al: The role of lipids and antioxidative factors for development of atherosclerosis. The Probucol Quantitative Regression Swedish Trial (PQRST). Am J Cardiol 1993; 71:15B.
54. Grundy SM, Mok HYI, Zech L, et al: Influence of nicotinic acid on metabolism of cholesterol and triglycerides in man. J Lipid Res 1981; 22:24.
55. Shepherd J, Packard CJ, Patsch JR, et al: Effects of nicotinic acid therapy on plasma high density lipoprotein subfraction distribution and composition and on apolipoprotein A metabolism. J Clin Invest 1979; 63:858.
56. Carlson LA, Hamsten A, Asplund A: Pronounced lowering of serum levels of lipoprotein Lp(a) in hyperlipidaemic subjects treated with nicotinic acid. J Intern Med 1989; 226:271.
57. Schmidt EB, Illingworth DR, Bacon S, et al: Hypolipidemic effects of nicotinic acid in patients with familial defective apolipoprotein B-100. Metabolism 1993; 42:137.
58. Rader JI, Calvert RJ, Hathcock JN: Hepatic toxicity of unmodified and time-release preparations of niacin. Am J Med 1992; 92:77.
59. Scott RS, Lintott CJ, Bremer JM, et al: Improvement in atherogenic risk factors with acipimox in non–insulin-dependent diabetic subjects. Atherosclerosis Reviews 1991; 22:201.
60. Alberti KGMM, Fulcher G, Walker M: Metabolic effects of acipimox in non–insulin-dependent diabetes mellitus. Atherosclerosis Reviews 1991; 22:193.
61. Walldius G, Tornvall P: Nicotinic acid and acipimox: similarities and differences. Atherosclerosis Reviews 1991; 22:197.
62. Coronary Drug Project Research Group: Clofibrate and niacin in coronary heart disease. JAMA 1975; 231:360.
63. Canner PL, Berge KG, Wenger NK, et al: Fifteen year mortality in Coronary Drug Project patients: long-term benefit with niacin. J Am Coll Cardiol 1986; 8:1245.
64. Carlson LA, Rosenhamer G: Reduction of mortality in the Stockholm Ischaemic Heart Disease Secondary Prevention Study by combined treatment with clofibrate and nicotinic acid. Acta Med Scand 1988; 223:405.
65. Simpson HS, Williamson CM, Olivecrona T, et al: Postprandial lipemia, fenofibrate and coronary artery disease. Atherosclerosis 1990; 85:193.
66. Beil FU, Schrameyer-Wernecke A, Beisiegel U, et al: Lovastatin versus bezafibrate: efficacy, tolerability, and effect on urinary mevalonate. Cardiology 1990; 77(suppl 4):22.
67. Illingworth DR: Fibric acid derivatives. *In* Rifkind BM (ed): Drug Treatment of Hyperlipidemia, p 103. New York: Marcel Dekker, 1991.
68. Tilly-Kiesi M, Tikkanen MJ: Low density lipoprotein density and composition in hypercholesterolaemic men treated with HMG CoA reductase inhibitors and gemfibrozil. J Intern Med 1991; 229:427.
69. Todd PA, Ward A: Gemfibrozil: a review of its pharmacodynamic and pharmacokinetic properties, and therapeutic use in dyslipidaemia. Drugs 1988; 36:314.
70. Davignon J: Fibrates: a review of important issues and recent findings. Can J Cardiol 1994; 10(suppl B):61B.
71. Andersen P, Smith P, Seljeflot I, et al: Effects of gemfibrozil on lipids and haemostasis after myocardial infarction. Thromb Haemost 1990; 63:174.
72. Nordoy A, Illingworth DR, Connor WE, et al: Increased activity of factor VII and factor VII–phospholipid complex measured using a Normotest system in subjects with hyperlipidemia. Haemostasis 1990; 20:65.
73. Committee of Principal Investigators: A co-operative trial in the primary prevention of ischaemic heart disease using clofibrate. Br Heart J 1978; 40:1069.
74. Committee of Principal Investigators: WHO cooperative trial on primary prevention of ischaemic heart disease with clofibrate to lower serum cholesterol: final mortality follow-up. Lancet 1984; 2:600.
75. Huttunen JK, Manninen V, Mänttäri M, et al: The Helsinki Heart Study: central findings and clinical implications. Ann Med 1991; 23:155.
76. Kannel WB: Metabolic risk factors for coronary heart disease in women: perspective from the Framingham Study. Am Heart J 1987; 114:413.
77. Stampfer MJ, Colditz GA, Willett WC, et al: Postmenopausal estrogen therapy and cardiovascular disease: ten-year follow-up from the Nurses' Health Study. N Engl J Med 1991; 325:756.
78. Nabulsi AA, Folsom AR, White A, et al: Association of hormone-replacement therapy with various cardiovascular risk factors in postmenopausal women. N Engl J Med 1993; 328:1069.
79. Bush TL, Barrett-Connor E, Cowan LD, et al: Cardiovascular mortality and noncontraceptive use of estrogen in women: results from the Lipid Research Clinics Program Follow-up Study. Circulation 1987; 75:1102.
80. Wilson PWF, Garrison RJ, Castelli WP: Postmenopausal estrogen use, cigarette smoking, and cardiovascular morbidity in women over 50: the Framingham Study. N Engl J Med 1985; 313:1038.
81. Granfone A, Campos H, McNamara JR, et al: Effects of estrogen replacement on plasma lipoproteins and apolipoproteins in postmenopausal, dyslipidemic women. Metabolism 1992; 41:1193.
82. Wagner JD, St Clair RW, Schwenke DC, et al: Regional differences in arterial low density lipoprotein metabolism in surgically postmenopausal cynomolgus monkeys. Effects of estrogen and progesterone replacement therapy. Arterioscler Thromb 1992; 12:717.
83. Gotto AM Jr: Postmenopausal hormone-replacement therapy, plasma lipoprotein[a], and risk for coronary heart disease [Editorial]. J Lab Clin Med 1994; 123:800.

84. Soma MR, Osnago-Gadda I, Paoletti R, et al: The lowering of lipoprotein[a] induced by estrogen plus progesterone replacement therapy in postmenopausal women. Arch Intern Med 1993; 153:1462.
85. Writing Group for the PEPI Trial: Effects of estrogen or estrogen/progestin regimens on heart disease risk factors in postmenopausal women: the Postmenopausal Estrogen/Progestin Interventions (PEPI) trial. JAMA 1995; 273:199.
86. Sullivan JM, Vander Zwaag R, Hughes JP, et al: Estrogen replacement and coronary artery disease. Effect on survival in postmenopausal women. Arch Intern Med 1990; 150:2557.
87. Gruchow HW, Anderson AJ, Barboriak JJ, et al: Postmenopausal use of estrogen and occlusion of coronary arteries. Am Heart J 1988; 115:954.
88. Bang HO, Dyerberg J: Plasma lipids and lipoproteins in Greenlandic west coast Eskimos. Acta Med Scand 1972; 192:85.
89. Newman WP, Middaugh JP, Propst MT, et al: Atherosclerosis in Alaska natives and non-natives. Lancet 1993; 341:1056.
90. Dolecek TA: Epidemiological evidence of relationships between dietary polyunsaturated fatty acids and mortality in the Multiple Risk Factor Intervention Trial. Proc Soc Exp Biol Med 1992; 200:177.
91. Murthy S, Albright E, Mathur SN, et al: Apolipoprotein B mRNA abundance is decreased by eicosapentaenoic acid in CaCo-2 cells. Arterioscler Thromb 1992; 12:691.
92. Braden GA, Knapp HR, FitzGerald GA: Suppression of eicosanoid biosynthesis during coronary angioplasty by fish oil and aspirin. Circulation 1991; 84:679.
93. Lehr HA, Hubner C, Nolte D, et al: Dietary fish oil blocks the microcirculatory manifestations of ischemia-reperfusion injury in striated muscle in hamsters. Proc Natl Acad Sci USA 1991; 88:6726.
94. Bairati I, Roy L, Meyer F: Double-blind, randomized, controlled trial of fish oil supplements in prevention of recurrence of stenosis after coronary angioplasty. Circulation 1992; 85:950.
95. Esterbauer H, Dieber-Rotheneder M, Striegl G, et al: Role of vitamin E in preventing the oxidation of low-density lipoprotein. Am J Clin Nutr 1991; 53(suppl 1):314S.
96. Gey KF, Puska P, Jordan P, et al: Inverse correlation between plasma vitamin E and mortality from ischemic heart disease in cross-cultural epidemiology. Am J Clin Nutr 1991; 53(1 suppl):326S.
97. Harats D, Ben-Naim M, Dabach Y, et al: Effect of vitamin C and E on susceptibility of plasma lipoproteins to peroxidation induced by acute smoking. Atherosclerosis 1990; 85:47.
98. Harats D, Dabach Y, Hollander G, et al: Fish oil ingestion in smokers and nonsmokers enhances peroxidation of plasma lipoproteins. Atherosclerosis 1991; 90:127.
99. Berry EM, Eisenberg S, Harats D, et al: Effects of diets rich in monounsaturated fatty acids on plasma lipoproteins—the Jerusalem Nutrition Study: high MUFAs vs high PUFAs. Am J Clin Nutr 1991; 53:899.
100. Newman WP III, Freedman DS, Voors AW, et al: Relation of serum lipoprotein levels and systolic blood pressure to early atherosclerosis. The Bogalusa Heart Study. N Engl J Med 1986; 314:138.
101. PDAY Research Group: Relationship of atherosclerosis in young men to serum lipoprotein cholesterol concentrations and smoking. A preliminary report from the Pathobiological Determinants of Atherosclerosis in Youth (PDAY) Research Group. JAMA 1990; 264:3018.
102. National Cholesterol Education Program: Report of the Expert Panel on Blood Cholesterol Levels in Children and Adolescents. Pediatrics 1992; 39(3, part 2):525.
103. Bao W, Srinivasan SR, Wattigney WA, et al: The relation of parental cardiovascular disease to risk factors in children and young adults: the Bogalusa Heart Study. Circulation 1995; 91:365.
104. Khachadurian AK, Uthman SM: Experiences with the homozygous cases of familial hypercholesterolemia. A report of 52 patients. Nutrition and Metabolism 1973; 15:132.
105. Rubin SM, Sidney S, Black DM, et al: High blood cholesterol in elderly men and the excess risk for coronary heart disease. Ann Intern Med 1990; 113:916.
106. Krumholz HM, Seeman TE, Merrill SS, et al: Lack of association between cholesterol and coronary heart disease mortality and morbidity and all-cause mortality in persons older than 70 years. JAMA 1994; 272:1335.
107. SHEP Cooperative Research Group: Prevention of stroke by antihypertensive drug treatment in older persons with isolated systolic hypertension. Final results of the Systolic Hypertension in the Elderly Program (SHEP). JAMA 1991; 265:3255.
108. Dahlof B, Lindholm LH, Hansson L, et al: Morbidity and mortality in the Swedish Trial in Old Patients with Hypertension (STOP-Hypertension). Lancet 1991; 338:1281.
109. Castelli WP: Epidemiology of triglycerides: a view from Framingham. Am J Cardiol 1992; 70:3H.
110. American Diabetes Association: Detection and management of lipid disorders in diabetes [American Diabetes Association Consensus Development Conference on the Detection and Management of Lipid Disorders in Diabetes, 11–13 January 1993, Dallas, Texas]. Diabetes Care 1993; 16(suppl 2):106.
111. Pyörälä K, Laakso M, Uusitupa M: Diabetes and atherosclerosis: an epidemiologic view. Diabetes Metab Rev 1987; 3:463.
112. Hulley SB, Walsh JM, Newman TB: Health policy on blood cholesterol: time to change directions [Editorial]. Circulation 1992; 86:1026.

26 The Steps Beyond Diet and Drug Therapy for Severe Hypercholesterolemia

9/18/98

Bruce R. Gordon, MD
Stuart D. Saal, MD

A small subset of patients with hypercholesterolemia have an inadequate lipid-lowering response to maximal diet and drug treatment and should be considered for additional therapy to come as close as possible to the therapeutic targets of the National Cholesterol Education Program (NCEP). Candidates for treatment beyond diet and drugs include (1) patients with homozygous familial hypercholesterolemia (FH), (2) patients with coronary artery disease (CAD) and a low-density lipoprotein cholesterol (LDL-C) level above 200 mg/dL, and (3) patients without CAD but with multiple risk factors for CAD including an LDL-C level greater than 300 mg/dL.

Treatment options either alone or in combination include plasmapheresis, low-density lipoprotein (LDL) apheresis, portacaval shunt, liver transplantation, partial ileal bypass (PIB), and gene therapy. The most commonly used and least invasive method for lowering

LDL-C in these patients is LDL apheresis. Methods for performing LDL apheresis include dextran sulfate–cellulose adsorption, immunoadsorption, and heparin-induced extracorporeal precipitation. Time-averaged LDL lowering of 40% to 50% is achieved with weekly or every other week LDL apheresis therapy. Portacaval shunts have been used to achieve LDL-C lowering of about 30% and should be considered in patients with homozygous FH who respond inadequately or cannot tolerate LDL apheresis. Liver transplantation, although capable of producing near-normalization of LDL-C, is associated with considerable morbidity and mortality. PIB surgery has slowed the progression of CAD but is probably not appropriate for patients with homozygous FH. Gene transfer has been used in a few patients with homozygous FH with limited success. Ex vivo gene transfer requires a partial hepatic resection and therefore has limited applicability. In vivo methods for gene transfer, although attractive, are not ready for routine clinical use.

DEFINITION OF TARGET POPULATION

Because nondietary, nonpharmacologic therapy for hypercholesterolemia entails a major commitment from the patient and medical community, and in some instances substantial risk, clear guidelines for considering such therapy are imperative. Unlike the NCEP guidelines[1] for instituting diet and drug therapy, there are no accepted guidelines for these patients. The patient should be on an American Heart Association Step II Diet or a more restrictive diet and maximal combination lipid-lowering drug therapy, including as tolerated a reductase inhibitor equivalent to lovastatin 80 mg daily, 6 scoops daily of a bile acid sequestrant, and nicotinic acid 1500 mg or more daily.

Criteria for additional therapy should include the degree of LDL-C elevation and whether the patient has CAD or multiple risk factors for CAD. It is reasonable to consider the addition of nondietary, nonpharmacologic therapy for the management of (1) all patients with homozygous FH, (2) patients with CAD and LDL-C levels above 200 mg/dL, and (3) patients without CAD but with an LDL-C level above 300 mg/dL and high risk for disease. Table 26–1 summarizes this approach and incorporates selection criteria with those from the NCEP. Individuals with extremely high triglyceride levels or secondary causes for hypercholesterolemia are generally not candidates for the therapies described in this chapter.

RATIONALE AND JUSTIFICATION FOR THIS POPULATION

Homozygous Familial Hypercholesterolemia

The clearest indication for nondietary, nondrug therapy is in patients with homozygous FH. This disorder is caused by the inheritance of two mutant genes at the LDL receptor locus. The clinical expression occurs in approximately 1 in 1 million individuals. The defect in LDL receptor function causes a marked elevation in the plasma concentration of LDL-C, which typically exceeds 500 mg/dL but can reach as high as 1000 mg/dL.[2] High-density lipoprotein cholesterol (HDL-C) levels tend to be substantially below normal. Clinical features include the presence of xanthomas, severe aortic root disease including aortic stenosis, and the premature onset of CAD. Angina pectoris, myocardial infarction, or sudden death frequently occurs between the ages of 5 and 20 years. Mabuchi and colleagues[3] observed 10 patients with homozygous FH for a period of approximately 14 years. During this time, six of the patients died of sudden death or heart failure at an average age of 26 years. Similar observations were reported in patients from South Africa.[4]

The severity of the clinical expression depends to a great extent on the percentage of functioning LDL receptors. In Goldstein and Brown's study of 57 homozygotes,[5] more than one fourth of receptor-absent patients died before the age of 25 years compared with 1 of 26 individuals with residual LDL receptor activity. Similar findings were reported by Sprecher and coworkers.[6] Because of very high risk for premature CAD and the poor response to diet and drug therapy, all patients with homozygous FH are candidates for alternative therapy.

TABLE 26–1. LOW-DENSITY LIPOPROTEIN CHOLESTEROL LEVELS AND THERAPY*

	Diet	Diet + Drugs	Beyond Diet + Drugs
Homozygous FH	All levels	All levels	All levels
CAD present	100 mg/dL	130 mg/dL	200 mg/dL
CAD not present			
≥ 2 risk factors	130 mg/dL	160 mg/dL	300 mg/dL
< 2 risk factors	160 mg/dL	190 mg/dL	—

Abbreviations: CAD, coronary artery disease; FH, familial hypercholesterolemia.

*The guidelines of the second Adult Treatment Panel of the National Cholesterol Education Program for instituting diet and drug therapy are combined with suggested recommendations for treating patients with severe hypercholesterolemia as described in the text. Because of the additional risks and substantial cost, the decision to pursue therapy beyond diet and drugs must be individualized.

Patients With Low-Density Lipoprotein Cholesterol Levels Above 200 mg/dL and Coronary Artery Disease

The majority of patients with LDL-C above 200 mg/dL and CAD have the heterozygous form of FH. This disorder has a prevalence of approximately 1 in 500 individuals and is typically manifested by the occurrence of premature CAD by the fifth decade for men and the sixth decade for women. The presence of CAD and elevated LDL-C levels are important risk factors for subsequent coronary events, and therefore patients with CAD need intensive LDL-C control. The reinfarction rate found in seven secondary-prevention trials reviewed by Rossouw and colleagues[7] was about 6% annually in contrast to a 1% to 2% rate of first infarction in four primary-prevention trials. Several trials[8–10] have reported regression or a lower rate of progression of coronary lesions when the elevated LDL-C concentration is lowered with diet or with diet and drugs.

Patients With Low-Density Lipoprotein Cholesterol Levels Above 300 mg/dL Without Coronary Artery Disease

The decision whether to use nondietary, nondrug therapy for primary prevention in asymptomatic adults is never as easy as it is in homozygotes. The risk for premature CAD is most apparent in patients with FH due to the presence of lifelong elevated LDL-C levels, typically above 300 mg/dL. In addition to the LDL-C level, the presence of risk factors as defined by the second report of the NCEP Adult Treatment Panel helps determine which patients are most susceptible to the development of CAD. It is also worthwhile to consider the lipoprotein(a) (Lp[a]) level in these patients because an elevated Lp(a) level (>20 mg/dL) has been recognized as an independent risk factor in patients with FH.[11, 12] In a trial of 115 patients with heterozygous FH, the median Lp(a) level was 57 mg/dL in patients with CAD versus 18 mg/dL in patients without CAD.[11]

In summary, it is reasonable to consider nondietary, nondrug therapy for primary prevention in patients with an LDL-C level above 300 mg/dL despite diet and maximal tolerated lipid-lowering drug therapy and two additional risk factors for CAD.

EXTRACORPOREAL THERAPIES FOR TREATING SEVERE HYPERCHOLESTEROLEMIA

Background

Plasmapheresis and the more specific LDL apheresis procedures have provided a safe and efficient method for LDL-C lowering in patients with severe hypercholesterolemia. These techniques are widely available around the world and have become the most common mode of therapy for patients with refractory hypercholesterolemia. The first report of plasma exchange for FH was published by de Gennes and coworkers[13] in 1967. The procedure was performed manually and was too cumbersome for prolonged use. In 1975, Thompson and associates[14] described plasmapheresis with an automated cell separator to treat patients with homozygous FH. Plasmapheresis therapy has been shown to improve survival of treated homozygotes compared with their untreated sibling controls.[15]

The nonselectivity of plasmapheresis led to the development of more specific procedures for removing LDL called LDL apheresis. Specific removal of apolipoprotein B–containing lipoproteins was first described in 1976 by Lupien and colleagues,[16] who used heparin-agarose beads. LDL apheresis has grown from a cumbersome laboratory procedure to a routine therapy with automated equipment. Several LDL apheresis methods are available. These include (1) columns containing dextran sulfate–cellulose,[17] (2) columns containing immobilized antibodies to apolipoprotein B,[18] and (3) heparin-induced extracorporeal LDL precipitation (HELP).[19]

Practical Considerations Common to All Therapies

Vascular Access. The primary consideration is achieving a sufficient blood flow rate with low morbidity for the patient. A major difference among extracorporeal therapies is whether artificial access (e.g., fistula or shunt for hemodialysis) needs to be inserted to perform the procedure. Fortunately, venous access from an antecubital fossa vein is most often sufficient for plasmapheresis and LDL apheresis because of the lower blood flow rates required (50 to 100 mL/min) compared with hemodialysis (400 mL/min). Consequently, a low frequency of difficulties with vascular access has been observed. In a study of 64 patients treated with 3023 LDL apheresis procedures,[20] only one patient required a fistula and four patients had one or more treatments with a femoral puncture. Difficulties with the access site occurred in less than 5% of treatments and were related to needle infiltration, poor blood flow, or pain around the needle site.

Anticoagulation. Some form of anticoagulation is necessary for all extracorporeal procedures. Heparin alone, heparin with acid citrate dextrose (ACD), and ACD alone are the anticoagulants most commonly used in extracorporeal therapies. Heparin is typically used for extracorporeal procedures that use a membrane to separate whole blood into plasma and cells. Typically, a bolus of 50 to 75 U/kg is given followed by a continuous infusion of approximately 1000 U/h. Although heparin is an effective anticoagulant, its effects are apparent several hours after completion of the procedure. ACD, also an effective anticoagulant, has the advantage of rapid metabolism and little residual effect after the procedure. Side effects due to ACD administration include symptoms of hypocalcemia, which may include perioral tingling, hypotension, or rarely tetany.

Blood Separation. Once vascular access is achieved and the blood anticoagulated, an automated cell separator uses a membrane or centrifuge to separate blood into plasma and cellular elements. Membrane separation of blood tends to be simpler and to require less extracorporeal volume, but it is less efficient than centrifugal techniques. The current membranes and centrifugation systems are biocompatible, and therefore hemolysis is rarely seen. The systems are sterile and self-contained, and the parts that come into contact with blood are disposable.

Lipid Lowering and Plasma Processed/ Treatment Frequency

Lowering of total cholesterol or LDL-C level can be quantified by measuring either the acute lowering or the time-averaged lowering achieved (Fig. 26–1). The acute lowering is the difference in preprocedure and postprocedure lipid values as a percentage of the initial value and is a function of the amount of plasma (number of plasma volumes) processed during a single treatment. The plasma volume is calculated from the total blood volume (estimated from the patient's sex, height, and weight) and hematocrit. Most plasmapheresis treatments process about 1.0 plasma volumes and achieve about a 50% reduction in lipid levels. Because nonspecific depletion of plasma proteins is not a problem, LDL apheresis procedures can process 1.5 to 2.0 plasma volumes and reduce LDL-C by 60% to 75%. For a blood flow of 50 to 80 mL/min, it takes about 3 h to process 1.5 to 2.0 plasma volumes. Three hours is also close to the limit that most patients will sit or recline comfortably.

Although acute lipid lowering is helpful in determining treatment efficiency, the time-averaged lipid value is a better indicator of the lipid level that the patient's arteries are exposed to over time. The time-averaged lowering takes into consideration the treatment frequency and rate of rebound. The relationship between treatment frequency and LDL-C lowering is shown in Figure 26–2. The time-averaged lipid value is arrived at by performing daily lipid determinations after a treatment. The time-averaged LDL-C lowering is usually between 40% and 50%.

Effects on HDL. LDL apheresis has been reported to maintain or increase HDL levels over time.[21] Plasmapheresis lowers HDL owing to nonspecific depletion.

Plasmapheresis

Plasmapheresis was the original extracorporeal method for lowering LDL-C levels in individuals with FH. It has the advantages of being simple and safe. Unfortunately, HDL and beneficial plasma proteins are also removed. This limitation makes plasmapheresis useful only when LDL apheresis is not available. Plasmapheresis should be used only in homozygous FH because it has not been shown to be of benefit in individuals with heterozygous FH and nonfamilial forms of hypercholesterolemia. Because of the clear advantages of LDL apheresis compared with plasmapheresis, the remainder of this section is devoted to LDL apheresis.

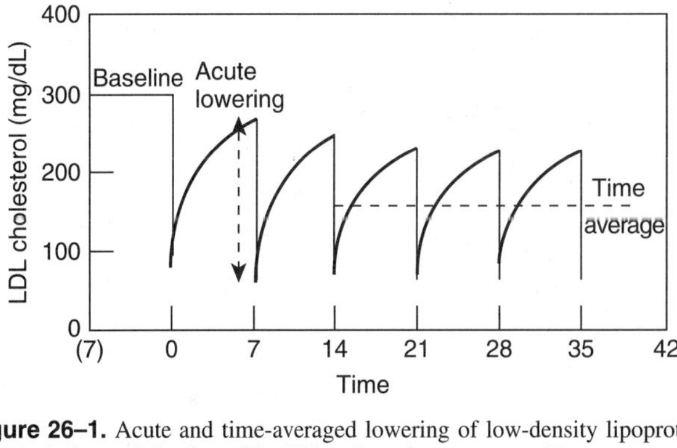

Figure 26–1. Acute and time-averaged lowering of low-density lipoprotein (LDL) cholesterol for 6 weekly LDL apheresis treatments. The acute lowering is the difference in pretreatment and posttreatment values as a percentage of the pretreatment value. The time-averaged level is determined by measuring a "rebound" after a treatment.

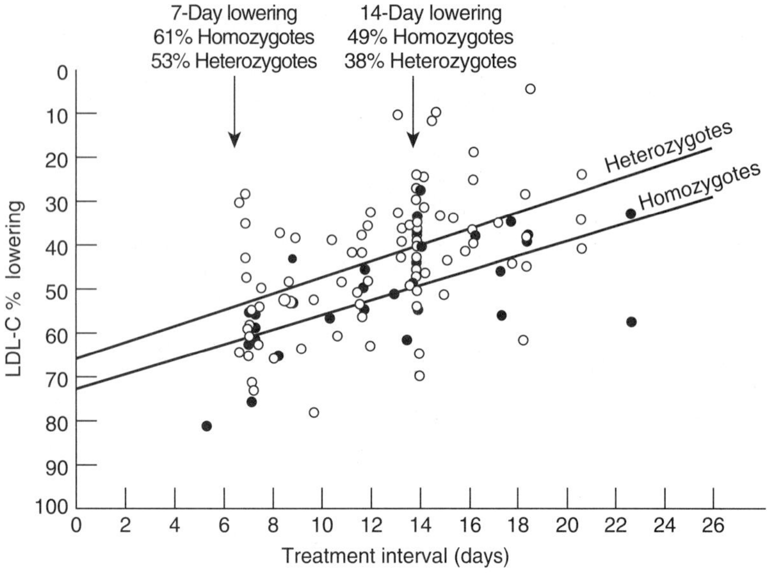

Figure 26–2. Relation between treatment frequency and low-density lipoprotein cholesterol (LDL-C) level for patients with homozygous (closed circles) and heterozygous (open circles) familial hypercholesterolemia (FH). Most patients will require weekly or every other week therapy to maintain adequate cholesterol lowering. (From Gordon BR, Kelsey SF, Bilheimer DW, et al: Treatment of refractory familial hypercholesterolemia by low-density lipoprotein apheresis using an automated dextran sulfate cellulose adsorption system. Am J Cardiol 1992; 70:1010–1016.)

Low-Density Lipoprotein Apheresis With Dextran Sulfate–Cellulose Columns

Dextran sulfate–cellulose selectively binds apolipoprotein B–containing lipoproteins on the basis of a charge attraction. Dextran sulfate–cellulose columns were initially single, large-volume, nonregenerable columns that could be attached to any cell separator. Limited LDL-binding capacity resulted in the development of dual regenerable columns in a system that included a hollow-fiber primary cell separator (Fig. 26–3). Plasma is alternately perfused through each 150-mL column, permitting regeneration of the off-line column with hypertonic sodium chloride solution. The process is controlled by a computerized unit. The plasma, after passing through the adsorbent column, is recombined with the cells and returned to the patient. The advantage of this system is the almost unlimited LDL-binding capacity due to the on-line regeneration of the columns. The columns are discarded after each treatment.

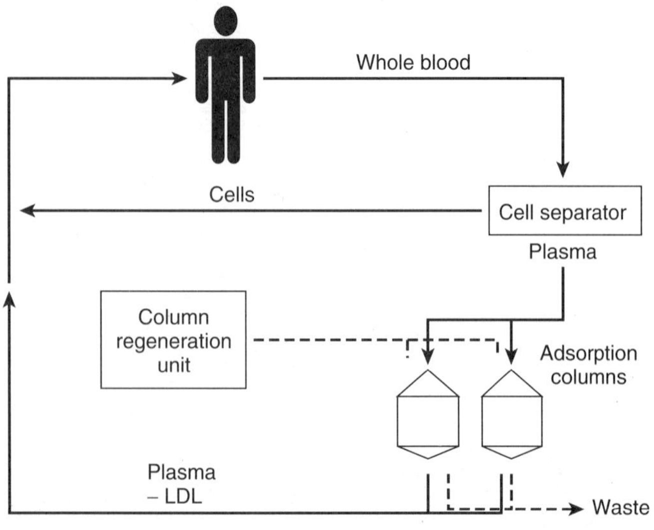

Figure 26–3. Schematic representation of dextran sulfate–cellulose and immunoadsorption low-density lipoprotein (LDL) apheresis systems.

Low-Density Lipoprotein Apheresis With Immunoadsorption Columns

Immunoadsorption for performing LDL apheresis has been used to treat patients for approximately 15 years. Polyclonal monospecific or monoclonal antibodies to apolipoprotein B are immobilized on a support, typically sepharose beads, and packed into glass columns. A column with antibodies specific for Lp(a) has also been developed. Each patient has two columns that are reused during each procedure and reused from one procedure to the next because of the expense of making these columns. On-line regeneration of the columns is controlled by a column control unit (see Fig. 26–3). The columns are typically eluted with an acid glycine solution, neutralized with a buffer solution, and then rinsed with saline. The procedure requires storage of the columns between treatments and thorough rinsing of the columns before each use to remove the storage solution. All apolipoprotein B–containing lipoproteins are removed—LDL, very low density lipoprotein (VLDL), and Lp(a). Because the columns are reused multiple times, they must be monitored for loss of activity, which may occur after several months. In addition, sensitization of the patient to small quantities of shed antibody has been demonstrated.[22]

Low-Density Lipoprotein Apheresis With Heparin-Induced Extracorporeal Precipitation

LDL apheresis with HELP specifically removes LDL, VLDL, and Lp(a) while minimally affecting HDL and most plasma proteins.[19] HELP differs from other procedures in that it removes a substantial quantity of fibrinogen. The technique is based on the precipitation of positively charged LDL and other beta lipoproteins when heparin is added at a low pH (Fig. 26–4). Few plasma proteins precipitate with heparin, primarily fibrinogen, plasminogen, C3, and C4. The initial step is the processing of whole blood by a cell separator to obtain plasma. The plasma is mixed continuously with a 0.3 M acetate buffer at pH 4.85 that contains 100 units of heparin per milliliter. The precipitation of the beta lipoproteins occurs at a pH just above 5.0. This suspension is perfused through a polycarbonate filter to remove the precipitated LDL, Lp(a), and fibrinogen. An anion exchange column removes excess heparin. The plasma is then treated with bicarbonate dialysis and ultrafiltration to return the pH to normal and to remove excess fluid. The entire process is controlled by a microprocessor.

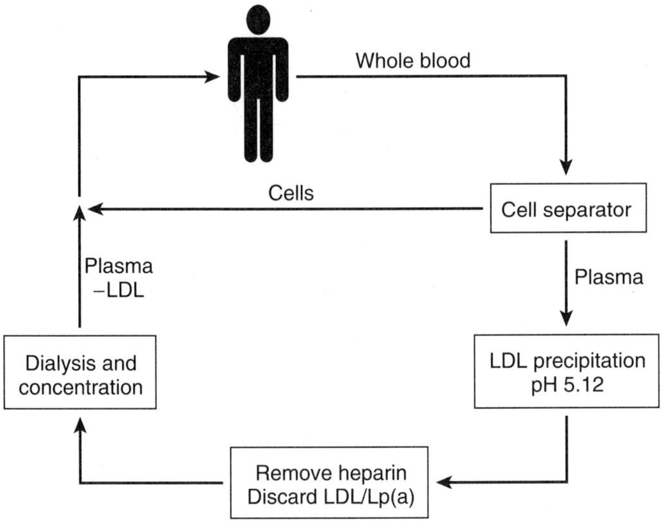

Figure 26–4. Schematic representation of the heparin-induced extracorporeal low-density lipoprotein (LDL) precipitation (HELP) system of LDL apheresis.

Risks/Benefits of Low-Density Lipoprotein Apheresis

Adverse reactions due to LDL apheresis have been few. The extracorporeal volume is well tolerated even in patients with severe CAD. Hypotension requiring infusion of saline occurs in less than 5% of treatments. Unusual side effects include angina, hemolysis, and allergic or anaphylactic reactions. In immunoadsorption treatments, possible causes for these reactions include complement activation and sensitization of the patient to column constituents. An anaphylactoid reaction during LDL apheresis with dextran sulfate–cellulose has been described in patients taking angiotensin converting enzyme (ACE) inhibitors.[23] It is recommended that patients taking ACE inhibitors be switched to alternative drugs before LDL apheresis with dextran sulfate–cellulose is initiated.

Regression of tendinous xanthomas and improvement in CAD have been demonstrated in patients with severe hypercholesterolemia when the LDL-C level is lowered by use of LDL apheresis–containing protocols. In the LDL Apheresis Regression Study,[24] angiographic evidence for regression of CAD was observed in 10 of 30 patients treated with LDL apheresis and lipid-lowering drugs despite a baseline LDL-C level of 311 mg/dL. The HELP-LDL Apheresis Multicenter Study[25] was a 2-year investigation in 51 patients treated with weekly LDL apheresis and lipid-lowering drugs. Computer-assisted analysis of paired angiograms from 33 evaluable patients revealed that 23 patients had regression, 1 patient had little change, and 9 patients had progression. The German Multicenter LDL Apheresis Trial[26] was a four-center, 3-year prospective trial of 32 patients with FH. All patients who had symptomatic CAD had improvement in their symptoms by the end of the study. Improvement in electrocardiographic stress testing was demonstrated in 17 patients. Analysis of the paired angiograms did not reveal regression of disease, although definite progression of disease was observed in only five patients in a 3-year period. Analysis of data from the Familial Hypercholesterolaemia Regression Study[27] revealed equivalent angiographic changes when similar LDL-C levels were achieved with either dual-drug therapy or a combination of single-drug therapy and LDL apheresis.

Availability

LDL apheresis has been used in Western Europe, the United States, and Japan. Approval by regulatory agencies and indications for approval vary from country to country. Approval by the U.S. Food and Drug Administration was received in February 1996 for patients with homozygous FH and LDL-C above 500 mg/dL, for patients with heterozygous FH and LDL-C of 300 mg/dL or higher (CAD absent), and for patients with heterozygous FH and LDL-C of 200 mg/dL or higher (CAD present).

SURGICAL PROCEDURES

Portacaval Shunt

Background. In 1963, a portacaval diversion was used to treat a child with a glycogen storage disease.[28] The observation by Starzl and coworkers[29] that the hyperlipidemia observed in these patients was improved by portacaval shunting provided the basis for using the procedure starting in 1973 to treat severe forms of hypercholesterolemia.[30] By 1983, a National Institutes of Health–sponsored registry included 45 patients.[31] Although the exact number of shunted hypercholesterolemic patients is not known, the majority have had homozygous FH[32, 33]; a few severe heterozygotes have also been reported.

Technique. With the exception of the earliest procedures, all patients have received end-to-side portacaval anastomoses. This type of anastomosis between the portal vein and the inferior vena cava prevents any portal blood from perfusing the liver (Fig. 26–5).

Cholesterol Lowering and Mechanisms. As shown in Table 26–2, total cholesterol and LDL-C levels are consistently lowered after a successful procedure. The percentage of lowering is similar in all groups, although it varies considerably among patients. Varying degrees of technical success may explain some of the differences. HDL-C levels may increase, especially for receptor-defective homozygotes and heterozygote patients. Cholesterol lowering is evident within a week of surgery; levels generally reach a new plateau within the first 6 months. Follow-up reports, although generally limited to less than 5 years, suggest that these new levels are usually maintained.[33] Evaluation of patients whose lipid levels returned to baseline values revealed shunt occlusion or revascularization of the portal stump with splanchnic collateral vessels.

The hypocholesterolemic effect is coincidental with a marked decrease in whole-body cholesterol and bile acid synthesis[34, 35] and a decrease in cholesterol pool size. Exogenous cholesterol absorption remained unchanged. In a receptor-negative homozygote patient,[36] a liver biopsy after portacaval shunt revealed a decrease in hepatocyte size, including a marked decrease in the cytoplasmic fat and rough and smooth endoplasmic reticulum area. There was a 56% decrease in 3-hydroxy-3-methylglutaryl coenzyme A (HMG-CoA) reductase

TABLE 26–2. CHOLESTEROL LOWERING IN PATIENTS TREATED WITH A PORTACAVAL SHUNT

	Percentage Reduction (Range)		
Diagnosis*	**Total Cholesterol**	**LDL-C**	**HDL-C**
Homozygous FH			
Receptor-negative	37 (23–55)	28 (22–44)	9 (32 to −26)
Receptor-defective	19 (11–33)	20 (11–32)	−23 (−11 to −78)
Heterozygous FH	30 (20–39)	33 (22–44)	−40 (−11 to −69)

Abbreviations: FH, familial hypercholesterolemia; HDL-C, high-density lipoprotein cholesterol; LDL-C, low-density lipoprotein cholesterol.

*There were 9 patients with receptor-negative homozygous FH, 12 patients with receptor-defective homozygous FH, and 2 patients with heterozygous FH. The data were obtained from references 32 and 33.

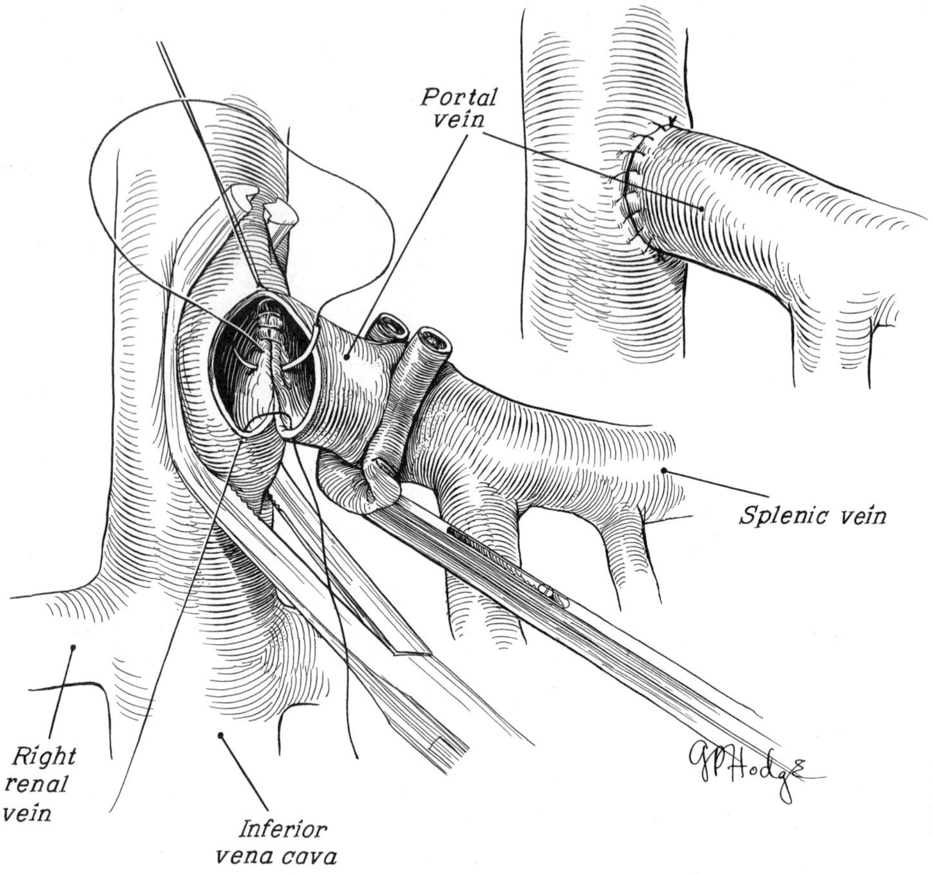

Figure 26–5. End-to-side portacaval shunt. (From Zuidema GD, Cameron JL, Zeppa R: Portal hypertension. 11: Operative procedures. *In* Nora PF: Operative Surgery: Principles and Techniques, p 694. Philadelphia: Lea & Febiger, 1980.)

activity, and hepatic LDL binding was significantly increased. Enhanced LDL clearance has been independently observed.

Risks/Benefits. The follow-up of patients undergoing the procedure has demonstrated that disease stabilization and improvement are possible. Starzl and coworkers[32] reported two cases of improved aortic stenosis, as evidenced by decreased aortic gradients, 13 and 16 months after surgery. Coronary angiography in five patients from 7 months to 7 years after the procedure suggested improvement in one patient and disease stabilization in two. Disease stabilization during a similar time frame for two patients who had also undergone coronary artery bypass grafting has also been reported.[37] These results are impressive considering the natural course of homozygous FH. Another observation is the uniform postprocedure regression of xanthomas.

A portacaval shunt is generally well tolerated, but some risk is present, particularly in patients with symptomatic cardiac disease. In two of the larger series, there was one perioperative death (myocardial infarction) in 25 patients (ages 2 to 52 years), the majority of whom had valvular disease and/or atherosclerosis at the time of surgery. A registry of 45 shunted, hypercholesterolemic patients reported three deaths within 30 days of surgery.[31] These three patients had symptomatic cardiac disease at the time of surgery. For the follow-up periods reported (generally <5 years), no evidence of renal or progressive hepatic dysfunction has been observed. However, transient liver enzyme abnormalities, elevated ammonia levels with and without encephalopathy,[32] and splenomegaly[33] have been described. Quality of life has generally improved, including improvement or disappearance of angina and increased exercise tolerance.

Guidelines for Use. A portacaval shunt *is not* satisfactory as a sole therapy but should be considered as part of the therapeutic regimen for the homozygote or refractory heterozygote patient. Timing should be before clinical coronary atherosclerosis or valvular heart disease develops, that is, between the ages of 5 and 10 years (although at times even earlier). LDL apheresis should be added when the patient reaches reasonable age and weight (e.g., 5 years, 30 to 35 kg).

Liver Transplantation

Background. The possibility that liver transplantation might be a reasonable therapy for patients with homozygous FH was based on the liver's having up to three quarters of the body's LDL receptors and the improvement in technical and immunologic methods for liver transplantation.[38] The first liver transplantation for homozygous FH was reported by Starzl and colleagues[39] in 1984. Because of diffuse coronary atherosclerosis, heart transplantation was performed at the same time. The number of patients treated in this manner and the data available for evaluation are extremely limited.

Technique. For a description of the liver transplantation technique, the reader is referred to an overview.[40] A simultaneous or staged liver-heart transplantation may be performed,[41] or liver transplantation may be undertaken after coronary artery bypass grafting.

Cholesterol Lowering. Provision of hepatic LDL receptors markedly enhances LDL clearance, suppresses LDL synthesis, and can provide dramatic cholesterol lowering. An increase in HDL-C may also be seen. Reports of the cholesterol-lowering response to liver transplantation generally describe data obtained less than 2 years after transplantation.[42–44] After transplantation, homozygous FH patients become more responsive to cholesterol-lowering medication (Table 26–3) and approach the cholesterol levels outlined by the NCEP. These results are in spite of steroids and cyclosporine therapy, which may increase total cholesterol and LDL-C levels.

TABLE 26–3. RESPONSE TO LIVER TRANSPLANT AND LOVASTATIN IN A PATIENT WITH HOMOZYGOUS FAMILIAL HYPERCHOLESTEROLEMIA

	Baseline	Liver Transplant	Transplant + Lovastatin
Total cholesterol (mg/dL)	1079	302	171
LDL-C (mg/dL)	988	184	107
Triglyceride (mg/dL)	238	218	121
HDL-C (mg/dL)	35	41	39
Catabolic rate (pools/day)	0.12	0.31	0.30
Production (mg/kg/day)	36.4	16.7	10.9

Abbreviations: HDL-C, high-density lipoprotein cholesterol; LDL-C, low-density lipoprotein cholesterol.

From Bilheimer DW: Portacaval shunt surgery and liver transplantation in the treatment of homozygous familial hypercholesterolemia. *In* Widhalm K, Niato HK (eds): Recent Aspects of Diagnosis and Treatment of Lipoprotein Disorders: Impact on Prevention of Atherosclerotic Disease, pp 295–304. New York: Alan R Liss, 1988.

Risks/Benefits. The limited number of patients receiving transplants makes it difficult to provide a risk/benefit analysis. When combined with a simultaneous heart transplantation, liver transplantation has been associated with an extremely high mortality rate.[45] As liver transplantation becomes more common and successful, survival of patients should improve. Long-term follow-up (>5 years) has not been reported. Long-term immunosuppression has some risk, including nephrotoxicity.

Treatment Guidelines. In an era of evolving therapies, recommendations to perform liver transplantation for treatment of patients with homozygous FH are difficult to make. Portacaval shunting and LDL apheresis have less risk and are effective in the majority of patients.

Partial Ileal Bypass

Background. The PIB surgical procedure was introduced for the management of hypercholesterolemia in 1963.[46] More than 600 PIB procedures have been performed for this purpose.[47–49] The procedure results in a lower serum cholesterol level by increasing fecal loss of normally absorbed endogenous (biliary and intestinally secreted) and exogenous dietary cholesterol and increasing hepatic conversion of body cholesterol stores to replenish the depleted bile acid reservoir.[50, 51] Its use is most appropriate in patients with heterozygous FH.

Technique. The PIB operation for lowering cholesterol bypasses the distal 200 cm or the distal third of the small intestine, whichever is greater, and is different from the weight-losing procedure, which includes a more extensive 90% jejunal-ileal bypass. Bowel continuity is restored by an end-to-side ileocecostomy. A more detailed description of the procedure is provided in Figure 26–6.

Cholesterol Lowering. The cholesterol lowering that was achieved in three series of patients undergoing PIB is summarized in Table 26–4. The Program on the Surgical Control of the Hyperlipidemias (POSCH) series[47] included approximately 400 patients randomized to cholesterol-lowering therapy using PIB and represents the largest, unified experience. These series began before the general availability of HMG-CoA reductase inhibitors. Overall, comparable cholesterol lowering was achieved in all three series, that is, approximately a 30% decrease in total cholesterol, a 40% decrease in LDL-C, and variable changes in HDL-C. The responses were generally sustained for as long as surgical bypass was maintained. Synergy with reductase inhibitors has been reported.[48]

Risks/Benefits. The operative and perioperative mortality is extremely low. The principal side effect of PIB surgery is more frequent and looser stools. During the first 5 years of follow-up, 6% to 8% of the surgically treated patients in the POSCH trial reported watery or frothy stools, compared with 0% to 1% of control subjects. A similar comparison includes an analysis of the incidence of kidney stones (4% per year in surgically treated patients versus 0.7% per year in control subjects) and gallstones (surgery required in 14 surgical patients versus 4 control patients). Fifty-seven (13.5%) of PIB patients had symptoms of bowel obstruction (the majority within the first year), and 15 (3.6%) required surgical intervention. Twenty-three (6%) of the POSCH patients underwent reversal of surgery between 2 and 11 years postoperatively. Similarly, 2 of 11 patients in the British series underwent surgical reversal.[48] The POSCH trial

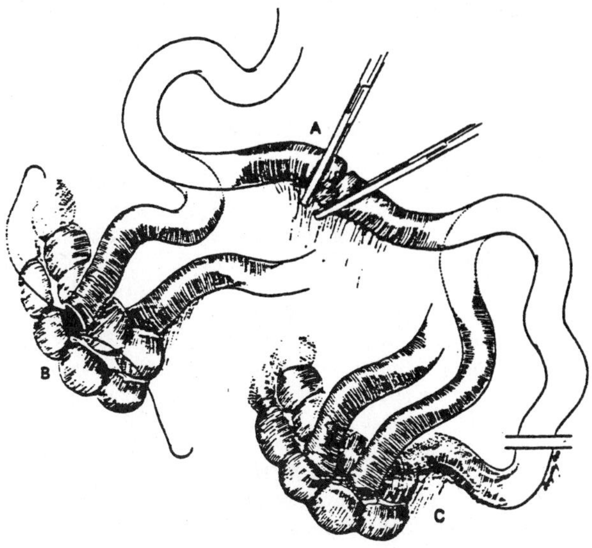

Figure 26–6. Partial ileal bypass. *A,* Division of the ileum 200 cm proximal to the ileocecal valve, or one third of the total small bowel length proximal to the ileocecal valve if the total small intestinal length is greater than 600 cm. *B,* End-to-side anastomosis of the proximal segment into the anterior taenia of the cecum, 6 cm distal to the appendiceal stump. *C,* Tacking of the closed distal segment to the anterior taenia of the cecum placed midway between the anastomosis and the appendiceal stump. (From Buchwald H, Stoller DK, Campos CT, et al: Partial ileal bypass for hypercholesterolemia: 20- to 26-year follow-up of the first 57 consecutive cases. Ann Surg 1990; 212:318–331.)

TABLE 26–4. CHOLESTEROL RESPONSE* TO PARTIAL ILEAL BYPASS SURGERY

	Buchwald et al[47] (5 years)	Ohri et al[48] (20–24 months)	Defraigne et al[49]
Number of patients	421	11	8
Percentage change			
Total cholesterol	−28	−20	−36
LDL cholesterol	−42	—	—
HDL cholesterol	+5	+21	—

Abbreviations: HDL, high-density lipoprotein; LDL, low-density lipoprotein.

*The long-term beneficial effect of partial ileal bypass surgery on the lipid profile is shown.

demonstrated that lipid lowering by PIB results in less progression of coronary and peripheral vascular atherosclerosis in treated versus control individuals.[47]

GENE THERAPY

Progress in molecular biology has provided hope for fixing the basic error in patients with severe FH by use of a technique called gene transfer. The foundation for this work was established by Goldstein and Brown's demonstration that in the majority of patients, an absent or defective LDL receptor was the cause for the marked elevation in LDL-C.[5] Gene therapy for FH provides a normal copy of the missing or defective gene for the LDL receptor. This therapy is specific for the genetic disorder being treated. For example, individuals with defective apolipoprotein B would require introduction of the normal apolipoprotein B gene rather than the LDL receptor gene.

There are two general approaches for gene therapy of hypercholesterolemia (see references 52 and 53 for review). Already in human trials is ex vivo gene therapy. For this treatment, liver tissue is harvested, the normal LDL receptor gene is transduced into the cells, and the hepatocytes are reinfused into the patient. The second method, in vivo gene transfer, has many theoretical advantages compared with the ex vivo technique. It involves the injection of the LDL receptor gene within its vector into the liver through its circulation.

Ex Vivo Gene Therapy

The details of the first patient treated with this process have been reported.[54] A summary of this procedure is shown in Figure 26–7. The patient chosen was a 28-year-old woman with homozygous FH due to a missense mutation for the LDL receptor. The patient had a myocardial infarction at age 16 years and coronary artery bypass surgery by age 26 years. Her baseline LDL-C concentration was 482 mg/dL with minimal response to drugs.

The initial step of gene therapy involved removal of the left lateral segment of the liver, which composed approximately 15% of her hepatic mass. At the time of surgery, a catheter was left in the inferior mesenteric vein and externalized to allow reinfusion of hepatocytes. The resected liver was perfused with collagenase to disperse hepatocytes. The recombinant retrovirus containing the LDL receptor was incubated with the cultured hepatocytes for 12 to 18 h. By use of a fluorescent-labeled LDL probe, approximately 20% of the cells were found to express the LDL receptor. The hepatocytes were slowly reinfused into the portal circulation. The patient tolerated the surgical procedure and cell infusion well with only a transient tachycardia and low-grade fever.

Lipid lowering, although statistically significant, did not reach levels that would be expected to halt progression of this patient's disease. Her LDL-C concentration decreased from 482 mg/dL to 404 mg/dL and her HDL-C level improved from 43 mg/dL to 51 mg/dL after the procedure. The addition of lovastatin resulted in further LDL-C lowering to 356 mg/dL. A liver biopsy and in situ hybridization using an RNA probe specific for the recombinant-derived LDL receptor transcript revealed relatively few hepatocytes containing the transgene (only 1:1000 to 1:10,000 cells). A possible explanation for some of these results is regional variation of LDL receptor–expressing cells within the liver that are not adequately sampled from a percutaneous biopsy.

A theoretical concern was the development of an immune response by the patient to the LDL receptor. There was no evidence for this occurrence: there was no antibody development to the LDL receptor and no autoimmune hepatitis pathologically. This first patient was to be part of a series of approximately three to five patients with homozygous FH treated with ex vivo gene therapy.[53] The results for the remainder of these patients have not been published.

In Vivo Gene Transfer

The morbidity inherent in ex vivo gene therapy will greatly limit its potential clinical application in FH. More appealing is delivery of the gene specifically to the liver. Efficient and safe in vivo gene transfer has been difficult primarily because hepatocytes rarely divide without a stimulus, such as a partial hepatic resection. Fortunately, other viral vectors and nonviral approaches for gene transfer may be applicable. Adenoviruses have the capability of transducing genes into hepatocytes that are not dividing. In vivo LDL receptor gene transfer using the adenovirus has been accomplished in rodents[55] and Watanabe heritable hyperlipidemic rabbits,[56] an animal model that lacks the LDL receptor. Other approaches for incorporating and delivering the LDL receptor transcript, such as the use of liposomes, are under development.

CONCLUSIONS AND RECOMMENDATIONS FOR THERAPY

The treatment of patients with hypercholesterolemia who respond inadequately to diet and lipid-lowering drug therapy remains a chal-

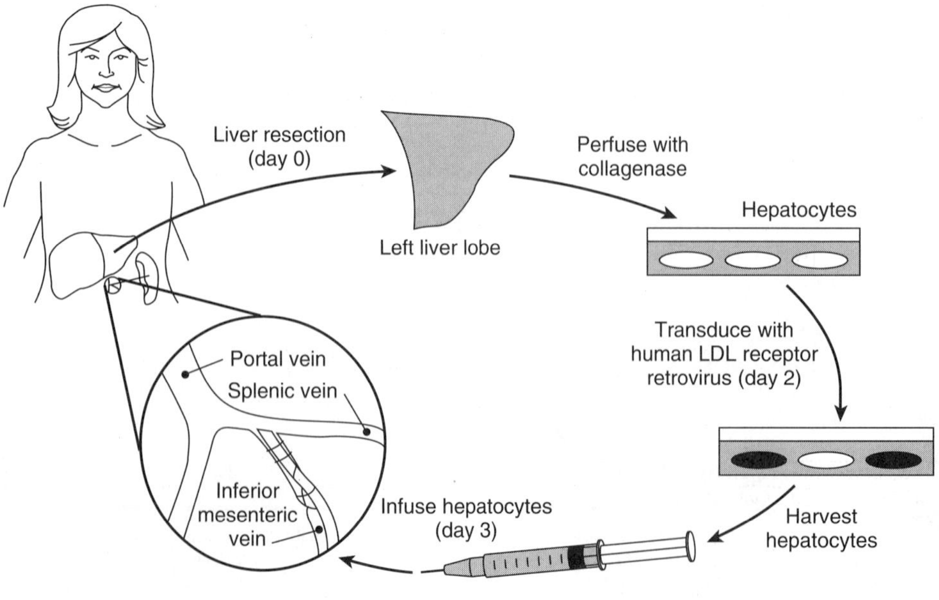

Figure 26–7. Schematic representation of ex vivo gene therapy for patients with homozygous FH. (From Grossman M, Raper SE, Kozarsky K, et al: Successful ex vivo gene therapy directed to liver in a patient with familial hypercholesterolemia. Nat Genet 1994; 6:335–341.)

TABLE 26–5. RECOMMENDATIONS FOR THERAPY

	Homozygous FH	Heterozygous FH and Non-FH
Whom to treat	All patients	LDL-C >200 mg/dL (+CAD) LDL-C >300 mg/dL (−CAD with multiple risk factors)
Treatment options	LDL apheresis* Portacaval shunt Gene transfer Liver transplanation	LDL apheresis or partial ileal bypass

Abbreviations: FH, familial hypercholesterolemia; CAD, coronary artery disease; LDL-C, low-density lipoprotein cholesterol; LDL, low-density lipoprotein.

*Use plasmapheresis if LDL apheresis is not available to treat patients with homozygous FH. If LDL apheresis cannot be performed for technical reasons (e.g., the patient's size or inability to tolerate extracorporeal therapy), a portacaval shunt should be considered.

lenge. Treatment recommendations and alternatives are summarized in Table 26–5.

Patients with homozygous FH are the clearest candidates for additional therapy because of their poor response to standard treatments. LDL apheresis has been the most commonly used treatment modality and is the safest alternative. The therapy should be initiated as soon as technically feasible, but age 5 years or 30 kg is generally the lower limit because of difficulties with vascular access and the 200- to 250-mL extracorporeal blood volume of the procedure. Portacaval shunting should be considered if, by age 5 years, LDL apheresis is inadequate for controlling the LDL-C level or technically difficult. Liver transplantation or gene transfer currently involves significant morbidity and should be reserved for the most refractory patients.

Individuals with CAD and primary hypercholesterolemia with LDL-C levels above 200 mg/dL despite maximal diet and drug therapy are also candidates for additional lipid-lowering therapy. The best alternatives are LDL apheresis and PIB. These patients may also be candidates for in vivo gene therapy should the technology continue to improve to a point at which safe and effective therapy is possible.

The use of nondietary, nonpharmacologic therapy as primary prevention in patients with hypercholesterolemia inadequately responsive to standard measures is more problematic. The standard risk factors should be used to segregate a small subset of individuals at highest risk for the development of atherosclerosis in whom additional therapy is reasonable. The best alternatives include LDL apheresis and PIB. Particularly for these patients, the decision to provide additional therapy must be individualized.

REFERENCES

1. Summary of the second report of the National Cholesterol Education Program (NCEP) Expert Panel on Detection, Evaluation, and Treatment of High Blood Cholesterol in Adults (Adult Treatment Panel II). JAMA 1993; 269:3015–3023.
2. Goldstein JL, Brown MS: Familial hypercholesterolemia. *In* Scriver CR, Beaudet AL, Sly WS, Valle D (eds): The Metabolic Basis of Inherited Disease, 6th ed, pp 1215–1250. New York: McGraw-Hill, 1989.
3. Mabuchi H, Koizumi J, Shimizu M, Takeda R, and the Hokuriku FH-CHD Study Group: Development of coronary heart disease in familial hypercholesterolemia. Circulation 1989; 79:225–332.
4. Haitis B, Baker SG, Meyer TE, et al: Natural history and cardiac manifestations of homozygous familial hypercholesterolemia. Q J Med 1990; 76:731–740.
5. Goldstein JL, Brown MS: The LDL receptor defect in familial hypercholesterolemia. Implications for pathogenesis and therapy. Med Clin North Am 1982; 66:335–362.
6. Sprecher DL, Schaefer EJ, Kent KM, et al: Cardiovascular features of homozygous familial hypercholesterolemia: analysis of 16 patients. Am J Cardiol 1984; 54:20–30.
7. Rossouw JE, Lewis B, Rifkind BM: The value of lowering cholesterol after myocardial infarction. N Engl J Med 1990; 323:1112–1119.
8. Brown G, Albers JJ, Fisher LD, et al: Regression of coronary artery disease as a result of intensive lipid-lowering therapy in men with high levels of apolipoprotein B. N Engl J Med 1990; 323:1289–1298.
9. Watts GF, Lewis B, Brunt JNH, et al: Effects on coronary artery disease of lipid-lowering diet, or diet plus cholestyramine, in the St. Thomas' Atherosclerosis Regression Study (STARS). Lancet 1992; 339:563–569.
10. Kane JP, Malloy MJ, Ports TA, et al: Regression of coronary atherosclerosis during treatment of familial hypercholesterolemia with combined drug regimens. JAMA 1990; 264:3007–3012.
11. Seed M, Hoppichler F, Reaveley D, et al: Relation of serum lipoprotein(a) concentration and apolipoprotein(a) phenotype to coronary heart disease in patients with familial hypercholesterolemia. N Engl J Med 1990; 322:1494–1499.
12. Wiklund O, Angelin B, Olofsson SO, et al: Apolipoprotein(a) and ischaemic heart disease in familial hypercholesterolaemia. Lancet 1990; 335:1360–1363.
13. de Gennes JL, Touraine R, Maunand B, et al: Homozygous cutaneotendinous forms of hypercholesterolemic xanthomatosis in an exemplary familial case. Trial of plasmapheresis as an heroic treatment. Bull Mem Soc Hosp (Paris) 1967; 118:1377–1402.
14. Thompson GR, Lowenthal R, Myant NB: Plasma exchange in the management of homozygous familial hypercholesterolaemia. Lancet 1975; 1:1208–1211.
15. Thompson GR, Miller JP, Breslow JL: Improved survival of patients with homozygous familial hypercholesterolaemia treated with plasma exchange. Br Med J 1985; 291:1671–1673.
16. Lupien PJ, Moorjani S, Awad J: A new approach to the management of familial hypercholesterolemia: removal of plasma cholesterol based on the principle of affinity chromatography. Lancet 1976; 1:1261–1264.
17. Yokoyama S, Hayashi R, Satani M, Yamamoto A: Selective removal of low density lipoprotein by plasmapheresis in familial hypercholesterolemia. Arteriosclerosis 1985; 5:613–622.
18. Stoffel W, Borberg H, Greve V: Application of specific extracorporeal removal of low density lipoprotein in familial hypercholesterolaemia. Lancet 1981; 2:1005–1007.
19. Schuff-Werner P, Armstrong VW, Eisenhauer TH, et al: Treatment of severe hypercholesterolemia by heparin-induced extracorporeal LDL precipitation (HELP). Contrib Infus Ther 1988; 23:118–126.
20. Gordon BR, Kelsey SF, Bilheimer DW, et al: Treatment of refractory familial hypercholesterolemia by low-density lipoprotein apheresis using an automated dextran sulfate cellulose adsorption system. Am J Cardiol 1992; 70:1010–1016.
21. Parker TS, Gordon BR, Saal SD, et al: Plasma high density lipoprotein is increased in man when low density lipoprotein (LDL) is lowered by LDL-pheresis. Proc Natl Acad Sci U S A 1986; 83:777–781.
22. Gordon BR, Sloan BJ, Parker TS, et al: Humoral immune response following extracorporeal immunoadsorption therapy of patients with hypercholesterolemia. Transfusion 1990; 30:318–321.
23. Olbricht CJ, Schaumann D, Fischer D: Anaphylactoid reactions, LDL apheresis with dextran sulphate, and ACE inhibitors. Lancet 1992; 340:908–909.
24. Tatami R, Inoue N, Itoh H, et al: Regression of coronary atherosclerosis by combined LDL apheresis and lipid-lowering drug therapy in patients with familial hypercholesterolemia: a multicenter study. Atherosclerosis 1992; 95:1–13.
25. Schuff-Werner P, Gohlke H, Bartmann U, et al: The HELP-LDL Apheresis Multicenter Study, an angiographically assessed trial on the role of LDL apheresis in the secondary prevention of coronary heart disease. II. Final evaluation of the effect of regular treatment on LDL-cholesterol plasma concentrations and the course of coronary heart disease. Eur J Clin Invest 1994; 24:724–732.
26. Borberg H, Oette K: Experience with and conclusions from three different trials on low density lipoprotein apheresis. *In* Agishi T, Kawamura A, Mineshima M (eds): Therapeutic Plasmapheresis (XII), pp 13–20. Utrecht: VSP, 1993.
27. Thompson GR, Maher VMG, Matthews S, et al: Familial Hypercholesterolaemia Regression Study: a randomised trial of low-density-lipoprotein apheresis. Lancet 1995; 345:811–816.

28. Starzl TE, Marchioro TL, Sexton AW, et al: The effect of portacaval transposition on carbohydrate metabolism: experimental and clinical observations. Surgery 1965; 57:687–697.
29. Starzl TE, Putnam CW, Porter KA, et al: Portal diversion for the treatment of glycogen storage disease in humans. Ann Surg 1973; 178:525–539.
30. Starzl TE, Chase HP, Putnam CW, Porter KA: Portacaval shunt in hyperlipoproteinaemia. Lancet 1973; 2:940–944.
31. Mitchell SC: Portacaval shunt in familial hypercholesterolaemia [Letter]. Lancet 1983; 1:193.
32. Starzl TE, Chase HP, Ahrens EH Jr, et al: Portacaval shunt in patients with familial hypercholesterolemia. Ann Surg 1983; 198:273–283.
33. Forman MB, Baker SG, Mieny CJ, et al: Treatment of homozygous familial hypercholesterolaemia with portacaval shunt. Atherosclerosis 1982; 41:349–361.
34. McNamara DJ, Ahrens EF Jr, Kolb R, et al: Treatment of familial hypercholesterolemia by portacaval anastomosis: effect on cholesterol metabolism and pool size. Proc Natl Acad Sci U S A 1983; 80:564–568.
35. Bilheimer DW, Goldstein JL, Grundy SM, Brown MD: Reduction in cholesterol and low density lipoprotein synthesis after portacaval shunt surgery in a patient with homozygous familial hypercholesterolemia. J Clin Invest 1975; 56:1420–1430.
36. Hoeg JM, Demosky SJ Jr, Schaefer EJ, et al: The effect of portacaval shunt on hepatic lipoprotein metabolism in familial hypercholesterolemia. J Surg Res 1985; 39:369–377.
37. Reeves F, Gosselin F, Herbert Y, Lambert M: Long term follow-up after portacaval shunt and internal mammary coronary bypass graft in homozygous familial hypercholesterolemia: report of two cases. Can J Cardiol 1990; 6:171–174.
38. Bilheimer DW, Goldstein JL, Grundy SM, et al: Liver transplantation to provide low-density lipoprotein receptors and lower plasma cholesterol in a child with homozygous familial hypercholesterolemia. N Engl J Med 1984; 311:1658–1664.
39. Starzl TE, Bilheimer DW, Bahnson HT, et al: Heart-liver transplantation in a patient with familial hypercholesterolemia. Lancet 1984; 1:1382–1383.
40. Simmons RL, Ildstad ST, Smith CR, et al: Transplantation. *In* Schwartz SI, Schires GT, Spencer FC (eds): Principles of Surgery, 6th ed, pp 414–419. New York: McGraw-Hill, 1994.
41. Figuera D, Ardaiz J, Martin-Judez V, et al: Combined transplantation of heart and liver from two different donors in a patient with familial type IIa hypercholesterolemia. J Heart Transplant 1986; 5:327–329.
42. Valdivielso P, Escolar JL, Cuevas-Mons V, et al: Lipids and lipoprotein changes after heart and liver transplantation in a patient with homozygous familial hypercholesterolemia. Ann Intern Med 1988; 108:204–206.
43. Cienfugos JA, Pardo F, Turrion VS, et al: Metabolic effects of liver replacement in homozygous familial hypercholesterolemia. Transplant Proc 1987; 19:3815–3817.
44. Brush JE Jr, Leon MB, Starzl TE, et al: Successful treatment of angina pectoris with liver transplantation and bilateral internal mammary bypass graft surgery in familial hypercholesterolemia. Am Heart J 1988; 116:1365–1367.
45. Shaw BW, Bahnson HT, Hardesty RL, et al: Combined transplantation of the heart and liver. Ann Surg 1985; 202:667–672.
46. Buchwald H: Surgical operation to lower circulating cholesterol. Circulation 1963; 28:649.
47. Buchwald H, Varco RL, Matts JP, et al, and the POSCH Group: Effect of partial ileal bypass surgery on mortality and morbidity from coronary heart disease in patients with hypercholesterolemia: report of the Program on the Surgical Control of the Hyperlipidemias (POSCH). N Engl J Med 1990; 323:946–955.
48. Ohri SK, Keane PF, Swift I, et al: Reappraisal of partial ileal bypass for the treatment of familial hypercholesterolemia. Am J Gastroenterol 1989; 84:740–743.
49. Defraigne JO, Pirenne P, Swinnen JC, et al: Interets et limites du bypass de l'ileon distal dans le traitement de l'hypercholesterolemie. J Chir (Paris) 1990; 127:77–82.
50. Buchwald H, Fitch LL, Campos CT: Partial ileal bypass in the treatment of hypercholesterolemia. J Fam Pract 1992; 35:69–76.
51. Moore RB, Frantz ID Jr, Buchwald H: Changes in cholesterol pool size, turnover rate, and fecal bile acid and sterol excretion after partial ileal bypass in hypercholesterolemic patients. Surgery 1969; 65:98–108.
52. Raper SE, Wilson JM: Cell transplantation in liver-directed gene therapy. Cell Transplant 1993; 2:381–400.
53. Wilson JM, Grossman M, Raper SE, et al: Clinical protocol. Ex vivo gene therapy of familial hypercholesterolemia. Hum Gene Ther 1992; 3:179–222.
54. Grossman M, Raper SE, Kozarsky K, et al: Successful ex vivo gene therapy directed to liver in a patient with familial hypercholesterolemia. Nat Genet 1994; 6:335–341.
55. Ishibashi S, Brown MS, Goldstein JL, et al: Hypercholesterolemia in low density lipoprotein receptor knockout mice and its reversal by adenovirus-mediated gene delivery. J Clin Invest 1993; 92:883–893.
56. Kozarsky KF, McKinley DR, Austin LL, et al: In vivo correction of low density lipoprotein receptor deficiency in the Watanabe heritable hyperlipidemic rabbit with recombinant adenoviruses. J Biol Chem 1994; 269:13695–13702.

SECTION FIVE

Thrombosis/Thrombolysis

27 Aspirin and Antiplatelet Agents in Cardiovascular Disease

Andrew I. Schafer, MD

Aspirin has been used medicinally since antiquity. It was first demonstrated to be an effective antithrombotic agent in 1953, when Dr. Lawrence L. Craven reported in the *Mississippi Valley Medical Journal* his personal 7-year clinical experience of administering "one aspirin a day" to 1465 healthy males "who were overweight and known to lead a sedentary life," finding that "not one of them developed coronary occlusion or coronary insufficiency."[1] Since then, aspirin has stood the test of time as an effective, inexpensive, and relatively safe drug in the prophylaxis of a variety of thrombotic and vascular disorders, particularly in the arterial circulation where platelets are predominant participants in the thrombotic process. Until recently, aspirin remained essentially the only available, clinically effective antiplatelet agent. However, despite its efficacy in ischemic coronary and cerebrovascular disease, aspirin is only partially effective in some clinical thrombotic disorders and is virtually ineffective in others. The surge in the development of new antiplatelet drugs has been based rationally on our evolving understanding of platelet function.

This chapter briefly outlines the sequence of events involved in platelet activation, each of which potentially serves as a target for antiplatelet intervention, and then provides detailed discussions of specific available and investigational agents. The chapter emphasizes the pharmacology and pharmacokinetics of these drugs, drug interactions, safety, and efficacy in experimental, preclinical, and clinical trials. Their therapeutic use in specific ischemic disorders is discussed in more detail in Section I of the book.

NORMAL MECHANISMS OF PLATELET ACTIVATION AS TARGETS OF ANTIPLATELET INTERVENTION[2, 3]

Endothelial cells, which line the intimal surface of the entire circulatory tree, possess metabolic properties that are designed to preserve blood fluidity under normal circumstances. Two endothelium-derived factors that passivate platelets are prostacyclin (prostaglandin I_2 [PGI_2]) and nitric oxide (also known as endothelium-derived relaxing factor). These potent inhibitors of platelet activation, shown in Figure 27–1*A*, are labile molecules that act only in the immediate vicinity of their sites of production. Their mechanisms of antiplatelet action are to stimulate platelet adenylyl cyclase (with prostacyclin) and guanylyl cyclase (with nitric oxide), thereby raising intraplatelet levels of cyclic adenosine monophosphate (cAMP) and cyclic guanosine monophosphate (cGMP), respectively. Because these endothelial autacoids are not only released into blood but also secreted abluminally, they likewise elevate cAMP and cGMP levels in subendothelial smooth muscle cells and thus also act as potent vasorelaxants and mediators of vascular tone.

Vascular intimal injury leads to the disruption of the antithrombotic properties of endothelium and exposure of blood to prothrombotic subendothelial structures. Circulating platelets adhere to the vessel wall at sites of intimal damage. Platelet adhesion is mediated by von Willebrand factor, a macromolecule that binds to specific platelet receptors localized on platelet membrane glycoprotein Ib (GpIb). Adherent platelets are also anchored to the injured vascular surface through the binding of subendothelial collagen to specific platelet surface collagen receptors (Fig. 27–1*B*). A variety of other platelet stimuli in blood, such as thrombin, serotonin, and epinephrine, can bind to their respective platelet surface receptors (Fig. 27–1*B*). Occupancy of these receptors on adherent platelets probably acts in concert to trigger a cascade of intracellular reactions that leads to the activation and subsequent aggregation of platelets. These intracellular events include the secretion of platelet granule constituents, such as adenosine diphosphate (ADP), fibrinogen, and von Willebrand factor itself, which in turn can bind to their own respective platelet receptors to amplify the process of platelet activation and thrombus formation. Platelet agonist receptor occupancy also induces the release of arachidonic acid from membrane phospholipid pools. Free arachidonic acid is then rapidly metabolized by cyclooxygenase (prostaglandin-G/H synthase) to the labile prostaglandin endoperoxides PGG_2 and PGH_2, and subsequently by thromboxane synthase to thromboxane A_2 (TXA_2). Released PGG_2/PGH_2 and TXA_2 bind to a common platelet receptor to further amplify the platelet activation process (Fig. 27–1*C*).

Activated and degranulated platelets can then adhere to each other in the process of aggregation, leading to the formation of an occlusive thrombus at the site of vascular injury. The ligand for platelet aggregation in lower shear stress regions of the circulation is fibrinogen; in higher shear stress regions, it is von Willebrand factor. The source of fibrinogen and von Willebrand factor for binding to platelets is released platelet granule contents as well as circulating plasma. The platelet receptor for both fibrinogen and von Willebrand factor to mediate this final aggregation process (as opposed to the initial adhesion process) is located on the platelet membrane glycoprotein IIb/IIIa (GpIIb/IIIa) complex. The heterodimeric GpIIb/IIIa receptor, which can bind to fibrinogen or von Willebrand factor, is formed on the platelet surface by the complexing of its individual components, (GpIIb and GpIIIa), only after platelet activation has occurred (Fig. 27–1*D*). The binding of fibrinogen and von Willebrand factor to

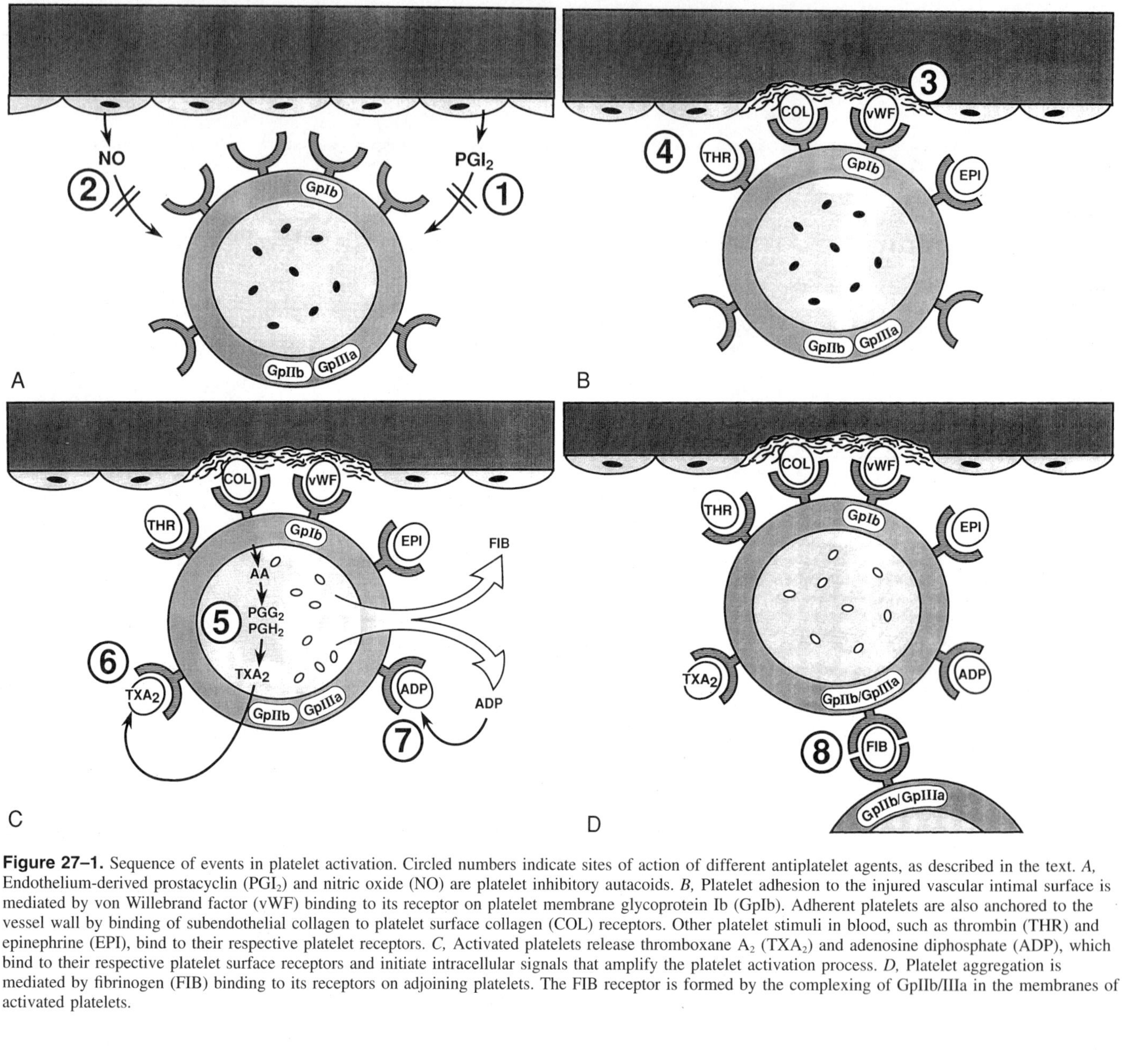

Figure 27–1. Sequence of events in platelet activation. Circled numbers indicate sites of action of different antiplatelet agents, as described in the text. *A,* Endothelium-derived prostacyclin (PGI_2) and nitric oxide (NO) are platelet inhibitory autacoids. *B,* Platelet adhesion to the injured vascular intimal surface is mediated by von Willebrand factor (vWF) binding to its receptor on platelet membrane glycoprotein Ib (GpIb). Adherent platelets are also anchored to the vessel wall by binding of subendothelial collagen to platelet surface collagen (COL) receptors. Other platelet stimuli in blood, such as thrombin (THR) and epinephrine (EPI), bind to their respective platelet receptors. *C,* Activated platelets release thromboxane A_2 (TXA_2) and adenosine diphosphate (ADP), which bind to their respective platelet surface receptors and initiate intracellular signals that amplify the platelet activation process. *D,* Platelet aggregation is mediated by fibrinogen (FIB) binding to its receptors on adjoining platelets. The FIB receptor is formed by the complexing of GpIIb/IIIa in the membranes of activated platelets.

GpIIb/IIIa is mediated by the tripeptide amino acid sequence arginine-glycine-aspartic acid (abbreviated RGD), a motif that is present in these adhesive molecules. Fibrinogen binding to platelet GpIIb/IIIa involves recognition not only of the RGD sequence in its alpha-chain but also of a dodecapeptide sequence at the C terminus of its gamma-chain. The intravascular platelet aggregate that results from this sequence of activation events is anchored by fibrin. Although platelets tend to be the predominant components of arterial thrombi, whereas fibrin predominates in venous thrombi, platelet activation and fibrin formation (coagulation) are interdependent and inseparable processes in the pathophysiologic mechanism of thrombosis.

ANTIPLATELET AGENTS

Antiplatelet agents are discussed in this section in the sequence of their individual actions on the process of platelet activation outlined earlier. However, aspirin is reviewed first, out of order, because it remains the major noninvestigational antiplatelet drug presently available. Furthermore, its proven clinical efficacy, long-lasting effects on platelet function, satisfactory safety profile, and low cost make it the "gold standard" by which other antiplatelet agents are judged.

Aspirin (Acetylsalicylic Acid)

Mechanisms of Action

After its ready absorption from the stomach and upper small intestine, aspirin is hydrolyzed by esterases in the gut wall, plasma, red cells, liver, and lungs to liberate free acetyl groups.[4] These released molecules then acetylate serine residues at position 529 of cyclooxygenase (prostaglandin-G/H synthase), leading to irreversible inactivation of the enzyme.[5–7] As shown in Figures 27–1*C* (circled number 5) and 27–2, this action of aspirin on cyclooxygenase leads to inhibition of TXA_2 synthesis by platelets. Because prostacyclin is also a cyclooxygenase metabolite of arachidonic acid, aspirin likewise blocks its production in vascular endothelial cells. An "aspirin dilemma"[8] is thus created theoretically if aspirin inhibition of the

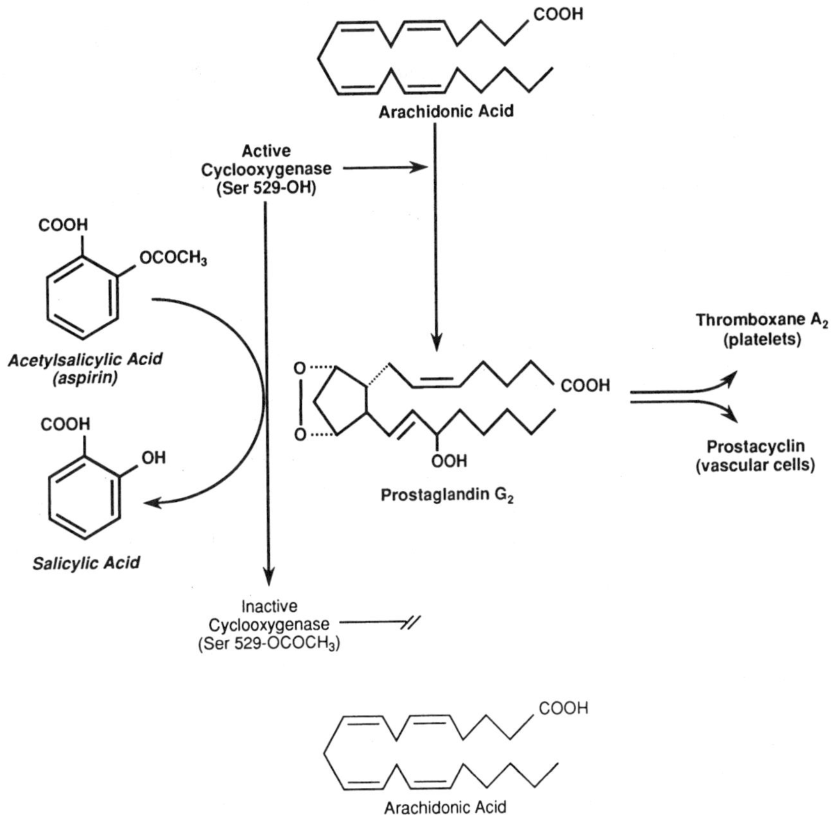

Figure 27–2. Aspirin (acetylsalicylic acid) inhibition of cyclooxygenase (prostaglandin-G/H synthase). Aspirin acetylates serine at position 529 of cyclooxygenase, rendering the enzyme inactive. Acetylated cyclooxygenase does not function to catalyze the oxygenation of arachidonic acid to prostaglandin G_2. Aspirin thereby blocks the formation of thromboxane A_2 (in platelets) and prostacyclin (in vascular cells). (From Loscalzo J, Schafer AI: Anticoagulants, antiplatelet agents, and fibrinolytics. *In* Loscalzo J, Creager MA, Dzau MV [eds]: Vascular Medicine, 2nd ed. Boston: Little, Brown, in press.)

platelet-derived proaggregatory/vasoconstrictor substance, TXA_2, is offset by its simultaneous inhibition of the endothelium-derived antiaggregatory/vasodilator substance, prostacyclin.

Because acetylation irreversibly inhibits cyclooxygenase, the ability of a cell to recover from its effect requires de novo synthesis of nonacetylated enzyme. Since platelets can synthesize only minimal amounts of new protein, aspirin blocks their function for their remaining lifetime (normally 7 to 10 days) in the circulation, even though the drug has only a 20-min half-life in the systemic circulation. In contrast, vascular cells are capable of new protein synthesis, and therefore they can resume prostacyclin synthesis after disappearance of aspirin from the circulation.

Effects on Hemostasis

Inhibition of TXA_2 formation does not affect the initial process of platelet adhesion but does partially inhibit the final step of platelet aggregation. Aspirin blocks platelet aggregation in vitro in response to arachidonic acid, which depends entirely on TXA_2 production, but interferes with platelet responses to other stimuli only to the extent to which their activating actions are mediated by TXA_2 production. For example, as shown in Figure 27–3, platelet aggregation induced in vitro by ADP or epinephrine is partially dependent on the ability of these agonists to stimulate TXA_2 formation, and therefore aspirin partially inhibits aggregation in response to them. High concentrations of thrombin, in contrast, aggregate platelets independently of TXA_2, and therefore aspirin does not impair thrombin-induced aggregation. The widely used cutaneous template bleeding time tests the integrity of platelet plug formation at a site of capillary injury. Therefore, the bleeding time is typically prolonged after aspirin administration. Aspirin may cause an exaggerated prolongation of the bleeding time in individuals with underlying defects of systemic hemostasis, such as von Willebrand disease. Alcohol consumption, which by itself does not prolong the bleeding time, can potentiate aspirin-induced prolongation of the bleeding time.[9]

Clinical Pharmacology

The inhibitory effects of aspirin on platelet thromboxane production and ex vivo aggregation are rapid; maximal effects are achieved within 15–30 min of ingestion of a dose as low as 81 mg.[10] The rapid inhibitory action of aspirin on platelets, which occurs even before the appearance of the drug in the systemic circulation, probably results from presystemic inhibition of platelet cyclooxygenase in the portal circulation.[11]

A single oral dose of 100 mg of aspirin almost completely blocks platelet thromboxane synthesis in normal individuals and in patients with atherosclerotic cardiovascular disease.[12, 13] Daily administration of only 30–50 mg of aspirin likewise results in almost complete suppression of thromboxane production after 7–10 days.[12–14] The maximal inhibitory effects on platelet thromboxane synthesis that are achieved by these regimens of aspirin correlate well with maximal suppression of thromboxane-dependent ex vivo platelet aggregation and prolongation of the bleeding time. Impairment of ex vivo platelet aggregation persists for about 4 to 7 days after a single oral dose of aspirin,[13] reflecting the life span of irreversibly inhibited platelets, whereas the prolonged bleeding time returns to normal within 24–48 h of aspirin ingestion. This discrepancy is probably due to the emergence in the circulation of a sufficient cohort of uninhibited platelets from the bone marrow after the disappearance of blood salicylate levels to support normal in vivo hemostasis even before there is restoration of completely normal ex vivo platelet function.

In view of the indiscriminate actions of aspirin on both platelet and vascular endothelial cell cyclooxygenase, attempts have been made to find a "platelet-selective" regimen of aspirin that spares endothelial prostacyclin synthesis. One approach has been based on

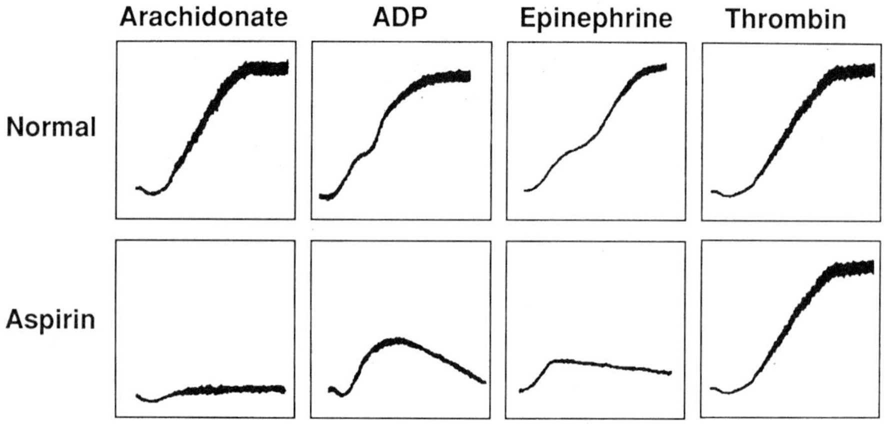

Figure 27–3. Platelet aggregation patterns in normal individuals *(upper panels)* and individuals after aspirin administration *(lower panels).*

the possibility of differential sensitivity of platelet and endothelial cyclooxygenase to aspirin. A single low dose of aspirin (40–80 mg) can nearly completely block thromboxane production and platelet aggregation while largely sparing vascular prostacyclin-forming capacity.[13, 16, 17] However, long-term administration of conventionally formulated aspirin at low doses also partially suppresses endothelial prostacyclin synthesis.[18, 19] Another strategy has been to administer aspirin on alternate days, on the basis of the premise that the rapid and selective recovery of vascular cyclooxygenase function would permit intermittent restoration of prostacyclin production while maintaining continuous suppression of thromboxane synthesis.[20–22] However, this assumption is not borne out by prolonged, alternate-day dosing regimens.[23] Finally, it has been proposed that slow release of low doses of enteric-coated aspirin preparations may selectively inhibit platelets recirculating in the portal system (presystemic inhibition), without reaching the systemic circulation to interfere with prostacyclin formation throughout the vascular tree.[23, 24] The practical feasibility of dose-selective inhibition of platelet cyclooxygenase remains unsettled; however, regardless of dose or regimen, there is ample clinical evidence that the antithrombotic effects of aspirin predominate, possibly involving mechanisms other than only TXA_2 inhibition.[6]

Clinical Use

Aspirin appears to have clinical efficacy in unstable angina, myocardial infarction, aortocoronary bypass grafts, and transient cerebrovascular ischemic attacks. The optimal regimens of aspirin in these clinical situations remain unsettled. In certain situations, the concurrent use of other antiplatelet agents may exert additive or synergistic beneficial actions. Meta-analyses, combining patient data across all methodologically sound trials of prophylactic antiplatelet therapy available for review before March 1990, have been published by the Antiplatelet Trialists' Collaboration.[25] Although trials of different antiplatelet drugs were included, the most widely tested regimen was aspirin, 75–325 mg daily. It was concluded that antiplatelet agents given to patients at increased risk for occlusive vascular disease reduced all-cause mortality, vascular mortality, vascular events (including nonfatal myocardial infarction, nonfatal stroke, and vascular death), and nonfatal myocardial infarction. Benefit was observed among patients with unstable angina, suspected acute myocardial infarction, past history of myocardial infarction, nonfatal stroke, transient ischemic attack (TIA), peripheral vascular disease, and in those having vascular procedures. Low-risk patients receiving antiplatelet agents had reduced nonfatal myocardial infarction only.

As discussed in the following, well-designed randomized trials have demonstrated that aspirin is effective as an antithrombotic agent when it is used in doses between 1.5 g/day and 75 mg/day, and possibly even in doses as low as 30 mg/day.[26] It has been concluded that there is no evidence that low doses (75 to 325 mg/day) are either more or less effective than high doses (900–1500 mg/day).[26] However, the risk of gastric side effects does appear to be dose related (see later). Recommendations for the use of aspirin are summarized in Table 27–1.

Primary Prevention. These trials are discussed in detail in Chapter 51. In the Physicians' Health Study of 22,000 male U.S. physicians 40–84 years of age, randomized to 325 mg of aspirin on alternate days or placebo, a significant 44% reduction in the risk of myocardial infarction was found in the aspirin group after an average follow-up of 5 years.[27] Significant benefits of aspirin were found on both nonfatal and fatal myocardial infarction. Another study of a smaller number of British physicians on a different aspirin regimen (500 mg daily) for 6 years failed to demonstrate a significant beneficial effect

TABLE 27–1. SUMMARY OF RECOMMENDATIONS FOR USE OF ASPIRIN AND TICLOPIDINE

Aspirin is probably effective for the following clinical indications:
- Primary prevention, especially for high-risk subjects
- Stable angina
- Secondary prevention, especially when started promptly after acute myocardial infarction
- Coronary artery bypass graft surgery, when started within 36 h after surgery
- Transient ischemic attacks, in which it is superior to warfarin
- Mechanical or high-risk tissue valves, when added to warfarin

Aspirin is possibly effective for the following clinical indications:
- Peripheral vascular disease
- Prevention of spontaneous abortion in patients with lupus anticoagulant
- Shunt thrombosis
- Prevention of complications of pregnancy-induced hypertension
- Nonrheumatic atrial fibrillation, although warfarin is more effective

Low doses (75 to 325 mg daily) are no more or less effective than high doses (900 to 1500 mg daily) of aspirin in antithrombotic prophylaxis.

The risks of gastrointestinal bleeding and other side effects of aspirin appear to be dose related. The frequency of these side effects can be reduced by treatment with H_2 antagonists or antacids as well as by use of enteric-coated or buffered aspirin.

Preoperative aspirin use does not cause clinically significant excessive perioperative bleeding, unless patients have a coexisting systemic coagulopathy.

Ticlopidine (250 mg twice daily) should be substituted for aspirin in patients with transient ischemic attacks and possibly also for other indications for aspirin listed above in cases of aspirin intolerance, allergy, or recurrence of thromboembolism on aspirin therapy.

of the drug on the incidence of first myocardial infarction, stroke, and total cardiovascular mortality.[28] Both studies found an increased risk of hemorrhagic strokes, which was statistically significant only in the American study, among those in the aspirin group. Nevertheless, when all nonfatal myocardial infarctions, strokes, and vascular deaths from all causes were combined in the U.S. study, those receiving aspirin still showed a significant reduction in risk.[29] Additional studies, some of which are in progress, will be required to resolve whether the beneficial effects of aspirin outweigh its hazards, particularly intracranial hemorrhage, in the primary prevention of myocardial infarction in either healthy or high-risk subjects. The role of aspirin in primary prevention in women is presently unclear; this problem is currently being addressed by the Nurses' Health Study of 40,000 nurses older than 50 years with no previous history of cardiovascular disease.[30]

Stable Angina. A subgroup of the subjects in the Physicians' Health Study with chronic stable angina had a reduced risk of first myocardial infarction with aspirin to at least the same degree as did the asymptomatic men in the trial.[31] The Swedish Angina Pectoris Aspirin Trial randomized patients with chronic stable angina (and without a history of prior myocardial infarction) to aspirin, 75 mg daily, or placebo: aspirin reduced the incidence of myocardial infarction and sudden death by 34%.[32]

Unstable Angina. Several studies have clearly established the efficacy of aspirin in patients with unstable angina. In the Veterans Administration Cooperative Study, death and myocardial infarction were halved after 12 weeks in men with unstable angina given a daily dose of 325 mg buffered aspirin, compared with placebo.[33] The beneficial effects persisted up to 1 year after completion of the 12-week trial, and the concurrent use of beta blockers was found to have an additive effect. A subsequent study confirmed that the incidence of cardiac death or nonfatal myocardial infarction was halved by aspirin.[34] Sulfinpyrazone, either alone or in addition to aspirin, provided no benefit. In this latter trial, men and women with unstable angina derived equal benefit from the use of aspirin, 325 mg four times daily.[34] The Research Group on Instability in Coronary Artery Disease in Southeast Sweden (RISC) reported similar findings: aspirin, 75 mg daily, significantly reduced the risk of myocardial infarction and death in patients with unstable angina or non–Q wave myocardial infarction after both 3 months[35] and 1 year of study.[36] The RISC study showed a beneficial effect of aspirin in patients with symptomatic and silent ischemia, the latter being detected by predischarge exercise testing.[37] Whereas this trial found that aspirin (75 mg daily) reduced the risk of myocardial infarction and death after treatment for 5 days but not during the first 2 days of treatment,[35] the risk of nonfatal and fatal myocardial infarction was markedly reduced in the early phase of unstable angina in patients receiving aspirin, 325 mg twice daily, in another study.[38, 39]

Secondary Prevention. Several trials of aspirin (in daily doses ranging from 300 mg to 2000 mg) have evaluated the efficacy of aspirin in secondary prevention after myocardial infarction.[40–48] Most of these studies reported a trend toward reduced mortality in patients treated with aspirin. When data from six of these trials were combined, the overall reduction in total mortality was estimated to be between 8% and 15%.[40] The Second International Study of Infarct Survival (ISIS-2) in more than 17,000 patients found that aspirin, 162.5 mg daily started within 24 h of acute myocardial infarction, reduced the occurrence of cardiovascular mortality at 5 weeks. The combination of aspirin and streptokinase was significantly more effective than either drug alone.[49] In a preliminary report of another trial, aspirin, 50 mg daily started 8 days after first myocardial infarction, significantly decreased the frequency of reinfarction in combination with either dipyridamole or ticlopidine in comparison with no antiplatelet therapy.[50]

Coronary Artery Bypass Graft Surgery. When aspirin (100 mg daily) was started 24 h after aortocoronary bypass surgery, graft patency was significantly improved at 4 months from 68% to 90% in a placebo-controlled, prospective, double-blind trial.[51] Subsequent studies of coronary artery bypass graft surgery have confirmed the efficacy of antiplatelet therapy, specifically aspirin, provided that treatment is initiated before surgery or within 36 h after operation.[52] Dipyridamole has not been found to add to the beneficial effect of aspirin in maintaining bypass graft patency.[53] Antiplatelet prophylaxis appears to lose its benefit if it is started more than 48 h after surgery.[41]

Cerebrovascular Disease. Aspirin is effective in preventing stroke or death in patients with TIAs and has been found to be superior to oral anticoagulants for this indication.[40, 41, 54, 55] Several large-scale trials have documented the efficacy of aspirin[56–59] as well as the lack of efficacy of dipyridamole or sulfinpyrazone in preventing these end points in patients with TIAs. The Swedish Aspirin Low-dose Trial (SALT) found an 18% reduction in stroke or death in patients who began to take aspirin compared with placebo within 4 months of an initial TIA.[60] The benefit of aspirin in cerebrovascular ischemic syndromes was confirmed as a coincidental finding in some secondary prevention trials after myocardial infarction.[61, 62] Whereas aspirin decreases the risk of stroke or death in patients with TIAs, its effect in reducing the frequency of further TIAs is less convincing. Two trials have failed to confirm a reduction in TIAs, stoke, or death by aspirin in patients with TIAs.[63, 64] The Dutch TIA Trial Study Group found no difference in vascular outcomes for a period of 2.6 years in patients with TIA treated with 30 mg/day versus 283 mg/day of aspirin,[65] but this study did not include a placebo group or a group randomized to take higher doses of aspirin. A critical analysis has concluded that, to date, no study of patients with cerebrovascular disease has established that aspirin doses of 325 mg/day or less are better than or even comparable with 975 mg/day or more.[66] This review raised the possibility that until the appropriate studies are done, high-dose aspirin might be better than low-dose aspirin for cerebrovascular disease. Aggregate meta-analysis of the large antiplatelet trials does not indicate a difference in the efficacy of aspirin according to gender.[67]

Other Vascular and Thromboembolic Disorders. Aspirin (900 mg/day) has been shown to retard the progression of atherosclerotic peripheral vascular diseases in one double-blind, placebo-controlled randomized trial[68]; the addition of dipyridamole (225 mg/day) enhanced the beneficial effect of aspirin. Other studies have also demonstrated that aspirin improves the clinical course of peripheral vascular disease in some patients.[25, 69] Aspirin has been shown to limit reocclusion after successful thrombolysis.[70] Aspirin (160 mg daily) has been found to be effective in preventing shunt thrombosis in patients undergoing chronic hemodialysis.[71] There is anecdotal evidence that aspirin, administered in conjunction with corticosteroids, may reduce the risk of spontaneous abortion in patients with lupus anticoagulants.[72] Pregnancy-induced hypertension, which may manifest clinically as preeclampsia, eclampsia, isolated hypertension, or fetal growth retardation, has been considered to be caused by placental arterial vasoconstriction or thrombosis: low-dose aspirin reduces the risk of severe low birth weight among newborns and the risk of cesarean section in mothers with pregnancy-induced hypertension.[73, 74]

Although lifelong high-intensity prophylactic anticoagulation with warfarin is now routinely used in patients with mechanical cardiac valves and in patients with tissue valves complicated by atrial fibrillation or previous embolism, major systemic embolism still occurs at a rate of 2% to 3% per year.[75] Earlier studies found that the addition of aspirin at doses of up to 1200 mg daily significantly reduced embolic complications but caused an increased risk of serious bleeding.[76, 77] A randomized, double-blind, placebo-controlled trial found that the addition of aspirin (100 mg daily) to warfarin (target International Normalized Ratio [INR] of 3.0 to 4.5) reduced major systemic embolism as well as mortality, particularly mortality from vascular causes, in 370 patients with mechanical heart valves or with high-risk tissue valves. Although there was some increase in bleeding, the risk of the combined treatment was more than offset by the considerable benefit.[78]

Warfarin is the established prophylactic therapy to prevent systemic embolism in patients with nonrheumatic atrial fibrillation. However, the Stroke Prevention in Atrial Fibrillation II (SPAF-II) trial[79], which compared warfarin (adjusted to an INR of 2.0 to 4.5) with aspirin (325 mg daily) in 1100 patients with atrial fibrillation, found that although warfarin appeared to be more effective than aspirin for the prevention of ischemic strokes, it was associated with more hemorrhagic strokes. Although the study suggested that aspirin can be recommended for younger, low-risk patients, warfarin remains clearly indicated in higher risk groups (e.g., including patients with previous TIA or strokes and those with cardiac abnormalities), in whom the study found the risk of thromboembolism during aspirin treatment to be almost twice as high as for those taking warfarin.[80] Antithrombotic prophylaxis of systemic embolism in patients with atrial fibrillation is discussed in detail in Chapter 30.

Limitations

Although many major clinical trials have established the efficacy of aspirin in a variety of vascular and thrombotic disorders, particularly in primary and secondary prevention of ischemic events in the coronary and cerebral circulations, the drug does have important limitations.[81] It has been shown that catecholamines, which may be important endogenous modulators of platelet reactivity,[82] can overcome the inhibitory effect of aspirin on coronary platelet thrombus formation in experimental models of myocardial ischemia.[83] Furthermore, in vitro studies have demonstrated that platelet aggregation induced by high levels of shear stress, which are attained in stenosed arteries, is not significantly inhibited by aspirin.[84] These experimental observations, combined with the relative lack of clinical potency of aspirin as an antiplatelet agent, are probably due to the site of inhibitory action of aspirin in the cascade of platelet activation events. Platelets can be activated by various strong stimuli (e.g., thrombin, collagen, shear stress) through pathways that are completely or partially independent of arachidonic acid metabolism and cyclooxygenase. In addition, aspirin-treated platelets can potentially replace the vasoconstrictor effect of thromboxane (which is abolished by aspirin) with other products (e.g., leukotriene C_4, which is metabolized by platelets in vitro from neutrophil-derived leukotriene A_4).[85, 86] It is somewhat surprising, in fact, that aspirin provides as much protection against atherothrombotic events as has been demonstrated in numerous clinical trials.[81] It is possible, therefore, that the therapeutic benefit of aspirin resides in actions above and beyond cyclooxygenase inhibition, which have not yet been elucidated.[87]

Safety

Bleeding Complications. Regular aspirin use has been associated with an increased incidence of spontaneous bleeding complications. Two trials for the primary prevention of cardiovascular disease showed that the regular use of aspirin (325 mg every other day or 75 mg/day) among healthy male physicians was associated with an increase in disabling hemorrhagic stroke.[27, 28] However, these results were not supported by a meta-analysis of 31 randomized secondary prevention trails.[88] Furthermore, an analysis of 124 antiplatelet trials indicated that a probable small increase in hemorrhagic strokes was outweighed by a larger and definite reduction in other strokes.[25]

An aspirin dose-related increase in occult fecal blood loss has been convincingly measured.[89, 90] The risk of overt gastrointestinal bleeding is likewise increased with the regular use of aspirin (75 to 250 mg/day).[91, 92] Although the incidence of clinically evident gastrointestinal hemorrhage is probably related to the dose of aspirin, even doses as low as 75 mg/day predispose to these events.[93] The risk of gastrointestinal bleeding from low-dose aspirin appears to be particularly pronounced in elderly patients, the population expected to derive greatest benefit from its regular administration for the prevention of atherothrombotic complications. In a 12-month, double-blind, placebo-controlled, randomized trial of 400 subjects older than 70 years, clinical gastrointestinal hemorrhage occurred in 3% of those taking low-dose enteric-coated aspirin (100 mg daily), whereas no such events were noted in the placebo group; this was associated with a significantly greater decrease in hemoglobin levels in the aspirin-treated subjects.[94]

Aspirin use also probably predisposes patients to excessive traumatic and surgical bleeding. It is associated with increased risk for the development of chronic subdural hematoma after head injury.[95] Ingestion of aspirin during pregnancy may be associated with excessive bleeding in both mother and neonate during the peripartum period,[96–98] but more recent analysis indicates that aspirin use during pregnancy is safe and is not associated with fetal or maternal complications.[74]

Numerous reports provide conflicting results regarding the relationship between aspirin use and surgical bleeding complications.[99] For different types of noncardiac surgery, both increased[100, 101] and no increase in[102] perioperative blood loss has been found in patients taking aspirin preoperatively. There are likewise conflicting data for the association of aspirin use preoperatively with risk of bleeding with cardiac surgery. Some studies have reported increased operative blood loss and increased risk of reoperation for bleeding in patients taking aspirin before undergoing coronary artery bypass graft surgery.[103–108] However, results of other studies have failed to demonstrate increased coronary artery bypass graft surgical bleeding with preoperative aspirin use.[109–111] It can be concluded from this information that if preoperative aspirin use does cause excessive perioperative bleeding, it is of marginal clinical significance in most patients. Indeed, many patients requiring cardiac surgery will be on prescribed aspirin therapy to prevent coronary events. Delaying surgery in these patients until discontinuation of aspirin permits restoration of normal hemostasis would not only increase cost but also carry a potentially undesirable clinical result.[111] A history of preoperative aspirin ingestion should not cause emergency surgery to be delayed. The decision whether to delay elective surgery for up to 1 week after stopping aspirin should be individually assessed for each patient, taking into consideration the risk (if any) of excessive bleeding, the urgency of the operation, and the type of surgery planned. It is probably advisable to discontinue aspirin for at least 1 week before elective surgery if the patient has a coexisting systemic coagulopathy (e.g., von Willebrand disease) that might enhance the risk of aspirin-provoked bleeding or if the surgery involves sites where even small amounts of bleeding are potentially dangerous (e.g., neurosurgery).

Gastrointestinal Side Effects. Aspirin and other nonsteroidal anti-inflammatory drugs (NSAIDs) are associated with an increased risk of not only gastrointestinal bleeding but also other serious gastrointestinal complications, such as ulceration and perforation, which may result in hospitalization or death.[112] Long-term aspirin use is associated with an increased incidence of gastric, but not duodenal, ulcers.[91] As reviewed by Patrono,[6] the incidence of upper gastrointestinal symptoms, such as abdominal pain, heartburn, and nausea, during prolonged aspirin therapy depends on dose and dosing interval as well as on the type of formulation (plain or enteric-coated) used. There is evidence that the gastrointestinal side effects of aspirin can be reduced by treatment with antacids or H_2 blockers as well as by the use of enteric-coated or buffered aspirin.[26]

Stimuli of Platelet cAMP and cGMP

Agents that increase platelet levels of cAMP or cGMP inhibit platelet activation and aggregation in response to any agonist; cGMP-elevating agents may also inhibit platelet adhesion to the vessel wall. The major endogenous stimuli of these platelet cyclic nucleotides are endothelium-derived prostacyclin (to induce cAMP) and nitric oxide (to induce cGMP), as shown in Figure 27–1*A* (circled numbers 1 and 2, respectively).

Prostacyclin is the most potent naturally occurring platelet inhibitor currently identified. Its clinical use has been limited by its extreme lability and its potent vasoactive effects. In vivo desensitization of platelet responsiveness with prolonged infusions of prostacyclin might also limit its therapeutic potential.[113, 114] The clinical use of prostacyclin is currently largely restricted to extracorporeal circuits, such as cardiopulmonary bypass, charcoal hemoperfusion, and hemodialysis. In these settings, the regional administration of prostacyclin prevents extracorporeal platelet consumption and reduces the risk of platelet embolization and bleeding.[115] Some studies have demonstrated transient beneficial effects of intravenous prostacyclin infusion in coronary artery disease,[116, 117] peripheral obliterative arterial and vasospastic disorders (including primary pulmonary hypertension),[118, 119] and thrombotic thrombocytopenic purpura.[120]

Prostacyclin's chemical instability, short in vivo half-life, and adverse hemodynamic actions have led to the development of stable synthetic analogues of the prostanoids. One such compound is iloprost, a synthetic prostacyclin analogue that is a more potent inhibitor of platelet aggregation than are prostacyclin or PGE_1,[121] has less pronounced vasoactive properties than the natural prostanoid,[122] and can be administered orally. Iloprost infusion (0.5 to 2 ng/kg/mL) has been reported to exert long-lasting beneficial clinical effects in patients with ischemia of the extremities.[123] However, hypercoagulability and enhanced platelet reactivity have been observed during and sometimes after iloprost infusion.[124] The development of a well-tolerated, orally effective analogue of long duration of activity and high selectivity for antiplatelet actions is still awaited.[125]

Organic nitrates have platelet inhibitory properties, mediated by an increase in platelet GMP.[126, 127] Nitric oxide donors inhibit both platelet adhesion and platelet thrombus formation in vivo[128] as well as have vasodilatory properties. Preliminary results of human trials comparing continuous infusion of a nitric oxide donor, linsidomine (SIN-1), with isosorbide nitrate in unstable angina, and of nitric oxide donors to diltiazem with percutaneous transluminal coronary angioplasty, have not demonstrated superior clinical benefit of the nitric oxide donors.[129] The platelet inhibitory mechanisms of nitric oxide and nitrates are described in detail in Chapter 2.

Dipyridamole

Mechanism of Action

Dipyridamole has been considered to act as an antiplatelet agent by directly stimulating the synthesis of prostacyclin by vascular cells,[130] although this has been disputed[131]; by potentiating the platelet inhibitory effects of prostacyclin[132] and blocking platelet TXA_2 formation[133]; by inhibiting phosphodiesterase, thereby raising platelet cAMP levels[134, 135]; and by interfering with the uptake of adenosine into endothelial cells, red cells, and leukocytes, resulting in the local accumulation of this platelet-inhibitory and vasodilating compound in the thrombotic microenvironment.[136, 137] However, these effects may not occur at concentrations of dipyridamole that are attained in plasma during therapy. Therefore, the mechanism of antithrombotic action of dipyridamole remains unclear and is probably multifactorial.[40, 136]

Effects on Hemostasis

Unlike aspirin, dipyridamole does not prolong the bleeding time.[138] It has been found to inhibit platelet adhesion in some but not all studies.[139–142] The drug inhibits platelet aggregation in vitro only at concentrations that are considerably higher than those attained in blood with therapeutic use.[143] Dipyridamole prolongs platelet survival in various thrombotic and vascular disorders that are characterized by rapid platelet turnover, such as arterial and venous thrombosis, prosthetic heart valves, prosthetic grafts, and possibly coronary artery disease.[144] These effects of dipyridamole contrast with those of aspirin, the use of which is associated with prolongation of bleeding time and impaired platelet aggregation but no changes in platelet survival.

Clinical Use

The dose of dipyridamole used in clinical trials has ranged from 75 to 400 mg/day, without apparent rationale. In general, controlled clinical studies have failed to demonstrate any antithrombotic efficacy by dipyridamole when it is used alone.[136] In fact, dipyridamole has not been found to add to the beneficial effects of aspirin in the secondary prevention of myocardial infarction,[42, 43] the maintenance of coronary bypass graft patency,[53] or the reduction in the incidence of stroke in patients with prior TIA or stroke.[57, 145] Dipyridamole may exert additive or synergistic effects in combination with aspirin or warfarin in certain selected situations. It may be effective in preventing the progression of peripheral occlusive arterial disease when it is combined with aspirin.[68] Combined with warfarin, dipyridamole significantly reduces the incidence of major systemic embolism in patients with mechanical heart valves.[146–148] Direct benefit and risk comparisons between aspirin[78] and dipyridamole as additions to oral anticoagulants in patients with high-risk cardiac valve prostheses are unknown.

Safety

The main side effects of dipyridamole are nausea and abdominal discomfort, which occur in a dose-related manner and are noted in about 10% of patients taking 400 mg daily.[149] The vasodilating action of dipyridamole can cause headache or, rarely with oral dosing, produce a coronary artery "steal" phenomenon, an effect that is currently used with thallium imaging as an alternative to exercise testing. Dipyridamole dose not cause an increased risk of bleeding, even when it is combined with anticoagulants.[149, 150] In a comprehensive review of clinical trials involving dipyridamole, FitzGerald concluded that, particularly in view of the drug's highly variable absorption kinetics and its cost and dose-related side effects, the emerging consensus does not support its use as an antiplatelet agent.[136]

Inhibitors of Platelet Adhesion

Drugs that block the interaction of von Willebrand factor with its platelet receptor on GpIb (circled number 3 in Figure 27–1*B*) should produce a global antiplatelet defect by interfering with the initial event of platelet activation, that is, their adhesion to the injured vessel wall. Such a therapeutic strategy offers the additional theoretic advantage of inhibiting the entire downstream cascade of platelet-activating events that follows adhesion, including secretion of mitogens from platelet granules into the vessel wall, as well as subsequent platelet aggregation. Agents under study that interfere with the interaction of von Willebrand factor with platelet GpIb include monoclonal antibodies against von Willebrand factor, monoclonal antibodies against GpIb, recombinant von Willebrand factor fragments (which bind to GpIb and inhibit the binding of von Willebrand factor multimers to the receptor), and aurin tricarboxylic acid (which binds to von Willebrand factor multimers and prevents their interaction with the receptor).[151, 152] The pig model of homozygous von Willebrand disease has provided experimental support for the pivotal role of von Willebrand factor–mediated platelet-vessel wall interactions in the pathogenesis and progression of spontaneous atherosclerosis as well as in the syndromes of accelerated atherosclerosis.[153] Therefore, although there are concerns that platelet adhesion inhibitors would also significantly interfere with normal hemostasis, this area is a highly promising target for the design of potent antiplatelet agents. There is presently no experience with the use of these drugs in humans.

Inhibitors of Specific Platelet Agonist-Receptor Interactions

The most potent platelet stimulus is thrombin. Therefore, direct antithrombins (e.g., hirudin) would be expected to not only prevent the formation of fibrin but also concurrently inhibit thrombin-induced platelet aggregation.[154, 155] This site of action on platelets is shown in Figure 27–1*B* (circled number 4). Hirudin, unlike heparin, does not need to form a complex with antithrombin III to inhibit thrombin, and therefore it can more effectively inhibit fibrin-bound thrombin. Direct antithrombins are considerably more potent than heparin in reducing platelet thrombus formation in animal models of thrombosis.[156, 157] Clinical trials are currently attempting to determine the relative efficacy and safety of heparin and direct antithrombins in arterial thrombotic disorders. It is not yet known, however, whether the optimal antiplatelet regimen will also be the optimal anticoagulant regimen of direct thrombin inhibitors.[154] Furthermore, although the important role of antithrombins as antiplatelet agents has been established in some experimental animal models of thrombosis, it is presently premature to extrapolate these findings to the treatment of human arterial thrombosis.

Specific inhibitors of platelet thromboxane and ADP receptors are discussed in the following because the actions of these mediators are exerted after the platelet release reaction and their roles are mainly to amplify the platelet activation and aggregation process. A general theoretic limitation of inhibitors of specific platelet agonist-receptor interactions is their capacity to interfere with the initiation of only one of several pathways of platelet activation.

Inhibitors of Arachidonic Acid

Omega-3 Fatty Acids

A reduced incidence of coronary atherosclerosis, myocardial infarction, and occlusive vascular disease in Greenland Eskimos, compared with mainland Danes, has been attributed to their distinctive, marine lipid-rich diets.[158] Cod liver oil supplementation of the atherogenic diets of hyperlipidemic swine has been associated with striking pathologic evidence of the retardation of the development and progression of coronary atherosclerosis.[159] The consumption of fish by a cohort of middle-aged Dutch men observed for 20 years lowered their mortality from coronary heart disease by more than 50%.[160] The Western Electric Study likewise demonstrated an inverse correlation between fish ingestion and mortality from coronary artery disease.[161] This protective effect was observed with an average daily intake of as little as 30 g of fish (equivalent to one or two fish dishes per week). Several randomized trials of fish oil supplementation to prevent restenosis after coronary angioplasty, using up to 6 g/day of omega-3 fatty acids, have shown mixed results.[162]

The predominant polyunsaturated fatty acids in the Eskimo diet belong to the family of omega-3 (or n-3) fatty acids, so designated because the first double bond is always located on the third carbon atom from the methyl (omega) terminus.[163] The major omega-3 fatty acids in fish oils are eicosapentaenoic acid (EPA) and docosahexaenoic acid (DHA). EPA is a 20-carbon polyunsaturated fatty acid with 5 double bonds and is therefore abbreviated C20:5, omega-3. DHA is a 22-carbon fatty acid with 6 double bonds, abbreviated C22:6, omega-3. In contrast, arachidonic acid (C20:4) belongs to the omega-6 family of fatty acids. Cold-water fish contain the largest amounts of EPA and DHA.

The mechanism of the protective effect of fish oils on atherosclerotic cardiovascular disease is probably multifactorial.[164–166] Omega-3 polyunsaturated fatty acids in fish oils have hypolipidemic effects, lowering serum cholesterol and low-density lipoprotein (LDL) cholesterol and triglyceride levels without affecting high-density lipoprotein (HDL) cholesterol,[167, 168] although other studies have reported elevations in LDL cholesterol concentrations in some cases.[169] The antithrombotic effects of fish oils may also be partly attributed to favorable alterations in blood rheology, cell membrane fluidity,[170] and their anti-inflammatory effects.[171] The antiplatelet effects of fish oils are clinically demonstrable in individuals ingesting diets rich in these marine lipids who have a mild bleeding tendency, prolonged bleeding times, mild thrombocytopenia, and abnormalities in platelet aggregation ex vivo.

The antithrombotic alterations in platelet-vascular interactions promoted by fish oils are due, at least in part, to competition between EPA and arachidonic acid for cyclooxygenase. Ingested EPA is incorporated into cell membrane phospholipids, raising the ratio of membrane EPA to arachidonic acid; both of these fatty acids are released by phospholipase in activated cells, and both become available as substrates for cyclooxygenase. TXA_2, formed by the action of cyclooxygenase on platelet arachidonic acid, is a potent activator of platelets and vasoconstrictor; however, TXA_3, produced from EPA, has virtually no biologic activity. In contrast, both PGI_2 (derived from arachidonic acid) and PGI_3 (derived from EPA) produced by endothelial cells have comparable actions as vasodilators and platelet inhibitors.[172] Thus, diets rich in omega-3 fatty acids promote the formation of TXA_3 and PGI_3 over TXA_2 and PGI_2 by platelets and blood vessels, respectively, favorably shifting the balance of these eicosanoids toward an antithrombotic effect. These relationships are shown in Figure 27–4. It has been emphasized that large (at least 10 g EPA daily) and potentially unpalatable doses of medicinal fish oil supplements are required to alter cell membrane fatty acid contents (ratios of EPA to arachidonic acid in platelet membranes approximating unity) that simulate those attained with Eskimo diets.[172]

The most extensively studied use of fish oils as antithrombotic agents has been in preventing restenosis after coronary angioplasty. Meta-analyses of several of these trials,[173, 174] which have yielded mixed results, have concluded that there might be a small to moderate benefit of fish oils on restenosis. A large trial of 470 patients randomized to receive placebo or 8 g/day of omega-3 fatty acids for 6 months after percutaneous transluminal coronary angioplasty failed to demonstrate a beneficial effect of fish oils on restenosis.[175]

Cyclooxygenase Inhibitors Other Than Aspirin

Other Nonsteroidal Anti-Inflammatory Drugs. Nonaspirin NSAIDs, such as indomethacin, phenylbutazone, ibuprofen, naproxen, piroxicam, diclofenac, meclofenamic acid, and sulindac, inhibit platelet function through a mechanism similar to that of aspirin.[143, 176, 177] However, these drugs are reversible rather than irreversible inhibitors of cyclooxygenase (circled number 5 in Figure 27–1*C*). Therefore, their antiplatelet actions are short lived, generally lasting no longer than 6 h, depending on the half-life of the drug in the circulation.[99] The effects of nonaspirin NSAIDs on clinical bleeding and gastrointestinal side effects are similar to, although less pronounced than those of aspirin. As with aspirin, there are conflicting reports regarding the effects of nonaspirin NSAIDs on perioperative blood loss.[99] Nonaspirin NSAIDs have not been tested rigorously in clinical trials as antithrombotic agents. Extrapolating their clinical efficacy from that of aspirin would be justified only if aspirin was clearly known to exert its antiplatelet action solely through cyclooxygenase blockade.

Sulfinpyrazone. Sulfinpyrazone is a uricosuric drug that has structural similarity to phenylbutazone.[4, 178] After gastrointestinal absorption, the drug is slowly metabolized from its sulfoxide form to a

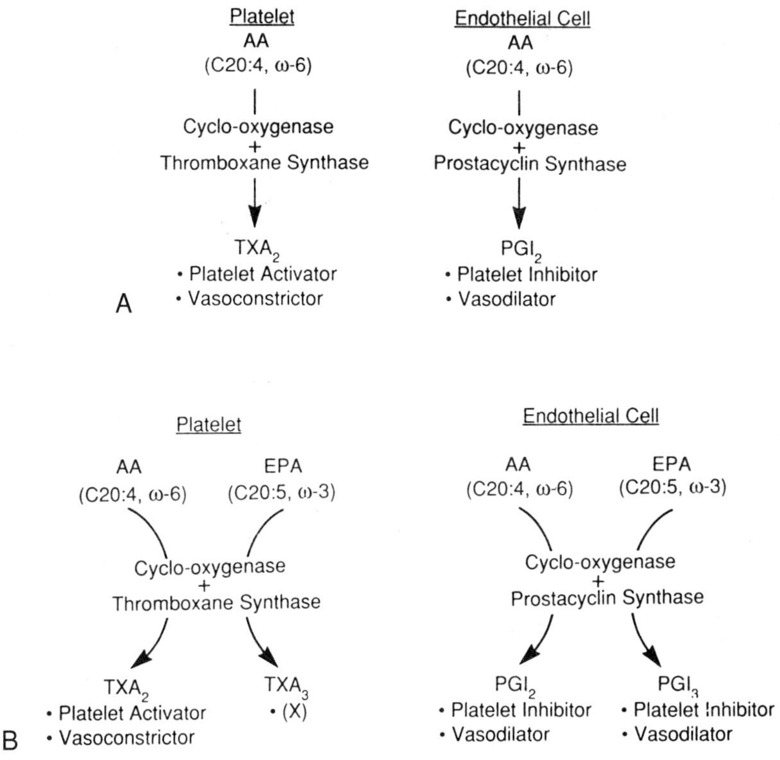

Figure 27–4. Platelet and endothelial cell cyclooxygenase metabolism with Western diet *(A)* and Eskimo diet *(B)*. *A,* With Western diet, the predominant substrate for cyclooxygenase is arachidonic acid (AA), leading to the production of biologically active thromboxane A_2 (TXA_2) and prostacyclin (PGI_2) in platelets and endothelial cells, respectively. *B,* With Eskimo diet or administration of omega-3 fatty acids, eicosapentaenoic acid (EPA) competes with AA for cyclooxygenase. The cyclooxygenase metabolites of EPA are biologically inactive TXA_3 and biologically active PGI_3 in platelets and endothelial cells, respectively. (From Schafer AI: The platelet life cycle: normal function and qualitative disorders. *In* Handin RI, Stossel TP, Lux SE [eds]: Blood: Principles and Practice of Hematology, p 1111. Philadelphia: JB Lippincott, 1995.)

sulfide.[179] In vitro, the sulfide metabolite is considerably more active than the parent compound in its antiplatelet actions.[180] The formation of a slowly formed active metabolite may account for the finding that the effects of sulfinpyrazone on platelets take several days to appear and disappear.[63]

Sulfinpyrazone acts as an incomplete and reversible inhibitor of platelet cyclooxygenase,[181] but this effect is unlikely to account entirely for the antiplatelet actions of the drug. Similar to dipyridamole and unlike aspirin, sulfinpyrazone normalizes the shortened platelet survival in various clinical situations.[182] There is equivocal evidence that sulfinpyrazone also inhibits platelet adhesion in vitro.[183, 184]

The clinical efficacy of sulfinpyrazone in the secondary prevention of myocardial infarction was the subject of considerable controversy.[185, 186] Interpretation of study results was complicated by the possible antiarrhythmic effects of the drug and the beneficial effects of the concomitant use of beta blockers. Sulfinpyrazone, used either alone or in combination with aspirin, has been found to have no beneficial effects in patients with TIAs[56] or unstable angina.[34] As has been reported with aspirin, sulfinpyrazone appears to prevent arteriovenous shunt thrombosis.[187]

Thromboxane Synthase Inhibitors and Thromboxane Receptor Antagonists. The lack of complete platelet specificity of aspirin and other cyclooxygenase inhibitors could be circumvented by the use of platelet thromboxane synthase inhibitors. Theoretically, as shown in Figure 27–5, such agents would offer the additional advantage of redirecting platelet-derived endoperoxide intermediates to neighboring endothelial cells to provide substrates for enhanced prostacyclin synthesis.[188, 189] Dazoxiben has emerged from a series of substituted imidazoles as a potentially useful orally administered thromboxane synthase (TxS) inhibitor.[190] Administration of dazoxiben to human subjects leads, as expected, to marked suppression of TXA_2 formation.[191] However, in vitro platelet aggregation is not consistently inhibited by TxS inhibitors.[192, 193] This may be due to the direct agonist effects of endoperoxides, which accumulate with TxS inhibition and themselves occupy and activate the platelet TXA_2 receptor. The additive inhibitory effect on platelet aggregation of TxS inhibitors and endoperoxide-thromboxane receptor antagonists supports this explanation.[194]

Despite their theoretical attractiveness, clinical experience with TxS inhibitors has been generally disappointing to date. These reversible TxS inhibitors have short plasma half-lives and provide only incomplete suppression of TXA_2 production during long-term dosing.[194] Dazoxiben has failed to produce improvement in the objective parameters of Raynaud phenomenon in various trials.[195–197] Another imidazole analogue has been found to be ineffective in improving renal or liver function in the hepatorenal syndrome.[198] Short-term administration of dazoxiben has failed to influence the time to exercise-induced angina,[199, 200] and beneficial effects of the drug on the hemodynamic response to atrial pacing in patients with chronic stable angina have been, at best, marginal.[201, 202]

Antagonists of thromboxane-endoperoxide receptors (circled number 6 in Figure 27–1*C*) represent a potentially valuable antiplatelet therapeutic approach.[203] Thromboxane receptor antagonists have the advantage over TxS inhibitors of blocking the effects of both TXA_2 and the endoperoxide PGH_2, whereas TxS inhibitors do not prevent the agonist effects of endoperoxides that accumulate.

The possibility of the combined use of a TxS inhibitor and a thromboxane receptor antagonist has particular appeal as clinical antiplatelet therapy. By blocking thromboxane receptors, the proaggregatory actions of the endoperoxides should be prevented while endoperoxide diversion to endothelial cells (see Fig. 27–5) is permitted and, hence, so is augmented vascular prostacyclin production.[204] Initial studies with ridogrel, a dual thromboxane synthase inhibitor and thromboxane-endoperoxide receptor blocker, found it to be a more potent antiplatelet agent than aspirin in human volunteers.[205] However, in a trial of 907 patients with myocardial infarction receiving streptokinase thrombolytic therapy, adjunctive ridogrel was not superior to aspirin in potentiating fibrinolysis and preventing rethrombosis.[206] These results suggest that ridogrel's effects on thromboxane receptor antagonism are relatively modest or that pathways of platelet activation or stimuli to thrombosis or rethrombosis that

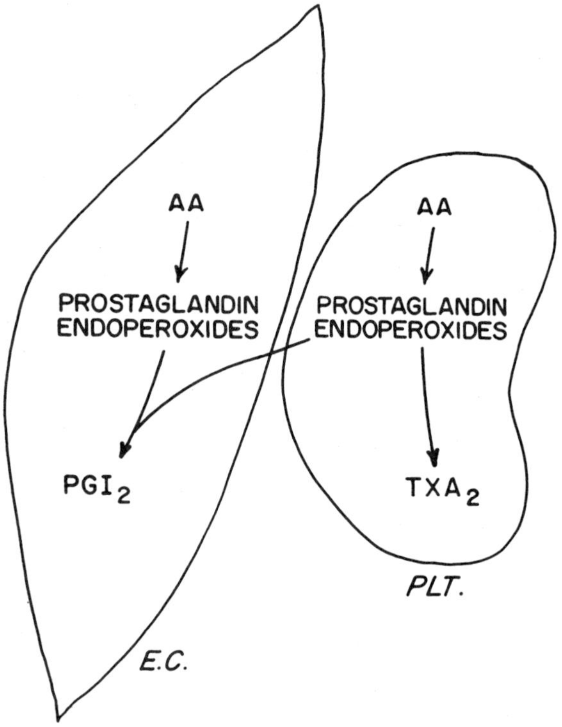

Figure 27–5. Prostaglandin endoperoxide diversion ("steal") from platelets (PLT.) to endothelial cells (E.C.). Endoperoxides (PGG_2 and PGH_2) produced in platelets by the action of cyclooxygenase on arachidonic acid (AA) can be further metabolized in platelets to thromboxane A_2 (TXA_2) by thromboxane synthase or transferred to nearby endothelial cells for conversion to prostacyclin (PGI_2) by prostacyclin synthase.

are not affected by aspirin or ridogrel may be operative in this clinical setting.

Ticlopidine

Ticlopidine[207] and its analogue, clopidogrel, are thienopyridine derivatives that cause potent inhibition of ADP-induced platelet aggregation. As shown in Figure 27–1*C* (circled number 7), these drugs exert their antiplatelet action primarily by inhibiting the binding of ADP to its specific platelet receptors.[208, 209] They also cause lesser degrees of inhibition of aggregation in response to other stimuli that act in part by releasing endogenous ADP from platelet dense granules.[210, 211] Therefore, earlier studies demonstrating inhibition by ticlopidine of fibrinogen binding to its platelet membrane GpIIb/IIIa receptor[212] probably reflected a downstream event after ADP receptor blockade. Unlike aspirin, ticlopidine also inhibits shear stress–induced platelet aggregation, which is partially mediated by released ADP.[213]

Full antiplatelet activity is obtained only 3 to 5 days after ticlopidine administration; the bleeding time is not maximally prolonged until 5 to 6 days after ticlopidine is started.[214] The effects of ticlopidine persist for 4 to 8 days after drug discontinuation, which suggests an irreversible antiplatelet effect. Maximal platelet antiaggregatory action is found only after oral administration and cannot be reproduced in vitro at pharmacologic concentrations of the drug. These findings suggest that antiplatelet activity is mediated by a metabolite of ticlopidine.[211]

Prevention of stroke is the most established clinical indication for the use of ticlopidine. The Ticlopidine versus Aspirin Stroke Study (TASS)[215] compared aspirin (650 mg twice daily) and ticlopidine (250 mg twice daily) in more than 3000 randomized patients with a history of TIA or minor ischemic stroke. Ticlopidine was superior to aspirin for preventing stroke, with significant relative risk reductions for the primary end points of nonfatal stroke or death from any cause (12%) as well as fatal and nonfatal stroke (21%) at 3 years. Subgroup analysis during a 5-year follow-up period also showed that ticlopidine is more effective than aspirin for the prevention of recurrent TIAs.[216] However, because many patients enrolled in TASS were "aspirin failures" at the time of their qualifying events, the relative efficacy of ticlopidine versus aspirin for preventing stroke or TIA in patients not previously treated with aspirin remains uncertain.[217] In the Canadian-American Ticlopidine study, ticlopidine was found to be superior to placebo in the secondary prevention of stroke,[218] but ticlopidine and aspirin have not yet been directly compared for this indication.

Although ticlopidine appears to be more effective than aspirin, at least for the prevention of cerebrovascular ischemic episodes, its advantage may be partially offset by its considerably higher expense and the complications of infrequent (less than 1%) but severe neutropenia and very rare thrombocytopenia. At this time, ticlopidine is generally considered to be indicated (at a recommended dose of 250 mg twice daily) for patients with TIA or stroke who have aspirin intolerance or who fail with aspirin treatment.

Ticlopidine has also been shown to be effective in placebo-controlled clinical trials to prevent coronary artery bypass graft reocclusion,[219] to prevent death or myocardial infarction in patients with unstable angina,[220] to treat patients with intermittent claudication,[221] and to reduce progression of nonproliferative diabetic retinopathy.[222] However, the efficacy and safety of ticlopidine in direct comparison with other antiplatelet agents remain to be demonstrated in these and other atherothrombotic disorders.

Inhibitors of Platelet Aggregation: Platelet Membrane GpIIb/IIIa Antagonists

The limited clinical efficacy of many of the antiplatelet drugs described has been attributed in part to their targeting of only single specific platelet receptors or platelet metabolic pathways. One potential solution to this problem is to use combinations of drugs, a strategy that has been inadequately explored to date. Alternatively, broad inhibition of platelet function by a single agent should provide greater antithrombotic efficacy. To this end, a number of agents have been developed to interrupt the final common pathway of platelet aggregation, the binding of fibrinogen (or von Willebrand factor) to its platelet membrane GpIIb/IIIa receptor (circled number 8 in Figure 27–1*D*). As described at the beginning of the chapter, platelet activation by any stimulus leads to the transition of the GpIIb/IIIa receptor to a high-affinity ligand-binding state. The multivalent adhesive glycoproteins, fibrinogen (at sites of lower shear stress) and von Willebrand factor (at sites of high shear stress), can then bind and form bridges between platelets in the process of platelet cohesion or aggregation.[154, 155, 223] The RGD recognition sequence, which is common to these adhesive molecules, mediates their binding to the GpIIb/IIIa receptor. Two general strategies to develop inhibitors of fibrinogen-GpIIb/IIIa interactions have used (1) monoclonal antibodies to GpIIb/IIIa and (2) small-molecule RGD analogues that compete with fibrinogen (or von Willebrand factor) for binding to platelet GpIIb/IIIa.

Monoclonal antibodies that block the GpIIb/IIIa receptor are potent inhibitors of platelet aggregation, both in vitro and in vivo. The monoclonal antibody known as 7E3, originally developed by Coller,[224] has been most extensively investigated in animal and human antithrombotic trials. Clinical studies have used either the Fab fragment of the mouse antibody or the Fab fragment of a chimeric antibody containing the variable regions of the mouse antibody and the constant regions of a human antibody.[154, 225]

The Evaluation of 7E3 for the Prevention of Ischemic Complications (EPIC) investigators have reported that a chimeric monoclonal antibody Fab fragment of 7E3 (c7E3 Fab), administered as a bolus and infusion to more than 2000 patients undergoing high-risk coronary angioplasty or atherectomy, resulted in a 35% reduction in the composite-event rate, primarily in the rate of nonfatal myocardial infarction and the need for emergency repeated angioplasty or bypass surgery.[226] Substantial blood loss was observed in this trial, particularly at sites of femoral puncture, requiring a significant increase in the use of blood products. The increased bleeding complications found in the EPIC trial may have been due to the relatively high doses of heparin that were used concomitantly; a follow-up study is currently testing the safety of lower doses of heparin used in conjunction with c7E3 Fab. The European Cooperative Study Group randomized 60 patients with unstable angina to either c7E3 Fab (by bolus and infusion) or placebo.[227] (All patients concomitantly received aspirin, intravenous nitroglycerin, and heparin.) Results of this pilot trial demonstrated a trend in the c7E3 Fab–treated patients to reduced rates of ischemia, reduced major events (deaths, infarcts, urgent interventions) during hospital stay, and angiographically demonstrated improvement in Thrombolysis in Myocardial Infarction (TIMI) flow and quantitative improvement of the lesions. Although the doses of 7E3 used were the same as in the EPIC trial, no excess bleeding complications were observed. The Thrombolysis and Angioplasty in Myocardial Infarction (TAMI) 8 pilot study reported improved coronary artery patency and a trend for fewer ischemic events with the use 7E3 (in conjunction with heparin and aspirin) after thrombolytic therapy for acute myocardial infarction.[228] Administration of the nonchimeric murine 7E3 Fab antibody, used in bolus injections, did not result in increased bleeding in this trial. The major limitations of monoclonal antibodies are their lack of reversibility and their immunogenicity. The latter problem may, to some extent, be circumvented by the use of "humanized" chimeric antibodies.

Peptides containing RGD or an analogous amino acid sequence have been developed that compete with fibrinogen (or von Willebrand factor) and thus reversibly prevent platelet aggregation in response to any stimulus. Several of these RGD-containing peptides (also called disintegrins) are derived from snake venoms or leeches.[229–232] Ornatin and decorsin, two RGD-containing GpIIb/IIIa inhibitors from leeches, possess the same protein scaffold but different binding epitopes as two other leech-derived antithrombotic proteins, hirudin (a thrombin inhibitor) and antistasin (a factor Xa inhibitor), which affect hemostasis by different mechanisms.[233] To increase the metabolic stability, potency, and selectivity of disintegrins, a number of cyclic peptides, peptidomimetics, and nonpeptide RGD mimetics have been synthesized.[234–241] Integrelin, which improves thrombolysis when administered with hirudin in a canine model of coronary thrombosis,[242] is currently in human clinical trials. A platelet GpIIb/IIIa antagonist has been isolated from tick salivary gland that does not contain the RGD recognition sequence, or a conservative substitution, and has no structural homology with the RGD-containing disintegrins.[243]

Differences among the various platelet GpIIb/IIIa inhibitors that will be examined in future clinical trials include routes of administration, pharmacokinetics, duration of effect, affinity for GpIIb/IIIa, integrin specificity (including cross-reactivity with the endothelial cell vitronectin receptor), potential antigenicity, and cost. There are several general problems with the clinical use of all platelet GpIIb/IIIa antagonists currently available. First, all of these GpIIb/IIIa inhibitors require intravenous administration, which limits their use to acute situations of thrombosis and reocclusion. Orally active compounds will be needed for use as long-term preventive therapy. Second, the restenosis effects and the need for repeated angioplasty will require investigation. Initial experience with 7E3 suggests that a 12-h infusion after bolus injection of the monoclonal antibody may promote "passivation" of the vascular intimal surface, thereby exerting long-term antithrombotic effect and reducing the need for repeated angioplasty. Third, standards of dose monitoring for these agents will have to be established. Finally, some of the early clinical experience with these drugs has emphasized the need for careful assessment of the risk of bleeding, particularly when treatment is combined with invasive procedures, such as arterial puncture. Pharmacologic blockade of platelet GpIIb/IIIa theoretically mimics the inherited bleeding disorder of Glanzmann thrombasthenia.[244] The limitation of bleeding risk, which is common to all potent antiplatelet drugs in current use, is due to the inability of any known antithrombotic agent to discriminate in its target of action between a pathologic thrombus and a protective hemostatic plug.

REFERENCES

1. Craven LL: Experiences with aspirin (acetylsalicylic acid) in the nonspecific prophylaxis of coronary thrombosis. Miss Valley Med J 1953; 75:38–44.
2. Schafer AI: The platelet life cycle: normal function and qualitative disorders. *In* Handin RI, Stossel TP, Lux SE (eds): Blood: Principles and Practice of Hematology, pp 1095–1127. Philadelphia: JB Lippincott, 1995.
3. Kroll MH, Schafer AI: Biochemical mechanisms of platelet activation. Blood 1989; 74:1181–1194.
4. Pedersen AK, FitzGerald GA: The human pharmacology of platelet inhibition: pharmacokinetics relevant to drug action. Circulation 1985; 112:1164–1176.
5. Roth GJ, Majerus PW: The mechanism of the effect of aspirin on human platelets. I: Acetylation of a particulate fraction protein. J Clin Invest 1975; 56:624–632.
6. Patrono C: Aspirin as an antiplatelet drug. N Engl J Med 1994; 330:1287–1294.
7. Funk CD, Funk LB, Kennedy ME, et al: Human platelet–erythroleukemia cell prostaglandin G/H synthase: cDNA cloning, expression, mutagenesis and gene chromosomal assignment. FASEB J 1991; 5:2304–2312.
8. Marcus AJ: Editorial perspective: aspirin as an antithrombotic medication. N Engl J Med 1983; 309:1515–1517.
9. Deykin D, Janson P, McMahon L: Ethanol potentiation of aspirin-induced prolongation of the bleeding time. N Engl J Med 1982; 306:852–854.
10. Dabaghi SF, Kamat SG, Payne J, et al: Effects of low-dose aspirin on in vitro platelet aggregation in the early minutes after ingestion in normal subjects. Am J Cardiol 1994; 74:720–723.
11. Pedersen AK, FitzGerald GA: Dose-related kinetics of aspirin: presystemic acetylation of platelet cyclooxygenase. N Engl J Med 1984; 311:1206–1211.
12. Patrignani P, Filabozzi P, Patrono C: Selective cumulative inhibition of platelet thromboxane production by low-dose aspirin in healthy subjects. J Clin Invest 1982; 69:1366–1372.
13. Weksler BB, Pett SB, Alonso D, et al: Differential inhibition by aspirin of vascular and platelet prostaglandin synthesis in atherosclerotic patients. N Engl J Med 1983; 308:800–805.
14. DeCaterina R, Giannessi D, Bernini W, et al: Low-dose aspirin in patients recovering from myocardial infarction: evidence for a selective inhibition of thromboxane-related platelet function. Eur Heart J 1985; 6:409–417.
15. FitzGerald GA, Oates JA, Hawiger J, et al: Endogenous biosynthesis of prostacyclin and thromboxane and platelet function during chronic administration of aspirin in man. J Clin Invest 1983; 71:676–688.
16. DeCaterina R, Giannessi D, Boem A, et al: Equal antiplatelet effects of aspirin 50 or 324 mg/day in patients after acute myocardial infarction. Thromb Haemost 1985; 54:528–532.
17. Hanley SP, Bevan J, Cockbill SR, et al: Differential inhibition by low-dose aspirin of human venous prostacyclin synthesis and platelet thromboxane synthesis. Lancet 1981; 1:969–971.
18. Ciabattoni G, Boss AH, Daffonchio L, et al: Radioimmunoassay measurement of 2,3-dinor metabolites of prostacyclin and thromboxane in human urine. Adv Prostaglandin Thromboxane Leukotriene Res 1987; 17:598–602.
19. Braden GA, Knapp HR, FitzGerald GA: Suppression of eicosanoid biosynthesis during coronary angioplasty by fish oil and aspirin. Circulation 1991; 84:679–685.
20. FitzGerald GA, Oates JA: Selective and nonselective inhibition of thromboxane formation. Clin Pharmacol Ther 1984; 35:633–640.
21. Heavey DJ, Barrow SE, Hickling NE, et al: Aspirin causes short-lived

inhibition of bradykinin-stimulated prostacyclin production in man. Nature 1985; 318:186–188.
22. Ritter JM, Cockroft JR, Doktor HS, et al: Differential effect of aspirin on thromboxane and prostaglandin biosynthesis in man. Br J Clin Pharmacol 1989; 28:573–579.
23. Clarke RJ, Mayo G, Price P, FitzGerald GA: Suppression of thromboxane A_2 but not of systemic prostacyclin by controlled-release aspirin. N Engl J Med 1991; 325:1137–1141.
24. Stampfer MJ, Jakubowski JA, Deykin D, et al: Effect of alternate-day regular and enteric-coated aspirin on platelet aggregation, bleeding time, and thromboxane A_2 levels in bleeding-time blood. Am J Med 1986; 81:400–404.
25. Antiplatelet Trialists' Collaboration: Collaborative overview of randomised trials of antiplatelet therapy—I: prevention of death, myocardial infarction, and stroke by prolonged antiplatelet therapy in various categories of patients. Br Med J 1994; 308:81–106.
26. Hirsh J, Dalen JE, Fuster V, et al: Aspirin and other platelet-active drugs. The relationship between dose, effectiveness, and side effects. Chest 1992; 102(suppl):327S–336S.
27. Steering Committee of the Physicians' Health Study Research Group: Final report on the aspirin component of the ongoing Physicians' Health Study. N Engl J Med 1989; 321:129–135.
28. Peto R, Gray R, Collins R, et al: Randomised trial of prophylactic daily aspirin in British male doctors. Br Med J 1988; 296:313–316.
29. Relman AS: Aspirin for the primary prevention of myocardial infarction. N Engl J Med 1988; 318:245–246.
30. Manson JE, Stampfer MJ, Colditz GA, et al: A prospective study of aspirin use and primary prevention of cardiovascular disease in women. JAMA 1991; 266:521–527.
31. Ridker PM, Manson JE, Gaziano JM, et al: Low-dose aspirin therapy for chronic stable angina: a randomized, placebo-controlled clinical trial. Ann Intern Med 1991; 114:835–839.
32. Juul-Möller S, Edvardsson N, Jahnmatz B, et al: Double-blind trial of aspirin in primary prevention of myocardial infarction in patients with stable chronic angina pectoris. Lancet 1992; 340:1421–1425.
33. Lewis HD, Davis JW, Archibald DG, et al: Protective effects of aspirin against acute myocardial infarction and death in men with unstable angina: results of a Veterans Administration Cooperative Study. N Engl J Med 1983; 309:396–403.
34. Cairns JA, Gent M, Singer J, et al: Aspirin, sulfinpyrazone, or both in unstable angina. N Engl J Med 1985; 313:1369–1375.
35. The RISC Group: Risk of myocardial infarction and death during treatment with low dose aspirin and intravenous heparin in men with unstable coronary artery disease. Lancet 1990; 336:827–830.
36. Wallentin LC, Research Group on Instability in Coronary Artery Disease in Southeast Sweden: Aspirin (75 mg/day) after an episode of unstable coronary artery disease: long-term effects on the risk for myocardial infarction, occurrence of severe angina and the need for revascularization. J Am Coll Cardiol 1991; 18:1587–1593.
37. Nyman I, Larsson H, Wallentin L, Research Group on Instability in Coronary Artery Disease in Southeast Sweden: Prevention of serious cardiac events by low-dose aspirin in patients with silent myocardial ischemia. Lancet 1992; 340:497–501.
38. Théroux P, Ouimet H, McCans J, et al: Aspirin, heparin, or both to treat acute unstable angina. N Engl J Med 1988; 319:1105–1111.
39. Théroux P, Waters D, Lam J, et al: Reactivation of unstable angina after the discontinuation of heparin. N Engl J Med 1992; 327:141–145.
40. Webster J, Douglas AS: Aspirin and other antiplatelet drugs in the prophylaxis of thrombosis. Blood Rev 1987; 1:9–20.
41. Gallus AS: The use of antithrombotic drugs in artery disease. Clin Hematol 1986; 15:509–559.
42. Persantine-Aspirin Reinfarction Study Research Group: Persantine and aspirin in coronary heart disease. Circulation 1980; 621:449–461.
43. Klimt CR, Knatterud GL, Stamler J, et al: Persantine-aspirin reinfarction study. II: Secondary coronary prevention with Persantine and aspirin. J Am Coll Cardiol 1986; 7:251–269.
44. Elwood PC, Cochrane AL, Burr ML, et al: A randomised controlled trial of acetyl salicylic acid in the secondary prevention of mortality from myocardial infarction. Br Med J 1974; 1:436–440.
45. Coronary Drug Project: Aspirin in coronary heart disease. J Chronic Dis 1976; 29:625–642.
46. Breddin K, Loew D, Lechner K, et al: Secondary prevention of myocardial infarction. Comparison of acetylsalicylic acid, phenprocoumon and placebo. A multicenter two-year prospective study. Thromb Haemost 1979; 41:225–236.
47. Elwood PC, Sweetman PM: Aspirin and secondary mortality after myocardial infarction. Lancet 1979; 2:1313–1315.
48. Aspirin Myocardial Infarction Study (AMIS) Research Group: A randomized controlled trial of aspirin in persons recovered from myocardial infarction. JAMA 1980; 243:661–669.
49. ISIS-2 (Second International Study of Infarct Survival) Collaborative Group: Randomised trial of intravenous streptokinase, oral aspirin, both, or neither among 17,187 cases of suspected acute myocardial infarction: ISIS-2. Lancet 1988; 2:349–360.
50. Ishikawa K, Kanamasa K, Ogawa I: Aspirin 50 mg per day combined with either dipyridamole or ticlopidine is effective to prevent recurrent myocardial infarction. Circulation 1992; 86(suppl)1:643.
51. Lorenz RL, Schacky CV, Weber M, et al: Improved aortocoronary bypass patency by low-dose aspirin (100 mg daily). Lancet 1984; 1:1261–1264.
52. Sanz G, Parajon A, Alegria E, et al: Prevention of early aortocoronary bypass occlusion by low-dose aspirin and dipyridamole. Circulation 1990; 82:765–773.
53. Brown BG, Cukingnan RA, DeRouen T, et al: Improved graft patency in patients treated with platelet-inhibiting therapy after coronary bypass surgery. Circulation 1985; 72:138–146.
54. Matchar DB, McCrory DC, Barnett HJM, Feussner JR: Medical treatment for stroke prevention. Ann Intern Med 1994; 121:41–53.
55. American College of Physicians: Guidelines for medical treatment for stroke prevention. Ann Intern Med 1994; 121:54–55.
56. Canadian Cooperative Study Group: A randomized trial of aspirin and sulfinpyrazone in threatened stroke. N Engl J Med 1978; 299:53–59.
57. American-Canadian Cooperative Study Group: Persantine aspirin trial in cerebral ischemia. II: Endpoint results. Stroke 1985; 16:406–415.
58. Fields WS, Lemak NA, Frankowski RF, et al: Controlled trial of aspirin in cerebral ischaemia. Stroke 1977; 8:301–314.
59. Fields WS, Lemak NA, Frankowski RF, et al: Controlled trial of aspirin in cerebral ischaemia. Part II: Surgical group. Stroke 1978; 9:309–319.
60. The SALT Collaborative Group: Swedish Aspirin Low-dose Trial of 75 mg aspirin as secondary prophylaxis after cerebrovascular ischemic events. Lancet 1991; 338:L345–L349.
61. Assessment of short term anticoagulant administration after cardiac infarction: report of the Working Party on Anticoagulant Therapy in Coronary Thrombosis to the Medical Research Council. Br Med J 1969; 1:335–342.
62. Telford AM, Wilson C: Trials of heparin vs. atenolol in prevention of myocardial infarction in intermediate coronary syndrome. Lancet 1981; 1:1225–1228.
63. Sorensen PS, Pedersen H, Marquardsen J, et al: Acetylsalicylic acid in the prevention of stroke in patients with reversible cerebral ischemic attacks. A Danish Cooperative Study. Stroke 1983; 14:15–22.
64. Guirand-Chaumeil B, Rascol A, David J, et al: Prevention des recidives des accidents vasculaires cerebraux ischemiques par les anti-aggregants plaquettaires. Neurology (Paris) 1982; 138:368–385.
65. The Dutch TIA Trial Study Group: A comparison of two doses of aspirin in patients after a transient ischemic attack or minor ischemic stroke. N Engl J Med 1991; 325:1261–1266.
66. Dyken ML, Barnett HJM, Easton D, et al: Low-dose aspirin and stroke: "it ain't necessarily so." Stroke 1992; 23:1395–1399.
67. Sivenius J, Laakso M, Pettila I, et al: The European Stroke Prevention Study: results according to sex. Neurology 1991; 41:1189–1192.
68. Hess H, Mietaschk A, Deichsel G: Drug-induced inhibition of platelet function delays progression of peripheral occlusive arterial disease: a prospective double-blind angiographically controlled trial. Lancet 1985; 1:415–419.
69. Clagett GP, Graor RA, Salzman EW: Antithrombotic therapy in peripheral arterial occlusive disease. Chest 1992; 102(suppl):516S–528S.
70. Roux S, Christeller S, Ludin E: Effects of aspirin on coronary reocclusion and recurrent ischemia after thrombolysis: a meta-analysis. J Am Coll Cardiol 1992; 19:678–680.
71. Harter HR, Burch JW, Majerus PW, et al: Prevention of thrombosis in patients on hemodialysis by low-dose aspirin. N Engl J Med 1979; 301:577–579.
72. Branch DW, Scott JR, Kochenous NK, et al: Obstetric complications associated with the lupus anticoagulant. N Engl J Med 1985; 313:1322–1326.
73. Uzan S, Beavfils M, Breart G, et al: Prevention of fetal growth retardation with low-dose aspirin: findings of the EPREDA trial. Lancet 1991; 337:1427–1431.
74. Imperiale TF, Stollenwerk-Petrulis A: A meta-analysis of low-dose

aspirin for the prevention of pregnancy-induced hypertensive disease. JAMA 1991; 266:260–264.
75. Bloomfield P, Wheatley DJ, Prescott RJ, Miller HC: Twelve-year comparison of a Bjork-Shiley mechanical heart valve with porcine bioprostheses. N Engl J Med 1991; 324:573–579.
76. Dale J, Myhre E, Storstein O, et al: Prevention of arterial thromboembolism with acetylsalicylic acid: a controlled clinical study in patients with aortic ball valves. Am Heart J 1977; 94:101–111.
77. Altman R, Boullon F, Rouvier J, et al: Aspirin and prophylaxis of thromboembolic complications in patients with substitute heart valves. J Thorac Cardiovasc Surg 1976; 72:127–129.
78. Turpie AGG, Gent M, Laupacis A, et al: A comparison of aspirin with placebo in patients treated with warfarin after heart-valve replacement. N Engl J Med 1993; 329:524–529.
79. SPAF-II Investigators: Warfarin versus aspirin for prevention of thromboembolism in atrial fibrillation: Stroke Prevention in Atrial Fibrillation II Study. Lancet 1994; 343:687–691.
80. White HD: Aspirin or warfarin for non-rheumatic atrial fibrillation? Lancet 1994; 343:683–684.
81. Folts JD, Loscalzo J, Muller JE, et al: Shortcomings of aspirin as an antithrombotic agent. Submitted.
82. Tofler GH, Brezinski D, Schafer AI, et al: Concurrent morning increase in platelet aggregability and the risk of myocardial infarction and sudden cardiac death. N Engl J Med 1987; 316:1514–1518.
83. Folts JD, Rowe GG: Epinephrine potentiation of in vivo stimuli reverses aspirin inhibition of platelet thrombus formation in stenosed canine coronary arteries. Thromb Res 1988; 50:507–516.
84. Moake JL, Turner NA, Stathopoulos NA, et al: Shear-induced platelet aggregation can be mediated by vWF released from platelets, as well as by endogenous large or unusually large vWF multimers, requires adenosine diphosphate and is resistant to aspirin. Blood 1988; 71:1366–1374.
85. Nicosia S, Patrono C: Eicosanoid biosynthesis and action: novel opportunities for pharmacological intervention. FASEB J 1989; 3:1941–1948.
86. Maclouf J, Murphy RC, Henson PM: Transcellular biosynthesis of sulfidopeptide leukotrienes during receptor-mediated stimulation of human neutrophil/platelet mixtures. Blood 1990; 76:1838–1844.
87. Marcus AJ: Thrombosis and inflammation as multicellular processes: significance of cell-cell interactions. Semin Hematol 1994; 31:261–269.
88. Antiplatelet Trialists' Collaboration: Secondary prevention of vascular disease by prolonged antiplatelet treatment. Br Med J 1988; 296:320–331.
89. Grossman MI, Matsumoto KK, Lichter RJ: Fecal blood loss produced by oral and intravenous administration of various salicylates. Gastroenterology 1961; 40:383–388.
90. Green D, Davies RO, Holmes GI, et al: Effects of diflunisal on platelet function and fecal blood loss. Clin Pharmacol Ther 1981; 30:378–384.
91. Prichard PJ, Kitchingman GK, Walt RP, et al: Human gastric mucosal bleeding induced by low dose aspirin but not warfarin. BMJ 1989; 298:493–496.
92. Naschitz JE, Yeshurun D, Odeh M, et al: Overt gastrointestinal bleeding in the course of chronic low-dose aspirin administration for secondary prevention of arterial occlusive disease. Am J Gastroenterol 1990; 85:408–411.
93. The SALT Collaborative Group: Swedish aspirin low-dose trial (SALT) of 75 mg aspirin as secondary prophylaxis after cerebrovascular ischaemic events. Lancet 1991; 338:1345–1349.
94. Silagy CA, McNeil JJ, Donnan GA, et al: Adverse effects of low-dose aspirin in a healthy elderly population. Clin Pharmacol Ther 1993; 54:84–89.
95. Reymond MA, Marbet G, Radu EW, Gratzl O: Aspirin as a risk factor for hemorrhage in patients with head injuries. Neurosurg Rev 1992; 15:21–25.
96. Bleyer WA, Breckenridge RT: Studies on the detection of adverse drug reactions in the newborn. II. The effects of prenatal aspirin on newborn hemostasis. JAMA 1970; 213:2049–2053.
97. Rumack CM, Guggenheim MA, Rumack BH, et al: Neonatal intracranial hemorrhage and maternal use of aspirin. Obstet Gynecol 1981; 58(suppl 5):52S–56S.
98. Stuart MJ, Gross SJ, Elrad H, Graeber JE: Effects of acetylsalicylic-acid ingestion on maternal and neonatal hemostasis. N Engl J Med 1982; 307:909–912.
99. Schafer AI: Effects of nonsteroidal anti-inflammatory drugs on platelet function and systemic hemostasis. J Clin Pharmacol, in press.
100. Amrein PC, Ellman L, Harris WH: Aspirin-induced prolongation of bleeding time and perioperative blood loss. JAMA 1981; 245:1825–1828.
101. Flordal PA, Sahlin S: Use of desmopressin to prevent bleeding complications in patients treated with aspirin. Br J Surg 1993; 80:723–724.
102. Ferraris VA, Swanson E: Aspirin usage and perioperative blood loss in patients undergoing unexpected operations. Surg Gynecol Obstet 1983; 156:439–442.
103. Michelson EL, Morganroth J, Torosian M, et al: Relation of preoperative use of aspirin to increased mediastinal blood loss after coronary artery bypass graft surgery. J Thorac Cardiovasc Surg 1978; 76:694–697.
104. Torosian M, Michelson EL, Morganroth J, et al: Aspirin- and coumadin-related bleeding after coronary-artery bypass graft surgery. Ann Intern Med 1978; 89:325–328.
105. Ferraris VA, Ferraris SP, Lough FC, et al: Preoperative aspirin ingestion increases operative blood loss after coronary artery bypass grafting. Ann Thorac Surg 1988; 45:71–74.
106. Goldman S, Copeland J, Moritz T, et al: Improvement in early saphenous vein graft patency after coronary artery bypass surgery with antiplatelet therapy: results of a Veterans Administration Cooperative Study. Circulation 1988; 77:1324–1332.
107. Bashein G, Nessly ML, Rice AL, et al: Preoperative aspirin therapy and reoperation for bleeding after coronary artery bypass surgery. Arch Intern Med 1991; 151:89–93.
108. Sethi GK, Copeland JG, Goldman S, et al: Implications of preoperative administration of aspirin in patients undergoing coronary artery bypass grafting. Department of Veterans Affairs Cooperative Study on Antiplatelet Therapy. J Am Coll Cardiol 1990; 15:15–20.
109. Karwande SV, Weksler BB, Gay WA Jr, et al: Effect of preoperative antiplatelet drugs on vascular prostacyclin synthesis. Ann Thorac Surg 1987; 43:318–322.
110. Giordano GF, Giordano GF Jr, Rivers SL, et al: Determinants of homologous blood usage utilizing autologous platelet-rich plasma in cardiac operations. Ann Thorac Surg 1989; 47:897–902.
111. Rawitscher RE, Jones JW, McCoy TA, et al: A prospective study of aspirin's effect on red blood cell loss in cardiac surgery. J Cardiovasc Surg 1991; 32:1–7.
112. Gabriel SE, Jaakkimainen L, Bombardier C: Risk of serious gastrointestinal complications related to use of nonsteroidal anti-inflammatory drugs: a meta-analysis. Ann Intern Med 1991; 115:787–796.
113. Bertele V, Stemerman M, Schafer A, et al: Refractoriness of platelets to prostaglandins after prolonged infusion in rabbits. J Lab Clin Med 1985; 106:551–561.
114. MacDermot J: Desensitization of prostacyclin responsiveness in platelets. Biochem Pharmacol 1986; 35:2645–2649.
115. Lewis PJ, Dollery CT: Clinical pharmacology and potential of prostacyclin. Br Med Bull 1983; 39:281–284.
116. Bergmann G, Daly K, Atkinson L, et al: Prostacyclin: haemodynamic and metabolic effects in patients with coronary artery disease. Lancet 1981; 1:569–572.
117. Henriksson P, Edhag O, Wennmalm A: Prostacyclin infusion in patients with acute myocardial infarction. Br Heart J 1985; 53:173–179.
118. Szczeklik A, Skawinski A, Gluszko P: Successful therapy of advanced arteriosclerosis obliterans with prostacyclin. Lancet 1979; 1:1111–1114.
119. Belch JJF, McKay A, McArdle B, et al: Epoprostenol (prostacyclin) and severe arterial disease. Lancet 1983; 1:315–317.
120. FitzGerald GA, Maas RL, Stein R, et al: Intravenous prostacyclin in thrombotic thrombocytopenic purpura. Ann Intern Med 1981; 95:319–322.
121. Fisher CA, Kappa JR, Sinha AK, et al: Comparison of equimolar concentrations of iloprost, prostacyclin, and prostaglandin E_1 on human platelet function. J Lab Clin Med 1987; 109:184–190.
122. Schror K, Darius H, Matzky R, et al: The antiplatelet and cardiovascular actions of a new carbacyclin derivative (ZK 36 374)—equipotent to PGI_2 in vitro. Naunyn Schmiedebergs Arch Pharmacol 1981; 316:252–255.
123. Fiessinger JN, Schafer M: Trial of iloprost versus aspirin treatment for critical limb ischemia of thromboangiitis obliterans. Lancet 1990; 1:555–557.
124. Kovacs IB, Mayo SC, Kirby JD: Infusion of a stable prostacyclin analogue, iloprost, to patients with peripheral vascular disease: lack of antiplatelet effect but risk of thromboembolism. Am J Med 1991; 90:41–46.
125. Whittle BJR, Moncada S: Platelet actions of stable carbocyclic analogues of prostacyclin. Circulation 1985; 72:1219–1225.

126. Schafer AI, Alexander RW, Handin RI: Inhibition of platelet function by organic nitrate vasodilators. Blood 1980; 55:649–654.
127. Stamler J, Loscalzo J: The antiplatelet effects of organic nitrates and nitroso-derivatives and their importance in cardiovascular disorders. J Am Coll Cardiol 1991; 18:1529–1536.
128. Groves PH, Lewis MJ, Cheadle HA, et al: SIN-1 reduces platelet adhesion and platelet thrombus formation in a porcine model of balloon angioplasty. Circulation 1993; 87:590–597.
129. Ferguson JJ: Meeting highlights: nitric oxide donors. Circulation 1994; 90:4.
130. Masotti G, Poggesi L, Galanti G, et al: Stimulation of prostacyclin by dipyridamole. Lancet 1979; 1:1412.
131. Boeynaems JM, Van Coevorden A, Demolle D: Dipyridamole and vascular prostacyclin production. Biochem Pharmacol 1986; 35:2897–2902.
132. Moncada S, Korbut R: Dipyridamole and other phosphodiesterase inhibitors act as anti-thrombotic agents by potentiating endogenous prostacyclin. Lancet 1978; 1:1286–1289.
133. Best LC, McGuire MB, Jones PB, et al: Mode of action of dipyridamole on human platelets. Thromb Res 1979; 16:367–379.
134. Tsien W-H, Sheppard H: The lack of correlation between inhibition of platelet aggregation and cAMP levels. Fed Proc 1981; 40:809.
135. Lam SC-T, Guccione MA, Packham MA, et al: Effect of cAMP phosphodiesterase inhibitors on ADP-induced shape change, cAMP and nucleoside diphosphokinase activity of rabbit platelets. Thromb Haemost 1982; 47:90–95.
136. FitzGerald GA: Dipyridamole. N Engl J Med 1987; 316:1247–1257.
137. Gresele P, Arnout J, Deckmyn H, et al: Mechanism of the antiplatelet action of dipyridamole in whole blood: modulation of adenosine concentration and activity. Thromb Haemost 1986; 55:12–18.
138. Dale J, Myhre E, Rostwelt K: Effects of dipyridamole and acetylsalicylic acid on platelet functions in patients with aortic ball-valve prosthesis. Am Heart J 1975; 89:613–618.
139. Sullivan JM, Kagnoff MF, Gorlin R: Reduction of platelet-adhesiveness in patients with coronary artery disease. Am J Med Sci 1968; 255:292–285.
140. Rajah SM, Crow MJ, Penny AF, et al: The effects of dipyridamole on platelet function: correlation with blood levels in man. Br J Clin Pharmacol 1979; 4:129–133.
141. Weiss HJ, Turrito VT, Vicic WJ, et al: Effect of aspirin and dipyridamole on the interaction of human platelets with subendothelium: studies using citrated and native blood. Thromb Haemost 1981; 45:136–141.
142. Graves HM, Kinlough-Rathbone RL, Cazenave JB, et al: Effect of dipyridamole and prostacyclin on rabbit platelet adherence in vitro and in vivo. J Lab Clin Med 1982; 99:548–558.
143. Weiss HJ: Platelets. *In* Pathophysiology and Antiplatelet Drug Therapy. New York: Alan R Liss, 1982.
144. Ritchie JL, Harker LA: Platelet and fibrinogen survival in coronary atherosclerosis: response to medical and surgical therapy. Am J Cardiol 1977; 39:595–598.
145. Bousser MG, Eschwege E, Haguenau M: "AICLA" controlled trial of aspirin and dipyridamole in the secondary prevention of athero-thrombotic cerebral ischemia. Stroke 1983; 14:5–14.
146. Sullivan JM, Harken DE, Gorlin R: Pharmacologic control of thromboembolic complications of cardiac-valve replacement. N Engl J Med 1971; 284:1391–1394.
147. Chesebro JH, Fuster V, Elveback LR, et al: Trial of combined warfarin plus dipyridamole or aspirin therapy in prosthetic heart valve replacement: danger of aspirin compared with dipyridamole. Am J Cardiol 1983; 1:1537–1541.
148. Stein PD, Kantrowitz A: Antithrombotic therapy in mechanical and biological prosthetic heart valves and saphenous vein bypass grafts. Chest 1989; 95(suppl):107S–117S.
149. Webster MWI, Chesebro JH, Fuster V: Platelet inhibitor therapy. Agents and clinical implications. Hematol Oncol Clin North Am 1990; 4:265–289.
150. Chesebro JH, Fuster V, McGoon DC, et al: Trial of combined warfarin plus dipyridamole or aspirin therapy in prosthetic heart valve replacement: danger of aspirin compared with dipyridamole. Am J Cardiol 1983; 51:1537–1541.
151. Alevriadou BR, Moake JL, Turner NA, et al: Real-time analysis of shear-dependent thrombus formation and its blockade by inhibitors of von Willebrand factor binding to platelets. Blood 1993; 81:1263–1276.
152. Ikeda Y, Handa M, Kawano K, et al: The role of von Willebrand factor and fibrinogen in platelet aggregation under varying shear stress. J Clin Invest 1991; 87:1234–1240.
153. Fuster V, Badimon L, Badimon JJ, et al: The porcine model for the understanding of thrombogenesis and atherogenesis. Mayo Clin Proc 1991; 66:818–831.
154. Coller BS: Antiplatelet agents in the prevention and therapy of thrombosis. Annu Rev Med 1992; 43:171–180.
155. Harker LA: Platelets and vascular thrombosis. N Engl J Med 1994; 330:1006–1007.
156. Chesebro JH, Fuster V: Dynamic thrombosis and thrombolysis: role of antithrombins. Circulation 1991; 83:1815–1817.
157. Lumsden AB, Kelly AB, Schneider PA, et al: Lasting safe interruption of endarterectomy thrombosis by transiently infused antithrombin peptide D-Phe-Pro-ArgCH_2Cl in baboons. Blood 1993; 81:1762–1770.
158. Bang HO, Dyerberg J: The bleeding tendency in Greenland Eskimos. Dan Med Bull 1980; 27:202–205.
159. Weiner BH, Ockene IS, Levine PH, et al: Inhibition of atherosclerosis by cod-liver oil in a hyperlipidemic swine model. N Engl J Med 1986; 315:841–846.
160. Kromhout D, Bosscheiter EB, de Lezenne Coulander C: The inverse relation between fish consumption and 20-year mortality from coronary heart disease. N Engl J Med 1985; 312:1205–1209.
161. Shekelle RB, Missell L, Paul O, et al: Fish consumption and mortality from coronary heart disease [Letter]. N Engl J Med 1985; 313:820.
162. Franklin SM, Faxon DP: Pharmacologic prevention of restenosis after coronary angioplasty: review of the randomized clinical trials. Coronary Artery Disease 1993; 4:232–242.
163. Leaf A, Weber PC: Cardiovascular effects of n-3 fatty acids. N Engl J Med 1988; 318:549–557.
164. Fish oil for the heart. Med Lett 1987; 29:7–9.
165. Kantha SS: Dietary effects of fish oils on human health: a review of recent studies. Yale J Biol Med 1987; 60:37–44.
166. Israel DH, Gorlin R: Fish oils in the prevention of atherosclerosis. J Am Coll Cardiol 1992; 19:174–185.
167. Harris WS, Connor WE, McMurry MP: The comparative reductions of the plasma lipids and lipoproteins by dietary polyunsaturated fats: salmon oil vs. vegetable oils. Metabolism 1983; 32:179–184.
168. Phillipson BE, Rothrock DW, Connor WE, et al: Reduction of plasma lipids, lipoproteins, and apoproteins by dietary fish oil in patients with hypertriglyceridemia. N Engl J Med 1985; 312:1210–1216.
169. Sullivan DR, Sanders TA, Trayner IM, et al: Paradoxical elevation of LDL apoprotein B levels in hypertriglyceridaemic patients and normal subjects ingesting fish oil. Atherosclerosis 1986; 61:129–134.
170. Spector AA, Yorek MA: Membrane lipid composition and cellular function. J Lipid Res 1985; 26:1015–1035.
171. Lee TH, Hoover RL, Williams JD, et al: Effects of dietary enrichment with eicosapentaenoic and docosahexaenoic acids on in vitro neutrophil and monocyte leukotriene generation and neutrophil function. N Engl J Med 1985; 312:1217–1224.
172. Knapp HR, Reilly IA, Alessandrini P, et al: In vivo indexes of platelet and vascular function during fish-oil administration in patients with atherosclerosis. N Engl J Med 1986; 314:937–942.
173. O'Connor GT, Malenka DJ, Olmstead EM, et al: A meta-analysis of randomized trials of fish oil in prevention of restenosis following coronary angioplasty. Am J Prev Med 1992; 8:186–192.
174. Gapinski JP, VanRuiswyk JV, Heudebert GR, et al: Preventing restenosis with fish oils following coronary angioplasty: a meta-analysis. Arch Intern Med 1993; 153:1595–1601.
175. Leaf A, Jorgensen MB, Jacobs AK, et al: Do fish oils prevent restenosis after coronary angioplasty? Circulation 1994; 90:2248–2257.
176. Simon LS, Mills JA: Nonsteroidal anti-inflammatory drugs. N Engl J Med 1980; 302:1179–1185.
177. Patrono C, et al: Clinical pharmacology of platelet cyclooxygenase inhibition. Circulation 1985; 72:1177–1184.
178. Margulies EH, White AM, Sherry S: Sulfinpyrazone: a review of its pharmacological properties and therapeutic use. Drugs 1980; 20:179–197.
179. Kirstein Pederson A, Jackobsen P: Sulphinpyrazone metabolism during long-term therapy. Br J Clin Pharmacol 1981; 11:597.
180. Wallis RB: Mechanisms of actions of sulfinpyrazone. Thromb Res 1983; S-IV:31.
181. Ali M, McDonald JWD: Effects of sulphinpyrazone on platelet prostaglandin synthesis and platelet release of serotonin. J Lab Clin Med 1977; 89:868–875.
182. Steele P, Carroll J, Overfield D, et al: Effect of sulfinpyrazone on platelet survival time in patients with transient cerebral ischemic attacks. Stroke 1977; 8:396–398.

183. Baumgartner HR: Effects of acetylsalicylic acid, sulfinpyrazone and dipyridamole on platelet adhesion and aggregation in flowing native and anticoagulated blood. Haemostasis 1979; 8:340–352.
184. Essien EM, Mustard JF: Inhibition of platelet adhesion to rabbit aorta by sulphinpyrazone and acetylsalicylic acid. Atherosclerosis 1977; 27:89–95.
185. The Anturane Reinfarction Trial Policy Committee: The Anturane Reinfarction Trial: reevaluation of outcome. N Engl J Med 1982; 306:1005–1008.
186. Sulphinpyrazone in post-myocardial infarction: report from the Anturane Reinfarction Italian Study. Lancet 1982; 1:237–242.
187. Kaegi A, Pineo GF, Shimizu A, et al: Arteriovenous shunt thrombosis. Prevention by sulfinpyrazone. N Engl J Med 1974; 290:304–306.
188. Deckmyn H, VanHoutte E, Verstraete M, et al: Manipulation of the local thromboxane and prostacyclin balance in vivo by the antithrombotic compounds dazoxiben, acetylsalicylic acid and nafazatrom. Biochem Pharmacol 1983; 32:2757–2762.
189. FitzGerald GA, Oates JA: Selective and nonselective inhibition of thromboxane formation. Clin Pharmacol Ther 1984; 35:633–640.
190. Smith JB: Pharmacology thromboxane synthetase inhibitors. Fed Proc 1987; 46:139–143.
191. Vermylen J, Defreyn G, Carreras LO, et al: Thromboxane synthetase inhibition as antithrombotic strategy. Lancet 1981; 1:1073–1075.
192. Bertele V, Cerletti C, Schieppati A, et al: Inhibition of thromboxane synthetase does not necessarily prevent platelet aggregation. Lancet 1981; 1:1057–1058.
193. Gresele P, Deckmyn H, Huybrechts, E, et al: Serum albumin enhances the impairment of platelet aggregation with thromboxane synthase inhibition by increasing the formation of prostaglandin D_2. Biochem Pharmacol 1984; 33:2083–2088.
194. FitzGerald GA, Reilly IAG, Pedersen AK: The biochemical pharmacology of thromboxane synthase inhibition in man. Circulation 1985; 72:1194–1201.
195. Belch JJF, Cormie J, Newman P, et al: Dazoxiben, a thromboxane synthetase inhibitor, in the treatment of Raynaud's syndrome: a double blind trial. Br J Clin Pharmacol 1983; 15:113S–116S.
196. Luderer JR, Nichols GG, Neumyer MM, et al: Dazoxiben, a thromboxane synthetase inhibitor in Raynaud's phenomenon. Clin Pharmacol Ther 1984; 36:105–115.
197. Ettinger WH, Wise RA, Schaffhauser D, et al: Controlled double-blind trial of dazoxiben and nifedipine in the treatment of Raynaud's phenomenon. Am J Med 1984; 77:451–456.
198. Zipser RD, Kronborg I, Rector W, et al: Therapeutic trial of thromboxane synthesis inhibition in the hepatorenal syndrome. Gastroenterology 1984; 87:1228–1232.
199. McGibney D, et al: Effects of UK 37,248, a thromboxane synthetase inhibitor, on platelet behavior in patients with coronary heart disease undergoing exercise to angina. Clin Sci 1983; 12:138.
200. Reuben SR, Kuan P, Cairns J, et al: Effects of dazoxiben and exercise performance in chronic stable angina. Br J Clin Pharmacol 1983; 15:83S–86S.
201. Kiff PS, Bergman G, Atkinson L, et al: Hemodynamic and metabolic effects of dazoxiben at rest and during atrial pacing. Br J Clin Pharmacol 1983; 15:73S–77S.
202. Thaulow E, Dale J, Myhre E: Effects of a selective thromboxane synthetase inhibitor, dazoxiben, and acetyl salicylic acid on myocardial ischemia in patients with coronary heart disease. Am J Cardiol 1984; 53:1255–1258.
203. Lefer AM, Darius H: A pharmacological approach to thromboxane receptor antagonism. Fed Proc 1987; 46:144–148.
204. Ritter JM, Dollery CT: Therapeutic opportunities in vasoocclusive disease. Circulation 1986; 73:240–243.
205. Hoet B, Falcon C, De Reys S, et al: R68070, a combined thromboxane/endoperoxide receptor antagonist and thromboxane synthase inhibitor, inhibits human platelet activation in vitro and in vivo: a comparison with aspirin. Blood 1990; 75:646–653.
206. The RAPT Investigators: Randomized trial of ridogrel, a combined thromboxane A_2 synthase inhibitor and thromboxane A_2/prostaglandin endoperoxide receptor antagonist, versus aspirin as adjunct to thrombolysis in patients with acute myocardial infarction. Circulation 1994; 89:588–595.
207. Hass WK, Easton JD (eds): Ticlopidine, Platelets, and Vascular Disease. New York: Springer-Verlag, 1993.
208. Defreyn G, Gachet C, Savi P, et al: Ticlopidine and clopidogrel (SR 25990C) selectively neutralize ADP inhibition of PGE_1-activated platelet adenylate cyclase in rats and rabbits. Thromb Haemost 1991; 65:186–190.
209. Mills DCB, Puri R, Hu C-J, et al: Clopidogrel inhibits the binding of ADP analogues to the receptor mediating inhibition of platelet adenylate cyclase. Arterioscler Thromb 1992; 12:430–436.
210. Sattiel E, Ward A: Ticlopidine: a review of its pharmacodynamic and pharmacokinetic properties, and therapeutic efficacy in platelet-dependent disease states. Drugs 1987; 34:222–262.
211. Murray JC, Kelly MA, Gorelick PB: Ticlopidine: a new antiplatelet agent for the secondary prevention of stroke. Clin Neuropharmacol 1994; 17:23–31.
212. Di Minno G, Cerbone AM, Mattioli PL: Functionally thrombasthenic state in normal platelets following the administration of ticlopidine. J Clin Invest 1985; 75:328–338.
213. Cattaneo M, Lombardi R, Bettega D, et al: Shear-induced platelet aggregation is potentiated by desmopressin and inhibited by ticlopidine. Arterioscler Thromb 1993; 13:393–397.
214. Defreyn G, Bernat A, Delebassee D, et al: Pharmacology of ticlopidine: a review. Semin Thromb Hemost 1989; 15:159–166.
215. Hass WK, Easton JD, Adams HP Jr, et al: Ticlopidine Aspirin Stroke Study group—a randomized trial comparing ticlopidine hydrochloride with aspirin for the prevention of stroke in high-risk patients. N Engl J Med 1989; 321:501–507.
216. Bellavance A, for the Ticlopidine Aspirin Stroke Study Group: Efficacy of ticlopidine and aspirin for prevention of reversible cerebrovascular ischemic events. Stroke 1993; 24:1452–1457.
217. Rothrock JF, Hart RG: Ticlopidine hydrochloride use and threatened stroke. West J Med 1994; 160:43–47.
218. Gent M, Blakeley JA, Easton JD, and the CATS Group: The Canadian-American Ticlopidine Study (CATS) in thromboembolic stroke. Lancet 1989; 1:1215–1220.
219. Limet R, David JL, Magotteaux P, et al: Prevention of aortocoronary bypass graft occlusion—beneficial effect of ticlopidine on early and late patency rates of venous coronary bypass grafts: a double-blind study. J Thorac Cardiovasc Surg 1987; 94:773–783.
220. Balsano F, Rizzon P, Violi F, et al, and the STA I Group: Antiplatelet treatment with ticlopidine in unstable angina, a controlled multicenter trial. Circulation 1990; 82:17–24.
221. Balsano F, Coccheri S, Libretti A, et al: Ticlopidine in the treatment of intermittent claudication: a 21-month double-blind trial. J Lab Clin Med 1989; 114:84–91.
222. TIMAD Study Group: Ticlopidine treatment reduces the progression non-proliferative diabetic retinopathy. Arch Ophthalmol 1990; 108:1577–1583.
223. Phillips DR, Charo IF, Scarborough RM: GP IIb-IIIa: the responsive integrin. Cell 1991; 65:359–362.
224. Coller BS: A new murine monoclonal antibody reports an activation-dependent change in the conformation and/or microenvironment of the platelet glycoprotein IIb/IIIa complex. J Clin Invest 1985; 76:101–108.
225. Coller BS, Scudder LE, Beer J, et al: Monoclonal antibodies to platelet GP IIb/IIIa as antithrombotic agents. Ann N Y Acad Sci 1991; 614:193–213.
226. The EPIC Investigators: Use of a monoclonal antibody directed against the platelet glycoprotein IIb/IIIa receptor in high-risk coronary angioplasty. N Engl J Med 1994; 330:956–961.
227. Simoons ML, de Boer MJ, van den Brand MJBM, et al, and the European Cooperative Study Group: Randomized trial of a GP IIb/IIIa platelet receptor blocker in refractory unstable angina. Circulation 1994; 89:596–603.
228. Kleiman NS, Ohman ME, Califf RM, et al: Profound inhibition of platelet aggregation with monoclonal antibody 7E3 Fab following thrombolytic therapy: results of the TAMI 8 pilot study. J Am Coll Cardiol 1993, 22:381–389.
229. Huang TF, Holt JC, Lukasiewicz H, et al: Trigramin: a low molecular weight peptide inhibiting fibrinogen interaction with platelet receptors expressed on glycoprotein IIb/IIIa complex. J Biol Chem 1987; 262:16157–16163.
230. Gan ZR, Gould RJ, Jacobs JW, et al: Echistatin: a potent platelet aggregation inhibitor from the venom of the viper *Echis carinatus*. J Biol Chem 1988; 262:19827–19832.
231. Gould RJ, Polokoff MA, Friedman PA, et al: Disintegrins: a family of integrin inhibitory proteins from viper venoms. Proc Soc Exp Biol Med 1990; 195:168–171.
232. Mazur P, Henzel WJ, Seymour JL, Lazarus RA: Ornatins: potent

glycoprotein IIb/IIIa antagonists and platelet aggregation inhibitors from the leech *Placobdella ornata.* Eur J Biochem 1991; 202:1073–1082.
233. Krezel AM, Wagner G, Weymour-Ulmer J, et al: Structure of the RGD protein decorsin: conserved motif and distinct function in leech proteins that affect blood clotting. Science 1994; 264:1944–1947.
234. Ruggeri ZM, Houghton RA, Russel SR, et al: Inhibition of platelet function with synthetic peptide designed to be high affinity antagonists of fibrinogen binding to platelets. Proc Natl Acad Sci U S A 1986; 83:5708–5712.
235. Nicholson NS, Panzer-Knodle SG, Salyers AK, et al: In vitro and in vivo effects of a peptide mimetic (SC-47643) of RGD as an antiplatelet and antithrombotic agent. Thromb Res 1991; 62:567–578.
236. Nichols AJ, Ruffolo RR, Huffman WF, et al: Development of GP IIb/IIIa antagonists as antithrombotic drugs. Trends Pharmacol Sci 1992; 13:413–417.
237. Hartman GD, Egbertson MS, Halczenko W, et al: Non-peptide fibrinogen receptor antagonists: I. Discovery and design of exosite inhibitors. J Med Chem 1992; 36:4640–4642.
238. Roux SP, Tschopp TB, Kuhn H, et al: Effects of heparin, aspirin, and a synthetic platelet glycoprotein IIb-IIIa receptor antagonist (Ro 43-5054) on coronary artery reperfusion and reocclusion after thrombolysis with tissue-type plasminogen activator in the dog. J Pharmacol Exp Ther 1992; 264:501–508.
239. Kouns WC, Kirchofer D, Hadvary P, et al: Reversible conformational changes in glycoprotein IIb-IIIa by a potent and selective peptidomimetic inhibitor. Blood 1991; 80:2539–2547.
240. Peerlinck K, De Lepeleire I, Goldberg M, et al: MK-383 (L-700, 462), a selective nonpeptide platelet glycoprotein IIb/IIIa antagonist, is active in man. Circulation 1993; 88:1512–1517.
241. Mousa SA, Bozarth JM, Forsythe MS, et al: Antiplatelet and antithrombotic efficacy of DMP 728, a novel platelet GP IIb/IIIa receptor antagonist. Circulation 1994; 89:3–12.
242. Nicolini FA, Lee P, Rios G, et al: Combination of platelet fibrinogen receptor antagonist and direct thrombin inhibitor at low doses markedly improves thrombolysis. Circulation 1994; 89:1802–1809.
243. Karczewski J, Endris R, Connolly TM: Disagregin is a fibrinogen receptor antagonist lacking the Arg-Gly-Asp sequence from the tick *Ornithodoros moubata.* J Biol Chem 1994; 269:6702–6708.
244. Mousa SA, De Grado WF, Reilly TM: Platelet GP IIb/IIIa antagonists: how safe is this antithrombotic approach? [Letter]. Am J Med 1994; 96:300.

28 Anticoagulation in Venous Thromboembolism

Clive Kearon, MB, FRCP(C), PhD
Jack Hirsh, MD, FRCP(C)

The long-established practice of anticoagulation with heparin followed by vitamin K antagonists remains the mainstay of treatment for deep venous thrombosis (DVT) and pulmonary embolism. However, prospective studies continue to refine the optimal doses, durations, and routes of administration of these familiar agents. In addition, the 1980s spanned the development of low-molecular-weight heparins (LMWH), which may improve on the efficacy and safety of standard (unfractionated) heparin for both the prevention and treatment of venous thromboembolism (VTE). Although still at the investigational stage of development, hirudin and related compounds that directly inhibit thrombin may lead to further improvements in the treatment of arterial and venous thrombosis.

In this chapter, advances in the use of warfarin and standard heparin are reviewed, the interrelationship between structure and function of heparin molecule which have spurred the development of LMWHs is outlined, the clinical applications of these new agents are reviewed, and the pharmacology and potential clinical role of the direct thrombin inhibitors in patients with VTE is considered. Although this chapter concentrates on the therapeutic use of anticoagulants, the key to successful management of venous thromboembolic disease also lies with use of primary prophylaxis in high-risk patients and with appropriate use of objective tests to confirm or rule out VTE when this diagnosis is considered.

In contrast to the arterial circulation, in which high flow rates and vessel wall abnormalities are the dominant pathogenic mechanisms for thrombosis, blood stasis is pivotal in the development of venous thrombosis.[1, 2] Venous thrombi, which are rich in red blood cells and fibrin content, generally start in the valve cusps of the deep veins of the calf and may extend to involve the larger proximal veins (popliteal or more proximal), in which they are much more likely to be associated with clinically important pulmonary embolism. It is now recognized that pulmonary embolism and DVT are not distinct entities; rather, they represent different manifestations and stages of the same process.[1, 3] Seventy percent of patients with pulmonary embolism have been found at venography to have DVT, even though leg symptoms are present in no more than 25% of these patients. Conversely, the majority of patients with proximal DVT and without respiratory symptoms have perfusion scan defects compatible with asymptomatic pulmonary embolism, and in 40% of patients the lung scans conform to a "high probability" pattern. In recognition of the inseparable relationship between pulmonary embolism and DVT, the term *venous thromboembolism* has been adopted to refer to these conditions, either singly or in combination. Consequently, prevention of pulmonary embolism is achieved primarily by preventing or treating DVT in the legs.

Improved understanding of the natural history of VTE in individual patients has important implications for patient management. The presence of risk factors necessitates primary prophylaxis and provides circumstantial evidence supporting a diagnosis of pulmonary embolism or DVT in patients with nonspecific clinical manifestations. Anticoagulation and definitive diagnostic testing (venography) can be withheld in patients with suspected DVT who do not exhibit proximal DVT on noninvasive testing (e.g., impedance plethysmography, venous ultrasonography), provided that serial testing remains normal over 7–10 days, because symptomatic isolated calf DVT is uncommon (occurring in approximately 15% of patients with symptomatic DVT) and rarely leads to clinically important pulmonary embolism in the absence of early extension.[4] Demonstration of DVT in patients with suspected pulmonary embolism who have nondiagnostic lung scans strongly suggests that pulmonary embolism has occurred and establishes the need for anticoagulation. Conversely, there is now evidence that anticoagulation or definitive diagnostic testing (e.g., pulmonary angiography) can be withheld in patients with suspected pulmonary embolism who have nondiagnostic lung scans if results of serial noninvasive testing for DVT remain negative over a 2-week period.[5]

In this chapter, therapeutic issues in VTE are considered, first with a review of the pharmacology of standard heparin, LMWHs, and warfarin (which is relevant to the use of these agents in the management of all thrombotic disorders) and then with specific consideration of their role in the prevention and treatment of venous disease. The discussion is confined to the use of anticoagulants; the role of thrombolytic agents in VTE is addressed in Chapter 30.

HEPARIN

Historical Highlights

The anticoagulant effects of heparin were first identified in 1916 by McLean, a medical student, who incidentally discovered that an extract of liver, "heparphosphatid," was a potent inhibitor of coagulation.[6] By the late 1930s, purified preparation of heparin had been used successfully in the prophylaxis and treatment of various thrombotic disorders. In 1939, Brinkhous and associates demonstrated that heparin required a plasma cofactor, which they termed "heparin cofactor," for its anticoagulant activity.[7] In 1968, Abildgaard isolated a substance from human plasma which had both antithrombin and heparin cofactor activity, which he named antithrombin III (AT-III).[8] Studies by Rosenberg and Lam and by Lindahl's group, in the 1970s, established that binding of heparin to AT-III converts it from a progressive slow inhibitor to a very rapid inhibitor of coagulation.[9, 10]

Structure and Function

Heparin is made up of a heterogeneous group of highly sulfated glycosaminoglycans, which are large linear carbohydrates composed of repeating disaccharide units (D-glycosamine and a uronic acid, either glucuronic or iduronic).[2, 11, 12] The anticoagulant effect of heparin is mediated largely through its ability to bind to AT-III and catalyzes its anticoagulant effect. Binding of heparin to AT-III requires the presence of a specific pentasaccharide sequence containing a particular glucosamine unit that combines with lysine sites on the AT-III molecule, thereby producing a conformational change that exposes an arginine reactive site on the heparin/AT-III complex. This arginine site can then inhibit the active center serine site of thrombin and a number of other coagulation factors.

In addition to thrombin (factor II_a), the heparin/AT-III complex inhibits factors X_a, XII_a, and IX_a. Of these, thrombin and factor X_a are most sensitive to inactivation; on average, inhibition of thrombin is about 10 times greater than the inhibition of factor X_a, but relative sensitivities vary with the length of heparin molecules. The inhibition of thrombin requires that heparin bind to both AT-III and thrombin (ternary complex formation), whereas the inhibition of factor X_a requires that heparin bind to AT-III alone. Heparin molecules with fewer than 18 saccharide residues are unable to bind to thrombin and AT-III simultaneously and thus cannot catalyze the inhibition of thrombin (Fig. 28–1). In contrast, heparin fragments with as few as five saccharide units are able to catalyze the inhibition of factor X_a by AT-III, provided that they contain the high-affinity pentasaccharide sequence. A large part of heparin's inhibitory effect on coagulation appears to be mediated by the inhibition of thrombin-induced activation of factors V and VIII. After the heparin/AT-III complex has produced its anticoagulant effect, heparin can disassociate and activate other AT-III molecules.

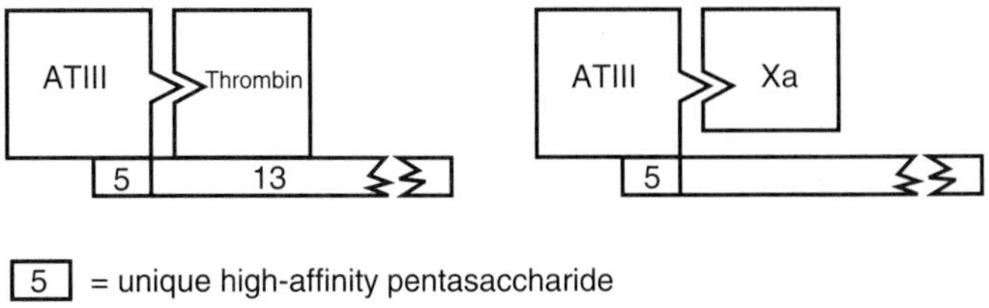

Figure 28–1. Inhibition of thrombin requires simultaneous binding of heparin to antithrombin III (ATIII), through the unique pentasaccharide sequence, and binding to thrombin through a minimum of 13 additional saccharide units. Inhibition of factor Xa (Xa) requires binding of heparin to ATIII through the unique pentasaccharide without the additional requirement for binding to Xa.

At high concentrations, heparin also catalyzes the inhibition of thrombin by a second plasma protease inhibitor, heparin cofactor II, but at the concentrations at which heparin is used clinically, this interaction is thought to be of little importance.

Heparin molecules vary according to (1) size/length, depending on the number of disaccharide residues; (2) constituents, depending on which uronic acid is present; and (3) sulfation and charge, depending on the extent and positioning of sulfate residues. All of these factors contribute to functional heterogeneity among heparin molecules.

Commercially, standard heparin is most commonly obtained from the lungs or intestinal mucosa of cows or pigs, from which it is extracted as either the sodium or the calcium salt, respectively. These heparin preparations are heterogeneous, with molecular weights ranging from 3000 to 30,000 (mean, 15,000). Only one third of standard heparin molecules have the specific pentasaccharide sequence required for binding with AT-III.

In addition to the anticoagulant effects of heparin outlined earlier, heparin has a number of non-anticoagulant actions, which include influences on vessel wall permeability, inhibition of platelet function, and antiproliferative effects on vascular smooth muscle cells with modulation of angiogenesis. These effects are not confined to heparin molecules that contain the active pentasaccharide sequence responsible for binding to AT-III and can account for some of heparin's side effects, particularly bleeding.

Pharmacokinetics and Pharmacodynamics

Heparin is not absorbed orally and therefore must be given parenterally, by either the intravenous or subcutaneous route. Intramuscular injection is discouraged because it may produce large hematomas. With intravenous administration, continuous infusion is preferred because intermittent intravenous injection is associated with increased bleeding complications.[13] After its passage into the blood stream, heparin binds to a number of plasma proteins, a phenomenon that contributes to its reduced bioavailability at low concentrations, the variability of the anticoagulant response to fixed doses in different patients, and the laboratory phenomenon of heparin resistance.

Heparin is cleared through a combination of a rapid, saturable, and much slower first-order mechanism (Fig. 28–2). The rapid, saturable phase of heparin clearance is thought to result from binding of heparin to endothelial cells and macrophages, where it is internalized and depolymerized. The slower, nonsaturable mechanism of heparin clearance is largely renal. The relative contribution of each of these mechanisms to heparin clearance depends on the dose and size of the heparin fractions administered. Low doses of standard heparin are eliminated predominantly by highly efficient but low-capacity saturable mechanisms. Larger doses of heparin exceed the capacity of the saturable mechanism, resulting in predominantly renal

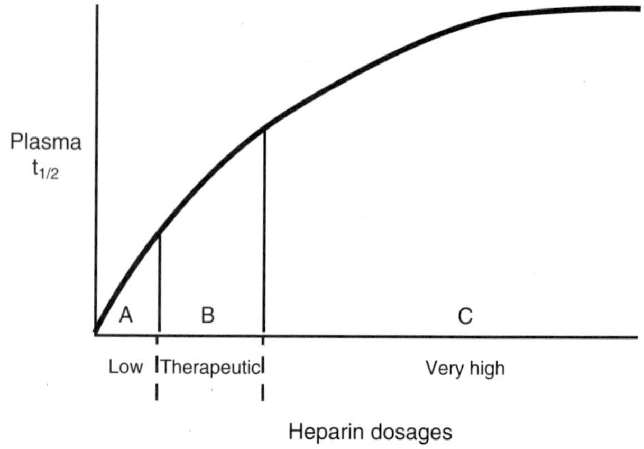

Figure 28–2. Plasma half-life ($t_{1/2}$) of heparin. Low doses of heparin are cleared rapidly through saturable (cellular) mechanism of clearance (A). Therapeutic doses of heparin are cleared by a combination of the rapid saturable mechanism and the slower, nonsaturable, dose-independent mechanism of renal clearance (B). Very high doses of heparin are cleared predominantly through the slower, nonsaturable mechanism of clearance (C).

clearance. Consequently, the apparent half-life of heparin increases from approximately 30 min with an intravenous bolus of 25 units/kg (approximately 2000 units) to 60 min with an intravenous bolus of 100 units/kg (approximately 8000 units) and to 150 min with a bolus of 400 units/kg (approximately 32,000 units). The requirement that heparin-binding proteins are occupied before therapeutic heparin levels are attained, in combination with the differential clearance mechanisms outlined earlier, results in a linear dose-response curve in individual patients. Large increments in heparin dose are required in order to increase heparin effects at lower dosages, but at higher dosages, further small increments in dose achieve large increases in both the intensity and the duration of heparin activity. The form of this dose-response relationship translates into a narrow therapeutic window for heparin administration and calls for close monitoring.

Monitoring Heparin

Heparin dose and effect are quantified in terms of units of anticoagulant activity against specific clotting factors (usually thrombin or factor X_a) or the effect of heparin on more global clotting assays, usually the aPTT. Specific clotting factor assays are performed by adding the clotting factor to the test (heparin-containing) plasma and measuring the residual activity of the factor after a period of incubation. Residual activity can be measured with a clotting assay or a chromogenic assay. The therapeutic range for the anti-X_a assay is 0.3–0.7 units/mL. Alternatively, heparin activity can be measured by determining the amount of protamine, a highly basic, naturally occurring protein that combines with and neutralizes heparin on a one-to-one basis, which must be added to the test plasma to return the thrombin clotting time to normal. The therapeutic range for the protamine titration heparin assay is 0.2–0.4 units/mL.

The anti-X_a and anti-II_a activity of different heparin preparations (standard heparin or LWMH) can be measured through these and other assays. The ratio of anti-X_a:anti-II_a activity has been arbitrarily defined as 1:1 for a reference standard heparin preparation, against which other heparin preparations are compared. Heparin preparations with low mean molecular weight distributions have higher anti-X_a:anti-II_a ratios, because a larger proportion of the molecules that have the AT-III binding pentasaccharide sequence contain less than the minimum 18 saccharide units required for binding and inhibition of thrombin (see Fig. 28–1). Similarly, as the higher molecular weight components of standard heparin are cleared more rapidly, anti-II_a activity decreases faster than anti-X_a activity after a bolus of heparin.

In clinical practice, the anticoagulant effect of heparin is usually monitored by the aPTT, a test that provides a global assessment of the intrinsic coagulation pathway and is sensitive to the inhibitory effects of heparin on thrombin, factor X_a, and factor XI_a. Unfortunately, different commercial aPTT reagents vary considerably in responsiveness to heparin, and consequently the same heparinized patient sample will yield different aPTT values and aPTT ratios (measured by dividing the observed aPTT by the mean of the laboratory control aPTT) with different assays.[14] For many reagents, a therapeutic effect is achieved with aPTT ratios of 1.5–2.5. For more sensitive aPTT reagents, the therapeutic range is higher than those ratios; for insensitive reagents, the therapeutic range is lower. The aPTT reagents can be standardized by calibrating them against heparin levels (e.g., anti-X_a or protamine titration) in a plasma system.

The recommended therapeutic range for the treatment of venous thrombosis was originally based on a study performed in rabbits demonstrating that thrombus extension was prevented by a heparin dose that resulted in a protamine titration heparin level of 0.2–0.4 units/mL, which corresponded to an aPTT ratio of 1.5–2.5.[15] The results of subsequent randomized, controlled trials confirmed that a relationship exists between the clinical effectiveness of heparin and its ex vivo affect on the aPTT.[16–18]

Maintaining the aPTT above 1.5 is associated with protection against thrombosis; unfortunately, bleeding complications may occur within the therapeutic range. The risk of heparin-associated bleeding increases with heparin dose (which in turn is related to the anticoagulant response), concomitant use of thrombolytic therapy, recent surgery, trauma, invasive procedures, generalized hemostatic abnormality, associated comorbid conditions (e.g., peptic ulceration, previous stroke), or poor functional status.[13, 19]

In addition to being influenced by technical or laboratory factors, the anticoagulant response to fixed doses of heparin in individual patients may be influenced by a number of other factors, including the patient's weight, the heparin preparation administered, the presence of comorbid conditions that increase circulating levels of heparin binding proteins or procoagulants, and the route of heparin administration (Table 28–1).

The mean dose of continuously infused heparin required to achieve a therapeutic aPTT in patients with acute VTE is approximately 31,000 units/24 h. However, approximately one third of patients with acute VTE require doses of heparin in excess of 35,000 units/24 h to achieve therapeutic aPTT ratios, and these patients are often

TABLE 28–1. FACTORS THAT MAY INFLUENCE THE aPTT OR HEPARIN LEVELS IN PATIENTS RECEIVING THE SAME DOSE OF HEPARIN

	Expected Effect On	
Factor	**aPTT**	**Heparin Level***
Increased weight	Low	Low
Systemic illness	Low	Low or no effect
Subcutaneous injection	Low	Low
Pregnancy	Low	No effect
Streptokinase	High	No effect
Warfarin	High	No effect
Responsive thromboplastin	High	No effect
aPTT test performance	Variable	No effect
High anti-Xa:IIa activity of heparin preparation	Low	High

Abbreviation: aPTT, activated partial thromboplastin time.

*Measured using an anti-Xa heparin assay. Similar results can be observed with a protamine titration heparin level, except for heparin preparations with a high anti-Xa:IIa ratio, in which the heparin level may also be low.

considered to be heparin resistant.[20] The mechanism for this apparent heparin resistance is multifactorial, one or more factors having a dominant influence in individual patients. In about half of these patients, the normal relationship between the aPTT and the heparin level is maintained; emerging evidence suggests that differences in patients' weights and increased levels of proteins that compete with AT-III for heparin binding are often responsible.[21] In the other half of patients who are resistant to heparin, there is a dissociation between the two measures of anticoagulation, the aPTT being inappropriately low for the anti-X_a heparin level. This phenomenon may be related to elevated levels of factor VIII and possibly other procoagulants.

The results of a trial in which patients were randomized to dose adjustment according to aPTT or heparin level established that it is not necessary to continue escalating the dose of heparin to achieve a therapeutic aPTT in patients who are receiving large doses of heparin (greater than 35,000 units/day), provided that the heparin level is therapeutic.[20] Low rates of recurrent VTE were seen in both groups (approximately 5%) despite a subtherapeutic average aPTT in patients monitored by anti-X_a heparin level. Patients monitored by heparin level received approximately 40,000 units/day, in comparison with approximately 44,000 units in patients monitored by the aPTT. The study was not large enough to establish whether monitoring according to the heparin level was a safer approach, although limiting heparin dose would be expected to reduce bleeding. Theoretically, AT-III deficiency may be responsible for heparin resistance; however, this is very rarely seen in practice.

Achieving a Therapeutic Effect With Heparin

Prolonged therapeutic anticoagulation with heparin is best achieved by either continuous intravenous infusion or subcutaneous injection. An initial intravenous bolus is required with both routes of administration to achieve a rapid onset of effect. This bolus occupies a large proportion of the plasma protein heparin-binding sites, allowing the subsequent infusion or subcutaneous injection to maintain heparin levels in the desired range. A logical approach to selecting the size of this bolus and an initial infusion rate (or subcutaneous dose) would be according to the patient's size. However, because of the many factors that influence heparin dose-response relationships (see Table 28–1), indexing heparin dosage to actual or ideal body weight is of limited value. In practice, a simpler and yet satisfactory approach is to give an initial bolus of 5000 units intravenously (unless this is contraindicated, e.g., within 24 h of surgery), followed by an infusion of 31,000 units over 24 h. This is the average dose required to achieve therapeutic anticoagulation. Weight adjustment with a bolus of 80 units/kg and an initial infusion rate of 18 units/kg/h has been prospectively evaluated and may be worthwhile in unusually large or small patients.[22]

Because of the short half-life of heparin at therapeutic doses, infusion rates should be adjusted on the basis of aPTT measurements as little as 6 h apart, the first being performed 6 h after heparin is initiated. A number of dose-adjustment nomograms have been developed, one of which is shown in Table 28–2. This nomogram adjusts heparin infusion rates to achieve a target aPTT of 60–85 sec, corresponding to 1.9–2.7 times the control aPTT in the authors' laboratory (specific to reagent used), which in turn corresponds to a protamine titration heparin level of 0.2–0.4 units. Therefore, this nomogram is not applicable to all aPTT reagents and should be adapted to the heparin responsiveness of the thromboplastin in local use. In one study with this protocol, the aPTT was therapeutic in 66% of patients after 24 h and in 81% after 48 h; these proportions were significantly better than in a historical control group.[23] Use of a more complex, weight-adjusted nomogram resulted in therapeutic heparin levels in 89% of patients at 24 h and all patients at 48 h.[22] The authors' practice is to use the locally developed nomogram shown in Table 28–2 in most patients but to modify the initial infusion rate on the basis of weight in unusually large or small patients. Many audits of heparin therapy have shown that in the absence of nomogram use, initial inadequate heparin dosing and a low frequency of infusion rate adjustment commonly contribute to delays in achieving therapeutic anticoagulation.

Subcutaneous heparin is usually administrated every 12 h, and monitoring of the aPTT is performed mid-interval (6 h after injection). The first aPTT is generally checked after the second dose, at which time a more stable level of anticoagulation is expected. The authors target the same therapeutic range as that used when heparin is given by continuous intravenous infusion. Because of the reduced bioavailability of subcutaneous heparin and fluctuation in heparin effect during each 24-h cycle, approximately 7% more heparin is required with intermittent subcutaneous injection than with continuous infusion (e.g., 33,800 vs. 31,700 units/day).[24] If therapeutic anticoagulation is initiated with subcutaneous heparin, the authors generally start with 17,500 units (0.7 mL of 25,000 units/mL heparin) every 12 h.

Clinical Studies of Heparin in VTE

Prevention of VTE

In addition to the use of heparin for the treatment of acute thrombotic episodes, subcutaneous low-dose heparin provides an effective and safe form of prophylaxis in medical and surgical patients who are at risk of thromboembolism.[25, 26] It is usually administered in a fixed dose of 5,000 units every 8 or 12 h. With these regimens, the aPTT rarely rises beyond the normal range, and heparin levels do not exceed 0.1 anti-X_a units/mL, and so monitoring of coagulation parameters is not required. For patients at particularly high risk of VTE, a number of studies have demonstrated that the efficacy of low-dose heparin can be improved without compromising safety by adjusting the dose to achieve a minimal heparin effect. Such adjustment generally results in a daily heparin dosage of 15,000–20,000 units. The adjusted dose regimen has limitations for routine use, because it requires careful monitoring.

Treatment of VTE

The first randomized control trial establishing the effectiveness of anticoagulation for the treatment of VTE was reported by Barritt and Jordan in 1960.[27] They randomized 35 patients with clinically diagnosed pulmonary embolism to heparin (10,000 units intravenously every 6 h for six doses [1.5 days]) or to oral anticoagulants for a minimum of 14 days. None of the sixteen patients randomized to anticoagulation were judged to have had recurrent pulmonary embolism, whereas there were five fatal and five nonfatal recurrences of pulmonary embolism in the 19 control patients. Randomization was discontinued, and of 38 additional patients treated with anticoagulants, none developed recurrent pulmonary embolism during the course of treatment. The all-cause mortality rate was significantly lower among the 54 treated patients (2) than among the 19 untreated patients (5).[27] At presentation, 27% of the patients studied had electrocardiographic changes that were considered diagnostic for massive pulmonary embolism, all of whom were also hypotensive, which suggests that the patients in this study were at the severe end of the nonfatal pulmonary embolism spectrum.

Over the next 30 years, the requirement for an initial course of heparin was based on results of laboratory studies, historical comparisons, and indirect evidence from randomized studies that demonstrated high recurrence rates for VTE in patients with proximal DVT who failed to rapidly achieve therapeutic heparin doses. The need for initial heparin therapy was confirmed in one study that found a recurrence rate for symptomatic VTE of 20% in patients with DVT who were randomized to receive oral anticoagulants alone, in comparison with a rate of 6.8% among those who received heparin for 7 days in addition to oral anticoagulation.[28]

TABLE 28–2. HEPARIN DOSE ADJUSTMENT PROTOCOL

	Dosing Instructions*			
Patient's aPTT†	**Repeat Bolus Dose**	**Stop Infusion (minutes)**	**Change Rate (Dose) of Infusion mL/h (units/24 h)‡**	**Timing of Next aPTT**
<50	5000 units	0	+3 (+2880)	6 h
50–59	0	0	+3 (+2880)	6 h
60–85§	0	0	0	Next morning
86–95	0	0	−2 (−1920)	Next morning
96–120	0	30	−2 (−1920)	6 h
>120	0	60	−4 (−3840)	6 h

Abbreviation: aPTT, activated partial thromboplastin time.
*Starting dose of 5000–unit intravenous bolus, followed by 32,000 units/24 h as a continuous infusion.
†Normal range for aPTT with Dade Actin FS reagent is 27–35 sec.
‡40 units/mL. First aPTT performed 6 h after the bolus injection; dosage adjustments made according to protocol and the aPTT repeated as indicated in the far right column.
§Therapeutic range of 60–85 sec is equivalent to a heparin level of 0.2–0.4 units/mL by protamine titration or 0.35–0.7 units/mL as an anti–factor Xa level. The therapeutic range varies with the responsiveness of the aPTT reagent to heparin.

The effectiveness of heparin when given by intermittent intravenous injections or high-dose subcutaneous injection has been compared with continuous intravenous infusion in each of six studies.[2, 29] Provided that adequate doses of heparin are given, there is no apparent difference in efficacy among these three methods of administration. However, as previously noted, intermittent intravenous injection is discouraged because of higher rates of associated bleeding.[13] Heparin has traditionally been administered for 10–14 days, but two studies established that the duration of heparin therapy can safely be reduced from 10 to 5 days.[30, 31] However, one of these studies excluded patients with large iliac vein thrombi or pulmonary embolism,[30] and this group made up a small proportion of the patients in the other study.[31]

The most reliable estimates of the incidence of recurrence during adequate heparin treatment and over the subsequent 3 months of less intense warfarin therapy (international normalized ratio [INR] of 2.0–3.0) come from three contemporary prospective studies of a total of 523 patients to whom heparin was administered by continuous infusion.[17, 30, 31] The 3-month incidence of recurrent venous thromboembolism, diagnosed by reliable objective tests, varied from 4.7% to 7.1%. No patients died of pulmonary embolism.

The need for and efficacy of an initial course of heparin for the treatment of VTE is therefore established, but heparin is not without its limitations (Table 28–3). The suboptimal pharmacokinetic and antihemostatic profile of standard heparin can be, at least partially, overcome by LMWH preparations that therefore have the potential to simplify and improve the safety of treatment. However, the biophysical limitations of heparin are not overcome by LMWH; improved efficacy is probably dependent on achieving higher anti-X_a heparin levels, which may compromise the safety advantages of these preparations.

TABLE 28–3. LIMITATIONS OF HEPARIN

Effect	Consequences
Pharmacokinetics	
Binding to plasma proteins and endothelium	Variability in dose response between patients Dose-dependent mechanism of clearance Responsible for phenomenon of heparin resistance
Biophysical	
Inability to access factors II_a and X_a bound to surfaces	Incomplete inactivation of fibrin-bound thrombin and platelet-bound factor X_a
Antihemostatic	
Binds to platelets and inhibits platelet function	Contributes to hemorrhagic effect

LOW-MOLECULAR-WEIGHT HEPARINS (LMWHs)

It has been noted that standard heparin is heterogeneous with respect to molecular weight (length) and that pharmacokinetic and pharmacodynamic properties vary between heparin molecules of different sizes. In particular, smaller heparin molecules bind less to plasma proteins and endothelial cells; are cleared predominantly by slower nonsaturable renal mechanisms rather than by the rapid saturable cellular route; inhibit platelet function to a lesser extent; have little affect on vascular permeability; and have a higher anti-X_a:anti-II_a ratio than do larger heparin molecules.[32] These observations provided the stimulus to develop LMWHs for clinical use. Having already been in widespread use in Europe, LMWHs have been approved in North America for prophylaxis of VTE in high-risk patients and for treatment of patients with DVT (Canada). Their therapeutic role in coronary artery disease is currently being evaluated.

Pharmacology of LMWHs

LMWHs are fragments of heparin, produced by either chemical or enzymic depolymerization. They are approximately one-third the size of standard heparin molecules and, like standard heparin, they are heterogeneous with regard to molecular size, with a molecular weight distribution of 1000–10,000 and a mean molecular weight of 4000–5000. Depolymerization of heparin results in a change in the pharmacokinetic and anticoagulant profile of the resulting low-molecular-weight fractions (Table 28–4). In addition to LMWHs produced by depolymerization, two other glycosaminoglycans have also been developed for clinical use: dermatan sulfate and the heparinoid danaparoid, which is a mixture of heparin sulfate (80% of the mixture), dermatan sulfate, and chondroitin sulfate.

LMWHs produce their anticoagulant effect by binding to AT-III through the same unique pentasaccharide sequence as that of standard heparin, which is present on less than one third of LMWH molecules. Because a minimal chain length of 18 saccharides (includ-

TABLE 28–4. COMPARISON OF PROPERTIES OF STANDARD HEPARIN (SH) AND LOW-MOLECULAR-WEIGHT HEPARINS (LMWHs)

	Differences	
Property	**SH**	**LMWHs**
Size		
Molecular Weight (Weight-average)	15,000	5,000*
Saccharide Units (Mean)	45	15
Anticoagulant Profile		
Ratio of Anti-Factor Xa to Anti-Factor IIa Activity	1:1	3:1
Binding Characteristics		
Plasma Proteins	+ + +	+
Vascular Wall Matrix Proteins	+ + +	+
Endothelial Cells & Macrophages	+ +	+
Binding to Platelets	+ +	+
Experimental Microvascular Bleeding	+ + +	+
Experimental Antithrombotic Effects	+ + +	+ +

*Approximate. + + +, Marked. + +, Moderate. +, None or minimal.

ing the pentasaccharide sequence) is required for AT-III–mediated inhibition of thrombin by heparin, and because only 25%–50% of different LMWH molecules contain fragments of this or greater length, LMWHs have low antithrombin activity in comparison with standard heparin. In contrast, all heparin molecules that contain the high-affinity pentasaccharide sequence catalyze the inactivation of factor X_a. Consequently, whereas standard heparin has an anti-X_a:anti-II_a activity ratio of 1:1, the various commercial LMWHs have anti-X_a:anti-II_a ratios that vary between 4:1 and 2:1, depending on their molecular weight distribution.[32]

The pharmacokinetics of LMWHs differ from those of standard heparin largely owing to their reduced binding and clearance by plasma proteins, macrophages, and endothelial cells. These differences cause them to have a longer plasma half-life, which is approximately two to four times that of standard heparin. Minimal protein binding contributes to excellent bioavailability of LMWHs at low doses and a predictable anticoagulant dose response. Because they are cleared principally by the kidneys, the half-life of LMWHs is largely independent of the dose administered and, unlike that of standard heparin, it is prolonged with renal failure.

When compared with standard heparin in experimental models of thrombosis and hemorrhage, LMWHs are slightly less effective as antithrombotic agents but produce less bleeding. The improved antithrombotic:bleeding ratio with LMWHs is thought to be a result of less impairment of platelet function, reduced binding of von Willebrand factor, and reduced effects on vascular permeability.

Like standard heparin, LMWHs do not cross the placenta, and descriptive studies suggest that they are safe and effective during pregnancy.[33] Results of a randomized trial suggest that osteoporosis, an infrequent but serious complication of long-term administration of standard heparin in high doses (i.e., ≥20,000 units/24 h for ≥5 months), occurs less often with LMWH (1 of 40 subjects) than with standard heparin (6 of 40 subjects).[34]

Clinical Studies of LMWH in VTE

Prevention of VTE

LMWHs are effective at preventing VTE in general and in orthopedic surgical patients, resulting in an approximately 75% risk reduction in comparison with untreated controls.[25, 35, 36] Once-daily administration is usual, the first dose being given preoperatively. LMWHs have also been shown to provide effective prophylaxis when started postoperatively in high-risk orthopedic patients,[37] usually being administered twice per day in this setting. LMWHs provide more effective prophylaxis than does fixed low-dose standard heparin, with an additional risk reduction of approximately 25% for DVT.[35, 38] They appear to be particularly effective in preventing proximal DVT[39] and pulmonary embolism[35, 38] and are emerging as the prophylactic method of choice for patients at high risk of VTE. Experience with LMWHs for VTE prophylaxis in nonsurgical patients is less extensive; however, they have been shown to be effective in preventing DVT in patients with stroke, patients with spinal cord injury, and general medical patients.[25, 36] Although there is some evidence that bleeding is less extensive with LMWHs than with fixed low-dose standard heparin,[40] this difference has not been marked;[35, 38, 40] major postoperative bleeding is uncommon with both classes of heparin (approximately 3%). The optimal approach to the administration of LMWH (e.g., preoperative vs. postoperative initiation, once vs. twice per day, total daily dose), particularly in high-risk patients, has yet to be determined. In the absence of direct comparison, it is not known whether different LMWH preparations are equally effective.

Treatment of VTE

LMWH has been compared with standard heparin in 16 randomized trials involving more than 2000 patients with venographically confirmed DVT.[36, 41] In these trials, LMWH was generally given by twice-per-day subcutaneous injection, and standard heparin was generally administered as a continuous intravenous infusion, although this was not invariable. The results of these trials have been combined in two separate meta-analyses that used somewhat different criteria for the inclusion of individual studies.[36, 41] One of these meta-analyses, which included all 16 randomized trials, determined common odds ratios for the following outcomes, all of which favored the LMWH: 0.51 for thrombus extension, as determined by routine repeat venography; 0.66 for recurrence of thromboembolic events; 0.65 for major hemorrhage; and 0.72 for total mortality.[41] The confidence intervals around these estimates were wide, and the reduction in thrombus extension was the only outcome that achieved statistic significance. This analysis found no evidence that the route of administration of LMWH, or dose adjustment on the basis of anti-X_a heparin levels, influenced efficacy or safety. Eleven of these studies used a weight-adjusted dose of LMWH; the remaining trials used a fixed daily dose ranging from 15,000 to 17,500 IU. Overall, the dose of LMWH corresponded to approximately 200 anti-X_a IU/kg/day.

A recent European study compared two doses of the low-molecular-weight heparinoid danaparoid (1250 units or 2000 units, intravenously and subcutaneously twice a day) with standard heparin, in patients with acute DVT or pulmonary embolism.[41a] Clinical evidence of recurrent VTE was rare in all three groups. However, evidence of asymptomatic extension or recurrence was less frequent in the high-dose danaparoid group.

The second meta-analysis, which combined the results of nine of these trials, found statistically significant improvement in post-treatment venograms, reductions in symptomatic thromboembolic complications during long-term follow-up (risk reduction, 62%), and reductions in major bleeding during heparin therapy (risk reduction, 68%).[36]

There are few available data on the efficacy of LMWHs for the treatment of patients presenting with pulmonary embolism. One of the earlier studies that found that LMWH was safe and effective for the treatment of acute VTE included a large number of patients (70 of 194 patients) with a primary diagnosis of pulmonary embolism.[42] In a randomized trial of 101 patients in which an LMWH preparation given in three doses either twice or three times per day was compared with standard heparin given by continuous intravenous infusion, no difference in angiographic improvement was seen among the four groups after 8 days of treatment, and there were no confirmed episodes of recurrent pulmonary embolism.[43] However, the two high-dose LMWH regimens, which used doses markedly in excess of those currently used for the treatment of DVT, were associated with excessive bleeding. In view of the current understanding of the relationship of pulmonary embolism to DVT, it is reasonable to extrapolate from studies of DVT treatment that LMWH will also be effective in patients presenting with pulmonary embolism.

Because of their favorable and predictable pharmacokinetic profile and evidence of superior efficacy and safety, it may soon become feasible to treat clinically stable patients with acute DVT and/or pulmonary embolism (with LMWHs) as outpatients. Such studies are currently in progress.

Heparins and Bleeding

Bleeding is the most important complication of heparin therapy, occurring in approximately 5% of patients who receive heparin for 5–7 days.[13, 19] If clinically important bleeding occurs during the initial period of heparin therapy, anticoagulants are usually discontinued and an inferior vena caval filter is inserted. In occasional patients with major bleeding and therapeutic levels of heparin, or in patients who are bleeding and who have received supratherapeutic doses of heparin, protamine sulfate may be given to reverse the effect of heparin. The full neutralizing dose is 1 mg of protamine sulfate for 100 units of heparin. Because of the short half-life of standard heparin, the dose of protamine must be reduced to half this amount at 1 h and to a quarter of this at 2 h after the heparin has been given. Protamine should be infused over 10 min to avoid hypotension and may need to be repeated because of its rapid clearance. Smaller repeated doses of protamine are required to reverse the effects of therapeutic doses of heparin that have been given subcutaneously.

Protamine sulfate only partly neutralizes the anticoagulant effect of LMWHs. It is probable that protamine complexes with the larger molecules, but not the very low molecular weight fractions. Nevertheless, there is evidence from animal experiments that protamine also reduces bleeding caused by LMWHs.

Heparins and Thrombocytopenia

A fall in platelet count beginning 5–15 days after heparin is started (median, 10 days; earlier in patients who have previously received heparin) may be a result of heparin-induced thrombocytopenia, the most serious consequence of which is associated arterial and venous thrombosis.[44–46] In the absence of a convincing alternative explanation for thrombocytopenia in this setting, all sources of heparin are stopped (including line flushes), and if indications for therapeutic anticoagulation persist, an alternative agent is used. If warfarin treatment has already been started and the INR is approaching or in the therapeutic range, warfarin can be continued without addition of an alternative treatment. Two alternative antithrombotic agents have been evaluated in descriptive studies, the defibrinating agent ancrod[47] and the heparinoid danaparoid.[46] Dosage regimens for ancrod and danaparoid are shown in Table 28–5. Alternatively, danaparoid can be administered as 2000 units intravenously and subcutaneously initially, followed by 2000 units subcutaneously twice a day, as previously noted.[41a] Preliminary evidence suggests that heparin-induced thrombocytopenia occurs less commonly with LMWHs, but if it occurs in association with standard heparin, LMWH preparations cannot be substituted because of a high frequency of immunologic cross-reactivity between LMWHs and standard heparin. Danaparoid, which is a mixture of 80% heparin sulfate and smaller amounts of dermatan sulfate and chondroitin sulfate, exhibits minimal cross-reactivity.[46]

Other side effects of heparin, which include skin necrosis, alopecia, hypersensitivity reactions, and hypoaldosteronism, rarely occur during short courses of heparin.

TABLE 28–5. ANTITHROMBOTIC ALTERNATIVES IN HEPARIN-INDUCED THROMBOCYTOPENIA

Ancrod

Initial Infusion

70 units (one vial) in 250 mL of normal saline over 6 h

Subsequent Infusion

based on fibrinogen levels (Clauss method) assayed approximately 6 hrs after completion of infusions. The following protocol acts as a guideline, to be modified according to response.

Fibrinogen, g/L	*Infusion*
<0.5	0 units for 24 hrs
0.5 to 1.0	70 units over 24 hrs
1.0 to 1.5	70 units over 18 hrs
1.5 to 2.0	70 units over 12 hrs
> 2.0	70 units over 8 hrs

Danaparoid

Bolus

2500 units

Infusion

400 units/hr for 2 h, then 300 units/h for 2 h, followed by 150–200 units/h, adjusted to achieve an anti-X_a activity level of 0.5–0.8 units/mL

ORAL ANTICOAGULANTS

Historical Highlights

The hemorrhagic consequences of vitamin K deficiency were inadvertently discovered in the late 1920s when H. Dam observed that a fat-soluble factor was required in order to maintain normal blood coagulant functions and that the defect produced by its absence could be corrected with a lipid abstract of alfalfa.[48] Vitamin K was subsequently isolated and its structure determined in the late 1930s. In parallel with these developments, ingestion of improperly cured sweet clover hay was found to be responsible for a hemorrhagic disease of cattle. Link and coworkers established that dicoumarol, formed in the spoilage process of sweet clover, was the responsible agent, that its ingestion resulted in "hypoprothrombinemia," and that this effect could be reversed by vitamin K.[49] In the early 1940s, oral anticoagulants were introduced into clinical practice, the predominant initial indication being the treatment of myocardial infarction and cerebral embolism. A derivative of dicoumarol, warfarin (named after the Wisconsin Alumni Research Foundation and the terminal syllable of coumarin), was promoted as a rodenticide in the late 1940s. Because of its predictable onset, predictable duration of action, and excellent bioavailability, warfarin is the most widely used oral anticoagulant in North America. In addition to the coumarins, indandione derivatives are also vitamin K antagonists, but they are no longer used because of a higher frequency of nonhemorrhagic complications.

Mechanism of Action

Oral anticoagulants produce their effects by causing a deficiency of the reduced form of vitamin K, vitamin K H_2, which is a necessary cofactor for the carboxylation of glutamic acid residues to form gamma carboxyglutamates on clotting factors II, VII, IX, and X[48, 50, 51] (Fig. 28–3). The formation of gamma carboxyglutamates is a prerequisite for the calcium-dependent complexing of these coagulation proteins with their cofactors on phospholipid surfaces. In the absence of vitamin K H_2, incompletely carboxylated forms of these factors, which are largely inactive, are produced by the liver. In the process of carboxylation, vitamin K H_2 undergoes oxidation to vitamin K epoxide, which must be recycled to vitamin K H_2 before it can facilitate further carboxylation reactions. The recycling of vitamin K

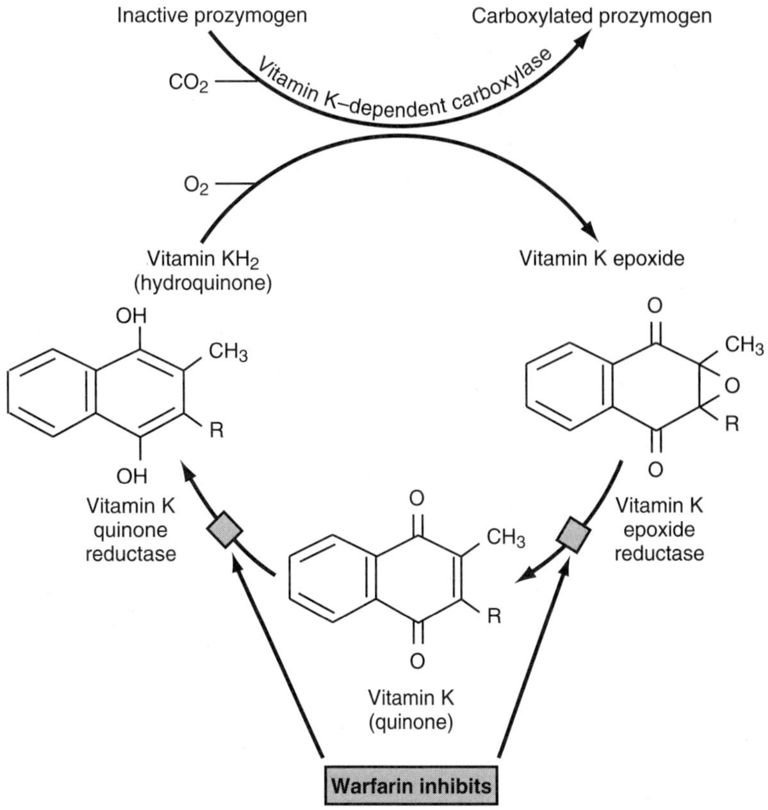

Figure 28–3. Vitamin K cycle and its inhibition by warfarin. Warfarin inhibits vitamin K epoxide reductase and vitamin K quinone reductase and so blocks the conversion of vitamin K epoxide to vitamin KH_2. Vitamin KH_2 is a cofactor for the carboxylation of inactive proenzymes (Factors II, VII, IX, and X) to their active forms. (From Furie B, Furie BC: Molecular basis of vitamin K–dependent γ-carboxylation. Blood 1990; 75:1753–1762.)

epoxide to vitamin K H_2 occurs in a number of steps, each of which is controlled by a reductase enzyme. In a manner not yet fully understood, oral anticoagulants block these reductase enzymes, particularly vitamin K epoxide reductase, resulting in deficiencies of vitamin K H_2 and reduced levels of functional coagulation factors.

Pharmacokinetics and Pharmacodynamics of Warfarin

Warfarin, like dicoumarol, is a 4-hydroxycoumarin compound. It is a racemic mixture of approximately equal amounts of optical isomers, the R and S forms, which have somewhat different drug interactions and different pharmacokinetic and pharmacodynamic properties.[52, 53] It is almost always administered orally, although an injectable preparation is available. Absorption is rapid, maximal blood concentrations occur after 90 min, and it has a plasma half-life of approximately 40 h. It is a weak acid that circulates bound to plasma proteins and rapidly accumulates in the liver, where it interferes with coagulation factor production. The dose-response relationship between warfarin and the intensity of anticoagulation induced is influenced by both pharmacokinetic factors (because of differences in absorption or clearance) and pharmacodynamic factors (because of differences in the hemostatic response to given concentrations of warfarin). Consequently, there is a highly variable between-subject and within-subject (temporal) dose-response relationship, necessitating close monitoring of the anticoagulant response. Nonpharmacologic factors also contribute to apparent variability in dose response; these include differences or inaccuracies in laboratory testing and reporting of anticoagulant effects, poor patient compliance, and poor communication between the patient and physician.

Drugs can influence the pharmacokinetics of warfarin by altering its absorption and metabolic clearance, or they can influence its pharmacodynamics by altering the rate of synthesis or clearance of the vitamin K–dependent coagulation factors.[53] The antithrombotic and hemorrhagic potential of warfarin can also be potentiated by drugs that interfere with other pathways of hemostasis or that disrupt mucosal integrity in the gastrointestinal tract.[54] The effects that drugs and other factors may have on the action of warfarin are summarized in Table 28–6. This list is not exhaustive; interactions between warfarin and other drugs have been questioned, but as the supporting evidence is not convincing, they have not been included in this review.[53] As a general rule, special care should be taken when any new drug is given in combination with oral anticoagulants; monitoring of prothrombin time should be more frequent to ensure that potential interactions are identified and appropriate dose adjustments made. Independently of pharmacologic interactions, drugs may also potentiate the antihemostatic effect of warfarin by interfering with other hemostatic pathways (Table 28–7).

Monitoring Oral Anticoagulation

In the 1930s, Quick developed and standardized a test of coagulation in which the time required for decalcified plasma to clot was determined after the addition of calcium and tissue thromboplastin.[55] A single plasma factor, prothrombin, was thought to be crucial for clot formation, and the test was therefore called the prothrombin time. Quick's prothrombin time was found to be prolonged in obstructive jaundice and vitamin K deficiency, and it soon became the measure of choice for monitoring oral anticoagulation, a position that it still holds. Thromboplastin, which is an extract of animal tissue, provides a rich source of tissue factor and the phospholipid necessary for the activation of factor X by factor VII_a.[51, 52] It is now recognized that the prothrombin time is sensitive to depression of three of the four vitamin K–dependent clotting factors (prothrombin, factor VII, and factor X).

Commercially available thromboplastins vary markedly in their ability to promote clotting of blood from oral anticoagulated patients, and so prothrombin times determined through the use of different

TABLE 28–6. DRUGS AND OTHER FACTORS THAT ALTER THE ANTICOAGULANT RESPONSE TO WARFARIN

Prolongs Prothrombin Time	Reduces Prothrombin
Pharmacokinetic	
Increases Warfarin Levels	**Decreases Warfarin Levels**
Phenylbutazone*	Cholestyramine*
Sulfinpyrazone*	Barbiturates*
Metronidazole*	Rifampin*
Cotrimoxazole*	Carbamazepine*
Erythromycin*	Griseofulvin*
Fluconazole*	Dextropropoxyphene†
Miconazole*	
Nafcillin*	
Cimetidine*	
Omeprazole*	
Amiodarone*	
Disulfiram†	
Pharmacodynamic‡	
Clofibrate*	High vitamin K intake* (certain vegetables, nutritional supplements)
Low vitamin K intake*	
Malabsorption	
Liver disease	
Hypermetabolic states	
Coagulopathies	
Mechanism Not Established	
Isoniazid*	Chlordiazepoxide*
Propafenone*	Sucralfate*
Propranolol*	Dicloxacillin†
Piroxicam*	
Acetaminophen†	
Anabolic steroids†	
Aspirin†	
Chloral hydrate†	
Ciprofloxacin†	
Itraconazole†	
Quinidine†	
Phenytoin†	
Simvastatin†	
Tamoxifen†	
Tetracyclines†	
Influenza vaccine†	

*Highly probable interaction. †Probable interaction as defined by Wells and colleagues.[53]
‡No effect on warfarin levels.

reagents are not interchangeable.[52] This greatly complicates monitoring of oral anticoagulant therapy; the "therapeutic range" for the prothrombin time may differ between and within laboratories with changes in the batch of thromboplastin used. Expressing the prothrombin time as a ratio of the patient's prothrombin time to normal prothrombin time (determined from normal pooled plasma) fails to correct for these differences, because the prothrombin time of non-anticoagulated blood varies little with the different thromboplastins used, whereas the prothrombin time of anticoagulated blood varies markedly.

A standardized method of prothrombin time reporting, the INR, has been introduced to circumvent this potentially dangerous situation by correcting for the effect of different thromboplastins on the prothrombin time.[52, 56–58] The INR is calculated by raising the patient's prothrombin time ratio to the power of a constant (i.e., prothrombin time ratio^{c}), where the constant (c) is the international sensitivity index (ISI) for each thromboplastin. The weaker the thromboplastin is at promoting clotting, the more responsive the prothrombin time assay is to oral anticoagulation and the lower the ISI value is.

Two additional technical factors add to variability in coagulation studies, and these factors are not fully overcome by knowing the ISI of the thromboplastin used and using the INR system of reporting. First, prothrombin time may vary according to the equipment used for clot detection; second, the larger the ISI of the thromboplastin (i.e., >2.0, as is commonly used in North America) and hence the shorter the prothrombin time ratio, the less reliable the calculated INR (i.e., with an ISI of 3.0, a prothrombin time ratio of 1.2 yields an INR of 1.7; a prothrombin time ratio of 1.3 yields an INR of 2.2). It is therefore better to use more responsive thromboplastins with a lower ISI (i.e., 1.0–1.2), particularly when low-intensity warfarin (i.e., target INR of 2.0–3.0) is used. Although the INR system of prothrombin time reporting is not without limitations,[59] it represents a major improvement over direct reporting of prothrombin time results or prothrombin time ratios. Improved laboratory methods for monitoring oral anticoagulation that are not based on the prothrombin time may be developed.[60] Because warfarin exerts its effect in the liver rather than in the blood, and because of the many pharmacodynamic factors that influence this response, warfarin levels are not valuable for monitoring oral anticoagulant therapy. However, in the occasional patient who is unexpectedly sensitive or resistant to warfarin, levels may be valuable for assessing pharmacokinetic variables or drug compliance.

Optimal Therapeutic Range

On the basis of expert opinion, prothrombin time ratios of 2.0–2.5 were recommended as the therapeutic range for oral anticoagulation in the 1950s and 1960s and were widely accepted in Great Britain and North America.[56] Responsive thromboplastins were in widespread use at that time, and although the INR system had yet to be to introduced, the ISI for these early preparations is likely to have been close to 1.0. Therefore, a prothrombin time ratio of 2.0–2.5 with these thromboplastins would correspond to a latter-day INR of 2.0–2.5. Whereas responsive thromboplastins continue to be used in much of Europe, use of less responsive thromboplastins became widespread in North America, and because the target prothrombin time ratio remained at approximately 2.0–2.5, the level of anticoagulation used in clinical practice in North America and Great Britain unwittingly diverged markedly. With a prothrombin time ratio of 2.0–2.5, therapeutic anticoagulation corresponded to an INR of 2.0 to 2.5 in Britain, but with a thromboplastin with an ISI of 2.3 in North America, therapeutic anticoagulation corresponded to an INR of 4.9–8.2.

TABLE 28–7. DRUGS THAT POTENTIATE THE ANTIHEMOSTATIC EFFECT OF WARFARIN BY INTERFERING WITH OTHER HEMOSTASIS PATHWAYS

Antiplatelet Effect
Aspirin
Other nonsteroidal anti-inflammatory drugs
Ticlopidine
Moxalactam
Carbenicillin
Indirect Antithrombin Effect
Heparins
Direct Antithrombin Effect
Hirudin
Hirulog
Systemic Fibrinolytic Effect
Streptokinase
Ancrod

A number of randomized studies have been performed to determine the optimal intensity of oral anticoagulation for different indications.[52] These studies have shown that an INR of 2.0–3.0 is as effective as an INR of 3.0–4.5 at preventing venous and arterial thrombosis and is associated with a greatly reduced frequency of bleeding.[61–64] Guidelines for the intensity of oral anticoagulation and the evidence supporting these recommendations have been published,[52] and an INR of 2.0–3.0 is currently recommended for the prevention and treatment of VTE, although there is evidence that a lower INR may be effective in patients receiving primary prophylaxis.[65–67] The clinical studies that have established the current role of oral anticoagulants in the management of VTE are reviewed in a subsequent section.

Achieving Therapeutic Coagulation With Warfarin

Warfarin has a rapid onset of action after oral administration. However, because the effects of warfarin on anticoagulation are indirect (first requiring a depletion of circulating vitamin K–dependent clotting factors) and because the half-life of most of these factors is long (generally 1–3 days), a 1- to 2-day delay is usual before the INR starts to rise. The initial increase in the INR is predominantly caused by decreases in factor VII, and because isolated decreases in factor VII may have little antithrombotic effect, it may take longer (i.e., an additional 1–2 days) to achieve affective anticoagulation than it takes to achieve a therapeutic INR. Because warfarin also causes rapid depletion of the naturally occurring anticoagulants protein C and protein S, which also have short half-lives, there is the potential for a paradoxical early prothrombotic period after oral anticoagulants are started. This has led to recommendation that warfarin be overlapped with heparin until the INR is therapeutic for 2 consecutive days (minimum of 5 days of heparin).

In addition to the lag phase between starting warfarin and achieving anticoagulation, there is a similar lag between stopping warfarin and reversing anticoagulation. This occurs because warfarin's antagonism of vitamin K persists because of its long half-life; subsequently, functional levels of coagulation factors need to be regenerated before normalization of coagulation occurs. These temporal sequences have to be considered when warfarin is prescribed; changes in warfarin dose depend as much on the rate of change of the INR in the preceding days as it does on the actual INR value. For example, a patient with an INR of 2.0 may not require any warfarin that day if the INR was 1.4 on the previous day, but an increase in warfarin dose may be required if the previous day's INR was 2.8. These considerations are particularly important when warfarin is started, and they largely preclude the use of simple dose adjustment nomograms. Computer programs may overcome these limitations.

The average daily maintenance dose of warfarin required to achieve an INR of 2.0 to 3.0 is 4–5 mg. When an early onset of affect is desired, warfarin should be started at approximately 10 mg; subsequent daily doses depend on INRs, which initially should be performed daily. If treatment is not urgent (e.g., VTE prophylaxis or chronic atrial fibrillation), therapy can begin with the anticipated maintenance dose, with the expectation of steady-state anticoagulation in 5–7 days. Depending on the stability of the anticoagulant response, the interval between INR measurements can be progressively increased to approximately once every 4 weeks

Reversing the Anticoagulant Effect of Warfarin

Depending on the current INR, warfarin maintenance dose, nutritional status, and additional factors that may influence pharmacodynamic responses (see Table 28–6), stopping warfarin usually causes the INR to return to normal in about 3 days. If more rapid reversal is required, vitamin K should be administered, preferably orally or by subcutaneous injection. Intravenous vitamin K need be given only if peripheral absorption may be poor as a result of shock or when a rapid lowering or reversal of anticoagulation is required. It should be administered slowly to minimize the risk of anaphylactic reactions. Very low doses of vitamin K (0.5–1.0 mg) should be used if moderate lowering of the INR is required (e.g., if the INR is 6.0–10.0 in a patient who is not bleeding), because this often causes the INR to return to the therapeutic range in 24 h.[68] If the INR is between 10.0 and 20.0, 3–5 mg of vitamin K can be given intravenously. Higher doses of vitamin K can be given for an INR higher than 20.0, for life-threatening bleeding, or for serious warfarin overdosage. Replacement of vitamin K–dependent coagulation factors with plasma (e.g., 2–4 units) or factor concentrates may be required in order to achieve more rapid reversal of anticoagulation in these situations.

Clinical Studies of Oral Anticoagulation for VTE

The efficacy of oral anticoagulants for the prevention and treatment of VTE was established by a series of randomized control trials, many of which were performed in the late 1970s and early 1980s. More recent studies of oral anticoagulants in patients with VTE focused on optimizing the intensity and duration of anticoagulation and on the identification of additional groups of patients who would benefit from this therapy.

Prevention of VTE

The classic studies of Sevitt and Gallagher provided strong evidence that oral anticoagulants were effective at preventing DVT and pulmonary embolism in trauma and burn patients.[69] Subsequent randomized control trials have confirmed that oral anticoagulants, generally with an INR of 2.0–3.0, achieve a risk reduction of approximately 60% for DVT after orthopedic or major general surgery, when started either before surgery or on the first postoperative day.[25] The risk of clinically important bleeding with this relatively low-intensity regimen is small, but because warfarin prophylaxis is more complicated than fixed low-dose heparin for patients at moderate risk of postoperative VTE and appears to be less effective than LMWH for prophylaxis in patients at very high risk, its use is now generally confined to patients who have an additional indication for oral anticoagulation (e.g., atrial fibrillation) or who will require long-term prophylaxis (e.g., recurrent VTE, prolonged immobilization).

In addition to prophylaxis of surgical patients, randomized control trials have established that very low intensity anticoagulation with warfarin is effective at preventing thrombosis of indwelling venous lines (INR, <1.3)[66] and VTE in patients with metastatic breast cancer who are being treated with systemic chemotherapy (INR, 1.3–1.9).[67]

Treatment of VTE

Three randomized trials provide evidence that oral anticoagulants are effective in the treatment of patients with acute VTE.[27, 70, 71] The first of these studies, reported by Barritt and Jordan and described previously, established that a minimum of 14 days of the oral anticoagulant nicoumalone (prothrombin time ratio, 2.0–3.0), in combination with heparin, reduced the incidences of symptomatic and fatal recurrent pulmonary embolism.[27]

Subsequently, Hull and colleagues randomized patients with isolated calf or proximal DVT to either 5000 units of standard heparin, subcutaneously, every 12 h, or warfarin (INR 2.5–4.5), for 3 months after an initial course of intravenous heparin.[70] Evidence of recurrence developed in 9 (47%) of the 19 patients with proximal DVT who were treated with subcutaneous heparin, whereas there were no recurrences in the 17 patients who were treated with warfarin; this difference was highly significant. Regardless of treatment, none of the patients with isolated calf vein thrombosis (predominantly asymptomatic, postoperative, clots detected by screening venography) experienced recurrence.

In a subsequent study of patients with venographically confirmed symptomatic calf vein thrombosis who were randomly assigned to warfarin (INR, 2.5–4.2) or placebo, with 5 days of initial heparin, none of the 23 warfarin patients experienced recurrence, whereas 8 (29%) of the 28 control patients manifested recurrence during the first 3 months (one vs. nine recurrences after 1 year). Bleeding was much more common among patients with DVT who were treated with warfarin (INR 2.5–4.5) than among those who received adjusted-dose heparin,[72] and the intensity of therapeutic anticoagulation used in North America was higher than that used in Britain and other parts of Europe; these two observations led to a subsequent study designed to determine the optimal intensity of anticoagulation with warfarin for patients with VTE. Less intense anticoagulation (INR, 2.0–2.5) was found to be as effective at preventing recurrent VTE as the traditional intensity of anticoagulation (INR, 2.5–4.5) but was associated with a greatly reduced risk of bleeding (risk reduction, 81%).[61]

A number of small studies in the 1970s and 1980s evaluated the optimal duration of oral anticoagulant therapy for VTE, but their results were inconclusive.[51] Three larger studies have addressed this question.[73, 74, 74a] The British Thoracic Society study randomized 712 patients with a clinical diagnosis of pulmonary embolism or DVT (confirmed by objective testing in 71%) to 4 weeks or 12 weeks of anticoagulation. The recurrence rate was higher among patients who were treated with anticoagulants for 4 weeks (7.8%) than among those treated for 12 weeks (4.0%).[73] Lack of blind comparisons and infrequent use of objective tests to diagnose recurrent VTE undermine the strength of the conclusions that can be drawn from this study. In the second study, 220 patients with proximal DVT who had normal findings on impedance plethysmography after 4 months of treatment were randomized either to 8 more weeks of warfarin or to placebo.[74] In this double-blind study, recurrence was significantly less common during the 8 weeks on study medication in patients randomized to warfarin; however, the difference in recurrence rates during the 11 months after randomization (a more clinically relevant period of follow-up), although less in patients treated with 3 months of therapy (11.2% vs. 6.2%), was not statistically significant.[74]

In the third study, 897 patients with a first episode of DVT or pulmonary embolism were randomized, in an open design, to 6 weeks or 6 months of anticoagulation.[74a] Recurrence rates during 2 years of follow-up were twice as high (18.1%) in patients treated for 6 weeks as in those treated for 6 months (9.5%).

Together, the results of these studies suggest that the duration of anticoagulation for proximal DVT and pulmonary embolism should not be shortened to less than 3 months. A possible exception may be feasible for patients with a first episode of VTE that has occurred as a complication of surgery; the three studies found that such patients had a low recurrence rate for VTE, regardless of the duration of anticoagulation. This finding needs to be evaluated prospectively.

DIRECT THROMBIN INHIBITORS

The limitations of heparin are based on its pharmacokinetic, biophysical, and non-anticoagulant antihemostatic properties (see Table 28–3). Whereas LMWHs can substantially overcome heparin's suboptimal pharmacokinetic and antiplatelet properties, the biophysical limitations are common to forms of both lower and higher molecular weight.[2, 75–78] In particular, heparin is a weak inhibitor of thrombin, which is bound to fibrin, both within thrombi and in solution.[78] LMWH preparations, which also inhibit thrombosis via AT-III and which specifically have low antithrombin activity, offer no advantages in this regard. A large number of new agents that inhibit thrombosis independently of AT-III have been discovered[75, 76] (see Chapter 30); the direct thrombin inhibitors hirudin and Hirulog are considered further, inasmuch as these agents have been the best studied and preliminary results are available from clinical trials.

Hirudin is a potent and specific thrombin inhibitor, originally isolated from the saliva of the medicinal leech (*Hirudo medicinalis*) and now available through recombinant DNA technology. It is a 65–amino acid protein that makes extensive contact with thrombin when the two combine, including binding to the active center (cleavage) and substrate recognition sites.[75–77, 79] Hirudin inhibits many functions of thrombin, including cleavage of fibrinogen to form fibrin, activation of platelets, and positive feedback on clotting factors V and VIII (which are strong promoters of coagulation) and factor XIII (which is responsible for crosslinking of fibrin to form a stable clot). Its major potential advantages over heparin are that it has a stable and predictable anticoagulant response and that it effectively blocks thrombin that is bound to fibrin or subendothelial matrix. Potential limitations include its inability to prevent initial thrombin generation, the possibility that it reduces the negative feedback functions of thrombin (e.g., activation of protein C via thrombomodulin), and the fact that its effects cannot be reversed in the event of bleeding. Hirudin has to be administered parenterally; intravenous infusion or twice-a-day subcutaneous injection appears to be most suitable. It has a predictable dose response with the activated partial thromboplastin time (aPTT) up to a value of approximately 100 sec, after which there is a plateau effect with little further increase in the aPTT. It is not known whether the aPTT response to hirudin has the same therapeutic implications as the aPTT response to standard heparin. Data from animal studies suggest that for an equivalent antithrombotic effect, the aPTT is less prolonged with hirudin. There is some evidence from clinical studies that patients with higher hirudin-induced aPTTs may be at greater risk for bleeding.[80, 81]

Hirugen is a synthetic 12–amino acid peptide (carboxy-terminal region of hirudin) that binds only to the substrate recognition site of thrombin. It is a less potent inhibitor of thrombin and has not been developed for clinical use. The covalent addition to hirugen of D-Phe-Pro-Arg-Pro-$(GLY)_4$, the amino acid sequence that binds to thrombin's catalytic site, yields Hirulog (bivalirudin). Like hirugen, Hirulog blocks both the active center and the substrate recognition site of thrombin.[75, 76, 79]

Clinical Studies With the Direct Antithrombin Inhibitors in VTE

The major impetus for the development of hirudin and related compounds has been to improve the management of acute ischemic coronary syndromes. A large number of mostly small-phase II studies have been performed in patients with acute myocardial infarction, unstable angina, and percutaneous transluminal coronary angiography and are reviewed elsewhere[76] (Chapter 29). Large multicenter trials involving patients with acute myocardial infarction are in progress. Although preliminary results relating to efficacy have been encouraging, enthusiasm has been tempered by the finding of higher-than-expected spontaneous bleeding rates among patients who received hirudin in combination with thrombolytic agents in the setting of acute myocardial infarction.[80–83]

A small number of studies have evaluated the direct thrombin inhibitors for the prevention and treatment of VTE. After an initial study of 48 patients,[84] Eriksson and colleagues compared three doses of hirudin (10, 15, and 20 mg, subcutaneously, b.i.d.) with heparin (5000 units, t.i.d.), the first dose given preoperatively in all arms, for the prevention of DVT in 1119 patients undergoing total hip replacement.[85] DVT, particularly proximal DVT, occurred much less frequently among patients treated with the two higher doses of hirudin (all DVT, ~18%; proximal DVT, ~3%) than with heparin (all DVT, 34%; proximal DVT, 20%). There was no difference in bleeding among the four groups. These results, particularly with regard to proximal DVT, compare favorable with those of studies using LMWHs.

A dose-finding cohort study found similar low rates of all and proximal DVTs in 46 patients who received 1 mg/kg of Hirulog three times per day, the first dose of which was given postoperatively.[86] In this study, much higher rates of DVT were seen among patients who received this dose twice per day, which suggests that subcutaneous Hirulog may need to be given more frequently than hirudin.

Two small pilot studies, each with 10 patients, have evaluated continuous intravenous hirudin (0.07 mg/kg as a bolus, followed by 0.05 mg/kg/h)[87] and subcutaneous hirudin (0.75 mg/kg, b.i.d.)[88] for the treatment of patients presenting with acute DVT, most of whom also had confirmed, and often major, pulmonary embolism. Recurrent pulmonary embolism was suspected clinically and angiographically in only one of these patients during treatment,[88] and there was evidence of asymptomatic extension of DVT at routine venography in another.[87] One patient experienced minor bleeding,[87] but no major bleeds occurred in either study. Although preliminary, this evidence suggests that hirudin may be safe and effective for the treatment of acute VTE and may provide a therapeutic option if heparin is contraindicated.

Putting Anticoagulant Drugs for VTE in Perspective

When used optimally, anticoagulation with standard heparin and warfarin is effective at preventing recurrent VTE. Venographic evidence of thrombus extension occurs in 10%–20% of patients with proximal DVT who are treated with standard heparin, of which only a small minority (10%–20%) are symptomatic. New perfusion scan defects occur in fewer than 10% of patients with proximal DVT who are treated with standard heparin, and symptomatic pulmonary embolism is extremely rare. The in-hospital mortality rate among patients with pulmonary embolism who are treated with standard heparin is approximately 8% and is closely related to the severity of cardiopulmonary compromise at presentation. This is determined by both baseline cardiopulmonary status and the severity of the initial pulmonary embolism. Although there is some room for improvement in these results, the potential for more effective antithrombotic agents (e.g., LMWH or direct antithrombins) to reduce morbidity and mortality from VTE is limited. It may therefore seem surprising that pulmonary embolism is considered the most common avoidable cause of death in hospitalized patients. The explanation for this is that most of these deaths occur within an hour of embolization or as a consequence of recurrent pulmonary embolism in patients in whom the initial event was not diagnosed. Despite unequivocal evidence that primary prophylaxis is effective and leans to overall savings in health care expenditure, a minority of hospitalized patients who are at high risk for VTE receive effective prophylaxis.[89]

Similarly, it has been estimated that VTE is diagnosed in less than a third of the symptomatic patients.[90] The proportion of patients with untreated symptomatic DVT who progress to fatal pulmonary embolism is uncertain, but it may be of the order of 15%. The proportion of patients with untreated symptomatic pulmonary embolism who progress to fatal recurrence has been estimated at approximately 30%. It is therefore clear that widespread use of primary prophylaxis, together with better recognition and evaluation of suspected DVT and pulmonary embolism, has the potential to greatly reduce rates of morbidity and mortality from this condition. The knowledge and means of achieving this are currently available. The development of new and more effective antithrombotic agents that are safer and require less monitoring will facilitate this process. In addition, such agents have the potential to reduce health care expenditure by allowing out-patient treatment of acute DVT and pulmonary embolism.

REFERENCES

1. Salzman EW, Hirsh J: Clinical aspects of thrombotic disorders: the epidemiology, pathogenesis, and natural history of venous thrombosis. *In* Colman RW, Hirsh J, Marder VJ, Salzman EW (eds): Hemostasis and Thrombosis: Basic Principles and Clinical Practice, 3rd ed, pp 1275–1296. Philadelphia: JB Lippincott, 1994.
2. Hirsh J, Fuster V: Guide to anticoagulant therapy part 1: heparin. Circulation 1994; 89:1449–1468.
3. Alpert JS, Dalen JE: Epidemiology and natural history of venous thromboembolism. Progr Cardiovasc Dis 1994; 36:417–422.
4. Lensing AWA, Hirsh J, Buller H: Diagnosis of venous thrombosis. *In* Coleman RW, Hirsh J, Marder VJ, Salzman EW (eds): Hemostasis and Thrombosis: Basic Principles and Clinical Practice, 3rd ed, pp 1297–1321. Philadelphia: Lippincott, 1994.
5. Hull RD, Raskob GE, Ginsberg JS, et al: A noninvasive strategy for the treatment of patients with suspected pulmonary embolism. Arch Intern Med 1994; 154:289–297.
6. McLean J: The discovery of heparin. Circulation 1959; 19:75–78.
7. Brinkhous KM, Smith HP, Warner ED, Seegers WH: The inhibition of blood clotting: an unidentified substance which acts in conjunction with heparin to prevent the conversion of prothrombin into thrombin. Am J Physiol 1939; 125:683–687.
8. Abildgaard U: Highly purified antithrombin III with heparin cofactor activity prepared by disc electrophoresis. Scand J Clin Lab Invest 1968; 21:89–91.
9. Rosenberg RD, Lam L: Correlation between structure and functional of heparin. Proc Natl Acad Sci USA 1979; 76(2):1218–1222.
10. Lindahl U, Backstrom G, Hook M, et al: Structure of the antithrombin-binding site of heparin. Proc Natl Acad Sci USA 1979; 76(4):3198–3202.
11. Rosenberg RD, Bauer KA: The heparin-antithrombin system: a natural anticoagulant mechanism. *In* Colman RW, Hirsh J, Marder VJ, Salzman EW (eds): Hemostasis and Thrombosis: Basic Principles and Clinical Practice, 3rd ed, pp 837–860. Philadelphia: JB Lippincott, 1994.
12. Hirsh J: Heparin. N Engl J Med 1991; 324(22):1565–1574.
13. Levine MN, Hirsh J, Landefelt S, Raskob G: Hemorrhagic complications of anticoagulant therapy. Chest 1992; 102:352S–363S.
14. Brill-Edwards P, Ginsberg JS, Johnston M, Hirsh J: Establishing a therapeutic range for heparin therapy. Ann Intern Med 1993; 119:104–109.
15. Chiu HM, Hirsh J, Yung WL, et al: Relationship between the anticoagulant and antithrombotic effects of heparin in experimental venous thrombosis. Blood 1977; 49(2):171–184.
16. Basu D, Gallus AS, Hirsh J, Cade J: A prospective study of the value of monitoring heparin treatment with the activated partial thromboplastin time. N Engl J Med 1972; 287:324–327.
17. Hull RD, Raskob GE, Hirsh J, et al: Continuous intravenous heparin compared with intermittent subcutaneous heparin in the initial treatment of proximal-vein thrombosis. N Engl J Med 1986; 315:1109–1114.
18. Turpie AGG, Robinson JG, Doyle DJ, et al: Comparison of high-dose with low-dose subcutaneous heparin to prevent left ventricular mural thrombosis in patients with acute transmural anterior myocardial infarction. N Engl J Med 1989; 320:352–357.
19. Landefeld CS, Beyth FJ: Risk for anticoagulant-related bleeding: a meta-analysis. Am J Med 1993; 95:315–328.
20. Levine MN, Hirsh J, Gent M, et al: A randomized trial comparing the activated thromboplastin time with the heparin assay in patients with acute venous thromboembolism requiring large daily doses of heparin. Arch Intern Med 1994; 154:49–56.
21. Young E, Prins MH, Levine MN, Hirsh J: Heparin binding to plasma proteins, an important mechanism for heparin resistance. Thromb Haemost 1992; 67(6):639–643.
22. Raschke RA, Reilly BM, Guidry JR, et al: The weight-based heparin dosing nomogram compared with a "standard care" nomogram. Ann Intern Med 1993; 119:874–881.
23. Cruickshank MK, Levine MN, Hirsh J, et al: A standard heparin nomogram for the management of heparin therapy. Arch Intern Med 1991; 151:333–337.
24. Pini M, Pattacini C, Quintavalla R, et al: Subcutaneous vs intravenous heparin in the treatment of deep venous thrombosis-a randomized clinical trial. Thromb Haemost 1990; 64(2):222–226.
25. Clagett GP, Anderson FA, Levine MN, et al: Prevention of venous thromboembolism. Chest 1992; 102:391S–407S.
26. Collins R, Scrimgeour A, Yusuf S, et al: Reduction in fatal pulmonary embolism and venous thrombosis by perioperative administration of subcutaneous heparin. N Engl J Med 1988; 318:1162–1173.
27. Barritt DW, Jordan SC: Anticoagulant drugs in the treatment of pulmonary embolism: a controlled trial. Lancet 1960; 1:1309–1312.
28. Brandjes DPM, Heijboer H, Buller HR, et al: Acenocoumarol and heparin compared with acenocoumarol alone in the initial treatment of proximal-vein thrombosis. N Engl J Med 1992; 327:1485–1489.

29. Hommes DW, Bura A, Mazzolai L, et al: Subcutaneous heparin compared with continuous intravenous heparin administration in the initial treatment of deep vein thrombosis. Ann Intern Med 1992; 116:279–284.
30. Gallus AS, Jackaman J, Tillett J, et al: Safety and efficacy of warfarin started early after submassive venous thrombosis or pulmonary embolism. Lancet 1986; 2:1293–1296.
31. Hull RD, Raskob GE, Rosenbloom D, et al: Heparin for 5 days as compared with 10 days in the initial treatment of proximal venous thrombosis. N Engl J Med 1990; 322:1260–1264.
32. Hirsh J, Levine MN: Review: low molecular weight heparin. Blood 1992; 79(1):1–17.
33. Melissari E, Parker CJ, Wilson NV, et al: Use of low molecular weight heparin in pregnancy. Thromb Haemost 1992; 68(6):652–656.
34. Monreal M, Lafoz E, Olive A, et al: Comparison of subcutaneous unfractionated heparin with a low molecular weight heparin (fragmin) in patients with venous thromboembolism and contraindications to coumarin. Thromb Haemost 1994; 71(1):7–11.
35. Leizorovicz A, Haugh MC, Chapuis F-R, et al: Low molecular weight heparin in prevention of perioperative thrombosis. Br Med J 1992; 305:913–920.
36. Green D, Hirsh J, Heit J, et al: Low molecular weight heparin: a critical analysis of clinical trials. Am Soc Pharmacol Exp Ther 1994; 46:89–109.
37. Kearon C, Hirsh J: Starting prophylaxis for venous thromboembolism postoperatively. Arch Intern Med 1995; 155:366–372.
38. Nurmohamed MT, Rosendaal FR, Buller HR, et al: Low-molecular-weight heparin versus standard heparin in general and orthopaedic surgery: a meta-analysis. Lancet 1992; 340:152–156.
39. Anderson DR, O'Brien BJ, Levine MN, et al: Efficacy and cost of low-molecular-weight heparin compared with standard heparin for the prevention of deep vein thrombosis after total hip arthroplasty. Ann Intern Med 1993; 119:1105–1112.
40. Kakkar VV, Cohen AT, Edmonson RA, et al: Low molecular weight versus standard heparin for prevention of venous thromboembolism after major abdominal surgery. Lancet 1993; 341:259–265.
41. Leizorovicz A, Simonneau G, Decousus H, Boissel JP: Comparison of efficacy and safety of low molecular weight heparins and unfractionated heparin in initial treatment of deep venous thrombosis: meta-analysis. Br Med J 1994; 309:299–304.
41a. De Valk HW, Banga JD, Wester JWJ, et al: Comparing subcutaneous danaparoid with intravenous unfractionated heparin for the treatment of venous thromboembolism. A randomized controlled trial. Ann Intern Med 1995; 123:1–9.
42. Albada J, Nieuwenhuis HK, Sixma JJ: Treatment of acute venous thromboembolism with low molecular weight heparin (fragmin). Results of a double-blind randomized study. Circulation 1989; 80:935–940.
43. Thery C, Simonneau G, Meyer G, et al: Randomized trial of subcutaneous low-molecular-weight heparin CY 216 (Fraxiparine) compared with intravenous unfractionated heparin in the curative treatment of submassive pulmonary embolism. Circulation 1992; 85(4):1380–1389.
44. Warkentin TE, Kelton JG: Heparin-induced thrombocytopenia. Annu Rev Med 1989; 40:31–44.
45. Boshkov LK, Warkentin TE, Hayward CPM, et al: Heparin-induced thrombocytopenia and thrombosis: clinical and laboratory studies. Br J Haematol 1993; 84:322–328.
46. Magnani HN: Heparin-induced thrombocytopenia (HIT): an overview of 230 patients treated with orgaran (Org 10172). Thromb Haemost 1993; 70:554–561.
47. Demers C, Ginsberg JS, Brill-Edwards P, et al: Rapid anticoagulatin using ancrod for heparin-induced thrombocytopenia. Blood 1991; 78:2194–2197.
48. Suttie JW: Vitamin K antagonists. *In* Colman RW, Hirsh J, Marder VJ, Salzman EW (eds): Hemostasis and Thrombosis: Basic Principles and Clinical Practice, 3rd ed, pp 1562–1566. Philadelphia: JB Lippincott, 1994.
49. Link KP: The discovery of dicoumarol and its sequels. Circulation 1959; 19:97–107.
50. Hirsh J: Oral anticoagulant drugs. N Engl J Med 1991; 324:1865–1875.
51. Hirsh J, Fuster V: Guide to anticoagulant therapy part 2: oral anticoagulants. Circulation 1994; 89:1469–1480.
52. Hirsh J, Dalen JE, Deykin D, Poller L: Oral anticoagulants: mechanism of action, clinical effectiveness, and optimal therapeutic range. Chest 1992; 102:312S–326S.
53. Wells PS, Holbrook AM, Crowther NR, Hirsh J: Interactions of warfarin with drugs and food. Ann Intern Med 1994; 121:676–683.
54. Shorr RI, Ray WA, Daugherty JR, Griffin MR: Concurrent use of nonsteroidal anti-inflammatory drugs and oral anticoagulants places elderly persons at high risk for hemorrhagic peptic ulcer disease. Arch Intern Med 1993; 153:1665–1670.
55. Quick AJ: The development and use of the prothrombin tests. Circulation 1959; 19:92–96.
56. Hirsh J, Poller L, Deykin D, et al: Optimal therapeutic range for oral anticoagulants. Chest 1989; 95(suppl):5S–11S.
57. Bussey HI, Force RW, Bianco TM, Leonard AD: Reliance on prothromin time ratios causes significant errors in anticoagulation therapy. Arch Intern Med 1992; 152:278–282.
58. Le DT, Weibert RT, Sevilla BK, et al: The international normalized ratio (INR) for monitoring warfarin therapy: reliability and relation to other monitoring methods. Ann Intern Med 1994; 120:552–558.
59. Hirsh J, Poller L: The international normalized ratio: a guide to understanding and correcting its problems. Arch Intern Med 1994; 154:282–288.
60. Kornberg A, Francis CW, Pellegrini VD, et al: Comparison of native prothrombin antigen with the prothrombin time for monitoring oral anticoagulant prophylaxis. Circulation 1993; 88:454–460.
61. Hull R, Hirsh J, Jay R, et al: Different intensities of oral anticoagulant therapy in the treatment of proximal-vein thrombosis. N Engl J Med 1982; 307:1676–1681.
62. Turpie AGG, Gunstensen J, Hirsh J, et al: Randomised comparison of two intensities of oral anticoagulant therapy after tissue heart valve replacement. Lancet 1988; 1:1242–1245.
63. Saour JN, Sieck JO, Mamo LAR, Gallus AS: Trial of different intensities of anticoagulation in patients with prosthetic heart valves. N Engl J Med 1990; 322:428–432.
64. Altman P, Rouvier J, Gurfinkel E, et al: Comparison of two levels of anticoagulant therapy in patients with substitute heart valves. J Thorac Cardiovasc Surg 1991; 101:427–431.
65. Poller L, McKernan A, Thomson JM, et al: Fixed minidose warfarin: a new approach to prophylaxis against venous thrombosis after major surgery. Br Med J 1987; 295:1309–1312.
66. Bern MM, Lokich JJ, Wallach SR, et al: Very low doses of warfarin can prevent thrombosis in central venous catheters. Ann Intern Med 1990; 112:423–428.
67. Levine M, Hirsh J, Gent M, et al: Double-blind randomised trial of very-low-dose warfarin for prevention of thromboembolism in stage IV breast cancer. Lancet 1994; 343:886–889.
68. Shetty HGM, Backhouse G, Bentley DP, Routledge PA: Effective reversal of warfarin-induced excessive anticoagulation with low dose vitamin K1. Thromb Haemost 1992; 67:13–15.
69. Sevitt S: Venous thrombosis and pulmonary embolism: their prevention by oral anticoagulants. Am J Med 1962; 33:703.
70. Hull RD, Delmore TJ, Genton E, et al: Warfarin sodium versus low dose heparin in the long-term treatment of venous thrombosis. N Engl J Med 1979; 301:855–858.
71. Lagerstedt CI, Olsson CG, Fagher BO, et al: Need for long-term anticoagulant treatment in symptomatic calf-vein thrombosis. Lancet 1985; 1:515–518.
72. Hull R, Delmore T, Carter C, et al: Adjusted subcutaneous heparin versus warfarin sodium in the long-term treatment of venous thrombosis. N Engl J Med 1982; 306:189–194.
73. Research Committee of the British Thoracic Society: Optimum duration of anticoagulation for deep-vein thrombosis and pulmonary embolism. Lancet 1992; 340:873–876.
74. Levine MN, Hirsh J, Gent M, et al: Optimal duration of oral anticoagulant therapy: a randomized trial comparing four weeks with three months of warfarin in patients with proximal deep vein thrombosis. Thromb Haemost 1995; 74:606–611.
74a. Schulman S, Rhedin A-S, Lindmarker P, et al: A comparison of six weeks with six months of oral anticoagulant therapy after a first episode of venous thromboembolism. N Engl J Med 1995; 332:1661–1665.
75. Weitz J: New anticoagulant strategies: current status and future potential. Drugs 1994; 48:485–497.
76. Lefkovits J, Topol EJ: Direct thrombin inhibitors in cardiovascular medicine. Circulation 1994; 90:1522–1536.
77. Johnson PH: Hirudin: clinical potential of a thrombin inhibitor. Annu Rev Med 1994; 45:165–177.
78. Weitz JI, Hudoba M, Massel D, et al: Clot-bound thrombin is protected from inhibition by heparin-antithrombin III but is susceptible to inactivation by antithrombin III–independent inhibitors. J Clin Invest 1990; 86:385–391.
79. Maraganore JM: Thrombin, thrombin inhibitors, and the arterial thrombotic process. Thromb Haemost 1993; 70:208–211.

80. Antman EM: Hirudin in acute myocardial infarction: safety report from the Thrombolysis and Thrombin Inhibition in Myocardial Infarction (TIMI 9A) trial. Circulation 1994; 90:1624–1630.
81. GUSTO IIa Investigators: Randomized trial of intravenous heparin versus recombinant Hirudin for acute coronary syndromes. Circulation 1994; 90:1631–1637.
82. Sobel BE: Intracranial bleeding, fibrinolysis, and anticoagulation: causal connections and clinical implications. Circulation 1994; 90:2147–d2152.
83. Neuhaus KL, Essen RV, Tebbe U, et al: Safety observations from the pilot phase of the randomized r-Hirudin for improvement of thrombolysis (HIT-III) study. Circulation 1994; 90:1638–1642.
84. Eriksson BI, Kălebo P, Ekman S, et al: Direct thrombin inhibition with rec-Hirudin CGP 39393 as prophylaxis of thromboembolic complications after total hip replacement. Thromb Haemost 1994; 72:227–231.
85. Eriksson BI, Kălebo P, Ekman S, et al: A dose-finding trial evaluating the efficacy and safety of three different doses of recombinant hirudin, CGP 39393, (TMRervasc-Ciba), in patients undergoing total hip replacement [Abstract]. Thromb Haemost 1995; 73:1108.
86. Ginsberg JS, Nurmohamed MT, Gent M, et al: Use of Hirulog in the prevention of venous thrombosis after major hip or knee surgery. Circulation 1994; 90:2385–2389.
87. Parent F, Bridey F, Dreyfus M, et al: Treatment of severe venous thrombo-embolism with intravenous Hirudin (HBW 023): an open pilot study. Thromb Haemost 1993; 70:386–388.
88. Schiele F, Vuillemenot A, Kramarz Ph, et al: A pilot study of subcutaneous recombinant Hirudin (HBW 023) in the treatment of deep vein thrombosis. Thromb Haemost 1994; 71:558–562.
89. Anderson FA, Wheeler HB, Goldberg RJ, et al: Physician practices in the prevention of venous thromboembolism. Ann Intern Med 1991; 115:591–595.
90. Bell WR, Simon TL: Current status of pulmonary embolic disease: pathophysiology, diagnosis, prevention, and treatment. Am Heart J 1982; 103:239–261.

29 Acute Coronary Syndromes: Thrombosis and Thrombolysis

Ronald Freudenberger, MD
Valentin Fuster, MD, PhD

PATHOGENESIS OF ATHEROTHROMBOSIS

Early Atherosclerotic Lesions

Nineteenth century scientific theory regarding the pathogenesis of atherosclerosis involved two schools of thought: the lipid theory of Virchow and the encrustation theory of von Rokitansky.[1] Virchow suggested that lipid accumulation in the arterial wall is secondary to emigration from the blood; the lipids then form complexes with the glycosaminoglycans. Von Rokitansky suggested that fibrin deposition and subsequent organization by the fibroblast lead to intimal thickening; this process of thickening then leads to secondary lipid accumulation. A combination of these two hypotheses encompasses today's view of the initiation of the atherosclerotic process.

Vascular injury and thrombus formation are central events in the initiation and progression of the atherosclerotic process and of the initiation of the acute coronary syndromes (Fig. 29–1). Chronic mild injury to the coronary endothelium caused by disturbances in the pattern of the blood flow, local shear forces enhanced by hypertension, and circulating factors such as hypercholesterolemia, oxidized lipoproteins, glycosylated end products in diabetes, vasoactive amines, possibly chemical irritants in tobacco smoke, immune complexes, and infection potentiate this mild, chronic injury, which in turn leads to lipid and macrophage accumulation.[2] Further endothelial damage of the vessel wall leads to lipid and macrophage accumulation, attracting platelets and activates endothelial cells, which in turn leads to release of growth factors. The release of growth factors then produce migration of the smooth muscle cells.[3–5] If the entrance of lipid predominates over the efflux and over the fibrointimal response, the total composition of the lesion changes to one that has significant extracellular lipids, foam cells, and smooth muscle cells.

Advanced Atherothrombotic Lesions and Acute Coronary Syndromes

These lesions might be expected to expand in a linear manner; however, angiographic studies have shown this not to be the case. Many high-grade lesions appear in segments of the coronary artery that were previously normal.[6] It is thought that this erratic and unpredictable growth is caused by plaque disruption or fissuring, thrombosis, and fibrous organization. This leads to changes in the geometry of the plaque, intermittent plaque growth and acute occlusive or ischemic syndromes.[1] Fuster and associates[1] classified the progression of coronary atherosclerotic disease into five phases (Fig. 29–2). Phase 1 represents a small plaque that is present in most people under the age of 30 and usually progresses very slowly (the types I, II, and III lesions). Phase 2 is represented by a plaque with high lipid content that is very prone to rupture (types IV and Va lesions). This type of plaque may rupture and become substrate for thrombus formation; this process is by definition phase 3 (the type IV lesion). The same rupture of the phase 2 plaque may lead to an acute coronary syndrome, which represents phase 4 (type VI lesion).

Pathologic, angiographic, and angioscopic studies prove the association between plaque rupture and the development of unstable angina, acute myocardial infarction, and sudden ischemic death.[7–9] Perhaps of more importance, several studies have demonstrated that lesions responsible for acute coronary syndromes are more often than not lesions that are less than 50%–70% occlusive.[6, 10, 11] The plaques that are prone to rupture are those with an eccentrically placed mass of lipid covered by a fibrous cap (types IV and Va); thinning of this cap often precedes the plaque rupture (phase 3).[12] Plaque rupture exposes a thrombogenic surface to flowing blood and stimulates the development of an occlusive thrombus (phase 4).

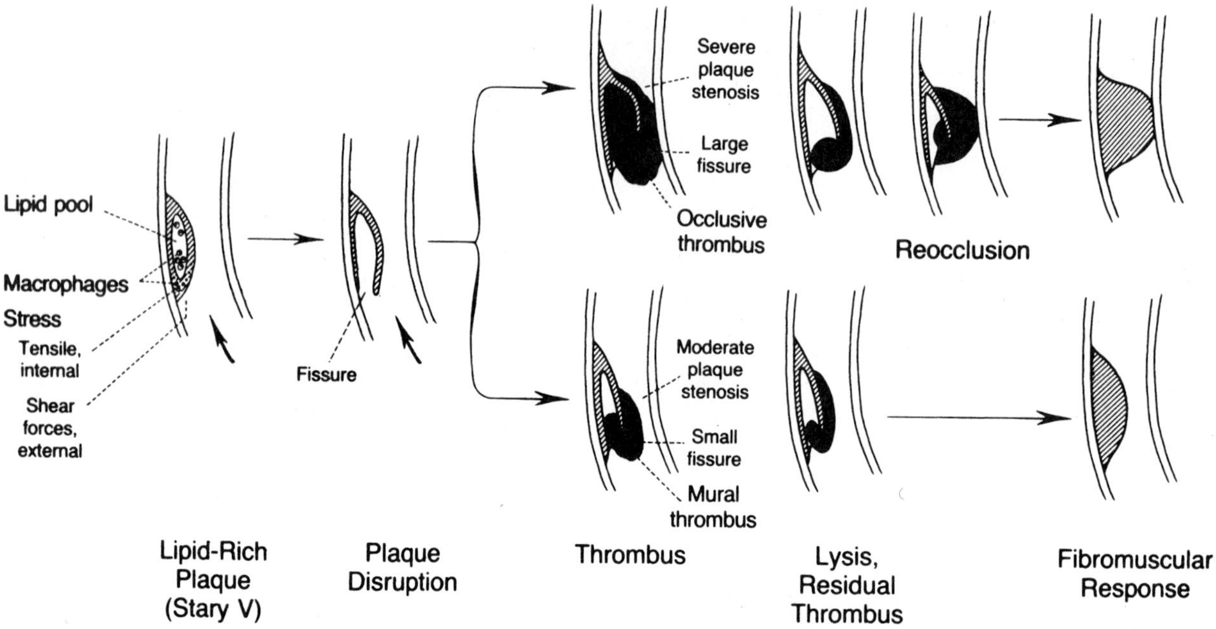

Figure 29–1. Typical dynamic evolution of the complicated disrupted plaque. (From Fuster V, Badimon L, Badimon J, Chesebro J: The pathogenesis of coronary artery disease and the acute coronary syndromes. N Engl J Med 1992; 326:242–250.)

Organization of the phases 3 and 4 thrombi may lead to progression of the atherosclerotic process (phase 5) and cause complete occlusion of the artery.

The activation of platelets, release of vasoactive substances, and impairment of vasodilator response lead to vasoconstriction, which further impairs coronary perfusion.[13] In unstable angina, there is transient or subtotal occlusion of the coronary artery, usually lasting only 10–20 minutes, with subsequent reperfusion of the vessel. In non–Q wave myocardial infarction, there is more severe plaque damage and more persistent occlusion of the vessel, often as long as 1 h in duration. As many as one fourth of the patients with non–Q wave infarction have occlusion of the infarct related vessel for more than 1 h, but the distal territory is usually supplied by collateral vessels.[14, 15] In Q wave infarctions, there is persistent occlusion of the coronary artery, which leads to cessation of blood flow for more than 1 h, resulting in transmural cellular necrosis. As discussed later, intermittent occlusion occurs because the occlusive thrombus may undergo spontaneous lysis, in the form of channels that run through the thrombus. This may restore some degree of blood flow. However, as can be expected, a very thrombogenic surface still exists in the intra-arterial surface—that is, the ruptured plaque and the thrombus itself. There are other conditions that promote rethrombosis, including the presence of activated platelets, exposed thrombin bound to fibrin and activation of other coagulation factors. These conditions also contribute to rethrombosis after successful pharmacologic thrombolysis.

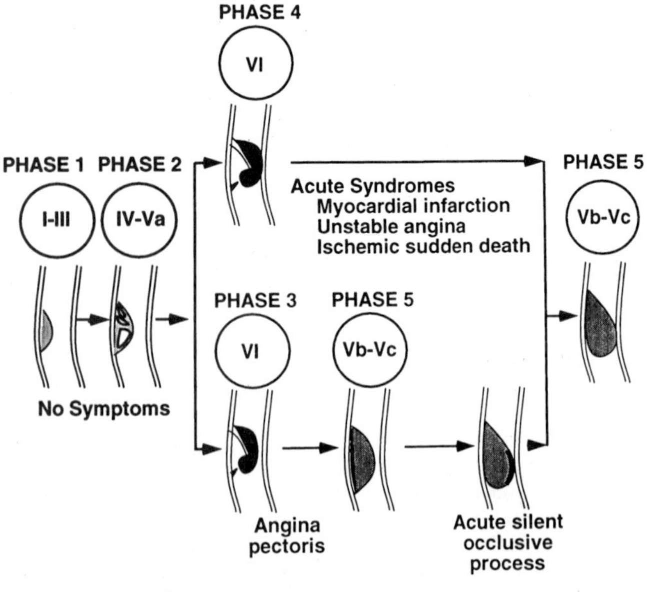

Figure 29–2. Schematic of staging (phases) and lesion morphology of the progression of coronary atherosclerosis according to the gross pathologic and clinical findings. (Modified from Fuster V, Badimon L, Badimon J, Chesebro J: The pathogenesis of coronary artery disease and the acute coronary syndromes. N Engl J Med 1992; 326:242–250.)

ACTIVATION OF PLATELETS AND COAGULATION

As mentioned, the presence of a ruptured plaque leads to thrombus formation. Several other conditions lead to thrombus formation, including platelet activation and aggregation, as well as activation of the coagulation system (Fig. 29–3). These conditions are examined as follows.

When there is superficial endothelial injury, the platelets form a monolayer to cover the exposed subendothelium. If injury is more severe, the lipid pool activates the platelets and subsequently activates the coagulation system, leading to thrombus formation. Platelet receptors are vital in the process of adhesion and aggregation. Glycoprotein Ia binds directly to exposed collagen and serves as a binding site for subendothelial von Willebrand factor. Glycoprotein IIb/IIIa is the receptor for fibrinogen and, at high shear rates, von Willebrand factor, which supports platelet-platelet interactions and aggregate formation. Platelet adhesion is determined primarily by the degree of vascular injury. Also, the wall shear rate, which is the difference between blood velocity at the center of the vessel and blood velocity along the vessel wall, is a major contributor to platelet deposition. Medium-sized stenotic lesions have the highest wall shear rate, which results in a high degree of platelet activation and deposition.[16, 17]

Once the initial platelet monolayer is formed, various factors

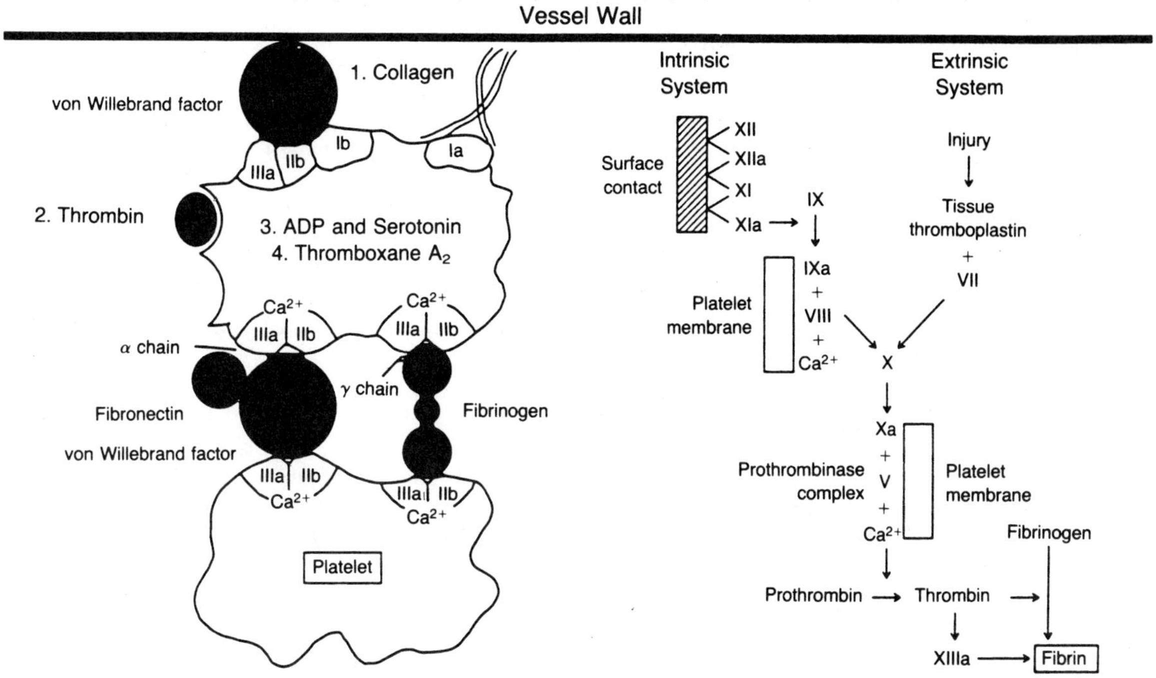

Figure 29–3. Interactions among platelet membrane receptors (Glycoproteina Ia, Ib, and IIb/IIIa). Adhesive macromolecules and the disrupted vessel wall (left panel) and a flow chart of the extinsic and intrinsic systems of the coagulation cascade (right panel). On the left panel arabic numerals indicate the pathways of platelet activation that are dependent on collagen, thrombin, ADP and serotonin, and thromboxane A2; there are also some reports that suggest the binding of von Willebrand factor to collagen or heparin. Note the interaction on the right panel between clotting factors (XII, XIIa, XI, XIa, VII, VIII, X, Xa, V and XIIIa) and the platelet membrane. (From Fuster V, Badimon L, Badimon J, Chesebro J: The pathogenesis of coronary artery disease and the acute coronary syndromes. N Engl J Med 1992; 326:242–250.)

accelerate subsequent platelet deposition. Collagen, thrombin, and the release of platelet adenosine diphosphate and thromboxane A_2 cause ongoing propagation of platelet deposition and aggregation.

Platelet aggregation in turn provides a surface for the localization and interaction of coagulation factors and accelerates the conversion of prothrombin to thrombin. This process involves activation of the intrinsic coagulation system. In addition to this system, the extrinsic pathway is activated through the release of tissue factor from the damaged endothelium. Factor X is the focal point of convergence of the intrinsic and extrinsic coagulation pathways. Once activated, factor X_a converts prothrombin to thrombin, which, as mentioned earlier, further accelerates platelet deposition. Thrombin cleaves fibrinogen to form fibrin, which activates factor XII, which in turn stabilizes the clot and induces additional platelet activation.

Several endogenous mechanisms that limit thrombus formation are important in the ongoing balance between coagulation and anticoagulation. The most important endogenous inhibitors of thrombosis are antithrombin III (AT-III), protein C, and protein S. AT-III functions by inhibiting thrombin and activated factors IX, X, XI, and XIII. Heparin, as discussed later, accelerates these inhibitory effects. Protein C is a potent anticoagulant. It functions by neutralizing a circulating inhibitor of tissue-type plasminogen activator (t-PA) and activates plasminogen.[18] Plasminogen in turn, becomes converted to plasmin, which degrades fibrinogen, prothrombin, and factors VIII and V. Plasmin also cleaves fibrin into soluble fragments on the surface of the fibrin complex. Plasmin is subsequently inactivated by α_2 plasmin inhibitor.

ANTITHROMBOTIC THERAPY IN ACUTE CORONARY SYNDROMES AND UNSTABLE ANGINA

Anticoagulants

Interest in the use of anticoagulants and antiplatelet agents varied over time in accordance with the prevailing theories of acute coronary syndromes. Initial interest in the use of these agents concerned the predominant etiologic theories about thrombus formation. However, as these theories came into question, so did the use of anticoagulants in the treatment of these syndromes. With the reemergence of the theory of thrombosis as a cause of acute coronary syndromes, interest in treatment of these syndromes with anticoagulants was renewed (Tables 29–1, 29–2).

The use of heparin for the treatment of unstable angina was suggested by Telford and Wilson.[19] In a 2 × 2 factorial design, 400 patients were randomized to atenolol, heparin, both, or neither. A 80% reduction in myocardial infarction was demonstrated in patients with unstable angina treated with heparin for 7 days. The most convincing evidence comes from the Montreal Heart Institute Study.[20] In this double-blind placebo-controlled 2 × 2 factorial design study, patients were randomized to heparin alone, aspirin alone, both, or neither. Endpoints of death, myocardial infarction, and severe unstable angina refractory to medical treatment were measured 6 ± 3 days after randomization. Heparin reduced the total event rate by 57% (p = .001). Aspirin also reduced the incidence of fatal and nonfatal myocardial infarction by 63% (p = .04) without affecting the total event rate because there was no effect on refractory angina. The combination of aspirin and heparin produced no increased benefit in comparison with heparin alone. There was a trend toward less frequent myocardial infarction in the heparin group than in the aspirin group. In a subsequent extension of this study, patients were randomized to either aspirin or heparin. The combined results of these studies demonstrated the superior reduction in the rate of myocardial infarction with heparin over aspirin.[21]

The Research Group on Instability in Coronary Artery Disease (RISC)[22] study examined patients with unstable angina or non–Q wave myocardial infarction. Patients were randomized to receive aspirin and or intermittent intravenous heparin. Aspirin therapy, in comparison with no-aspirin therapy, significantly reduced the risk ratios of fatal and nonfatal myocardial infarction. Heparin did not

TABLE 29–1. MAJOR ANTITHROMBOTIC TRIALS IN UNSTABLE ANGINA

Trial	Follow-Up	Drug	Reduction in Death or Myocardial Infarction (%)	*p*
Telford and Wilson[19]	7 days	Heparin	80	<.05
Theroux et al.[20]	6 days	Heparin		<.001
		Aspirin + heparin	88	.001
RISC[22]	3 months	Heparin	5	Nonsignificant
		Aspirin + heparin	68	<.0005
ATACS[24]	3 months	Aspirin + heparin	25	.06

Abbreviations: RISC, Research Group on Instability in Coronary Artery Disease; ATACS, Antithrombotic Therapy in Acute Coronary Syndromes Study Group.

show such benefit. However, the group treated with the combination of heparin and aspirin showed the lowest event rate at 5 days.

It is important to be aware of a rebound phenomenon (recrudescence of ischemia) that may occur when heparin is discontinued. This effect may be blunted when aspirin is given as concomitant therapy.[23]

Antiplatelet Agents

Antiplatelet agents have been found to reduce rates of acute myocardial infarction and death over the short term and long term in four large trials of unstable angina.[23] In the Veterans Administration Cooperative Study, 1266 men with unstable angina were randomized to receive 325 mg/day of aspirin or placebo for 12 weeks. During the treatment period, the aspirin group demonstrated a risk reduction of 51%, and the overall benefits of aspirin were maintained during the 1-year follow-up period.[24] In the Canadian Multicenter Trial, 55 patients with unstable angina were randomized to receive aspirin (1300 mg/day), sulfinpyrazone (800 mg/day), the combination of both, or placebo. After 18 months, the incidence of myocardial infarction and death was reduced in the aspirin groups from 17% to 8.6%; sulfinpyrazone demonstrated no benefit.[25]

The Montreal Heart Institute Study randomized 479 patients with unstable angina to aspirin (325 mg b.i.d.), intravenous heparin, the combination of both, or placebo. After 6 days the final medical regimen for individual patients was based on the results of cardiac catheterization. Aspirin reduced the rate of myocardial infarction by 72% in comparison with placebo, and heparin reduced the rate by 89%.[20] In the European RISC study group, 794 men with unstable angina or non–Q wave infarction were randomized to receive 75 mg/day of aspirin for 3 months, intravenous heparin for 5 days, both, or neither. At the end of 3 months the incidence of death or myocardial infarction was significantly reduced by aspirin and, to a greater extent, by the combination of aspirin and heparin. The more recent Antithrombotic Therapy in Acute Coronary Syndromes Study Group (ATACS)[26] trial (Fig. 29–4) randomized 214 patients, who were not prior aspirin users, with either unstable angina or non–Q wave myocardial infarction, to receive aspirin alone or aspirin plus anticoagulants. The trial was begun by a mean of 9.5 h after the onset of chest pain and continued for 12 weeks. There was a significant reduction in total ischemic events in the combination group vs. aspirin-alone group (10.5% vs. 27%, $p = .004$) at the end of 14 days. At the end of 12 weeks, there was a trend toward reduction in total ischemic events (13% vs. 25%, $p = .06$).

TABLE 29–2. MAJOR ASPIRIN TRIALS IN UNSTABLE ANGINA

Study	No. of Patients	Dose (mg/day)	Duration of Follow-Up	Relative Risk Reduction
Lewis et al.[24]	1338	324	3 months	51%
Cairns et al.[25]	555	1300	24 months	51%
Theroux et al.[20]	479	650	6 days	72%
RISC[22]	796	75	5 days	57%
			30 days	46%

Abbreviation: RISC, Research Group on Instability in Coronary Artery Disease.

Ticlopidine in unstable angina was examined in patients with unstable angina.[27] The administration of ticlopidine in a dose of 250 mg twice a day for 6 months was found to reduce the incidence of death and myocardial infarction by 46%. The potential side effects of neutropenia and (rarely) thrombocytopenia warrant careful monitoring.

In summary, ample evidence suggests that the use of aspirin in unstable angina reduces the incidence of myocardial infarction and death. The combination of aspirin and heparin in unstable angina and non–Q wave myocardial infarction reduces total ischemic events in the early phase of unstable angina.

Direct Thrombin Inhibitors

In view of the central role of thrombin in the coagulation process, there is much enthusiasm for the development of direct thrombin inhibitors for use in acute coronary syndromes. Several small studies have examined the efficacy of these agents in treating unstable angina. Sharma and associates administered Hirulog to 20 patients with unstable angina for 5 days. They found a more favorable outcome, in terms of death, myocardial infarction, intractable angina, intracoronary thrombus, and bleeding, in patients who received Hirulog than in those who received heparin infusion (by historical comparison).[28]

The seventh Thrombolysis in Myocardial Infarction (TIMI-7) study examined 400 patients with unstable angina who received Hirulog infusion for 72 h at one of four escalating doses. The patients who received the three highest doses, in comparison with the patients who received the lowest dose, had significant reductions in rates of death and nonfatal myocardial infarction in the hospital, at discharge, and 6 weeks after discharge.[29]

Topol and associates studied 363 patients with rest pain, an abnormal electrocardiogram (ECG), and angiographically visible thrombus at the culprit lesion. These patients were randomized to one of four escalating doses of hirudin or to the heparin control group. The endpoints were predetermined angiographic characteristics of the culprit lesion. Patients treated with hirudin showed greater improvement in these characteristics. There were seven procedure-related major hemorrhages and three spontaneous hemorrhages that did not necessitate transfusion in the hirudin group.[30]

Results of these studies are encouraging. However, further studies to determine optimal dosing and the optimal protocol are needed.

Thrombolytics

There is little current experimental evidence to support the use of thrombolytic therapy in unstable angina. Many small and inconclu-

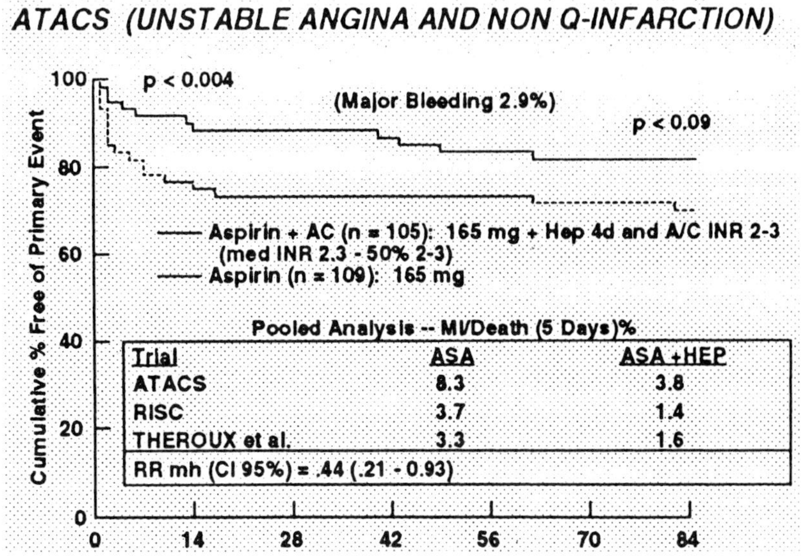

Figure 29–4. Data from the ATACS[27] trial examining the use of aspirin versus aspirin plus anticoagulation in unstable angina and non Q-wave myocardial infarction, demonstrates an improvement in event free survival in the combination therapy group. Pooled analysis from the ATACS,[27] the RISC,[23] and the Theroux[20] study groups demonstrate a relative risk reduction (RR) of .44 in the combination group.

sive studies conducted between 1980 and 1990 evaluated the use of thrombolytic therapy in unstable angina.[18] Many of these studies are difficult to evaluate because of the different patient populations, timing of angiography, dose, and route of administration of the thrombolytic agent.

Two large trials evaluating thrombolytics give important insight into the issue of thrombolytic agents in unstable angina. The Unstable Angina Study Using Eminase (anistreplase) (UNASEM) trial was a large, randomized, placebo-controlled trial designed to evaluate both the angiographic and clinical outcomes of the use of Eminase in unstable angina. One hundred fifty-nine patients with either crescendo angina or rest pain of less than 4 weeks' duration and with ischemic ECG changes were randomized to receive intravenous anisoylated plasminogen streptokinase activator complex (APSAC) or placebo. All patients were randomized before angiography and within 12 h of the last ischemic episode. All patients received aspirin and heparin. Angiography was performed within 3 h of randomization and 12–28 h later.[31] The APSAC group was found to have a significantly decreased lesion severity in comparison with the placebo group ($p = .002$). However, of importance is that 26% of the APSAC group and only 18% of the placebo group had total occlusion of the artery. APSAC opened 70% of the occluded arteries, and placebo opened none. The improvement in the occluded arteries accounted for the entire difference in degree of stenosis before and after therapy. Despite a possible difference between the two groups in angiographic appearance, there was no significant difference in clinical outcome.

The TIMI-IIIB study was designed to evaluate the use of t-PA and early angiography and revascularization for patients with unstable angina. All patients received heparin and aspirin; 606 patients also received t-PA, and 706 received placebo. At 42 days and at 1 year, there were no differences between the two groups in rates of myocardial infarction and death.[79]

Some evidence suggests that thrombolytic therapy in unstable angina may be detrimental. In UNASEM the incidence of recurrent ischemia and myocardial infarction tended to be higher in the group receiving thrombolytic agents than in the group receiving placebo ($p = .06$). Some of the smaller studies had similar results.

Possible reasons for the failure of thrombolytic therapy to improve outcome in unstable angina as opposed to acute infarction relate to pathophysiologic observations in unstable angina. In unstable angina, the incidence of total occlusion of the culprit vessel is significantly lower than in acute myocardial infarction.[18] In addition, Falk[32] found partial organization and layering of the thrombus in patients with unstable angina. Thus much of the thrombus formation in unstable angina may be beneath the fibrous cap, rather than within the lumen of the artery. This may allow only small amounts of thrombus to be accessible to the thrombolytic agent.

Current Recommendations

All patients with unstable angina should immediately receive at least 75 mg of chewable aspirin and intravenous heparin (bolus followed by continuous infusion in doses sufficient to raise the partial thromboplastin time 1.5–2 times higher than control levels). The combination of aspirin and heparin is probably more efficacious than either agent alone. This is particularly true in view of aspirin's ability to blunt the rebound phenomenon when heparin is discontinued. There is little current experimental evidence to support the administration of thrombolytic therapy to patients with unstable angina.

MYOCARDIAL INFARCTION

Antithrombotic agents used in acute myocardial infarction may have these important benefits: (1) prevention of rethrombosis, reinfarction, and mortality after thrombolysis, either endogenous or pharmacologic; (2) prevention of mural thrombus formation and embolization; and (3) prevention of venous thromboembolism. In addition, antithrombotic agents are of benefit in the prevention of late thrombosis or reinfarction and mortality (i.e., secondary prevention).

Acute Myocardial Infarction, Reinfarction, and Mortality

Thrombolytics

Goals of Thrombolytic Therapy. The goal of thrombolytic therapy during acute myocardial infarction is to restore patency as quickly as possible with the lowest rate of bleeding complications and rethrombosis (Table 29–3). Factors correlated with reperfusion of the infarct-affected vessel relate to the age and location of the occluded vessel and the concentration of plasminogen and plasmin inhibitors on the thrombus. The use of a loading dose was developed to overcome natural or acquired inhibitors, and the subsequent use of a maintenance infusion was developed to maintain a large enough concentration of the fresh plasminogen activator to the thrombus

TABLE 29–3. CLINICAL USE OF THROMBOLYTIC AGENTS

Indications for Thrombolytic Therapy
Patients presenting with substernal chest pain lasting at least 20 min accompanied by 0.1 mV ST segment elevation in the limb leads or >0.2 mV ST segment elevation in two contiguous limb leads
Patients presenting within 12 h of symptom onset
Absolute Contraindications to Thrombolytic Therapy
Acute pericarditis
Possible aortic dissection
Active internal bleeding
Recent (<2 months) cerebrovascular accident
Intracranial disease (neoplasm, arteriovenous fistula, aneurysm, hemorrhage)
Relative Contraindications to Thrombolytic Therapy
Recent craniospinal surgery
Pregnancy
Severe uncontrolled hypertension (SBP >200 or DBP >110)
Bleeding diathesis
Thrombocytopenia or coagulopathy
Major surgery in the preceding 10 days
Puncture of a noncompressible vessel
Prolonged CPR with evidence of resulting chest trauma

Abbreviations: SBP, systolic blood pressure; DBP, diastolic blood pressure; CPR, cardiopulmonary resuscitation.

surface to promote dissolution. Once dissolution has occurred, the risk of rethrombosis reappears as a result of the continued presence of a thrombogenic surface (i.e., the ruptured plaque). Regimens to minimize the risk of rethrombosis include the use of prolonged infusions, the use of agents with longer half-lives, and the concomitant use of antithrombotics such as heparin and possibly hirudin and related compounds.

Reperfusion. The principal mechanism by which thrombolytic therapy confers benefit is by lysis of the occlusive coronary thrombus. Accordingly, several studies have used angiography to document patency rates with various thrombolytic regimens. The following findings have emerged from these studies: (1) coronary angiography performed within the first 6 h of a myocardial infarction in evolution will reveal completely occlusive thrombosis in 85% of cases; (2) the spontaneous reperfusion rate is about 10% during acute coronary angiographic evaluation,[33] and the spontaneous patency rate is about 35% among patients undergoing angiography at 12–24 h and up to 83% by 3 weeks; (3) reocclusion occurs in 5%–30% of vessels that are initially reperfused, most of it by 24 h but with additional reocclusions over subsequent days; and (4) bedside markers of reperfusion often are not correlated with true reperfusion.

These observations highlight the need for careful use of terminology in reports of angiographic outcome. Reperfusion and reocclusion rates can be determined only when pretreatment angiography has been performed. The reocclusion rate is the proportion of initially occluded vessels that are subsequently open; reocclusion is the proportion of vessels observed to reperfuse that then reocclude. Patency rate is assessed by obtaining an angiogram at a given time and is an aggregate of the rates of initial patency, reperfusion after thrombolytics and spontaneously, and reocclusion. Because pretreatment angiograms are usually omitted to avoid delay in the use of intravenous thrombolytics, true reperfusion and reocclusion rates have been determined in relatively few studies and were routinely available only when intracoronary thrombolytics were commonly used.

Bedside markers of reperfusion have been suggested.[34] These include ST segment normalization; symptom resolution; and ventricular arrhythmias, particularly accelerated idioventricular rhythm. Califf and associates[34] studied 386 patients given t-PA and found that of those with complete resolution of the ST segment elevation before the 90-min angiogram, 97% showed perfusion on the angiogram. Of those with partial improvement, 84% showed perfusion, but this finding occurred in only 6% and 38% of patients with complete resolution and those with partial resolution, respectively. Of patients in whom chest pain resolved completely before the angiogram, 84% showed perfusion. However, this finding occurred in only 29% of all patients. Although arrhythmias occurred frequently in the first 90% of therapy, no particular type of arrhythmia or the occurrence of an arrhythmia was associated with a higher rate of patency. Christian and colleagues[35] found that the subjective response of chest pain to thrombolysis was significantly associated with myocardial salvage, as assessed by Sestamibi injection before thrombolysis and at hospital discharge. Complete relief was associated with the greatest degree of salvage, but this finding was present in only 45% of patients. Shah and associates[36] found that rapid and progressive decrease in pain and ST elevation is a reliable marker of perfusion with TIMI grade 3 flow. Accelerated idioventricular rhythm and bradycardia, although specific to perfusion, do not occur in all patients with reperfusion.

Factors relating to success of thrombolysis include optimal selection of patients, optimal timing of thrombolytic therapy, and optimal dosing regimens. In most clinical trials, only 33% of patients screened for thrombolytic therapy received it. Factors relating to exclusion include timing, age, equivocal ECG changes, and other general medical contraindications.[37] Part of the reason why only a small percentage of patients presenting with acute myocardial infarction receive thrombolytic therapy concerns certain characteristics of the patients who are assumed to be at high risk of bleeding such as what was initially thought to be the case with the elderly. The Gruppo Italiano per lo Studio della Sopravivenza nell'Infarto Miocardico (GISSI), the second International Study of Infarct Survival (ISIS-2), and Global Utilization of Streptokinase and Tissue Plasminogen Activator for Occluded Coronary Arteries (GUSTO) did not exclude patients on the basis of age. In spite of a higher incidence of hemorrhagic stroke, the highest absolute mortality-related benefit in all three of these studies was in the elderly. Therefore, in the absence of other reasons to exclude the patient, age should not be an exclusionary criterion for the use of thrombolytic therapy. However, the relative benefit of t-PA in the GUSTO trial was less in the elderly group than in those less than 75 years of age.

Many patients do not receive thrombolytic therapy because of a lack of specific electrocardiographic changes. The classical ECG criteria for the administration of thrombolytics that were used in many of the clinical trials are at least 0.1 mV of ST segment elevation in two contiguous limb leads and more than 0.2 mV of ST segment elevation in two contiguous precordial leads. Many questions have arisen concerning the use of thrombolytic therapy in ST segment depression and the presence of a new left bundle branch block pattern on the ECG. In an effort to answer these questions, the Thrombolytic Therapy Trialists Group published a meta-analysis of nine large controlled clinical trials of thrombolytic agents. These investigators found that new bundle branch block was associated with a high risk of death, and administration of thrombolytic therapy resulted in a 25% reduction in mortality ($p < .05$). There was no evidence of decreased mortality in patients with ST segment depression or normal ECGs in the presence of clinical findings that were consistent with acute myocardial infarction.[38]

Some clinicians raise concerns over administration of thrombolytic agents to patients with diabetic retinopathy because of a concern of possible retinal hemorrhage. No cases of this complication have been reported despite administration of thrombolytic therapy to thousands of patients with diabetes mellitus in many large clinical trials; resultant decrease in mortality has been associated with thrombolysis.

The *timing* of thrombolytic therapy has received considerable attention (Tables 29–4, 29–5). It was originally thought that there was little benefit in patients who presented more than 4 h after the onset of chest pain. However, the ISIS-2 trial demonstrated a signifi-

TABLE 29–4. EFFECT OF INTRAVENOUS THROMBOLYTIC THERAPY ON MORTALITY

Study	No. of Patients	Drug	Time (Hours)	Follow-Up	Mortality With Drug (%)	Mortality in Control Group (%)	*p*
GISSI-2[46]	11,806	Streptokinase	<12	Hospital	10.7	13.0	0.002
ISAM	1741	Streptokinase	<6	21 days	6.3	7.1	Nonsignificant
ISIS-2[39]	17,187	Streptokinase	<24	5 weeks	9.3	12.0	0.0001
W. Wash	368	Streptokinase	<6	14 days	6.3	9.6	0.23
GAMIS[73]	313	APSAC	<4	28 days	5.6	12.6	0.032
LATE[40]	5711	t-PA	6–24	8.9 months	8.9	10.3	Nonsignificant
	5711	t-PA	6–12	8.9 months	8.9	12.0	0.02
EMERAS[41]	4534	Streptokinase	6–24	11.9 months	11.9	12.4	Nonsignificant
	4534	Streptokinase	7–12	11.7 months	11.7	13.2	Nonsignificant

Abbreviations: GISSI, Gruppo Italiano per lo Studio della Sopravivenza nell'Infarto Miocardico; ISAM, Intravenous Streptokinase in Acute Myocardial Infarction; ISIS-2, second International Study of Infarct Survival; W. Wash, Western Washington Myocardial Infarction Registry and Emergency Department Tissue Plasminogen Activator Treatment Trial; GAMIS, German-Austrian Myocardial Infarction Study; LATE, Late Assessment of Thrombolytic Efficacy; EMERAS, Estudios Multicentrico Estreptoquinasa Republica Americas Sud; APSAC, anisoylated plasminogen streptokinase activator complex; t-PA, tissue plasminogen activator.

cant reduction in mortality among patients treated with thrombolytic therapy between 5 and 24 h after the onset of chest pain (Fig. 29–5).[39] Two randomized studies were subsequently performed to directly address this issue. The Late Assessment of Thrombolytic Efficacy (LATE) trial administered t-PA or placebo to 5709 patients 6–24 h after acute infarction.[40] The 35-day mortality rate was reduced in patients receiving thrombolytic therapy 6–12 h after symptom onset. However, there was only a nonsignificant trend toward reduction of mortality in those receiving t-PA after 12 h. In the Estudios Multicentrico Estreptoquinasa Republica Americas Sud (EMERAS) trial,[41] there was a nonsignificant mortality-related benefit among patients receiving streptokinase 6–12 h after infarction and no trend toward mortality reduction in those treated later.

Those patients who continue to have ST segment elevation but in whom chest pain resolves nevertheless benefit from administration of thrombolytic therapy. By using technetium-99m Sestamibi injection before administering thrombolytic agents and at hospital discharge, Christian and associates demonstrated that patients who had continued ST segment elevation and resolution of chest discomfort showed a significant degree of myocardial salvage (11%) with the use of thrombolytic therapy.[35]

Thus the indications for thrombolytic therapy (i.e., *optimal selection of patients)* are as follows:

1. Patients presenting with substernal chest pain lasting at least 20 min and accompanied by >0.1 mV ST segment elevation in two contiguous limb leads or >0.2 mV ST segment elevation in two or more contiguous leads.
2. Those presenting within 6 h after the onset of chest pain and who have unequivocal indications for thrombolytic therapy.
3. Those presenting 6–12 h after the onset of chest pain who may benefit from use of these agents.

Patients presenting 12–24 h after the onset of chest pain probably should not receive these agents. Patients of all ages may benefit from thrombolytics agents, but there is an increase in hemorrhagic cerebral infarctions with increasing age.

Contraindications to thrombolytic agents can be separated into absolute and relative contraindications. Absolute contraindications include possible aortic dissection, acute pericarditis, and active bleeding. Relative contraindications include intracranial neoplasm, arteriovenous fistula or aneurysm, recent craniospinal surgery or trauma, cerebral hemorrhage at any time, pregnancy, severe uncontrolled hypertension (systolic blood pressure > 200 or diastolic blood pressure > 120), bleeding diathesis, thrombocytopenia or coagulopathy, major surgery in the previous 2–4 weeks, puncture of a noncompressible vessel, and administration of prolonged cardiopulmonary resuscitation (CPR) with evidence of resulting chest trauma.

Optimal Dosing Regimens. Various dosing regimens have been proposed for the use of thrombolytic therapy, and regimens for combination therapy have been suggested. Dosing regimens with the

TABLE 29–5. INTRAVENOUS THROMBOLYTIC THERAPY: COMPARISON OF AGENTS AND MORTALITY

Trial	No. of Patients	Drugs	Time (Hours)	Follow-Up	Mortality With Streptokinase (%)	Mortality With t-PA (%)	Mortality With t-PA + Streptokinase (%)	Mortality With APSAC (%)	*p*
GISSI-2[46]	20,891	t-PA	<6	Hospital	8.5	8.0			Nonsignificant
GUSTO[48]	41,021	t-PA	<6	30 days	7.3	6.3			.001
		t-PA + streptokinase					7.0		
ISIS-3[47]	46,091	t-PA,	<24						
		APSAC		35 days	10.6	10.3		10.5	Nonsignificant

Abbreviations: t-PA, tissue plasminogen activator; APSAC, anisoylated plasminogen streptokinase activator complex; GISSI-2, Gruppo Italiano per lo Studio della Sopravivenza nell'Infarto Miocardico (second study); GUSTO, Global Utilization of Streptokinase and Tissue Plasminogen Activator for Occluded Coronary Arteries; ISIS-3, third International Study of Infarct Survival.

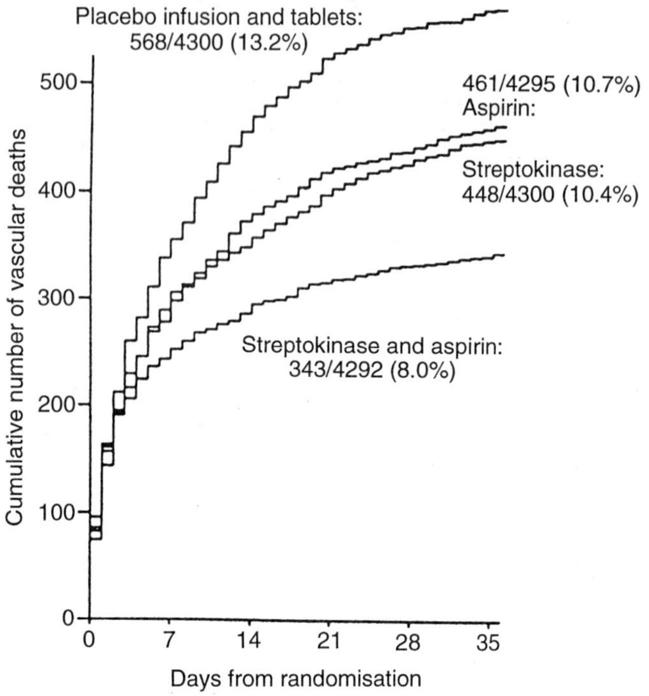

Figure 29–5. Cumulative vascular mortality within 35 days after suspected acute myocardial infarction. Odds reduction in mortality were 23 percent for aspirin alone, 25 percent for streprokinase alone, and 42 percent for the combination of aspirin and streptokinase. (From the ISIS-2 Collaborative group: Randomized trial of intravenous streptokinase, oral aspirin, both or neither in 17,187 cases of suspected acute myocardial infarction: ISIS-2. Lancet 2:349–360, 1988. By permission from the Lancet, Ltd.)

use of t-PA, including the use of weight-adjusted dosing, front-loading, and double-bolus t-PA, have been written. Patency rates have been reported in several angiographic studies in which various dosage regimens were used; the most efficacious, as assessed by the 90-min patency rate, is the front-loaded regimen.[42–45] The GUSTO trial[48] compared accelerated t-PA and the combination of t-PA and streptokinase. The findings—that accelerated t-PA in a regimen of 15-mg bolus, 0.75 mg/kg over the next 30 min, and 0.5 mg/kg over the next 60 min was superior to streptokinase and to the combination of the two lytic agents—suggest that using both front-loaded and weight-adjusted regimens offer superior mortality-related benefits over standard regimens of streptokinase.

Which Agent, Which Patient: An Algorithm for Treatment. Much accumulated information irrefutably demonstrates a reduction in mortality rates after acute myocardial infarction with the use of intravenous streptokinase, t-PA, or APSAC.[33] The GISSI-2,[46] the International Study Group, and the third International Study of Infarct Survival (ISIS-3)[47] compared these agents and found no difference in survival. GISSI-2 and ISIS-3 received some criticism concerning the timing and route of administration of heparin therapy. The GUSTO study examined new strategies of administration and dosing by combining different thrombolytic agents and by changing the route in which heparin was given as adjunctive therapy.

The GUSTO[48] trial attempted to address these questions. It enrolled 41,021 patients with acute myocardial infarctions from 1081 centers in 15 countries, all of which made it one of the largest and best executed clinical trials ever performed. The patients were randomly assigned to one of four treatment groups: (1) accelerated t-PA (a bolus followed by a conventional infusion dose with the highest concentration given during the first 30 min and the total dose given over a 1.5-h period rather than the conventional 3-h infusion) plus intravenous heparin; (2) streptokinase plus subcutaneous heparin; (3) streptokinase plus intravenous heparin; or (4) both thrombolytic agents, whereby t-PA was given in a conventional dose but over 1 h rather than 3 h and a lower dose of streptokinase was administered with intravenous heparin. All patients received 160–325 mg of aspirin daily.

In contrast to GISSI-2 and ISIS-3, the GUSTO investigators found that at 30 days, accelerated t-PA and heparin significantly reduced the mortality rate to 6.3%, in comparison with 7.3% with the two streptokinase-only strategies. The combination strategy was accompanied by an intermediate mortality rate of 7.0%. Thus, accelerated t-PA appeared to save one additional life per 100 people treated, but it was also associated with a higher risk of in-hospital stroke (0.2–0.3 per 100), a rate similar to that seen in GISSI-2 and ISIS-3. In analyses of prespecified subgroups, there appeared to be a smaller net benefit or none for t-PA over streptokinase in patients over age 75, in those with inferior myocardial infarctions, and in those presenting more than 4 h after the onset of myocardial infarction. The group aged over 75 had smaller or no net benefit of accelerated t-PA because of a particularly high rate of intracranial hemorrhage. Of importance is that even in this very large study, there was a lack of statistical significance to rule out a definitive benefit in these subgroups.

The rationale for using accelerated t-PA was to achieve earlier and more complete recanalization of the infarct-related artery. An angiographic substudy of GUSTO appeared to support the hypothesis that earlier reperfusion leads to improved survival. The results of GISSI-2, ISIS-3, and GUSTO suggest that for streptokinase, the addition of heparin to full-dose aspirin produces no benefit. These studies did not assess the results of intravenous heparin in comparison with no heparin with the use of t-PA in the setting of adequate-dose heparin.

Although definitive recommendations about the most cost-effective thrombolytic regimen must await further analysis of the GUSTO data and data from other large trials, the following guidelines may provide a reasonable framework for therapy and are compatible with the available data.

Patients with acute myocardial infarctions who are seen within the first 6 h of the onset of symptoms or within 12 h of large or anterior infarctions and who have no contraindications should receive chewable aspirin (160–325 mg) and an intravenous thrombolytic agent. It is of paramount importance that the many patients who are eligible for thrombolytic therapy receive a thrombolytic agent. The authors believe that administration of any agent is of greater importance than which agent is given. Adjunctive intravenous heparin should be considered when t-PA is used, but when streptokinase or APSAC is used, there is little evidence of additional benefit when heparin is added to full-dose aspirin. Second, on the basis of subgroup analysis in the GUSTO trial, which is limited by lack of statistical power, streptokinase may be an appropriate thrombolytic agent for patients over age 75, for patients with small inferior infarctions, and for patients presenting more than 4 h after the onset of symptoms.[49] Third, the GUSTO trial shows that accelerated t-PA is preferable to streptokinase for patients under age 75 who have anterior or large infarctions and who present within 4 h of symptom onset and for those who have previous exposure to streptokinase or APSAC, because antibodies against these agents may develop after the first exposure. Finally, patients with contraindications to thrombolytic therapy or severe hemodynamic compromise should be considered for immediate coronary angioplasty.

Antiplatelet Agents

The use of aspirin in acute myocardial infarction is proved.

Aspirin Without Thrombolytic Therapy. For patients with acute myocardial infarction, the landmark ISIS-2 study,[39] which included more than 17,000 patients, randomized patients to receive aspirin (160 mg/day for 30 days), intravenous streptokinase, both, or neither. In the group taking aspirin alone, there was a 23% reduction in mortality in comparison with the group taking neither streptokinase nor aspirin (see Figure 29–5); the risk reduction for nonfatal reinfarction was 49%, and that for nonfatal stroke was 46%.

Treatment With Thrombolytic Therapy. In ISIS-2, when aspirin was combined with streptokinase, a 42% reduction in mortality was seen. Aspirin alone, as previously stated, resulted in a 23% reduction in mortality, and streptokinase alone yielded a 25% reduction in mortality (see Figure 29–5). Thus the effects of aspirin and thrombolytic agents appear to be additive. No significant difference in major hemorrhage necessitating transfusion was seen. However, there was a small but significant increase in minor hemorrhage in the aspirin group. Aspirin reduced the rate of nonfatal reinfarction and stroke by 49% and 46%, respectively. A follow-up study of ISIS-2 found that at 4 years, there was a persistent mortality benefit.[50]

Since ISIS-2, aspirin has become the accepted adjunctive therapy for acute myocardial infarction. Most clinical trials involving patients with acute myocardial infarction include full-dose aspirin; any new agent must further improve the efficacy beyond that of aspirin in order to be used routinely.

Anticoagulants

There have been no trials of aspirin vs. heparin during acute myocardial infarction in the absence of thrombolytic therapy. However, there are studies examining anticoagulants in conjunction with thrombolytic agents.

Heparin in the presence of streptokinase was examined in many studies, including GISSI-2, ISIS-3, Studio Sulla Calciparina nell'Angina e nella Thrombosi Ventriculare nell'Infarto (SCATI), and GUSTO (Table 29–6). In GISSI-2, patients who received streptokinase and heparin beginning 12 h after the infusion of the thrombolytic agent demonstrated a trend ($p < .02$) toward a decrease in mortality in comparison with those who received streptokinase alone. The mortality rate for those receiving t-PA was the same regardless of whether heparin was added to the regimen.[46] ISIS-3[47] found that heparin (given subcutaneously, 12,500 units every 12 h starting 4 h after the start of thrombolytic therapy) and aspirin, given with t-PA or streptokinase, resulted in a nearly significant decrease in mortality during heparin therapy ($p = .06$). There was a trend toward a decrease in hospital reinfarction rate in the heparin group ($p = .09$). This early benefit was lost when the primary endpoint of 35 days was reached. Also, heparin produced a small excess of extracerebral hemorrhages (1.0% in comparison with 0.8%, $p < .01$) and intracerebral hemorrhages (0.056% in comparison with 0.40%, $p < .05$).

The SCATI[51] group randomized 711 patients to either heparin or no heparin. These patients, unlike the patients in GISSI-2, ISIS-3 and GUSTO, did not receive aspirin. This study found a 44% reduction in mortality when 12,500 units of subcutaneous heparin was given to patients with acute myocardial infarction. This reduction in mortality was significant both in the patients who received streptokinase and in those who did not receive the thrombolytic agent. The GUSTO study provided great insight into the issue of anticoagulation as therapy adjunctive to thrombolysis.[48] It enrolled 41,021 patients with myocardial infarctions who were randomized to four treatment groups: (1) streptokinase and subcutaneous heparin, (2) streptokinase and intravenous heparin, (3) accelerated t-PA and intravenous heparin, or (4) the combination of both agents with intravenous heparin. The results were a significant reduction in mortality in the accelerated t-PA and intravenous heparin groups in comparison with the streptokinase groups ($p < .001$). The rates of hemorrhagic stroke were 0.49%, 0.54%, 0.72%, and 0.94%, respectively. The difference in the t-PA group in comparison with the streptokinase group was statistically significant ($p = .03$). There was no difference between the t-PA and the streptokinase groups in extracranial bleeding. The combined end incidence of nonfatal hemorrhagic stroke and death was significantly reduced for the t-PA group in comparison with the streptokinase group. The lessons learned from GUSTO are that there is a small but significant increase in hemorrhagic stroke among patients who receive t-PA and high-dose heparin. This group also demonstrated significantly improved survival rates. There was no advantage to the use of intravenous heparin with streptokinase.

As might be suspected, there were similar findings with the use of APSAC. The Duke University Clinical Cardiology Studies–1 found no difference in coronary artery patency between patients who received APSAC with heparin and patients who received APSAC alone.[1]

Heparin in the Presence of t-PA. Several smaller studies examining the use of heparin in conjunction with t-PA have been conducted. In Thrombosis And Myocardial Infarction–3 (TAMI-3), 134 patients were randomized to receive non–front-loaded t-PA with or without heparin (10,000-unit intravenous bolus).[52] Aspirin was not

TABLE 29–6. ADJUNCTIVE HEPARIN THERAPY WITH STREPTOKINASE

	GISSI-2[46]	ISIS-3[47]	GUSTO[48]
No. of patients	12,490	41,299	41,021
Design	2 × 2 factorial	3 × 2 factorial	Four arms
Lytic agent		t-PA vs. streptokinase vs. alteplase	Streptokinase vs. accelerated t-PA vs. t-PA + streptokinase
Heparin arm	Streptokinase vs. alteplase	12,500 units subcutaneously q 12 h vs. no heparin	12,500 units subcutaneously q 12 h vs. 5000 units intravenous bolus, then 1000 units/h (in streptokinase patients)
Heparin start	12,500 units subcutaneously q 12 h vs. no heparin	4 h after thrombolytic	Subcutaneously 4 h after thrombolytic; intravenously after streptokinase infusion
Heparin duration	12 h after thrombolytic	7 days	Subcutaneously: 7 days; intravenously: ≥48 h
Primary endpoint	To hospital discharge Death, severe LV dysfunction at hospital discharge	Death at 35 days	Death at 30 days
Heparin effect on primary endpoint	None	None	None

Abbreviations: GISSI-2, Gruppo Italino per lo Studio della Sopravivenza nell'Infarto Miocardico (second study); ISIS-3, third International Study of Infarct Survival; GUSTO, Global Utilization of Streptokinase and Tissue Plasminogen Activator for Occluded Arteries; t-PA, tissue plasminogen activator; LV, left ventricular.

given until after angiography at 90 min was performed. At 90 min, angiographic patency was 79% in both groups. The Heparin Aspirin Reperfusion Trial compared heparin with aspirin (80 mg/day) after t-PA administration.[53] Coronary artery patency at 18 hours was 82% in the heparin group, in comparison with 52% in the aspirin alone group ($p < .002$). Bleich and colleagues found that in patients not receiving aspirin (80 mg a day) during acute myocardial infarction after t-PA administration, patency (as assessed by angiography) of the infarct related artery at 2–3 days was improved by heparin therapy (71% vs. 44%, $p = .04$).[80] In the European Cooperative Study Group–6, 687 patients received aspirin and t-PA. Half of this group were randomized to receive heparin; the other half received no heparin. Patency at 81 h was 80% in the heparin group and 75% in the no-heparin group ($p < .01$).[54] The Australian Coronary Thrombolysis Group determined that there was no difference in patency at 1 week between patients receiving continuous heparin infusion after an initial bolus and patients receiving a combination of 300 mg of aspirin and 300 mg of dipyridamole after the initial heparin bolus that followed t-PA infusion.[55]

In summary, to date no large trials have evaluated heparin alone or heparin as the sole adjunctive therapy; in GISSI-2, ISIS-3, and GUSTO, all patients received aspirin. The SCATI study excluded aspirin and showed a decrease in mortality after thrombolysis, but heparin was not compared with aspirin. GUSTO showed no benefit of intravenous heparin over subcutaneous heparin. No study has yet supported the use of either intravenous or subcutaneous heparin as adjunctive therapy to streptokinase when an adequate dose (162–325 mg/day) of aspirin is used. This is probably also true of the use of heparin in conjunction with APSAC. As discussed later, heparin should be used in conjunction with aspirin and streptokinase in patients who would otherwise benefit from anticoagulation.

On the basis of the trials of angiographic patency as a primary endpoint, heparin appears to improve early (18 h) infarct-related artery patency in patients who receive t-PA. These angiographic studies have been unable to link decreased mortality to earlier patency resulting from adjunctive heparin, perhaps because of small sample sizes. Nevertheless, until results of further trials are available, it is prudent to recommend the adjunctive use of heparin in patients receiving t-PA and aspirin.

Current Recommendations. From the aforementioned studies, heparin in combination with t-PA appears to reduce mortality acutely, reduce the incidence of rethrombosis, and reduce the incidence of mural thrombus formation. The use of heparin in conjunction with streptokinase does not add a mortality benefit, but use of heparin beginning within 24 h does reduce the incidence of mural thrombus formation (Table 29–7).[51]

Direct Thrombin Inhibitors

Several small studies using thrombin inhibitors as adjuncts to thrombolysis in acute myocardial infarction have been published (Table 29–8). Lidon and colleagues randomized 42 patients with acute myocardial infarction to heparin or Hirulog as an adjunct to thrombolytic therapy.[56] The patients in the Hirulog group had significantly greater 90- and 120-min patency rates with no increase in bleeding complications. The Hirudin for the Improvement in Thrombolysis (HIT) study[57] used increasing doses of recombinant Hirudin as an adjunct to front-loaded t-PA in the treatment of acute myocardial infarction. Patency rates were determined at 30, 60, and 90 min; at 36 and 48 h; and after discharge. The 90-min patency rate and reocclusion rate increased with increasing doses of hirudin. Among 143 patients, there were only three spontaneous hemorrhages; in 5 of the 83 patients in the highest dose group, there was an increase in puncture site bleeding.

The TIMI-5[58] study randomized 246 patients to heparin or hirudin after accelerated t-PA for acute myocardial infarction. At 90 min there was a trend toward improved patency in the hirudin group. At 18–36 h there was significantly improved patency in the hirudin group; there was also less reocclusion, a lower incidence of death, and a lower incidence of recurrent myocardial infarction during hospitalization. There was no increase in bleeding in the hirudin group. TIMI-6[59] reported the initial experience with hirudin vs. heparin in patients treated with streptokinase for acute myocardial infarction. This study found a trend toward lower event rates in the hirudin group with the use of a composite endpoint of death, reinfarction, new congestive heart failure, and shock.

Studies using hirudin, including TIMI-9A,[60] GUSTO-IIA,[61] and HIT-III,[62] examined the safety and efficacy of hirudin as therapy adjunctive to thrombolytic therapy. TIMI-9A compared the efficacy and safety of intravenous hirudin with weight-adjusted heparin as therapy adjunctive to thrombolysis and aspirin in patients with acute myocardial infarction. After 757 patients were enrolled, the randomization was suspended because of a higher rate of intracranial bleeding in both the heparin (1.7%) and hirudin (1.9%) arms in comparison with the bleeding rates in previous studies such as GUSTO-I (0.7%). GUSTO-IIA compared intravenous heparin with intravenous hirudin in patients presenting within 12 h of onset of ischemic chest pain. After 2564 patients were enrolled, the trial was suspended because of an excess of intracerebral hemorrhagic events. The overall incidence of hemorrhagic stroke was higher in the patients receiving hirudin (1.3%) than in those receiving heparin (0.7%) (Table 29–9). The events were particularly high in those receiving these agents in combination with thrombolytic therapy (overall hemorrhagic stroke rate, 1.8%). The hemorrhagic stroke rate varied by the thrombolytic and antithrombin combination. All of the rates were higher than the overall incidence of hemorrhagic stroke in patients receiving heparin and thrombolytic therapy in the GUSTO-I trial. After 302 patients were enrolled in the HIT-III trial, the study was stopped because of an increase in intracranial bleeding in the hirudin group (3.4%) in comparison with the weight-adjusted heparin group (0%) when given in combination with front-loaded t-PA and aspirin. These three studies indicate that hirudin may have a narrower therapeutic range than was previously thought (Table 29–10).

TABLE 29–7. ANGIOGRAPHIC TRAILS OF ADJUNCTIVE HEPARIN PLUS t-PA

	TAMI-3[52]	Bleich et al.[80]	HART[53]	ECSG-6[54]	NHSA[55]
No. of patients	134	83	205	652	241
Heparin dose	10,000 units IV bolus	5000 units IV bolus; 1000 units/h	5000 units IV bolus; 1000 units/h	5000 units IV bolus; 1000 units/h	5000 units IV bolus; 1000 units/h
Timing of heparin	With t-PA	With t-PA	With t-PA	With t-PA	After t-PA
Mean time to angiography	90 min	57 h	18 h	81 h	7 days
Patency with heparin	79%	71%	82%	83%	80%
Patency without heparin	79%	44%	51%	75%	82%
ASA given	No	Yes	Yes	Yes	Yes

Abbreviations: t-PA, tissue plasminogen activator; TAMI-3, Thrombolysis And Myocardial Infarction–3; HART, Heparin-Aspirin Reperfusion Trial; ECSG-6, European Cooperative Study Group–6; NHSA, Australian Coronary Thrombolysis Group; IV, intravenous; ASA, acetylsalicylic acid.

TABLE 29–8. CURRENT STATUS OF ADJUNCTIVE THERAPY FOR THROMBOSIS

Adjunctive Strategy	Thrombolytic Agent	Mortality Benefit	Angiographic Benefit
Aspirin vs. no aspirin	Streptokinase	*(ISIS-2[39])	*
	t-PA	‡	‡
Heparin vs. no heparin	Streptokinase	*†(SCATI[51])	‡
	t-PA	‡	*(HART[53])
Heparin vs. full-dose aspirin	Streptokinase	‡	‡
	t-PA	‡	‡
Subcutaneous heparin + aspirin vs. aspirin alone	Streptokinase	†(GISSI-2[46], ISSI-3[47])	‡
	t-PA	†(GISSI-2[46], ISSI-3[47])	‡
Intravenous heparin + aspirin vs. aspirin alone	Streptokinase	†(GUSTO[48])	†(GUSTO[48])
	t-PA	‡§	*†(ECSG-6[54])
Specific antithrombins + aspirin vs. heparin + aspirin	Streptokinase	‡§	*(Hirulog pilot)
	t-PA	‡§	*(Hirulog pilot)
Anti-factor IIb/IIIa + heparin + aspirin vs. heparin + aspirin	Streptokinase	‡§	‡
	t-PA	‡§	*(TAMI-8 pilot)

*Effective.
†Not effective.
‡Not studied.
§Should be studied.
Abbreviations: t-PA, tissue plasminogen activator; ISIS-2, second International Study of Infarct Survival; SCATI, Studio Sulla Calciparina nell'Angina e nella Thrombosi Ventriculate nell'Infarto; GISSI-2, Gruppo Italiano per lo Studio della Sopravivenza nell'Infarto Miocardico (second study); ISIS-3, third International Study of Infarct Survival; GUSTO, Global Utilization of Streptokinase and Tissue Plasminogen Activator for Occluded Arteries; HART, Heparin-Aspirin Reperfusion Trial; ECSG-6, European Cooperative Study Group–6; TAMI-8, Thrombolysis and Myocardial Infarction–8.

Acute Myocardial Infarction: Left Ventricular Thrombus

The use of heparin in acute myocardial infarction may prevent the formation of left ventricular thrombus (Table 29–11). Left ventricular thrombus develops in approximately 30% of patients with anterior myocardial infarction and is associated with increased risk of subsequent arterial embolization.[63] Thrombi form in fewer than 5% of patients with infarctions in other areas. Other factors predictive of left ventricular thrombus formation are low ejection fraction, large infarct, and atrial fibrillation. Thrombi almost always form in the anterior, particularly anteroapical, area of akinesis or dyskinesis.[64, 65] When thrombi form, they usually do so by the end of the first week, with peak incidence at 4–5 days after the infarction.[66–69] Echocardiography has a 90% specificity and 75%–90% sensitivity for detection of thrombus. The risk of embolization from a detected thrombus is particularly high when the thrombus is mobile or protuberant.[64] Most emboli that embolize do so within the first 3 months of the infarction.[65] The effect of subcutaneous heparin on the incidence of intracardiac thrombosis was evaluated in two clinical trials in which patients receiving 12,500 units every 12 h were compared with either an untreated group or patients taking 5000 units subcutaneously every 12 h. In these two studies, the incidence of mural thrombosis detected by two-dimentional echocardiography was 72% and 58% lower, respectively, in patients taking 12,500 units of heparin.[51, 70]

Thus the authors currently recommend the use of heparin in all patients with anterior myocardial infarctions, with long-term (3 months) anticoagulants in patients with large anterior myocardial infarctions and with patients in whom thrombi are visible on echocardiograms. Use of long-term anticoagulants in patients with postinfarction cardiomyopathy is controversial. Use of anticoagulants in patients with left ventricle aneurysms and mural thrombi is generally not indicated.

TABLE 29–9. PERCENTAGES OF TREATED PATIENTS SUFFERING HEMORRHAGIC STROKE*

	GUSTO-I[47]	GUSTO-IIA[61]	TIMI-9A[60]	HIT-III[63]	Statistical Significance
Overall					Trend
Heparin	0.7	0.7	1.9	0.0	
Hirudin	—	1.3	1.7	2.7	
Nonthrombolytic					
Heparin	—	0.0	—	—	
Hirudin	—	0.5	—	—	
Thrombolytic					$p < .001$
Heparin	0.7	1.5	1.9	0.0	
Hirudin	—	2.2	1.7	2.7	
t PA					$p < .06$
Heparin	0.7	0.9	1.9	0.0	
Hirudin	—	1.7	1.7	3.4	
Streptokinase					
Heparin	0.6	2.7	—	—	
Hirudin	—	3.2	—	—	

*For Hirudin, mortality ranges from 1.3% (TIMI-9A) to 2.7% (HIT-III), 75% of intracranial hemorrhage, most within 24 h.
Abbreviations: GUSTO, Global Utilization of Streptokinase and Tissue Plasminogen Activator for Occluded Arteries; TIMI, Thrombolysis in Myocardial Infarction; HIT, Hirudin for Improvement in Thrombolysis; t-PA, tissue plasminogen activator.

Acute Myocardial Infarction: Prevention of Venous Thromboembolism

Patients who are not ambulatory and are expected to be at prolonged bed rest are at increased risk for deep venous thrombosis (DVT) and pulmonary embolism. Other factors that increase risk of DVT and pulmonary embolism are age greater than 40, congestive heart failure, cancer, chronic pulmonary disease, and significant infection. In patients with myocardial infarction, subcutaneous heparin, intravenous heparin, and oral anticoagulants all are effective in preventing DVT and pulmonary embolism.

After Myocardial Infarction: Anticoagulant Therapy

Survivors of acute myocardial infarction are at medium risk of recurrent infarction or cardiac death. Because morbidity and mortal-

TABLE 29–10. STUDIES USING DIRECT THROMBIN INHIBITORS IN CONJUNCTION WITH THROMBOLYTIC AGENTS

	GUSTO-I[47]	GUSTO-II Pilot,[61] TIMI-5 Pilot,[58] HIT[57]	GUSTO-IIA,[61] TIMI-9A,[58] HIT-III[62]	GUSTO-IIB[61] TIMI-5B,[58] HIT-II (Streptokinase)
Heparin				
aPPT	60–85 sec Titration, 6–12 H	60–90 sec Titration, 6–12 h	60–90 sec (2–3.5 times) No titration 6–24 h*	60–85 sec (GUSTO-IIB, HIT-II) 55–85 sec (TIMI-5B) Titration, 6–12 h
Dose	5000-unit bolus; 1000 units/h	5000-unit bolus; 1000 units/h	5000-unit bolus; 1000 units/h if <80 kg, 1300 units/h if >80 kg	5000-unit bolus; 1000 units/h
Hirudin				
aPTT	—	No titration	>150 sec, no titration (GUSTO-IIA, TIMI-9A) 2–3.5 times, titration after 24 h (HIT-III)	60–85 sec (GUSTO-IIB, HIT-II) 55–85 sec (TIMI-5B) Titration, 6–12 h
Dose (mg/kg bolus/h IV)	—	0.1–0.05 to 0.6–0.2	0.6–0.2; (GUSTO-IIA, TIMI-9A) 0.40–0.15 (HIT-III)	0.1–0.1
Risks Other Than aPTT	Age Sex (female) Systolic blood pressure	Similar	Similar	Prior stroke Blood pressure >200/150; Cr >2.0 (higher in ICH)
No. Patients	31,148	166 (GUSTO-II) 246 (TIMI-5) 143 (HIT)	2564 (GUSTO-IIA) 757 (TIMI-9A) 302 (HIT-III)	12,000 (GUSTO-IIB)

*ICH in 12–24 h: 110 (GUSTO-IIA), 100 (TIMI-9A), and 106 (HIT-III). No ICH in 12–24 h: 87 (GUSTO-IIA), 85 (TIMI-9A), and 76 (HIT-III).

Abbreviations: GUSTO, Global Utilization of Streptokinase and Tissue Plasminogen Activator for Occluded Arteries; TIMI, Thrombolysis in Myocardial Infarction; HIT, Hirudin for Improvement in Thrombolysis; aPTT, activated partial thromboplastin time; Cr, creatinine; ICH, intracranial hemorrhage.

ity after a myocardial infarction may be related to arrhythmias, to left ventricular dysfunction, and to recurrent myocardial infarction, proving that antithrombotic therapy is beneficial in these patients has been difficult.

Antiplatelet Agents

Multiple trials examining the use of aspirin for the secondary prevention of myocardial infarction have been conducted; however, no single study has provided definitive results (Table 29–12). The results of a meta-analysis that included more than 18,000 patients revealed that platelet inhibitor therapy reduced cardiovascular mortality by 13%, nonfatal reinfarction by 31%, and nonfatal stroke by 42%.[71] Aspirin alone was at least as effective as the combination of aspirin and dipyridamole and more effective than sulfinpyrazone. Available data do not justify the additional cost and frequency of administration of drugs other than aspirin in this group of patients.[71] Medium-dose (75–325 mg) aspirin was as efficacious as high-dose aspirin.[36] No studies on the use of ticlopidine for secondary prevention are available.

TABLE 29–11. EFFECT OF SUBCUTANEOUS HEPARIN ON MURAL THROMBOSIS AFTER MYOCARDIAL INFARCTION

Study	Experimental Dose	Control Dose	%Reduction in Incidence of Mural Thrombosis in Treatment Group	*p*
Turpie et al.[70]	12,500 units SQ q 12 h	5000 units SQ q 12 h	58%	<.05
SCATI[51]	12,500 units SQ q 12 h	No treatment	72%	<.05

Abbreviations: SQ, subcutaneous; SCATI, Studio Sulla Calciparina nell'Angina e nella Thrombosi Ventriculare nell'Infarto.

Anticoagulants

Numerous studies have assessed the usefulness of anticoagulants in the secondary prevention of cardiovascular disease after myocardial infarction. The Warfarin and Reinfarction Study (WARIS) is the largest study to date of anticoagulants in the secondary prevention of myocardial infarction.[72] In this placebo-controlled double-blind trial, 1214 patients aged 75 or less were randomized, on average, 27 days after initial acute myocardial infarction to warfarin (target International Normalized Ratio [INR], 2.8–4.8) or placebo. Only 1% of patients received thrombolytic therapy for the initial acute myocardial infarction. Patients were advised not to take aspirin during the trial. At follow-up (mean, 37 months), warfarin resulted in significant reductions of mortality, total reinfarctions, nonfatal infarctions, and total strokes. Although four fatal intracranial hemorrhages occurred in the warfarin group, in comparison with none in the placebo group, 10 nonhemorrhagic fatal strokes occurred in the placebo group, in comparison with none in the warfarin group. Efficacy analysis showed even greater benefit from warfarin.

Two clinical trials compared warfarin therapy with antiplatelet therapy in secondary prevention of myocardial infarction. In the German-Austrian Myocardial Infarction Study (GAMIS), 946 patients were randomized 38–42 days after acute myocardial infarction to open-label phenprocoumon (target INR, 2.5–5.0), aspirin (1.5 g/day), or placebo.[73] No difference in mortality or reinfarction was observed between groups. The French Enquete de Prevention Secondaire de l'Infarctus de Myocarde (EPSIM) study[74] revealed no difference in death or reinfarction among patients receiving either oral anticoagulants or aspirin. However, 54% more patients suffered gastrointestinal events with aspirin and four times as many severe hemorrhagic events with warfarin. In the Aspirin Versus Coumadin

TABLE 29–12. ASPIRIN (ASA) AND ANTICOAGULANTS (A/C): SECONDARY PREVENTION EFFICACY IN PATIENTS WITH CAD

	No Lysis		Lysis		MI >1 Month to 3 Years		Chronic Stable CAD	
Events	**ASA***	**A/C†**	**ASA***	**A/C‡**	**ASA§**	**A/C‖ ¶**	**ASA**, ††**	**A/C‡‡**
Nonfatal cardiovascular event	46	51	50	—	42	63	25	—
Nonfatal MI	49	22	53	—	31	38	39	56
Death	23	16	42	—	13	22	26	26

*ISIS-II. Lancet 1988; 2:342. †Yusuf S, Sleight P, Held P, McMahon S: Routine medical management of acute myocardial infarction. Circulation 1990; 82(suppl II):117. ‡Bleich S, et al: Heparin-Aspirin Reperfusion Trial (HART), European Cooperative Study Group–6 (ECSG-6). §Trialists. Br Med J 1994; 308:81. ‖WARIS.[72] ¶Swedish Angina Pectoris Aspirin Trial (SAPAT). Lancet 1992; 340:1421. **Mayo Study. Circulation 1989; 80(2):266. ††Physicians Health Study. Ann Intern Med 1991; 114:835. ‡‡SAPAT. Lancet 1990; 340:1421. Sixty Plus Study. Lancet 1980; 2:989.

Abbreviations: CAD, coronary artery disease; MI, myocardial infarction; ISIS, International Study of Infarct Survival; WARIS, Warfarin and Reinfarction Study.

in the Prevention of Reocclusion and Recurrent Ischemia After Successful Thrombolysis (APRICOT) trial, 300 patients were randomized to either 325 mg of aspirin/day or to heparin followed by warfarin (target INR, 2.8–4.0) after an initial angiogram less than 48 h after acute myocardial infarction revealed a patent infarct-related artery.[75] At 3 months there was no significant difference in reocclusion rates among the warfarin, aspirin, and placebo groups. Aspirin significantly reduced reinfarction in comparison with placebo but not in comparison with warfarin. Mortality rates did not differ between the groups.

Two randomized studies are currently examining the unsolved issue of anticoagulant and antiplatelet regimens after acute myocardial infarction. The Coronary Artery Reinfarction Study (CARS) trial is studying 6000 patients randomized to three treatment regimens: (1) 160 mg/day of aspirin, (2) 80 mg/day aspirin plus 3 mg/day of warfarin, and (3) a combination pill consisting of 80 mg of aspirin plus 1 mg warfarin/day. An ongoing Veterans Affairs trial (CHAMP) will randomize 4000 patients to receive either 160 mg/day of aspirin or 80 mg of aspirin plus warfarin (Coumadin) to achieve an INR of 1.5–2.5. Results of these studies may definitively settle some of the unanswered questions regarding the use of anticoagulants and antiplatelets for the secondary prevention of acute myocardial infarction.

FUTURE DIRECTIONS

Four approaches may improve the effectiveness of thrombolytic therapy in the future. In order of priority, they are as follows: (1) to improve the identification of evolving myocardial infarction and minimize delays in initiation of thrombolytic therapy; (2) to identify the most appropriate thrombolytic approach, in view of the patient's characteristics, the expected benefit and risks, and the cost; (3) to evaluate specific antithrombins; and (4) to continue to search for new thrombolytic agents and strategies that result in safe, timely, and complete reperfusion.

It is well recognized that early initiation of thrombolytic therapy is essential. In spite of this, in the GUSTO trial conducted in 1990–1993, only 3% of patients received thrombolytic therapy within the first hour after myocardial infarction.[48] The average time delay is 3.7 h when a patient with symptoms of acute myocardial infarction achieves coronary reperfusion.[76] The Mayo Clinic examined the components of this time delay. Approximately 22%, or 45 min, of the delay occurs from the onset of symptoms to the time when patients seek medical attention. On average, an additional 48 min is required for transportation to the hospital. The longest delay before reperfusion took place, the "door-to-needle time," was an average of 84 ± 55 minutes. Only 19%, or 45 min, of the delay was between administration of the agent and clot lysis. Therefore, to improve effectiveness of coronary reperfusion and minimize time delays, particularly within the hospital, efforts must be made to improve on all aspects of this delay, with particular attention to rapid triage of these patients.

Efforts must be continued to elucidate the most appropriate individualized approach to the patient with acute myocardial infarction through further analysis of the current clinical trials and conducting of future trials.

Continued evaluation of specific antithrombins and new antiplatelet agents is currently under way. GUSTO-IIA in acute ischemic syndromes, TIMI-9, and ISIS-5 in acute myocardial infarction. TAMI-8 is examining the use of glycoprotein IIb/IIIa antibody as adjunctive treatment with t-PA in acute myocardial infarction. The antithrombin agent DuP-714 is an orally administered agent with high thrombin affinity that is in the preclinical phase of investigation. Hirulog, a hirudin-like peptide, is being tested as adjunctive therapy with streptokinase.

Several new thrombolytic agents are currently under development. These agents may prove to possess improved fibrinolytic potency and greater clot specificity. Recombinant plasminogen activator (r-PA) is a mutant of t-PA with greater thrombolytic potency and prolonged half-life, which will allow bolus administration.[77] Vampire bat salivary plasminogen activator (bat-PA) is related to t-PA but exhibits greater specificity for clot bound fibrin because of its requirement for polymeric fibrin as a cofactor for plasminogen cleavage.[78] This agent is also relatively resistant to circulating inhibitors of t-PA and has a half-life of 190 min, allowing for potential bolus administration. Recombinant staphylokinase is able to lyse platelet-rich thrombi, which are relatively resistant to lysis by conventional agents. This agent will be compared with accelerated t-PA in an upcoming clinical trial.

The results of the CARS and CHAMP studies may provide answers to the issue of anticoagulant and antiplatelet therapy after myocardial infarction as well as the possibility of using novel prostacyclin-sparing antiplatelet agents in conjunction with oral anticoagulants.

Studies evaluating the use of direct thrombin inhibitors are currently under way. These studies may provide definitive recommendations for optimal dose, monitoring, and method of administration of these agents.

CURRENT RECOMMENDATIONS

All patients experiencing an acute myocardial infarction should immediately receive 75–325 mg of chewable aspirin. Aspirin should be administered regardless of whether thrombolytic therapy is planned. As mentioned previously, patients receiving streptokinase need not receive initial anticoagulant therapy with heparin. Patients receiving t-PA should receive concurrent heparin therapy with an intravenous bolus of 5000 units and a maintenance dose of 1000 units/h. In patients without a large or anterior myocardial infarct, the heparin may be discontinued once the patient begins to ambulate. If the patient is nonambulatory or if prolonged bed rest is anticipated, the patient should be either maintained on heparin or switched over to warfarin or subcutaneous heparin for prevention of DVT. If the patient received t-PA, streptokinase, or APSAC and had a large or anterior myocardial infarct, the patient should be placed on or should continue heparin therapy and switched to warfarin for the prevention of left ventricular thrombus formation.

All patients should be maintained on 75–325 mg/day of aspirin indefinitely for secondary prevention of recurrent myocardial infarction. All patients with documented left ventricular thrombi should receive anticoagulants indefinitely. Current data suggest that anticoagulants are of benefit in patients after a myocardial infarction. The results of the CARS and the CHAMP studies are awaited to address these important issues.

REFERENCES

1. Fuster V, Badimon L, Badimon J, Chesebro J: The pathogenesis of coronary artery disease and the acute coronary syndromes. N Engl J Med 1992; 326:242–250.
2. Fuster, V: Lewis Conner Memorial Lecture—mechanisms leading to myocardial infarction: insights from studies of vascular biology. Circulation 1994; 90:2126–2146.
3. Ross R: The pathogenesis of atherosclerosis a perspective for the 1990's. Nature 1993; 362:801–808.
4. Rosenfeld M, Pestel E: Cellularity of atherosclerotic lesions. Coron Artery Dis 1994; 5:189–197.
5. Willerson J, Yao S, McNatt J, et al: Frequency and severity of cyclic flow alterations and platelet aggregation predict the severity of neointimal proliferation following experimental coronary stenosis and endothelial injury. Proc Natl Acad Sci USA 1991; 88:10624–10628.
6. Ambrose J, Tannenbaum M, Alexopoulos D, et al: Angiographic progression of coronary artery disease and development of myocardial infarction. J Am Coll Cardiol 1988; 12:56–62.
7. Ambrose J, Winters S, Stern A, et al: Angiographic morphology and the pathogenesis of unstable angina pectoris. J Am Coll Cardiol 1985; 5:609–616.
8. Sherman C, Litvack F, Grundfest W, et al: Coronary angioscopy in patients with unstable angina pectoris. N Engl J Med 1986; 315:913–919.
9. Levin D, Fallon J: Significance of the angiographic morphology of localized coronary stenosis: histopathologic correlations. Circulation 1982; 66:316–320.
10. Ambrose J, Winters S, Arora R, et al: Angiographic evolution of coronary artery morphology in unstable angina. J Am Coll Cardiol 1986; 7:472–478.
11. Little W, Constantinescu M, Applegate R, et al: Can coronary angiography predict the site of subsequent myocardial infarction in patients with mild to moderate coronqary artery disease? Circulation 1988; 78:1157–1166.
12. Richardson R, Davies M, Born G: Influence of plaque configuration and stress distribution on fissuring of coronary atherosclerotic plaques. Lancet 1989; 2:941–944.
13. Bogaty P, Hackett D, Davies G, Maseri A: Vasoreactivity of the culprit lesion in unstable angina. Circulation 1994; 90:5–11.
14. DeWood M, Stifter W, Simpson C, et al: Coronary arteriographic findings soon after non–Q wave myocadial infarction. N Engl J Med 1986; 315:417–423.
15. Fuster V, Frye R, Kennedy M, et al: The role of collateral circulation in various coronary syndromes. Circulation 1979; 59:1137–1144.
16. Badimon L, Badimon J, Galvez A, et al: Influence of artrial damage and wall shear rate on platelet deposition: ex vivo study in a swine model. Arteriosclerosis 1986; 6:312.
17. Badimon L, Badimon J: Mechanism of arterial thrombosis in nonparallel streamlines: platelet thrombi grew on the apex of stenotic severely injured vessel wall: experimental study in the pig model. J Clin Invest 1989; 84:1134.
18. Fuster V, Ip J, Jang I, et al: Antithrombotic therapy in cardiac disease. *In* Parmley W, Chatterjee K (eds): Cardiology—Physiology, Pharmacology, Diagnosis, pp 1–40. Philadelphia: JB Lippincott, 1990.
19. Telford A, Wilson C: Trial of heparin versus atenolol in prevention of myocardial infarction in intermediate coronary syndromes. Lancet 1981; 1:1225.
20. Theroux P, Ouimet H, McCanu T: Aspirin, heparin or both to treat acute unstable angina. N Engl J Med 1988; 319:1105.
21. Hirsh J, Fuster V: AHA Medical/Scientific Statement Guide to Anticoagulant Therapy Part 1: heparin. Circulation 1994; 89:1449–1468.
22. RISC Investigators: Risk of myocardial infarction and death during treatment with low dose aspirin and intravenous heparin in men with unstable coronary artery disease. Lancet 1990; 336:827–830.
23. Theroux P, Walters D, Lam J, et al: Reactivation of unstable angina after discontinuation of heparin. N Eng J Med 1992; 327:141–145.
24. Lewis H, Davis J, Archibald D, et al: Protective effects of aspirin against acute myocardial infarction and death in men with unstable angina: results of a Veterans Administration Cooperative Study. N Engl J Med 1983; 309:396–403.
25. Cairns J, Gent M, Singer J, et al: Aspirin sulfinpyrazone or both in unstable angina. N Engl J Med 1985; 313:1369–1375.
26. Cohen M, Adams P, Parry G, et al: Combination antithrombotic therapy in unstable rest angina and non–Q-wave infarction in nonprior aspirin users. Primary end points analysis from the ATACS trial. Circulation 1994; 89:81–88.
27. Balsano F, Rizzon P, Violoi F, et al: Antiplatelet treatment with ticlopidine in unstable angina: a controlled multicenter clinical trial. The Studio della Ticlopidina nell'Angina Instabile Group. Circulation 1990; 82:17–26.
28. Sharma G, Lapsely D, Vita J, et al: Safety and efficacy of Hirulog in patients with unstable angina. Circulation 1992; 86:1–386.
29. Fuchs J, McCabe C, Antman E, et al: Hirulog in the treatment of unstable angina:results of the TIMI-7 trial. J Am Col Cardiol 1994; 23:56A.
30. Topol E, Fuster V, Harrington R, et al: Recombinant Hirudin for unstable angina pectoris: a multicenter, randomized angiographic trial. Circulation 1994; 89:1557–1566.
31. Bar F, Verheugt F, Col J, et al: Thrombolysis in patients with unstable angina improves the angiographic but not the clinical outcome. Results of UNASEM. Circulation 1992; 86:131–137.
32. Falk E: Unstable angina with fatal outcome: dynamic coronary thrombosis leading to infarction and/or sudden death: autopsy evidence of recurrent mural thrombosis and peripheral embolization culminating in total vascular occlusion. Circulation 1985; 71:699–708.
33. Cairns J, Fuster, V, Kennedy J: Coronary thrombolysis. Chest 1992; 102:482S–507S.
34. Califf R, O'Neil W, Stack R, et al: Failure of simple clinical measurements to predict perfusion status after intrvaenous thrombolysis. Ann Intern Med 1988; 108:658–662.
35. Christian T, Gibbons R, Hopfenspirger M, Gersh B: Severity and response of chest pain during thrombolytic therapy for acute myocardial infarction: a useful indicator of myocardial salvage and infarct size. J Am Coll Cardiol 1993; 22:1311–1316.
36. Shah P, Cercek B, Lew A, Ganz W: Angiographic validation of bedside markers of reperfusion. J Am Coll Cardiol 1993; 21:55–61.
37. Muller D, Topol E: Selection of patients with acute myocardial infarction for thrombolytic therapy. Ann Intern Med 1980; 113:949–960.
38. Fibrinolytic Trialists' Collaborative Group: Indications for fibrinolytic therapy in suspected acute myocardial infarction: collaborative overview of early mortality and major morbidity results from all randomised trial of more than 1000 patients. Lancet 1994; 343:311–322.
39. ISIS-2 Collaborative Group: Randomized trial of intravenous streptokinase, oral aspirin, both or neither among 17,187 cases of suspected acute myocardial infarction: ISIS-2. Lancet 1988; 2:349–360.
40. LATE Study Group: Late Assessment of Thrombolytic Efficacy (LATE) study with alteplase 6–24 hours after onset of acute myocardial infarction. Lancet 1993; 342:759–766.
41. EMERAS: Randomized trial of late thrombolysis in patients with suspected acute myocardial infarction. Lancet 1993; 342:767–772.
42. Carney R, Murphy G, Brandt T, et al: Randomized angiographic trial of recombinant t-PA in myocardial infarction. J Am Coll Cardiol 1992; 20:17–23.
43. Neuhaus K, Von Essen R, Tebbe U, et al: Improved thrombolysis in acute myocardial infarction with front-loaded administration of alteplase: results of the rt–PA-APSAC patency study (TAPS). J Am Coll Cardiol 1992; 19:885–891.
44. Neuhaus K, Feuerer W, Jeep-Tebbe S, et al: Improved thrombolysis with a modified dose regimen of recombinant tisuues type plasminogen activator. J Am Coll Cardiol 1989; 14:1566–1569.
45. Smalling R, Schumacher R, Morris D, et al: Improved infarct related arterial patency after high dose, weight adjusted, rapid infusion of tissue type plasminogen activator in myocardial infarction: results of a multicenter randomized trial of two dosage regimens. J Am Coll Cardiol 1990; 15:915–921.

46. GISSI-2: A factorial randomized trial of alteplase versus streptokinase and heparin versus no heparin among 12,490 patients with acute myocardial infarction. Lancet 1990; 336:65–71.
47. ISIS-3 Collaborative Group: ISIS-3: a randomized comparison of streptokinase vs t-PA vs anistreplase and of aspirin plus heparin vs aspirin alone among 41,229 cases of suspected acute myocardial infarction. Lancet 1992; 339:753–770.
48. The GUSTO Investigators: An international randomized trial comparing four thrombolytic strategies for acute myocardial infarction. N Engl J Med 1993; 329:678–682.
49. Fuster V: Coronary thrombolysis—a perspective for the practicing physician. N Engl J Med 1993; 329:723–725.
50. Baigent C, Collins R: ISIS-2: 4 year mortality follow-up of 17187 patients after fibrinolytic and antiplatelet therapy in suspected acute myocardial infarction. Circulation 1993; 88:I-291.
51. The SCATI Group: Randomized controlled trial of subcutaneous calcium heparin in acute myocardial infarction. Lancet 1989; 2:182–186.
52. TAMI Study Group: A randomized controlled trial of intravenous tissue plasminogen activator and early intravenous heparin in acute myocardial infarction. Circulation 1989; 79:281.
53. Hsia J, Hamilton W, Kleiman N, et al: A comparison between heparin and low dose aspirin as adjunctive therapy with tissue plasminogen activator for acute myocardial infarction: Heparin-Aspirin Reperfusion Trial (HART) Investigators. N Engl J Med 1990; 323:1433–1437.
54. de Bono D, Simoons M, Tijssen J, et al: Effect of early intravenous heparin on coronary patency, infarct size, and bleeding complications after alteplase thrombolysis: results of double blind European Cooperative Study Group trial. Br Heart J 1992; 67:122–128.
55. Australian Coronary Thrombolysis Group: A randomized comparison of oral aspirin/dipyridamole versus intravenous intravenous heparin after rt-PA for acute myocardial infarction. Circulation 1989; 80S:114.
56. Lidon R, Theroux P, Bonan R, et al: Hirulog as adjunctive therapy to streptokinase in acute myocardial infarction. J Am Coll Cardiol 1993; 21:419A.
57. Neuhaus K, Niederer W, Wagner J, et al: HIT (Hirudin for Improvement of Thrombolysis) results of a dose escalation study. Circulation 1993; 88:292A.
58. Cannon C, McCabe C, Henry T, et al: A pilot trial of recombinant desulfatohirudin compared with heparin in conjunction with t-PA and aspirin for acute myocardial infarction: results of TIMI-5 trial. J Am Coll Cardiol 1994; 23:993–1003.
59. Lee L, McCabe C, Antman E, et al: Initial experience with Hirudin and streptokinase in acute myocardial infarction: results of TIMI-6 trial. J Am Coll Cardiol 1994; (special issue):344A.
60. Antman E: Hirudin in acute myocardial infarction. Safety report from the thrombolysis and thrombin inhibition in myocardial infarction (TIMI) 9A Trial. Circulation 1994; 90:1624–1630.
61. GUSTO IIa Investigators: Randomized trial of intravenous heparin versus recombinant Hirudin for acute coronary syndromes. Circulation 1994; 90:1631–1637.
62. Neuhaus K, van Essen R, Tebbe U, et al: Safety observations from the pilot phase of the randomized r-Hirudin for improvement of thrombolysis (HIT-III) study. Circulation 1994; 90:1638–1642.
63. Kontny F, Dale J, Hegren L, et al: Left ventricular thrombosis and arterial embolism after thrombolysis in acute anterior myocardial infarction: predictors and effects of adjunctive antithrombotic therapy. Eur Heart J 1993; 14:1489–1492.
64. Visser C, Kan G, David K, et al: Two-dimensional echocardiography in the diagnosis of left ventricular thrombus. Chest 1983; 83:228–232.
65. Penny W, Chesebro J, Heras M, Fuster V: Antithrombotic therapy for patients with cardiovascular disease. Curr Prob Cardiol 1988; 13:464–469.
66. Asinger R, Mikell F, Elsperger J, Hodges M: Incidence of left ventricular thrombosis after acute myocardial infarction: serial evaluation by two dimensional echicardiography. N Engl J Med 1981; 305:297–302.
67. Spirito P, Bellotti P, Chiarella F, et al: Prognostic significance and natural history of left ventricular thrombi in patients with acute anterior myocardial infarction: a 2D echocardiographic study. Circulation 1985; 72:774–780.
68. Domenicucci S, Chiarella F, Bellotti P, et al: Early appearance of left ventricular thrombi after anterior myocardial infarction: a marker of higher in-hospital mortality of patients not treated with antithrombotic drugs. Eur Heart J 1990; 11:51–58.
69. Visser C, Kan G, Lie K, Durrer D: Left ventricular thrombus following acute myocardial infarction: a prospective serial echocardiographic study of 96 patients. Eur Heart J 1983; 4:333–337.
70. Turpie A, Robinson J, Doyle D: A comparison of high dose with low dose subcutaneous heparin to prevent left ventricular mural thrombosis in patients with acute transmural anterior myocardial infarction. N Engl J Med 1989; 320:352–357.
71. Antiplatelet Trialists Collaborative: Secondary prevention of vascular disease by prolonged antiplatelet treatment. Br Med J 1988; 296:320.
72. Smith P, Arnesen H, Holme I: The effect of warfarin on mortality and reinfarction after myocardial infarction. N Engl J Med 1990; 323:147.
73. Breddin D, Loew D, Lechner K, et al: The German-Austrian Aspirin Trial: a comparison of aspirin, placebo and phenprocoumon in secondary prevention of myocardial infarction. Circulation 1980; 62:63.
74. The EPSIM Research Group: A controlled comparison of aspirin and oral anticoagulants in prevention of death after myocardial infarction. N Engl J Med 1982; 307:701.
75. Meijer A, Verheug F, Werter C: Aspirin versus coumadin in the prevention of reocclusion and recurrent ischemia after successful thrombolysis: a prospective placebo-controlled angiographic study: results of the APRICOT study. Circulation 1993; 87:1524.
76. Gersh B, Anderson J: Thrombolysis and myocardial salvage. Circulation 1993; 88:296–306.
77. Martin U, Sponer G, Strein K: Evaluation of thrombolytic and systemic effects of the novel recombinant plasminogen activator BM 06.022 compared with alteplase, anistreplase, streptokinase and urokinase in a canine model of coronary artery thrombosis. J Am Coll Cardiol 1992; 19:433–440.
78. Gardell S, Duong L, Diehl R, et al: Isolation characterization and cDNA cloning of vampire bat salivary plasminogen activator. J Biol Chem 1989; 264:17947–17952.
79. TIMI IIIB: Effects of tissue plasminogen activator and a comparison of early invasive and conservative strategies in unstable angina and non–Q-wave myocardial infarction. Results of the TIMI IIIB study. Circulation 1994; 89:1545–1556.
80. Bleich S, Nichols T, Schumacher R, et al: The effect of heparin on coronary arterial patency after thrombolysis with tissue plasminogen activator in acute myocardial infarction. Am J Cardiol 1990; 66:1412–1417.

30 Arterial and Venous Thrombotic Disease: Thrombolytic and Antithrombotic Therapies

Jane E. Freedman, MD
Joseph Loscalzo, MD, PhD

Clinical sequelae of arterial or venous thrombosis are important causes of cardiovascular morbidity and mortality. Treatment of these common disorders involves the use of agents that prevent thrombosis, limit the extension of thrombus, or dissolve pre-existing thrombus, such as platelet inhibitors, anticoagulants, and plasminogen activators. All of these agents have the potential to interfere with normal hemostasis. Thus, all antithrombotic and fibrinolytic therapies have low toxic/therapeutic indices and must be used with care to ensure optimal clinical benefit.

FIBRINOLYTIC AGENTS

Fibrinolytic agents lead to the dissolution of thrombi by converting the plasma zymogen plasminogen to its active form, plasmin (Fig. 30–1). Plasmin then mediates fibrin degradation directly by cleaving fibrin into soluble proteolytic fragments. Currently, streptokinase (SK), urokinase (UK), and tissue-type plasminogen activator (t-PA) are available for treatment of venous and arterial thromboembolic diseases. The mechanism of action of these agents is briefly reviewed, and the benefits and risks of their general use are then discussed.

Streptokinase

SK is a 47,000-D protein derived from beta-hemolytic streptococci. SK does not convert plasminogen to plasmin enzymatically but instead binds to plasminogen in a stoichiometric manner, forming a complex that has plasmin activity (see Fig. 30–1). Equimolar SK and plasminogen combine to form this complex in which a conformational change in plasminogen occurs that enables the zymogen to express catalytic activity. This activity is manifested by the conversion of plasminogen to plasmin as well as by the conversion of the SK-plasminogen complex to an SK-plasmin complex. SK has a comparatively low affinity for the plasminogen bound to fibrin and, therefore, predominantly leads to systemic fibrinogenolysis. Given intravenously, SK has a half-life of approximately 23 min.

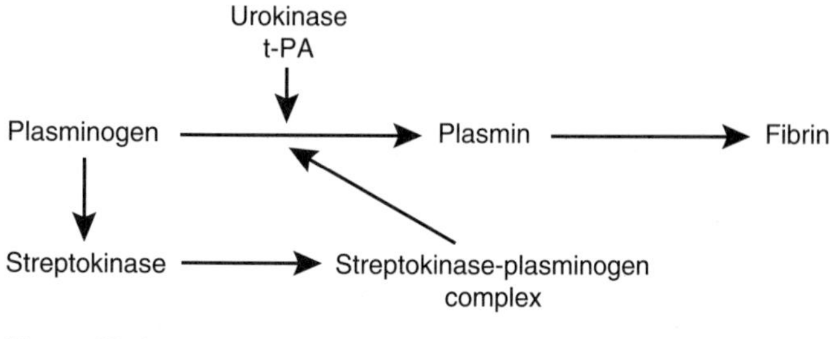

Figure 30–1. Site of action of fibrinolytic agents. Urokinase, streptokinase, and tissue-type plasminogen activator (t-PA) convert plasminogen into plasmin.

Because SK is of bacterial origin, it can elicit allergic reactions and antibody formation. This is a specific side effect of SK that occurs with a frequency estimated between 1.7% and 18%.[1]

Although the SK-plasmin complex efficiently converts fibrin-bound plasminogen to plasmin, its potency is limited by its rapid inactivation in plasma. Owing to this limitation, derivatives of SK have been synthesized that become activated in vivo. Anisoylated plasminogen SK activator complex (APSAC) is one such approved form of SK in which the active site of plasminogen is acylated and complexed to SK. APSAC is given as a rapid intravenous bolus and immediately undergoes spontaneous deacylation in vivo; this process generates the active SK-plasminogen complex. The half-life of APSAC in vivo is approximately 90 min. Like SK, APSAC is of bacterial origin and is, therefore, potentially allergenic.

Urokinase

UK is a 34,000-D protein isolated from mammalian urine and derived from kidney cells that converts plasminogen to plasmin directly. Also elaborated by endothelial cells, it is synthesized as a proenzyme known as single-chain urokinase-type plasminogen activator (scu-PA) or prourokinase.[2] On exposure to plasmin, proteolytic cleavage of scu-PA occurs, leading to the generation of high-molecular-weight and, subsequently, low-molecular-weight forms of UK, both of which contain the active site and manifest plasminogen activator activity. After UK undergoes these two successive cleavages, it does not discriminate between circulating and fibrin-bound plasminogen and can, therefore, lead to systemic fibrinogenolysis. UK, a nonantigenic protein, is removed by hepatic clearance and has an estimated half-life of 14 min. A disadvantage to the use of UK is its cost, which is approximately 10 times that of SK.

Tissue-Type Plasminogen Activator

t-PA is a major endogenous fibrinolytic molecule. Synthesized in single-chain form by endothelial cells,[3] t-PA is converted to a two-chain form by the action of plasmin, factor X_a, or kallikrein. t-PA is relatively fibrin selective and has greater catalytic efficiency toward plasminogen bound to fibrin than toward circulating unbound plasminogen.[4] Despite its fibrin selectivity, t-PA has been reported to cause systemic bleeding complications similar to those of other fibrinolytic agents,[5] and this side effect is largely a consequence of the doses needed to achieve rapid thrombolysis. The single-chain form of t-PA has an initial plasma half-life of 4 min and a terminal half-life of 46 min; the two-chain form has an initial half-life of 5 min and a terminal half-life of 46 min. There is a direct relationship between hepatic blood flow and t-PA clearance,[6] which must be considered when this agent is given to patients with liver disease or significant congestive heart failure.

Contraindications to Thrombolytic Therapy

Patients must be carefully selected for thrombolytic therapy because of the great potential for hemorrhagic complications. Contraindications to thrombolytic therapy and guidelines for selection of patients are listed in Table 30–1.[7] Absolute contraindications include active internal bleeding, recent cerebrovascular accident, or known intracranial disease. In addition, specific contraindications to treatment with SK include known allergy, recent streptococcal infection, or SK treatment within the previous 6 months. With the use of any thrombolytic agent, invasive procedures, including intramuscular injections, should be avoided; puncture of noncompressible arteries is contraindicated.

ANTITHROMBOTIC AGENTS

Heparin

The primary anticoagulants currently in use for treatment of venous and arterial thrombotic diseases are heparin and warfarin, which act to inhibit thrombin generation and fibrin formation. Heparin and warfarin are used to treat patients with established thrombosis and to prevent the occurrence of thrombus in high-risk patients; more recently, heparin (with aspirin) has been used as an adjunct to fibrinolytic therapy.

Heparin is a sulfated glycosaminoglycan polymer derived from porcine intestinal mucosa or beef lung. Commercially available heparin is a heterogeneous preparation consisting of both active and inactive polydispersed polymers. Because usually less than 30% of the heparin polymers possess anticoagulant activity, each lot must be calibrated against a standard. When administered intravenously, this complex carbohydrate functions by catalyzing the complexation of the plasma serine protease inhibitor (serpin) antithrombin III to thrombin (factor II_a) and the activated coagulation factors XII_a, XI_a, X_a, and IX_a. In addition, heparin catalyzes the inhibition of thrombin by a related serine protease inhibitor, heparin cofactor II. The inhibition of thrombin and other coagulation factors by heparin produces a systemic state of anticoagulation. Heparin sulfate glycosaminoglycans expressed on the surface of endothelial cells and heparins released from mast cells represent endogenous sources of this anticoagulant catalyst.

Heparin is not absorbed orally and thus must be administered by the intravenous or subcutaneous route; it should not be given intramuscularly because of the possibility of local hematoma formation. Heparin action is immediate after intravenous infusion but delayed 20–60 min after subcutaneous injection. After intravenous administration, the average half-life of heparin is 90 min; however, the time needed to achieve a steady-state plasma concentration may vary considerably from individual to individual.

Heparin is usually administered by continuous intravenous infusion with the aid of a constant-infusion pump. To ensure rapid anticoagulation, patients should be given an initial bolus of 5000 U followed by a continuous infusion of approximately 1000 units/h. Initial dosing can also be estimated on a unit-per-weight basis. An initial loading dose of 75 units/kg is followed by a continuous infusion of 10–25 units/kg/h. When heparin is given by intermittent bolus, the usual dose is 4000–8000 units every 4 h. Subcutaneous dosing requires approximately 7500–15,000 units every 12 h. The anticoagulant effect of equivalent doses of heparin may vary from patient to patient and during the course of therapy; thus, careful monitoring of the anticoagulant action of the drug is required throughout the course of therapy.

During therapy, heparin is not routinely measured directly in plasma; however, its effects can be monitored by analyzing the whole blood clotting time, the thrombin time, or, most commonly, the activated partial thromboplastin time. Monitoring of heparin should begin shortly after the initiation of intravenous therapy because inadequate initial dosing may permit progression of the underlying thrombotic process; the activated partial thromboplastin time should be checked and the infusion rate adjusted approximately every 4–6 h until steady-state levels are achieved.

The weight–average molecular weight of standard heparin preparations is approximately 15,000. Fractions of heparin enriched in low-molecular-weight oligosaccharides (4000–9000) have primarily anti–factor X_a activity and little antithrombin activity. Several of these preparations have been evaluated clinically, including tedelparin (Fragmin), Fraxiparine, enoxaparin, and logiparin. Their potential advantages compared with standard heparin preparations are a reduced frequency of administration (once or twice daily subcutaneously) and improved antithrombotic efficacy (cf. Chapter 28).

TABLE 30–1. CONTRAINDICATIONS TO THROMBOLYTIC THERAPY

Absolute Contraindications

Active internal bleeding
Recent cerebrovascular event (<2 months)
Intracranial disease (neoplasm, arteriovenous fistula, aneurysm, hemorrhage)
Acute pericarditis
Possible aortic dissection

Relative Contraindications: Major

Recent gastrointestinal bleeding
Recent (<10 days) major trauma, major surgery, previous puncture of noncompressible vessel, recent cardiopulmonary resuscitation with resulting chest trauma
Uncontrolled severe hypertension (>200 mm Hg systolic or >110 mm Hg diastolic)
Bleeding diathesis

Relative Contraindications: Minor

Recent minor surgery or trauma (including cardiopulmonary resuscitation)
Active bacterial endocarditis
Pregnancy
Diabetic hemorrhagic retinopathy

Oral Anticoagulants

Oral anticoagulants are commonly used in clinical practice to prevent primary or recurrent episodes of thromboembolic disorders. Oral anticoagulants are vitamin K antagonists and exert their actions by inhibiting vitamin K epoxide reductase and, thus, the gamma-carboxylation of the vitamin K–dependent coagulation factors: prothrombin (factor II); factors VII, IX, and X; and anticoagulant proteins C and S. Of the oral anticoagulants available, racemic warfarin sodium is most commonly used in the United States owing to its favorable pharmacokinetic and safety profile.[8] Racemic warfarin has nearly 100% oral bioavailability and a mean half-life of 40 h, which permits once-daily dosing and a minimal side effect profile. Warfarin action is not immediate, however, because warfarin has no effect on the function of preformed, active coagulation factors. After a single oral dose, maximal plasma warfarin levels are achieved in approximately 90 min, with a range of 30 min to 4 h.[9] Warfarin is usually administered orally, and doses range between 1 and 20 mg/day. A loading dose is not recommended; rather, 5–10 mg should be given daily until a steady state is reached. Resistant patients can be given larger doses, and dosages can be adjusted as indicated by the prothrombin time. In general, the clinical effect of warfarin is directly related to the vitamin K status of the patient.

Appropriate warfarin dosing by indication has not been well established, and recommendations vary for venous disease, arterial disease, and valvular heart disease. The adequacy of anticoagulation achieved with warfarin is monitored by measuring the prothrombin time. In general, prolongation of the prothrombin time does not correlate well with antithrombotic efficacy, and undue emphasis on prothrombin time prolongation may place patients at increased risk for bleeding. To standardize warfarin monitoring, many laboratories report prothrombin time results as the International Normalized Ratio (INR). This system is based on the use of thromboplastin reagents that are standardized for activity against an international reference preparation provided by the World Health Organization. Each lot of thromboplastin is assigned an international sensitivity index (ISI) value that relates its activity to the standard. The locally measured prothrombin time (PT) is converted to the INR by using the formula

$$\text{INR} = (\text{observed PT/control PT})^{\text{ISI}}$$

Until recently in the United States, most laboratories have not reported INRs, which resulted in significant but often unappreciated variability in prothrombin times and increased bleeding risk.[10]

ANTIPLATELET AGENTS

See Chapter 27.

THROMBOLYTIC AND ANTITHROMBOTIC TREATMENT OF ARTERIAL THROMBOTIC DISEASE

Coronary Artery Disease

See Chapter 29.

Peripheral Intra-Arterial Thrombosis

Arterial thrombosis frequently manifests as a catastrophic event complicating the course of patients with chronic arterial occlusive disease. Although there is significant morbidity and mortality associated with intra-arterial thrombosis, catheter-directed intra-arterial administration of thrombolytic agents can effectively treat this disease with a low complication rate when small doses of these drugs are given.[11, 12] Rates of reperfusion after local administration (50%–80%) are somewhat higher than with systemic therapy, although no large, conclusive studies have prospectively compared local with systemic therapy. There have been numerous reports of successful arterial thrombolytic regimens using SK or UK in doses ranging from 1000–250,000 units/h for continuous periods that range from several hours to 2 weeks. Typical regimens for local administration of UK and t-PA are summarized in Table 30–2. t-PA has been used in the treatment of intra-arterial thrombosis and found to achieve vessel patency more rapidly than SK.[13, 14] A randomized trial comparing t-PA with UK in peripheral arterial and graft occlusion in a small group of patients found equivalent numbers of lysed lesions in t-PA and UK groups, but more rapid thrombolysis in the t-PA group;[15] however, t-PA was also associated with an increased frequency of hemorrhagic complications in this trial (t-PA, 31%; UK, 13%).

Owing to its lower frequency of hemorrhagic complications and greater catalytic efficiency, UK is generally accepted as the drug of choice for catheter-directed intra-arterial thrombolysis. Thrombolytic agents are typically administered directly into the thrombus by use of catheters with multiple side holes. A commonly accepted regimen involves the administration of a transthrombus bolus of 150,000–250,000 IU UK, followed by a continuous infusion of 4000 IU/min for 2 h, then 2000 IU/min for 2 h, and finally 1000 IU/min for the duration of treatment, which not infrequently lasts 24 h. When t-PA is used, 5–10 mg is administered as a transthrombus bolus, followed by a continuous infusion of 0.5–3.0 mg/h for the remainder of the treatment schedule. These types of approaches yield higher local concentrations and lower systemic levels. Indwelling arterial catheterization for long periods, however, has been associated with bleeding or thromboembolism in up to 20% of patients.[16]

TABLE 30–2. TREATMENT PROTOCOLS FOR INTRA-ARTERIAL THROMBOLYSIS

Agent	Loading Dose	Infusion Rate
Urokinase	60,000 U IV	240,000 units/h for 2 h 120,000 units/h for 2 h Followed by 60,000 units/h for up to 25 h
t-PA[123]	0.1 mg/kg IV	1–6 h of 0.05–0.1 mg/kg/h

Abbreviation: t-PA, tissue-type plasminogen activator.

Treatment by intra-arterial thrombolysis can also allow concurrent angiographic study. As thrombus is lysed, the extent of underlying vascular disease and effectiveness of therapy can be defined. Only in a minority of patients will thrombolytic therapy alone be sufficient to optimize restoration of limb perfusion. Most patients with focal stenoses can be treated with percutaneous transluminal angioplasty, and others require surgical revascularization. Although information obtained during angiography may be helpful in planning operative intervention, thrombolysis followed by surgery has not been shown to decrease mortality or limb loss compared with surgery alone and, on average, adds $20,000 to the cost of a patient's hospitalization.[17]

The principles used in the treatment of intra-arterial thrombosis can be applied to the treatment of thrombosed prosthetic arterial grafts as well. Whereas surgical embolectomy or thrombectomy with graft revision is typically the treatment of choice, catheter-directed thrombolytic therapy has been reported to produce comparable results in selected patients.[18]

Antithrombotic therapy is important in the management of peripheral arterial thrombosis, both during the acute event as well as long term. After the diagnosis of acute arterial thromboembolism is made, heparin is administered (5000- to 10,000-unit bolus followed by a continuous infusion to maintain the activated partial thromboplastin time at 1.5–1.7 times the control value) to prevent thrombus propagation. After successful revascularization or embolectomy, heparin is given systemically to prevent thrombotic complications and preserve vessel patency. Currently, there is no conclusive evidence that antithrombotic therapy alters the clinical course of vascular insufficiency from atherothrombosis; prophylactic administration of antithrombotic agents in these patients is currently under investigation.

Thrombolytic therapy has also found a role in the treatment of drug-induced intra-arterial vascular injury, a condition that often causes vascular insufficiency and necessitates further treatment. Most often a consequence of illegal drug use, this form of intra-arterial injury often presents with swelling, ulceration, or infection. Therapy includes pain relief, improved venous drainage, and assessment of vessel patency. Thrombolytic therapy may be considered a reasonable option, especially in the presence of a poor response to vasodilating agents and persistent vessel occlusion.

Treatment of acute central retinal artery occlusion with intra-arterial fibrinolytic therapy has also met with some early success.[19] Initiation of therapy within 6–8 h of the onset of symptoms led to marked improvement in visual acuity in this early trial. Controlled, prospective trials have yet to be completed, however, and this therapeutic approach thus remains experimental.

Atherothrombotic Cerebrovascular Disease

Thrombolytic Therapy

Cardiac sources of embolism are believed to account for more than 30% of ischemic strokes. Emergent restoration of flow may lessen the sequelae of acute cerebral ischemia, and thus attempts to restore vessel patency rapidly have included the use of thrombolytic agents. Early studies using fibrinolytic agents for the treatment of stroke were fraught with severe hemorrhagic complications producing disastrous results, including extremely high mortality rates.[20] Although many subsequent studies showed no significant improvement or clinical benefit,[21, 22] thrombolytic treatment of ischemic stroke continues to be an active area of investigation.

Local, early intra-arterial infusions in patients with acute stroke have had some limited success in limiting cerebral infarct size.

Recanalization of carotid or vertebrobasilar territory was demonstrated with only a 17% rate of minor hemorrhage, and in the patients who were recanalized early, there were no severe residual cerebrovascular deficits.[23] t-PA has been evaluated in patients with acute cerebrovascular accident and produced some clinical improvement without causing excessive bleeding.[24] A composite review of the cerebral thrombolytic trials, which excluded patients with spontaneous intraparenchymal hemorrhage, demonstrated a 37% decrease in the risk of death and an overall 56% improvement in neurologic symptoms and residual deficit.[25] These encouraging initial results notwithstanding, large placebo-controlled trials show modest benefit in patients treated early (<3 h) with t-PA[25a] and lethal hemorrhagic events in patients treated later.[25b]

The major problem with the use of thrombolytic agents for the treatment of stroke is the risk of converting bland into hemorrhagic (parenchymatous) infarcts, especially because many nonhemorrhagic infarcts have been shown at autopsy to have some degree of microscopic hemorrhage. Approximately 5% of untreated ischemic stroke lesions spontaneously convert to symptomatic hemorrhagic infarcts. Treatment within 6 h, and especially within 90 min, after the onset of symptoms is associated with a lower risk of hemorrhagic conversion.[26] The risk of hemorrhagic extension is reduced when no infarct is visible by computed tomography immediately before the initiation of thrombolytic therapy.[27]

Antithrombotic Therapy

Antithrombotic therapy is commonly used in the treatment of acute cerebral ischemic syndromes, namely, transient (reversible) ischemic attack and stroke in evolution, and to prevent the occurrence of pulmonary embolism and deep venous thrombosis, which are commonly known to complicate the recovery of these patients. Antithrombotic treatment may prevent ongoing thrombosis, which often continues after the onset of a cerebral event.[28] Antiplatelet agents, such as aspirin, have been widely studied and have been shown to reduce the risk of stroke in patients with transient ischemic attacks or completed stroke by 22%. They are fully discussed in Chapter 27. Although intravenous heparin is commonly used to treat patients with ongoing cerebral ischemia or with symptomatic vertebrobasilar disease,[29] there are no conclusive data demonstrating any clear benefit of heparin for either of these indications.[30, 31]

The use of anticoagulation to treat the sequelae of cardioembolic stroke and prevent recurrent embolism carries a risk of hemorrhagic (parenchymatous) transformation of the infarction. Recurrent embolism occurs in approximately 10% of cardioembolic stroke patients during the 2 weeks after the acute event. Estimates of the frequency of hemorrhagic transformation after antithrombotic therapy range widely from 1.4% to 24%.[32] This risk is increased in the elderly and in the presence of large infarcts involving greater than 30% of the cerebral hemisphere.[33] Currently, heparin treatment is recommended for transient ischemic attack and for acute, small to moderate-sized cardioembolic strokes; this treatment should be followed by warfarin treatment, targeting the prothrombin time to an INR of 2.0–3.0. Patients receiving antithrombotic treatment should have a computed tomographic scan of the head 48 h after the onset of symptoms to ensure that spontaneous hemorrhagic transformation has not occurred. For patients with large embolic strokes, anticoagulation should be postponed for 5–14 days.

Antithrombotic Therapy in Atrial Fibrillation

Atrial fibrillation is associated with an increased risk of embolic stroke. For patients with atrial fibrillation, risk factors associated with an increased frequency of cerebral ischemia include increasing age and a history of hypertension, diabetes mellitus, previous transient ischemic attack, or stroke. In the past several years, five randomized, multicenter trials have investigated the efficacy of oral anticoagulant treatment for patients with nonvalvar atrial fibrillation[34–38] (Table 30–3). All of these studies reported that anticoagulant treatment consistently decreases the risk of stroke. Analysis of pooled data from the completed randomized controlled trials demonstrated an overall 68% reduction in risk of stroke for patients with atrial fibrillation treated with warfarin compared with control subjects.[39] This reduction in embolic events was not associated with a significant increase in major hemorrhagic events (1% per year vs. 0.9% per year on average). Patients younger than 65 years who had no history of hypertension, diabetes, or previous transient ischemic attack or stroke had a low risk of having a stroke even if not treated and may not warrant long-term anticoagulation with its inherent risks.

Secondary prevention in patients with transient ischemic attack or minor ischemic stroke with use of warfarin or aspirin has also been addressed in patients with atrial fibrillation.[40] Ninety vascular events (mainly stroke) were prevented for every 1000 patients anticoagulated for 1 year. Aspirin was a safe, although less effective, therapy in this group of patients, preventing 40 vascular events per 1000 patients treated per year. The bleeding rate was 2.8% per year in patients treated with warfarin and 0.9% per year in patients treated with aspirin.

Patients with lone atrial fibrillation were also shown to have a low risk for stroke; no events were reported in those younger than 60

TABLE 30–3. EVENT RATES COMPARING WARFARIN WITH PLACEBO IN NONRHEUMATIC ATRIAL FIBRILLATION

	AFASAK[34]		SPAF[35]		BAATAF[36]		CAFA[37]		SPINAF[38]	
	W	P	W	P	W	P	W	P	W	P
Total										
(Patients/Year)	423	417	271	259	487	435	239	251	456	440
% Patients/Year										
Stroke	1.9	4.8	2.3	7.0	0.4	0.3	2.1	3.7	0.9	4.3
Embolism	0	0.2	0	0.8	0	0	0.4	0.8	0.8	0.4
ICH	0.2	0	0.4	0	0	0	0.4	0	0.2	0
TIA	0.2	0.7	1.5	2.4	0.8	0.9	0.8	0.8	1.5	2.6
Death	4.7	6.5	2.2	3.1	2.3	6.0	4.2	3.2	3.3	5.0
Death (vasc.)	3.3	4.1	1.5	1.9	1.4	3.2	3.8	4.2	—	—
Hemorrhage	0.3	0	0.4	0.8	1.0	1.9	1.7	0.8	1.5	1.9

Abbreviations: W, warfarin-treated patients; P, placebo-treated patients. Embolism, systemic embolism; ICH, intracerebral hemorrhage; TIA, transient ischemic attack; Death, all-cause death; Death (vasc.), death from vascular causes; Hemorrhage, major hemorrhage.

TABLE 30–4. THERAPY FOR PATIENTS WITH LONE ATRIAL FIBRILLATION[124]

Age	Stroke Rate	Therapy
Younger than 60 years and no clinical risk factors	<0.5%/year	None
60–75 years and no clinical risk factors	1.6%/year	Aspirin
Older than 75 years and no clinical risk factors	2.1%/year	Anticoagulants

years, compared with a 3% frequency in patients older than 80 years. The annual incidence of major hemorrhagic events was 1.3% in the warfarin-treated patients compared with 1.0% in the control patients. The target range for oral anticoagulation treatment varied in each of these studies. Although some patients with intracranial hemorrhage were within the targeted range set by the study, most had an INR of greater than 3.0. Current anticoagulant recommendations for treatment of patients with lone atrial fibrillation are summarized in Table 30–4.

Aspirin treatment, discussed in Chapter 27, is currently under investigation to determine its effectiveness relative to warfarin for the treatment of thromboembolism in atrial fibrillation. Evidence suggests that the additive effect of warfarin, although real, may be minimal.[41]

THROMBOLYTIC AND ANTITHROMBOTIC TREATMENT OF VENOUS THROMBOTIC DISEASE

See also Chapter 28.

Pulmonary Embolism

Pulmonary embolism is responsible for as many as 50,000 deaths in the United States each year.[42] For this reason and the expectation that timely administration of appropriate therapy can markedly lower mortality, aggressive therapeutic approaches to this common disease have been emphasized. The initial treatment of pulmonary embolism with heparin and subsequent treatment with warfarin for long-term anticoagulation are discussed in Chapter 28. For selected patients, thrombolytic therapy may be a reasonable alternative therapeutic option.

Briefly, after the diagnosis of pulmonary embolism, heparin is given, usually administered as a 5000- to 10,000-unit bolus followed by a continuous infusion of approximately 35,000 units/day.[43] Initial dosing may also be administered on a unit-per-weight basis with an initial loading dose of 80 units/kg followed by a continuous infusion of 18 units/kg/hr or according to a titration nomogram.[43a] The heparin dosage should be adjusted to maintain the activated partial thromboplastin time between 1.5 and 2.0 times the control value. Heparin treatment interrupts the thrombotic process, permitting the endogenous fibrinolytic system to dissolve the thrombus.

Certain patients require more rapid intervention to correct the presence of a potentially profound thrombus burden and its associated pathophysiologic complications, such as acute cor pulmonale. Thrombolytic agents lead to rapid dissolution of thrombus and may quickly restore cardiopulmonary function to normal. Thrombolytic therapy promotes faster clot lysis than is possible by anticoagulation alone and, as a result, rapidly improves right ventricular failure.[44] The administration of fibrinolytic agents also reduces the frequency of chronic pulmonary hypertension that results from pulmonary emboli.[45] The initial studies of thrombolytic treatment of pulmonary embolism included the Urokinase and Urokinase-Streptokinase Pulmonary Embolism Trials (UPET and UPSET).[46, 47] In these trials, patients treated with UK or SK in conjunction with heparin achieved more rapid pulmonary reperfusion and decreases in pulmonary artery pressures than did patients treated with heparin alone. Similar benefits have been shown with t-PA.[48]

Thrombolytic agents were approved for the treatment of pulmonary emboli in 1977, but their use has not become as widespread as originally predicted.[49] Although the results appear encouraging, decreases in death or recurrent pulmonary embolism with thrombolytic treatment have not been documented; several large, multicenter clinical trials have failed to demonstrate a significant reduction in mortality with the use of these agents. In addition, hemorrhagic complications impede the routine use of thrombolytic therapy for pulmonary embolism with high rates of bleeding at sites of catheter insertion for pulmonary angiography. Thus, in patients with suspected pulmonary embolism who are candidates for thrombolytic therapy, it is safer to use only nondiagnostic testing before therapy.[50]

Despite these shortcomings, thrombolytic agents have been recommended for patients with massive pulmonary embolism to prevent acute cor pulmonale and sudden death.[51] Thrombolytic therapy appears to benefit patients who have pulmonary embolism in the presence of significant hemodynamic disturbances and/or have obstructed blood flow to a whole lung or to multiple lung segments. Thus, it is currently recommended that thrombolytic therapy be used for patients with massive pulmonary embolism associated with hypotension in the absence of standard contraindications.[52]

Three thrombolytic regimens are currently approved for the treatment of pulmonary embolism in the United States, and these employ intravenous administration of SK, UK, or t-PA (Table 30–5). These protocols have been found to lyse thrombus effectively and require no dosage adjustments during the infusion of the plasminogen activator. The t-PA regimen involves the shortest infusion time and can rapidly reduce clot burden. Shorter infusion times are believed to reduce hemorrhagic risk; however, t-PA use has not been shown to reduce morbidity or mortality in clinical trials, compared with other thrombolytic regimens. Heparin treatment is not given concurrently with the thrombolytic agents but should be started on completion of the infusion without a bolus.

Deep Venous Thrombosis

Deep venous thrombosis[53] is a spectrum of diseases ranging from asymptomatic calf vein thrombosis to venous gangrene. The most important acute complication of deep venous thrombosis is pulmonary embolism; the long-term effect is the post-thrombotic (postphlebitic) syndrome. Thrombolytic agents have been used in many trials to treat deep venous thrombosis, but unlike their known efficacy in the treatment of myocardial infarction, thrombolytic therapy for venous thromboembolism lacks proven mortality benefit.[54] The role of heparin in the treatment of deep venous thrombosis is discussed in Chapter 28.

Ideally, the treatment of deep venous thrombosis should prevent acute embolic complications as well as the long-term sequela of post-thrombotic syndrome. The frequency of residual venous insuf-

TABLE 30–5. SYSTEMIC THROMBOLYTIC TREATMENT FOR PULMONARY EMBOLISM

Agent	Loading Dose	Infusion Rate
t-PA	None	50 mg/h for 2 h IV
Streptokinase	250,000 units/30 min IV	100,000 units/h for 24 h
Urokinase	4400 units/kg/10 min IV	4400 units/kg/h for 12 h

Abbreviations: t-PA, tissue-type plasminogen activator; IV, intravenously.

ficiency and recurrent thrombosis during antithrombotic-treated deep venous thrombosis suggests that heparin may not prevent the progression of local disease. Studies have shown that thrombus can propagate even when full anticoagulation is achieved.[55, 56] With thrombus extension and persistence of residual thrombus, loss of venous function can develop with altered venous hemodynamic return as well as postphlebitic syndrome, including pigmentation changes, swelling, and ulceration. Therefore, whereas antithrombotic treatment is adequate for most patients, it may not protect some patients against the late sequelae of venous thrombosis.

The development of post-thrombotic syndrome may be reduced by thrombolytic therapy. Studies have shown that approximately 50% of patients achieve rapid lysis of greater than 75% of the thrombus with fibrinolytic therapy.[57] A pooled analysis of the randomized trials comparing intravenous SK with heparin in the treatment of deep venous thrombosis demonstrated that thrombolysis is achieved approximately four times more often for those patients treated with SK than for those treated with heparin;[58] however, bleeding complications were three times more prevalent in the SK-treated group. Trials with UK have shown similar rates of clot lysis but somewhat fewer bleeding complications.[59] Most investigators using thrombolytic agents for the treatment of deep venous thrombosis have reported an increase in clot lysis and decreased frequency of postphlebitic syndrome.[60] Nonetheless, the more than doubled hemorrhagic risks accompanying SK and t-PA[61] have tempered the overall enthusiasm for the broad use of plasminogen activators in patients with deep venous thrombosis.

Owing to the overall benefits of fibrinolysis, thrombolytic treatment is currently recommended in patients with deep venous thrombosis to reduce the occurrence of the postphlebitic syndrome.[62] Currently, only a 24- to 72-h continuous infusion of SK is approved by the U.S. Food and Drug Administration for the treatment of deep venous thrombosis (Table 30–6). With use of this method, lysis is achieved in about two thirds of the patients; shorter infusion times may also have clinical benefit.[63]

The optimal duration of treatment for deep venous thrombosis depends on the rate of lysis and quantity of clot. Intravascular thrombolysis has also been used with success in the treatment of deep venous thrombosis particularly in the iliofemoral vein.[64] A guide wire is inserted into the thrombus, and UK is given as a 250,000- to 500,000-unit bolus followed by an infusion of 250,000 units/h. Catheter-directed thrombolysis with UK for the treatment of iliofemoral deep venous thrombosis has also been shown to achieve lysis in more than two thirds of treated patients.[65]

Subclavian-Axillary Venous Thrombosis

Other venous disorders that have been shown to benefit from thrombolytic therapy include upper extremity venous thrombosis[66] as well as thrombosis of the axillary and subclavian veins. Venous thrombosis in the upper extremity may be either primary or secondary. Primary thrombosis results from decreased venous flow rates, with flow abnormalities caused by intrinsic (webs or valves) or extrinsic (subclavian muscle, anterior scalene muscle, fibrous bands, or first rib compression) structural abnormalities. Symptoms are commonly associated with repetitive arm movements; thus, patients commonly have a history of recent physical exertion or trauma. Secondary thrombosis occurs after iatrogenic trauma, such as that which results from placement of catheters or pacemakers and other types of central venous manipulation. Patients usually present with significant upper extremity swelling, pain, and occasional prominence of the superficial veins. Patients are evaluated by venography of the affected upper extremity to confirm the diagnosis and then treated acutely with heparin, followed by warfarin for 3 months. The decision about the need for thrombolytic therapy is based on the initial extent of thrombosis and evidence for ongoing thrombus propagation despite adequate anticoagulation. First rib resection or muscle release may be considered when extrinsic compression is identified on venography.

For thrombosis of the subclavian or axillary vein, improved results have been demonstrated with local thrombolytic therapy compared with systemic treatment.[67] A typical high-dose regimen involves traversing the thrombus with a guidewire and then administering a transthrombus loading dose of 4000 units/min UK for 1–2 h followed by 1000 units/min for up to 24 h.[68] After completion of the infusion, systemic heparin is given to maintain the activated partial thromboplastin time at 1.5–2 times the control value. Oral anticoagulation is recommended thereafter for 3 months.

TABLE 30–6. SYSTEMIC THROMBOLYTIC TREATMENT FOR DEEP VENOUS THROMBOSIS

Agent	Loading Dose	Infusion Rate
t-PA	None	40–50 mg/h for 2 h IV
Streptokinase[125]	250,000 units/30 min IV	100,000 units/h for 24–72 h
Urokinase	2000–4000 units/kg	2000 to 4000 units/kg/hr for 12–48 h

Abbreviations: t-PA, tissue-type plasminogen activator; IV, intravenous.

THROMBOLYTIC AND ANTITHROMBOTIC TREATMENT OF VALVULAR DISEASE

Arterial thromboembolic events may complicate prosthetic heart valve placement and are often a consequence of ineffective anticoagulant therapy. The incidence of thrombosis of prosthetic heart valves is reported to range from 0.5% to 6% per patient-year in the aortic and mitral positions[69] to as high as 20% for valves in the tricuspid position.[70] Fibrinolytic therapy has been used as an alternative to surgery and is especially useful in critically ill patients. Despite an overall efficacy of 73%, there remains a significant risk of cerebral embolism complicating valvular fibrinolytic therapy for thrombosed left-sided prosthetic valves (14.6%).[71]

In general, native valvular heart disease is not treated with antithrombotic therapy. In certain situations, however, anticoagulant therapy may be beneficial. Long-term anticoagulant therapy is recommended for patients with rheumatic mitral valvular heart disease who have either paroxysmal or chronic atrial fibrillation or a history of systemic embolism. Warfarin therapy should be targeted to prolong the INR to 2.0–3.0.[72] Long-term anticoagulant therapy has also been suggested for patients with rheumatic mitral valve disease who are in sinus rhythm if the left atrial diameter exceeds 5.5 cm,[73] although this recommendation is not based on published data. There is a low frequency of systemic thromboembolism in patients with isolated aortic valvular disease, and long-term antithrombotic therapy is not recommended for these patients unless there is a history of coexisting mitral valve disease, atrial fibrillation, or past systemic embolism.

Antithrombotic therapy is not necessary for patients with mitral valve prolapse unless there is a concomitant history of atrial fibrillation or systemic embolism.[74] If patients have either of these conditions in the presence of mitral valve prolapse, anticoagulant therapy is advised with long-term warfarin to maintain an INR of 2.0–3.0. No antithrombotic therapy is advised for patients with mitral annular calcification unless there is a history of atrial fibrillation or embolism.[75] Anticoagulant therapy is not recommended for patients with uncomplicated infective endocarditis, owing to the increased frequency of hemorrhage in such patients. Patients who have endocarditis in the presence of a mechanical prosthetic valve should have their antithrombotic therapy continued because there is a high frequency of embolic complications on cessation of therapy;[76] these patients are also at significant risk for intracerebral events.[77]

Mechanical Prosthetic Heart Valves

In general, it has been recommended that all patients with mechanical prosthetic heart valves be treated with long-term warfarin at a dose that will prolong the prothrombin time ratio to approximately 2.0 times the control value according to North American guidelines for thromboplastin.[78] Levels less than this (INR ≤ 1.8) appear to be associated with a high frequency of thromboembolic events,[79] whereas levels producing an INR of greater than 4.5 are associated with excessive bleeding. Tilting disk valves should have an INR maintained at 2.5 to 3.5; INR levels of 2.2 to 3.3 are recommended for ball valves.[80, 81]

Bioprosthetic Heart Valves

Patients with bioprosthetic valves in the mitral position may be treated with smaller doses of warfarin. In one study, an INR of 2.0–2.25 was found to be as effective as an INR of 2.5–4.5, but with a lower rate of hemorrhagic complications.[82] On the basis of this study, the current recommendation is that such patients be treated for the first 3 months after bioprosthetic valve insertion with warfarin therapy (INR of 2.0–3.0). For patients with bioprosthetic valves who are in atrial fibrillation or have documented left atrial thrombus, long-term anticoagulation is recommended (INR of 2.0–3.0). Patients with bioprosthetic valves and a history of systemic embolism may need long-term anticoagulant therapy (3–12 months) at an INR of 2.0–3.0.

COMPLICATIONS OF THROMBOLYTIC THERAPY

The major complications of thrombolytic therapy that often lead to a decrease in the use of these agents are hemorrhage and reocclusion. Hemorrhagic complications have been reduced by using new regimens with shorter infusion times, minimizing the number of invasive vascular procedures, and excluding patients with significant hypertension or a history of stroke. Despite these guidelines, bleeding continues to be a significant complication of thrombolytic therapy; major hemorrhagic complications occur in up to 15% of patients.[83] It was initially hoped that fibrin-selective agents would reduce hemorrhagic complications, but the somewhat decreased lytic state noted with t-PA, for example, has not translated into a reduced frequency of bleeding complications compared with fibrin-nonspecific agents (SK). This lack of clinical benefit may be caused by the failure of clot-selective agents to discriminate between an occlusive thrombus and a protective hemostatic plug.[84] Therefore, minimizing thrombolytic use in patients with possible hemostatic plugs, such as those with prior stroke or recent gastrointestinal hemorrhage, can be an effective means of decreasing hemorrhagic complications of therapy. Invasive procedures, as well as the duration of therapy, greatly influence the frequency of bleeding complications. Owing to the devastating consequences of central nervous system hemorrhage, the neurologic status of patients receiving thrombolytic therapy should be carefully observed.

Other complications of thrombolytic therapy include reocclusion and allergic reactions. Reocclusion is an important problem of thrombolytic therapy and occurs with both SK (19%)[85] and t-PA (24%)[86] and to a lesser extent with UK (4%)[87] in myocardial infarction trials. Although SK is immunogenic and febrile reactions may occur in up to 30% of patients receiving SK, serious allergic reactions are rare.

COMPLICATIONS OF ANTITHROMBOTIC THERAPY

Heparin

Bleeding is the most common complication of heparin use. Heparin should be administered with caution to patients who have recently undergone surgery; who have bleeding disorders or severe hypertension; and who have a recent or past history of cerebrovascular, gastrointestinal, or genitourinary hemorrhage or metastatic cancer. The frequency of bleeding has been reported to vary with the mode of administration and ranges from approximately 7% for patients receiving continuous infusion to 14% for patients given intermittent bolus doses.[88] However, the total dose administered in a 24-h period may be the most important determinant of bleeding risk.[89]

Minor bleeding can be treated by simply stopping heparin therapy. Significant hemorrhage may necessitate additional therapy, including blood transfusion. The effect of heparin can be immediately reversed by infusion of protamine sulfate. Protamine is a strongly basic low-molecular-weight protein that forms complexes with and inactivates heparin.[90] One milligram of protamine neutralizes approximately 90 USP units of bovine-derived heparin or 115 USP units of porcine-derived heparin. Thus, for every 100 units of heparin estimated to be in the circulation, 1 mg of protamine should be given. Protamine should be infused slowly during several minutes to avoid potential adverse reactions, such as hypotension, dyspnea, and flushing. Protamine use should also be avoided in diabetics receiving NPH insulin because of the risk of allergic reaction.

Another important complication of heparin administration is thrombocytopenia. Heparin may cause a benign, transient thrombocytopenia at the time of initiation of therapy. More important, heparin use can cause a significant clinical disorder, heparin-induced thrombocytopenia, beginning 3 to 10 days after the start of drug administration and earlier in patients previously sensitized. The former is thought to result from temporary sequestration of platelets in the spleen, possibly the result of mild heparin-initiated platelet activation; whereas the latter is believed to be a manifestation of a heparin-dependent immune effect that can persist for days, even after heparin is discontinued.[91]

Heparin-induced thrombocytopenia poses a significant problem for management of patients. The frequency of heparin-induced thrombocytopenia has been reported in the past to range from 5% to 30%, although recent analysis suggests that the true frequency is less than 3%.[92] There is no clear relationship between heparin dose and the risk of heparin-induced thrombocytopenia; the disorder has even been described in patients whose exposure to heparin is as minimal as that from an indwelling heparin-coated pulmonary artery catheter.[93] Some data suggest that this disorder is more likely to occur in patients receiving bovine-derived heparin than in patients receiving porcine-derived heparin.[94]

Although not commonly associated with bleeding, heparin-induced thrombocytopenia is paradoxically implicated as a cause of life-threatening venous and/or arterial thrombosis. Thrombosis complicating heparin-induced thrombocytopenia may occur in as many as 20% of affected patients. The development of thrombosis is not predictable and is not related to platelet count nadir. Any patients having new or progressive thrombosis during heparin therapy should, therefore, be evaluated for the possibility of heparin-induced thrombocytopenia. Common sites of thrombosis include the distal aorta and the iliofemoral artery.

Other adverse reactions associated with prolonged heparin use include accelerated bone loss and osteoporosis. Most patients with symptomatic osteoporosis have received greater than 20,000 units/day for longer than 6 months.[95] Heparin does not cross the placenta and is considered the drug of choice for long-term anticoagulation in pregnant patients. It has no known teratogenic effects and is not found in maternal milk. In a review of 186 studies of anticoagulant use during pregnancy, no increased risk of prematurity was found for heparin-treated patients;[96] however, heparin use is accompanied by an increase in maternal bleeding.

Patients receiving heparin should be monitored for the development of thrombocytopenia. A baseline platelet count should be obtained at the initiation of heparin therapy and repeated every other day while heparin is administered. Occurrence of a significant decline in platelet count, even if it is still within the normal range, should be confirmed. Primary therapy for heparin-induced thrombocytopenia is cessation of heparin. In most patients, platelet counts will return to normal within 4 days. Alternative anticoagulant therapy with dextran and/or warfarin should be considered. Low-molecular-weight heparin preparations cannot be uniformly substituted for conventional heparin in this setting because they have also been associated with thrombocytopenia.[97]

Warfarin

Complications of warfarin therapy are, in part, influenced by the degree of anticoagulation, existing disease, concomitant drug administration, and the patient's reliability. Particular attention must be paid to patients receiving concurrent platelet-inhibiting agents. Anticoagulation must proceed with caution in patients with recent surgery; bleeding disorders; severe hypertension; a recent or past history of cerebrovascular, gastrointestinal, or genitourinary hemorrhage; metastatic cancer; or motion disorders associated with an increased risk of falling.

Warfarin should be avoided during pregnancy. Oral anticoagulants can cross the placenta, and warfarin use during the first trimester has been implicated in a specific malformation syndrome referred to as the fetal warfarin syndrome.[98] In addition, warfarin use at any time during pregnancy may increase the risk of central nervous system abnormalities in the fetus. Finally, anticoagulation during labor and delivery can result in devastating neonatal hemorrhage.

Many prescription drugs and over-the-counter medications interact with or alter warfarin action, resulting in enhanced or diminished anticoagulant effects. Interfering mechanisms include alterations in absorption, metabolism, and excretion. Variation in vitamin K intake affects a patient's response to warfarin and complicates dosing. Patients should be aware that vitamin K is plentiful in leafy green vegetables.

As with heparin, the major complication of warfarin therapy is bleeding. The risk of hemorrhage is estimated at 4%–5% per treatment year, and major bleeding events are estimated to occur at 1%–2% per year; the risk of anticoagulant-induced intracranial hemorrhage is between 0.07% and 1.5% per treatment year. Seventy-five percent of bleeding complications occur in patients with a prothrombin time within the targeted therapeutic range. It is possible that universal adoption of reduced dosing levels will result in diminished rates of hemorrhage. Another complication of oral anticoagulant therapy, the unusual syndrome of warfarin-associated skin necrosis, can occur 3–8 days after initiation of therapy. This disorder is believed to be a consequence of inadequate activated protein C, a naturally occurring vitamin K–dependent anticoagulant.

To treat hemorrhage, the most common complication of oral anticoagulation, fresh-frozen plasma and red blood cells can be transfused. Fresh-frozen plasma, rich in vitamin K–dependent coagulation factors, immediately corrects the warfarin-induced coagulation defect. However, clinical and laboratory parameters must be observed closely in patients treated only with fresh-frozen plasma because the effect of warfarin, still present in the plasma, may cause recurrent hemorrhage. In patients with serious hemorrhage or profound overanticoagulation, vitamin K should be administered either subcutaneously or intravenously at doses of 0.5–10 mg. Correction of the prothrombin time requires at least 24 h. Large doses of vitamin K should be avoided in patients who will require further anticoagulation because a state of resistance may occur when warfarin therapy is reinstituted. Cholestyramine can also be given to reduce absorption of warfarin still in the gut.

FUTURE DIRECTIONS IN THROMBOLYTIC AND ANTITHROMBOTIC THERAPY

Thrombolytic Therapy

Thrombolytic therapies are currently being given as combinations of available agents[99–101] in the hope of optimizing efficacy while minimizing hemorrhagic complications and cost. However, results from these trials have shown no improvement in benefit and an increased hemorrhagic risk for patients treated with t-PA and SK in combination. The use of scu-PA in combination with t-PA has shown some promise.[102]

The duration of thrombolytic treatment for pulmonary embolism and deep venous thrombosis continues to be investigated, because shorter infusion times may limit hemorrhagic events. In deep venous thrombosis, 48–72 h is usually necessary for successful clot lysis; for pulmonary embolism, shorter infusion times may be successful. Newer ways of administering these agents have already been tested for coronary ischemia as a means of improving fibrinolysis and preserving patency.[101]

The goal of future thrombolytic therapy is to develop new agents that will produce fewer hemostatic alterations and, consequently, cause less bleeding while at the same time maintaining lytic efficacy; many investigators are attempting to achieve this end by producing mutants (deletion or inclusion) of t-PA as an initial strategy. Chimeric thrombolytic agents are being developed that may have greater thrombolytic potency or fibrin specificity. Chimeric proteins that incorporate t-PA and UK have been created and have been shown to have increased fibrin specificity.[103] A recombinant t-PA variant has been shown to have increased fibrin specificity and a decreased plasma clearance rate without producing a severe systemic lytic state.[104]

Antithrombotic Therapy

New direct and indirect inhibitors of thrombin are being developed with the goal of identifying an agent with greater specificity and fewer hemostatic complications than the traditional antithrombotic drugs, warfarin and heparin (Fig. 30–2). Specifically, the inhibition of thrombin formation may be an important approach for preventing vessel occlusion in cardiovascular disorders.

Low-Molecular-Weight Heparin

Low-molecular-weight heparin regimens and preparations are currently being developed in the United States; some forms are already marketed and in use in Europe. Low-molecular-weight heparins can be produced from conventional heparin by enzymatic or chemical depolymerization; the resulting preparations have heterogeneous molecular masses and varied anticoagulant activities. The molecular mass of current preparations ranges from 1000 to 15,000 D with an average molecular weight of 4000–5000; these preparations include heparin species of 2500–15,000 D.

Currently, low-molecular-weight heparin is formulated only for subcutaneous administration. The pharmacokinetic profile of low-molecular-weight heparin is different from that of conventional heparin. After subcutaneous injection, the bioavailability of low-molecular-weight heparin preparations approaches 90%, compared with 20% for unfractionated heparin.[105] The plasma half-life of low-molecular-weight heparin varies with preparation and ranges from 100 to 200 min. Low-molecular-weight heparins are cleared primarily through renal excretion, and thus their biologic half-life is increased with renal failure.

Low-molecular-weight heparins have been shown to be highly effective and safe for postsurgical and medical prophylaxis of deep venous thrombosis.[106] In patients with acute ischemic stroke, low-molecular-weight heparin prevents the formation of deep venous thrombosis compared with standard heparin preparations, without significantly increasing bleeding complications.[107] Low-molecular-weight heparin has also been shown to be beneficial in the prevention of arterial thrombosis. Patients undergoing femorodistal reconstructive surgery were given enoxaparin, a low-molecular-weight heparin (75 anti–factor Xa/kg intravenously), or heparin (50 units/kg intravenously) before surgery, then b.i.d. subcutaneously for 10 days.[108] Arterial thrombosis developed in 8 patients given low-molec-

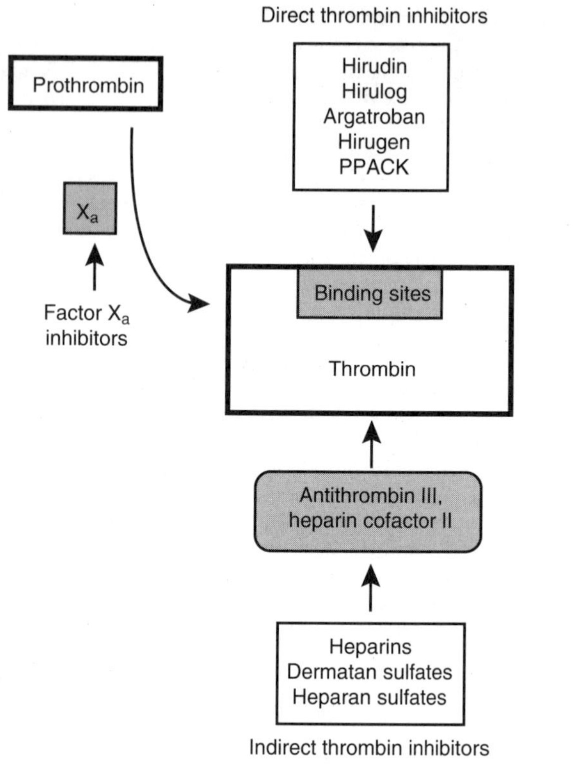

Figure 30–2. Direct and indirect inhibitors of thrombin. Direct thrombin inhibitors inactivate thrombin by interacting with one or more binding sites. Indirect thrombin inhibitors require the serpins antithrombin III or heparin cofactor II to inactivate thrombin. Inhibitors of factor X_a prevent the generation of thrombin.

ular-weight heparin and 20 patients given unfractionated heparin (p = .02) with similar rates of major hemorrhage.

Hirudin

Hirudin, a direct thrombin inhibitor, is a polypeptide originally extracted from the salivary gland of the leech *Hirudo medicinalis* and now available in the recombinant form. Hirulog is a synthetic peptide that, like hirudin, contains two distinct domains with antithrombin activity.[109] Hirudin forms a complex with thrombin, inhibiting the enzyme's proteolytic function. This inhibition prevents fibrin formation as well as the activation of clotting factors V, VIII, and XIII and thrombin-induced platelet aggregation. Therefore, compared with heparin, hirudin does not require the presence of endogenous cofactors, like antithrombin III. In addition, hirudin is not bound to or inactivated by proteins acting as antiheparin substances, such as platelet factor 4.[110] Hirudin is primarily excreted by the kidneys with a plasma half-life of approximately 1 h.[111]

In experimental models of arterial and venous thrombosis, hirudin is a more effective antithrombotic than heparin.[112] Recombinant desulfatohirudin (CG 39393) is nearly identical in structure to natural hirudin and has also begun clinical testing. Hirudin has been compared with heparin in patients undergoing coronary angioplasty. Infusions of hirudin (20 mg as a bolus before angioplasty followed by a continuous infusion of 0.16 mg/kg/h given for 24 h) resulted in complete maintenance of perfusion and fewer acute cardiac or procedural complications than with heparin.[113] Hirudin was compared with heparin as adjunctive therapy to t-PA for treatment of acute myocardial infarction in a pilot trial (Thrombolysis In Myocardial Infarction [TIMI]–5) and was found to carry a reduced rate of in-hospital death or reinfarction as well as a trend toward fewer major hemorrhagic events.[114] More recently, a larger trial (TIMI-9) has failed to show a significant difference between adjunctive heparin and hirudin in patients with acute myocardial infarction treated with thrombolytic therapy.[114a] Hirulog has also been shown to reduce the progression to infarction after angioplasty compared with heparin, and to do so with half the rate of hemorrhagic complications as that of heparin.[115]

Factor X_a Inhibitors

Factor X_a inhibitors are a new class of antithrombotic agents that inhibit thrombin generation indirectly by preventing its generation from prothrombin. The best studied of these agents is tick anticoagulant peptide (TAP), a potent and highly selective direct inhibitor of factor X_a.[116] This peptide is available in recombinant form[117] and has been studied in animal models of disseminated intravascular coagulation as well as venous and arterial thrombosis. TAP has been shown to enhance vessel patency, compared with heparin, in a model of canine coronary thrombosis.[118] Recombinant antistasin also directly inhibits factor X_a and has been shown to prevent platelet-dependent thrombus formation in a baboon model without significantly altering the bleeding time.[119]

Antithrombin III

Recombinant antithrombin III has mainly been studied as replacement therapy for patients with a congenital or acquired deficiency of this glycoprotein.[120] It has also been administered to patients as prophylaxis for postoperative venous thromboembolism. Patients given antithrombin III (1500–3000 units intravenously 2 h preoperatively and 1000–2000 units postoperatively for 5 days) with low-dose subcutaneous heparin had a significantly decreased frequency of venous thrombosis compared with a group given dextran. In addition, the antithrombin III treatment had no significant side effects.

Activated Protein C and Factor IX_a Inhibitors

Activated protein C has been studied in a primate graft model.[121] Recombinant activated protein C significantly reduced occlusion in Dacron grafts compared with that of controls. Deposition of platelets labeled with indium IN III concomitantly decreased.

Inhibitors of factor IX_a have also been shown to block intravascular thrombosis without impairing extravascular hemostasis.[122]

REFERENCES

1. Sharma GV, Cella G, Parisi AF, et al: Thrombolytic therapy. N Engl J Med 1982; 306:1268–1272.
2. Hussain SS, Gurewich B, Lipinski B: Purification and partial characterization of single-chain high-molecular-weight form of urokinase from human urine. Arch Biol Biophys 1983; 280:31–38.
3. Levin EG: Latent tissue plasminogen activation produced by human endothelial cells in cultures: evidence for an enzyme inhibitor complex. Proc Natl Acad Sci USA 1983; 80:6804–6808.
4. Rijken DC, Hoylaerts M, Collen D: Fibrinolytic properties of one-chain and two-chain human extrinsic (tissue-type) plasminogen activator. J Biol Chem 1982; 257:2920–2925.
5. TIMI Study Group: Thrombolysis in Myocardial Infarction (TIMI) trial. Phase I findings. N Engl J Med 1985; 312:932–936.
6. Bounameaux H, Stassen HM, Seghers C, Collen D: Influence of fibrin and liver blood flow on the turnover and systemic fibrinogenolytic effects of recombinant human tissue-type plasminogen activator. Blood 1986; 67:1493–1497.
7. Nurmohamed MT, Rosendaal FR, Buller HR, et al: Low molecular weight heparin in the prophylaxis of venous thrombosis: a meta-analysis. Lancet 1992; 340:152–156.
8. Hirsh J: Oral anticoagulant drugs. N Engl J Med 1991; 324:1865–1875.
9. Gallus A, Jackson J, Tillett J, et al: Safety and efficacy of warfarin started early after submassive venous thrombosis or pulmonary embolism. Lancet 1986; 2:1293–1296.

10. Bussey HI, Force RW, Bianco TM, Leonard AD: Reliance on prothrombin time ratios causes significant errors in anticoagulant therapy. Arch Intern Med 1992; 152:278–282.
11. Avery A, Deloof W, Vermylen J, Verstraete M: Outcome of recent thromboembolic occlusions of limb arteries treated with streptokinase. Br Med J 1970; 4:639–644.
12. Belkin M, Belkin B, Bucknam CA, et al: Intra-arterial fibrinolytic therapy: efficacy of streptokinase vs. urokinase. Arch Surg 1986; 121:769–773.
13. Earnshow JJ: Thrombolytic therapy in the management of acute limb ischaemia. Br J Surg 1991; 78:261–269.
14. Juhan C, Haupert S, Miltgen G, et al: A new intra-arterial rt-PA dosage regimen in peripheral arterial occlusion: bolus followed by continuous infusion [Letter]. Thromb Haemost 1991; 65:635.
15. Risius B, Graor RA, Geisinger MA: Thrombolytic therapy with recombinant tissue-type plasminogen activator: a comparison of two doses. Radiology 1987; 164:465–468.
16. Hofling B, Backa D, Lauterjung L, et al: Percutaneous removal of atheromatous plaque in peripheral arteries. Lancet 1988; 1:384–385.
17. Hoch JR, Tullis MJ, Acher CW, et al: Thrombolysis versus surgery as the initial management for native artery occlusion: efficacy, safety, and cost. Surgery 1994; 116:649–657.
18. Graor RA, Risius B, Young JR, et al: Thrombolysis of peripheral arterial bypass grafts: surgical thrombectomy compared with thrombolysis. J Vasc Surg 1988; 7:347–353.
19. Schumacherts M, Schmidt D, Wakhloo AK: Intra-arterial fibrinolytic therapy in central retinal artery occlusion. Neuroradiology 1993; 35:600–605.
20. Herndon RM: Thrombolytic treatment in cerebrovascular thrombosis. *In* MacMillan RL, Mustard JF (eds): Anticoagulants and Fibrinolysis, pp 154–164. Philadelphia: Lea & Febiger, 1961.
21. Fletcher AP, Alkjaersig N, Lewis M, et al: A pilot study of urokinase therapy in cerebral infarction. Stroke 1976; 7:135–142.
22. Del Zoppo GJ, Zeumer H, Hortier A: Thrombolytic therapy in stroke: possibilities and hazards. Stroke 1986; 17:595–607.
23. Zeumer H, Hundgen R, Ferbert A, Ringelstein EB: Local intraarterial fibrinolytic therapy in inaccessible intracranial carotid occlusion. Neuroradiology 1984; 26:315–317.
24. Puca A: Thrombolysis in cerebral ischemia. J Neurosurg Sci 1993; 37:63–70.
25. Wardlaw JM, Warlow CP: Thrombolysis in acute ischemic stroke: does it work? Stroke 1992; 23:1826–1839.
25a. The National Institute of Neurological Disorders and Stroke rt-PA Stroke Study Group: Tissue plasminogen activator for acute ischemic stroke. N Engl J Med 1995; 333:1581–1587.
25b. Hommel M, Boissel JP, Cornu C, et al: Termination of a trial of streptokinase in severe acute ischemic stroke. Lancet 1995; 345:57.
26. Haley ED, Levy DE, Brott TG, et al: Urgent therapy for stroke. Part II. Pilot study of tissue plasminogen activator administered 92–180 minutes from onset. Stroke 1992; 23:641–645.
27. Okada Y, Sadoshima S, Nakane H, et al: Early computed tomographic findings for thrombolytic therapy in patients with acute brain embolism. Stroke 1992; 23:20–23.
28. Britton M, Rodin A: Progression of stroke after arrival to the hospital. Stroke 1985; 16:629–632.
29. Estol CJ, Pessin MS: Anticoagulation: is there still a role in atherothrombotic stroke? Stroke 1990; 21:820–824.
30. Rothrock JR, Hart RG: Antithrombotic therapy in cerebrovascular disease. Ann Intern Med 1991; 115:885–895.
31. Wityk RJ, Stern BJ: Ischemic stroke. Crit Care Med 1994; 22:1278–1293.
32. Sherman DG, Dyken ML, Fisher M, et al: Antithrombotic therapy for cerebrovascular disorders. Chest 1992; 102:529S–537S.
33. Okada Y, Yamaguchi T, Minematsu K, et al: Hemorrhagic transformation in cerebral embolism. Stroke 1989; 20:598–603.
34. Petersen P, Boysen G, Godtfredsen J, et al: Placebo-controlled, randomized trial of warfarin and aspirin for prevention of thromboembolic complications in chronic atrial fibrillation: the Copenhagen AFASAK study. Lancet 1989; 1:175–178.
35. Stroke Prevention in Atrial Fibrillation Investigators: Stroke Prevention in Atrial Fibrillation Study; final results. Circulation 1991; 84:527–530.
36. The Boston Area Anticoagulation Trial for Atrial Fibrillation Investigators: The effect of low-dose warfarin on the risk of stroke in patients with nonrheumatic atrial fibrillation. N Engl J Med 1990; 323:1505–1509.
37. Connolly S, Laupacis A, Gent M: Canadian Atrial Fibrillation Anticoagulation (CAFA) study. J Am Coll Cardiol 1991; 18:349–355.
38. Ezekowitz M, Bridgers S, James K, et al: VA cooperative study of warfarin in the prevention of stroke associated with nonrheumatic atrial fibrillation. N Engl J Med 1992; 327:1406–1412.
39. Atrial Fibrillation Investigators: Risk factors for stroke and efficacy of antithrombotic therapy in atrial fibrillation. Arch Intern Med 1994; 154:1449–1457.
40. European Atrial Fibrillation Trial (EAFT) Study Group: Secondary prevention in nonrheumatic atrial fibrillation after transient ischemic attack or minor stroke. Lancet 1993; 342:1255–1262.
41. Stroke Prevention in Atrial Fibrillation Investigators: Warfarin versus aspirin for prevention of thromboembolism in atrial fibrillation: Stroke Prevention in Atrial Fibrillation II Study. Lancet 1994; 343:687–691.
42. Moser KM: Venous thromboembolism: state of the art. Am Rev Respir Dis 1990; 141:235–249.
43. Hirsch J: Heparin. N Engl J Med 1991; 324:1565–1574.
43a. Raschke RA, Reilly BM, Guidrey JR, et al: The weight-adjusted heparin nomogram compared with a standard care nomogram: a randomized controlled trial. Ann Intern Med 1993; 119:874–881.
44. Come PC, Kim D, Parker JA, et al: Early reversal of right ventricular dysfunction in patients with acute pulmonary embolism after treatment with intravenous tissue plasminogen activator. J Am Coll Cardiol 1987; 10:971–978.
45. Sharma GVRK, Burleson VA, Sasahara AA: Effective thrombolytic therapy on pulmonary capillary blood volume in patients with pulmonary embolism. N Engl J Med 1980; 303:842–845.
46. The Urokinase Pulmonary Embolism Trial: A national cooperative study. Circulation 1973; 47(suppl II):1–108.
47. Urokinase-Streptokinase Embolism Trial: Phase 2 results: a comparative study. JAMA 1974; 229:1606–1613.
48. Goldhaber SZ, Marks JE, Meyerovitz MF, et al: Acute pulmonary embolism treated with tissue plasminogen activator. Lancet 1986; 2:886–889.
49. Marder VJ: Are we using fibrinolytic agents often enough? Ann Intern Med 1980; 93:136–137.
50. Stein PD, Hull RD, Raskob G: Risks for major bleeding from thrombolytic therapy in patients with acute pulmonary embolism. Ann Intern Med 1994; 121:313–317.
51. Urokinase–Pulmonary Embolism Trial: Phase I results: a comparative study. JAMA 1970; 214:2163–2172.
52. Witty LA, Krichman A, Tapson VF: Thrombolytic therapy for venous thromboembolism. Arch Intern Med 1994; 154:1601–1604.
53. Weinmann EE, Salzman EW: Deep-vein thrombosis. N Engl J Med 1994; 331:1630–1641.
54. Hyers TM, Hull RD, Weg JG: Antithrombotic therapy for venous thromboembolic disease. Chest 1992; 102:408S–425S.
55. Strandness DE, Langlois Y, Cramer M, et al: Long-term sequelae of acute venous thrombosis. JAMA 1983; 250:1289–1292.
56. O'Donnell TF, Brose NL, Burnand KG, et al: The socioeconomic factors of an iliofemoral thrombosis. J Surg Res 1977; 22:483–486.
57. Immelman EV, Jeffery PC: The postphlebitic syndrome; pathophysiology, prevention and management. Clin Chest Med 1984; 5:537–550.
58. Goldhaber SZ, Buring JE, Lipnick RJ, et al: Pooled analyses of randomized trials of streptokinase and heparin and phlebographically documented acute deep vein venous thrombosis. Am J Med 1984; 76:393–397.
59. Graor RA, Young JR, Risius B, Ruschhaupt WF: Cost-effective comparison of streptokinase and urokinase in the treatment of deep vein thrombosis. Ann Vasc Surg 1987; 1:524–528.
60. Arnesen H, Heilo A, Jakobsen E, et al: A prospective study of streptokinase and heparin in the treatment of deep vein thrombosis. Act Med Scand 1978; 203:457–460.
61. Levine MN, Goldhaber SZ, Califf RM, et al: Hemorrhagic complications of thrombolytic therapy in the treatment of myocardial infarction and venous thromboembolism. Chest 1992; 102:364S–373S.
62. Kakkar VV, Howe CT, Lawa JW, Flanc C: Late results of treatment of deep vein thrombosis. Br Med J 1969; 1:810–811.
63. Goldhaber SZ, Pollak JF, Feldstein ML, et al: Efficacy and safety of repeated boluses of urokinase in the treatment of deep venous thrombosis. Am J Cardiol 1994; 73:75–79.
64. Hill S, Martin D, Evans P: Massive vein thrombosis of the extremity. Am J Surg 1989; 158:131–134.
65. Semba CP, Dake MD: Iliofemoral deep venous thrombosis: aggressive therapy with catheter-directed thrombolysis. Radiology 1994; 191:487–494.
66. Druy EM, Trout HH, Giordano JM, Hix WR: Lytic therapy with treatment of axillary and subclavian vein thrombosis. J Vasc Surg 1985; 2:821–827.
67. Becker GJ, Holden RW, Rabe FE, et al: Local thrombolytic therapy for subclavian and axillary vein thrombosis. Radiology 1983; 59:419–423.

68. McNamara TO, Fischer JR: Thrombolysis of peripheral arterial and graft occlusions: improved results using high-dose urokinase. Am J Radiol 1985; 144:769–775.
69. Edmunds LH: Thromboembolic complications of current cardiac valvular prosthesis. Ann Thorac Surg 1982; 34:96–104.
70. Thorburn CW, Morgan JJ, Shanaban MX, Chang VP: Long-term results of tricuspid valve replacement and the problem of prosthetic valve thrombosis. Am J Cardiol 1983; 51:1128–1132.
71. Roudaut R, Labbe T, Lorient-Roudaut M-F, et al: Mechanical cardiac valve thrombosis: is fibrinolysis justified. Circulation 1992; 86(suppl II):8–15.
72. Stroke Prevention in Atrial Fibrillation Study Group Investigators: Preliminary report of the Stroke Prevention in Atrial Fibrillation Study. N Engl J Med 1990; 322:863–868.
73. Levine HJ, Pauker SG, Salzman EW, Eckman MH: Antithrombotic therapy in valvular heart disease. Chest 1992; 102:434S–444S.
74. Hart RG, Easton JD: Mitral valve prolapse and cerebral infarction. Stroke 1982; 13:420–430.
75. Fulkerson PK, Beaver BM, Ausen J, et al: Calcification of the mitral annulus: etiology, clinical associations, complications and therapy. Am J Med 1979; 66:967–977.
76. Wilson WR, Geraci JE, Danielson GK, et al: Anticoagulant therapy and central nervous system complications in patients with prosthetic valve endocarditis. Circulation 1978; 57:1004–1007.
77. Lieberman A, Hass WE, Pinto R, et al: Intracranial hemorrhage and infarction in anticoagulated patients with prosthetic heart valves. Stroke 1978; 9:18–24.
78. Stein PD, Alpert JS, Copeland J, et al: Antithrombotic therapy in patients with mechanical and biological prosthetic heart valves. Chest 1992; 102:445S–455S.
79. Saour JN, Sieck JO, Rahim L, et al: Trial of different intensities of anticoagulation in patients with prosthetic heart valves. N Engl J Med 1990; 322:428–432.
80. Sethia B, Turner MA, Lewis S, et al: Fourteen years' experience with the Bjork-Shiley tilting disc prosthesis. Thorac Cardiovasc Surg 1986; 91:350–361.
81. DiSesa VJ, Collins JJ Jr, Cohn LH: Hematological complications with the St. Jude valve and reduced-dose coumadin. Ann Thorac Surg 1989; 48:280–283.
82. Turpie AGG, Gunstensen J, Hirsh J, et al: Randomized comparison of two intensities of oral anticoagulant therapy after tissue heart valve replacement. Lancet 1988; 1:1242–1245.
83. Rao AK, Pratt C, Berke A, et al: Thrombolysis in Myocardial Infarction (TIMI) trial—phase I: hemorrhagic manifestations and changes in plasma fibrinogen and the fibrinolytic system in patients treated with recombinant tissue plasminogen activator. J Am Coll Cardiol 1988; 11:1–11.
84. Marder VJ, Sherry S: Thrombolytic therapy: current status. N Engl J Med 1988; 318:1512–1520, 1585–1595.
85. Sherry S: Appraisal of various thrombolytic agents in the treatment of acute myocardial infarction. Am J Med 1987; 83(suppl 27):31–46.
86. Chesebro JH, Knatterud G, Roberts R, et al: Thrombolysis in Myocardial Infarction (TIMI) trial phase I: a comparison between intravenous tissue plasminogen activation and intravenous streptokinase. Circulation 1987; 76:142–154.
87. Mathey DG, Schofer J, Sheehan FH, et al: Intravenous urokinase in acute myocardial infarction. Am J Cardiol 1985; 55:878–882.
88. Glazier RL, Crowell EB: Randomized prospective trial of continuous vs. intermittent heparin therapy. JAMA 1976; 236:1365–1367.
89. Morabia A: Heparin doses and major bleedings. Lancet 1986; 1:1278–1279.
90. Wessler S, Gitel SN: Pharmacology of heparin and warfarin. J Am Coll Cardiol 1986; 8:10B–20B.
91. Warkentin TE, Keiton JG: Heparin and platelets. Hematol/Oncol Clin North Am 1990; 4:243–264.
92. Schmitt BP, Adelman B: Heparin associated thrombocytopenia; a critical review and pooled analysis. Am J Med Sci 1993; 305:208–215.
93. Laster JL, Nichols K, Silver D: Thrombocytopenia associated with heparin-coated catheters in patients with heparin-associated antiplatelet antibodies. Arch Intern Med 1989; 149:2285–2287.
94. Bell WR, Royall RM: Heparin-associated thrombocytopenia: a comparison of three heparin preparations. N Engl J Med 1980; 303:902–907.
95. Ginsberg JS, Hirsh J: Use of anticoagulants during pregnancy. Chest 1989; 95:156S–160S.
96. Hall JG, Pauli RM, Wilson KM: Maternal and fetal sequelae of anticoagulation during pregnancy. Am J Med 1980; 68:122–130.
97. Leroy J, Leclerc MH, Delahousse B: Treatment of heparin-associated thrombocytopenia and thrombosis with low-molecular weight heparin (CY 216). Semin Thromb Hemost 1985; 11:326–329.
98. Stevenson RE, Burton OM, Ferlauto GJ, Taylor HA: Hazards of oral anticoagulants during pregnancy. JAMA 1980; 243:1549–1551.
99. Collen D, Stassen J-M, Stump DC, Verstraete M: Synergism of thrombolytic agents in vivo. Circulation 1986; 74:838–842.
100. Cannon CP, McCabe CH, Diver DJ, et al: Comparison of front-loaded recombinant tissue-type plasminogen activator, anistreplase, and combination thrombolytic therapy for acute myocardial infarction: results of the Thrombolysis in Myocardial Infarction (TIMI) 4 trial. J Am Coll Cardiol 1994; 24:1602–1610.
101. The GUSTO Investigators: An international randomized trial comparing four thrombolytic strategies for acute myocardial infarction. N Engl J Med 1993; 329:673–682.
102. Zarich SW, Kowalchuk GJ, Weaver WD, et al: Sequential combination thrombolytic therapy for acute myocardial infarction: results of the pro-urokinase and t-PA enhancement of thrombolysis (PATENT) trial. J Am Coll Cardiol 1995; 26:374–379.
103. Haber E, Quertermous T, Matsueda GR, Engle MS: Innovative approaches to plasminogen activator therapy. Science 1989; 243:51–56.
104. Refino CJ, Paoni NF, Keyt BA, et al: A variant of t-PA (T103N, KHRR 296–299 AAA) that, by bolus, has increased potential and decreased systemic activation of plasminogen. Thromb Haemost 1993; 70:313–319.
105. Ambrosioni E, Strocchi E: Pharmacokinetics of heparin and low molecular weight heparin. Haemostasis 1990; 20:94–97.
106. Wolf H: Low-molecular-weight heparin. Med Clin North Am 1994; 78:733–743.
107. Turpie AGG, Gent M, Cote R, et al: A low-molecular-weight heparinoid compared with unfractionated heparin in the prevention of deep venous thrombosis in patients with acute ischemic stroke. Ann Intern Med 1992; 117:353–357.
108. Samama CM: Low-molecular weight heparin (enoxaparin) versus unfractionated heparin during and after arterial reconstructive surgery: a multicenter randomized study. Thromb Haemost 1993; 69:546–550.
109. Maraganore JM, Bourdon P, Jablonski J, et al: Design and characterization of hirulogs: a novel class of bivalent peptide inhibitors of thrombin. Biochemistry 1990; 29:7095–7101.
110. Markwardt F: The development of Hirudin as an antithrombotic drug. Thromb Res 1994; 74:1–23.
111. Johnson PH, Sze P, Winant R, et al: Biochemistry and genetic engineering of hirudin. Semin Thromb Hemost 1989; 15:302–315.
112. Heras M, Chesebro JH, Penny WJ, et al: Clot bound thrombus is protected from inhibition by heparin–antithrombin III but is susceptible to inactivation by antithrombin III–independent inhibitors. Circulation 1989; 79:657–665.
113. van den Bos AA, Deckers JW, Heyndricks GR, et al: Safety and efficacy of recombinant hirudin (CGP 39 393) vs heparin in patients with stable angina undergoing coronary angioplasty. Circulation 1993; 88:2058–2066.
114. Cannon CP, McCabe CH, Henry TD, et al: A pilot trial of recombinant desulfatohirudin compared with heparin in conjunction with tissue-type plasminogen activator and aspirin for acute myocardial infarction: results of the Thrombolysis in Myocardial Infarction (TIMI) 5 trial. J Am Coll Cardiol 1994; 23:993–1003.
114a. Cannon CP, Braunwald E: Hirudin: initial results in acute myocardial infarction, unstable angina, and angioplasty. J Am Coll Cardiol 1995; 25:305–375.
115. Meckel CR, Ahmed W, Ferguson JJ, et al: Angiographic predictors of severe dissection during balloon angioplasty: a report from the Hirulog Angioplasty Study [Abstract]. Circulation 1994; 90:I-64.
116. Vlasuk GP: Structural and functional characterization of tick anticoagulant peptide (TAP): a potent and selective inhibitor of blood coagulation factor Xa. Thromb Haemost 1993; 70:212–216.
117. Waxman L, Smith DE, Arcuri KE, Vlasuk GP: Tick anticoagulant peptide (TAP) is a novel inhibitor of blood coagulation factor Xa. Science 1990; 248:593–599.
118. Sitko GR, Ramjit DR, Stabilito II, et al: Conjunctive enhancement of enzymatic thrombolysis and prevention of thrombotic reocclusion with the selective factor Xa inhibitor tick anticoagulant peptide: comparison to hirudin and heparin in a canine model of acute coronary thrombosis. Circulation 1992; 85:805–815.
119. Schaffer LW, Davidson JT, Vlasuk GP, et al: Selective factor Xa inhibition by recombinant antistasin prevents vascular graft thrombosis in baboons. Arterioscler Thromb 1992; 12:879–885.
120. Pratt CW, Church FC: Antithrombin: structure and function. Semin Hematol 1991; 3:28–33.

121. Gruber A, Hanson SR, Kelly AB, et al: Inhibition of thrombus formation by activated recombinant protein C in a primate model of arterial thrombosis. Circulation 1990; 82:578–585.
122. Benedict CR, Ryan J, Wolitzky B, et al: Active site-blocked factor IXa prevents intravascular thrombus formation in the coronary vasculature without inhibiting extravascular coagulation in a canine thrombosis model. J Clin Invest 1991; 88:1760–1765.
123. Graor RA, Risius B, Lucas FV, et al: Thrombolysis with recombinant human tissue-type plasminogen activator in patients with peripheral artery and bypass graft occlusions. Circulation 1986; 74(suppl I):I-15–I-21.
124. Albers GW: Atrial fibrillation and stroke. Arch Intern Med 1994; 154:1443–1448.
125. Watz R, Savidge GF: Rapid thrombolysis and preservation of valvular venous function of high deep vein thrombosis. Acta Med Scand 1979; 293:205–207.

SECTION SIX **Hypertension**

31 Management of Essential Hypertension: An Overview

Norman K. Hollenberg, MD, PhD

It is interesting to contrast the following chapters on the treatment of hypertension with the earlier chapters on the treatment of cardiac arrhythmias and conduction disturbances. For the latter, the nature of the arrhythmia is ascertained from the electrocardiogram and detailed electrophysiologic studies; then an attempt is made to choose an appropriate antiarrhythmic agent on the basis of the pharmacologic characteristics of the agent in relation to the disordered electrophysiologic findings. In the field of electrophysiology, however, evidence that the natural history of the process can be changed with these agents in many situations remains marginal,[1] and the concerns engendered by the Cardiac Arrhythmia Suppression Trial (CASS)[2] are referred to in detail in that section.

The contrast with hypertension is striking. In the case of hypertension, abundant data indicate that the natural history can be changed with the drugs available. A meta-analysis performed in 1990 summarized the results of 14 studies involving thousands of patients.[3, 4] The results were unambiguous. There was a reduction in both stroke rate and stroke mortality that was sufficient to indicate that the entire burden imposed by hypertension had been reversed. The news with coronary events—not surprising in view of their multifactorial pathogenesis—was more ambiguous. It took the power of the meta-analysis to indicate that coronary event and mortality rates could be reduced, although only by 25%.[3, 4] If there was doubt, it involved the extremes of age. There are still no data involving the influence on natural history of treatment in pediatric populations, but there is now an abundance of information about the elderly.[5–7]

One concern raised by the marginal effects of treatment in reducing coronary events in comparison with stroke involved the possibility that antihypertensive therapy could not overcome the influence of long-standing hypertension. The damage, it was thought, was already done and irreversible; therefore, it was reasonable to suspect that treatment of the hypertension in the elderly would be less rewarding in terms of improved natural history. The opposite has proved to be the case.[5–7] Treatment of hypertension in patients up to the age of 80 years not only reduces stroke frequency and stroke-related mortality but also reduces the rates of coronary events and coronary-related mortality to a degree never recognized in younger patients. There is no clear explanation for this interesting observation. Possibilities range from the rather pedestrian (that the event rate is sufficiently high in the elderly that it is easy to recognize a reduction) to potentially fascinating biologic processes (that hypertensive patients at risk of coronary events who have managed to live to an advanced age differ in coronary pathophysiology from those in whom the event occurs early and thus are more responsive to antihypertensive treatment). Whatever the explanation, all of the currently available information favors treatment for the elderly more strongly than for any other group.

Again, to contrast the problems of electrophysiology and hypertension, the success in antihypertensive therapy does not reflect the depth of the understanding. In the field of hypertension, there is no equivalent to the classification of cardiac arrhythmias. Chapter 37 introduces a series of "secondary forms of hypertension" involving the kidney (Chapter 38), endocrine causes (Chapter 39), diabetes and obesity (Chapter 40), and pregnancy (Chapter 41). Although the pathogenesis of hypertension remains uncertain even in the secondary forms involving the kidneys, the adrenal glands, and so forth, it is even more mysterious in the 90% or more of patients in whom the hypertension cannot be labeled secondary.

The results of studies of the natural history strongly support treatment of hypertension, and the treatment trials have included a wide variety of agents, including diuretics, potassium-sparing combination diuretics, beta blockers, centrally acting agents, and vasodilators.[4] Less is known about the influence of calcium channel blocking agents and angiotensin converting enzyme (ACE) inhibitors on the natural history, but the wide range of agents effective in reducing stroke rate suggests that efficacy does extend to the newer classes of agents as well. How shall physicians choose among the available agents—over 80 in seven drug classes marketed in the United States today? The problem of choice is complicated further by the fact that behavioral changes, including weight reduction in obese patients, a reduction in salt intake in patients who abuse salt, or a reduction in alcohol intake in those taking more than six standard drinks a day, can reduce blood pressure in selected persons.[8, 9] Chapter 32 addresses these issues.

Another determinant of treatment involves the severity of the process. Severe hypertension mandates emergency treatment and can represent a true emergency that allows no delay in the patient with a dissecting aneurysm, hypertensive encephalopathy, severe heart failure, or rapidly progressive azotemia. Chapter 33 addresses treatment of those problems.

Concomitant medical problems are an important force shaping antihypertensive therapy. Indeed, in most cases they are the major determinants. The Fifth Joint National Committee on Hypertension Treatment published a broad series of recommendations.[9] In brief, the committee concluded that diuretics and beta blockers should be the first choice, in the absence of alternative indications that would shape treatment, because they had been employed in the therapeutic trials. In fact, centrally active agents, including reserpine and methyldopa, have also been used but did not receive attention. The committee[9] did acknowledge that concomitant medical conditions would influence choice of treatment, but the tables and abstract did not provide detailed information on the frequency with which concomitant medical problems are found.[10] In one study of unselected patients, a concomitant medical problem that would shape antihypertensive therapy was found in more than 50% of patients.[11] In the elderly, the incidence of concomitant medical problems approaches 80%.[12] In view of the prevalence of cardiovascular disease in the community and the increase in prevalence among patients with hypertension, it is not surprising that cardiac disease is the leading cause of concomitant medical problems in patients with hypertension. Chapter 34 addresses the issue of the treatment of hypertension in patients with heart disease.

The fact that the natural history of hypertension in the elderly is improved by antihypertensive therapy is, as mentioned, the most recent expansion in knowledge. The specifics of the treatment of hypertension in the young and the elderly are covered in Chapters 35 and 36, respectively, by experts in the field.

There are special circumstances that are not covered in any specific chapter. In 1993, for example, mounting evidence that ACE inhibitor treatment could modify the progression of renal disease transport was presented in a definitive policy-making study on type I diabetes mellitus.[13, 14] Shortly thereafter, the U.S. Food and Drug Administration made type I diabetic nephropathy a specific indication for treatment with captopril, the ACE inhibitor employed in the trial. There are substantial reasons for suspecting that the ACE inhibitor is effective not because of better blood pressure regulation but by virtue of its ability to reduce the formation of angiotensin II in the kidney.

The future should entail progressive growth in the list of specific patient populations with a specific problem in whom a specific class of agent is most likely to be effective. What is currently a rather short list will become progressively longer as insight into pathophysiology grows. Perhaps in the not-too-distant future, the introductory overview on hypertension will divide chapters, not by demographics or concomitant medical problems, but rather by pathogenesis and mechanisms, as in the section on cardiac arrhythmias.

REFERENCES

1. Roden DM: Risks and benefits of antiarrhythmic therapy. Drug Therapy 1994; 331:785–791.
2. Echt DS, Liebson PR, Mitchell LB, et al: Mortality and morbidity in patients receiving encainide, flecainide, or placebo: the Cardiac Arrhythmia Suppression Trial. N Engl J Med 1991; 324:781–788.
3. MacMahon S, Peto R, Cutler J, et al: Blood pressure, stroke, and coronary heart disease. Part 1, Prolonged differences in blood pressure; prospective observational studies corrected for the regression dilution bias. Lancet 1990; 335:765–774.
4. Collins R, Peto R, MacMahon S, et al: Blood pressure, stroke, and coronary heart disease. Part 2, Short-term reductions in blood pressure; overview of randomized drug trials in their epidemiological context. Lancet 1990; 335:827–838.
5. SHEP Cooperative Research Group: Prevention of stroke by antihypertensive treatment in older persons with isolated systolic hypertension. Final results of the Systolic Hypertension in the Elderly Program (SHEP). JAMA 1991; 265:3255–3264.
6. Dahlof B, Lindholm L, Hansson L, et al: Morbidity and mortality in the Swedish Trial in Old Patients with Hypertension (STOP-Hypertension). Lancet 1991; 338:1281–1285.
7. MRC Working Party: Medical Research Council Trial of treatment of hypertension in older adults: principal results. Br Med J 1992; 1304:405–412.
8. Neaton JD, Grimm RH, Prineas RJ, et al: Treatment of Mild Hypertension Study (TOMHS): final results. Treatment of Mild Hypertension Study Research Group. JAMA 1993; 270:713–724.
9. The Fifth Report of the Joint National Committee on Detection, Evaluation, and Treatment of High Blood Pressure. Arch Intern Med 1993; 153:154–183.
10. Case DB: Patient population as consideration for antihypertensive therapy. *In* Hollenberg NK (ed): Management of Hypertension: A Multifactorial Approach, pp 101–120. Stoneham, MA: Butterworths, 1987.
11. Materson BJ: Hypertension and concomitant disease: guidelines for treatment. Drug Therapy 1985; 15:177–188.
12. Anderson RJ, Reed G, Kirk LM: Therapeutic considerations for elderly hypertensives. Clin Ther 1982; 5:25–38.
13. Lewis EJ, Hunsicker LG, Bain RP, Rohde RD: The effect of angiotensin-converting-enzyme inhibition on diabetic nephropathy. The Collaborative Study Group. N Engl J Med 1993; 329:1456–1462.
14. Hollenberg NK, Raij L: Angiotensin-converting enzyme inhibition and renal protection. An assessment of implications for therapy. Arch Intern Med 1993; 153:2426–2435.

32 Nonpharmacologic and Pharmacologic Treatment of Hypertension

Stephen L. Swartz, MD
Thomas J. Moore, MD

Patients with hypertension are at increased risk of developing end-organ damage, such as coronary artery disease, stroke, congestive heart failure, renal insufficiency, and peripheral vascular disease.[1–3] This end-organ damage increases progressively with higher levels of both systolic and diastolic blood pressure and with increasing age, both in males and in females.[4–6] Approximately 15% of patients with mild diastolic hypertension proceed to develop moderate or severe hypertension within 3–5 years of diagnosis,[7] with a less favorable prognosis; the remaining patients continue to have mild hypertension. It is now well established that lowering even mildly elevated blood pressures will significantly reduce rates of cardiovascular morbidity and mortality.[8] Drug therapy has been shown to reduce the risk of stroke by 35%–40% and to reduce the risk of nonfatal and fatal myocardial infarction by 15%–20%.[9]

Because cardiovascular risk associated with the level of blood pressure is on a continuum of severity, the dividing line between normal and high blood pressure is somewhat arbitrary. The most recent reclassification of high blood pressure definitions is from the fifth report on the treatment of high blood pressure by the Joint National Committee on Detection, Evaluation, and Treatment of High Blood Pressure (JNC-V).[10] Normal blood pressure is now defined as less than 130/85. A new category of high-normal blood pressure (130/85–139/89) has been added because persons with blood pressures in this range are at increased risk both of proceeding to develop definite high blood pressure and of experiencing nonfatal and fatal cardiovascular events, in comparison with persons with lower blood pressures. Patients with high-normal blood pressure are usually given instructions on lifestyle modifications rather than prescriptions for pharmacologic therapy.

The range of blood pressures for patients with mild, moderate, severe, and very severe hypertension is unchanged but has been relabeled as Stages 1, 2, 3, and 4 hypertension, respectively. This change in terminology was instituted to prevent any patient previously identified as having mild hypertension or the physician from thinking that the risk of nonfatal and fatal cardiovascular disease is also mild. All stages of hypertension warrant long-term therapy. The JNC-V also points out that the risk of cardiovascular disease related to high blood pressure increases in association with other concomitant cardiovascular risk factors and is also increased severalfold for patients who already have end-organ damage. In such patients, blood pressure should be reduced to levels of 130/85 rather than 140/90. How far the diastolic blood pressure should be reduced below 85 mm Hg is unclear at the present time.[11]

The therapeutic approach to a patient with hypertension must therefore take into account the severity of the hypertension, the presence of other cardiovascular risk factors, and the question of whether end-organ damage already exists. In the following discussion, therapies are divided into nonpharmacologic (Fig. 32–1) and pharmacologic (Fig. 32–2).

MODIFICATION OF DIETARY FACTORS

Electrolytes

Dietary Sodium/Salt Restriction

Evidence for the blood pressure–lowering effect of sodium restriction was first noted in observational studies that demonstrated that populations with lower salt intake had lower average blood pressure than populations with liberal salt intake.[12–16] In the Intersalt study,[16] the relationship between salt intake and blood pressure was assessed in 52 populations worldwide. Sodium intake was estimated from 24-h urinary sodium excretion, which varied from 0.2–240 mEq/day. In these populations, there were highly significant relationships between sodium intake and the rate at which blood pressure rose as subjects aged. The relationship was also significant for sodium intake and the actual level of systolic blood pressure across populations (although not significant for diastolic blood pressure). Law and associates[14] analyzed the relationship between salt intake and blood pressure from previously published reports of 24 communities (47,000 subjects). They confirmed that lower sodium intake was associated with a lower level of blood pressure, that the effect of salt intake was greater in older than in younger subjects, and that the effect was greater in subjects with higher than with lower levels of blood pressure. On average, reducing sodium intake by 100 mEq/day was

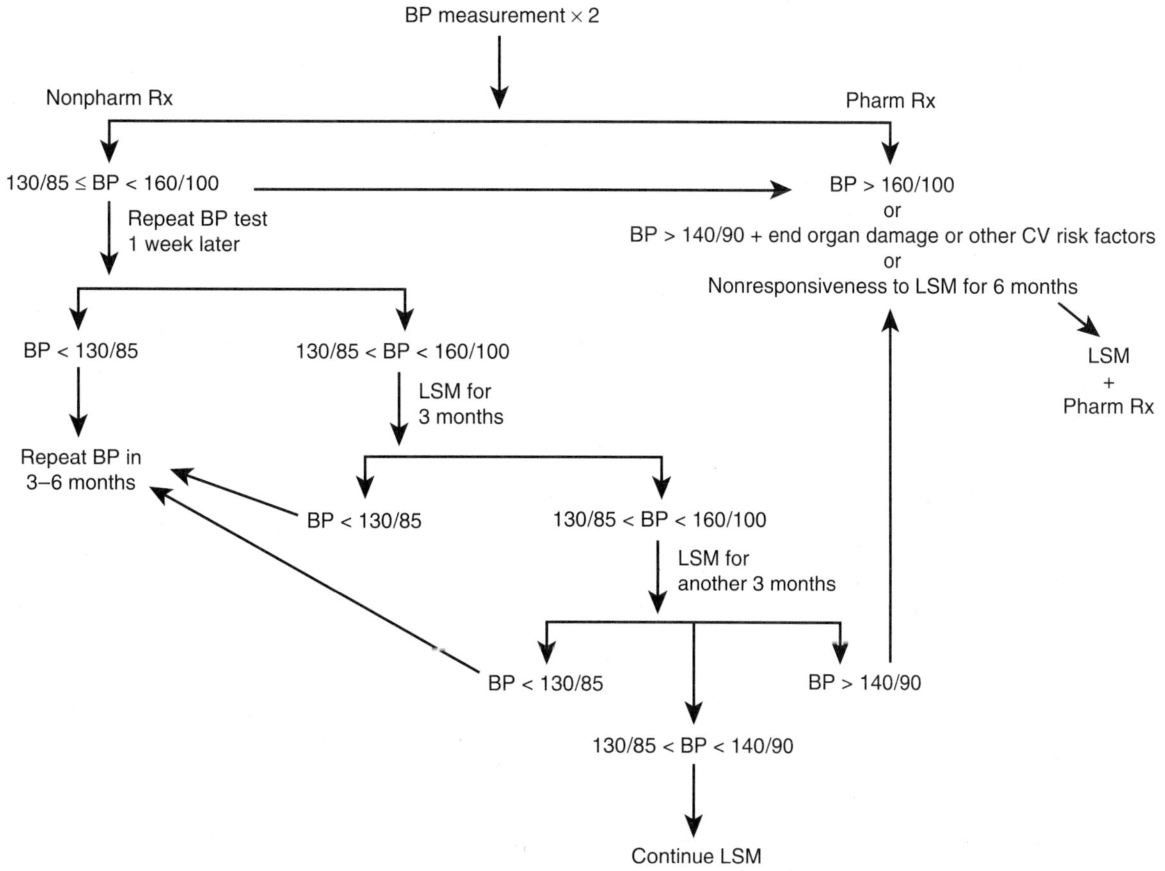

Figure 32–1. Nonpharmacologic treatment of hypertension. *Abbreviations*: BP, blood pressure; Nonpharm Rx, nonpharmacologic treatment; Pharm Rx, pharmacologic treatment; LSM, life style modifications; CV, cardiovascular.

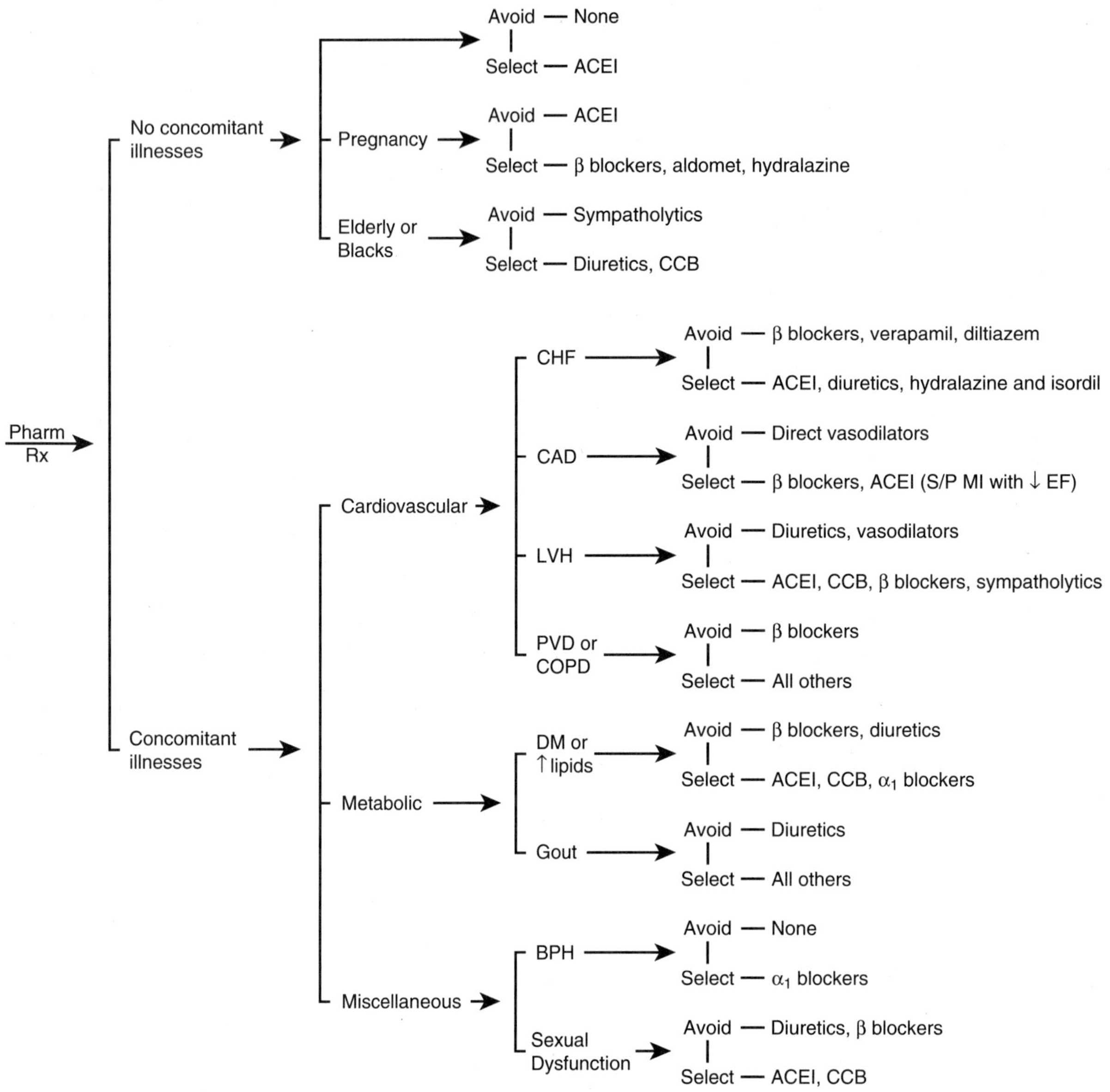

Figure 32–2. Pharmacologic treatment of essential hypertension. *Abbreviations*: ACEI, angiotensin converting enzyme inhibitors; CCB, calcium channel blockers; MI, myocardial infarction; EF, ejection fraction; CHF, congestive heart failure; CAD, coronary artery disease; LVH, left ventricular hypertrophy; PVD, peripheral vascular disease; COPD, chronic obstructive pulmonary disease; DM, diabetes mellitus; BPH, benign prostatic hypertrophy.

associated with a 5–mm Hg lower systolic blood pressure during adolescence and a 10–mm Hg reduction at ages 60–69.

Beyond this epidemiologic evidence, the effect of restricting sodium intake as a treatment for hypertension also has been extensively tested. Law and associates[17] summarized 78 trials of dietary sodium restriction. They found that trials longer than 4 weeks revealed the greatest blood pressure–lowering effect. The blood pressure response to sodium in these intervention trials correlated closely with the blood pressure change predicted from previous epidemiologic studies. Again, the blood pressure response was greater in older than in younger subjects and greater in hypertensive than in normotensive subjects, although normotensive subjects also displayed a significant blood pressure decline with sodium restriction. Cutler and colleagues[18] summarized the results of 23 randomized, controlled trials of sodium restriction (1536 subjects). In comparison with the respective control groups, sodium-restricted hypertensive subjects lowered blood pressure by 5 mm Hg systolic and 2.6 mm Hg diastolic. Both reductions were highly significant. In normotensive subjects, the reductions were smaller (1.7 mm Hg systolic, 1.0 mm Hg diastolic; both significant). The median reduction in 24-h sodium excretion in these trials was 76 mEq/day.

Although sodium restriction across a broad range of subjects lowers blood pressure significantly, it is equally clear that some hypertensive subjects are particularly sensitive to sodium restriction and others are insensitive. Subgroups that appear to be particularly salt-sensitive include older subjects, patients with renal insufficiency, black subjects,[19] patients with low plasma renin levels,[20] overweight subjects,[19, 21] and nonmodulators (subjects with abnormal renal and adrenal responses to angiotensin II and a family history of hypertension).[22]

Beyond its effect as first-line therapy, sodium restriction also enhances the effect of antihypertensive medications. In view of these many lines of evidence supporting the efficacy of sodium restriction, JNC-V[10] recommended moderate sodium restriction (to a level of <100 mEq/day) in all subjects with hypertension.

Potassium Supplementation

Higher potassium intake or potassium supplementation has also been reported to lower blood pressure. The Intersalt study[16] noted an inverse relationship between potassium excretion and blood pressure: overall, a 60-mEq increase in dietary potassium was associated with a decrease in systolic blood pressure of 2.7 mm Hg.

There are many reports of the effect of potassium supplementation (or restriction) on blood pressure, both as a solitary intervention and in conjunction with antihypertensive medications. Krishna and Kapoor[23] studied potassium restriction vs. supplementation (16 vs. 96 mEq/day potassium intake) in 12 untreated hypertensive subjects in a double-blind, randomized crossover study. In comparison with the potassium-restricted state, potassium supplements lowered systolic blood pressure by 7 mm Hg and diastolic blood pressure by 6 mm Hg. In a meta-analysis of trials of potassium supplementation, Cappuccio and MacGregor[24] found that potassium supplementation significantly lowered blood pressure (5.9 mm Hg systolic; 3.4 mm Hg diastolic) in 19 trials involving 586 participants. Potassium supplementation ranged from 48 to 120 mEq/day. The blood pressure–lowering effect was greatest in subjects with hypertension and was greater in trials of longer duration. Siani and coworkers[25] studied the interaction between potassium supplementation and antihypertensive medications. They divided subjects controlled on medications into a potassium supplementation group and a control group and followed a strict protocol for discontinuing antihypertensive medications. At the end of 1 year, they found that potassium-supplemented subjects required only 24% of the medication that they had required before supplementation; the control group required 60%. Siani and coworkers concluded that increasing dietary potassium intake provided an effective means of reducing other antihypertensive medications.

Thus, although a significant benefit is not seen in every trial, potassium supplementation appears overall to lower blood pressure in both normotensive and hypertensive patients and may reduce the need for antihypertensive medication.

Calcium

Many epidemiologic studies have associated lower blood pressures with higher levels of calcium intake, although this has not been a totally consistent finding.[26–28] These epidemiologic studies have been reviewed by Cutler and Brittain.[29] Interventional studies of calcium supplementation have been pooled and meta-analyzed. Cutler and Brittain[29] found a 1.8–mm Hg reduction in systolic blood pressure with calcium supplementation but no significant diastolic effect. Cappuccio and associates found a significant blood pressure decrement in standing pressure only.[30]

Because of this marginal blood pressure response, there is no clear reason for recommending increasing calcium intake beyond the level of 800–1200 mg/day recommended by the U.S. Food and Drug Administration (FDA).

Magnesium

Observational epidemiologic studies have demonstrated significant inverse associations between the level of blood pressure and magnesium intake.[31, 32] However, dietary magnesium supplementation was not found to decrease blood pressure in two studies of unselected hypertensives.[33, 34] Lind and colleagues[35] reported that blood pressure did fall with magnesium supplementation in magnesium-depleted (diuretic-treated) subjects. The large, well-designed Trials of Hypertension Prevention found no blood pressure–lowering effect of potassium, calcium, or magnesium supplementation in adults with normal blood pressure.[36]

Macronutrients

Dietary Fat Intake

Dietary fat intake is inversely correlated with level of blood pressure in studies comparing populations (reviewed by Sacks[37]). The populations compared, however, differ in many ways other than the level of dietary fat intake. In 11 observational studies, Sacks examined the relationship between fat intake and blood pressure within a population. No relationship was found in six studies, a positive relationship was found in two, and an inverse relationship was found in four.[37] Attempts to uncover a relationship between the type of fat intake (e.g., saturated or unsaturated fatty acids) and blood pressure have been unsuccessful.

Sacks also reviewed randomized, controlled trials of modifying dietary fat intake.[37] Only one trial[38] demonstrated a significant blood pressure–lowering effect of fat restriction. Most of these trials were small and so had the power only to detect blood pressure changes in the range of 3 to 5 mm Hg. However, the actual effect size of the trials was so close to zero that it is unlikely that even meta-analysis would uncover any significant blood pressure effect.

Dietary Protein Intake

Epidemiologic studies of stroke in Japanese men suggest that a liberal dietary protein intake may be protective.[39, 40] Prospective studies of modifying protein intake have not found significant effects on blood pressure.[41, 42] However, there have been no large-scale, well-controlled trials of protein intake in the general population to test the blood pressure effect of protein intake.

Vegetarian Dietary Pattern

Members of nonindustrialized societies tend to have lower blood pressure that increases more slowly with age than in members of industrialized societies. Such societies often consume a largely vegetarian diet. Within industrialized societies, vegetarians typically have lower blood pressure levels than comparable nonvegetarian populations.[43, 44] The lowest blood pressures are typically found in strict vegetarians who consume no animal products.[45]

In two studies, vegetarian diets were given to nonvegetarians. In both cases, consumption of animal fat decreased. In one case it was replaced with an increase in vegetable products, including vegetable oil; in the other, animal fat was replaced with carbohydrates.[46, 47] Only the vegetable-substituted diet lowered blood pressure. Vegetarian diets are typically low in animal fat, low in protein, and rich in green leafy vegetables, root vegetables, whole grains, and beans. This combination of foods generally increases the intake of magnesium, potassium, and calcium. The fact that trials of these nutrients given individually as supplements have not been impressive suggests that the mixture of micronutrients and macronutrients in the vegetarian diet may be responsible for its hypotensive effect. An alternative possibility is that some as-yet-untested component of a vegetarian diet may be responsible for its blood pressure–lowering effect.

Weight Reduction

Overweight individuals have, on average, higher blood pressures and a higher prevalence of hypertension. Two controlled clinical trials indicate that weight reduction can significantly lower blood pressure, both in subjects with high-normal blood pressure and in patients with stage I hypertension.

In the Trial of Antihypertensive Interventions and Management

Study (TAIM), 878 subjects were randomly assigned to one of three dietary interventions: usual diet, weight loss diet, or low sodium/high potassium diet. These subjects were then further divided into three medication treatments: placebo, chlorthalidone, and atenolol.[48] In the subjects not given antihypertensive medication, the weight-loss group lost 4.4 kg over the 6-month study (in comparison with a loss of 0.71 kg in the usual-diet group), and the diastolic pressure declined by 2.5 mm Hg more than in the usual-diet group ($p < .001$). The blood pressure decrement in the weight-loss group was marginally better than that in the sodium-restriction group, whose decrement in this study was not better than that of the usual-diet group. In addition, weight loss increased the effectiveness of both chlorthalidone and atenolol. In fact, weight loss showed a greater drug-enhancing effect than did sodium restriction.

In the Trials of Hypertension Prevention Study (TOHP), participants with high-normal diastolic blood pressure (80–89 mm Hg) and excess body weight (115%–165% of ideal body weight) were assigned to either a weight-loss program or a usual diet (control).[49] The study was conducted for 18 months, and 564 subjects were randomized. In comparison with the control group, the weight-loss group lost 3.9 kg at the end of the study. Their diastolic blood pressures fell 2.3 mm Hg and systolic pressures 2.9 mm Hg more than those of the control group (both $ps < .001$). Men in the study lost more weight than did women (4.7 kg vs. 1.8 kg). Women did not display a significant blood pressure decrement, probably because of their smaller weight loss.

These two well-controlled trials demonstrate that weight loss can be an effective long-term strategy for lowering blood pressure in subjects with high-normal pressure or stage I hypertension.

The mechanism of the blood pressure–lowering effect of weight loss remains unclear. Short-term studies of rigorous caloric restriction (600–800 calories/day) have demonstrated water diuresis, natriuresis, and reductions in activity of the sympathetic nervous system.[50–52] To what extent any of these mechanisms plays a role in the hypotensive effect of more gradual, long-term weight loss remains uncertain.

PHARMACOLOGIC THERAPY

Reducing high blood pressure to normotensive levels even before the development of end-organ damage is of proven benefit in reducing the incidences of cardiovascular morbidity and mortality.[8] If the blood pressure stays at levels higher than 140/90 mm Hg despite a 6-month period of compliance with lifestyle modifications, antihypertensive therapy should be started (see Fig. 32–2). This is especially recommended for patients with severe hypertension (stage III or IV), patients with other known cardiovascular risk factors, and patients with end-organ damage. The five classes of antihypertensive medications that are currently available are listed in Table 32–1.[53]

Adverse Effect on Concomitant Illness

At present, there is no strong evidence from randomized clinical trials that the benefits of lowering blood pressure are attributable to any particular class of antihypertensive drug rather than to the lowering of the blood pressure per se. For stage I and stage II hypertension, initial drug therapy should start with a single drug. In view of the Hippocratic oath ("Above all else, do no harm"), the first consideration in the selection of an antihypertensive agent should be the potential of that drug to adversely affect the patient with a concomitant illness. Some of the more common adverse drug effects are noted as follows:

1. *Beta blockers* should not be used in patients with chronic obstructive pulmonary disease, congestive heart failure, peripheral vascular disease, or heart block of greater than first degree (see Table 32–1 and Fig. 32–2). They should be used with caution in patients with hyperlipidemia or diabetes; in patients with non–insulin-dependent diabetes mellitus (NIDDM), beta blockers have the potential to aggravate glucose intolerance. They also have the potential to prolong insulin-induced hypoglycemia and thus may mask the adrenergically mediated symptoms of hypoglycemia.
2. *Combined alpha/beta blockers* have the same profile as do beta blockers.
3. *Alpha blockers* should be used with caution in elderly patients because of the possibility of postural hypotension.
4. *Diuretics* may precipitate gout, worsen glucose intolerance, raise cholesterol, lower serum potassium, and cause sexual dysfunction (see Table 32–1). Fortunately, these undesirable adverse effects can be reduced if the diuretic dosage is kept as low as possible.
5. *ACE inhibitors* can cause reversible acute renal insufficiency in approximately 50% of patients with pre-existing bilateral renal artery stenosis or stenosis in a solitary functioning or transplanted kidney (as a result of decreased renal perfusion pressure) and in patients with congestive heart failure with volume depletion from prior diuretic use. They should be used with caution in patients with hyperkalemia, especially in patients with concomitant diabetes mellitus and/or renal insufficiency, and in patients who are also taking nonsteroidal anti-inflammatory drugs (NSAIDs) and/or potassium-sparing diuretics. They are contraindicated for use during the second and third trimesters of pregnancy.
6. *Calcium channel blockers* should be used with caution in patients with congestive heart failure. Thebenzothiazepine and phenylalkylamine derivatives (diltiazem and verapamil, respectively) are contraindicated in patients with second- or third-degree heart block or sick sinus syndrome.
7. *Reserpine* is contraindicated in patients with a history of mental depression or active peptic ulcer disease.
8. *Direct vasodilators*, when used as monotherapy, may cause tachycardia and sodium and water retention and, as such, may precipitate angina in patients with pre-existing coronary heart disease (see Fig. 32–2). Therefore, they should be used in conjunction with beta blockers. *Minoxidil* may cause pleural and/or pericardial effusions, especially in patients with congestive heart failure.

Positive Effect on Concomitant Illness

The next consideration in the selection of initial therapy is the presence of concomitant diseases that may be ameliorated by the antihypertensive agent chosen. Selection of an antihypertensive agent that also treats a coexisting disease may simplify therapeutic regimens and reduce costs. These agents are described as follows:

1. *Beta blockers* are also useful in patients with angina pectoris, hypertrophic cardiomyopathy with diastolic dysfunction, and vascular headaches (see Fig. 32–2). They have also been shown to prevent fatal and nonfatal coronary events in patients with a previous myocardial infarction.[54]
2. *Calcium channel blockers* are also useful in patients with angina pectoris (see Fig. 32–2). Diltiazem and verapamil are of value in treating patients with hypertrophic cardiomyopathy with diastolic dysfunction, and these drugs have been reported to reduce rates of morbidity and mortality in post–myocardial infarction patients, provided that heart failure and left ventricular dysfunction are absent.[55] In patients with atherosclerotic arterial disease, the calcium channel antagonists may reduce the development of new plaques.[56]
3. *ACE inhibitors* are of proven value in reducing rates of cardiovascular morbidity and mortality among patients with congestive heart failure[57, 58] and among patients with a reduced ejection fraction after a myocardial infarction[59, 60] and are the drugs of choice in diabetic patients with proteinuria.[61]
4. *Diuretics* have been shown to be effective in the prevention of fatal and nonfatal stroke in older persons with isolated systolic hypertension.[62] They are also of value in the treatment of patients with congestive heart failure (see Fig. 32–2).

TABLE 32–1. ANTIHYPERTENSIVE AGENTS GROUPED BY SITE OF ACTION

Site of Action	Drug	Dosage	Indications	Contraindications	Frequent or Peculiar Side Effects
Diuretics					
Renal tubule	Thiazides E.g., hydrochlorothiazide	Depends on specific drug Oral: 25 mg/day or b.i.d.	Mild hypertension, as adjunct in treatment of moderate to severe hypertension	Diabetes mellitus, hyperuricemia, primary aldosteronism	Potassium depletion, hyperglycemia, hyperuricemia, hypercholesterolemia, dermatitis, purpura, depression, hypercalcemia
	Loop acting: E.g., furosemide	Oral: 40–80 mg b.i.d. or t.i.d.	Mild hypertension, as adjunct in severe or malignant hypertension particularly with renal failure	Hyperuricemia, primary aldosteronism	Potassium depletion, hyperuricemia, hyperglycemia, hypocalcemia, blood dyscrasias, rash, nausea, vomiting, diarrhea
	Potassium-sparing: Spironolactone	Oral: 25 mg b.i.d. to q.i.d.	Hypertension due to hypermineralocorticoidism, adjunct to thiazide therapy	Renal failure	Hyperkalemia, diarrhea, gynecomastia, menstrual irregularities
	Triamterene	Oral: 50–100 mg s.i.d. or b.i.d.	Hypertension due to hypermineralocorticoidism, adjunct to thiazide therapy		Hyperkalemia, nausea, vomiting, leg cramps, nephrolithiasis, GI disturbances
	Amiloride	Oral: 5–10 mg/day		Renal failure	
Antiadrenergic Agents					
Central nervous system	Clonidine Guanabenz Guanfacine	Oral: 0.05–0.6 mg b.i.d. Oral: 4–16 mg b.i.d. Oral: 1–3 mg/day	Mild to moderate hypertension, renal disease with hypertension		Postural hypotension, drowsiness, dry mouth, rebound hypertension after abrupt medication withdrawal, insomnia
	Methyldopa (also acts by blocking sympathetic nerves)	Oral: 250–1000 mg b.i.d. IV: 250–1000 mg every 4–6 h (tolerance may develop)	Mild to moderate hypertension (oral), malignant hypertension (IV)	Pheochromocytoma, active hepatic disease (IV), during MAO inhibitor administration	Postural hypotension, sedation, fatigue, diarrhea, impaired ejaculation, fever, gynecomastia, lactation, positive Coombs test results (occasionally associated with hemolysis), chronic hepatitis, acute ulcerative colitis, lupus-like syndrome
Autonomic ganglia	Trimethaphan	IV: 1–6 mg/min	Severe or malignant hypertension	Severe coronary artery disease, cerebrovascular insufficiency, diabetes mellitus (on hypoglycemic therapy), glaucoma, prostatism	Postural hypotension, visual symptoms, dry mouth, constipation, urinary retention, impotence
Nerve endings	Rauwolfia alkaloids: Reserpine	Oral: 0.05–0.25 mg/day	Mild to moderate hypertension in young patients	Pheochromocytoma, peptic ulcer, depression, during MAO inhibitor administration	Depression, nightmares, nasal congestion, dyspepsia, diarrhea, impotence
	Guanethidine Guanadrel	Oral: 10–150 mg/day Oral: 5–75 mg b.i.d.	Moderate to severe hypertension	Pheochromocytoma, severe coronary artery disease, cerebrovascular insufficiency, during MAO inhibitor administration	Postural hypotension, bradycardia, dry mouth, diarrhea, impaired ejaculation, fluid retention, asthma
Alpha receptors	Phentolamine	IV: 1–5 mg	Suspected or proven pheochromocytoma	Severe coronary artery disease	Tachycardia, weakness, dizziness, flushing
	Phenoxybenzamine	Oral: 10–50 mg s.i.d. or b.i.d. (tolerance may develop)	Proven pheochromocytoma		Postural hypotension, tachycardia, miosis, nasal congestion, dry mouth
	Prazosin Terazosin	Oral: 1–10 mg b.i.d. Oral: 1–20 mg s.i.d.	Mild to moderate hypertension	Use with caution in the elderly	Sudden syncope, headache, sedation, dizziness, tachycardia, anticholinergic effect, fluid retention
Beta receptors	Propranolol Metoprolol Carteolol Nadolol Atenolol Timolol	Oral: 10–120 mg b.i.d. to q.i.d. Oral: 25–150 mg b.i.d. Oral: 2.5–10 mg/day Oral: 20–120 mg/day Oral: 25–100 mg/day Oral: 5–15 mg b.i.d.	Mild to moderate hypertension (especially with evidence of hyperdynamic circulation), adjunct to hydralazine therapy	Congestive heart failure, asthma, diabetes mellitus (on hypoglycemic therapy), during MAO inhibitor administration, COPD, sick sinus syndrome, second- or third-degree heart block	Dizziness, depression, bronchospasm, nausea, vomiting, diarrhea, constipation, heart failure, fatigue, Raynaud's phenomenon, hallucinations, hypertriglyceridemia, hypercholesterolemia, psoriasis; sudden withdrawal may precipitate angina or myocardial injury in patients with heart disease
	Pindolol Acebutolol Labetalol	Oral: 5–30 mg b.i.d. Oral: 200–600 mg b.i.d. Oral: 100–600 mg b.i.d. IV: 2 mg/min			Less resting bradycardia than other beta blockers

Table continued on following page

TABLE 32–1. ANTIHYPERTENSIVE AGENTS GROUPED BY SITE OF ACTION *Continued*

Site of Action	Drug	Dosage	Indications	Contraindications	Frequent or Peculiar Side Effects
Vasodilators					
Vascular smooth muscle	Hydralazine	Oral: 10–75 mg q.i.d. IV or IM: 10–50 mg every 6 h (tolerance may develop)	As adjunct in treatment of moderate to severe hypertension (oral), malignant hypertension (IV or IM), renal disease with hypertension	Lupus erythematosus, severe coronary artery disease	Headache, tachycardia, angina pectoris, anorexia, nausea, vomiting, diarrhea, lupus-like syndrome, rash, fluid retention
	Minoxidil	Oral: 2.5–40 mg b.i.d.	Severe hypertension	Severe coronary artery disease	Tachycardia, aggravation of angina, marked fluid retention, hair growth on face and body, coarsening of facial features, possible pericardial effusions
	Diazoxide	IV: 1–3 mg/kg up to 150 mg, rapidly	Severe or malignant hypertension	Diabetes mellitus, hyperuricemia, congestive heart failure	Hyperglycemia, hyperuricemia, sodium retention
	Nitroprusside	IV: 0.5–8 μg/kg/min	Malignant hypertension		Apprehension, weakness, diaphoresis, nausea, vomiting, muscle twitching, cyanide toxicity
ACE Inhibitors					
Converting enzyme	Captopril	Oral: 12.5–75 mg b.i.d.	Mild to severe hypertension, renal artery stenosis	Renal failure (reduction of dose), bilateral renal artery stenosis, pregnancy	Leukopenia, pancytopenia, hypotension, cough, angioedema, urticarial rash, fever, loss of taste, acute renal failure in bilateral renal artery stenosis, hyperkalemia
	Benazepril Enalapril Enalaprilat Fosinipril Lysinopril Quinapril Ramipril	Oral: 10–40 mg/day Oral: 2.5–40 mg/day IV: 0.626–1.25 mg over 5 min every 6–8 h Oral: 10–40 mg/day Oral: 5–40 mg/day Oral: 10–80 mg/day Oral: 2.5–20 mg/day			Same as captopril but little evidence of leukopenia, but perhaps increased frequency of cough and angioedema; all can be given s.i.d., but side effects are reduced if half dose is given b.i.d.; fosinipril is excreted in bile more than the others
Calcium Channel Antagonists					
Vascular smooth muscle	Nifedipine	Oral: 10–30 mg q.i.d. or, as XL form, 30–90 mg/day	Mild to moderate hypertension	Heart failure, second- or third-degree heart block	Tachycardia, flushing, gastrointestinal disturbances, hyperkalemia, edema, headache
	Amlodipine Felodipine XL Isradipine Nicardipine	Oral: 2.5–10 mg/day Oral: 5–10 mg/day Oral: 2.5–10 mg/day Oral: 20–40 mg t.i.d.			
	Diltiazem Verapamil	Oral: 30–90 mg q.i.d. or, as CD form, 180–300 mg/day Oral: 30–120 mg q.i.d. or, as SR form, 120–480 mg/day			Same as nifedipine except no tachycardia, but can cause heart block, constipation, and liver dysfunction

Modified from Williams GH: Hypertensive vascular disease. *In* Isselbacher KJ, Braunwald E, Wilson JD, et al (eds): Harrison's Principles of Internal Medicine, 13th ed, pp 1116–1131. New York: McGraw-Hill, 1994.

Abbreviations: GI, gastrointestinal; IV, intravenous; MAO, monoamine oxidase; COPD, chronic obstructive pulmonary disease; IM, intramuscular; ACE, angiotensin converting enzyme.

5. *Alpha blockers* have been shown to reduce insulin resistance[63] (and as such may be of benefit in patients with glucose intolerance) and serum cholesterol levels, especially the low-density lipoprotein subfraction (see Fig. 32–2). Alpha blockers are also of value in relieving the symptoms of urinary tract obstruction in males with benign prostatic hypertrophy.

A reanalysis of the Framingham data[64] indicated that the presence of left ventricular hypertrophy (LVH) represents an independent risk factor for fatal and nonfatal myocardial infarction. Because LVH occurs in response to increased afterload imposed by elevated blood pressure, it follows that an antihypertensive drug that reduces left ventricular mass as well as blood pressure has the potential to produce an even greater reduction in rates of cardiovascular morbidity and mortality (although this point is at present still unproved). All of the major drug classes except diuretics and direct vasodilators may reduce LVH (see Fig. 32–2).[65]

Drug-Drug Interactions

Another consideration in the choice of an antihypertensive agent is the potential interaction between a particular antihypertensive drug and other concomitant medications which the patient is taking. These drug-drug interactions are usually not absolute contraindications, because dosage titration or more careful monitoring of potential side effects may allow the simultaneous use of both drugs. For example, NSAIDs may decrease the effectiveness of angiotensin converting enzyme (ACE) inhibitors, beta blockers, and diuretics. Diuretics, ACE inhibitors, and methyldopa may increase serum lithium levels and thereby increase the possibility of lithium toxicity. Cimetidine may increase the pharmacologic effect of beta blockers and calcium channel blockers by inhibiting hepatic metabolism, thereby increasing serum levels. Beta blockers and diltiazem or verapamil may have additive inhibitory effects on the sinoatrial and atrioventricular nodes, as well as negative inotropic effects on the failing myocardium. Beta blockers and reserpine may result in marked bradycardia and syncope. Beta blockers may increase serum levels of theophylline, lidocaine, and chlorpromazine due to reduced hepatic clearance. Bile acid resins decrease absorption of diuretics. Antacids may decrease the bioavailability of ACE inhibitors. Rifampin, carbamazepine, phenobarbital, and phenytoin may decrease the serum levels of verapamil. Verapamil, and possibly diltiazem, may increase serum levels of digoxin and carbamazepine. Verapamil may increase serum levels of prazosin, quinidine, and theophylline. Serum levels of cyclosporine may be increased by diltiazem, nicardipine, and verapamil. Tricyclic antidepressants may decrease the effects of centrally acting and peripheral norepinephrine depleters. Finally, sympathomimetics, amphetamines, phenothiazines, and cocaine may interfere with the antihypertensive effects of guanethidine.

Demographics

In hypertensive patients who have no concomitant illnesses and are not taking any supplemental medications, demographic considerations may help in the selection of initial drug therapy. It is important to remember that gender, age, and race are not sufficient reasons to exclude a particular class of drugs, inasmuch as efficacy differences can usually be overcome with the addition of a diuretic or another antihypertensive agent. However, in general, black patients and older patients are usually more responsive to diuretics and calcium channel blockers than to beta blockers or ACE inhibitors (see Fig. 32–2).[66] Older patients are more likely to develop systolic hypertension, which is now recognized as an independent risk factor for coronary heart disease and stroke. The Systolic Hypertension in the Elderly Program (SHEP) trial[62] demonstrated the protective effect of treatment with low-dosage diuretic and, if needed, atenolol or reserpine in elderly patients with systolic hypertension. Younger patients with resting tachycardia usually respond well to beta blockers or ACE inhibitors.[66]

Hypertension is more common among women taking oral contraceptive pills (OCP) for 5 or more years.[67] The risk increases with age and with duration of use. In a small number of patients, OCP may cause accelerated or malignant hypertension.[68] The mechanism of the increase in blood pressure is unclear, but it may involve an increase in the level of the vasoconstrictor angiotensin II, which results from estrogenic stimulation of hepatic angiotensinogen synthesis. If hypertension develops in a woman taking OCP, discontinuation of the OCP is recommended, and blood pressure usually returns to normal within 3 months. Of interest is that the use of conjugated estrogens as replacement therapy in postmenopausal women may have a beneficial effect on blood pressure.[69] However, some women may experience a rise in blood pressure with estrogen replacement therapy, and therefore blood pressures should be monitored more frequently in women taking estrogen replacement therapy.

The choice of initial antihypertensive drug therapy for a patient with uncomplicated mild essential hypertension (who has no concomitant illnesses and is not taking any medications) is a challenge for the physician. Therapeutic trials with antihypertensive drugs have provided clear evidence that the treatment of high blood pressure greatly reduces the frequency of congestive heart failure, stroke, renal failure, and accelerated hypertension; however, events related to atherosclerosis, especially coronary artery disease, did not respond as dramatically to the antihypertensive therapy.[7–9]

Several possibilities account for the failure of the large "global" studies (i.e., studies in which no restrictive patient entry characteristics were imposed on the eligible patient population) to demonstrate a reduction in coronary events. First, because of the global nature of these studies, the event rate in these relatively healthy middle-aged patients was not high enough for researchers to detect a significant reduction in morbidity and mortality. Second, these trials may have focused on controlling blood pressure without correction of other cardiovascular risk factors (e.g., cholesterol elevation and smoking). Also, patient compliance and the efficacy of the antihypertensive drugs themselves may have contributed to the failure to reduce coronary events. It is instructive to examine carefully the Medical Research Council (MRC) trial[7] and the Multiple Risk Factor Intervention Trial (MRFIT)[70] because they are two of the largest, most widely quoted global studies that have provided insight into the use of thiazide diuretics and beta blockers, two of the most commonly used antihypertensive drugs in the 1980s, with specific emphasis on coronary events.

The MRC trial involved more than 17,000 patients, aged 35–64 years, with mild hypertension treated for more than 85,000 patient-years with either a thiazide (bendrofluazide, 10 mg/day) or the beta blocker propranolol (up to 240 mg/day), in comparison with placebo. Approximately 70%–75% of bendrofluazide-treated patients and 65%–70% of propranolol-treated patients achieved goal diastolic blood pressure of less than 90 mm Hg. A fairly high percentage of patients (33%–34% for bendrofluazide- and propranolol-treated patients) dropped out from the study; 20%–25% withdrew because of side effects. There was no influence of propranolol on the frequency of myocardial infarction in women; in men, a modest benefit was seen only in nonsmokers. In male smokers, the frequency of myocardial infarction was actually slightly higher when patients were treated with propranolol, although this frequency did not achieve statistical significance.

In the MRFIT trial, almost 13,000 men aged 35–57 years with mild hypertension, elevation in serum cholesterol, and cigarette-smoking habit were studied for a 7-year period. Patients were randomized to either (1) a special intervention (SI) program of stepped-care treatment for hypertension, counseling for smoking cessation, and dietary advice for lowering blood cholesterol levels or (2) their usual sources of health care in the community (UC). Antihypertensive drugs were prescribed according to a stepped-care protocol, beginning with the use of either hydrochlorothiazide or chlorthalidone. Reserpine, hydralazine, or guanethidine was subsequently added if goal diastolic blood presure (90 mm Hg) had not been achieved. Eighty-eight percent of the SI patients achieved goal blood pressure. The dropout rate was less than 10%. Despite the expenditure of vast resources, the MRFIT study failed to show a statistically significant reduction in rates of mortality from coronary heart disease in the SI patients (17.9 deaths per 1000) in comparison with the UC group (19.3 per 1000), despite the fact that risk factors declined to a greater degree for the SI patients. The probable explanation for this is that the comparison group (UC), prompted by changes in the social milieu (educational programs), also reduced blood pressure, cholesterol levels, and cigarette use. As a consequence, both the treatment and comparison groups showed a progressive reduction in morbid events, with one exception. Although analysis of mortality based on separation by resting electrocardiographic (ECG) abnormalities was not part of the original working hypotheses and, as such, suffers from the weakness of a post hoc analysis, hypertensive patients in the SI group who had baseline ECG abnormalities exhibited an increase in mortality from coronary heart disease. These data have been interpreted to suggest that the more aggressive intervention in the SI group, particularly with regard to thiazide diuretics, increased the risk for death related to coronary heart disease in the subset of patients who were hypertensive and had ECG abnormalities at baseline. The implication is that the diuretic treatment itself was responsible for the increase in mortality.

Because of the failure of these studies to show a clear benefit in reduction in cardiovascular mortality with the use of diuretics and beta blockers (and the fact that these antihypertensive agents may have actually increased mortality in certain subgroups of patients, as mentioned), the Joint National Committee on Detection, Evaluation, and Treatment of High Blood Pressure in 1988 backed away from their previous recommendation of using only diuretics and beta blockers as first-line agents for the treatment of hypertension. In the 1988 report,[71] diuretics, beta blockers, ACE inhibitors, and calcium channel blockers were recommended as initial therapy.

Since that report, additional studies of selected patient groups with a higher risk of developing adverse cardiovascular events have been published. The European Working Party on High Blood Pressure in the Elderly trial[72] was a double-blind, placebo-controlled study in which hydrochlorothiazide and triamterene were used for active treatment of patients over age 60 with mild hypertension. Methyldopa was added for patients who failed to respond to the initial therapy. Among the patients who were treated, there was a significant (38%) reduction in cardiac mortality combined with a nonsignificant decrease in mortality from cerebrovascular events. In the SHEP study,[63] 4736 patients aged 60 years and over with isolated systolic hypertension were randomized to chlorthalidone (to which atenolol was added if goal blood pressure was not achieved) or placebo for a 5-year period. Incidences of both stroke (fatal and nonfatal) and coronary heart disease were significantly reduced in the patients who received antihypertensive drug treatment. Partly on the basis of these data, the JNC-V report in 1993 recommended that diuretics and beta blockers were preferred as initial antihypertensive therapy but acknowledged that there were not sufficient data available in 1993 to determine whether ACE inhibitors and/or calcium channel blockers could also reduce the incidence of cardiovascular mortality. Data in other high-risk patient populations are available to address, in part, this issue.

In the Survival and Ventricular Enlargement (SAVE) study,[59] hypertensive patients who survived a myocardial infarction (and had a reduced ejection fraction but no evidence of congestive heart failure) were randomized to receive captopril, an ACE inhibitor, or placebo. The patients were allowed to receive any other cardiovascular drugs that their physicians would normally prescribe (e.g., beta blockers). Among the hypertensive patients with left ventricular dysfunction who were randomized to the captopril group, there was a significant reduction in subsequent morbidity and mortality from cardiovascular events (in comparison with the placebo group), which was comparable with that seen in the hypertensive patients who received only beta blockers. In the landmark trial of 409 patients with insulin-dependent diabetes and nephropathy (urinary protein excretion > 500 mg per 24 h), there was a 50% reduction in death, dialysis, and transplantation among patients treated with captopril, in comparison with the placebo-controlled patients. This was true for both hypertensive and normotensive patients. Of importance is that the hypertensive patients who were randomized to the placebo group were treated with conventional antihypertensive regimens and achieved comparable reductions in blood pressure, as did the captopril-treated patients. The beneficial effect of captopril on subsequent morbidity and mortality could therefore not be explained by the difference in blood pressure control between the two groups.

The situation with calcium channel blockers is unresolved. Although verapamil and diltiazem have been reported to reduce rates of reinfarction after non–Q wave myocardial infarctions (in the absence of heart failure or left ventricular dysfunction), their ability to reduce the incidence of cardiovascular events in hypertensive patients has not been proved in controlled clinical trials. In the Danish Verapamil Infarction Trial II (DAVIT II) trial,[73] the results showed a favorable trend for the risk of reinfarction for verapamil and for diltiazem in comparison with placebo. However, an overview of all mortality data does not provide evidence of either benefit or harm with either agent. There is preliminary evidence that dihydropyridine derivatives (e.g., nifedipine) may increase the risk of myocardial infarction in patients with hypertension or ischemic heart disease. The use of nifedipine in patients with threatened and acute myocardial infarction not only showed no prevention of myocardial infarction but also demonstrated a significant increase in the 2-week mortality rate among the nifedipine-treated patients.[74]

It is possible that tracking "hard" endpoints (fatal and nonfatal myocardial infarction and stroke) of cardiovascular morbidity and mortality in young or middle-aged patients may not be as relevant as after the progression of cardiovascular lesions over decades. Because such a study would be financially prohibitive, it may be useful to follow surrogate endpoints. In 1984, it was demonstrated that angiotensin II receptors were present on platelets and that platelet activation was enhanced in the presence of angiotensin II.[75] Platelet activation results in the release of platelet-derived growth factor, which is an atherogenic stimulus. In addition, angiotensin II increases the plasma level of plasminogen activator/inhibitor-1 (PAI-1), which is an important physiologic inhibitor of tissue-type plasminogen activator.[76] Elevated levels of PAI-1 appear to constitute a marker of risk for recurrent coronary thrombosis.[77] Thus, ACE inhibitors could reduce angiotensin II–mediated platelet activation and PAI-1 stimulation and thereby lessen the progression of atherosclerotic disease.

Because ACE inhibitors are not associated with the adverse metabolic effects seen with diuretics and/or beta blockers (potassium depletion, reduced glucose tolerance, ventricular ectopic beats) that may have limited their efficacy in lowering cardiovascular events in the two "global" studies mentioned earlier, and in view of their effectiveness in reducing morbidity and mortality among specialized populations of post–myocardial infarction and diabetic patients, in addition to their ability to lower surrogate endpoints of atherogenesis, it is reasonable to consider ACE inhibitors as initial antihypertensive drug therapy in any patient with uncomplicated essential hypertension (see Fig. 32–2).

Side Effects

The side effect profile of the antihypertensive drugs is an important consideration with regard to both compliance and the quality of life of the patient. It is impossible to predict a priori whether a potential side effect that has been associated with an antihypertensive drug will occur in an individual patient. ACE inhibitors and long-acting calcium channel blockers are very well tolerated and have been correlated with preservation of a good quality of life, but they are also the most expensive of the available drugs. Diuretics frequently cause impotence, weakness, and fatigue. Beta blockers may also cause sexual dysfunction and fatigue, as well as insomnia, vivid dreams, and nightmares. Alpha blockers are associated with postural dizziness, as are α_2 agonists. The α_2 agonists can also cause dry mouth, sedation, and drowsiness. Direct peripheral vasodilators result in headaches, palpitations, and fluid retention. In addition, significant hypertrichosis frequently occurs with minoxidil and is therefore not well tolerated by female patients.

Headaches, palpitations, dizziness, and fluid retention also can occur with the short-acting calcium channel blockers, but fortunately these side effects occur much less frequently with the long-acting calcium channel antagonists. Significant constipation appears to be limited to the use of verapamil. Cough, rash, pruritus, dysgeusia, and, in rare instances, angioneurotic edema have been described with use of the ACE inhibitors. Of these potential side effects, a nonproductive cough is the most frequent reason for discontinuation of the drug. A persistent cough can develop immediately or after months of therapy. Although the incidence of cough may be as high as 15% (the longer the duration of action of the ACE inhibitor, the greater the likelihood of cough), it actually limits therapy in only 2%–5% of patients.

Follow-Up

It is customary to start with a low dosage of whichever drug is chosen, and then see the patient in follow-up evaluation 2 or 3 weeks later (unless the initial blood pressure is higher than 179/109, in which case an earlier return appointment is warranted). If the blood pressure has not returned to normal levels at this point, the dosage should be increased. If, after 2 or 3 months of titrating the dosage upward, the antihypertensive drug is still ineffective in lowering blood pressure in a given patient (and the patient is faithfully adhering to the prescribed regimen), it is reasonable to substitute a drug from a different class. If moderate dosages of a single drug have been partly effective in lowering blood pressure, it may be preferable to add a small dosage of a second drug with a different mode of action. This helps minimize the hemodynamic compensations that occur with a single drug and thereby limit its antihypertensive effectiveness. Thus, combining antihypertensive drugs from different classes allows the use of smaller dosages of drugs, thereby minimizing the potential for dosage-dependent side effects.

In general, if a diuretic was not chosen as the first drug, using it as the second drug tends to be helpful because diuretics usually enhance the effects of all other antihypertensive drugs. If the addition of a second drug produces a satisfactory response, tapering and eventually withdrawing the first drug should be considered, because monotherapy with most antihypertensive drugs provides adequate blood pressure control in about 50% of patients. In patients with stage III or IV hypertension, a three-drug combination may be required. Examples of effective three-drug combinations include (1) minoxodil, a diuretic, and a beta blocker and (2) an ACE inhibitor, a calcium channel blocker, and a diuretic.

As a rule, antihypertensive therapy should be maintained indefinitely. Once blood pressure is stabilized, follow-up visits at 3- to 6-month intervals are warranted in order to check for adequacy of blood pressure control, the degree of patient compliance, and the presence of adverse side effects. Associated medical problems such as the presence of end-organ damage or other major cardiovascular risk factors should be treated accordingly. Cessation of therapy in hypertensive patients is usually followed by return of blood pressure to pretreatment levels. Nevertheless, after prolonged blood pressure control, it may be possible to carefully reduce the dosages of the drugs used, especially in patients strictly adhering to lifestyle modifications. Attempts at step-down treatment should be done slowly and progressively, and the patients should continue to have frequent follow-up evaluations because blood pressure may rise again to hypertensive levels, sometimes even months or years after the dosages have been lowered or discontinued.

REFERENCES

1. MacMahon S, Peto R, Cutler J, et al: Blood pressure, stroke, and coronary heart disease: part 1. Prolonged differences in blood pressure: prospective observational studies corrected for the regression dilution bias. Lancet 1990; 335:765–774.
2. Whelton PK, Klag MJ: Hypertension as a risk factor for renal disease. Review of clinical and epidemiological evidence. Hypertension 1989; 13(suppl I):19–27.
3. Kannel WB, Sorlie P: Hypertension in Framingham. *In* Paul O (ed): Epidemiology and Control of Hypertension, pp 553–592. Miami, FL: Symposia Specialists, 1975.
4. Kannel WB, Dawber TR, McGee DL: Perspectives on systolic hypertension: the Framingham study. Circulation 1986; 61:1179–1182.
5. Kannel WB, Sorlie P: Hypertension in Framingham. *In* Paul O (ed): Epidemiology and Control of Hypertension, pp 553–592. Miami, FL: Symposia Specialists, 1975.
6. Whelton PK: Blood pressure in adults and the elderly. *In* Birkenhager WH, Reid JL (eds): Handbook of Hypertension, pp 51–69. Amsterdam: Elsevier, 1985. (Bulpitt CJ, ed. Epidemiology of hypertension; vol 6).
7. Medical Research Council Working Party: MRC trial of treatment of mild hypertension: principal results. Br Med J 1985; 291:97–104.
8. Hypertension Detection and Follow-Up Program Cooperative Group: The effect of treatment on mortality in "mild" hypertension: results of the Hypertension Detection and Follow-up Program. N Engl J Med 1982; 307:976–980.
9. Collins R, Peto R, MacMahon S, et al: Blood pressure, stroke and coronary heart disease: Part 2. Short-term reductions in blood pressure: overview of randomised drug trials in their epidemiological context. Lancet 1990; 335:827–838.
10. Joint National Committee on Detection, Evaluation, and Treatment of High Blood Pressure: The fifth report of the Joint National Committee on Detection, Evaluation, and Treatment of High Blood Pressure (JNC-V). Arch Intern Med 1993; 153:154–183.
11. Fletcher AE, Bulpitt CJ: How far should blood pressure be lowered? N Engl J Med 1992; 326:251–254.
12. Thomas WA: Health of a carnivorous race: a study of the Eskimo. JAMA 1927; 88:1559–1560.
13. Hunt JC: Sodium intake and hypertension: a cause for concern. Ann Intern Med 1983; 98:724–728.
14. Law MR, Frost CD, Wald NJ: By how much does dietary salt reduction lower blood pressure? I. Analysis of observational data among populations. Br Med J 1991; 302:811–815.
15. Law MR, Frost CD, Wald NJ: By how much does dietary sodium restriction lower blood pressure? II. Analysis of observational data within populations. Br Med J 1991; 302:815–818.
16. Intersalt Cooperative Research Group: Intersalt: an international study of electrolyte excretion and blood pressure. Results of 24 hour urinary sodium and potassium excretion. Br Med J 1988; 297:319–330.
17. Law MR, Frost CD, Wald MJ: III. Analysis of data from trials of salt reduction. Br Med J 1991; 302:819–824.
18. Cutler JA, Follmann D, Elliott P, Suh I: An overview of randomized trials of sodium reduction and blood pressure. Hypertension 1991; 17(suppl I):27–33.
19. Dimsdale JE, Ziegler M, Mills P, Berry C: Prediction of salt sensitivity. Am J Hypertens 1990; 3:429–435.
20. Weinberger MH, Miller JZ, Luft FC, et al: Definitions and characteristics of sodium sensitivity and blood pressure resistance. Hypertension 1986; 8(suppl II):127–134.
21. Rocchini AP, Key J, Bondie D, et al: The effect of weight loss on the sensitivity of blood pressure to sodium in obese adolescents. N Engl J Med 1989; 321:580–585.
22. Williams GH, Hollenberg NK: Non-modulating hypertension: a subset of sodium-sensitive hypertension. Hypertension 1991; 17(suppl I):81–85.
23. Krishna GG, Kapoor SC: Potassium depletion exacerbates essential hypertension. Ann Intern Med 1991; 115:77–83.
24. Cappuccio FP, MacGregor GA: Does potassium supplementation lower blood pressure? A meta-analysis of published trials. J Hypertens 1991; 9:465–473.
25. Siani A, Strazzullo P, Garcia A, et al: Increasing the dietary potassium intake reduces the need for antihypertensive medication. Ann Intern Med 1991; 115:753–759.
26. Garcia-Palmieri MR, Costas R Jr, Cruz-Vidal M, et al: Milk consumption, calcium intake, and decreased hypertension in Puerto Rico: Puerto Rico Heart Health Program study. Hypertension 1984; 6:322–328.
27. Kesteloot H, Joossens JV: Relationship of dietary sodium, potassium, calcium, and magnesium with blood pressure: Belgian Interuniversity Research on Nutrition and Health. Hypertension 1988; 12:594–599.
28. McCarron DA, Morris CD, Henry HJ, et al: Blood pressure and nutrient intake in the United States. Science 1984; 224:1392–1398.
29. Cutler JA, Brittain E: Calcium and blood pressure: an epidemiological prospective. Am J Hypertens 1990; 3(8, pt 2):137S–146S.
30. Cappuccio FP, Siani A, Strazzullo P: Oral calcium supplementation and blood pressure: an overview of randomized controlled trials. J Hypertens 1989; 7:941–946.
31. Joffres MR, Reed DM, Yano K: Relationship of magnesium intake and other dietary factors to blood pressure. The Honolulu Heart Study. Am J Clin Nutr 1987; 45:469–475.
32. Whelton PK, Klag MJ: Magnesium and blood pressure: review of the epidemiologic and clinical trial experience. Am J Cardiol 1989; 63:26G–30G.
33. Cappuccio FP, Markandu ND, Beynon GW, et al: Lack of effect of oral magnesium on high blood pressure: a double-blind study. Br Med J 1985; 291:235–238.
34. Dyckner T, Wester PO: Effect of magnesium on blood pressure. Br Med J 1983; 286:1847–1849.

35. Lind L, Lithell H, Pollare T, et al: Blood pressure response during long-term treatment with magnesium is dependent on magnesium status. Am J Hypertens 1991; 4(8):674–679.
36. The Trials of Hypertension Prevention Collaborative Research Group: The effects of nonpharmacologic interventions on blood pressure of persons with high-normal levels. Results of the trials of hypertension prevention, phase I. JAMA 1992; 267:1213–1220.
37. Sacks FM: Dietary fats and blood pressure: a critical review of the evidence. Nutr Reviews 1989; 47(10):291–300.
38. Puska P, Iacono JM, Nissinen A, et al: Controlled, randomised trial of the effect of dietary fat on blood pressure. Lancet 1983; 1:1–5.
39. Kagan A, Popper JS, Rhoads G, Yano K: Dietary and other risk factors for stroke in Hawaiian-Japanese men. Stroke 1995; 16:390–396.
40. Kimura ON: Atherosclerosis in Japan. Atheroscler Rev 1977; 2:209–221.
41. Sacks FM, Wood PG, Kass EH: Stability of blood pressure in vegetarians receiving dietary protein supplements. Hypertension 1984; 6:99–201.
42. Prescott SL, Jenner EA, Beilin LJ, et al: A randomized, controlled trial of the effect on blood pressure of dietary non-meat protein vs. meat protein in normotensive omnivores. Clin Sci 1988; 74:665–672.
43. Kean BH: The blood pressure of the Cuna Indians. Am J Trop Med Hyg 1944; 24:341–343.
44. Sacks FM, Kass EH: Low blood pressure in vegetarians: effects of specific foods and nutrients. Am J Clin Nutr 1988; 48:795–800.
45. Sacks FM, Rosner B, Kass EH: Blood pressure in vegetarians. Am J Epidemiol 1974; 100:390–398.
46. Sacks FM, Wood PG, Kass EH: Stability of blood pressure in vegetarians receiving dietary protein supplements. Hypertension 1984; 6:199–201.
47. Rouse IL, Armstrong BK, Beilin LJ: The relationship of blood pressure to diet and lifestyle in two religious populations. J Hypertens 1983; 1:65–71.
48. Langford HG, Davis BR, Blaufox, D, et al: Effect of drug and diet treatment of mild hypertension on diastolic blood pressure. Hypertension 1991; 17:210–217.
49. Stevens VJ, Corrigan SA, Obarzanek E, et al: Weight loss intervention in phase I of the trials of hypertension prevention. Arch Intern Med 1993; 153:849–858.
50. Yang M, VanItalle TB: Composition of weight loss during short-term weight reduction. JCI 1976; 58:722–730.
51. Jacobs D, Sowers JR, Hmeidan A, et al: Effects of weight reduction on cellular cation metabolism and vascular resistance. Hypertension 1993; 21:308–314.
52. Kushiro T, Kobayashi F, Osada H, et al: Role of sympathetic activity in blood pressure reduction with low calorie regimen. Hypertension 1991; 17:965–968.
53. Williams GH: Hypertensive vascular disease. *In* Isselbacher KJ, Braunwald E, Wilson JD, et al (eds): Harrison's Principles of Internal Medicine, 13th ed, pp 116–1131. New York: McGraw-Hill, 1994.
54. Yusuf S, Peto R, Lewis J, et al: Beta-blockade during and after myocardial infarction. An overview of the randomized trials. Progr Cardiovasc Dis 1985; 27:335–371.
55. Yusuf S, Held P, Furberg C: Update of effects of calcium antagonists in myocardial infarction or angina in light of the Second Danish Verapamil Infarction Trial (DAVIT-II) and the other recent studies. Am J Cardiol 1991; 67:1295–1297.
56. Zanchetti A: The antiatherogenic effects of antihypertensive drugs: experimental and clinical evidence. Clin Exper Hypertens 1992; A14:307–331.
57. Captopril Multicenter Research Group I: A cooperative multicenter study of captopril in congestive heart failure: hemodynamic effects and long-term response. Am Heart J 1985; 110:439–447.
58. The SOLVD Investigators: Effect of enalapril on survival in patients with reduced left ventricular ejection fractions and congestive heart failure. N Engl J Med 1991; 325:293–301.
59. Pfeffer MA, Braunwald E, Moye L, et al: Effects of captopril on mortality and morbidity in patients with left ventricular dysfunction after myocardial infarction. Results of the Survival and Ventricular Enlargement trial. N Engl J Med 1992; 327:669–677.
60. The SOLVD Investigators: Effects of enalapril on mortality and the development of heart failure in asymptomatic patients with reduced left ventricular ejection fraction. N Engl J Med 1992; 327:685–691.
61. Lewis EJ, Hunsicker LG, Bain RP, Rohde RD: The effect of angiotensin-converting-enzyme inhibition on diabetic nephropathy. N Engl J Med 1993; 329:1456–1462.
62. SHEP Cooperative Research Group: Prevention of stroke by antihypertensive drug treatment in older persons with isolated systolic hypertension. JAMA 1991; 265:3255–3264.
63. Lithell H: Insulin resistance and cardiovascular drugs. Clin Exper Hypertens 1992; A14:151–162.
64. Levy D, Garrison RJ, Savage DD, et al: Prognostic implications of echocardiographically determined left ventricular mass in the Framingham Heart Study. N Engl J Med 1990; 322:1561–1566.
65. Frohlich ED, Apstein C, Chobanian AV, et al: The heart in hypertension. N Engl J Med 1992; 327:998–1008.
66. Materson BJ, Reda DJ, Cushmen WC, et al: Single-drug therapy for hypertension in men. A comparison of six antihypertensive agents with placebo. N Engl J Med 1993; 328:914–921.
67. Layde PM, Beral V, Kay CR: Further analyses of mortality in oral contraceptive users. Royal College of General Practioners' Oral Contraceptive Study. Lancet 1981; 1:541–546.
68. Lim KG, Isles CG, Hodsman GP, et al: Malignant hypertension in women of child bearing age and its relation to the contraceptive pill. Br Med J 1987; 294:1057–1059.
69. Wren BG, Routledge DA: Blood pressure changes: oestrogens in climacteric women. Med J Aust 1981; 2:528–531.
70. Multiple Risk Factor Intervention Trial: Risk factor changes and mortality results. JAMA 1982; 248:1465–1477.
71. The 1988 report of the Joint National Committee on Detection, Evaluation, and Treatment of High Blood Pressure. Arch Intern Med 1988; 148(5):1023–1038.
72. Amery A, Birkenhager W, Brixko P, et al: Mortality and morbidity results from the European Working Party on High Blood Pressure in the Elderly trial. Lancet 1985; 1:1349–1354.
73. The Danish study on verapamil in myocardial infarction: The effect of verapamil on mortality and major events after myocardial infarction. The Danish Verapamil Infarction Trial II (DAVIT II). Am J Cardiol 1990; 66:779–785.
74. Muller JE, Morrison J, Stone PH, et al: Nifedipine therapy for patients with threatened and acute myocardial infarction: a randomized, double-blind, placebo-controlled comparison. Circulation 1984; 69:740–747.
75. Moore TJ, Taylor T, Williams GH: Human platelet angiotensin II receptors: regulation by the circulating angiotensin level. J Clin Endocrinol Metab 1984; 58:778–782.
76. Ridker PM, Gaboury CL, Conlin PR, et al: Stimulation of plasminogen activator inhibitor in vivo by infusion of angiotensin II. Circulation 1993; 87:1969–1973.
77. Hamsten A, DiFaire U, Wallidus G, et al: Plasminogenbactivator-inhibitor in plasma: risk factor for recurrent myocardial infarction. Lancet 1987; 2:3–9.

33 Treatment of Hypertensive Emergencies

Randall M. Zusman, MD

The terms *hypertensive crisis, hypertensive emergency, hypertensive urgency*, and *severe accelerated and/or malignant hypertension* have been applied to the clinical setting characterized by a marked elevation in blood pressure and associated pathophysiologic abnormalities.[1–7] In fact, these terms describe a continuum of clinical disease states in which the absolute value of blood pressure elevation, the rapidity of blood pressure elevation, the patient's history of hypertension, and the patient's underlying concomitant medical illnesses determine the need for an immediate, prompt, or gradual reduction in blood pressure to normal values. The absolute blood pressure elevation alone does not necessarily reflect the critical nature of the clinical condition of the patient; underlying illness complicated by the elevation in blood pressure may necessitate immediate blood pressure reduction at lower initial values, whereas a more marked elevation in blood pressure in a patient in whom hypertension has gradually developed without associated pathophysiologic disturbances may necessitate only gradual blood pressure control. The initial goal of pharmacologic therapy might be, not the normalization of blood pressure, but rather the amelioration of the associated medical complications that accompany the hypertensive episode.

A true hypertensive crisis mandates immediate blood pressure reduction; that is, antihypertensive therapy must be initiated within minutes of recognition of the clinical condition in order to protect life or sustain vital organ functions. In this setting, the drugs chosen should have an immediate onset of action, be effective regardless of the underlying cause of blood pressure elevation, and be titratable with a short half-life.

Blood pressure monitoring in an intensive care unit setting with continuous intra-arterial blood pressure recording, which provides instantaneous measurement of the blood pressure response, permits maximal use of the blood pressure–lowering benefits of a drug that can be given intravenously and titrated to any blood pressure level. Although this ideal situation maximizes the likelihood of prompt, controlled, and safe blood pressure reduction, it is often difficult to achieve ideal circumstances in the real clinical setting. Most patients have hypertensive emergencies outside the intensive care unit setting. Frequently, immediate-acting antihypertensive medications are not readily available, the time required to transfer the patient to an intensive care unit is excessive, and acquisition of the ideal antihypertensive agent and placement of an intra-arterial catheter would introduce an unacceptable delay in treating the patient. Under these conditions, a pharmacologic agent more commonly used in less emergent settings can, in fact, become the drug of choice because of its ease of access and delivery and the likelihood of successful blood pressure reduction in the shortest possible time. Thus, although the patient's underlying physiologic abnormalities and concomitant medical illnesses often suggest an ideal approach to the patient's blood pressure reduction, practical issues of the clinical setting may direct that therapy be initiated through alternative and acceptable, if not perfect, treatment. The varied manifestation of hypertensive emergencies prevents completion of randomized clinical trials in which alternative therapies have been subjected to scientific testing. Thus, the treatment of patients who have accelerated hypertension is often based on principles and outcomes gathered from the treatment of patients with less severe blood pressure elevations.

CLINICAL CONDITIONS NECESSITATING IMMEDIATE BLOOD PRESSURE REDUCTION

(Table 33–1)

Hypertensive Encephalopathy

Hypertensive encephalopathy, an alteration in cerebral/neurologic function in the setting of a severe elevation in blood pressure, can occur regardless of the underlying cause of the blood pressure elevation. Often, hypertensive encephalopathy accompanies an abrupt rise

TABLE 33–1. CLINICAL CONDITIONS ASSOCIATED WITH HYPERTENSIVE EMERGENCY

Adrenergic Crisis
Pheochromocytoma
Acute withdrawal from antihypertensive therapy
Ingestion of monoamine oxidase inhibitors and tyramine-containing foods
Ingestion of alpha-adrenergic agonists
Cardiac/Vascular
Acute left ventricular failure
Unstable angina pectoris
Acute myocardial infarction
Dissecting aortic aneurysm
Cerebrovascular
Head injury
Hypertensive encephalopathy (of any cause)
Intracerebral hemorrhage
Subarachnoid hemorrhage
Atherothrombotic/embolic brain infarction
Intracranial mass
Eclampsia
Postoperative Complications
After coronary artery bypass surgery
After peripheral vascular reconstruction
After renal transplantation
Renal
Renovascular hypertension (especially associated with acute renal artery occlusion)
Acute glomerulonephritis
Acute/chronic renal failure
Miscellaneous Conditions
Severe burns
Quadriplegia
Vasculitis

in blood pressure occurring either in a patient previously known to be hypertensive or in association with another medical illness in a patient who has no history of blood pressure elevation.[8–11] Manifestations of hypertensive encephalopathy include minimal neurologic disturbances such as headache or lethargy but can progress to more severe alterations in mental function, including confusion, delirium or coma, visual impairment, and/or generalized seizures.[8, 9, 12, 13] Focal neurologic findings rarely accompany hypertensive encephalopathy, because hypertensive encephalopathy is a more generalized cerebral dysfunction; but when they do occur, the physician should entertain the possibility that a localized neurologic lesion is complicating the hypertensive event, such as a cerebrovascular accident or intracranial hemorrhage.

Cerebral blood flow is normally maintained by an autoregulatory mechanism that sustains cerebral perfusion over a wide range of arterial perfusion pressures.[12, 14] As blood pressure rises to levels beyond the autoregulatory range, localized hyperperfusion and edema can result in the generalized central nervous system dysfunction that accompanies the encephalopathic process.[15, 16] Alternatively, encephalopathy can result from vascular narrowing, spasm, and/or occlusion leading to cerebral ischemia.[17–19]

In patients with hypertensive encephalopathy, concomitant evidence of systemic non-neurologic manifestations of severe blood pressure elevation has resulted in the application of the term *malignant hypertension.* Vascular damage in these patients is indicated on physical examination by retinal hemorrhages or exudates and, in the extreme, by papilledema.[20] Vascular lesions associated with malignant hypertension, as it is used in this context, are myointimal proliferation and fibrinoid necrosis of the vessel wall.[13] These pathologic changes lead to areas of vascular dilation or spasm, with resultant hyperperfusion or hypoperfusion and associated endothelial cell damage.[21] Disruption of vascular integrity then leads to the diffusion of plasma proteins into the extracellular space and to edema, fibrin deposition, and intravascular thrombus formation. When these changes occur in the kidney, acute renal failure ensues; blood pressure control does not always restore renal function in these patients, and they can become dialysis dependent.[22, 23] Microangiopathic hemolytic anemia, another manifestation of vascular disruption, is associated with intravascular hemolysis, coagulation, fibrin deposition, and thrombocytopenia.[24] The presence of retinal changes, accelerating renal dysfunction, and microangiopathic hemolytic anemia is an indication of the severity of blood pressure elevation and mandates immediate reduction in blood pressure.

Left Ventricular Failure

Hypertension alters left ventricular function through mechanisms involving both systolic and diastolic ventricular performance.[25] In patients with systolic ventricular failure, the increase in systemic vascular tone impairs left ventricular emptying and increases left ventricular end-diastolic filling pressure, which results in orthopnea, paroxysmal nocturnal dyspnea, and dyspnea on exertion. An acute increase in systemic vascular resistance associated with a marked elevation in blood pressure accelerates this physiologic process, limits ventricular emptying, and leads to premature closure of the aortic valve, which further compromises cardiac performance and results in acute pulmonary edema.[26]

In hypertensive patients without left ventricular systolic dysfunction, severe diastolic dysfunction can account for the development of congestive heart failure in the presence of a marked blood pressure elevation. The acute physiologic response in such patients to an increase in systemic vascular tone is ventricular dilation, which enables cardiac output to be sustained in the setting of an increased vascular resistance. Depending on the diastolic properties of the ventricle, the presence or absence of left ventricular hypertrophy, and the intravascular volume in the patient, this can result in a precipitous increase in left ventricular end-diastolic pressure without associated systolic dysfunction.[26, 27]

The symptoms of congestive heart failure in the setting of a marked elevation in blood pressure are probably secondary to both systolic and diastolic dysfunction in most patients. Patients with predominantly systolic dysfunction generally respond best to diuretic and vasodilator therapy, whereas those with predominantly diastolic dysfunction often respond best to agents that improve left ventricular diastolic relaxation. Initially, however, the treatment modalities of patients with either of these physiologic mechanisms are similar in that a prompt reduction in blood pressure improves left ventricular systolic function in the patient with compromised cardiac contractility and also allows improved diastolic filling in the patient who has a stiff, noncompliant ventricle. Although not specifically indicated for the treatment of hypertensive emergencies, rapidly acting diuretic agents can be valuable in the treatment of patients with congestive heart failure due to intravascular volume overload and systolic ventricular dysfunction.

Myocardial Ischemia

An elevation in blood pressure markedly increases myocardial oxygen consumption and exacerbates angina pectoris in patients with coronary artery disease or increases myocardial damage in patients with acute myocardial infarction.[28, 29] In this setting, any attempt to lower blood pressure must take into account the need to sustain myocardial perfusion and to concomitantly reduce myocardial oxygen consumption. Peripheral vasodilating agents, which diminish coronary artery blood flow while lowering blood pressure or increase heart rate as a reflex response to the decrease in vascular tone, can exacerbate myocardial ischemic syndromes. Excessive blood pressure reduction can lead to exacerbation of myocardial ischemia if diastolic pressure falls below critical values for coronary perfusion. Beta-adrenergic receptor blockers, although rarely used primarily for the treatment of marked hypertension, can be helpful in this setting because their negative chronotropic effect improves the relationship between myocardial oxygen supply and demand.

A detailed discussion of the treatment of the patient with hypertension and cardiac disease can be found in Chapter 34.

Dissecting Aortic Aneurysm

A rapid reduction in blood pressure in the patient with dissecting aortic aneurysm is necessary to reduce the shear forces that propagate the dissection of the damaged aorta.[30] When blood pressure in these patients is lowered, the reflex sympathetic activation that often accompanies the use of peripheral vasodilating agents must be avoided; the vasodilation associated with the use of such agents can increase heart rate and the velocity of left ventricular ejection, which is associated with further vascular disruption. Thus, when an acutely acting vasodilating drug is used, the reflex activation of the sympathetic nervous system must be simultaneously blocked to minimize aortic dissection. This is usually accomplished by the concomitant use of a beta-adrenergic receptor blocker, which decreases cardiac contractility in the setting of the falling blood pressure.

Intracranial Hemorrhage

Acute management of the elevation in blood pressure that accompanies intracranial hemorrhage is the most controversial area in the management of a hypertensive emergency.[31, 32] Few controlled studies have addressed the question of the benefit of blood pressure reduction in patients with accelerated hypertension accompanying subarachnoid hemorrhage[33] and/or intracerebral hematoma. Ideally, acute blood pressure control will prevent edema formation and decrease the extent of hemorrhage in such patients. However, blood pressure reduction may lead to ischemia of marginally perfused border zones, thus extending the area of damage, and may compromise blood flow in patients with increased intracranial pressure. An excessive reduction in blood pressure in patients with carotid stenoses may further compromise cerebral blood flow in this population of patients. In such patients with severely elevated blood pressure values, the value is generally reduced to a more acceptable range in the hope of preserving central nervous system function. However, clearly demonstrable benefits of this approach have not been proved, and care must be taken to monitor the patient for deteriorating central nervous system function in the setting of blood pressure reduction. Evaluating the effects of blood pressure control in the patient with an intracerebral hemorrhage is further complicated by the possibility that the underlying neurologic disorder has progressed independently of the reduction in blood pressure, and thus the fall in blood pressure has neither contributed to nor prevented the progression of neurologic damage.

Thrombotic/Lacunar Cerebral Infarcts

Marked blood pressure elevation is generally associated with lacunar and thrombotic stroke, especially in view of the role of chronic hypertension as a risk factor for the development of cerebrovascular accidents.[31, 34, 35] The mechanism leading to the marked increase in blood pressure that often accompanies cerebrovascular events is unclear but may relate to activation of the sympathetic nervous system. As in the case of intracranial hemorrhage, the benefits of immediate blood pressure control in this setting are unclear. On the one hand, the elevation in systemic blood pressure may increase cerebral blood flow through a stenotic vessel or by perfusion of collateral channels; however, it may also lead to further edema in the region of the damaged neurologic tissue and to intracerebral pressure elevations.

In light of the unconfirmed benefits of immediate blood pressure control in this setting, a conservative approach to blood pressure elevation in patients with mild increases in systemic pressure, especially in patients with chronic hypertension, is generally accepted. In patients with acute or severe elevations in blood pressure, a gradual reduction in blood pressure to less markedly elevated (diastolic blood pressure less than 100 mm Hg) but not necessarily normal values over an extended time (60–120 min) is desirable. Rapidly acting agents whose effect can be quickly reversed are clearly ideal in this population of patients because deteriorating neurologic function associated with blood pressure reduction can be reversed, it is hoped, by discontinuation of the antihypertensive therapy with a resultant increase in blood pressure.

Adrenergic Crises

The term *adrenergic crises* refers to a variety of clinical states associated with a marked increase in plasma catecholamine levels. Adrenergic crises may occur after acute discontinuation of antihypertensive therapy with clonidine and/or beta-adrenergic receptor blockers, with ingestion of alpha-adrenergic agonists such as phenylpropanolamine, with ingestion of monoamine oxidase inhibitors and tyramine-containing foods, or in association with increased catecholamine levels in patients with pheochromocytoma.

Recognition of the hyperadrenergic state is particularly important in the treatment of these patients. Although they may respond to antihypertensive agents used more generally in the treatment of accelerated hypertension, the use of an alpha-adrenergic blocking drug will provide more specific and often more prompt reduction in blood pressure in this setting.

Eclampsia

The development of accelerated hypertension in the pregnant patient poses unique problems in treating the high blood pressure of the mother while maintaining the viability of the fetus. For a detailed discussion of the treatment of hypertension in pregnancy and eclampsia, see Chapter 41.

Miscellaneous Conditions

Sudden, marked blood pressure elevations may occur in the setting of severe vasculitides (including acute glomerulonephritis), severe burns, or quadriplegia. Similarly, hypertension may become more marked after coronary artery bypass surgery, renal transplantation, or vascular surgical reconstruction owing to either changes in underlying physiologic control mechanisms or discontinuation of preoperative antihypertensive therapy. In these settings, the selection of drugs that are appropriate (not contraindicated) and perhaps therapeutic for the underlying clinical condition should direct therapy.

PRINCIPLES OF TREATMENT (Table 33–2)

The availability of a variety of potent, immediately acting antihypertensive agents has led to virtually complete success in the reduction in blood pressure of patients with hypertensive emergencies. However, the danger of complications associated with rapid blood pressure reduction requires that the risks and benefits of blood pressure reduction be considered in each patient. How quickly the blood pressure must be controlled and to what level it should be reduced are the most immediate questions to be addressed. In general, complete normalization of the blood pressures is not necessary and should not be attempted. Among the factors to be considered are concomitant medical illnesses that are being worsened by the elevation in blood pressure or that may be worsened through the use of an agent that has an inappropriate mechanism of action (e.g., the development of tachycardia in a patient with coronary artery disease or dissecting aortic aneurysm). In general, elderly patients are at greater risk for development of an adverse effect of acute blood pressure reduction because of compromised autoregulatory responses and the prolonged duration of action of antihypertensive drugs in the elderly. Thus, lower initial doses of medications and higher target blood pressure values may be appropriate in this setting. The patient's intravascular volume status is a third factor that may affect the outcome of attempted blood pressure reduction. In patients who have previously received diuretic agents and in whom intravascular volume is suspected to be low, an inordinate blood pressure reduction may occur after the administration of potent vasodilating drugs. In this setting, the potential need for intravascular volume expansion through intravenous fluid infusion must be recognized and lower doses of medications used for initial treatment. Prior ingestion of antihypertensive medications must also be considered in the patient presenting with a hypertensive emergency. Patients who have taken antihypertensive drugs orally before presenting for emergency treatment may not have absorbed those agents because of vasoconstriction and inadequate gastrointestinal function. With a reduction in blood pressure and mesenteric vasodilation, these agents may then

TABLE 33–2. FACTORS AFFECTING INITIAL TREATMENT OF PATIENTS WITH A HYPERTENSIVE EMERGENCY

Urgency of need for blood pressure reduction
Availability of intensive care unit monitoring
Concomitant medical illness
Mechanism of action of the antihypertensive agent
Route of administration of the antihypertensive agent
Age of the patient
Intravascular volume status
Prior ingestion of antihypertensive medications

be absorbed, resulting in an "overdose" of antihypertensive therapy that leads to precipitous reductions in blood pressure.

Perhaps the most important decision to be made in the treatment of patients presenting with a hypertensive crisis is whether to use parenteral or orally active antihypertensive drugs. Although the onset of action of orally active agents is generally later than that of intravenous drugs, the use of some oral drugs—for example, nifedipine or captopril—is associated with a measurable reduction in blood pressure within 15–30 min of administration and in some cases within only a few minutes of drug ingestion. Thus, it is not always necessary to use a parenteral agent with the associated need for intra-arterial blood pressure monitoring. However, parenteral agents offer the potential safety factor of the ability to immediately discontinue administration of the drug in the event of an untoward and excessive reduction in blood pressure. In contrast, the physician must be prepared to treat a hypotensive response to an orally active agent for a prolonged time until the activity of the orally administered drug has completely resolved.

DRUG SELECTION (Table 33–3)

Sodium Nitroprusside

Sodium nitroprusside is generally considered the drug of choice in the treatment of hypertensive emergencies because of its almost universal effectiveness in the treatment of elevated blood pressure regardless of the underlying cause.[36, 37] The drug is characterized by rapid onset and offset of action; ease of titratability, which permits the selection of a precise goal blood pressure response; and moment-to-moment regulation of blood pressure values. The blood pressure reduction that follows nitroprusside administration is caused by both arterial and venous dilatation, which results in both decreased systemic vascular resistance and cardiac preload; these effects decrease myocardial oxygen consumption and prevent reflex tachycardia associated with direct arterial vasodilation. In general, cardiac output is unaffected after sodium nitroprusside therapy except in patients with left ventricular systolic dysfunction; in such patients, decreased systemic vascular resistance/afterload usually leads to improved ventricular systolic performance.

Although often used in the treatment of patients with coronary artery disease, sodium nitroprusside does not specifically dilate the coronary vasculature, and thus a decrease in coronary perfusion may accompany its use; this decrease in coronary flow may be caused by either decreased diastolic perfusion pressure or "coronary steal" effects.[38]

Owing to the potency of sodium nitroprusside's antihypertensive effect, it should be administered only in an intensive care unit setting with continuous arterial blood pressure monitoring by an indwelling arterial catheter. Because of the photosensitivity of nitroprusside, the infusion solution and the intravenous lines must be protected from light. Toxicity associated with nitroprusside administration is caused by the accumulation of thiocyanate. Signs of thiocyanate toxicity include blurred vision, tinnitus, confusion, lethargy, and/or seizures and usually accompany prolonged administration of the drug at levels greater than 200 μg/min. Ideally, it should not be necessary to use high doses of sodium nitroprusside for prolonged periods; once blood pressure control has been achieved, an attempt to convert therapy to an appropriate long-term antihypertensive regimen should be initiated immediately. Blood thiocyanate levels should be monitored whenever high-dose or prolonged treatment is necessary; levels in excess of 10 mg/dL are generally associated with toxic effects.

Nitroglycerin

Intravenous nitroglycerin effectively lowers blood pressure through both arterial and venous dilatation.[39, 40] The associated reduction in blood pressure is accompanied by decreases in left ventricular filling pressure and myocardial oxygen consumption. In comparison with an equivalent reduction in blood pressure accompanying nitroprusside therapy, there is a greater reduction in myocardial oxygen consumption and maintenance of coronary artery perfusion with nitroglycerin; thus, nitroglycerin is often considered the drug of choice in the treatment of patients with hypertension associated with unstable angina pectoris, acute myocardial infarction, or left ventricular dysfunction associated with myocardial ischemia. Although nitroglycerin is free of toxic side effects, tolerance to nitrate-induced vasodilatation occurs in patients receiving long-term nitroglycerin infusions. Thus, once adequate blood pressure control has

TABLE 33–3. CHARACTERISTICS OF DRUGS USED FOR TREATMENT OF HYPERTENSIVE EMERGENCIES

Drug	Method of Administration	Initial Dose	Dosage Range or Interval	Onset	Peak Effect	Duration
Direct Vasodilators						
Nitroprusside	IV infusion	0.5 μg/kg/min	0.5–10 μg/kg/min	Immediately	1–2 min	2–3 min
Nitroglycerin	IV infusion	50 μg/min	50–1000 μg/min	Immediately	1–2 min	1–2 min
ACE Inhibitors						
Captopril	PO	6.25–50 mg	12.5–50 mg at 30–45 min intervals	10–15 min	45–90 min	2–6 h
Enalaprilat	IV	1.25 mg	1.25–5 mg q6h	15 min	4–6 h	6 h
Adrenergic Inhibitors						
Phentolamine	IV infusion	0.5–1 mg bolus or 1 mg/min infusion	1–5 mg/min	1–2 min	3–5 min	15–60 min
Labetalol	IV bolus	20 mg	40–80 mg at 5- to 10-min intervals	5 min	5 min	2–6 h
Calcium Channel Blocker						
Nifedipine	SL	10 mg	10–20 mg q 15 min	2–5 min	5–10 min	3–6 h
	PO	10 mg	10–20 mg q 30–45 min	15–30 min	30–60 min	3–6 h
Beta-Adrenergic Receptor Blocker						
Esmolol	IV infusion	200–500 μg/kg/min	50–300 μg/kg/min	1–2 min	4–8 min	10–20 min
Propranolol	IV infusion	1–10 mg	1–5 mg/h	1–2 min	5–10 min	3–6 h

Abbreviations: ACE, angiotensin converting enzyme; IV, intravenous; PO, oral; SL, sublingual.

been achieved, the transition to long-term antihypertensive therapy should be initiated.

Phentolamine

Phentolamine, a nonselective alpha-adrenergic receptor blocking agent, is particularly effective owing to prevention of catecholamine-induced vasoconstriction[2, 41] in the treatment of patients with adrenergic crises. It is useful in the treatment of patients with a hypertensive emergency secondary to pheochromocytoma; however, its use may be associated with precipitous reductions in blood pressure in this setting. Before long-term administration of phentolamine is initiated, a test dose of between 0.5 and 1 mg should be infused in a short time interval to assess the patient's sensitivity to the drug. A precipitous reduction in blood pressure to the test dose infusion should prompt suspicion of an underlying pheochromocytoma. Phentolamine may be particularly appropriate, however, in the treatment of patients with hypertensive emergencies resulting from abrupt withdrawal of prior antihypertensive therapy, particularly clonidine or beta-adrenergic blockade, or hypertension resulting from the ingestion of alpha-adrenergic agonists.

Angiotensin Converting Enzyme Inhibitors

Although not available in a parenteral form, captopril[37, 42] produces a rapid reduction in blood pressure in patients with hypertensive emergencies when it is given orally in doses up to 50 mg. The use of captopril by sublingual administration has also been reported with some success.[43–47] The onset of action is within 15–30 min. Although the response to converting enzyme inhibition may be dependent on elevations in plasma renin activity, captopril is effective in lowering the blood pressure of subjects ingesting a high-salt diet. This suggests that the antihypertensive response to captopril therapy is mediated in part through non–renin-dependent mechanisms of action, the potentiation of the vasodilatory response to bradykinin, and/or the enhanced synthesis of vasodilatory prostanoids.[43] Captopril's utility in the treatment of patients with chronic congestive heart failure makes it highly desirable for the treatment of patients with hypertensive emergencies and associated left ventricular systolic dysfunction.

Enalaprilic acid, the biologically active metabolite of enalapril, is available for intravenous infusion.[48] It has a rapid onset of action after an initial bolus and can be infused over a long term for a prolonged antihypertensive response. An extensive experience with enalaprilic acid (enalaprilat) in the treatment of patients with hypertensive emergencies is not available.

Although angiotensin converting enzyme inhibition is effective in the treatment of a majority of hypertensive patients, a predictable response to the administration of captopril or enalaprilat is questionable; thus, the use of more rapidly acting, intravenously active agents may be preferable for initial treatment. However, in settings in which agents such as nitroprusside are not immediately available or when monitoring facilities are not present, the use of either of these agents may be desirable.

Calcium Channel Entry Blockers

The calcium channel antagonist nifedipine is highly effective and is widely used in the treatment of marked blood pressure elevations.[49] It is effective in the capsule formulation when given orally or chewed ("bite and swallow") or when the contents of the capsule are aspirated and placed sublingually.[47, 50–56] As with other calcium channel antagonists, the greater the initial elevation in blood pressure, the greater the blood pressure response that has been reported after nifedipine administration in the acute setting; however, the reduction in pressure is generally gradual and to "normal" values. Nifedipine is generally effective after a single dose, with a gradual reduction in blood pressure that avoids the need for invasive blood pressure monitoring. Precipitous reductions in blood pressure have been reported, however, particularly in patients who are volume depleted and/or who have received other antihypertensive medications before recognition of the antihypertensive emergency. Precipitous reductions in blood pressure may result in acute myocardial ischemia in patients with underlying coronary artery stenoses or in the development of neurologic dysfunction in patients with carotid artery disease. When given in the capsule formulation, reflex sympathetic activation with resultant tachycardia may exacerbate unstable angina pectoris or myocardial infarction; the potential development of reflex tachycardia is a contraindication to the use of this agent in the patient with a dissecting aortic aneurysm.

Although calcium channel antagonists have inherent negative inotropic activity and, thus, would generally be considered undesirable in the treatment of patients with left ventricular failure, the marked peripheral vasodilating effect in a patient with severe hypertension may result in improved cardiac performance in patients with pulmonary congestion. The improvement in left ventricular performance is dependent on the degree to which the reduction in blood pressure accompanying nifedipine therapy improves contractility and the extent to which its favorable effect on cardiac diastolic relaxation overcomes the inherent negative inotropic activity associated with the drug.[57]

Labetalol

Labetalol has both alpha-adrenergic and beta-adrenergic blocking activity; after intravenous administration, it has an early onset of action, a high degree of efficacy, and low toxicity. It can be administered by either repeated bolus injection or continuous infusion and offers the advantage of reduced peripheral vascular resistance without reflex sympathetic activation.[41, 58–60] The hemodynamic characteristics of labetalol are particularly desirable in the treatment of hyperadrenergic states associated with pheochromocytoma or clonidine withdrawal. In patients with pheochromocytoma, the possibility of excessive beta-adrenergic stimulation after the use of labetalol must be considered in the patient more "sensitive" to its alpha-blocking activity. Thus, it is probably preferable in the patient with known or suspected pheochromocytoma to initially establish selective alpha-adrenergic blockade with an agent such as phentolamine, followed by administration of a selective beta-adrenergic receptor blocker.

Beta-Adrenergic Receptor Blocking Agents

Intravenous administration of beta-adrenergic receptor blocking drugs such as propranolol or esmolol rarely results in an acute blood pressure–lowering response in patients with hypertensive emergencies. However, beta-adrenergic receptor blockers are valuable adjuncts to the use of a vasodilating agent such as nitroprusside in treating patients with acute aortic dissection, myocardial infarction, and/or unstable angina pectoris to prevent reflex sympathetic activation in these patients.[37, 41]

Other Vasodilators and Sympatholytic Agents

The vasodilating agents hydralazine, diazoxide, trimethaphan, and minoxidil as well as the sympatholytic agents clonidine, methyldopa, and reserpine and the alpha-adrenergic blocker prazosin have been used for the treatment of hypertensive emergencies. The unpredictable response to these agents, their lack of an immediate onset of action, and/or the toxic effects of these drugs have rendered them second-line therapies in the treatment of hypertensive emergencies at this time.

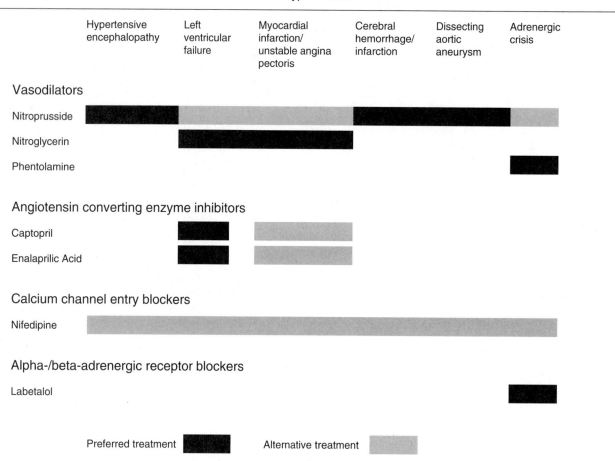

Figure 33–1. Preferential drug selection for the treatment of hypertensive emergencies. In the treatment of patients with a dissecting aortic aneurysm with nitroprusside, a beta-adrenergic receptor blocker (esmolol, propranolol) should be added to prevent reflex sympathetic activation.

SUMMARY AND CONCLUSIONS

Figure 33–1 depicts the drugs of choice for the treatment of particular hypertensive emergencies. These recommendations are generalizations for the treatment of populations of patients and do not necessarily reflect ideal choices for the treatment of an individual patient. To establish the most advantageous approach to the treatment of an individual patient with a hypertensive emergency, careful consideration must be given to the underlying medical illnesses present in that patient, the need for rapid reduction in blood pressure,

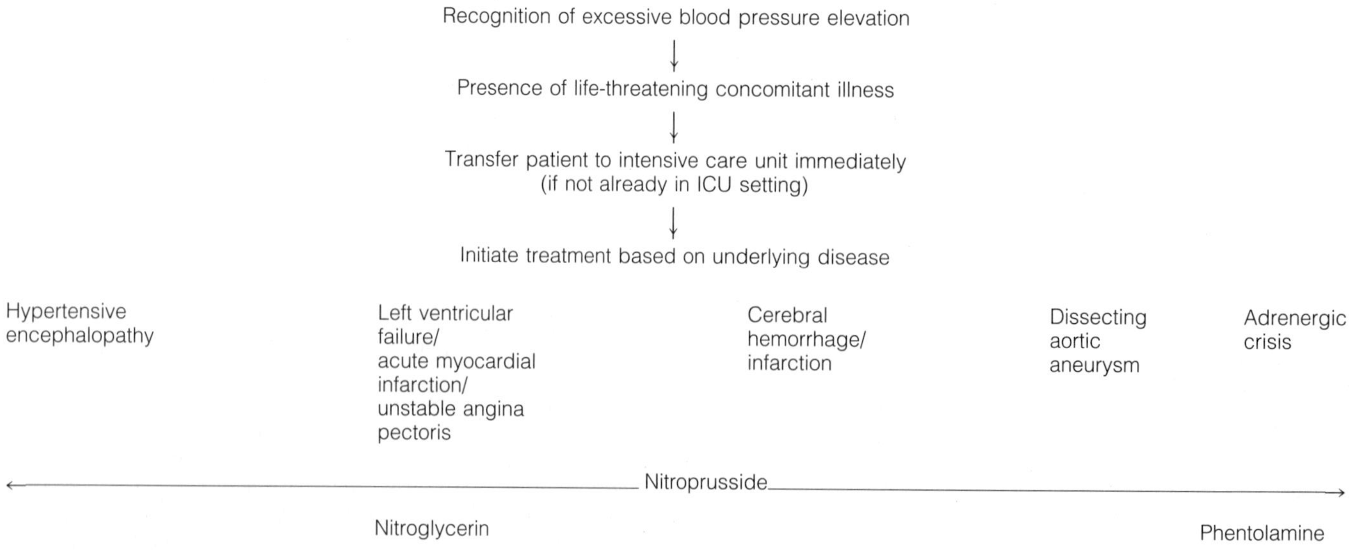

Figure 33–2. Flow diagram for the idealized treatment of a hypertensive emergency. In the treatment of patients with a dissecting aortic aneurysm with nitroprusside, a beta-adrenergic receptor blocker (esmolol, propranolol) should be added to prevent reflex sympathetic activation.

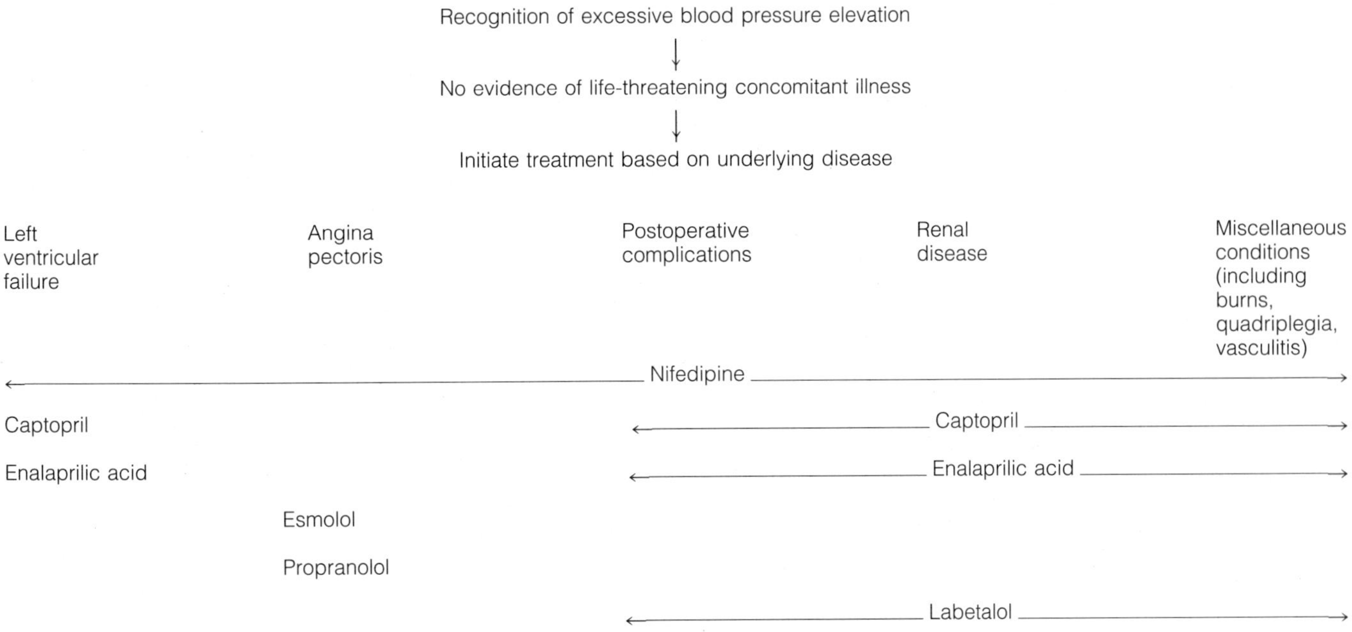

Figure 33–3. Flow diagram for the treatment of a hypertensive urgency.

and the extent of blood pressure reduction that is desired. Figures 33–2 and 33–3 outline the sequence of decisions to be made in treating a patient with a true hypertensive emergency in whom immediate blood pressure reduction is needed to preserve life or organ function and a patient with a hypertensive urgency that necessitates more gradual blood pressure control. Only after careful consideration of these three factors can an initial plan of action be designed and a drug chosen for the treatment of the patient. After initial control of blood pressure, it is important that a plan for long-term blood pressure control be formulated and treatment initiated according to the principles outlined in Chapter 32.

Finally, although secondary causes of hypertension are infrequent in a generalized population of hypertensive patients, the frequency of correctable forms of hypertension is considerably higher in patients with marked elevations in blood pressure. In particular, the presence of renovascular hypertension must be considered in any patient who has a marked elevation in blood pressure, especially in those with previously well-controlled disease, in elderly patients, and in patients with evidence of renal dysfunction.[61, 62]

REFERENCES

1. Kaplan NM: Systemic hypertension: mechanisms and diagnosis. *In* Braunwald E (ed): Heart Disease, pp 817–851. Philadelphia: WB Saunders, 1992.
2. Burris JF, Freis ED: Hypertensive emergencies. *In* Messerli FH (ed): Cardiovascular Drug Therapy, pp 58–74. Philadelphia: WB Saunders, 1990.
3. Kaplan NM. Etiologies and treatment of systemic arterial hypertension. *In* Willerson JT (ed): Treatment of Heart Diseases, pp 7.1–7.106. London: Gower Medical Publishing, 1994.
4. Mann SJ, Atlas SA: Hypertensive emergencies. *In* Laragh JH, Brenner BM (eds): Hypertension: Pathophysiology, Diagnosis, and Management, pp 2275–2290. New York: Raven Press, 1990.
5. Kaplan NM: Hypertensive crises. *In* Clinical Hypertension, pp 281–298. Baltimore: Williams & Wilkins, 1994.
6. Houston MC: Pathophysiology, clinical aspects, and treatment of hypertensive crises. Prog Cardiovasc Dis 1989; 32:99–148.
7. Calhoun DA, Oparil S: Treatment of hypertensive crisis. N Engl J Med 1990; 223:1177–1183.
8. Dinsdale HB: Hypertensive encephalopathy. *In* Barnett HJM, Mohr JP, Stein BM, et al (eds): Stroke: Pathophysiology, Diagnosis, and Management, pp 787–792. New York: Churchill Livingstone, 1992.
9. Chester EM, Agamanolis DP, Banker BQ: Hypertensive encephalopathy: a clinicopathologic study of 20 cases. Neurology 1978; 28:928–939.
10. Healton EB, Brust JC, Feinfeld DA, Thompson GE: Hypertensive encephalopathy and the neurological manifestations of malignant hypertension. Neurology 1982; 32:127–132.
11. Kontos HA, Wei E, Dietrich WD, et al: Mechanism of cerebral arteriolar abnormalities after acute hypertension. Am J Physiol 1981; 240:H511–H527.
12. Johansson B, Strandgaard S, Lassen NA: On the pathogenesis of hypertensive encephalopathy. The hypertensive "breakthrough" of autoregulation of cerebral blood flow with forced vasodilatation, flow increase, and blood-brain-barrier damage. Circ Res 1974; 34 & 35 (suppl 1):I-167–I-171.
13. Kincaid-Smith P, McMichael J, Murphy EA: The clinical course and pathology of hypertension with papilledema. Q J Med 1958; 27:117–154.
14. Strangaard S, Haunso S: Why does antihypertensive treatment prevent stroke but not myocardial infarction? Lancet 1987; 2:658–662.
15. Kwong YL, Yu YL, Lam KSL, et al: CT appearance in hypertensive encephalopathy. Neuroradiology 1987; 29:215.
16. Weingarten KL, Zimmerman RD, Pinto RS, Whelan MA: Computed tomographic changes of hypertensive encephalopathy. Am J Neuroradiol 1985; 6:395–398.
17. Byrom FB: Pathogenesis of hypertensive encephalopathy and its relation to malignant phase of hypertension; experimental evidence in the hypertensive rat. Lancet 1954; 2:201–211.
18. Dinsdale HB, Robertson DM, Haas RA: Cerebral blood flow in acute hypertension. Arch Neurol 1974; 31:80–87.
19. Kincaid-Smith P: Malignant hypertension: mechanisms and management. Pharmacol Ther 1980; 9:245–269.
20. McGregor E, Isles CG, Jay JL, et al: Retinal changes in malignant hypertension. Br Med J 1986; 292:233–234.
21. Schwartz GI, Strong CG: Renal parenchymal involvement in essential hypertension. Med Clin North Am 1987; 71:843–858.
22. McCormack LJ, Beland JE, Schneckloth RE, Corcoran AC: Effects of antihypertensive treatment on the evolution of the renal lesions in malignant nephrosclerosis. Am J Pathol 1958; 34:1011–1022.
23. Pitcock JA, Johnson JH, Hatch FE: Malignant hypertension in blacks. Malignant intrarenal arterial disease as observed by light and electron microscopy. Hum Pathol 1976; 7:333–346.
24. Gavras H, Oliver N, Aitchison J, et al: Abnormalities of coagulation and the development of malignant phase hypertension. Kidney Int 1975; 8:S252–S261.

25. Braunwald E, Sonnenblick EH, Ross J Jr: Mechanisms of cardiac contraction and relaxation. *In* Braunwald E (ed): Heart Disease, pp 351–392. Philadelphia: WB Saunders, 1992.
26. Braunwald E: Pathophysiology of heart failure. *In* Braunwald E (ed): Heart Disease, pp 393–418. Philadelphia: WB Saunders, 1992.
27. Katz AM: Heart failure. *In* Fozzard HA, Haber E, Jennings RB, et al (eds): The Heart and Cardiovascular System: Scientific Foundations, pp 333–353. New York: Raven Press, 1992.
28. Braunwald E, Sobel BE: Coronary blood flow and myocardial ischemia. *In* Braunwald E (ed): Heart Disease, pp 1161–1199. Philadelphia: WB Saunders, 1992.
29. Pasternak RC, Braunwald E, Sobel BE: Acute myocardial infarction. *In* Braunwald E (ed): Heart Disease, pp 1200–1291. Philadelphia: WB Saunders, 1992.
30. Eagle KA, DeSanctis RW: Diseases of the aorta. *In* Braunwald E (ed): Heart Disease, pp 1528–1557. Philadelphia: WB Saunders, 1992.
31. Kistler JP, Ropper AH, Martin JB: Cerebrovascular diseases. *In* Isselbacher KJ, Wilson J, Braunwald E, et al (eds): Harrison's Principles of Internal Medicine, pp 2233–2256. New York: McGraw-Hill, 1994.
32. Kase CS, Mohr JP, Caplan LR: Intracranial hemorrhage. *In* Barnett HJM, Mohr JP, Stein BM, et al (eds): Stroke: Pathophysiology, Diagnosis, and Management, pp 561–616. New York: Churchill Livingstone, 1992.
33. Mohr JP, Kistler JP, Fink ME: Intracranial aneurysms. *In* Barnett HJM, Mohr JP, Stein BM, et al (eds): Stroke: Pathophysiology, Diagnosis, and Management, pp 617–636. New York: Churchill Livingstone, 1992.
34. Mohr JP, Gantier JC, Pessin MS: Internal carotid artery disease. *In* Barnett HJM, Mohr JP, Stein BM, et al (eds): Stroke: Pathophysiology, Diagnosis, and Management, pp 285–336. New York: Churchill Livingstone, 1992.
35. Mohr JP: Lacunes. *In* Barnett HJM, Mohr JP, Stein BM, et al (eds): Stroke: Pathophysiology, Diagnosis, and Management, pp 539–560. New York: Churchill Livingstone, 1992.
36. Murphy J, Lavie CJ, Bresnahan D: Nitroprusside. *In* Messerli FH (ed): Cardiovascular Drug Therapy, pp 861–870. Philadelphia: WB Saunders, 1990.
37. Gerber JG, Nies AS: Antihypertensive agents and the drug therapy of hypertension. *In* Gilman AG, Rall TW, Nies AS, Taylor P (eds): Goodman and Gilman's The Pharmacological Basis of Therapeutics, pp 784–813. New York: Pergamon Press, 1990.
38. Chiarello M, Gold HK, Leinbach RC: Comparison between the effects of nitroprusside and nitroglycerin on ischemic injury during acute myocardial infarction. Circulation 54:766–774, 1976.
39. Charash B, Scheidt S: Nitroglyercin. *In* Messerli FH (ed): Cardiovascular Drug Therapy, pp 871–880. Philadelphia: WB Saunders, 1990.
40. Murad F: Drugs used for the treatment of angina: organic nitrates, calcium channel blockers, and beta-adrenergic antagonists. *In* Gilman AG, Rall TW, Nies AS, Taylor P (eds): Goodman and Gilman's The Pharmacological Basis of Therapeutics, pp 764–783. New York: Pergamon Press, 1990.
41. Hoffman BB, Lefkowitz RJ: Adrenergic receptor antagonists. *In* Gilman AG, Rall TW, Nies AS, Taylor P (eds): Goodman and Gilman's The Pharmacological Basis of Therapeutics, pp 221–243. New York: Pergamon Press, 1990.
42. Punzi HA, Zusman RM: Captopril. *In* Messerli FH (ed): Cardiovascular Drug Therapy, pp 770–791. Philadelphia: WB Saunders, 1990.
43. Karachalios GN, Georgiopoulos AN: Treatment of hypertensive crisis with sublingual captopril. Clin Pharm 1989; 8:90–91.
44. Komsuoglu B, Sengun B, Bayram A, Komsuoglu SS: Treatment of hypertensive urgencies with oral nifedipine, nicardipine, and captopril. Angiology 1991; 42:447–454.
45. Angeli P, Ghiesa M, Caregaro L, et al: Comparison of sublingual captopril and nifedipine in immediate treatment of hypertensive emergencies: a randomized, single-blind clinical trial. Arch Intern Med 1991; 151:678–682.
46. Hasdai D: Sublingual captopril and nifedipine in immediate treatment of hypertensive emergencies. Arch Intern Med 1992; 152:1725–1726.
47. Leeman M, Degaute JP: Invasive hemodynamic evaluation of sublingual captopril and nifedipine in patients with arterial hypertension after abdominal aortic surgery. Crit Care Med 1995; 23:843–847.
48. Gavras I, Gavras H: Enalapril. *In* Messerli FH (ed): Cardiovascular Drug Therapy, pp 792–799. Philadelphia: WB Saunders, 1990.
49. Resnekov L: Nifedipine. *In* Messerli FH (ed): Cardiovascular Drug Therapy, pp 926–938. Philadelphia: WB Saunders, 1990.
50. Jaker M, Atkin S, Soto M, et al: Oral nifedipine vs. oral clonidine in the treatment of urgent hypertension. Arch Intern Med 1989; 149:260–265.
51. Phillips RA, Ardeljan M, Shimabukuro S, et al: Normalization of left ventricular mass and associated changes in neurohormones and atrial natriuretic peptide after one year of sustained nifedipine therapy for severe hypertension. J Am Coll Cardiol 1991; 17:1595–1602.
52. Gonzalez-Carmona V, Ibarra-Perez C, Jerjes-Sanchez C: Single-dose sublingual nifedipine as the only treatment in hypertensive urgencies and emergencies. Angiology 1991; 42:908–913.
53. Schwartz MP, Taylor AT: Nifedipine: use of an oral antihypertensive agent in the emergency department setting. J Fam Pract 1992; 34:98–100.
54. Diker E, Erturk S, Akgun G: Is sublingual nifedipine administration superior to oral administration in the active treatment of hypertension? Angiology 1992; 43:477–481.
55. McDonald AJ, Yealy DM, Jacobson S: Oral labetalol versus oral nifedipine in hypertensive urgencies in the ED. Am J Emerg Med 1993; 11:460–463.
56. Hirschl MM, Seidler D, Zeiner A, et al: Intravenous urapidil versus sublingual nifedipine in the treatment of hypertensive urgencies. Am J Emerg Med 1993; 11:653–656.
57. Guazzi MD, Polese A, Fiorentini C, et al: Treatment of hypertension with calcium antagonists. Hypertension 1983; 5(suppl II):II-85–II-90.
58. Graves JW: Prolonged continuous infusion labetalol: a new alternative for parenteral antihypertensive therapy. Crit Care Med 1989; 17:759–761.
59. Zell-Kanter M, Leikin JB: Oral labetalol in hypertensive urgencies. Am J Emerg Med 1991; 9:136–138.
60. Atkin S, Jaker MA, Beaty P, et al: Oral labetalol versus oral clonidine in the emergency treatment of severe hypertension. Am J Med Sci 1992; 303:9–15.
61. Davis BA, Crook JE, Vestal RE, Oates JA: Prevalence of renovascular hypertension in patients with grade III or IV hypertensive retinopathy. N Engl J Med 1978; 301:1273–1276.
62. Vetrovec GW, Landwehr DM, Edwards VL: Incidence of renal artery stenosis in hypertensive patients undergoing coronary angiography. J Interven Cardiol 1989; 2:2–9.

34 Treatment of Hypertension in the Patient With Cardiovascular Disease

William G. Haynes, MD
J. Antonio G. Lopez, MD
Allyn L. Mark, MD

Hypertension, which occurs in 15%–20% of the adult population, is an important risk factor for the development of atherosclerosis. Hypertension therefore frequently causes cardiovascular target organ disease, including stroke, myocardial infarction, congestive heart failure, and sudden death. Treatment of hypertension can minimize these cardiovascular complications; a reduction of 5 mm Hg in diastolic pressure in 5 years reduces stroke by 38% and coronary artery disease by 16%.[1] Although the decrease in coronary artery disease mortality appears small, the 95% confidence limits for this reduction (8%–23%) overlap the 20%–25% decrease that, according to epidemiologic data, would occur if the risk of hypertension were fully reversible.

The management of hypertensive patients with coexisting cardiovascular disease differs in many respects from standard management. These patients require more detailed assessment and investigation. Because they are at higher risk for future complications, both the threshold for treatment and the blood pressure target are lower than in uncomplicated cases. The choice of drug therapy is influenced by the usual considerations of the efficacy in clinical trials, side effect profile, and cost but is also based on the particular actions of the antihypertensive agent on the specific coexisting cardiovascular disease. This chapter addresses the management of hypertension, taking account of these considerations, in patients with angina pectoris, myocardial infarction, left ventricular hypertrophy, chronic heart failure, cardiac dysrhythmias, valvular heart disease, peripheral vascular disease, aortic aneurysm, and cerebrovascular disease.

GENERAL PRINCIPLES

General Approach to the Patient

It is easy to focus on one problem, such as hypertension, and ignore other more pressing problems in these complicated patients. A holistic approach is to be preferred in such patients, who often possess multiple cardiovascular risk factors and have evidence of multiorgan disease. For example, attempts should be made to modify risk factors for development of atherosclerosis, with advice given regarding smoking, exercise, and diet. *Patients who smoke should be strongly encouraged to stop. Stopping smoking will produce a greater reduction in morbidity and mortality in this group than most pharmacologic interventions.*[2] Nicotine replacement therapy doubles the 6-month abstinence rate in patients who attempt to quit; transdermal patches are about twice as effective as nicotine gum.[3] Weight loss and salt restriction may reduce blood pressure substantially in obese patients.[4] Reduction in saturated fat intake may improve the plasma lipid profile. Patients should be screened for the presence of dyslipidemia, which should be treated appropriately. Antiplatelet therapy is almost always indicated. A meta-analysis of trials in ischemic heart disease, stroke, peripheral vascular disease, and valvular disease has shown that low-dose aspirin (75–300 mg/day) reduces vascular events and total mortality by 27% and 17%, respectively.[5] If low-dose aspirin cannot be tolerated, an alternative antiplatelet agent, such as ticlopidine, should be considered.[5]

If antihypertensive therapy is necessary, it should be started at low doses; in most cases, at least 1 month should be allowed for the full effects of one drug to become apparent before another drug is added. This will help prevent abrupt decreases in blood pressure that may be deleterious to patients with disturbed coronary or cerebral circulatory autoregulation.

Threshold for Pharmacologic Therapy

The risk of cardiovascular events in patients with hypertension is strikingly dependent on the level of blood pressure and on the presence of other risk factors, such as smoking, dyslipidemia, and diabetes. However, the adverse risk associated with hypertension is even more marked in the presence of target organ disease, such as left ventricular hypertrophy and atherosclerosis affecting the coronary, cerebral, or peripheral circulation. In the presence of hypertension, risks of future cardiovascular complications are increased at least twofold above the risk in comparable subjects with no evidence of such disease.[6]

The recommended thresholds for treatment of uncomplicated hypertension are systolic pressures above 140–150 mm Hg or diastolic pressures above 90–95 mm Hg, the exact level depending on age and the presence of other risk factors.[7, 8] Furthermore, it is usually recommended that lifestyle modification be tried for 3–6 months before drug therapy is initiated. *The adverse risk associated with the presence of target organ damage lowers these thresholds to a systolic pressure of 140 mm Hg and a diastolic pressure of 90 mm Hg.* Because the Treatment of Mild Hypertension Study (TOMHS) demonstrated fewer events in patients randomized to drug therapy than to lifestyle modification alone, drug therapy should be initiated as soon as the presence of sustained hypertension is confirmed in these high-risk patients.[9]

"White coat" hypertension is sometimes observed in patients with evidence of cardiovascular disease. There may be doubt about the need for pharmacologic reduction in blood pressure in such patients. However, the thresholds for "normal" ambulatory blood pressure have not been tested in an outcome trial, and there is no conclusive evidence that white coat hypertension is innocuous. Indeed, some studies have shown that white coat hypertension is associated with increased left ventricular mass in these patients compared with normotensive subjects.[10] On the basis of these considerations, we recommend that patients with cardiovascular disease and white coat hypertension be treated in a manner similar to other hypertensive patients with cardiovascular disease. It is worthwhile monitoring such patients carefully for evidence of excessively low daytime blood pressures when they are receiving treatment. Measurement of left ventricular mass may be useful in determining the adequacy of treatment in this population.[10]

The authors' research in hypertension has been supported through a NIH Specialized Center of Research in Hypertension grant (HL 44546). Dr. William Haynes was a recipient of a Wellcome Trust Advanced Training Fellowship (No. 042145/114) during the writing of this chapter.

Target Blood Pressure

The optimal level to which blood pressure should be reduced for prevention of cardiovascular complications is still not known. The usual blood pressure goal in patients with uncomplicated hypertension is 140/90 mm Hg or less.[8] In view of the fact that antihypertensive therapy is recommended at a threshold of only 140/90 mm Hg in patients with target organ disease, and that these patients are at particularly high risk for further events, the therapeutic blood pressure goal is usually set somewhat lower than 140/90 mm Hg. However, on the basis of retrospective analyses of epidemiologic and clinical trial data, there has been some concern about the finding that diastolic blood pressures below 85 mm Hg are associated with higher coronary mortality.[11] This J-shaped relationship between diastolic pressure and coronary mortality has been postulated to be due to reduced coronary blood flow during diastole, which precipitates myocardial ischemia.

Although a J-curved relationship between diastolic blood pressure and mortality has not been found in all studies,[12] the J curve hypothesis has led to suggestions that diastolic blood pressure should not be reduced pharmacologically below 85 mm Hg. Parenthetically, if such advice were followed, many patients with systolic hypertension would not be given antihypertensive therapy despite mounting evidence that treatment for systolic hypertension is beneficial. No J-shaped relationship has ever been found between diastolic blood pressure and renal failure or stroke; maximal protection from these complications is found at diastolic pressures below 80 mm Hg. There is also no evidence whatsoever for a J curve between systolic blood pressure and total or coronary mortality. In addition, the J curve hypothesis has not been tested in a prospective treatment trial, although trials examining the effects of different target diastolic pressures on outcome are under way. Furthermore, the Systolic Hypertension in the Elderly Program (SHEP) showed that reducing diastolic blood pressure from 77 to 68 mm Hg, during treatment of systolic hypertension, reduced the myocardial infarction rate by 27%.[13] This occurred in a population in which 60% had abnormal electrocardiograms and thus should have been susceptible to the risk of decreased diastolic coronary blood flow. Indeed, a meta-analysis has suggested that the lowest overall risk of stroke and myocardial infarction is achieved by pharmacologically reducing blood pressure to 125/85 mm Hg or lower.[14] Finally, because the increased mortality at low levels of diastolic blood pressure has also been observed in patients receiving no treatment or receiving placebo, the J curve is probably unrelated to drug therapy. Thus, this phenomenon probably reflects the low levels of diastolic pressure found in people who are already seriously ill from heart disease.

In summary, even if the J curve relationship is found to be relevant to therapeutic reduction of blood pressure, the benefits of reducing systolic pressure and the favorable effects of reducing diastolic blood pressure on stroke should far outweigh the theoretical adverse effects. This is particularly true in the high-risk population under consideration here. *The authors therefore suggest a blood pressure goal of 130/85 mm Hg in patients with coexisting cardiovascular disease.* This is similar to the blood pressure goal recommended for diabetic patients in Chapter 40. However, it is important that blood pressure be reduced gradually toward this goal and that any new or worsening symptoms of myocardial ischemia in association with blood pressure reduction prompt modification of therapy.

Principles Underlying the Choice of Antihypertensive Therapy

Two main principles underlie the recommendations regarding antihypertensive drugs in this chapter. The first is the strength of evidence from primary outcome trials using low-dose thiazide diuretics and beta blockers in hypertension,[13, 15–17] along with the lack of similar evidence for newer agents, such as calcium antagonists, angiotensin converting enzyme (ACE) inhibitors, or alpha antagonists. These results have led to the recommendation by the U.S. Joint National Committee that thiazides and beta blockers are preferred for first-line use in uncomplicated hypertension.[7] This subject is reviewed in detail in Chapter 32. *The second main principle that the authors have followed is to take advantage of the "dual" actions of some of the main classes of antihypertensive drugs on hypertension and the coexisting cardiovascular disease.* Where possible, given the evidence of positive effects on outcome in hypertension for the accepted first-line drugs, the authors have based their choice of alternative agents on similar outcome evidence for the coexisting disease. For example, the beneficial effects of ACE inhibitors on mortality in chronic heart failure justify the use of these drugs as first-line antihypertensive agents in such patients.

ISCHEMIC HEART DISEASE

General Management

Patients should be advised to modify their lifestyle where appropriate: for example, by stopping smoking, reducing saturated fat intake, and increasing exercise. There is a theoretical risk of exacerbation of angina by nicotine replacement therapy in patients with ischemic heart disease, so more frequent follow-up is recommended for these patients; however, this should also help improve their abstinence rate. Antiplatelet therapy should be instituted. There is compelling evidence that treatment of dyslipidemia is beneficial in patients with ischemic heart disease. For example, simvastatin therapy in patients with ischemic heart disease and total cholesterol level more than 220 mg/dL increases the regression rate of coronary atheroma by 50%[18] and reduces coronary and total mortality by 42% and 34%, respectively.[19] *Patients with ischemic heart disease should therefore be screened and treated for dyslipidemia.*

In most cases, lifestyle modification alone does not reduce blood pressure to the desired goal (130/85 mm Hg). However, adequate control of blood pressure is essential, because not only is there an increased chance of myocardial infarction, but prognosis after infarction is also worse if there is poorly controlled hypertension. This may be related to increased afterload causing greater myocardial oxygen demand during coronary occlusion or to a propensity to fatal ventricular arrhythmias. Therefore, it is usually recommended that antihypertensive drugs be started concurrently with lifestyle modification in these patients. *The key to treatment of hypertensive patients with ischemic heart disease is the avoidance of rapid decreases in blood pressure.* Coronary autoregulation is profoundly disturbed in experimental left ventricular hypertrophy.[20] Therefore, abrupt reductions in blood pressure should be avoided because pressure may be reduced below the limits of coronary autoregulation and this may thus lead to precipitous decreases in coronary blood flow. Careful titration of doses and addition of new agents over a period of several months allows coronary autoregulatory mechanisms to gradually adapt to a lower perfusion pressure.

Angina Pectoris

Pathophysiology

There are two pathophysiologic mechanisms for angina in hypertension; these often occur concurrently. First, hypertension is an important risk factor in the development of atherosclerosis. Thus obstructive coronary artery atheroma commonly occurs in patients with hypertension, which leads to angina. Second, patients with hypertension, particularly those with left ventricular hypertrophy, frequently have ischemic symptoms in the absence of obstructive atheroma in the epicardial conduit coronary vessels. This is probably a result of impaired function of the coronary microcirculation caused by extrinsic vascular compression, inadequate vascular growth, and impaired endothelial dilator function.[21, 22]

Investigation

Evaluation of hypertensive patients with angina should follow the same broad direction as for nonhypertensive patients, with the following exceptions. First, hypertension should usually be controlled as well as possible before detailed investigations, because this may improve anginal symptoms and possibly reduce the need for more invasive assessment. Second, it is helpful to accurately quantify left ventricular mass and function; evidence of left ventricular hypertrophy or diastolic dysfunction might suggest microvascular dysfunction causing, or exacerbating, ischemia. Third, the presence of left ventricular hypertrophy or left bundle branch block on the electrocardiogram makes interpretation of exercise electrocardiography difficult and may require other noninvasive procedures, such as nuclear perfusion scans and stress echocardiography.[23]

Therapy

Lowering blood pressure improves symptoms and prognosis in hypertensive patients with angina in several ways. First, it will decrease afterload and preload and thus decrease myocardial workload and oxygen demand. Second, regression of left ventricular hypertrophy will improve microvascular perfusion and thus oxygen supply. Third, long-term antihypertensive therapy may help prevent coronary atheroma progression or even encourage regression. Fourth, several antihypertensive agents, such as beta blockers, calcium antagonists, and organic nitrates, possess additional antianginal actions.

Beta blockers, by antagonizing cardiac β-receptors, attenuate exercise-induced increases in heart rate and contractility, thereby decreasing myocardial oxygen demand. They also reduce central sympathetic outflow, decreasing total peripheral resistance and afterload. Beta blockers therefore have direct antianginal actions in addition to their antihypertensive effects. Although beta blockers tend to decrease plasma levels of high-density lipoprotein and insulin sensitivity in some patients,[24] these drugs reduce mortality in primary prevention trials.[16] The proven efficacy of beta blockers in patients after myocardial infarction (see later section), together with recent doubts regarding calcium channel blockers (see later section), helps strengthen the case for their first-line use in hypertensive patients with angina.

The calcium channel blockers diltiazem and verapamil reduce heart rate during exercise, thereby decreasing myocardial oxygen demand, and are also peripheral and coronary vasodilators. The dihydropyridine class of calcium channel blockers (nifedipine, isradipine, nicardipine, felodipine, and amlodipine) has no direct actions on cardiac conduction pathways. However, their potent vasodilator actions tend to cause a reflex sympathetic activation with increases in heart rate, and thus myocardial oxygen demand, which may be deleterious in patients with angina. Indeed, nifedipine has been shown in one trial to cause no improvement in angina symptoms or exercise duration in patients already receiving a beta blocker.[25] Although calcium channel antagonists have been widely used in the management of hypertensive patients with angina, studies raise concern about their safety in such patients.[26] First, increases of approximately 20% in cardiovascular event rates have been reported in two secondary prevention trials of dihydropyridines with use of nifedipine[27] or nicardipine.[28] Second, a meta-analysis has confirmed an adverse effect of dihydropyridines on combined mortality and infarction in patients with ischemic heart disease.[29, 30] *Thus, dihydropyridine calcium antagonists should be used cautiously and certainly not without concomitant use of a beta blocker.* Heart rate–slowing calcium antagonists (such as diltiazem and verapamil) do not appear to possess such adverse effects and may prevent reinfarction after non–Q wave myocardial infarction. However, there is no evidence that these drugs, unlike beta blockers, significantly reduce mortality in either hypertensive or ischemic heart disease patients.

Organic nitrates are the third group of drugs with anti-ischemic and antihypertensive actions, although they are less efficacious than beta blockers and calcium antagonists in reduction of blood pressure. Nitrates reduce preload by venodilatation and, at higher doses, reduce afterload by arteriolar dilatation; both actions decrease myocardial oxygen demand. Nitrates also increase myocardial oxygen supply by dilating first-order (epicardial) and second-order (penetrating) conduit coronary vessels,[31] thereby increasing collateral flow and redistributing blood flow to the ischemic endocardium.[32] In patients taking a beta blocker, addition of isosorbide mononitrate causes a significantly greater improvement in exercise duration than does the addition of nifedipine.[25] Mortality benefits have not been shown for nitrates; but in comparison with calcium antagonists, these agents appear safe in patients with ischemic heart disease.[33, 34]

Thiazide diuretics are not widely used in patients with ischemic heart disease, partly because they do not possess anti-ischemic actions. It also reflects a concern that these agents possess adverse metabolic effects that may worsen atheroma and predispose to arrhythmias.[24] There is evidence, from a case-control study, that high-dose thiazide therapy (100 mg of chlorthalidone or equivalent) may predispose to cardiac arrest in hypertensive patients without known cardiac disease.[35] However, in this study, lower doses of a thiazide (25 and 50 mg) were associated with a risk similar to that seen in patients receiving beta blockers alone. In addition, the risk of cardiac arrest in patients taking 25 mg of thiazide with a potassium-sparing agent was 70% less than for those taking a beta blocker alone. Furthermore, in the TOMHS trial, low doses of thiazide diuretics, like the other classes of drugs, did not adversely alter the biochemical profile, even after 4 years of treatment.[9] In view of the fact that thiazides appear to cause a greater reduction in ischemic heart disease mortality than beta blockers do,[2, 17] these agents should remain part of the therapeutic armamentarium in patients with coronary artery disease. Thiazides appear be more effective in black and obese patients and may therefore be particularly useful in these groups.

A number of direct vasodilator drugs cause reflex tachycardia, which may worsen angina. Such agents include the alpha-adrenoceptor antagonists prazosin and doxazosin as well as minoxidil and hydralazine. When possible, these drugs should be avoided in patients with angina. If direct vasodilator drugs are used, for example, in refractory hypertension, patients should also be receiving a beta blocker.

Management Plan

Management of the hypertensive patient with angina is outlined in Figure 34–1. These patients should be strongly encouraged to stop smoking, be started on low-dose aspirin, and have evaluation and treatment if they are dyslipidemic. Some hypertensive patients with angina will not have obstructive coronary artery disease. Therefore, if possible, investigations aimed at delineating the extent of myocardial ischemia should be deferred until blood pressure and left ventricular size have been normalized. *First-line therapy should consist of a beta blocker.* A negatively chronotropic calcium antagonist, such as diltiazem or verapamil, could be used if beta blockers are not tolerated or contraindicated. If both angina and hypertension persist, we recommend the addition of a calcium antagonist or nitrate; the choice depends on the relative severity of hypertension (calcium antagonist) as opposed to angina (nitrate). If a calcium antagonist is used here, a cardiac-slowing agent is preferable. If ischemic symptoms have abated with beta blocker therapy but blood pressure is still elevated, we believe that these patients should not be deprived of the proven beneficial effects of thiazide diuretics. A low dose should be used, with the addition of a potassium-sparing agent if there is any concern regarding arrhythmias, such as the presence of left ventricular hypertrophy, systolic dysfunction, or electrolyte disturbance. An ACE inhibitor could be used in patients with hypertension resistant to these agents. Continuing angina with adequately controlled blood pressure on beta blocker therapy is an indication for an oral nitrate; persistent angina suggests the need for coronary angiography.

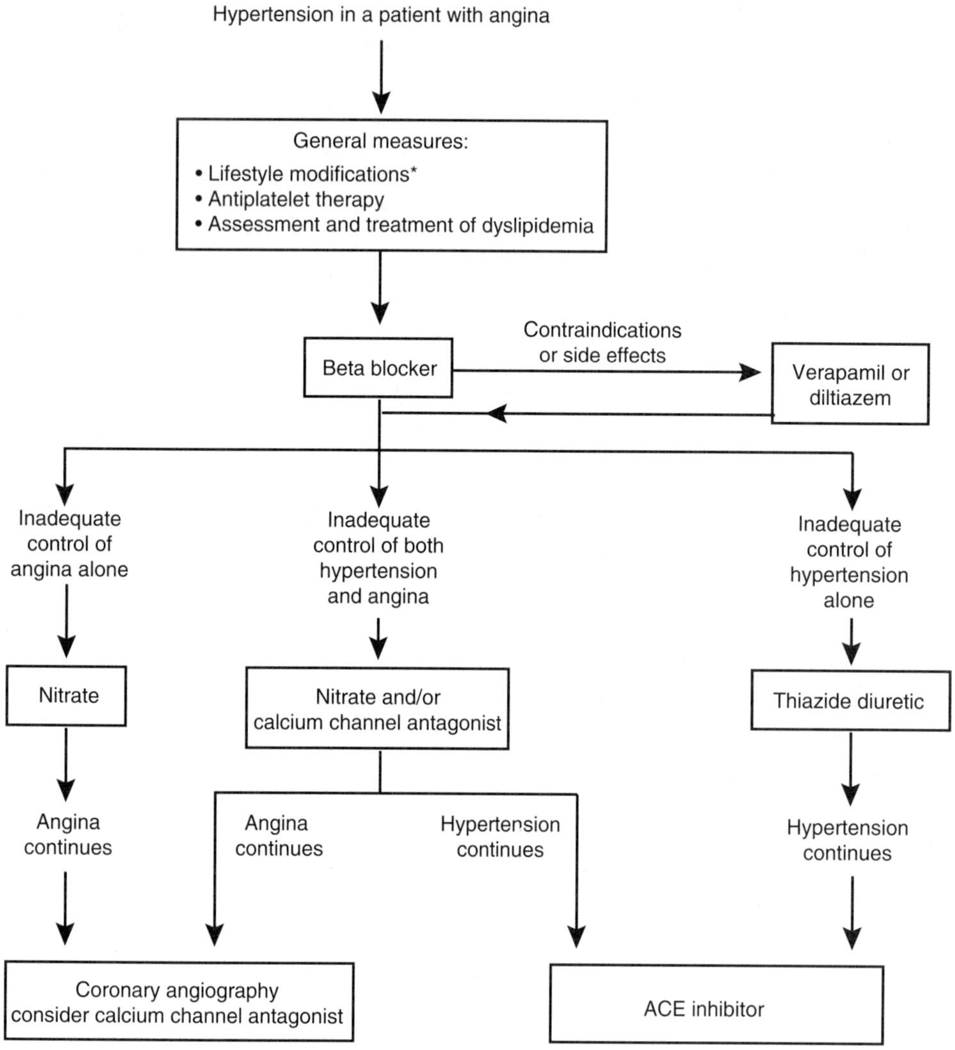

Figure 34–1. Algorithm for the management of a patient who presents with hypertension and angina. Doses of drugs should normally be titrated to the usual maximal dose before a second agent is tried. The recommended calcium antagonists are cardiac-slowing agents such as verapamil or diltiazem. Inadequate control of angina is defined as continuing limiting symptoms. Inadequate control of hypertension is defined as a blood pressure above goal (130/85 mm Hg). *See text.

Myocardial Infarction

Therapy

Five percent to 10% of patients with hypertension have suffered a myocardial infarction in the past. Although these patients may be asymptomatic, certain classes of drugs appear to possess favorable properties and should therefore be preferred in these patients. A meta-analysis has shown that oral beta blockers reduce total mortality by approximately 20% and the risk of nonfatal reinfarction by about 25% in survivors of acute myocardial infarction in periods up to 3 years.[36] Much of the reduction in mortality is due to a decrease in sudden cardiac death. These results are applicable to patients with hypertension because approximately 40% of subjects included in the trials had a history of hypertension. The true reduction in mortality risk may be as much as 30%, if the results of trials of drugs possessing intrinsic sympathomimetic activity (practolol, oxprenolol, pindolol, and alprenolol), from which there was no overall benefit, are excluded. The protective effect of beta blockers is apparent even in patients with a prior history of diuretic-treated mild chronic heart failure.[37] *Thus, if there are no contraindications, hypertensive patients with a history of myocardial infarction should receive a beta blocker without intrinsic sympathomimetic activity, such as atenolol or metoprolol.*

The effect of ACE inhibitors on outcome in unselected survivors of myocardial infarction has also been examined.[33, 34, 38, 39] Like the beta blocker trials, these studies included patients with history of hypertension, who accounted for 30%–40% of subjects. *A meta-analysis of these four trials of early oral ACE inhibitor therapy in all patients with myocardial infarction has shown a mortality benefit of approximately 7%.*[34] This reduction in mortality is somewhat less than that observed after beta blockers (about 20%).[36] However, ACE inhibitors cause more marked decreases in mortality (about 25%) in postinfarction patients with evidence, at some point during hospitalization, of left ventricular dysfunction on history, physical examination, or chest radiography.[40] Asymptomatic patients with left ventricular dysfunction on echocardiography also appear to benefit substantially from ACE inhibitor therapy, with a 17%–19% reduction in mortality.[41, 42] These findings have led to suggestions that routine post–myocardial infarction ACE inhibitor therapy be reserved solely for those patients with left ventricular dysfunction. Because many hypertensive postinfarction patients will have poorly controlled blood pressure with a beta blocker alone, it would appear worthwhile to use an ACE inhibitor as the next step in therapy if blood pressure is still high. In addition, evidence of transient clinical or radiographic heart failure during hospital admission for myocardial infarction, or a left ventricular ejection fraction under .40, is an indication for first-line long-term ACE inhibition, even if there is no current clinical evidence of overt heart failure.[40–42] Obviously, given the strength of evidence from the heart failure trials, all hypertensive patients with overt heart failure should receive an ACE inhibitor if possible (see later).

In contrast to beta blockers and ACE inhibitors, calcium antago-

nists appear to have detrimental effects in patients with a history of myocardial infarction. Short-acting dihydropyridine calcium antagonists tend to worsen mortality and reinfarction in patients with previous myocardial infarction.[29, 30] Verapamil and diltiazem appear to lack similar detrimental effects and may prevent reinfarction in selected groups, although there is no clear evidence of a mortality benefit.[30] Thus, dihydropyridines should be avoided in hypertensive postinfarction patients, whereas diltiazem and verapamil are useful alternatives if other agents are contraindicated or not tolerated. Unlike beta blockers, which reduce mortality even in postinfarction patients with chronic heart failure, diltiazem causes more cardiac events in such patients and should therefore be avoided in these circumstances.[43]

Management Plan

The management plan for hypertensive patients with a history of myocardial infarction is outlined in Figure 34–2. These patients should be strongly encouraged to stop smoking, be started on antiplatelet therapy, and undergo evaluation and treatment of dyslipidemia. Left ventricular function should be assessed. *All patients without left ventricular dysfunction or other contraindications should receive standard doses of a beta blocker without intrinsic sympathomimetic activity.* If blood pressure is not controlled, an ACE inhibitor should be added. Again, as with angina, the benefits of thiazides should not be ignored and a thiazide should be added if blood pressure is still above goal on the combination of a beta blocker and ACE inhibitor. If there is even transient clinical evidence of heart failure, or asymptomatic left ventricular dysfunction, then an ACE inhibitor is the first-line drug of choice. A diuretic should be added if there is an inadequate response. A beta blocker may be cautiously added to this regimen, given the evidence of benefit to postinfarction patients with mild heart failure[37] and the preliminary results in heart failure trials (see later). Dihydropyridine calcium antagonists should be avoided in hypertensive postinfarction patients, whereas diltiazem and verapamil are useful alternatives in patients without heart failure if beta blockers, ACE inhibitors, and thiazides are contraindicated or not tolerated.

LEFT VENTRICULAR HYPERTROPHY

Pathophysiology

Left ventricular hypertrophy, measured echocardiographically, is present in approximately 20% of middle-aged hypertensives.[44] The most important causative factor in the development of left ventricular hypertrophy is the level of blood pressure, particularly systolic. However, hormonal influences (catecholamines and angiotensin II), sex (male), age (younger), and race (African-American) may contribute. Left ventricular hypertrophy increases the risk of future cardiovascular events by twofold, compared with hypertensive subjects without left ventricular hypertrophy.[6] These events include sudden death, angina, myocardial infarction, and chronic heart failure. The risks associated with left ventricular hypertrophy are probably due to reduced coronary microvascular flow reserve,[21, 22] impaired coronary autoregulation,[20] diastolic dysfunction, systolic dysfunction, and increased arrhythmic potential.[44]

Investigation

Left ventricular hypertrophy can be detected by clinical examination, chest radiography, electrocardiography, and echocardiography. Clinical examination and chest radiography are not sufficiently sensitive for routine detection of hypertrophy. Electrocardiography is more sensitive at detection of left ventricular hypertrophy and, particularly when there are repolarization abnormalities, electrocardiographic left ventricular hypertrophy is a powerful predictor of cardiovascular events. Thus, electrocardiography remains the most cost effective investigation for the routine detection of left ventricular hypertrophy in the hypertensive patient. However, electrocardiography detects only 20%–50% of autopsy-proven left ventricular hypertrophy. Echocardiography is the most sensitive routinely available test for detection of left ventricular hypertrophy. Therefore, echocardiography is preferred when it is important to be certain of the presence of left ventricular hypertrophy. However, because sustained hypertension should be treated irrespective of the presence of left ventricular hypertrophy and because there is no evidence that reversal of hypertrophy, as opposed to hypertension, reduces mortality, echocardiographic evaluation of the hypertensive patient should be restricted to specific indications. These indications are borderline or white coat elevation of blood pressure, which would, otherwise, go untreated[10]; dyspnea or other evidence of heart failure; and systolic murmurs.[44]

Therapy

It is not known whether reduction of left ventricular mass decreases cardiovascular risk beyond that achieved by lowering of blood pressure alone. Therefore, the best current therapy for left ventricular hypertrophy is rigorous control of hypertension, to the same blood pressure goal as for patients without left ventricular hypertrophy. Antihypertensive agents have a varied time course in reduction of left ventricular mass. Beta-adrenergic antagonists, centrally acting sympatholytics, calcium channel antagonists, and ACE inhibitors will regress LVH in 3 to 8 weeks.[44] These rapid effects probably reflect inhibition of growth-promoting mechanisms, including the sympathetic nervous system and the renin-angiotensin system. Diuretics and direct vasodilators reduce left ventricular hypertrophy more slowly in a period of many months. This slow regression is presumably purely secondary to the reduction in blood pressure caused by these agents. At present, the authors do not know whether rapid or slow reversal of left ventricular hypertrophy is best. In the TOMHS trial, the only drug to significantly lower left ventricular mass by more than placebo after 12 months of treatment was chlorthalidone.[45] The results of the Medical Research Council trials, in which thiazides were as good as if not better than beta blockers in reducing event rates, suggest that slow reversal of left ventricular hypertrophy may be perfectly adequate.[2, 17] Some patients with left ventricular hypertrophy have manifestations of heart failure (see later), and this may suggest the need for an ACE inhibitor. However, many of these patients have diastolic dysfunction with preserved systolic function. Beta blockers may be indicated in this situation because they aid left ventricular relaxation and thus filling.

In summary, the presence of left ventricular hypertrophy signals that the patient is at high risk for cardiovascular events. This suggests the need for rigorous control of hypertension. Although certain drugs cause more rapid regression of left ventricular hypertrophy than others do, all antihypertensive agents will ultimately reduce left ventricular mass. Therefore, given the known beneficial mortality effects of thiazides and beta blockers, these agents are usually to be preferred, unless there is heart failure or a myocardial infarction, when an ACE inhibitor may be a better choice.

CHRONIC HEART FAILURE

Pathophysiology

Untreated hypertension causes chronic heart failure and also exacerbates cardiac failure caused by other diseases. Thus, 20%–40% of patients with chronic heart failure have a history of hypertension.[46, 47] In most cases of purely hypertensive heart failure, the earliest pathophysiologic abnormality is impaired diastolic filling, which may occur even in the absence of apparent left ventricular hypertrophy.[44] Less frequently, hypertension can cause systolic dysfunction, although this is more common in the presence of obstructive coronary artery disease.

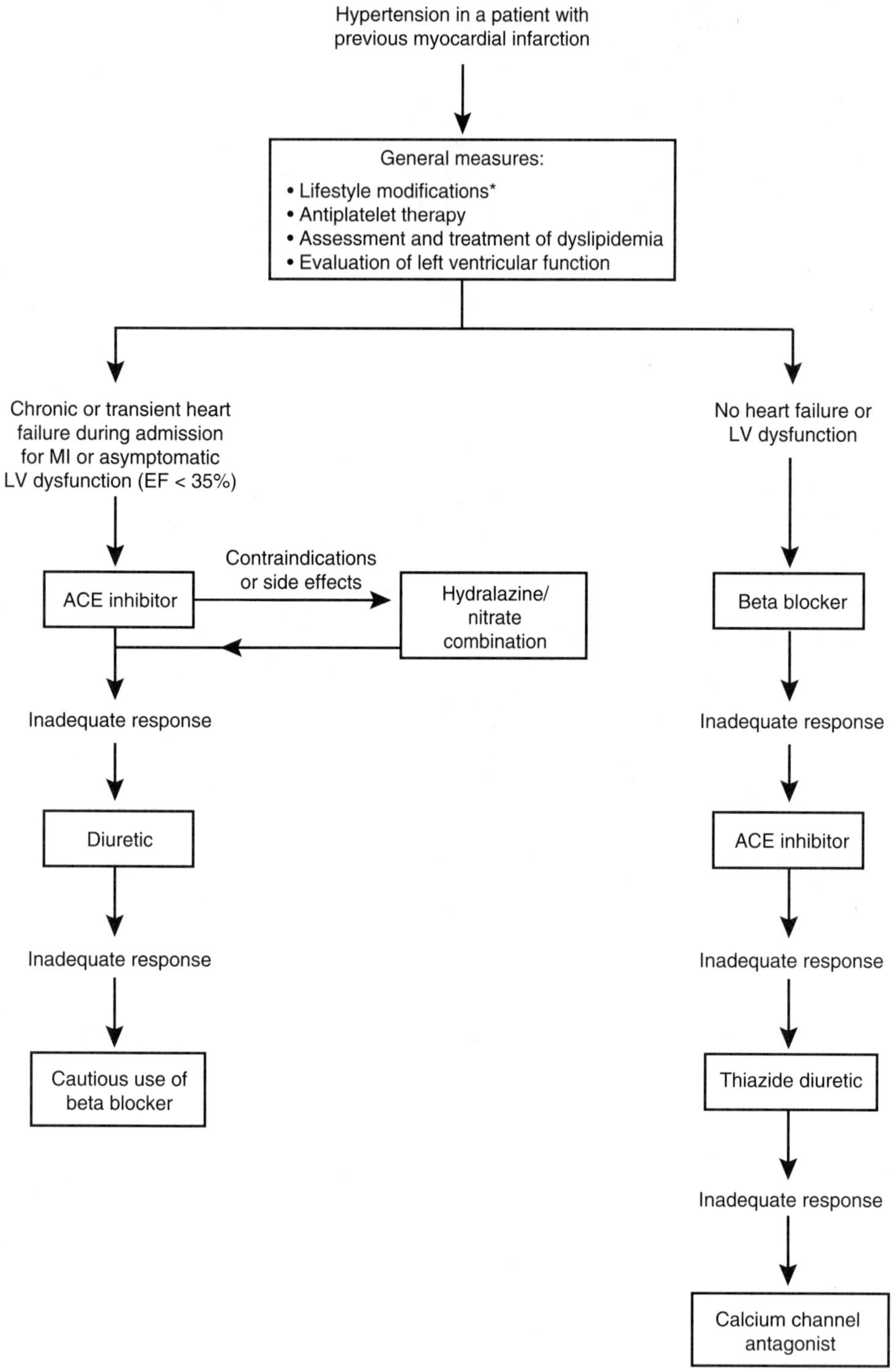

Figure 34–2. Algorithm for the management of hypertension in a patient with a previous myocardial infarction. Doses of drugs should normally be titrated to the usual maximal dose before a second agent is tried. The recommended calcium antagonists are cardiac-slowing agents such as verapamil or diltiazem. Inadequate control of hypertension is defined as a blood pressure above goal (130.85 mm Hg). *See text. *Abbreviations*: EF, ejection fraction; LV, left ventricle; MI, myocardial infarction.

Investigation

Echocardiography is the cornerstone of the evaluation of the hypertensive patient with heart failure. It allows assessment of left ventricular mass as well as left ventricular systolic and diastolic function and should also detect clinically occult valve lesions. As noted before, obstructive atherosclerotic coronary artery disease frequently occurs in hypertensive patients and commonly causes impaired left ventricular systolic function and dilation. In patients with angina and moderate to severe left ventricular dysfunction, coronary bypass grafting has been shown to substantially improve survival compared with medical therapy.[48] It is therefore particularly important to investigate hypertensive patients with heart failure and angina for coronary artery disease. It may also be useful to screen patients without angina for occult coronary ischemia; myocardial perfusion scintigraphy may be necessary.[23] In addition, rare causes of heart failure should also be excluded, including alcohol-related and thyrotoxic, both of which may also cause hypertension. Furthermore, iatrogenic factors should be excluded. Drugs such as nonsteroidal anti-inflammatory agents and corticosteroids increase blood pressure, in part through sodium retention, and may therefore aggravate left ventricular dysfunction; nonsteroidal anti-inflammatory agents also predispose patients receiving ACE inhibitors to renal failure. Beta blockers and calcium antagonists have negative inotropic properties and may exacerbate heart failure in some patients. Finally, renovascular disease can cause a syndrome that resembles heart failure, with systemic and pulmonary edema in association with hypertension.[49] The absence of systolic dysfunction and the presence of resistant hypertension, with or without renal dysfunction, should suggest the need for appropriate investigations, most commonly captopril renography or renal angiography, in such patients.

Therapy

Lifestyle modifications may improve symptoms in the hypertensive patient with chronic heart failure. Cigarette smoking causes peripheral vasoconstriction, and patients should be encouraged to stop. Extreme thirst may occur in heart failure and lead to excessive fluid intake, causing hyponatremia in some patients. Fluid intake should therefore be restricted to approximately 2000 mL/day. Salt intake should be assessed, although there is no need for salt restriction unless intake is high. Regular graded exercise causes symptomatic improvements in heart failure and reduces blood pressure; exercise should therefore be encouraged in these patients. Weight loss in obese patients reduces both blood pressure and cardiac workload and is strongly recommended.

Reduction in blood pressure in the hypertensive patient with heart failure will reduce afterload and thus tend to improve left ventricular function. More specifically, substantial morbidity and mortality benefits have been obtained with vasodilator therapy in chronic heart failure. In the Vasodilator Heart Failure Trial (V-HeFT-1), in which 40% of patients had a history of hypertension, high doses of hydralazine (300 mg/day) and isosorbide dinitrate (160 mg/day) reduced mortality by 34%.[46] Therapy with the ACE inhibitor enalapril reduced mortality by 40% in the Cooperative North Scandinavian Enalapril Survival Study (CONSENSUS) trial, in which 20% of patients had a history of hypertension.[47] Therapy with enalapril improved mortality by 28% compared with a hydralazine-nitrate combination in the V-HeFT-2 trial.[50] It appears to be important that vasodilator therapy reduces both preload and afterload because prazosin, which is predominantly an arteriolar dilator, was no better than placebo in its effects on mortality in V-HeFT-1.[46] Even so, because alpha blockers are not negatively inotropic, these drugs may be useful in the hypertensive heart failure patient when other agents have failed to control blood pressure.

Beta blockers are negatively inotropic and therefore are conventionally contraindicated in chronic heart failure due to systolic dysfunction. However, there is evidence of benefit from beta blockers in both dilated cardiomyopathy[51] and chronic heart failure due to ischemic heart disease.[37, 52] This may reflect blockade of the deleterious effects of increased sympathetic nerve activity in this condition. For example, the Metoprolol in Dilated Cardiomyopathy trial demonstrated an improved quality of life, exercise tolerance, and a substantially reduced requirement for transplantation, although without improvement in survival.[51] This study was not designed to have power to detect an improvement in survival, and transplantation of control subjects may have obscured a beneficial effect; further studies are under way. At the very least, the metoprolol trial provides reassurance that when appropriate care is exercised, beta blockers can be symptomatically useful in heart failure without adverse mortality effects. Beta blockers are also useful when diastolic dysfunction exists (see section on left ventricular hypertrophy). If beta blockers are used in patients with heart failure, it is important to start with a low dose (e.g., metoprolol 5 mg twice daily) and titrate this carefully, against the patient's response, to a maximally tolerated dose (i.e., metoprolol 50 mg twice daily) in the next 6 to 8 weeks.

Diuretics are usually necessary in hypertensive patients with heart failure; loop diuretics are often used initially because of their greater efficacy. Addition of a thiazide diuretic or spironolactone may produce a clinically useful additional diuresis in patients with continuing evidence of fluid retention. Digoxin improves symptoms and reduces hospitalization in chronic heart failure, although mortality benefits have not yet been demonstrated. Digoxin does not lower blood pressure and should probably be reserved for those patients in atrial fibrillation or flutter or who still have symptoms or signs of heart failure when blood pressure is normalized. Short-acting dihydropyridine calcium antagonists, and cardiac-slowing calcium antagonists such as diltiazem, appear to worsen mortality in patients after myocardial infarction who have impaired left ventricular dysfunction and should probably be avoided.[30, 43] The treatment of heart failure is an evolving area and it is likely that new approaches to treatment will arise. Most of these are likely to be applicable to the hypertensive patient with heart failure. For example, the beta blocker carvedilol, which possesses vasodilator properties, may be beneficial in chronic heart failure.[53] Amlodipine, a long-acting dihydropyridine calcium antagonist, appears to cause symptomatic improvement in chronic heart failure.[54] Finally, endothelin receptor antagonists have been shown to cause peripheral vasodilatation in patients with essential hypertension[55] and chronic heart failure.[56]

Management Plan

The management plan for hypertensive patients with heart failure is outlined in Figure 34–3. The presence of heart failure in a hypertensive patient should prompt careful echocardiographic and Doppler evaluation of left ventricular mass, systolic and diastolic function, and valve morphology and function. Myocardial ischemia secondary to obstructive coronary atheroma should be excluded, by coronary angiography if necessary. Thyrotoxicosis, alcohol excess, and iatrogenic factors should be considered. *It is imperative to reduce blood pressure to as near to normal as possible in this group. ACE inhibitors have proven mortality benefits; if these are contraindicated or not tolerated, a hydralazine-nitrate combination should be used.* Therapy with loop diuretics is usually also necessary. In those patients with persistent hypertension, with or without continuing evidence of heart failure, alpha blockers or a hydralazine-nitrate combination should be used. Cautious use of beta blockers may also be beneficial if there is poorly controlled hypertension, particularly when there is evidence of left ventricular hypertrophy or diastolic dysfunction. Patients with atrial fibrillation, or continuing heart failure despite adequate control of blood pressure, should receive digoxin. Persistent heart failure in such patients will require thiazide diuretics or spironolactone if fluid retention is present; a hydralazine-nitrate combination or beta blocker is recommended if there is no fluid retention. Calcium antagonists should not normally be used in hypertensive patients with heart failure.

CARDIAC ARRHYTHMIAS

Atrial fibrillation and flutter are sometimes precipitated by left ventricular hypertrophy. Treatment of hypertension, by reducing afterload and left ventricular hypertrophy, may help prevent recurrent atrial fibrillation and flutter. Beta blockers, diltiazem, and verapamil decrease atrioventricular conduction and control the ventricular response to atrial fibrillation or flutter. Therefore, in the absence of heart failure, they are preferred in hypertensive patients with these rhythm disturbances. These agents are contraindicated in patients with sinoatrial nodal disease (sick sinus syndrome). If conduction abnormalities are present in the hypertensive patient, then antihypertensive medications that affect conduction, such as beta blockers, verapamil, or diltiazem, should be avoided.

Patients with hypertension, particularly those with left ventricular hypertrophy, are more likely to die suddenly,[57] possibly because of their propensity for ventricular arrhythmias.[58] Hypokalemia and hypomagnesemia secondary to diuretic use have been suggested to contribute to this risk of sudden cardiac death.[35, 59] However, these

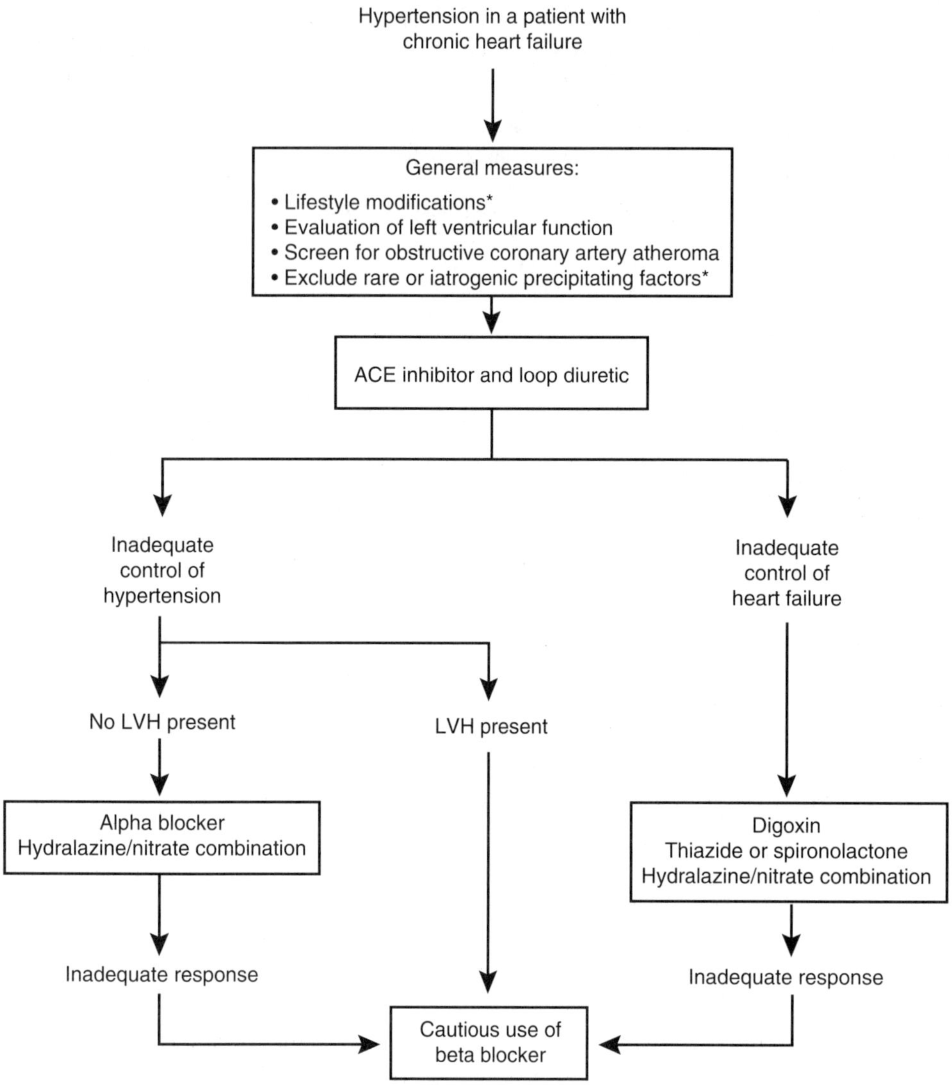

Figure 34–3. Algorithm for the management of hypertension in a patient with chronic heart failure. Doses of drugs should normally be titrated to the usual maximal dose before a second agent is tried. Inadequate control of hypertension is defined as a blood pressure above goal (130/85 mm Hg). Inadequate control of heart failure is defined as continuing symptoms (dyspnea/fatigue) or signs (pulmonary or peripheral edema). *See text. *Abbreviation*: LVH, left ventricular hypertrophy.

observations are only relevant at much higher doses of thiazide diuretics than are now recommended, and low-dose thiazides do reduce coronary event rates in elderly hypertensives.[13, 15, 17] Thus, the best preventive measure for sudden death in patients with hypertension is adequate treatment of hypertension. In a hypertensive patient with ventricular arrhythmias, beta blocker therapy is indicated. Low-dose thiazide diuretics can be used once any electrolyte disturbances are corrected. The presence of recurrent supraventricular and ventricular arrhythmias in a hypertensive patient, particularly if the blood pressure is labile, should suggest a catecholamine-secreting pheochromocytoma. Appropriate screening tests should be performed.

VALVULAR HEART DISEASE

Aortic and mitral stenosis may limit cardiac output. The effects of antihypertensive agents may not, therefore, be buffered by reflex compensatory increases in stroke volume, and marked decreases in blood pressure may result. Because such decreases can precipitate myocardial ischemia and syncope, antihypertensive agents should be used with caution; peripheral vasodilators, including ACE inhibitors, should be particularly avoided. Diuretics and beta blockers are already used in some patients with mitral stenosis for control of pulmonary edema and heart rate, respectively. Therefore, if treatment of hypertension is necessary before surgery, or if surgery is contraindicated, we suggest cautious use of thiazides and beta blockers.

Patients with aortic regurgitation often remain asymptomatic for many years despite severe valvular incompetence. Ultimately, however, there is an increase in left ventricular volume and mass, leading to decompensated left ventricular function. The aim of management is to delay the need for surgical valve replacement for as long as possible by preventing left ventricular dilatation. Arteriolar vasodilators, by reducing afterload, may increase forward flow and thereby decrease the degree of regurgitation and improve cardiac performance. The ACE inhibitor enalapril,[60] the direct-acting vasodilator hydralazine,[60, 61] and the dihydropyridine calcium antagonist nifedipine[62] all have favorable effects on left ventricular stress and volume, although the effects of hydralazine were least convincing. Nifedipine also appears to reduce or delay the need for surgery in these patients.[62] Vasodilator therapy in chronic mitral regurgitation also improves cardiac performance.[61]

Thus, in hypertensive patients with aortic or mitral valve regurgitation, nifedipine and ACE inhibitors should be used as first-line agents, with the ACE inhibitor preferred when there is evidence of left ventricular dysfunction. Thiazide diuretics should be used next and may also relieve edema, although loop diuretics will be necessary in some cases for this indication. Beta blockers should be avoided because of their negative inotropic actions.

PERIPHERAL VASCULAR DISEASE

Atherosclerotic peripheral vascular disease affects approximately 12% of the general population and is symptomatic in about 2%. There is a 15-fold increase in rates of mortality from cardiovascular disease in patients with severe and symptomatic large-vessel peripheral vascular disease.[63] Hypertension, along with smoking and impaired glucose tolerance, is a major risk factor for peripheral vascular disease. A substantial proportion of patients investigated for peripheral artery disease have concomitant renovascular occlusive disease.[64] Consequently, there should be a low threshold for requesting renal angiography in a hypertensive patient with peripheral vascular disease. In addition, occult, surgically correctable coronary artery disease is common in these patients and they should be screened noninvasively for evidence of myocardial ischemia.[65]

Although vasodilator agents might be expected to be beneficial, ACE inhibitors, alpha-adrenergic antagonists, calcium channel antagonists, and direct vasodilators do not improve walking distance, calf blood flow, or claudication in patients with peripheral vascular disease.[66–68] There are several possible reasons for this disappointing outcome. First, during exercise, the diseased and distal vessels may be maximally dilated so that vasodilator drugs do not decrease vascular resistance. Second, these diseased vessels may dilate, but blood flow through them remains unchanged because nearby nondiseased vessels dilate more and receive a relatively greater proportion of leg blood flow (a "steal" phenomenon). Third, any improvement in vascular resistance may be offset by a reduction in systemic blood pressure or "driving" pressure, so that blood flow does not increase. Indeed, in one trial, addition of calcium channel antagonists to beta blocker therapy worsened walking distance and claudication,[69] despite the fact that these drugs given alone had no adverse effects on these parameters.

Beta-adrenergic antagonists may precipitate peripheral vasoconstriction and increase the frequency of intermittent claudication in some patients.[66] However, a meta-analysis of nine trials revealed that claudication distance and calf blood flow are not reduced by beta blockers.[70] Because many patients with peripheral vascular disease have concomitant coronary artery disease and/or hypertension, beta-adrenergic antagonists may be important agents to use. If a patient notices the onset of intermittent claudication after institution of a beta blocker or if the symptoms worsen, an alternative agent should be used, but beta blockers should not necessarily be avoided in patients with peripheral vascular disease and intermittent claudication.

In view of the high frequency of renal artery stenosis in peripheral vascular disease,[64] and with the propensity of ACE inhibitors to cause acute renal failure in bilateral renal artery stenosis, ACE inhibitors must be used with caution in these patients. In practical terms, if an ACE inhibitor is being considered because there is hypertension resistant to beta blockers, diuretics, calcium channel antagonists, and alpha blockers, renal artery disease is likely and appropriate investigations are warranted. Similarly, although ACE inhibitors are specifically indicated in patients with chronic heart failure (see earlier), the association of hypertension, peripheral vascular disease, and peripheral or pulmonary edema should prompt investigation for renal artery stenosis before an ACE inhibitor is started.[49]

Management Plan

The management of hypertensive patients with peripheral vascular disease is outlined in Figure 34–4. *No agent offers specific dual actions in hypertensive patients with peripheral vascular disease.* If the patient is free of coronary artery disease, a thiazide diuretic is probably best, followed by a beta blocker. In the presence of coronary artery disease, a beta blocker followed by a diuretic is recommended. A calcium channel antagonist could be tried if the patient is intolerant of, or resistant to, one or both of these agents; in this circumstance, a cardiac-slowing drug (i.e., verapamil or diltiazem) is to be preferred. Calcium channel blockers and beta blockers should be used only in combination if other drugs have been tried or are contraindicated, and the patient needs to be monitored to detect any exacerbation of claudication symptoms. Alpha blockers may also be useful if these drugs fail or cause side effects. *The possibility of renovascular occlusive disease should be considered carefully before use of ACE inhibitors in hypertensive patients with peripheral vascular disease.* As with other atherosclerotic diseases, cessation of smoking, low-dose aspirin, and evaluation and treatment of dyslipidemia are recommended.

If a patient has hypertension and Raynaud phenomenon, beta-adrenergic antagonists may increase the frequency of vasospasm. Calcium channel blockers and an alpha-adrenergic antagonist appear to improve symptoms of Raynaud syndrome as well as reduce blood pressure. Thiazide diuretics and ACE inhibitors do not worsen Raynaud symptoms and may be used if these agents fail.

ABDOMINAL AORTIC ANEURYSM

Atherosclerosis is the main cause of abdominal aortic aneurysm. Hypertension is present in approximately 60% of patients with abdominal aortic aneurysm.[71] Aneurysms grow more rapidly in experimental animals with hypertension than in normotensive animals.[72] In humans, there is evidence that the rate of expansion of abdominal aortic aneurysm is decreased by about 50% in patients receiving beta-adrenergic antagonists.[73, 74] This may be true for other antihypertensive agents, but these have not yet been tested. *Therefore, if no contraindications exist, beta blockers are preferable for management of hypertension in patients with abdominal aortic aneurysms.*

CEREBROVASCULAR DISEASE

Hypertension is a major risk factor for development of cerebrovascular disease, with a fourfold increased risk of cerebral infarction, lacunar softenings, and hemorrhages. Antihypertensive therapy with diuretics or beta-adrenergic antagonists is effective in primary prevention of stroke.[1] Despite these positive findings, a substantial proportion of patients presenting with stroke have untreated or undertreated hypertension,[75] which emphasizes the need for continued attention to the detection and management of hypertension.

Hypertensive patients with symptoms and signs of cerebrovascular disease should be examined for the presence of an embolic source, particularly from the heart or carotid vessels. Long-term low-dose aspirin therapy is usually indicated after cerebral infarction; full anticoagulation is beneficial in the presence of atrial fibrillation. Treatment of hypertension in patients with a history of cerebrovascular disease has been shown to reduce the 10% annual risk of recurrent stroke by approximately 70%.[76] Therefore, hypertensive patients with known cerebrovascular disease should have their blood pressure rigorously controlled, with pharmacologic therapy started at a lower threshold and blood pressure reduced to a goal of less than 130/85 mm Hg.

Diseased cerebral blood vessels are less capable of maintaining cerebral blood flow by autoregulation than are nondiseased vessels. Reduction of blood pressure must therefore be done cautiously to maintain cerebral blood flow.[77] Cerebral blood flow is preserved during reductions in blood pressure induced by diuretic therapy, calcium channel antagonists, alpha-adrenergic antagonists, labetalol, and ACE inhibitors.[78–81] Thus, these agents probably cause cerebral vasodilatation in proportion to the decrease in blood pressure. Clonidine decreases cerebral blood flow as blood pressure decreases, probably by causing cerebral vasoconstriction.[79] Diazoxide lowers blood pressure without causing cerebral vasodilation; consequently, it decreases cerebral blood flow if blood pressure falls below the lower limit of autoregulation. On the other hand, hydralazine and sodium nitroprusside are cerebral vasodilators, increasing cerebral

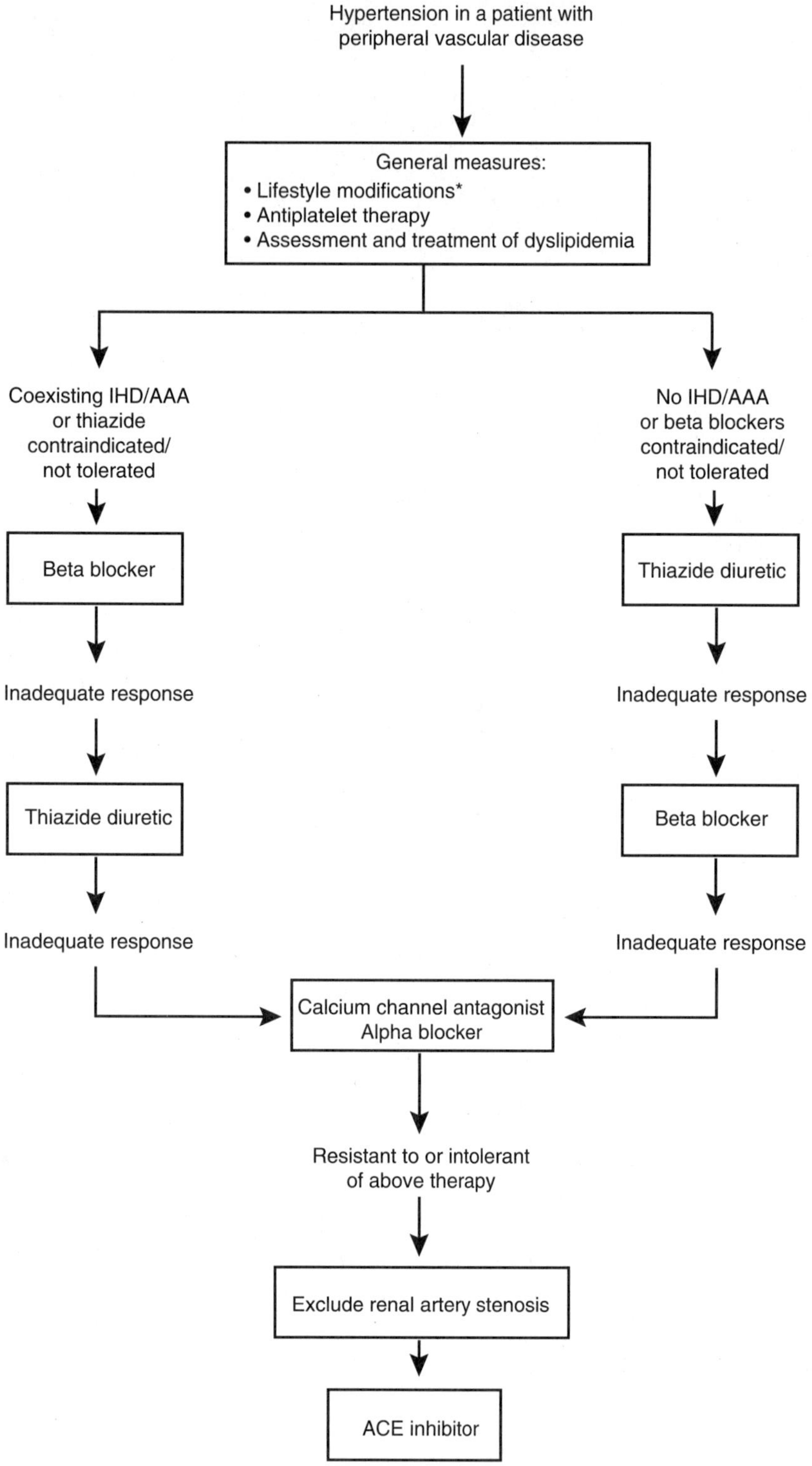

Figure 34–4. Algorithm for the management of hypertension in a patient with hypertension and peripheral vascular disease. Doses of drugs should normally be titrated to the usual maximal dose before a second agent is tried. The recommended calcium antagonists are cardiac-slowing agents such as verapamil or diltiazem. Inadequate control of hypertension is defined as a blood pressure above goal (130/85 mm Hg). *See text. *Abbreviations*: AAA, abdominal aortic aneurysm; IHD, ischemic heart disease.

blood flow even as blood pressure decreases.[82, 83] However, because increased cerebral blood flow raises intracranial pressure, these agents should be used with caution when there may be increased intracranial pressure. These situations include hypertensive encephalopathy and acute stroke.

The management of hypertension in acute stroke has been controversial. Blood pressure is transiently increased in acute stroke, usually falling to premorbid levels in a few days.[84] Such hypertension may help maintain adequate cerebral perfusion pressure in the face of raised intracranial pressure caused by cerebral edema. Antihypertensive treatment in this setting may provoke cerebral ischemia because of decreased cerebral perfusion pressure, a steal phenomenon, or an increase in intracranial pressure secondary to vasodilatation that reduces cerebral perfusion pressure. Therefore, rapid lowering of blood pressure is best avoided in acute ischemic stroke. If blood pressure remains high after the first few days, oral therapy with diuretics or beta blockers can be commenced. The situation is somewhat different in hemorrhagic stroke, in which very high blood pressure may increase the risk of rebleeding. Here, it may be worthwhile to lower blood pressure if it is above 210/120 mm Hg. This must be done gradually with the pressure reduced by no more than 25% in the first 24 hours.[85] Sodium nitroprusside has been commonly used because it allows precise blood pressure control. This agent has the disadvantage that it may increase intracranial pressure, whereas labetalol appears to reduce blood pressure without adversely affecting cerebral blood flow. In any case, it wise to monitor such patients invasively, including intracranial pressure recording.

In summary, hypertensive patients with a history of cerebrovascular disease should receive advice about lifestyle modifications and have preventable causes of stroke remedied. Hypertension must be controlled rigorously, although abrupt falls in blood pressure should be avoided. The choice of drug is similar to that for other hypertensive patients; it is best to avoid clonidine, along with diazoxide and related drugs (minoxidil and nicorandil). In acute ischemic stroke, urgent blood pressure reduction is not advised. In acute hemorrhagic stroke, gradual reduction of very high blood pressure may be beneficial, although patients require intensive monitoring.

REFERENCES

1. Herbert R, Moser M, Mayer J, et al: Recent evidence on drug therapy of mild to moderate hypertension and decreasing risk of coronary artery disease. Arch Intern Med 1993; 153:378.
2. Medical Research Council Working Party: MRC trial of treatment of mild hypertension: principal results. Br Med J 1985; 291:97–104.
3. Silagy C, Mant D, Fowler G, Lodge M: Meta-analysis on efficacy of nicotine replacement therapies in smoking cessation. Lancet 1994; 343:139.
4. Reisin E: Treatment of obese hypertensive patients. *In* Izzo JL, Black HR (eds): Hypertension Primer, Chapter E16, p 323. Dallas: American Heart Association, 1993.
5. Antiplatelet Trialists' Collaboration: Collaborative overview of randomised trials of antiplatelet therapy—I: prevention of death, myocardial infarction, and stroke by prolonged antiplatelet therapy in various categories of patients. Br Med J 1994; 308:81.
6. Lackland DT: Left ventricular hypertrophy and cardiac risks. *In* Izzo JL, Black HR (eds): Hypertension Primer, Chapter C14, p 183. Dallas: American Heart Association, 1993.
7. Joint National Committee on the Detection, Evaluation and Treatment of High Blood Pressure: Fifth Report. Arch Intern Med 1993; 153:154.
8. Gifford RW: Approach to treatment of hypertension. *In* Izzo JL, Black HR (eds): Hypertension Primer, Chapter E1, p 285. Dallas: American Heart Association, 1993.
9. Neaton JD, Grimm RH, Prineas RJ, et al: Treatment of Mild Hypertension Study. Final results. JAMA 1993; 270:713.
10. Weber MA, Neutel JM, Smith DH, Graettinger WF: Diagnosis of mild hypertension by ambulatory blood pressure monitoring. Circulation 1994; 90:2291.
11. Cruickshank JM, Thorp JM, Zacharias FJ: Benefits and potential harm of lowering blood pressure. Lancet 1987; 1:581.
12. Glynn RJ, Field TS, Rosner B, et al: Evidence for a positive linear relation between blood pressure and mortality in elderly people. Lancet 1995; 345:825.
13. SHEP Cooperative Research Group: Prevention of stroke by antihypertensive drug treatment in older persons with isolated systolic hypertension: final results of the Systolic Hypertension in the Elderly Program (SHEP). JAMA 1991; 255:3255.
14. Fletcher AE, Bulpitt CJ: How far should blood pressure be lowered? N Engl J Med 1992; 326:251.
15. Amery A, Birkenhäger W, Brixko P, et al: Mortality and morbidity results from the European Working Party on High Blood Pressure in the Elderly trial. Lancet 1985; 1:8442.
16. Dahlöf B, Lindholm LH, Hansson L, et al: Morbidity and mortality in the Swedish Trial in Old Patients with Hypertension (STOP-Hypertension). Lancet 1991; 338:1281.
17. Medical Research Council Working Party: MRC trial of treatment of hypertension in older adults: principal results. Br Med J 1992; 304:405.
18. Multicenter Anti-Atheroma Study Investigators: Effect of simvastatin on coronary atheroma: the Multicenter Anti-Atheroma Study (MAAS). Lancet 1994; 344:633.
19. Scandinavian Simvastatin Survival Group: Randomised trial of cholesterol lowering in 4444 patients with coronary artery disease: the Scandinavian Simvastatin Survival Study (4S). Lancet 1994; 344:1383.
20. Harrison DG, Florentine MS, Brooks LA, et al: The effect of hypertension and left ventricular hypertrophy on the lower range of coronary autoregulation. Circulation 1988; 77:1108.
21. Marcus ML, Harrison DG, Chilian WM, et al: Alterations in the coronary circulation in hypertrophied ventricles. Circulation 1987; 75(suppl I):I-19.
22. Treasure CB, Klein JL, Vita JA, et al: Hypertension and left ventricular hypertrophy are associated with impaired endothelium-mediated relaxation in human coronary resistance vessels. Circulation 1993; 87:86.
23. Tubau JF, Szlachcic J, Hollenberg M, et al: Usefulness of thallium-201 scintigraphy in predicting the development of angina pectoris in hypertensive patients with left ventricular hypertrophy. Am J Cardiol 1989; 64:45.
24. Pinkney JH, Yudkin JS: Antihypertensive drugs: issues beyond blood pressure control. Prog Cardiovasc Dis 1994; 36:397.
25. Akras F, Jackson G: Efficacy of nifedipine and isosorbide mononitrate in combination with atenolol in stable angina. Lancet 1991; 338:1036.
26. Psaty BM, Heckbert SR, Koepsell TD, et al: The risk of incidental myocardial infarction associated with anti-hypertensive drug therapies. Circulation 1995; 91:925.
27. Litchlen PR, Hugenholtz PD, Rafflenbeul W, et al, on behalf of the INTACT group: Retardation of angiographic progression of coronary artery disease by nifedipine. Results of the International Nifedipine Trial on Atherosclerotic Therapy (INTACT). Lancet 1990; 335:1109–1113.
28. Waters D, Lesperance J, Francetich M, et al: A controlled clinical trial to assess the effect of a calcium channel blocker upon the progression of coronary atherosclerosis. Circulation 1990; 82:1940.
29. Held PH, Yusuf S, Furberg CD: Calcium channel blockers in acute myocardial infarction and unstable angina: an overview. Br Med J 1989; 299:1187.
30. Yusuf S, Held P, Furberg C: Update of effects of calcium antagonists in myocardial infarction or angina in light of the second Danish verapamil trial (DAVIT II) and other recent studies. Am J Cardiol 1991; 67:1295.
31. Harrison DG, Bates JN: The nitrovasodilators: new ideas about old drugs. Circulation 1993; 87:1461.
32. Fallen EL, Nahmias C, Scheffel A, et al: Redistribution of myocardial blood flow with topical nitroglycerin in patients with coronary artery disease. Circulation 1995; 91:1381–1388.
33. GISSI-3: Effects of lisinopril and transdermal glyceryl trinitrate singly and together on 6-week mortality and ventricular function after acute myocardial infarction. Lancet 1994; 343:1115.
34. Fourth International Study of Infarct Survival Collaborative Group: ISIS-4: a randomised factorial trial assessing early oral captopril, oral mononitrate, and intravenous magnesium sulphate in 58 050 patients with suspected acute myocardial infarction. Lancet 1995; 345:669.
35. Siscovick DS, Raghunathan TE, Psaty BM, et al: Diuretic therapy for hypertension and the risk of primary cardiac arrest. N Engl J Med 1994; 330:1852.
36. Yusuf S, Peto R, Lewis J, et al: Beta blockade during and after myocardial infarction: an overview of randomized trials. Prog Cardiovasc Dis 1985; 27:335.
37. Chadda K, Goldstein S, Byington R, et al: Effect of propranolol after acute myocardial infarction in patients with congestive heart failure. Circulation 1986; 73:503.
38. Swedberg K, Held P, Kjekshus J, et al, on behalf of the CONSENSUS II study group: Effects of the early administration of enalapril on mortality in patients with acute myocardial infarction. Results of the Cooperative New Scandinavian Enalapril Survival Study II (CONSENSUS II). N Engl J Med 1992; 327:678.
39. Chinese Cardiac Study Collaborative Group: Oral captopril versus placebo among 13 634 patients with suspected acute myocardial infarction: interim report from the Chinese Cardiac Study (CCS-1). Lancet 1995; 345:686.
40. The Acute Infarction Ramipril Efficacy Study Investigators: Effect of ramipril on mortality and morbidity of survivors of acute myocardial infarction with clinical evidence of heart failure. Lancet 1993; 342:821.
41. Pfeffer MA, Braunwald E, Moye LA, et al: Effect of captopril on mortality and morbidity in patients with left ventricular dysfunction after myocardial infarction. Results of the Survival and Ventricular Enlargement trial. N Engl J Med 1992; 327:669.
42. The SOLVD Investigators: Effect of enalapril on mortality and the

development of heart failure in asymptomatic patients with reduced left ventricular ejection fractions. N Engl J Med 1992; 327:685.
43. Goldstein RE, Boccuzzi SJ, Cruesj D, et al: Diltiazem increases late-onset congestive heart failure in post infarction patients with early reduction in ejection fraction. Circulation 1991; 83:52.
44. Frohlich ED, Apstein C, Chobanian AV, et al: The heart in hypertension. N Engl J Med 1992; 327:998.
45. Liebson PR, Grandits GA, Dianzumba S, et al: Comparison of five antihypertensive monotherapies and placebo for change in left ventricular mass in patients receiving nutritional-hygienic therapy in the Treatment of Mild Hypertension Study (TOMHS). Circulation 1995; 91:698.
46. Cohn JN, Archibald DG, Ziesche S, et al: Effect of vasodilator therapy on mortality in chronic congestive heart failure: results of a Veterans Administration cooperative study. N Engl J Med 1986; 314:1547.
47. The CONSENSUS Trial Study Group: Effects of enalapril on mortality in severe congestive heart failure: results of the Cooperative North Scandinavian Enalapril Survival Study (CONSENSUS). N Engl J Med 1987; 316:1429.
48. Bounous EP, Mark DB, Pollock BG, et al: Surgical survival benefits in coronary disease patients with left ventricular dysfunction. Circulation 1988; 78:I-151.
49. Missouris CG, Buckenham T, Vallance PJ, MacGregor GA: Renal artery stenosis masquerading as congestive heart failure. Lancet 1993; 341:152.
50. Cohn JN, Johnson G, Ziesche S, et al: A comparison of enalapril with hydralazine-isosorbide dinitrate in the treatment of chronic congestive heart failure. N Engl J Med 1991; 325:303.
51. Waagstein F, Bristow MR, Swedberg K, et al: Beneficial effects of metoprolol in idiopathic dilated cardiomyopathy. Lancet 1993; 342:1441.
52. Woodley SL, Gilbert EM, Anderson JL, et al: β-Blockade with bucindolol in heart failure caused by ischemic versus idiopathic dilated cardiomyopathy. Circulation 1991; 84:2426.
53. Metra M, Nardi M, Giubbini R, Dei Cas L: Effects of short- and long-term carvedilol administration on rest and exercise hemodynamic variables, exercise capacity and clinical conditions in patients with idiopathic dilated cardiomyopathy. J Am Coll Cardiol 1994; 24:1678.
54. Packer M, Nicod P, Khandheria BR, et al: Randomised multi-center, double-blind, placebo-controlled evaluation of amlodipine in patients with mild-to-moderate heart failure [Abstract]. J Am Coll Cardiol 1991; 17(suppl 1):274A.
55. Haynes WG, Webb DJ: Generation of endothelin contributes to vascular tone in man [Abstract]. Hypertension 1994; 24:380.
56. Love MP, Haynes WG, Webb DJ, McMurray JJV: Anti-endothelin therapy is of potential benefit in heart failure [Abstract]. Circulation 1994; 90:I-547.
57. Kannel WB, Doyle JT, McNamara PM, et al: Precursors of sudden cardiac death: factors related to the incidence of sudden death. Circulation 1975; 51:606.
58. Messereli FH, Ventura HO, Elizardi DJ, et al: Hypertension and sudden death: increased ventricular ectopic activity in left ventricular hypertrophy. Am J Med 1984; 77:18.
59. Multiple Risk Factor Intervention Trial Research Group: Baseline rest electrocardiographic abnormalities, antihypertensive treatment, and mortality in the Multiple Risk Factor Intervention trial. Am J Cardiol 1985; 55:1.
60. Lin M, Chiang H-T, Lin S-L, et al: Vasodilator therapy in chronic asymptomatic aortic regurgitation: enalapril versus hydralazine therapy. J Am Coll Cardiol 1994; 24:1046.
61. Greenberg B, Massie B, Bristow JD, et al: Long-term vasodilator therapy of chronic aortic insufficiency. A randomized double-blinded, placebo-controlled trial. Circulation 1988; 78:92.
62. Scognamiglio R, Rahimtoola SH, Fasoli G, et al: Nifedipine in asymptomatic patients with severe aortic regurgitation and normal left ventricular function. N Engl J Med 1994; 331:689.
63. Criqui MH, Langer RD, Fronek A, et al: Mortality over a period of 10 years in patients with peripheral vascular disease. N Engl J Med 1992; 326:381.
64. Choudhri AH, Cleland JG, Rowlands PC, et al: Unsuspected renal artery stenosis in peripheral vascular disease. Br Med J 1990; 301:1197.
65. Olin JW: Treatment of hypertensive patients with peripheral arterial disease. *In* Izzo JL, Black HR (eds): Hypertension Primer, Chapter E28, p 352. Dallas: American Heart Association, 1993.
66. Coffman JD: Drug therapy: vasodilator drugs in peripheral vascular disease. N Engl J Med 1979; 300:713.
67. Roberts DH, McLoughlin GA, Tsao Y, et al: Placebo-controlled comparison of captopril, atenolol, labetalol, and pindolol in hypertension complicated by intermittent claudication. Lancet 1987; 1:650.
68. Creager MA, Ruddy MA: The effect of nifedipine on calf blood flow and exercise capacity in patients with intermittent claudication. J Vasc Med Biol 1990; 2:94.
69. Solomon SA, Ramsay LE, Yeo WW, et al: β Blockade and intermittent claudication: placebo controlled trial of atenolol and nifedipine and their combination. Br Med J 1991; 303:100.
70. Radack K, Deck C: Beta-adrenergic blocker therapy does not worsen intermittent claudication in subjects with peripheral vascular disease. A meta analysis of randomized controlled trials. Arch Intern Med 1991; 151:1769.
71. Roberts WC: The hypertensive diseases. Evidence that systemic hypertension is a greater risk factor to the development of other cardiovascular diseases than previously expected. Am J Med 1975; 59:523.
72. Gadowski GR, Ricci MA, Hendley ED, et al: Hypertension accelerates the growth of experimental aortic aneurysms. J Surg Res 1993; 54:431.
73. Leach SD, Toole AI, Stern H, et al: Effect of β-adrenergic blockade on the growth rate of abdominal aortic aneurysms. Arch Surg 1988; 123:606.
74. Gadowski GR, Pilcher DB, Ricci MA: Abdominal aortic aneurysm expansion rate: effect of size and beta-adrenergic blockade. J Vasc Surg 1994; 19:727.
75. Reid JL: Hypertension and stroke: opportunities for prevention and prospects for protection. J Hypertens 1993; 11(suppl 5):S2.
76. Marshall J: A trial of long-term hypotensive therapy in cerebrovascular disease. Lancet 1964; 1:10.
77. Mori S, Sadoshima S, Fujii K, et al: Decrease in cerebral blood flow with blood pressure reductions in patients with chronic stroke. Stroke 1993; 24:1376.
78. Traub YM, Shapiro AP, Dusovny M, et al: Cerebral blood flow changes with diuretic therapy in elderly subjects with diastolic hypertension. Clin Exp Hypertens 1982; A4:1193.
79. Conen D, Ruttmann S, Noll G, et al: Short- and long-term cerebrovascular effects of nitrendipine in hypertensive patients. J Cardiovasc Pharmacol 1988; 12(suppl 14):S64.
80. Ram CVS, Meese R, Kaplan NM, et al: Antihypertensive therapy in the elderly: effects on blood pressure and cerebral blood flow. Am J Med 1987; 82(suppl 1A):53.
81. Frei A, Muller-Brand J: Cerebral blood flow and antihypertensive treatment with enalapril. J Hypertens 1986; 4:365.
82. Rowe GG, Maxwell GM, Crumpton CW: The cerebral haemodynamic response to administration of hydralazine. Circulation 1962; 25:970.
83. Turner JM, Powell D, Gibson RM, et al: Intracranial pressure changes in neurosurgical patients during hypotension induced with sodium nitroprusside or trimethaphan. Br J Anesthesiol 1977; 49:419.
84. Britton M, Carlsson A, de Faire U: Blood pressure course in patients with acute stroke and matched controls. Stroke 1986; 17:861.
85. Phillips SJ, Whisnant JP: Treatment of hypertensive patients with cerebrovascular disease. *In* Izzo JL, Black HR (eds): Hypertension Primer, Chapter E24, p 343. Dallas: American Heart Association, 1993.

35 Evaluation and Treatment of Hypertension in Children

Julie R. Ingelfinger, MD

Blood pressure in childhood increases with the child's age and size, and elevated blood pressure is found in diverse settings with varied significance. The aware physician must keep this in mind, along with the potential causes, when elevated blood pressure is observed or reported. The goals of this chapter are (1) to provide pragmatic paradigms for evaluation of the infant, child, or adolescent with hypertension; (2) to outline likely causes of hypertension in childhood; and (3) to provide a rational management approach. The likelihood of finding a definable cause for elevated blood pressure is increased the younger the child is or the higher the blood pressure is for the age of the child.[1] Normative data must always be kept in mind (Fig. 35–1) as well as cutoff levels for hypertension defined by age group, as seen in Table 35–1. Thus, a child of 2 years might well have a hypertensive crisis at a blood pressure level that would be only mildly elevated for an adult.

The question of a normal blood pressure value at any given age is still debated, since in addition to age, other factors (such as height, weight, and time of day) are contributors. Rosner and colleagues[3] have reanalyzed the blood pressure data sets that gave rise to the normal blood pressure graphs used in the 1987 Task Force Report[1] and have generated some easy-to-use tables that take height into account.

TRACKING OF BLOOD PRESSURE

If a child has high-normal blood pressure in early childhood, is this predictive of the development of hypertension in later childhood or adult life? Although many studies have addressed this question, the answer is still elusive, although it is probably "yes." *Tracking* is a term to describe the observation that children tend to maintain their relative blood pressure percentiles over time, starting at about 6 months of age. Thus a child with a systolic blood pressure of 112 mm Hg at age 7 years (90th percentile for age—high-normal blood pressure) has a strong likelihood of having a systolic blood pressure at that same percentile at age 14 years (122 mm Hg). Such a child with high-normal blood pressure would be one to follow closely, yet the link between tracking during childhood and adolescence and subsequent adult hypertension has not truly been established as yet. However, several studies have reported tracking of systolic[4–7] but not diastolic[6] blood pressure in the first decade of life.

WHAT CONSTITUTES CHILDHOOD HYPERTENSION?

As is true in adult populations, sustained hypertension may be grouped into several etiologic categories. Secondary or definable hypertension is far more common in children than it is in adults. Consequently, much effort is spent (often with the reward of finding a cause) in evaluating a child with elevated blood pressure for secondary hypertension.

Definable (Secondary) Hypertension

Most definable causes of hypertension in children are due to renal parenchymal disease (80% of definable hypertension), renovascular disease (10%), or coarctation of the aorta (2%).[8] Endocrinologic and neurologic conditions account for some of the remaining causes of secondary hypertension. It should also be borne in mind that iatrogenic hypertension, most frequently related to drugs or toxins, is not uncommon. The most common categories of hypertension for each age group in childhood are helpful "flags" for subsequent evaluation and therapy (Table 35–2). Secondary hypertension may be sustained over a relatively short time (days, weeks, or months) or may be virtually permanent. The blood pressure elevation seen in the course of acute postinfectious nephritis or neurologic insults often abates after a time. In contrast, nonresolving glomerular disease and chronic pyelonephritis are situations in which hypertension will likely remain a long-term problem.

Renal Parenchymal Hypertension

Many glomerular and small artery diseases affecting the kidney are associated with hypertension[9–16] Hemolytic uremic syndrome, acute postinfectious glomerulonephritis, the acute presentation of other glomerulonephritides, and polyarteritis may be accompanied by severe hypertension. With an adequate glomerular filtration rate, the hypertension in ongoing glomerulonephritis is variable. As glomerular disease progresses, however, nearly all patients experience hypertension, regardless of the cause of the glomerular disease. Primary nephrotic syndrome in childhood, which is most commonly due to minimal lesion disease, is associated with some blood pressure elevation in about one fourth of children at presentation.[14] In minimal lesion disease, the patients with blood pressure elevation usually have mild hypertension, whereas other forms of nephrotic syndrome, such as focal segmental glomerulosclerosis, as noted earlier, are present in a higher percentage of patients with hypertension, which can be severe.[11]

Hemolytic uremic syndrome is often accompanied by hypertension—in half of the children presenting in the first 3 years of life and in three quarters of those older than that.[9, 17] The hypertension usually resolves after the acute illness but can recur. Nonresolving or recurring hypertension constitutes a harbinger of progression, suggesting that the renal lesion has not resolved or that chronic scarring has occurred. In addition, a substantial number of patients with tubulointerstitial disease experience hypertension, as reported by Vendemia and colleagues (Fig. 35–2).[13]

Renovascular Hypertension

The spectrum of renovascular disease in childhood differs substantially from that seen in adults in that a number of systemic diseases may contribute to the stenosis.[18, 19] A great number of such children have neurofibromatosis and stenosis associated with abnormal ves-

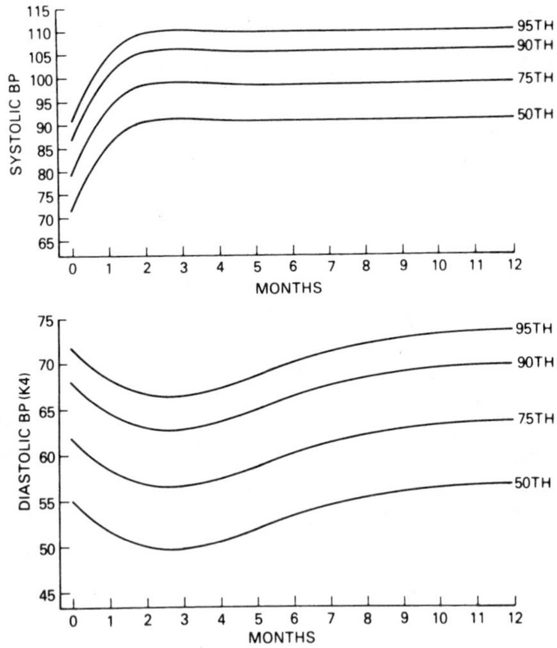

A: 90TH PERCENTILE													
SYSTOLIC BP	87	101	106	106	106	105	105	105	105	105	105	105	105
DIASTOLIC BP	68	65	63	63	63	65	66	67	68	68	69	69	69
HEIGHT CM	51	59	63	66	68	70	72	73	74	76	77	78	80
WEIGHT KG	4	4	5	5	6	7	8	9	9	10	10	11	11

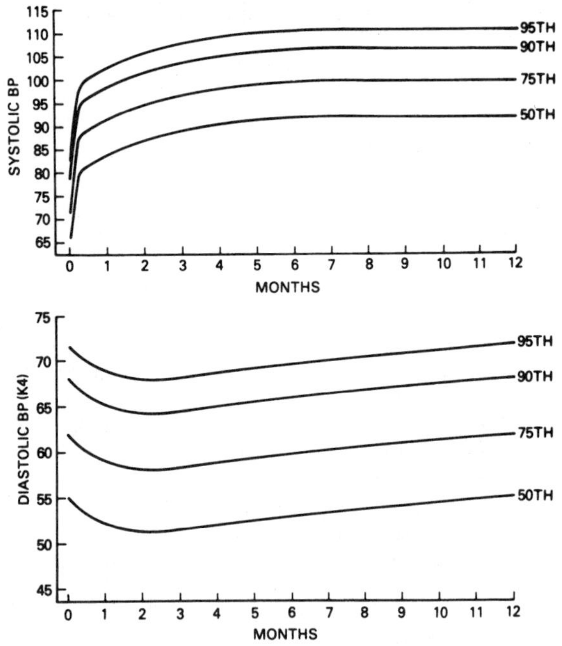

B: 90TH PERCENTILE													
SYSTOLIC BP	76	98	101	104	105	106	106	106	106	106	106	105	105
DIASTOLIC BP	68	65	64	64	65	65	66	66	66	67	67	67	67
HEIGHT CM	54	55	56	58	61	63	66	68	70	72	74	75	77
WEIGHT KG	4	4	4	5	5	6	7	8	9	9	10	10	11

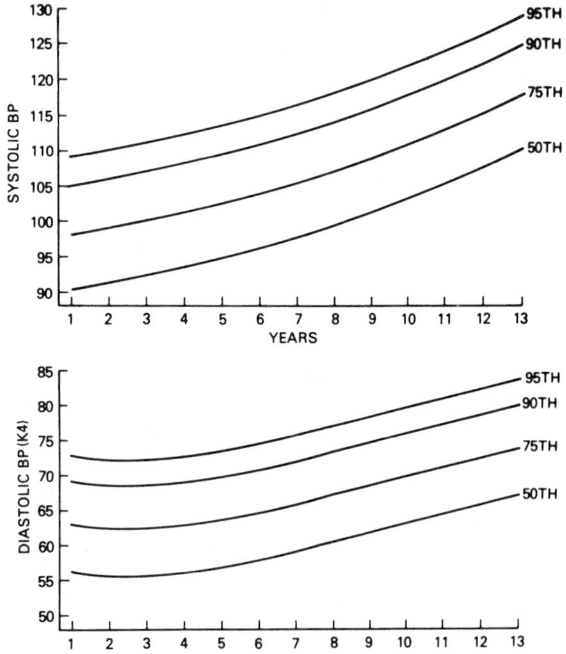

C: 90TH PERCENTILE													
SYSTOLIC BP	105	106	107	108	109	111	112	114	115	117	119	121	124
DIASTOLIC BP	69	68	68	69	69	70	71	73	74	75	76	77	79
HEIGHT CM	80	91	100	108	115	122	129	135	141	147	153	159	165
WEIGHT KG	11	14	16	18	22	25	29	34	39	44	50	55	62

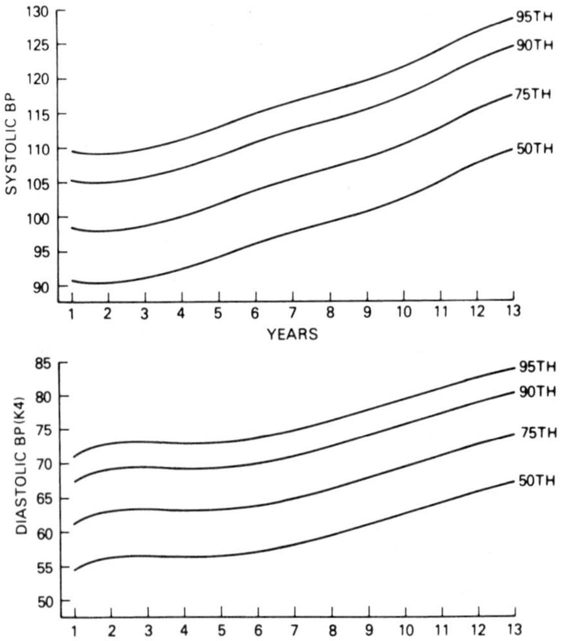

D: 90TH PERCENTILE													
SYSTOLIC BP	105	105	106	107	109	111	112	114	115	117	119	122	124
DIASTOLIC BP	67	69	69	69	69	70	71	72	74	75	77	78	80
HEIGHT CM	77	89	98	107	115	122	129	135	142	148	154	160	165
WEIGHT KG	11	13	15	18	22	25	30	35	40	45	51	58	63

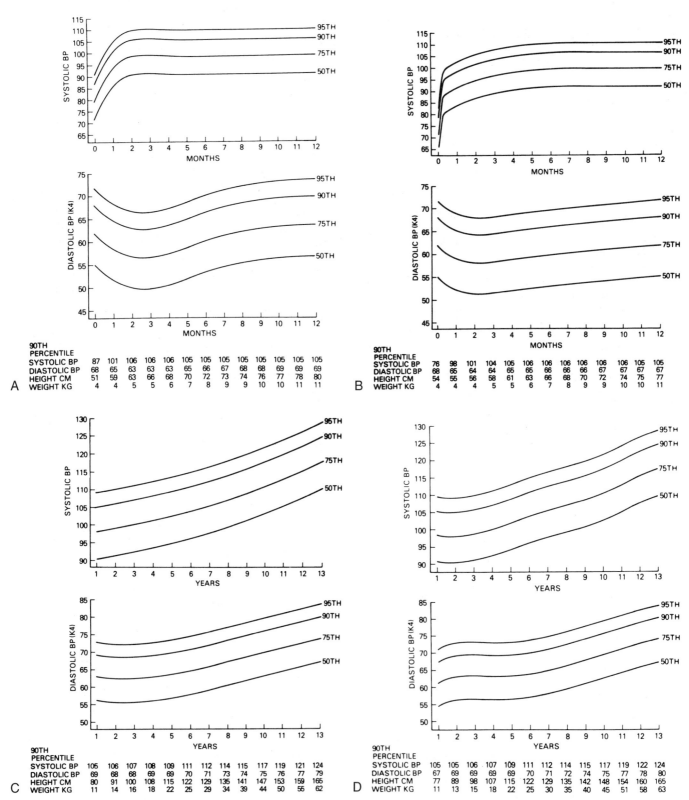

Figure 35–1. *A–D,* Age-specific percentiles of blood pressure from birth to age 18 years. The 90th percentile for systolic blood pressure, the diastolic blood pressure, height, and weight are shown beneath each panel. (From Report of the Second Task Force on Blood Pressure Control in Children—1987. Pediatrics 1987; 79:1–25.)

TABLE 35–1. CUTOFF LEVELS FOR HYPERTENSION BY AGE

Age	Significant Hypertension	Severe Hypertension	Hypertensive Crisis
Neonate			
1 week	SBP > 96 mm Hg	SBP > 106 mm Hg	?
2–4 weeks	SBP > 104 mm Hg	SBP > 110 mm Hg	?
Infant (<2 years)	>112/74 mm Hg	>118/82 mm Hg	145/95 mm Hg
3–5 years	>116/76 mm Hg	>124/84 mm Hg	150/95 mm Hg
6–9 years	>122/78 mm Hg	>130/86 mm Hg	160/100 mm Hg
10–12 years	>126/82 mm Hg	>134/90 mm Hg	165/105 mm Hg
13–15 years	>136/86 mm Hg	>144/92 mm Hg	175/110 mm Hg
16–18 years	>142/92 mm Hg	>150/98 mm Hg	185/120 mm Hg

Abbreviation: SBP, systolic blood pressure.

Data from Report of the Second Task Force on Blood Pressure Control in Children—1987. Pediatrics 1987; 79:1–25 and Burg FB, Ingelfinger JR, Wald ER: Current Pediatric Therapy, vol 14, pp 158–164. Philadelphia: WB Saunders, 1993.

sels, with Schwann cells proliferating in the arterial wall or compression of the vasculature from without. In neurofibromatosis, there is frequently progressive stenosis as well as involvement of multiple vessels and the abdominal aorta.[18] Renovascular hypertension also occurs in Williams syndrome, also known as idiopathic hypercalcemia of infancy.[20] Viral infection may lead to renovascular disease, for example, rubella syndrome in utero[21] or current severe systemic varicella.[18]

Coarctation of the Aorta

The menu of diagnostic and therapeutic modalities to deal with coarctation of the aorta is increasing.[22] Because of recent diagnostic technology, most individuals with coarctation are now discovered in infancy or early childhood, although an occasional patient will be discovered later in childhood. Diagnosis is based on finding an upper- to lower-extremity blood pressure differential, radial femoral pulse delay, and presence of collaterals. The classic therapy for many years has been surgical.[23–25] Recently, however, balloon angioplasty has been used for primary repair or for repair of residual or recurrent coarctation. Medical therapy is often used to stabilize infants with coarctation who have congestive heart failure. Such therapy may permit delay of surgery to a later time. With acute and severe heart failure in infants related to closure of a previously patent ductus arteriosus, prostaglandin E_1 may effect relief of obstruction until surgery or balloon catheterization can take place.[26] Otherwise, usual anticongestive heart failure therapy is important in concert with judicious antihypertensive therapy.

Mendelsohn and colleagues recently reported balloon angioplasty in 59 children with coarctation of the aorta.[27] Ninety percent of the patients had follow-up cardiac catheterization. Of these individuals, 64% had a satisfactory result. Restenosis occurred in six patients, more often in infants less than 12 months of age. Such reports are encouraging to those engaged in relatively noninvasive therapy. Although there is a high percentage of patients in whom intimal damage develops in the form of tears, there is angiographic evidence of healing.[28] Hypertension after coarctation correction is common in the immediate postoperative period.[29] This elevation in blood pressure is ascribed to activation of the sympathetic nervous system and renin-angiotensin system. In addition, hypertension persists in about one quarter of patients after coarctation repair.[22] The older the patient at the time of initial repair, the more likely this is to occur.

Endocrine Hypertension

Several forms of endocrine hypertension have distinct presentations in childhood as compared with the presentation in adult life (see Chapter 39).

Pheochromocytoma

Pheochromocytoma is unusual in children and most often presents clinically as sustained rather than intermittent hypertension.[30, 31] Cardiovascular symptoms are far more rare in children than in adults.[30] Extra-adrenal tumors are more common in childhood than in adulthood. Familial pheochromocytoma may occur in multiple endocrine neoplasia type II. Recurrence is common in children, and lifetime screening, even in the absence of signs or symptoms, is important. Adrenocorticotropic hormone and/or adrenocortical hormones may occasionally be secreted by pheochromocytomas in children, so Cushing syndrome may develop.[30] Thus children with pheochromocytoma who appear with cushingoid symptoms should have their adrenal cortical function evaluated (and the obverse).

Other Catecholamine-Secreting Tumors

Neuroblastoma, ganglioneuroblastoma, and ganglioneuroma may also cause hypertension in children.[32, 33] Of these tumors, neuroblastoma is the most common solid tumor in childhood, and it is often associated with hypertension.

Adrenocortical Hypertension in Children

Primary aldosteronism is rare in children and is usually caused by bilateral adrenal hyperplasia as opposed to an aldosteronoma.[34] In addition to primary aldosteronism, Cushing syndrome, congenital adrenal hyperplasia (usually 11 α-hydroxylase or 17 α-hydroxylase/17,20-lyase deficiency) and glucocorticoid-remediable hypertension (or dexamethasone-suppressible hypertension)[35, 36] can rarely cause hypertension in children.

Renin-Secreting Tumors

Tumors within the kidney that secrete renin are rare,[37] but the hypertension that accompanies them is potentially curable if a diagnosis is made. Occasionally, a Wilms tumor or other tumors have been reported to secrete renin.

Central Hypertension

Although far more is now known about the central nervous system and hypertension, there are few entities in which centrally mediated hypertension is well understood.[38, 39] In children, there are a number of diagnoses in which centrally mediated hypertension should be considered; for example, in many conditions involving infection

TABLE 35–2. CAUSES OF HYPERTENSION IN CHILDHOOD

Renal	*Vascular System*
Glomerular diseases	Coarctation
Acute glomerulonephritis	Patient ductus arteriosus (systolic only)
Acute presentation of chronic nephritides	Anemia (systolic only)
Hemolytic uremic syndrome (HUS)	Polycythemia
Anaphylactoid purpura	Cardiac problems (heart block, aortic insufficiency)
Focal segmental glomerulosclerosis	*Endocrine*
IgA nephropathy	Aldosteronism
Membranoproliferative glomerulonephritis	GRA
Familial nephritis	Congenital adrenal hyperplasia
Membranous nephropathy	Catecholamine-secreting tumors (pheochromocytoma, neuroblastoma, and so on)
Nephritis with systemic diseases	Cushing syndrome or disease
Systemic lupus erythematosus	Hyperthyroidism (systolic only)
Other collagen diseases	Hyperparathyroidism
Vasculitides	Renin-secreting tumors (reninoma, other)
Fabry disease (angiokeratoma corporis diffusum)	Liddle syndrome
Amyloidosis	*Neurologic*
Tubulointerstitial	Increased intracranial pressure (of any cause, particularly infection, tumors, trauma)
Acute or chronic pyelonephritis	Guillain-Barré syndrome
Heavy metal poisoning	Dysautonomia (Riley-Day syndrome)
Renal tubular acidosis with nephrocalcinosis	Myelodysplasia and other neurodevelopmental abnormalities
Acute renal failure	Neurofibromatosis
Post-transplant hypertension (rejection, recurrence, steroid-related, cyclosporine-related)	?Anxiety
After genitourinary surgery	*Metabolic*
After renal biopsy	Diabetes mellitus
Obstructive uropathy	Gouty nephropathy
Cystic kidney diseases	Acute intermittent porphyria
Autosomal dominant PKD	Hypercalcemia
Autosomal recessive PKD	Hypernatremia
Nephronophthisis	Cyclic vomiting syndrome
Multicystic dysplastic kidney	*Iatrogenic*
Cystic hamartomatous disease (in tuberous sclerosis)	Steroids
Radiation nephritis	Heavy metals
Infiltrative (e.g., leukemia)	Sympathomimetics
Infectious (e.g., SBE-related)	Oral contraceptives
Renovascular	Rebound hypertension (e.g., with clonidine withdrawal)
Renal artery stenosis	Drug-drug interaction
Fibromuscular disease	Licorice ingestion
Related to systemic disease (e.g., neurofibromatosis)	Tobacco chewing
After viral disease	Street drugs
Syndrome-related (Turner, Williams)	Sodium-containing drugs in renal-impaired individuals
After transplantation	After surgery (genitourinary, orthopedic, gastroschisis repair)
Vasculitides	*Miscellaneous*
Collagen-vascular (e.g., periarteritis)	Burns
Moyamoya disease	Stevens-Johnson syndrome
Kawasaki disease	Primary hypertension
Takayasu disease	
Radiation aortitis or vasculitis	
Page kidney (compression)	

Abbreviations: GRA, glucocorticoid-responsive aldosteronism; PKD, polycystic kidney disease; SBE, subacute bacterial endocarditis.

of the central nervous system (including meningitis, encephalitis, poliomyelitis, and Guillain-Barré syndrome), blood pressure is elevated acutely. Hypertension is also seen following convulsions, in diencephalic epilepsy, with hypothalamic lesions or brainstem lesions, as well as in tumors. Unknown peripheral neural factors may be present to cause hypertension in polyneuropathy and familial dysautonomia.

Iatrogenic Hypertension

Iatrogenic causes of hypertension are important to consider in the evaluation of a child with hypertension.[1, 2] A history of prescribed drugs and the possibility of ingestion of agents that could lead to hypertension are important in the diagnosis.

Primary (Essential) Hypertension

There are still few data that specifically discriminate childhood factors influencing the onset or development of primary hypertension. Sinaiko and associates examined plasma catecholamines and plasma renin activity (PRA) in 8-year-olds with high and low blood pressure.[40] They found no difference in plasma norepinephrine in any position or activity. PRA was significantly lower, as was 24-hour urinary kallikrein excretion, in the group with high blood pressure. However, sodium intake, which can influence each parameter, was not controlled. In contrast, McCrory and colleagues earlier found that catecholamine response was accentuated in adolescents with hypertension as well as in their siblings.[41] In additional, Falkner and colleagues found that adolescents with borderline hypertension have a marked response to mental stress, suggesting a role for the

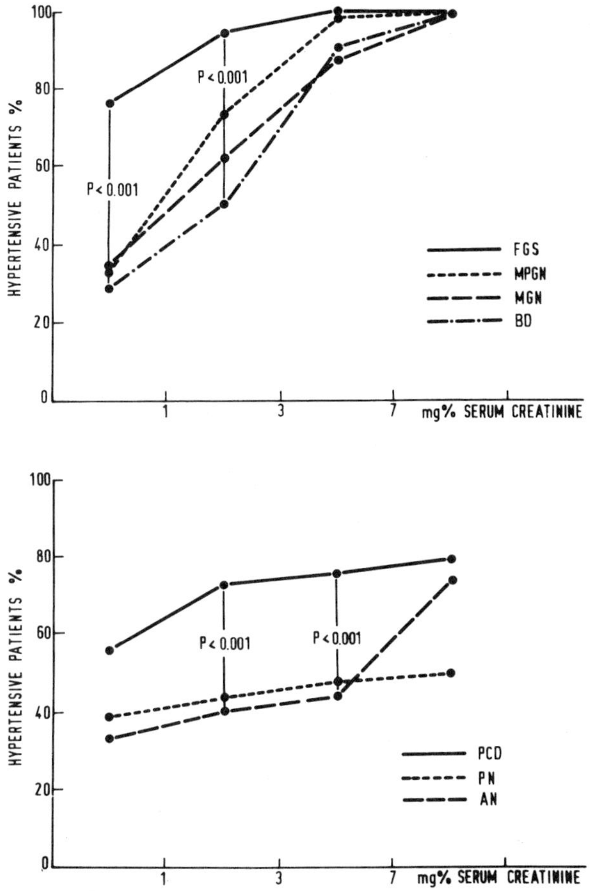

Figure 35–2. The upper panel shows the relationships among the type of glomerulopathy, the level of plasma creatinine, and blood pressure. The lower panel shows the relationships among the type of tubulointerstitial disease, plasma creatinine levels, and blood pressure. *Abbreviations:* MPGN, membranoproliferative glomerulonephritis; MGN, membranous glomerulonephritis; FGS, focal glomerulosclerosis; BD, Berger disease (same as IgA nephropathy); PCD, polycystic kidney disease; PN, pyelonephritis; AN, analgesic nephropathy. (From Vendemia F, Fornasiera A, Velis O, et al: Different prevalence rates of hypertension in various reno-parenchymal diseases. *In* Blaufox MD, Bianchi C [eds]: Secondary Forms of Hypertension: Current Diagnosis and Management, p 92. New York: Grune & Stratton, 1981.)

sympathetic nervous system.[42] Rocchini examined the relationships among insulin levels, insulin resistance, and hypertension.[43] He found a positive correlation between insulin levels and blood pressure in obese adolescents. Perhaps the most interesting correlation between the onset of hypertension and childhood is the increasing number of studies that show a correlation between low birth weight and subsequent hypertension.[44, 45] A possibility is that small infants are among those individuals who have a decreased complement of nephrons and that such individuals are prone to both hypertension and nephrosclerosis. Examination of early data on the range of glomeruli seen in apparently normal individuals suggests that rather than the figure generally used of 1 $\times$ 10^6 nephrons per kidney, there is a range of 400,000–1,400,000 nephrons. It has been hypothesized that those individuals with a low number of nephrons are especially at risk for the development of future hypertension.[46] Whether the decreased nephron complement theory proves indicative of future hypertension or not, it seems likely that primary hypertension develops in more than one way and is, in fact, more than one condition. At present, however, there are no particularly pediatric features, although hypertension without a definable cause may be found in many patients, even very young ones.

EVALUATION OF HYPERTENSION IN CHILDREN

Evaluation of Neonates With Hypertension

Associated clinical circumstances should direct the evaluation of a newborn infant noted to have elevated blood pressure.[47, 48] Blood pressure elevation in the first month of life is usually detected because the neonate has been found to have an anatomic problem involving the kidneys or cardiovascular system or because the baby has been receiving in-hospital therapy related to prematurity, small-for-gestational-age status, or birth asphyxia. Hypertension in these latter categories may be related to thromboembolic events (e.g., umbilical artery catheterization or spontaneous arterial and/or renal venous thrombosis) or to increased intracranial pressure (related to intraventricular hemorrhage or cerebral infarct). Table 35–3 lists causes of hypertension in the first month of life, and Figure 35–3 shows blood pressure in the first month of life in infants of low birth weight. Because iatrogenic events may be associated with hypertension in the neonate, attention should be focused on the circumstances of perinatal events, medications given to both mother and baby, and intrapartum history. Direct physical examination may be especially useful in this age group for making a diagnosis and assessing the baby for end-organ effects of hypertension. Blood pressure determination in all four extremities may be helpful in diagnosing coarctation of the aorta, although in the setting of complicated cardiac lesions and heart failure, hypertension may not develop in the newborn period. The baby's general physical status may suggest syndromes associated with hypertension, including congenital infections (e.g., toxoplasmosis, rubella, or cytomegalovirus), after which renovascular disease may occur. Palpation of the kidneys in the neonate is relatively easy, so large kidneys or masses may easily be felt. Thus autosomal recessive polycystic kidney disease is often detected on physical examination (if it has not already been suspected after viewing prenatal sonograms). Severe hypertension in the neonate often leads to retinopathy, so a careful examination of the baby's fundus is important; a pediatric ophthalmologist should be consulted. Heart failure may occur because of hypertension, and a careful cardiac examination is essential.

TABLE 35–3. HYPERTENSION IN THE FIRST YEAR OF LIFE

Renovascular
Thromboembolic
Catheter
Renal vein/renal artery thrombosis
Small vessel—birth asphyxia–related
Renal parenchymal
Polycystic kidney disease
Pyelonephritis (acute)
Hydronephrosis
Glomerulopathy
Acute renal failure
Perirenal compression (infectious, hematoma, other)
Coarctation of the aorta
Simple
Combined defect
Double aortic arch
Centrally mediated
Intraventricular hemorrhage
Hydrocephalus
Increased intracranial pressure—any cause
Tumor
Wilms
Neuroblastoma
Other
Iatrogenic
Medication
Volume expansion

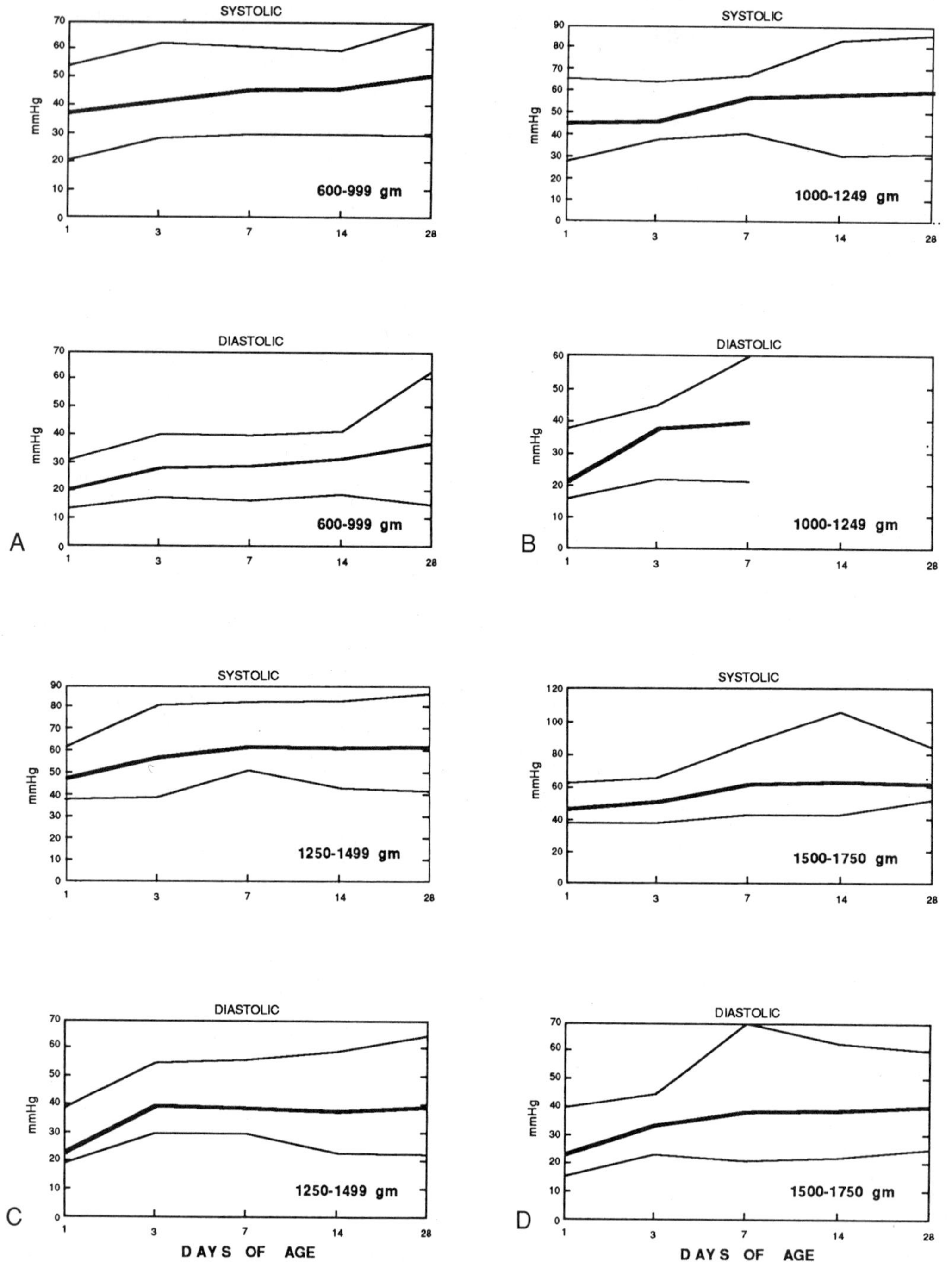

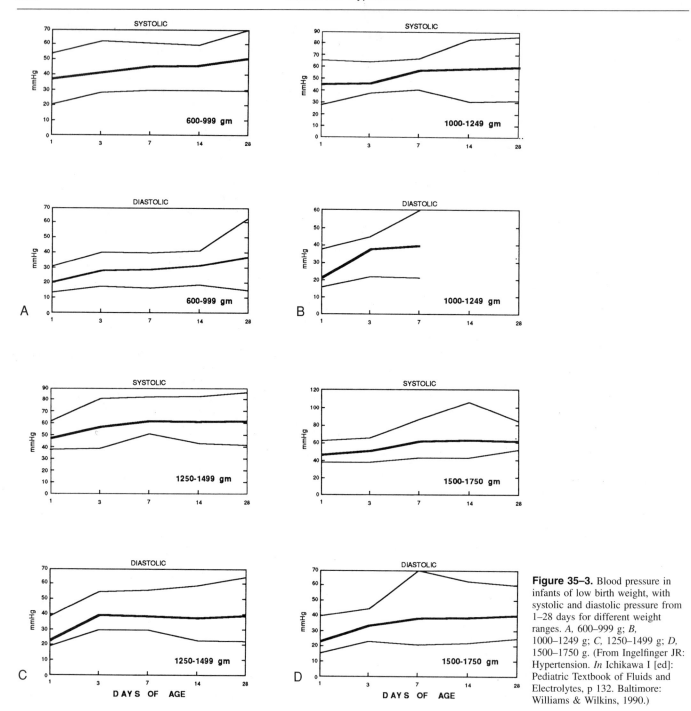

Figure 35–3. Blood pressure in infants of low birth weight, with systolic and diastolic pressure from 1–28 days for different weight ranges. *A,* 600–999 g; *B,* 1000–1249 g; *C,* 1250–1499 g; *D,* 1500–1750 g. (From Ingelfinger JR: Hypertension. *In* Ichikawa I [ed]: Pediatric Textbook of Fluids and Electrolytes, p 132. Baltimore: Williams & Wilkins, 1990.)

Hypertension may lead to end-organ damage quickly in the neonate, so *severe elevations should be treated while the investigation proceeds.* The very ill neonate with hypertension should have an evaluation for presumptively ruling in or ruling out renovascular disease and renal parenchymal disease. Ultrasonography with Doppler flow studies may be most helpful, as this provides both good renal anatomy and some view of the renal artery and vein as well as the great vessels. The most feasible study for looking at segmental vascular flow is usually a radionuclide renal scan, which provides an estimate both of arterial perfusion and tissue uptake. (Although "pull-out" arteriograms have been performed to find clots in umbilical vessel catheters or to detect emboli, arteriography may pose a problem, owing to the need for the administration of contrast material. In addition, magnetic resonance [MR] angiography, although appealingly noninvasive, is not easily applied to a neonate, who may well be attached to life support systems. Thus vascular studies per se may best be deferred.) When coarctation of the aorta is suspected, echocardiography is usually diagnostic, and unless complex lesions are suspected, cardiac catheterization may not be necessary. Similarly, an endocrine evaluation should be undertaken only when there is reason to suspect endocrinologic disease. In the neonatal period, congenital adrenal hyperplasia, usually found for other reasons, would be the most common reason for hypertension.

Hypertension Evaluation in Infancy (1 Month to 2 Years)

After the neonatal period, blood pressure measurement in infants and toddlers is a challenge. Babies usually wiggle, and getting an accurate blood pressure routinely proves time-consuming and challenging. Thus, blood pressure often is not measured at well-baby check-ups in the first year of life and, indeed, the 1987 Task Force did not recommend routine blood pressure checks for children in this age group.[1] However, blood pressure in the very young child should be measured and monitored when the cause of illness is not evident, when a child is hospitalized, or when the family or individual history is likely to be associated with hypertension. If an infant is found to have elevated blood pressure, one should be sure it is an actual blood pressure reading (a common error is to use a blood pressure cuff that is far too small, which artifactually elevates the pressure). Use of a plethysmograph machine, such as the Dinamap, or a finger-pulse machine permits reasonably accurate measurement when standard classic measurement with auscultation proves difficult.

When hypertension is documented in the very young child, there is a high chance that a secondary cause will appear. Thus a full evaluation is appropriate, but it must be tailored to the size of the child and the severity and duration of the hypertension. Careful attention to the child's neonatal course, the family history, and present medications may point the way to diagnosis. Screening laboratory examinations and renal imaging are both important. Increasingly, imaging for renovascular hypertension can be noninvasive; but the use of MR angiography in the very young child is still not sufficiently sensitive to replace formal angiography in most cases. In this age group, it is reasonable to perform renal ultrasonography with Doppler flow and then to consider whether an isotopic renal radioscintiscan is needed before arteriography. If there is severe hypertension for the age of the child, arteriography usually is warranted, and skipping the scintigram may be reasonable. The use of angiotensin-converting enzyme (ACE) inhibitors before performing a scan is controversial in this age group, and in any event results are less clear than in adults.

Evaluation of Children Past Toddlerhood

There is often definable secondary hypertension after toddlerhood, and the older the child the less difficult the technical aspects of the evaluation. Thus a common sense approach should be advocated. A careful history, a careful evaluation for end-organ involvement, and a fastidious search for iatrogenic causes will dictate which children should get full evaluations. A child with severe hypertension must be evaluated while blood pressure control is initiated and maintained; such children should have a complete evaluation, including vascular imaging, unless a defined cause is evident otherwise. Conversely, a child with only occasional blood pressure readings above the 95th percentile for age need not have a detailed investigation, at least initially.

THE INVESTIGATION OF HYPERTENSION

Investigation of the pediatric patient is tailored as noted earlier and is usually phased (Fig. 35–4).[1, 2] Certain parts of the evaluation should be repetitious. Family history and signs and symptoms must be sought repetitively. Not only should the presence or absence of familial hypertension be sought but also the age of onset as well as sequelae such as renal, cardiovascular, and peripheral vascular problems. It may also be important to ask whether medication was needed and which drug was used. Recent blood pressure levels of family members should be documented by history or by taking them directly. A positive family history may direct the evaluation to rule out familial renal disease, phacomatoses, familial pheochromocytoma in multiple endocrinopathy type II, glucocorticoid-responsive aldosteronism and, by exclusion, primary hypertension. It may be worthwhile to note the mode of blood pressure control in family members. Other historical information of importance includes obtaining a neonatal history in that the use of umbilical arterial catheters may be associated with renovascular hypertension secondary to thromboembolic events, and infants with bronchopulmonary hyperplasia may have high blood pressure. Medication history, including over-the-counter medications, is important, as is learning or getting a sense of whether the patient is taking any illicit drugs. One must elicit a detailed dietary history because the salt and caloric requirements of the patient may be relevant, suggesting, for example, salt sensitivity or a hypermetabolic state. Symptoms suggesting severe hypertension or a particular diagnosis should be sought. For instance, headaches, dizziness, nosebleeds, or visual problems, although nonspecific, may suggest severe hypertension or central causes of hypertension. It has been reported that some children with renovascular hypertension have relative polyuria, polydipsia, and growth failure. Signs that may suggest renal disease include dysuria, frequency, nocturia, and enuresis (although most cases of enuresis are idiopathic and not related to renal disease). Edema may be associated with various glomerulonephritides, and joint pain or swelling may suggest systemic or glomerular disease. Muscle cramps, weakness, and/or constipation may suggest low potassium, as seen in aldosteronism. If the patient is a girl, the age of menarche is important, as this may suggest 17α-hydroxylase deficiency. It is time-consuming to seek answers to all these questions, but the answers can lead to a far more efficient hypertension evaluation. The physical examination, too, is important.[49] Stigmata of syndromes associated with hypertension should be sought: webbed neck, widely spaced nipples, wide carrying angle (Turner syndrome); café au lait spots (neurofibromatosis); fibroma or shagreen patches (tuberous sclerosis); elfin facies (Williams syndrome); retinal changes (von Hippel–Lindau disease); and striae, moon facies, buffalo hump, hirsutism (Cushing syndrome). Pallor may suggest anemia, which may be common in renal insufficiency; such individuals may also have edema. Thyroid enlargement may suggest either hyperthyroidism or hypothyroidism. Circulatory examination is important.[50] An arm and leg pressure differential is suggestive of coarctation as decreased femoral pulses or radial femoral pulse delay. A heart murmur best heard over the back may be revealing of coarctation. Rapid pulse rate, as well as arrhythmia and postural hypotension, may be indicative of pheochromocytoma. Bruits over the great vessels, head, or flank may suggest arterial stenosis. The abdomen should be examined for masses, some of which cause hypertension (as noted previously). Neurologic signs such as Bell palsy or hemiparesis suggest severe hypertension, which is generally chronic. End-organ damage must be sought by careful funduscopic examination to rule out changes in the ocular fundus and by careful cardiovascular examination.

Laboratory Screening Studies

All children with documented hypertension should undergo some initial studies.[1] A careful urinalysis performed by the physician, if possible, is invaluable for directing further evaluation at defining renal disease. An early-morning urine specimen may be most helpful, if examined fresh, in that a concentrated early-morning specimen is reassuring in terms of renal function. A urine culture should be performed. Hemoglobin, blood urea nitrogen, creatinine, electrolyte, and bicarbonate determinations are also helpful, and determining uric acid has also been thought to be important. If primary hypertension is suspected, lipoprotein electrophoresis as a risk factor selector is helpful.

Further Studies

Additional studies should be performed on a selected-case basis. When blood pressure elevation is mild, renal imaging studies may be deferred for a short time. Since most definable pediatric hypertension is renal or renovascular, however, screening ultrasonography should be performed if hypertension persists.[51–53] Adding Doppler flow studies is important if blood pressure elevation is moderate to severe. Radionuclide renal scans with an ACE inhibitor may be

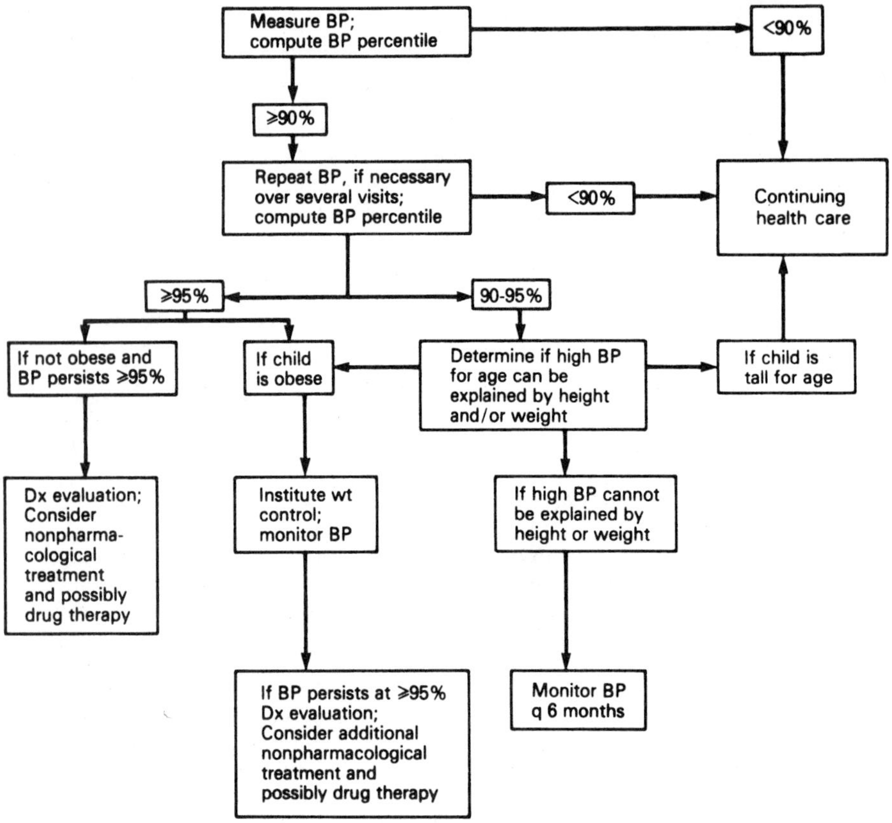

Figure 35–4. Flow diagram for evaluation of blood pressure in children. Note that at least two blood pressure measurements should be used for each nodal point. In the case of severe hypertension, evaluation and therapy should proceed immediately. (From Report of the Second Task Force on Blood Pressure Control in Children—1987. Pediatrics 1987; 79:1–25.)

helpful in patients whose blood pressure is not so elevated that arteriography should be performed right away but who do not seem to be responding to conventional therapy. If blood pressure elevation is severe, it may be most cost-effective to proceed early to arteriography and renal vein renin sampling. Excretory urography should be reserved for individuals who appear to have renal structural abnormalities. Computed tomography (CT) usually is not indicated, although it may be useful when small renal tumors are being sought. MR angiography has been successful in detecting renal artery abnormalities in transplant recipients, but experience with it is limited in children.

Whether to measure peripheral renin activity and/or aldosterone is unclear.[54, 55] PRA values change with age and salt state, so it is important that (1) the normal values for various ages of children are run by the laboratory and (2) the salt balance is known. Furthermore, unless the peripheral PRA value is very high (suggesting renal or renovascular disease) or low (suggesting aldosteronism or familial glucocorticoid-responsive aldosteronism), it is not clinically helpful. Finally, as in adults, if renovascular disease is suspected, imaging studies are performed anyway. Primary aldosteronism is rare in children, so it is not cost-effective to measure aldosterone levels in all children. If PRA is low, aldosterone may be worth measuring if hypokalemia is also present. In clinical practice, it makes sense to determine PRA in the setting of moderately severe or severe hypertension before pharmacotherapy, since finding a renal cause for such hypertension is likely.

In addition, in children with early onset of difficult to control hypertension and a family history of the same, glucocorticoid-responsive aldosteronism (GRA) is likely[35, 36] (see Chapter 31). In such cases, a low PRA, with or without high aldosterone levels, would render a work-up for GRA important. The evaluation for GRA includes measurement of urinary steroid metabolites (which few laboratories now perform) or determining whether the gene is abnormal using DNA extracted from leukocytes.

Evaluation for pheochromocytoma, which is extremely rare in childhood, should be undertaken when patients declare themselves likely to have the tumor. A 24-hour urine collection for measurement of norepinephrine, epinephrine, dopamine, vanillylmandelic acid, and metanephrine should be performed.[30, 31] It has been suggested that a 24-hour urine specimen should be collected in several fractionated subunits of 24 hours if there is paroxysmal hypertension (unusual in children) to include the times around an attack and times from the rest of the day, since in this scenario, the total 24-hour collection may be normal, whereas the amount excreted around the attack may be very high.[30] However, rare as it is, pheochromocytoma presents in many guises. Thus, before undertaking any other invasive tests in evaluating hypertensive patients, it is important to be certain that plasma or urine catecholamine levels are normal. If so, further studies are indicated. For instance, if plasma catecholamine levels are elevated, clonidine suppression testing should be normal if there is no tumor. CT or magnetic resonance imaging (MRI) of the abdomen and chest should be carried out to try to locate a tumor. Whether an iodine-131 metaiodobenzylguanidine (MIBG) scan, with the amount of radioactivity required, should be performed at this point is debated. Comparison of MIBG scanning with other modalities has not been carried out in children, although studies in adults suggested that CT and MRI are about equivalent to MIBG in identifying adrenal pheochromocytomas and that MRI and MIBG were slightly better than CT for detecting extrarenal pheochromocytoma.[32] Other possible testing includes caval sampling for catecholamines. Provocative testing with phentolamine and arteriography are rarely carried out any longer. Other catecholamine-secreting tumors, most often neuroblastoma, are usually detected because of mass effect and, therefore, hypertension management is more important than studies. In neuroblastoma, determining cystathionine levels may be worthwhile. With other conditions associated with hypertension, the evaluation should proceed based on the condition that is suspected. A toxic screen should be performed if it is possible that elevated blood pressure is due to street drugs such as phencyclidine, amphetamines, or crack cocaine.[1, 2]

MANAGEMENT OF THE HYPERTENSIVE CHILD OR ADOLESCENT

Management depends on the age of the child and the severity of the hypertension. If pharmacotherapy is being used in a child, the aim of making this a time-limited exposure to a pharmacotherapeutic agent always makes sense. Thus, after a period of blood pressure control, it is important to try to decrease the dosage and number of agents required. Whenever possible, nonpharmacologic therapy should be used as primary and/or adjunctive therapy. Whatever the type of therapy, the goal should be to reduce blood pressure to levels at or below the 95th percentile for age. Progressive, steady lowering of pressure is preferred, unless there is a hypertensive crisis. Even in that situation, blood pressure should be lowered in steps to avoid too rapid a decrease, which can lead to renal, cardiac, or central nervous system compromise.

The following sections summarize pediatric aspects of the therapy of hypertension.

Nonpharmacologic Therapy

As in adults, if the blood pressure is significantly but mildly elevated, a nonpharmacologic regimen should be initiated.[1, 56, 57] It is helpful to introduce the concept of this type of program in the context of cardiovascular risk, discussing family history, hyperlipidemia, tobacco use, weight control, and exercise. Because compliance is difficult to obtain, proposing this approach necessitates patient education not only verbally but also with printed information and practical staff support. To monitor progress, it may be helpful to have the patient and family measure blood pressure, keeping a record, and to set up positive reinforcements.

Weight Loss

If the child is overweight, a weight-loss program can be helpful.[58–60] When weight loss is successful, the decrease in blood pressure is proportional to the prediet weight, with the heaviest patients having the greatest decrement in blood pressure. Other cardiovascular risk parameters also improve with weight loss. Having the child and family see a nutritionist in a supportive environment can be instrumental to successful weight loss.

Modification of Salt Intake

Sodium restriction is difficult to carry out, since it takes several months for the appetite for salt to change. Generally, the effect of lowering sodium intake in hypertensive children is successful if (1) compliance occurs and (2) the patient is salt-sensitive. Mixed reports of significant blood pressure reduction[61] and little change[62] have been published. In general, the concept of a salt "allowance" can help teenagers with compliance. It *can* be stated that sodium intake in most children and adolescents in the Western world is far greater than the recommended daily allowance for normal growth and development. Thus, moderate salt restriction in most individuals carries no adverse risk. Whether or not salt restriction alone is beneficial, it is thought that adding other cations to the diet may be helpful. For example, potassium and calcium supplementation have been advocated, but there is little information about how well this works in the long term in children and adolescents. In the study of Geleijnse and colleagues, adding potassium supplementation to sodium restriction was successful in lowering blood pressure.[62] Thus, although sodium restriction alone was ineffective, the combination of sodium restriction and added potassium to a salt-restricted diet apparently was efficacious. However, increasing potassium intake sufficiently with diet alone is not an easy matter. Table 35–4 lists foods with high sodium content (foods to avoid or take in moderation) and foods with high potassium content (foods to include in the diet).

TABLE 35–4. FOODS CONTAINING HIGH SODIUM AND HIGH POTASSIUM

Foods with high sodium content (limited list)
Meats: Bacon, pork, hotdogs, most sausage, ham, bologna, salami, smoked turkey, and so on
Fish: smoked salmon (lox)
Cheese: most "yellow" cheese, feta cheese
Special types of food:
Pizza
Mexican food
Chinese food
Fast food (Burger King, McDonald's, Roy Rogers, Arby's, Wendy's, and so on)
Processed food: spaghetti sauces, canned vegetables, canned soups
Snacks: salted crackers, pretzels, potato chips, nacho chips
Bread crumbs (if salted)
Cereals: many contain a lot of salt
Condiments: pickles, olives, many relishes, salad dressing
Foods with high potassium content (limited list)
Very high: potatoes with skins, tomato juice, orange juice, beans, bananas, avocados, meats
High: raisins/grapes, grapefruit juice, oranges, pineapple juice, raw tomatoes, milk, yogurt, cheese

Salt Restriction

In general, salt restriction should consist of a no-salt-added diet.[63] It is important for the health care provider to go over this diet with the child and family so that dietary habits can be combined with a program most likely to encourage compliance. Extra sources of sodium intake should be elicited (e.g., canned foods that the family does not realize contain a lot of sodium). Indeed, with current, more stringent labeling regulations, the salt content of most foods is listed on the package and should help in effecting compliance.

Exercise

Many children with hypertension are overweight and tend to be sedentary. In these youngsters, a program of exercise is a useful adjunct to blood pressure control. Indeed, aerobic exercise lowers blood pressure in teenagers and also has a salutary effect on blood lipids. Limited studies have also demonstrated that weight training lowers resting blood pressure in teenagers with hypertension, but because of the questions concerning static exercise and cardiac fitness, aerobic exercise is preferable.

Exercise in the Hypertensive Athletic Child or Teenager

Exercise is important in hypertensive athletic children.[64, 65] Strenuous dynamic exercise increases systolic blood pressure in normal individuals as well as in those with hypertension, whereas it does not generally increase diastolic pressure significantly. Data to this point indicate that there is no increased risk from exercise to the child or teenager with mild hypertension. It is worthwhile to assess cardiovascular response to exercise if there is any question concerning the level of blood pressure. Children with severe hypertension should not participate in strenuous sport activity until blood pressure levels have been normalized with therapy. Whether controlling blood pressure to normal levels lowers the risk in the child with severe hypertension to that of a normotensive individual is not known, and what recommendation to make is controversial. Since exercise reduces both blood pressure and cardiovascular risk, it makes sense to control blood pressure and then institute an exercise program even in the child with severe hypertension. Whether such individuals should be barred from competitive sports should depend on cardiac evaluation and, perhaps, exercise tolerance testing. An issue with such testing is that a significant incidence of false-positive ST segment changes can occur in maximal graded exercise testing (ST segment values are subsequently found to be normal on radionuclide exercise testing).[65] This kind of finding limits the value of such testing for cardiac function, although the blood pressure documented at maximal stress may be helpful. Another issue is that the choice of medication for the athlete is problematic. Many cardiovascular agents affect cardiac output and thus performance. In general, the agents that facilitate normal cardiovascular response include clonidine, methyldopa, calcium channel blockers, angiotensin converting enzyme (ACE) inhibitors, and diuretics. The long-term effects of some of these agents rule out diuretics for most athletes. For this reason, ACE inhibitors or calcium channel blockers may be helpful.

Behavioral Modification Techniques

Modifying behavior has been considered efficacious in lowering blood pressure according to some studies.[66] In order for biofeedback, relaxation techniques, or meditation to be successful, however, the patient needs to be motivated. Although some school-aged children are interested in this approach, most are not able to carry it out. Among adolescents, few in our experience are interested in pursuing this avenue. When we have found a motivated individual, this approach can be most helpful.

DRUG TREATMENT OF HYPERTENSION IN CHILDREN

Pharmacotherapy for childhood hypertension is based on limited data, as many potent antihypertensive agents are never formally tested in infants or children with hypertension.[2, 67, 68] Of the recently developed antihypertensive agents, such as ACE inhibitors, none of the many now available in the US has been formally approved for use in children or been used in sufficient patient numbers for one to be confident concerning specific recommendations about pediatric dosing. For many drugs, then, the pediatric dosing is based on scaling down the dose for adults and then modifying that based on clinical experience as garnered from case reports or compilations of such reports.

General Approach

In children and adolescents, monotherapy is to be preferred over multiple agents. Adolescence is a time during which compliance is particularly difficult, so the fewer agents given, the more likely it is that a given regimen will be successful.

Hypertensive Crisis

Table 35–5 lists medications (and doses) used for treating hypertensive crisis in children. For pediatric usage, nifedipine is especially attractive, since it can be given sublingually and with little delay. When nifedipine is used for a small child, the capsule must be punctured and the appropriate amount of medication withdrawn for administration (a 10-mg capsule contains approximately 0.33 mL of fluid, so 1 mg = 0.033 mL). Intravenous labetalol or nitroprusside is also being used increasingly with good success in children. The other agents listed in the table are also used, although with decreasing enthusiasm, given the success of the more recently available preparations.

TABLE 35–5. ANTIHYPERTENSIVE AGENTS IN HYPERTENSIVE CRISIS*

Drug	Dose
Sodium nitroprusside	0.5–8 μg/kg/min IV
Labetalol	1–3 mg/kg/hr IV
Diazoxide	2–5 mg/kg IV
Hydralazine	0.2–0.4 mg/kg IV
Nifedipine	0.25–0.5 mg/kg sublingually
Minoxidil	0.1–0.2 mg/kg orally
Phentolamine	0.1–0.2 mg/kg IV

*See text for details.
Abbreviation: IV, intravenously.

Suggested Order of Medications

Moderate Hypertension

If no contraindications exist, for most patients we would suggest using ACE inhibitors or calcium channel blockers as first-line drugs in chronic hypertension, recognizing that there is no formal approval for their use in children. If blood pressure does not promptly come under control, adding a thiazide diuretic may help. Vasodilators and beta blockers, although recommended by many texts and by the Report of the Second Task Force on Blood Pressure in Children,[1] are often not well tolerated and are used as a second choice if there is a contraindication to ACE inhibitors or calcium channel blockers. Alpha-adrenergic blockade—for example, with prazosin—is not often used in children. Central α_2-agonists may make children sleepy but may be useful in centrally mediated hypertension. In addition, clonidine as a skin patch (Catapres TTS) is often useful in otherwise noncompliant adolescents in our experience.

Severe Hypertension

When hypertension is severe, the same first-line drugs may be used after initial blood pressure control with emergency use of hypotensive medications. It is likely in such situations that monotherapy will *not* suffice. Therefore, combinations may be used initially. ACE inhibitors or calcium channel blockers may be useful in concert with diuretics. Oral labetalol may be effective in treating severe hypertension, although experience in children and adolescents is not extensive. Combinations and order of medication as recommended in earlier publications[1]—for example, using diuretics and adding a beta-adrenergic blocker as first-line therapy—should be modified, given the larger number of medications now available.

Severe hypertension seen in children with primary renal disease can be difficult to control, needing multiple agents.[69–71] Thus, drug-drug interaction and pharmacokinetics need special consideration. Doses for hypertensive emergencies/urgencies in children are listed in Table 35–5; for infants, the doses are listed in Table 35–6; and for chronic therapy, they are listed in Table 35–7.

Treatment of Hypertension in Infancy

With the high percentage of infants with hypertension having a renovascular cause, ACE inhibitors are useful. However, the dosage needed is far less than that needed for older individuals (roughly one tenth the dose). Fetuses exposed to ACE inhibitors in utero suffer renal failure, and other abnormalities such as hypocalvaria have been described. The calcium channel blocker nifedipine is useful for treatment of neonatal hypertension, and in this case (as for small children generally) the capsule needs to be punctured and the drug withdrawn, given the small amount needed in the neonatal period. Diuretic therapy in the hypertensive infant, especially the newborn, may be indicated. When using loop diuretics, which increase calcium excretion, it must be considered that sick infants are often hypercalciuric and prone to nephrocalcinosis. Thus, use of thiazides as adjunct medication may be preferable to loop diuretics, although even with thiazides there has been a question of hypercalciuria.

TABLE 35–6. ANTIHYPERTENSIVE MEDICATIONS FOR NEONATES*

Medication Class	Route	Dose	Comment
Diuretic			
Furosemide	IV or PO	0.5–1 mg/kg/dose	Possible hyponatremia, hypokalemia, hypercalciuria
Chlorothiazide	PO	20–30 mg/kg/24 hr	Possible hyponatremia, hypokalemia
Adrenergic blockers			
Beta-adrenergic blocker†			
Propranolol	PO	0.5–2.0 mg/kg/day	Avoid in lung disease
	IV	0.05–0.15 mg/kg/dose	Avoid in lung disease; beware of possible arrhythmias
Alpha-adrenergic blocker			
Phentolamine	IV	0.1–0.2 mg/kg/dose	Little experience in newborn
Alpha/beta-adrenergic blocker			
Labetalol	IV	1–3 mg/kg/hr	Limited experience
Vasodilators			
Hydralazine	PO, IV	1–9 mg/kg/24 hr	Reflex tachycardia may occur
Sodium nitroprusside	IV	1–5 μg/kg/min	Check for thiocyanate toxicity, protect infusate from light
Diazoxide	IV	2–5 mg/kg/dose	Unpredictable degree of blood pressure lowering
Calcium channel blockers			
Nifedipine	SL or PO	0.5–1 mg/dose	Effective rapidly
Central nervous system agents			
Methyldopa	PO	5–40 mg/kg/day	May be sedating
Angiotensin-converting enzyme inhibitors			
Captopril	PO	0.05–0.5 mg/kg/dose	May cause marked oliguria, renal failure, or hyperkalemia
Enalaprilat	IV	5–28 μg/kg/day	May cause marked oliguria, renal failure, or hyperkalemia

*See text for details.
†Other β-adrenergic blockers have rarely been used in the neonatal period.

TABLE 35–7. ANTIHYPERTENSIVE MEDICATIONS FOR CHILDREN

Drug Class	Examples	Dosage	Comments
Thiazide diuretics	Chlorothiazide	20–30 mg/kg/day	Not very effective with GFR <30 mL/min/1.73m²
	Hydrochlorothiazide	2–3 mg/kg/day	
	Metolazone	2.5–5 mg once daily to start in adult; ? in child	
Loop diuretics	Furosemide	0.5–2 mg/kg/dose	May potentiate other antihypertensives
	Bumetanide	0.5–2 mg in adult; ? in child	May cause hypokalemia, hyperuricemia
Vasodilators	Hydralazine	0.1–3 mg/kg/day	Not good monotherapy; salt retention and reflex tachycardia
	Minoxidil	0.2 mg/kg to start; maximum 30–40 mg	Not good monotherapy; salt retention and reflex tachycardia; hirsutism
Beta-adrenergic blockers	Propranolol	0.5 mg/kg to start	Problematic if history of asthma
	Nadolol	40 mg once daily to start in adult; ? in child	
	Atenolol	50 mg once daily to start in adult; ? in child	
Alpha-adrenergic blocker	Prazosin	1 mg 2–3 × day in adult; ? in child	First dose may cause hypotension
Alpha- and beta-adrenergic blocker	Labetalol	0.25–0.5 mg/kg to start	
Central α_2-adrenergic agonists	Methyldopa	10 mg/kg/day	May cause sleepiness
	Clonidine	0.05–2.4 mg BID	May cause sleepiness; may cause rebound hypertension
ACE inhibitors	Captopril	0.5 mg/kg/day	Use ACE inhibitors with great caution in patients with single kidney
	Enalapril	2.5–5 mg once/day in adult to start; ? in child	
Calcium channel blockers	Verapamil	40 mg TID in adult to start; ? in child	
	Nifedipine	0.25–0.5 mg/kg to start	For older children, consider sustained release forms

Note: This table presents *examples* of various classes of antihypertensives used in treating hypertension. It is *not* meant to be exhaustive.
*See text for approach to the hypertensive child.
Abbreviations: GFR, glomerular filtration rate; ACE, angiotensin converting enzyme.

Chronic Antihypertensive Therapy

The therapy of sustained hypertension in children should follow several principles.[67, 68] The lowest dose, the fewest number of drugs, and the fewest side effects should be the aim of the prescriber. The typical pediatric patient requiring medication for hypertension is a teenager, and compliance with prescribed therapy is often problematic. Thus, close follow-up is recommended. The use of long-acting ACE inhibitors, combined with thiazides, is especially attractive for use in the athletic child or adolescent. However, there is little information on which to base doses. If a teenager receiving antihypertensive therapy becomes pregnant, it is critical that any ACE inhibitor therapy be stopped, given the occurrence of ACE fetopathy. The reader is referred to Chapter 41, Hypertension in Pregnancy.

Step-Down Therapy

Hypertension often becomes easier to manage in the hypertensive child after the blood pressure has been well controlled for a time. Thus, after a period of good blood pressure control, decreasing the dose to a minimum is important. If blood pressure has been fully normal for a substantial period, a trial without medication is indicated. The drugs listed in Tables 35–5 to 35–7 have had some history of safe and successful use in pediatric patients.

REFERENCES

1. Report of the Second Task Force on Blood Pressure Control in Children—1987. Pediatrics 1987; 79:1-25.
2. Feld LG: Hypertension. *In* Burg FB, Ingelfinger JR, Wald ER: Current Pediatric Therapy 14, pp 158–164. Philadelphia: WB Saunders, 1993.
3. Rosner B, Prineas RJ, Loggie JMH, Daniels SR: Blood pressure nomograms for children and adolescents, by height, sex and age, in the United States. J Pediatr 1993; 123:871–886.
4. Zinner SH, Rosner B, Oh W, Kass EH: Significance of blood pressure in infancy. Familial aggregation and predictive effect on later blood pressure. Hypertension 1985; 7:411–416.
5. Schacter J, Cutler LH, Perfetti C: Blood pressure during the first two years of life. Am J Epidemiol 1982; 116:29–41.
6. Burke GL, Voors AW, Shear CL, et al: Blood pressure: the Bogalusa Heart Study. Pediatrics 1987; 80(suppl):784–788.
7. Lauer RM, Anderson AR, Beaglehole R, Burns TL: Factors related to tracking of blood pressure in children. U.S. National Center for Health Statistics Health Examinations Surveys Cycles I and II. Hypertension 1984; 6:307–314.
8. Londe S: Causes of hypertension in the young. Pediatr Clin North Am 1978; 25:55–65.
9. Boineau FG, Lewy JE: Renal parenchymatous disease causes hypertension. *In* Loggie JMH (ed): Pediatric and Adolescent Hypertension, pp 202–216. Boston: Blackwell Scientific, 1992.
10. Jacobson SH, Eklof O, Eriksson CF, et al: Development of hypertension and uraemia after pyelonephritis in childhood: 27-year follow-up. Br Med J 1989; 299:703–706.
11. Southwest Pediatric Nephrology Study Group: Focal segmental glomerulosclerosis in children with idopathic nephrotic syndrome. Kidney Int 1985; 27:442–449.
12. Ramirez F, Brouhard BH, Travis LB, Ellin EN: Idiopathic membranous nephropathy in children. J Pediatr 1982; 101:677–681.
13. Vendemia F, Fornasiera A, Velis O, et al: Different prevalence rates of hypertension in various reno-parenchymal diseases. *In* Blaufox MD, Bianchi C (eds): Secondary Forms of Hypertension: Current Diagnosis and Management, pp 89–94. New York: Grune & Stratton, 1981.
14. International study of kidney disease in children. Nephrotic syndrome in children: prediction of histopathology from clinical and laboratory characteristics at time of diagnosis. Kidney Int 1978; 13:159–165.
15. West CD: Childhood membranoproliferative glomerulonephritis: an approach to managment. Kidney Int 1973; 29:1077–1093.
16. Habib R, Kleinknecht C, Gubler MC: Extramembranous glomerulonephritis in children: report of 50 cases. J Pediatr 1973; 82:754–756.
17. Siegler RL, Milligan MK, Burningham TH, et al: Long-term outcome and prognostic indicators in the hemolytic uremic syndrome. J Pediatr 1991; 118:195–200.
18. Ingelfinger JR: Renovascular disease in children [Clinical Conference]. Kidney Int 1993; 43:493–505.
19. McGrath BP, Clarke K: Renal artery stenosis: current diagnosis and treatment. Med J Aust 1993; 158:343–346.
20. Daniels SR, Loggie JMH, Schwartz DC, et al: Systemic hypertension secondary to peripheral vascular anomalies in patients with Williams syndrome. J Pediatr 1985; 106:249–251.
21. Menser MA, Dorman DC, Reye RDK, Reid RR: Renal-artery stenosis in the rubella syndrome. Lancet 1966; 1:790–792.
22. Marcus B, Hohn AR: Coarctation of the aorta. *In* Loggie JMH (ed): Pediatric and Adolescent Hypertension, pp 288–300. Boston: Blackwell Scientific, 1992.
23. Hesslein PS, McNamara DG, Morriss MJH, et al: Comparison of resection versus patch aortoplasty for repair of coarctation in infants and children. Circulation 1981; 64:164–168.
24. Maron BJ, Humphries JO, Rowe RD, Mellits ED: Prognosis of surgically corrected coarctation of the aorta: a 20 year post-operative appraisal. Circulation 1973; 47:119–126.
25. Waldhausen JA, Nahrwold DL: Repair of coarctation of the aorta with a subclavian flap. J Thorac Cardiovasc Surg 1966; 51:532–533.
26. Heymann MA, Berman W Jr, Rudolf A, Whitman V: Dilatation of the ductus arteriosus by prostaglandin E_1 in aortic arch abnormalities. Circulation 1979; 59:169–173.
27. Mendelsohn AM, Lloyd TR, Crowley DC, et al: Late follow-up of balloon angioplasty in children with a native coarctation of the aorta. Am J Cardiol 1994; 74:696–700.
28. Sohn S, Rothman A, Shiota T, et al: Acute and follow-up intravascular ultrasound findings after balloon dilation of coarctation of the aorta. Cirulation 1994; 90:340–347.
29. Rocchini AP, Rosenthal A, Barger AC, et al: Pathogenesis of paradoxical hypertension after coarctation resection. Circulation 1976; 54:382–387.
30. Loggie JMH: Catecholamine-producing tumors that cause hypertension: diagnosis and management. *In* Loggie JMH (ed): Pediatric and Adolescent Hypertension, pp 301–313. Boston: Blackwell Scientific, 1992.
31. Stackpole RH, Melicow MM, Uson AC: Pheochromocytoma in children. Report of 9 cases and review of the first 100 published cases with follow-up studies. J Pediatr 1963; 63:315–330.
32. Quint LE, Glazer GM, Francis IR, et al: Pheochromocytoma and paraganglioma: comparison of MR imaging with CT and I-131 MIBG scintigraphy in diagnosing pheochromocytoma. Am J Radiol 1983; 141:719–735.
33. Weinblatt ME, Heisel MA, Siegel SE: Hypertension in children with neurogenic tumors. Pediatrics 1883; 71:947–951.
34. Rodd CJ, Sockalosky JJ: Endocrine causes of hypertension in children. Pediatr Clin North Am 1993; 40:149–164.
35. Curnow KM, Slutsker L, Vitek J, et al: Mutations in the CYP11B1 gene causing congenital adrenal hypertension and hypertension cluster in exons 6, 7, and 8. Proc Natl Acad Sci USA 1993; 90:4552–4556.
36. Lifton RP, Dluhy RG, Powers M, et al: A chimaeric 11-beta hydroxylase/aldosterone synthase gene causes glucocorticoid-remediable aldosteronism and human hypertension. Nature 1992; 355:262–266.
37. Abbi RK, McVicar M, Teichberg S, et al: Pathologic characterization of a renin-secreting juxtaglomerular cell tumor in a child and review of the pediatric literature. Pediatr Pathol 1993; 13:443–451.
38. Dickinson CJ: Hypertension and central nervous system disease. *In* Swales JD (ed): Textbook of Hypertension, pp 980–986. Oxford: Blackwell Scientific, 1994.
39. Pranzatelli MR, De Vivo DC: The role of the central nervous system in blood pressure regulation. *In* Loggie JMH (ed): Pediatric and Adolescent Hypertension, pp 52–63. Cambridge: Blackwell Scientific, 1992.
40. Sinaiko AR, Gillum RF, Jacobs DR, et al: Renin angiotensin and sympathetic nervous system activity in grade school children. Hypertension 1982; 4:299–306.
41. McCrory WW, Klein AA, Fallo F: Predictors of blood pressure: humoral factors. *In* Loggie JMH, Horan MJ, Gruskin AB, et al (eds): NHLBI Workshop on Juvenile Hypertension, pp 181–202. New York: Biomedical Information, 1984.
42. Falkner B, Kushner H, Onesti G, Angelakos ET: Cardiovascular characteristics in adolescents who develop essential hypertension. Hypertension 1981; 3:521–527.
43. Rocchini AP: Adolescent obesity and hypertension. Pediatr Clin North Am 1993; 40:81–92.
44. Law CM, de Swiet M, Osmond C, et al: Initiation of hypertension in utero and its amplification in adult life. Br Med J 1993; 306:24–27.

45. Whicup PH, Papacosta O, Cook DH: Letters: initiation of hypertension in utero. Br Med J 1993; 306:6877.
46. Brenner BM, Garcia DL, Anderson S: The renal abnormality in hypertension: a proposed defect in glomerular filtration surface area. *In* Laragh JH, Brenner BM (eds): Hypertension: Pathophysiology Diagnosis and Management, pp 1151–1161. New York: Raven Press, 1990.
47. Goble MM: Hypertension in infancy. Pediatr Clin North Am 1993; 40:105–122.
48. Adelman RD: Long term follow-up of neonatal renovascular hypertension. Pediatr Nephrol 1987; 1:35–41.
49. Loggie JMH: Evaluation of the hypertensive child and adolescent. *In* Loggie JMH (ed): Pediatric and Adolescent Hypertension, pp 1112–1118. Cambridge: Blackwell Scientific, 1992.
50. Finta KM: Cardiovascular manifestations of hypertension in children. Pediatr Clin North Am 1993; 40:51–59.
51. Hillman BJ: Imaging advances in the diagnosis of renovascular hypertension. Am J Roentgenol 1989; 153:5–14.
52. Abernethy LF, Hendry GMA, Reid JH: Fibromuscular dysplasia of the renal artery in a child: detection by Doppler ultrasound and correction by percutaneous transluminal anigoplasty. Pediatr Radiol 1989; 19:539–540.
53. Zerin JM, Hernandez RJ: Renal imaging in children with persistent hypertension. Pediatr Clin North Am 1993; 40:165–178.
54. Guillery EN, Robillard JE: The renin-angiotensin system and blood pressure regulation during infancy and childhood. Pediatr Clin North Am 1993; 40:61–79.
55. Harshfield GA, Alpert BS, Pulliam DA: Renin angiotensin aldosterone system in healthy subjects aged ten to eighteen years. J Pediatr 1993; 122:563–567.
56. Gillman MW, Cook NR, Rosner B, et al: Identifying children at high risk for the development of essential hypertension. J Pediatr 1993; 122:837–846.
57. Sinaiko AR, Gomez-Marin O, Prineas RJ: Effect of low sodium diet or potassium supplementation on adolescent blood pressure. Hypertension 1993; 21:989–994.
58. Becque MD, Katch VL, Rocchini AP, et al: Coronary risk incidence of obese adolescents: reduction by exercise plus diet intervention. Pediatrics 1988; 81:605–612.
59. Rocchini AP, Katch V, Anderson J, et al: Blood pressure in obese adolescents: effect of weight loss. Pediatrics 1988; 82:16–23.
60. Brownell KD, Kelaren JH, Stunkard AJ: Treatment of obese children with and without their mothers: changes in weight and blood pressure. Pediatrics 1983; 71:515–523.
61. Hofman A, Hazebroek A, Valkenburg HA: A randomized trial of sodium intake and blood pressure in newborn infants. JAMA 1983; 250:370–373.
62. Geleijnse JM, Grobbee DE, Hofman A: Sodium intake and blood pressure change in childhood. Br Med J 1990; 300:899–902.
63. Sinaiko AR, Gomez-Marin O, Prineas RJ: Effect of low sodium diet or potassium supplementation on adolescent blood pressure. Hypertension 1993; 21:989–994.
64. Christiansen JL, Strong WB: Blood pressure in young athletes. *In* Loggie JMH (ed): Pediatric and Adolescent Hypertension, pp 323–332. Boston: Blackwell Scientific, 1995.
65. Spirito P, Maron BJ, Bonow RO, Epstein SE: Prevalence and significance of an abnormal S-T segment response to exercise in a young athletic population. Am J Cardiol 1983; 51:1663–1666.
66. Eisenberg DM, Delbanco TL, Berkey CS, et al: Review: cognitive behavioral techniques for hypertension: are they effective? Ann Intern Med 1993; 118:964–972.
67. Sinaiko AR: Pharmacologic management of childhood hypertension. Pediatr Clin North Am 1993; 40:195–212.
68. Bunchman TE, Lynch RE, Wood EG: Intravenously administered labetalol for treatment of hypertension in children. J Pediatr 1992; 120:140–144.
69. Angeli P, Chieza M, Caregaro L, et al: Comparison of sublingual captopril and nifedipine in immediate treatment of hypertensive emergencies. Arch Intern Med 1991; 151:678–682.
70. Deal JE, Barratt TM, Dillon MJ: Management of hypertensive emergencies. Arch Dis Child 1992; 67:1089–1092.
71. Houston M: Pathophysiology, clinical aspects and treatment of hypertensive crises. Prog Cardiovasc Dis 1989; 232:99–148.
72. Calhoun DA, Oparil S: Treatment of hypertensive crisis. N Engl J Med 1990; 323:1177–1183.

36 Evaluation and Treatment of Hypertension in the Elderly Patient

James A. Schoenberger, MD

SCOPE OF THE PROBLEM

Although there is no precise definition of "elderly," in current use the term applies to persons 65 years of age or older. This segment of the U.S. population is the most rapidly growing, increasing to 13% (31.2 million) by 1990. Furthermore, people over the age of 85 constitute an even more rapidly growing part of the elderly population, and more than 16 million will be that age by 2050.[1]

This trend of an aging population is of tremendous importance from a public health standpoint and will have a major impact on health care costs.[2] The trend will also be of major importance to primary care physicians because a high percentage of elderly persons are hypertensive and their treatment will be a part of those costs.

The proposed classification of blood pressure by both systolic and diastolic values is shown in Table 36–1.[3] It differs from previous classifications in that systolic hypertension is defined for the first time. This is an important change based on the recognition that systolic hypertension is an independent and significant risk factor for cardiovascular disease. Isolated systolic hypertension (ISH) is defined as a systolic blood pressure (SBP) of 140 mm Hg or higher with a diastolic blood pressure (DBP) of less than 90 mm Hg. With use of these criteria, the prevalence of high blood pressure in the elderly can be seen in Table 36–2. It is higher in African-Americans of both genders and comparable in whites and Mexican-Americans. It is clear that blood pressure greater than 140/90 mm Hg is common among the elderly, affecting more than half of that population. The prevalence of ISH in the general population as defined by a SBP of 160 mm Hg or higher is 6% among persons aged 65–69 years, 11%

TABLE 36–1. CLASSIFICATION OF BLOOD PRESSURE FOR ADULTS AGED 18 YEARS AND OLDER*

Category	Systolic (mm Hg)	Diastolic (mm Hg)
Normal†	<130	<85
High-normal	130–139	85–89
Hypertension‡		
Stage 1	140–159	90–99
Stage 2	160–179	100–109
Stage 3	180–209	110–119
Stage 4	≥210	≥120

*Not taking antihypertensive drugs and not acutely ill. When systolic and diastolic pressures fall into different categories, the higher category should be selected to classify the individual's blood pressure status. For instance, 160/92 mm Hg should be classified as stage 2, and 180/120 mm Hg should be classified as stage 4. Isolated systolic hypertension is defined as a systolic blood pressure of 140 mm Hg or more and a diastolic blood pressure below 90 mm Hg and staged appropriately (e.g., 170/85 mm Hg is defined as stage 2 isolated systolic hypertension). In addition to classifying stages of hypertension on the basis of average blood pressure levels, the clinician should specify presence or absence of target organ disease and additional risk factors. For example, a patient with diabetes and a blood pressure of 142/94 mm Hg plus left ventricular hypertrophy should be classified as having "stage 1 hypertension with target organ disease (left ventricular hypertrophy) and with another major risk factor (diabetes)." This specificity is important for risk classification and management.

†Optimal blood pressure with respect to cardiovascular risk is less than both 120 mm Hg systolic and 80 mm Hg diastolic. However, unusually low readings should be evaluated for clinical significance.

‡Based on the average of two or more readings taken at each of two or more visits after an initial screening.

From the Joint National Committee on the Detection, Evaluation, and Treatment of High Blood Pressure: Fifth Report of the Joint National Committee on Detection, Evaluation, and Treatment of High Blood Pressure. Arch Intern Med 1993; 153:154–183.

in those aged 70–79 years, and 22% in those aged 80 years and older. Rates are higher among women and nonwhites.[4] Among hypertensive patients, ISH was present in 58.9% of men aged 60–74 years and in 74.6% of men 75 years of age and older. For women, the comparable prevalence was 61% and 73.7%.[1]

In summary, the U.S. population is aging, and more than half older than 65 years are hypertensive, as defined by a SBP of 140 mm Hg or a DBP of 90 mm Hg or higher. Of this hypertensive population, almost two thirds have ISH.

RELATIONSHIP OF BLOOD PRESSURE TO MORBIDITY AND MORTALITY

The relationship of DBP and SBP to cardiovascular events has been demonstrated in the 30-year follow-up of the Framingham Heart Study, as shown in Figure 36–1.[5] The risk is greater for those aged 65–94 years than in those aged 35–64 years for both men and women. SBP is as predictive of risk as is DBP, and the increase in risk becomes evident at levels below 140 mm Hg. At any level of SBP or DBP, women are at lower risk than are men, presumably because of the role of other factors in the cause of cardiovascular disease. In nine prospective observational studies, similar relationships have been shown to exist for DBP.[6] There is a log-linear relationship between DBP and the risk of stroke and coronary heart disease (CHD). The risk begins to increase significantly well below 90 mm Hg (Fig. 36–2).

These relationships underscore the difficulty in defining hypertension. At present, the definition of 140/90 mm Hg or greater[3] serves as a guideline for initiation of therapeutic measures that have been shown in clinical trials to be effective and beneficial. Future studies may establish the value of treatment of lower levels of elevated blood pressure, especially in high-risk groups such as those with renal disease[7] or diabetes.[8] This supports the concept of identifying SBP levels in the range of 140–159 mm Hg and DBP levels in the range of 85–89 mm Hg as high-normal.

The pathogenesis of hypertension is discussed in other chapters. In the elderly, rigidity of the major arterial tree is considered to be one of the main causes of elevated blood pressure. Accompanying this is a fall in cardiac output.[9] In these circumstances, the major characteristic of hypertension in the elderly is an increase in peripheral resistance. Therapy designed to lower peripheral resistance should be the most appropriate physiologic way to lower blood pressure in the elderly. This may not always be possible in the presence of rigid and sclerotic major blood vessels.

EVALUATION OF HYPERTENSION IN THE ELDERLY

The evaluation of hypertension in an elderly person is similar in many respects to that of any hypertensive patient (see Chapter 32 for details) and the methods of measurement have now been standardized,[10] with several important caveats.

Orthostatic Effects

Postural and postprandial falls in blood pressure are common in the elderly, and evaluation of the elderly patient must include a measurement of blood pressure after the patient has been standing for 3 min. It has been estimated that nearly 20% of elderly persons experience a fall in SBP of 20 mm Hg or more while standing.[11] Normal orthostatic changes are a mean fall in SBP of 6.5 mm Hg and a mean rise in DBP of 5.6 mm Hg.[12] After treatment is initiated, standing blood pressure measurements should be repeated at regular intervals. The risk of syncope and injury caused by falling is real and must be avoided.

Pseudohypertension

In the face of sclerotic peripheral arteries, an excessive elevation in cuff pressure may be necessary to determine the blood pressure, but it gives rise to falsely high readings. This phenomenon may be

TABLE 36–2. TRENDS IN HYPERTENSION* PREVALENCE BY GENDER AND ETHNICITY IN THE CIVILIAN, NONINSTITUTIONALIZED POPULATION, AGED 65–74 YEARS, DURING 1976–1980 AND 1988–1991

Gender and Ethnic Group	1976–1980 (%)	1988–1991 (%)
Women	67.5	52.5
African-Americans	82.9	71.9†
Whites	66.2	51.2†
Mexican-Americans	—	53.1
Men	60.2	56.4
African-Americans	67.1	71.6†
Whites	59.2	54.9†
Mexican-Americans	—	56.9
Total	64.3	54.3
African-Americans	76.1	71.8†
Whites	63.1	52.9†
Mexican-Americans	—	54.9

*Defined as the average of three blood pressure measurements ≥140 mm Hg (systolic) and/or ≥90 mm Hg (diastolic) on a single occasion or taking antihypertensive medication. Estimates based on three blood pressure measurements taken by physicians in the Health and Nutrition Examination Survey mobile examination center.

†Non-Hispanics.

From the Centers for Disease Control and Prevention, National Center for Health Statistics: The Second National Health and Nutrition Examination Survey (NHANES II), 1976–1980 (Vital Health Stat [11], 1986. US Dept of Health and Human Services publication PHS 86–1684); and unpublished data from Hispanic HANES, 1982–1984, and NHANES III, 1988–1991. Totals include racial and/or ethnic groups not shown separately.

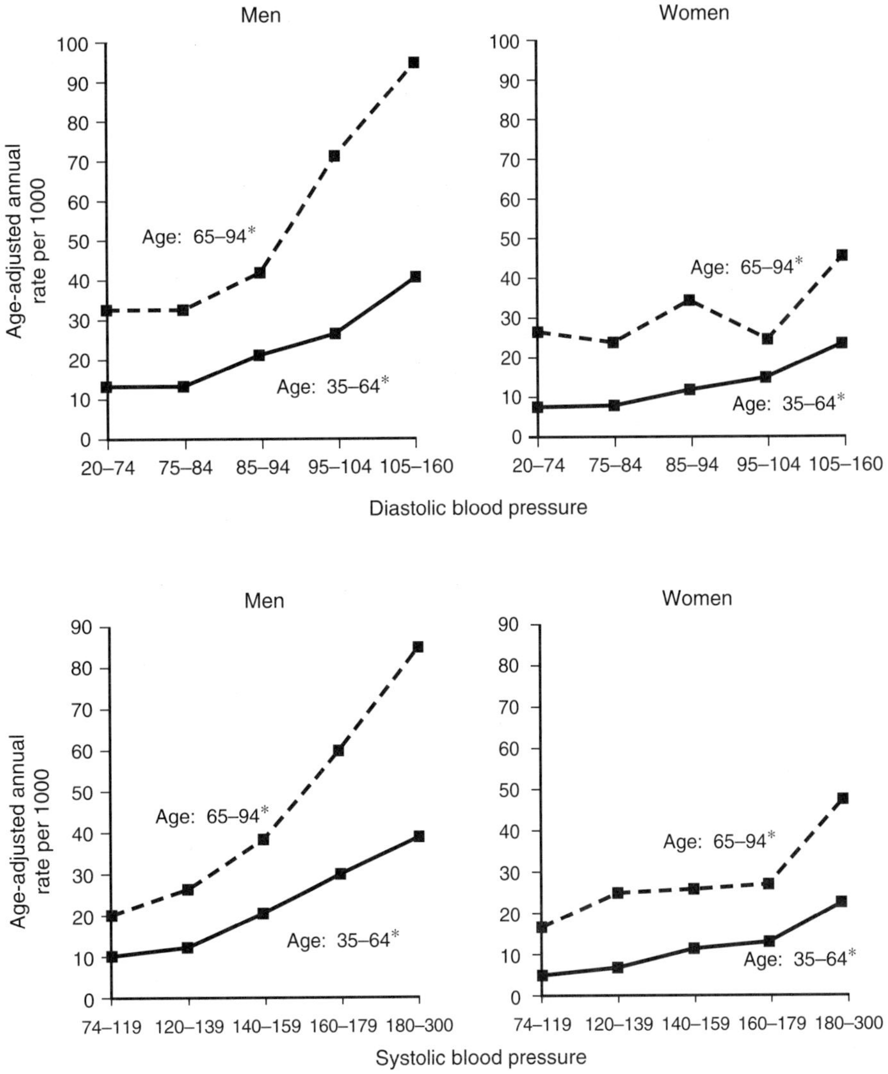

Figure 36–1. Risk of cardiovascular disease, by age, sex, and level of diastolic or systolic blood pressure, from a 30-year follow-up in the Framingham Heart Study. The relation of systolic and diastolic blood pressures to cardiovascular events is generally more pronounced in people aged 65 to 94 years than in those aged 35 to 64 years. Increased evidence of cardiovascular disease occurs at a higher diastolic blood pressure of 75 mm Hg or greater in men but is not definitively evident until 95 mm Hg in women. $^{***}p < .001$ (Wald statistic for logistic regression analysis). (From Vokonas PS, Kannel WB, Cupples LA: Epidemiology and risk of hypertension in the elderly: the Framingham Study. J Hypertens Suppl 1988; 6:S3–S9.)

suspected if the brachial artery remains palpable after SBP in the cuff is exceeded (Osler maneuver). The prevalence of pseudohypertension was found to be 7.1% in a geriatric clinic population.[13] Pseudohypertension should be suspected when there is no evidence of target organ damage in the presence of high levels of blood pressure.

Use of Ambulatory Monitoring

The persistence of elevated blood pressure measurements in the clinic setting and normal values elsewhere has been termed *white-coat hypertension*. It may be present in up to 20% of patients with mild hypertension.[14] However, its frequency among elderly patients is unknown. It is important to identify such patients to avoid unnecessary treatment. Portable devices are available for determining blood pressure during a 24-h period. Their expense, with lack of coverage by insurance carriers, has precluded their widespread use. Therefore, at present, despite their proven reliability, ambulatory blood pressure monitors are not recommended,[3] even though they may be especially useful in the elderly because the blood pressure is often labile. For most purposes, home blood pressure measurement with relatively inexpensive devices permit better evaluation of blood pressure than do clinical measurements alone, and their use in elderly patients should be encouraged. They should be monitored by office personnel to ensure accuracy of home measurements, and patients should be instructed to record the time and blood pressure reading so that the measurement can be made available to the physician.

Important Physical Findings

A careful physical examination of the patient is an essential component of care of the elderly hypertensive. Special attention should be focused on the cardiovascular system to determine the presence of target organ damage. Examination of the ocular fundi should always be carried out. Although there can be some lack of agreement about early changes (arteriolar narrowing or spasm), definite changes such as arteriovenous compression, hemorrhage, exudates, and papilledema when present confirm the existence of clinically important hypertension. Modern, effective treatment has rendered such findings to a lesser degree of prognostic significance than was once the case. In the elderly, cataracts may prevent adequate ophthalmoscopic examination.

The presence of bruits confirms the existence of significant arteriosclerosis. When present in the neck, bruits may indicate the risk of transient ischemic attacks or stroke. When present in the lower extremities, a bruit may be accompanied by ischemia and intermittent claudication. In any event, the widespread presence of bruits is indirect evidence that coronary arteriosclerosis may also be present. A continuous systolic-diastolic abdominal bruit suggests renal artery

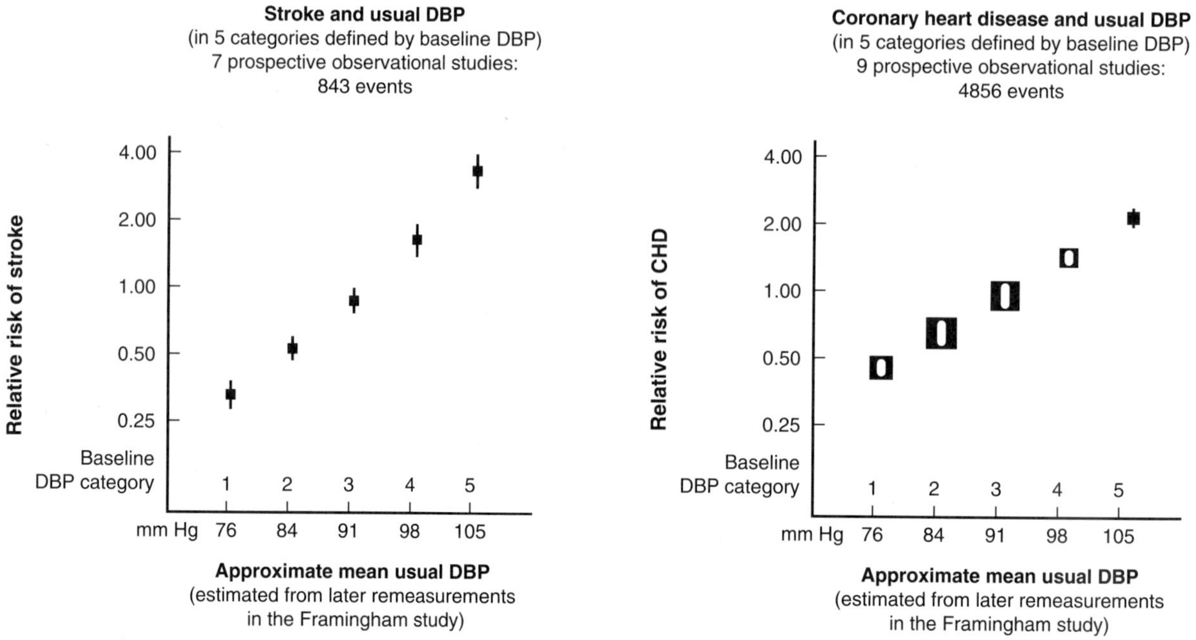

Figure 36–2. Relative risks of stroke and of coronary heart disease, estimated from combined results. Estimates of the usual diastolic blood pressure (DBP) in each baseline DBP category are taken from mean DBP values 4 years after baseline in the Framingham Study. Solid squares represent disease risks in each category in relation to risk in the whole study population; sizes of squares are proportional to number of events in each DBP category; 95% confidence intervals for estimates of relative risk are denoted by vertical lines. (From MacMahon S, Peto R, Cutler J, et al: Blood pressure, stroke, and coronary heart disease: Part 1. Prolonged differences in blood pressure: prospective observational studies corrected for the regression and dilution bias. Lancet 1990; 335:765–774.)

stenosis. The existence of an abdominal aneurysm, more common in the elderly, should also be ruled out by careful palpation.

In addition to the physical examination, a careful history should be obtained. Recent onset of hypertension or sudden resistance to previously effective treatment suggests hypertension secondary to renal artery stenosis. Cardiac symptoms, such as fatigue and dyspnea on exertion, suggest coronary artery disease even in the absence of angina. Transient ischemic attacks are also of great importance.

Important Laboratory Findings

Evidence of target organ damage in the elderly can also be obtained from certain laboratory studies. Left ventricular hypertrophy is a common sequela of sustained hypertension because of pressure overload. However, other factors, including hormonal agents such as catecholamines and angiotensin, play a role. It has been shown that left ventricular hypertrophy is an independent risk factor for cardiovascular disease. Left ventricular hypertrophy can be detected by electrocardiography or echocardiography. Electrocardiography is relatively insensitive; echocardiography is much more likely to detect left ventricular hypertrophy. With use of echocardiography, it has been shown that the prevalence of left ventricular hypertrophy rises with age to as high as 50%, thereby increasing its predictive value in the elderly. The risk attached to left ventricular hypertrophy determined by echocardiography is similar to that previously demonstrated for left ventricular hypertrophy detected by electrocardiography.[15] Although the routine use of echocardiography in evaluation of the hypertensive patient is not recommended,[3] it does provide useful information in confirming the existence of target organ damage to the myocardium. Because the frequency of arrhythmias increases with the existence of left ventricular hypertrophy, it is important to monitor serum electrolyte levels carefully in hypertensive patients with left ventricular hypertrophy treated with a diuretic or digitalis.[16]

The presence of renal impairment is other evidence of target organ damage. Hypertension is the most important cause of loss of renal function along with diabetes. Evidence for renal damage may be found if proteinuria is present. The routine dipstick is a relatively insensitive method for detecting proteinuria. Excretion of minute amounts of protein can be detected by tests for microalbuminuria.[17] In addition, the level of serum creatinine is useful in detecting renal insufficiency. In older adults, muscle mass declines, and a creatinine concentration still within the normal range may mask significant renal insufficiency. Levels above 1.3 mg/dL should arouse suspicion.[1]

In summary, the laboratory evaluation of the elderly hypertensive patient need not be extensive or expensive. The cause of the hypertension is primary in the majority of cases, so it is not cost effective to routinely rule out hypertension secondary to other underlying conditions. The laboratory studies necessary before initiation of treatment are shown in Table 36–3.[3]

TREATMENT

Therapeutic Choices

Once the patient has been found to be hypertensive, several options are available for treatment as detailed in Chapter 32. These include lifestyle modification alone or in combination with antihypertensive medication. All the currently available drugs have been found to be effective in the elderly. The choice of which drug to use may depend on concurrent conditions, such as known CHD, diabetes, or serum lipid abnormalities. The choice can also be influenced by the results of clinical trials that have evaluated the ability of these drugs to prevent the cardiovascular morbidity and mortality resulting from hypertension in the elderly.

Levels for Initiation of Treatment

The guidelines of the Fifth Report of the Joint National Committee on the Detection, Evaluation, and Treatment of High Blood Pressure (JNC-5) recommend initiation of pharmacologic treatment when the blood pressure is persistently above 140/90 mm Hg despite lifestyle modification.[3] The decision is strengthened by evidence of target

TABLE 36–3. RECOMMENDED LABORATORY TESTS AND DIAGNOSTIC PROCEDURES

Routine
Complete blood count
Urinalysis
Serum electrolytes
Creatinine
Total cholesterol
High-density lipoprotein cholesterol
Triglyceride
Electrocardiogram
Optional
24-h urine for microalbuminuria
Echocardiogram

From the Joint National Committee on the Detection, Evaluation, and Treatment of High Blood Pressure: Fifth Report of the Joint National Committee on the Detection, Evaluation, and Treatment of High Blood Pressure. Arch Intern Med 1993; 153:154–183.

organ damage or the presence of CHD risk factors. Evidence from clinical trials also supports the action. Delay in initiating treatment in mildly elevated blood pressure without target organ damage or other risk factors may permit the blood pressure to become more severe. Also, it has been shown that the benefits of treatment are greater if treatment is initiated before there is target organ damage,[18] although no data specifically support this conclusion in the elderly.

In the case of ISH, the guidelines recommend treatment when SBP is persistently above 160 mm Hg. This recommendation is based on the results of clinical trials in the elderly. In the absence of trial results, the guidelines advise only lifestyle modification for the treatment of ISH in the range of 140–159 mm Hg.[3]

Lifestyle Modification

Lifestyle or nonpharmacologic intervention in the treatment of hypertension has been found to be successful in lowering blood pressure.[3] It has not been proved that reduction of elevated blood pressure achieved in this manner will prolong life or prevent the complications of hypertension. Lifestyle changes are discussed in detail in Chapter 32. Of importance is that there have been no studies to support or reject this approach in the elderly. However, in the absence of such data, it seems prudent to encourage appropriate lifestyle modifications, including any necessary weight reduction, reduction of alcohol intake, and particularly salt restriction and exercise.[19, 20]

SBP appears to be more responsive to salt restriction, and older and black patients have greater reductions. The JNC-5 recommends reducing salt intake to 100 mmol (6 g) per day.[3] Reductions greater than this are hard to achieve because of the high salt content of processed foods. Salt labeling, now required, may help the consumer to make appropriate choices.

Exercise is useful as an adjunct to weight reduction and improving quality of life. There are no data to support the use of exercise to prolong life in elderly patients. Because of the frequency of associated arthritic problems, only mild exercise is advised for elderly patients. Walking 3–4 miles at a brisk pace three or four times a week probably confers maximal benefit. Isometric exercise, such as weightlifting, should be avoided.

In the Treatment of Mild Hypertension Study (TOMHS), patients were provided sustained nutritional-hygienic advice[21] designed to induce weight loss, reduce alcohol and sodium intake, and increase physical activity. At the end of 4 years, the average weight loss was 2.6 kg, urinary sodium level was reduced by about 10%, and alcohol consumption was decreased by an average of one drink a day. Even with intensive and sustained counseling throughout the 4 years, maximal improvement was noted after the first year for weight loss and sodium excretion. SBP fell 9.1 mm Hg and DBP fell 8.6 mm Hg at the end of 4 years. These findings confirm the value of lifestyle modification. The mean age of TOMHS participants was 55 years; age range on entry was 45–69 years. Thus, whether the benefit from these measures in reducing elevated blood pressure would apply to elderly hypertensives is uncertain.

Antihypertensive Drugs

There is extensive literature on antihypertensive drugs, and their use is discussed in Chapter 32. In this section, the discussion is confined to the efficiency and safety of these drugs in the elderly hypertensive.

Diuretics

Diuretics enhance the secretion of salt and water, reducing plasma volume and cardiac output initially. Within 6 to 8 weeks, plasma volume and cardiac output return toward normal, and the persistent reduction in blood pressure results from a fall in peripheral resistance.[3] Many adverse side effects of diuretics are increased in the elderly and are generally related to the dose. Excess mortality was seen in the Multiple Risk Factor Intervention Trial when doses of chlorthalidone or hydrochlorothiazide were 50 mg or higher,[22] and since that report, lower doses have been recommended. Despite that, there are still some adverse metabolic effects of diuretic therapy: hypokalemia, hyperglycemia, increased insulin resistance, and increase in low-density lipoprotein cholesterol.[1] The clinical importance of these effects is unknown, but they do tend to increase the risk of atherogenesis and possibly detract from the full benefit of blood pressure reduction. Because of these changes, patients must be monitored for effects on potassium, glucose, and lipids. In clinical practice, diuretics have been found to be particularly effective in the elderly and in black patients.[1] However, they must be used with caution when renal impairment is present or plasma volume is depleted, both of which are more common among the elderly. The recommended starting dose for hydrochlorothiazide is 12.5 mg.[3]

Beta Blockers

Beta blockers lower blood pressure by reducing cardiac output.[23] They have adverse metabolic effects on glucose and lipid metabolism, increasing insulin resistance and glucose intolerance. Lipid changes include an increase in triglycerides and a fall in high-density lipoprotein. These lipid changes are not seen in beta blockers possessing intrinsic sympathomimetic activity. Beta blockers are contraindicated in patients with chronic obstructive lung disease and in congestive heart failure due to systolic dysfunction. In general, older patients do not respond as well to beta blockers[24] and have an increased risk of side effects.

Calcium Channel Blockers

The three classes of calcium channel blockers are all equally effective in reducing elevated blood pressure but differ in cardiac and hemodynamic effects. Blood pressure is reduced by vasodilatation,[25] and they may be particularly useful in elderly patients. The dihydropyridine calcium channel blockers are more likely to cause headache and edema, and the others are likely to be associated with gastrointestinal side effects such as constipation. However, each of these side effects may be exaggerated in the elderly.

Angiotensin Converting Enzyme Inhibitors

These drugs lower blood pressure by blocking the conversion of angiotensin I to angiotensin II, thereby causing vasodilatation.[3] The angiotensin converting enzyme (ACE) inhibitors do not have adverse effects on serum lipids and have been shown to exert a beneficial effect on insulin resistance.[26] The ACE inhibitors have a favorable effect on quality of life, but their use is associated with a troublesome dry cough. This is thought to be caused by an accumulation of bradykinin and prostaglandins. It has been reported to occur in 5%–20% of patients,[27] but the percentage of patients who quit or are removed from ACE therapy is not precisely known. Although elderly hypertensives have low plasma renin levels, the ACE inhibitors are highly effective.[28]

Alpha Blockers

The alpha blockers reduce peripheral resistance by selectively blocking the α_1-receptors, thereby lowering blood pressure.[29] They have a beneficial effect on blood lipids[29] and may also have a beneficial effect on the symptoms of prostatic hypertrophy. Alpha blockers have been shown to improve insulin resistance. Some caution in their use in the elderly is appropriate because they may cause first-dose syncope or postural hypotension.

Findings From Clinical Trials

It has been shown that hypertension is extremely common among the elderly and that it is associated with an increase in cardiovascular disease, especially heart attack, stroke, and renovascular damage. Measures for reducing elevated blood pressure in the elderly are effective and well tolerated. All classes of antihypertensive agents lower elevated blood pressure to a comparable degree.

From a therapeutic standpoint, there are two questions: (1) Is there a benefit to the patient from blood pressure reduction? (2) What is the best regimen for achieving the desired goal of preventing the morbidity and mortality from hypertension in the elderly?

The clinical trials to be reviewed here convincingly answer the first question. Because not all of the antihypertensive drugs in use have been tested in clinical trials, the second question remains unanswered. As stated previously, lifestyle modification has not yet been shown to be effective in preventing the complications of hypertension. Nevertheless, effective lifestyle modification should be employed in the overall management of every elderly hypertensive patient.

A review of the literature on antihypertensive drug treatment of elderly hypertensive patients published from 1980 to 1992 revealed nine major trials involving 15,559 patients older than 59 years.[30] The nine trials are described individually, and the results of a meta-analysis are presented. In all of the trials, diuretics and beta blockers were the main drugs used.

The Australian National Blood Pressure Study

In this study, 582 patients with a mean age of 63 years were studied for an average of 3.4 years.[31] Chlorothiazide, methyldopa, propranolol, pindolol, hydralazine, and clonidine were compared with placebo. At entry, the SBP was 166.3 mm Hg and the DPB was 100.9 mm Hg. DBP fell 6.7 mm Hg. The fall in SBP was not reported. The death rate was 2.4% in the treatment group, compared with 3.1% in the control group.

Systolic Hypertension in the Elderly Program

This is the only study in which the patients had ISH.[32] The 4736 patients were mainly white and had a mean age of 71.6 years. The drugs used included chlorthalidone, atenolol, and reserpine compared with placebo. On entry, the SBP was 170.5 mm Hg and the DBP was 76.7 mm Hg. SBP fell 11.1 mm Hg, and DBP fell 3.4 mm Hg. The 5-year incidence of total stroke was 5.2% in treated patients vs. 8.2% in the control subjects, a 36% reduction. Nonfatal myocardial infarction plus coronary death was reduced by 37%, all major cardiovascular events were reduced by 32%, and total mortality was reduced by 13% (10.2% in the control group to 9.0% in the treated group). This trial is one of few trials to demonstrate a statistically significant reduction in coronary heart disease.

Hypertension Detection and Follow-Up Program

In this study, 2376 participants with a mean age of 63.9 years, 44% of whom were black, were randomized to special care or referred care in the community.[33] Treatment in the special care consisted of chlorthalidone, hydralazine, spironolactone, reserpine, and methyldopa. At entry, SBP was 170.9 mm Hg and DBP was 101.6 mm Hg. At the end of the study, the difference in DBP between the special care group and the referred care group was 5.1 mm Hg. Total mortality was reduced from 15.8% to 12.7%. Stroke was reduced by 44%; CHD, by 15%.

Medical Research Council

In this study, 4396 patients with a mean age of 70.3 years received atenolol, hydrochlorothiazide, nifedipine, or placebo.[34] At entry, the SBP was 184.5 mm Hg and the DBP was 91.0 mm Hg. At the end of the trial, SBP was reduced by 6.3 mm Hg and DBP by 5.9 mm Hg. Total mortality fell from 14.2% to 13.8%. Stroke was reduced by 25%; CHD, by 19%.

The Practice in Primary Care

In this study, 884 patients with a mean age of 68.8 years were randomized to atenolol, bendroflumethiazide, or methyldopa or to an observational control group.[35] Entry SBP was 196.7 mm Hg, and entry DBP was 98.7 mm Hg. A fall of 11 mm Hg in DBP and a fall of 18 mm Hg in SBP were noted. Mortality was 14.3% in the treatment group and 14.8% in the control group. Stroke was reduced by 42%, but no benefit for CHD was observed.

European Working Party on High Blood Pressure in the Elderly

The 840 patients in this study had a mean age of 72.0 years. They received hydrochlorothiazide with triamterene and methyldopa or placebo.[36] Entry SBP was 183.0 mm Hg, and entry DBP was 101.0 mm Hg. A fall of 10 mm Hg in DBP and a fall of 22 mm Hg in SBP were noted. Total mortality fell from 35.1% to 32.5%. Stroke was reduced by 36%.

Swedish Trial in Old Patients With Hypertension

In this study, 1627 patients with a mean age of 75.6 years received atenolol, hydrochlorothiazide with amiloride, metoprolol, and pendolol or placebo.[37] Entry SBP was 195 mm Hg, and entry DBP was 102 mm Hg. A fall of 10 mm Hg in DBP and a fall of 27.0 mm Hg in SBP were observed. Mortality in the treatment group was 4.4%, compared with 7.7% in the control group. Stroke was reduced by 47%.

Veterans Administration

In this early trial, 380 men with an age range of 60–75 years were randomized to treatment with a chlorothiazide, reserpine, and hydralazine or placebo.[38] Entry SBP was 165.1 mm Hg, and entry DBP was 104.7 mm Hg. A fall of 18.6 mm Hg in DBP was noted.

With use of the criteria in the meta-analysis,[30] the mortality rate was not determinable.

Sprackling

The final trial entered into the meta-analysis involved 120 patients treated with methyldopa or observation.[39] Entry SBP was 190.1 mm Hg, and entry DBP was 106.7 mm Hg. DBP fell 7.5 mm Hg, and SBP fell 18.4 mm Hg. The death rate fell from 80.7% to 73.7%.

Meta-Analysis of Trial Results

The results of these nine trials are summarized in Table 36–4. A meta-analysis of the results revealed a 12% reduction in all-cause mortality (p = .009), a 36% reduction in stroke mortality (p < .001), and a 25% reduction in CHD mortality (p < .001). Coronary morbidity was reduced by 15% (p = .036) and stroke morbidity by 35% (p < .001). These results offer convincing evidence of the benefit of treating hypertension in the elderly in regard to total mortality, stroke-related mortality, and CHD-related mortality. Treatment was based predominantly on the use of diuretics and beta blockers, but in subgroup analyses, most or all of the benefit was seen with the use of diuretics.[32, 34] The meta-analysis for mortality is shown in Figure 36–3, and the meta-analysis for morbidity is shown in Figure 36–4.

In a similar meta-analysis of essentially the same trials,[40] the pooled data on 15,990 patients were highly significant. The odds-ratios comparing control and treatment groups were .64 for fatal or nonfatal stroke, .62 for fatal stroke, .81 for fatal or nonfatal CHD, .77 for fatal CHD, and .88 for all-cause mortality. These results closely confirm the results of the first meta-analysis.[30]

In contrast to the findings of trials in the elderly, trials of antihypertensive treatment in middle-aged hypertensives have yielded different findings. The major drugs used were diuretics and beta blockers, as in the elderly trials. A meta-analysis[41] of the trials demonstrated a significant benefit for prevention of stroke (42%), which confirmed the predicted benefit based on the prospective epidemiologic data.[6] For CHD, the reduction in CHD (14%) was only half of the predicted benefit. Why antihypertensive treatment with diuretics and beta blockers is not fully protective against CHD in middle-aged hypertension is unknown. The adverse effects of these drugs on glucose and lipid metabolism are one possible explanation. On the other hand, the benefit of diuretics in prevention of both stroke and CHD in the elderly seems to be clearly established. It may be that hypertension is the major risk factor for CHD in the elderly, outweighing the contribution of blood lipid and glucose levels.

Recommended Treatment

The optimal management of the elderly hypertensive is shown in Figure 36–5. It may not always be possible to obtain 24-h blood pressure monitoring data because of cost, but this is the best method of determining average blood pressure and correctly identifying hypertensive persons. Similarly, the echocardiogram is much superior to the electrocardiogram in detecting left ventricular hypertrophy and stratifying the risk. Determination of microalbuminuria is more sensitive than determination of proteinuria by the dipstick method. The evidence at this time supports the use of diuretics as first-choice antihypertensive drugs because of their proven efficacy in prevention of the CHD- and stroke-related morbidity and mortality among elderly hypertensives.

TABLE 36–4. HYPERTENSION RESULTS

	Study (Reference)								
	ANBP (31)	SHEP (32)	HDFP (33)	MRC (34)	PPC (35)	EWPHE (36)	Sprackling and Colleagues (39)	VA (38)	STOP-H (37)
Severity ranking	1	2	3	4	5	6	7	Not ranked	Not ranked
Mean follow-up, years	3.4	4.5	5.0	5.8	4.4	4.7	4.0	3.8	2.1
Mean blood pressure at entry, mm Hg									
Treatment group									
Systolic	166.3	170.5	170.9	184.5	196.7	183.0	190.1	165.1*	195.0
Diastolic	100.7	76.7	101.6	91.0	98.7	101.0	106.7	104.7*	102.0
Control group									
Systolic	163.9	170.1	169.1	184.5	196.1	182.0	197.7	162.1*	195.0
Diastolic	100.9	76.4	100.9	90.5	98.0	101.0	108.5	103.6*	102.0
5-year follow-up									
Difference in diastolic blood pressure (treatment group − control group), mm Hg	−6.7	−3.4	−5.1	−5.9	−11	−10	−7.8	−18.6	−10.0
Difference in systolic blood pressure (treatment group − control group), mm Hg	ND	−11.1	ND	−6.3	−18	−22	−18.4	ND	−27.0
Death rate, %									
Treatment group	2.4	9.0	12.7	13.8	14.3	32.5	80.7	ND	4.4
Control group	3.1	10.2	15.8	14.2	14.8	35.1	73.7	ND	7.7

Abbreviations: ANBP, Australian National Blood Pressure Study; EWPHE, European Working Party on High Blood Pressure in the Elderly; HDFP, Hypertension Detection and Follow-Up Program; MRC, Medical Research Council; PPC, Practice in Primary Care; SHEP, Systolic Hypertension in the Elderly Program; STOP-H, Swedish Trial in Old Patients With Hypertension; VA, Veterans Administration Cooperative Study on Antihypertensive Agents; ND, not determinable.

*Refers to entire study population.

From Insua JT, Sacks HS, Lau T, et al: Drug treatment of hypertension in the elderly: a meta-analysis. Ann Intern Med 1994; 121:355–362.

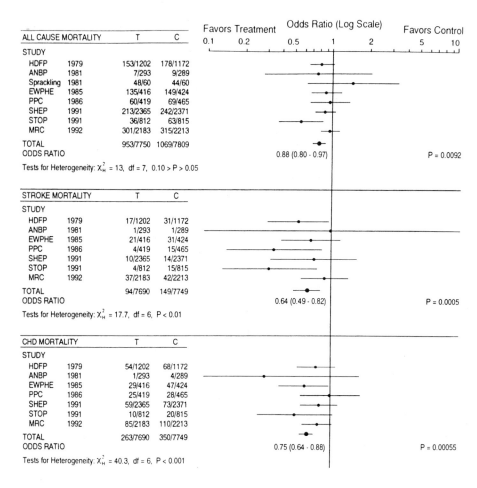

ALL CAUSE MORTALITY		T	C
STUDY			
HDFP	1979	153/1202	178/1172
ANBP	1981	7/293	9/289
Sprackling	1981	48/60	44/60
EWPHE	1985	135/416	149/424
PPC	1986	60/419	69/465
SHEP	1991	213/2365	242/2371
STOP	1991	36/812	63/815
MRC	1992	301/2183	315/2213
TOTAL		953/7750	1069/7809
ODDS RATIO			

Tests for Heterogeneity: $\chi^2_H = 13$, df = 7, 0.10 > P > 0.05

STROKE MORTALITY		T	C
STUDY			
HDFP	1979	17/1202	31/1172
ANBP	1981	1/293	1/289
EWPHE	1985	21/416	31/424
PPC	1986	4/419	15/465
SHEP	1991	10/2365	14/2371
STOP	1991	4/812	15/815
MRC	1992	37/2183	42/2213
TOTAL		94/7690	149/7749
ODDS RATIO			

Tests for Heterogeneity: $\chi^2_H = 17.7$, df = 6, P < 0.01

CHD MORTALITY		T	C
STUDY			
HDFP	1979	54/1202	68/1172
ANBP	1981	1/293	4/289
EWPHE	1985	29/416	47/424
PPC	1986	25/419	28/465
SHEP	1991	59/2365	73/2371
STOP	1991	10/812	20/815
MRC	1992	85/2183	110/2213
TOTAL		263/7690	350/7749
ODDS RATIO			

Tests for Heterogeneity: $\chi^2_H = 40.3$, df = 6, P < 0.001

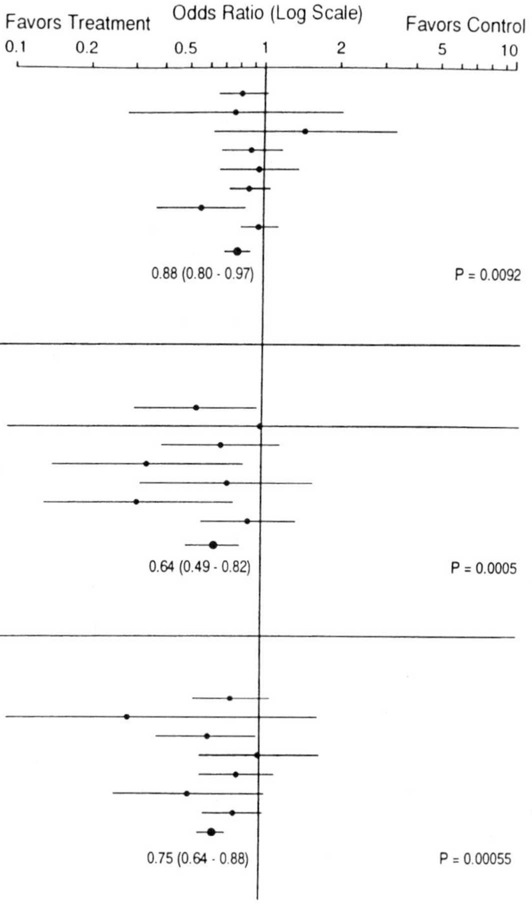

Figure 36–3. Results of meta-analysis of mortality end points. *Left*, Absolute numbers. *Right*, Odds-ratios and 95% confidence intervals. *Abbreviations*: ANBP, Australian National Blood Pressure Study; EWPHE, European Working Party on High Blood Pressure in the Elderly; HDFP, Hypertension Detection and Follow-Up Program; MRC, Medical Research Council; PPC, Practice in Primary Care; SHEP, Systolic Hypertension in the Elderly Program; STOP, Swedish Trial in Old Patients With Hypertension. (From Insua JT, Sacks HS, Lau T, et al: Drug treatment of hypertension in the elderly: a meta-analysis. Ann Intern Med 1994; 121:355–362.)

STROKE MORBIDITY		T	C
STUDY			
VA	1970	3/38	10/43
HDFP	1979	19/1202	31/1172
ANBP	1981	6/293	8/289
EWPHE	1985	17/416	27/424
PPC	1986	16/419	24/465
SHEP	1991	96/2365	149/2371
STOP	1991	26/812	41/815
MRC	1992	64/2183	92/2213
TOTAL		247/7728	382/7792
ODDS RATIO			

Tests for Heterogeneity: $\chi^2_H = 23.6$, df = 7, P < 0.01

CHD MORBIDITY		T	C
STUDY			
VA	1970	5/38	5/43
HDFP	1979	100/1202	105/1172
ANBP	1981	22/293	24/289
EWPHE	1985	19/416	12/424
PPC	1986	10/419	10/465
SHEP	1991	99/2365	143/2371
STOP	1991	27/812	31/815
MRC	1992	43/2183	49/2213
TOTAL		325/7728	379/7792
ODDS RATIO			

Tests for Heterogeneity: $\chi^2_H = 8.1$, df = 7, P > 0.10

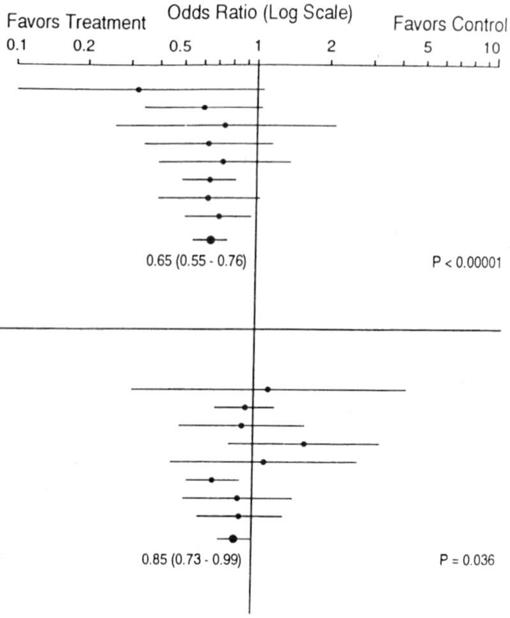

Figure 36–4. Results of meta-analysis of morbidity end points. *Left*, Absolute numbers. *Right*, Odds-ratios and 95% confidence intervals. *Abbreviations*: ANBP, Australian National Blood Pressure Study; EWPHE, European Working Party on High Blood Pressure in the Elderly; HDFP, Hypertension Detection and Follow-Up Program; MRC, Medical Research Council; PPC, Practice in Primary Care; SHEP, Systolic Hypertension in the Elderly Program; STOP, Swedish Trial in Old Patients With Hypertension; VA, Veterans Administration Cooperative Study on Antihypertensive Agents. (From Insua JT, Sacks HS, Lau T, et al: Drug treatment of hypertension in the elderly: a meta-analysis. Ann Intern Med 1994; 121:355–362.)

Establish the blood pressure level:
1. Repeated office measurements over several days
2. Home blood pressure measurements
3. 24-h blood pressure monitoring

↓

Treatable hypertension is present if all readings average
1. SBP ≥ 160 mm Hg
2. DBP ≥ 90 mm Hg

↓

Complete physical examination with emphasis on
1. Eye grounds
2. Bruits

↓

Laboratory findings with emphasis on
1. ECG or echocardiogram for evidence of LVH
2. Proteinuria or microalbuminuria
3. Creatinine
4. Blood lipids, glucose, and electrolytes

↓

Institute lifestyle modifications:
1. *Weight loss* if more than 10% overweight
2. *Salt restriction* to 6 g/day
3. *Alcohol restriction* to 1 oz/day
4. *Aerobic exercise* (e.g., walking 20–30 min three times/week)

↓

If goal BP (SBP 140 mm Hg and/or DBP 90 mm Hg) not achieved, initiate pharmacologic treatment:
1. Diuretic (e.g., hydrochlorothiazide starting at 12.5 mg/day)
2. Titrate the dose gradually
3. Check for orthostatic hypotension
4. Monitor creatinine, glucose, and electrolytes

↓

If goal BP not achieved, substitute another drug (e.g., calcium channel blocker) or add a second drug (e.g., ACE inhibitor)

Figure 36–5. A proposed flowchart for the confirmation of hypertension, physical and laboratory examination, and treatment of hypertension in the elderly.

Unresolved Issues

Because other drugs in wide use for the treatment of hypertension have not been tested by clinical trial methodology, it is possible that future studies may reveal that ACE inhibitors, calcium channel blockers, and alpha blockers are equally effective as or more or less effective than diuretics in the treatment of the elderly hypertensive.

Another unresolved issue is to define the numeric goal of blood pressure reduction. In patients with known ischemic heart disease, a U-shaped relationship between blood pressure reduction and mortality has been reported (the J curve), which suggests that reduction of DBP below 85 mm Hg increases mortality.[42] Similar results were not seen in either the Systolic Hypertension in the Elderly Program trial[32] or the TOMHS trial.[21] In both of these trials, diastolic blood pressure was reduced considerably below 85 mm Hg with no ill effect. Furthermore, in a prospective observational study, there was no evidence of a J curve.[6]

The issue is of considerable importance because limited blood pressure reduction to a DBP level of 85 mm Hg may not confer full benefit of antihypertensive treatment. In managing elderly hypertensives, however, it is best to start with low doses and carefully monitor the patient as the dose is increased. In patients with known CHD, treatment should be less aggressive.

In patients with ISH, whose SBP is 140–159 mm Hg, the JNC-5 recommends only lifestyle modification,[3] yet a study of the natural history of people with borderline ISH revealed both short-term and long-term risk of progression to definite hypertension and the development of cardiovascular disease.[43] The prevalence of borderline ISH rose with age, and by age 70 years, almost 20% of both men and women were affected. Progression to definite hypertension was twice that in normotensive participants in the Framingham Study, and the risk for development of cardiovascular disease was increased by 47%. Whether pharmacologic treatment would be of benefit in this high-risk group is unknown. If the conservative approach of the JNC-5 is followed, those patients should be closely monitored.

REFERENCES

1. National High Blood Pressure Education Program Working Group report on hypertension in the elderly. Hypertension 1994; 23:275–285.
2. Schneider EL, Gurainik JM: The aging of America; impact on health care costs. JAMA 1990; 263:2335–2340.
3. Joint National Committee on the Detection, Evaluation, and Treatment of High Blood Pressure: Fifth Report of the Joint National Committee on the Detection, Evaluation, and Treatment of High Blood Pressure (JNC V). Arch Intern Med 1993; 153:154–183.
4. Perry HM, Smith WM, McDonald RH, et al: Morbidity and mortality in the Systolic Hypertension in the Elderly Program (SHEP). Stroke 1989; 20:4–13.
5. Vokonas PS, Kannel WB, Cupples LA: Epidemiology and risk of hypertension in the elderly: the Framingham Study. J Hypertens Suppl 1988; 6:S3–S9.
6. MacMahon S, Peto R, Cutler J, et al: Blood pressure, stroke, and coronary heart disease. Part 1. Prolonged differences in blood pressure: prospective observational studies corrected for the regression and dilution bias. Lancet 1990; 335:765–774.
7. National High Blood Pressure Education Program: National High Blood Pressure Education Program Working Group report on hypertension and chronic renal failure. Arch Intern Med 1991; 151:1280–1287.
8. Epstein M, Sowers JR: Diabetes mellitus and hypertension. Hypertension 1992; 19:403–418.
9. Weisfeild MR, Lekatta EG, Gerstenblith G: Aging and the heart. *In* Braunwald E (ed): Heart Disease, 4th ed, pp 1656–1669. Philadelphia: WB Saunders, 1992.
10. Grim CM, Grim CE: Blood pressure measurement. *In* Izzo JL, Black HR (eds): Hypertension Primer, pp 217–226. Dallas: American Heart Association, 1993.
11. Rutan GA, Hermann B, Bild DE: Orthostatic hypotension in older adults. The Cardiovascular Heart Study. Hypertension 1992; 19:508–519.
12. Streeten DHP: Orthostatic hypotension and hypertension. *In* Izzo JL, Black HR (eds): Hypertension Primer, pp 224–225. Dallas: American Heart Association, 1993.
13. Tsapatsris NP, Nepolitana GT, Rothchild JR: Osler's maneuver in an outpatient clinic setting. Arch Intern Med 1991; 151:2209–2211.
14. Pickering TG, Preper C, Schechter CB: Ambulatory Monitoring and Blood Pressure Variability. London: UK Science Press, 1991.
15. Levy D, Garrison RJ, Savage DD, et al: Prognostic implications of echocardiographically determined left ventricular mass in the Framingham Heart Study. N Engl J Med 1990; 322:1561–1566.
16. Frohlich ED, Epstein C, Chobanian AV, et al: The heart in hypertension. N Engl J Med 1992; 327:998–1008.
17. National High Blood Pressure Education Program: National High Blood Pressure Education Program Working Group report on hypertension and chronic renal failure. Arch Intern Med 1991; 151:1280–1287.
18. Hypertension Detection and Follow-up Groups: the effects of treatment on mortality in "mild" hypertension; results of the Hypertension Detection and Follow-up Program. N Engl J Med 1982; 307:976–980.
19. World Hypertension League: Alcohol and hypertension—implications for management: a consensus statement by the World Hypertension League. J Hum Hypertens 1991; 5:1854–1856.
20. Cutler JA, Folkmann D, Elliot P, Suh D: An overview of randomized tricks of sodium reduction and blood pressure. Hypertension 1991; 17(suppl I):I-27–I-33.
21. Neaton JD, Grimm RH, Prineas RJ, et al: Treatment of Mild Hypertension Study: final results. JAMA 1993; 270:713–724.
22. Multiple Risk Factor Intervention Trial Research Groups: Coronary heart disease death, non-fatal acute myocardial infarction and other chemical outcomes in the Multiple Risk Factor Intervention Trial. Am J Cardiol 1986; 55:1–13.
23. Frishman WH: Beta-adrenergic blockers. Med Clin North Am 1988; 72:37–81.
24. Buhler F: Antihypertensive treatment according to age, plasma renin, and race. Drugs 1988; 35:495–502.
25. Epstein M: Calcium antagonists in the management of hypertension. *In*

Epstein M (ed): Calcium Antagonists in Clinical Medicine, pp 213–230. Philadelphia: Hanley & Belfus, 1992.
26. Pollare T, Lithell H, Berne C: A comparison of the effects of hydrochlorothiazide and captopril on glucose and lipid metabolism in patients with hypertension. N Engl J Med 1989; 321:868–874.
27. Israli ZH, Hall WD: Cough and angioneurotic edema associated with angiotensin converting enzyme inhibitor therapy: a review of the literature and pathophysiology. Ann Intern Med 1992; 117:234–242.
28. Schoenberger JA, Zesta M, Ross AD, et al: Efficacy and quality-of-life assessment of captopril antihypertensive therapy in clinical practice. Arch Intern Med 1990; 150:301–309.
29. Grimm RH Jr: Alpha blockers in the treatment of hypertension. Hypertension 1989; 1B(suppl 1):131–137.
30. Insua JT, Sacks HS, Lau T, et al: Drug treatment of hypertension in the elderly: a meta-analysis. Ann Intern Med 1994; 121:355–362.
31. Treatment of mild hypertension in the elderly: a study initiated and administered by the National Heart Foundation of Australia. Med J Aust 1981; 2:398–402.
32. SHEP Cooperative Research Group: Prevention of stroke by antihypertensive drug treatment in old persons with isolated systolic hypertension: final results of the Systolic Hypertension in the Elderly Program (SHEP). JAMA 1991; 265:3255–3264.
33. Maxwell MH, Ford CE: Cardiovascular morbidity and mortality in HDFP patients 50–69 years old at entry. J Cardiovasc Pharmacol 1985; 7(suppl 2):55–59.
34. MRC Working Party: Medical Research Council trial of treatment of hypertension in older adults: principal results. Br Med J 1992; 304:405–416.
35. Coope J, Warrender TS: Randomized Trial of Hypertension in the Elderly Patients in Primary Care. Br Med J 1986; 293:1145–1151.
36. Amery A, Birkenhager W, Brixko W, et al: Efficacy of antihypertensive treatment according to age, sex, blood pressure, and previous cardiovascular disease in patients over the age of 60. Lancet 1986; 2:589–592.
37. Dalhof B, Lundholm LH, Hanson L, et al: Morbidity and mortality in the Swedish Trial in Old Patients with Hypertension (STOP, Hypertension). Lancet 1991; 338:1281–1285.
38. Veterans Administration Cooperative Study Group on Antihypertensive Agents: Effect of treatment on morbidity in hypotension: III. Influence of age, diastolic pressure and prior cardiovascular disease: further analyses of side effects. Circulation 1972; 45:991–1004.
39. Sprackling ME, Mitchell JR, Short AH, et al: Blood pressure reduction in the elderly: a randomized controlled trial of methyldopa. Br Med J 1981; 283:1151–1153.
40. Pearce KA, Furburg CD: Meta-analysis of hypertension treatment trials in the elderly: short-term effects of treatment on cardiovascular events and mortality [Abstract]. Am J Hypertens 1994; 7(pt 2):1018.
41. Collins R, Peto R, MacMahon S, et al: Blood pressure, stroke and coronary heart disease. Part 2. Short-term reductions in blood pressure; overview of randomized drug trials in their epidemiological context. Lancet 1990; 335:827–838.
42. Cruickshank JM: Coronary blood flow reserve and the J curve relation between diastolic blood pressure and myocardial infarction. Br Med J 1988; 297:1227–1234.
43. Sagie A, Larson MG, Levy D: The natural history of borderline isolated systolic hypertension. N Engl J Med 1993; 329:1912–1917.

37 Secondary Hypertension: Causes and Treatment

Gordon H. Williams, MD

The preceding five chapters have provided an assessment of the pathophysiology of essential hypertension and the evaluation and treatment of patients with this condition. As discussed in those chapters, the cause of hypertension in the vast majority of patients with elevated blood pressure is unknown. Thus, individual treatment programs are usually developed from generalized concepts that apply to large numbers of hypertensive patients but may not apply, in particular, to the individual in the physician's examination room.[1]

Most of the diagnostic studies reviewed in the previous chapters are directed toward uncovering the secondary effects of the elevated blood pressure or concomitant diseases, which may modify the selection of therapy. Tests usually are not used to define the underlying pathophysiology, unless a suspicion is raised by history or physical examination that a secondary form of hypertension might be present. The percentage of patients with secondary forms of hypertension, that is, those patients in whom the underlying cause of the elevated blood pressure is known, varies widely depending on whether one surveys tertiary or primary care facilities. It is likely that in the general population, however, the frequency is approximately 6%.

Most forms of secondary hypertension fall into one of two broad categories: renal abnormalities or endocrine dysfunction (Table 37–1). As pointed out in Chapter 38, various renal diseases are associated with an increase in blood pressure. In most, the hypertension appears to be secondary to either an alteration in the production of the vasoconstrictor hormone angiotensin II (AII) or a defect in the renal excretory capacity, or both.

Either an increase or decrease in hormone production can lead to a rise in blood pressure. However, the most common "endocrine" form of hypertension is secondary to oral contraceptive use. It is of interest that some pregnant women who had no indication of hypertension before pregnancy acquire hypertension—some progressing to the point of eclampsia.[2] Again, the relationship between the changes in hormonal milieu and volume status of these patients in producing the increase in blood pressure is variable. The various hypotheses, and how one should treat hypertension in pregnancy, are explored in Chapter 41.

Perhaps the most common endogenous endocrine form of hypertension is that associated with diabetes mellitus.[3] The metabolic disturbances present in diabetes mellitus provide an environment that likely predisposes some subjects with certain genetic traits to acquire hypertension. In other cases, hypertension is likely secondary to the complications of diabetes, the most relevant being those associated with renal damage. One of the most intriguing recent aspects in this field is the apparent relationship among diabetes, AII production,

TABLE 37–1. CAUSES OF SECONDARY HYPERTENSION

Renal
Renal vascular stenosis or renal infarction
Polycystic kidney disease
Acute and chronic glomerulonephritis
Chronic pyelonephritis
Renin-producing tumors
Diabetic nephropathy
End-stage renal disease
Endocrine
Thyroid dysfunction
Hypothyroidism
Hyperthyroidism
Pheochromocytoma
Acromegaly
Adrenocortical hyperfunction
Cushing syndrome and disease
Primary aldosteronism
Congenital adrenal hyperplasia (17 α-hydroxylase and 11 β-hydroxylase defects)
Genetic dysregulation of aldosterone function or secretion
Glucocorticoid-remediable aldosteronism
11 β-hydroxysteroid dehydrogenase deficiency or licorice ingestion
Liddle syndrome
Hypertension Associated With Pregnancy or Hormones Related to Pregnancy
Oral contraceptives
Pregnancy-induced hypertension
Toxemia of pregnancy
Neurogenic
Increased intracranial pressure (acute)
Spinal cord section (acute)
"Diencephalic syndrome"
Reilly-Day syndrome (familial dysautonomia)
Acute porphyria or lead poisoning with polyneuritis

renal failure, and hypertension.[4] The implications of these various pathophysiologic mechanisms for therapy are explored in Chapter 40.

Finally, Chapter 39 explores a variety of more classic endocrine forms of hypertension. Most of these are related to alterations in the secretion of adrenal hormones, although abnormalities in thyroid hormone production and growth hormone can lead to an increase in blood pressure.[5] Intriguingly, the first genetic forms of hypertension recognized have been associated with alterations in adrenocortical hormone production. Although the classic congenital adrenal hyperplasia syndromes that also produce alterations in androgen production have been appreciated for several decades, the advances in molecular biologic techniques recently have identified other genetic forms, most notably, glucocorticoid-remediable aldosteronism, reviewed in Chapter 39.[6]

Identifiable, specific renal and endocrine causes of hypertension are infrequent. Nevertheless, evaluating hypertensive patients for them is important. First, to date, patients with secondary forms of hypertension are the only ones with potentially correctable lesions. Second, insights into the pathogenesis of the much larger essential hypertensive population have come, and presumably will continue to come, from analyses of the pathophysiology of hypertension in patients with secondary forms. Third, the development of specific therapeutic programs often has occurred as a result of analyses of the causes of hypertension in patients with secondary forms of the syndrome. For example, the classes of drugs termed *converting enzyme inhibitors* and *AII antagonists* were developed as a result of an assessment of the role of AII in producing an increase in blood pressure in individuals with renal vascular hypertension.

Thus, the following four chapters provide a critical assessment of the pathophysiology, evaluation, and treatment of patients with secondary forms of hypertension. Equally important is an assessment of when such an evaluation should be performed in patients with elevated blood pressure.

REFERENCES

1. Williams GH: Hypertensive vascular disease. *In* Isselbacher KJ, Braunwald E, Wilson JD, et al (eds): Harrison's Principles of Internal Medicine, 13th ed, pp 1116–1131. New York: McGraw-Hill, 1994.
2. Seely EW, Graves SW: Hormonal control of sodium and volume in the non-pregnant and pregnant state. Res Staff Phys 1994; 40:23–32.
3. Epstein M, Sowers JR: Diabetes mellitus and hypertension. Hypertension 1992; 19:403–418.
4. Lewis EJ, Hunsicker LG, Bain RP, Rohder D: The effect of angiotensin converting enzyme inhibition on diabetic nephropathy. The Collaborative Study Group. N Engl J Med 1993; 329:1456–1462.
5. Irony I, Kater CE, Biglieri EG, et al: Correctable subsets of primary aldosteronism. Am J Hypertens 1990; 3:576–582.
6. Lifton RP, Dluhy RG, Powers M, et al: A chimeric 11 β-hydroxylase/aldosterone synthase gene causes glucocorticoid-remediable aldosteronism and human hypertension. Nature 1992; 355:262–265.

38 Management of Hypertension in Patients With Renal Disease

Christopher S. Wilcox, MD, PhD

The presence of renal disease has an important impact on the management of patients with hypertension. Hypertension itself can cause nephrosclerosis and, especially in patients with proteinuria or diabetic nephropathy, can determine the rate of progression of renal disease. Antihypertensive agents may affect renal function, and the presence of renal insufficiency can have clinically important effects on drug kinetics and hence on drug dosing. The cause of the renal disease can influence the best choice of drugs. This chapter reviews the approach to the management of a patient with hypertension and renal disease.

INTERRELATIONSHIPS BETWEEN HYPERTENSION AND RENAL DISEASE

Patients with acute renal failure resulting from glomerulonephritis characteristically have a sharp rise in blood pressure associated with fluid retention. In contrast, those with acute renal failure from acute tubular necrosis characteristically have low blood pressure even in the presence of marked fluid retention.

The prevalence of hypertension in patients with chronic renal disease increases progressively with the development of renal insufficiency. At the time of end-stage renal disease, when patients are prepared for dialysis, the prevalence of hypertension increases to 80%–90%. However, the prevalence of hypertension also depends on the category of renal disease.[1] Diseases that predominantly affect the tubules, such as tubulointerstitial nephritis, have a low prevalence of hypertension because there is normally an impaired tubular reabsorption of sodium chloride (NaCl) and fluid. Indeed, occasional patients can experience salt-losing nephropathy with episodes of hypovolemia and hypotension. More commonly, the renal disease involves the glomerulus. In patients with glomerular diseases that lead to relatively little impairment of renal function, such as minimal-change glomerulonephritis or IgA nephropathy, the prevalence of hypertension is approximately 30%. In contrast, when the glomerular disease leads to more severe functional impairment, as is typical of focal segmental glomerulosclerosis, the prevalence of hypertension is approximately 75%. Patients with type I diabetes have a 70% prevalence of hypertension as they develop nephropathy, whereas almost all patients with type II diabetes have hypertension at the time that nephropathy develops. In patients with renal insufficiency and vasculitis, the hypertension is particularly prevalent and prone to progress to a malignant phase.[1]

Hypertension is an important factor contributing to end-stage renal disease. More than two thirds of patients entering dialysis programs have hypertension or diabetes mellitus as the primary diagnosis for renal failure.[2] African-American patients are particularly prone to nephrosclerosis and renal failure as a consequence of hypertension. Currently, African-Americans make up 29% of the patients with end-stage renal disease in the U.S. but comprise only about 12% of the population. Much of this increased prevalence of end-stage renal disease can be accounted for by hypertension and diabetes. Overall, the incidence rate of end-stage renal disease associated with hypertension in the U.S. is approximately sixfold greater in African-Americans than in white subjects. This disparity is even greater in younger age groups.[2]

The death rate from myocardial infarction and stroke has been declining progressively, but end-stage renal disease, and especially that attributable to hypertension and diabetes, is increasing despite the wide availability of antihypertensive treatment. The reason for this trend, and the apparent susceptibility of African-Americans to nephrosclerosis, is currently unclear.

Analysis of data in the Hypertension Detection and Follow-up Program[3] shows that the development of an increase in serum creatinine concentration with time was significantly more common in African-Americans, males, and patients older than 60 years of age.[3] Additionally, those with hypertension or higher levels of serum creatinine were more likely to demonstrate evidence of progressive renal impairment. In a prolonged follow-up study of patients with essential hypertension and normal renal function initially, African-American patients were twice as likely as white patients to have elevations in serum creatinine concentration.[4] Some patients experience an increase in serum creatinine concentration despite apparently good control of diastolic blood pressure to less than 90 mm Hg at clinic visits.[4] In a follow-up analysis of hypertensive members of the Multiple Risk Factor Intervention Trial, effective blood pressure control was associated with stable or improved renal function in non–African-Americans but not in African-Americans.[5] Such data have led some authors to question whether renal failure due to hypertension can be prevented, at least in some subsets of patients.[6]

The reason for the failure of antihypertensive therapy to prevent progression of renal disease in some patients is not established. In the spontaneously hypertensive rat, however, treatment that is apparently successful in normalizing blood pressure throughout life does not prevent the development of glomerulosclerosis and proteinuria.[7] Conversely, some studies have been more reassuring about the protective effect of successful antihypertensive therapy. Pettinger and associates[8] studied a group of patients with hypertension and renal function impairment, most of which was probably due to nephrosclerosis. They found that after an aggressive initial 2- to 4-month period of antihypertensive therapy to reduce the diastolic blood pressure to levels less than 80 mm Hg, followed by control of diastolic blood pressure to less than 90 mm Hg, the patients in this group had an improvement in renal function, as shown by a reduction in serum creatinine levels and/or an increase in the glomerular filtration rate over a 36-month period. These beneficial effects were apparent in those with mild and more severe degrees of renal failure and did not appear to be dependent on the choice of antihypertensive agent. In other studies of patients who progressed to end-stage renal disease, blood pressure and racial background have been found to be important predictors of the progression of renal disease.[9] Those with diastolic blood pressures less than 90 mm Hg had approximately half the rate of decline of renal function (as assessed from the reciprocal of serum creatinine concentration against time) compared with those with higher diastolic values.

Recently, radiotelemetric techniques have been developed that allow more accurate and less invasive methods for measuring blood pressure in conscious rats over prolonged periods. This method was used to study rats with renal failure due to renal ablation.[10] This model is relevant to the development of progressive nephrosclerosis in humans, since these rats experience progressive renal failure because of sclerosis of the remaining glomeruli in association with hypertension. Groups of rats received one of three different antihypertensive regimens or no therapy. There was a close correlation between the blood pressure achieved during the final 2 months of observation and the development of glomerulosclerosis. There was no particular advantage of angiotensin II inhibitor therapy over other forms of treatment that were equally effective in reducing blood pressure.

In the recently completed Modification of Diet in Renal Disease (MDRD) study, patients with moderate or severe renal disease were followed with regular measurements of the glomerular filtration rate over 36 months.[11] One group's treatment consisted of a usual blood pressure goal of a mean arterial pressure of 107 mm Hg; another group's treatment consisted of a lower goal of 92 mm Hg (equivalent to approximately 130/75 mm Hg). In patients who had more proteinuria at baseline, those whose treatment included the lower blood pressure goal had a slower rate of decline in the glomerular filtration rate. This effect was most pronounced in those with proteinuria exceeding 3 g/24 h.

Overall, these data suggest that hypertension not only can contribute to nephrosclerosis and progressive renal destruction, especially in African-American patients, but also may increase the rate of progression of other categories of renal disease.[12] The relationship between blood pressure and loss of renal function is complicated, and some patients or animal models show progression of renal failure despite apparently adequate control of hypertension. The reason for some of these discordant results is not yet clear.[6] Evolving information suggests that the goals of antihypertensive therapy may have been too conservative and that lower values for blood pressure may be required in some patients—for example, in those with heavy proteinuria—to prevent progressive loss of renal function. These lower levels of arterial pressure cannot be achieved safely in all patients, however, especially in those with a high-grade stenosis affecting blood vessels to critical organs such as the heart or brain. Therefore, care and judgment are required, with close follow-up in titrating individual blood pressures down to the levels suggested in the MDRD study.[11]

PATHOPHYSIOLOGIC MECHANISMS CONTRIBUTING TO HYPERTENSION IN RENAL DISEASE

A brief discussion of the pathophysiology of hypertension in renal disease is required to provide a rational basis for different forms of antihypertensive therapy.[1, 13, 14] A reduction in renal function, associated with a fall in the glomerular filtration rate, necessarily restricts excretion of sodium and fluid. Early in the development of renal failure, patients generally have an increase in cardiac output with a relatively low peripheral resistance. As renal failure progresses, the blood pressure rises because of a rise in peripheral resistance.[1, 15] This occurs despite the development of anemia that normally leads to reduced peripheral resistance. The increase in peripheral resistance may reflect, in part, an autoregulatory response to a sustained increase in cardiac output. However, activation of the specific vasoconstrictor mechanism and inhibition of vasodilator mechanisms make important contributions. The retention of fluid is more marked in patients with primarily glomerular or vascular disease when compared with individuals having tubulointerstitial disease in which frank salt-wasting nephropathy can occur. Prolonged expansion of the extracellular fluid volume appears to be the major factor underlying hypertension in end-stage renal disease, since scrupulous control of body fluid volume by dialysis can reverse hypertension in the majority of patients.[14, 16]

There have been many studies of body fluid volume in patients with renal insufficiency. As shown in Figure 38–1, there is generally an expansion of plasma, extracellular and intracellular fluid volumes, and total body sodium in patients with advanced renal failure.[14]

Some patients with renal insufficiency experience a stimulus to the renin-angiotensin-aldosterone system. This is especially likely when the underlying condition is renal artery stenosis, malignant hypertension, vasculitis, polycystic kidney disease, or some condition in which there is interference with the transmission of arterial pressure to the afferent arteriole. In the majority of patients, however, the renin-angiotensin system likely is not the major cause of hypertension, at least until end-stage renal disease develops.[16]

Recent studies have emphasized the importance of increased sympathetic nervous system activity in the maintenance of hypertension in patients with advanced renal disease. By direct recording of postganglionic sympathetic nerve activity to blood vessels in skeletal muscle using implanted microelectrodes, Converse and coworkers[17] showed that sympathetic nerve discharge was nearly three times higher in patients with end-stage renal disease receiving hemodialysis than in normal subjects. Interestingly, a group of hemodialysis patients who had been subjected to bilateral nephrectomy were found to have lower blood pressure and normal rates of sympathetic nerve discharge. These authors concluded that chronic renal failure may be accompanied by sympathetic activation that appears to be mediated by an afferent signal arising in the failing kidney.

A number of other factors may contribute to vasoconstriction, reduction in renal blood flow, and hypertension in patients with renal failure.[1, 16] Some investigators have detected evidence of a circulating inhibitor of Na/K-ATPase in human subjects with renal failure or animal models of reduced renal mass hypertension.[18] Such a compound could increase blood pressure by increasing intracellular sodium concentration in vascular smooth muscle cells, thereby diminishing sodium-calcium exchange and raising the intracellular calcium concentration. There is also evidence for increased production of the vasoconstrictor prostaglandins thromboxane and PGH_2 and of endothelin.[19] Asymmetric dimethyl arginine had been detected in the plasma of patients with chronic renal disease.[20] This substance is a circulating inhibitor of nitric oxide synthase and might thereby contribute to hypertension by blunting endogenous nitric oxide production, contributing to vasoconstriction. These pathophysiologic mechanisms, and some of the major points of their interaction, are summarized in Figure 38–2.

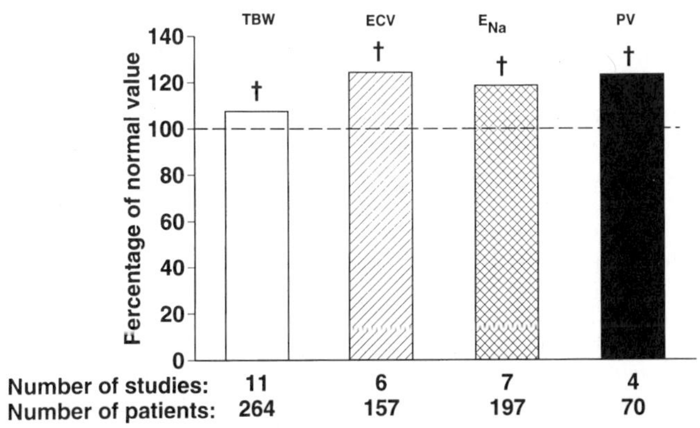

Figure 38–1. Compilation from published studies of mean values for body fluid volumes in patients with advanced renal failure who were not receiving dialysis therapy. Data are shown as percentage of normal values. †$p < .005$, compared with normal subjects. *Abbreviations:* TBW, total body water; ECV, extracellular fluid volume; E_{Na}, exchangeable sodium; PV, plasma volume. (Data from Mitch WE, Wilcox CS: Disorders of body fluids, sodium and potassium in chronic renal failure. Am J Med 1982; 72:536–550.)

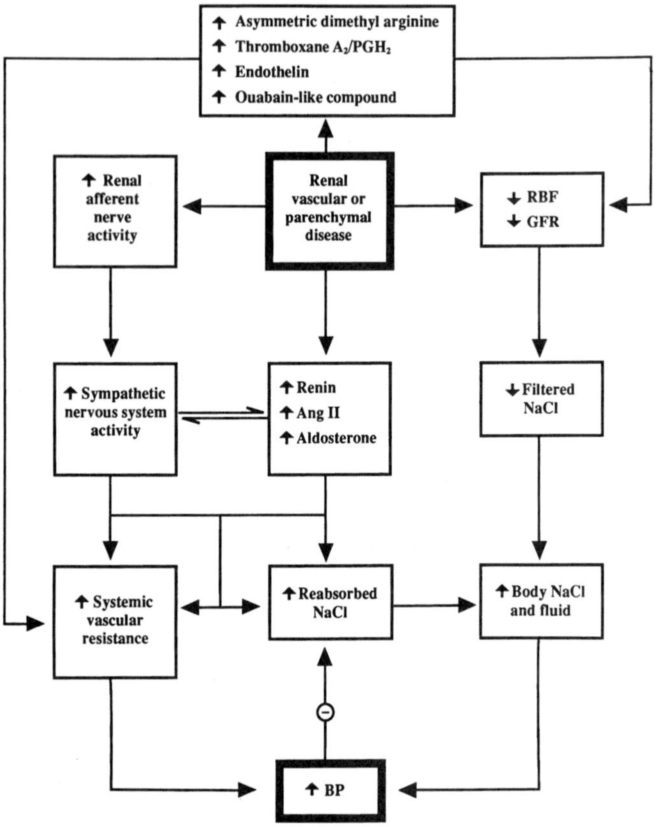

Figure 38–2. Summary of some pathophysiologic mechanisms leading to hypertension and their interactions in patients with renal failure. For explanation, see text. *Abbreviations:* PGH_2, prostaglandin H_2; RBF, renal blood flow; GFR; glomerular filtration rate; Ang II, angiotensin II; NaCl, sodium chloride; BP, blood pressure.

ANTIHYPERTENSIVE DRUG USE IN RENAL FAILURE

Some special considerations are required in selecting a drug to treat hypertension in patients with renal failure (Table 38–1). Drugs that are excreted by the kidney require major dosage reduction.[21] Generally, a metabolized drug of the same class is preferable because the potential for accumulation in renal failure is greatly diminished.

Drugs that increase plasma potassium concentration should generally be avoided, or prescribed only under very close supervision, in patients with renal insufficiency. Diuretics that block aldosterone receptors (e.g., spironolactone) and those acting in the collecting duct (e.g., amiloride and triamterene) are particularly hazardous and can cause life-threatening hyperkalemic metabolic acidosis by preventing renal secretion of potassium and hydrogen ions. Angiotensin converting enzyme inhibitors (ACEIs) reduce plasma angiotensin II and aldosterone concentrations and may thereby exacerbate hyperkalemia. Beta blockers inhibit the disposition of a potassium load and may thereby lead to some increase in serum potassium concentration especially if intake is not restricted. Heparin can inhibit aldosterone secretion and can precipitate hyperkalemia in some patients, for example, those with borderline hyporeninemic hypoaldosteronism. ACEIs, beta blockers, and heparin are used in patients with renal insufficiency because the changes that they make in serum potassium concentration are usually small. Clearly, close surveillance is required, especially during times of alteration in renal function or fluid volume status (e.g., concurrent gastrointestinal illness) that could lead to an abrupt hyperkalemia.

Thiazide diuretics when used alone become increasingly ineffective with the development of moderate to severe renal insufficiency. In contrast, loop diuretics retain efficacy even in patients with advanced renal insufficiency, but they have to be used in increasing doses.

Diuretics

Table 38–2 contains information pertinent to the use of diuretics in treating hypertension in patients with renal insufficiency. The diuretics of choice for patients with renal insufficiency are loop diuretics because, with appropriate increases in dosage, they retain efficacy even in patients with advanced renal failure.[22, 23] Distal tubular agents are not recommended because of the danger of precipitating hyperkalemic metabolic acidosis. The blood pressure of patients with high degrees of renal insufficiency is generally closely dependent on body fluid status. Therefore, loop diuretics and restriction of dietary salt intake are important components of management in most patients with hypertension and renal insufficiency. The appropriate dose of diuretics is hard to predict and will depend on other factors, such as dietary salt intake. Therefore, these drugs should be introduced in moderate dosage—for example, furosemide, 40 mg twice per day—and the dose increased at approximately 2-week intervals until the desired effect is achieved or some adverse effect such as worsening azotemia dictates a reduction in dose.

The first step should be to assess salt intake by a 24-hour urine collection. Urine creatinine excretion should be measured concurrently to ensure adequacy of collection (12–20 mg/kg for females and 15–25 mg/kg for males). During regular diuretic therapy, 24-hour sodium excretion can still be used as an index of sodium intake provided that diuretic dosage has not been adjusted recently and the patient is in a steady state. The aim should normally be to reduce dietary salt intake to 100 mEq/24 h in a hypertensive patient with renal insufficiency. Thereafter, loop diuretics can be prescribed and further reductions in dietary salt intake attempted to control residual hypertension. Care is required, however, because some patients experience worsening azotemia that necessitates liberalizing salt intake and/or withdrawing diuretics. As the need for dialysis approaches, patients frequently require large doses of loop diuretics (e.g., furosemide, 80–400 mg per day) and greater restrictions of dietary salt (75–100 mEq/24 h). High doses of loop diuretics in patients with impaired renal function can cause deafness that is not always reversible on withdrawal of the drug. Therefore, patients should be warned of this potential problem and advised to report any impairment of hearing to their physicians without delay.

TABLE 38–1. ANTIHYPERTENSIVE DRUGS FOR PATIENTS WITH RENAL FAILURE

Drugs excreted by the kidney require major dosage reduction
Nadolol (Corgard)
Atenolol (Tenormin)
Captopril (Capoten)
Initiate therapy with low dosages to avoid abrupt falls in blood pressure that can worsen azotemia
Drugs that increase plasma potassium concentration should be avoided or prescribed under close supervision
Spironolactone (Aldactone)
Amiloride (Midamor)
Triamterene (Dyrenium)
ACEIs
Beta blockers
Heparin
Thiazide diuretics used alone are ineffective at a serum creatinine level >2–3 mg/dL
Dosage of loop diuretics has to be increased in proportion to the fall in creatinine clearance

Abbreviation: ACEIs, angiotensin-converting enzyme inhibitors.

TABLE 38–2. USE OF DIURETICS FOR HYPERTENSION IN PATIENTS WITH RENAL FAILURE

Drugs	Loop diuretics: bumetanide, ethacrynic acid, furosemide, indapamide, piretanide Thiazides: bendroflumethiazide, chlorothiazide, chlorthalidone, hydrochlorothiazide, metolazone (not recommended as single agents in moderate/severe renal failure) Distal agents: amiloride, spironolactone, triamterene (not recommended in renal failure)
Efficacy	Concurrent salt restriction is required to achieve full efficacy. Thiazides and distal agents are relatively ineffective, and more toxic, when used alone in patients with moderate/severe renal failure (serum creatinine concentration >2–3 mg/dL; creatinine clearance <30–40 mL/min)
Adverse effects in renal failure	Volume depletion, orthostatic hypotension, prerenal azotemia, cramps, impaired carbohydrate metabolism. Loop diuretics and thiazides can cause hypokalemia and alkalosis (unusual in renal failure); distal agents can cause life-threatening hyperkalemia and acidosis. Diuretics worsen hyperuricemia and can occasionally precipitate gout. Loop diuretics can cause deafness when used in high doses in patients with renal failure.
Interactions	Enhances antihypertensive efficacy of other agents (except calcium antagonists); nonsteroidal anti-inflammatory drugs in full dosage can blunt or prevent diuretic and antihypertensive actions
Special indications	Edema, hyperkalemia (loop diuretics), and hyporeninemic hypoaldosteronism
Dosage modifications for advanced end-stage renal disease	Loop diuretics require increased dosage with advancing renal insufficiency

Thiazide diuretics used alone lose much of their efficacy in patients with renal failure and a creatinine clearance less than 30–40 mL/min. These drugs may still cause diuresis and a fall in blood pressure when prescribed concurrently with loop diuretics. However, the concurrent use of two or more diuretics, although promoting efficacy, also enhances the potential for electrolyte disturbances and azotemia.[23] Therefore, combined therapy mandates that the physician see the patient regularly and monitor closely for adverse electrolyte changes, such as hypokalemia, hypomagnesemia, hyponatremia and alkalosis, or worsening azotemia.

Some degree of hypokalemic metabolic alkalosis is common in patients with normal renal function who are receiving thiazide or loop diuretics. It is unusual in those with renal insufficiency. Hyperurocemia is frequent in patients with renal impairment, however, and may be worsened by concurrent therapy with diuretics and sodium depletion. Diuretics may also exacerbate carbohydrate intolerance and lead to frank diabetes mellitus on occasion. They also may cause hyperlipidemia, but this effect is usually transient. Therefore, diuretics are best avoided when possible in patients with diabetes mellitus or pre-existing lipid abnormalities. Nevertheless, in practice, many such patients do require therapy with diuretic agents to provide adequate control of blood pressure or edema, especially with advancing renal insufficiency. In these circumstances, the benefits of diuretic use can outweigh its disadvantages. The development of worsening azotemia can signify a diuretic dose that is too high and should prompt a trial of reduced dosage or a more liberal salt intake.

Diuretics enhance the antihypertensive efficacy of other agents, with the exception of calcium antagonists. Moreover, in the treatment of severe and drug-resistant hypertension that requires more than two antihypertensive agents, there is frequently an element of salt and fluid retention that limits the reduction in blood pressure.[22] Therefore, diuretics should be included in the prescription for most hypertensive patients requiring two or more antihypertensive agents, unless there are specific contraindications.

Nonsteroidal anti-inflammatory drugs, when used in full dosage, can blunt or prevent the diuretic and antihypertensive action of diuretics. Moreover, these drugs can worsen renal function impairments and can themselves lead to an increase in blood pressure. Therefore, nonsteroidal anti-inflammatory drugs should be withdrawn whenever possible in patients with hypertension and renal disease, or their dosage should be reduced. Small, intermittent doses of aspirin, as used to inhibit platelet aggregation in patients with vascular disease, do not have this adverse effect on renal function, blood pressure, or diuretic efficacy.[23]

Special indications for diuretic use include patients with edema, those with hyperkalemia, and those with hypertension and hyporeninemic hypoaldosteronism. The diuretic promotes an increase in delivery of fluids and solutes to the distal nephron, thereby potentiating secretion of potassium and hydrogen ions that help correct hyperkalemic acidosis.

Loop diuretics are effective only from the luminal aspect of the tubule. They gain access to the tubule lumen largely by secretion in the proximal tubule. The secretory system for diuretics in the proximal tubule is shared with other organic anions, many of which accumulate in renal insufficiency. Renal disease limits renal mass, impairs proximal tubule function, and leads to the accumulation of substances that compete for proximal tubule secretion. These effects combine to limit the secretion of diuretics into the tubular lumen. Thus, increasing doses are necessary in patients with advanced renal insufficiency.[21]

Beta Blockers

Nonselective and B_1-selective agents and those with intrinsic sympathomimetic activity or alpha blocking actions are available for treatment of hypertension (Table 38–3). Antihypertensive efficacy in general is greater in white than in African-American subjects, greater in the young than in the old, and greater in those with high- compared with low-renin hypertension. Beta blockers are effective in patients with renal insufficiency, although in those with marked fluid retention and renin suppression, their efficacy is reduced. Special toxicities in patients with renal failure include exacerbation of hyperkalemia and hyperlipidemia. These drugs should be used with special caution in patients with diabetes mellitus, heart failure, or bronchospasm. They can lead to dangerous bradyarrhythmias when used in combination with verapamil or diltiazem. Beta blockers are particularly useful for the management of hypertension in patients with coexisting angina pectoris or those who have had a prior myocardial infarction. They have proven efficacy in the prevention of recurrent myocardial infarction, although this has not been tested in the setting of renal failure.

Despite some initial reservations, beta blockers have generally been well tolerated in patients with chronic renal failure and usually do not affect renal function adversely. There are significant differences, however, among beta blockers with regard to the need for dosage modification in patients with end-stage renal disease (see Table 38–3). Those drugs that are eliminated predominantly by metabolism need little or no dosage modification. In contrast, major dosage reductions are required for atenolol and nadolol, because they are excreted largely unmetabolized in the urine, and for acebutolol, because its active metabolites accumulate in renal failure.[21]

Central Sympatholytic Agents and Adrenergic Antagonists

Central sympatholytic agents include clonidine, methyldopa, and guanfacine. These drugs are generally well tolerated in patients with

TABLE 38–3. SUMMARY OF USE OF BETA BLOCKERS FOR HYPERTENSION IN PATIENTS WITH RENAL FAILURE

Drugs	Nonselective: labetalol (with alpha blocking action), nadolol, pindolol (with ISA), propranolol, timolol β_1-selective: acebutolol (with ISA), atenolol, esmolol, metoprolol
Efficacy	Greater antihypertensive efficacy in whites than in African-Americans, in young than in old patients, and in high- than in low-renin hypertensives; efficacy is increased by salt restriction and diuretics
Adverse effects in renal failure	Exacerbates hyperkalemia and hyperlipidemia; special precaution required in patients with diabetes mellitus, cardiac failure, bronchospasm, or bradycardia
Interactions	Can cause cardiac conduction defects, especially when used with verapamil or diltiazem
Special indications	Patients with angina pectoris or those who have had a myocardial infarction
Dosage modifications in advanced end-stage renal disease	Little or no dosage adjustments required with metabolized drugs, e.g., propranolol, labetalol, metoprolol, timolol, or esmolol; reduction of 50%–75% required for excreted drugs, e.g., acebutolol, atenolol, and nadolol

Abbreviation: ISA, intrinsic sympathetic activity.

renal failure. They are effective in reducing blood pressure and do not adversely affect renal function. Clonidine and guanfacine are metabolized and do not require dosage modification, whereas methyldopa should be given once daily in patients with advanced renal failure.[21] Clonidine can be prescribed as a skin patch, which is particularly useful in poorly compliant patients. This can provide a useful background antihypertensive action in patients undergoing hemodialysis. These drugs do not impair cardiovascular reflexes and therefore do not usually promote dialysis-induced hypotension.

Alpha-adrenergic antagonists include doxazosin, prazosin, and terazosin. These drugs are generally well tolerated in patients with renal insufficiency and do not require dosage modification.[21] These agents may be particularly useful in patients with metabolic disturbances, such as diabetes mellitus, hyperlipidemia, or electrolyte disturbances because they do not normally cause adverse changes in these parameters.

Calcium Antagonists

Calcium antagonists are particularly effective in patients with severe hypertension (Table 38–4). Verapamil or diltiazem may cause dangerous bradyarrhythmia, especially in patients treated with beta blockers. This can be a particular problem in renal failure because certain beta blockers are cumulative (see Table 38–2). Calcium antagonists can cause ankle edema that is not related to renal sodium retention but rather to partitioning of plasma fluid into the interstitial space. These agents generally do not adversely affect renal function. Indeed, long-term studies in patients with mildly impaired renal function have indicated that blood pressure and renovascular resistance are reduced and the glomerular filtration rate is increased.[24] These drugs are eliminated by metabolism, and therefore major dosage modifications are not required in patients with renal disease.[21]

Calcium antagonists are an important part of the antihypertensive prescription of many patients with severe hypertension and renal failure. They may be particularly useful for patients with renal artery stenosis in whom they generally do not cause a fall in the glomerular filtration rate in the poststenotic kidney, as can occur with ACEIs.[25] Their long-term effects on progression of renal failure have yet to be properly evaluated. In patients with heavy proteinuria, dihydropyridines (e.g., nifedipine) generally have little effect on reducing the protein excretion. This is in contrast to ACEIs, which generally diminish proteinuria by a clinically significant degree.[26, 27] Therefore, calcium antagonists may be preferable in patients with renal artery stenosis, whereas ACEIs are drugs of first choice in patients with diabetes mellitus and heavy proteinuria.

Angiotensin Converting Enzyme Inhibitors

ACEIs are effective antihypertensive agents in most patients with renal insufficiency (Table 38–5).[26, 27] Special adverse effects encountered in renal failure include hypotension and azotemia in certain patients who are treated vigorously by concurrent salt restriction and diuretic therapy. This is especially likely to occur in patients receiving multiple other antihypertensive agents. A significant, and reversible, increase in serum creatinine or blood urea nitrogen (BUN) concentration in a patient who is not obviously salt-depleted should raise the possibility of underlying renal artery stenosis.[25, 28] Occasionally, ACEIs can precipitate serious hyperkalemia and metabolic acidosis resulting from inhibition of angiotensin II generation and aldosterone secretion. A dry cough is the most frequently encountered adverse effect.

The efficacy of ACEIs is increased by concurrent use of diuretics and a low salt intake. This can also lead to the development of prerenal azotemia, however, and therefore requires careful monitoring. These drugs are indicated in patients with diabetes mellitus, especially those with microalbuminuria or heavy proteinuria, and in patients with congestive heart failure or left ventricular hypertrophy.

Fosinopril and quinapril are eliminated largely by metabolism and require little or no dosage modification in patients with renal insufficiency. At the other extreme, captopril can be markedly cumulative in advanced renal failure, in which case its dosage should be reduced by 50%–75%, and it should be given once daily. Other agents in this class usually require some reduction in dosage in patients with end-stage renal disease.[29]

Data from animal models indicate that ACEIs may have special benefits in preventing the development of compensatory glomerular hyperfiltration, glomerulosclerosis, proteinuria, and progressive renal failure in models of renal functional impairment. Long-term, properly

TABLE 38–4. SUMMARY OF USE OF CALCIUM ANTAGONISTS TO TREAT HYPERTENSION IN PATIENTS WITH RENAL FAILURE

Drugs	Amlodipine, diltiazem, felodipine, isradipine, nicardipine, nifedipine, nimodipine, nisoldipine, nitrendipine, verapamil
Efficacy	Most effective in severe hypertension; efficacy not increased by diuretics
Adverse effects in renal failure	Bradyarrhythmia and constipation (verapamil and diltiazem), ankle edema
Interactions	Dangerous bradyarrhythmia can occur with concurrent use of verapamil or diltiazem and beta blockers
Special indications	Patients with angina pectoris
Dosage modifications in advanced end-stage renal disease	None required

TABLE 38–5. ANGIOTENSIN-CONVERTING ENZYME INHIBITORS TO TREAT HYPERTENSION IN PATIENTS WITH RENAL FAILURE

Drugs	Benazepril, captopril, enalapril, fosinopril, lisinopril, quinapril, ramipril
Efficacy	Greater in patients with high renin levels; efficacy enhanced by concurrent salt restriction and diuretic use
Adverse effects in renal failure	Hypotension and azotemia exacerbated by salt restriction and diuretics; can cause serious hyperkalemia and metabolic acidosis; azotemia (usually reversible) in patients with bilateral renal artery stenosis or stenosis of a single kidney; dry cough the most frequent adverse effect
Interactions	Antihypertensive action curtailed by nonsteroidal anti-inflammatory drugs
Special indications	Patient with diabetes mellitus, especially those with microalbuminuria; patients with moderate or severe proteinuria (>1–13 g/24 h) or the nephrotic syndrome; patients with congestive heart failure or left ventricular hypertrophy
Dosage modifications in advanced end-stage renal disease	Little or none required with fosinopril or quinapril; 50%–75% reduction with benazepril, enalapril, lisinapril and ramipril; captopril dose should be reduced by 50%–75% and given once daily

controlled crossover trials comparing ACEIs with other agents in patients with renal failure are not yet available. Nevertheless, these agents are widely prescribed in patients with renal failure to combat hypertension and progressive renal insufficiency and may have special efficacy in patients with heavy proteinuria. [27]

Vasodilators

Minoxidil has a spectrum of adverse effects that include hirsutism, fluid retention, tachycardia and sympathetic excitation, and orthostatic hypotension. In addition, it can cause pericardial effusion in occasional patients with renal failure. Despite these adverse effects, minoxidil remains an important drug for the treatment of severe, refractory renal hypertension. Concurrent therapy with salt restriction and a diuretic and beta blockers is required in most patients. The drug is eliminated by metabolism and does not require significant dosage alterations in end-stage renal disease. Sodium nitroprusside can be used as a parenteral agent in patients with renal failure. It is highly effective but its metabolite, thiocyanate, can accumulate in renal failure, leading to central nervous system disturbances, seizure, or coma.[21]

MANAGEMENT OF HYPERTENSION IN PATIENTS WITH RENAL FAILURE

The first step in managing hypertension in renal failure is to decide on the need for antihypertensive therapy and to set the target goals. Maneuvers that decrease blood pressure and glomerular capillary pressure can slow the rate of progression of renal failure in certain categories of patients, notably those with diabetic nephropathy or heavy proteinuria.[30] Patients with malignant hypertension have a rapid loss of renal function that can be halted, and to some extent reversed, by appropriate antihypertensive therapy. There remains a large group with renal disease, sometimes a consequence of the hypertension, in whom it is prudent to institute closely regulated antihypertensive therapy, although firm evidence that blood pressure control to normal or below average levels will slow the rate of progression of renal disease is currently lacking.

An important adaptive response to renal injury or loss of renal mass is a compensatory hypertrophy of the glomerulus associated with glomerular capillary hypertension. These structural and functional changes accompany the development of progressive proteinuria and glomerulosclerosis in animal models.[30] Full reversal of glomerular capillary hypertension may require a lower target blood pressure than is customarily recommended. Indeed, in the MDRD trial, patients with proteinuria had a slower rate of progression of renal insufficiency if they were assigned to the low blood pressure group compared with the conventional blood pressure group. This beneficial effect was not seen in those without significant proteinuria.[11] Therefore, in patients with more than 1 g/day of proteinuria, and especially those whose proteinuria is in the nephrotic range, it is prudent to set a target blood pressure of approximately 125/70–75 mm Hg. Abrupt reductions in blood pressure in patients with chronic renal disease can lead to a temporary worsening of renal function, however, with a rise in serum creatinine and BUN levels. The aim should be to introduce antihypertensive therapy in a gradual but escalating manner to control blood pressure to the target level while monitoring for adverse effects from the reduced blood pressure.

The next step in a patient with chronic renal disease is to assess proteinuria, creatinine clearance, and salt intake from a 24-hour urine collection and to provide dietary advice for restriction of salt intake when this is needed. For those with mild hypertension, restriction of sodium intake to the range 100 mEq/24 h is reasonable, but for those with severe or drug-resistant hypertension, more severe restriction to 75 mEq/24 h is often necessary. Once salt restriction has been achieved, if blood pressure is not adequately controlled, diuretics should be considered as the next step provided that there are no specific contraindications. Subsequent choices for antihypertensive therapy are often governed by considerations of cost, convenience, and the presence of coexisting indications or contraindications to the use of specific agents (see Tables 38–2 to 38–5).

Patients Receiving Dialysis Treatment

The key to controlling blood pressure in patients receiving dialysis is effective normalization of body fluids by appropriate dialysis management.[16] Therefore, the therapy for hypertension in these patients should be coordinated closely with the patient's nephrologist. Even among compliant patients who are appropriately dialyzed to maintain a near-normal dry body weight, approximately 10%–25% have significant hypertension. In this group, the renin-angiotensin-aldosterone axis is often activated, and blood pressure can respond well to ACEI or calcium antagonist therapy.

Some patients experience large swings of blood pressure during dialysis. They may start dialysis with hypertensive levels of blood pressure but experience hypotension after fluid removal. In this group, antihypertensive agents are best given after dialysis, with the patient instructed not to take the agents on the morning of the dialysis treatment. For other patients, a drug that provides a background antihypertensive action, while not interrupting cardiovascular reflexes, is often useful. This can be achieved by several regimens; a clonidine skin patch is often effective.

Some drugs are removed by hemodialysis or peritoneal dialysis. Drug removal is restricted by protein binding or a large volume of distribution.[21]

Renal Artery Stenosis

The ideal management of patients with renal artery stenosis and renovascular hypertension is percutaneous transluminal renal artery angioplasty or surgical bypass of the stenosis. There are some patients in whom interventions are not possible, however, because they are at high risk or the renal artery has been stenosed to the point of complete occlusion. Moreover, elderly patients and those with long-established hypertension or with a small, shrunken poststenotic kidney usually do not derive much antihypertensive benefit from correction of renal artery stenosis.[25] In these situations, the physician may elect for medical therapy to control the hypertension.

The best choice of drug for hypertension in a patient with renal insufficiency and known renal artery stenosis presents a therapeutic dilemma (Table 38–6). On the one hand, these patients have an activated renin-angiotensin system and a good antihypertensive response to drugs, such as ACEIs, that act by interrupting the system. On the other hand, the glomerular filtration rate in the poststenotic kidney is unusually dependent on angiotensin II. Downstream from a renal artery stenosis, the reduction in renal perfusion pressure stimulates release of renin within the kidney with generation of angiotensin II. A predominant site of action for angiotensin II is the efferent arteriole, where vasoconstriction maintains an effective glomerular capillary pressure. Therefore, blockade of angiotensin II generation, although lowering blood pressure and often increasing renal blood flow, can lead to a sharp reduction in glomerular capillary pressure and thereby in glomerular filtration rate. Moreover, if renal artery stenosis is extreme, occasional patients experience a thrombosis of the artery with total loss of function to that kidney.[28]

Despite these adverse effects on renal function, ACEIs have been found to be effective antihypertensive agents and generally well tolerated in patients with renal artery stenosis.[31] Patients who experience clinically significant increases in serum creatinine or BUN levels are typically those treated concurrently with diuretics and volume-depleting therapy or those with bilateral renal artery stenosis or stenosis of a single or transplanted kidney. Therefore, if the clinician elects ACEI therapy in a patient with renal artery stenosis, the treatment must be monitored carefully with serial measurements of renal function and intermittent measurements of renal size (by ultrasound measurement). Therapy should be discontinued if the serum creatinine level rises abruptly or if there is a significant reduction of size in the poststenotic kidney.

Calcium antagonists can block many of the actions of angiotensin II and are effective in lowering blood pressure in animal models of angiotensin-dependent hypertension.[32] Unlike ACEIs, calcium antagonists have a predominant vasodilator action on the afferent rather than the efferent arteriole and thereby maintain glomerular capillary pressure despite a fall in blood pressure. Therefore, calcium antagonists are less likely to produce a sharp decline in renal function in patients with renovascular hypertension, although the control of blood pressure may not be as effective as with ACEIs.[33]

Blood pressure in renovascular hypertension characteristically is not closely dependent on body fluid volume. With the development of renal insufficiency, however, and especially in patients with bilateral renal artery stenosis, fluid retention can be substantial and may lead to episodes of recurrent pulmonary edema. Indeed, recurrent pulmonary edema with a relatively well-preserved ejection fraction in the context of hypertension and renal insufficiency should always raise the possibility of bilateral renal artery stenosis. In these circumstances, attention to dietary salt intake and diuretic therapy is important.

TABLE 38–6. ANTIHYPERTENSIVE THERAPY FOR PATIENTS WITH RENOVASCULAR HYPERTENSION

Ideal therapy is percutaneous transluminal renal artery angioplasty or reconstructive surgery
Blood pressure
Is responsive to beta blockers, ACEIs, or calcium antagonists
Becomes responsive to salt deletion when renal failure develops
The GFR in the poststenotic kidney may be reduced by
A precipitous fall in BP
Vigorous ECV depletion and diuretic therapy
ACEIs

Abbreviations: ACEIs, angiotensin-converting enzyme inhibitors; ECV, extracellular fluid volume; GFR, glomerular filtration rate.

Polycystic Kidney Disease

Most patients with polycystic kidney disease experience hypertension that progresses in parallel with the development of renal failure. The cause is multifactorial. Studies have indicated that during the early phases of polycystic kidney disease, hypertension is related predominantly to tubular sodium and fluid retention with volume expansion. Circulating levels of plasma renin are usually normal. However, after correction of the volume excess with dietary salt restriction and diuretic therapy, plasma renin activity levels may rise, and the blood pressure becomes responsive to angiotensin antagonists or ACEIs. Care is necessary with the use of ACEIs because some patients experience an abrupt decline in renal function.[34]

Renal Transplant Recipients

Hypertension in the transplant recipient is multifactorial.[35, 36] There are factors intrinsic to the graft, which include delayed graft function, acute and chronic rejection, cyclosporine nephropathy, or recurrent primary renal disease. Additionally, there may be effects of cyclosporine and corticosteroids on blood vessels, the influence of the native kidneys, the presence of a transplant renal artery stenosis, or metabolic derangements such as hypercalcemia that can contribute to hypertension. It is important to work closely with the nephrologist supervising the patient to assess the importance of the diverse causes of hypertension. Cyclosporine-induced renal vasoconstriction is of considerable importance in the development of hypertension. Calcium antagonists are effective in cyclosporine-induced hypertension and renal vasoconstriction. They usually maintain renal function in cyclosporine-treated hypertensive patients, whereas in the short term, ACEIs may reduce the glomerular filtration rate.[37] In a 3-year study, however, ACEIs and calcium antagonists produced similar control of blood pressure without a clear-cut advantage of one agent over another.[38] Moreover, ACEIs have the potential to produce hyperkalemia and anemia in patients with more severe renal function impairment. Indeed, ACEI therapy is indicated to control post-transplant erythrocytosis that can occur in some patients with well-functioning grafts after renal transplantation.[36]

In general, ACEIs are best avoided in the immediate post-transplant period, at which time calcium antagonists are often effective. ACEIs can be introduced under close supervision in patients who are otherwise stable at a later stage after transplantation. The presence of refractory hypertension should raise the possibility of a transplant renal artery stenosis. When diagnosed, the therapy of choice is angioplasty because long-lasting remission can be expected in many patients. Finally, there is a group of patients with good graft function and absence of renal artery stenosis but severe or uncontrolled hypertension. Some of these subjects benefit from native kidney nephrectomy. This situation is less common, however, in the modern era of wide availability of powerful antihypertensive medications.[36]

REFERENCES

1. Smith MC, Dunn MJ: Hypertension in renal parenchymal disease. *In* Laragh JH, Brenner BM (eds): Hypertension: Pathophysiology, Diagnosis and Management, pp 1583–1599. New York: Raven Press, 1990.
2. U.S. Renal Data System: USRDS 1993 Annual Data Report. Bethesda, MD: The National Institutes of Health, National Institute of Diabetes and Digestive Kidney Diseases, April 1993.
3. Shulman NB, Ford CE, Hall WD, et al: Prognostic value of serum creatinine and effect of treatment of hypertension on renal function; results from the Hypertension Detection and Follow-up Program. Hypertension 1989; 13:I-80–I-93.

4. Rostand SG, Brown G, Kirk KA, et al: Renal insufficiency in treated essential hypertension. N Engl J Med 1989; 320:684–688.
5. Walker WG, Neaton JD, Cutler JA: Renal function change in hypertensive members of the Multiple Risk Factor Intervention Trial. JAMA 1992; 268:3085–3091.
6. Luke RG: Can renal failure due to hypertension be prevented? Hypertension 1991; 18:I-139–I-142.
7. Feld LG, VanLien JB, Brantjens JR, et al: Renal function and proteinuria in the spontaneously hypertensive rat made normotensive by treatment. Kidney Int 1981; 20:606–614.
8. Pettinger WA, Lee HC, Reisch J, et al: Long-term improvement in renal function after short-term strict blood pressure control in hypertensive nephrosclerosis. Hypertension 1989; 13:766–772.
9. Brazy PC, Fitzwilliam JF: Progressive renal disease: role of race and antihypertensive medications. Kidney Int 1990; 37:1113–1119.
10. Griffin KA, Picken M, Bidani AK: Radiotelemetric BP monitoring, antihypertensives and glomeruloprotection in remnant kidney model. Kidney Int 1994; 46:1010–1018.
11. Klahr S, Levey AS, Beck GJ, et al: The effects of dietary protein restriction and blood-pressure control on the progression of chronic renal disease. N Engl J Med 1994; 330:877–884.
12. Becker GJ, Whitworth JA, Ihle BU, et al: Prevention of progression in non-diabetic chronic renal failure. Kidney Int 1994; 45:S-167–S-170.
13. Zucchelli P, Zuccala A: Hypertension in advanced renal failure. *In* Cameron S, Davison AM, Grunfeld JP, et al (eds): Oxford Textbook of Clinical Nephrology, vol 3, pp 2117–2123. Oxford: Oxford University Press, 1992.
14. Mitch WE, Wilcox CS: Disorders of body fluids, sodium and potassium in chronic renal failure. Am J Med 1982; 72:536–550.
15. Brod J, Bahlmann J, Cachovan M, et al: Development of hypertension in renal disease. Clin Sci 1983; 64:141–152.
16. London GM, Marchais SJ, Guerin AP: Blood pressure control in chronic hemodialysis patients. *In* Winchester JF, Jacobs C, Kjellstrand CM, et al (eds): Replacement of Renal Function by Dialysis, 4th ed. Dordrecht: Kluwer Academic, in press.
17. Converse RL, Jacobsen TN, Toto RD, et al: Sympathetic overactivity in patients with chronic renal failure. N Engl J Med 1992; 327:1912–1918.
18. Huot SJ, Pamnani MB, Clough DL, et al: Sodium-potassium pump activity in reduced renal-mass hypertension. Hypertension 1983; 5:I-94–I-100.
19. Wilcox CS, Lin L: Vasoconstrictor prostaglandins in angiotensin-dependent and renovascular hypertension. J Nephrol 1993; 6:124–133.
20. Vallance P, Leone A, Calver A, et al: Accumulation of an endogenous inhibitor of nitric oxide synthesis in chronic renal failure. Lancet 1992; 339:572–575.
21. Golper TA, Marx MA, Shuler C, et al: Drug dosage in dialysis patients. *In* Winchester JF, Jacobs C, Kjellstrand CM, et al (eds): Replacement of Renal Functions by Dialysis, 4th ed. Dordrecht: Kluwer Academic, in press.
22. Unwin RJ, Liguros M, Shakelton C, et al: Role of diuretic treatment for hypertension. *In* Laragh JH, Brenner BM (eds): Hypertension: Pathophysiology, Diagnosis and Management. New York: Raven Press, in press.
23. Wilcox CS: Diuretics. *In* Brenner BM, Rector FC (eds): The Kidney, 5th ed. New York: Raven Press, in press.
24. Eliahou HE, Cohen D, Hellberg B, et al: Effect of the calcium channel blocker nisoldipine on the progression of chronic renal failure in man. Am J Nephrol 1988; 8:285–290.
25. Wilcox CS: Renovascular hypertension. *In* Glassock R, Klahr S (eds): Textbook of Nephrology, 3rd ed, pp 1218–1228. Baltimore: Williams & Wilkins, 1994.
26. Bauer JH, Reams GP, Lal SM: Renal protective effect of strict blood pressure control with enalapril therapy. Arch Intern Med 1987; 147:1397–1400.
27. Ruilope LM, Miranda B, Morales JM, et al: Converting enzyme inhibition in chronic renal failure. Am J Kidney Dis 1989; 8:120–126.
28. Wilcox CS: Use of angiotensin-converting-enzyme inhibitors for diagnosing renovascular hypertension. Kidney Int 1993; 44:1379–1390.
29. Hoyer J, Schulte K, Lenz T: Clinical pharmacokinetics of angiotensin converting enzyme (ACE) inhibitors in renal failure. Clin Pharmacokinet 1993; 24:230–254.
30. Brenner BM: Nephron adaptation to renal injury or ablation. Am J Physiol 249:F324–F337, 1985.
31. Hollenberg N: A buoyant view of the value of angiotensin-converting enzyme inhibition in renovascular disease. *In* Robertson JIS, Nichols MG (eds): The Renin-Angiotensin System: Pathophysiology and Therapeutics, vol 2, pp 90.1–90.8. London: Gower Medical, 1993.
32. Huelseman JL, Sterzel RB, McKenzie DE, et al: Effect of a calcium entry blocker on blood pressure and renal function during angiotensin-induced hypertension. Hypertension 1985; 7:374–379.
33. Menard J, Michel JB, Plouin PF: A cautious view of the value of angiotensin-converting enzyme inhibition in renovascular disease. *In* Robertson JIS, Nichols MG (eds): The Renin-Angiotensin System: Pathophysiology and Therapeutics, vol 2, pp 89.1–89.8. London: Gower Medical, 1993.
34. Gabow PA, Grantham JJ: Polycystic kidney disease. *In* Schrier RW, Goottschalk CW (eds): Diseases of the Kidney, 5th ed, pp 535–570. Boston: Little, Brown, 1993.
35. Curtis JJ: Management of hypertension after transplantation. Kidney Int 1993; 44(43):S45–S49.
36. Gaston RS, Curtis JJ: Hypertension following renal transplantation. *In* Massry SG, Glassock RJ (eds): Textbook of Nephrology, vol 2, pp 1694–1699. Baltimore: Williams & Wilkins, 1995.
37. Curtis JJ, Laskow DA, Jones PA, et al: Captopril induced fall in glomerular filtration rate in cyclosporine-treated patients. J Am Soc Nephrol 1993; 3:1570–1574.
38. Mourad G, Ribstein J, Mimran A: Converting enzyme inhibitor versus calcium antagonist in cyclosporine-treated renal transplants. Kidney Int 1993; 43:419–425.

39 Endocrine Causes of Hypertension

Caren G. Solomon, MD
Robert G. Dluhy, MD

Endocrine diseases are uncommon causes of hypertension, accounting for fewer than 3% of cases (Table 39–1). Nonetheless, they are important to recognize, as treatment of an underlying endocrinopathy may cure or improve hypertension as well as other associated metabolic abnormalities. Because the vast majority of hypertension is of the essential type rather than secondary to another disorder, a search for an endocrine cause of hypertension should not be routinely pursued but rather should be predicated on suggestive symptoms or signs (e.g., early onset of hypertension, family history, or features of endocrine disease such as cushingoid appearance, suggesting cortisol excess). This chapter reviews endocrinologic causes of hypertension, with particular emphasis on therapeutic approaches to these disorders.

GLUCOCORTICOID EXCESS STATES

Presentation and Diagnosis

Glucocorticoid excess results from either endogenous overproduction of cortisol or exogenous glucocorticoids given in supraphysiologic doses (see discussion of exogenous glucocorticoids further on). Disorders causing Cushing syndrome can be viewed as adrenocorticotropic hormone (ACTH)-independent (adrenal neoplasms) or ACTH-dependent (ectopic ACTH production or pituitary ACTH hypersecretion).[1] Hypertension occurs in up to 80% of patients with hypercortisolism; postulated causes include increased plasma renin activity, increased cardiac output, inhibitory effects on vasodilatory prostaglandins, and possibly, in small part, mineralocorticoid effects. High blood pressure is particularly common in patients who have ACTH-dependent hypercortisolism or adrenal carcinoma, probably because of overproduction of other steroids such as desoxycorticosterone (DOC) in addition to cortisol in this setting.

Symptoms and signs suggestive of cortisol excess include truncal obesity and other manifestations of central fat accumulation (moon facies, supraclavicular fat pad, "buffalo hump"); purple striae; proximal muscle weakness; and osteopenia/fracture. Hyperglycemia is common, and hypokalemic alkalosis may be noted, especially in the setting of ectopic ACTH secretion. Measurement of 24-h urine-free cortisol is an excellent screening test for Cushing syndrome and is particularly useful in differentiating simple obesity from hypercortisolism.

TABLE 39–1. ENDOCRINE CAUSES OF HYPERTENSION

Adrenal Disease
Cushing syndrome
Hyperaldosteronism
DOC-secreting tumor
Congenital adrenal hyperplasia
Pheochromocytoma
Thyroid Disease
Hypothyroidism
Hyperthyroidism
Hyperparathyroidism
Acromegaly
Renin-Secreting Tumor
Exogenous Hormones/Hormone-Like Agents
Oral contraceptives
Anabolic steroids
Glucocorticoids
Mineralocorticoids/mineralocorticoid-like agents
Fludrocortisone
Licorice
Sympathomimetic agents
Thyroid-related agents
Thyroxine
Amiodarone

Abbreviation: DOC, desoxycorticosterone.

Therapy

Adrenal Neoplasms

Therapy should be directed at the cause of Cushing syndrome.[2] When an adrenal adenoma underlies the syndrome, surgical resection is the treatment of choice in the absence of major contraindications.[3] Because the contralateral adrenal gland is expected to be atrophic in the setting of chronic glucocorticoid excess, intra- and perioperative glucocorticoid treatment is mandatory. On the operative day, hydrocortisone should be administered continuously at a rate of 10 mg/h or, alternatively, as intravenous bolus therapy (80–100 mg q8h). Postoperatively, the dose of cortisol is reduced in 20%–30% daily decrements to maintenance levels (25–30 mg of hydrocortisone per day in divided doses) if the patient is afebrile and not hypotensive. In cases of cortisol-producing adenomas, recovery of the pituitary adrenal axis may take up to 6–9 months. During this time, the steroid dose should be gradually reduced while clinical symptoms of steroid withdrawal, such as severe fatigue and arthralgias, are observed. An early morning cortisol level before dosing can be used to gauge the recovery of endogenous cortisol production. A morning cortisol level greater than 10 μg/dL suggests recovery of the pituitary adrenal axis, allowing discontinuation of cortisol replacement therapy. Because responsiveness of the axis may remain blunted for up to 12 months, however, "stress" doses of cortisol should be reinstituted for severe, acute illness or surgery during this period.

Adrenocortical carcinoma has a poor prognosis and has often metastasized at the time of diagnosis. Beyond surgical resection, radiation to the operative bed and chemotherapy are commonly needed as adjunctive modalities, when possible.[4]

When surgical control of disease is not possible or is ineffective, medical therapy is indicated to reduce cortisol overproduction and its associated metabolic effects (Table 39–2). The agent that is often the first choice is ketoconazole, which interferes with adrenal

TABLE 39–2. TREATMENT ALTERNATIVES FOR HYPERALDOSTERONISM AND CUSHING SYNDROME

	Medications	Usual Daily Dosage
Hyperaldosteronism	Spironolactone	100–400 mg (b.i.d.–t.i.d.)
	Amiloride	5–20 mg (b.i.d.)
Cushing syndrome	Aminoglutethimide	1–2 g (q.i.d.)
	Mitotane	2–6 g (q.i.d.)
	Ketoconazole	400–1200 mg (b.i.d.)
	Octreotide*	300 μg (b.i.d.)

*Useful in reducing adrenocorticotropic hormone (ACTH) secretion in some patients with ectopic ACTH production; other agents inhibit cortisol biosynthesis.

steroidogenesis by inhibiting the side chain cleavage enzyme of cholesterol as well as inhibiting 11β-hydroxylase.[5] High doses (800–1200 mg daily) taken orally in divided doses are generally required to control hypercortisolism. Side effects include hepatic toxicity and hypocalcemia. Because this agent also inhibits testosterone production, additional side effects in male patients include impotence, loss of libido, and gynecomastia. A serious complication of this agent, as well as of all therapies designed to inhibit cortisol production, is adrenal insufficiency. Therefore, serum cortisol levels should be carefully monitored and concomitant glucocorticoid replacement therapy instituted as steroid levels are reduced to the normal range. Dexamethasone (0.75 mg/day orally) should be used initially while titrating the ketoconazole dose to allow assessment of endogenous cortisol production. Subsequently, the shorter acting glucocorticoid hydrocortisone is preferable as chronic replacement therapy. Doses of 25–30 mg/day in two divided doses (15–20 mg every morning, 10 mg every evening) are generally appropriate, whereas higher doses are indicated in the setting of acute stress.

Other agents known to inhibit steroidogenesis include aminoglutethimide, metyrapone, and mitotane. Aminoglutethimide inhibits several steps in steroid biosynthesis, including 11β-hydroxylase, aldosterone synthase, and 21-hydroxylase, as well as the conversion of cholesterol to pregnenolone. Aminoglutethimide is started at 250 mg orally every 6 h and may be increased in increments of 250 mg/day every several weeks to a maximal dose of 2 g/day. Mineralocorticoid deficiency may also occur with this agent, necessitating treatment with fludrocortisone. Metyrapone, which blocks 11β-hydroxylase in the adrenal cortex, is given in divided doses four times daily at a daily dosage of 1–4 g. Mitotane likewise inhibits adrenal steroidogenesis and may in some cases result in objective tumor regression, although it does not prolong survival. Starting dosages range between 2 and 6 g/day in three to four daily doses at mealtimes. Adverse effects, especially at high doses, include gastrointestinal and neurologic toxicity, such as drowsiness and ataxia. A novel agent that should still be considered experimental therapy is RU-486, which acts as a glucocorticoid receptor antagonist. Its major use at this time has been pregnancy termination caused by its antiprogestin activity.

Adrenocorticotropic Hormone–Dependent Cushing Syndrome

As for adrenal neoplasms, surgical resection is the preferred treatment for ACTH-dependent Cushing syndrome. Many neoplasms producing ectopic ACTH (e.g., small cell carcinomas of lung) are malignant, however, and are not amenable to surgical cure. In pituitary-dependent Cushing disease, transsphenoidal resection of a pituitary microadenoma can be accomplished in 85% of cases.[6–9] If pituitary tumors are large and not completely resectable, radiation therapy may be considered as adjunctive treatment.[10, 11] Hypopituitarism is a common complication of radiation treatment, and thus annual evaluation of hormones that are regulated by the pituitary gland is required.

If treatment directed at the pituitary gland is not successful, an alternative is bilateral surgical adrenalectomy. One major disadvantage of this approach is the subsequent lifelong requirement for replacement therapy with both glucocorticoids and mineralocorticoids. A second concern is the potential for growth of a pituitary tumor after adrenalectomy (i.e., Nelson syndrome), a phenomenon attributed to lack of feedback suppression by high cortisol levels. Tumors developing in this setting are characteristically associated with hyperpigmentation from high levels of ACTH or its precursor proopiomelanocortin and are frequently aggressive, requiring surgery and often adjunctive radiation therapy.

Pharmacologic therapies discussed previously for the treatment of unresectable adrenal cancer can also be used to advantage in selected patients with ACTH-dependent Cushing syndrome to control hypercortisolism, for example, in patients who are not surgically cured or as adjunctive therapy after radiation treatment.[11] An additional pharmacologic treatment for selective patients is octreotide, a long-acting somatostatin analog that may reduce ectopic tumor ACTH production in cases of pancreatic tumor or bronchial carcinoid. This agent is administered subcutaneously at a usual dose of 300 μg/day in divided doses. In some patients, this agent may also reduce tumor mass. The major side effects of this therapy include the need for multiple injections and the long-term complication of gallstone formation in more than half of patients, probably related to bile stasis as a result of cholecystokinin inhibition. To date, responsiveness to this agent in patients with excess ectopic ACTH secretion is variable and unpredictable.

When an antihypertensive agent is required, awaiting more definitive treatment of cortisol excess, potassium-wasting diuretics are relatively contraindicated because of the underlying tendency toward hypokalemia associated with steroid excess. Potassium-sparing diuretics or angiotensin-converting enzyme inhibitors may be particularly useful in this setting.

MINERALOCORTICOID EXCESS STATES

Presentation and Diagnosis

Mineralocorticoid excess states include hyperaldosteronism as well as the overproduction of other mineralocorticoids, such as DOC. Hallmark features of mineralocorticoid excess include hypertension, which is sometimes severe, suppression of the renin-angiotensin system (often to undetectable levels), and hypokalemia.[12, 13] Autonomous overproduction of aldosterone is confirmed by the failure to suppress aldosterone production in response to a volume-expanding maneuver such as intravenous saline loading. Hyperaldosteronism may result from a neoplasm, commonly an adenoma but rarely an aldosterone-producing carcinoma. Other causes include bilateral idiopathic hyperplasia and glucocorticoid-remediable aldosteronism (GRA). DOC may also be overproduced as a result of neoplastic disease or more commonly a congenital adrenocortical enzyme deficiency (11β-hydroxylase or 17α-hydroxylase). Apparent mineralocorticoid excess may occur secondary to exogenous agents such as excessive licorice ingestion (discussed later in this chapter).

Therapy

Therapy varies with the cause of mineralocorticoid excess, as described in the following sections.

Hyperaldosteronism

Aldosterone-Secreting Tumors. Surgery is indicated for aldosterone-secreting adenomas or carcinomas when there are no contraindications to this approach, such as severe cardiovascular disease or metastatic disease.[14] Results are most gratifying for patients with solitary adenomas, in which cure or improvement of hypertension and resolution of hypokalemia are seen in the majority of individuals within 3–6 months; however, as many as a third of patients will remain hypertensive, a result of coexistent essential hypertension or renal damage secondary to antecedent uncontrolled hypertension.

Preoperatively these patients should undergo repletion with exogenous administration of potassium and should maintain a low-salt diet (<2 g sodium) to minimize renal potassium secretion. Spironolactone, an aldosterone antagonist, also may be used preoperatively (its use is detailed in the following section discussing the management of bilateral adrenal hyperplasia). Some investigators have transiently administered stress doses of glucocorticoids (as outlined in the discussion of glucocorticoid excess) as a precaution in case the remaining adrenal gland is not functionally normal. Because the cortisol axis should logically remain unaffected by mineralocorticoid excess, this practice should not be routine, although careful clinical monitoring for any signs of cortisol deficiency is prudent. A complication that is far more common than glucocorticoid insufficiency in this setting is postoperative hypoaldosteronism, a consequence of long-standing suppression of the renin-angiotensin system. Adequate sodium intake is imperative during this time to prevent hyperkalemia as well as to counter possible salt-wasting. Use of the mineralocorticoid fludrocortisone is not recommended in this setting, however, since it will perpetuate suppression of the renin-angiotensin system. Prolonged preoperative treatment with spironolactone decreases the likelihood of this complication because the renin-angiotensin system will be activated by the reversal of the mineralocorticoid excess state. This medication must be discontinued on hospital admission, however, to minimize the risk of postoperative hyperkalemia.

Bilateral Adrenal Hyperplasia. In contrast to hypertension secondary to adenomas, that due to bilateral adrenal hyperplasia responds poorly to adrenalectomy, resolving in only 15% of cases despite correction of the hypokalemia and hyperaldosteronism. The preferred therapy for patients with bilateral hyperplasia, as in patients with an adenoma awaiting surgery, is the aldosterone antagonist spironolactone.[15] The starting dosage is 50 mg twice daily, and dosing may be increased at weekly intervals up to a maximum dosage of 200 mg twice daily. The treatment goals are control of blood pressure as well as correction of hypokalemia. To avoid gastrointestinal side effects, this drug should be administered at mealtimes. Up to 20% of patients, primarily males, reject this therapy because of the androgen-antagonizing effects of spironolactone, including gynecomastia, loss of libido, and impotence. Females may also experience intermenstrual spotting or menstrual irregularity. If spironolactone is poorly tolerated, an alternative agent is amiloride. This medication blocks the apical distal tubule Na^+/K^+ channel, thereby decreasing sodium and potassium exchange. A starting dose is 10 mg daily, which can be increased at 2-week intervals to a maximum of 40 mg/day. It is safe and without antiandrogen side effects, although gastrointestinal side effects have been reported. Although comparative studies have not been performed, most clinicians sense that amiloride is less effective than spironolactone in states of hyperaldosteronism. As with spironolactone, the goals of therapy include normalization of potassium levels as well as reduction of blood pressure.

Glucocorticoid-Remediable Aldosteronism. GRA is a disorder inherited in an autosominal dominant fashion and characterized by sole regulation of aldosterone secretion by ACTH rather than by the renin-angiotensin system.[16] Hypertension characteristically presents early in life, and a family history of early-onset hypertension is common. The genetic mutation causing this disorder has been identified—a gene duplication fusing the promoter region of 11β-hydroxylase (regulated by ACTH) to the coding sequence of aldosterone synthase.[17, 18] This leads to ectopic expression of aldosterone synthase in the cortisol-producing zona fasciculata. Glucocorticoid suppression of ACTH reverses the mineralocorticoid excess state and logically would be considered first-line therapy for this disorder. In adults, glucocorticoid suppression of ACTH has been accomplished with dexamethasone (0.5–1 mg/day) or prednisone (5 mg at bedtime or 5 mg twice per day) as in the treatment of congenital hyperplasia (see later discussion). Excessive glucocorticoid dosing is unnecessary and may produce cushingoid side effects, including severe complications such as aseptic necrosis of the head of the femur. When dosing of glucocorticoids required to control hyperaldosteronism is associated with significant steroid side effects, therapy with amiloride or spironolactone should be instituted, as described in the Bilateral Adrenal Hyperplasia section. Dihydropyridine calcium channel blockers, such as the extended release nifedipine formulation, 30–90 mg/day, have also been used successfully in this setting. As in all mineralocorticoid excess states, dietary sodium restriction will minimize potassium-wasting and enhance pharmacologic therapy.

The preferred treatment for children with GRA remains controversial. Pediatricians agree that children with blood pressure levels exceeding the 95th percentile for age and sex on three occasions merit therapy for their hypertension, but no studies have compared different therapies in children affected with GRA. If glucocorticoids are used, the dose should be calculated in regard to body surface area to avoid overtreatment. Some clinicians prefer the shorter acting glucocorticoid hydrocortisone in divided doses at 10 mg/m^2/day to accomplish suppression. Long-acting glucocorticoids (dexamethasone or prednisone) may be associated with greater compliance but also with greater risks of growth retardation and other manifestations of glucocorticoid excess. Growth should be regularly charted in any child treated with glucocorticoids because excessive treatment retards linear skeletal growth. For the preceding reasons, some clinicians prefer spironolactone, amiloride, or other antihypertensive agents such as calcium channel blockers, although the long-term effects of such medications in children are uncertain.

Desoxycorticosterone-Secreting Tumors

Benign or malignant neoplasms rarely secrete DOC as an end product rather than aldosterone. Overproduction of this potent mineralocorticoid leads to suppression of plasma renin activity and a low aldosterone level. Pre- and perioperative management of such neoplasms is identical to that outlined for aldosterone-secreting tumors (see earlier discussion).

Congenital Adrenal Hyperplasia

Congenital adrenal hyperplasia may be evident at birth or early in life (classic case) or during puberty and early adulthood (late onset).[19] Hypertension results from specific deficiencies in enzymes involved in cortisol biosynthesis, with accumulation of steroid precursors that have mineralocorticoid activity.[20] Either of two enzyme deficiencies, 11β-hydroxylase or 17α-hydroxylase, may result in hypertension secondary to overproduction of the potent mineralocorticoid DOC (Fig. 39–1). Volume expansion results in hypertension and leads to suppression of renin activity and a resultant low aldosterone level. In 11β-hydroxylase deficiency, there is also overproduction of adrenal androgens, leading to virilization in females or an early growth spurt with premature epiphyseal closure and short stature; less severe manifestations such as mild hirsutism, acne, or oligomenorrhea may also occur. In 17α-hydroxylase deficiency, there is a lack of secondary sexual characteristics because of a deficiency in the production of androgens and estrogens.

Treatment of these disorders involves glucocorticoid suppression, as outlined previously for GRA, with a short-acting glucocorticoid such as hydrocortisone in divided dosages or the longer acting steroids prednisone or dexamethasone. Steroid side effects should be minimized or avoided by titration of the dosage to body surface area;

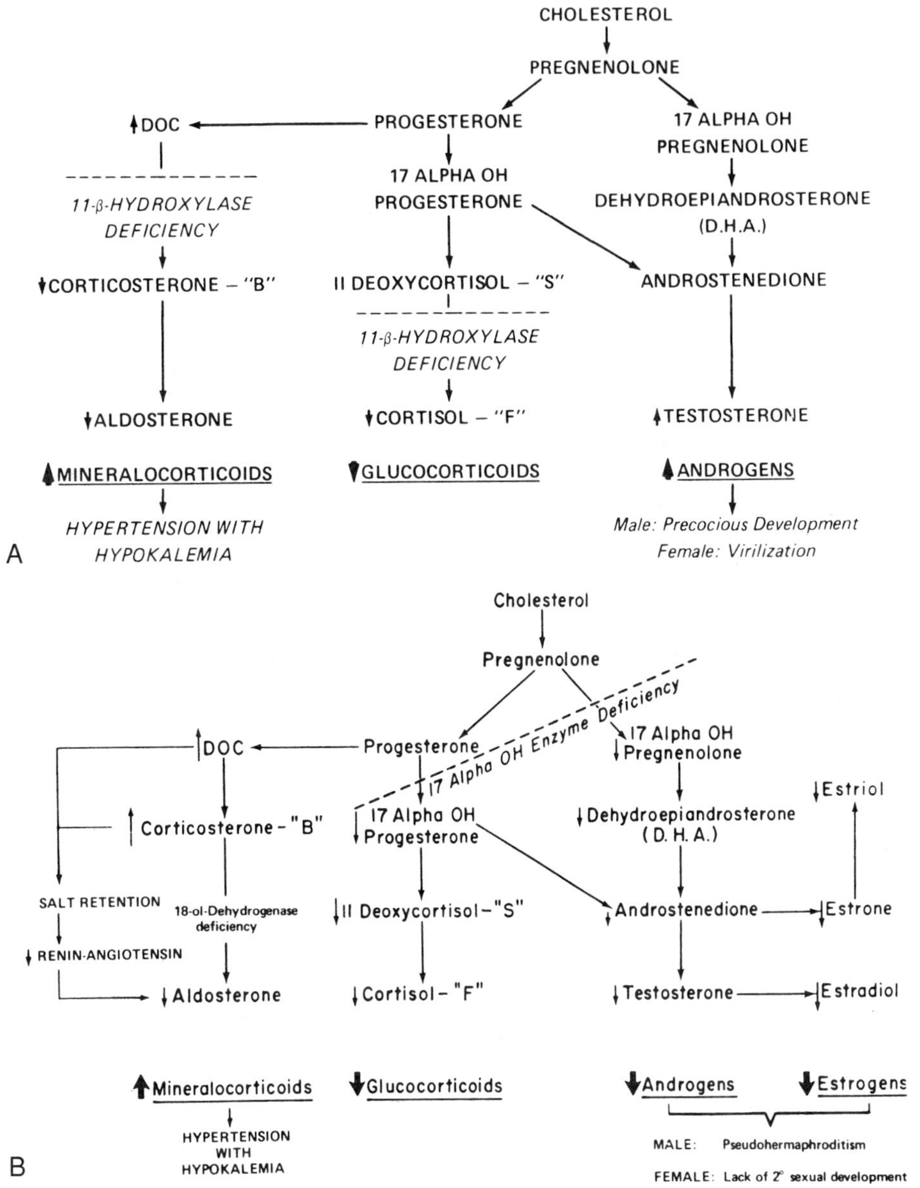

Figure 39–1. Adrenal enzyme deficiencies of 11β-hydroxylase (*A*) and 17α-hydroxylase (*B*). Both syndromes result in a mineralocorticoid excess state. The former is also associated with adrenal androgen overproduction, whereas in the latter there is a deficiency in production of androgens and estrogens. (From Kaplan NM [ed]: Clinical Hypertension, p 431. Baltimore: Williams & Wilkins, 1986.)

as discussed in the section on GRA, this is particularly important in children.

PHEOCHROMOCYTOMA

Presentation and Diagnosis

Pheochromocytoma, a tumor of chromaffin cells of sympathetic nervous system origin, has an estimated incidence of less than 1 per 100,000 population. However, its lethal potential if unrecognized underscores the importance of considering this tumor in appropriate clinical settings. Paroxysmal increases in blood pressure represent the classic presentation of this disorder, but half of patients have sustained rather than episodic hypertension.[21] Typical symptoms include episodic headaches, palpitations, and sweats; pheochromocytoma is rarely identified in someone with none of these symptoms, although many patients will manifest only one or two of them. Pheochromocytoma may be associated with orthostatic hypotension, a result of the volume depletion that accompanies chronic vasoconstriction, although this finding may be less common and less often symptomatic than was once thought.[1] A family history of pheochromocytoma or other tumors (e.g., parathyroid adenomas or medullary carcinoma of the thyroid; neurofibromas; or renal cell, retinal, or cerebellar hemangiomas) should raise suspicion of a familial syndrome, that is, multiple endocrine neoplasia type IIa or IIb, neurofibromatosis, or von Hippel–Lindau disease.

When the diagnosis of pheochromocytoma is suspected, biochemical confirmation should be obtained before pursuing radiologic imaging because incidental, usually benign, adrenal tumors are found on almost 1% of computed tomography scans. Testing should involve a 24-h urine specimen for unmetabolized or free catecholamines (norepinephrine and epinephrine) and metabolites (metanephrines and vanillylmandelic acid [VMA]); creatinine should be measured as well to ensure adequacy of collection. Total catecholamines should routinely be fractionated into their two components, as pure epinephrine-secreting tumors may be missed on a composite measure. If only one test is to be ordered, measurement of metanephrines is most sensitive, whereas measurement of VMA is most specific.[21] Measurement of both fractionated free catecholamines and catecholamine metabolites is routinely recommended, however, as some cases of pheochromocytoma will present with an abnormality in only one of these measures, whereas other tests are within normal limits.

Certain medications—for example, methyldopa and labetalol—may interfere with test results, and such medications should ideally be discontinued at the time of testing. Normal results on all measures in the setting of symptoms and/or blood pressure elevation essentially excludes the diagnosis. A positive test result should be followed up with radiologic imaging, either computed tomography or magnetic resonance imaging. A tumor of one adrenal gland is most common, but familial bilateral adrenal tumors or extra-adrenal tumors may also occur.

Therapy

Preoperative Management

Definitive therapy of pheochromocytoma is surgical in the vast majority of cases, but adjunctive medical management is critical pre- and perioperatively (Table 39–3). Alpha blockade should be started at least several days before surgery. Phenoxybenzamine is classically used for this purpose, but there is also recent experience with more selective α_1 blockers, for example, doxazosin.[22] The alpha blocker dosage should be increased every 2–3 days until blood pressure is controlled; therapeutic end points include a supine blood pressure no greater than 160/90 mm Hg, orthostatic hypotension not in excess of 80/45 mm Hg, and absence of ischemic changes on electrocardiography. Preoperative volume repletion has been shown to minimize the risk of intraoperative hypotension and also to facilitate upward titration of alpha blocker dosage. The patient should be instructed to consume a high-salt diet before hospital admission. Volume expansion with intravenous normal saline may be needed in selected patients, and associated hemodynamic monitoring is warranted when there is heart disease or renal insufficiency. A preoperative echocardiogram may assist in the management of patients with suspected cardiac disease, including catecholamine cardiomyopathy. Beta blockers are indicated for persistent tachycardia or ectopy but must be withheld until a patient has received adequate alpha blockade, since premature initiation of beta blockade carries the risk of hypertensive crisis secondary to inhibition of beta receptor–mediated vasodilation. Calcium channel blockers have also been effectively used to reduce blood pressure in the setting of pheochromocytoma; all classes appear to reduce blood pressure largely by blocking norepinephrine-mediated calcium transport into vascular smooth muscle.[23] Metyrosine, an inhibitor of catecholamine synthesis, has also been used in preoperative management; however, because of frequent side effects, including neurotoxicity (extrapyramidal signs) and diarrhea, its use is more common in the setting of inoperable or metastatic pheochromocytoma with retracting hypertension.

TABLE 39–3. MEDICAL MANAGEMENT OF PHEOCHROMOCYTOMA

	Recommended Dosages	
Medications	**Starting**	**Maximal**
Alpha blockers		
Phenoxybenzamine	10 mg b.i.d.	40 mg t.i.d.
Doxazosin	1 mg daily	16 mg daily
Terazosin	1 mg daily	20 mg daily
Beta blockers (*after* alpha blockade)		
Propranolol	10 mg q.i.d.	40 mg q.i.d.
Metoprolol	50 mg b.i.d.	100 mg q.i.d.
Calcium channel blockers		
Nifedipine (Procardia XL)	30 mg daily	60 mg b.i.d.
Nicardipine	20 mg t.i.d.	40 mg t.i.d.
Catecholamine synthesis inhibitor		
Metyrosine*	250 mg q.i.d.	1 g q.i.d.

*More commonly used in setting of inoperable or metastatic disease.

TABLE 39–4. USUAL MEDICATIONS FOR SURGICAL MANAGEMENT OF PHEOCHROMOCYTOMA

Drug	Recommended Dosage Range
Nitroprusside	2–10 μg/kg/min*
Phentolamine	5 mg IV p.r.n.
Labetalol	1–2 mg IV bolus, drip at 0.5–2 mg/min
Esmolol	80 mg IV bolus over 30 seconds, then 150–300 μg/kg/min

*Risk of cyanide toxicity increased at doses >4 μg/kg/min.
Abbreviations: IV, intravenous; p.r.n., as needed.

Intraoperative Management

Intraoperatively, hemodynamic monitoring is mandatory. A central venous line is generally considered adequate in patients without cardiac or pulmonary disease, whereas monitoring with a pulmonary artery line is preferred in patients with these conditions. As at the time of tumor manipulation, blood pressure elevations are best managed with sodium nitroprusside or phentolamine; labetalol has also been used effectively, although, as noted previously, there is theoretic concern about beta blockade before effective alpha blockade. Cardiac arrhythmias generally respond to esmolol or lidocaine (Table 39–4). The type of anesthesia (spinal or general) and the specific anesthetic agents appear of less import than appropriate preoperative preparation and intraoperative monitoring, although some investigators have suggested that certain agents, such as halothane and droperidol, are best avoided. Removal of the tumor may result in hypotension. Primary therapy for this complication is fluid resuscitation, generally with lactated Ringer solution; large volumes are often required. In rare cases of hypotension secondary to catecholamine withdrawal, alpha agonists may also be indicated, but this is never the first-line approach.

Postoperative Management

Postoperatively, blood pressure and glucose levels should be followed. Hypoglycemia may occur for 2 days or more after surgery. This complication, which has been attributed to sudden catecholamine withdrawal and previous depletion of glycogen stores, is a particular risk in patients receiving beta blockade, which can also diminish warning symptoms of hypoglycemia. Intravenous dextrose should be given as needed. As is true during surgery, hypotension may occur postoperatively and is volume-sensitive. Alternatively, hypertension may occur secondary to volume overload. In the absence of persistent tumor or underlying essential hypertension, blood pressure is expected to return to normal within days after surgery. As already described, 24-h urine catecholamine and metabolite levels should be rechecked 2–4 weeks after surgery to confirm complete tumor removal. Yearly urine tests are indicated indefinitely to exclude recurrence or a second pheochromocytoma. Serum levels of chromogranin A, a peptide secreted by pheochromocytomas, may also be useful as a marker of recurrent disease, although this test is nonspecific and levels may be high in the setting of renal insufficiency or other tumors.[22]

Nonsurgical Management

Approximately 10% of pheochromocytomas are estimated to be malignant, a figure that may be higher with long-term follow-up. In malignant disease, metastases occur most commonly to the lungs, liver, and bones and are frequently unresectable. In such cases, hypertension and associated symptoms should be managed medically using medications typically used preoperatively in operable cases—phenoxybenzamine or other alpha blockers, with or without a beta blocker, or calcium channel blockers, most commonly long-acting nifedipine. Metyrosine, described in the Preoperative Management section, is indicated for refractory hypertension not controlled by these medications.

Combination chemotherapy with cyclophosphamide, vincristine, and dacarbazine has also been used for malignant pheochromocytoma and may cause partial or complete remission but has not been curative.[24] Methyliodobenzoguanidine (MIBG), a radioactive tracer taken up by chromaffin cells and sometimes used in imaging of pheochromocytoma, has been used therapeutically, but results have been discouraging. The usual radioresistance of pheochromocytomas makes external radiation rarely useful, although it may have a role in painful bone metastases or impending spinal cord compression. There are isolated reports of long-term survival after resection of solitary bone metastases[25]; in general, tumor debulking is unlikely to induce remission but may improve response to medical therapy.

HYPERPARATHYROIDISM

Presentation and Diagnosis

Hyperparathyroidism has an incidence of approximately 1 per 1000 population and may be present in up to 1% of hypertensive patients. One study has suggested a shift to the right in blood pressure distribution as great as 15/10 mm Hg in the setting of hyperparathyroidism.[26] This disorder—caused most often by a solitary parathyroid adenoma, less frequently by multigland hyperplasia, and in rare cases by parathyroid carcinoma—is most often identified after hypercalcemia is detected incidentally on routine blood testing. Associated symptoms and signs include renal stones, renal insufficiency, bone pains or fractures, dyspepsia, peptic ulcer disease, fatigue, constipation, and depression. Diagnosis is based on an elevated serum calcium level in the setting of a high or inappropriately "normal" intact parathyroid hormone level; low serum phosphate and elevated bicarbonate levels are also frequently noted. Measurement of the serum calcium level is reasonable in any hypertensive individual; however, it is important to recognize that although treatment of hyperparathyroidism may improve several of its associated complications, blood pressure may not improve with therapy (see following sections).

Therapy

Surgical Therapy

Definitive therapy for hyperparathyroidism is surgical, and this approach is clearly indicated for all symptomatic patients in the absence of significant contraindications. A relatively recent National Institutes of Health (NIH) consensus also recommended surgery for many asymptomatic patients, including all premenopausal women (at risk of osteoporosis); anyone with a serum calcium level of 11.4 12 mg/dL or greater; and all patients with evidence of end-organ damage or deterioration secondary to hyperparathyroidism. Criteria for the latter included bone density more than 2 SD below age-matched controls, creatinine clearance reduced by 30% or more versus age-matched norms, 24-h urine calcium levels greater than 400 mg/24 h, or deteriorations in these parameters over time.[27] As noted previously, hypertension is *not* considered an indication for surgical therapy, largely because of the inconsistent effects of parathyroidectomy on blood pressure. Although some investigators have reported improvement in hypertension after such surgery,[26] others have found no significant benefit.[28]

Medical Therapy

In patients who decline surgery or who are not surgical candidates, medical management is possible. In hypophosphatemic patients, phosphate supplementation may lower calcium levels; however, its use is frequently complicated by diarrhea and carries a risk of calcium phosphate salt precipitation if the calcium-phosphate product exceeds 70. In postmenopausal women, premarin (0.625 mg by mouth per day) may reduce the serum calcium level slightly by inhibiting osteoclastic bone resorption and may also lower blood pressure slightly (see discussion of exogenous hormones further on).

THYROID DISEASE

Hypothyroidism

Presentation and Diagnosis

Hypertension has been reported in approximately 15% of hypothyroid individuals. Elevations in diastolic blood pressure are characteristic and are attributed to an increase in total peripheral resistance. Hypothyroidism is more common in women than in men, and suggestive symptoms and signs include fatigue, weight gain, edema, dry skin, menorrhagia, and sometines galactorrhea. The thyroid gland may be enlarged, and deep tendon reflexes are characteristically delayed. The best screening test for primary thyroid failure is an elevated thyroid-stimulating hormone (TSH) level measured with a supersensitive assay. In the rare case of secondary thyroid insufficiency due to hypothalamic or pituitary disease, the TSH level is not useful in diagnosis, and levels of thyroxine and thyroid hormone binding (e.g., triiodothyronine [T_3] resin uptake or thyroid hormone binding ratio) should be measured.

Therapy

Hypothyroidism and associated hypertension are effectively treated with thyroid hormone replacement. Usual replacement doses are in the range of 0.8 μg/lb body weight. Thyroid replacement may precipitate cardiac ischemia in susceptible individuals and thus should be started cautiously in the elderly hypothyroid patient or in those with known or suspected coronary artery disease; suspected concomitant adrenal insufficiency also warrants cautious replacement, as thyroid hormone replacement may precipitate adrenal crisis through an effect of thyroxine that accelerates the hepatic clearance of cortisol. In the preceding situations, the starting dose of thyroxine should be 0.025 mg, and the dosage should be gradually increased by 0.025 mg at intervals of every 3–4 weeks, observing for any adverse effects. In healthy, young individuals, replacement can be started at or near the dose expected to be fully therapeutic. Clinical assessment and thyroid function tests should be performed after 4 weeks of therapy when there is full metabolic expression of a given thyroid dose. Therapy is primarily targeted to a TSH level in the normal range; overreplacement with thyroid hormone, as evidenced by low or undetectable TSH levels, may result in accelerated bone loss and osteopenia[29] and may increase the risk of atrial fibrillation.[30] With appropriate replacement, blood pressure is expected to fall to the normal range in the absence of other causes of hypertension, such as concomitant essential hypertension.

Hyperthyroidism

Presentation and Diagnosis

Hyperthyroidism increases the risk of systolic hypertension, particularly in younger individuals, whereas diastolic blood pressures in hyperthyroid individuals tend to be normal or reduced. Symptoms of hyperthyroidism include sweating, palpitations, weight loss, and difficulty sleeping. Signs, in addition to a widened pulse pressure, include sinus tachycardia, lid lag, staring, hyperreflexia, tremor, ophthalmopathy (if hyperthyroidism is caused by Graves disease), and often thyroid enlargement. As with hypothyroidism, the supersensitive TSH assay is the key to diagnosis; it is suppressed in the vast majority of patients with this disorder (secondary hyperthyroidism due to a pituitary tumor is a notable but exceedingly rare exception).

Therapy

Successful treatment of hyperthyroidism routinely results in normalization of the heart rate and resolution of systolic hypertension. Therapy depends on the cause of hyperthyroidism.

Thyroiditis

There are two forms of thyroiditis classically associated with transient hyperthyroidism: (1) subacute (painful) thyroiditis, which commonly follows upper respiratory infection, and (2) lymphocytic (painless) thyroiditis, which may occur at any time but is particularly common postpartum. In either situation, hyperthyroidism is due to leakage of thyroid hormone from an inflamed gland and is self-limited; therapy is recommended only to control bothersome symptoms. There is no role for medications that inhibit thyroid hormone synthesis. Beta blockers (e.g., propranolol, 10–40 mg q.i.d; metoprolol, 50–100 mg b.i.d) are the treatment of choice, improving palpitations, tremor, and anxiety and reducing the pulse and blood pressure. Neck discomfort in the setting of subacute thyroiditis is generally responsive to aspirin or nonsteroidal anti-inflammatory agents.

Graves Disease

Graves disease is an autoimmune disease in which hyperthyroidism is due to stimulation of thyroxine production by antibodies directed against the TSH receptor (thyroid-stimulating immunoglobulins). Thyrotoxicosis in this setting is often severe and long-lasting, with relapse common even when disease temporarily remits. First-line treatment is generally with antithyroid medications, either propylthiouracil (PTU) or methimazole. Both agents inhibit thyroid hormone synthesis and, at high doses, PTU may also inhibit conversion of thyroxine to the more active triiodothyronine. Methimazole has the advantage of less frequent dosing—once or at most twice a day as compared with three times daily dosing of PTU. The usual starting dose of PTU is approximately 100 mg t.i.d., and that of methimazole is 10–15 mg/day (or b.i.d.). The dosage of these agents is adjusted every 4 weeks or so based on results of thyroid function tests. Both medications have the rare but potentially fatal side effect of agranulocytosis, which occurs idiosyncratically; any patient taking these medications must be warned to inform the physician in the setting of persistent sore throat or fever so that the white blood cell count can be checked. Both agents also may produce liver toxicity. Medical therapy with either agent results in resolution of thyrotoxicosis in the majority of patients with Graves disease, but up to two thirds of patients will have recurrence of disease when therapy is discontinued, generally after 1 year of treatment. Recent data have suggested that initiation of thyroid hormone replacement in combination with antithyroid drug therapy, once euthyroidism has been achieved, may improve long-term remission rates[31]; this remains to be confirmed by further studies. Until hyperthyroidism is controlled with antithyroid drugs, beta blockers may be used to treat blood pressure and some other manifestations of hyperthyroidism, as described in the discussion of thyroiditis.

Radioactive iodine ablation is generally recommended for individuals with recurrent hyperthyroidism after antithyroid drug therapy as well as for those who are unable to tolerate antithyroid drugs or who have contraindications to their use. The usual dose of radioactive iodine is 10–15 millicuries, calculated depending on iodine uptake, with the aim of delivering 6–8 millicuries to the thyroid gland. For pregnant patients who are intolerant of or refractory to antithyroid medications (pregnancy is a contraindication to the use of radioactive iodine) or patients who are unwilling to take radioactive iodine, subtotal thyroidectomy is indicated. Both radioactive iodine and surgery generally result in hypothyroidism (discussed further on), requiring lifelong thyroxine replacement therapy.

Toxic Adenoma/Multinodular Goiter

Hyperthyroidism due to one or more autonomously functioning nodules may be treated transiently with antithyroid drug therapy, as already described, but unlike Graves disease, it ultimately requires definitive therapy, as remissions do not occur. As noted previously, radioactive iodine is generally preferred to surgery. Effective treatment of multinodular goiters usually requires higher doses of radioactive iodine than does the treatment of Graves disease, since the radioactive iodine uptake is characteristically lower in the former compared with the latter disorder. Nonetheless, hypothyroidism is uncommon after such treatment, as thyroid tissue suppressed in the setting of autonomous nodule function fails to take up significant radioactive iodine.

ACROMEGALY

Presentation and Diagnosis

A diagnosis of acromegaly is suspected from the progressive physical signs and symptoms resulting from an excess of chronic growth hormone: coarsening of facial features; enlargement of the tongue, hands, and feet; prognathism; and excessive sweating and oiliness of the skin. The diagnosis is confirmed by glucose tolerance testing with measurement of growth hormone levels or, alternatively, by assessment of somatomedin C (insulin-like growth factor ([IGF]–I) level.[32] Hypertension is present in at least 20%–30% of patients with active acromegaly, at least in part attributed to excessive sodium retention in the majority of patients, with resultant expansion of the extracellular fluid volume.

Therapy

When possible, resection of a growth hormone–secreting pituitary adenoma is the treatment of choice. In rare instances, ectopic production of growth hormone–releasing hormone (GHRH) from a lung or pancreatic neoplasm may underlie the growth hormone elevation, and resection of such lesions is also indicated when possible.

When surgery is contraindicated, or fails to control disease, medical therapy is indicated. Octreotide is the preferred therapy and is effective in virtually all cases of growth hormone overproduction.[33, 34] In rare cases of ectopic GHRH secretion, octreotide treatment also inhibits secretion of the releasing hormone as well as reducing pituitary responsiveness to GHRH. As discussed earlier, octreotide therapy is associated with a high risk of gallstone formation. Hypothyroidism also occurs in approximately 10% of patients. This agent is a good choice for patients in whom surgical cure has failed but who require medical treatment after adjunctive pituitary irradiation. After irradiation, growth hormone levels fall gradually over months to years; thus, octreotide may be used until growth and somatomedin C (IGF-I) hormone levels have returned to the normal range. The usual starting dose of octreotide is 50 μg b.i.d. or t.i.d. subcutaneously. Higher doses, generally 100 μg t.i.d., are usually required for adequate growth hormone suppression, with a maximum dose of 500 μg t.i.d.

The ergot alkaloid bromocriptine, a dopamine agonist, may also paradoxically decrease growth hormone secretion in up to 50% of acromegalic cases. Its use may be associated with nausea and transient hypotension; these effects can be minimized by starting with small doses, such as 1.25–2.5 mg, at bedtime with a snack. The dose should then be increased in small increments until growth hormone secretion is controlled. In general, and in comparison with prolactin-secreting tumors, relatively large doses of bromocriptine (20–40 mg/day) are required to diminish growth hormone secretion in responsive patients. These doses are almost universally associated with the side effects already mentioned; the cost of chronic administration at high dosage also is significant.

Although the treatments indicated are aimed at reducing growth hormone secretion, treatment of the blood pressure elevation per se can also be accomplished with standard therapies. Since this is a volume-expanded low-renin state, diuretic therapy is a logical choice. Large doses of diuretics should be avoided to maintain normal potassium homeostasis, however, especially since many patients with acromegaly have accelerated cardiovascular disease and/or cardiomyopathy and thus may be at increased risk for arrhythmia and sudden death. Other agents that have been used successfully include the dihydropyridine calcium channel blockers and in some instances, the angiotensin-converting enzyme inhibitors. Caution should be exercised in prescribing agents that reduce cardiac performance because of the higher risk of cardiac disease in these patients. Electrocardiography, appropriate in all hypertensive patients, is particularly relevant in patients with acromegaly. Echocardiography is useful in patients with suspected cardiomyopathy.

RENIN-SECRETING TUMORS

Presentation and Diagnosis

A diagnosis of a renin-secreting tumor (also called primary reninism) should be suspected in a young patient with severe hypertension, hypokalemia, and extremely high levels of plasma renin activity in whom a diagnosis of renovascular disease has been excluded by prior angiography. In most cases, the tumor is of renal origin, but extrarenal renin-secreting tumors have also been reported.

Corvol and associates recommend computed tomography scanning as the best means of tumor localization of renal neoplasms, although renal arteriography and selective measurement of renal vein renin levels may be useful in selected patients.[35]

Therapy

Surgical resection of renal renin-secreting tumors usually cures the hypertension. Moreover, these generally benign tumors are usually superficial and can be dissected from adjacent renal tissue; thus nephrectomy is not necessary.

Characteristically, the hypertension in patients with renin-secreting tumors is resistant to most conventional drugs except those agents that interrupt the renin-angiotensin system. Although a major blood pressure response to angiotensin-converting enzyme inhibitors is not specific for primary reninism, it may provide a clue to the diagnosis in a young hypokalemic hypertensive subject.

EXOGENOUS HORMONES AND HORMONE-LIKE AGENTS

There are a number of medications that share features in common with endogenous hormones and, correspondingly, may raise blood pressure. Table 39–1 lists relevant agents. Hypertension is effectively treated by discontinuing or, in selected situations, reducing the dose of the offending medication.

Oral Contraceptives

Older preparations of oral contraceptives routinely raised blood pressure slightly, with average increases of 5 mm Hg in systolic blood pressure and 1–2 mm Hg in diastolic blood pressure; correspondingly their use was associated with a threefold or greater increased risk of hypertension, particularly in women aged 35 years or older.[36] Increases in blood pressure appear related to both estrogen[37] and progestin[38] dosages. Hypertension appears less common with currently used oral contraceptive preparations but still remains a risk. With discontinuation of oral contraceptives, hypertension is expected to resolve, although this may take 3–6 months, paralleling the time course for the stimulated renin-angiotensin system to return to normal.[39]

Postmenopausal Hormones

There is little evidence to warrant a concern that postmenopausal estrogen replacement will induce or aggravate hypertension. Although hypertension has rarely been reported as a complication of estrogen replacement therapy, such therapy is far more commonly associated with slight decreases in systolic and diastolic blood pressure.[40] Furthermore, observational data consistently indicate a 40%–50% lower risk of coronary heart disease among women taking estrogen replacement as compared with untreated women.[41]

Anabolic Steroids

Although endogenous testosterone levels have been inversely associated with blood pressure levels,[42] available data indicate a significant increase in blood pressure with anabolic steroid use.[43] These steroids also have an adverse impact on lipids and may increase coagulability[1]; their use should be confined to the rare clinical situations in which their benefits outweigh associated risks.

Glucocorticoids

Analogous to the effects of endogenous glucocorticoid excess (see earlier discussion of Cushing syndrome), supraphysiologic doses of exogenous glucocorticoids (e.g., more than 5–7.5 mg/day of prednisone) may likewise cause hypertension, which appears to be less common in the latter setting, however, and is reported in 20% of individuals treated with glucocorticoids as compared with 80% of individuals with Cushing disease. Renal insufficiency also appears to predispose patients to hypertension in those treated with exogenous glucocorticoids. In all cases in which exogenous glucocorticoids are required, therapy should be maintained at the lowest effective dose to minimize risks of hypertension and other adverse steroid effects.

Mineralocorticoids or Mineralocorticoid-Like Agents

Fludrocortisone

Fludrocortisone, a synthetic mineralocorticoid used in the therapy of both primary adrenal insufficiency and orthostatic hypotension, may result in significant recumbent hypertension. This agent should routinely be initiated at the lowest dose (0.05 mg/day orally) and increased gradually with attention to both recumbent and standing blood pressures. Attempts should be made to use other approaches to orthostasis, such as support stockings and a high sodium intake, in an attempt to minimize the dosage of fludrocortisone.

Licorice

Excessive intake of licorice has been associated with a syndrome of "apparent mineralocorticoid excess." It appears that the glycyrrhizic acid present in licorice inhibits the renal 11β-hydroxysteroid dehydrogenase enzyme, preventing the intrarenal inactivation of cortisol to the biologically inactive cortisone. As a result, high local concentrations of cortisol can bind to the type I mineralocorticoid receptor, causing hypertension and hypokalemia in the setting of suppressed levels of renin and aldosterone.

Sympathomimetic Agents

Appetite suppressants such as ephedrine and phenylpropanolamine, nasal decongestants such as pseudoephedrine and phenylephrine, and some illicit drugs such as cocaine and amphetamines have sympathetic agonist effects that may elevate blood pressure. Although development of significant hypertension is extremely unlikely when usual doses are ingested by normotensive individuals, significant pressor effects have rarely been reported, possibly more so with ephedrine and phenylpropanolamine.[44] If hypertensive crisis occurs, as with overdosage of these agents, treatment with an intravenous alpha blocker, such as intravenous phentolamine (5 mg), is indicated; beta blockers should theoretically be withheld until alpha blockade is complete, as described for pheochromocytoma, although case reports have reported the successful use of intravenous propranolol in this setting.[45] Individuals who have a hypertensive response to sympathomimetic agents should be evaluated for the presence of a pheochromocytoma (see discussion of pheochromocytoma).

Thyroid-Related Agents

Thyroxine Overreplacement

Many patients with hypothyroidism are inadvertently overtreated with thyroxine, and some other individuals overmedicate themselves with the aim of weight reduction. Supraphysiologic doses of thyroxine are also routinely prescribed to patients after a diagnosis of thyroid cancer or in an attempt to shrink a thyroid nodule or multinodular goiter. In any of these settings, systolic hypertension may occur in association with other symptoms and signs of hyperthyroidism. Discontinuation of thyroid hormone in those who do not need it, and reduction in the thyroxine dose to maintain normal TSH levels in hypothyroid individuals and low but detectable levels in patients with thyroid neoplasms, should result in normalization of blood pressure in the majority of patients.

Amiodarone

The antiarrhythmic medication amiodarone characteristically causes changes in thyroid function test results (decreased triiodothyronine, mildly elevated thyroxine, normal or elevated TSH) in the setting of clinical euthyroidism. In up to 5% of patients, however, this agent results in true thyroid dysfunction as a result of its high iodine content. Either hypo- or hyperthyroidism may occur, with associated blood pressure elevations, although the former is more common in the United States, where diets are characteristically replete with iodine. Although discontinuation of amiodarone would logically be expected to result in restoration of euthyroidism and normalization of any asssociated hypertension, effects may last for months because of the drug's long half-life. Furthermore, cardiac disease often necessitates its use despite this side effect. Treatment of hypothyroidism associated with amiodarone is thus generally no different from that for other causes of hypothyroidism, that is, levothyroxine, started at a low dose and increased cautiously because of coexisting cardiac disase (see earlier discussion of hypothyroidism). Amiodarone-induced hyperthyroidism is treated with the antithyroid drugs methimazole or PTU (see earlier discussion of hyperthyroidism) but with the expectation that they may be required indefinitely. Treatment with radioactive iodine generally is not possible because of the usually low iodine uptake in this condition. As with other causes of hyperthyroidism, beta blockers may have a role in controlling hypertension and symptoms, but this depends on the underlying cardiac status.

REFERENCES

1. Williams GH, Dluhy RG: Diseases of the adrenal cortex. *In* Isselbacher KJ, Braunwald E, Wilson JD, et al (eds): Harrison's Principles of Internal Medicine, 13th ed, pp 1953–1976. New York: McGraw-Hill, 1994.
2. Atkinson AB: The treatment of Cushing's syndrome. Clin Endocrinol 1991; 34:507.
3. Bertagna C, Orth DN: Clinical and laboratory findings and results from therapy in 58 patients with adrenocortical tumors admitted to a single medical center (1957–1978). Am J Med 1981; 71:855–875.
4. Greenberg PH, Marks C: Adrenal cortical carcinoma: a presentation of 22 cases and a review of the literature. Am Surg 1978; 44:81–85.
5. Sonino N: The use of ketoconazole as an inhibitor of steroid production. N Engl J Med 1987; 317(13):812–818.
6. Chandler WF, Schteingard DE, Lloyd RV, McKeever PE: Surgical treatment of Cushing's disease. J Neurosurg 1987; 66:204–212.
7. Melby JC: Therapy of Cushing's disease: a consensus for pituitary microsurgery. Ann Intern Med 1988; 109:455–456.
8. Laws ER: Pituitary tumors—therapeutic considerations: surgical. Concepts in Neurosurgery. Neuroendocrinology 1992; 5:395–400.
9. Tindall GT, Herring CJ, Clark RV, et al: Cushing's disease: results of transsphenoidal microsurgery with emphasis on surgical failures. J Neurosurg 1990; 363–369.
10. Degerbald M, Rahn T, Bergstrand G, Thoren M: Long-term results of stereotactic radiosurgery to the pituitary gland in Cushing's disease. Acta Endocrinol 1986; 112:310–314.
11. Schteingart DE, Tsao HS, Taylor CI, et al: Sustained remission of Cushing's disease with mitotane and pituitary irradiation. Ann Intern Med 1980; 92:613.
12. Young WF, Hogan MJ, Klee GG, et al: Primary aldosteronism: diagnosis and treatment. Mayo Clin Proc 1990; 65:96–110.
13. Bravo E, Tarazi R, Dustan H, et al: The changing clinical spectrum of primary aldosteronism. Am J Med 1983; 74:641–651.
14. Lim RC, Nakayama DK, Biglieri EG, et al: Primary aldosteronism: changing concepts in diagnosis and management. Am J Surg 1986; 152:116–127.
15. Melby JC: Diagnosis and treatment of primary aldosteronism and isolated hypoaldosteronism. Clin Endocrinol Metab 1985; 14:977–981.
16. Dluhy RG, Lifton RP: Glucocorticoid-remediable aldosteronism. *In* Mazzaferri EI (ed): Advances in Endocrinology and Metabolism, vol 5, pp 203–218. St. Louis: Mosby–Year Book, 1994.
17. Lifton RP, Dluhy RG, Powers M, et al: A chimeric 11-hydroxylase/aldosterone synthase gene causes glucocorticoid-remediable aldosteronism and human hypertension. Nature 1992; 355:262–265.
18. Lifton RP, Dluhy RG, Powers M, et al: Hereditary hypertension caused by chimeric gene duplications and ectopic expression of aldosterone synthase. Nature 1992; 2:66–74.
19. Levine LS, Pang S: Prenatal diagnosis and treatment of congenital adrenal hyperplasia. *In* Milunsky CA (ed): Genetic Disorders and the Fetus, 2nd ed, p 425. New York: Plenum Press, 1992.
20. Miller WI, Levine LS: Molecular and clinical advances in congenital adrenal hyperplasia. J Pediatr 1987; 111:1–17.
21. Bravo EL, Gifford RW: Current concepts. Pheochromocytoma: diagnosis, localization, and management. N Engl J Med 1984; 311:1298.
22. Taylor SH: Efficacy of doxazosin in specific hypertensive patient groups. Am Heart J 1991; 121:286–292.
23. Bravo EL: Evolving concepts in the pathophysiology, diagnosis, and treatment of pheochromocytoma. Endocrinol Rev 1994; 15:356–368.
24. Averbuch SD, Steakley CS, Young RC, et al: Malignant pheochromocytoma: effective treatment with a combination of cyclophosphamide, vincristine, and dacarbazine. Ann Intern Med 1988; 109:267–273.
25. McCarthy EF, Bonfiglio M, Lawton W: A solitary functioning osseous metastasis from a malignant pheochromocytoma of the organ of Zuckerkandl. Cancer 1977; 40:3092–3096.
26. Nainby-Luxmoore JC, Langford HG, Nelson NC, et al: A case-comparison study of hypertension and hyperparathyroidism. J Clin Endocrinol Metab 1982; 55:303–306.
27. Consensus Development Conference Panel: Diagnosis and management of asymptomatic primary hyperparathyroidism: Consensus Development Conference statement. Ann Intern Med 1991; 114:593–597.
28. Lafferty FW, Hubay CA: Primary hyperparathyroidism. A review of the long-term surgical and non-surgical morbidities as a basis for a rational approach to treatment. Arch Intern Med 1989; 149:789–796.
29. Faber J, Galloe AM: Changes in bone mass during prolonged subclinical

hyperthyroidism due to L-thyroxine treatment: a meta-analysis. Eur J Endocrinol 1994; 130:350–356.
30. Sawin CT, Geller A, Wolf PA, et al: Low serum thyrotropin concentrations as a risk factor for atrial fibrillation in older persons. N Engl J Med 1994; 331:1249–1252.
31. Hashizume K, Ichikawa K, Sakurai A, et al: Administration of thyroxine in treated Graves' disease. Effects on the level of antibodies to thyroid-stimulating hormone receptors and on the risk of recurrence of hyperthyroidism. N Engl J Med 1991; 324:947–953.
32. Melmed S: Acromegaly. N Engl J Med 1990; 322:966–977.
33. Frohman LA: Therapeutic options in acromegaly. J Clin Endocrinol Metab 1991; 72:1175–1181.
34. vonWerder K, Faglia G: Potential indications for octreotide in acromegaly. Metabolism 1992; 41:91–98.
35. Corvol P, Pinet F, Plouin P-F, et al: Renin-secreting tumors. Endocrinol Metab Clin North Am 1994; 23:255–270.
36. Ramcharan S, Pellegrin FA, Hoag EJ: The occurrence and course of hypertensive disease in users and non-users of oral contraceptive drugs. *In* Ramcharan S (ed): The Walnut Creek Contraceptive Drug Study: a prospective study of the side effects of oral contraceptives, vol 2, pp 1–16. Washington, DC: Government Printing Office, 1976 (DHEW publication no. [NIH] 76–563).
37. Briggs M, Briggs M: Oestrogen content of oral contraceptives. Lancet 1977; 2:1233.
38. Effect on hypertension and benign breast disease of progestogen component in combined oral contraceptives: Royal College of General Practitioners' Oral Contraception Study. Lancet 1977; 1:624.
39. Speroff L, Glass RH, Kase NL: Clinical Gynecologic Endocrinology and Infertility, pp 461–498. Baltimore: Williams & Wilkins, 1989.
40. Mashchak CA, Lobo RA: Estrogen replacment therapy and hypertension. J Reprod Med 1985; 30(suppl10): 805–810.
41. Stampfer MJ, Colditz GA: Estrogen replacment therapy and coronary heart disease: a quantitative assessment of the epidemiologic evidence. Prev Med 1991; 20:47–63.
42. Khaw KT, Barrett-Connor E: Blood pressure and endogenous testosterone in men: an inverse relationship. J Hypertens 1988; 6:329–332.
43. Freed DLJ, Banks AJ, Logson D, Burley DM: Anabolic steroids in athletics: crossover double-blind trial on weightlifters. Br Med J 1975; 2:471–473.
44. Chua SS, Benrimoj SI: Non-prescription sympathomimetic agents and hypertension. Med Toxicol Adverse Drug Exp 1988; 3:387–417.
45. Burkhart KK: Intravenous propranolol reverses hypertension after sympathomimetic overdose: two case reports. J Toxicol Clin Toxicol 1992; 30:109–114.

40 Hypertension in Diabetes Mellitus and Obesity

Michael L. Tuck, MD

Hypertension and diabetes are interrelated disorders that greatly increase the risk of atherosclerotic cardiovascular disease.[1] It is estimated that hypertension is twice as common in diabetic as in nondiabetic persons and that about 3 million people in the United States have both diabetes and hypertension.[2] Both conditions are more common among the socioeconomically disadvantaged and in African-Americans and Mexican-Americans.[3] Non–insulin-dependent diabetes mellitus (NIDDM) is 10 times as frequent as insulin-dependent diabetes mellitus (IDDM), accounting for more than 90% of people with diabetes and hypertension. However, when the incidence rates of hypertension in IDDM and NIDDM are age adjusted, its incidence is as great as if not greater in IDDM.[4]

The concurrence of hypertension and diabetes is associated with a higher frequency of other atherosclerotic risk factors, including dyslipidemia, hyperuricemia, elevated fibrinogen levels, and left ventricular hypertrophy.[5–8] Hypertension is one of the leading contributors to macrovascular complications in diabetes, such as coronary heart disease, stroke, peripheral vascular disease, and conditions necessitating lower extremity amputations. Hypertension is also a major risk factor for microvascular complications in diabetes, as is well documented in diabetic nephropathy.[9] Findings also show that blood pressure may be a predictor of the incidence and progression of diabetic retinopathy.[10, 11]

PATHOPHYSIOLOGY OF HYPERTENSION IN DIABETES

The most common cause of hypertension in IDDM is diabetic nephropathy; the rise in blood pressure parallels the onset of renal disease in the 30%–40% of IDDM patients in whom nephropathy develops. The hypertension in NIDDM is more diverse in etiology; it may occur in subjects with normal renal function and reflects the concurrence of several conditions, such as essential hypertension, obesity, and atherosclerosis. Because up to 80% of NIDDM subjects are obese, body weight is an important contributor to the hypertension of NIDDM. The prevalence of hypertension in NIDDM also increases with age. Volume expansion, sodium retention, and increased vascular reactivity are frequently noted in subjects with diabetes, and these abnormalities may contribute to their hypertension.

Volume and Sodium

Volume expansion is commonly found in patients with diabetes mellitus, as shown by measurements of total exchangeable sodium, which are 10% higher in diabetics than in nondiabetic subjects.[12–15] Volume expansion is probably caused by sodium retention because both glucose and ketones are actively reabsorbed in the kidney as sodium salts, increasing the sodium pool in diabetics.[16, 17] Several markers of volume status are abnormal in diabetes. Atrial natriuretic peptide levels are increased in diabetic subjects, probably in response to volume excess.[17–19] Elevated levels of a digitalis-like substance, a factor often associated with hypervolemic states, have also been described in experimental[20] and human[21] diabetic hypertension.

The Renin-Angiotensin-Aldosterone System

The sodium excess in diabetes does not result from an overt increase in mineralocorticoid activity, and normal or low levels of plasma renin activity (PRA) and aldosterone are usually found.[12, 22] The low PRA level in diabetics results from impairment of renin release secondary to autonomic neuropathy, microvascular complications, and reduced prostaglandin synthesis.[12, 22, 23] Reduced levels of aldosterone in diabetes parallel reductions in PRA. The syndrome of hyporeninemic hypoaldosteronism is often seen in diabetics with chronic renal insufficiency, and both the hypertension and accompanying hyperkalemia are best controlled with diuretic therapy.

Measurement of the precursor to renin, prorenin, shows that levels are high in diabetes, and the high prorenin levels signal the presence of microvascular complications.[24, 25] In experimental diabetes, tissue levels of renin are high,[26] as is expression of the renin[27] and angiotensin converting enzyme (ACE)[28] genes. In human diabetes, circulating levels of ACE are high.[29] The high tissue activity of the renin-angiotensin system may explain the excellent blood pressure and renal response to ACE inhibitors in diabetes.[22]

Renal Function and Volume

In diabetics with impaired renal function, there is further sodium retention and hypervolemia,[30, 31] and normalization of volume status and blood pressure in diabetic nephropathy with diuretics corrects the hypertension.[30, 31] Elevated levels of the erythrocyte sodium-lithium countertransport are found in diabetic subjects with renal disease,[32, 33] and this assay may indicate increased sodium reabsorption in the proximal tubule in this condition.[34]

Insulin and Hypertension

Hypertension is associated with insulin resistance, as seen in three common hypertensive conditions: essential hypertension, NIDDM, and obesity.[35–38] The three conditions share several abnormalities in insulin secretion, metabolism, and peripheral tissue actions but differ in their patterns of insulin resistance for various target organs[36] (Table 40–1). Essential hypertension, NIDDM, and obesity are characterized by a decreased whole-body insulin-mediated glucose disposal and compensatory hyperinsulinemia but differ in the effects of insulin in specific tissues.[38] In normotensive NIDDM, reduced insulin action in extrahepatic tissues may predict future hypertension.[39] The etiology of insulin resistance in these conditions is only partly understood but is known to be related to both insulin receptor and postreceptor defects.[38]

The hemodynamic link between insulin and hypertension may reside in abnormal activity of the sympathetic nervous system, abnormal sodium metabolism, or direct effects on the vasculature.[40] Insulin infusion in normal subjects increases plasma norepinephrine levels and other indices of sympathetic nervous system activity.[41, 42] Obese subjects have increased insulin levels and increased sympathetic nervous system activity.[43] In addition, there are positive correlations among body weight, blood pressure, insulin, and norepinephrine in obesity.[44] Insulin administration also increases sodium reabsorption, probably through direct effects on tubule sodium transport by the sodium-hydrogen exchange system or the Na^+,K^+-ATPase pump.[12]

TABLE 40–1. CHOICES OF ANTIHYPERTENSIVE MEDICATION IN DIABETES MELLITUS WITH COMPLICATIONS

Complication	Choices	Precautions
Orthostatic hypotension	ACE inhibitors Beta blockers Calcium channel antagonists	Methyldopa Prazosin Guanethidine
Poor glucose/lipid control	ACE inhibitors Calcium channel antagonists Clonidine Prazosin	Beta blockers Diuretics
Hypoglycemia		Beta blockers
Coronary artery disease History of recent MI	Calcium channel antagonists Beta blockers	
Left ventricular hypertrophy	ACE inhibitors Calcium channel antagonists Beta blockers Alpha-adrenoceptor blockers	Diuretics Direct vasodilators
Concentric ventricular hypertrophy in older patients	Beta blockers Calcium channel antagonists	ACE inhibitors Vasodilators
Peripheral vascular disease	ACE inhibitors Calcium channel antagonists Clonidine Prazosin	Beta blockers
Impotence	ACE inhibitors Calcium channel antagonists Prazosin	Adrenergic inhibitors
Renal impairment		
Microalbuminuria	ACE inhibitors	
Proteinuria	ACE inhibitors	
Sodium retention (creatinine <2 mg/dL)	Thiazide diuretics Calcium channel antagonists ACE inhibitors	Vasodilators
Sodium retention (creatinine >2 mg/dL)	Loop diuretics	
Hyporeninemic hypoaldosteronism (borderline hyperkalemia)	Diuretics Beta-blockers	ACE inhibitors Calcium channel antagonists

Abbreviations: ACE, angiotensin converting enzyme; MI, myocardial infarction.

Insulin has direct effects on the vasculature to alter blood vessel tone and structure. In experimental models, insulin enhances atherosclerosis and alters vascular wall structure; these effects could increase blood pressure through structural irregularity in the arterial bed.[45, 46] Many studies in humans and experimental animals show that insulin administration causes vasodilation and increased blood flow. In NIDDM, the action of insulin to increase skeletal muscle flow is impaired, which suggests a novel mechanism for insulin resistance and possibly for hypertension.[47] Insulin also directly stimulates several growth and hypertensive factors in vascular tissue, including insulin-like growth factor-1 expression[48] and endothelin-1 gene expression.[49]

Glucose and Hypertension

Epidemiologic surveys in both diabetic and nondiabetic subjects show a positive correlation between blood pressure and plasma glucose that is independent of age, body weight, and heart rate.[50] The correlation between glucose and blood pressure may be related to coexisting hyperinsulinemia. However, glucose can have direct effects on vascular tissue to impair endothelium-dependent relaxation[51] and to increase endothelin-1.[52] Insulin removal worsens hypertension in NIDDM,[53] and in general, tight metabolic control should help control blood pressure.[54]

Vascular Reactivity

Blood pressure responses to various stimuli (angiotensin II, norepinephrine) are accentuated in both normotensive and hypertensive IDDM and NIDDM subjects.[12, 15] For example, the venous response to norepinephrine-induced vasoconstriction is hypersensitive in IDDM patients with microalbuminuria, which suggests enhanced activity of the alpha-adrenergic system.[55] Insulin could be a factor in the accentuated vascular responses because its effect on vascular reactivity is through the adrenergic nervous system.[56, 57] A generalized peripheral hyperperfusion is also found in diabetes as best described in the glomerular capillary circulation of diabetic animal models.[58] Vasodilatation in the microcirculation has been proposed as a precursor to hypertension and vascular disease in diabetes.[58]

HYPERTENSION IN DIABETIC NEPHROPATHY

(see also Chapter 38)

Hypertension is the hallmark of overt diabetic nephropathy, being found in more than 90% of patients.[30] In IDDM, hypertension parallels the degree of diabetic nephropathy, and an inverse correlation is found between creatinine clearance and arterial pressure.[30] Hypertension may precede or occur early in the course of diabetic renal disease. Arterial pressure is already elevated at an early phase of diabetic nephropathy: IDDM patients with microalbuminuria and proteinuria have higher blood pressure than those free of renal impairment.[59] Patients with overt proteinuria but normal glomerular filtration rate show a progressive increment in blood pressure associated with the decline in this rate over time.[60] Ambulatory blood pressure monitoring may better detect early hypertension in diabetics with proteinuria.[61]

In IDDM, microalbuminuria, mesangial cell hypertrophy, and blood pressure are highly correlated and predict the development of nephropathy.[62] Two indicators of genetic susceptibility to hypertension have been linked to diabetic nephropathy: parental hypertension and increased maximal velocity of the erythrocyte sodium-lithium countertransport system. Elevated erythrocyte countertransport is found in IDDM subjects with nephropathy[32] and in NIDDM subjects independently of hypertension or renal disease.[63] Poor glycemic control is also an important risk factor for nephropathy, and tight metabolic control will retard nephropathy.[54]

TREATMENT

Hypertension and diabetes are independent cardiovascular risk factors, and when they are combined, the result is a much higher incidence of coronary and cerebral vascular disease. For example, the mortality rate among diabetics with systolic pressure exceeding 160 mm Hg is four times that among diabetics with lower blood pressure.[3] However, evidence that pharmacologic control of blood pressure reduces overall mortality in diabetes mellitus is limited. In both the Hypertension Detection and Follow-up Program (HDFP)[64] and the Systolic Hypertension in the Elderly Program (SHEP),[65] about 10% of participants had diabetes. In the HDFP trial, which was a diuretic-based stepped care study, the effect on total mortality in the diabetic subset did not differ from that of the overall cohort. In the SHEP study, the relative risk reduction for all major end points in diabetics was similar to that in the total cohort.

In 1994, the National High Blood Pressure Education Program (NHBPEP) Working Group on Hypertension in Diabetes issued its second consensus statement advocating an algorithm approach (Fig. 40–1) to treatment of hypertension in diabetes.[1] The report emphasized the need to start with lifestyle changes and, if they are not sufficient, to begin drug monotherapy, but not using the traditional stepped care approach. Initial monotherapy could include thiazide diuretics, converting enzyme inhibitors, calcium channel blockers, or α-adrenergic blockers. The role of beta blockers in treatment of hypertension in diabetes remains controversial because of their multiple metabolic side effects, and they were not advocated as first-line therapy except in special situations.[1] Other expert reports including the American Diabetes Association Consensus Statement on the Treatment of Hypertension in Diabetes[7] and the Report of the Canadian Hypertension Consensus Conference on Hypertension and Diabetes[8] have recommended avoiding diuretics and beta blockers in hypertensive diabetic patients except under special conditions. The NHBPEP Working Group on Hypertension in Diabetes defined goal blood pressure as less than 135/85 mm Hg in hypertension and diabetes.[1]

Lifestyle Modifications

Lifestyle modification is considered as an initial treatment modality or as an adjunct to pharmacologic therapy in most forms of hypertension. The Treatment of Mild Hypertension Study (TOMHS) documented that initial therapy of mild hypertension with lifestyle interventions was effective in controlling blood pressure.[66]

Weight Management

Control of body weight is perhaps the most important nonpharmacologic means to reduce blood pressure because its hypotensive effect is pronounced even with modest amounts of weight loss.[1, 66–68] Weight reduction has the additional advantage of correcting the underlying metabolic disorders that occur in hypertensive patients. A 1-year study in Dalby, UK, using lifestyle modifications such as diet and exercise, showed that nonpharmacologic treatment could reduce insulin resistance in hypertensive patients.[69] Fagerberg and colleagues[70] reported that diet treatment was inferior to drug treatment in controlling hypertension but superior in lowering plasma insulin and lipid levels.

The diet recommended for obese NIDDM patients should be hypocaloric but with a balanced intake of less than 30% of calories from fat, 15% from protein, and 55%–60% from carbohydrate (preferably complex carbohydrates). In IDDM patients receiving exogenous insulin, the diet should be adjusted so that calories cover periods of peak insulin action. The Diabetes Complications and Control Study showed that dietary control coupled with intensive insulin administration could help attain euglycemia in IDDM subjects.[54] Because tight metabolic control reduces fluid volume and hyperfiltration, it should help in blood pressure control.

Sodium Restriction

Because a high proportion of hypertensive diabetics have salt-sensitive hypertension[71] and sodium retention,[12] it could be predicted that sodium restriction would be effective in blood pressure control. This issue has not been studied in detail, but one report showed that sodium restriction in hypertensive NIDDM subjects is effective.[72] A diet moderately restricting sodium chloride to 100 mmol/day (2.3 g sodium/day, 6 g sodium chloride/day) is recommended for patients with diabetic hypertension.

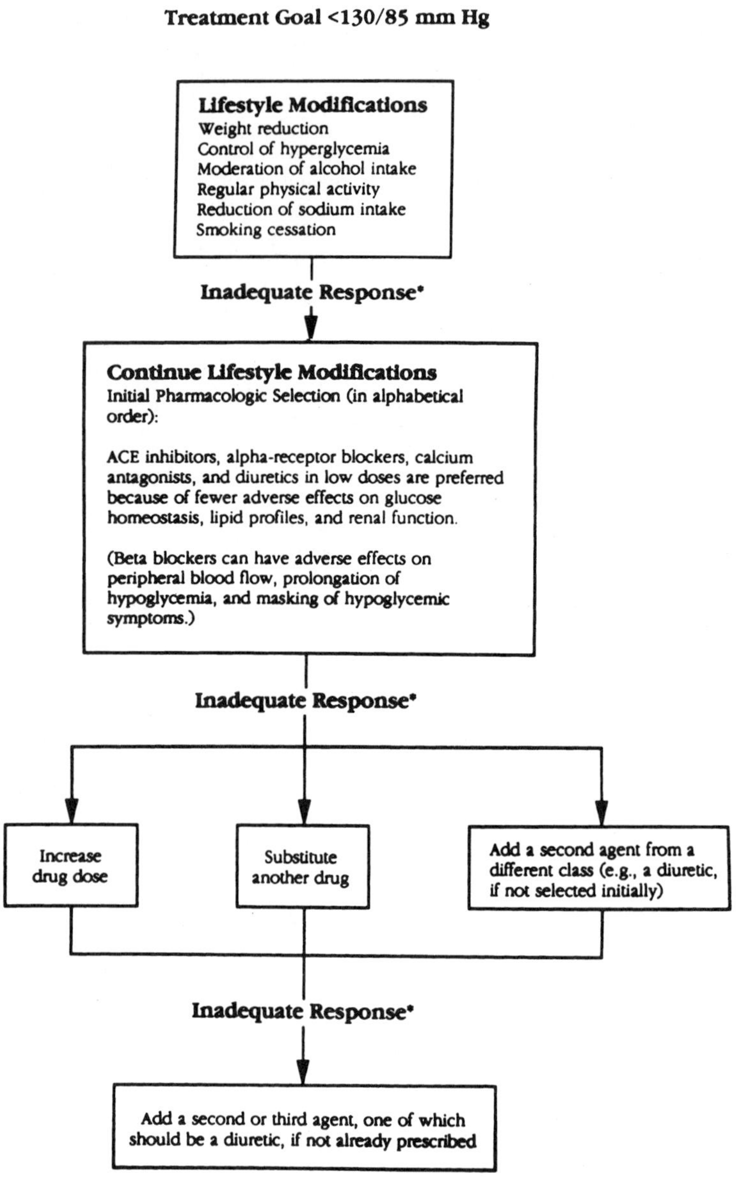
Treatment Goal <130/85 mm Hg
Lifestyle Modifications
Weight reduction
Control of hyperglycemia
Moderation of alcohol intake
Regular physical activity
Reduction of sodium intake
Smoking cessation
Inadequate Response*
Continue Lifestyle Modifications
Initial Pharmacologic Selection (in alphabetical order):
ACE inhibitors, alpha-receptor blockers, calcium antagonists, and diuretics in low doses are preferred because of fewer adverse effects on glucose homeostasis, lipid profiles, and renal function.
(Beta blockers can have adverse effects on peripheral blood flow, prolongation of hypoglycemia, and masking of hypoglycemic symptoms.)
Inadequate Response*
Increase drug dose
Substitute another drug
Add a second agent from a different class (e.g., a diuretic, if not selected initially)
Inadequate Response*
Add a second or third agent, one of which should be a diuretic, if not already prescribed

Figure 40–1. Algorithm for the treatment of hypertension in diabetes. (From the National High Blood Pressure Education Program Working Group on Hypertension in Diabetes. Hypertension 1990; 23:145.)

The NHBPEP Working Group on Hypertension in Diabetes also recommended alcohol moderation, daily exercise, and smoking cessation programs for hypertension control in diabetes.[1] For those with stage 1 hypertension, a 3-month period of lifestyle modification is indicated. For individuals in whom lifestyle modification does not lower blood pressure to the goal of 130/85 mm Hg, drug therapy should be added.

Drug Therapy

There is little evidence that efficacy rates for classes of antihypertensive agents differ between diabetic and nondiabetic subjects. Thus, the major treatment decisions in selection of drugs for hypertension in patients with diabetes mellitus are special considerations such as glycemia control, lipid levels, and cardiovascular and renal complications (see Table 40–1).

Diuretics (Table 40–2)

Glycemic Control. Thiazide diuretics are reported to decrease insulin release,[73] worsen glycemic control,[73] and decrease tissue sensitivity to insulin.[73, 75] Other reports have questioned the significance of these adverse metabolic effects on long-term glycemic control and complications.[74, 83] Significant increments in fasting glucose can be encountered in up to 50% of hypertensive diabetic patients during thiazide diuretic therapy and can be substantial (increments in glucose from 48 to 270 mg/dL).[76] Low-dose thiazide diuretic therapy (12.5–25 mg hydrochlorothiazide) is noted to have less effect on glucose or HbA_{1c}.[77] Hypokalemia decreases insulin secretion and tissue sensitivity, and this can be reversed with potassium supplemen-

TABLE 40–2. SUMMARY OF DIURETICS IN HYPERTENSION AND DIABETES

Correct the excess volume and vascular reactivity associated with diabetes and hypertension
Increase insulin resistance and glucose intolerance
Increase total and low-density lipoprotein cholesterol
Hypokalemia may predispose to ventricular ectopy
Useful in hyporeninemic hypoaldosteronism

tation or potassium-sparing diuretics.[78] With use of insulin clamp methodology, it was found that thiazide diuretics decrease insulin action by 20%–30%,[75] and this adverse effect persists during long-term (2–3 years) therapy.[79] However, a retrospective study of prescribing patterns in hypertension showed that thiazide diuretics did not increase the rate for new prescriptions for hypoglycemic agents to a greater extent than any other of the classes of antihypertensive drugs did.[80] Fries[83] emphasized that there is no evidence from several major diuretic-based antihypertensive trials (Multifactorial Primary Prevention of Cardiovascular Disease, the Heart Attack Primary Prevention in Hypertension, and the Medical Research Council trials) of long-term changes in plasma glucose.

Lipid Control. Multiple linear regression analysis of 474 clinical trials with antihypertensive agents showed that diuretics increase cholesterol levels and that the effect was greater with higher doses and in black hypertensive subjects.[81] Occasionally, total cholesterol levels increase substantially (i.e., >70 mg/dL) with diuretic therapy.[82] It has been argued that in the short term, diuretics may increase cholesterol, but long-term trials show that cholesterol returns to pretreatment levels.[83]

Cardiovascular Complications. The fact that the increased total exchangeable sodium[12] and vascular hyperreactivity found in diabetic patients can be normalized by diuretic therapy[15] suggests that these agents are highly selective for this condition. However, it has been argued that the cardiovascular risks of diuretic therapy, including hypokalemia, increased ectopy, and arrhythmias, may outweigh any beneficial effects. Yet, it is not certain that hypokalemia increases the electrical instability of the heart or that diuretic therapy alters rates of morbidity and mortality from coronary heart disease, especially in low doses.[83] Diuretics have also been shown to reduce left ventricular hypertrophy in some but not all trials.[84]

Renal Complications. Although not studied in sufficient detail, these agents have been reported to reduce proteinuria and progression of renal disease in diabetic nephropathy.[9, 91] One report shows equal beneficial effects of hydrochlorothiazide and the converting enzyme inhibitor enalapril on slowing the progression of diabetic nephropathy.[85]

Beta Blockers (Table 40–3)

Glycemic Control. Insulin secretion is enhanced by β_2-adrenergic stimulation, and beta-adrenergic blockade impairs insulin release by up to 50%. Because NIDDM patients rely on insulin release, the adverse effects of beta blockers on glycemic control can be significant.[75] The beta blockers atenolol, metoprolol, propranolol, and pindolol have all been shown to reduce insulin sensitivity by up to 25% with short-term (2–3 months)[86] and long-term (2–3 years)[79] treatment. The glycemic effect of beta blockers is amplified when they are used with thiazide diuretics. One study of 300 elderly hypertensives showed a twofold increase in new-onset NIDDM in the patients receiving beta blocker and diuretic treatment.[87] These findings are at odds with the recommendations of the Joint National Committee on Detection, Evaluation, and Treatment of Hypertension (JNC-5), which advocated use of diuretics and beta blockers as preferred initial therapy in hypertension.[88]

Lipid Control. Blood pressure therapy in diabetic patients with agents that increase triglyceride levels and decrease high-density lipoprotein (HDL) cholesterol is highly undesirable. Both selective and nonselective beta blockers increase triglyceride levels and decrease HDL_2 cholesterol.[81, 89] However, the effect of beta blockers on HDL appears to diminish with duration of treatment. In a meta-analysis of 474 studies of antihypertensive agents, it was found that when combined with cardioselectivity, beta blockers with intrinsic sympathomimetic activity favorably affected lipids and reduced both total and low-density lipoprotein (LDL) cholesterol levels.[81] It was also found that cardioselective beta blockers were more beneficial among patients with diabetes.[81]

Cardiovascular Complications. All classes of beta-blocking agents have proven efficacy in the treatment of hypertension in diabetes mellitus.[73, 74] Beta-blocking agents are particularly effective in younger diabetic patients with active coronary heart disease, tachyarrhythmias, or concentric ventricular hypertrophy or who have suffered recent myocardial infarction. Nonselective beta blockers that reduce cardiac output and increase peripheral resistance may precipitate congestive heart failure. Beta blockers have been reported to reduce left ventricular mass.[84]

Renal Complications. Beta blockers reduce blood pressure and slow the progression of diabetic renal disease, as reported in diabetic patients with overt renal disease.[90] Meta–regression analysis of studies using beta blockers in diabetic nephropathy indicate that they can reduce urinary protein excretion in patients with hypertension.[91] Their effect on protein excretion in normotensive patients with increased albumin excretion is less certain. The adverse effect of beta blockers on metabolic factors and their negative effect on renal blood flow suggest that these agents may not be the best choice as initial monotherapy for diabetic patients with nephropathy.

Converting Enzyme Inhibitors (Table 40–4)

Glycemic Control. Converting enzyme inhibitors have proven efficacy in the control of hypertension in diabetes and may have the most beneficial metabolic profile of all classes of antihypertensives.[73] Captopril and enalapril have been shown to improve insulin sensitivity in hypertensive subjects,[75, 78, 91] and other converting enzyme inhibitors may have beneficial effects on insulin and glucose.[92] Paolisso and coworkers[93] noted that five converting enzyme inhibitors, including captopril, enalapril, quinapril, ramipril, and lisinopril, improved insulin sensitivity in elderly hypertensive subjects. Fosino-

TABLE 40–3. SUMMARY OF BETA BLOCKERS IN HYPERTENSION AND DIABETES

Indicated in diabetic patients with a history of myocardial infarction or younger diabetic patients with evidence of hyperadrenergic activity
Increase insulin resistance and glucose intolerance
Increase triglycerides and decrease high-density lipoprotein cholesterol
Increase symptoms in peripheral vascular disease
Can cause hypoglycemia
Reduce left ventricular hypertrophy

TABLE 40–4. SUMMARY OF ANGIOTENSIN CONVERTING ENZYME INHIBITORS IN HYPERTENSION AND DIABETES

Preferred first choice in hypertension and diabetes
Reduce peripheral resistance by vasodilation without sodium retention
Have favorable effects on intermediary metabolism and insulin-mediated glucose disposal
Have neutral effect on serum lipid profile
In diabetic nephropathy
Reduce protein excretion
Retard renal failure
Reduce left ventricular hypertrophy
Contraindications
In hyperkalemia
In bilateral renal artery stenosis

pril[94] and cilazapril[95] may improve glucose tolerance, and ramipril[96] does not alter insulin and glucose. In hypertensive, high-risk metabolic subjects, switching from a beta blocker to a converting enzyme inhibitor improves glucose tolerance by 60%.[97] Studies examining blood glucose levels in diabetic patients treated with converting enzyme inhibitors show either no change[98] or improvement.[76, 99, 100] In a report of 130 hypertensive NIDDM patients, 4 months' treatment with captopril was associated with a significant reduction in fasting blood glucose levels in a stepwise manner during each month.[100] Converting enzyme inhibitors added to diuretic therapy can partially offset diuretic-induced hyperglycemia.[101]

Lipid Control. Converting enzyme inhibitors have been shown to reduce triglycerides, especially in younger hypertensives and, in patients with diabetes, to reduce total cholesterol levels.[81, 102] Their beneficial effect on insulin and glucose may explain the positive effects on lipids.[76, 81] Captopril has been shown to reduce cholesterol deposition in the aorta of the experimental hypercholesterolemic rabbit.[103]

Cardiovascular Complications. As vasodilators, these agents lower total peripheral resistance and exert a positive effect on cardiac performance. They do not cause sodium retention, as do the direct-acting vasodilators. ACE inhibitors have well-documented beneficial effects on survival in congestive heart failure[104] and in the reduction of left ventricular hypertrophy.[84]

Renal Complications. Converting enzyme inhibitors reduce urinary albumin excretion by selective relaxation of the glomerular efferent arterioles, leading to a reduction in glomerular filtration pressure.[105] This action may be unique to converting enzyme inhibitors and is independent of systemic hemodynamic changes, as demonstrated by their reducing of albuminuria and slowing of renal disease in normotensive subjects with diabetes.[105] A meta–regression analysis of antihypertensive agents in diabetic nephropathy substantiated that converting enzyme inhibitors were superior to other classes of agents in reducing proteinuria, with effects independent of blood pressure reduction.[91] Further evidence of their renal protective effects was provided by Lewis and the Collaborative Study Group,[106] who showed that in IDDM patients with established renal failure, captopril reduced by 50% the rate to doubling of serum creatinine concentration and the combined endpoints of progression to end-stage renal disease (dialysis, transplantation, death). Because blood pressure changed little during the trial period, it appears that converting enzyme inhibitors have renal protective effects independent of blood pressure. The adverse effects of these agents are few. Borderline hyperkalemia during converting enzyme inhibitor therapy may occur in diabetic patients with type IV renal tubular acidosis. Converting enzyme inhibitors are contraindicated in bilateral renal artery stenosis.

Calcium Channel Antagonists (Table 40–5)

Glycemic Control. Calcium channel blockers are highly effective in control of hypertension in diabetes and exert neutral effects on glucose and insulin metabolism. Diltiazem has little effect on peripheral insulin sensitivity,[107] verapamil may improve insulin sensitivity in renal failure,[108] and nifedipine has been reported to diminish insulin sensitivity.[109] In the Modern Treatment of Hypertension Trial, nifedipine GITS had no adverse effects on blood glucose in 926 obese hypertensive and 157 diabetic hypertensive subjects.[110] Most 1,4-dihydropyridine agents have no adverse effects on insulin and glucose,[73] and amlodipine may show improved glucose tolerance.[111]

Lipid Control. Numerous studies show that calcium channel blockers have few effects on serum lipids,[112] and a few studies have noted mild favorable effects.[73] Calcium channel blockers retard experimentally induced atherogenesis.[81]

Cardiovascular Complications. The calcium channel blocker verapamil has significant negative inotropic effects, which may accelerate heart failure in the hypertensive diabetic patient. Some calcium channel blockers diminish cardiac hypertrophy.[84]

Renal Complications. These agents have been shown to enhance, to decrease, or to not change urinary albumin excretion in diabetic subjects.[105] One report demonstrates an additive effect of calcium channel blockers and converting enzyme inhibitors to reduce albumin excretion and slow the morphologic progression of diabetic nephropathy.[105] The nondihydropyridine agents (verapamil, diltiazem) have proved more effective than did the dihydropyridine agents in reducing protein excretion and slowing the progression of diabetic renal disease.[105]

TABLE 40–5. SUMMARY OF CALCIUM CHANNEL BLOCKERS IN HYPERTENSION AND DIABETES

Proven antihypertensive efficacy in hypertension and diabetes
Have neutral effect on serum lipid profile
Reduce protein excretion in diabetic nephropathy (?)
Reverse left ventricular hypertrophy
Have neutral effect on intermediary metabolism
Indicated in peripheral vascular disease
Indicated in coronary heart disease

Alpha-Adrenergic Antagonists (Table 40–6)

Glycemic Control. Alpha blockers have beneficial effects on insulin and glucose. The agent prazosin has been shown to increase insulin-mediated glucose disposal in obese hypertensive subjects.[113] The longer-acting agent doxazosin improves glucose tolerance in diabetic hypertensive subjects.[114] The Finnish Multicenter Study Group[115] found that an alpha blocker reduced insulin and lipid levels in obese hypertensive subjects.

Lipid Control. Alpha blockers beneficially affect triglyceride levels, total and LDL cholesterol, and, in younger persons, HDL cholesterol.[81] In the TOMHS trial, an alpha blocker (doxazosin) was the only one of the six classes of antihypertensives to have significant beneficial effects on the total cholesterol:HDL cholesterol ratio.[66]

Cardiovascular Complications. The alpha-adrenergic receptor antagonists prazosin, terazosin, and doxazosin effectively lower diastolic blood pressure to 90 mm Hg or less in 70% of hypertensive patients and are effective in diabetic patients with hypertension.[73] Alpha blockers have been shown to reverse left ventricular hypertrophy.[84] Although orthostatic hypotension occurring with alpha blockers is considered a first-dose phenomenon, it may persist in diabetic patients with autonomic neuropathy.

Renal Complications. By lowering blood pressure, the alpha blockers should reduce proteinuria in patients with hypertension and diabetic nephropathy.

TABLE 40–6. SUMMARY OF ALPHA BLOCKERS IN HYPERTENSION AND DIABETES

Neutral to beneficial effect on insulin and glucose
Have beneficial effect on serum lipids
Can cause orthostatic hypotension

Effect of Antihypertensive Agents on Pre-Existing Diabetic Conditions

Orthostatic Hypotension

A significant fall in standing blood pressure (i.e., diastolic drop of 10 mm Hg or greater) is observed in up to 12% of diabetic subjects. Diabetic autonomic neuropathy represents the most common underlying mechanism,[1] and impaired baroreflex sensitivity leads to reduced sympathetic activation and low circulating catecholamine levels.[116] Reduced levels of renin also contribute to orthostatic hypotension secondary to low circulating angiotensin II levels. Intravascular hypovolemia in diabetes may be caused by a relative deficiency of aldosterone (hyporeninemic hypoaldosteronism),[12] by hypoalbuminemia, or by diuretic therapy. Orthostatic hypotension can be encountered in both normotensive and hypertensive diabetic patients. Symptoms are dizziness, lightheadedness, and inability to assume the upright position. Drugs known to aggravate orthostatic hypotension include methyldopa, alpha-adrenergic blockers, calcium channel blockers, and diuretics.[117] One of the most difficult treatment conditions is supine hypertension with orthostatic hypotension because the physician must try to simultaneously increase upright and decrease supine blood pressure levels. The mineralocorticoid 9α-fluorohydrocortisone in small doses (0.05–0.2 mg/day) lessens orthostatic hypotension by volume expansion. Converting enzyme inhibitors or calcium channel blockers given at bedtime help lower supine pressure.

Sexual Dysfunction

Erectile dysfunction occurs in up to 50%–75% of male diabetic patients,[118] and the incidence increases with age so that by the age of 70 years, the prevalence of impotence may exceed 95%.[118] Neural, vascular, hormonal, and psychological factors all contribute to erectile dysfunction in diabetes.[118] Contrary to common belief, neuropathy alone accounts for only one third of impotence in diabetic men. Impotence is not related to duration of diabetes and, once it appears, is affected little by glycemic control. Several antihypertensive agents, such as methyldopa, alpha-adrenergic blockers, and spironolactone, are known for their adverse effects on erectile function.[119, 120] However, sexual dysfunction occurs in up to 10%–20% of people using thiazide diuretics because of direct effects on smooth muscle relaxation or by reduction of free testosterone levels.[119] Beta blockers cause fewer problems than do thiazide diuretics, but their impairment of sexual function can be significant.[121, 122] Converting enzyme inhibitors and calcium channel antagonists are less frequently associated with impotence.[1]

Hypoglycemia

Beta blockers have known aggravating effects on insulin-induced hypoglycemia in diabetic subjects.[73] Beta-blocking agents mask the palpitations, tremor, and anxiety (but not diaphoresis) elicited by epinephrine and norepinephrine during hypoglycemia.[1, 73] In addition, blood pressure may rise during hypoglycemia in patients receiving beta-blocking agents because of an "unopposed" alpha-adrenergic effect. When hypoglycemia is induced in normal subjects, epinephrine has a more minor role than does glucagon in counteracting hypoglycemia. However, IDDM subjects with long-standing disease lack the glucagon response and rely on epinephrine to restore euglycemia. Propranolol, metaprolol, and atenolol, by blocking the epinephrine response, can delay hypoglycemia recovery in diabetes.

Peripheral Vascular Disease

Macrovascular disease is common in diabetes mellitus. Aggravation of intermittent claudication, Raynaud phenomenon, or diminished blood supply to the extremities is observed in diabetics treated with nonselective beta blockers.[1] In theory, cardioselective β_1 blockers should have fewer of these side effects, but these agents can act on the β_2-adrenergic receptors when high doses are administered.[1]

REFERENCES

1. The National High Blood Pressure Education Program Working Group: National High Blood Pressure Education Program Working Group report on hypertension in diabetes. Hypertension 1994; 23:145.
2. American Diabetes Association: Diabetes 1993 Vital Statistics. Alexandria, VA: American Diabetes Association, 1993.
3. Haffner SM, Mitchell BD, Pugh JA, et al: Proteinuria in Mexican Americans and non-Hispanic whites with NIDDM. Diabetes Care 1989; 12:530.
4. National Diabetes Data Group: Summary. *In* Harris MI, Hamman RF (eds): Diabetes in America, p 1. Washington, DC: Government Printing Office, 1985. US Department of Health and Human Services publication NIH 85–1468.
5. Bild D, Teutsch SM: The control of hypertension in persons with diabetes: a public health approach. Public Health Rep 1987; 102:522.
6. Horan M: Diabetes in hypertension. *In* Harris MI, Hamman RF (eds): Diabetes in America, p 17. Washington, DC: Government Printing Office, 1985. US Department of Health and Human Services publication NIH 85–1468. Diabetes data compiled 1984.
7. American Diabetes Association: Consensus statement on the treatment of hypertension in diabetes. Diabetes Care 1993; 16:1394.
8. Dawson KG, McKenzie JK, Ross SA, et al: Report of the Canadian Hypertension Consensus Conference: 5, hypertension and diabetes. Can Med Assoc J 1993; 149:821.
9. National High Blood Pressure Education Program Working Group: Working group report on hypertension and chronic renal failure. Arch Intern Med 1991; 151:1280.
10. Klein R, Klein BEK, Moss SE, et al: Is blood pressure a predictor of the incidence or progression of diabetic retinopathy? Arch Intern Med 1989; 149:2427.
11. Tuetscher A, Schnell H, Wilson PWF: Incidence of diabetic retinopathy and relationship to baseline plasma glucose and blood pressure. Diabetes Care 1988; 11:246.
12. Stern N, Tuck ML: Mechanisms of hypertension in diabetes mellitus. *In* Laragh JH, Brenner BM (eds): Hypertension: Pathophysiology, Diagnosis, and Management, p 1689. New York: Raven Press, 1995.
13. Tuck ML, Corry DB: Pathophysiology and management of hypertension in diabetes. Annu Rev Med 1991; 42:533.
14. Epstein M, Sowers JR: Diabetes mellitus and hypertension. Hypertension 1992; 19:403.
15. Weidmann P: Pathogenesis of hypertension accompanying diabetes mellitus. Contrib Nephrol 1988; 73:73.
16. O'Hare JA, Roland JM, Walters G, Corrall RJM: Impaired sodium excretion in response to volume expansion induced by water immersion in insulin-dependent diabetes mellitus. Clin Sci 1986; 71:403.
17. Nosadini R, Floretto P, Trevisan R, et al: Insulin-dependent diabetes mellitus and hypertension. Diabetes Care 1991; 14:210.
18. Ortola FV, Ballermann BJ, Anderson S, et al: Elevated plasma atrial natriuretic peptide levels in diabetic rats: potential mediator of hyperfiltration. J Clin Invest 1987; 80:670.
19. Abonchacra S, Baines AD, Zinman BK, et al: Insulin blunts the natriuretic action of atrial natriuretic peptide in hypertension. Hypertension 1994; 23(pt 2):1054.
20. Chen S, Yeen C, Clough D, et al: Role of digitalis-like substance in the hypertension of reduced renal mass rats. Am J Hypertens 1994; 6(pt 1):397.
21. Takahashi H, Matsusawa M, Nishimura M, et al: Digoxin-like immunoreactivity may contribute to hyperinsulinemia-associated hypertension in patients with glucose intolerance. J Cardiovasc Pharmacol 1993; 22(suppl 2):S22.
22. Hseuh WA: Effect of renin-angiotensin system in the vascular disease of type II diabetes mellitus. Am J Med 1992; 92(suppl):13s.
23. Trujillo A, Eggena P, Barrett J, et al: Renin regulation in type II diabetes mellitus: influence of dietary sodium. Hypertension 1989; 13:200.
24. Danenman D, Crompton CH, Bolfe JW, et al: Plasma prorenin as an early marker of nephropathy in diabetic (IDDM) adolescents. Kidney Int 1994; 46:1154.

25. Franken AAM, Derkx FHM, Blankestein JAMJL, et al: Plasma prorenin as an early marker of microvascular disease in patients with diabetes mellitus. Diabete Med 1992; 18:137.
26. Ubeda M, Hernandez I, Fenoy F, et al: Vascular and adrenal renin-like activity in chronically diabetic rats. Hypertension 1988; 11:339.
27. Corrila-Rotter R, Hostetter TH, Rosenberg ME: Renin and angiotensin gene expression in experimental diabetes mellitus. Kidney Int 1992; 41:796.
28. Doria M, Warram JH, Krolewski AS: Genetic predisposition to diabetic nephropathy. Evidence for a role of angiotensin I converting enzyme gene. Diabetes 1994; 43:690.
29. Feman SS, Mericle RA, Reed GW, et al: Serum angiotensin converting enzyme in diabetic patients. Am J Med Sci 1993; 305:280.
30. Ritz E, Hasslacher C, Guo J-Z, et al: Role of hypertension in diabetic nephropathy. Contrib Nephrol 1989; 73:91.
31. Corry D, Tuck ML: Hypertension and diabetes. Semin Nephrol 1991; 11:561.
32. Krolewski AS, Canessa M, Warram J, et al: Predisposition to hypertension and susceptibility to renal disease in insulin-dependent diabetes mellitus. N Engl J Med 1988; 381:140.
33. Mangili R, Bending JJ, Scoot G, et al: Increased sodium-lithium countertransport activity in red cells of patients with insulin-dependent diabetes and nephropathy. N Engl J Med 1988; 318:146.
34. Weder AB: Red cell lithium-sodium countertransport and renal lithium clearance in hypertension. N Engl J Med 1986; 314:1986.
35. Modan M, Halkin H, Almog S, et al: Hyperinsulinemia: a link between hypertension, obesity and glucose intolerance. J Clin Invest 1985; 75:809.
36. Ferrannini E, Buzzigoli G, Bonadonna R, et al: Insulin resistance in essential hypertension. N Engl J Med 1987; 317:350.
37. Reaven GM, Hoffman BB: Hypertension as a disease of carbohydrate and lipoprotein metabolism. Am J Med 1989; 87(suppl 6A):2s.
38. DeFronzo RA, Ferrannini E: Insulin resistance: a multifaceted syndrome responsible for NIDDM, obesity and hypertension, dyslipidemia and atherosclerotic cardiovascular disease. Diabetes Care 1991; 14:173.
39. Nosadini R, Solini A, Velussi M, et al: Impaired insulin-induced glucose uptake by extrahepatic tissue is the hallmark of NIDDM patients who have or will develop hypertension and microalbuminuria. Diabetes 1994; 43:491.
40. Julius S, Gundrandsson T, Jamerson K, et al: The hemodynamic link between insulin resistance and hypertension. J Hypertens 1991; 9:983.
41. Rowe JW, Young JB, Minaker KL, et al: Effect of insulin and glucose infusions on sympathetic nervous system activity in normal man. Diabetes 1981; 30:219.
42. Anderson EA, Hoffman RP, Balon TW, et al: Hyperinsulinemia produces both sympathetic neural activation and vasodilation in normal humans. J Clin Invest 1991; 87:2246.
43. Tuck ML: Obesity, the sympathetic nervous system and essential hypertension. Hypertension 1992; 19(suppl 1):I-67.
44. Maxwell M, Heber D, Tuck M: Role of insulin and norepinephrine in the hypertension of obesity. Am J Hypertens 1994; 7:402.
45. Stout RW: Insulin and atheroma: a 20-year perspective. Diabetes Care 1990; 53:631.
46. Epstein M, Sowers JR: Diabetes mellitus and hypertension. Hypertension 1992; 19:403.
47. Baron AO, Laakso M, Brechtel G, et al: Mechanism of insulin resistance in insulin dependent diabetes mellitus: a major role for reduced skeletal muscle blood flow. J Clin Endocrinol Metab 1991; 73:637.
48. Murphy LJ, Ghahary A, Chakrabart S: Insulin regulation of IGF-I expression in rat aorta. Diabetes 1990; 39:657.
49. Frank HJ, Levin ER, Hu RM, et al: Insulin stimulates endothelin binding and action in cultured vascular smooth muscle cells. Endocrinology 1993; 133:1092.
50. Ferris JB, O'Hare JA, Kelleher CCM, et al: Diabetic control and the renin angiotensin system, catecholamines and blood pressure. Hypertension 1985; 7(suppl 2): II-58.
51. Gupta S, Sussman I, McArthur CVS, et al: Endothelium-dependent inhibition of Na^+K^+ ATPase activity in rabbit aorta by hyperglycemia. Possible role of endothelium-derived nitric oxide. J Clin Invest 1992; 90:727.
52. Yamauchi T, Ohnaka K, Takayanagi R, et al: Enhanced secretion of endothelin-I by elevated glucose levels from cultured bovine aortic endothelial cells. FEBS Lett 1990; 267:16.
53. Randeree HA, Omar MAK, Motala AA, et al: Effect of insulin therapy on blood pressure in NIDDM patients with secondary failure. Diabetes Care 1992; 15:1258.
54. The Diabetes Control and Complication Trial Research Group: The effect of intensive treatment of diabetes on the development and progression of long term complications in insulin dependent diabetes mellitus. N Engl J Med 1993; 329:977.
55. Bodmaer CW, Patrick AW, How TV, Williams G: Exaggerated sensitivity to NE-induced vasoconstriction in IDDM patients with microalbuminuria. Diabetes 1994; 1241:209.
56. Gans ROB, Bilo HJG, Maarschalkerweerd Heine RJ, et al: Exogenous insulin augments in healthy volunteers the cardiovascular reactivity to noradrenaline but not to angiotensin II. J Clin Invest 1991; 88:512.
57. Gros R, Borkowski KR, Feldman RD: Human insulin-mediated enhancement of vascular β-adrenergic responsiveness. Hypertension 1994; 23:551.
58. Zatz R, Brenner BM: Pathogenesis of diabetic microangiopathy: the hemodynamic view. Am J Med 1986; 80:443.
59. Mathiesen ER, Ronn B, Jensen T, et al: Relationship between blood pressure and urinary albumin excretion in development of microalbuminuria. Diabetes 1990; 39:245.
60. Chase HP, Sarg SK, Harris S, et al: High-normal blood pressure and early diabetic nephropathy. Arch Intern Med 1990; 150:639.
61. Poulsen PL, Hansen KW, Mogensen CE: Ambulatory blood pressure in transition from normo- to micro-albuminuria: a longitudinal study in IDDM patients. Diabetes 1994; 43:1248.
62. Chavers BM, Bilous RW, Ellis EN, et al: Glomerular lesions and urinary albumin excretion in type I diabetes without overt proteinuria. N Engl J Med 1989; 320:966.
63. Gall MA, Rossing P, Jensen JS, et al: Red cell Na^+ countertransport in non–insulin-dependent diabetics with diabetic nephropathy. Kidney Int 1991; 39:135.
64. Hypertension Detection and Follow-up Program Cooperative Group: Five-year findings of the Hypertension Detection and Follow-up Program, I: reduction in mortality of persons with high blood pressure, including mild hypertension. JAMA 1979; 242:2562.
65. Systolic Hypertension in the Elderly Program Cooperative Research Group: Implications of the Systolic Hypertension in the Elderly Program. Hypertension 1993; 21:335.
66. Neaton JD, Grimm RH, Prineas RJ, et al: Treatment of Mild Hypertension Study Research Group: Treatment of Mild Hypertension Study: final results. JAMA 1993; 270:713.
67. Tuck M: Obesity. *In* Swales JD (ed): Textbook of Hypertension, p 576. London: Blackwell Scientific Publications, 1994.
68. Daly PA, Landsberg L: Pathogenesis of hypertension in NIDDM: lessons from obesity. J Hum Hypertens 1991; 5:277.
69. Barnard RJ, Ugianskis EJ, Martin DA, et al: Role of diet and exercise in the management of hyperinsulinemia and associated atherosclerotic risk factors. Am J Cardiol 1992; 69:440.
70. Fagerberg B, Berglund A, Anderson OK, et al: Cardiovascular effects of weight reduction versus antihypertensive drug treatment: a comparative, randomized, 1-year study of obese men with mild hypertension. J Hypertens 1991; 9:431.
71. Tuck ML, Corry D, Trujillo A: Salt-sensitive blood pressure and exaggerated vascular reactivity in the hypertension of diabetes mellitus. Am J Med 1990; 88:210.
72. Dodson PM, Beevers M, Hallworth R, et al: Sodium restriction and blood pressure in hypertensive type II diabetics: randomised blind controlled and crossover studies of moderate sodium restriction and sodium supplementation. Br Med J 1989; 298:227.
73. Stern N, Tuck M: Drug therapy of hypertension in diabetic patients. J Hum Hypertens 1991; 5:295.
74. Moser M, Ross H: The treatment of hypertension in diabetic patients. Diabetes Care 1993; 16:542.
75. Pollare T, Lithell H, Berne C: A comparison of the effects of hydrochlorothiazide and captopril on glucose and lipid metabolism in patients with hypertension. N Engl J Med 1989; 321:868.
76. Prince MJ, Stuart CA, Padia M, et al: Metabolic effects of hydrochlorothiazide and enalapril during treatment of the hypertensive diabetic patient. Arch Intern Med 1988; 148:2363.
77. Carlsen JE, Koober L, Torp-Pedersen C, Johansen P: Relation between dose of bendrofluazide, antihypertensive effect, and adverse biochemical effects. Br Med J 1990; 300:975.
78. Andersson OK, Gudbrandsson T, Jamerson K: Metabolic adverse effects of thiazide diuretics: the importance of normokalemia. J Intern Med 1991; 229:89.
79. Lund L, Pollare T, Berne C, et al: Long-term metabolic effects of antihypertensive drugs. Am Heart J 1994; 128:1177.

80. Gurwitz JH, Bohn RL, Glynn RJ, et al: Antihypertensive drug therapy and the initiation of treatment for diabetes mellitus. Ann Intern Med 1992; 118:273.
81. Kasiske BL, Ma JZ, Kalil RSN, Louis SA: Effects of antihypertensive therapy on serum lipids. Ann Intern Med 1995; 122:133.
82. Bloomgarden AT, Gienzberg-Fellner F, Rayfield EJ, et al: Elevated hemoglobin A_{1c} and low density lipoprotein cholesterol levels in thiazide treated diabetic patients. Am J Med 1984; 77:823.
83. Fries ED: The efficacy and safety of diuretics in treating hypertension. Ann Intern Med 1995; 122:223.
84. Hachamivitz S, Sonnenblick EH, Storm JA, et al: Left ventricular hypertrophy in hypertension and the effects of antihypertensive drug therapy. Curr Probl Cardiol 1988; 13:369.
85. Walker WG, Hermann JA, Anderson JE: Randomized doubly blinded trial of enalapril (E) versus hydrochlorothiazide (H) on glomerular filtration rate (GFR) in diabetic nephropathy: early vs late results. Hypertension 1993; 22:410.
86. Pollare T, Lithell H, Selinus I, et al: Sensitivity to insulin during treatment with atenolol and metoprolol: a randomized double blind study of effects on carbohydrate and lipoprotein metabolism in hypertensive patients. Br Med J 1989; 298:1152.
87. Mykkanen L, Haffner SM, Kuusisto V, et al: Hypertensives with beta blocker or diuretic therapy have an increased risk of developing type II diabetes. Diabetologia 1993; 36:A212.
88. Joint National Committee: The Fifth Report of the Joint National Committee on Detection, Evaluation, and Treatment of High Blood Pressure. Arch Intern Med 193; 153:154.
89. Ames RP: The effects of antihypertensive drugs on serum lipids and lipoprotein. II. Non-diuretic drugs. Drugs 1986; 32:335.
90. Parving HH, Andersen AR, Smidt UM, et al: Early aggressive antihypertensive treatment reduces rate of decline in kidney function in diabetic nephropathy. Lancet 1983; 1:1176.
91. Kasiske BL, Kalil RSN, Ma JZ, et al: Effect of antihypertensive therapy on the kidney in patients with diabetes: a meta-regression analysis. Ann Intern Med 1993; 118:129.
92. Donnelly R: Angiotensin-converting enzyme inhibitors and insulin sensitivity: metabolic effects in hypertension, diabetes, and heart failure. J Cardiovasc Pharmacol 1992; 20(suppl II): S38.
93. Paolisso G, Gambardella A, Verza M, et al: ACE inhibition improves insulin sensitivity in aged insulin-resistant hypertensive patients. J Hum Hypertens 1992; 6:175.
94. Allemann Y, Baumann S, Jost M, et al: Insulin sensitivity in normotensive subjects during angiotensin converting enzyme inhibition with fosinopril. Eur J Clin Pharmacol 1992; 42:275.
95. Shionoiri H, Sugimoto K, Minamisawa K, et al: Glucose and lipid metabolism during long-term treatment with cilazapril in hypertensive patients with or without impaired glucose metabolism. J Cardiovasc Pharmacol 1990; 15:33.
96. Ludvik B, Kueenburg E, Brunnbauer M, et al: The effects of ramipril on glucose tolerance, insulin secretion, and insulin sensitivity in patients with hypertension. J Cardiovasc Pharmacol 1991; 18(suppl 2):S157.
97. Bjorntorp K, Lingarde F, Mattiasson I: Long-term effects on insulin sensitivity and sodium transport in glucose-intolerant hypertensive subjects when beta-blockade is replaced by captopril treatment. J Hum Hypertens 1992; 6:291.
98. Lithell HO: Effects of antihypertensive drugs on insulin, glucose, and lipid metabolism. Diabetes Care 1991; 14:203.
99. Torlone E, Britta M, Rambotti AM, et al: Improved insulin action and glycemic control after long-term angiotensin-converting enzyme inhibition in subjects with arterial hypertension and type II diabetes. Diabetes Care 1993; 16:1347.
100. Alkarouf J, Narinikumari K, Corry DB, Tuck ML: The effect of captopril on blood pressure and blood glucose in hypertensive patients with noninsulin dependent diabetes mellitus. Am J Hypertens 1993; 6:337.
101. Weinberger MH: Optimizing cardiovascular risk reduction during antihypertensive therapy. Hypertension 1990; 16:201.
102. Costa EV, Borghi C, Mussi A, et al: Use of captopril to reduce serum lipids in hypertensive patients with hyperlipidemia. Am J Hypertens 1988; 1:221S.
103. Chobanian AV, Haudenschild CC, Nickerson C, et al: Antiatherogenic effect of captopril in the Watanabe heritable hyperlipidemic rabbit. Hypertension 1990; 15:327.
104. Yusuf S, for the SOLVD Investigators: Effect of enalapril on survival in patients with reduced left ventricular ejection fractions and congestive heart failure. N Engl J Med 1991; 325:293.
105. Bakris GL, Barnhill BW, Sadler R: Treatment of arterial hypertension in diabetic humans: importance of therapeutic selection. Kidney Int 1993; 41:912.
106. Lewis EJ, Hunsicker LG, Bain RP, et al: The effect of angiotensin converting enzyme inhibition in diabetic nephropathy. N Engl J Med 1993; 323:1456.
107. Pollare T, Lithell H, Morlin C, et al: Metabolic effects of diltiazem and atenolol: results from a randomized, double-blind study with parallel groups. J Hypertens 1989; 7:551.
108. Faddo GZ, Admal M, Soliman AR, et al: Correction of glucose intolerance and the impaired insulin release of chronic renal failure by verapamil. Kidney Int 1989; 36:773.
109. Sheu WH, Swislocki AL, Hoffman B, et al: Comparison of the effects of atenolol and nifedipine on glucose, insulin, and lipid metabolism in patients with hypertension. Am J Hypertens 1991; 4:199.
110. Tuck ML, Bravo EL, Krakoff LR, Friedman CP, and the Modern Approach to the Treatment of Hypertension Study Group: Endocrine and renal effects of nifedipine gastrointestinal therapeutic system in patients with essential hypertension: results of a multicenter trial. Am J Hypertens 1990; 3:333S.
111. deCourten M, Ferrari P, Bohlen L, et al: Lack of effect of long-term amlodipine on insulin sensitivity and plasma insulin in obese patients with essential hypertension. Eur J Clin Pharmacol 1993; 44:457.
112. Trost BN, Weidmann P: Effects of calcium antagonists on glucose homeostasis and serum lipids in non-diabetic and diabetic subjects: a review. J Hypertens 1987; 5(suppl 4):81.
113. Pollare T, Lithell H, Selinus I, Berne C: Application of prazosin is associated with an increase in insulin sensitivity in obese patients with hypertension. Diabetologia 1988; 31:415.
114. Shieh SM, Sheu WH, Shen DC, et al: Glucose, insulin, and lipid metabolism in doxazosin-treated patients with hypertension. Am J Hypertens 1992; 5:827.
115. Lehtonen A: Doxazosin effects on insulin and glucose in hypertensive patients. The Finnish Multicenter Study Group. Am Heart J 1991; 121(pt 2):1307.
116. Eckberg DL, Harkins SW, Fritsch JM, et al: Baroreflex control of plasma norepinephrine and heart period in healthy subjects and diabetic patients. J Clin Invest 1986; 78:366.
117. Onrot J, Goldberg MR, Hollister AS, et al: Management of chronic orthostatic hypotension. Am J Med 1986; 80:454.
118. Kaiser FE, Korenman SG: Impotence in diabetic men. Am J Med 1988; 85:147.
119. Carrier S, Zvara P, Lue TF: Erectile dysfunction. Endocrinol Metab Clin North Am 1994; 23:773.
120. Bullum J: Pharmacosexuology update: prescription drugs and sexual function. J Psychoactive Drugs 1986; 18:99.
121. Murray FT, Wyss HU, Thomas RG, et al: Gonadal dysfunction in diabetic men with and without organic impotence. J Clin Endocrinol Metab 1987; 65:127.
122. The IPPPSH Collaborative Group: Cardiovascular risks and risk factors in a randomized trial of treatment based on the beta blocker oxprenolol: the International Prospective Primary Prevention Study in Hypertension (IPPPSH). J Hypertens 1985; 3:379.

41 Hypertension During Pregnancy

Ellen W. Seely, MD
Steven W. Graves, PhD
John T. Repke, MD

ETIOLOGY OF PREECLAMPSIA AND OTHER HYPERTENSIVE COMPLICATIONS OF PREGNANCY

Pregnancy-induced hypertension (PIH), particularly preeclampsia, is one of the most studied medical problems, and yet has no definitive etiology. Two features of this medical complication have contributed substantially to this continued uncertainty. The first is that PIH is not a homogeneous disorder. The precise number of differing diseases is unclear, as are the specific genetic, biochemical, or functional features that underlie each. Efforts have been made to distinguish one from another. Recent definitions subdividing hypertension in pregnancy are based on the Working Group Report on High Blood Pressure in Pregnancy and endorsed by the American College of Obstetrics and Gynecology.[1] These definitions allow for the categorization of hypertension in pregnancy into six groups: (1) chronic hypertension, (2) transient hypertension of pregnancy (THP) or gestational hypertension, (3) preeclampsia, (4) preeclampsia superimposed on chronic hypertension, (5) severe preeclampsia, and (6) eclampsia. Definitions of these terms are provided in Table 41–1. However, each criterion represents a cutoff point that occurs within a continuum; none is specific or etiologic. This allows for overlaps and heterogeneity. Nevertheless, some biochemical abnormalities appear to segregate reasonably well according to some of the six classifications, which suggests that the divisions are not meaningless. Nonetheless, careful studies suggest that many, if not all, of these current subgroups are heterogeneous. The second challenge is that many hypertensive pregnant women, especially those with more severe disease, have multiorgan and multisystem involvement, which makes it difficult to know which response is primary vs. secondary.

Hypotheses

A thorough discussion of all abnormalities associated with hypertensive complications of pregnancy is beyond the scope of this chapter. Some evidence suggests that transient or gestational hypertension may be part of the same hypertensive process that is seen in essential hypertension: specifically, women with THP have a higher incidence of later essential hypertension;[2] hence, hypotheses advanced to explain essential hypertension may apply to THP. Current theories invoke abnormalities in the renin-angiotensin system,[3] the vascular sodium pump,[4] insulin resistance,[5] endothelial damage,[6] and specific genetic abnormalities.[7] Some of these abnormalities are discussed in more detail later. In contrast, the incidence of hypertension later in life appears to be lower among women with preeclampsia than among women in general.[2]

APPROACHES TO THE PREVENTION OF HYPERTENSION DURING PREGNANCY

In the absence of a complete understanding of THP or preeclampsia, the inability to prevent both is not surprising. Nevertheless, when biochemical abnormalities have been consistent and well documented, efforts to correct the observed abnormality as an attempt to prevent or treat the disease have usually followed. None has proved to be particularly effective in the prevention of THP or preeclampsia. However, several of these are discussed, because of their currency or their occasional or modest benefits.

Historical Approaches to Prevention

Protein Restriction. Observations that higher socioeconomic class was associated with a higher incidence of PIH[8] and that rates of PIH fell with starvation[9] led to restriction of meat consumption as a means of treating PIH. A more vegetarian diet was typically implemented. However, later data also emerged to suggest that PIH is accompanied by protein deficiency.[10] Careful studies of protein restriction do not exist, existing studies are inconclusive, and there is no evidence that either approach has a preventive effect.

TABLE 41–1. DEFINITIONS OF HYPERTENSIVE DISORDERS AND DIABETES

Hypertension	SBP > 140 mm Hg; DBP > 90 mm Hg; or SBP increase of ≥30 mm Hg and DBP increase of ≥15 mm Hg over first-trimester or prepregnancy values
Proteinuria	Protein > 0.3 g/dL/24 h or >1 g/L on dipstick test*
Chronic Hypertension	Hypertension before 20 weeks of gestation in the absence of neoplastic trophoblastic disease
Transient Hypertension of Pregnancy	Hypertension after 20 weeks of gestation, not accompanied by other signs of preeclampsia (also called *gestational hypertension)*
Preeclampsia	Development of hypertension with proteinuria, edema, or both after 20 weeks of gestation
Superimposed Preeclampsia	Development of preeclampsia in a woman with pre-existing hypertension
Severe Preeclampsia	Blood pressure > 160/110 mm Hg with significant end-organ manifestations†

Abbreviations: SBP, systolic blood pressure; DBP, diastolic blood pressure.
*At least two urine specimens, collected 6 or more h apart.
†Proteinuria (>5 g/dL in 24 h), oliguria (<500 mL in 24 h), rising serum creatinine concentration, persistent visual disturbances, epigastric or right upper quadrant pain, pulmonary edema or right upper quadrant pain, pulmonary edema or cyanosis, thrombocytopenia or overt hemolysis, hepatocellular damage, and intrauterine growth retardation.

Caloric Reduction. Another early but largely untested premise was that preeclampsia resulted from overeating during pregnancy. General caloric restriction as an approach to prevention has not been shown to have a positive effect.

Sodium Restriction. Abnormalities in both sodium homeostasis[11] and plasma volume[12] have been well documented in preeclampsia and THP. Severely restricting sodium intake prophylactically in women has been and continues to be advocated by some authors.[13] The results of trials of sodium restriction to prevent PIH are few and in conflict.[13, 14] Compliance with such diets is difficult to achieve even in the most closely monitored studies and would be unlikely to occur in the absence of such monitoring.

Contemporary Prophylactic Approaches

Antioxidants

Tocopherols (Vitamin E), Ascorbic Acid (Vitamin C), and Carotenes/Retinol (Vitamin A). One hypothesis suggests that endothelial damage early in the pregnancy initiates a cascade of changes that ultimately result in the development of preeclampsia. Many lines of evidence support endothelial damage in established disease,[15] and some data suggest that these changes predate the development of clinical findings.[15] Endothelial damage is thought to increase the levels of lipid peroxides, which in turn may consume the body's protective antioxidants. Inadequate free radical scavenging could then lead to further vascular and cellular damage, perpetuating the series of events. Indeed, in preeclampsia most studies have revealed increased levels of lipid peroxides[16, 17] and reductions of a number of antioxidants, including tocopherols,[16–18] retinol/carotenes,[17, 18] and ascorbic acid.[18] Therapeutic trials with vitamin E have been very limited and have shown no improvement in maternal or fetal outcome among patients with established preeclampsia.[19] The prophylactic use of these antioxidants has not been assessed.

Omega-3 Fatty Acids

Research during the 1980s and 1990s indicated that increased consumption of certain fish products, which are rich in omega-3 fatty acids, has beneficial cardiovascular effects in the general population, including reduction of blood pressure.[20] The exact mechanisms remain uncertain. Results of several studies suggest that moderate consumption of these oils tends to prolong bleeding times, lower serum triglyceride levels, and shift prostaglandin synthesis to favor vasodilatory as opposed to pressor products. Other studies have demonstrated that the antihypertensive effect of these oils is independent of changes in prostaglandin synthesis.[21] The possibility of a comparable antihypertensive effect in the setting of PIH and, in particular, preeclampsia has been entertained. Study findings have been very limited but suggest that fish oil may reduce the incidence of preeclampsia and early delivery.[22, 23] However, well-controlled prospective studies have yet to be performed to assess both risks and benefits, and consequently no recommendation can be made.

Arachidonic Acid Metabolism and Aspirin

It has been long recognized that both thrombocytopenia and disseminated intravascular coagulation are common features of preeclampsia. Their presence suggests a disturbance in clotting mechanisms in preeclamptic women. Treatment with antiplatelet medications such as heparin or dipyridamole has produced no reduction in morbidity in preeclampsia and has in some cases led to hemorrhage.[24, 25] Nevertheless, in 1985 and early 1986, two reports suggested that the platelet abnormalities might be caused by changes in the prostaglandin-thromboxane series and, in addition, that they not only accompany preeclampsia but may cause it.[26, 27] Moreover, the investigators found that early treatment with aspirin might actually prevent the disease.

In the most compelling of these reports, the researchers studied second-trimester primigravida in whom a susceptibility to preeclampsia was suggested by an enhanced blood pressure sensitivity to angiotensin II, the potent vasoconstrictor.[27] The women were then randomized to a treatment group receiving 60 mg of aspirin per day or to a control group receiving placebo. The treatment group showed a marked reduction in the incidence of preeclampsia (0 of 21) in comparison with the control group (8 of 23). The women with THP were not affected.[27] This report galvanized a large research effort that has convincingly demonstrated a dysregulation of prostanoid synthesis in women with preeclampsia, seen as a relative increase in the circulating levels of thromboxane A_2 (TXA_2), a vasoconstrictor, and a relative reduction in prostacyclin (prostaglandin I_2 [PGI_2]), a potent vasorelaxant.[16, 28] Low-dose aspirin was found to reduce TXA_2 significantly while preserving PGI_2 levels, thereby reversing their ratio.[29] These findings resulted in the initiation of several large, multiyear, randomized, placebo-controlled, double-blind prospective studies. In the interim, many smaller trials of low-dose aspirin were performed and reported. A meta-analysis of these studies suggested that among 394 women total at risk for PIH, low-dose aspirin resulted in a 65% reduction in PIH.[30] This reduction appeared to be limited to preeclampsia and was not seen in women with THP. The reduction in preeclampsia was accompanied by a significant reduction in the incidence of very low birth weight.

The completion and publication of the two largest low-dose aspirin trials, however, has been disappointing.[31, 32] The National Institutes of Health (NIH)–sponsored U.S. study of 2985 healthy nulliparous women[31] found a modest reduction in the incidence of preeclampsia in the treatment group (60 mg/day of aspirin) in comparison with the control group (69 of 1485 vs. 94 of 1500, which approached significance). However, no benefit on fetal outcome and an increased risk of placental abruption were found. Of interest is that the women who had systolic blood pressures of 120 mm Hg or higher at the time of randomization showed a significant reduction in the development of preeclampsia. Typically, these women would be suspected of having chronic hypertension. The larger European trial appeared in 1994 and included 9364 women, enrolled because they were considered to be at increased risk for developing preeclampsia or for treatment of suspected preeclampsia.[32] Rates of preeclampsia were comparable for either the prophylaxis or the treatment group in comparison with the control group (6.7% for prophylaxis or treatment with 60 mg/day of aspirin; 7.6% with placebo). There was no improvement in overall infant mortality nor a reduction in complications. However, for women who delivered before 28 weeks, aspirin significantly reduced the incidence of preeclampsia. This study found no increased risk with aspirin.

The rates of other hypertensive complications of pregnancy were equivalent for treatment and control groups in both studies. Other agents such as indomethacin or TXA_2 antagonists provide no advantage over aspirin. None of these agents corrected the blood pressure elevation, which suggests that once the disease is established, TXA_2 does not mediate the hypertension.[31–33] In summary, there is no evidence to support the general use of low-dose aspirin in healthy pregnant women. There is some evidence to suggest that in some women at high risk for the development of preeclampsia, aspirin may have a benefit but this must be weighed against a possible small increase in some complications.

Linoleic Acid (Primrose Oil). Linoleic acid, including its natural sources such as primrose oil, represents the precursor of arachidonic acid, which in turn is converted to both vasodilatory (prostaglandins I_2 and E_2 [PGI_2 and PGE_2]) and vasocontractile (TXA_2 and prostaglandin F_{2a} [PGF_{2a}]) prostanoids. Imbalance in these groups is seen in preeclampsia.[28] Some authors have noted a decrement in linoleic acid in preeclampsia,[34] whereas others have found increased levels.[35] Because linoleic acid was found by some researchers to have an antihypertensive effect in essential hypertension,[21] others explored the effect of enriching the diet of preeclamptic women with linoleic acid.[36] This produced no effects on PGI_2 or TXA_2 synthesis, blood pressure, or features of the disease.

Elemental Nutrients

Zinc. There has been interest in the relationship between nutritional factors and preeclampsia and THP. Zinc is an essential constituent of a number of human enzymes. Pregnancy is a period of increased zinc demand by the body. In the majority of studies, women with severe (and in some studies mild) preeclampsia have lower circulating zinc levels in comparison with normotensive pregnant women.[37, 38] Zinc levels among pregnant women with chronic hypertension do not appear to differ.[37, 38] Because cadmium competes with zinc, some authors have suggested that cadmium toxicity was responsible for the low zinc levels. Indeed, cadmium toxicity manifests with hypertension, proteinuria, and edema.[39] However, studies have demonstrated zinc deficiency independent of excess cadmium.[38] A double-blind prospective study in which 494 women were randomized to zinc or placebo showed no difference in the incidence of maternal hypertension or in fetal outcome.[40]

Magnesium. Short-term magnesium sulfate infusion has long been the standard of care in the United States for anticonvulsive therapy in the setting of preeclampsia. Low serum levels of magnesium have been found in some studies of essential hypertension and PIH, but there are no persuasive data to support a marked or consistent reduction of serum magnesium in THP or preeclampsia.[41] Prolonged magnesium therapy may have a modest antihypertensive effect.[42] When given acutely to preeclamptic women for anticonvulsive coverage, it typically has little or no antihypertensive effect,[42, 43] despite data that suggest that it reduces levels of endothelin (a potent vasoconstrictor)[44] and increases prostacyclin[45] and cyclic guanosine monophosphate (cGMP) (both of which are vasodilators).[46] Magnesium has also been used for tocolysis, usually in conjunction with other agents.[47] Among women who received magnesium tocolysis, the later incidence of either THP or preeclampsia was found to be lower.[47] However, prospective studies of magnesium supplementation to reduce the incidence of THP or preeclampsia have shown no general benefit,[48, 49] and recommendation for its use as such is limited to prophylaxis of seizure (eclampsia).

Calcium Supplementation. Most forms of hypertension, including THP and preeclampsia, represent states of increased vasoconstriction.[12] Calcium is acknowledged to be the primary cellular mediator of the vascular contractile process. There exists substantial research on the specific systems that transport calcium across the cell membrane and their interface with the body's broader calcium homeostasis. In pregnancy, the increased demand for calcium as a result of fetal bone mineralization leads to dramatic adaptations in calcium homeostasis. This increased demand in turn puts women at risk, either for inadequate dietary intake, especially in some cultures, or for consequences of an incomplete adaptation. Studies of areas with endemically low dietary calcium demonstrate markedly higher incidences of THP and preeclampsia.[50] Population studies suggest a close reciprocal relationship between dietary calcium and hypertensive complications of pregnancy.[50] Pregnant animals maintained on a low-calcium diet develop hypertension and proteinuria.[51]

When calcium and calcium-regulatory hormones have been studied in normotensive pregnant women, women with preeclampsia, and women with THP, significant abnormalities in the women with preeclampsia have been seen. These include lower levels of ionized[52] and urinary calcium,[52, 53] an elevated serum parathyroid hormone concentration,[52] and reduced 1,25-dihydroxyvitamin D levels.[52] These results are most easily explained by a reduction in the 1,25-dihydroxyvitamin D, which leads to decreased calcium absorption, which in turn results in lower ionized calcium levels. In response, parathyroid hormone (PTH) increases, reducing calcium loss in the urine. These abnormalities are not present in pregnant women with THP[54] or chronic hypertension.[53]

As a consequence of these findings, calcium supplementation has been considered for prophylactic use during pregnancy. In patients with essential hypertension, a week or more is required for calcium supplementation to produce any reduction in blood pressure, and the changes are very modest; hence dietary calcium is not useful for acute blood pressure management. There have been numerous small trials of calcium supplementation as prophylaxis for THP and preeclampsia. A current meta-analysis,[55] limited to randomized, controlled trials, found that among 1728 healthy pregnant women enrolled in six studies, there was a significant reduction in the incidence of both THP (56%) and preeclampsia (66%). Preterm delivery was also significantly lowered by 34%. The amount of calcium administered was typically 2000 mg/day, even though normal pregnant women excrete 200–500 mg of calcium in urine before supplementation.[55] It is not clear why the women with THP, who have no observable abnormalities related to calcium or calciotropic hormones, should benefit as much or more than women with preeclampsia. Perhaps the benefit in this latter group would be amplified if 1,25-dihydroxyvitamin D, which is abnormally low, were augmented as well. Large trials of calcium supplementation are currently nearing completion, and thus final recommendations regarding the use, dose, and form of calcium remain open issues.

Future Approaches

Data implying that vascular endothelial dysfunction accompanies preeclampsia have generated a great deal of interest. Evidence at present suggests strongly that the endothelium mediates some portion of the maintenance and potentially the pathologic elevation of blood pressure in essential hypertension.[6] Pharmacologic modification of endothelial function in animals to produce or correct hypertension[56] suggests that this is an area that will be pursued, especially as more specific agents become available.

Another approach to prevention might be prenatal counseling. One of the unanticipated findings of the large aspirin trials[31] as well as of other studies[57] was that increased prepregnancy weight conferred a significantly higher risk of preeclampsia. Therefore, education resulting in the implementation of weight control among women anticipating pregnancy might produce reductions in preeclampsia.

Finally, there is substantial evidence for a strong genetic component in preeclampsia.[58] Findings from preliminary genetic association studies have suggested a possible abnormality in the coding for angiotensinogen.[59] If genetic markers that tracked with a single diagnosis were developed, research into the specific underlying abnormality would be greatly facilitated. Ultimately, if the gene or genes that cause a specific hypertensive disease during pregnancy were identified, specific therapy might be employed. Research clearly must continue until the actual mechanisms for specific hypertensive diseases during pregnancy are identified.

NONACUTE MANAGEMENT OF HYPERTENSION DURING PREGNANCY

Women with hypertension during pregnancy require increased monitoring for symptoms and signs suggestive of the development or worsening of preeclampsia. Areas that deserve particular attention on physical examination are summarized in Table 41–2. Laboratory evaluation of the end-organ systems that may be involved in preeclampsia allows for potential early detection of complications that may necessitate intervention. Laboratory tests useful in observing a hypertensive pregnant women are summarized in Table 41–3. These tests provide a basis both for a diagnosis of preeclampsia and for the assessment of deterioration in a women with established pre-

TABLE 41–2. PHYSICAL EXAMINATION OF THE HYPERTENSIVE PREGNANT PATIENT

Organ or System	Finding/Comment
Eyes	Segmental arteriolar narrowing suggests vasospasm
	Papilledema suggests cerebral edema
Heart	Hyperdynamic
Lungs	Rule out congestive heart failure
Neuromuscular	Look for clonus
Epigastric/right upper quadrant	Liver congestion
Uterus	Rule out evolving placental abruption
Extremities	Nondependent edema
Cervix	Cervical examination aids in delivery planning

eclampsia. In general, women with THP or preeclampsia may be managed until term and the spontaneous onset of labor or until the cervix becomes favorable for induction of labor. Any evidence of worsening preeclampsia or any suggestion of maternal or fetal compromise, as assessed by ultrasonography and biophysical profile, should prompt intervention with hospitalization and consideration of delivery regardless of gestational age (Table 41–4). Delivery is the definitive curative treatment of preeclampsia. However, when pregnancy can be prolonged to allow for greater fetal maturity, three main options are currently used: bed rest, dietary sodium manipulation, and antihypertensive medications.

Bed Rest

Bed rest in the hospital is the most universally used therapy for hypertension during pregnancy and is considered an established therapy for preeclampsia by the NIH National High Blood Pressure Education Working Group.[1] It is thought that bed rest increases uteroplacental blood flow and promotes diuresis. Despite the widespread use of bed rest, few studies have addressed its actual benefit. Existing studies have often focused on different types of hypertension in pregnancy, and so it is difficult to compare them. The published controlled randomized studies that exist are therefore discussed.

TABLE 41–3. EVALUATION OF THE PREGNANT HYPERTENSIVE PATIENT: LABORATORY TESTS

Complete Blood Count (With Platelets)

Chemistry Panel
Electrolytes
Blood urea nitrogen (BUN)
Creatinine
Uric acid
Transaminases
Total protein, albumin
Calcium, magnesium

24-h Urine
Protein
Creatinine
Calcium

Electrocardiogram

PT/PTT, Fibrinogen

Abbreviations: PT, prothrombin time; PTT, partial thromboplastin time.

TABLE 41–4. MATERNAL AND FETAL GUIDELINES FOR EXPEDITED DELIVERY IN SEVERE PREECLAMPSIA

Maternal Clinical Findings
One or more of the following:
- Uncontrolled severe hypertension*
- Eclampsia
- Platelet count < 100,000/μL
- AST or ALT > 2 times upper limit of normal with epigastric pain or RUQ tenderness
- Pulmonary edema
- Compromised renal function†
- Persistent severe headache or visual changes

Fetal Clinical Findings
One or more of the following:
- Fetal distress by FHR tracing or BPP
- Amniotic fluid index ≤2
- Ultrasound-estimated fetal weight ≤ fifth percentile
- Reverse umbilical artery diastolic flow

Abbreviations: AST, aspartate aminotransferase; ALT, alanine aminotransferase; RUQ, right upper quadrant; FHR, fetal heart rate; BPP, biophysical profile.

*Blood pressure persistently ≥160 mm Hg systolic or ≥110 mm Hg diastolic despite maximal recommended doses of two antihypertensive medications.

†Persistent oliguria (<0.5 mL/kg/h) or rise in serum creatinine of 1 mg/dL over baseline.

Adapted from Schiff E, Friedman SA, Sibai B: Conservative management of severe preeclampsia remote from term. Obstet Gynecol 1994; 84:626–630.

Mathews performed a controlled randomized study of 135 women with pregnancy-induced hypertension to see whether bed rest decreased the incidence of the later development of preeclampsia.[60] There was no difference between the experimental and control groups in the numbers of women who developed preeclampsia or in birth weight. Because the majority of the women were more than 35 weeks pregnant when treatment was initiated, one criticism of the study is that the pregnancies may have been too far advanced for bed rest to be beneficial. In another study, Mathews and associates examined whether bed rest could be beneficial in 40 women with established preeclampsia.[61] All women in this study had diastolic blood pressures between 90 and 110 mm Hg and urine albumin levels greater than trace amounts on dipstick testing. Gestational age at entry was not specified. All subjects received 500 mg of clomethiazole daily. Women admitted to the hospital were randomized to bed rest vs. free ambulation. There was no statistical difference between the two groups in human placental lactogen or estriol levels (measured to reflect placental well-being). Five pregnancies in each group were accompanied by hyperuricemia and intrauterine growth retardation. Other studies on the effect of bed rest on the development or improvement of preeclampsia have not been controlled.

In a randomized study of women with an elevation of blood pressure during pregnancy (≥140/90 mm Hg and no proteinuria), Crowther and colleagues examined the effect of bed rest on pregnancy outcome.[62] One hundred ten women were admitted to a clinic and rested as much as possible, whereas 108 were sent home to maintain normal activity and perform self-monitoring with a daily urine dipstick. Women were admitted to the hospital for blood pressures of 160/110 mm Hg and higher. Both groups included similar numbers of primigravidae, multigravidae, and multigravidae with histories of chronic hypertension. Significantly fewer women in the bed rest group developed "severe hypertension" (defined by the authors as ≥160/110 mm Hg) and proteinuria (levels ≥ 3+) than in the normal activity group. However, despite the differences, there was no benefit of bed rest with regard to mean blood pressure, the overall incidence of proteinuria, length of gestation, the number of women who required labor induction, mode of labor, mean birth weight, number of infants of low birth weight or who were small for gestational age, or neonatal morbidity. Crowther and colleagues concluded that although bed rest can decrease the incidence of severe hypertension, it does not have any impact on the underlying disease process of preeclampsia. Much of the benefit attributed to bed rest may come from the close monitoring that these women get once they are admitted to the hospital.

Despite the increasing financial impetus to minimize the number of days of hospitalization, it remains to be determined whether hypertension during pregnancy can be managed as effectively in an outpatient setting. A study of 54 women with THP compared day unit management (to allow for close outpatient follow-up) with management by their own obstetricians (controls). The group receiving day unit care required fewer and shorter inpatient admissions than did the controls. There was no improvement in pregnancy outcome in the group who spent more time hospitalized, which suggests that intensive outpatient management may be equivalent to inpatient management.[63] A more recent study of 592 women, comparing inpatient with outpatient management of mild THP, revealed similar maternal and fetal outcomes. There was a decrease in the number of days of maternal hospitalization with outpatient management.[64]

Further studies are necessary in order to determine the role of and approach to outpatient management of hypertension during pregnancy, even preeclampsia. Until then, continued inpatient management is recommended by some authors.[65]

Dietary Sodium Intake

It remains unclear how to counsel women with pregnancy-induced hypertension as to dietary sodium intake. There is debate as to whether such women should increase or decrease sodium intake. Gallery and coworkers found volume expansion beneficial in pregnancy-induced hypertension.[66] In that study, women received 500 mL of a volume expander and demonstrated decreases in both systolic and diastolic blood pressure. This response was seen in all groups of women studied (Figure 41–1). A meta-analysis of nine randomized diuretic trials showed that although there was a decrease in the incidence of preeclampsia, there was no benefit with regard to perinatal mortality.[67] Preeclampsia was not defined by the same criteria across these studies, and it is not clear that women with essential hypertension were excluded.

Again, as with bed rest, there are few controlled studies of dietary sodium intake available. In 1958, Robinson reported the results of a study of 2019 women who were counseled to follow either a high- or a low-salt diet during pregnancy.[14] Of interest is that only 4% (38/1019) of the women counseled to follow a high-salt diet developed toxemia, whereas 10% (97/1000) of those counseled to follow a low-salt diet developed toxemia. This difference was also found in examination of only the primiparous women (1% of high-salt consumers vs. 6% of low-salt consumers). In addition, perinatal complications were reported to be lower among the women who had been counseled to follow the high-salt diet.[14] Critics of this study have pointed out that the amount of sodium consumed was not specified and that compliance could not be assessed.

Bower compared the effects of three levels of dietary sodium intake on hospitalized women with preeclampsia: 2 g/day (N = 341), 10 g/day (N = 201), and 25 g/day (N = 197) for up to 10 days.[68] Blood pressures from the first half of the study were averaged, and the mean of these pressures was compared with the mean of blood pressures from the second half of the study, and each mean was divided by the number of days on a given diet (termed *mean BP* [blood pressure] *index*). Bower concluded that a low-salt diet was not beneficial, because the mean BP index of the low-salt group was not lower than those of the two high-salt groups. Although no absolute blood pressures were reported, women on the 10-g/day

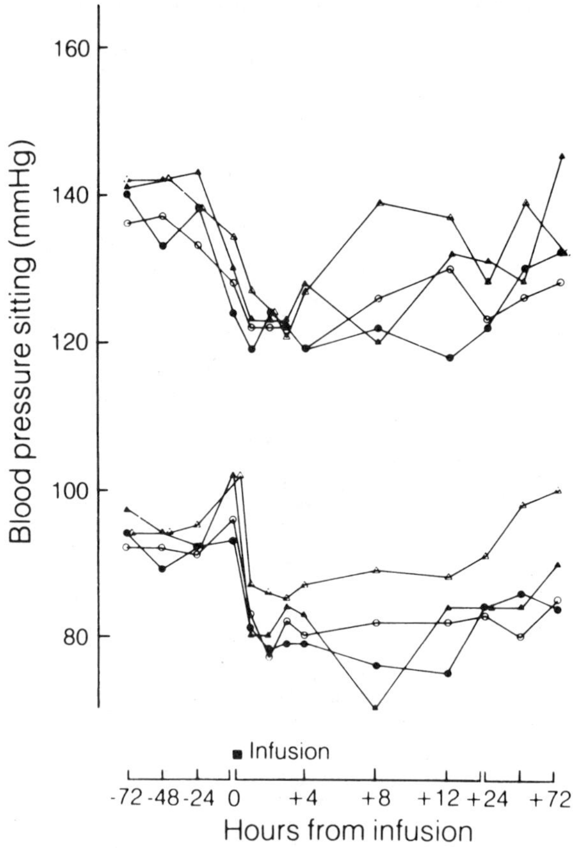

Figure 41–1. Systolic and diastolic blood pressure response to volume expansion in pregnancy-induced hypertension (PIH). *Closed circles*, PIH alone; *open circles*, PIH with edema; *closed triangles*, PIH with proteinuria; *open triangles*, PIH with edema and proteinuria. (From Gallery EDH, Mitchell MDM, Redman CWG: Fall in blood pressure in response to volume expansion in pregnancy-associated hypertension. J Hypertens 1984; 2:177–182.)

sodium diet had a significantly lower mean systolic blood pressure index than did those on the 2-g/day sodium diet.

In the United States, there is no consensus on the appropriate amount of dietary sodium for pregnant women with hypertension. In view of the available data, the authors recommend that pregnant women not be sodium restricted and that women with hypertension induced or exacerbated by pregnancy have a liberal salt intake.

Antihypertensive Medications

Although many of the drugs used to treat hypertension in pregnancy are similar to those used to treat nonpregnant patients, at least two considerations in management differ for pregnant women: different goals of treatment and consideration of the effects of antihypertensive agents on the fetus.

Goals of Treatment

The usual goal of lowering blood pressure in a nonpregnant patient is an attempt to decrease the long-term risks of cardiovascular, cerebrovascular, and renal disease. In this regard, blood pressures over 140/90 mm Hg are usually treated. However, during pregnancy the concern is not the long-term effect of elevated blood pressure but the regulation of blood pressure to a level that reduces the risk for acute complications in the mother and fetus while maintaining adequate perfusion to the fetus. The most dire maternal complication related to hypertension is a cerebrovascular accident. Hypertensive complications to the fetus include placental abruption (separation of the placenta from the uterus, which results in loss of perfusion to the fetus) and intrauterine growth retardation (IUGR). However, a decrease in placental and fetal perfusion caused by lowering of the maternal systemic pressure by antihypertensive medications can further compromise the fetus, leading to greater IUGR. Therefore, drug therapy is instituted at different and usually higher levels of blood pressure during pregnancy.

Overall, women with mild to moderate hypertension (diastolic blood pressure of 90–110 mm Hg) do well during pregnancy without the institution of antihypertensive treatment. If a woman is already receiving treatment, it may be possible to taper the medication. As discussed later, it is important to consider the potential effect of the medication on the fetus. For a woman whose medication cannot be stopped, it may be important to change the medication to one that has been used frequently during pregnancy and whose potential side effects on the fetus are well known. It is when women with chronic hypertension develop superimposed preeclampsia that morbidity and mortality occur.[69] However, antihypertensive agents have not been shown to reduce the risk of the development of preeclampsia in women with chronic hypertension; nor will they decrease most of the sequelae of preeclampsia once it has developed, regardless of whether a woman has preceding hypertension. Therefore, many physicians will not treat women with blood pressures in the aforementioned range. However, a benefit to the mother in terms of decreased morbidity from cerebrovascular accident has been demonstrated for diastolic blood pressures of 110 mm Hg or higher.[70]

Medications Used During Pregnancy

A variety of medications have been used to treat hypertension during pregnancy. Some of the most commonly used drugs are depicted in Table 41–5. These drugs and others used during pregnancy are discussed in further detail as follows.

Methyldopa. The first-line agent of therapy is usually methyldopa (Aldomet). This agent has lost popularity in the treatment of nonpregnant patients because of its side effects (sedation, dizziness, and depression) and the development of more potent antihypertensives; however, it remains the agent most commonly used during pregnancy because experience during pregnancy has been greatest with this drug. Existing data show no long-term developmental or intellectual impairment in the offspring (observed up to 7.5 years of age) of mothers who took methyldopa during pregnancy.[71]

Diuretics. Although women with preeclampsia appear to suffer volume overload manifesting peripheral edema, invasive measurement of intravascular volume indicates that they are suffering intravascular volume depletion.[12] As discussed earlier, volume expansion may be helpful in treatment of pregnancy-induced hypertension; therefore, the use of diuretics in pregnancy has been questioned. Indeed, diuretics have been shown to inhibit the normal volume expansion that occurs during pregnancy;[72] in addition, they lower placental perfusion.[73] Furthermore, no prophylactic benefit of hydrochlorothiazide in reducing the incidences of preeclampsia, prematurity, or perinatal mortality was seen in a double-blind study of 1030 pregnant women.[74] Therefore, diuretics are not widely used in the nonacute management of hypertension during pregnancy and have no established role in the prevention of preeclampsia. Although there have been no well-controlled studies on diuretic use during pregnancy, the National High Blood Pressure Education Working Group concluded that diuretics could be used if they were started before pregnancy or before midpregnancy.[1] However, they should not be used in situations in which there is pre-existing decreased placental perfusion, such as preeclampsia or IUGR.

Beta Blockers. These drugs are commonly used in the nonpregnant population. Early reports on the use of propranolol during pregnancy showed an association with fetal and neonatal bradycardia and neonatal hypoglycemia, as well as IUGR. Further studies have not confirmed any of these side effects except IUGR, which is commonly but inconsistently reported with the various beta blockers. Atenolol (100–200 mg/day), when compared with placebo in 85 pregnant women (mean gestational length, 34 weeks) with mild to moderate hypertension (systolic blood pressure $>$ 140 and $<$ 170 mm Hg, or diastolic blood pressure $>$ 90 and $<$ 110 mm Hg) in pregnancy (THP N = 69, preeclampsia N = 16), produced no difference in birth weight. Furthermore, the atenolol-treated group had lower blood pressures, a lower incidence of proteinuria, and a decreased number of hospital admissions.[75] Labetalol, when compared with placebo, has been shown to lower systolic and diastolic blood pressure but not to produce a benefit with regard to inpatient days, gestational age at delivery, or need for early delivery.[76] Atenolol, when compared with labetalol, has been linked to lower birth weight.[77]

Calcium Channel Blockers. Nifedipine is increasingly used during pregnancy to inhibit uterine contractions. Its use during pregnancy to treat hypertension has increased as well. In a study of 200 women (gestational length, 26–36 weeks) with severe preeclampsia randomized to bed rest alone (N = 100) or bed rest and nifedipine (N = 100), blood pressures were significantly lowered only in the group that received nifedipine in doses ranging from 40 to 120 mg/day.[78] Despite the beneficial maternal blood pressure decrease, there was no improvement in perinatal outcome in comparison with bed rest alone. Nifedipine has also been compared with hydralazine in the treatment of preeclampsia and is easier to titrate.[79] Other agents of the dihydropyridine class have been studied as well. In a small study of 9 women with chronic hypertension or THP, isradipine was started between 26 and 33 weeks of gestation and continued until delivery.[80] Maternal blood pressure was lowered with maintenance of uteroplacental perfusion, as measured by pulsed Doppler ultraso-

TABLE 41–5. MEDICATIONS USED IN THE TREATMENT OF THE PREGNANT HYPERTENSIVE PATIENT

Drug	Usual Dose	Disadvantages
First-Line Agent		
Methyldopa	250 mg t.i.d. to 500 mg q.i.d.	Depression, sedation; rare: drug-induced hepatitis, positive result of Coombs test
Second-Line Agents		
Beta blockers: labetalol	100 mg b.i.d. to 300 mg q.i.d.	Possible: decreased fetal growth, fetal bradycardia (avoid in asthmatics)
Calcium channel blockers: nifedipine	10–30 mg q.i.d.	Headache, flushing
Hydralazine	50 mg q.d. to 10 mg t.i.d.	Postural hypotension; rare: lupus-like syndrome

nography. Another dihydropyridine, nicardipine, has also been shown to lower maternal pressure with maintenance of placental perfusion.[81]

Hydralazine. Hydralazine is a direct vasodilator that is much more effective intravenously (see the following section on acute management) than orally because of its low bioavailability. In addition, when given orally in a continuous manner, its vasodilatory action leads to compensatory tachycardia and fluid retention, which decrease its effectiveness.

Converting Enzyme Inhibitors. Drugs of this class have become extremely popular antihypertensives for treating essential hypertension because of their efficacy and few side effects. They are considered the drugs of choice in treating hypertensive diabetic patients with nephropathy. Therefore, many women of childbearing age now receive these drugs for hypertension control. However, converting enzyme inhibitors are contraindicated in pregnancy because they have been linked to neonatal hypotension, renal failure, and neonatal death (only in the mothers who had developed renal failure).[82] Women being treated for hypertension should be asked about future pregnancy plans, and if a pregnancy is planned, an alternative antihypertensive should be substituted.

ACUTE MANAGEMENT OF THE HYPERTENSIVE CRISIS COMPLICATING PREGNANCY

Hypertensive crisis (blood pressure > 200/115 mm Hg) is not an uncommon event in a high-risk delivery unit. As stated earlier, preeclamptic patients have enhanced vascular reactivity and are at particular risk for labile hypertension. In turn, the preeclamptic patient with uncontrolled blood pressure is at great risk for cerebral vascular accident and placental abruption.

A number of pharmacologic agents are available for the management of patients in hypertensive crisis (Table 41–6). Because of long experience with hydralazine demonstrating efficacy and safety, it generally remains the drug of first choice for the acute management of blood pressure emergencies in the antepartum or intrapartum patient. Intravenous hydralazine is given initially as a 5-mg bolus, followed by an additional 5-mg bolus after 10 min. If significant hypotension has not occurred, 10-mg intravenous boluses may be administered at 20-min intervals until blood pressure control is achieved. The goal of therapy is maintenance of blood pressure in the range of 140–150 mm Hg systolic and 90–100 mm Hg diastolic to avoid uterine hypoperfusion.

Another approach is continuous infusion of sodium nitroprusside or hydralazine. Either of these agents may be started at a rate of 0.5 μg/kg/min and increased by 0.5 μg/kg/min every 5–10 min until blood pressure control is achieved. The more gradual lowering of blood pressure may also maintain uteroplacental perfusion. Intravenous hydralazine has a longer half-life than does nitroprusside and is therefore less easily titrated. There are, however, hypothetical concerns associated with the use of sodium nitroprusside; it may be selectively concentrated in the fetal compartment as cyanide and thiocyanate, theoretically poisoning the electron transport chain and resulting in subsequent fetal asphyxia. Despite these theoretical risks, sodium nitroprusside has been used successfully in antepartum, intrapartum, and postpartum patients and has been particularly useful in controlling arterial pressure before and during Cesarean section. An alternative approach is to use nitroglycerin, although this agent is used primarily in the intraoperative setting to control acute hypertension (see Chapter 33 for additional details).

Intravenous labetalol may also be used for the antepartum management of acute hypertension, although there is less experience with the parenteral administration of labetalol in this setting. Although any of these agents may be used in the postpartum patient who undergoes a hypertensive crisis, all should be used with great caution in the antepartum patient because of the risk of uncontrolled hypotension and consequent fetal distress. The importance of prompt recognition and management of the hypertensive crisis in the pregnant patient cannot be overemphasized. The most common direct cause of death in hypertensive pregnant patients is cerebral vascular accident; hence hypertension remains one of the leading causes of maternal mortality.

TABLE 41–6. PHARMACOLOGIC MANAGEMENT OF HYPERTENSIVE CRISIS (PERSISTENT BLOOD PRESSURE >200/115)

Drug	Administration
Hydralazine	5 mg IV; repeat in 10 min; then 10 mg IV every 20 min until stable blood pressure (140–140/90–110 mm Hg) achieved
Labetalol	5- to 15-mg IV push; repeat every 10–20 min by doubling dose to a maximum of 300 mg total
Sodium nitroprusside*†	Controlled infusion, 0.5–3 μg/kg/min, not to exceed 800 μg/min (best used for refractory hypertension)
Nifedipine	10 mg sublingual; repeat in 30 min; then 10–20 mg PO every 4–6 h
Nitroglycerin*	Should be used only by practitioners thoroughly familiar with its use in obstetrics

Abbreviations: IV, intravenous; PO, per os (oral).
*Requires arterial line for continuous blood pressure monitoring.
†Avoid use in antepartum patients. Profound hypotension may result.

Eclampsia

Eclampsia is defined as the occurrence of a grand mal tonic clonic seizure in a woman exhibiting symptoms of preeclampsia without underlying neurologic disease. Eclampsia is relatively rare, occurring in approximately 1 of every 1000 deliveries. The maternal and fetal consequences of eclampsia have been recognized and feared since antiquity. Some serious sequelae of an eclamptic seizure include maternal apnea, which results in fetal asphyxia; maternal cerebral edema, which can lead to coma; maternal intracerebral hemorrhage; aspiration of gastric contents; placental abruption; and maternal and fetal death. Until the introduction of magnesium sulfate therapy in the 1930s, nearly 30% of women with eclampsia died.

Prevention of Eclampsia

Once preeclampsia has progressed to the point that delivery is deemed necessary, an immediate priority becomes prevention of progression of preeclampsia to eclampsia. Magnesium sulfate remains the drug most commonly used for this in the United States. Because eclampsia is potentially life-threatening, and because seizures can occur either intrapartum or within the first 24 h postpartum, magnesium sulfate therapy is usually employed during this entire period.

Although there is continuing controversy over whether all patients with mild preeclampsia require magnesium sulfate or even whether magnesium sulfate should be used at all, it is currently the drug most predominantly employed. Magnesium competes with calcium for specific ion channels and may reduce cellular excitability. Clinically, magnesium also exerts a peripheral effect at the neuromuscular junction. For seizure prophylaxis, magnesium sulfate is generally administered as an intravenous regimen, although an intramuscular regimen may be used if intravenous access cannot be obtained (Table 41–7).

Magnesium sulfate has a relatively wide margin of safety; how-

TABLE 41–7. MAGNESIUM SULFATE ADMINISTRATION FOR SEIZURE PROPHYLAXIS

Intramuscular

10 g (5 g deep IM in each buttock)

5 g deep IM in one buttock every 4 h, alternating sides; made up as 50% solution

Intravenous

6 g bolus over 15 min

1–3 g/h by continuous infusion pump; may be mixed in 100 mL of crystalloid; if given as intravenous push, make up as 20% solution and push at maximal rate of 1 g/min

40 g $MgSO_4 \cdot 7\ H_2O$ in 1000 mL of Ringer's lactate; infuse at 25–75 mL/h (1–3 g/h)

ever, because serious complications have been associated with its use, it has become increasingly common to monitor serum magnesium levels in patients receiving magnesium sulfate. Levels between 4 and 8 mEq/L have generally been accepted as therapeutic, although there are few data to support this choice. Levels above 6 mEq/L may be associated with lethargy and loss of the patellar reflex, and respiratory depression may occur at levels in excess of 8 mEq/L. Cardiotoxicity, though extraordinarily rare, may occur at therapeutic levels of magnesium sulfate but typically does not develop until levels exceed 15 mEq/L. Although magnesium levels may be useful in helping to establish a steady rate for magnesium infusion and as an adjunct to clinical assessment, these levels cannot serve as a substitute for the frequent clinical evaluation of the patient. Women receiving magnesium sulfate should be monitored for maintenance of the patellar reflex and a respiration rate at least 12 breaths/min, for absence of oxygen desaturation, for arrhythmia, and for widened QRS or prolonged QT interval on electrocardiogram. In addition, magnesium sulfate can interfere with uterine contractions in such a way that many patients receiving this therapy may require oxytocin for augmentation of labor. This finding, as well as other issues regarding the central nervous system, has led some authors to suggest alternative therapeutic regimens for the management of this condition.[83]

Outside the United States, a number of other agents have been employed for prevention of eclampsia, including phenytoin and diazepam.[84] A study of over 2000 hypertensive women compared magnesium sulfate with phenytoin (Dilantin) for the prevention of eclampsia. In the group randomized to receive magnesium sulfate, no women had seizures, whereas in the group that received Dilantin, 10 had seizures, which was a significant difference.[85]

Management of the Eclamptic Patient

The best management of eclampsia would be its prevention. Unfortunately, the ability to predict which preeclamptic patients will progress to eclampsia is poor. A study of 186 cases of eclampsia at the University of Tennessee revealed that seizures occurred in the postpartum period in 28% of patients, and half of these occurred more than 48 h after delivery.[86] In fact, only one third of eclamptic events occurred during labor. Almost half of all convulsions happened before admission to the delivery unit.[86]

When an eclamptic seizure occurs, the initial management is extremely important. Prevention of maternal injury and protection of the maternal airway are the most crucial first steps. Nearly all eclamptic seizures are self-limited and resolve without sequelae. Seizures may recur, however, resulting in maternal cardiovascular collapse, intercerebral hemorrhage, fetal asphyxia, or placental abruption. As with most grand mal seizures, the seizure event is characterized by maternal apnea and transient hypoxia. It is important to also recognize that an eclamptic seizure has consequences for the fetus. When an eclamptic seizure occurs, fetal bradycardia is nearly invariable. Maintenance of the maternal airway and administration of oxygen postictally will result in eventual in utero resuscitation of the fetus with resolution of fetal bradycardia.

For patients brought to the hospital after an eclamptic seizure and for hospitalized patients who suffer a seizure without having received magnesium sulfate, the first step in the management should be initiation of magnesium sulfate therapy (see Table 41–7). Patients suffering eclamptic seizures while being treated with magnesium sulfate or who have an otherwise atypical presentation should be considered for additional or alternative anticonvulsant therapy. This latter recommendation is based on reports that pathologic central nervous system abnormalities are more common than might otherwise be expected among patients who experience seizures while receiving magnesium sulfate.[87]

If phenytoin therapy is instituted, close monitoring of the patient is essential to prevent potentially life-threatening cardiotoxicity. This is extremely uncommon in young healthy women who receive intravenous phenytoin infusion at rates less than 50 mg/min. A regimen for phenytoin administration is presented in Table 41–8.

A study comparing the effectiveness of magnesium sulfate to Dilantin in preventing recurrent eclamptic seizures showed magnesium sulfate to be the superior agent.[88]

In general, once an eclamptic seizure has occurred, plans must be made for delivery regardless of gestational age. This requires stabilization of mother and fetus and determination of their suitability for surgery. Once the decision to deliver is made, vaginal delivery is generally preferred because it causes less physiologic stress on the mother. However, when circumstances do not favor a prolonged labor and delivery process, Cesarean section is indicated. Cesarean section requires close collaboration between the perinatal and anesthesiology teams. Coagulation factors should be checked, and the means to normalize them should be available before surgery is undertaken. In the authors' institution, epidural anesthesia is generally considered the method of choice in patients with severe preeclampsia or eclampsia because of its minimal effects on maternal and fetal physiology in comparison with either general or spinal anesthesia.[89] Epidural anesthesia requires intravenous access, means of accurate blood pressure determination, ample time for stepwise preblock maternal hydration, a normal coagulation profile, and an anesthesiology team skilled in the administration of epidural anesthesia to these types of critically ill patients. If these requirements cannot be fulfilled, general anesthesia is preferred with meticulous blood pressure control at the time of induction of anesthesia and endotracheal intubation.

HELLP Syndrome

The HELLP (hemolysis, elevated liver enzymes, low platelets) syndrome frequently complicates the clinical course of patients with

TABLE 41–8. PROTOCOL FOR INTRAVENOUS ADMINISTRATION OF PHENYTOIN

Initial Dosage Based on Weight of Patient		Further Dosing Based on Serum Phenytoin Levels	
Weight of Patient	**Dosage***	**Serum Level**	**Additional Dosage**
<50 kg	1000 mg	<10 mg/L	500 mg
50–70 kg	1250 mg	10–12 mg/L	250 mg
>70 kg	1500 mg	>12 mg/L	None

*Note: first 750 mg of phenytoin administered at 25 mg/min. Remainder of dose administered at 12.5 mg/min. Electrocardiographic tracing (lead II) obtained for 1 min of every 10 min during the first 750 mg.

Adapted from Repke JT, Friedman SA, Kaplan PW: Prophylaxis of eclamptic seizures: current controversies. Clin Obstet Gynecol 1992; 35:365–374.

severe preeclampsia. Although considered a variant of severe preeclampsia, HELLP syndrome may appear without hypertension or proteinuria. The management is essentially the same as for severe preeclampsia. Data collected in 1994 have suggested that under proper circumstances, and with close observation in a tertiary center, HELLP syndrome may be managed expectantly.[90] The objective is to stabilize the mother and fetus and to allow appropriate decisions regarding timing and route of delivery.

Postpartum Management

When the patient with severe preeclampsia or eclampsia has delivered, postpartum management consists of careful observation of blood pressure, intravascular volume, and urine output. Seizure prophylaxis should continue for at least 24 h postpartum. In general, signs of disease resolution include a brisk and profound diuresis, generally accompanied by a resolution of proteinuria and a gradual (but in some cases, rapid) reduction in blood pressure.

Transient thrombocytopenia is observed in many postpartum preeclamptic women and can generally be managed expectantly. The platelet count typically reaches a nadir on postpartum day 2 or 3 and then gradually returns to normal. Platelets should be available for immediate use in such patients. Platelet transfusion may be useful if surgery was complicated, with markedly abnormal bleeding times, or if there is venous oozing from intravenous sites. In most cases, however, platelet transfusion is not necessary, even with platelet counts as low as 20,000/μL. In severe cases of thrombocytopenia, normalization of the platelet count may take up to 7 days.[91]

SUMMARY

Despite the existence of many biochemical abnormalities associated with preeclampsia and THP, none has pointed to an incontrovertible approach to prevention of either disorder. The early promise of low-dose aspirin has not been confirmed in large clinical trials, and its benefits, if any, are limited to some but not all high-risk patients. The outcome of similar clinical studies on calcium supplementation, although currently promising, is awaited; thus management of hypertension during pregnancy continues to be important. Bed rest, although commonly employed, may not be as effective as close monitoring of blood pressure, urine protein, and other indices of worsening disease. Recommendations regarding dietary sodium intake are debated, but available data suggest that women with preeclampsia are relatively hypovolemic and may benefit from a sodium-rich diet. Antihypertensive medications do not modify the progression of preeclampsia; however, they do protect the mother from potential cerebral vascular events. Typical goals for diastolic blood pressure are 90–100 mm Hg. Newer and less widely used medications such as some calcium channel blockers and labetalol may lower maternal blood pressure without significantly compromising uteroplacental perfusion. For worsening preeclampsia, delivery is the only known cure. Antiseizure prophylaxis with magnesium sulfate during and after the peripartum period is the standard of practice in the United States and supported by the recent randomized study.[85] Blood pressure should be carefully monitored during this period, and several medications have been used safely for its acute reduction.

REFERENCES

1. National High Blood Pressure Education Working Group Report on High Blood Pressure in Pregnancy. Am J Obstet Gynecol 1990; 163:1689–1712.
2. Adams EM, MacGillivray I: Long-term effect of pre-eclampsia on blood pressure. Lancet 1961; 2:1373–1375.
3. Shoback DM, Williams GH, Moore TJ, et al: Defect in the sodium-modulated tissue responsiveness to angiotensin II in essential hypertension. J Clin Invest 1983; 72:2115–2124.
4. Graves SW: The sodium pump in hypertension. Curr Opinion Nephrol Hypertens 1994; 3:107–111.
5. Ferrannini E, Buzzigoli G, Bonnadonna R, et al: Insulin resistance in essential hypertension. N Engl J Med 1987; 317:350–357.
6. Rees DD, Palmer RMJ, Moncada S: Role of endothelium-derived nitric oxide in the regulation of blood pressure. Proc Natl Acad Sci 1989; 86:3375–3378.
7. Jeunemaitre X, Soubrier F, Kotelevtsev YV, et al: Molecular basis of human hypertension: role of angiotensinogen. Cell 1992; 71:169–180.
8. Fitzgibbon G: The relationship of eclampsia to the other toxemias of pregnancy. J Obstet Gynaecol 1922; 29:402–415.
9. Smith CA: The effect of wartime starvation in Holland upon pregnancy and its product. Am J Obstet Gynecol 1947; 53:599–608.
10. Briend A, Carles C: Protein deficiency and pregnancy toxaemia in Africa [Letter]. Lancet 1978; 1:146.
11. Seely EW, Williams GH, Graves SW: Markers of sodium and volume homeostasis in pregnancy-induced hypertension. J Clin Endocrinol Metab 1992; 74:150–156.
12. Wallenburg HCS: Hemodynamics in hypertensive pregnancy. *In* Rubin PC (ed): Handbook of Hypertension, Vol 10: Hypertension in Pregnancy, pp 66–101. Amsterdam: Elsevier, 1988.
13. Steegers EAP, Eskes TKAB, Jongsma HW, Hein PR: Dietary sodium restriction during pregnancy; a historical review. Eur J Obstet Gynecol Reprod Biol 1991; 40:83–90.
14. Robinson M: Salt in pregnancy. Lancet 1958; 1:178–181.
15. Roberts JM, Taylor RN, Goldfien A: Clinical and biochemical evidence of endothelial cell dysfunction in the pregnancy syndrome preeclampsia. Am J Hypertens 1991; 4:700–708.
16. Wang YP, Walsh SW, Guo JD, Zhang JY: The imbalance between thromboxane and prostacyclin in preeclampsia is associated with an imbalance between lipid peroxides and vitamin E in maternal blood. Am J Obstet Gynecol 1991; 165:1695–1700.
17. Uotila JT, Tuimala RJ, Aarnio TM, et al: Findings on lipid peroxidation and antioxidant function in hypertensive complications of pregnancy. Br J Obstet Gynaecol 1993; 100:270–276.
18. Mikhail MS, Anyaegbunam A, Garfinkel D, et al: Preeclampsia and antioxidant nutrients: decreased plasma levels of reduced ascorbic acid, alpha-tocopherol, and beta-carotene in women with preeclampsia. Am J Obstet Gynecol 1994; 171:150–157.
19. Stratta P, Canavese C, Porcu M, et al: Vitamin E supplementation in preeclampsia. Gynecol Obstet Invest 1994; 37:246–249.
20. Bonaa KH, Bjerve KS, Straume B, et al: Effect of eicosapentaenoic and docosahexaenoic acids on blood pressure in hypertension. A population-based intervention trial from the Tromso study. N Engl J Med 1990; 322:795–801.
21. Hui R, St. Louis J, Falardeau P: Antihypertensive properties of linoleic acid and fish oil omega-3 fatty acids independent of the prostaglandin system. Am J Hypertens 1989; 2:610–617.
22. Olsen SF, Secher NJ: A possible preventive effect of low-dose fish oil on early delivery and pre-eclampsia: indications from a 50-year-old controlled trial. Br J Nutr 1990; 64:599–609.
23. D'Almeida A, Carter JP, Anatol A, Prost C: Effects of a combination of evening primrose oil (gamma linoleic acid) and fish oil (eicosapentaenoic + docosahexaenoic acid) versus magnesium, and versus placebo in preventing pre-eclampsia. Women Health 1992; 19:117–131.
24. Howie PW, Prentice CR, Forbes CD: Failure of heparin to affect the clinical course of severe pre-eclampsia. Br J Obstet Gynaecol 1975; 82:711–717.
25. Uzan S, Beaufils M, Greart G, et al: Prevention of fetal growth retardation with low-dose aspirin: findings of the EPREDA trial. Lancet 1991; 337:1427–1431.
26. Beaufils M, Uzan S, Donsimoni R, Calau JC: Prevention of pre-eclampsia by early antiplatelet therapy. Lancet 1985; 1:840–842.
27. Wallenburg HCS, Dekker GA, Makowitz JW, Rotmans P: Low-dose aspirin prevents pregnancy-induced hypertension and preeclampsia in angiotensin-sensitive primigravidae. Lancet 1986; 1:1–3.
28. Walsh SW: Preeclampsia: an imbalance in placental prostacyclin and thromboxane production. Am J Obstet Gynecol 1985; 152:335–340.
29. Benigni A, Gregorini G, Frusca T, et al: Effect of low-dose aspirin on fetal and maternal generation of thromboxane by platelets in women at risk for pregnancy-induced hypertension. N Engl J Med 1989; 321:357–362.

30. Imperiale TF, Petrulis AS: A meta-analysis of low-dose aspirin for the prevention of pregnancy-induced hypertensive disease. J Am Med Assoc 1991; 266:261–265.
31. Sibai BM, Caritis SN, Thom E, et al: Prevention of preeclampsia with low-dose aspirin in healthy, nulliparous pregnant women. N Engl J Med 1993; 329:1213–1218.
32. Collaborative Low-Dose Aspirin Study in Pregnancy Collaborative Group: CLASP: a randomized trial of low-dose aspirin for the prevention and treatment of pre-eclampsia among 9364 pregnant women. Lancet 1994; 343:619–629.
33. Viinikka L, Hartikainen-Sorri AL, Lumme R, et al: Low dose aspirin in hypertensive pregnant women: effect on pregnancy outcome and prostacyclin-thromboxane balance in mother and newborn. Br J Obstet Gynaecol 1993; 100:809–815.
34. Wang Y, Kay HH, Killam AP: Decreased levels of polyunsaturated fatty acids in preeclampsia. Am J Obstet Gynecol 1991; 164:812–818.
35. Erskine KJ, Iversen SA, Davies R: An altered ratio of 18:2 (9,11) to 18:2 (9,12) linoleic acid in plasma phospholipids as a possible predictor of pre-eclampsia. Lancet 1985; 1:554–555.
36. Laivouri H, Hovatta O, Viikikka L, Ylikorkala O: Dietary supplementation with primrose oil or fish oil does not change urinary excretion of prostacyclin and thromboxane metabolites in pre-eclamptic women. Prostagland Leukot Essent Fatty Acids 1993; 49:691–694.
37. Bassiouni BA, Foda AI, Rafei AA: Maternal and fetal plasma zinc in pre-eclampsia. Eur J Obstet Gynecol Reprod Biol 1979; 9:75–80.
38. Lazebnik N, Kuhnert BR, Kuhnert PM: Zinc, cadmium, and hypertension in parturient women. Am J Obstet Gynecol 1989; 161:437–440.
39. Chisolm JC, Handorf CR: Zinc, cadmium, metallothionein, and progesterone: do they participate in the etiology of pregnancy induced hypertension? Med Hypotheses 1985; 17:231–242.
40. Mahomed K, James DK, Golding J, McCabe R: Zinc supplementation during pregnancy: a double blind randomized controlled trial. Br Med J 1989; 299:826–830.
41. Skajaa K, Dorup I, Sandstrom BM: Magnesium intake and status and pregnancy outcome in a Danish population. Br J Obstet Gynaecol 1991; 98:919–928.
42. Rudnicki M, Frolich A, Rasmussen WF, McNair P: The effect of magnesium on maternal blood pressure in pregnancy-induced hypertension. Acta Obstet Gynecol Scand 1991; 70:445–450.
43. Boston JL, Beauchene RE, Cruikshank DP: Erythrocyte and plasma magnesium during teenage pregnancy: relationship with blood pressure and pregnancy-induced hypertension. Obstet Gynecol 1989; 2:69–74.
44. Mastrogiannis DS, Kalter CS, O'Brien WF, et al: Effect of magnesium sulfate on plasma endothelin-1 levels in normal and preeclamptic pregnancies. Am J Obstet Gynecol 1992; 167:1554–1559.
45. Watson KN, Moldow CF, Ogburn PL, Jacob HS: Magnesium sulfate: rationale for its use in preeclampsia. Proc Natl Acad Sci 1986; 83:1075–1078.
46. Barton JR, Sibai BM, Ahokas RA, et al: Magnesium sulfate therapy in preeclampsia is associated with increased urinary cyclic guanosine monophosphate excretion. Am J Obstet Gynecol 1992; 167:931–934.
47. Conradt A, Weidinger H, Algayer H: On the role of magnesium in fetal hypotrophy, pregnancy induced hypertension and pre-eclampsia. Magnesium Bull 1984; 2:68–76.
48. Spatling L, Spatling G: Magnesium supplementation in pregnancy. A double-blind study. Br J Obstet Gynaecol 1988; 95:120–125.
49. Sibai BM, Villar MA, Bray E: Magnesium supplementation during pregnancy: a double-blind randomized controlled clinical trial. Am J Obstet Gynecol 1989; 161:115–119.
50. Belizan JM, Villar J: The relationship between calcium intake and edema, proteinuria, and hypertension-gestosis: an hypothesis. Am J Clin Nutr 1980; 33:2202–2210.
51. Prada JA, Ross R, Clark KE: Hypocalcemia and pregnancy-induced hypertension produced by maternal fasting. Hypertens 1992; 20:620–626.
52. Seely EW, Wood RJ, Brown EM, Graves SW: Lower serum ionized calcium and abnormal calciotropic hormone levels in preeclampsia. J Clin Endocrinol Metab 1992; 74:1436–1440.
53. Taufield PA, Ales KL, Resnick LM, et al: Hypocalciuria in preeclampsia. N Engl J Med 1987; 316:715–718.
54. Graves SW, Wood RJ, Brown EM, Seely EW: Calcium and calciotropic hormones in transient hypertension of pregnancy versus preeclampsia. Hypertens Pregnancy 1994; 13:87–95.
55. Carroli G, Duley L, Belizan JM, Villar J: Calcium supplementation during pregnancy: a systematic review of randomized controlled trials. Br J Obstet Gynaecol 1994; 101:753–758.
56. Baylis C, Mitruka B, Deng A: Chronic blockade of nitric oxide synthesis in the rat produces systemic hypertension and glomerular damage. J Clin Invest 1992; 90:278–281.
57. Solomon CA, Graves SW, Seely EW: Glucose intolerance as a predictor of hypertension in pregnancy. Hypertens 1994; 23:717–721.
58. Adams EM, Finlayson A: Familial aspects of pre-eclampsia and hypertension in pregnancy. Lancet 1961; 2:1375-1378.
59. Ward K, Hata A, Jeunemaitre X, et al: Molecular variant of angiotensinogen associated with preeclampsia. Nature Genetics 1993; 4:59–61.
60. Mathews DD: A randomized controlled trial of bed rest and sedation or normal activity of non-sedation in the management of non-albuminuric hypertension in late pregnancy. Br J Obstet Gynecol 1977; 84:108–114.
61. Mathews DD, Agarwal V, Shuttleworth TP: The effect of rest and ambulation on plasma urea and urate levels in pregnant women with proteinuric hypertension. Br J Obstet Gynecol 1980; 87:1095–1098.
62. Crowther CA, Bouwmeester AM, Ashurst HM: Does admission to hospital for bed rest prevent disease progression or improve fetal outcome in pregnancy complicated by non-proteinuric hypertension? Br J Obstet Gynecol 1992; 99:13–17.
63. Tuffnell DJ, Lilford RJ, Buchan PC, et al: Randomized controlled trial of day care for hypertension in pregnancy. Lancet 1992; 339:224–227.
64. Barton JR, Stanziano GJ, Sibai BM: Monitored outpatient management of mild gestational hypertension remote from term. Am J Obstet Gynecol 1994; 170:765–769.
65. Nathan L, Gilstrap LC 3rd: Management of mild pregnancy-induced hypertension remote from term. Semin Perinatol 1994; 18:79–93.
66. Gallery EDH, Mitchell MDM, Redman CWG: Fall in blood pressure in response to volume expansion in pregnancy-associated hypertension. Why does it occur? J Hypertens 1984; 2:177–182.
67. Collins R, Yusuf S, Peto R: Overview of randomized trials of diuretics in pregnancy. Lancet 1985; 290:17–23.
68. Bower D: The influence of dietary salt intake on preeclampsia. J Obstet Gynecol Brit Comm 1964; 71:123–125.
69. Sibai BM, Abdella TN, Anderson GD: Pregnancy outcome in 211 patients with mild chronic hypertension. Obstet Gynecol 1983; 61:571–576.
70. Sibai BM, Anderson GD: Pregnancy outcome of intensive therapy in severe hypertension in first trimester. Obstet Gynecol 1986; 67:5178–5222.
71. Cockburn J, Moar VA, Ounsted, Redman CWG: Final report of study on hypertension during pregnancy: the effects of specific treatment on the growth and development of the children. Lancet 1982; 1:647–649.
72. Sibai BM, Grossman RA, Grossman HG: Effects of diuretics on plasma volume in pregnancies with long-term hypertension. Am J Obstet Gynecol 1984; 150:831–835.
73. Suonio S, Saarikoski S, Tahvanainen K, et al: Acute effects of dihydralazine mesylate, furosemide, and metoprolol on maternal hemodynamics in pregnancy-induced hypertension. Am J Obstet Gynecol 1986; 155:122–125.
74. Kraus GW, Marchase JR, Yen SSC: Prophylactic use of hydrochlorothiazide in pregnancy. JAMA 1966; 198:1150.
75. Rubin PC, Butters L, Clark DM, et al: Placebo-controlled trial of atenolol in treatment of pregnancy associated hypertension. Lancet 1983; 1:431–434.
76. Pickles CJ, Broughton-Pipkin F, Symonds EM: A randomized placebo controlled trial of labetalol in the treatment of mild to moderate pregnancy induced hypertension. Br J Obstet Gynecol 1992; 99:964–968.
77. Lardoux H, Gerard J, Blazquez G, et al: Hypertension in pregnancy; evaluation of two beta blockers atenolol and labetalol. Eur Heart J 1983; 4:35–40.
78. Sibai BM, Barton JR, Akl S, et al: A randomized prospective comparison of nifedipine and bed rest versus bed rest alone in the management of preeclampsia remote from term. Am J Obstet Gynecol 1992; 167:879–884.
79. Fenakel K, Fenakel G, Appelman Z, et al: Nifedipine in the treatment of severe preeclampsia. Obstet Gynecol 1991; 77:331–337.
80. Feiks A, Grunberger W, Meisner W: Influence of isradipine on the maternal and fetal cardiovascular system in hypertensive disorders in pregnancy. Am J Hypertens 1990; 4:200S–202S.
81. Carbonne B, Jannet D, Touboul C, et al: Nicardipine treatment of hypertension during pregnancy. Obstet Gynecol 1993; 81:908–914.
82. Hanssens M, Keirse AJNC, Vankelecom F, Van Assche FA: Fetal and neonatal effects of treatment with angiotensin-converting enzyme inhibitors in pregnancy. Obstet Gynecol 1991; 78:128–143.
83. Repke JT, Friedman SA, Kaplan PW: Prophylaxis of eclamptic seizures: current controversies. Clin Obstet Gynecol 1992; 35:365–374.

84. Crowther C: Magnesium sulfate versus diazepam in the management of eclampsia: a randomized controlled trial. Br J Obstet Gynecol 1990; 97:110–117.
85. Lucas MJ, Leveno KJ, Cunningham FG: A comparison of magnesium sulfate with phenytoin for the prevention of eclampsia. N Engl J Med 1995; 333:201–205.
86. Sibai BM, Schneider JM, Morrisson JC: The late postpartum eclampsia controversy. Obstet Gynecol 1980; 55:75–78.
87. Dunn R, Lee W, Cotton DB: Evaluation by computed axial tomography of eclamptic women with seizures refractory to magnesium sulfate therapy. Am J Obstet Gynecol 1986; 155:267–268.
88. The Eclampsia Trial Collaborative Group: Which anticonvulsant for women with eclampsia? Evidence from the Collaborative Eclampsia Trial. Lancet 1995; 345:1455–1463.
89. Ramanathan J, Coleman P, Sibai BM: Anesthetic modification of hemodynamic and neuroendocrine responses to Cesarean delivery in women with severe preeclampsia. Anesth Analges 1991; 73:772–776.
90. Schiff E, Friedman SA, Sibai B: Conservative management of severe preeclampsia remote from term. Obstet Gynecol 1994; 84:626–630.
91. Martin JN, Blake PG, Lowry SL, et al: Pregnancy complicated by preeclampsia/eclampsia with the syndrome of hemolysis, elevated liver enzymes, and low platelet count: how rapid is postpartum recovery? Obstet Gynecol 1990; 76:737–742.

SECTION SEVEN

Interventional Cardiology/Cardiac Surgery

42 Percutaneous Coronary Intervention for Stable Angina

Stephen G. Ellis, MD

For any given patient or lesion, the results of balloon angioplasty and other forms of percutaneous coronary intervention (e.g., atherectomy, laser) can appear to be frustratingly unpredictable. However, a considerable body of knowledge has been acquired over the past several years that allows estimation of the likelihood of success and complications in most clinical situations. This stratification is dependent on a thorough understanding of the patient's clinical presentation and anatomy, the device approaches available, and the physician's own skill in the particular situation.

ALTERNATIVES TO PERCUTANEOUS REVASCULARIZATION: MEDICAL THERAPY AND BYPASS SURGERY

It is important to remember that angioplasty and related techniques are only a few of several approaches available to treat the patient with coronary disease. Angioplasty and related techniques have been demonstrated to decrease angina compared with medical therapy in patients with limited disease,[1] but in general, they are not as effective as bypass surgery in decreasing symptoms in patients with advanced disease.[2–4] These techniques have never been shown to decrease the risk of infarction, despite the intuitive treatment of the high-grade stenosis known as the "oculostenotic reflex", nor have they been shown to extend survival.

Randomized clinical trials should be used to guide treatment approach, particularly given the disparity between results in registries compared with carefully monitored trials[5–7] and the recent failure of some meta-analyses to predict the outcome of randomized trials.[8–10] However, such trial results are limited by narrow focus and changing techniques and technology. In cases in which trials are limited, large-scale, unbiased registries (e.g., The Duke Cardiovascular Database[11]) can provide useful information.

For the patient with limited disease, medical therapy remains an important option. Only two randomized trials, both of modest size, have addressed the relative merit of medical therapy compared with percutaneous transluminal coronary angioplasty (PTCA). In the ACME trial,[1] 212 patients with stable angina, limited disease, maintained left ventricular function, and no prior PTCA or bypass surgery were randomly assigned to PTCA or medical therapy. Although PTCA led to a reduction of angina (at 6 months after angioplasty, 64% of PTCA patients were angina-free compared with 46% of the medically treated patients; $p < .01$) and an improvement in exercise time (increased by 2.1 vs. 0.5 minutes; $p < .0001$), it also led to an increased referral for bypass surgery (7% vs. 0% at 6 months after angioplasty; $p < .01$). In a study limited to patients with single-vessel disease of the left anterior descending artery, Hueb and colleagues[12] showed a higher rate of treatment failure for PTCA compared with either medical therapy or bypass surgery. The Duke database,[11] despite following more than 3700 patients with single-vessel disease for 5 years, failed to show a survival advantage for PTCA over medical therapy. Thus, it appears that PTCA and related techniques can reasonably be recommended over medical therapy to reduce symptoms in patients with limited disease, at the possible risk of an increased need for bypass surgery.

Several ongoing randomized trials are assessing the relative utility of PTCA vs. bypass surgery for patients with more advanced disease; however, these studies usually exclude patients with very advanced and diffuse disease. A review of published data from the Randomised Intervention Treatment of Angina (RITA) trial,[3] the Coronary Angioplasty Bypass Revascularization Investigation (CABRI),[13] and the German Angioplasty Bypass Surgery Intervention (GABI)[2] study and partial data from the Emory Angioplasty versus Surgery Trial (EAST)[14] shows no difference between PTCA and coronary artery bypass graft (CABG) for in-hospital mortality (2.1% vs. 2.1%; for PTCA and CABG, respectively) or infarction (4.1% vs. 4.9%) and a possible advantage for PTCA for stroke (0.2% vs. 1.0%). At 1 year after the procedure, infarct-free survival is the about the same (92% vs. 93%), but infarct- and CABG-free survival is dramatically worse for patients randomized to PTCA (69% vs. 92%). Costs equalize by 3 years after the procedure.[15] In the Duke database,[11] PTCA shows, in general, superior survival over that for CABG for patients with single-vessel disease (odds ratio [OR] = 1.6), equivalent survival for patients with two-vessel disease (OR = 0.8–1.5) and worse survival for patients with three-vessel disease (OR = 0.4–0.7). Thus, PTCA appears to be well suited for patients with limited multivessel disease. It should be remembered, however, more so for percutaneous techniques than for surgery, that the results are highly lesion specific and that the randomized trials have used only PTCA and not the newer techniques that appear to give better results for some of the more complex lesions (vide infra).

MAJOR COMPLICATIONS OF PERCUTANEOUS TREATMENT

As a result of advances in operator experience and technique, as well as the availability of new devices and an improving understanding of how and when to use them, the results of percutaneous intervention have improved considerably compared with those reported in the 1980s.[16–18] Treatment choice should take these factors, as well as local skills and results, into consideration.

Experienced institutions using a variety of technologies report overall procedural success in 90%–95% of patients and major complications in only 3%–4% of procedures. Particularly with the availability of stents, the need for bypass surgery at some centers has now fallen to less than 1%–1.5%.[17, 18] It would be a mistake, however, to assume that all lesions can be as adequately treated at all centers. Despite the availability of new devices, results remain highly dependent on morphology,[19–21] and low-volume centers generally have a higher rate of complications.[22] In addition, when considering percutaneous therapy vs. medical or surgical options, the physician must not forget the 25%–30% chance of restenosis sufficiently severe to require further revascularization.[23, 24]

Factors Affecting Risk of Ischemic Complications

Andreas Gruentzig taught that "the first thing you always should consider (in assessing a patient's suitability for angioplasty) is what should happen if the vessel should close." To this important assessment this author would add, "what is the likelihood of the vessel closing with any of several devices available, by what mechanism or mechanisms might it be likely to close, and what is the likelihood that the closure can be corrected by stenting?"

The consideration of what will happen if the vessel should close partly determines whether or not a patient should be considered for percutaneous treatment. The likelihood of the vessel closing with each device governs device choice. Consideration of what mechanisms might produce closure guide the choice of adjunctive pharmacology; lesions at heightened risk of thrombotic closure may best be treated with higher than usual doses of heparin and activated clotting times (ACTs) or with newer antiplatelet or antithrombin drugs (e.g., c7E3 or hirudin). The likelihood that the closure can be corrected by stenting guides catheter choice; lesions with a moderate to high likelihood of dissection should be approached with guide catheters

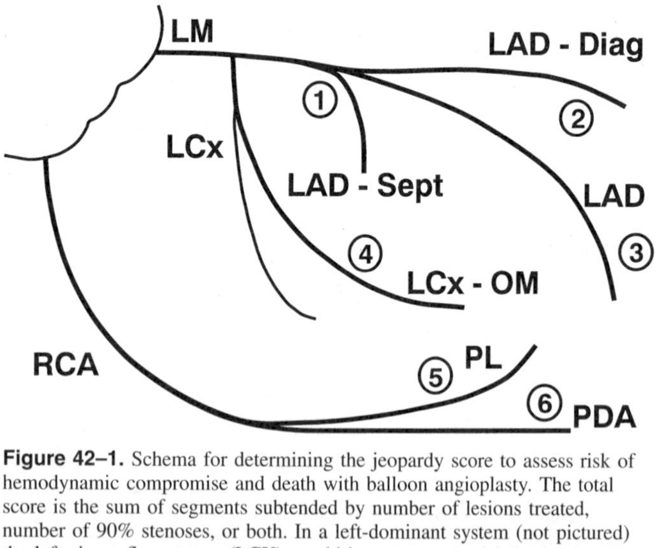

Figure 42–1. Schema for determining the jeopardy score to assess risk of hemodynamic compromise and death with balloon angioplasty. The total score is the sum of segments subtended by number of lesions treated, number of 90% stenoses, or both. In a left-dominant system (not pictured) the left circumflex system (LCX) would have two potential "points" and the right coronary artery (RCA) only one "point." *Abbreviations:* LAD, left anterior descending artery; LAD-Diag, left anterior descending diagonal artery; LAD-Sept, left anterior descending septal artery; OM, obtuse marginal; PDA, posterior descending artery; PL, posterolateral branch. (From Ellis SG, Myler RK, King SB III, et al: Causes and correlates of cardiac death after unsupported coronary angioplasty—implications for the use of advanced support techniques in high-risk settings. Am J Cardiol 1991; 68:1447–1451.)

TABLE 42–1. CORRELATION OF JEOPARDY SCORE WITH RISK OF DEATH AFTER ABRUPT CLOSURE

Jeopardy Score	Mortality
≤2	2.3%
2.5–3	10.0%
3.5–5	11.5%
5.5–6	33.3%

From Ellis SG, Myler RK, King SB III, et al: Causes and correlates of death after unsupported coronary angioplasty: implications for use of angioplasty and advanced support techniques in high-risk settings. Am J Cardiol 1991; 68:1447–1451.

large and supportive enough to allow placement of perfusion balloons, stents, or atherectomy devices.

Risk of Death or Severe Hemodynamic Compromise

At least two systems have been devised to supplement intuition to predict the likelihood of hemodynamic collapse in the event of vessel closure. In the first of these systems, Ellis and colleagues[25] studied 8052 consecutive patients (32 deaths) treated from 1984 through 1989 at three institutions. Hemodynamic collapse was strongly and independently correlated with female gender, with a jeopardy score (an estimate of the amount of left ventricular mass likely to become dysfunctional in the event of vessel closure; Fig. 42–1), and closure of a proximal right coronary artery lesion. The effect of gender and jeopardy score on death and hemodynamic compromise in this series is shown in Tables 42–1 and 42–2. Closures with jeopardy scores of 4/6 for men and 3/6 for women were highly likely to lead to cardiogenic shock. Of importance, pre-PTCA left ventricular ejection fraction was a poor predictor of outcome. In the second system, Bergelson and colleagues[26] studied 157 patients with closure treated at Boston University. Multivessel disease, diffuse disease, the percent of myocardium "at risk" and the pre-PTCA percent stenosis were independent correlates of hemodynamic collapse. These factors were amalgamated into a 13-point scoring system (Table 42–3), which was well correlated with risk (Fig. 42–2).

Of importance, both systems were devised before widespread use of intracoronary stents and the availability of percutaneous cardiopulmonary bypass as means of treatment and support after vessel closure. My colleagues and I recently analyzed the results of 283 consecutive patients with closure or threatened closure treated with stents (age = 59 ± 11 years; 69% men; 58% threatened closure) and found that the occurrence of death or Q wave infarction was independently correlated only with true closure (TIMI flow ≤ 2; OR = 6.3; $p < .001$), age (OR/decade = 1.4; $p = .02$) and jeopardy score ≥ 3 (OR = 2.3; $p = .06$; Fig. 42–3). Multivessel disease, baseline ejection fraction, vessel size, and gender were not found to be important in predicting death or Q wave infarction.

TABLE 42–2. CORRELATION OF JEOPARDY SCORE WITH BLOOD PRESSURE AFTER ABRUPT ARTERIAL CLOSURE

Jeopardy Score	Men	Women
≤2	113 ± 20	109 ± 15
2.5–3	117 ± 13	81 ± 24
3.5–4.5	96 ± 7	65 ± 4
5–6	75 ± 5	68 ± 13

Adapted from Ellis SG, Myler RK, King SB III, et al: Causes and correlates of death after unsupported coronary angioplasty: implications for use of angioplasty and advanced support techniques in high-risk settings. Am J Cardiol 1991; 68:1447–1451.

TABLE 42–3. BOSTON UNIVERSITY SCORING SYSTEM FOR ASSESSING RISK OF HEMODYNAMIC COMPROMISE WITH BALLOON ANGIOPLASTY

Angiographic Characteristic	Score
Myocardium at risk (%)	
6–14	−2
15–23	−1
24–32	0
33–41	1
42–50	2
51–59	3
60–68	4
Multivessel disease	3
Pre-PTCA stenosis (%)	
50–57	3
58–65	2
66–73	1
74–81	0
82–89	−1
90–97	−2
98–100	−3
Diffuse disease	3

Abbreviation: PTCA, percutaneous transluminal coronary angioplasty.
From Bergelson BA, Jacobs AK, Cupples A, et al: Prediction of risk for hemodynamic compromise during percutaneous transluminal coronary angioplasty. Am J Cardiol 1992; 20:1540–1545.

Risk of Vessel Closure: Balloon Angioplasty and Newer Devices

The likelihood of success and the risk of complications with current balloon angioplasty techniques and new devices are 85%–95% and 3%–8%, respectively, but these numbers must not be applied indiscriminately. Results are patient and lesion dependent.

Published results for different clinical situations are not always available. Furthermore, the source of these results must be considered. In general, results from nonaudited registries, which may be funded by device industries or collected by device enthusiasts, are typically more optimistic than those for the same device applied in randomized trials.[5–7] Often, device evaluation progresses in four stages: (1) excitement and unrealistic expectations, often from initial registry data and often with subgrouping and searching for groups that appear to do well; (2) sobering reality, sometimes during the registry phase, sometimes during the randomized trial stage; (3) better understanding of mechanisms, disturbingly, often only after the first randomized trials; and (4) refinement of technique, indications, or both. For these reasons, results from industry registries are clearly identified and presented separately from those generated by randomized trials.

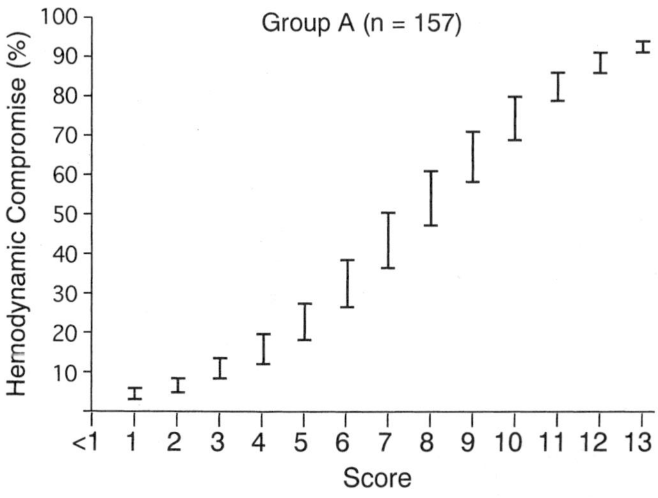

Figure 42–2. Risk of hemodynamic compromise on the basis of the Boston University risk assessment system (see Table 42–3).[26] (From Bergelson BA, Jacobs AK, Cupples A, et al: Prediction of risk for hemodynamic compromise during percutaneous transluminal coronary angioplasty. Am J Cardiol 1992; 70:1540–1545.)

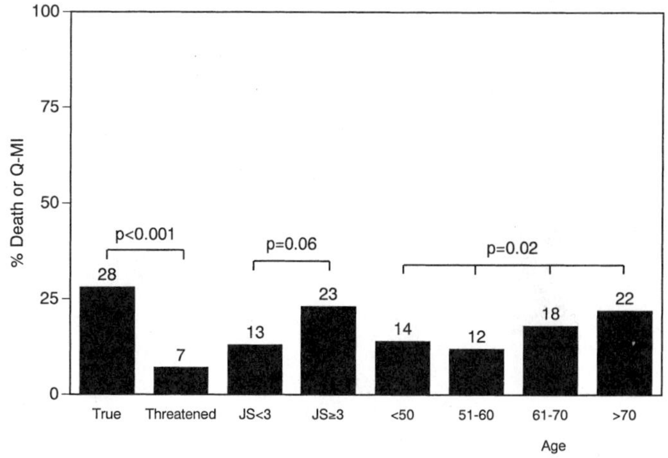

Figure 42–3. Risk of periprocedural death or Q wave infarction with true or threatened closure in the stent era. *Abbreviation:* JS, jeopardy score.

Fortunately, standard balloon angioplasty, perfusion balloon angioplasty, directional and rotational atherectomy, stents, and excimer laser therapy have all been studied in trials performed since 1991. Unfortunately, lesion-specific results are not always available; therefore, data regarding lesion-specific results for the various devices often relies on registry data. In addition, refinements in technique may produce improved results compared with those noted in early randomized trials. Data from patients with stable angina as opposed to unstable angina are even more difficult to find; therefore, in general, both are given together.

BALLOON ANGIOPLASTY VS. NEW DEVICES: RANDOMIZED TRIALS

Key results from eight major trials are highlighted in Figures 42–4 to 42–9.

Perfusion Balloon Angioplasty

Two trials have assessed the short- and long-term impact of perfusion balloon angioplasty compared with standard PTCA and their results are concordant. Ohman and colleagues[27] randomized 478 patients to either two to four 1-min (standard) inflations, or one to two 15-min inflations using a balloon allowing passive blood flow during dilatation. Patients with angulated, ostial, side branch–associated or vein graft lesions longer than 15 mm were excluded. Perfusion angioplasty was associated with improved primary success (95% vs. 89%; $p = .02$) and a lessened incidence of major dissections (3% vs. 9%; $p = .003$) but no difference in clinical complications (death, infarction, or bypass surgery) or restenosis (see Fig. 42–4). Patients with complex (B2 or C)[28] lesions appeared to benefit most.[29]

Cribier and colleagues[30] randomized 259 patients with 278 lesions to either standard (three <1-min) or prolonged (three to four 4- to 5-min) inflations. Results were virtually identical to those of the first

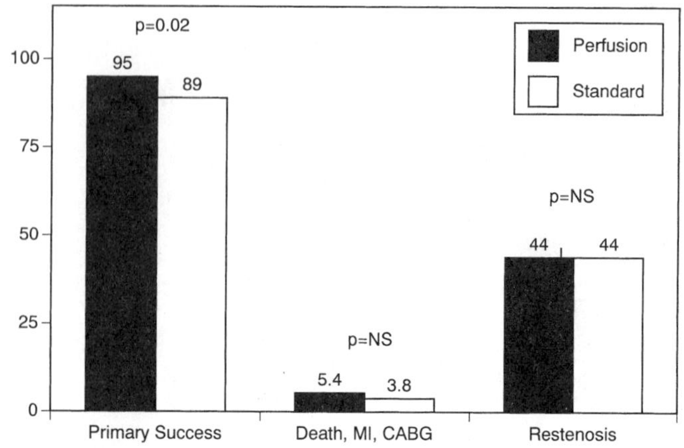

* 1 min. x 2 - 4 vs 15 min. x 1- 2
n = 478

Ohman Circ 1994

Figure 42–4. Results of a North American randomized trial of perfusion versus standard balloon angioplasty.[27] *Abbreviations:* CABG, coronary artery bypass graft; MI, myocardial infarction; NS, not significant.

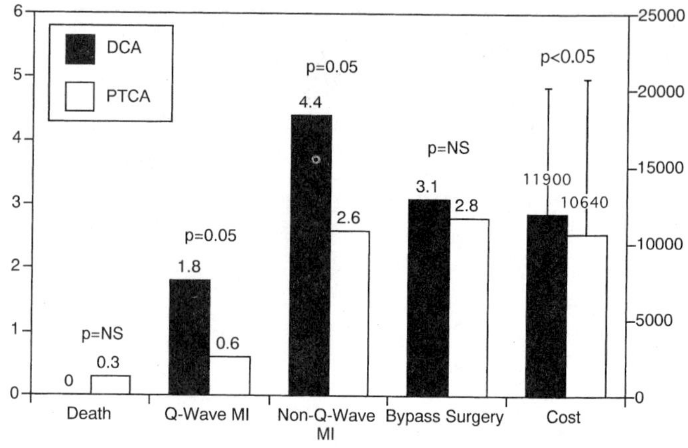

Figure 42–6. Periprocedural complications and cost of directional coronary atherectomy (DCA) and balloon angioplasty (PTCA) in de novo native coronary arteries from CAVEAT I[7] and CCAT.[31] *Abbreviations:* MI, myocardial infarction; NS, not significant.

study (see Fig. 42–5). Both studies, however, may be criticized in that they used rather short (by current standards) inflations in their "standard" arm, and the difference in results between the 2- and 4-minute inflations can be obtained with nonperfusion balloons, and results with inflations of 5–10 min or more using perfusion balloons may not be as marked. Nonetheless, long inflations (>5 min), typically requiring balloons with passive or active blood perfusion, appear to offer an improved initial result, especially for higher-risk lesions. In addition, advances in balloon technology allow perfusion balloons to be used for longer (20–40 mm), and hence probably angulated, lesions. Lesions with adjacent large side branches or major tortuosity still present often insurmountable obstacles, because the balloons are still rather bulky. Of importance, these results also cast some shadow over any results purporting to show a short-term benefit of a new nonballoon device over standard angioplasty (vide infra).

Directional Coronary Atherectomy

Although directional coronary atherectomy (DCA) was designed primarily to reduce the risk of restenosis compared with angioplasty, early studies suggested a reduction in complications with DCA. This has been called into question by the results of three more recent randomized trials.

The Coronary Angioplasty versus Excisional Atherectomy Trial (CAVEAT) I[7] and Canadian Coronary Atherectomy Trial (CCAT)[31] randomized patients with de novo native vessel lesions "suitable" for either PTCA or DCA. Although these studies were designed with a primary end point of restenosis, valuable information also was obtained for procedural success and complications. When the results of these two studies are combined (see Fig. 42–6), it can be seen that there were higher rates of both Q wave and non–Q wave infarction for patients treated with DCA (both $p < .05$) but no difference in the likelihood of death or bypass surgery; however, in-hospital cost was higher with DCA. The exact cause of the increase in infarction has not been fully elucidated. Prolonged ischemia as a result of the bulky nature of the DCA device, tissue emboli, and enhanced platelet activation as a result of the "unroofing" of thrombogenic substances have been suggested as causative factors. Fernandez-Ortiz and colleagues[32] found an atheromatous plaque "core" with cholesterol crystals to be much more thrombogenic than collagen or matrix, supporting this concept. Interestingly, use of the glycoprotein IIb/IIIa inhibitor c7E3 in the Evaluation of 7E3 for the Prevention of Ischemic Complications (EPIC) trial[33] appeared to

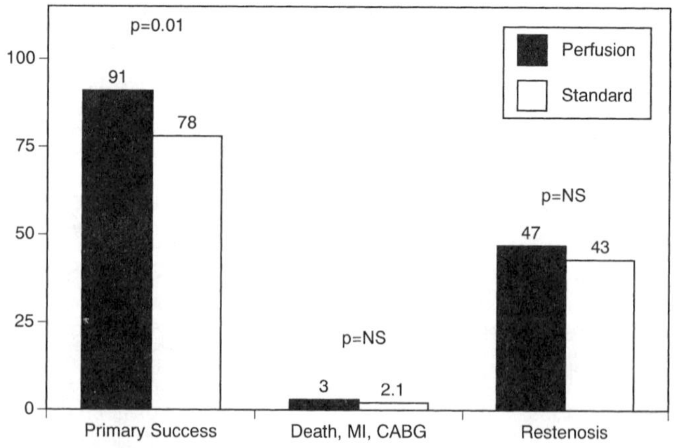

* ≤ 1 min. x 3 vs 4 - 5 min. x 3 - 4
n = 259

Figure 42–5. Results of a European-Asian randomized trial of perfusion versus standard balloon angioplasty.[30] *Abbreviations:* CABG, coronary artery bypass graft; MI, myocardial infarction; NS, not significant.

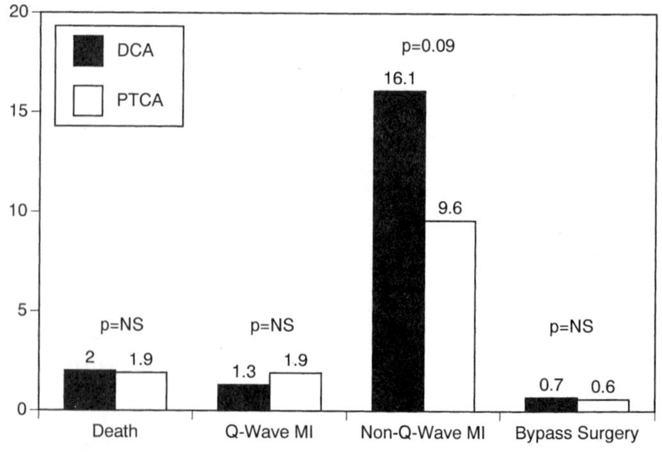

Figure 42–7. Periprocedural complications with directional coronary atherectomy (DCA) and balloon angioplasty (PTCA) in de novo saphenous graft lesions from CAVEAT II.[34] *Abbreviations:* MI, myocardial infarction; NS, not significant.

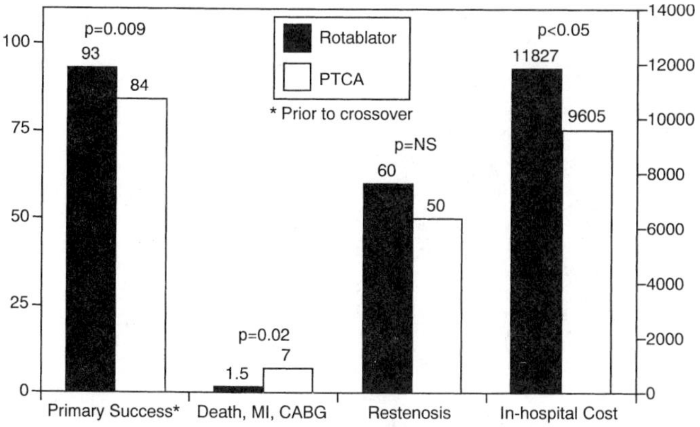

Figure 42–8. Periprocedural results and cost in the ERBAC study: Rotablator versus balloon angioplasty (PTCA).[36] *Abbreviations:* CABG, coronary artery bypass graft; MI, myocardial infarction; NS, not significant.

equalize the incidence of myocardial infarction between patients treated with DCA and those treated with PTCA, whereas in those patients receiving heparin and aspirin, a disparity between DCA and PTCA was confirmed, suggesting platelet activation as a cause.

The results of these two means of treatment in de novo saphenous vein graft lesions in CAVEAT II[34] were similar (see Fig. 42–7). The results of these trials have been criticized by "DCA advocates" who claim that DCA was not used effectively enough (i.e., the residual stenosis was too large). Although it is possible that the larger residual stenosis left in CAVEAT and CCAT compared with that which might be left with more aggressive debulking or the use of adjunct PTCA might lead to a decrease in platelet deposition as a result of increased shear forces,[35] it seems equally likely that more aggressive therapy would lead to more exposure of lipid-rich material and more platelet activation.

Rotational Atherectomy With the Rotablator

Similar to the Simpson directional device, the Rotablator has been reported to reduce complications in some groups of patients and the evolution of many technique changes may or may not alter the results it can achieve. In general, both "European" and "North American" techniques have emerged; only the former has been tested against balloon angioplasty. With the European technique, a single burr is passed, often fairly quickly, through the lesion, and the balloon is used at 5–10 atm to complete the procedure. Some practitioners, notably the Rotablator's inventor, David Auth, would argue that debulking and differential cutting are not well achieved by this technique, and that this technique is really "Rotablator-assisted balloon angioplasty." The other approach involves the use of two or three burrs of increasing size passed slowly (advancement such that rotations per minute drop no more than 4000), followed by a low-pressure (≤3 atm) balloon inflation to "touch up."

The Excimer Laser Rotational Atherectomy Balloon Angioplasty Comparison (ERBAC) trial[36] assessed the use of the single-burr approach compared with both balloon angioplasty and excimer laser in complex lesions. The results (see Fig. 42–8) show an increase in immediate success and decrease in complications with the Rotablator compared to PTCA but higher cost and late restenosis rate are associated with the Rotablator.

Primary Stenting

The Palmaz-Schatz–design slotted-tube stainless-steel stent, recently approved for use in the United States, has been formally studied as a means to decrease restenosis in de novo native vessel lesions in the Stent Restenosis Study (STRESS)[37] and Belgium-Netherlands Stent Study (BENESTENT)[24] (Table 42–4). In the STRESS trial, 407 patients with single-vessel disease (66%), well-preserved left ventricular function (61% ± 11%), unstable angina (47%), and de novo lesions in 3-mm vessels (by visual assessment) were randomly assigned to stenting or standard PTCA. Aspirin, dipyridamole (Persantine), dextran, and heparin were given as initial anticoagulants, with later institution of warfarin. Procedural success was achieved more commonly in the stent group (92% vs. 83%; $p = .006$), but there was no difference in acute ischemic complications, although 7% of PTCA patients received a "bailout" stent. Stent thrombosis occurred in 3% of patients, predominantly on days 5–6 but as late as day 15 after the procedure. Bleeding or vascular complications occurred somewhat more frequently in the stent group (10% vs. 5%; $p = .05$). The BENESTENT results were similar except for a greater excess of bleeding in the stent group (15% vs. 2%). Their results should be viewed in the context that more recently, with an emphasis on high-pressure poststent dilatation to optimize stent-wall apposition, less vigorous anticoagulation has been used without an apparent increase in stent thrombosis.[38, 39] The restenosis results are discussed later in this chapter.

Excimer Laser

Based on registry data, excimer laser has also been suggested to decrease complications compared with PTCA in complex lesions.[40] The technique of application of excimer laser therapy also has varied. Two approaches have evolved in an attempt to reduce the somewhat unpredictable occurrence of shock wave–induced coronary dissection: the "fast-pass" approach and the "saline-flush" approach. Nei-

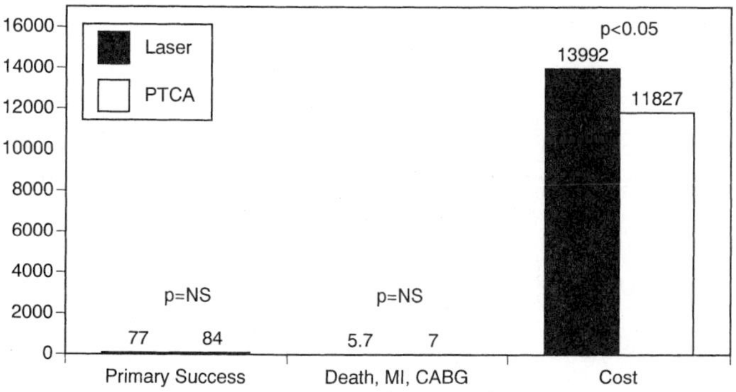

Figure 42–9. Periprocedural results and cost in the ERBAC study: Excimer laser versus balloon angioplasty.[36]

TABLE 42–4. ELECTIVE STENTING TO PREVENT RESTENOSIS

	Stress[37] (n = 407)		Benestent[24] (n = 520)	
	Stent	PTCA	Stent	PTCA
Procedural success (%)	96	90**	93	90
Final percent stenosis	35	19**	22	33**
In-hospital bleeding (%)	7	4	15	2**
Angiographic restenosis (%)	32	42*	22	32*
Event-free survival at 6 months (%)	81	76	79	67*

*$p<0.05$.
**$p<0.01$.
Abbreviation: PTCA, percutaneous transluminal coronary angioplasty.

ther of these approaches were used in the ERBAC trial, the only randomized trial of laser therapy vs. PTCA.[36] In that study (see Fig. 42–9), laser was found to be more costly than PTCA but did not yield appreciably better results. It remains to be seen whether a different technical approach will yield different results, although complications may be reduced with the saline flush technique in particular.[41] The results with laser energy using a near infrared source (holmium) have also been tested clinically in an ongoing registry[42] and appear generally similar to those reported for excimer laser energy.

LESION-SPECIFIC DEVICE APPLICATION

It has become abundantly clear that lesion morphology plays a key role in determining the response of a lesion to balloon angioplasty and to many other newer devices designed to overcome the limitations of angioplasty. The first large-scale analysis demonstrating this relation came from the 1981–1985 Emory University experience reported by Ellis and colleagues.[43] Since this study, other risk factors have been added,[17, 44] and these analyses have been extended to other devices.[19–21, 45] Comparisons of nonrandomized lesion-specific data have driven many researchers to advocate a lesion-specific approach such as that outlined in Table 42–5. It must be remembered, however, that a lesion's response to therapy is still rather capricious and that clinical and angiographic factors can only explain about 12% of the variance in the likelihood of complications with PTCA (Cleveland Clinic Interventional Database, unpublished observations, 1994; Fig. 42–10). It is likely that other forms of lesion examination such as intravascular ultrasonography will allow the outcomes of various therapies to be more predictable. Preliminary data suggests that this may indeed be true.[46]

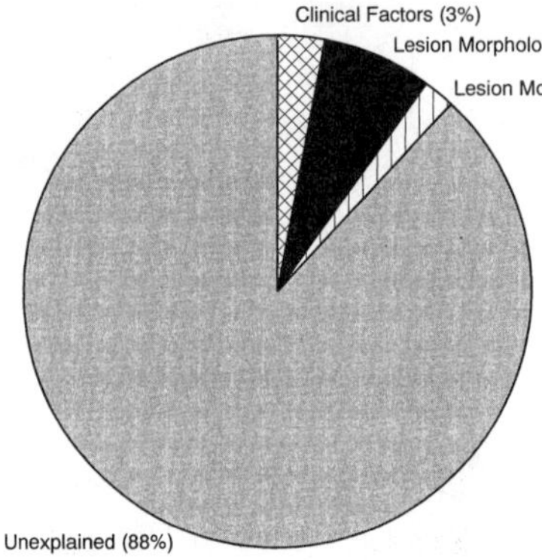

Figure 42–10. Variance in complications of balloon angioplasty, as assessed by McFadden's rho square testing, "explained" by clinical factors and lesion morphology. Although statistically powerful in large numbers of patients, these factors are limited in their predictive capacity for a given lesion to be treated. *Abbreviation:* ACC/AHA, American College of Cardiology/American Heart Association.

RESTENOSIS

Any decision regarding therapy for coronary disease must account for the progressive nature of the condition and the long-term impact of the recommended therapy. Unfortunately, angiographically determined restenosis continues to occur after 40%–50% of percutaneous interventions,[23, 47] although further revascularization is required in only 50%–60% of these cases.[23]

The literature on restenosis is extensive, and several good reviews are available.[23, 48] The likelihood of restenosis is largely dependent on the adequacy of the initial luminal result and also on the late loss of the initial arterial distension as a result of neointimal hyperplasia, recoil, and remodeling.[23, 48, 49]

Maximizing the initial gain in lumen diameter is therefore desirable, although in general, late loss increases nearly linearly with acute gain,[49] and oversizing balloon diameter relative to vessel size at a ratio of more than 1.1:1 leads to a higher incidence of complications.[50] Nonetheless, an improved initial result is undoubtedly a large part of the explanation for the beneficial results of stent placement in selected patients (see Table 42–4).[24, 37]

Lesion recoil may also be reduced by stent placement and by debulking the lesion via atherectomy or laser. Debulking alone, however, may increase late loss and in general has only been shown to very modestly decrease restenosis[7, 31] (Fig. 42–11).

Numerous attempts to decrease neointimal hyperplasia by systemic application of antiplatelet, antiproliferative, or other agents has largely proven futile[48] and has led to increased interest in local drug therapy to enhance drug concentrations and minimize side effects.[51]

TABLE 42–5. DEVICE-SPECIFIC TREATMENT FOR LESIONS SUBOPTIMALLY TREATED WITH STANDARD PTCA TO IMPROVE PRIMARY OUTCOME

	Long Balloon PTCA	Perfusion PTCA	DCA	Rotablator	Primary Stent	ELCA	TEC
Calcified	*	*	†	‡	*	*	†
Length ≥ 10 mm	§	§	†	‖	*¶	§	*
Bend ≥ 60 degrees	§	§	†	**	†	†	†
Thrombus	*	§	§	†	†	*	§
Ostial	*	*	§	§	§	§	†
Bifurcation	*	*	§	†	†	††	†
Diffuse disease	§	§	†	*	†	§	*
Degenerated SVG	*	*	†	†	*	*	§

*Results comparable to standard PTCA.
†Worse results compared to standard PTCA by registry, "consensus," or both.
‡Better results compared to standard PTCA by randomized trial.
§Better results compared to standard PTCA by registry, "consensus," or both.
‖Requires further evaluation. Early results were poor, but more recent results appear to be comparable to those achieved with long balloons.
¶Up to 15 mm.
**Requires further evaluation. Actively "flexing" stenoses and those with an abrupt bend just after the most severe portion of the stenosis appear to be at heightened risk of perforation with the Rotablator; otherwise, results may be better than with standard PTCA.
††Using directional laser. Concentric laser therapy has an increased risk of perforation with bifurcation lesions.
Abbreviations: DCA, directional coronary atherectomy; ELCA, excimer laser coronary angioplasty; PTCA, percutaneous transluminal coronary angioplasty; SVG, saphenous vein graft; TEC, transluminal extraction catheter.

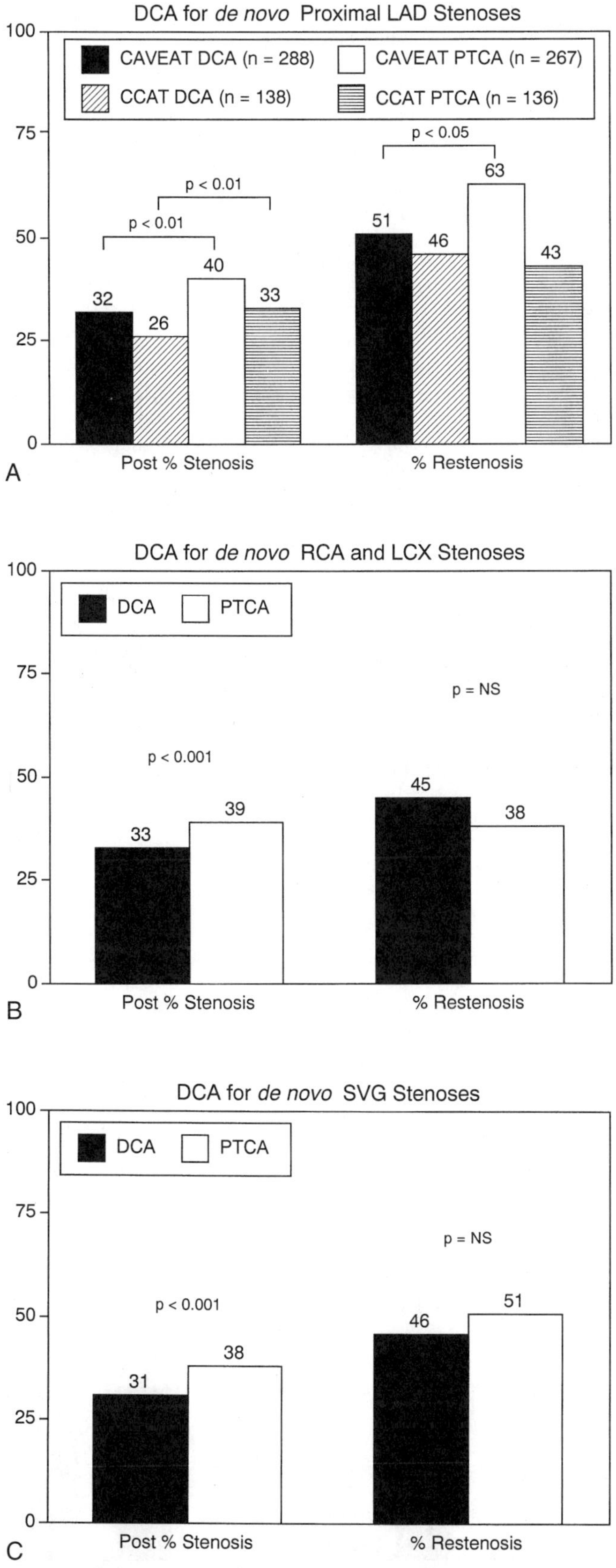

Figure 42–11. Restenosis rates for directional coronary atherectomy (DCA) and balloon angioplasty (PTCA) from the Coronary Angioplasty Versus Excisional Atherectomy Trials (CAVEAT) I[7] and II[34] and the Canadian Coronary Atherectomy Trial.[31]

An important exception, however, seems to be the use of the powerful platelet glycoprotein IIb/IIIa inhibitor, c7E3, which in the large-scale EPIC trial, decreased the need for recurrent revascularization by 26% (Fig. 42–12).[52] Whether this decrease is the result of a true reduction in restenosis is currently under study in the Evaluation in PTCA to Improve Long-term Outcome with GPIIb/IIa blockade (EPILOG) trial, as well as other trials using similar agents.

ADJUNCTIVE PHARMACOLOGY

The intimal disruption caused by balloon inflation and the tearing or ablation caused by other devices leads to rapid and exuberant platelet and fibrin deposition at the injured site.[53] Of importance, most platelet activation appears to occur in the first 2 hours after balloon inflation.[53] If unchecked, this platelet activation can lead to prompt vessel occlusion. Both antiplatelet (usually aspirin) and antithrombin (usually heparin) medications are given as standard prophylactic countermeasures, but when given in excess, they can promote unwanted bleeding.

The optimal dose of aspirin and the possible need for adjunctive dipyridamole were evaluated by Lembo and Mufson and colleagues from the Emory group, who found no difference in the incidence of complications for patients treated with 80 mg vs. 1500 mg aspirin daily or between those treated with or without dipyridamole.[54a, 54b] Ticlopidine may also be used and has been shown to be at least as effective as dipyridamole.[54] Before 1988, heparin was usually administered as a 10,000-unit bolus, followed by 5000 units every 30–60 min if the procedure was prolonged. The need for postprocedural heparinization in uncomplicated angioplasty was disproved in randomized trials,[56] although it is likely to be beneficial for patients with suboptimal results. In 1988, Dougherty and colleagues[57] and others[58] reported that 5% of patients with stable angina and 15% of patients with unstable angina had ACTs of less than 300 sec with "standard" procedural heparin regimens and appeared to be at heightened risk of thrombotic complications. Most physicians titrate heparin administration to the ACT, although the optimal ACT remains controversial. Because the risk of both thrombotic coronary closure and vascular bleeding (Table 42–6) vary from patient to patient, there is probably not one "best" ACT. It should also be noted that the ACT is also device dependent and may vary by 20–30 sec depending on the measurement device used.

According to data from the Duke Cardiovascular Database,[59] the risk of bleeding appears to be linearly related to the in-laboratory maximal ACT, ranging from about 5% with an ACT of 250 sec, to about 18% with an ACT of 500 sec, as measured using Hemochron.

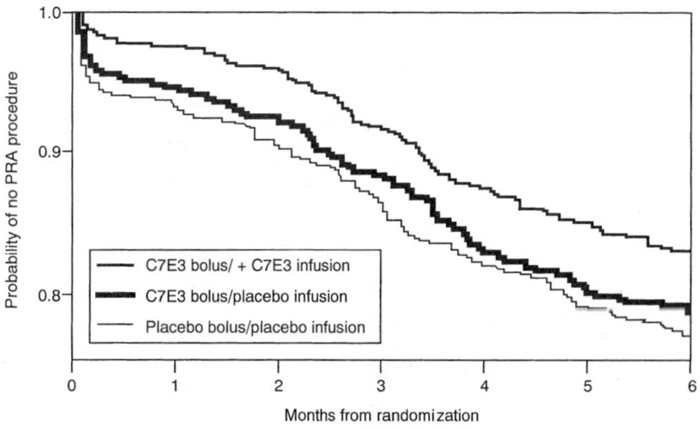

Figure 42–12. Need for subsequent bypass surgery or percutaneous intervention in the EPIC trial, showing a reduction in events with treatment bolus plus 12-h infusion of c7E3.[52] (From Topol EJ, Califf RM, Weisman HF, et al: Randomised trial of coronary intervention with antibody against platelet IIb/IIIa integrin for reduction of clinical restenosis: results at six months. Lancet 1994; 343:881–886.)

TABLE 42–6. FACTORS ASSOCIATED WITH INCREASED RISK OF BLEEDING

Patient	Procedure
Advanced age	High ACT
Creatinine elevation	Prolonged aPTT (>100 sec)
Female gender	Repeat PTCA
Nadir platelet count	Stent usage
	Use of thrombolytics
	Use of c7E3

Abbreviations: ACT, activated clotting time; PTCA, percutaneous transluminal coronary angioplasty; aPTT, activated partial thromboplastin time.

The probability of abrupt closure was almost linear and was inversely related to the ACT (14% risk of closure with ACT of 250 sec; 4% risk of closure with ACT of 500 sec). On the basis of this data, Hillegass and colleagues[59a] argue that the "optimal" ACT in their laboratory is 425–525 sec, although most laboratories attempt to achieve an ACT of 350–400 sec.

More recently, the possible benefit of more powerful and possibly more predictable antiplatelet (platelet glycoprotein IIb/IIIa receptor blockers such as c7E3) and antithrombin (e.g., hirudin, Hirulog) agents have been tested. In the EPIC study,[59b] 2099 patients determined to be high risk by virtue of lesion morphology or unstable clinical syndrome were randomized to conventional aspirin-plus-heparin therapy, aspirin-plus-heparin therapy supplemented by a bolus injection of c7E3 (0.25 mg/kg), or bolus plus 12-h infusion of c7E3 (10 μg/min IV). Heparin was titrated in an attempt to achieve an activated partial thromboplastin time 1.5–2.5 times the laboratory control. Early ischemic events (i.e., death, infarction, further intervention) were decreased by 35% with the bolus plus infusion (there was no benefit with bolus alone), but the early benefit was largely limited to patients with unstable angina or acute infarction and was seen to a much lesser extent in patients with stable angina (Fig. 42–13). A long-term improvement in event-free survival has been noted for all groups, however (data pending review). As might be expected, bleeding risk was also increased with this treatment regimen (14% with bolus plus infusion vs. 7% with standard therapy). This was largely the result of major access site bleeding (8%), bleeding during bypass surgery (4%), and gastrointestinal bleeding (1.5%). Pending closer analysis of the long-term data and full consideration of the cost of this therapy, it is probably best reserved for patients with unstable rather than stable angina.

The value of direct thrombin inhibitors in the setting of angioplasty has also been evaluated, in the Hirudin in a European Trial versus Heparin in the Prevention of Restenosis after PTCA (HELVETICA)[60] and Hirulog[61] trials. In HELVETICA,[60] in which the heparin dose may have been low compared with U.S. standards, hirudin (bolus + 3 days of SC injections) decreased early ischemic events (11% vs. 6%, $p < .01$) but had no effect on long-term outcome. In the Hirulog study,[61] in which an aggressive intraprocedural heparin policy was applied, there was no improvement in early ischemic events with Hirulog compared with heparin therapy, except for patients with postinfarction angina.

IN-HOSPITAL COST OF PERCUTANEOUS INTERVENTION

With U.S. spending on medical care now consuming 13% of the gross national product, the relative cost of percutaneous intervention must also be considered. Current patterns of reimbursement focusing on short-term outcomes force an emphasis on reducing in-hospital costs at the exclusion and sometimes at the expense of long-term costs. My colleagues and I recently completed a study of the in-hospital cost (not charges) of caring for 1154 consecutive patients with percutaneous intervention.[62] Cost could be very well explained ($r^2 = .80$) by major complications (multiple $p < .0001$), decision delays ($p < .001$), overall length of stay ($p < .001$), number of diseased vessels ($p < .001$), and use of nonballoon technology ($p < .001$; Fig. 42–14). Such studies fail to take into consideration the long-term reduction in cost from reductions in restenosis (e.g., stents[63]) or improvements in technique likely to reduce cost (e.g., stenting via brachial–radial technique or without attendant warfarinization, or disposable Rotablator burrs).

SUMMARY

Improved techniques of balloon angioplasty and related devices compared with those available even a few years ago have led to a dramatic increase in the use of this form of therapy, such that 410,000 procedures were performed in the United States alone in 1994.[64] The capacity to perform a procedure does not mean that it should be performed. The results of trials testing percutaneous interventions against other forms of therapy and testing one device against another are just becoming available. Additional data are needed to adequately define the proper roles of many of these

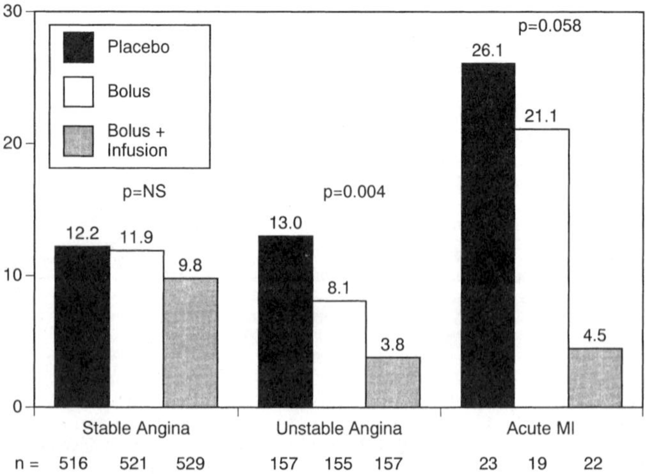

Figure 42–13. Relation of clinical presentation to periprocedural benefit of c7E3 from the EPIC trial. Patients with unstable angina or acute myocardial infarction benefited most.

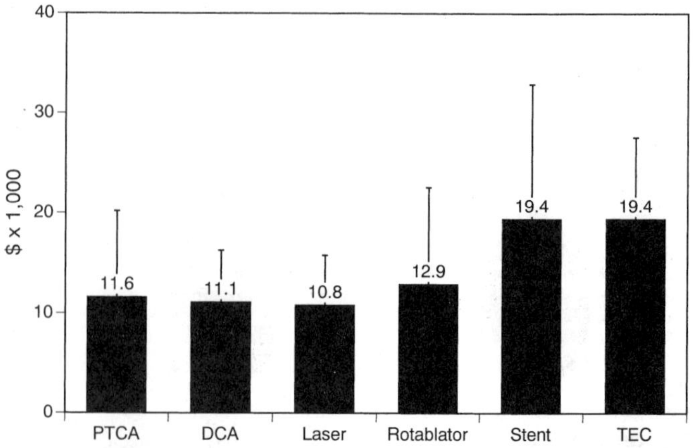

Figure 42–14. Relation of in-hospital costs to first treatment device used. (From Ellis SG, Miller DP, Brown KJ, et al: The in-hospital cost of percutaneous coronary revascularization: critical determinants and implications. Circulation 1995; 92:741–747.)

techniques. At the same time, however, advances in technology are still occurring rapidly, and researchers must be very careful not to conclude that a device or treatment is not beneficial when it has only been tested in a primitive phase of development. Numerous advances can be foreseen for the near future, and with them lies the hope that the inexorable progression of coronary disease can be further delayed.

REFERENCES

1. Parisi AF, Folland ED, Hartigan P, Veterans Affairs ACME Investigators: A comparison of angioplasty with medical therapy in the treatment of single-vessel coronary artery disease. N Engl J Med 1992; 326:10–16.
2. Hamm CW, Reimers J, Ischinger T, et al: Angioplasty vs bypass-surgery in patients with multivessel disease: results of the GABI Trial. Circulation 1993; 88:I–594.
3. RITA Trial Participants: Coronary angioplasty versus coronary artery bypass surgery: the Randomised Intervention Treatment of Angina (RITA) trial. Lancet 1993; 341:573–580.
4. Rodriguez A, Boullon F, Perez-Balino N, et al: Argentine Randomized Trial of Percutaneous Transluminal Coronary Angioplasty Versus Coronary Artery Bypass Surgery in Multivessel Disease (ERACI): in hospital results and 1-year follow-up. J Am Coll Cardiol 1993; 22:1060–1067.
5. Hinohara T, Robertson GC, Selmon MR, et al: Restenosis after directional coronary atherectomy. J Am Coll Cardiol 1992; 20:623–632.
6. Popma JJ, Topol EJ, Hinohara T, et al: Abrupt vessel closure after directional coronary atherectomy. J Am Coll Cardiol 1992; 19:1372–1379.
7. Topol EJ, Leya F, Pinkerton CA, et al: A comparison of directional atherectomy with coronary angioplasty in patients with coronary artery disease. N Engl J Med 1993; 329:221–227.
8. Lau J, Antman EM, Jimenez-Silva J, et al: Cumulative meta-analysis of therapeutic trials for myocardial infarction. N Engl J Med 1992; 327:248–254.
9. Pipilis A, Flather M, Collins R, et al: ISIS-4 pilot study: serial hemodynamic changes with oral captopril and oral isosorbide mononitrate in a randomized double-blind trial in acute myocardial infarction. J Am Coll Cardiol 1991; 17:115A.
10. GISSI: GISSI-3: effects of lisinopril and transdermal glyceryl trinitrate singly and together on 6-week mortality and ventricular function after acute myocardial infarction. Lancet 1994; 343:1115–1122.
11. Mark DB, Nelson CL, Califf RM, et al: Continuing evolution of therapy for coronary artery disease. Initial results from the era of coronary angioplasty. Circulation 1994; 89:2015–2025.
12. Hueb WA, Arie S, Almeida Oliveira S, et al: Randomized trial of surgery, angioplasty or medical therapy for single vessel proximal left anterior descending artery stenosis. Results of long term follow-up [Abstract]. J Am Coll Cardiol 1994; p 268A.
13. Rickards AF: Data presented at European College of Cardiology Symposia, Nice, France, 1993.
14. King SB III, Lembo NJ, Weintraub WS, et al: A randomized trial comparing coronary angioplasty with coronary bypass surgery. N Engl J Med 1994; 331:1044–1050.
15. Weintraub WS, Mauldin PD, Becker E, King SB III: The impact of additional procedures on the cost at three years of coronary angioplasty and coronary surgery in the EAST trial. Circulation 1994; 90:I–91.
16. Detre K, Holubkov R, Kelsey S, et al: Percutaneous transluminal coronary angioplasty in 1985–1986 and 1977–1981. N Engl J Med 1988; 318:265–270.
17. Myler RK, Shaw RE, Stertzer SH, et al: Lesion morphology and coronary angioplasty: current experience and analysis. J Am Coll Cardiol 1992; 19:1641–1652.
18. Ellis SG, Cowley MJ, Whitlow PL, et al: Prospective case control comparison of percutaneous transluminal coronary revascularization in patients with multivessel disease in 1986-87 and 1991: improved in-hospital and 12 month results. J Am Coll Cardiol 1995; 25:1137–1142.
19. Ellis SG, DeCesare NB, Pinkerton CA, et al: Relation of stenosis morphology and clinical presentation to the procedural results of directional coronary atherectomy. Circulation 1991; 84:644–653.
20. Ellis SG, Popma JJ, Buchbinder M, et al: Relation of clinical presentation, stenosis morphology and operator technique to the procedural results of rotational atherectomy. Circulation 1994; 89:882–892.
21. Bittl JA, Sanborn TA. Excimer laser-facilitated coronary angioplasty. Relative risk analysis of acute and follow-up results in 200 patients. Circulation 1992; 86:71–80.
22. Ritchie JL, Phillips KA, Luft HS: Coronary angioplasty. Statewide experience in California. Circulation 1993; 88:2735–2743.
23. Popma JJ, Califf RM, Topol EJ: Clinical trials of restenosis after coronary angioplasty. Circulation 1991; 84:1426–1436.
24. Serruys PW, de Jaegere P, Kiemeneij F, et al: A comparison of balloon-expandable-stent implantation with balloon angioplasty in patients with coronary artery disease. N Engl J Med 1994; 331:489–495.
25. Ellis SG, Myler RK, King SB III, et al: Causes and correlates of cardiac death after unsupported coronary angioplasty—implications for the use of advanced support techniques. Am J Cardiol 1991; 68:1447–1451.
26. Bergelson BA, Jacobs AK, Cupples A, et al: Prediction of risk for hemodynamic compromise during percutaneous transluminal coronary angioplasty. Am J Cardiol 1992; 70:1540–1545.
27. Ohman EM, Marquis J-F, Ricci DR, et al: A randomized comparison of the effects of gradual prolonged versus standard primary balloon inflation on early and late outcome. Results of a multicenter clinical trial. Circulation 1994; 89:1118–1125.
28. Ellis SG, Vandormael MG, Cowley MJ, et al: Coronary morphologic and clinical determinants of procedural outcome with angioplasty for multivessel coronary disease. Implications for patient selection. Circulation 1990; 82:1193–1202.
29. Kereiakes DJ, Knudtson ML, Ohman EM, et al: Prolonged dilatation improves initial results during PTCA of complex coronary stenoses: results from a randomized trial [Abstract]. J Am Coll Cardiol 1993; 21:290A.
30. Cribier A, Eltchaninoff H, Chan C, et al: Comparative effects of long (>12 min) versus standard (3 min) sequential balloon inflations in PTCA. Preliminary results of a prospective randomized study: immediate results and restenosis rate [Abstract]. J Am Coll Cardiol 1994; p 58A.
31. Adelman AG, Cohen EA, Kimball BP, et al: A comparison of directional atherectomy with balloon angioplasty for lesions of the left anterior descending coronary artery. N Engl J Med 1993; 329:228–233.
32. Fernandez-Ortiz A, Badimon JJ, Falk E, et al: Characterization of the relative thrombogenicity of atherosclerotic plaque components: implications for consequences of plaque rupture. J Am Coll Cardiol 1994; 23:1562–1569.
33. Lefkovits J, Anderson K, Weisman H, et al: Increased risk of non-Q MI following DCA: evidence for a platelet dependent mechanism from the EPIC trial. Circulation 1994; 90:I–214.
34. Holmes DR Jr, Topol EJ, Califf RM, et al: A multicenter, randomized trial of coronary angioplasty versus directional atherectomy for patients with saphenous vein bypass graft lesions. Circulation 1995; 91:1966–1974.
35. Chien S: Transport across arterial endothelium. *In* Spaet TH (ed): Progress in Hemostasis and Thrombosis, vol. 4, pp 1–36. New York, Grune and Stratton, 1978.
36. Vandormael M, Reifart N, Preusler W, et al: Six months follow-up results following excimer laser angioplasty, rotational atherectomy and balloon angioplasty for complex lesions: ERBAC Study. Circulation 1994; 90:I-213.
37. Fischman DL, Leon MB, Baim D, et al: A randomized comparison of coronary stent placement and balloon angioplasty in the treatment of coronary artery disease. New Engl J Med 1994; 331:496–501.
38. Columbo A, Hall P, Almagor Y, et al: Results of intravascular ultrasound guided coronary stenting without subsequent anticoagulation [Abstract]. J Am Coll Cardiol 1994; p 335A.
39. Barragan PT, Silvestri MA, Sainsous JB, et al: Coronary stenting without Coumadin [Abstract]. J Am Coll Cardiol 1994; p 336A.
40. Litvack F, Eigler N, Margolis J, et al: Percutaneous excimer laser coronary angioplasty: results in the first consecutive 3,000 patients. J Am Coll Cardiol 1994; 23:323–329.
41. Deckelbaum LI, Strauss BH, Bittl JA, et al: Effect of intracoronary saline infusion on dissection during excimer laser coronary angioplasty: a randomized trial. J Am Coll Cardiol 1995; 26:1264–1269.
42. Topaz O, McIvor M, Stone G, et al: Solid state laser coronary angioplasty: multicenter registry report. Circulation 1994; 90:I-330.
43. Ellis SG, Roubin GS, King SB III, et al: Angiographic and clinical predictors of acute closure after native vessel coronary angioplasty. Circulation 1988; 77:372–379.
44. Tenaglia AN, Fortin DF, Califf RM, et al: Predicting the risk of abrupt vessel closure after angioplasty in an individual patient. J Am Coll Cardiol 1994; 24:1004–1011.
45. Popma JJ, Leon MB, Mintz GS, et al: Results of coronary angioplasty

using the transluminal extraction catheter. Am J Cardiol 1992; 70:1526–1532.
46. DeFranco AC, Nissen SE, Tuzcu SE, et al: Ultrasound plaque morphology predicts major dissections following stand-alone and adjunctive balloon angioplasty. Circulation 1994; 90:I-59.
47. Nobuyoshi M, Kimura T, Nosaka H, et al: Restenosis after successful percutaneous transluminal coronary angioplasty: serial angiographic follow-up of 2229 patients. J Am Coll Cardiol 1988; 12:616–623.
48. Hillegass WB, Ohman EM, Califf RM: Restenosis: the clinical issues. *In* Topol EJ (ed): Textbook of Interventional Cardiology, pp 415–435. Philadelphia: WB Saunders, 1994.
49. Kuntz RE, Gibson CM, Nobuyoshi M, Baim DS. Generalized model of restenosis after conventional balloon angioplasty, stenting and directional atherectomy. J Am Coll Cardiol 1993; 21:15–25.
50. Roubin GS, Douglas JS Jr, King SB III, et al: Influence of balloon size on initial success, acute complications, and restenosis after percutaneous transluminal coronary angioplasty. A prospective randomized study. Circulation 1988; 78:557–565.
51. Lincoff AM, Topol EJ, Ellis SG. Local drug delivery for the prevention of restenosis—fact, fancy and future. Circulation 1994; 90:2070–2084.
52. Topol EJ, Califf RM, Weisman HF, et al: Randomised trial of coronary intervention with antibody against platelet IIb/IIIa integrin for reduction of clinical restenosis: results at six months. Lancet 1994; 343:881–886.
53. Wilentz JR, Sanborn TA, Haudenschild CC, et al: Platelet accumulation in experimental angioplasty: time course and relation to vascular injury. Circulation 1987; 75:636–642.
54a. White CW, Chaitman B, Lassar TA, The Ticlopidine Study Group: Antiplatelet agents are effective in reducing the immediate complications of PTCA: results from the Ticlopidine Multicenter Trial. Circulation 1987; 76:IV-400.
54b. Lembo NJ, Black AJR, Roubin GS, et al: Effect of pretreatment with aspirin versus aspirin plus dipyridamole on frequency and type of acute complications of percutaneous coronary angioplasty. Am J Cardiol 1990; 65:422–426.
55. Mufson L, Black A, Roubin G, et al: A randomized trial of aspirin in PTCA: effect of high vs. low dose aspirin on major complications and restenosis. J Am Coll Cardiol 1988; 11:236A.
56. Ellis SG, Roubin GS, Wilentz J, et al: Effect of 18- to 24-hour heparin administration for prevention of restenosis after uncomplicated coronary angioplasty. Am Heart J 1989; 117:777–782.
57. Dougherty KG, Gaos CM, Bush HS, et al: Activated clotting times and activated partial thromboplastin times in patients undergoing coronary angioplasty who receive bolus doses of heparin. Catheter Cardiovasc Diagn 1992; 26:260–263.
58. Ferguson JJ, Dougherty KG, Gaos CM, et al: Relation between procedural activated coagulation time and outcome after percutaneous transluminal coronary angioplasty. J Am Coll Cardiol 1994; 23:1061–1065.
59a. Hillegass WB, Narins CR, Brott BC, et al: Activated clotting time predicts bleeding complications from angioplasty. J Am Coll Cardiol 1994; 23:184A.
59b. EPIC Investigators: Use of a monoclonal antibody directed against the platelet glycoprotein IIb/IIIa receptor in high-risk coronary angioplasty. N Engl J Med 1994; 330:956–961.
60. Serruys PW, Herrman J-PR, Simon R, et al: A comparison of hirudin with heparin in the prevention of restenosis after coronary angioplasty. N Engl J Med 1995; 333:757–763.
61. Bittl JA, Strony J, Brinker JA, et al: Treatment with bivalirudin (Hirulog) as compared with heparin during coronary angioplasty for unstable or postinfarction angina. N Engl J Med 1995; 333:764–769.
62. Ellis SG, Miller DP, Brown KJ, et al: The in-hospital cost of percutaneous coronary revascularization: critical determinants and implications. Circulation 1995; 92:741–747.
63. Cohen DJ, Breall JA, Ho KKL, et al: Evaluating the potential cost-effectiveness of stenting as a treatment for symptomatic single-vessel coronary disease—use of a decision-analytic model. Circulation 1994; 89:1859–1874.
64. Industry survey. Billerica, MA: United States Cardiac Instruments (USCI), 1994.

43 Interventional Approaches for Unstable Angina

John A. Bittl, MD

For the patient with unstable angina, the primary goal of therapy is to stabilize the culprit coronary artery lesion and prevent myocardial infarction. Before 1980, the treatment strategy for unstable angina involved managing the acute ischemic syndrome with intensive medical therapy and reserving coronary artery bypass surgery for the patient who continued to show evidence of ischemia.[1, 2] This approach was challenged by the first reports of successful coronary angioplasty for unstable angina.[3] Since 1985, unstable angina has become one of the most important indications for interventional cardiovascular therapy.

This chapter identifies which patients require invasive evaluation and interventional treatment for unstable angina. New adjunctive antithrombotic therapies are discussed after a brief review of the pathogenesis of unstable angina and a summary of recent clinical trials. The practical discussion of interventional techniques in this chapter is organized into separate sections on the basis of common clinical and angiographic subjects such as clinical risk factor profiles, the timing of interventional therapy, and the management of filling defects and bypass graft lesions.

PATHOGENESIS OF UNSTABLE ANGINA AND RATIONALE FOR CORONARY INTERVENTION

The basis for the interventional treatment of unstable angina comes from an understanding of the pathophysiology of acute coronary syndromes and the identification of the role of arterial injury and the influence of shear rates on arterial thrombus formation. Coronary artery thrombosis is a high-shear, platelet-dependent process that occurs on exposure of blood to sites of deep arterial injury[4–8] or plaque rupture.[9, 10] At sites of vessel injury,[11] exposed tissue factor protein combines with factors VIIa and Xa to form the prothrombinase complex, which catalyzes the conversion of prothrombin to thrombin (Fig. 43–1). Thrombin plays the dual role of cleaving fibrin to fibrinogen and activating platelets.[12] Platelet activation leads to aggregation through the externalization of glycoprotein IIb/IIIa receptors for cross-linking adhesive macromolecules such as fibrinogen.[13] Although platelets become activated on adhesion to subintimal collagen, fibronectin, or von Willebrand factor, thrombin is the strongest agonist of platelet activation, and it exerts its effects independent of the pathways inhibited by aspirin.

Several angiographic,[14–18] angioscopic,[19–21] and histologic[22–27] studies have identified the pathogenic mechanisms of unstable angina. It is postulated that plaque inflammation, plaque rupture, and intracoronary thrombus formation precipitate unstable angina in many patients (Fig. 43–2), but there is wide variability in the detection of these pathogenic events using angiographic and angioscopic methods. Ten to twenty-six percent of patients with unstable angina have angiographic evidence of thrombus,[15–18, 28–30] and the majority of these patients show angioscopic findings of intracoronary thrombus.[19–21]

Histologic examination of atherectomy specimens has confirmed coronary thrombus formation in a significant proportion of patients with unstable angina[26, 31] and established the importance of tissue factor protein in the pathogenesis of intracoronary thrombus[32] but raised important questions about the pathogenesis of unstable angina in the remaining patients. Thrombus or hemorrhage were observed in 34% of patients with unstable angina, compared with 8% of patients with restenosis and none with stable angina.[26] It is possible, however, that plaque healing may have taken place by the time atherectomy was performed or thrombus was missed because of a sampling error.

Although many episodes of unstable angina are undoubtedly caused by plaque rupture and thrombus formation, other causes potentially amenable to interventional therapy must be considered. The similarity between unstable angina and restenosis in some patients, as assessed by histologic examination of atherectomy specimens, suggests that the pathogenic mechanisms responsible for both syndromes may also be similar. Smooth muscle cell proliferation,[33–35] arterial remodeling,[36] and secretion of glycosaminoglycans may increase the absolute or relative mass of the atheroma after restenosis,[37] reducing the diameter of the coronary lumen and thus precipitating an ischemic syndrome.

Observations from experimental models have identified why angioplasty is a successful treatment for unstable angina (Fig. 43–3). In a canine model of arterial stenosis, the synergistic effects of arterial injury and the coexistence of vessel narrowing on arterial thrombus formation were quantified in the presence of heparin.[38] Although balloon injury resulted in a twofold increase in platelet deposition in the dilated segment compared with the normal arterial segment, the presence of a constriction induced by a vascular ring resulted in an additional threefold increase in platelet deposition.[38] Thus, angioplasty is beneficial in unstable angina because of its ability to enlarge the lumen of the narrowed coronary artery, lower the shear rate in the dilated coronary segment, and reduce platelet activation at the site of the ruptured or inflamed plaque.[39] This beneficial effect is opposed by the capacity of the injured vessel to form thrombus[40, 41] in the presence of activated platelets,[42] endothelial denudation,[9] exposed thrombogenic subintimal elements,[10] and occasional deep medial dissections.[43] Although localized intracoronary thrombus formation occasionally overwhelms the systemic anticoagulant action of heparin, the attainment of a large postprocedural lumen in the presence of intense systemic anticoagulation guided by measurements of activated clotting time maximizes the likelihood of success and reduces the risk of thrombotic vessel occlusion during angioplasty for unstable angina.

ANTICOAGULANT THERAPY DURING CORONARY INTERVENTION FOR UNSTABLE ANGINA

Heparin

The goal of systemic anticoagulant therapy during angioplasty for unstable angina is to inhibit further activation of the coagulation system within a localized segment of the coronary artery. In combination with aspirin, heparin is the mainstay of anticoagulant therapy during angioplasty because of its ability to potentiate the capacity of antithrombin III to inhibit thrombin and block the conversion of fibrinogen to fibrin.[44] Despite its mechanisms of action, heparin has several theoretical limitations: (1) the nonspecific binding of heparin to plasma proteins and acute phase reactants,[45] leading to reduced

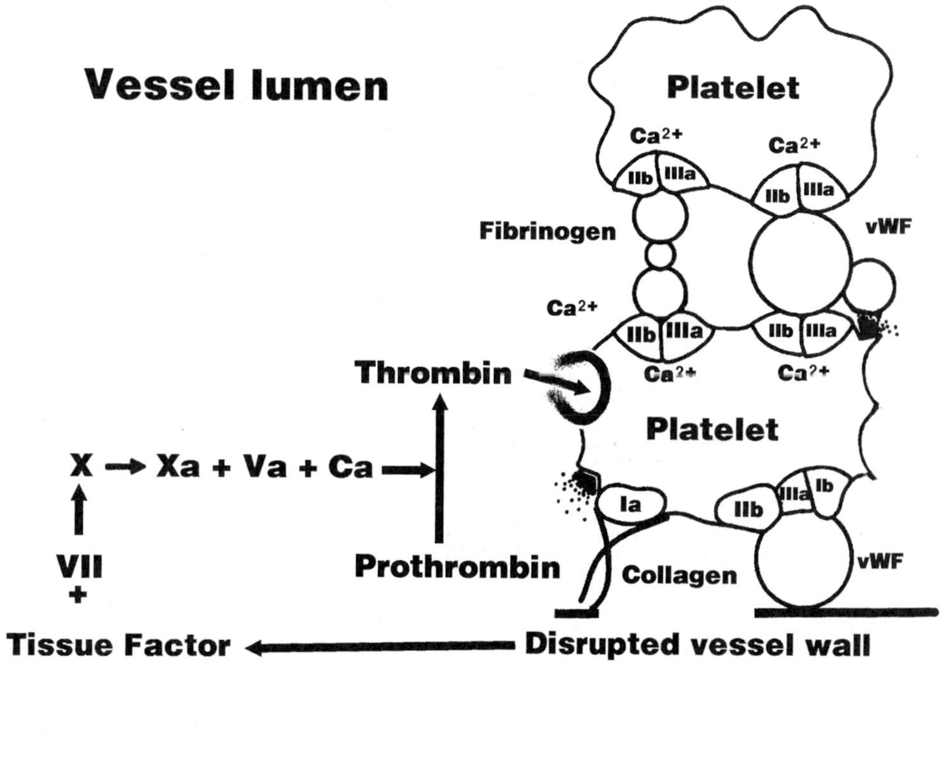

Figure 43–1. Schematic representation of adhesion and activation of platelets causing arterial thrombus formation. Vessel injury leads to the exposure of collagen and tissue factor. Tissue factor combines with factors Xa and VIIa to form the prothrombinase complex, which generates thrombin. Thrombin plays a dual role in arterial thrombus formation by converting fibrinogen to fibrin (not shown) and by activating platelets. Activated platelets externalize the glycoprotein IIb/IIIa receptor, which binds to adhesive macromolecules such as fibrinogen or von Willebrand factor (vWF) and thus mediates the process of platelet aggregation. (Data from Chesebro JH, Webster MWI, Zoldhelyi P, et al: Antithrombotic therapy and progression of coronary artery disease: antiplatelet versus antithrombins. Circulation 1992; 86(suppl III):100–111. Reproduced with permission of the American Heart Association.)

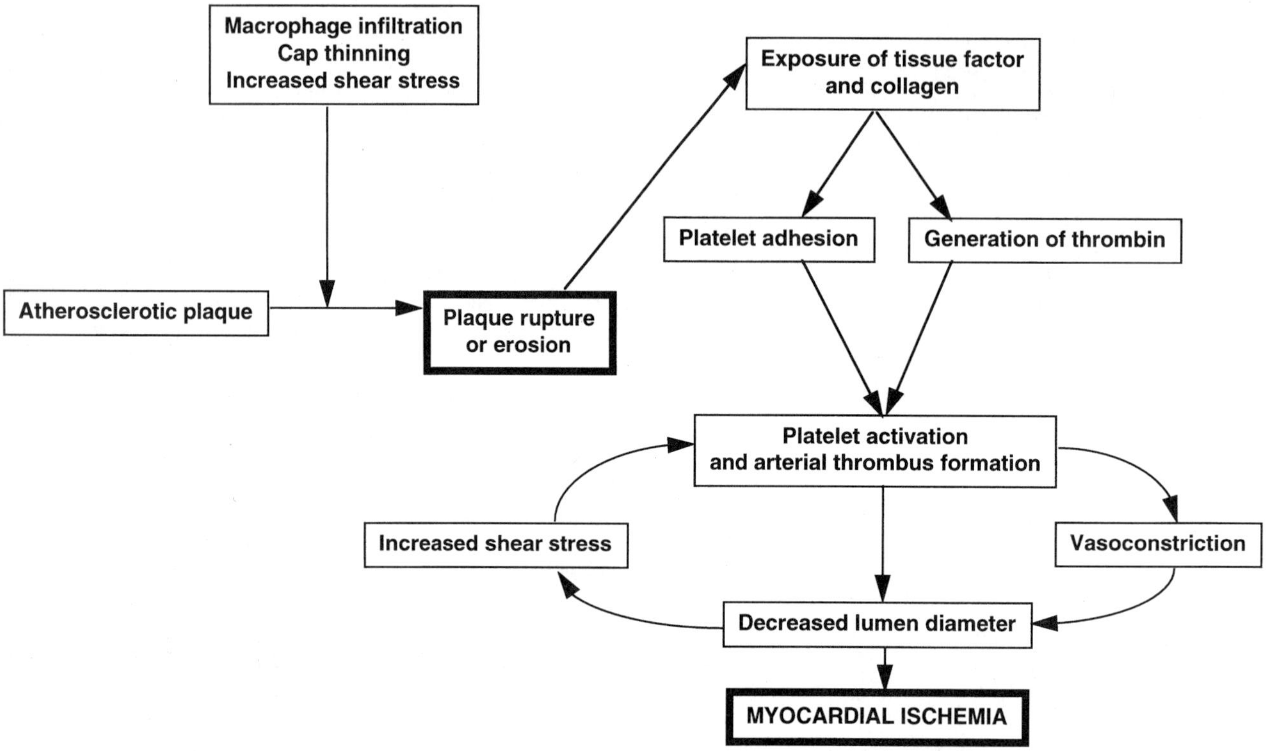

Figure 43–2. Schematic representation of the pathogenesis of unstable angina. Evidence from pathologic, angiographic, and angioscopic studies suggests that inflammation and macrophage infiltration of an atherosclerotic plaque, in combination with alteration in shear stress, leads to plaque rupture or erosion. This is followed by the formation of arterial thrombi, as mediated by the action of tissue factor, thrombin, and the activation of platelets. Critical narrowing of the coronary artery lumen results in myocardial ischemia.

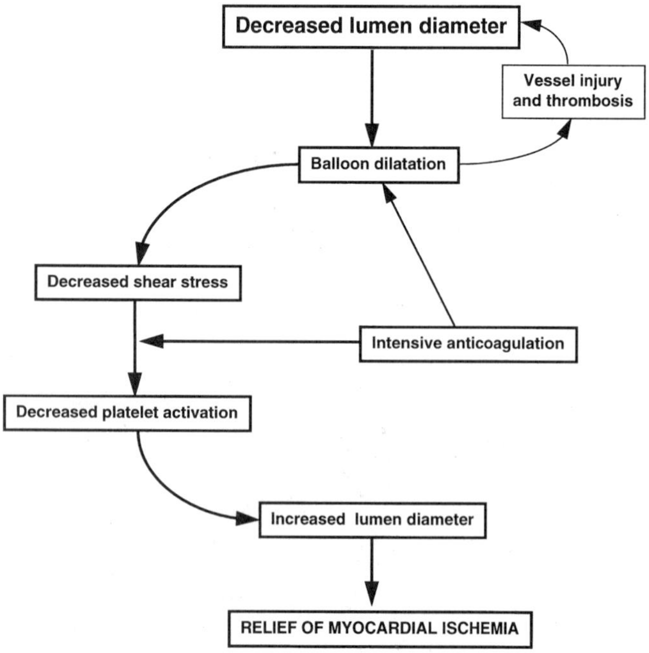

Figure 43–3. Schematic representation of the mechanism of benefit of coronary angioplasty in unstable angina. The deleterious effect of balloon-induced vessel injury and thrombosis is balanced by the beneficial effect of lumen enlargement. The decrease in shear stress and use of intensive antithrombotic therapy decreases the extent of platelet aggregation, resulting in a stable arterial lumen and relief from myocardial ischemia.

bioavailability and a nonlinear relation between dose and the intensity of anticoagulation[46]; (2) localized heparin resistance arising within platelet-rich thrombi within the coronary artery as a result of the presence of platelet factor 4[47]; and (3) a conformational change in fibrin-bound thrombin, rendering it inaccessible to the heparin-antithrombin III complex.[48] Because clot-bound thrombin is extremely thrombogenic and yet resists heparin therapy, high systemic doses of heparin are commonly used in angioplasty.

Thrombin Inhibitors

To overcome the limitations of heparin, powerful inhibitors of platelet aggregation have been developed.[49] These agents exert their effects either through inhibition of the thrombin-dependent steps of platelet activation or through the ultimate step in platelet aggregation mediated by the platelet glycoprotein IIb/IIIa receptor (see Fig. 43–1). Compared with heparin, direct thrombin inhibitors such as hirudin or Hirulog produce more consistent levels of anticoagulation,[50] are effective against clot-bound thrombin,[48] do not require a cofactor such as antithrombin III, and have no known natural inhibitors such as platelet factor 4.[47] Thus, the direct thrombin inhibitors specifically select a forming thrombus by combining antithrombotic activity with thrombus-targeting properties in a single hybrid molecule. The direct antithrombins may have an additional effect because they concurrently, yet reversibly, interrupt the recruitment of platelets and the formation of fibrin.

In clinical studies, Hirulog has been used as a substitute for heparin. In 258 patients undergoing elective coronary angioplasty, Hirulog was used in an open-label, dose-escalation study. Compared with lower doses, bolus doses of 1.8–2.2 mg/kg significantly reduced the incidence of ischemic events and abrupt vessel closure from 10.2% to 3.9% without an increase in bleeding complications.[51] In the Hirulog Angioplasty Study,[52] 4098 patients undergoing coronary angioplasty for postinfarction or unstable angina were enrolled at 121 clinical centers in a randomized, double-blind comparison of Hirulog vs. heparin. The primary end point was procedural failure, defined as in-hospital death, myocardial infarction, abrupt vessel closure, or clinical deterioration of cardiac origin requiring bypass surgery, intra-aortic balloon pumping, or repeat angioplasty. The safety end point was major hemorrhage, defined as overt blood loss associated with a decrease in hemoglobin of more than 3 g/dL, blood transfusion, or intracranial or retroperitoneal hemorrhage. For the entire 4098-patient cohort, Hirulog therapy was not associated with a significant reduction in ischemic complications compared with heparin therapy. The incidence of in-hospital death (0.4% vs. 0.2%), myocardial infarction (3.2% vs. 3.9%), emergency bypass surgery (1.7% vs. 1.7%), and other ischemic complications was similar between the two treatment groups (all probabilities nonsignificant). For the prospectively defined cohort of patients undergoing coronary angioplasty for postinfarction angina, Hirulog was associated with a significant reduction in ischemic events compared with heparin therapy. Hirulog reduced the incidence of myocardial infarction (2% vs. 5.1%; odds ratio [OR] = 0.4; 95% confidence interval 0.2–0.9; p = .04) or any major or minor ischemic complication (9.1% vs. 14.2%; OR = 0.6; 95% confidence interval 0.4–0.9; p = .04). For the cohort of patients undergoing angioplasty for unstable angina without recent myocardial infarction, Hirulog did not reduce the incidence of death, myocardial infarction, or bypass surgery (5% vs. 4.9%; OR = 1; 95% confidence interval 0.7–1.4; p = 1) or major or minor ischemic complications (11.9% vs. 11.8%; OR = 1; 95% confidence interval 0.8–1.2; p = 1). For the entire cohort of patients treated with either anticoagulant, Hirulog was associated with lower bleeding complications than heparin. Hirulog reduced the incidence of retroperitoneal hemorrhage (0.2% vs. 0.7%; OR = 0.3; 95% confidence interval 0.1–0.9; p = .02), need for transfusion (3.7% vs. 8.6%; OR = 0.4; 95% confidence interval 0.3–0.6; $p < .001$), and major hemorrhage 3.8% vs. 9.8%; OR = 0.4; 95% confidence interval 0.3–0.5; $p < .001$).

Hirudin has also been compared with heparin in angioplasty studies. In the Hirudin Angioplasty Study,[53] 1141 patients were randomized to treatment with heparin, hirudin infusion, or hirudin infusion plus prolonged subcutaneous therapy for 72 h in an effort to reduce clinical and angiographic restenosis at 7 months. The use of hirudin was associated with a significant reduction in the secondary end point, which consisted of a composite of death, myocardial infarction, or need for repeat revascularization at 96 h (11% vs. 5.6% in the group of patients treated with prolonged hirudin therapy), but hirudin did not improve the primary end point of restenosis.[53]

Platelet Glycoprotein IIb/IIIa Receptor Inhibitors

The final common pathway for platelet aggregation is mediated by the platelet glycoprotein IIb/IIIa receptor. Chimeric 7E3, the monoclonal antibody Fab fragment directed against the platelet glycoprotein IIb/IIIa receptor, binds to this receptor irreversibly and potentially reduces the extent of arterial thrombus formation. In the Evaluation of 7E3 for the Prevention of Ischemic Complications (EPIC) study,[54] 2099 patients undergoing coronary angioplasty for acute myocardial infarction, refractory unstable angina, or high-risk coronary stenosis were randomly assigned to three treatment groups: heparin, heparin plus a bolus of c7E3, or heparin plus a bolus and infusion of 7E3. The use of c7E3 reduced the occurrence of the primary end point of death, nonfatal myocardial infarction, bypass surgery, repeat angioplasty, stent placement, or use of intra-aortic balloon pumping within 30 days of treatment (12.8%, 11.4%, and 8.3% in the three study groups; p = .009). Six months after angioplasty,[55] patients treated with bolus plus infusion had a lower incidence of major ischemic complications or need for revascularization of the initially treated vessel than those treated with heparin alone (35.1% vs. 27.0%; p = .001). This favorable long-term effect was predominantly due to a lower need for bypass surgery or repeat angioplasty (16.5% vs. 22.3%; p = .007), which was consistent with a reduction in clinical restenosis. The use of c7E3 in the EPIC study, however, was associated with increased bleeding during the initial hospitalization (7.0%, 13.2%, and 15.4% in the three study groups).[54] Because bleeding may have been increased by the concomitant use of fixed-dose heparin irrespective of body weight, a pilot study was carried out to evaluate the safety of using lower doses of heparin and removing femoral catheter sheaths on the day of the angioplasty procedure. In this pilot study, transfusions during c7E3 therapy were reduced to as low as 2.0% (heparin bolus, 70 U/kg) to 7.7% (heparin bolus, 100 U/kg) without an increase in ischemic events.[56] The strategy of using c7E3 with weight-adjusted, lower dose heparin was confirmed in the larger study Evaluation in PTCA to Improve Long-term Outcome with c7E3 Glycoprotein IIb/IIIa Blockade (EPILOG),[56a] which was initially planned to enroll 4500 patients with stable angina or unstable angina. The EPILOG study was stopped prematurely after a preplanned interim safety analysis revealed a striking reduction in death or myocardial infarction in patients treated with c7E3 (8.1% vs. 2.6%; $p < .001$) without an increase in bleeding. In a separate study evaluating the ability of c7E3 to reduce ischemic events in patients with refractory unstable angina awaiting coronary angioplasty, pretreatment with c7E3 one to two days before angioplasty was associated with a reduction in acute myocardial infarction, from 9.4% to 4.4%.[57]

Other large clinical trials have evaluated reversible IIb/IIa receptor inhibitors such as integrelin or tirofiban during angioplasty for unstable angina. In a study involving 4010 patients undergoing angioplasty, high-dose integrelin (135 μg/kg bolus plus 0.75 μg/kg/h infusion) was associated wih a lower incidence of major ischemic complications or emergency revascularization at 24 h (6.8% vs. 5.1%; p = .01) but a smaller difference at 30 days (11.4% to 9.9%; p = .18).[57a] Similarly, in a study involving 2139 patients undergoing angioplasty for unstable angina, therapy with tirofiban was associated with a lower incidence of major ischemic complications or emergency revascularization at 2 days (8.7% vs. 5.4%; $p = .005$) but not at 30 days (12.2% vs. 10.3%; p .16).[58]

Current Recommendations

During angioplasty for unstable angina, heparin should be administered to achieve an activated clotting time of 350 sec. This can be achieved by giving a 10,000-unit bolus to female patients and a 12,500-unit bolus to male patients. If the initial bolus is not associated with an activated clotting time of 350 sec, additional boluses of 2500–5000 units of heparin should be given. An alternative dosing regimen adjusted to patient body weight and to baseline activated clotting time is presented in Table 43–1.

After an uncomplicated angioplasty procedure, heparin can be discontinued and the sheaths removed when the activated clotting time falls to less than 180 sec. Prolonged heparinization after angioplasty increases the need for red blood cell transfusion (3.8% vs. 8.2%; $p = .09$) but provides no benefit for patients undergoing angioplasty for unstable angina in the absence of filling defects, significant dissection, or abrupt vessel closure.[59] If prolonged heparinization is required, heparin should be administered to achieve an aPTT of 55–90 sec, measured approximately 6 hours after the initial bolus.

Aspirin in a dose of 325 mg PO q.d. must be administered with heparin to reduce the risk of periprocedural myocardial infarction.[60] Aspirin is also effective in reducing the likelihood of ischemic rebound after abrupt cessation of heparin in patients requiring prolonged infusions.[61] Ischemic rebound after heparin withdrawal may be caused by persistence of the underlying thrombogenic substrate, dissociation of the thrombin-antithrombin complexes, or reduced clearance of thrombin. An additional measure to avoid ischemic rebound after discontinuation of heparin involves decreasing the infusion in half for 2 h before discontinuation.

For aspirin-intolerant patients, dipyridamole, 75 mg PO t.i.d., or ticlopidine, 250 mg PO b.i.d., can be used. Because of the 1% risk of neutropenia from ticlopidine, complete blood counts should be obtained every 2 weeks during the first 3 months of therapy.

The use of c7E3 can be considered for patients with severe unstable angina associated with complex thrombus-containing lesions or unstable angina refractory to therapy with heparin and aspirin.

CORONARY ARTERIOGRAPHY IN UNSTABLE ANGINA

Goals

Coronary arteriography is important for managing patients with unstable angina who are judged to be at high risk for cardiac complications on the basis of their presentation or results of noninvasive testing.[62] The aim of cardiac catheterization is to optimize therapy by providing measurements of right and left heart filling pressures, to support the systemic circulation with intra-aortic balloon counterpulsation for patients with hemodynamic compromise or refractory pain, and most importantly, to define the coronary anatomy for possible revascularization.

For many patients with significant stenoses associated with refractory ischemia despite medical therapy, coronary angioplasty will be recommended. For patients with left main coronary artery or three-vessel coronary artery disease, bypass surgery is the preferred method of treatment.[63] At the other end of the spectrum, a significant proportion of patients who present with unstable angina have no significant coronary artery disease. In the Thrombolysis in Myocardial Ischemia Trial IIIA (TIMI-IIIA) of patients with unstable angina or possible non–Q wave myocardial infarction,[64] 14% had no luminal diameter stenosis of 60% or greater at diagnostic coronary arteriography. Compared with patients with unstable angina and an identifiable culprit lesion, patients without significant coronary artery disease were more likely to be women and nonwhite and less likely to have ST shifts on the presenting electrocardiogram. Patients with unstable angina and no significant coronary artery disease had an excellent short-term prognosis with fewer deaths or myocardial infarctions compared with patients with significant disease (2% vs. 18%, respectively).[64]

TABLE 43–1. NOMOGRAM FOR ADDITIONAL BOLUSES OF HEPARIN FOR PATIENTS PREVIOUSLY TREATED WITH HEPARIN

	Heparin, 10,000 U (1,000 U/mL)	
ACT (sec)	<70 kg (Units)	≥70 kg (Units)
150–200	7000	10,000
201–250	5000	7500
251–300	1500	2500
301–350	1000	1500
>350	0	0

Abbreviations: ACT, activated clotting time.

Indications

Recurrent symptoms after initial medical management are an indication of failure of medical therapy and should prompt referral for urgent cardiac catheterization. Cardiac catheterization should also be carried out in most patients judged to be at high risk for complications of unstable angina, including those with prolonged ischemic chest pain lasting more than 20 min, pulmonary edema, new mitral regurgitation, dynamic ST changes, S_3 or rales, hypotension, impaired left ventricular function with ejection fraction less than 0.50, or significant ventricular arrhythmias or atrioventricular block.[62] Cardiac catheterization should also be carried out in most patients with unstable angina if they have had prior angioplasty or bypass surgery.

Patients with active comorbid illness such as rapidly worsening renal function, active infection, significant cerebrovascular impairment, or other contraindication to revascularization should not undergo cardiac catheterization until these problems are stable or improving.

Medical therapy has substantially diminished the risk of progression of unstable angina to myocardial infarction; myocardial infarction has been reduced by 44% with intravenous heparin, by 40% with aspirin, and by 13% with beta blockers.[65] At the time of hospital admission, however, it is not possible to predict whether unstable angina will remit or progress to myocardial infarction, because the causes of instability and the mechanisms underlying its evolution are not fully known. In patients with persistent or worsening symptoms and signs of ischemia despite full medical therapy, prognosis is poor. Thus, many patients who present with unstable angina currently undergo interventional therapy or surgical revascularization. In 104 consecutive patients with unstable angina admitted to two coronary care units, 41% underwent angioplasty, 46% had coronary artery bypass surgery, and only 13% had continued medical therapy.[66]

Despite the widespread use of coronary arteriography and revascularization, it has been difficult until recently to define the role of early invasive evaluation in patients with unstable angina. The TIMI-IIIB study[29] has provided important insights into the value of coronary arteriography for unstable angina. This study evaluated the rationale for using an early aggressive strategy consisting of catheterization and angioplasty vs. a conservative strategy in patients with unstable angina. The study found that the major end points of death, myocardial infarction, or positive exercise tolerance test at 6 weeks occurred with similar frequencies in patients assigned to each of the two groups. However, more postdischarge procedures and hospitalizations were required in patients assigned to the early conservative strategy (7.8% vs. 14.1%; $p < .001$). By comparing TIMI-IIB[67] and TIMI-IIIB,[29] it was found that invasive strategies were ultimately required in more patients initially assigned to conservative therapy with unstable angina or non–Q wave myocardial infarction than in those with Q wave myocardial infarction. This implies that patients with unstable angina or non–Q wave myocardial infarction have an incomplete ischemic event that frequently requires additional invasive evaluation and revascularization.

The TIMI-IIIB results suggest that an early aggressive strategy provides more rapid and complete relief of angina than the early conservative strategy without increasing the risk of major clinical events such as death or myocardial infarction.[29] Thus, angiography is useful in assessing the severity of coronary artery disease and in defining a treatment plan. About 15% of patients with "unstable angina" will have more stenoses and a good prognosis on medical therapy. Conversely, patients with left main or multivessel coronary artery disease or severe left ventricular dysfunction can be identified and referred for bypass surgery. Other patients can be treated with coronary angioplasty to reduce the need for anti-anginal treatment and early rehospitalization.

TECHNICAL ASPECTS

Upon arrival in the cardiac catheterization laboratory, the patient with unstable angina should have vital signs measured, electrocardiographic monitoring established, and the femoral area draped and prepared to allow placement of femoral arterial and venous access. At the same time, attention must be given to the ongoing discomfort experienced by the patient. Pain refractory to intravenous nitroglycerin should be treated with 2–4 mg morphine sulfate or 25–50 μg fentanyl IV. If heart rate control has not been achieved, 5 mg metoprolol should be given intravenously, when there are no contraindications, to achieve a target heart rate of less than 75 bpm. Previous doses of heparin can be safely augmented with an additional empiric dose of 5000 units of heparin intravenously without increasing the risk of hemorrhage during arterial access. For the patient with ongoing chest pain, oxygen should be administered. A single-wall puncture needle may minimize bleeding complications in patients at increased risk if the operator is skilled at such an approach. Otherwise, the routine technique for femoral artery puncture should be used. It is reasonable to place a 6-French arterial sheath initially in the femoral artery for diagnostic coronary arteriography. The 6-French sheath can then be replaced by a 7- or an 8-French sheath if coronary angioplasty is performed.

The adequacy of oxygenation should be confirmed by continuous transcutaneous pulsed oximetry. In the patient with hypotension accompanying ischemia refractory to inotropic agents and intravenous fluid administration, the contralateral femoral artery can be punctured for intra-aortic balloon counterpulsation.

In the unstable patient, the primary objective of coronary arteriography is to identify the coronary anatomy responsible for ischemia and to determine suitability for acute intervention such as angioplasty or emergency bypass surgery.

The selection of contrast agents for coronary arteriography in unstable angina is the subject of controversy. Diatrizoate sodium may be less well tolerated than an agent with lower osmolarity because of the undesirable hemodynamic effects of a high-osmolar contrast agent. The advantage of diatrizoate, however, is that it provides better anticoagulant properties than the nonionic agents. Ioxaglate, a low-ionic agent that retains most of the anticoagulant properties of diatrizoate sodium,[68–70] may have advantages in the unstable patient with hemodynamic compromise. It has been suggested that the nonionic agents such as iopamidol result in increased platelet activation, but a recent study suggested that the intensity of platelet aggregation after balloon dilatation was similar for diatrizoate sodium, ioxaglate, and iopamidol.[71] Although the slopes of the aggregation responses were accentuated in the presence of iopamidol, balloon dilatation and arterial injury were more important than the specific contrast agent used in inducing platelet activation during coronary angioplasty.

Coronary arteriography of the suspected ischemia-related vessel, selected on the basis of electrocardiographic localization, is generally performed first. While angiography of the contralateral coronary artery is being performed, an angioplasty balloon can be prepared. The left coronary artery is generally evaluated first in either the anteroposterior-caudal view or left anterior oblique-cranial view. The right coronary artery is initially evaluated with the nonangulated or mildly cranially angulated left anterior oblique view, with subsequent views taken to maximize visualization of the offending stenosis or stenoses.

Angiographic Detection of Thrombus

Because coronary angiography provides a silhouette of lesion edges, it has only a limited ability to identify an intracoronary thrombus compared with other imaging modalities such as angioscopy.[19–21] Despite its limitations, the angiographic detection of complex lesions or thrombus in unstable angina has important prognostic and therapeutic implications. Angiographic-pathologic correlations have suggested that an eccentric stenosis with a narrow neck, overhanging edge, or scalloped border corresponds to plaque rupture or hemorrhage with superimposed partially occlusive or recanalized thrombus.[14] In unstable angina, the angiographic detection of thrombus in the setting of unstable angina has varied from 6% to 17% in angioplasty series, and from 16% to 57% in angiographic series (Table 43–2).[17, 18, 28, 30, 31, 72–76] The variation in the reporting of coronary thrombus in angiography has been attributed to the type of study performed, the patient population studied, and definitions used. Patients in angioplasty series have a lower incidence of intracoronary thrombus than those in angiographic series, because angioplasty is often postponed when thrombus is detected.[30, 73–79] Patients with resting or postinfarction angina have been found to have a higher likelihood of intracoronary thrombus than those with crescendo angina.[17, 30] Angiographic detection of complex or ulcerated lesions in unstable angina is associated with an increased likelihood of thrombosis and risk of adverse cardiac events.[15]

CORONARY ANGIOPLASTY IN UNSTABLE ANGINA

Goals

The primary goal of angioplasty for unstable angina is to enlarge the lumen diameter and thereby reduce the activation of platelets from the effects of shear rates inherent in severe stenoses.

Indications

Coronary angioplasty is recommended for patients with severe ischemia refractory to initial therapy when a suitable lesion for interventional therapy can be identified. The preceding section identifies the selection of patients for invasive evaluation and interventional therapy. The following sections define the technical approach and timing of angioplasty in patients with unstable angina.

Technical Aspects

The interventional procedure is performed after coronary arteriography has defined the location and physical characteristics of the culprit lesion in the ischemia-related artery. If angioplasty immediately follows diagnostic coronary arteriography, the 6-French arterial

TABLE 43–2. DEFINITION AND INCIDENCE OF THROMBUS AT ANGIOGRAPHY PERFORMED FOR UNSTABLE ANGINA

Investigators	Definition of Thrombus	No. of Patients (%)	Setting
Ahmed et al.[17]	Radiolucent filling defect surrounded by contrast on three sides	37/238 (16%)	Diagnostic study of unstable and postinfarction angina
Gotoh et al.[18]	Shaggy or irregular margins	21/37 (57%)	Diagnostic study of unstable angina
1985–1986 NHLBI Registry[30]	Filling defect	71/679 (10%)	Angioplasty for rest unstable angina
1985–1986 NHLBI Registry[30]	Filling defect	11/178 (6%)	Angioplasty for unstable angina without rest pain
1985–1986 NHLBI Registry[30]	Filling defect	24/140 (17%)	Angioplasty for postinfarction angina
Ellis et al.[78]	Discrete luminal filling defect or an area of contrast staining	48/451 (11%)	Angioplasty for stable and unstable angina
Bär et al.[155]	Filling defect located proximal to, within, or distal to a stenosis with contrast medium on at least three sides; or occluded arteries	39/119 (33%)	Thrombolysis for unstable angina
Sullivan et al. (CAVEAT)[31]	Histologic evidence	101/281 (36%)	Unstable angina patients undergoing atherectomy
Sutton et al. (elective Cook stent)[73]	Discrete intraluminal filling defects with convex curvature, presence of irregular lesion borders with hazy lumen, or frank contrast staining	13/224 (6%)	Elective stenting
Sutton et al. (acute Cook stent placement)[73]	Discrete intraluminal filling defects with convex curvature, presence of irregular lesion borders with hazy lumen, or frank contrast staining	78/415 (19%)	Emergency stent placement
Popma et al. (transluminal extraction catheter)[74]	Discrete, mobile intraluminal filling defects	19/51 (37%)	Interventional series
Safian et al. (transluminal extraction catheter)[75]	Definite circumscribed filling defect	45/158 (28%)	Interventional series
TIMI IIIA[28]	Globular intraluminal radiolucency	80/306 (26%)	Unstable angina or non–Q wave myocardial infarction
Mabin et al.[76]	Intraluminal central filling defect, contrast retention	15/238 (6%)	Angioplasty series

sheath is exchanged for an 8-French sheath that can accommodate an angioplasty guiding catheter, which is then advanced to the target coronary artery. Heparin is administered to achieve an activated clotting time of 350 sec (see Table 43–1). If blood pressure is higher than 100 mm Hg, intravenous nitroglycerin in a dose of 25 μg/min should be administered. If the ischemia-related artery is totally occluded, a floppy guide wire is frequently successful in recanalization, because a new thrombus is soft and easily penetrated. For similar reasons, a balloon catheter selected to match the size of the artery is relatively easy to advance through the occlusion. The guide wire should be extended to permit unimpeded angiography with contrast medium in multiple views and easy access to the dilated site if acute closure occurs. If more than a small, focal dissection with impairment of flow is seen, the segment can be redilated with a standard angioplasty balloon. In some cases, repeat dilatation with a perfusion catheter or coronary stenting will be needed to repair dissections. After uncomplicated angioplasty, the arterial and venous sheaths are removed after heparin has been discontinued for 3–4 h. The heparin infusion can be restarted without a loading dose 1–4 h after sheath removal if no hemorrhagic complication is encountered. In extremely high-risk individuals, prophylactic intra-aortic balloon pumping is recommended because of the benefit that has been achieved with this therapy for patients with acute myocardial infarction.[80]

Timing of Angioplasty

The timing of interventional therapy for unstable angina is critical, because any benefit in delaying interventional therapy will be lost if the patient requires an emergency procedure as a result of failure of medical therapy to stabilize a lesion with increased thrombus burden and reduced flow. Because angioplasty performed early for patients with unstable angina and thrombus-containing lesions may be associated with increased complication rates, angioplasty delayed until a more propitious time after stabilization and "passivation" of the ischemia-related stenosis with prolonged heparin and aspirin may be associated with lower complication rates. This strategy has been retrospectively evaluated in several studies. The procedural success rate was higher (91% vs. 81%; $p = .02$) and the abrupt closure rate lower (2% vs. 8%; $p < .01$) for patients with unstable angina who were treated with heparin for 24 h or longer before coronary angioplasty than for those patients who did not receive heparin.[81] Other investigators have observed a trend toward improved outcome if angioplasty can be deferred for about 2 weeks after the onset of unstable angina.[82]

In a prospective study in 53 patients with unstable angina and intracoronary thrombus, pretreatment with heparin before angioplasty was associated with high success (61% vs. 94%; $p < .05$) and lower abrupt closure rates (33% vs. 6%; $p < .05$) than was proceeding immediately to angioplasty without pretreatment.[83] In a randomized double-blind study of platelet inhibition with c7E3 administered 24–48 h before angioplasty, pretreatment with c7E3 was associated with a reduction in acute myocardial infarction, from 9.4% to 4.4%.[57]

Information about the timing of angioplasty for postinfarction angina can be obtained from serial angiographic studies after thrombolytic therapy. Globular filling defects, present initially at angiography in patients with postinfarction angina, may disappear at a second angiographic study 2–10 days after streptokinase and heparin therapy.[84] In 14 of 98 patients with significant stenoses during an emergency coronary arteriogram performed for acute myocardial infarction, insignificant lesions were observed 1 week later.[85] Deferring angioplasty and administering antithrombotic therapy with heparin or c7E3 may thus prove to be superior to angioplasty without pretreatment in patients with unstable angina and large globular filling defects seen on initial angiography.

Patients With Saphenous Vein Bypass Grafts

The optimal timing of interventional therapy for thrombotic lesions in bypass grafts is difficult to define. Delays in definitive treatment often lead to total thrombotic occlusion (Fig. 43–4), which is frustratingly resistant to therapy. In 107 patients with occluded bypass grafts (64% with rest angina),[86] an infusion of urokinase and angioplasty resulted in patency in 74 patients (69%) but was associated with a high incidence of death (7%), Q wave myocardial infarction (5%), or stroke (3%). Graft patency at 6 months was documented in only 16 patients. Patients with unstable angina associated with subtotally occluded bypass grafts thus require prompt action to avoid progression to graft occlusion.

In the Second Coronary Angioplasty Versus Excisional Atherectomy Trial (CAVEAT-II),[87] 305 patients (89% with unstable angina) were randomized to treatment with directional atherectomy or balloon angioplasty. The acute rates of death (2.0% vs. 1.9%) and myocardial infarction (17.4% vs. 11.5%) were similar for both treatments, but the rate of distal embolization was higher for directional atherectomy (13.4% vs. 5.1%; p = .01). Stenting for vein graft lesions in 589 patients (72% with unstable angina) was associated with a low rate of major ischemic complications (2.9%) or stent thrombosis (1.4%).[88] Thus when the decision is made to proceed with angioplasty for saphenous vein graft lesions, a treatment plan often involving stenting and possibly IIb/IIIa receptor blockers should be instituted promptly to reduce the risk of graft occlusion or embolization (Fig. 43–5).

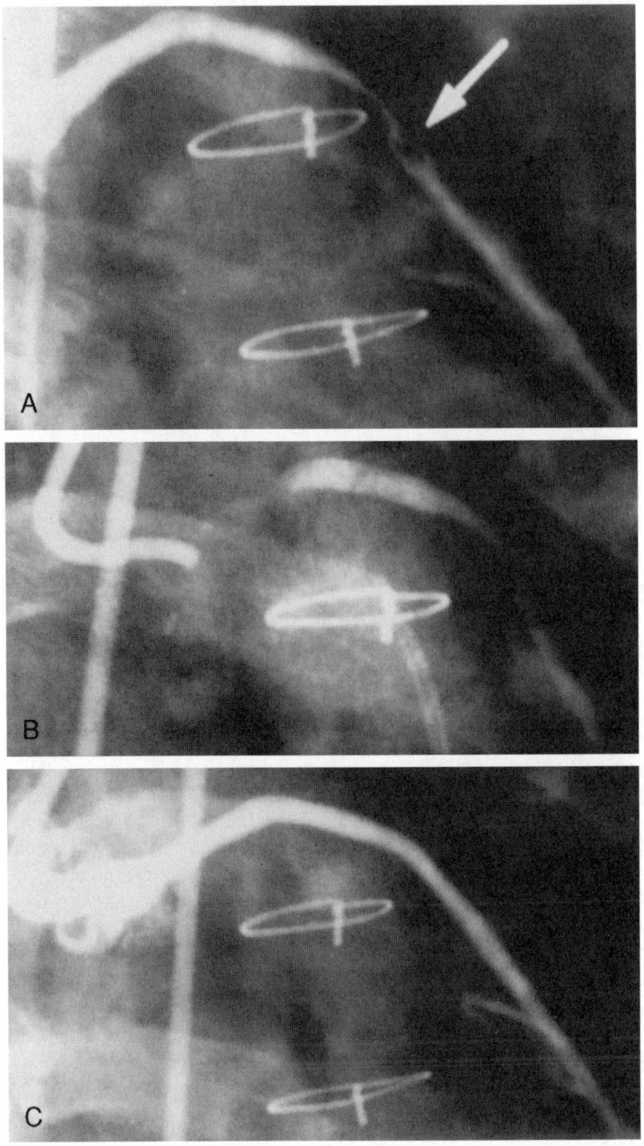

Figure 43–4. Delay in treatment of saphenous vein graft lesion. *A,* A 56-year-old man presented with rest pain and anterior ST depression associated with a filling defect in an 11-year-old saphenous vein graft to the left anterior descending artery (*arrow*). *B,* A strategy of prolonged anticoagulation therapy followed by angioplasty was considered, but the patient developed rest pain associated with ST depression and reduced flow in the graft despite a therapeutic activated partial thromboplastin time of 64 sec. *C,* Emergency balloon dilatation and stent implantation was required to achieve an adequate result.

Procedural Outcome of Angioplasty Performed for Unstable Angina

Despite the increased proportion of patients with advanced age and multivessel disease in several large angioplasty series,[51, 89–92] procedural success has improved (Table 43–3). The assessment of procedural outcome for the specific subgroup of patients with unstable angina, however, is more difficult to define.

Although the term "unstable angina" was originally introduced 25 years ago to denote a syndrome whose risk to the patient is intermediate between that of stable angina and acute myocardial infarction,[93, 94] the diagnosis of unstable angina has been increasingly applied to a wide range of clinical syndromes[11] ranging from low-risk presentations consisting of atypical chest pain at rest and no significant coronary stenoses to high-risk presentations consisting of postinfarction angina and hemodynamic compromise.[95] For example, patients with restenosis after a prior coronary intervention are often diagnosed as having "unstable angina." Although such patients present with "crescendo" or "new-onset" angina in relation to their immediate postintervention asymptomatic status, it is clear that these patients experience a better prognosis when treated with repeat intervention than do patients with stable angina and no prior angioplasty.[96–99]

Several studies have revealed that the outcome of angioplasty performed for unstable angina is determined by the severity and acuity of clinical presentation,[100] baseline clinical characteristics such as patient age,[77] and angiographic features such as lesion complexity.[77, 101] A gradient of success and complication rates is seen across the spectrum of patients with unstable angina.[100] The success rates (Fig. 43–6) are approximately 85% for patients with refractory unstable angina,[101–108] 88% for patients with postinfarction angina,[82, 87, 109–114] 89% for patients with unstable angina stabilized on medical therapy,[82, 106, 115–117] 92% for patients with stable angina,[90, 118–123] and 98% for patients undergoing angioplasty for restenosis.[96–99] The complication rates vary reciprocally across these groups of patients. The rates of acute myocardial infarction after angioplasty (Fig. 43–7) are approximately 6.3% for patients with refractory unstable angina,[101–108] 6.3% for patients with postinfarction angina,[82, 87, 109–114] 5.1% for patients with unstable angina stabilized on medical therapy,[82, 106, 115–117] 1.6% for patients with stable angina,[90, 118–123] and 1% for patients undergoing angioplasty for symptomatic restenosis.[96–99] Thus, the various pathophysiologic factors underlying the coronary syndromes, ranging from symptomatic restenosis to the acute coronary syndromes, are associated with a range of angioplasty-related complications that spans almost an order of magnitude.

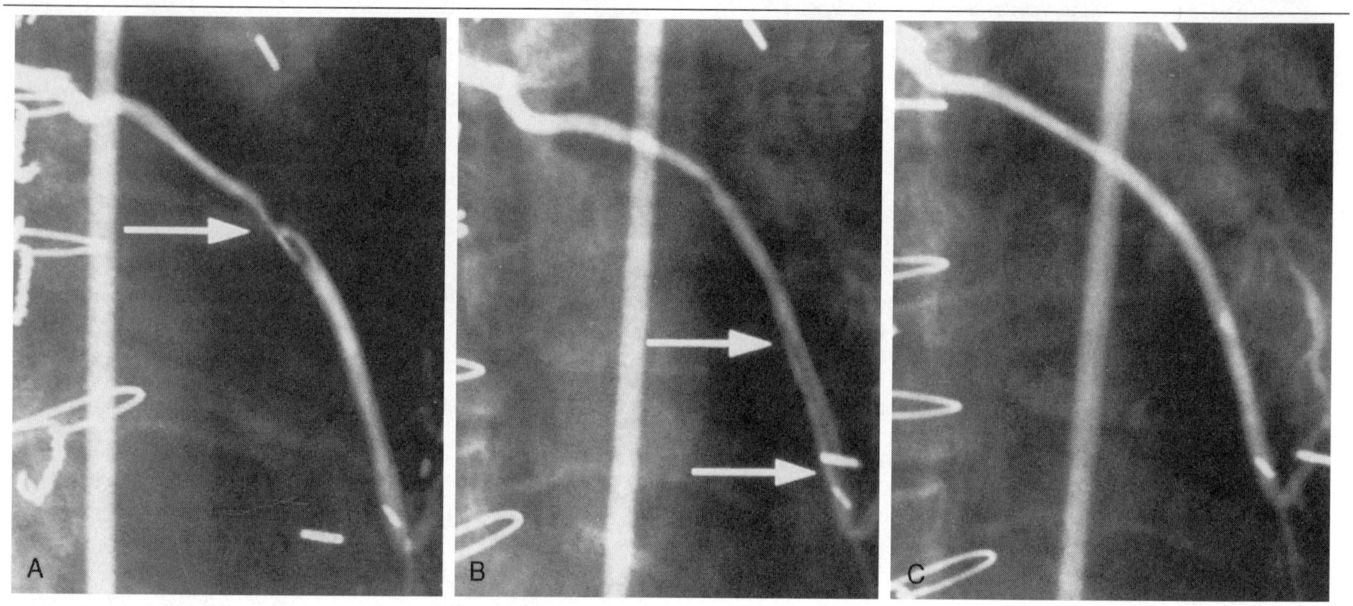

Figure 43–5. Embolization in a saphenous vein graft. *A,* A 52-year-old woman presented with unstable angina associated with a complex lesion (*arrow*) in the midportion of the graft to the left anterior descending artery. Angioplasty was successful in dilating the target lesion, but embolization of thrombus occurred (*B, arrows*), requiring additional heparin and repeat balloon inflations to achieve a good result (*C*).

The electrocardiographic changes associated with ischemic rest pain also have important predictive value. Patients with unstable angina and ST segment elevations have a worse prognosis than those with ST depressions.[124] Patients with unstable angina associated with electrocardiographic changes are more likely than those with stable angina to have thrombus detectable by histologic examination of atherectomy specimens.[31] Nevertheless, in a series of patients with unstable angina and ST elevations, the initial success rate of coronary angioplasty was 87%, and there were no deaths or incidences of urgent coronary bypass surgery, although two patients (13%) sustained a myocardial infarction.[125]

Other predictors of procedural outcome in patients with unstable angina undergoing angioplasty have been evaluated in the Heparin Registry.[77] A total of 386 consecutive patients with unstable angina undergoing coronary angioplasty of 487 lesions with conventional balloon angioplasty were evaluated at nine clinical centers in North America. Strong predictors of any complication (i.e., death, myocardial infarction, emergency bypass surgery, or abrupt vessel closure) included age (OR = 1.04; 95% confidence interval 1.02–1.07; for each additional year of age, $p < .001$), number of diseased vessels (OR = 1.58; 95% confidence interval 1.16–2.15; per additional vessel, $p = .012$), the number of lesions treated (OR = 1.72; 95% confidence interval 1.11–2.66; $p = .014$), and angiographic evidence of filling defects preceding angioplasty (OR = 3.3; 95% confidence interval 1.11–9.75).[77] Thus, the outcome of PTCA performed for unstable angina is influenced by a combination of clinical, angiographic, and procedural variables. This suggests that PTCA performed for lesions associated with filling defects or for more than one lesion at the time of the procedure carries an increased risk of complication.

Filling Defects

Angiographic evidence of thrombus is one of the most important determinants of the clinical success with interventional therapy for unstable angina (Table 43–4).[30, 78] In the 1985–1986 National Heart, Lung & Blood Institute (NHLBI) registry,[30] angioplasty performed for thrombus-containing lesions was associated with greater 5-year mortality than angioplasty performed without these angiographic findings (13.9% vs. 8.9%, respectively; $p < .05$). The success rate for balloon angioplasty ranged from 27% to 50%.[76, 77] Thus, the outcome of interventional therapy for unstable angina may be improved by identifying new treatments for lesions associated with filling defects. New strategies may involve delaying angioplasty so that prolonged therapy with heparin and aspirin or novel anticoagulation regimens may be used (see Timing of Angioplasty section).

TABLE 43–3. INCREASING INCIDENCE OF UNSTABLE ANGINA IN LARGE STUDIES OF ANGIOPLASTY

	NHLB-II[89]	NHLBI-II[89]	Hirulog[51]	Myler et al[90]*	Topol et al. (CAVEAT)[91]†	Wolfe et al.[92]
Inclusive years	1977–1981	1985–1986	1991–1992	1990–1992	1991–1992	1992
Number of patients	1155	1802	258	533	500	591
Average age (y)	54	58	57	61	59	61
Unstable angina (%)	37	49	44	58	70	65
Multivessel CAD (%)	25	53	20	53	35	55
Success (%)‡	61	78	89	92	79	87

*No core angiographic laboratory.
†Data only for patients undergoing balloon angioplasty in the Coronary Angioplasty Versus Excisional Atherectomy Trial.
‡Success = <50% residual stenosis or 20% improvement in target lesion, as assessed in a core angiographic laboratory, without major complication.

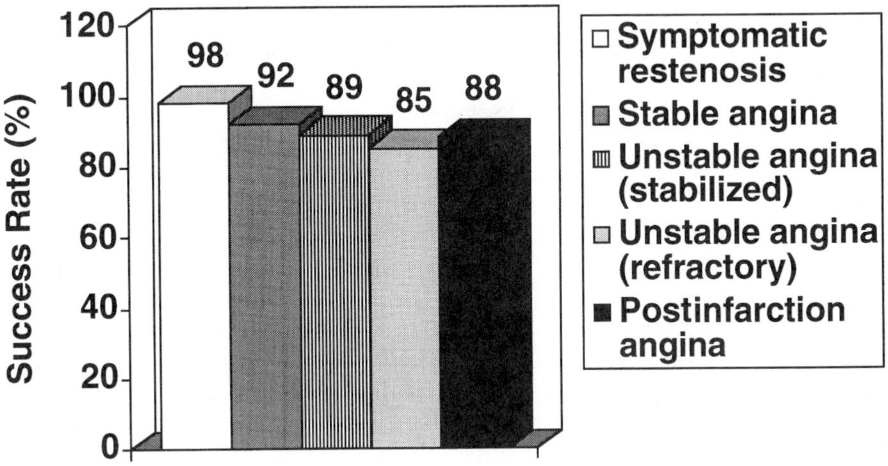

Figure 43–6. Success rates for angioplasty performed for unstable angina. The success rates are influenced by the severity and acuity of the clinical presentation. (Data from de Feyter PJ, Serruys PW: Percutaneous transluminal coronary angioplasty for unstable angina. *In* Topol EJ [ed]: Textbook of Interventional Cardiology, pp 272–291. Philadelphia: WB Saunders, 1994.)

Abrupt Vessel Closure

Abrupt vessel closure continues to be a common and serious problem despite the introduction of perfusion balloon angioplasty, coronary stenting, and novel anticoagulant regimens. Abrupt vessel closure is attributed to a combination of vessel dissection and thrombus formation.[92, 126] In a retrospective study of 1423 consecutive patients undergoing elective angioplasty between 1986 and 1988, abrupt vessel closure developed in 104 patients (7.3%).[127] The rate of fatal outcome was 6%, that of myocardial infarction was 36%, and that of emergency bypass surgery was 30%. Multivariable analysis identified that unstable angina increased the likelihood of abrupt vessel closure almost twofold.[127] In the 1985–1986 NHLBI Registry,[128] abrupt vessel closure developed in 9.9% of patients with unstable angina.

Strategies for the management of patients with abrupt vessel closure involve the use of several interventional devices. Although repeat balloon dilatation is the most common strategy, other strategies include prolonged balloon inflation with a perfusion balloon catheter,[129] directional coronary atherectomy for inadequate dilatation, use of adjunctive thrombolytic therapy, or placement of intracoronary stents.[73, 130] Whereas it is reasonable to conclude that the second-line devices are superior to conventional balloon angioplasty for the treatment of abrupt vessel closure, it is difficult to identify

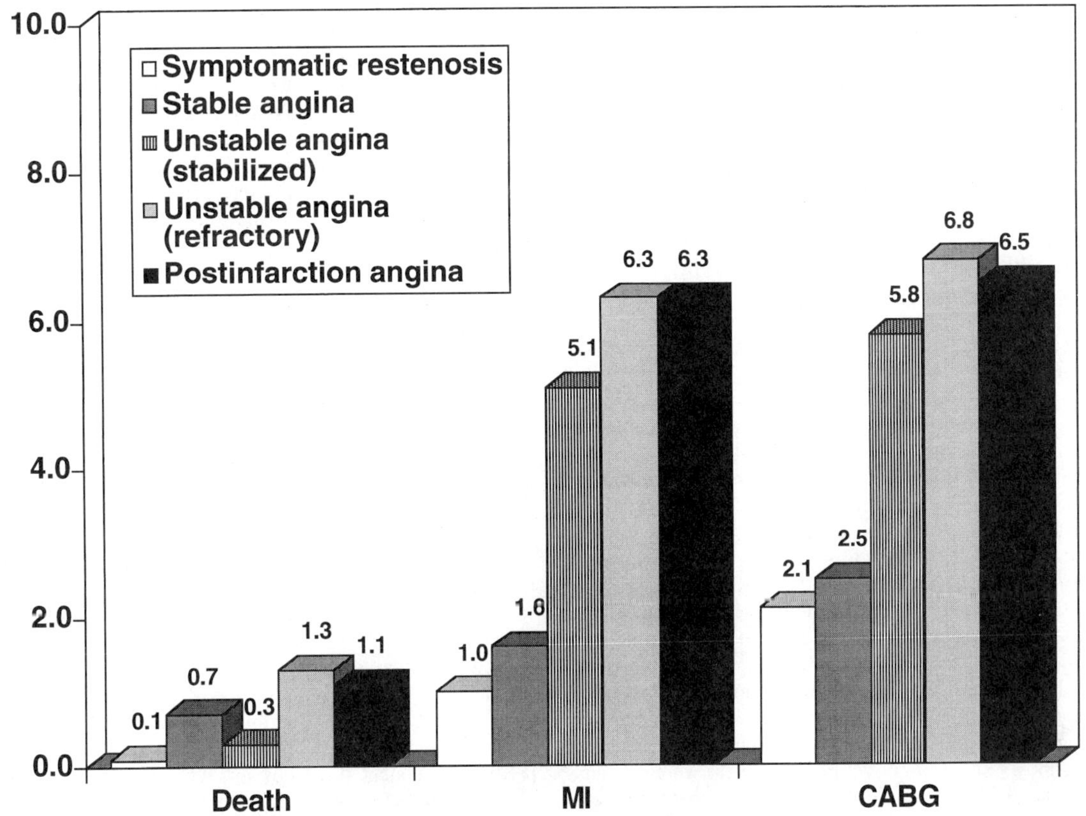

Figure 43–7. Complication rates for angioplasty performed for unstable angina. The incidence of death, myocardial infarction (MI), and emergency coronary artery bypass graft (CABG) are influenced by the type and severity of unstable angina. (Data from de Feyter PJ, Serruys PW: Percutaneous transluminal coronary angioplasty for unstable angina. *In* Topol EJ [ed]: Textbook of Interventional Cardiology, pp 272–291. Philadelphia: WB Saunders, 1994.)

TABLE 43–4. INTERVENTIONAL APPROACHES FOR LESIONS ASSOCIATED WITH FILLING DEFECTS

Device	No. of Patients	Thrombus Definition	Success	Death	MI	CABG	AVC
Balloon[77]	14	FD/CR	7 (50%)	2 (14%)	2 (14%)	0 (0%)	3 (21%)
Balloon[30]	82	FD	NR	NR	NR	5 (6%)	NR
Balloon[78]	48	FD/CR	NR	NR	NR	NR	20 (11%)
Balloon[76]	15	FD	7 (27%)	NR	NR	11 (73%)	11 (73%)
Excimer laser[79]	12	FD/CR	7 (57%)	0 (0%)	4 (33%)	0 (0%)	2 (17%)
Transluminal extraction atherectomy[74]	91	FD/haziness	70 (77%)	6 (7%)	4 (4%)	11 (12%)	NR
Gianturco-Roubin stent[73]	19	FD	12 (63%)	2 (10%)	4 (21%)	NR	NR

Abbreviations: AVC, abrupt vessel closure; CABG, coronary artery bypass graft; CR, contrast retention; FD, filling defect; MI, myocardial infarction; NR, not reported.

which of the devices is the superior one. In a prospective, nonrandomized evaluation of treatments for acute closure, defined as reduced TIMI flow associated with ischemic chest pain and electrocardiographic changes, 61 patients were treated with a perfusion balloon and 34 patients were treated with a coronary stent.[131] Although the procedural success rate (70% vs. 94%; $p = .02$) and emergency bypass rate (21% vs. 0%; $p < .001$) favored stenting, this factor was offset by subacute stent thrombosis leading to death in 3 patients (0% vs. 8%; $p = .05$) or rehospitalization (0% vs. 22%, $p < .001$). At 3-month follow-up, there was no difference in event-free survival between the two groups.[131] In the recent experience from the Hirulog Angioplasty Study,[52] abrupt vessel closure occurred in 378 of 4098 patients (9.2%). Patients treated with stents had lower rates of emergency bypass (10% vs. 19%; $p = .01$) and major ischemic complications or repeat revascularization at 6 months (54% vs. 71%; $p < .001$) than did matched patients treated with repeat balloon angioplasty.[132]

Culprit-Vessel Angioplasty

In an effort to reduce the consequences of abrupt vessel closure during interventional therapy for unstable angina, several studies have recommended the strategy of culprit-vessel angioplasty in patients with unstable angina and multivessel disease. Identification of the culprit lesion depends on the results of electrocardiography, myocardial perfusion scanning, or coronary angiography. Lesions associated with unstable angina have complex angiographic morphology or are associated with filling defects.[16] Quantitatively, lesions responsible for unstable angina are severe but not totally occluded. Only 8% of patients undergoing angioplasty for unstable angina had a total occlusion identified as the culprit lesion in the Heparin Registry.[77]

The success of the approach of culprit-vessel angioplasty has been evaluated in several studies. One study[133] compared the culprit-vessel strategy with a multivessel approach for 153 patients with unstable angina. Angioplasty of the ischemia-related artery alone in 43 patients with multivessel disease and unstable angina was associated with an 88% success rate, 12% risk of emergency coronary artery bypass surgery, and 9% incidence of myocardial infarction. These results were not different from those in a group of 111 patients with unstable angina who had angioplasty for single-vessel coronary artery disease. However, recurrence of angina and noninvasive evidence of provocable ischemia was greater in the multivessel disease group. In a prospective, randomized study of 43 patients comparing culprit vessel angioplasty with multivessel angioplasty for patients with unstable angina, event-free survival rates at 1 year were similar between the two treatment groups.[134] The results of these studies suggest that if a culprit lesion can be identified, angioplasty targeted to that site can be undertaken. Because the major limitation of culprit-vessel angioplasty is incomplete revascularization, symptoms may recur. If angina recurs, a staged angioplasty procedure can be performed.

The strategy of culprit-vessel angioplasty can be further refined by an assessment of the patient's overall risk. The strategy of culprit-vessel angioplasty is recommended for patients who are at increased risk for the likelihood or consequences of abrupt vessel closure. Patients at increased risk are those with refractory unstable angina, postinfarction angina, or other high-risk clinical variables such as decreased left ventricular function.

Use of Second-Generation Interventional Devices

Although it was anticipated that the success and complication rates of balloon angioplasty for unstable angina would be improved by alternative interventional devices that ablate atherosclerotic plaque and thrombus, the totality of information suggests that the overall incidence of ischemic complications has not been reduced by new devices. Directional atherectomy,[91, 135, 136] rotational atherectomy,[137] and excimer laser angioplasty[138, 139] have not been shown to reduce complication rates of interventional treatment. Although two randomized studies have shown that the elective use of coronary stenting has reduced the need for repeat intervention more than 2 weeks after the initial coronary intervention, patients with unstable angina were excluded in one study,[141] and procedural complications were not reduced in either study.[140, 141] Coronary stenting may be effective, however, for the management of acute coronary dissections complicating angioplasty for unstable angina.[132] In this setting, small residual dissections are frequently seen but have a good outcome and disappear at follow-up. Large residual dissections may have a good outcome if coronary flow is not impaired and no residual stenosis is seen.[142]

The presence of unstable angina may reduce the likelihood of success with new interventional devices. For example, in 100 consecutive patients with resting or postinfarction angina treated with directional atherectomy, complications resulting in death, Q wave myocardial infarction, or emergency bypass occurred in 7%, exceeding the rates for stable angina and new-onset angina.[143] In 142 patients treated with excimer laser angioplasty, the presence of thrombus was the strongest predictor of poor outcome.[79] With excimer laser angioplasty, the success rate was sharply reduced in lesions associated with filling defects vs. those without this finding (58% vs. 94%).[79]

In an early study evaluating the safety of the flexible coil stent, the presence of unstable angina was identified as one of the strongest predictors of stent thrombosis.[144] The use of coronary stenting has also been associated with increased complications in the presence of intracoronary thrombus.[73] In a multicenter registry, the use of the Gianturco-Roubin stent in the presence of intracoronary thrombus was associated with a success rate of 77%. Major complications included death in 7%, myocardial infarction in 4%, and need for emergency surgery in 12%.[73] Although transluminal extraction atherectomy has been proposed for the treatment of thrombus-containing lesions, this therapy has been associated with reduced success rates in thrombus-containing lesions and unstable angina[75] and is associated with a success rate of 63% in the presence of filling defects.[74] The use of rotational atherectomy is not recommended for the clinical setting of unstable angina or the angiographic finding of intracoronary thrombus.[137]

Although primary use of the second-generation devices cannot be recommended over conventional balloon angioplasty for the broad group of patients with unstable angina, the conditional use of certain devices is critical to the success of the angioplasty procedure in selected patients. For example, if balloon angioplasty results in an inadequate dilatation, other second-generation devices should be used to achieve an improved result. Directional coronary atherectomy should be considered as a salvage procedure in coronary arteries with a reference diameter larger than 2.75 mm if balloon dilatation is associated with residual stenosis of more than 50% or a focal type A or B dissection[145] that persists despite repeat balloon inflations (Fig. 43–8). Rotational atherectomy or excimer laser angioplasty can be used for undilatable calcific or fibrotic lesions in coronary arteries of any size,[146] but these angiographic features are not typically associated with unstable angina. Transluminal extraction atherectomy may be used if filling defects are present. If balloon dilatation results in a severe dissection with decreased coronary flow refractory to treatment with a perfusion balloon catheter, bailout coronary stenting should be strongly considered (see Fig. 43–4).

THROMBOLYTIC THERAPY FOR UNSTABLE ANGINA

Because coronary thrombus formation and abrupt vessel closure are increased in the setting of angioplasty performed for unstable angina, the use of thrombolytic therapy for unstable angina may be associated with improved outcome. This hypothesis has been tested in two large randomized trials.

In TIMI-IIIB,[6] 1473 patients seen within 24 h of ischemic chest discomfort at rest, representing either unstable or non–Q wave myocardial infarction, were randomized to compare tissue plasminogen activator (t-PA) plus heparin vs. heparin for initial therapy. In this setting, patients with unstable angina or non–Q wave myocardial infarction did not benefit from treatment with t-PA; fatal and nonfatal myocardial infarctions occurred more frequently in t-PA–treated patients than in controls. The rate of fatal or nonfatal myocardial infarction at 42 days after presentation was 7.4% for t-PA–treated patients and 4.9% for placebo-treated patients ($p = .04$).[2]

In the TAUSA Trial,[41] 469 patients with resting angina were randomized to treatment with placebo or intracoronary urokinase in two doses: 250,000 units of urokinase was used during the randomization phase in 257 patients, and 500,000 units of urokinase was used in 212 patients. Although the angiographic end point of thrombus showed a trend toward reduction with urokinase compared with placebo (13.8% vs. 18%), the incidence of abrupt vessel closure was increased with the adjunctive use of urokinase (10.2% vs. 4.3%; $p < .02$). This was associated with an increase in occurrence of the clinical end points of recurrent ischemia, myocardial infarction, or emergency bypass surgery (12.9% vs. 6.3%; $p < .02$). The occurrence of angiographic and clinical end points was worse with urokinase in patients with unstable angina than in those with unstable angina after recent myocardial infarction.[41]

Thus, both studies found no benefit of thrombolytic therapy for patients with unstable angina. It is known that thrombolytic agents simultaneously exert clot-dissolving and procoagulant actions.[147, 148] Thrombolytic therapy exposes fibrin-associated thrombin, which in turn is a potent stimulus of rethrombosis. Thrombolytic therapy also activates platelets directly. The thrombi of patients with unstable angina appear to be grayish white on angioscopy[20] and are composed

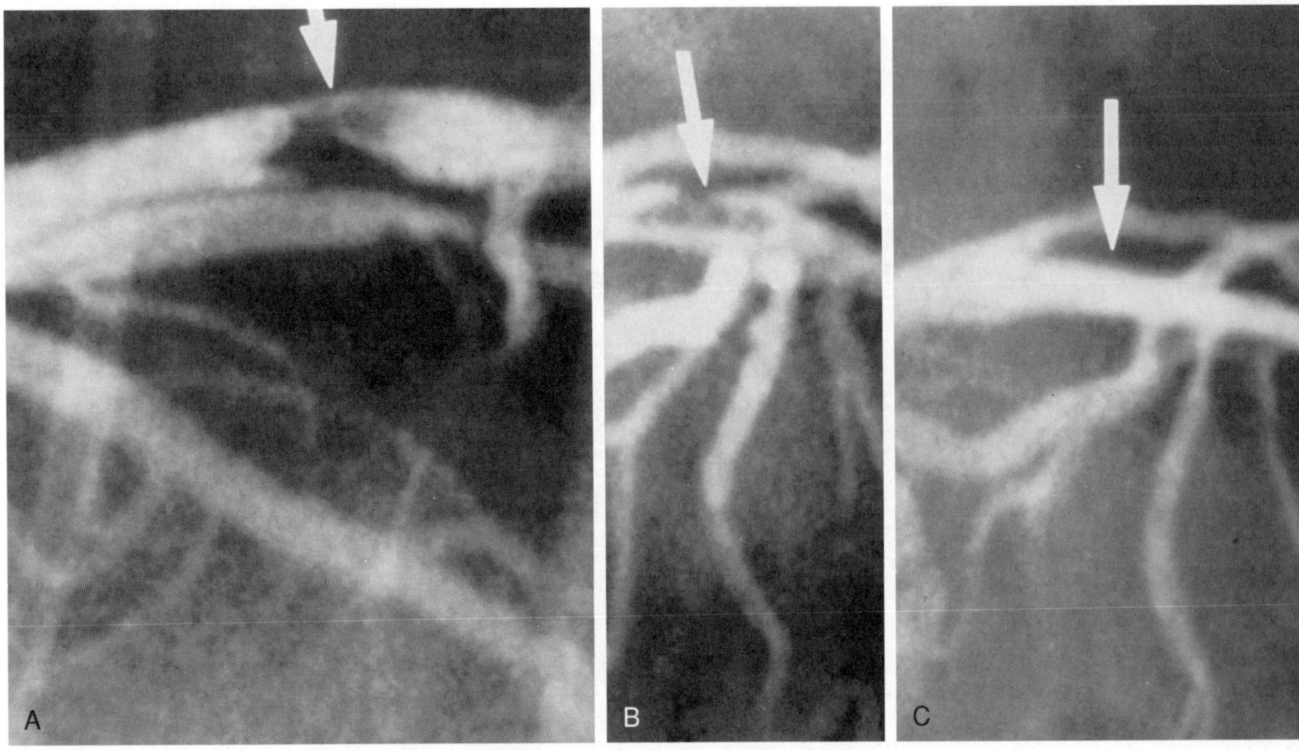

Figure 43–8. Salvage atherectomy for failed balloon angioplasty. *A,* Despite intensive anticoagulation, a 66-year-old patient developed postinfarction angina associated with hypotension, pulmonary congestion, and a thrombus-containing lesion in the proximal left anterior descending artery (*arrow*). *B,* After multiple prolonged inflations with a perfusion balloon catheter, the dilatation site (*arrow*) continued to degrade. *C,* The use of directional atherectomy was successful in achieving a large, stable lumen diameter (*arrow*).

predominantly of platelets rather than erythrocytes or fibrin. Platelet-rich thrombi are considerably more resistant to lysis by thrombolytic therapy than erythrocyte- or fibrin-rich thrombi. In addition, the subtotal occlusion of unstable angina provides a continued source of procoagulant substances for the activation of the blood coagulation system. It can be postulated that the consequences of the two opposing actions of thrombolytic therapy—clot-dissolving on the one hand and procoagulant on the other—result in a less favorable effect in patients with unstable angina who have subtotal occlusion and platelet-rich thrombi than in patients with evolving Q wave myocardial infarction and total coronary occlusion as a result of a fibrin-rich thrombus.

Although the two studies evaluating thrombolytic therapy used different protocols, they provide a consistent message about the limitations of adjunctive thrombolytic therapy for unselected patients with unstable angina. The success of angioplasty appears to be compromised when thrombolytic therapy is used for the broad range of patients presenting with unstable angina.[149] However, this does not rule out the potential importance of the selective use of adjunctive thrombolytic therapy for patients who have filling defects associated with the ischemia-related stenosis refractory to high-dose heparin (Fig. 43–9).

The selective use of adjunctive thrombolytic therapy associated with balloon angioplasty for unstable angina has been evaluated by several investigators. In one study, intracoronary streptokinase was used in 12 patients who experienced abrupt closure during balloon angioplasty for unstable angina.[113] Three patients had complete restoration of flow after intracoronary streptokinase alone. Four patients underwent repeat balloon angioplasty with a larger balloon, four patients required emergency bypass surgery (with one death), and one patient received conservative therapy for a persistently occluded vessel complicated by myocardial infarction. In a separate study, the selective use of intracoronary urokinase was evaluated in 10 patients with unstable angina who developed flow-limiting thrombus formation during angioplasty.[150] Intracoronary urokinase in a mean dose of 141,000 units (range, 100,000–250,000 units) and repeat balloon angioplasty were successful in restoring flow and relieving ischemia in 9 of 10 patients. No patient experienced acute myocardial infarction, needed bypass surgery, or had clinical or angiographic evidence of reocclusion.

For patients requiring immediate interventional treatment for unstable angina, it is reasonable to consider the use of intracoronary thrombolytic agents when large (>5-mm) intraluminal filling defects are encountered. A significant dissection, however, should be considered a contraindication to the use of thrombolytic agents because of the risk of lumen compromise from a mural hematoma. If adjunctive thrombolytic therapy is used, the recommended dose of intracoronary urokinase is a bolus dose of 50,000 units followed by 20,000 units/min for a total dose of 250,000 to 500,000 units. This approach may also be helpful for patients with thrombus-containing lesions in saphenous vein grafts.

RESTENOSIS

Patients undergoing angioplasty for unstable angina appear to have a greater risk of subsequent restenosis than patients with stable angina.[151] In patients undergoing double-vessel angioplasty in the setting of unstable angina, restenosis was seen in 67% of the stenoses identified as the culprit lesion responsible for the unstable syndrome but in only 32% of the nonculprit stenoses,[152] suggesting that local lesion-related factors such as thrombus or inflammatory cells are determinants of the high rates of restenosis in unstable angina. The angiographic risk factors for restenosis in unstable angina were analyzed in another study.[153] The lesion characteristics that predicted restenosis by multivariable analysis included the presence of luminal irregularities (complex lesion) and decreased TIMI flow. Other studies have identified the presence of collateral vessels, ST segment depression, multivessel disease, stenosis in the left anterior descending artery, and history of recent onset of symptoms as risk factors for restenosis after angioplasty performed for unstable angina.[101]

EMERGENCY BYPASS SURGERY FOR UNSTABLE ANGINA

For patients with left main coronary artery or three-vessel coronary artery disease, especially for those with left ventricular dysfunction, bypass surgery is the preferred method of treatment.[63] For patients with severe two-vessel coronary artery disease involving the proximal left anterior descending artery, coronary artery bypass surgery

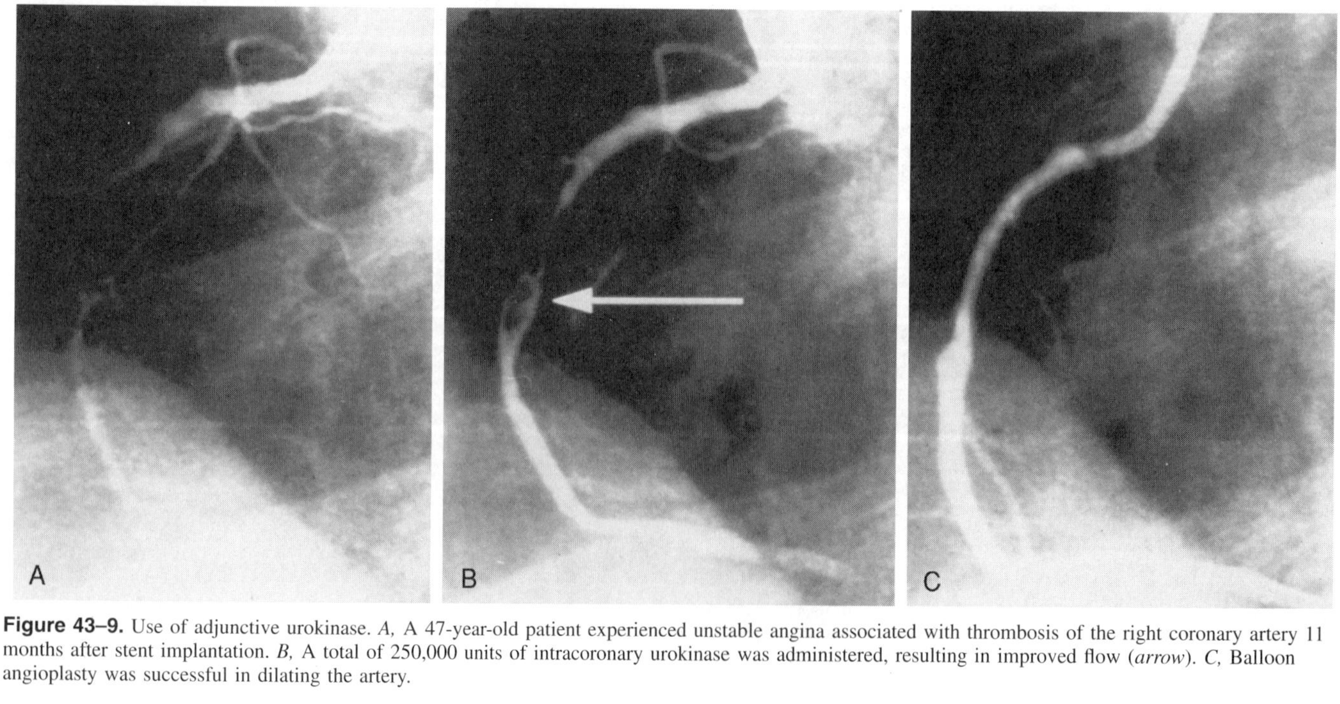

Figure 43–9. Use of adjunctive urokinase. *A,* A 47-year-old patient experienced unstable angina associated with thrombosis of the right coronary artery 11 months after stent implantation. *B,* A total of 250,000 units of intracoronary urokinase was administered, resulting in improved flow (*arrow*). *C,* Balloon angioplasty was successful in dilating the artery.

may offer a long-term survival advantage over angioplasty.[154] Because as many as 46% of patients with unstable angina are referred for coronary artery bypass surgery,[66] the catheterization and interventional team must work closely with their surgical colleagues. In selected patients, a sequential perfusion strategy of coronary angioplasty and urgent bypass surgery may be used to treat refractory unstable angina associated with extensive coronary artery disease. The use of angioplasty does not necessarily rule out the planned, coordinated use of bypass surgery for such patients. Instead, careful coordination between cardiologists and surgeons may permit successful implementation of a sequential revascularization strategy for patients with unstable angina associated with unprotected left main disease, severe three-vessel coronary artery disease, chronic total occlusions not amenable to angioplasty yet supplying viable myocardium, or severe coronary artery disease and impaired left ventricular function.

CONCLUSIONS

Patients at increased risk for complications of unstable angina should undergo coronary arteriography to determine whether they are candidates for revascularization therapy with conventional balloon angioplasty, coronary stenting, or other approaches. Thrombolytic therapy is not routinely recommended for patients with unstable angina, but newer antiplatelet agents such as c7E3 may reduce the likelihood of complications of interventional therapy for severe unstable angina. Improved methods are urgently needed, however, for more accurate identification of high-risk clinical and angiographic characteristics and for improved management of patients with unstable angina.

REFERENCES

1. Plotnick GD: Approach to the management of unstable angina. Am Heart J 1979; 98:243–255.
2. Silverman KJ, Grossman W: Angina pectoris: natural history and strategies for evaluation and management. N Engl J Med 1984; 310:1712–1717.
3. Williams DO, Riley RS, Singh AK, et al: Evaluation of the role of coronary angioplasty in patients with unstable angina pectoris. Am Heart J 1981; 102:1–9.
4. Faxon DP, Weber VJ, Haudenschild C, et al: Acute effects of transluminal angioplasty in three experimental models of atherosclerosis. Atherosclerosis 1982; 2:125–133.
5. Steele PM, Chesebro JH, Stanson AW, et al: Balloon angioplasty: natural history of the pathophysiologic response to injury in the pig model. Circ Res 1985; 57:105–112.
6. Lam JYT, Chesebro JH, Steele PM, et al: Deep arterial injury during experimental angioplasty: relation to a positive indium-111-labeled platelets scintigram, quantitative platelet deposition and mural thrombosis. J Am Coll Cardiol 1986; 8:1380–1386.
7. Badimon L, Badimon JJ, Turitto VT, et al: Platelet thrombus formation on collagen type I: a model of deep vessel injury: influence of blood rheology, von Willebrand factor, and blood coagulation. Circulation 1988; 78:1431–1442.
8. Heras M, Chesebro JH, Penny WJ, et al: Effects of thrombin inhibition on the development of acute platelet-thrombus deposition during angioplasty in pigs: heparin versus recombinant Hirudin, a specific thrombin inhibitor. Circulation 1989; 79:657–665.
9. Fuster V, Badimon L, Badimon JJ, et al: The pathophysiology of coronary artery disease and the acute coronary syndromes. N Engl J Med 1992; 326:242–250, 310–318.
10. Fernandez-Ortiz A, Badimon JJ, Falk E, et al: Characterization of the relative thrombogenicity of atherosclerotic plaque components: implications for consequences of plaque rupture. J Am Coll Cardiol 1994; 23:1562–1569.
11. Wilcox JN, Smith KN, Schwartz SM, et al: Localization of tissue factor in the normal vessel wall and in the atherosclerotic plaque. Proc Natl Acad Sci USA 1989; 86:2839–2843.
12. Coughlin SR, Vu THH, Hung DR, et al: Characterization of a functional thrombin receptor. J Clin Invest 1992; 89:351–355.
13. Coller BS, Peerschke EI, Scudder LE, et al: A murine monoclonal antibody that completely blocks the binding of fibrinogen to platelets produces a thrombasthenic-like state in normal platelets and binds to glycoprotein IIb and/or IIIa. J Clin Invest 1983; 72:325–338.
14. Holmes DR, Hartzler GO, Smith HC. et al: Coronary artery thrombosis in patients with unstable angina. Br Heart J 1981; 45:411–416.
15. Freeman MR, Williams AE, Chisholm RJ, et al: Intracoronary thrombus and complex morphology in unstable angina. Relation of timing of angiography and in-hospital cardiac events. Circulation 1989; 80:17–23.
16. Ambrose JA, Winters SL, Stern A, et al: Angiographic morphology and the pathogenesis of unstable angina pectoris. J Am Coll Cardiol 1985; 5:609–614.
17. Ahmed WH, Bittl JA, Braunwald E: Relation between clinical presentation and angiographic findings in unstable angina pectoris, and comparison with that in stable angina. Am J Cardiol 1993; 72:544–550.
18. Gotoh K, Minamino T, Katoh O, et al: The role of intracoronary thrombus in unstable angina: angiographic assessment and thrombolytic therapy during ongoing anginal attacks. Circulation 1988; 77:526–34.
19. Silva JA, Escobar A, Collins TJ, et al: Unstable angina: a comparison of angioscopic findings between diabetic and nondiabetic patients. Circulation 1995; 92:1731–1736.
20. Mizuno K, Satomura K, Miyamoto A, et al: Angioscopic evaluation of coronary-artery thrombi in acute coronary syndromes. N Engl J Med 1992; 326:287–291.
21. de Feyter PJ, Ozaki Y, Baptista J, et al: Ischemia-related lesion characteristics in patients with stable or unstable angina: a study with intracoronary angioscopy and ultrasound. Circulation 1995; 92:1408–1413.
22. Falk E. Unstable angina with fatal outcome: dynamic coronary thrombosis leading to infarction and/or sudden death. Circulation 1983; 71:699–708.
23. Davies MJ, Thomas AC: Plaque-fissuring—the cause of acute myocardial infarction, sudden ischaemic death, and crescendo angina. Br Heart J 1985; 53:363–373.
24. Davies MJ, Thomas AC, Knapman PA, et al: Intramyocardial platelet aggregation in patients with unstable angina suffering ischemic cardiac death. Circulation 1986; 73:418–427.
25. Lendon CL, Davies MJ, Born GV, et al: Atherosclerotic plaque caps are locally weakened when macrophage density is increased. Atherosclerosis 1991; 87:87–90.
26. Flugelman MY, Virmani R, Correa R, et al: Smooth muscle cell abundance and fibroblast growth factors in coronary lesions of patients with nonfatal unstable angina. Circulation 1993; 88:2493–2500.
27. van der Wal AC, Becker AE, van der Loos CM, et al: Site of intimal rupture or erosion of thrombosed coronary atherosclerotic plaques is characterized by an inflammatory process irrespective of the dominant plaque morphology. Circulation 1994; 89:36–44.
28. The TIMI-IIIA Investigators: Early effects of tissue-type plasminogen activator added to conventional therapy on the culprit coronary lesion in patients presenting with ischemia cardiac pain at rest: results of the Thrombolysis in Myocardial Ischemia (TIMI-IIIA) Trial. Circulation 1993; 87:38–52.
29. The TIMI-IIIB Investigators: Effects of tissue plasminogen activator and a comparison of early invasive and conservative strategies in unstable angina and non-Q-wave myocardial infarction. Circulation 1994; 89:1545–1556.
30. Bentivoglio LG, Detre K, Yeh W, et al: Outcome of percutaneous transluminal coronary angioplasty in subsets of unstable angina pectoris: a report of the 1985-1986 National Heart, Lung, and Blood Institute Percutaneous Transluminal Coronary Angioplasty Registry. J Am Coll Cardiol 1994; 24:1195–1206.
31. Sullivan E, Kearney M, Isner JM, et al: Pathology of unstable angina: analysis of biopsies obtained by directional coronary atherectomy. J Thromb Thrombolys 1994; 1:63–71.
32. Annex BH, Denning SM, Channon KM, et al: Differential expression of tissue factor protein in directional atherectomy specimens from patients with stable and unstable coronary syndromes. Circulation 1995; 91:619–622.
33. Farb A, Virmani R, Atkinson JB, et al: Plaque morphology and pathologic changes in arteries from patients dying after coronary balloon angioplasty. J Am Coll Cardiol 1990; 16:1421–1429.
34. Nobuyoshi M, Kimura T, Ohishi H, et al: Restenosis after percutaneous transluminal coronary angioplasty: pathologic observation in 20 patients. J Am Coll Cardiol 1991; 17:433–439.
35. Waller BF, Pinkerton CA, Orr CM, et al: Morphological observations late (>30 days) after clinically successful coronary balloon angioplasty. Circulation 1991; 81(suppl I):28–41.
36. Kakuta T, Currier J, Haudenschild C, et al: Differences in compensatory

vessel enlargement, not intimal formation, account for restenosis after angioplasty in the hypercholesterolemic rabbit model. Circulation 1994; 89:2809–2815.
37. Strauss BH, Chisholm RJ, Keeley FW, et al: Extracellular matrix remodeling after balloon angioplasty injury in a rabbit model of restenosis. Circ Res 1994; 75:650–658.
38. Merino A, Cohen M, Badimon JJ, et al: Synergistic action of severe wall injury and shear forces on thrombus formation in arterial stenosis: definition of a thrombotic shear rate threshold. J Am Coll Cardiol 1994; 24:1091–1094.
39. Badimon JJ, Badimon L, Turitto VT, et al: Platelet deposition at high shear rates is enhanced by high plasma cholesterol levels: an in vivo study in the rabbit model. Arterioscler Thromb 1991; 11:395–402.
40. Uchida Y, Hasegawa K, Kawamura K, et al: Angioscopic observation of the coronary luminal changes induced by percutaneous transluminal coronary angioplasty. Am Heart J 1989; 117:769–776.
41. Ambrose JA, Almeida OD, Sharma SK, et al: Adjunctive thrombolytic therapy during angioplasty for ischemic rest angina: results of the TAUSA Trial. Circulation 1994; 90:69–77.
42. Barnathan ES, Schwartz JS, Taylor L, et al: Aspirin and dipyridamole in the prevention of acute coronary thrombosis complicating coronary angioplasty. Circulation 1987; 76:125–134.
43. Block P, Myler R, Stertzer S, et al: Morphology after transluminal angioplasty in human beings. N Engl J Med 1981; 305:382–384.
44. Hirsh J, Fuster V: Guide to anticoagulant therapy. Part I: heparin. Circulation 1994; 89:1449–1468.
45. Young E, Prins M, Levine MN, et al: Heparin binding to plasma proteins, an important mechanism for heparin resistance. Thromb Haemost 1992; 67:639–643.
46. Hirsh J, van Aken WG, Gallus AS, et al: Heparin kinetics in venous thrombosis and pulmonary embolism. Circulation 1976; 53:691–695.
47. Eitzmann DT, Chi L, Saggin L, et al: Heparin neutralization by platelet-rich thrombi: role of platelet factor 4. Circulation 1994; 89:1523–1529.
48. Weitz JI, Hudoba M, Massel D, et al: Clot-bound thrombin is protected from inhibition by heparin-antithrombin III but is susceptible to inactivation by antithrombin III–independent inhibitors. J Clin Invest 1990; 86:385–391.
49. Lefkovits J, Topol EJ: Direct thrombin inhibitors in cardiovascular medicine (review). Circulation 1994; 90:1522–1536.
50. Cannon CP, McCabe CH, Henry TD, et al: A pilot trial of recombinant desulfatohirudin compared with heparin in conjunction with tissue-type plasminogen activator and aspirin for acute myocardial infarction: results of the Thrombolysis in Myocardial Infarction (TIMI) 5 Trial. J Am Coll Cardiol 1994; 23:993–1003.
51. Topol EJ, Bonan R, Jewitt D, et al: Use of a direct antithrombin, Hirulog, in place of heparin during coronary angioplasty. Circulation 1993; 87:1622–1629.
52. Bittl JA, Strony J, Brinker JA, et al: Treatment with bivalirudin (Hirulog) as compared with heparin during coronary angioplasty for unstable or post-infarction angina. N Engl J Med 1995; 333:764–769.
53. Serruys PW, Herrman J-PR, Simon R, et al: A comparison of hirudin with heparin in the prevention of restenosis after coronary angioplasty. N Engl J Med 1995; 333:757–763.
54. The EPIC Investigators: Use of a monoclonal antibody directed against the platelet glycoprotein IIb/IIIa receptor in high-risk coronary angioplasty. New Engl J Med 1994; 330:956–961.
55. Topol EJ, Califf RM, Weisman HF, et al: Randomised trial of coronary interventional with antibody against platelet IIb/IIIa integrin for reduction of clinical restenosis: results at six months. Lancet 1994; 343:881–886.
56. Lincoff AM, Tcheng JE, Bass TA, et al: A multicenter, randomized, double-blind pilot trial of standard versus low dose weight-adjusted heparin in patients treated with the platelet GP IIb/IIIa receptor antibody c7E3 during percutaneous coronary revascularization [Abstract]. J Am Coll Cardiol 1995; 25:80A.
56a. Lincoff AM: Evaluation of PTCA to Improve Long-Term Outcome by c7E3 Glycoprotein IIb/IIIa Receptor Blockade (EPILOG) [Abstract]. Presented at the Scientific Sessions of the American College of Cardiology, Orlando, FL, March 27, 1996.
57. Simoons ML: Refractory unstable angina: reduction of events by c7E3: the CAPTURE Study [Abstract]. Presented at the Scientific Sessions of the American College of Cardiology, Orlando, FL, March 25, 1996.
57a. Horrigan MCG, Tcheng JE, Califf RM, et al: Maximal benefit of integrelin platelet IIb/IIIa blockade 6–12 hours after therapy: results of the IMPACT-II Trial [Abstract]. J Am Coll Cardiol 1996; 27:55A.
58. King SB III: Administration of tirofiban (MK-0383) will reduce the incidence of adverse cardiac outcome following PTCA/PCA (RESTORE) [Abstract]. Presented at the Scientific Sessions of the American College of Cardiology, Orlando, FL, March 27, 1996.
59. Ellis SG, Roubin GS, Wilentz J, et al: Effect of 18- to 24-hour heparin administration for prevention of restenosis after uncomplicated coronary angioplasty. Am Heart J 1989; 117:777–782.
60. Schwartz L, Bourassa MG, Lesperance J, et al: Aspirin and dipyridamole in the prevention of restenosis after percutaneous transluminal coronary angioplasty. N Engl J Med 1988; 318:1714–1719.
61. Théroux P, Waters D, Lam J, et al: Reactivation of unstable angina after the discontinuation of heparin. N Engl J Med 1992; 327:141–145.
62. Braunwald E, Jones RH, Mark DB, et al: Diagnosing and managing unstable angina. Circulation 1994; 90:613–622.
63. Sharma GVRK, Deupree RH, Luchi RJ, et al: Identification of unstable angina patients who have favorable outcome with medical or surgical therapy (eight-year follow-up of the Veterans Administration Cooperative Study). Am J Cardiol 1994; 74:454–458.
64. Diver DJ, Bier JD, Ferreira PE, et al: Clinical and arteriographic characterization of patients with unstable angina without critical coronary arterial narrowing. Am J Cardiol 1994; 74:531–537.
65. Yusuf S, Wittes J, Friedman L: Overview of results of randomized clinical trials in heart disease. II. Unstable angina, heart failure, primary prevention with aspirin, and risk factor modification. JAMA 1988; 260:2259–2263.
66. Leeman DE, McCabe CH, Faxon DP, et al: Use of percutaneous transluminal coronary angioplasty and bypass surgery despite improved medical therapy for unstable angina pectoris. Am J Cardiol 1988; 61:38G–44G.
67. The TIMI Study Group: Comparison of invasive and conservative strategies after treatment with intravenous tissue plasminogen activator in acute myocardial infarction. Results of the thrombolysis in myocardial infarction (TIMI) phase II trial. N Engl J Med 1989; 320:618–627.
68. Levi M, Pascucci C, Agnelli G, et al: Effect on thrombus growth and thrombolysis of two types of osmolar contrast media in rabbits. Invest Radiol 1990; 25:533–535.
69. Ing JJ, Smith DC, Bull BS: Differing mechanisms of clotting inhibition by ionic and nonionic contrast agents. Radiology 1989; 172:345–348.
70. Rasuli P, McLeish WA, Hammond DI: Anticoagulant effects of contrast materials: in vitro study of iohexol, ioxaglate, and diatrizoate. Am J Roentgenol 1989; 152:309–311.
71. Gasparetti CM, Gonias SL, Gimple LW, et al: Platelet activation during coronary angioplasty in humans. Circulation 1993; 88:2728–2734.
72. Ellis SG, Topol EJ, Gallison L, et al: Predictors of success for coronary angioplasty performed for acute myocardial infarction. J Am Coll Cardiol 1988; 12:1407–1415.
73. Sutton JM, Ellis SG, Roubin GS, et al: Major clinical events after coronary stenting: The multicenter registry of acute and elective Gianturco-Roubin stent placement. Circulation 1994; 89:1126–1137.
74. Popma JJ, Leon MB, Mintz GS, et al: Results of coronary angioplasty using the transluminal extraction catheter. Am J Cardiol 1992; 70:1526–1532.
75. Safian RD, Grines CL, May MA, et al: Clinical and angiographic results of transluminal extraction coronary atherectomy in saphenous vein bypass grafts. Circulation 1994; 89:302–312.
76. Mabin TA, Holmes DR Jr, Smith HC, et al: Intracoronary thrombus: role in coronary occlusion complicating percutaneous transluminal coronary angioplasty. J Am Coll Cardiol 1985; 5:198–202.
77. Grassman ED, Leya F, Johnson SA, et al: Percutaneous transluminal coronary angioplasty for unstable angina: predictors of outcome in a multicenter study. J Thromb Thrombolys 1994; 1:73–78.
78. Ellis SG, Roubin GS, King SB III, et al: Angiographic and clinical predictors of acute closure after native vessel coronary angioplasty. Circulation 1988; 77:372–379.
79. Estella P, Ryan TJ Jr, Landzberg JS, et al: Excimer laser-assisted angioplasty for lesions containing thrombus. J Am Coll Cardiol 1993; 21:1550–1556.
80. Ohman EM, George BS, White CJ, et al: Use of aortic counterpulsation to improve coronary artery patency during acute myocardial infarction: results of a randomized trial. Circulation 1994; 90:792–799.
81. Laskey MA, Deutsch E, Barnathan E, et al: Influence of heparin therapy on percutaneous transluminal coronary angioplasty outcome in unstable angina pectoris. Am J Cardiol 1990; 65:1425–1429.
82. de Feyter PJ, Serruys PW, Soward A, et al: Coronary angioplasty for early postinfarction unstable angina. Circulation 1986; 74:1365–1370.
83. Laskey MA, Deutsch E, Hirshfeld JW Jr, et al: Influence of heparin therapy on percutaneous transluminal coronary angioplasty outcome in patients with coronary arterial thrombus. Am J Cardiol 1990; 65:179–182.
84. Davies SW, Marchant B, Lyons JP, et al: Coronary lesion morphology in acute myocardial infarction: demonstration of early remodeling after streptokinase treatment. J Am Coll Cardiol 1990; 16:1079–1086.

85. Topol EJ, Califf RM, George BS, et al: A randomized trial of immediate versus delayed elective angioplasty after intravenous tissue plasminogen activator in acute myocardial infarction. N Engl J Med 1987; 317:581–588.
86. Hartmann JR, McKeever LS, O'Neill WW, et al: Recanalization of chronically occluded aortocoronary saphenous vein bypass grafts with long-term, low dose direct infusion of urokinase (ROBUST): a serial trial. J Am Coll Cardiol 1996; 27:60–66.
87. Holmes DR Jr, Topol EJ, Califf RM, et al: A multicenter, randomized trial of coronary angioplasty versus directional atherectomy for patients with saphenous vein bypass graft lesions. CAVEAT-II Investigators. Circulation 1995; 91:1966–1974.
88. Wong SC, Baim DS, Schatz RS, et al: Immediate results and late outcomes after stent implantation in saphenous vein graft lesions: the multicenter U.S. Palmaz-Schatz Stent experience. J Am Coll Cardiol 1995; 26:704–712.
89. Detre K, Holubkov R, Kelsey S, et al: Percutaneous transluminal coronary angioplasty in 1985-1986 and 1977-1981. The National Heart, Lung, and Blood Institute Registry. N Engl J Med 1988; 318:265–270.
90. Myler RK, Shaw RE, Stertzer SH, et al: Lesion morphology and coronary angioplasty: current experience and analysis. J Am Coll Cardiol 1992; 19:1641–1652.
91. Topol EJ, Leya F, Pinkerton CA, et al: A comparison of balloon angioplasty with directional atherectomy in patients with coronary artery disease. N Engl J Med 1993; 329:221–227.
92. Wolfe MW, Roubin GS, Schweiger M, et al: Length of hospital stay and complications after percutaneous transluminal coronary angioplasty: clinical and procedural predictors. Circulation 1995; 92:311–319.
93. Conti CR, Greene B, Pitt B: Coronary surgery in unstable angina pectoris [Abstract]. Circulation 1971; 44(suppl II):154.
94. Fowler NO: "Preinfarctional" angina: a need for objective definition and for a controlled clinical trial of its management. Circulation 1971; 44:744–758.
95. Braunwald E: Unstable angina. A classification. Circulation 1989; 80:410–414.
96. Dimas AP, Grigera F, Arora RR, et al: Repeat coronary angioplasty as treatment for restenosis. J Am Coll Cardiol 1992; 19:1310–1314.
97. Weintraub WS, Ghazzal ZMB, Douglas JS, et al: Initial management and long-term clinical outcome of restenosis after initially successful percutaneous transluminal coronary angioplasty. Am J Cardiol 1992; 70:47–55.
98. Alfonso R, Macaya C, Iniquez A, et al: Repeat coronary angioplasty during the same angiographic diagnosis of coronary restenosis. Am Heart J 1990; 119:237–241.
99. Meier B, King SB III, Gruentzig AR, et al: Repeat coronary angioplasty. J Am Coll Cardiol 1984; 4:463–466.
100. de Feyter PJ, Serruys PW: Percutaneous transluminal coronary angioplasty for unstable angina. *In* Topol EJ (ed): Textbook of Interventional Cardiology, pp 274–291. Philadelphia: WB Saunders, 1994.
101. de Feyter PJ, Suryapranata H, Serruys PW, et al: Coronary angioplasty for unstable angina: immediate and late results in 200 consecutive patients with identification of risk factors for unfavorable early and late outcome. J Am Coll Cardiol 1988; 12:324–333.
102. Timmis AD, Griffin B, Crick JC, et al: Early percutaneous transluminal coronary angioplasty in the management of unstable angina. Int J Cardiol 1987; 14:25–31.
103. Thijs Plokker HW, Ernst SM, Bal ET, et al: Percutaneous transluminal coronary angioplasty in patients with unstable angina pectoris refractory to medical therapy: long-term clinical and angiographic results. Cath Cardiovasc Diagn 1988; 14:15–18.
104. Sharma B, Wyeth RP, Kilath GS, et al: Percutaneous transluminal coronary angioplasty of one vessel for refractory unstable angina pectoris: efficacy in single and multivessel disease. Br Heart J 1988; 59:280–286.
105. Perry RA, Seth A, Hunt A, et al: Coronary angioplasty in unstable angina and stable angina: a comparison of success and complications. Br Heart J 1988; 60:367–372.
106. Myler RK, Shaw RE, Stertzer SH, et al: Unstable angina and coronary angioplasty (review). Circulation 1990; 82(suppl II):88–95.
107. Morrison DA: Percutaneous transluminal coronary angioplasty for rest angina pectoris requiring intravenous nitroglycerin and intra-aortic balloon counterpulsation. Am J Cardiol 1990; 66:168–172.
108. Rupprecht HJ, Brennecke R, Kottmeyer M, et al: Short- and long-term outcome after percutaneous transluminal coronary angioplasty in patients with stable and unstable angina. Eur Heart J 1990; 11:964–969.
109. Holt GW, Sugrue DD, Bresnahan JF, et al: Results of percutaneous transluminal coronary angioplasty for unstable angina pectoris in patients 70 years of age and older. Am J Cardiol 1988; 61:994–997.
110. Gottlieb SO, Walford GD, Ouyang P, et al: Initial and late results of coronary angioplasty for early postinfarction unstable angina. Cath Cardiovasc Diagn 1987; 13:93–99.
111. Safian RD, Snyder LD, Snyder BA, et al: Usefulness of percutaneous transluminal coronary angioplasty for unstable angina pectoris after non-Q-wave acute myocardial infarction. Am J Cardiol 1987; 59:263–266.
112. Hopkins J, Savage M, Zalewski A, et al: Recurrent ischemia in the zone of prior myocardial infarction: result of coronary angioplasty of the infarct-related artery. Am Heart J 1988; 115:14–19.
113. Suryapranata H, Beatt K, de Feyter PJ, et al: Percutaneous transluminal coronary angioplasty for angina pectoris after a non-Q-wave acute myocardial infarction. Am J Cardiol 1988; 61:240–243.
114. TIMI Study Group: Phase II Trial: comparison of invasive and conservative strategies after treatment with intravenous tissue plasminogen activator in acute myocardial infarction. N Engl J Med 1989; 320:618–627.
115. Quigley PJ, Erwin J, Maurer BJ, et al: Percutaneous transluminal coronary angioplasty in unstable angina. Br Heart J 1986; 55:227–230.
116. Steffenino G, Meier B, Finci L, et al: Follow up results of treatment of unstable angina by coronary angioplasty. Br Heart J 1987; 57:416–419.
117. Stammen F, de Scheerder I, Glazier JJ, et al: Immediate and follow-up results of the conservative coronary angioplasty strategy for unstable angina pectoris. Am J Cardiol 1992; 69:1533–1537.
118. Bredlau CE, Roubin G, Leimgruber P, et al: In-hospital morbidity and mortality in patients undergoing elective coronary angioplasty. Circulation 1985; 72:1044.
119. Hartzler G: Complex coronary angioplasty: multivessel/multilesion dilatation. *In* Ischinger T (ed): Practice of Coronary Angioplasty, pp 250–267. New York, Springer-Verlag, 1986.
120. Holmes DR Jr, Holubkov R, Vlietstra RE, et al: Comparison of complications during percutaneous transluminal angioplasty from 1977 to 1981 and from 1985 to 1986: the National Heart, Lung, and Blood Institute Percutaneous Transluminal Coronary Angioplasty Registry. J Am Coll Cardiol 1988; 12:1149–1155.
121. Tuzcu EM, Simpfendorfer C, Badhwar K, et al: Determinants of primary success in elective percutaneous transluminal coronary angioplasty for significant narrowing of a single major coronary artery. Am J Cardiol 1988; 62:873–875.
122. de Feyter PJ, van den Brand M, Serruys PW: Increase of initial success and safety of single-vessel PTCA in 1371 patients: a seven-years' experience. J Intervent Cardiol 1988; 1:1–10.
123. O'Keefe JH Jr, Reeder GS, Miller GA, et al: Safety and efficacy of percutaneous transluminal coronary angioplasty performed at time of diagnostic catheterization compared with that performed at other times. Am J Cardiol 1989; 63:27–29.
124. Gerstenblith G, Ouyang P, Achuff SC, et al: Nifedipine in unstable angina: a double-blind, randomized trial. N Engl J Med 1982; 306:885–889.
125. de Feyter PJ, Serruys PW, van der Brand M, et al: Coronary angioplasty for treatment of unstable angina with transient marked ST-segment elevation. Eur Heart J 1987; 8:569–574.
126. Lincoff AM, Popma JJ, Ellis SG, et al: Abrupt vessel closure complicating coronary angioplasty: clinical, angiographic and therapeutic profile. J Am Coll Cardiol 1992; 19:926–935.
127. de Feyter PJ, van den Brand M, Jaarman G, et al: Acute coronary artery occlusion during and after percutaneous transluminal coronary angioplasty: frequency, prediction, clinical course, management, and follow-up. Circulation 1991; 83:927–936.
128. Detre KM, Holmes DR Jr, Holubkov R, et al: Incidence and consequences of periprocedural occlusion. The 1985–1986 National Heart, Lung, and Blood Institute Percutaneous Transluminal Coronary Angioplasty Registry. Circulation 1990; 82:739–750.
129. Jackman JD, Zidar JP, Tcheng JE, et al: Outcome after prolonged balloon inflations of >20 minutes for initially unsuccessful percutaneous transluminal coronary angioplasty. Am J Cardiol 1992; 69:1417–1421.
130. Roubin GS, Cannon AD, Agrawal SK, et al: Intracoronary stenting for acute and threatened closure complicating percutaneous transluminal coronary angioplasty. Circulation 1992; 85:916–927.
131. de Muinck ED, den Heijer P, van Dijk RB, et al: Autoperfusion balloon versus stent for acute or threatened closure during percutaneous transluminal coronary angioplasty. Am J Cardiol 1994; 74:1002–1005.
132. Meckel CR, Kjelsberg MA, Ahmed WH, et al: Bailout stenting for abrupt closure during coronary angioplasty [Abstract]. Circulation 1995; 92:I-688.
133. de Feyter PJ, Serruys PW, Arnold A, et al: Coronary angioplasty of the

unstable angina related vessel in patients with multivessel disease. Eur Heart J 1986; 7:460–467.
134. Kussmaul WG III, Krol J, Laskey WK, et al: One-year follow-up results of "culprit" versus multivessel coronary angioplasty trial. Am J Cardiol 1993; 71:1431–1433.
135. Adelman AG, Cohen EA, Kimball BP, et al: A comparison of coronary atherectomy with coronary angioplasty for lesions of the proximal left anterior descending coronary artery. N Engl J Med 1993; 329:228–233.
136. Holmes DR Jr, Topol EJ, Califf RM, et al: A multicenter, randomized trial of coronary angioplasty versus directional atherectomy for patients with saphenous vein bypass graft lesions. Circulation 1995; 91:1966–1974.
137. Safian RD, Niazi KA, Strzlelecki M, et al: Detailed angiographic analysis of high-speed mechanical rotational atherectomy in human coronary arteries. Circulation 1993; 88:961–968.
138. Litvack F, Eigler N, Margolis J, et al: Percutaneous excimer laser coronary angioplasty: results in the first consecutive 3,000 patients. J Am Coll Cardiol 1994; 23:323–329.
139. Bittl JA, Sanborn TA, Tcheng JE, et al: Clinical success, complications and restenosis rates with excimer laser coronary angioplasty. Am J Cardiol 1992; 70:1533–1539.
140. Fischman DL, Leon MB, Baim DS, et al: A randomized comparison of coronary-stent placement and balloon angioplasty in the treatment of coronary artery disease. N Engl J Med 1994; 331:496–501.
141. Serruys P, de Jaegere P, Kiemeneij F, et al: A comparison of balloon-expandable-stent implantation with balloon angioplasty in patients with coronary artery disease. N Engl J Med 1994; 331:489–495.
142. Alfonso F, Hernandez R, Goicolea J, et al: Coronary stenting for acute coronary dissection after coronary angioplasty: implications of residual dissection. J Am Coll Cardiol 1994; 24:989–995.
143. Abdelmeguid AE, Ellis SG, Sapp SK, et al: Directional coronary atherectomy in unstable angina. J Am Coll Cardiol 1994; 24:46–54.
144. Nath FC, Muller DWM, Ellis SG, et al: Thrombosis of a flexible coil coronary stent: frequency, predictors, and clinical outcome. J Am Coll Cardiol 1993; 21:622–627.
145. Huber MS, Mooney JF, Madison J, et al: Use of a morphologic classification to predict clinical outcome after dissection from coronary angioplasty. Am J Cardiol 1991; 68:467–471.
146. Bittl JA, Sanborn TA, Tcheng JE, et al: Excimer laser-facilitated angioplasty for undilatable coronary lesions: results of a prospective, controlled study [Abstract]. Circulation 1993; 88(suppl I):23.
147. Eisenberg PR, Sherman LA, Jaffe AS: Paradoxical elevation of fibrinopeptide A after streptokinase: evidence for continued thrombosis despite intense fibrinolysis. J Am Coll Cardiol 1987; 10:527–35.
148. Eisenberg PR, Sobel BS, Jaffe AS: Activation of prothrombin accompanying thrombolysis with recombinant tissue type plasminogen activator. J Am Coll Cardiol 1992; 19:1065–1069.
149. Vaitkus PT, Laskey WK: Efficacy of adjunctive thrombolytic therapy in percutaneous transluminal coronary angioplasty (review). J Am Coll Cardiol 1994; 24:1415–1423.
150. Schieman G, Cohen BM, Kozina J, et al: Intracoronary urokinase for intracoronary thrombus accumulation complicating percutaneous transluminal coronary angioplasty for acute ischemic syndromes. Circulation 1990; 82:2052–2060.
151. Faxon DP, for the Multicenter American Research Trial with Cilazapril after Angioplasty to Prevent Coronary Obstruction and Restenosis (MARCATOR) Study Group: Effect of high dose angiotensin-converting enzyme inhibition on restenosis: final results of the MARCATOR Study, a multicenter, double-blind, placebo-controlled trial of cilazapril. J Am Coll Cardiol 1995; 25:362–369.
152. de Groote P, Bauters C, McFadden EP, et al: Local lesion-related factors and restenosis after coronary angioplasty: evidence from a quantitative angiographic study in patients with unstable angina undergoing double-vessel angioplasty. Circulation 1995; 91:968–972.
153. Halon DA, Merdler A, Shefer A, et al: Identifying patients at high risk for restenosis after percutaneous transluminal coronary angioplasty for unstable angina. Am J Cardiol 1989; 64:289–293.
154. Mark DB, Nelson CL, Califf RM, et al: Continuing evolution of therapy for coronary artery disease: initial results from the era of coronary angioplasty. Circulation 1994; 89:2015–2025.
155. Bär FW, Raynaud P, Renkin JP, et al: Coronary angiographic findings do not predict clinical outcome in patients with unstable angina. J Am Coll Cardiol 1994; 24:1453–1459.

44 Angioplasty Strategies in Acute Myocardial Infarction

Mark C. G. Horrigan, MB, FRACP
Eric J. Topol, MD

Although Herrick described acute coronary thrombosis in 1912,[1] more than half a century elapsed before there was consensus concerning the pathogenesis of acute myocardial infarction. Only since the 1970s has plaque fissuring with overlying thrombus formation been widely recognized as the process underlying the majority of cases of myocardial infarction, unstable angina pectoris, and sudden cardiac death.[2–5] In 1980, DeWood and coworkers[6] demonstrated the high frequency of thrombotic coronary occlusion in the early hours of acute myocardial infarction; this led to the use of intracoronary streptokinase,[7] which was eventually superseded by intravenous administration of thrombolytic agents to allow wider application and less delay in administration. The use of percutaneous transluminal coronary angioplasty (PTCA) after intracoronary administration of streptokinase in the setting of acute myocardial infarction was reported in 1982 by Meyer and coworkers.[8] In 1983, Hartzler and coworkers[9] first described the use of angioplasty in acute myocardial infarction without prior thrombolytic therapy.

After the major thrombolytic trials of the last decade, early reperfusion is considered crucial for reduction of infarct size[10] and mortality[11] in the management of acute myocardial infarction. Contemporary thrombolytic regimens have notable deficiencies, including failure of clot lysis and incomplete reperfusion,[12] "early hazard,"[13] serious hemorrhagic complications, and frequent presence of contraindications to their use. Mechanical reperfusion strategies are in many respects complementary to the pharmacologic approach and may have much to offer in the broader context of reperfusion therapy for acute myocardial infarction. This chapter critically reviews mechanical approaches to the treatment of the patient with myocardial infarction with predominant emphasis on *acute* management. Controversial areas are addressed, and a set of clinical guidelines is provided.

CORONARY ANGIOGRAPHY

Emergency Angiography

In patients presenting with acute myocardial infarction, angiography may be performed at the time of presentation to confirm the diagnosis or with a view to primary mechanical reperfusion, or subsequently when indicated by clinical events punctuating the patient's course. Common indications in the latter category are when failure of thrombolytic reperfusion is suspected and a secondary mechanical approach to reperfusion is desirable or when reocclusion is suspected after initially successful thrombolysis. Other situations in which urgent angiography is indicated during the course of acute infarction include sustained hypotension, incipient or established cardiogenic shock, and the occurrence of ventricular septal rupture or acute mitral insufficiency; affected patients generally have a grave prognosis, which may improve markedly with aggressive intervention. Angiography is also performed electively after myocardial infarction as a tool in the processes of risk stratification and designing individualized reperfusion strategies.

The safety of coronary angiography in patients with evolving infarction was initially demonstrated by DeWood and coworkers.[6] Since then, the use of emergency angiography has been described in prospective multicenter trials of intracoronary thrombolysis,[14–16] in trials of combined thrombolysis and angioplasty,[17–30] and in trials of primary angioplasty.[31–35] Although this list is not exhaustive, the number of patients undergoing emergency angiography in this setting exceeds 10,000. Detailed review of this group[36] suggests that the safety profile of the procedure is impressive, with only slightly greater risk than elective catheterization.[14–30] The cumulative incidence of death and stroke is very low ($<0.5\%$), and the frequency of arrhythmias, nephrotoxic effects of contrast agents, and other adverse events remains acceptable.[36]

The most frequent complications of emergency catheterization relate to the vascular access site and include hemorrhage, pseudoaneurysm formation, and development of arteriovenous fistulas. The reported frequency of access site bleeding varies widely from 5% to 45%,[9, 14–35, 37, 38] and although somewhat dependent on definitions selected, it may be influenced by usage and dosage[39] of thrombolytic agents, concomitant use of antiplatelet and antithrombotic drugs, procedural and patient variables, and operator technique. Performance of vascular repair procedures is a common source of morbidity in this group of patients, and minimizing the risk of arterial trauma is a priority. In addition to the problems posed by bleeding complications, there are significant logistic impediments to wide provision of urgent angiography. Only a quarter of U.S. hospitals in a 1987 survey had cardiac catheterization facilities[40]; thus, in many cases, patients requiring urgent investigation would require rapid interhospital transport. Furthermore, providing 24-h coverage imposes significant burdens on institutions offering such services.

Despite its complications, emergency angiography has advantages that may prove crucial in some patients. As discussed in detail in the section on rescue angioplasty, several technologies have been applied to the noninvasive diagnosis of reperfusion without consistent success, and angiography remains the "gold standard" for rapid identification of patients with failed reperfusion; in clinical practice, this is the most common indication for urgent angiography. In addition to providing rapid diagnosis in most cases, immediate definition of the coronary anatomy allows stratification of patients according to risk and coronary anatomy. Triage to the most appropriate reperfusion strategy is thus facilitated, subsequent clinical decisions can be made with more information and less delay, and duration of hospitalization can be reduced in some cases.[41, 42]

In addition to these situations, other clinical settings exist in which early angiography may be beneficial. In patients at moderate to high risk with contraindications to systemic thrombolysis, triage to a cardiac catheterization laboratory is highly desirable and provides the option of mechanical reperfusion if this is required. Patients with prior contralateral Q wave infarction appear to derive specific benefit from early catheterization and angioplasty when appropriate.[43, 44] When symptoms suggest the diagnosis of acute myocardial infarction but the electrocardiogram is nondiagnostic, urgent catheterization confers the benefits outlined and may preclude inappropriate use of systemic thrombolytic agents. Finally, among patients presenting early to a center with a proficient invasive facility, angiography with a view to primary angioplasty may be the optimal management strategy.

Elective Angiography

The role of elective angiography in the management of patients with uncomplicated infarction is controversial, and a comprehensive review of the relevant medical and economic issues is beyond the scope of this chapter. There are two approaches to elective angiography. The *routine* approach refers to performance of coronary angiography as a standard part of the postinfarction risk stratification process; the *selective* approach uses angiography only for patients with spontaneously recurring ischemia or with evidence of ischemia on functional testing.

Routine Coronary Angiography

The rationale for routine angiography is that it usually defines the culprit lesion, evaluates the success of thrombolytic therapy if administered, identifies patients with "high-risk" coronary anatomy who may derive prognostic benefit from revascularization procedures, and may in selected cases facilitate early hospital discharge. The population of patients surviving myocardial infarction is diverse, and knowledge of coronary anatomy has value in prognostication and in formulation of individualized management strategies.

On the basis of data from the Thrombolysis and Angioplasty in Myocardial Infarction (TAMI) and the Thrombolysis in Myocardial Infarction (TIMI) studies,[17–25] patients undergoing elective catheterization after thrombolysis can be divided into five groups with differing prognoses and treatment requirements (Fig. 44–1). This population is restricted to those eligible for thrombolysis and excludes those with prior bypass surgery; thus, there is a selection bias

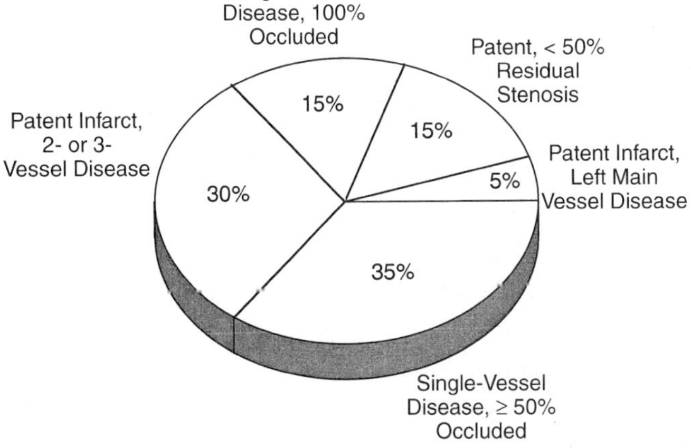

Figure 44–1. Anticipated angiographic subgroups in patients undergoing pre-discharge angiography after thrombolytic therapy. (Adapted from Topol EJ, Holmes DR, Rogers WJ: Coronary angiography after thrombolytic therapy for acute myocardial infarction. Ann Intern Med 1991; 114:877–885.)

against those with severe underlying coronary disease. Nonetheless, it provides a useful clinical model for risk stratification.

A small but significant proportion of patients have left main stenosis or its functional equivalent and will clearly benefit from bypass surgery. Approximately 30% of patients will have multivessel disease with stenoses of 70% or greater in one or more non–infarct-related vessels. In the TAMI cumulative experience, there was a threefold increase (11.4% vs. 4.2%) in hospital mortality among patients with multivessel disease; non–infarct zone wall motion and the number of diseased vessels are also independently predictive of in-hospital mortality. The presence of multivessel disease defined a group at increased risk in which each additional diseased vessel was equivalent in prognostic terms to 16 years of increased age or a 13-point reduction in ejection fraction.[45]

Fifteen percent have a persistently occluded artery, which may be subtended by viable or nonviable myocardium. As outlined in a subsequent section, *both* groups may stand to benefit from restoration of patency. Fourth is the group with patent vessels and residual stenosis of 50% or greater, who represent a third of the total. The management of this group is discussed in the section devoted to thrombolysis and angioplasty. Approximately 15% of patients fit into the group with "minimal lesion syndrome," defined as the presence of a low-grade infarct vessel stenosis after thrombolysis. In the TIMI-2 trial, 13% of 1326 patients had residual stenosis of less than 50% at an average of 30 h after thrombolysis.[25] In the TAMI database,[46] 15% had minimal lesions at 90 min; and in the TAMI-1 trial,[17] serial angiography demonstrated that 14% of patients with severe obstruction at 90 min had residual stenoses of less than 50% by 7 days. Those with minimal lesion syndrome tend to be younger, and there is a relative preponderance of females and cases of single-vessel disease; ventricular function is generally well preserved.[46] This group is probably heterogeneous; rupture of predominantly lipid plaques and a superadded primary or secondary predisposition to vasospasm or thrombosis are contributing factors in some cases.

Selective Coronary Angiography

Its proponents argue that the selective approach is more practical and that it is not associated with adverse short- or long-term outcomes. Because only a quarter of acute care hospitals in the United States have catheterization facilities, selective use of catheterization would allow continuity of care in community hospitals for the majority of patients, minimizing interhospital transfers for predischarge angiography.

In a retrospective analysis, Rogers and coworkers[47] compared the group assigned to the TIMI-2A strategy of conservative management and routine predischarge catheterization with patients from the TIMI-2B group assigned to conservative management with angiography reserved for those with spontaneous or inducible ischemia. At the end of a year, angiography had been performed at least once in 99% of those undergoing routine angiography and in 59% of those managed with the selective approach. Although the rate of subsequent angiography was greater in the selective catheterization group, rates of death, nonfatal infarction, and coronary revascularization procedures were similar.

Further indirect evidence favoring the selective approach comes from the TIMI-2[25] and Should We Intervene Following Thrombolysis (SWIFT)[48] trials, in which patients randomized to the conservative strategy of "watchful waiting" had outcomes identical with or superior to those of patients randomized to an invasive strategy of angiography and angioplasty. These trials were not specifically designed to compare routine and selective angiographic strategies and pertain exclusively to the post-thrombolytic population of patients.

Which Strategy?

In the United States, there is considerable controversy concerning the appropriate role of elective angiography after myocardial infarction; however, there are no data to mandate either approach, and no randomized trial is planned or likely. In reality, there are various clinical settings in which knowledge of coronary anatomy will not affect management (e.g., advanced age, comorbidity, or the patient's preference), which makes routine angiography superfluous. Equally, advocates of the selective approach must concede that considerable crossover occurs despite the initial intention to treat[25, 47, 49] and that unresolved difficulties exist with the interpretation[50, 51] and performance (in up to 45% of patients) of functional tests in the era of reperfusion therapy.[52–54] In practice, physicians recommending a selective approach may follow more flexible guidelines in specific situations, favoring elective investigation in subgroups at high risk who may benefit from revascularization, such as those with low ejection fractions or with previous contralateral infarction.

Economic factors are assuming ever-increasing importance, particularly in the managed care environment, and are comprehensively reviewed elsewhere.[36, 55] Predominant concerns regarding routine angiography center around issues of resource use and the potential for overzealous "reflex" dilatation of lesions based on anatomic rather than functional characteristics.[56] The potential for early hospital discharge stemming from prompt routine catheterization may offset the cost of "unnecessary" angiograms. The TIMI-2 investigators projected that the conservative strategy would result in an annual $750 million saving, but in a group of patients observed prospectively, this was not corroborated by cost and charge tracking.[25, 57] Thus, at this time, it is not clear whether the routine approach is less or more expensive than a policy of selective angiography.

It is the perspective of these authors that liberal use of elective catheterization can provide incisive clinical information, allowing accurate prognostication and decisive planning of postinfarction management for many patients. However, in the absence of compelling data favoring either approach and an increasingly cost-conscious environment, it is equally reasonable to recommend an individualized approach to elective catheterization determined by clinical factors and the results of functional testing.

PATHOLOGY OF ANGIOPLASTY IN ACUTE MYOCARDIAL INFARCTION: RECENT INSIGHTS INTO MECHANISMS OF VESSEL DILATATION

There are limited but important postmortem data describing the status of the infarct-related artery (IRA) and the myocardium in patients acutely reperfused with thrombolytic therapy, coronary angioplasty, or a combined approach. Waller and coworkers[58] described hemorrhagic infarction in patients receiving thrombolytic or combined forms of therapy, whereas patients treated with angioplasty alone had nonhemorrhagic or "anemic" infarcts. Angioplasty as sole therapy was associated with intimal and medial fissuring, but intramural hemorrhage was not observed. In those receiving combined therapy, there was intramural hemorrhage involving plaque, intima, and media (in some cases compromising flow) and subadventitial hemorrhage surrounding the angioplasty site (Fig. 44–2). Colavita and coworkers[59] described similar hemorrhagic changes in patients treated with a combined approach. In addition to hemorrhagic changes, activation of platelets and thrombin generation by thrombolytic agents[60, 61] may result in a prothrombotic milieu not favoring instrumentation of the ruptured plaque with further exposure of thrombogenic subendothelial tissue components. These findings are in keeping with the results of large clinical trials[17, 29, 62] (see later) in which, rather than improving clinical results, combined use of PTCA and thrombolytic agents was associated with a disturbing trend toward adverse outcomes.

Reports[63, 64] describe intravascular ultrasonographic findings before and after balloon angioplasty for acute myocardial infarction. Deep wall injury was uncommon, and luminal gains were largely produced by compression, dislodgment, or dissolution of thrombus. Kawagoe and coworkers[64] noted that in vessels with severe (>70%) underlying

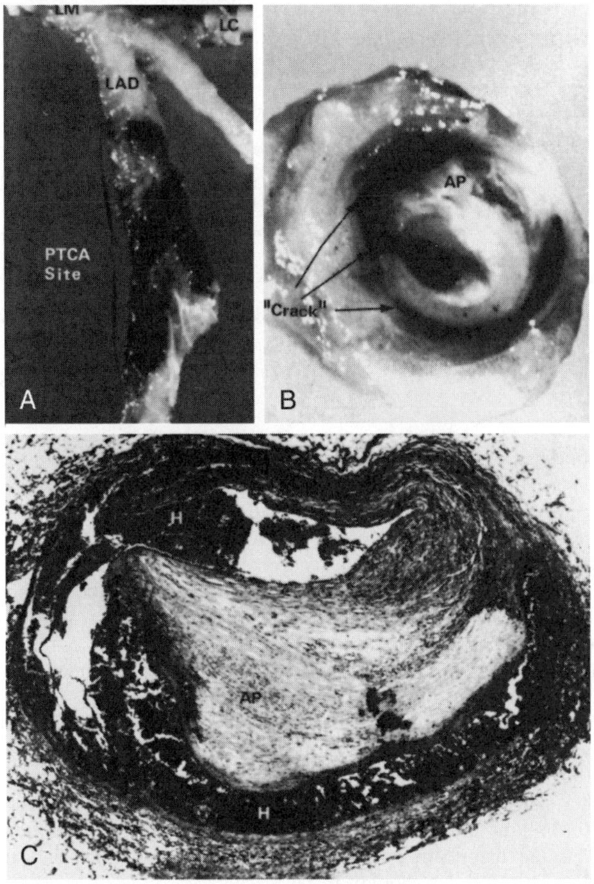

Figure 44–2. Gross and histologic findings in a patient treated with streptokinase and PTCA. *A*, External view of the left anterior descending artery, showing gross adventitial hemorrhage surrounding the angioplasty site. *B*, Transverse coronary section through the angioplasty site, showing a "crack" in the atherosclerotic plaque (AP) and gross intimal and medial hemorrhage. *C*, Histologic section, showing atherosclerotic plaque rupture and hemorrhage (H) into the media producing luminal compromise. (Adapted from Waller BF, Rothbaum DA, Pinkerton CA, et al: Status of the myocardium and infarct-related coronary artery in 19 necropsy patients with acute recanalization using pharmacologic (streptokinase, r-tissue plasminogen activator), mechanical (percutaneous transluminal coronary angioplasty) or combined types of reperfusion therapy. J Am Coll Cardiol 1987; 9:785–801.)

stenoses, luminal enlargement was associated with small but significant changes in lumen cross-sectional area but little change in plaque cross-sectional area. In lesions with only moderate plaque burden, the predominant mechanism of luminal enlargement was removal of thrombus. Interestingly, these investigators noted that luminal improvement assessed by ultrasonography was considerably less than that measured by conventional angiographic techniques.

CORONARY ANGIOPLASTY STRATEGIES

There are five distinct strategies for angioplasty in the treatment of myocardial infarction (Table 44–1). The different approaches vary with respect to timing, therapeutic goals, and whether they are associated with the use of thrombolytic agents.

Thrombolysis and Angioplasty

Immediate Angioplasty

Considerable investigative effort has been invested in the evaluation of angioplasty as an *immediate routine adjunct* to fibrinolytic therapy. The rationale underlying this application was that during acute thrombotic coronary occlusion, dissolution of thrombus *coupled* with dilatation of underlying plaque would be superior to either treatment used alone. The hypothesis that such treatment would increase preservation of myocardial function and reduce the frequency of subsequent reocclusion was tested in three trials[17, 29, 62] whose designs are summarized in Table 44–2. Despite differences in study design, these trials essentially compared immediate catheterization and PTCA with less aggressive management strategies after administration of tissue-type plasminogen activator (t-PA); in each trial, the primary end point was the left ventricular ejection fraction (LVEF) at discharge.

In the TAMI trial,[17] 386 patients presenting within 4 h of the onset of myocardial infarction underwent emergency angiography 90 min after administration of t-PA. After angiographic assessment of coronary anatomy, 99 were randomized to immediate PTCA and 98 to a strategy of elective angioplasty at 7–10 days. Of those not randomized, 96 (25%) with occluded culprit vessels were triaged to rescue angioplasty; in an additional 93 (24%), PTCA was precluded by severe multilesion or multivessel disease, cardiogenic shock, left main stem disease, or other factors. There was no significant difference in global or regional function 1 week after enrollment, and the mortality and reocclusion rates did not vary with the angioplasty strategy employed. Angioplasty was successful in 85% of those randomized to immediate angioplasty, with a 7% rate of emergency bypass surgery. Cumulatively, PTCA was actually performed in only half of those randomized to the elective strategy, with a 95% success rate and a 2% emergency bypass rate; the influence of patient selection bias in the elective group makes strict comparison impossible. Among patients randomized to the elective strategy, 18% crossed over emergency PTCA for recurrent ischemia, and 14% had a substantially reduced residual stenosis that obviated the need for intervention.

In the European Cooperative Study Group (ECSG) trial,[29] 367 patients who had received t-PA were randomized to immediate catheterization and PTCA (actually performed in 93%) or a conservative strategy with catheterization and intervention only for manifest or provocable ischemia. The invasive strategy did not reduce infarct size, improve left ventricular function, or reduce the reinfarction rate (see Table 44–2). However, patients randomized to the invasive strategy had significantly more recurrent ischemia (17% vs. 3%) and

TABLE 44–1. CORONARY ANGIOPLASTY STRATEGIES FOR ACUTE MYOCARDIAL INFARCTION

Strategy	Thrombolytic	Goal	Timing
Direct (primary)	No	Recanalization	As soon as possible
Immediate	Yes	Recanalization	As soon as possible
Rescue	Yes	Fallback-recanalization	60 to 120 min
Deferred (empirical)	Yes	Prophylaxis of recurrent ischemia	1 to 7 days
Elective	Yes	Treatment of angina/provocable ischemia	>1 week

From Topol EJ: Coronary Angioplasty for Acute Myocardial Infarction. Ann Intern Med 1988; 108:970–980.

TABLE 44–2. LEFT VENTRICULAR FUNCTION AND MORTALITY IN THE STUDIES OF THROMBOLYSIS AND IMMEDIATE ANGIOPLASTY FOR ACUTE MYOCARDIAL INFARCTION

	TIMI-2A		TAMI		ECSG	
	Immediate PTCA (n = 195)	PTCA at 18–48 h (n = 194)	Immediate PTCA (n = 99)	Elective PTCA (n = 98)	Immediate PTCA (n = 183)	Noninvasive ± PTCA (n = 184)
Discharge LVEF	50%	49%	53%	56%	51%	51%
In-hospital mortality	7.2%	5.7%	4%	1%	7%	3%

Abbreviations: ECSG, European Cooperative Study Group trial; LVEF, left ventricular ejection fraction; PTCA, percutaneous transluminal coronary angioplasty; TAMI, Thrombolysis and Angioplasty in Myocardial Infarction trial; TIMI-2A, Thrombolysis in Myocardial Infarction trial, phase 2A.

bleeding complications (41% vs. 23%). The study was terminated after an emerging trend toward increased early mortality became apparent among those randomized to the invasive strategy. In the TIMI-2A substudy,[62] 389 patients treated with t-PA were randomized before angiography to immediate angioplasty or to a delayed invasive strategy with PTCA at 18–48 h if the culprit lesion was deemed suitable for dilatation. Predischarge radionuclide LVEF and hospital mortality were similar in both groups. However, compared with patients randomized to the delayed strategy, those randomized to immediate angioplasty had a higher frequency of a composite clinical endpoint of major adverse events.

One-year follow-up data are available for two of these studies. In the ECSG study,[65] reinfarction was less frequent (6.6% vs. 11.2%) in the PTCA group, as was the frequency of revascularization procedures (16.9% vs. 25.5%). However, this benefit was offset by the high rate of immediate reocclusion and early recurrent ischemia in the PTCA group and by increased mortality at 1 year (9.3% vs. 5.4%). In the TIMI-2A study,[66] the cumulative 1-year bypass rate was similar in both groups, as was the frequency of PTCA between discharge and 1 year. The incidence of death and reinfarction during follow-up was similar in both groups.

There are notable differences in the design of these trials. In contrast to TIMI-2A and ECSG, randomization after angiography in TAMI selected only patients with patent vessels. All trials used t-PA, but dosing regimens differed within and between trials. In the ECSG trial, the deferred strategy was noninvasive compared with elective PTCA in TAMI and TIMI-2A. In spite of these differences, the common theme was a trend toward increased mortality and morbidity in the aggressively treated groups without improvement in left ventricular function. Although none of the trials was designed with sufficient statistical power to definitively assess mortality effects, the trend toward increased mortality approached significance in the ECSG trial. It has been argued that the results of these trials may have been distorted by early assessment of left ventricular function; however, data from the TAMI study group indicate no change in serial global ejection fraction from 7 days to 6 months.[67]

The studies discussed explore the role of immediate adjunctive PTCA in the thrombolytic treatment of acute myocardial infarction. In the only trial comparing direct PTCA with direct PTCA plus thrombolysis, O'Neill and coworkers[30] randomized 122 patients presenting within 4 h of the onset of acute myocardial infarction to primary PTCA or streptokinase plus immediate PTCA. The combination of streptokinase and PTCA did not improve outcome compared with PTCA alone. There was no difference in LVEF at 24 h or at 6 weeks. At 6 months, the group as a whole had improved LVEF (.54 to .60) and arterial patency and restenosis rates of 87% and 38%, respectively, but without differences according to treatment strategy. However, in the group receiving streptokinase, the rates of emergency bypass surgery (10.3% vs. 1.6%) and transfusion (39% vs. 8%) were markedly decreased, whereas the duration and expense of hospitalization were significantly increased. These results confirm the findings of the trials of immediate angioplasty[17, 29, 62] and suggest that unfavorable outcomes after PTCA combined with fibrinolytic therapy are not confined to fibrin-specific agents. Of interest, Ambrose and coworkers[68] randomized patients with rest angina to PTCA with or without adjunctive intracoronary urokinase. There was no significant difference in angiographic endpoints, but the frequency of acute closure and adverse clinical outcomes was increased in the group receiving urokinase, paralleling the results of PTCA for acute myocardial infarction and extending the paradigm to include unstable coronary syndromes.

Why is angioplasty in this setting associated with adverse outcomes? First, it was used nonselectively rather than in cases in which the risk/benefit ratio favored intervention. Histologic studies[58, 69] offer further insights. Ruptured atherosclerotic plaques (the usual substrate for thrombotic coronary occlusion) typically have a thinner fibrous cap and greater lipid content than stable plaques do,[70] and their lipid components are thought to be the most thrombogenic constituents [70, 71] of the system. Angioplasty may increase exposure of lipids and other thrombogenic vessel wall components by further disruption of plaque, intima, and media, causing increased platelet activation and thrombus propagation. As discussed subsequently, PTCA is more effective in the *absence* of thrombolytic agents, which suggests that they possess additive unfavorable effects in this situation. These may include a shift in the balance of procoagulant and fibrinolytic effects of t-PA and streptokinase[72] toward thrombosis, resulting in an increased occurrence of ischemic events.

If a patient is clinically stable and has achieved chemical patency of the infarct vessel, immediate PTCA cannot be justified. Many fissured plaques with superadded thrombus will remodel as thrombus is lysed and healing occurs.[73] Remodeling may render stenoses non–flow limiting, obviating the need for mechanical intervention. In the TAMI and TIMI-2A trials, 15% of patients required no intervention after delayed angiography because the culprit stenosis was less than 50%–60%.[17, 62] Furthermore, in TAMI, only 35% of patients in the delayed group underwent PTCA as planned. As well as favorable remodeling, 20% of patients had negative stress test results with no peri-infarct redistribution by thallium scintigraphy, and 11% were triaged to elective bypass surgery. Thus, by avoiding "reperfusion momentum"[74] early in the patient's course, immediate intervention with its attendant morbidity may be omitted without adverse sequelae in a significant proportion of cases. The optimal approach to the patient with persistent occlusion and ongoing ischemia despite thrombolytic intervention is unresolved and is discussed in the next section.

Rescue Angioplasty

The term *rescue angioplasty* refers to an emergency angioplasty procedure performed to re-establish patency after failure of thrombolytic therapy.

Rationale. Randomized trials of immediate PTCA after thrombolysis[17, 29, 62] clearly demonstrate that *routine* PTCA after successful thrombolysis is associated with unfavorable clinical outcomes. However, TIMI grade 0 or 1 flow 90 min after thrombolytic treatment portends increased morbidity and mortality,[75–78] and this population composing 15%–40% of patients stands to gain most from a secondary mechanical strategy aiming to re-establish patency after failure of thrombolysis. Although some patients with persistent occlusion 90 min after thrombolysis will eventually recanalize without PTCA,[77, 79] early reperfusion and myocardial salvage is thought to be of fundamental importance.

In the accelerated t-PA arm of the Global Utilization of Streptokinase and Tissue Plasminogen Activator for Occluded Coronary Arteries (GUSTO) angiographic substudy,[75] early patency of the IRA was established in 81% of patients with TIMI grade 3 flow in 54% only. Thus, despite use of the most effective thrombolytic regimen currently available, approximately 20% of patients have persisting occlusion at 90 min, with abnormal flow conditions in a third of those with "patent" vessels. Early TIMI flow grade has been shown to be a powerful predictor of survival after reperfusion therapy (Fig. 44–3). Furthermore, in addition to reperfusion of viable myocytes, achieving IRA patency may confer benefits independent of myocardial salvage relating to improved ventricular healing, dimensions and geometry, reduced risk of serious ventricular arrhythmias, and preservation of a potential future source of collateral flow (see later).

Series. Ellis and coworkers performed a meta-analysis of 12 reported series of rescue angioplasty.[17, 18, 43, 80–88] Addition of rescue data from the GUSTO angiographic substudy[89] describes cumulative experience in more than 750 cases summarized in Table 44–3. This experience has been conspicuously variable, with patency achieved in 83% (range, 71%–100%) overall. Success rates are lower than those reported in the randomized trials of direct angioplasty,[31–35, 90, 91] indicating that the "thrombolytic-resistant" occlusions are technically more challenging to the interventionalist. It is likely that the increased difficulty of angioplasty in this setting is related to two crucial differences in this population of vessels. Operators frequently find this group of lesions to be characterized by plaques that are more complex and extensive, often containing a greater thrombus burden. As discussed before, the platelet-activating effects of some thrombolytic agents and their association with intramural hemorrhage after PTCA are likely to further jeopardize the results of such procedures.

The reocclusion rate, ranging as high as 29% in some series, averaged 16% overall. In individual trials and within the combined experience, important differences were noted between rescue angioplasty after t-PA and rescue angioplasty after streptokinase, urokinase, or t-PA in combination with streptokinase or urokinase (see Table 44–3). In TAMI, 85 patients underwent rescue angioplasty for persistent occlusion after receiving t-PA.[17] Rescue was successful in 73%, with reocclusion in 29% and a 10.4% mortality rate. In contrast, in the TAMI-2[18] and TAMI-5[43] trials, the combination of t-PA and urokinase with rescue angioplasty was associated with a single case of reocclusion, improved cardiac function, and no mortality.

TABLE 44–3. REPORTED SERIES OF RESCUE ANGIOPLASTY: COMBINED RESULTS

Series	Patients	Thrombolytic Regimen	Success (%)	Reocclusion (%)	Mortality (%)
Topol et al.[17]	85	t-PA	73	29	10.4
Califf et al.[43]	15	t-PA	87	15	NR
	25	UK	84	12	NR
	12	t-PA + UK	92	0	NR
Belenkie et al.[80]	16	SK	81	NR	6.7
Fung et al.[81]	13	SK	92	16	7.6
Topol et al.[18]	22	t-PA + UK	86	3	0
Grines et al.[82]	12	t-PA + SK	100	8	NR
Holmes et al.[83]	34	SK	71	NR	11.0
Grines et al.[84]	10	t-PA + SK	90	12	10.0
O'Connor et al.[85]	90	SK	89	14	17.0
Baim et al.[86]	37	t-PA	92	26	5.4
Whitlow[87]	26	t-PA	81	29	NR
	18	UK	89	25	NR
Ellis et al.[88]	109	t-PA	79	20	10.1
	5	t-PA + UK	70	20	20.0
	59	SK	76	18	10.2
GUSTO (Ross et al.[89])	38	t-PA	92	15	NR
	44	t-PA + SK	91	12	NR
	132	SK	89	10	NR
Pooled UK, SK, or combination	484		417/484 (86.2)	48/380 (12.6)	11.2
Pooled t-PA	290		226/290 (77.9)	43/192 (22.4)	9.5
Total	774		643/774 (83.1)	91/572 (15.9)	10.6

Abbreviations: NR, not reported; SK, streptokinase; t-PA, tissue-type plasminogen activator; UK, urokinase.

Data from Ellis SG, Van de Werf F, Ribiero da Silva E, Topol EJ: Present status of rescue angioplasty: current polarization of opinion and randomized trials. J Am Coll Cardiol 1992; 19:681–686; and Ross AM, Reiner JS, Thompson MA, et al, for the GUSTO Investigators: Immediate and follow-up procedural outcome of 214 patients undergoing rescue PTCA in the GUSTO trial: no effect of the lytic agent [Abstract]. Circulation 1993; 88(suppl I):I-410.

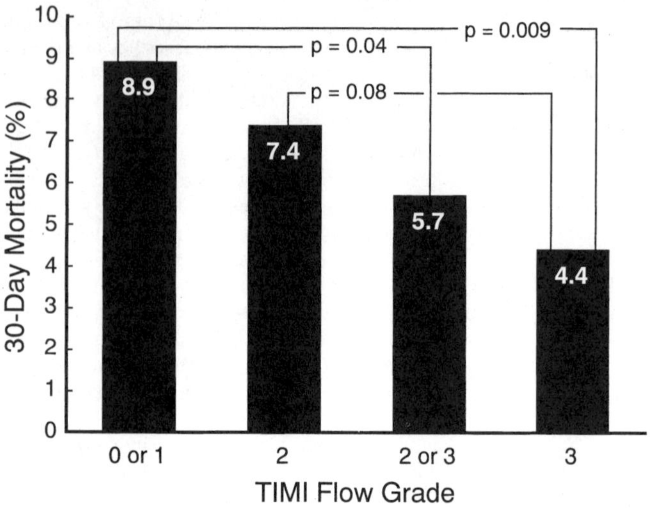

Figure 44–3. Mortality (%) according to TIMI flow grade at 90 minutes in the GUSTO angiographic substudy. (Based on data from The GUSTO Angiographic Investigators: The effects of tissue plasminogen activator, streptokinase, or both, on coronary artery patency, ventricular function and survival after acute myocardial infarction. N Engl J Med 1993; 329:1615–1622.)

This pattern is also evident in the pooled analysis, in which use of non–fibrin-selective agents was associated with a 10% increase in procedural success and a 44% reduction in the frequency of reocclusion (see Table 44–3).

The explanation for this dichotomy may reside in the marked elevation of fibrinogen degradation products in plasma after treatment with non–fibrin-selective agents.[18, 42] Their potent antiplatelet effects have been demonstrated in several studies.[92–96] A subgroup of the fibrinogen fragments bind to the platelet IIb/IIIa integrin (the fibrinogen receptor), which is the final common mediator of platelet aggregation. In this clinical setting, where persistent thrombus is the norm, interference with the IIb/IIIa receptor and platelet aggregation would be desirable and represents the likely mechanism for this effect. In the absence of randomized data, these data suggest that the use of a nonspecific plasminogen activator alone or in combination with t-PA may be the preferred option when rescue angioplasty is undertaken and that, in the future, the use of selective agents to block the IIb/IIIa receptor may have an important adjunctive role in this setting.

Larger Trials. In the TAMI-5 trial, 575 patients with acute myocardial infarction were first randomized to receive t-PA, urokinase, or a combination; within each thrombolytic arm, a second randomization was then made between emergency angiography with rescue angioplasty if the IRA was occluded and deferred angiography at 5–7 days, resulting in a 2 × 3 matrix design.[43] Although this was not primarily a trial of rescue angioplasty (patients with occluded vessels were not randomized to PTCA or no PTCA), it tested rescue angioplasty as part of a comprehensive revascularization strategy. Emergency angiography with rescue angioplasty resulted in an immediate patency rate of 96% and a predischarge patency rate of 94% compared with 90% among those randomized to deferred angiography ($p = .065$). The aggressively treated group had fewer episodes of recurrent ischemia (25% vs. 35%, $p < .005$) without an increase in bleeding complications and less adverse outcomes overall (55% vs. 67%, $p = .004$).

The RESCUE trial is the most important trial of rescue angioplasty to date.[97] Ellis and coworkers enrolled 151 patients within 8 h of the onset of chest pain; the group had angiographically demonstrated occlusion of the left anterior descending vessel persisting after intravenous thrombolytic therapy. Exclusion criteria included cardiogenic shock, significant left main stem disease, and prior myocardial infarction. Patients were randomized to "conservative" treatment with aspirin, heparin, and vasodilators or to rescue angioplasty. Those in the latter group received similar medical therapy and were treated with a non–fibrin-selective thrombolytic agent before angioplasty. Although there was no difference in the primary trial end point of resting LVEF at 30 days, rescue angioplasty was associated with less mortality and heart failure and an improvement in exercise LVEF at follow-up (Table 44–4). The results of the RESCUE trial at least support the use of rescue angioplasty in this group of patients who were at moderate to high risk with an initial anterior infarct.

Controversies and Areas of Continuing Research. The appropriateness, optimal use, and timing of angioplasty after failed thrombolysis continue to provoke heated debate among clinicians. Areas of controversy include the risks and benefits of rescue angioplasty in various clinical settings, whether risk/benefit ratios will be influenced favorably by the use of novel antithrombotic agents such as 7E3, the significance of IRA patency with abnormal flow in various settings, and if and when mechanical intervention will benefit patients with incomplete reperfusion. Whereas angiography is currently the gold standard for assessment of reperfusion status, an accurate noninvasive means for diagnosis of reperfusion status and myocardial viability will have a major impact on directing the appropriate deployment of mechanical intervention in this setting. The use of 12-lead and continuous monitoring criteria are notably inaccurate in the diagnosis of reperfusion; the only sign accurately predicting angiographic reperfusion is rapid and complete ST segment normalization, but this is seen in only 6% of cases.[98, 99] Several noninvasive methods involving the use of rapid measurement of creatine kinase isoforms[100–108] and myoglobin[109] and continuous digital ST segment[110–113] and/or QRS vector analysis are being investigated. At this time, however, the most promising approach is the bedside use of echocardiography with myocardial echo-contrast agents; this technique has potential to accurately localize and quantify the volume of myocardium at risk and to assess the degree of residual perfusion.[113, 114]

The TAMI study group[115] reviewed composite rescue angioplasty experience in 192 patients, comparing these with 607 patients in

TABLE 44–4. RESCUE TRIAL RESULTS

	PTCA (n = 78)	No PTCA (n = 73)	*p*
Age, years	59 ± 11	59 ± 11	
Male gender, %	79	85	
Time from MI, hours	4.5 ± 1.5	4.5 ± 1.9	
Killip class ≥2, %	21	26	
Proximal occlusion, %	45	51	
Multivessel disease, %	34	40	
Angiographic collaterals, %	32	37	
Angioplasty success, %	92	50*	
30-day LVEF, %			
Resting	40 ± 11	39 ± 12	
Exercise	45 ± 14	40 ± 11	.04
30-day outcomes, %			
Death	5.2	9.9	.18
Severe CHF	1.3	7.0	.11
Nonfatal VT	11.5	12.3	.88
Death or CHF	6.4	16.6	.05

Abbreviations: MI, myocardial infarction; LVEF, left ventricular ejection fraction; CHF, congestive heart failure; VT, ventricular tachycardia.

*Of two patients crossing over to urgent angioplasty.

Data from Ellis SG, Ribiero da Silva E, Heyndrickx G, et al: Randomized comparison of rescue angioplasty with conservative management of patients with early failure of thrombolysis for acute myocardial infarction. Circulation 1994; 90:2280–2284.

whom thrombolytic-mediated patency had been achieved. Those who achieved patency by either means had similar in-hospital mortality and event rates in a 20-month follow-up period. However, angioplasty was unsuccessful in 23 patients, and in-hospital mortality was 39% in this group compared with 6% among the 169 with successful rescue angioplasty.[115] Although a cause-and-effect relationship between failed PTCA and mortality has not been established, it is conceivable that an unsuccessful rescue angioplasty may in some instances have a worse outlook than conservative management in the same situation; such a scenario would be most likely to unfold in a patient at low risk even with persistent occlusion. This is illustrated by work of Gaioch and Topol[116] and the TAMI study group,[115] who examined outcome after rescue angioplasty of the right coronary artery. Compared with rescue angioplasty for occlusion of the left anterior descending vessel, there was an excess of hemodynamic instability, rhythm disturbances, abrupt closure, and subsequent reocclusion in patients undergoing right coronary rescue angioplasty. The in-hospital mortality rates were similar at 9% and 11%, respectively, and there was a notable increase in mortality in patients presenting with uncomplicated inferior wall infarction. This is a disturbing finding, when the low mortality reported with thrombolytic therapy in this situation is considered,[13] and supports the contention that the risk of persisting occlusion with the possibility of late spontaneous reperfusion[79] is equivalent to or less than the risk of a "rescue" procedure in certain instances. The use of 7E3 has shown promising initial results as adjunctive therapy in direct angioplasty,[117] which suggests that this and other novel antithrombotic agents may have similar potential to increase safety and efficacy of rescue angioplasty procedures.

Although there is general consensus that mechanical intervention in the setting of TIMI grade 3 flow is contraindicated,[29] it is now clear that patients with TIMI grade 2 flow early after thrombolysis have a less favorable outcome profile than those with normal flow[76–78]; however, the majority of available data on rescue angioplasty concerns the treatment of total occlusions. In some cases, abnormal flow is due to persisting high-grade obstruction at the lesion site; if flow is improving, PTCA may not be required; if it is stable or deteriorating, PTCA may be beneficial. When sluggish flow is due to microvascular damage or dysfunction—the "no reflow" phenomenon[118, 119]—PTCA may be ineffective or even harmful. A reanalysis of data from the TAMI trial[120] suggests that PTCA to infarct arteries with TIMI grade 2 flow may modestly improve recovery of left ventricular function. This important issue will be prospectively examined in the forthcoming RESCUE-2 trial; 240 patients with TIMI grade 2 flow after thrombolytic therapy will be randomized to rescue angioplasty or to a conservative strategy, and clinical outcomes up to 12 months will be compared.

Deferred and Elective Angioplasty

Deferred angioplasty is a procedure performed empirically after thrombolysis as prophylaxis against recurrent ischemia. Elective angioplasty is performed for the treatment of angina or ischemia provoked by functional testing.

The role of deferred empirical angioplasty compared with more conservative strategies was examined in the TIMI-2,[25] SWIFT,[48] and Streptokinase in Acute Myocardial Infarction (SIAM)[121] trials and in the studies of Barbash and coworkers[122] and van den Brand[123] and colleagues (Table 44–5). In the largest study, 3262 patients were randomized to an "invasive" strategy of deferred angioplasty (routinely performed 18–48 h after administration of t-PA), if the coronary anatomy was suitable, or to a "conservative" approach with cardiac catheterization or revascularization only for spontaneous or provocable ischemia. Catheterization was performed in 24% of the conservative group. Among patients assigned to the invasive strategy, 57% underwent angioplasty. Reasons for not performing angioplasty included unsuitable anatomy, minimal lesions, and occluded vessels. In contrast, at 6 weeks, PTCA had been required for only 16% of the conservative group, and coronary artery bypass graft (CABG) rates were similar in both groups (Fig. 44–4).

As shown in Table 44–5, there were no significant differences in mortality, reinfarction, or LVEF at 6 weeks or 1 year. These results are in keeping with the other trials, the one exception being an excess of reinfarction in the PTCA arm of the SWIFT[48] trial. Taken together, these data fail to demonstrate any benefit accruing from empirical post-thrombolytic PTCA and emphasize the need for objective evidence of ischemia before patients are exposed to the risks of the procedure.

In the Treatment of Post-Thrombolytic Stenosis (TOPS) trial,[124] Ellis and coworkers randomized 87 patients with negative exercise or functional test results after thrombolytic therapy to PTCA or medical therapy. All patients had a significant residual stenosis of the infarct vessel. In the PTCA group, there was a 9.5% incidence of non–Q wave myocardial infarction due to acute closure, no difference in LVEF at 6 weeks, and a trend toward reduced infarct-free survival at 1 year. These results indicate that regardless of the severity of the residual stenosis, when response to functional testing is negative, empirical PTCA is ill advised. The TOPS trial result underscores the importance of functional testing in the asymptomatic postinfarction patient and emphasizes the hazards of reacting too readily to angiographic findings in isolation.

Direct Angioplasty

Pooled angiographic data from trials of thrombolytic therapy[79] confirm earlier work[6, 125] documenting the frequency of infarct vessel occlusion during the first 24 h of myocardial infarction. Although approximately 60% of "control" patients in this large cohort achieved patency after 3 days without treatment, the rate of occlusion was approximately 80% during the first 24 h after the onset of infarction (Table 44–6). Direct or primary angioplasty refers to an initial mechanical strategy aiming to achieve early reperfusion without prior administration of thrombolytic agents.

Nonrandomized Series of Patients Treated With Direct Angioplasty for Acute Myocardial Infarction

After its introduction in 1983, direct angioplasty for the treatment of acute myocardial infarction emerged as an alternative to the use of intracoronary streptokinase or the use of thrombolysis combined with angioplasty. After the initial report from the Mid-America Heart Institute,[9] several large, consecutive series describing the use of direct angioplasty in acute myocardial infarction were published.

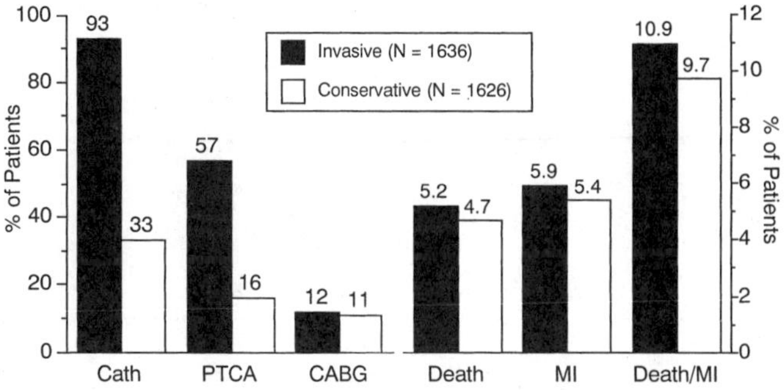

Figure 44–4. Revascularization procedures and primary endpoint at 42 days in patients assigned to invasive and conservative strategies in the TIMI-II trial. (Adapted from The TIMI Study Group: Comparison of invasive and conservative strategies following intravenous tissue plasminogen activator in myocardial infarction: Results of the Thrombolysis In Myocardial Infarction (TIMI) II Trial. N Engl J Med 1989; 320:618–627.)

TABLE 44–5. A SUMMARY OF RANDOMIZED TRIALS COMPARING DEFERRED ANGIOPLASTY WITH CONSERVATIVE MANAGEMENT FOLLOWING THROMBOLYSIS

Trial	No. Patients		Thrombolytic Agent Used	Timing of Angioplasty	Major Findings
	Invasive	Conservative			
TIMI-2 B[25]	1636	1626	t-PA	18–48 hours	No difference in mortality, reinfarction.
SWIFT[48]	397	403	APSAC	< 48 hours	Similar mortality, more reinfarction in invasive group.
SIAM[121]	158	166	SK	14–48 hours	No difference.
Barbash et al.[122]	97	104	t-PA	5 ± 2 days	Excess mortality with invasive strategy.
van den Brand et al.[123]	113	115	t-PA	2–5 days	Less recurrent angina at three months in invasive group.

Abbreviations: TIMI, Thrombolysis in Myocardial Infarction; SWIFT, Should We Intervene Following Thrombolysis; SIAM, Streptokinase Acute Myocardial Infarction; t-PA, tissue-type plasminogen activator; APSAC, anisoylated plasminogen streptokinase activator complex; SK, Streptokinase.

Modified from DeFranco AC, Topol EJ: Angiography and angioplasty. *In* Julian D, Braunwald E (eds.): Management of Acute Myocardial Infarction, pp 104–146. Philadelphia: WB Saunders, 1994.

Eckman and coworkers[126] performed a meta-analysis of direct angioplasty series; ten were analyzed,[127–136] forming a combined cohort of 2073 cases (Table 44–7), including patients with cardiogenic shock and those ineligible for thrombolytic therapy. Infarct vessel patency uniformly exceeded 83% and averaged 91%; in-hospital mortality was 8.3% overall and 1.0% in patients with single-vessel disease. In the largest series, investigators from Mid-America Heart Institute reported 95% survival at 1 year and a 5-year survival rate of 84%. The 3-year survival rate was 92% in those with single-vessel disease and 87% in patients with multivessel disease.[137]

The Primary Angioplasty Registry (PAR)[138, 139] was a multicenter investigation in which 271 prospectively enrolled patients underwent angioplasty as primary therapy for acute myocardial infarction. Entry criteria were designed to mimic contemporary selection criteria for trials of thrombolytic therapy; thus, there was no age limit,[140] the time limit was 12 h from onset of symptoms,[141] patients with previous revascularization procedures were eligible, and those with cardiogenic shock were excluded. Ten percent of patients were anatomically unsuitable for PTCA or had spontaneously reperfused by the time of angiography. The remainder underwent direct angioplasty; reperfusion was achieved in 98%, and 92% had a residual stenosis of less than 50%. Urgent CABG was required in 5% (in 3 for failed PTCA and in 11 for life-threatening anatomy), in-hospital mortality was 4%, recurrent ischemia occurred in 10%, and the reinfarction rate was 3%. Stroke occurred in 1% with a single intracranial hemorrhage and two embolic infarcts, which emphasizes that stroke may infrequently complicate direct angioplasty.

Of 258 patients observed for 6 months, 76% of those eligible for repeated angiography were restudied, and the infarct vessel was patent in 87%. Post-hospital clinical events were relatively infrequent (death 2%, nonfatal reinfarction 3%, recurrent ischemia 10%, repeated PTCA 20%, and bypass surgery 14%), with adverse outcomes more frequent in those with reocclusion. The 10% incidence of readmission for chest pain through 6 months of follow-up compared favorably with the 28% 1-year incidence reported by the TIMI-2 investigators.[142] In 133 patients with paired ventriculograms, there was a 6% improvement in ejection fraction, an 8% improvement in those with IRA patency, and no change in the group with reocclusion. This study demonstrated impressive early outcomes in a population meeting contemporary criteria for thrombolytic therapy. At 6-month follow-up, post-hospital and cumulative mortality rates of 2% and 6%, respectively, compared favorably with the best outcomes reported in thrombolytic trials.[141, 142]

The excellent results reported in these series established direct angioplasty as an attractive alternative to thrombolytic therapy in experienced centers. A therapeutic option for reperfusion of patients ineligible for thrombolytic therapy was introduced, and the stimulus for randomized trials comparing angioplasty with thrombolytic therapy in the setting of acute myocardial infarction was provided.

Randomized Trials Comparing Direct Angioplasty With Thrombolytic Therapy

To date, there have been six randomized trials[31–35, 143–145] comparing direct angioplasty with intravenous thrombolytic therapy. As summa-

TABLE 44–6. POOLED ANGIOGRAPHIC PATENCY RATES FROM THROMBOLYTIC THERAPY TRIALS

	No Therapy	SK	t-PA	Acc. t-PA
60 min	15%	48%	62%	74%
90 min	21%	51%	70%	84%
2–3 h	24%	70%	73%	—
1 day	21%	86%	84%	86%
3–21 days	61%	74%	80%	89%

Abbreviations: SK, streptokinase; t-PA, tissue-type plasminogen activator; Acc, accelerated.

Adapted from Granger CB, Ohman EM, Bates ER: Pooled analysis of angiographic patency rates from thrombolytic therapy trials [Abstract]. Circulation 1992; 86(suppl I):269.

TABLE 44–7. SERIES OF DIRECT ANGIOPLASTY FOR ACUTE MYOCARDIAL INFARCTION

Study	Study Period	No. Patients	In-Hospital Mortality (%)
Flaker et al.[127]	1985–1988	93	14.0
Marco et al.[128]	published 1987	43	14.0
Ellis et al.[129]	1983–1988	271	13.3
Rothbaum et al.[130]	1982–1986	271	13.3
Brodie et al.[131]	1984–1988	383	9.0
Kahn et al.[132]	1981–1989	614	8.0
Beauchamp et al.[133]	1982–1989	214	7.9
Bittl[134]	1989–1990	20	5.0
Grines et al.[135]	published 1991	58	5.0
Williams et al.[136]	published 1991	226	4.9
Pooled		2073	8.3

From Eckman MH, Wong JB, Salem DN, et al: Direct angioplasty for acute myocardial infarction. A review of outcomes in clinical subsets. Ann Intern Med 1992; 177:667–676.

TABLE 44–8. RANDOMIZED TRIALS OF DIRECT ANGIOPLASTY VERSUS THROMBOLYSIS IN ACUTE MYOCARDIAL INFARCTION

Trial	Number			Agent	% PTCA Success	In-Hospital Mortality %		Recurrent Ischemia %		% Unscheduled Revascularization	
	PTCA	Lysis	Total			PTCA	Lysis	PTCA	Lysis	PTCA	Lysis
PAMI[31]	195	200	395	t-PA	97	2.6	6.5	10.6	28.0	14.4	48.0
Netherlands[144]	152	149	301	SK	97	2.0	11.0	8.0	35.0	12.5	25.5
Mayo Clinic[33]	47	56	103	t-PA	96	4.2	3.6	15.0	36.0	14.9	23.2
Sao Paulo[34]	50	50	100	SK	80	6.0	2.0	8.0	10.0	2.0	6.0
Madrid[143]	23	29	52	t-PA	91	4.3	17.2	26.1	20.7	NR	
Spokane[35]	18	18	36	t-PA	72	0	0	NR		NR	
Pooled	485	502	987		94	2.9	6.4	10.7	28.7	12.2	31.9

Abbreviations: PTCA, percutaneous transluminal coronary angioplasty; PAMI, Primary Angioplasty in Myocardial Infarction; t-PA, tissue-type plasminogen activator; SK, streptokinase; NR, not reported.

rized in Table 44–8, an aggregate of 987 patients were randomized in these trials, three of which are discussed in detail.

The Primary Angioplasty in Myocardial Infarction Trial. The largest randomized trial to date was the PAMI trial,[31] which compared direct angioplasty with t-PA in 395 patients with acute myocardial infarction. Principal end points were LVEF at 6 weeks and the composite end point of death and nonfatal reinfarction. Two hundred patients received intravenous t-PA as initial therapy. Of 195 randomized to the interventional strategy, 175 patients (90%) underwent PTCA; 97% had a successful procedure, and none required CABG. Of the remaining 20 patients, 10 were triaged directly to CABG; the remainder did not require PTCA chiefly because of minimal residual stenoses. Antegrade flow was re-established in 193 of 195 (99%) of the PTCA group. Despite similar times from onset of pain to initiation of therapy, the duration of pain was significantly shorter (290 vs. 354 min) in the PTCA group. In the t-PA group, 4 (2.0%) had hemorrhagic stroke compared with none in the PTCA group. When nonhemorrhagic strokes were considered, there were seven strokes in the t-PA group (3.5%) and none in the PTCA group ($p = .024$).

Among those in the invasive group, the endpoints of reinfarction, death, or nonfatal infarction and recurrent ischemia were less frequent, and there was a trend toward reduced mortality with a total of five cardiac deaths compared with nine cardiac deaths plus four from intracranial bleeding in the t-PA group (Table 44–9). In a post hoc analysis, the mortality advantage of PTCA was greatest (2.0% vs. 10.4%, $p = .01$) in a high-risk subgroup of patients older than 70 years and with anterior infarction or a heart rate of more than 100 beats per minute on admission. Unscheduled catheterization (13.3% vs. 63.0%) and unscheduled PTCA (6.2% versus 36.0%) were less frequent in the PTCA group (both $ps < .001$); however, physicians were aware of initial triage and the results of catheterization in the invasive group. In the PTCA group, there was no fatal bleeding, and the most common source of bleeding was the vascular access site. Overall, the frequency of bleeding and transfusion was similar in both groups.

In 75% of patients, predischarge exercise testing was performed. In spite of a relative excess of unscheduled angioplasty among those randomized to t-PA (19.4% versus 2.7%), there was still an excess of positive test results (30% versus 20%, $p = .014$) in this group. Radionuclide ventriculography was used to assess ventricular function at 24 h and again at 6 weeks. Initial ejection fractions were similar, as were measurements at rest and during exercise repeated at 6 weeks (Table 44–10). During 6 months of follow-up, reinfarction or death occurred in 16.8% of the t-PA group and 8.5% of those treated with direct angioplasty ($p = .02$).

Notable features of the PAMI trial include the high rate of procedural success and the striking reduction in recurrent ischemia and revascularization procedures in the PTCA group. Certain clinical outcomes in the thrombolytic arm of the PAMI trial are at variance with the results of large contemporary thrombolytic trials. In particular, the rate of intracerebral hemorrhage was 2.0% compared with 0.7% in TIMI-2[25] and GUSTO,[146] the rate of catheterization for

TABLE 44–9. MORTALITY, RECURRENT ISCHEMIA, AND STROKE IN THE PRIMARY ANGIOPLASTY IN MYOCARDIAL INFARCTION (PAMI) TRIAL

	PTCA ($N = 195$)	Thrombolysis ($N = 200$)	p
Death	5 (2.6%)	13 (6.5%)	.06
Cardiac death	5 (2.6%)	9 (4.5%)	NS
Reinfarction	5 (2.6%)	13 (6.5%)	.06
Death or nonfatal reinfarction	10 (5.1%)	24 (12.0%)	.02
Recurrent ischemia	20 (10.3%)	56 (28.0%)	<.001
Stroke	0 (0.0%)	4 (2.0%)	.05

Abbreviation: NS, nonsignificant.

Data from: Grines CL, Browne KF, Marco J, et al: A comparison of immediate angioplasty with thrombolytic therapy for acute myocardial infarction. N Engl J Med 1993; 328:673–679.

TABLE 44–10. DIRECT ANGIOPLASTY VERSUS THROMBOLYSIS: LEFT VENTRICULAR EJECTION FRACTION RESULTS

Trial	Early Global LVEF		Early Infarct Zone LVEF		6-Week Global LVEF	
	PTCA	Lysis	PTCA	Lysis	PTCA	Lysis
PAMI[31]	53	53	—	—	53	53
Netherlands[144]	50*	45	42*	34	—	—
Mayo Clinic[33]	53	50	—	—	53	50
Sao Paulo[34]	59	57	—	—	—	—
Madrid[143]	45	52	—	—	—	—
Spokane[35]	51	56	—	—	46	50
Pooled	52.2%	50.7%			52.3%	51.8%

Abbreviations: PTCA, percutaneous transluminal coronary angioplasty; LVEF, left ventricular ejection fraction; PAMI, Primary Angioplasty in Myocardial Infarction.

*$p < .001$ favoring PTCA over thrombolytic therapy.

recurrent ischemia was markedly increased compared with GUSTO (23.5% versus 5.1%), and the reinfarction rate of 6.5% represented more than a 50% increase above the lower rates (≤14.0%) reported in several large thrombolytic trials.[25, 146, 147] Cognizance of these differences helps place the results of this important trial in the broader context of contemporary trials of reperfusion therapy.

The Mayo Clinic Series. Gibbons and coworkers[33] randomized 108 patients to receive direct angioplasty or treatment with intravenous t-PA. The primary study endpoint was the change in size of the perfusion defect between admission and discharge quantified by serial technetium Tc99m sestamibi imaging. Secondary endpoints included LVEF at discharge and 6 weeks, ischemic events and revascularization procedures during 6 months of follow-up, and a cost analysis. Of those randomized, 103 had complete data for analysis. Fifty-six patients received t-PA, and 47 were randomized to PTCA. In the latter group, the IRA was patent in two; among the remaining 45, PTCA was successful in 96% of patients. The percentage of left ventricular myocardium in jeopardy was similar in the two groups (27% in the PTCA group and 31% in the t-PA group), as was the degree of myocardial salvage (13% and 15%, respectively). Neither therapy conferred any advantage in patients with anterior or inferior wall infarction.

In the group randomized to thrombolytic therapy, 36% underwent revascularization procedures for recurrent ischemia, compared with 16% in the PTCA group. There were two deaths in each group, and no significant difference in LVEF was demonstrated at discharge or at 6 weeks. A trend toward greater hospital costs was noted in the thrombolytic group ($p = .09$), with failure to reach significance because of large variability in costs incurred. Patients randomized to PTCA had significantly shorter hospitalizations, fewer readmissions within 6 months, and lower 6-month follow-up costs than did patients who received t-PA. Thus, each strategy salvaged similar amounts of myocardium, but there was less recurrent ischemia, less requirement for revascularization procedures, and a trend toward reduced health care costs in those randomized to the invasive strategy.

The Netherlands Study. In the series of Zijlstra and coworkers,[32] 142 patients were randomized to direct angioplasty or to intravenous streptokinase therapy. Primary study end points were the in-hospital rate of recurrent ischemia, infarct vessel patency, and predischarge LVEF. Angioplasty was successful in 98% of the patients in whom it was attempted. The incidence of recurrent ischemia was 38% in the streptokinase group compared with 9% in the PTCA group ($p < .001$). Predischarge LVEF was .45 in the streptokinase group compared with .51 in the PTCA group ($p = .004$), and the infarct-related vessel was patent in 68% of the streptokinase group at 3 weeks and in 91% of the PTCA group at 2 h and again at 82 days. Angiography after discharge demonstrated residual stenoses of 76% and 36% in the streptokinase and PTCA groups, respectively. Thus, among those randomized to PTCA, there was increased patency, a reduction in the degree of residual stenosis, a lower rate of recurrent ischemia, and greater preservation of left ventricular function.

After completion of their initial series, the Netherlands group extended the study to a total of 301 patients,[144, 145] with essentially similar results. Infarct size estimated from cumulative enzyme release was significantly smaller in the PTCA group; the greatest benefits were observed in those with anterior infarction and in patients randomized less than 2 h after the onset of symptoms. In the PTCA group, there were significant improvements in global ejection fraction (.50 versus .45, $p < .001$), infarct-related wall motion (42% vs. 34%, $p < .001$), and non–infarct-related wall motion (55% vs. 51%, $p = .005$) compared with the streptokinase group. Differences were more pronounced in patients with anterior infarction, but patients with nonanterior infarct location also benefited from PTCA. Of 152 patients randomized to primary angioplasty, the procedure was successful in 97% of patients in whom it was attempted, with TIMI grade 3 flow in 92% of patients at 120 min. Again, in the PTCA group, the frequency of recurrent ischemia and revascularization procedures was significantly reduced.

Summary: Trials of Direct Angioplasty vs. Thrombolysis. Despite differences in study design and end points, the large randomized trials of direct angioplasty share common features. Approximately 10% of patients randomized to invasive strategies were unsuitable for PTCA and were rapidly triaged to CABG or medical treatment. Procedural success rates were uniformly high in keeping with results of published series, including the PAR study.[126, 138] Although none of the trials was designed to detect differences in mortality or reinfarction, there were consistent trends favoring PTCA, with the greatest benefits in those at high risk. Simari and coworkers[148] performed a meta-analysis of three trials,[31–33] examining the endpoints of in-hospital mortality and reinfarction; their analysis suggests that primary angioplasty is associated with lower in-hospital mortality rates and less reinfarction (Table 44–11). The meta-analysis by Michels and Yusuf[149] confirmed reduced mortality and reinfarction rates at 6 weeks but demonstrated smaller differences in these outcomes at 1 year.

In patients treated with PTCA, the impressive reductions in the frequency of recurrent and provocable ischemia and need for revascularization procedures persisted after hospital discharge; this may have been related to reduced residual stenosis and favorable plaque remodeling. Bleeding episodes in patients receiving PTCA were related chiefly to vascular access sites, and their frequency was similar to the frequency of bleeding episodes observed in those receiving intravenous thrombolytic drugs. In spite of the similar occurrence of bleeding, stroke is less frequent in mechanically reperfused patients but still complicates direct angioplasty as reported in some series.[138, 150]

There is discordance between trials regarding the influence of direct angioplasty on LVEF, a controversial end point that poses significant logistic problems.[151, 152] In the Netherlands study, improvement in ejection fraction with PTCA was associated with smaller enzymatic infarct size but may in part have been due to the relatively greater proportion of patients with Killip class 3 or class 4 status

TABLE 44–11. META-ANALYSIS OF RANDOMIZED TRIALS OF DIRECT ANGIOPLASTY VERSUS THROMBOLYSIS IN ACUTE MYOCARDIAL INFARCTION

	PTCA			Lysis		
		Events			Events	
Trial	**No. Patients**	*No.*	*%*	**No. Patients**	*No.*	*%*
PAMI[31]	195	5	2.6	200	13	6.5
Netherlands[32]	70	0	0.0	72	4	5.6
Mayo Clinic[33]	47	2	4.3	56	2	3.6
Total	312	7	2.2	328	19	5.8
In-Hospital Reinfarction†						
PAMI	195	5	2.6	200	13	6.5
Netherlands	70	0	0.0	72	9	12.5
Mayo Clinic	47	1	2.1	56	3	5.4
Total	312	6	1.9	328	25	7.6

Abbreviations: PTCA, percutaneous transluminal coronary angioplasty; PAMI, Primary Angioplasty in Myocardial Infarction.

*The odds ratio for in-hospital mortality with thrombolysis vs. angioplasty is 2.68 (95% confidence limits, 1.16 and 6.92; $p = .023$).

†The odds ratio for in-hospital reinfarction with thrombolysis vs. angioplasty is 4.22 (95% confidence limits, 1.82 and 11.46; $p = .0008$).

From Simari RD, Berger MD, Bell MR, et al: Coronary angioplasty in acute myocardial infarction: primary, immediate adjunctive, rescue or deferred adjunctive approach? Mayo Clin Proc 1994; 69:346–358.

and triple-vessel disease, reflecting the greater benefit of PTCA in severely compromised patients. In the PAMI trial, the 6-week LVEF data were derived from only 65% of survivors, and of the 34 patients who died or had nonfatal reinfarction, only 9 underwent follow-up testing. At present, there are insufficient data for firm conclusions to be reached regarding the effect of direct angioplasty on LVEF, and further large-scale randomized trials are required to provide definitive information about this end point. Other criticisms of the PAMI trial have included the lack of an independent clinical events committee and the universal use of diltiazem, a drug without proven benefit in Q wave myocardial infarction; the protocol did not specify the use of beta blocking drugs. As discussed before, comparisons should be made with the knowledge that those randomized to thrombolytic therapy fared poorly as a group compared with large cohorts in contemporary thrombolytic trials.

These trials stand in contradistinction to the trials of angioplasty as a routine adjunct to thrombolytic therapy,[17, 29, 62] in which combined therapy failed to improve outcome and was associated with increased morbidity. This suggests that the combination of thrombolysis with PTCA is inferior to PTCA alone, possibly reflecting the prothrombotic effects of fibrinolytic therapy in this setting. There is a small but relatively constant proportion of patients in the invasive arms of these trials who are better served by therapies other than PTCA; thus, these trials actually compared thrombolytic therapy with a strategy of urgent angiography and triage to the most appropriate form of therapy. Furthermore, the results of trials comparing PTCA with fibrinolytic agents can be generalized only to patients eligible for thrombolytic therapy and should not be freely extrapolated to the large group of patients for whom no randomized comparative data are available.

Infarct Vessel Patency. Although none of these trials compares angioplasty with the front-loaded t-PA regimen used in the GUSTO trial,[146] patency rates are generally superior (>90%) to the best reported in the thrombolytic literature[75] (Fig. 44–5). Even with the most effective regimen in the GUSTO trial, only 54% of patients had patency with TIMI grade 3 flow at 90 min, and it is this finding that is the strongest predictor of improved ejection fraction and of survival at 30 days.[75, 153] Using myocardial contrast echocardiography, Ito and coworkers[154] demonstrated the absence of tissue perfusion in 23% of a group of patients with "successfully recanalized" infarct vessels. Mismatch was associated with marked diminution in recovery of left ventricular function, highlighting the effects of the dissociation that may exist between IRA patency and myocardial perfusion. After thrombolysis, causes of abnormal tissue perfusion may also include critical residual stenosis with dynamically fluctuating thrombus load and vasomotor tone, distal embolism of platelet-fibrin aggregates, and, at the tissue level, myocardial and microvascular inflammation and edema.[155, 156] It is likely that less than 50% of patients receiving the best thrombolytic regimen currently available experience optimal reperfusion. PTCA may not be analogous to thrombolysis in the setting of acute myocardial infarction and cannot address problems at the microvascular or myocardial level; however, brisk epicardial coronary flow is a powerful predictor of favorable clinical outcomes, and direct angioplasty has the potential to achieve and sustain early TIMI grade 3 flow in a large proportion of patients.

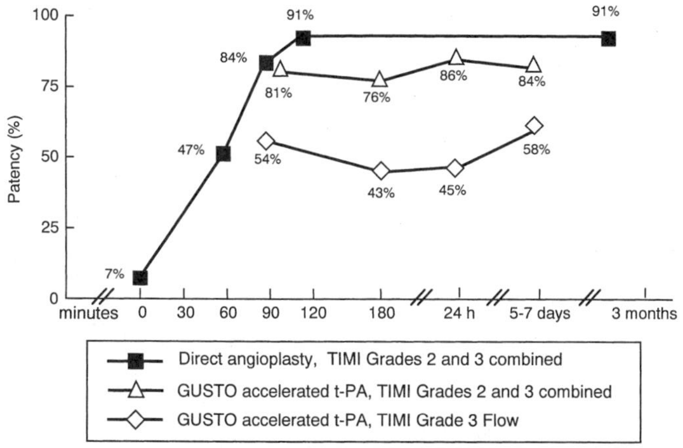

Figure 44–5. Patency rates comparing direct angioplasty and contemporary thrombolytic regimens. (Data from Zijlstra F, de Boer MJ, Hoorntje JCA, et al: A comparison of immediate coronary angioplasty with intravenous streptokinase in acute myocardial infarction. N Engl J Med 1993; 328:680–684; and The GUSTO Investigators: An international randomized trial comparing four thrombolytic strategies for acute myocardial infarction. N Engl J Med 1993; 329:673–682.)

The Angioplasty Strategy: Possible Mechanisms of Benefit

The potential physiologic advantages of a mechanical reperfusion strategy in acute myocardial infarction can be viewed as being related to myocardial salvage or independent of salvage. In the PAMI trial,[31] despite a greater delay to initiation of therapy in the PTCA group, complete relief of pain was achieved more rapidly, consistent with faster relief of ischemia. In the Netherlands study,[144] myocardial salvage was greater in the PTCA group when treatment was commenced in less than 2 h (31% vs. 14%), with a corresponding increase in LVEF.

Mechanisms unrelated to myocardial salvage include greater lesion stability, myocardial effects mediated by patency of the infarct-related vessel, and reduced risk of intracranial hemorrhage that is frequently lethal when it complicates thrombolytic therapy. The use of direct angioplasty creates a larger lumen possibly less susceptible to rethrombosis and reocclusion in the peri-infarct period; this is associated with a marked reduction in episodes of recurrent ischemia. In the PAR study,[138] 13% of patients had occluded infarct vessels at 6 months, but half had done so silently without clinically manifest events. In the Netherlands trial,[32] the incidence of occlusion at 3 months was 9%. Although there are few late patency studies and the post-thrombolytic reocclusion rates of 41% at 6 months in the TAMI-6 trial[157] and 25%–30% at 3 months in the Antithrombotics in the Prevention of Reocclusion in Coronary Thrombolytics (APRICOT) study[158] may represent the worst case scenario, the reported results of direct angioplasty compare favorably.

Patency of the infarct vessel may independently influence outcome by a mechanism unrelated to myocardial salvage. Pooled data from thrombolytic trials[13] suggest a highly significant mortality reduction in patients reperfused 7–12 h after the onset of infarction. The TAMI-6 trial compared angioplasty with conservative management after unsuccessful thrombolysis; however, no trial to date has directly compared late angioplasty with late thrombolytic therapy in acute myocardial infarction. In patients who had received thrombolytic therapy, Leung and Lau[159] observed that the severity of residual stenosis in the IRA was a determinant of the degree of left ventricular dilatation at 6 months and at 1 year. Contrary to the conventional view that ventricular dilatation is promoted by occlusion and prevented by patency, this study demonstrated a continuous relationship between the degree of residual stenosis in the IRA and the extent of ventricular dilatation.

The pathophysiologic mechanism underlying this phenomenon is unknown, but it occurs independently of myocardial salvage and is potentially a mechanism by which direct angioplasty could favorably influence outcome.[160] Hirayama and coworkers[161] demonstrated that reperfusion 6 h or more after onset of infarction limited ventricular dilatation without reducing infarct size. The series of Tison and colleagues[162] supports these findings; 200 patients underwent direct angioplasty for acute myocardial infarction with complete angiographic follow-up. At 6 months, restenosis and reocclusion were associated with left ventricular dilatation, whereas volumes remained unchanged in patients with patent infarct vessels.

In a pilot study, Dzavik and coworkers[163] observed a cohort of 44 patients with occluded infarct vessels after first Q-wave infarction. Patients were randomized to PTCA within the first 6 weeks after infarction or to conservative management; the mean baseline LVEF was .45 in both groups. Four-month angiographic follow-up was complete in 37, of whom 12 had persisting IRA patency. Numbers were too small to analyze according to intention to treat, but secondary analysis showed a significantly greater increase in ejection fraction in those with patent infarct vessels (+.094 vs. +.018, $p < .01$) and identified IRA patency as an independent predictor of improved LVEF. These studies suggest that severity of residual stenosis and patency of the IRA exert significant effects on left ventricular dilatation and systolic function beyond what has been traditionally perceived as the window for myocardial salvage. At this time, it remains to be seen whether these intriguing results will be duplicated in larger trials and whether late IRA patency achieved by PTCA improves survival after myocardial infarction.

Restenosis After Direct Angioplasty

There has been little formal, prospective assessment of the incidence of restenosis after direct angioplasty. Complete angiographic follow-up (>90%) is the exception rather than the rule,[164] and when follow-up is incomplete, results may be skewed by selection bias. If clinical assessments are relied on, underestimation of the true restenosis rate occurs.[165] Other problems include variability in definitions of restenosis and the timing of angiographic restudy, heterogeneity of patient populations, and varying frequency of conjunctive thrombolytic use. The results of six reports[130, 139, 162, 166–168] are summarized in Table 44–12. These data would suggest that the incidence of restenosis is similar to or slightly greater than the rate associated with elective PTCA. In the Evaluation of 7E3 for the Prevention of Ischemic Complications (EPIC) trial,[169] there was a reduction of coronary events at 6-month follow-up, suggesting that restenosis may be reduced after PTCA for unstable coronary syndromes (including acute myocardial infarction) by the use of a chimeric monoclonal antibody (c7E3) directed against the IIb/IIIa platelet surface receptor. This finding has particular relevance and provides rationale for the study of the use of c7E3 as an adjunct to direct angioplasty.

Subgroups of Patients

In the population of patients with acute myocardial infarction, several clinical subgroups warrant special consideration. These include patients in cardiogenic shock, patients ineligible for thrombolytic therapy, the elderly, and those with previous CABG. A major obstacle to determining the most appropriate management for these patients is the relatively small amount of data from randomized trials; because of variations in the populations studied, selection criteria, definitions, and end points used, data from published series cannot be generalized to allow comparison of treatment strategies.

TABLE 44–12. RESTENOSIS AFTER DIRECT ANGIOPLASTY

Study	Year	Restudy/ Eligible	Restenosis No.	Restenosis %	Months to Restudy
Brodie et al.[139]	1994	154/203	69/154	45	6
Tison et al.[162]	1991	204/204	92/204	45	6
Almany et al.[166]	1991	87/141	45/87	52	6
Simonton et al.[167]	1988	79/91	25/79	32	6.5
Miller et al.[168]	1987	76/100	27/76	36	4.6
Rothbaum et al.[130]	1987	85/121	34/85	40	3–6
Pooled		685/860 (80%)	292/685	43	

Angioplasty for Cardiogenic Shock and the Role of Support Devices. In 1954, Griffith and coworkers[170] reported an 80% hospital mortality in patients with cardiogenic shock. In the mid 1960s, Killip and Kimball[171] reported a mortality rate of 81% for patients with cardiogenic shock. Despite major subsequent advances in the management of acute myocardial infarction, Goldberg and coworkers[172] detected no improvement in the outcome of this condition for the years 1975 through 1988 and found its incidence to be remarkably constant at 7.5% of the infarcts in their cohort. Even with the advent of the thrombolytic era, neither intracoronary nor intravenous agents were shown to favorably affect outcome.[173–176] Several series describing the use of PTCA for the treatment of this condition are comprehensively reviewed elsewhere.[36, 177] In these series, reperfusion was achieved in more than 60% of patients. In-hospital survival after reperfusion exceeded 70%, whereas less than a quarter of patients survived without reperfusion. Short-term survival is rare in the elderly, and long-term survival is significantly greater among reperfused survivors than in the group who survive without reperfusion. Early therapy is desirable, but myocardial necrosis may be protracted,[178] and reperfusion may be effective up to 24 h after the onset of symptoms. Although it is not confirmed by a randomized trial, many clinicians believe that there is compelling collective evidence to support the use of PTCA in cardiogenic shock.[177] The SHOCK trial is currently in progress[179] and will prospectively examine the role of various reperfusion strategies including direct angioplasty in this high-risk group.

Direct angioplasty is the contemporary treatment of choice for cardiogenic shock complicating acute myocardial infarction. The use of various support devices is in evolution and promises to increase the potential for salvaging patients with extensive myocardial dysfunction and circulatory collapse.[180] Although it has little effect on distal flow in the presence of a critical stenosis, counterpulsation with the intra-aortic balloon pump (IABP) has been shown to augment coronary flow velocity[181] after angioplasty; whereas IABP counterpulsation is ineffective in preventing infarct expansion, its use as part of an aggressive afterload reduction strategy has been shown to prevent dilatation and remodeling of non–infarct-related segments in patients with extensive infarction.[182] Use of IABP counterpulsation has been shown in a retrospective study[183] and in a randomized trial[184] to reduce recurrent ischemic events in patients undergoing PTCA for acute myocardial infarction. Ohman and coworkers[184] demonstrated significant reductions in the incidence of reocclusion (8% vs. 21%) and in the frequency of a composite clinical end point (13% vs. 24%) among patients randomized to counterpulsation. The rates of bleeding and vascular complications were similar in both groups.

Although experience with percutaneous cardiopulmonary bypass has chiefly consisted of prophylactic use in elective high-risk angioplasty, Shawl and coworkers[185, 186] reported its efficacy in supporting patients with cardiogenic shock; PTCA was performed in 8 of 10 patients, all of whom survived at least 10 months. The use of the Nimbus Hemopump, a catheter-mounted percutaneous left ventricular assist device (Johnson & Johnson, New Brunswick, NJ), has been described to support PTCA in patients with cardiogenic shock.[187] The utility of these devices is currently limited by their size and potential for cardiovascular trauma; however, even with significant technical advances, there are many other factors that may limit their widespread use.

Patients Ineligible for Thrombolytic Therapy. Despite the energy invested in the development and use of intravenous thrombolytic agents during the last decade, little attention has been devoted to the general applicability of such therapy. In thrombolytic trials, a large majority of patients are excluded from randomization, with exclusion rates of 65% or more.[174] Cragg and coworkers[188] surveyed 1471 consecutive patients admitted to a large community-based hospital and found that only 22% received reperfusion therapy. Those ineligible for thrombolytic therapy were 11 years older, more likely to be female and hypertensive, and to have long-standing ischemic heart disease. The mortality rate was five times higher among ineligible patients (19% vs. 4%). Other workers have reported similar rates of thrombolytic ineligibility in large series[189] and similar mortality among such patients after direct angioplasty even with high procedural success rates.[150, 190] Such patients clearly constitute a high-risk group regardless of treatment, and the precise role of mechanical reperfusion therapy requires further randomized appraisal in the context of new broader indications for thrombolytic therapy.

Direct Angioplasty in the Elderly. With increasing age, the rates of mortality and morbidity associated with acute myocardial infarction rise steeply regardless of treatment. Despite the favorable risk/benefit ratio of thrombolytic therapy in this group, physicians remain reluctant to use this option, largely because of the increased frequency of catastrophic hemorrhage in these patients.[13, 191, 192] To date, there is a paucity of randomized data available, and most information concerning direct PTCA in the elderly is derived from published series. In the meta-analysis of Eckman and coworkers,[126] elderly patients receiving direct angioplasty had an average in-hospital mortality that was worse than that of similar patients receiving thrombolytic therapy and no better than that in the placebo arms of thrombolytic trials. From a large consecutive series of elderly thrombolytic candidates, Stuckey and coworkers[193] report increasing mortality with increasing age of the patient in spite of high procedural success rates. Randomized data from the PAMI trial showed a strong trend to reduced mortality (15.0% versus 5.7%) among patients older than 65 years and also in women of all ages.[194] It is clear that in this group, persistent occlusion of the IRA is a powerful predictor of mortality,[195] and as discussed previously, patients older than 75 years rarely survive cardiogenic shock regardless of treatment.[177] At present, it is not possible to confidently advocate a specific approach to reperfusion therapy in this fast-growing and fragile group of patients; further data from randomized trials will be helpful in guiding future efforts.

Patients With Previous Coronary Artery Bypass Surgery. Another group encountered with increasing frequency is patients with myocardial infarction who have had prior CABG. Grines and coworkers[196] first described the increased thrombus burden in occluded saphenous vein grafts and their resistance to intravenous thrombolytic therapy. Kavanaugh and Topol[197] studied a series of 40 patients with prior CABG and acute myocardial infarction, performing PTCA in 16. They noted that the group was angiographically and electrocardiographically difficult to assess. In the Coronary Artery Surgery Study Registry, 30-day mortality was 21% in patients admitted with acute myocardial infarction within 3 years of CABG surgery.[198] In a large multicenter analysis from the University of California, San Diego, database,[199] patients with CABG an average 7.1 years before infarction experienced increased in-hospital morbidity, and 1-year mortality was twice that of those without prior CABG.

From a subanalysis of the GUSTO trial,[200] it is apparent that patients with prior CABG (mean time from CABG to index infarction 8.6 years) had more advanced clinical coronary disease and worse short- and long-term outcomes (Table 44–13). Sixty percent of CABG patients had angiography within 30 days of infarction, mostly at the discretion of the attending physician. In patients with prior CABG, 35% of infarct vessels were saphenous vein grafts, and compared with patients without prior CABG, graft and native stenoses were more severe and the frequency of occlusion and abnormal flow was greater. Although potential sources of selection bias in this cohort were many, even in these thrombolytic-eligible patients (expected to have a better prognosis than ineligible patients), prior CABG was strongly associated with adverse outcomes. In the largest series of direct PTCA to date, 130 patients with prior CABG were treated with an 86% success rate in saphenous vein graft lesions compared with a 95% success rate in native vessels ($p < .0001$). In-hospital mortality rates were similar for patients with and without bypass grafts.[150]

TABLE 44–13. CLINICAL CHARACTERISTICS OF PATIENTS WITH AND WITHOUT PRIOR CABG SURGERY IN THE GUSTO TRIAL

	Prior CABG (N = 1784)	No CABG (N = 39,119)	p
Prior myocardial infarction	65.0	14.2	<.0001
Prior angina	77.8	35.0	<.0001
24-h mortality	3.5	2.6	<.03
Overall 30-day mortality	10.7	6.4	<.0001
1-year mortality	15.8	8.0	<.0001
Cardiogenic shock	9.0	5.8	<.0001
Pulmonary edema	22.3	16.0	<.0001
Recurrent ischemia	25.8	19.7	<.0001
Reinfarction	5.9	3.9	<.0001

Abbreviations: CABG, coronary artery bypass grafting; GUSTO, Global Utilization of Streptokinase and Tissue Plasminogen Activator for Occluded Coronary Arteries.

Data from De Franco AC, Abramowitz B, Krichbaum D, et al: Substantial (threefold) benefit of accelerated t-PA over standard thrombolytic therapy in patients with prior bypass surgery and acute MI: Results of the GUSTO trial [Abstract]. J Am Coll Cardiol 1994; 23:1A–484A.

The limited information available from diverse groups of patients does not provide clear guidelines for management of this complex population. However, given that this is a group at increased risk with demonstrated resistance to intravenous thrombolytic agents, a strong case can be made for urgent catheterization with a view to mechanical reperfusion. Performance of PTCA in thrombus-laden saphenous vein grafts is associated with the risk of distal embolism of thrombus and debris; however, this problem has not been evaluated in the context of acute graft occlusion. The use of extraction atherectomy[201] and laser angioplasty[202] has been reported in treatment of acute myocardial infarction without angiographic evidence of distal embolism and may represent a valuable future strategy for approaching acute vein graft thrombosis.

Reocclusion

Although angioplasty is highly effective in restoring vessel patency in acute myocardial infarction, subsequent reocclusion occurs in 10%–20% of patients (see Tables 44–3 and 44–8) and is a major limitation of the procedure in terms of morbidity. In the PAR registry,[139] reocclusion after discharge was silent in 65% but was associated with adverse outcomes whether it was silent or clinically apparent. Compared with reocclusion after successful thrombolytic therapy, which is reviewed elsewhere,[203, 204] clinical knowledge is sparse, and biologic processes await clarification. In the rescue angioplasty setting, initial use of non–fibrin-selective thrombolytic agents seems to be associated with a significant increase in the frequency of reocclusion (see Table 44–3). However, in the absence of randomized data, firm recommendations cannot be made.

Ohman and coworkers[184] randomized 182 patients in whom IRA patency had been mechanically restored to 48 h of IABP counterpulsation or to standard care. The use of intracoronary and prior intravenous thrombolytics was similar in both groups. Patients randomized to IABP counterpulsation had similar rates of severe bleeding complications, yet the frequency of IRA reocclusion was significantly reduced (8% versus 21%) compared with those receiving standard care. Lefkovits and coworkers[117] described a group of 64 patients enrolled in the EPIC trial who underwent PTCA within 12 h of the onset of infarction. In those treated with high-dose c7E3, there was a 5-fold reduction in the incidence of events at 30 days and a 10-fold reduction at 6 months. These findings indicate that potent inhibition of the platelet glycoprotein IIb/IIIa receptor may drastically reduce the frequency of ischemic complications in patients undergoing direct angioplasty. Reducing the rate of reocclusion after mechanical reperfusion is required to increase the overall efficacy of this strategy, and clinical advances will undoubtedly follow greater insights into the biology underlying this process.

Predictors of Outcome and the Price of Failure

Ellis and coworkers[205] analyzed a cohort of 300 patients undergoing direct angioplasty for acute myocardial infarction and identified preserved LVEF, absence of triple-vessel disease, bends of 45 degrees or greater, multilesion IRA disease, and small thrombus burden as predictors of successful procedural outcome. Independent predictors of adverse clinical outcome include persistent occlusion of the infarct vessel, the presence of multivessel coronary disease, and cardiogenic shock.[206, 207] Bedotto and coworkers[207] reported a 94% success rate in a group of 750 patients. Patients with failed direct PTCA had multiple high-risk characteristics and an in-hospital death rate of 31% compared with 4.8% in those with a successful procedure.

Current Status of Angioplasty for Acute Myocardial Infarction: Contemporary Trials

To date, the number of patients enrolled in prospective, randomized studies of angioplasty in myocardial infarction is small compared with the large number studied in trials of thrombolytic therapy. At present, there are no definitive data on mortality or clinical endpoints occurring during intermediate and long-term follow-up, and potential low-risk subsets in which the net effect of an invasive approach may be detrimental await identification. The GUSTO-2 substudy currently in progress will have the power to prospectively address the endpoints of death and reinfarction. A subgroup of 1200 patients with acute myocardial infarction will be studied in a protocol of factorial design comparing direct angioplasty with accelerated t-PA and comparing heparin with r-hirudin, which may facilitate PTCA more than thrombolysis. The PAMI-2 trial will consist of two arms; in high-risk patients, randomization will be to IABP or no IABP; in the low-risk group, early discharge will be compared with standard management. The results of the RESCUE-2 trial will provide further valuable information to guide future management of patients with failed thrombolysis. After the encouraging results of c7E3 combined with rescue angioplasty reported in the EPIC trial,[117] a further randomized trial, RAPPORT, is planned to prospectively assess the use of this drug as an adjunct to mechanical revascularization.

An area of increasing interest is the application of new device technologies in the acute infarct setting. Extraction and laser atherectomy have been described in the treatment of myocardial infarction,[191, 192, 208] particularly for the treatment of the complex lesion subset with large thrombus burdens. The selective use of stents (Fig. 44–6) may assist the operator confronted by recoil or persistent

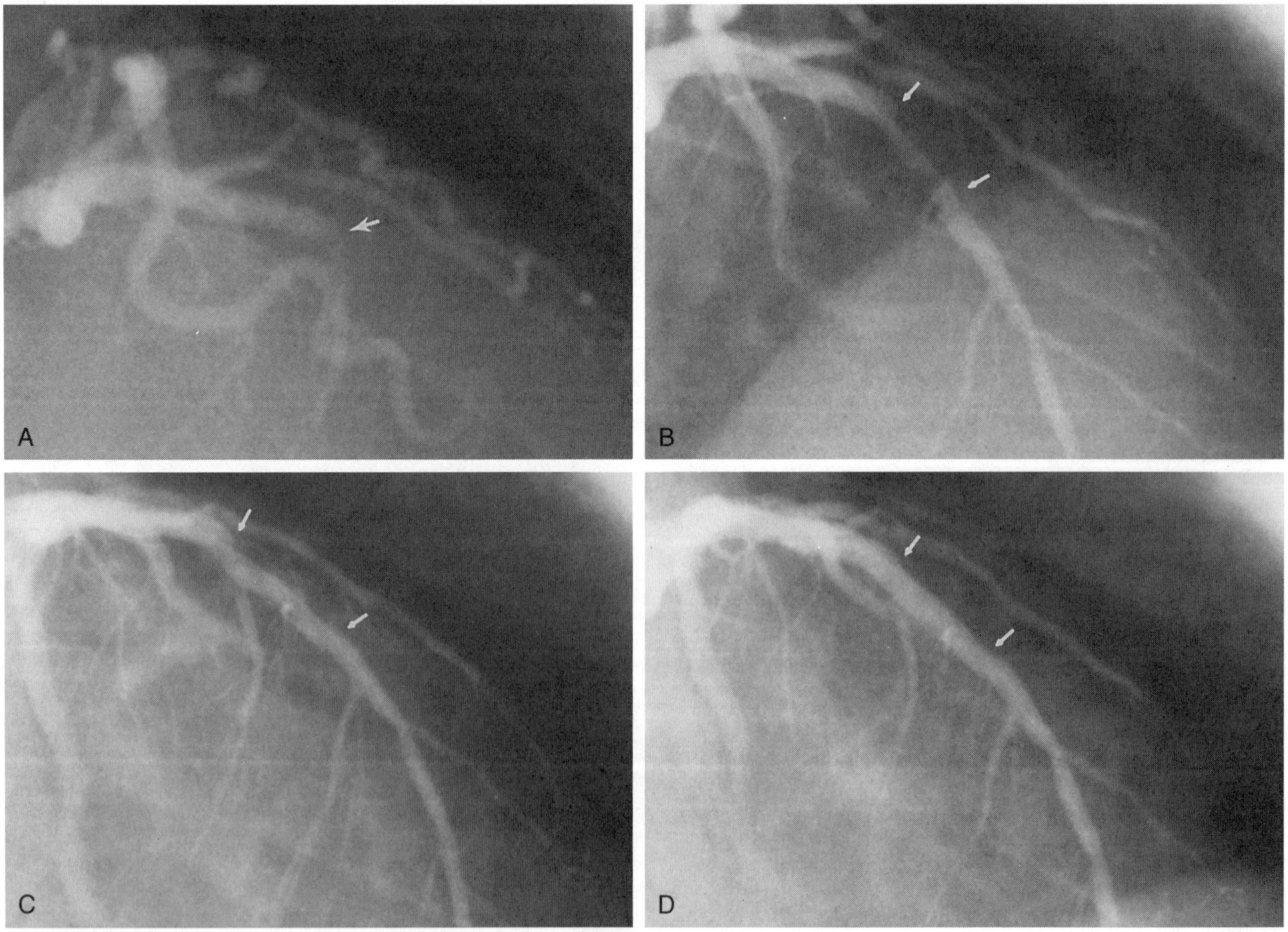

Figure 44–6. Stent deployment in acute anterior wall myocardial infarction. *A*, Left anterior descending artery occlusion (*arrow*) in a 72-year-old man. *B*, Patency reestablished after passage of guide wire. *C*, After PTCA, TIMI grade 3 flow is restored, but significant intimal disruption is present. *D*, Shortly after the patient left the catheterization laboratory, symptomatic reocclusion occurred; the patient returned to the laboratory, and a Johnson and Johnson Interventional Systems coronary stent (*arrows*) was deployed. The patient's subsequent hospital course was uncomplicated.

disruption of intima and plaque after clearance of luminal thrombus that follows initial dilatation. Local delivery of antithrombotic or anticoagulant agents may have a role in achieving "passivation" of prothrombotic surfaces acting as substrates for refractory thrombus formation.[209]

Current data suggest that direct angioplasty is able to establish and sustain TIMI grade 3 flow in the infarct vessel more quickly and more often than contemporary thrombolytic regimens. Life-threatening bleeding complications and recurrent ischemic events are less frequent, and late IRA patency is superior. Furthermore, those at greatest risk (patients with severe hemodynamic compromise, pulmonary edema, or cardiogenic shock) stand to benefit most from direct angioplasty. Given these considerations, direct angioplasty is at least equivalent to thrombolytic therapy overall, and in selected groups of patients, it is the preferred initial treatment.

There are major impediments to the widespread use of angioplasty in myocardial infarction. Direct angioplasty was used as first-line treatment in only 3.1% of patients surveyed in the most recent report from the National Registry of Myocardial Infarction.[210] The results of published series and trials emanate from institutions with high-volume catheterization laboratories staffed by physicians and support personnel with considerable experience and expertise in performance of direct angioplasty; obviously, these results cannot be extrapolated to all catheterization facilities. Data from the Alabama Registry of Myocardial Infarction[211] and the Myocardial Infarction Triage and Intervention (MITI) Project Registry[212] suggest that use of primary angioplasty in community hospitals results in 1-year mortality similar to thrombolytic therapy, but with reduced morbidity.

Provision of direct angioplasty in a timely and safe fashion requires physicians, call teams, and surgical back-up to be available at short notice on a 24-h basis; this clearly presents complex logistic and possible financial challenges. The need for surgical standby is controversial. The American College of Cardiology officially sanctions direct angioplasty in centers without on-site surgical support only as a last resort or if transfer to a more appropriate center is impossible or impractical.[213] However, in a large study from the MITI project in which more than 50% of direct angioplasty was performed in facilities without on-site cardiac surgery, the mortality rate was low and dependent on clinical factors but not on the presence of on-site surgery.[212]

Recommendations. Direct angioplasty is the treatment of choice in those with cardiogenic shock and Killip class 3 infarction. It should also be carefully considered in patients with previous contralateral Q wave infarction and those ineligible to receive thrombolytic therapy because of prior stroke, uncontrolled hypertension, or increased risk of serious bleeding. Patients whose diagnosis is uncertain but who have suggestive symptoms and a nondiagnostic electrocardiogram (e.g., left bundle branch block of unknown duration) may benefit from urgent catheterization. This obviates the risks of empirical thrombolytic administration, defines coronary anatomy, and will expedite management. Finally, it is arguable that any patient presenting early after the onset of symptoms in geographic proximity to a proficient interventional catheterization laboratory is best managed by prompt mechanical reperfusion—the "right time, right place" indication. As discussed previously, the benefits of reperfusion extend beyond the traditional thrombolytic "window," and direct angioplasty should be considered in any patient with "stuttering infarction" or protracted anginal chest pain with ST segment changes.

Rescue angioplasty is warranted in patients with persistent IRA occlusion, ST segment elevation, and ongoing symptoms. Its respective roles in patients with incomplete reperfusion and in individuals at low risk remain to be defined. It is the perspective of these authors that emergent interventions are optimally performed in facilities with on-site cardiac surgery unless the expected benefit clearly outweighs the risks of intervention or transfer of the patient. A hierarchy of indications for primary mechanical intervention in the acute infarct setting is summarized in Table 44–14.

Technical Aspects. If urgent catheterization is undertaken before treatment, thrombolytic therapy should be withheld because all available data suggest that it adversely affects the results of PTCA for acute myocardial infarction and may increase the risk of serious bleeding. In the hemodynamically unstable patient, dual femoral artery access is ideal, permitting rapid institution of IABP counterpulsation if necessary; placement of a pulmonary balloon wedge catheter allows measurement of the pulmonary capillary wedge pressure to optimize hemodynamic status and guide inotrope therapy. The use of non-ionic contrast agents has commonly been advocated to minimize negative inotropic effects, particularly in patients with significantly impaired left ventricular function. However, in an analysis of data from 1930 high-risk patients enrolled in the EPIC trial, Aguirre and coworkers[214] showed that use of ionic contrast agents was independently associated with a lower probability of Q wave infarction and death. These results are likely to be relevant in the direct angioplasty setting, where use of ionic media is traditionally preferred to the use of nonionic agents. After rapid assessment of the coronary anatomy, angioplasty of the infarct vessel is performed when appropriate. Because of the increased risk of thrombotic reocclusion in this setting, an "over-the-wire" technique is recommended to maintain access to the distal lumen of the vessel.

A non–infarct-related vessel should never be dilated in acute myocardial infarction unless a state of refractory cardiogenic shock exists. Inability to identify the culprit vessel is not uncommonly encountered in patients with multivessel disease and is a relative contraindication to percutaneous intervention because of the potentially catastrophic sequelae of abrupt closure of a non–infarct-related vessel. A left main trunk culprit lesion or a significant left main stenosis proximal to a left anterior descending or left circumflex culprit lesion should prompt consideration of urgent CABG surgery. Balloon counterpulsation should be instituted promptly in the compromised patient, and in view of the favorable effects of IABP counterpulsation on recurrent ischemic events even in the absence of cardiogenic shock,[184] this intervention should be considered in all patients, particularly those at risk for reinfarction in large infarct vessel territories.

THE FUTURE OF ANGIOPLASTY FOR MYOCARDIAL INFARCTION

Although the body of prospective randomized data is small in the larger context of trials of reperfusion therapy, procedural success rates reported for direct angioplasty are high, and it is clearly the treatment of choice for the majority of severely compromised patients with acute myocardial infarction. It appears at least equivalent to thrombolysis with respect to mortality reduction, preservation of left

TABLE 44–14. INDICATIONS FOR DIRECT ANGIOPLASTY IN ACUTE MYOCARDIAL INFARCTION

Absolute Indication	Cardiogenic shock, <75 years of age
Strong Indications	Killip class III or IV status
	Prior contralateral Q wave infarction
	Patients ineligible for thrombolysis
	"Right time, right place" indication
Relative Indication	Suggestive clinical presentation with nondiagnostic ECG
Uncertain Indications	Presentation >6 h after onset
	Patients with prior CABG surgery
	Cardiogenic shock, >75 years of age

Abbreviations: ECG, electrocardiogram; CABG, coronary artery bypass grafting.

ventricular function, and cost and seems superior with respect to infarct vessel patency and frequency of recurrent ischemic events. Further information to guide future efforts will be available from large patient cohorts in the near future as results become available from the PAMI-2, GUSTO-2, RESCUE-2, SHOCK, and RAPPORT trials currently in progress.

Although direct angioplasty may have been undervalued in the past, its utility in the treatment of acute coronary occlusion is now firmly established and it will unquestionably remain an integral component of myocardial reperfusion therapy. The role of rescue angioplasty requires further detailed study before definitive recommendations can be made. As refinements evolve in percutaneous revascularization equipment, cardiovascular support techniques, and pharmacologic adjunctive therapy, the challenge facing cardiologists in the 1990s will be to define the most effective role for mechanical reperfusion therapies in the management of acute myocardial infarction.

REFERENCES

1. Herrick JB: Clinical features of sudden obstruction of the coronary arteries. JAMA 1912; 59:2015–2020.
2. Davies M, Woolf N, Robertson W: Pathology of acute myocardial infarction with particular reference to occlusive coronary thrombi. Br Heart J 1976; 38:659–664.
3. Roberts WC, Buja LM: The frequency and significance of coronary arterial and other observations in fatal acute myocardial infarction: a study of 107 necropsy patients. Am J Med 1972; 52:425–443.
4. Falk E: Plaque rupture with severe pre-existing stenosis precipitating coronary thrombosis. Characteristics of coronary atherosclerotic plaques underlying fatal occlusive thrombi. Br Heart J 1983; 50:127–134.
5. Davies MJ, Thomas A: Thrombosis and acute coronary-artery lesions in sudden cardiac ischaemic death. N Engl J Med 1984; 310:1137–1140.
6. DeWood MA, Spores J, Notske R, et al: Prevalence of total coronary occlusion during the early hours of transmural myocardial infarction. N Engl J Med 1980; 303:897–902.
7. Rentrop P, Blanke H, Karsch KR, et al: Selective intracoronary thrombolysis in acute myocardial infarction and unstable angina pectoris. Circulation 1981; 63:307–317.
8. Meyer J, Merx W, Schmitz H, et al: Percutaneous transluminal coronary angioplasty immediately after intracoronary streptolysis of transmural myocardial infarction. Circulation 1982; 66:905–913.
9. Hartzler GO, Rutherford BD, McConahay DR, et al: Percutaneous transluminal coronary angioplasty with and without thrombolytic therapy for treatment of acute myocardial infarction. Am Heart J 1983; 106:965–973.
10. Weaver WD, Cerquiera M, Hallstrom AP, et al: Pre-hospital initiated vs hospital initiated thrombolytic therapy. The Myocardial Infarction Triage and Intervention trial. JAMA 1993; 270:1211–1216.
11. Kleiman NS, White HD, Ohman EM, et al, for the GUSTO Investigators: Mortality within 24 hours of thrombolysis for myocardial infarction: the importance of early reperfusion. Circulation 1994; 90:2658–2665.
12. Lincoff AM, Topol EJ: The illusion of reperfusion. Does anyone achieve optimal myocardial reperfusion? Circulation 1993; 87:1792–1805 (erratum 1993; 88:1361–1375).
13. Fibrinolytic Therapy Trialists' (FTT) Collaborative Group: Indications for fibrinolytic therapy in suspected acute myocardial infarction: collaborative overview of early mortality and major morbidity results from all randomised trials of more than 1000 patients. Lancet 1994; 343:311–322.
14. Kennedy JW, Ritchie JL, Davis KB, Fritz JK: Western Washington randomized trial of intracoronary streptokinase in acute myocardial infarction. N Engl J Med 1983; 309:1477–1482.
15. Simoons ML, van den Brand M, de Zwaan C, et al: Improved survival after early thrombolysis in acute myocardial infarction. Lancet 1985; 2:578–582.
16. Rentrop KP, Feit F, Blanke H, et al: Effects of intracoronary streptokinase and intracoronary nitroglycerin infusion on coronary angiographic patterns and mortality in patients with acute myocardial infarction. N Engl J Med 1984; 311:1458–1463.
17. Topol EJ, Califf RM, George BS, et al: A randomized trial of immediate versus delayed elective angioplasty after intravenous tissue plasminogen activator in acute myocardial infarction. N Engl J Med 1987; 317:581–588.
18. Topol EJ, Califf RM, George BS, et al: Coronary arterial thrombolysis with combined infusion of recombinant tissue-type plasminogen activator and urokinase in patients with acute myocardial infarction. Circulation 1988; 77:1100–1107.
19. Topol EJ, George BS, Kereiakes DJ, et al: A randomized controlled trial of intravenous tissue plasminogen activator and early intravenous heparin in acute myocardial infarction. Circulation 1989; 79:281–286.
20. Topol EJ, Ellis SG, Califf RM, et al: Combined tissue-type plasminogen activator and prostacyclin therapy for acute myocardial infarction. J Am Coll Cardiol 1989; 14:877–884.
21. Williams DO, Borer J, Braunwald E, et al: Intravenous recombinant tissue-type plasminogen activator in patients with acute myocardial infarction: a report from the NHLBI thrombolysis in myocardial infarction trial. Circulation 1986; 73:338–346.
22. The TIMI Study Group: The Thrombolysis in Myocardial Infarction (TIMI) trial. N Engl J Med 1985; 312:932–936.
23. Chesebro JH, Knatterud G, Roberts R, et al: Thrombolysis in Myocardial Infarction (TIMI) trial, phase I: a comparison between intravenous tissue-type plasminogen activator and intravenous streptokinase. Circulation 1987; 76:142–154.
24. Passamani E, Hodges M, Herman M, et al: The Thrombolysis in Myocardial Infarction (TIMI) phase II pilot study: tissue plasminogen activator followed by percutaneous transluminal coronary angioplasty. J Am Coll Cardiol 1987; 10:51B–64B.
25. The TIMI Study Group: Comparison of invasive and conservative strategies following intravenous tissue plasminogen activator in myocardial infarction: results of the Thrombolysis in Myocardial Infarction (TIMI) II trial. N Engl J Med 1989; 320:618–627.
26. Verstraete M, Brower RW, Collen D, et al: Double blind randomized trial of intravenous tissue-type plasminogen activator versus placebo in acute myocardial infarction. Lancet 1985; 2:965–969.
27. Verstraete M, Bory M, Collen D, et al: Randomized trial of intravenous tissue-type plasminogen activator versus intravenous streptokinase in acute myocardial infarction. Lancet 1985; 1:842–847.
28. Verstraete M, Arnold AER, Brower RW, et al: Acute coronary thrombolysis with recombinant human tissue-type plasminogen activator: initial patency and influence of maintained infusion on reocclusion rate. Am J Cardiol 1987; 60:231–237.
29. Simoons ML, Arnold AE, Betriu A, et al: Thrombolysis with tissue plasminogen activator in acute myocardial infarction: no additional benefit from immediate percutaneous transluminal coronary angioplasty. Lancet 1988; 1:197–203.
30. O'Neill W, Weintraub R, Grines CL, et al: A prospective, placebo-controlled, randomized trial of intravenous streptokinase and angioplasty versus lone angioplasty therapy of acute myocardial infarction. Circulation 1992; 86:1710–1717.
31. Grines CL, Browne KF, Marco J, et al: A comparison of immediate angioplasty with thrombolytic therapy for acute myocardial infarction. N Engl J Med 1993; 328:673–679.
32. Zijlstra F, de Boer MJ, Hoorntje JCA, et al: A comparison of immediate coronary angioplasty with intravenous streptokinase in acute myocardial infarction. N Engl J Med 1993; 328:680–684.
33. Gibbons RJ, Holmes DR Jr, Reeder GS, et al: Immediate angioplasty compared with the administration of a thrombolytic agent followed by conservative treatment for acute myocardial infarction. N Engl J Med 1993; 328:685–691.
34. Ribiero EE, Silva LA, Carniero R, et al: Randomized trial of direct coronary angioplasty versus streptokinase in acute myocardial infarction. J Am Coll Cardiol 1993; 22:376–380.
35. DeWood MA, Fisher MJ, for the Spokane Heart Research Group, Sacred Heart and Deaconess Medical Centers, Spokane, WA: Direct PTCA versus intravenous r-tPA in acute myocardial infarction: results from a prospective randomized trial [Abstract]. Circulation 1989; 80(suppl II):418.
36. Topol EJ: Mechanical interventions for acute myocardial infarction. *In* Topol EJ (ed): A Textbook of Interventional Cardiology, 2nd ed, pp 292–317, Philadelphia: WB Saunders, 1992.
37. Guerci AD, Gerstenblith G, Brinker JA, et al: A randomized trial of intravenous tissue plasminogen activator for acute myocardial infarction with subsequent randomization to elective coronary angioplasty. N Engl J Med 1987; 317:1613–1618.

38. Stack RS, O'Connor CM, Mark DB, et al: Coronary perfusion during acute myocardial infarction with a combined therapy of coronary angioplasty high-dose intravenous streptokinase. Circulation 1988; 77:151–161.
39. Topol EJ, George BS, Kereiakes DJ, et al: Comparison of two dose regimens of intravenous tissue plasminogen activator for acute myocardial infarction. Am J Cardiol 1988; 61:723–728.
40. Topol EJ, Bates ER, Walton JA, et al: Community hospital administration of intravenous tissue plasminogen activator in acute myocardial infarction: improved timing, thrombolytic efficacy and ventricular function. J Am Coll Cardiol 1987; 10:1173–1177.
41. Topol EJ, Holmes DR Jr, Rogers WJ: Coronary angiography after thrombolytic therapy for acute myocardial infarction. Ann Intern Med 1991; 114:877–885.
42. Bates ER, Topol EJ: Early hospital discharge in the myocardial reperfusion era. Clin Cardiol 1989; 12:III-65–III-70.
43. Califf RM, Topol EJ, Stack RS, et al, for the TAMI Study Group: Evaluation of combination thrombolytic therapy and timing of catheterization in acute myocardial infarction. Circulation 1991; 83:1543–1556.
44. Mueller HS, Cohen LS, Braunwald E, et al, for the TIMI Investigators: Predictors of early morbidity and mortality after thrombolytic therapy of acute myocardial infarction. Analyses of patient subgroups in the Thrombolysis In Myocardial Infarction (TIMI) trial, phase II. Circulation 1992; 85:1254–1264.
45. Muller DWM, Topol EJ, Ellis SG, et al, and the Thrombolysis and Angioplasty in Myocardial Infarction (TAMI) Study Group: Multivessel coronary artery disease: a key predictor of short-term prognosis following successful reperfusion therapy for acute myocardial infarction. Am Heart J 1991; 121:1042–1049.
46. Kereiakes DJ, Topol EJ, George BS, et al, and the Thrombolysis and Angioplasty in Myocardial Infarction (TAMI) Study Group: Myocardial infarction with minimal coronary atherosclerosis in the era of thrombolytic reperfusion. J Am Coll Cardiol 1991; 17:304–312.
47. Rogers W, Babb J, Baim D, et al, for the TIMI II Investigators: Selective versus routine pre-discharge coronary arteriography after therapy with tissue-type plasminogen activator, heparin and aspirin for acute myocardial infarction. J Am Coll Cardiol 1991; 17:1007–1016.
48. SWIFT (Should We Intervene Following Thrombolysis) Trial Study Group: SWIFT trial of delayed elective intervention vs conservative treatment after thrombolysis with anistreplase in acute myocardial infarction. Br Med J 1991; 302:555–560.
49. Muller DWM, Topol EJ, Ellis SG, et al: Determinants of the need for early acute intervention in patients treated conservatively after thrombolytic therapy for acute myocardial infarction. J Am Coll Cardiol 1991; 18:1594–1601.
50. Simoons ML, Vos J, Tijssen JG, et al: Long-term benefit of early thrombolytic therapy in patients with acute myocardial infarction: 5 year follow-up of a trial conducted by the Interuniversity Cardiology Institute of the Netherlands. J Am Coll Cardiol 1989; 14:1609–1615.
51. Chaitman BR, McMahon RP, Terrin M, et al: Exercise ECG tests in the TIMI II trial. Am J Cardiol 1993; 71:131–138.
52. American College of Physicians: Evaluation of patients after recent acute myocardial infarction. Ann Intern Med 1989; 110:485–488.
53. Theroux P, Waters D, Halphen C, et al: Prognostic value of exercise testing soon after myocardial infarction. N Engl J Med 1979; 301:341–345.
54. Hamm L, Crow R, Stull G, et al: Safety and characteristics of exercise testing early after myocardial infarction. Am J Cardiol 1989; 63:1193–1197.
55. DeFranco AC, Topol EJ: Angiography and angioplasty. *In* Julian DG, Braunwald E (eds): Management of Acute Myocardial Infarction, pp 107–146, Philadelphia: WB Saunders, 1994.
56. Topol EJ, Ellis SG, Cosgrove DM, et al: Analysis of coronary angioplasty practice in the United States using a private insurance database. Circulation 1993; 87:1489–1497.
57. Charles ED, Rogers W, Reeder GS, et al: Economic advantages of a conservative strategy for AMI management: t-PA without obligatory PTCA [Abstract]. J Am Coll Cardiol 1989; 13:152A.
58. Waller BF, Rothbaum DA, Pinkerton CA, et al: Status of the myocardium and infarct-related coronary artery in 19 necropsy patients with acute recanalization using pharmacologic (streptokinase, r-tissue plasminogen activator), mechanical (percutaneous transluminal coronary angioplasty) or combined types of reperfusion therapy. J Am Coll Cardiol 1987; 9:785–801.
59. Colavita PG, Ideker RE, Reimer KA, et al: The spectrum of pathology associated with percutaneous transluminal coronary angioplasty during myocardial infarction. J Am Coll Cardiol 1986; 8:855–860.
60. FitzGerald DJ, Catella F, Roy L, et al: Marked platelet activation in vivo after intravenous streptokinase in patients with acute myocardial infarction. Circulation 1988; 77:142–150.
61. Montrucchio G, Bergerone F, Bussolino F, et al: Streptokinase induces intravascular release of platelet-activating factor in patients with acute myocardial infarction and stimulates its synthesis by cultured human endothelial cells. Circulation 1993; 88:1476–1483.
62. The TIMI Research Group: Immediate versus delayed catheterization and angioplasty following thrombolytic therapy for acute myocardial infarction: TIMI II-A results. JAMA 1988; 260:2849–2858.
63. Boksch W, Schartl M, Beckman S, et al: PTCA for acute myocardial infarction: thrombus formation and vessel wall changes evaluated by intravascular ultrasound [Abstract]. Circulation 1993; 88(suppl I):410.
64. Kawagoe T, Sato H, Tateshi M, et al: Intravascular ultrasound assessment of the dilatation of infarct related artery after percutaneous transluminal coronary angioplasty in acute myocardial infarction. Eur Heart J 1994; 15(suppl):341.
65. Arnold AER, Simoons ML, Van de Werj F, et al: Recombinant tissue-type plasminogen activator and immediate angioplasty in acute myocardial infarction: one year follow-up. Circulation 1992; 86:111–120.
66. Rogers WJ, Baim DS, Gore JM, et al: Comparison of immediate invasive, delayed invasive, and conservative strategies after tissue type plasminogen activator. Results of the Thrombolysis in Myocardial Infarction (TIMI) phase II-A trial. Circulation 1990; 81:1457–1476.
67. Harrison JK, Califf RM, Harrelson-Woodleif L, et al, and the TAMI Study Group: Systolic left ventricular function after reperfusion therapy for acute myocardial infarction: an analysis of determinants of improvement. Circulation 1993; 89:1531–1541.
68. Ambrose JA, Almeida OD, Sharma SK, et al: Adjunctive thrombolytic therapy during angioplasty for ischemic rest angina: results of the TAUSA trial. Circulation 1994; 90:69–77.
69. Duber C, Jungbluth A, Rumpelt H, et al: Morphology of the coronary arteries after combined thrombolysis and percutaneous coronary angioplasty for acute myocardial infarction. Am J Cardiol 1986; 58:698–703.
70. Fernandez-Ortiz A, Badimon J, Falk E, et al: Characterization of the relative thrombogenicity of atherosclerotic plaque components: indications for consequences of plaque rupture. J Am Coll Cardiol 1994; 23:1562–1569.
71. MacIsaac AI, Thomas JD, Topol EJ: Toward the quiescent coronary plaque. J Am Coll Cardiol 1993; 22:1228–1241.
72. Coller BS: Platelets and thrombolytic therapy. N Engl J Med 1990; 322:33–42.
73. Schmidt WG, Uebis R, von Essen R, et al: Residual coronary stenosis after thrombolysis with rt-PA or streptokinase: acute results and three weeks follow up. Eur Heart J 1987; 8:1182–1188.
74. Holmes DR Jr, Topol EJ: Reperfusion momentum: lessons from the randomized trials of immediate coronary angioplasty for myocardial infarction. J Am Coll Cardiol 1989; 14:1572–1578.
75. The GUSTO Angiographic Investigators: The effects of tissue plasminogen activator, streptokinase, or both, on coronary artery patency, ventricular function and survival after acute myocardial infarction. N Engl J Med 1993; 329:1615–1622.
76. Lincoff AM, Ellis SG, Galeana A, et al, for the TAMI Study Group: Is a coronary artery with TIMI grade 2 flow "patent"? Outcome in the Thrombolysis and Angioplasty in Myocardial Infarction (TAMI) trials [Abstract]. Circulation 1992; 86(suppl I):268.
77. Vogt A, von Essen R, Tebbe U, et al: Impact of early perfusion status of the infarct-related artery on short term mortality after thrombolysis for acute myocardial infarction: retrospective analysis of four German multicenter studies. J Am Coll Cardiol 1993; 21:1391–1395.
78. Anderson JL, Karagounis LA, Becker LC, et al: TIMI perfusion grade 3 but not grade 2 results in improved outcome after thrombolysis for myocardial infarction. Ventriculographic, enzymatic, and electrocardiographic evidence from the TEAM-3 study. Circulation 1993; 87:1829–1839.
79. Granger CB, Ohman EM, Bates ER: Pooled analysis of angiographic patency rates from thrombolytic therapy trials [Abstract]. Circulation 1992; 86(suppl I):269.
80. Belenkie I, Knudston ML, Hall CA, et al: Vessel patency, rescue PTCA and mortality in acute myocardial infarction: results from a prospective randomized reperfusion trial [Abstract]. Clin Invest Med 1990; 13:157.
81. Fung AY, Lai P, Topol EJ, et al: Value of percutaneous transluminal coronary angioplasty after unsuccessful intravenous streptokinase therapy in acute myocardial infarction. Am J Cardiol 1986; 58:686–691.

82. Grines CL, Nissen SE, Booth DC, et al, and the KAMIT Study Group: A prospective, randomized trial comparing half dose tPA with streptokinase to full dose tPA in acute myocardial infarction: preliminary report [Abstract]. J Am Coll Cardiol 1989; 1990:154A.
83. Holmes DR Jr, Gersh BJ, Bailey KR, et al: "Rescue" percutaneous transluminal coronary angioplasty after failed thrombolytic therapy: 4 year follow-up [Abstract]. J Am Coll Cardiol 1989; 13:193A.
84. Grines CL, Nissen SE, Booth DC, et al, and the KAMIT Study Group: A new thrombolytic regimen for acute myocardial infarction using combination half dose tissue-type plasminogen activator with full dose streptokinase: a pilot study. J Am Coll Cardiol 1989; 14:573–580.
85. O'Connor CM, Mark DB, Hinohara T, et al: Rescue coronary angioplasty after failure of intravenous streptokinase in acute myocardial infarction: in-hospital and long term outcomes. J Invasive Cardiol 1989; 1:85–95.
86. Baim DS, Diver DJ, Knatterud GL, and the TIMI II-A Investigators: PTCA "salvage" for thrombolytic failures: implications from TIMI II-A [Abstract]. Circulation 1988; 78(suppl II):112.
87. Whitlow PL: Catheterization/Rescue Angioplasty Following Thrombolysis (CRAFT) Study: results of rescue angioplasty [Abstract]. Circulation 1990; 82(suppl III):308.
88. Ellis SG, Van de Werf F, Ribiero-daSilva E, Topol EJ: Present status of rescue coronary angioplasty: current polarization of opinion and randomized trials. J Am Coll Cardiol 1992; 19:681–668.
89. Ross AM, Reimer JS, Thompson MA, et al: Immediate and follow up procedural outcome of 214 patients undergoing rescue PTCA in the GUSTO trial: no effect of lytic agent [Abstract]. Circulation 1993; 88(suppl I):410.
90. de Boer MJ, Suryapranata H, Hoorntje JCA, et al: Limitation of infarct size and preservation of left ventricular function after primary angioplasty compared with intravenous streptokinase in acute myocardial infarction. Circulation 1994; 90:753–761.
91. Elizaga J, Garcia EJ, Bueno HJ, et al: Primary coronary angioplasty versus systemic thrombolysis in acute anterior myocardial infarction: in-hospital results from a prospective randomized trial. Eur Heart J 1993; 14(suppl):118.
92. Thorsen LI, Brosstad F, Gogstad G, et al: Competition between fibrinogen with its degradation products for interactions with the platelet-fibrinogen receptor. Thromb Res 1986; 44:611–623.
93. Buluk K, Malofiejew M: The pharmacological properties of fibrinogen degradation products. Br J Pharmacol 1969; 35:79–89.
94. Wilson PA, McNicol GP, Douglas AS, et al: Effect of fibrinogen degradation products on platelet aggregation. J Clin Pathol 1968; 21:147–153.
95. Barnhart MI, Cress DC, Henry RL, Riddle JM: Influence of fibrinogen split products on platelets. Thromb Diath Haemorrh 1967; 17:78–98.
96. Kopec M, Budzynski A, Stachurska J, et al: Studies on the mechanism of interference by fibrinogen degradation products (FDP) with the platelet function, role of fibrinogen in the platelet atmosphere. Thromb Diath Haemorrh 1966; 15:476.
97. Ellis SG, Ribiero da Silva E, Heyndrickx G, et al: Randomized comparison of rescue angioplasty with conservative management of patients with early failure of thrombolysis for acute anterior myocardial infarction. Circulation 1994; 90:2280–2284.
98. Kircher RJ, Topol EJ, O'Neill WW, Pitt B: Prediction of infarct coronary artery recanalization after intravenous thrombolytic therapy. Am J Cardiol 1987; 59:513–551.
99. Califf RM, O'Neill W, Stack RS, et al: Failure of simple clinical measurements to predict perfusion status after intravenous thrombolysis. Ann Intern Med 1988; 108:658–662.
100. Puleo PR, Guadagno PA, Roberts R, et al: Early diagnosis of acute myocardial infarction based on assay for subforms of creatine kinase-MB. Circulation 1990; 82:759–764.
101. Puleo PR, Perryman B, Bresser MA, et al: Creatine kinase isoform analysis in the detection and assessment of thrombolysis in man. Circulation 1987; 75:1162–1169.
102. Katus HA, Deiderich KW, Schwarz F, et al: Influence of reperfusion on serum concentrations of cytosolic creatine kinase and structural myosin light chains in acute myocardial infarction. Am J Cardiol 1987; 60:440–445.
103. Garabedian HD, Gold HK, Yasuda T, et al: Detection of coronary artery reperfusion with creatine kinase-MB determinations during thrombolytic therapy: correlation with acute angiography. J Am Coll Cardiol 1988; 11:729–734.
104. Tsukamoto H, Hashimoto H, Matsui Y, et al: Detection of myocardial reperfusion by analysis of serum creatine kinase isoforms. Clin Cardiol 1988; 11:287–291.
105. Seacord LM, Abendschein DR, Nohara R, et al: Detection of reperfusion within 1 hour after coronary recanalization by analysis of isoforms of the MM creatine kinase isoenzyme in plasma. Fibrinolysis 1988; 2:151–156.
106. Abendschein DR, Seacord LM, Nohara R, et al: Prompt detection of myocardial injury by assay of creatine kinase isoforms in initial plasma samples. Clin Cardiol 1988; 11:661–664.
107. van der Laarse A, van der Wall EE, van den Pol RC, et al: Rapid enzyme release from acutely infarcted myocardium after early thrombolytic therapy: washout or reperfusion damage? Am Heart J 1988; 115:711–716.
108. de Zwaan DH, Willems DM, Vermeer F, et al: Enzyme tests in the evaluation of thrombolysis in acute myocardial infarction. Br Heart J 1988; 59:175–183.
109. Ellis AK, Saran BR: Kinetics of myoglobin release and prediction of myocardial myoglobin depletion after coronary artery reperfusion. Circulation 1989; 80:867–883.
110. Krucoff MW, Croll MA, Pope JE, et al: Continuously updated 12-lead ST-segment recovery analysis for myocardial infarct patency assessment and its correlation with multiple simultaneous early angiographic observations. Am J Cardiol 1993; 71:145–151.
111. Dellborg M, Topol EJ, Swedberg K: Dynamic QRS complex and ST-segment vector-cardiographic monitoring can identify vessel patency in patients with acute myocardial infarction treated with reperfusion therapy. Am Heart J 1991; 122:943–948.
112. Kwon K, Freedman B, Wilcox I, et al: The unstable ST segment early after thrombolysis for acute infarction and its usefulness as a marker of recurrent coronary occlusion. Am J Cardiol 1991; 67:109–115.
113. Cotter B, Kriett J, Perricone T, et al: Detection of coronary artery occlusion by decreased myocardial opacification following intravenous injection of QW3600 (EchoGen) [Abstract]. Circulation 1994; 90(suppl I):67.
114. Xie F, Porter TR: Acute myocardial ischemia and reperfusion can be visually identified non-invasively with intravenous perfluoropropane-enhanced sonicated dextrose albumin ultrasound contrast. Circulation 1994; 90(suppl I):I-555.
115. Abbottsmith CW, Topol EJ, George BS, et al: Fate of patients with acute myocardial infarction with patency of the infarct-released vessel with successful thrombolysis versus rescue angioplasty. J Am Coll Cardiol 1990; 16:770–778.
116. Gacioch GM, Topol EJ: Sudden paradoxical clinical deterioration during angioplasty of the occluded right coronary artery in acute myocardial infarction. J Am Coll Cardiol 1989; 14:1202–1209.
117. Lefkovits J, Ivanhoe R, Anderson K, et al: Platelet IIb/IIIa receptor inhibition during PTCA for acute myocardial infarction: insights from the EPIC trial. Circulation 1994; 90(suppl I):564.
118. Kloner RA, Ganote CE, Jennings RB, et al: The "no reflow" phenomenon after temporary coronary occlusion in the dog. J Clin Invest 1974; 54:1496–1508.
119. Ito H, Tomooka T, Sakai N, et al: Lack of myocardial perfusion immediately after successful thrombolysis—a predictor of recovery of left ventricular function in anterior myocardial infarction. Circulation 1992; 85:1699–1705.
120. Ellis SG, Lincoff AM, George BS, et al: Randomized evaluation of coronary angioplasty for early TIMI 2 flow after thrombolytic therapy to treat acute myocardial infarction: a new look at an old study. Coronary Artery Disease 1994; 5:611–615.
121. Ozbek C, Dyckmans J, Sen S, et al: Comparison of invasive and conservative strategies after treatment with streptokinase in acute myocardial infarction: results of a randomized trial (SIAM) [Abstract]. J Am Coll Cardiol 1990; 15:63A.
122. Barbash GI, Roth A, Hod H, et al: Randomized controlled trial of late in-hospital angiography and angioplasty versus conservative management after treatment with recombinant tissue-type plasminogen activator in acute myocardial infarction. Am J Cardiol 1990; 66:538–545.
123. van den Brand MJ, Betrui A, Bescos LL, et al: Randomized trial of deferred angioplasty after thrombolysis after myocardial infarction. Coronary Artery Disease 1992; 3:393–401.
124. Ellis SG, Mooney MR, George BS, et al, for the Treatment of Post-Thrombolytic Stenosis (TOPS) Study Group: Randomized trial of late elective angioplasty versus conservative management for patients with residual stenoses after thrombolytic treatment of myocardial infarction. Circulation 1992; 86:1400–1406.
125. Bertrand ME, Lefebvre JM, Laisne CL, et al: Coronary arteriography in acute transmural myocardial infarction. Am Heart J 1979; 97:61–69.

126. Eckman MH, Wong JB, Salem DN, et al: Direct angioplasty for acute myocardial infarction. A review of outcomes in clinical subsets. Ann Intern Med 1992; 117:667–676.
127. Flaker GC, Webel RR, Meinhardt S, et al: Emergency angioplasty in acute anterior myocardial infarction. Am Heart J 1989; 118:1154–1160.
128. Marco J, Caster L, Szatmary LJ, et al: Emergency percutaneous transluminal coronary angioplasty without thrombolysis as initial therapy in acute myocardial infarction. Int J Cardiol 1987; 15:55–63.
129. Ellis SG, O'Neill WW, Bates ER, et al: Implications for patient triage from patient survival and left ventricular functional recovery analyses in 500 patients treated with coronary angioplasty for acute myocardial infarction. J Am Coll Cardiol 1989; 13:1251–1259.
130. Rothbaum DA, Linnemeier TJ, Landin RJ, et al: Emergency percutaneous transluminal coronary angioplasty in acute myocardial infarction: a 3 year experience. J Am Coll Cardiol 1987; 10:264–272.
131. Brodie BR, Weintraub RA, Stuckey TD, et al: Outcomes of direct coronary angioplasty for acute myocardial infarction in candidates and non-candidates for thrombolytic therapy. Am J Cardiol 1991; 67:7–12.
132. Kahn JK, Rutherford BD, McConahay DR, et al: Results of primary angioplasty in patients with multivessel coronary artery disease. J Am Coll Cardiol 1990; 16:1089–1096.
133. Beauchamp GD, Vacek JL, Robuck W: Management comparison for acute myocardial infarction: direct angioplasty versus sequential thrombolysis-angioplasty. Am Heart J 1990; 120:237–242.
134. Bittl JA: Indications, timing, and optimal technique for diagnostic angiography and angioplasty in acute myocardial infarction. Chest 1991; 99:150S–156S.
135. Grines CK, Meany TB, Weintraub R, et al: Streptokinase angioplasty myocardial infarction trial: early and late results [Abstract]. J Am Coll Cardiol 1991; 17:336A.
136. Williams DO, Holubkov AL, Detre KM, et al: Impact of pretreatment by thrombolytic therapy upon outcome of emergent direct coronary angioplasty for patients with acute myocardial infarction [Abstract]. J Am Coll Cardiol 1991; 17:337A.
137. O'Keefe J Jr, Rutherford BD, McConahay DR, et al: Early and late results of coronary angioplasty without antecedent thrombolytic therapy for acute myocardial infarction. Am J Cardiol 1989; 64:1221–1230.
138. O'Neill WW, Brodie BR, Ivanhoe R, et al: Primary coronary angioplasty for acute myocardial infarction (the Primary Angioplasty Registry). Am J Cardiol 1994; 73:627–634.
139. Brodie BR, Grines CL, Ivanhoe R, et al: Six month clinical and angiographic follow-up after direct angioplasty for acute myocardial infarction. Final results from the Primary Angioplasty Registry. Circulation 1994; 90:156–162.
140. Topol EJ, Califf RM: Thrombolytic therapy for elderly patients. N Engl J Med 1992; 327:45–47.
141. ISIS-2 (Second International Study of Infarct Survival) Collaborative Group: Randomized trial of intravenous streptokinase, oral aspirin, both or neither among 17,187 cases of suspected acute myocardial infarction. Lancet 1988; 2:349–360.
142. Williams DO, Braunwald E, Knatterud G, et al: One year results of the Thrombolysis in Myocardial Infarction investigation (TIMI) phase II trial. Circulation 1992; 85:533–542.
143. Elizaga J, Garcia EJ, Bueno H, et al: Primary coronary angioplasty versus systemic thrombolysis in acute anterior myocardial infarction: in-hospital results from a prospective randomized trial. Eur Heart J 1993; 14(suppl):118.
144. de Boer MJ, Suryapranata H, Hoorntje JCA, et al: Limitation of infarct size and preservation of left ventricular function after primary angioplasty compared with intravenous streptokinase in acute myocardial infarction. Circulation 1994; 90:753–761.
145. de Boer MJ, Hoorntje JCA, Ottervanger JP, et al: Immediate coronary angioplasty versus intravenous streptokinase in acute myocardial infarction: left ventricular ejection fraction, hospital mortality and reinfarction. J Am Coll Cardiol 1994; 23:1004–1008.
146. The GUSTO Investigators: An international randomized trial comparing four thrombolytic strategies for acute myocardial infarction. N Engl J Med 1993; 329:673–682.
147. ISIS-3 (International Studies of Infarct Survival) Collaborative Group: ISIS-3: a randomised comparison of streptokinase versus tissue plasminogen activator versus anistreplase and of aspirin plus heparin versus aspirin alone among 41299 cases of suspected acute myocardial infarction. Lancet 1992; 339:753–770.
148. Simari RD, Berger MD, Bell MR, et al: Coronary angioplasty in acute myocardial infarction: primary, immediate adjunctive, rescue or deferred adjunctive approach? Mayo Clin Proc 1994; 69:346–358.
149. Michels KB, Yusuf S: Does PTCA in acute myocardial infarction affect mortality and reinfarction rates? A quantitative overview (meta-analysis) of the randomized clinical trials. Circulation 1995; 91:476–485.
150. O'Keefe JH Jr, Bailey WL, Rutherford BD, et al: Primary angioplasty for acute myocardial infarction in 1,000 consecutive patients. Results in an unselected population and high-risk subgroups. Am J Cardiol 1993; 72:107G–115G.
151. Norris RM, White HD: Therapeutic trials in coronary thrombolysis should measure left ventricular function as primary end-point of treatment. Lancet 1988; 1:104–106.
152. Califf RM, Harrelson-Woodlief L, Topol EJ: Left ventricular ejection fraction may not be useful as a primary endpoint of thrombolytic therapy comparative trials. Circulation 1990; 82:1847–1853.
153. Simes R, Ross A, Simoons M, et al, for the GUSTO Investigators: Mortality reduction with accelerated tissue plasminogen activator is explained by early coronary patency [Abstract]. Circulation 1993; 88(suppl I):291.
154. Ito H, Tomooka T, Sakai N, et al: Lack of myocardial perfusion immediately after successful thrombolysis. A predictor of poor recovery of left ventricular function in anterior myocardial infarction. Circulation 1992; 85:1699–1705.
155. Lincoff AM, Topol EJ: Trickle down thrombolysis. J Am Coll Cardiol 1993; 21:1396–1398.
156. Lincoff AM, Topol EJ: The illusion of reperfusion. Does anyone achieve optimal myocardial reperfusion? Circulation 1993; 87:1792–1805 (erratum 1993; 88:1361–1375).
157. Topol EJ, Califf RM, Vandormael M, et al, for the TAMI-6 Study Group: A randomized trial of late reperfusion for acute myocardial infarction. Circulation 1992; 85:2090–2099.
158. Meijer A, Verheugt FW, Werter CJ, et al: Aspirin versus coumadin in the prevention of reocclusion and recurrent ischemia after successful thrombolysis: a prospective placebo-controlled angiographic study. Results of the APRICOT study. Circulation 1993; 87:1524–1530.
159. Leung WH, Lau CP: Effects of severity of the residual stenosis of the infarct related coronary artery on LV dilatation and function after acute myocardial infarction. J Am Coll Cardiol 1992; 20:307–313.
160. Kloner RA: Coronary angioplasty: a treatment option for left ventricular remodeling after myocardial infarction? J Am Coll Cardiol 1992; 20:314–316.
161. Hirayama A, Adachi T, Asada S, et al: Late reperfusion for acute myocardial infarction limits the dilatation of left ventricle without the reduction of infarct size. Circulation 1993; 88:2565–2574.
162. Tison E, Gommeaux A, Lablanche JM, et al: Long term risk/benefit of PTCA of infarct related vessel [Abstract]. J Am Coll Cardiol 1991; 17:266A.
163. Dzavik V, Beanlands DS, Davies RF, et al: Effects of late percutaneous transluminal coronary angioplasty of an occluded infarct-related artery on left ventricular function in patients with a recent (<6 weeks) Q-wave acute myocardial infarction (Total Occlusion Post-Myocardial Infarction Intervention Study [TOMIIS]—a pilot study). Am J Cardiol 1994; 73:856–861.
164. Kuntz RE, Keaney KM, Senerchia C, et al: A predictive method for estimating the late angiographic results of coronary intervention despite incomplete ascertainment. Circulation 1993; 87:815–830.
165. Nelson CL, Tcheng JE, Frid DJ, et al: Incomplete angiographic followup results in significant underestimation of true restenosis rates after PTCA [Abstract]. Circulation 1990; 82(suppl III):312.
166. Almany SL, Meany BE, Cragg DR, et al: Long term patency and incidence of restenosis after primary angioplasty for acute myocardial infarction [Abstract]. J Am Coll Cardiol 1991; (suppl 17 II):336.
167. Simonton CA, Mark DB, Hinohara T, et al: Late restenosis after emergent coronary angioplasty for acute myocardial infarction: comparison with elective coronary angioplasty. J Am Coll Cardiol 1988; 11:698–705.
168. Miller PF, Brodie BR, Weintraub RA, et al: Emergency coronary angioplasty for acute myocardial infarction. Results from a community hospital. Arch Intern Med 1987; 147:1565–1570.
169. Topol EJ, Califf RM, Weisman HF, et al: Randomised trial of coronary intervention with antibody against platelet IIb/IIIa integrin for reduction of clinical restenosis: results at six months. Lancet 1994; 343:881–886.
170. Griffith GC, Wallace WB, Cochran B, et al: The treatment of shock associated with myocardial infarction. Circulation 1954; 9:527–532.
171. Killip T 3d, Kimball JT: Treatment of myocardial infarction in a coronary care unit. A two year experience with 250 patients. Am J Cardiol 1967; 20:457–464.

172. Goldberg RJ, Gore JM, Alpert JS, et al: Cardiogenic shock after acute myocardial infarction: incidence and mortality from a community-wide perspective. N Engl J Med 1991; 325:1117–1122.
173. Kennedy J, Gensini G, Timmis G, et al: Acute myocardial infarction treated with intracoronary streptokinase: a case report for the society of cardiac angiography. Am J Cardiol 1985; 55:871–877.
174. Gruppo Italiano per lo Studio della Streptochinasi nell'Infarto Miocardico (GISSI): Effectiveness of intravenous thrombolytic treatment in acute myocardial infarction. Lancet 1986; 1:397–402.
175. Gruppo Italiano per lo Studio della Sopravvivenza nell'Infarto Miocardico (GISSI-2): A factorial randomized trial of alteplase versus streptokinase and heparin versus no heparin among 12,490 patients with acute myocardial infarction. Lancet 1990; 336:65–70.
176. Garrahy PJ, Henzlova MJ, Forman S, et al: Has thrombolytic therapy improved survival from cardiogenic shock? Thrombolysis in Myocardial Infarction (TIMI II) results [Abstract]. Circulation 989; 80(suppl II):623.
177. O'Neill WW: Angioplasty therapy of cardiogenic shock: are randomized trials necessary? J Am Coll Cardiol 1992; 19:915–917.
178. Gutovitz AL, Sobel BE, Roberts P: Progressive nature of myocardial injury in selected patients with cardiogenic shock. Am J Cardiol 1991; 17:770–780.
179. Hochman JS, Boland J, Sleeper LA, et al: Current spectrum of cardiogenic shock and effect of early revascularization on mortality. Results of an international registry. Circulation 1995; 91:873–881.
180. Lincoff AM, Popma JJ, Ellis SG, et al: Percutaneous support devices for high risk or complicated coronary angioplasty. J Am Coll Cardiol 1991; 17:770–780.
181. Kern MJ, Aguirre F, Bach R, et al: Augmentation of coronary blood flow by intra-aortic balloon pumping after coronary angioplasty. Circulation 1993; 87:500–511.
182. Flaherty JT, Becker LC, Weiss JL, et al: Results of a randomized prospective trial of intraaortic balloon counterpulsation and intravenous nitroglycerin in patients with acute myocardial infarction. J Am Coll Cardiol 1985; 6:434–436.
183. Ishihara M, Sato H, Tateishi H, et al: Intraaortic balloon pumping as the postangioplasty strategy in acute myocardial infarction. Am Heart J 1991; 122:385–389.
184. Ohman EM, George BS, White CJ, et al: Use of aortic counterpulsation to improve sustained coronary artery patency during acute myocardial infarction. Results of a randomized trial. Circulation 1994; 90:792–799.
185. Shawl FA, Domanski MJ, Hernandez TJ, et al: Emergency percutaneous cardiopulmonary bypass support in cardiogenic shock from acute myocardial infarction. Am J Cardiol 1989; 64:976–970.
186. Shawl FA, Domanski MJ, Punja S, et al: Emergency percutaneous cardiopulmonary support in cardiogenic shock: long-term follow-up [Abstract]. Circulation 1989; 80(suppl II):258.
187. Lincoff AM, Popma JJ, Bates ER, et al: Successful coronary angioplasty in two patients with cardiogenic shock using the Nimbus Hemopump support device. Am Heart J 1990; 120:970–972.
188. Cragg DR, Friedman HZ, Bonema JD, et al: Outcome of patients with myocardial infarction who are ineligible for thrombolytic therapy. Ann Intern Med 1991; 115:173–177.
189. Karlson BW, Herlitz J, Edvardsson N, et al: Eligibility for intravenous thrombolytic therapy in suspected acute myocardial infarction. Circulation 1990; 82:1140–1146.
190. Brodie BR, Weintraub RA, Stuckey TD, et al: Outcomes of direct coronary angioplasty for acute myocardial infarction in candidates and non-candidates for thrombolytic therapy. Am J Cardiol 1991; 67:7–12.
191. Krumholz HM, Pasternak RC, Weinstein MC, et al: Cost effectiveness of thrombolytic therapy with streptokinase in elderly patients with acute myocardial infarction. N Engl J Med 1992; 327:7–13.
192. Topol EJ, Califf RM: Thrombolytic therapy for elderly patients. N Engl J Med 1992; 327:45–47.
193. Stuckey T, Brodie B, Hansen C, et al: Primary angioplasty for acute myocardial infarction in elderly thrombolytic candidates: is it the best option? J Am Coll Cardiol February 1995; special issue:47A.
194. Stone GW, Grines CL, Vlietstra R, et al: Primary angioplasty is the preferred therapy for women and the elderly with acute myocardial infarction—results of the Primary Angioplasty in Myocardial Infarction (PAMI) trial [Abstract]. J Am Coll Cardiol 1993; 21:330A.
195. Holland KJ, O'Neill WW, Bates ER, et al: Emergency percutaneous transluminal coronary angioplasty during acute myocardial infarction for patients more than 70 years of age. Am J Cardiol 1989; 63:399–403.
196. Grines CL, Booth DC, Nissen SE, et al: Mechanism of acute myocardial infarction in patients with prior coronary artery bypass grafting and therapeutic implications. Am J Cardiol 1990; 65:1292–1296.
197. Kavanaugh KM, Topol EJ: Acute intervention during myocardial infarction in patients with acute myocardial infarction. Am J Cardiol 1990; 65:924–926.
198. Davis KB, Alderman EL, Kosinski AS, et al: Early mortality of acute myocardial infarction in patients with and without prior coronary revascularization surgery. A Coronary Artery Surgery Registry Study. Circulation 1992; 85:2100–2109.
199. Dittrich HC, Gilpin E, Nicod P, et al: Outcome after acute myocardial infarction in patients with prior coronary bypass surgery. Am J Cardiol 1993; 72:507–513.
200. De Franco AC, Abramowitz B, Krichbaum D, et al: Substantial (three-fold) benefit of accelerated t-PA over standard thrombolytic therapy in patients with prior bypass surgery and acute MI: results of the GUSTO trial [Abstract]. J Am Coll Cardiol 1994; 23:1A–484A.
201. Larkin TJ, Niemyski PR, Parker NA, et al: Primary and rescue extraction atherectomy in patients with acute myocardial infarction [Abstract]. Circulation 1991; 82(suppl II):537.
202. Topaz O, Minisi AJ, Luxenberg M, et al: Laser angioplasty for lesions unsuitable for PTCA in acute myocardial infarction: quantitative angiography and clinical results. Circulation 1994; 90(suppl I):434.
203. Ohman EM, Califf RM, Topol EJ, et al, and the TAMI Study Group: Consequences of reocclusion after successful reperfusion therapy in acute myocardial infarction. Circulation 1990; 82:781–791.
204. Ellis SG, Topol EJ, George BS, et al: Recurrent ischemia without warning. Analysis of risk factors for in-hospital ischemic events following successful thrombolysis with intravenous tissue plasminogen activator. Circulation 1989; 80:1159–1165.
205. Ellis SG, Topol EJ, Gallison L, et al: Predictors of success for coronary angioplasty performed for acute myocardial infarction. J Am Coll Cardiol 1988; 12:1407–1415.
206. Brodie BR, Stuckey TD, Hansen CJ, et al: Importance of a patent infarct-related artery for hospital and late survival after direct coronary angioplasty for acute myocardial infarction. Am J Cardiol 1992; 69:1113–1119.
207. Bedotto JB, Kahn JK, Rutherford BD, et al: Failed direct coronary angioplasty for acute myocardial infarction: in-hospital outcome and predictors of death. J Am Coll Cardiol 1993; 22:690–694.
208. Kaplan BM, O'Neill W, Safian RD, et al: Clinical and angiographic followup to a prospective study of transluminal extraction atherectomy in high risk patients with acute myocardial infarction [Abstract]. J Am Coll Cardiol February 1995; special issue:331A.
209. Hong MK, Wong SC, Popma JJ, et al: A dual-purpose angioplasty–drug infusion catheter for the treatment of intragraft thrombus. Cathet Cardiovasc Diagn 1994; 32:193–195.
210. Rogers WJ, Bowlby LJ, Chandra NC, et al, for the Participants in the National Registry of Myocardial Infarction: Treatment of myocardial infarction in the United States (1990–1993): observations from the National Registry of Myocardial Infarction. Circulation 1994; 90:2103–2114.
211. Rogers WJ, Dean LS, Moore PB, et al: Comparison of primary angioplasty versus thrombolytic therapy for acute myocardial infarction. Am J Cardiol 1994; 74:111–118.
212. Weaver WD, Litwin PE, Martin JS, et al, for The Myocardial Infarction Triage and Intervention Project Investigators: Use of direct angioplasty for treatment of myocardial infarction in hospitals with and without on-site cardiac surgery. Circulation 1993; 88:2067–2075.
213. AHA/ACC Taskforce Report: Guidelines for percutaneous transluminal coronary angioplasty. A report of the American College of Cardiology/American Heart Association Task Force on Assessment of Diagnostic and Therapeutic Procedures. J Am Coll Cardiol 1993; 22:2033–2054.
214. Aguirre FV, Topol EJ, Donohue TJ, et al: Impact of ionic and non-ionic contrast media on post-PTCA ischemic complications: results from the EPIC trial [Abstract]. J Am Coll Cardiol February 1995; 25:8A.

45 Intra-Aortic Balloon Counterpulsation

Gregory S. Couper, MD

Although several new mechanical devices have been developed for the management of circulatory collapse (see Chapter 15), intra-aortic balloon counterpulsation (IABC) remains the most widely used and easily applied device for the temporary support of patients with acute myocardial ischemic syndromes or reversible hypoperfusion caused by cardiac dysfunction. The concept of diastolic augmentation of coronary blood flow by devices was initially explored by Kantrowitz and Kantrowitz and reported in 1953.[1] Their first clinical applications of a balloon pump were in 1966, with the intent to provide permanent mechanical assistance in chronic terminal cardiac failure. Although both patients died in the early postoperative period, there was evidence of hemodynamic assistance.[2] In 1968, Kantrowitz and associates[3] reported the first successful human application of short-term IABC in cardiogenic shock. Over the next several years, additional series of patients supported for cardiogenic shock were reported. Unfortunately, survival was an uncommon end result. Despite such an inauspicious start, the technology and clinical application of IABC has grown dramatically, with an estimated greater than 70,000 procedures performed annually.[4] The spectrum of clinical syndromes amenable to treatment with IABC has expanded far beyond the initial intent to provide circulatory support in cardiogenic shock. The aim of this chapter is to review technical advances, complications, and outcomes in patients managed with IABC.

TECHNICAL ADVANCES AND COMPLICATIONS

Optimal IABC produces several physiologic effects. Balloon inflation provides augmentation of diastolic blood pressure and coronary perfusion. Deflation during isovolumic systole results in early systolic unloading of the left ventricle. The relative contribution of each effect to outcome differs depending on the cause of the underlying cardiac condition. Figure 45–1 depicts a typical arterial tracing during alternate beat support (1:2 timing) with proper timing. Current console technology allows automatic triggering of balloon cycles by native electrocardiographic signals, pacing spikes, or pulse pressure detection. The ability to pump effectively despite irregular or rapid rhythms has improved greatly in recent years.

Before 1980, IABC was exclusively a surgical procedure. Through a groin incision, a small polyester (Dacron) graft was anastomosed to the side of the common femoral artery. The intra-aortic balloon catheter was passed through the graft and advanced retrograde through the femoral artery to the descending thoracic aorta. An alternative route available in cardiac surgical procedures was the antegrade insertion via the ascending aorta.[5]

Although the Seldinger method of percutaneous cannulation of vessels was described in 1953, the preliminary report of percutaneous insertion of intra-aortic balloon catheters was not made until 1980 in separate publications by Bregman and associates and Subramanian and colleagues.[6, 7] This technical advance allowed rapid nonsurgical insertion and removal and greatly expanded the pool of operators capable of carrying out the insertion to include cardiologists and radiologists with vascular catheterization experience.

Until recent years, the most common percutaneous method used an indwelling sheath through which the catheter was advanced. Numerous reports have documented the high success rate of percutaneous insertion, ranging from 90%–98%, comparable to that seen with surgical insertion.[8, 9] The majority of complications seen with intra-aortic balloon catheters have been caused by local vascular compromise. In one of the largest IABC series reported, covering 872 surgical and percutaneous intra-aortic balloon procedures in 733 patients from 1967–1982, Kantrowitz and colleagues[9] observed a 22% incidence of vascular complications. In 1987, Iverson and colleagues[10] reported that percutaneous insertion of 10.5- to 12-French intra-aortic balloon catheters resulted in a lower incidence of vascular complications than did the older surgical insertion technique (19% vs. 32%).

In 1991, Kvilekval and associates[11] examined the relation between pre-existing vascular disease and complications from IABC in 144 patients. All procedures were performed percutaneously using 10.5-French catheters. Of 20 patients with vascular disease, 4 experienced

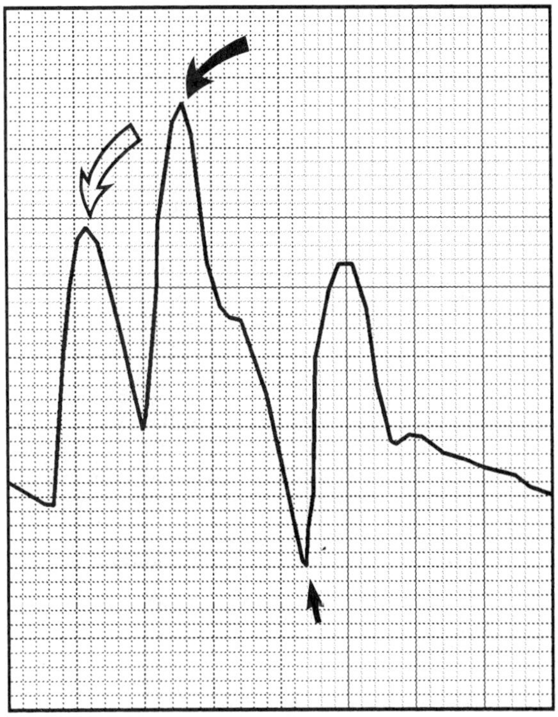

Figure 45–1. IABC in 1:2 mode. Balloon inflation after the first native heart beat *(open arrow)* results in an augmentation of diastolic pressure above systolic pressure *(closed arrow)*. Balloon deflation during isovolumic contraction of the second beat results in systolic unloading of the LV *(small arrow)*. Although the systolic pressure is lower, the stroke volume of unloaded beats is maintained or increased. *Abbreviations:* IABC, intra-aortic balloon counterpulsation; LV, left ventricle.

embolic complications (20%) and 5 had occlusive complications (25%). All the embolic complications occurred in patients with aneurysmal aortic disease. All the occlusive complications occurred in patients with occlusive peripheral vascular disease. In 124 patients without evidence of vascular disease undergoing 133 intra-aortic balloon insertions, only two embolic events (1.5%) and one occlusive complication (0.8%) occurred. Despite the small number of patients in the vascular disease group, this study demonstrated the potentially high risk of transfemoral retrograde insertion of intra-aortic balloons in the presence of aneurysmal or occlusive vascular disease.

Although improvements in balloon catheter technology resulted in smaller catheter shaft sizes of 9.5-French, vascular complications continued to be observed throughout the late 1980s. The use of a sheath of significantly greater diameter than the catheter shaft was recognized to be an important factor contributing to limb ischemia. In the late 1980s, a new balloon design allowed sheathless insertion of a 9.5-French catheter. In their initial report, Nash and coworkers[12] successfully inserted intra-aortic balloon catheters in 20 of 22 patients without a sheath. The remaining two patients had successful percutaneous insertion with a sheath. No patient had clinically important bleeding despite usual heparin therapy, but 2 of 20 patients had limb ischemia. One patient underwent intra-aortic balloon removal prematurely and the other required an axillofemoral bypass for ischemia caused by a low insertion through the superficial femoral artery. In 1993, Tatar and colleagues[13] reported a series of 126 IABC patients. Forty-four of 45 patients (98%) had successful sheathless insertion. Seventy of 81 patients (86%) had successful percutaneous insertion using a sheath. Limb ischemia occurred in 17 patients (22%) with a sheath but in only 3 patients (6%) with sheathless insertion ($p < .01$). As a result of these encouraging reports, many centers, including our own, have shifted to sheathless percutaneous insertion with excellent success.

INDICATIONS AND OUTCOMES OF INTRA-AORTIC BALLOON COUNTERPULSATION FOR CARDIAC SURGERY PROCEDURES

The majority of IABC procedures are performed for temporary management of acute myocardial ischemic syndromes or circulatory collapse secondary to cardiac dysfunction, with the intent to carry out definitive therapy. Often, the definitive therapy includes cardiac surgery. A number of centers have reported large series of patients requiring perioperative IABC[14–16] associated with a broad range of cardiac surgical procedures. Preoperative insertion of intra-aortic balloon catheters is recommended for patients with left main coronary artery disease, severe coronary disease associated with impaired left ventricular function with ejection fractions less than .30, or myocardial infarction complicated by cardiogenic shock, severe mitral regurgitation, or ventricular septal defect. Approximately 2%–11% of patients undergoing cardiac surgery will require preoperative, intraoperative, or postoperative IABC. In 1980, Golding and colleagues[14] from the Cleveland Clinic reported results in 197 patients requiring perioperative IABC out of 8879 patients undergoing coronary artery bypass grafting in 1975–1978. The overall hospital mortality rate for the IABC patients was 28.4%. Twelve years later, Creswell and coworkers[15] from Washington University in St. Louis reported results in 353 patients requiring IABPs for bypass surgery out of 7884 diverse cardiac surgical cases from 1986–1991. The operative mortality rate was 28.7%, quite similar to that reported many years earlier. Table 45–1 demonstrates the remarkable similarity in distribution of timing of IABC in isolated coronary artery bypass grafts in these two different institutions in two different eras of cardiac surgery. IABC was used intraoperatively and postoperatively when there was failure to wean the patient from cardiopulmonary bypass or low cardiac output syndromes, whereas approximately half the preoperative cases involved stabilization of acute myocardial ischemia without left ventricular dysfunction.

Prolonged circulatory assistance with IABC has been reported in small groups of patients and is best described as a bridge to recovery, primary cardiac surgery, or transplant operation. Lazar and associates[17] reviewed hemodynamic benefits of prolonged IABC support in 49 patients with end-stage ischemic or nonischemic cardiomyopathy treated for a mean of 11.3 days (range 5–46 days). Only 10 patients (20%) were weaned from IABC support. Twenty patients (40%) died while on the pump, 11 patients (22%) underwent cardiac transplantation, and 8 patients (16%) received another cardiac assist device. During the IABC support, the cardiac index rose from 1.6 ± 0.4 to 2.2 ± 0.5 L/min/m^2 acutely after balloon pump insertion. A further rise in cardiac index to 2.7 ± 0.5 L/min/m^2 occurred during the duration of support. Filling pressures rose slightly but remained below baseline. Rosenbaum and coworkers[18] used IABC as a bridge to cardiac transplantation in 55 patients with ischemic or nonischemic cardiomyopathies. Support ranged from 3 hours to 54 days. Hemodynamic indices of cardiac index, filling pressure, and systemic vascular resistance improved in both forms of cardiomyopathy acutely and over the duration of IABC support. In the nonischemic group, 33% were weaned from IABC, 33% underwent cardiac transplantation, 22% received a ventricular assist device or total artificial heart, and 11% died on IABC. In the ischemic group, 44% were weaned from IABC support, 13% underwent cardiac transplantation, 38% received a ventricular assist device or total artificial heart, and 6% died on IABC. This study demonstrated the hemodynamic efficacy of intra-aortic balloons in "bridging" potential transplant patients with ischemic or nonischemic cardiomyopathies.

INTRA-AORTIC BALLOON COUNTERPULSATION SUPPORT DURING CORONARY INTERVENTIONS

IABC is the mainstay of circulatory support for high-risk coronary interventions. Although every laboratory performing coronary interventions must have the ability to institute emergency IABC, prophylactic placement of IABC is desirable in certain patients undergoing high-risk angioplasty. Patients undergoing angioplasty for left main coronary artery disease, for left main equivalent disease, or in the

TABLE 45–1. OPERATIVE MORTALITY AND INTRA-AORTIC BALLOON COUNTERPULSATION DURING CORONARY ARTERY BYPASS SURGERY

	Cleveland Clinic Series[13] (n = 197)		Washington University Series[15] (n = 353)	
Time of Insertion	**Number (%)**	**Mortality (%)**	**Number (%)**	**Mortality (%)**
Preoperative	61 (31)	6 (10)	138 (39)	18 (13)
Intraoperative	98 (50)	26 (27)	166 (47)	43 (26)
Postoperative	37 (19)	17 (46)	49 (14)	19 (38)

setting of impaired left ventricular function with ejection fractions less than .30 may benefit from the prophylactic use of IABC.[19] Patients who experience abrupt vessel closure during angioplasty with hemodynamic compromise may require IABC support when attempts to restore perfusion to the target vessel are prolonged or unsuccessful.

IABC should be considered for all patients who require emergency coronary artery bypass surgery for failed angioplasty (see Chapter 43). Although IABC is commonly used for patients with refractory ischemia associated with a failed angioplasty,[20] support of the coronary and systemic circulations with IABC may avert unforeseen complications from hemodynamic compromise in these unstable patients during transport to the operating room, induction of anesthesia, and the postoperative period.

After successful coronary intervention for acute myocardial infarction (see Chapter 44), IABC has been shown to reduce the incidence of reocclusion.[21] In a randomized study, IABC for 48 hours was compared with standard care in 182 patients undergoing successful angioplasty within 24 hours of the onset of acute myocardial infarction. The rate of angiographically documented reocclusion was lower in patients treated with IABC than in those treated with standard care (8% vs. 21%). The composite end point of death, stroke, reinfarction, a need for emergency revascularization, or evidence of recurrent ischemia was also reduced with the use of IABC (13% vs. 24%). Bleeding rates were similar in the two treatment groups (2% vs. 1%). Thus, this study showed evidence that IABC can prevent reocclusion of the infarct-related artery and reduce clinical complications after successful angioplasty for acute myocardial infarction.[21]

REFERENCES

1. Kantrowitz A, Kantrowitz A: Experimental augmentation of coronary flow by retardation of the arterial pulse. Surgery 1953; 34:678.
2. Kantrowitz A, Akutsu T, Chaptal P-A, et al: A clinical experience with an implanted mechanical auxiliary ventricle. JAMA 1966; 197:525.
3. Kantrowitz A, Tjonneland S, Freed PS, et al: Initial experience with intra-aortic balloon pumping in cardiogenic shock. JAMA 1968; 203:135.
4. Kantrowitz A: Origins of intra-aortic balloon pumping. Ann Thorac Surg 1990; 50:672.
5. Pinkard J, Utley JR, Leyland SA, et al: Relative risk of aortic and femoral insertion of intra-aortic balloon pump after coronary artery bypass grafting procedures. J Thorac Cardiovasc Surg 1993; 105:721.
6. Bregman D, Nichols AB, Weiss MB, et al: Percutaneous intra-aortic balloon insertion. Am J Cardiol 1980; 46:261.
7. Subramanian VA, Goldstein JE, Sos TA, et al: Preliminary clinical experience with percutaneous intra-aortic balloon pumping. Circulation 1980; 62(suppl1):1–123.
8. Funk M, Gleason J, Foell D: Lower limb ischemia related to use of the intra-aortic balloon pump. Heart Lung 1989; 18:542.
9. Kantrowitz A, Wasfie T, Freed P, et al: Intra-aortic balloon pumping 1967–1982. Analysis of complications in 733 patients. Am J Cardiol 1986; 57:976.
10. Iverson LIG, Herfindahl G, Ecker RR, et al: Vascular complications of intra-aortic balloon counterpulsation. Am J Surg 1987; 154:99.
11. Kvilekval KH, Mason RA, Newton B, et al: Complications of percutaneous intra-aortic balloon pump use in patients with peripheral vascular disease. Arch Surg 1991; 126:621.
12. Nash IS, Lorell BH, Fishman RF, et al: A new technique for sheathless percutaneous intra-aortic balloon catheter insertion. Cathet Cardiovasc Diagn 1991; 23:57.
13. Tatar H, Cicek S, Demirkilic U, et al: Vascular complications of intra-aortic balloon pumping: unsheathed versus sheathed insertion. Ann Thorac Surg 1993; 55:1518.
14. Golding LAR, Loop FD, Mohan P, et al: Late survival following use of intra-aortic balloon pump in revascularization operations. Ann Thorac Surg 1980; 30:48.
15. Creswell LL, Rosenbloom M, Cox JL, et al: Intra-aortic balloon counterpulsation: patterns of usage and outcome in cardiac surgery patients. Ann Thorac Surg 1992; 54:11.
16. Naunheim KS, Swartz MT, Pennington DG, et al: Intra-aortic balloon pumping in patients requiring cardiac operations. J Thorac Cardiovasc Surg 1992; 104:1654.
17. Lazar JM, Ziady GM, Dummer SJ, et al: Outcome and complications of prolonged intra-aortic balloon counterpulsation in cardiac patients. Am J Cardiol 1992; 69:955.
18. Rosenbaum AM, Murali S, Uretsky BF: Intra-aortic balloon counterpulsation as a "bridge" to cardiac transplantation: effects in non-ischemic and ischemic cardiomyopathy. Chest 1994; 106:1683.
19. Kahn JK, Rutherford BD, McConahay DR, et al: Supported "high-risk" coronary angioplasty using intra-aortic balloon pump counterpulsation. J Am Coll Cardiol 1990; 15:1151.
20. Craver JM, Weintraub WS, Jones EL, et al: Emergency coronary artery bypass surgery for failed percutaneous coronary angioplasty: a 10-year experience. Ann Surg 1992; 215:425.
21. Ohman EM, George BS, White CJ, et al: Use of aortic counterpulsation to improve coronary artery patency during acute myocardial infarction: results of a randomized trial. Circulation 1994; 90:792.

46 Coronary Artery Bypass Surgery

Lawrence H. Cohn, MD

The surgical treatment of coronary artery disease by coronary artery bypass grafting (CABG) remains an important cornerstone of therapy for patients with acute and chronic syndromes of ischemic heart disease. As remarkable improvements in interventional cardiologic therapy have taken place since 1980, concomitant changes in indications, patient profiles, and techniques have also taken place in the surgical treatment of ischemic heart disease. In 1992, approximately 300,000 patients in the United States underwent coronary bypass. This chapter summarizes selection data for patients with coronary bypass, the indications for coronary bypass surgery, and the various subsets of acute and chronic myocardial ischemia. Technical details regarding the current operation for the surgical treatment of ischemic heart disease, perioperative and immediate postoperative therapy to prevent complications, and factors to promote the long-term success of surgical therapy of ischemic heart disease are also discussed.

INDICATIONS FOR CORONARY BYPASS GRAFT SURGERY

The indications for coronary bypass surgery (CABG) have evolved since the original operations performed by Falvaloro at the Cleveland Clinic Foundation in 1967.[1] At that time, patients underwent CABG for single- or double-vessel disease with moderate to severe angina pectoris and no compromise of left ventricular function. As natural history studies have evolved, the pathophysiologic subsets and indications for patient profiles have changed significantly since the early days of coronary bypass surgery. Indications for coronary artery bypass surgery are summarized in Table 46–1.

Chronic ischemia includes "silent" ischemia, in which there is no obvious angina pectoris, but a markedly positive stress electrocardiographic test result has been obtained. This suggests the lack of an anginal warning system present in most patients with ischemic heart disease. Patients in whom this syndrome exists are recommended for surgery should there be evidence of severe hemodynamic compromise during exercise testing along with electrocardiographic changes. Many of these patients have severe left main coronary disease that requires urgent intervention.

A typical patient with chronic stable angina who is a candidate for coronary bypass surgery would be one with triple-vessel disease who has had maximal medical therapy, including calcium channel blockers, vasodilators, and antiplatelet agents. Patients with single- or uncomplicated two-vessel disease would probably undergo percutaneous transluminal coronary angioplasty (PTCA).

The second major category is *acute myocardial ischemia*, with the largest group in this category being those with unstable angina. The latter condition has been defined in a number of different ways, but the recent publication by the Guideline Committee on the diagnosis and treatment of unstable angina has codified this definition.[2] The ability to differentiate acute myocardial ischemia from acute subendocardial myocardial infarction may not always be possible because of the similarity in presentation, but patients presenting for surgery are those who usually have multivessel disease and have become hemodynamically unstable in a coronary care unit, requiring stabilization with intravenous nitrates, anticoagulation, and possibly an intra-aortic balloon pump before surgery. Stabilization of the acutely ischemic patient has been enormously helpful in decreasing the risk of CABG surgery in this group so that a completely stable patient will have a lower risk and better long-term outlook than the unstable patient requiring emergency CABG.

Patients with a variety of syndromes resulting in acute myocardial necrosis and then requiring coronary bypass surgery have become increasingly frequent candidates for CABG. Those with evolving myocardial infarction who have a relatively short time from onset of chest pain to time of potential operative therapy do well, particularly if the ischemia is in the anterior myocardium. The current use of acute angioplasty for acute myocardial infarction has obviated the need for surgery in a great many patients with acute myocardial infarction and single-vessel disease.[3] There will be some in whom the interventional techniques or thrombolysis cannot open the acutely obstructed artery, however, and operation may be necessary. Many of these patients will have a severely stunned left ventricular myocardium so that depression of left ventricular function at the time of the diagnosis may be severe. At present, most patients undergoing surgery for evolving myocardial infarction have multivessel coronary disease and are treated with three or four bypass grafts.

Postinfarction angina is an important indication for CABG. Patients with this condition have had a transmural myocardial infarction and have continuing chest pain and ischemia in the same area or in a remote area of the myocardium. They are treated with intravenous nitroglycerin and a balloon pump. These patients are important candidates for CABG, which is performed on an urgent or emergent basis to prevent infarct extension. The increased use of coronary bypass in this setting appears to have decreased the incidence of sequelae of myocardial infarction, especially ventricular septal rupture.

Finally, in the patient with acute myocardial infarction with shock, therapeutic options are difficult and require a careful interplay among interventional cardiovascular techniques, intra-aortic balloon pumping, and coronary bypass surgery. Many patients with this syndrome require angioplasty and opening of an important artery that supplies a large area (perhaps as much as 40%) of left ventricular myocardium. Surgery in this syndrome is reserved for patients who are otherwise a reasonable risk, who have some evidence of viable residual left ventricular myocardium, and who have good distal target vessels for bypass.

TABLE 46–1. INDICATIONS FOR CORONARY ARTERY BYPASS SURGERY

Chronic Ischemia
"Silent ischemia"
Chronic stable angina

Acute Myocardial Ischemia
Unstable angina
Subendocardial infarction
Postinfarction angina
Acute evolving myocardial infarction
Myocardial infarction with shock

With Other Cardiac Operations
Valve surgery
Mechanical sequelae of myocardial infarction
- Ventricular septal defect
- Ruptured septal defect
- Left ventricular aneurysm

RISK STRATIFICATION AND CORONARY BYPASS SURGERY

With the increasing numbers of patients presenting with severe syndromes of ischemic heart disease, success rates for coronary bypass surgery using cardiopulmonary bypass vary depending on the presence or absence of multiple risk factors. The age of the patient is a primary consideration. In many publications describing experiences with the elderly, great emphasis is placed on the acute nature of the surgery. For example, elective coronary bypass in patients older than 75 years is as successful as it is in younger patients.[4] It is only when there are serious comorbidities that the patients in this age group do poorly, usually because of ventilator dependency, stroke, or renal failure. An elevated creatinine level, particularly in the elderly, can be the harbinger of serious problems postoperatively because of the well-known propensity of patients on cardiopulmonary bypass to experience worsening renal function if there is already pre-existing disease. Acute alterations related to hemodynamic compromise may be well tolerated, however.

Diabetes as a risk factor, per se, is not a significant problem. Only severe vascular disease in diabetics with extremely small-caliber vessels, especially those with juvenile diabetes, may pose a problem during CABG. No data have indicated difficulty with the diabetic patient who undergoes coronary bypass surgery. Bypass surgery is more likely than angioplasty to confer a survival advantage for the diabetic patient with multivessel disease.

Left ventricular dysfunction is the most important risk factor in CABG surgery, and success is inversely correlated with the degree of left ventricular dysfunction. From the Coronary Artery Surgery Study (CASS),[5] it is clear that despite the higher surgical risk, the long-term results of CABG in patients with severe depression of left ventricular function were better than those attained with medical therapy. Thus, the heart surgeon is faced almost daily with decisions regarding patients with low left ventricular systolic ejection fractions, caused primarily by previous myocardial infarction, who require complex multiple-vessel coronary revascularization. Often, this depression of left ventricular function may be so severe as to indicate cardiac transplantation for these patients. A number of current studies comparing coronary bypass surgery and transplantation for ischemic cardiomyopathy have been published, with varying results. With our present knowledge, it is still extremely difficult to tell which patient will benefit from coronary bypass operation when techniques such as positron emission tomography have not been able to differentiate the hibernating from scarified myocardium in all cases. One of the main adjunctive factors to consider when contemplating CABG for these patients is the state of the coronary vessels. A patient with severe left ventricular dysfunction and diffuse small coronary disease is at great risk for a nonsuccessful outcome, whereas a patient with equal depression of left ventricular function and excellent distal coronary vessels for bypass grafts will have a much better prognosis after CABG.[6]

NEWER CONCEPTS IN OPERATIVE TECHNIQUE

Arterial Conduits

The use of arterial conduits—namely, the internal thoracic (internal mammary) artery (IMA)—since 1985 has been a major change in the way surgeons perform coronary bypass surgery and has altered both the perioperative and late success rates after CABG. The IMA has been shown to be extremely effective in promoting the long-term revascularization of the left anterior descending artery, primarily because of the better size match-up, the lack of atherosclerosis in its wall, and the in situ nature of the graft so that no proximal anastomosis need be performed (Fig. 46–1). The right IMA, and more recently the gastroepiploic arteries, have also been used for some younger patients requiring arterial grafts, but the success rates have not been as clearly documented as they have been with the in situ left IMA to left anterior descending artery bypass. The use of this graft delays reoperations and has improved event-free survival when compared with matched controls in whom saphenous vein bypass grafts were used or with patients who have had PTCA to the left anterior descending coronary artery. The use of bilateral IMAs in the younger patient has been popular, but this approach is not considered for patients who have diabetes mellitus, since the mediastinal infection rate is much greater in this high-risk group. The efficacy of the "free" IMA bypass graft, which is disconnected from the proximal in situ connection, is not at all clear. Although some have suggested that the free graft is as good as the in situ graft, this fact has not been documented in terms of long-term patency. In the Brigham and Women's Hospital experience, 1993–1994, 97% of patients undergoing coronary bypass, both electively and urgently, received at least one IMA bypass graft.

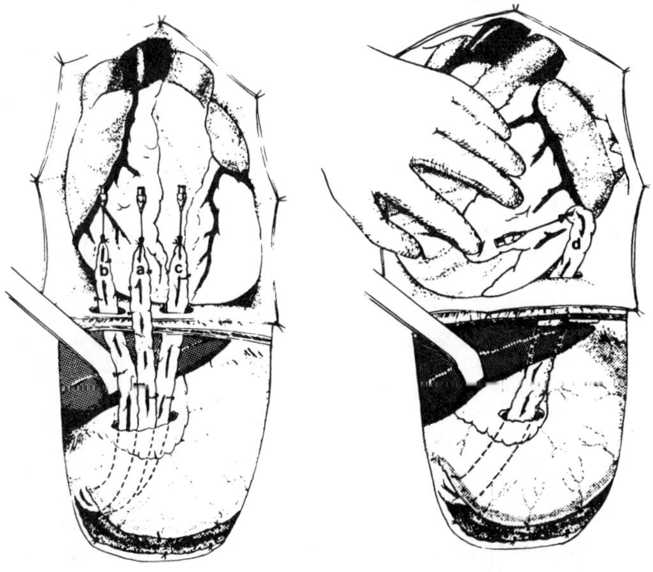

Figure 46–1. Gastroepiploic arterial bypass operation. The vascular pedicule of the gastroepiploic artery and its branches (b, a, c) are pulled through the diaphragm and attached to the distal right coronary artery (d). (Courtesy of Noel Mills, MD, New Orleans.)

Coronary Endarterectomy

Coronary endarterectomy is a technique that removes the atheromatous core from the vessel before a vein graft is sutured to the arteriotomy. Most recently, there has been a resurgence in this technique because of the diffuse nature of coronary vascular disease increasingly referred to surgeons in both primary and reoperative cases. A bypass graft into a diffusely diseased vessel is worse than not grafting this vessel at all and, in fact, can have catastrophic results, particularly in the left anterior descending artery. Thus, the improvement in open endarterectomy technique with either a vein graft or a mammary artery patch graft is a therapeutic option. This procedure accounted for 12% of grafted artery cases in 1993 at the Brigham and Women's Hospital, demonstrating the increasingly diffuse nature of coronary disease of patients admitted for surgery today. Early results have been excellent, with no increase in perioperative morbidity. Long-term patency, however, is not well documented, primarily because of an inability to perform postoperative angiography in asymptomatic patients. These techniques, however, do require extensive experience and skilled operators.

Saphenous Vein Grafts

The saphenous vein graft is still the cornerstone of CABG surgery (Fig. 46–2). In fact, with increased emphasis on saving time in the operating room to conform to managed care plans, there may actually be a swing back toward more frequent use of the saphenous vein rather than arterial conduits, which are much more time-consuming, particularly in the patient with multiple-vessel disease. Saphenous vein graft preparation is improved with the use of physiologic distention solutions, lack of overextension of these grafts, and finer suture material to connect the graft to the artery at the time of implantation. With improved surgical techniques, the patency rates of saphenous vein grafts have improved in the last 2 decades. The use of other alternative venous conduits, such as arm veins, has not been satisfactory, but there has been an increase in the use of commercially available homograft veins.

Myocardial Protection

Improvements in myocardial protection during CABG have led to decreases in perioperative morbidity despite an older population, more diffuse coronary disease, and more severe left ventricular dysfunction. The use of cardioplegia, delivered antegrade and more recently retrograde via the coronary sinus, using cold blood or cold crystalloid-containing potassium has been standard technique. Continuous warm cardioplegia has been advocated as a new form of myocardial protection, and some feel this is an improved technique.[7] More data are being obtained by prospective randomized studies, but an early vein graft study indicated that despite reasonable myocardial protection, the use of the warm technique resulted in a higher stroke

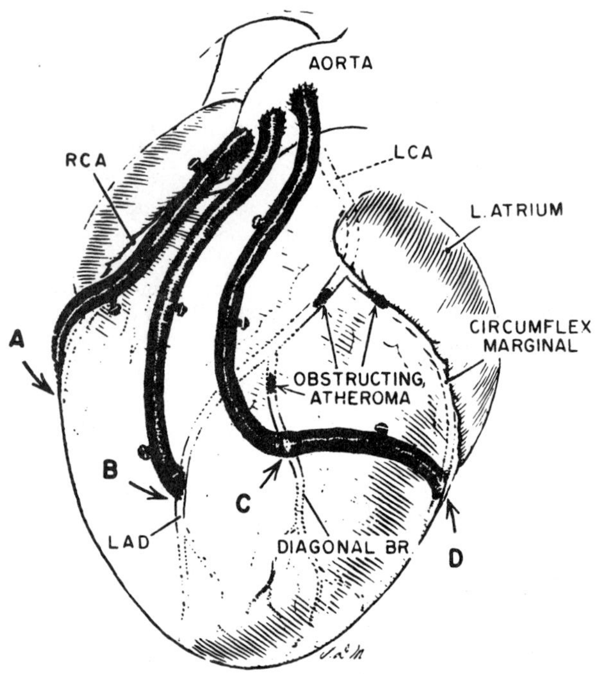

Figure 46–2. Saphenous vein bypass grafts. Aorto-coronary bypass grafts are placed on the posterior descending artery (A), left anterior descending artery (B), diagonal branch (C), and obtuse marginal (D). *Abbreviations:* RCA, right coronary artery; LCA, left coronary artery; LAD, left anterior descending (coronary artery); BR, branch.

rate postoperatively.[7] The use of the retrograde technique has been especially important in patients with severe left ventricular dysfunction. Laboratory and clinical evidence suggest a better dispersion of the cardioplegia solution and better overall cooling if both the antegrade and retrograde techniques are used.[8]

An interesting new concept has been to use the single aortic cross-clamp to perform all anastomoses, both proximal and distal. Traditionally the surgeon has performed the distal anastomoses first; the aortic cross-clamp is then removed, the heart is reperfused, and a partially occluding clamp is used for the aorta to construct the proximal anastomoses while the patient is being rewarmed. This was believed to aid in reperfusion while the patient was being rewarmed, helping him or her adjust to the circulatory load before coming off bypass. Evidence now shows that myocardial protection is better overall with the use of the single aortic cross-clamp. This has allowed a markedly decreased postoperative stroke rate, probably from the reduction of aortic manipulation.[9] The single aortic cross-clamp technique is also important in the patient with a calcified aorta, which is an increasingly common finding as the age of the patient and the extent of atherosclerosis increase in this patient population. The use of the single cross-clamp prevents embolization or fragmentation of the aortic atheromas and allows more precise and direct suturing of the proximal bypass grafts on the aorta. For the totally calcified aorta in which no cross-clamp use is possible, techniques have been devised for using saphenous vein grafts off the IMA.[10, 11]

Reoperative Coronary Bypass Surgery

CABG reoperations are increasing yearly, and the operative risks are also increased in this difficult group of patients. Patients requiring reoperation generally have vascular disease that has increased since the prior operation as well as worsening left ventricular function because of interim myocardial infarctions and decreased amounts of conduit available for the reoperative procedure. Documentation of patient risk in reoperative CABG 10 years ago indicated that a patient with patent grafts had a threefold increase in mortality over patients without a patent bypass graft. Additionally, a patent IMA bypass also provided some major challenges to surgeons when reoperations were indicated for inadequate posterior circulation.

Recent data would suggest that a total myocardial protection technique is important. Such a technique entails frequent use of femorofemoral bypass, occasional opening of the sternum on bypass so as not to injure the patent IMA, and preventing palpation of atheromatous grafts, which may cause embolization of atheromatous material into the distal coronary circulation and myocardial infarctions. Also, the meticulous use of hypothermic techniques with retrograde cardioplegia has been effective in reducing the operative mortality in this high-risk group to levels almost consistent with those seen in primary operation.[12]

EARLY AND LATE POSTOPERATIVE CARE

Early Postoperative Care

The recent trend toward "fast-tracking" patients after CABG has accelerated the traditional conservative postoperative care to one that includes early extubation in low-risk patients within 6 hours of surgery so that intensive care unit and intermediate care stays have become markedly reduced. These "critical pathway" patients have been used for cost savings by reducing the patient's postoperative stay to 5 or 6 days rather than the length of time of 8–10 days that was traditional even as recently as 1990. The use of prophylactic beta blockers seems to be important in the prevention of atrial fibrillation after coronary bypass. This particular complication is extremely expensive and has resulted in untold billions of wasted health care dollars resulting from prolonged hospital stays because of this aggravating complication. A recent prospective study by Aranki and associates[13] indicated that an adjusted hospital stay of 4.9 days has resulted because of this postoperative arrhythmia. Current protocols that discuss prophylactic and pharmacologic approaches as well as anticoagulation are ongoing, but no definitive conclusions have yet been reached about the management of this complication. It is estimated that about 25%–30% of all patients undergoing CABG, depending on the age of the patient, experience atrial fibrillation postoperatively.[14] It is also a common reason for readmission of patients after CABG.

Postoperative bleeding has also been decreased by routine use of antifibrinolytic agents,[15] the increasing use of aprotinine for reoperations, and the use of heparin-bonded surfaces in the cardiopulmonary bypass perfusion equipment. These techniques have resulted in decreased blood use postoperatively. Decreased blood use and a decreased stay in the intensive care unit have been two important factors that have decreased the length of stay and overall charges for CABG patients.

Immediate Graft Closure

Some patients may experience immediate graft closure for a variety of reasons in the immediate postoperative period, most commonly because of IMA spasm, especially in elderly women. In addition, there may be acute myocardial ischemia in patients exhibiting closure of a vein graft. The proposed method of management consists of insertion of an intra-aortic balloon, coronary and graft angiography, or re-exploration of the patient in the operating room to determine the patency of all graft sites. In most instances, surgeons will add a saphenous vein graft to the IMA graft in the left anterior descending artery for additional protection of this important artery. Prevention of IMA spasm is usually accomplished by placing a vasodilator such as papaverine around the mammary, and intraluminally.[16] The incidence of perioperative myocardial infarction has remained relatively stable over the several past decades despite the increasing complexity of the conditions requiring operation. In a recent analysis,[17] the overall perioperative myocardial infarction rate was 7%. Q wave infarction occurred in 5% of the patients and non–Q wave infarction occurred in 2%. In most centers, perioperative myocardial

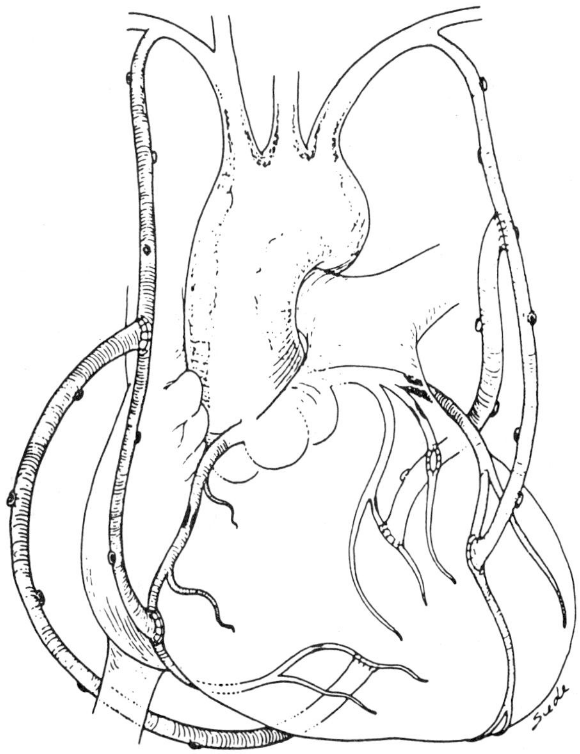

Figure 46–3. Internal mammary-coronary bypass grafts. Saphenous vein grafts are interposed between the internal mammary arteries and distal right coronary artery and obtuse marginal branch. (Courtesy of Noel Mills, MD, New Orleans.)

infarction ranges from 2%–7%. The magnitude of the CK enzyme leak is conjectural; whether this is actually an infarction or a massive elevation of enzymes, it is the diagnostic harbinger of a perioperative infarction.

Late Postoperative Complications

The most important late postoperative complication is coronary bypass graft closure. The use of antiplatelet-aggregating agents has been postulated by a number of investigators in this area[18] to retard or prevent this complication. Patients are given aspirin as soon as possible and maintained indefinitely on this agent. In many circumstances, dipyridamole (Persantine) is added as another agent. There is no compelling evidence that anticoagulation with warfarin enhances the long-term patency. Recurrence rates requiring reoperation have been estimated at approximately 1.1% per year.[19] Patients undergoing coronary bypass surgery should be enrolled in rehabilitation programs that include graded exercise, diet control, abstention from smoking, and hypertension control. These all seem to be factors that play a salutary role in promoting long-term graft patency and prevention of angina recurrence.

SUCCESS RATE OF CORONARY BYPASS SURGERY

Coronary bypass surgery is an effective technique for treating angina pectoris, particularly the unstable variety and that associated with acute myocardial infarction. Relief of angina, prevention of myocardial infarction, and improvement in long-term survival have been well documented and are discussed in other chapters. Coronary bypass surgery has the advantage of being able to accomplish complete revascularization in all patients and is a flexible treatment modality, using both arterial and venous conduits (Fig. 46–3). It is successful in patients with severe left ventricular dysfunction and provides a considerably better alternative than either interventional or medical therapy for this group of patients. As the patient mix becomes extremely diverse in terms of left ventricular function, coronary vascular disease, and the multiplicity of risk factors, the combination of total myocardial protection, flexibility of operative techniques, and the ability to define risk stratification adequately in patients will be of enormous value in optimizing surgical therapy for patients with ischemic heart disease.

REFERENCES

1. Favaloro RG: Saphenous vein autograft replacement of severe coronary artery occlusion. Operative technique. Ann Thorac Surg 1968; 5:334.
2. Unstable angina: diagnosis and management. (Clinical Practice Guideline No. 10, AA CPR Publication 94-0602.) Washington, DC: U.S. Department of Health and Human Services, Agency for Health Care Policy and Research, March 1994.
3. Grines CL, Browne KF, Marco J, et al: A comparison of immediate angioplasty with thrombolytic therapy for acute myocardial infarction. N Engl J Med 1993; 328:673.
4. Horvath KA, DiSesa VJ, Pelgh PS, et al: Favorable results of coronary artery bypass grafting in patients older than 75 years. J Thorac Cardiovasc Surg 1990; 99:92.
5. CASS Principal Investigators: Coronary Artery Surgery Study (CASS): a randomized trial of coronary artery bypass surgery: survival data. Circulation 1983; 68:939.
6. Cohn LH: Surgical treatment of coronary artery disease. *In* Wyngaarden JB, Smith LH, Bennett JC (eds): Cecil Textbook of Medicine, 19th ed, p 318. Philadelphia: WB Saunders, 1992.
7. Horsley WS, Whitlank JD, Hall JD, et al: Revascularization for acute regional infarct: superior protection with warm blood cardioplegia. Ann Thorac Surg 1993; 56:1228.
8. Sun S-C, Tam SKL, Hill SM, et al: Effects of antegrade cardioplegia with simultaneously controlled coronary sinus occlusion on preservation of regionally ischemic myocardium after acute coronary occlusion and reperfusion. Surg Forum 1987; 38:254.
9. Aranki SF, Rizzo RJ, Adams DH, et al: Single-clamp technique: an important adjunct to myocardial and cerbral protection in coronary operations. Ann Thorac Surg 1994; 58:296.
10. Peigh PS, DiSesa VJ, Collins JJ, et al: Coronary bypass grafting with totally calcified or acute dissected ascending aorta. Ann Thorac Surg 1991; 51:102.
11. Mills NL, Everson CT, Rigley CS, et al: Atherosclerosis of the ascending aorta and coronary artery bypass. Pathology clinical correlates and operative management. J Thorac Cardiovasc Surg 1991; 102:546.
12. Savage EB, Cohn LHC: "No touch" dissection, antegrade-retrograde blood cardioplegia, and single aortic cross clamp significantly reduce operative mortality of reoperative CABG. Circulation 1994; 90(part 2):140.
13. Aranki SF, Shaw DP, Adams DH, et al: Predictors of atrial fibrillation following coronary artery surgery: current trends and impact on hospital resources. Presented at the 67th Scientific Session of the American Heart Association, Dallas, TX, November 1994.
14. Andrews TC, Reimold SC, Antman EM, et al: Prevention of supraventricular arrhythmias after coronary artery bypass surgery. Circulation 1991; 84(suppl III):236.
15. Karski JM, Teasdale SJ, Norman PH, et al: Prevention of post bypass bleeding with tranexamic acid and epsilon-aminocaprioc acid. J Cardiothorac Vasc Anesth 1993; 7:431.
16. Mills NL, Bringaze WL: Preparation of internal mammary artery graft. J Thorac Cardiovasc Surg 1989; 98:73.
17. Greaves SC, Rutherford JD, Aranki SF, et al: Current incidence and determinants of perioperative myocardial infarction in coronary artery surgery [Abstract]. Circulation 1994; 90(4, part 2, suppl I):529.
18. Chesebro JH, Fuster V, Elveback LR, et al: Effect of dipyridamole and aspirin on late vein-graft patency after coronary bypass operations. N Engl J Med 1994; 310:209.
19. Cosgrove DM, Loop FD, Lytle BW, et al: Predictors of reoperation after myocardial revascularization. J Thorac Cardiovasc Surg 1986; 92:811.

47 The Timing of Valve Surgery

Blase A. Carabello, MD

Valvular heart disease inevitably places a hemodynamic overload on the left or right ventricle. If the valvular lesion is mild, the hemodynamic overload will be small and the disease may be tolerated indefinitely. However, severe valvular heart disease produces an overload that eventually causes circulatory decompensation and symptoms and, if untreated, produces irreversible myocardial damage. The definitive therapy for valvular heart disease is mechanical removal of the overload. The proper timing of this intervention is a complex clinical decision based on the severity of the lesion, the status of the symptoms, the risk of morbidity and mortality caused by the intervention, and the need to perform intervention before unwanted sequelae (including irreversible ventricular damage) occur. Intervention, therefore, should not be performed earlier or later than is necessary.

In the decision of the appropriate management strategy, three questions must be answered: (1) Is the lesion severe enough to cause the patient's symptoms or, if the patient is asymptomatic, to eventually result in left ventricular damage? (2) Has ventricular dysfunction already developed and, if so, how will it impact on the prognosis? (3) What intervention (valve replacement, percutaneous valvotomy, or valve repair) will be performed?

Since the early 1980s, the ability to answer these questions has increased dramatically. Markers of the severity of the lesion and of ventricular dysfunction can now be detected by longitudinal noninvasive follow-up, which is made possible by advances in Doppler echocardiography. The advent of Doppler interrogation of the cardiac valves changed the noninvasive evaluation of valvular heart disease from an anatomic description of the patient's heart to a physiologic examination of the importance and effect of the valvular lesion. For the two common stenotic lesions (aortic and mitral stenosis), noninvasive evaluation is often adequate to provide all the information needed for the proper timing of valve intervention and for the surgeon to plan the operation. However, this is frequently not true for valvular regurgitation. Although color-flow Doppler imaging provides an estimation of the severity of regurgitation that is usually accurate, this technique images regurgitant flow velocity, not actual volume of flow. It may therefore give the clinician an erroneous description of the amount of regurgitation present in a significant number of patients. Thus, invasive evaluation is usually required to assess the severity of the lesion in most cases of valvular regurgitation.

The following is an overview of the contribution of invasive hemodynamic analysis to noninvasive data in determining the severity of valve lesions and in assisting in the proper timing of valve surgery.

AORTIC STENOSIS

Timing of Surgery

The timing of surgery for the correction of aortic stenosis is the most straightforward for the common left-sided valvular lesions. In almost every case of aortic stenosis acquired in adulthood, the valve is too badly diseased to permit repair; therefore, an aortic valve replacement is always performed. Thus the clinician can anticipate that corrective surgery will entail the risks from valve replacement, which include the operative mortality, thromboembolism, the development of endocarditis, and prosthetic valve failure. These risks necessitate avoidance of valve replacement until it is definitely necessary.

Fortunately, the natural history for this disease is an excellent guide for timing surgery.[1] Figure 47–1 shows data, compiled by Ross and Braunwald, demonstrating that survival among asymptomatic patients with aortic stenosis is nearly the same as that among the general population. However, when the symptoms of angina, syncope, or congestive heart failure develop, there is an abrupt decrease in survival. Approximately 35% of patients who develop symptoms present with angina pectoris.[2] These patients have an average life expectancy of 5 years unless aortic valve replacement is performed. Of the 15% of patients who present with syncope, 50% survive only 3 years without aortic valve replacement; of the 50% of patients presenting with congestive heart failure, 50% survive only 2 years without aortic valve replacement. More recent studies confirm the low risk of cardiac death for the asymptomatic patient.[3, 4]

Because almost all patients with aortic stenosis receive a prosthetic valve, and because the prognosis for an asymptomatic patient is excellent, surgery should be avoided until the onset of symptoms, regardless of stenosis severity. Once symptoms develop, the abrupt increase in mortality rate mandates prompt aortic valve replacement. When the patient with aortic stenosis does develop symptoms, the clinician can be reasonably confident that aortic stenosis is responsible for those symptoms if the mean transvalvular gradient exceeds 50 mm Hg and the calculated aortic valve area is less than 0.7 cm^2. Both of these pieces of data can usually be obtained quite accurately through echocardiography.[5]

When surgery is performed, the results are usually excellent. As shown in Figure 47–2, survival after aortic valve replacement is close to that expected for the general population, especially in patients over 65 years of age.[6]

Exercise Testing

In patients who have classic symptoms of aortic stenosis, exercise testing is unnecessary and also carries increased risk.[7, 8] However, some patients experience vague symptoms that are not typical of those in the classic triad shown in Figure 47–1. Other patients may develop symptoms with valve areas slightly larger than 0.7 cm^2 or gradients lower than 50 mm Hg. In such patients, exercise testing is safe and may provide important information regarding exercise tolerance.[9, 10] For example, the patient who has only vague symptoms but who displays severe exercise intolerance is probably a candidate for aortic valve replacement, whereas a similarly symptomatic patient who can perform extended exercise probably does not require surgery.

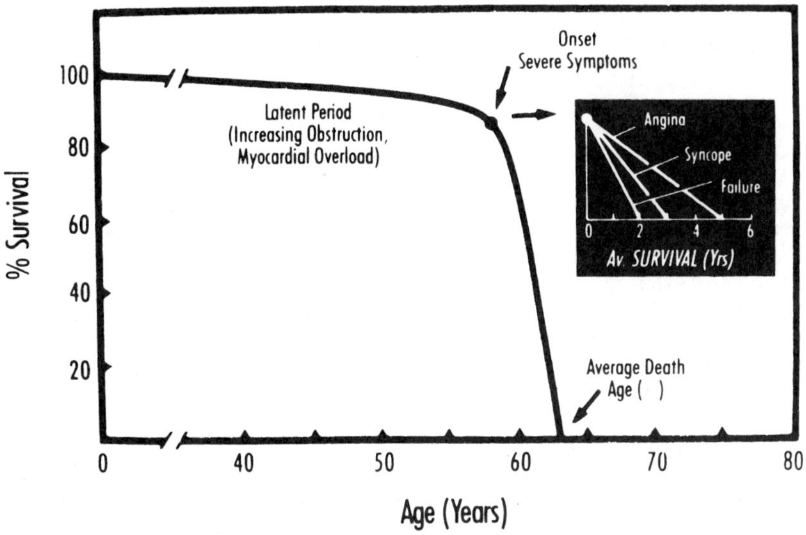

Figure 47–1. Survival for patients with aortic stenosis is plotted against age. There is an abrupt decrease in length of survival when the symptoms of angina, syncope or heart failure develop. (Adapted from Ross J Jr, Braunwald E: Aortic stenosis. Circulation 1968; 38[1, suppl V]:61.)

When Is Invasive Evaluation Required in Aortic Stenosis?

Despite the accuracy of assessing the severity of aortic stenosis noninvasively, invasive evaluation is still performed for two major reasons: (1) to assess coronary anatomy in patients who are usually at risk for having coronary disease because of their age and (2) to add further hemodynamic information in cases in which the severity of the disease is still in doubt after noninvasive testing.

Coronary Arteriography

In industrialized countries, the most common cause of aortic stenosis is valve degeneration rather than rheumatic heart disease.[11] Bicuspid aortic valve is the most common congenital cardiac abnormality, and stenotic degeneration of bicuspid aortic valves is a frequent occurrence. It is probably the flow characteristics of the bicuspid aortic valve that make it susceptible to develop stenosis early, usually in the fifth and sixth decades of life. When aortic stenosis develops in a previously normal tricuspid valve, the onset of symptoms is usually later, in the sixth and seventh decades of life. In both types of stenosis, the age at onset of symptoms for aortic stenosis puts patients at risk for also having coronary disease.

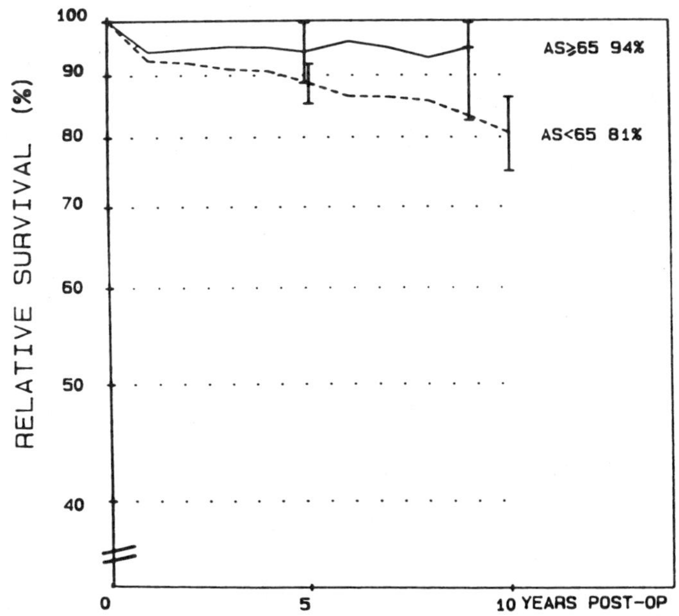

Figure 47–2. Relative (age-corrected) survival after aortic valve replacement is plotted for patients with aortic stenosis according to age. Length of survival among patients with aortic stenosis who undergo operation after the age of 65 is similar to that of the age-matched population of patients without aortic stenosis. (From Lindblom D, Lindblom U, Qvist J, Lundström H: Long-term relative survival rates after heart valve replacement. J Am Coll Cardiol 1990; 15[3]:566. Reprinted with permission of the American College of Cardiology.)

It is clear that the presence of coronary disease worsens the prognosis for aortic stenosis.[12, 13] Despite the remarkable difficulty in proving that concomitant revascularization of diseased coronary vessels at the time of aortic valve replacement enhances survival beyond that expected for aortic valve replacement alone,[13–17] the current wisdom is not to purposely leave correctable coronary disease untreated during aortic valve replacement. This is especially true if the patient has angina, a situation in which it would be impossible to know whether the angina was caused by the patient's severe aortic stenosis, by concomitant coronary disease, or by both. Thus most patients with aortic stenosis eventually undergo cardiac catheterization for coronary arteriography before surgery. Because the current array of catheters and guide wires allows retrograde passage of a catheter across even a severely stenotic aortic valve with relative ease, hemodynamic confirmation of the noninvasive studies is often made at the time of cardiac catheterization.

Invasive Evaluation of the Severity of Aortic Stenosis

Invasive evaluation of the severity of aortic stenosis is required in symptomatic patients in whom the noninvasive evaluation is ambiguous as to whether stenosis severity is enough to cause the symptoms. The severity of aortic stenosis is judged invasively by relating the mean transvalvular gradient to the patient's cardiac output (CO). The two formulas for drawing this relationship are the Gorlin formula for the derivation of aortic valve area (AVA cm^2) and the formula for aortic valve resistance (AVR dynes/sec/cm^{-5}), as shown below.[18]

$$AVA = \frac{CO/(SEP \cdot HR)}{44.3 \cdot C \cdot \sqrt{G}}$$

$$AVR = \frac{G \cdot SEP \cdot HR \cdot 1330}{CO}$$

where CO = cardiac output (mL/min), SEP = systolic ejection period (sec), HR = heart rate (beats per minute), C = empiric constant, and G = mean transvalvular gradient (mm Hg).

The Gorlin formula is usually accurate in assessing the true aortic valve area when valve flow exceeds 150 mL/sec, approximately equivalent to a cardiac output of 4.5 L/min.[19] At lower flows, the formula is less accurate because calculated aortic valve area varies directly with flow.[20–22] Thus as flow falls, calculated aortic valve area becomes smaller, regardless of the true severity of the aortic stenosis. Flow dependence at lower flows probably occurs because (1) the empiric constant for the aortic valve was never developed[18] and has been assumed erroneously to be 1.0 and (2) it is likely that at lower flows there is less mechanical force present to separate the aortic valve cusps. Thus the functional valve orifice is actually smaller at lower flows.

Aortic valve resistance is simply the mean gradient divided by the cardiac output and involves no discharge coefficients or empiric constant.[23] Resistance seems helpful in low-flow states in distinguishing patients who have truly stenotic valves from patients who have small calculated areas but in whom severe aortic stenosis is not present (Fig. 47–3).[24]

In either method of evaluation, the formulas are meaningless unless an accurate cardiac output and pressure gradient can be measured. Unfortunately, current procedures for obtaining both of these parameters are substandard in many catheterization laboratories. Consequently, basic hemodynamic data that are usually considered to provide the gold standard for evaluation may be actually less reliable than data that are obtained noninvasively.

The techniques available for measuring cardiac output include the Fick method, the thermodilution technique, the dye dilution technique, and the angiographic technique. Current practices in the use of the techniques leave much to be desired. The Fick method, which uses carefully measured oxygen consumption and arteriovenous oxygen difference, is the gold standard for measuring cardiac output. Because of the inconvenience of measuring oxygen consumption, some laboratories use algorithms that generate an assumed oxygen consumption. Such assumptions may produce as much as a 50% error in the estimation of cardiac output.[25, 26] Thus this practice should be abandoned in the assessment of aortic valve stenosis severity. The thermodilution technique for determining cardiac output is least accurate at low cardiac outputs at which the accuracy of the calculation of the aortic valve area is the most problematic.[27] The technique also tends to underestimate cardiac output when tricuspid regurgitation is present. Thus, use of thermodilution in some patients with aortic stenosis is inappropriate. The dye dilution technique may underestimate cardiac output if concomitant aortic regurgitation or mitral regurgitation is present.[28] The angiographic technique requires the accurate calculation of end-diastolic and end-systolic volumes. This condition can be met by paying careful attention to detail, especially in measuring the angiographic correction factor. However, these details are often overlooked.

Thus although cardiac output can be measured accurately, it frequently is not, a fact that probably causes few misdiagnoses when the degree of the aortic stenosis is obviously severe. However, in cases of intermediate severity and in the case of the patient with a low cardiac output in whom invasive data are the most important, the calculations should be based on the most accurate data available. Measurement of the cardiac output in such cases should be obtained from a properly performed Fick measurement that is corroborated by a second technique chosen because it is used accurately in a given laboratory.

Measurement of the transvalvular gradient is also fraught with difficulty.[29] Modern recording devices usually have standard internal calibration systems that are not entirely dependable. Therefore, there is no substitute for mercury calibration of the pressure transducers

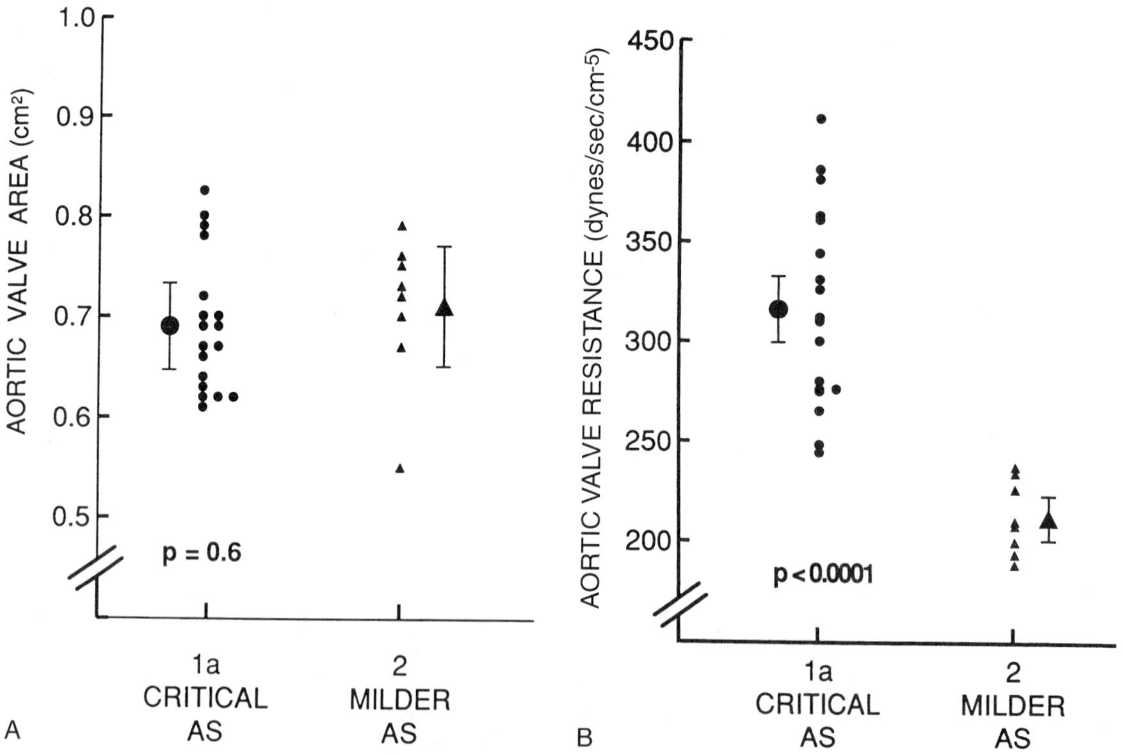

Figure 47–3. *A*, Aortic valve area for patients with critical aortic stenosis (AS) is plotted with valve area for patients who had milder disease but who had similar calculated valve areas. (From Cannon JD, Zile MR, Crawford FA Jr, Carabello BA: Aortic valve resistance as an adjunct to the Gorlin formula in assessing the severity of aortic stenosis in symptomatic patients. J Am Coll Cardiol 1992; 20[7]:1517. Reprinted with permission from the American College of Cardiology.) *B*, Aortic valve resistance is plotted for the same patients as in part *A*. Although aortic valve area did not separate the two groups of patients, aortic valve resistance did provide separation. (From Cannon JD, Zile MR, Crawford FA Jr, Carabello BA: Aortic valve resistance as an adjunct to the Gorlin formula in assessing the severity of aortic stenosis in symptomatic patients. J Am Coll Cardiol 1992; 20[7]:1517. Reprinted with permission from the American College of Cardiology.)

before the beginning of the case. However, a more serious source of error in gradient measurement arises from improper placement of the catheter. Figure 47–4 demonstrates five positions for catheter placement during cardiac catheterization of the patient with aortic stenosis.[30] Position 1 is with the ventricular catheter placed well into the body of the left ventricle. In position 2, the catheter is still inside the left ventricle but is now located in the aortic outflow tract. As shown in Figure 47–5, both recordings are typical of left ventricular pressure tracings. However, in most patients with aortic stenosis, there is a substantial gradient between the body of the left ventricle (which more accurately represents the pressure overload) and the outflow tract.[31] Thus it is important to confirm that the ventricular catheter is placed in position 1 before the pressure gradient is recorded.

The smallest gradient is that measured between position 2 and position 5 (femoral artery) when the tracings are manually realigned (5a in Fig. 47–4) to correct for the time delay inherent in the passage of the pulse wave from the left ventricle to the femoral artery.[30, 32] Overall, different combinations of catheter locations can yield differences in the measured gradient of up to 45 mm Hg in the same patient.[30] The magnitude of difference is shown graphically in Figure 47–6, in which it is obvious that variation in the pressure gradient recorded at different catheter positions might cause an erroneous diagnosis.

Once accurate cardiac output and pressure gradient data are obtained, these data are applied to the Gorlin formula for calculating aortic valve area. As noted earlier, valve area calculated by the Gorlin formula is flow-dependent, which presents a particular problem when a low gradient is measured at a cardiac output of less than 4.5 L/

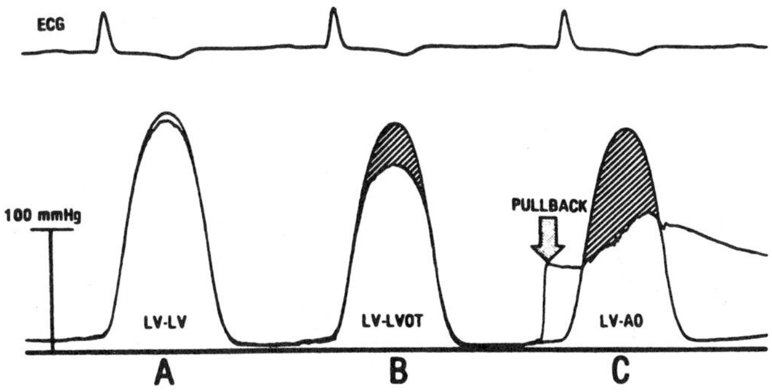

Figure 47–5. Pressure tracings made from Figure 47–4 at site 1 (*A*), sites 1 and 2 (*B*), and sites 1 and 3 (*C*). In *B*, both catheters record a left ventricular pressure tracing; however, there is a substantial drop in left ventricular pressure from the body of the left ventricle to the aortic outflow tract. This gradient is attributable to physiologic acceleration of blood as it enters the narrower outflow tract, and it does not represent an anatomic stenosis. (From Pasipoularides A: Clinical assessment of ventricular ejection dynamics with and without outflow obstruction. J Am Coll Cardiol 1990; 15[4]:859. Reprinted with permission from the American College of Cardiology.)

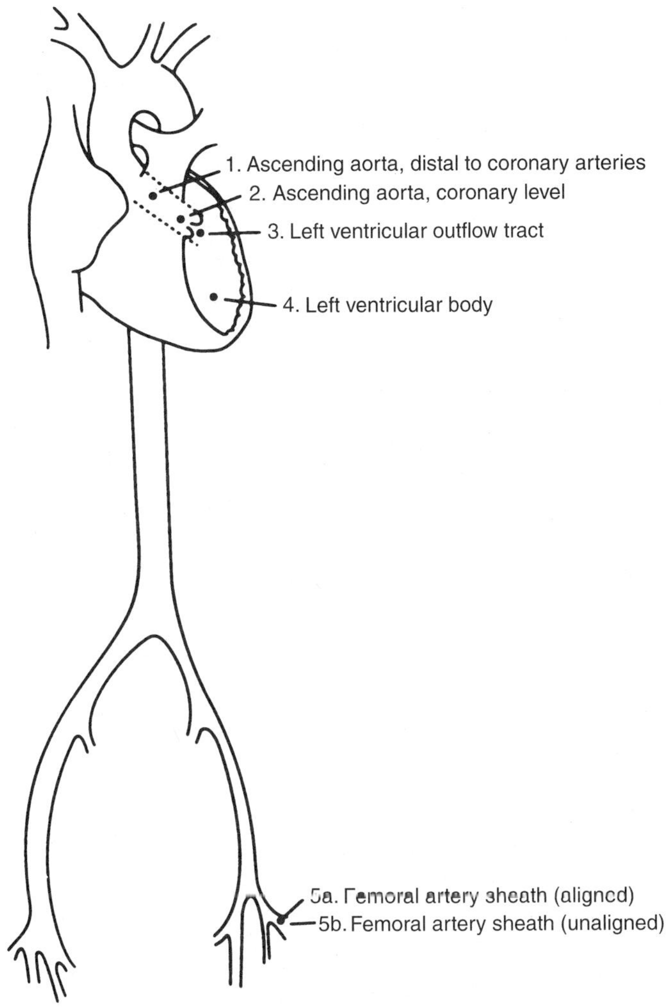

Figure 47–4. Shown is a schema of the arterial tree with various locations for placing catheters to measure the transvalvular gradient in aortic stenosis. Location 5a represents postrecording temporal alignment of the femoral artery tracing with the left ventricular tracing; 5b indicates that the femoral artery and left ventricular tracings are unaligned. (Adapted from Karavan MP, Carabello BA: Hemodynamic controversies in aortic stenosis. Mod Concepts Cardiovasc Dis 1991; 60[12]:65.)

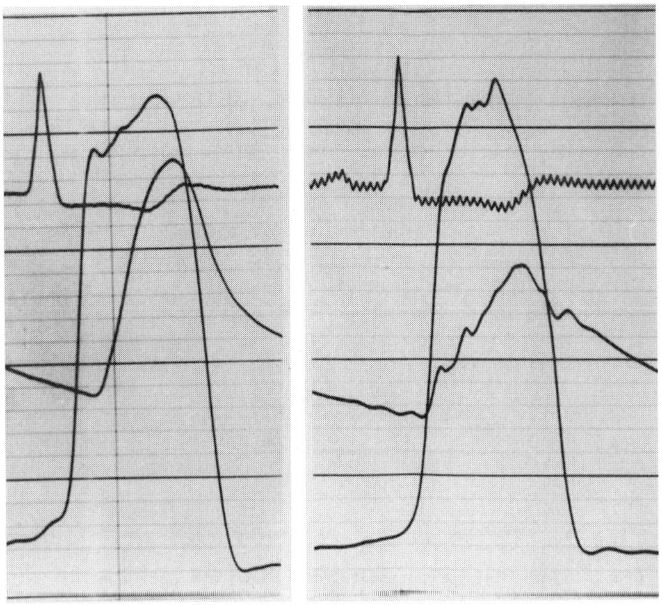

Figure 47–6. Pressure tracings recorded from Figure 47–4 at sites 2 and 5 (*left*) and sites 1 and 3 (*right*), made approximately 30 sec apart. There were no intercurrent physiologic changes in the patient's condition. In the left pair of tracings, the gradient appears small and would be consistent with mild or moderate aortic stenosis. However, the actual transvalvular gradient as shown on the right is much larger. On the left there has been substantial pressure recovery as the pulse wave moved down the arterial system. Although such recovery may reduce the total work required of the cardiovascular system, it no longer represents the transvalvular gradient and should not be used in calculation of either aortic valve area or aortic valve resistance.

min. For instance, a patient who presents for cardiac catheterization with a cardiac output of 3.0 L/min who has a transvalvular gradient of 20 mm Hg will have a calculated valve area of approximately 0.7 cm^2, a "critical" valve area that indicates severe aortic stenosis that requires surgical correction.

Many patients with low transvalvular gradients and low cardiac output do not have truly severe aortic stenosis despite the small calculated valve area.[24] This fact may be crucial in predicting the outcome for patients with impaired left ventricular performance. On one hand, patients with aortic stenosis and a low ejection fraction may have an excellent outcome after aortic valve replacement despite poor ejection performance.[33, 34] Good outcome is predicated on enhanced ejection once the obstruction to outflow is removed. A favorable prognosis does not pertain to the patient with a transvalvular gradient of less than 30 mm Hg,[33, 35, 36] although some patients with a low gradient do have satisfactory improvement after aortic valve replacement.[36] The difference in outcome for patients with a low gradient probably depends on the true severity of the aortic stenosis. Patients with a low transvalvular gradient who have only mild aortic stenosis despite a calculated severely stenotic valve area will probably not exhibit improvement after surgery. In these patients it is not severe aortic stenosis but rather a cardiomyopathy coexisting with mild aortic stenosis that causes the low cardiac output and a low gradient. On the other hand, patients with truly severe aortic stenosis might benefit from surgery by relief of severe outflow obstruction even if the gradient is low.

How can these two different pathophysiologic processes with opposite outcomes be separated? Two studies suggest that the distinction can be made in the catheterization laboratory by infusing nitroprusside or dobutamine to increase cardiac output.[24, 37] In the patient with only mild aortic stenosis, an infusion of nitroprusside causes peripheral vasodilatation that leads to an increase in forward cardiac output. Increased output across a mildly stenotic valve produces little increase in transvalvular gradient or even a decrease in gradient.[24] Instead, this change results in new hemodynamic parameters that, when applied in the Gorlin formula, cause a large increase in calculated valve area so that it is no longer in the "critical" range. The results of nitroprusside infusion in a patient who typified this problem are shown in Table 47–1. On the other hand, in patients with severe aortic stenosis, infusion of nitroprusside increases the gradient as downstream pressure decreases owing to vasodilatation, whereas cardiac output cannot increase through the severely stenotic valve. In this case, valve area increases only slightly.

Dobutamine, which is a positive inotropic agent, can cause the same change in hemodynamics by directly increasing cardiac output and promoting a reflex fall in total peripheral resistance. One advantage of nitroprusside infusion over dobutamine is that if nitroprusside is successful in improving hemodynamics, it usually indicates that it is safe to administer oral vasodilator drugs for chronic therapy of heart failure. Although vasodilators are contraindicated in true aortic stenosis, they may be beneficial in mild disease.[38] On the other hand, nitroprusside may cause transient hypotension when infused in patients with truly severe aortic stenosis. For this reason, it must be used with great caution with slowly incremented doses in the catheterization laboratory while hemodynamics are monitored. Dobutamine has an advantage over nitroprusside because it is unlikely to cause hypotension. Unfortunately, dobutamine may precipitate ischemia in patients who have concomitant coronary artery disease.

As noted earlier (see Fig. 47–3), aortic valve resistance may also be helpful in distinguishing the patients with calculated "critical" aortic valve areas who have truly severe aortic stenosis from patients with similarly calculated small valve areas who have milder disease.[24] Aortic valve resistance is the inverse of valve area with the square root sign removed. As such, it increases the importance of the gradient in the equation and decreases the importance of cardiac output, making the results less flow-dependent. Cannon and colleagues suggested that a transvalvular resistance of less than 275 dynes/sec/cm^{-5} indicates that the aortic stenosis is not severe.[24] However, before this figure can be used in clinical decision making, it must be validated in larger studies.

Evaluation of the patient with a low transvalvular gradient (≤30 mm Hg) and a cardiac output of less than 4.5 L/min should usually include hemodynamic manipulation in the catheterization laboratory; valve resistance should also be calculated. These data can help determine whether there is truly severe aortic stenosis or aortic "pseudostenosis," a situation in which the calculated valve area is critically small but the actual stenosis is mild. An algorithm outlining management for the patient with aortic stenosis is shown in Figure 47–7. It indicates that asymptomatic patients in whom physical examination findings are consistent with aortic stenosis should un-

TABLE 47–1. NITROPRUSSIDE'S EFFECTS ON VALVE AREA

	Baseline	Nitroprusside (0.5 μg/kg/min)
Cardiac output (L/min)	3.0	4.5
Left ventricular pressure (mm Hg)	130/30	120/20
Aortic pressure (mm Hg)	90/60	90/50
Aortic valve area (cm^2)	0.6	1.0
Valve resistance (dynes/sec/cm^{-5})	200	160

From Carabello BA, Ballard WL, Gazes PC (eds): Cardiology Pearls, p 142. Philadelphia: Hanley & Belfus, 1994.

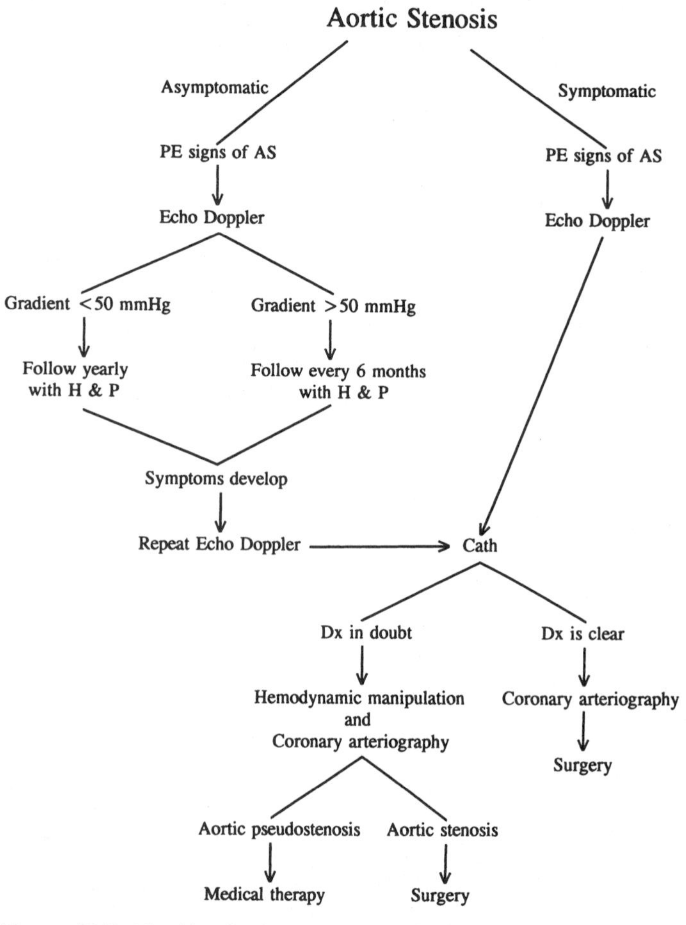

Figure 47–7. Algorithm for the management of patients with aortic stenosis. *Abbreviations*: AS, aortic stenosis; Dx, diagnosis; H & P, history and physical examination; PE, physical examination.

dergo an initial echocardiographic Doppler examination to establish the hemodynamic severity of the disease. Asymptomatic patients with relatively low gradients can be monitored yearly to look for a change in symptomatic status without repeat echocardiography, whereas patients with higher gradients should be observed more frequently. Once symptoms occur, a repeat echocardiographic Doppler study is performed to confirm a change in hemodynamic status. The patients are then usually referred for cardiac catheterization before surgery.

Patients in whom the physical examination yields findings of aortic stenosis and who present with typical symptoms are referred for a confirmatory echocardiographic Doppler study and then usually for catheterization before surgery. During catheterization of the patient with classic aortic stenosis, coronary arteriography is often all that is required. For patients with a low gradient, hemodynamic manipulation is performed to establish the severity of the stenosis.

MITRAL STENOSIS

Assessment of Severity

Although the noninvasive evaluation of the severity of mitral stenosis is usually precise, many patients with the disease nonetheless undergo hemodynamic evaluation. This usually occurs after noninvasive evaluation has indicated that mitral stenosis is severe and that balloon mitral valvotomy is warranted. During valvotomy, the left atrium is catheterized transseptally. At this time the transmitral pressure gradient is measured directly, and cardiac output is obtained. Unlike the calculated valve area in aortic stenosis, the calculated valve area in mitral stenosis is usually an accurate reflection of the true severity of mitral stenosis.[18] The difference in the accuracy of the valve area calculations for the two different valves probably arises from the fact that the Gorlin formula was validated for mitral stenosis and that an empiric constant was determined for the mitral valve.

Diagnostic hemodynamic evaluation of mitral stenosis before mitral valve surgery or balloon valvotomy is still performed occasionally, despite the availability of the usually accurate noninvasive evaluation of this condition. Diagnostic hemodynamics are either performed incidentally at the time of coronary arteriography or are necessary because of confusing and inconclusive noninvasive data. Confusion often arises when the magnitude of the stenosis does not appear to be severe enough to be causing the symptoms that brought the patient to clinical attention. For example, noninvasive evaluation might demonstrate a transmitral gradient of 6 mm Hg and a planimetered mitral valve area of 1.5 cm^2. These findings suggest that the mitral stenosis is mild and is not capable of limiting forward flow appreciably or of causing pulmonary congestion. In many cases, however, exercise performed during cardiac catheterization is quite revealing. Frequently, both the pulmonary capillary wedge pressure and the pulmonary artery pressure increase substantially during exercise but cardiac output fails to increase normally. This explains why the patient has dyspnea on exertion. Such patients usually show improvement after successful mitral valvotomy or mitral valve surgery.

An important pitfall to avoid in the hemodynamic evaluation of patients with mitral stenosis is improper wedging of the pulmonary artery catheter when pulmonary capillary wedge pressure is obtained.[39] It is clear that when the right-sided heart catheter is properly wedged, it reliably estimates left atrial pressure. However, frequent misinterpretation occurs when an improperly wedged catheter causes overestimation of the left atrial pressure and transmitral gradient. An example of improper wedging is shown in Figure 47–8. Confirmation that the catheter is properly wedged depends on the following criteria: (1) that the catheter appears wedged on fluoroscopy; (2) that the V wave of the pulmonary capillary wedge tracing follows the T wave of the electrocardiogram in time and precedes a well-defined y descent; (3) that the mean pulmonary artery pressure is greater than the mean pulmonary capillary wedge pressure; and (4) that blood obtained from the catheter when wedged is highly oxygenated left atrial blood, confirmed by oximetry. The last criterion is the most important. Adherence to these criteria prevents overestimation of left atrial pressure from a tracing that is assumed to be a pulmonary capillary wedge pressure but is in fact a damped pulmonary artery pressure tracing.

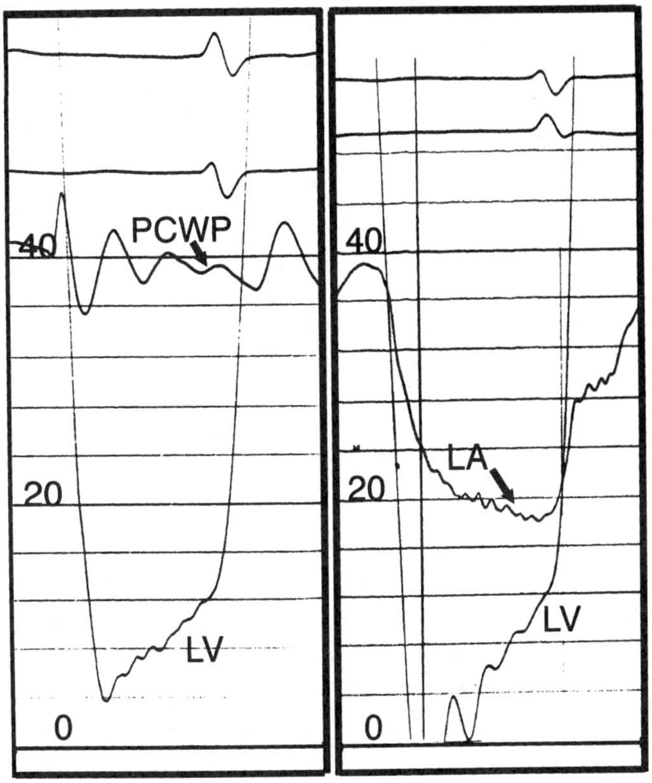

Figure 47–8. *Left*, Simultaneous recordings of an improperly obtained pulmonary capillary wedge pressure (PCWP) and a properly obtained left ventricular pressure tracing (LV). *Right*, Improper wedging led to complete obliteration of the y descent and considerable overestimation of the true transmitral valve gradient (LA-LV tracings). (Contributed by J. Bittl.)

Timing of Surgery

Figure 47–9 shows survival for patients with mitral stenosis according to therapy and symptom classification.[40] Both class III and class IV patients have longer survival after surgical relief of mitral stenosis than do patients who undergo medical management. Another prognosticator is the development of pulmonary hypertension, which increases operative mortality if surgery rather than balloon valvotomy must be performed. Thus symptom severity, pulmonary artery pressure, and the type of mechanical relief of the obstruction must all be taken into consideration in the timing of mechanical intervention. Equally effective relief of the obstruction can be provided by balloon valvotomy or open commissurotomy if valve anatomy is favorable for the success of these procedures.[41, 42] Neither of the procedures results in placement of a prosthesis, and thus relief of obstruction by these methods can be timed earlier than if a prosthesis with its attendant risks is required. Favorable valve anatomy for both balloon valvotomy and open commissurotomy includes (1) good valve mobility, (2) minimal leaflet thickening, (3) minimal calcification, (4) sparing of the subvalvular apparatus, and (5) minimal mitral regurgitation.[43] An example of the hemodynamic results of balloon valvotomy is shown in Figure 47–10. If valve anatomy is unfavorable, mitral valve replacement may be required.

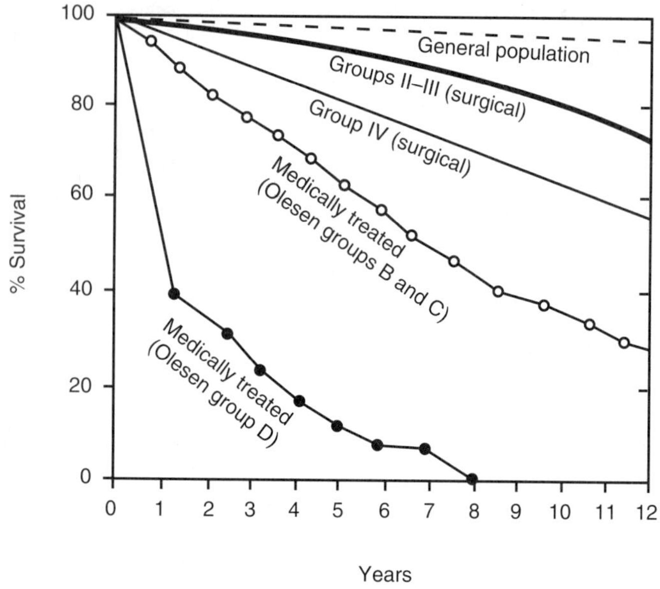

Figure 47–9. Comparison of surgically treated patients with medically treated patients with mitral stenosis. Groups II, III, and IV equivalent to New York Heart Association classifications II, III, and IV are approximately similar to the groups represented by letters B, C, and D, respectively. Class IV patients had much improved survival when treated surgically than did class D patients who were treated medically. Class II and III patients also had better survival when treated surgically than did the patients in groups B and C, although the difference is not as dramatic. (From Roy SB, Gopinath N: Mitral stenosis. Circulation 1968; 38[1, suppl V]:68.)

Regardless of the method used, mechanical correction should be provided after class II symptoms have appeared but before class III symptoms or pulmonary hypertension develops. Although pulmonary pressure can usually be estimated noninvasively, its invasive confirmation adds important data in the timing of surgery. When pulmonary hypertension has developed, balloon valvotomy is preferable if the valve characteristics are predictive of a good result from this procedure. Although pulmonary hypertension increases surgical risk, it is not a contraindication to surgery because pulmonary pressure usually falls dramatically after mechanical relief from the obstruction.[44]

A more controversial issue in the timing of mechanical intervention is the onset of atrial fibrillation that cannot be converted to sustained sinus rhythm in an otherwise asymptomatic or minimally symptomatic patient. In such a patient, if valve anatomy is favorable for a successful balloon valvotomy, valvotomy should probably be performed then. When performed early, relief of obstruction generally enhances the ability to return the patient to sinus rhythm and prevent the unwanted rhythm of atrial fibrillation from becoming permanent. On the other hand, in cases in which valve anatomy does not favor valvotomy, it may not be justified to take the increased risk associated with mitral valve replacement just to treat atrial fibrillation.

An algorithm outlining management of the patient with mitral stenosis is shown in Figure 47–11. It suggests that asymptomatic patients with the physical findings of mitral stenosis undergo initial Doppler echocardiography to quantify disease severity. The patients should then be followed yearly until symptoms become more severe than those of New York Heart Association class II or until pulmonary hypertension or recalcitrant atrial fibrillation develops. At that time, the patient should undergo balloon valvotomy if valve anatomy is favorable for success of this procedure. If valve anatomy is unfavorable and symptoms or pulmonary hypertension has developed, surgery to perform an open commissurotomy or mitral valve replacement is indicated. Patients who present with symptoms more severe than class II symptoms should be referred for valvotomy or surgery once ultrasonic or hemodynamic studies confirm that the degree of stenosis is severe enough to cause the patient's symptoms.

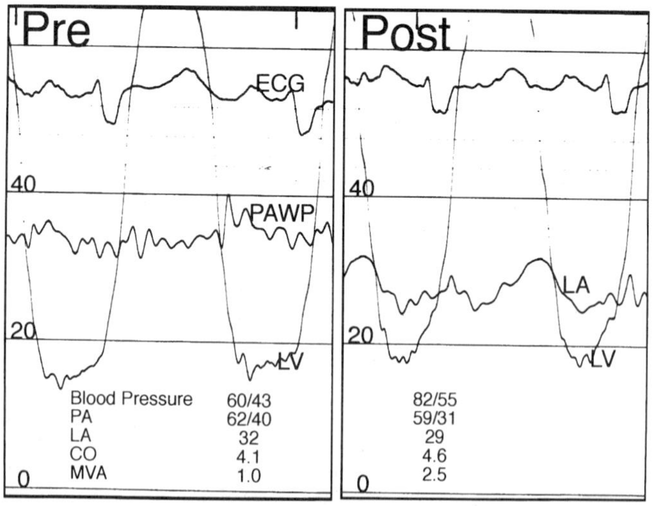

Figure 47–10. Emergency percutaneous balloon mitral valvotomy was performed in a hypotensive, intubated, pregnant 30-year-old with severe mitral stenosis. Hemodynamics are shown before (*Pre*) and after (*Post*) balloon mitral valvotomy. Transmitral gradient (between pulmonary artery wedge pressure [PAWP] and left ventricle [LV]) on the left was substantially decreased (left atrium [LA] and LV) on the right. At the same time, there was an increase in forward cardiac output, and mitral valve area increased from 1.0 to 2.5 cm^2. The patient improved, was discharged 3 days after valvotomy, and later gave birth uneventfully to a normal baby boy. (Contributed by J. Bittl.)

MITRAL REGURGITATION

Assessment of Severity

The noninvasive evaluation of regurgitant lesions is less accurate than the precise noninvasive evaluation for stenotic lesions. Although color-flow imaging detects the disturbed flow produced by the regurgitant lesion as blood enters the left atrium during systole, it is the velocity of flow, not actual flow, that is imaged. It is possible for a small high-velocity jet to entrain a large volume of blood, causing overestimation of the severity of regurgitation.[45] In some cases of mitral regurgitation in which the history, physical examination, chest radiograph, and echocardiogram are all concordant in the assessment of the severity of the disease, an invasive evaluation may not be necessary. However, in most cases, the severity of mitral regurgitation can be established only after all diagnostic modalities, including qualitative and quantitative ventriculography, are taken into consideration.[46]

Quantitative Left Ventriculography

During left ventriculography, radiopaque contrast is injected into the left ventricle, and a portion of it is regurgitated into the left atrium. Ventricular ectopy, which causes artifactual mitral regurgitation, must be avoided. A second error that must be avoided is injection of an amount of contrast that is inadequate to opacify the enlarged left atrium and ventricle. This flaw in technique can cause serious underestimation of the degree of regurgitation. As a rule, 60 mL of contrast should be injected over 4 sec. Inference regarding the severity of mitral regurgitation is made by observing the degree to which the left atrium becomes opacified in comparison with the left ventricle.

The standard system for grading the severity of mitral regurgitation

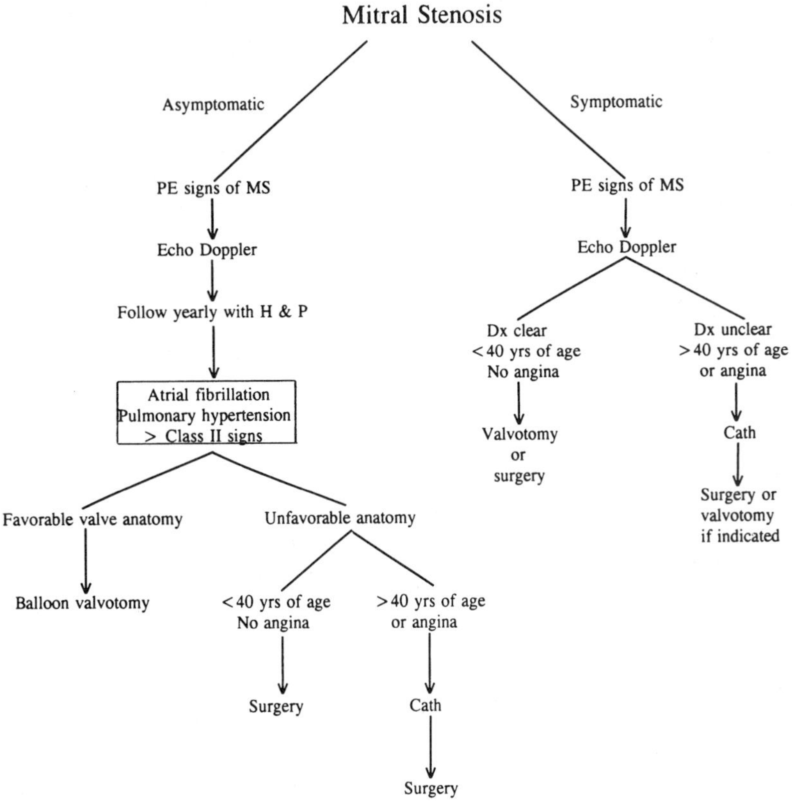

Figure 47–11. Algorithm for the therapy of mitral stenosis. *Abbreviations*: PE, physical examination; MS, mitral stenosis; H & P, history and physical examination.

is shown in Table 47–2. Grades 3+ and 4+ mitral regurgitation indicate severe disease that is capable of causing symptoms, severe hemodynamic overload, and left ventricular dysfunction. Therefore, these grades mandate corrective surgery. Conversely, grades 1+ and 2+ indicate that the mitral regurgitation is only mild to moderate and is probably not capable of causing symptoms or muscle dysfunction under most circumstances. Unfortunately, this semiquantitative system is often ambiguous. Frequently the diagnosis is 2+ to 3+ mitral regurgitation—that is, moderate to moderately severe disease.[47] The proper management for patients in this range of severity is unclear. More precise ways of evaluating the severity of mitral regurgitation at the time of cardiac catheterization are obviously desirable.

Qualitative Angiography

A better assessment of the severity of mitral regurgitation can be gained by measuring regurgitant volume in relationship to forward stroke volume (regurgitant fraction). Regurgitant fraction is formulated as

$$\frac{\text{Total stroke volume} - \text{forward stroke volume}}{\text{Total stroke volume}}$$

TABLE 47–2. QUALITATIVE GRADING OF MITRAL REGURGITATION

1+	Puff of contrast enters the left atrium without completely opacifying the chamber
2+	Left atrium completely but faintly opacified; left atrial opacification less dense than left ventricular opacification
3+	Early opacification of left atrium, equal to that of the left ventricle
4+	Left atrium more densely opacified than left ventricle; concomitant opacification of the pulmonary veins

in which the total stroke volume is the difference between end-diastolic volume and end-systolic volume measured angiographically, whereas forward stroke volume is that derived from the various techniques for measuring systemic cardiac output (i.e., the thermodilution technique or the Fick method). The exact regurgitant fraction that imparts a load on the heart severe enough to cause symptoms and eventual muscle dysfunction is unknown. However, most patients with mitral regurgitation who have required mitral valve surgery have regurgitant fractions of greater than .50, which suggests that at least this amount of regurgitation is required in order to precipitate enough decompensation to warrant surgical correction.[48, 49] Furthermore, there is evidence that after surgery, left ventricular function does not return to normal unless surgery reduces regurgitant fraction to lower than .40.[50] Thus, a regurgitant fraction in the 40%–50% range or greater is probably the severity required in order to cause symptoms and decompensation. Figure 47–12 demonstrates the discordance between angiographic grade and quantitative angiography for assessing mitral regurgitation.[51] Although in general angiographic grade increases as regurgitant volume (or regurgitant fraction) increases, there is much overlap between the angiographic grades when regurgitant volume is used as a gold standard.

Unfortunately, although quantitative angiography is more precise than either color-flow Doppler echocardiography or qualitative angiography in assessing mitral regurgitation, this technique has many drawbacks and has not gained widespread acceptance in the routine clinical assessment of mitral regurgitation, for the following reasons. First, in order to employ this technique, angiographic volumes and forward cardiac output must be measured accurately to measure total stroke volume and forward stroke volume, respectively. It is clear that with cautious attention to detail, angiographic volumes can be calculated accurately. However, variations in angiographic technique from one laboratory to another make it unwise to use published techniques for calculating cardiac volumes angiographically without laboratory-specific validation. Validation requires confirmation of the relation between calculated volumes and known phantom volumes.

Additional validation can be obtained by comparing angiographic stroke volume with stroke volume derived from the Fick or thermodilution cardiac method in patients who have no valvular regurgitation. Once established, revalidation of angiographic technique should be performed periodically to ensure that practice of the technique is not being degraded with the passage of time or with changes in laboratory personnel. Such validations are almost never made. Second, as noted earlier, the calculation of forward cardiac output has inherent problems that add further error to the calculation of regurgitant volume and regurgitant fraction. Finally, the technique cannot be used in patients with atrial fibrillation in which the stroke volume of a given beat is unlikely to represent average stroke volume. Thus quantitative angiography to establish the severity of mitral regurgitation is feasible and can be practiced accurately but, in reality, rarely is.

Other Hemodynamic Clues to the Severity of Mitral Regurgitation

In addition to the techniques noted earlier, two other invasive markers can be helpful in establishing the severity of mitral regurgitation in some cases: the end-diastolic volume and the pulmonary capillary wedge pressure. The ventricular response to volume overload is the development of eccentric hypertrophy in which sarcomeres are laid down in series. This type of hypertrophy causes the ventricle to dilate, a mechanism whereby it can pump more total stroke volume to compensate for that portion of the output that is regurgitated. If mitral regurgitation has been both chronic and severe, end-diastolic volume should be greatly increased.[52] Failure of end-diastolic volume to increase in mitral regurgitation suggests (1) that the mitral regurgitation is acute and there has not been enough time for dilatation to occur; (2) that the mitral regurgitation is not as severe as other markers have suggested and therefore dilatation has had no reason to occur; or (3) that other diseases such as constrictive pericarditis or antecedent concentric hypertrophy are preventing dilatation from occurring. All three give important insights into the patient's disease and may alter management. For instance, if dilatation is absent because the lesion is of acute onset and the patient is partially compensated, it is likely that in time, dilatation and better compensation will ensue. Thus it may be appropriate to delay surgery in such patients.

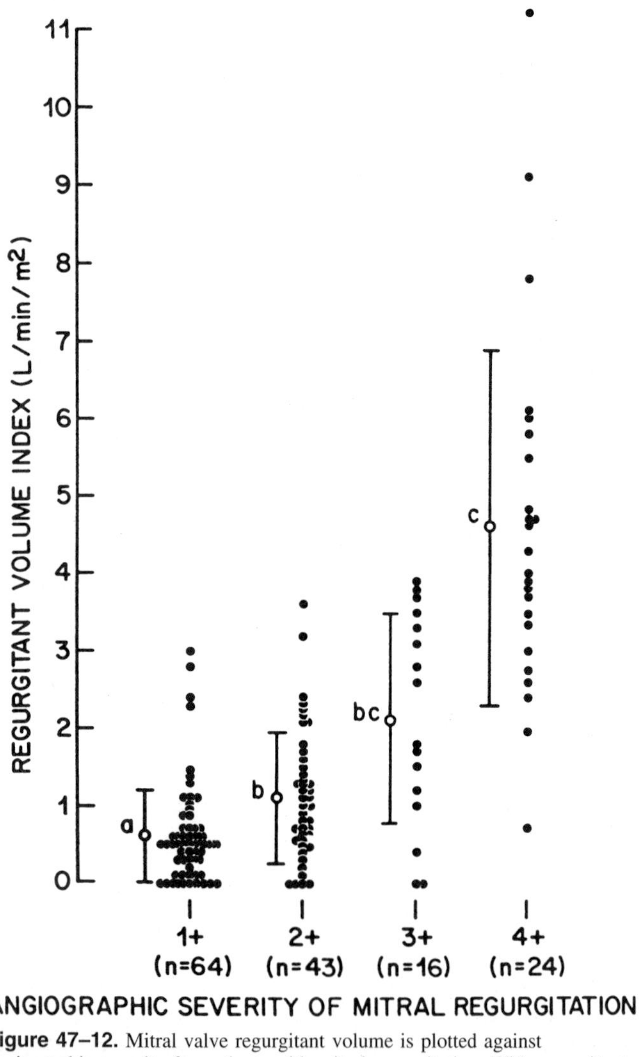

Figure 47–12. Mitral valve regurgitant volume is plotted against angiographic severity for patients with mitral regurgitation. With regurgitant volume used as the gold standard, there is a large variation of angiographic severity for any given regurgitant volume. Values for angiographic groups marked with the same letter are statistically indistinguishable. Values for groups marked with different letters are statistically different ($p < .05$). (From Croft CH, Lipscomb K, Mathis K, et al: Limitations of qualitative angiographic grading in aortic or mitral regurgitation. Am J Cardiol 1984; 53(11):1593. Reprinted with permission from the American College of Cardiology.)

The pulmonary capillary wedge pressure tracing may also give insight into the amount and duration of mitral regurgitation and the level of patient compensation. In the symptomatic patient with mitral regurgitation, the left atrial pressure should be elevated because pulmonary congestion is usually the source of the patient's symptoms. Failure of the pulmonary capillary wedge pressure to be elevated suggests (1) that the patient is well compensated, (2) that the mitral regurgitation is mild and symptoms may be coming from another source, or (3) that the patient is well compensated at rest but that during exercise, left atrial pressure rises, producing the symptom of dyspnea on exertion. Exercise performed during hemodynamic monitoring can often distinguish which of these mechanisms is operative.

A second feature of the wedge pressure tracing that should be examined is the size of the V wave. During systole in mitral regurgitation, the left atrium fills both with blood returning from the pulmonary veins and with blood regurgitated across the incompetent mitral valve. The large left atrial volume that this double-filling causes often increases left atrial pressure during ventricular systole, producing a large V wave. The presence of a V wave that is twice the mean pulmonary capillary wedge pressure is usually consistent with severe mitral regurgitation. When large V waves are found, they help confirm that the disease is severe. On the other hand, in many patients with chronic disease, the left atrium becomes compliant, accepting the increased systolic atrial volume with little increase in pressure, and thus a large V wave is absent.[53, 54] Therefore, although the V wave is of interest, few therapeutic decisions are made on the basis of its presence, especially in chronic mitral regurgitation.

Timing of Surgery

Although medical therapy for acute mitral regurgitation is beneficial in relieving symptoms, no studies have shown that the use of vasodilators retards the progression of muscle dysfunction or delays the need for surgery. On the basis of hemodynamic observations,[49, 52, 53, 56] it is reasonable to conclude that the left ventricle in chronic asymptomatic mitral regurgitation is exposed to low resistance, and vasodilators would not be expected to provide clinical or hemodynamic benefit. In contrast, data support chronic vasodilator use in patients with asymptomatic aortic insufficiency to forestall surgery.[55] Thus the only proven definitive therapy for severe mitral regurgitation is surgery.

Determining the timing of surgery for mitral regurgitation is a complex process because of the confusing effects that mitral regurgitation has on standard ejection phase indices of ventricular function (e.g., ejection fraction) and because three different operations can be used to correct the regurgitation[56]: (1) conventional mitral valve replacement, in which the mitral valve apparatus is destroyed; (2) mitral valve replacement, in which the chordal structures are preserved in the presence of a prosthetic valve; and (3) mitral repair, in which no prosthesis is used and in which the surgeon repairs the patient's native valve to restore valve competence. Outcome is significantly affected by sparing vs. destroying the valvular apparatus that is integral in the mechanism of ventricular contraction.[57] Shortening of the papillary muscles during isovolumic systole reduces the long axis of the left ventricle, which in turn increases the length of the short axis. It is probably this action that prepares the short axis (which performs the major portion of left ventricular ejection) for the ejection phase of systole by increasing short axis preload. Destruction of the mitral apparatus ablates this mechanism and may reduce left ventricular function by as much as 25%.[58] Thus if a patient is to undergo conventional mitral valve replacement that is, in effect, going to damage the ventricle, the patient must enter surgery with better ventricular function than if the chordal structures are ultimately preserved.

Because it is often impossible to know for certain which operation will actually be performed, the best policy is to ensure that preoperative ventricular function is adequate to sustain a conventional mitral valve replacement, the operation that causes the most amount of postoperative dysfunction.[59–61] Good preoperative ventricular function is indicated by an echocardiographic end-systolic dimension of less than 45 mm and by an echocardiographic shortening fraction of greater than .32.[62] The importance of the end-systolic dimension in predicting the outcome is demonstrated in Figure 47–13.[63]

During catheterization, three other indexes of ventricular function that have been predictive of outcome—ejection fraction, end-systolic volume index, and the ratio of end-systolic stress to end-systolic volume index—can be obtained. Increased preload and normal or decreased afterload in mitral regurgitation augment ventricular ejection performance and cause measures of ejection to overestimate ventricular contractile function. Thus an ejection fraction of greater than .60 should be present in order to ensure that contractile function

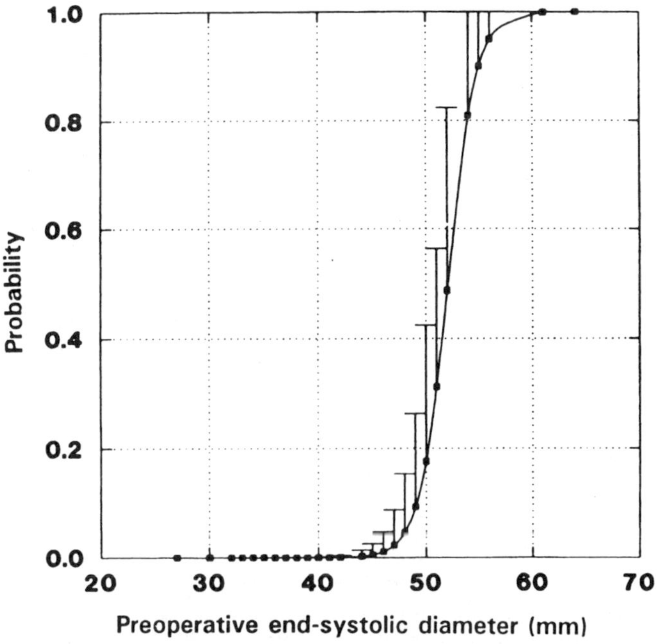

Figure 47–13. The probability of postoperative death or persistent severe heart failure is plotted against preoperative end-systolic diameter for patients with rheumatic mitral regurgitation. The risk of either of these poor outcomes begins to increase sharply as end-systolic dimension exceeds 45 mm. (From Wisenbaugh T, Skudicky D, Sareli P: Prediction of outcome after valve replacement for rheumatic mitral regurgitation in the era of chordal preservation. Circulation 1994; 89[1]:191.)

is adequate for withstanding a mitral valve replacement.[64, 65] In some cases, even an ejection fraction of .60 may be coincident with significant left ventricular dysfunction.[66]

Because of the vagaries of using ejection fraction to gauge muscle function in mitral regurgitation, end-systolic volume, which is independent of preload, has been used to factor out preload as a confounding influence. An end-systolic volume index of greater than 50–60 mL/m^2 is a good cutoff value for predicting outcome of mitral valve replacement.[67, 68] When end-systolic volume index exceeds 60 mL/m^2, the likelihood of a good outcome begins to diminish, and when end-systolic volume exceeds 90 mL/m^2, a poor postoperative outcome is likely.

The ratio of end-systolic stress to end-systolic volume index has been used to normalize end-systolic volume index for the afterload present at the end of systole.[66] This ratio has been useful in predicting outcome in mitral regurgitation but has not been employed widely, probably because the additional need for calculating wall stress makes its use cumbersome.[66, 69] A low ratio indicates that the left ventricle is large at the end of systole in relation to the load opposing contraction, which reflects contractile dysfunction. A ratio of less than 2.5 is a poor prognostic sign.

The values noted earlier for end-systolic dimension, ejection fraction, end-systolic volume index, and the ratio of end-systolic stress to end-systolic volume index are predictors for outcome of conventional mitral valve replacement but may not apply to operations that spare the mitral apparatus. If the mitral valve apparatus can be preserved, ejection fraction does not fall after surgery, whereas a fall in ejection fraction is expected after conventional mitral valve replacement.[59–61] If even the posterior chordal structures can be preserved, postoperative left ventricular function is better than if the entire apparatus is destroyed.[70] Thus the patient with mitral regurgitation and advanced disease who is a poor candidate for conventional mitral valve replacement, according to the indices cited earlier, may have an acceptable operative mortality risk and favorable postoperative course if the mitral apparatus can be spared.

One problem that frequently arises in evaluation of patients with left ventricular dysfunction for mitral valve replacement is whether the mitral regurgitation is primary or secondary. Did primary mitral regurgitation cause the left ventricular dysfunction, or did left ventricular dysfunction of another etiology lead to secondary mitral regurgitation? The answer to this question is crucial, because correction of primary mitral regurgitation may lead to improved muscle function when the offending cause has been removed.[71] On the other hand, correction of secondary mitral regurgitation may have only limited benefit, because the primary etiology of the ventricular dysfunction remains uncorrected.

The distinction between primary and secondary mitral regurgitation can often be made on the basis of one or more of the following factors: severity of mitral regurgitation, clinical history, and valve anatomy. For the mitral regurgitation to have caused left ventricular dysfunction, the amount of mitral regurgitation should be severe. Milder mitral regurgitation suggests that it is secondary in nature. Another clue to the nature of the mitral regurgitation can be gleaned from the patient's history. If it is clear that severe mitral regurgitation antedated the development of ventricular dysfunction, it indicates that the mitral regurgitation is primary. Finally, if it is obvious during echocardiography that the valve itself is anatomically abnormal, the mitral regurgitation is probably primary.

An algorithm outlining the management for the patient with mitral regurgitation is shown in Figure 47–14. It indicates that asymptomatic patients with the physical findings of mitral regurgitation should undergo an echocardiographic Doppler study, both to assess the severity of mitral regurgitation and to assess left ventricular size and function. The patient should be monitored until symptoms develop, recalcitrant atrial fibrillation develops or left ventricular dimension approaches 45 mm, at which time mitral valve surgery preceded by cardiac catheterization is indicated.

For both asymptomatic and symptomatic patients with severe

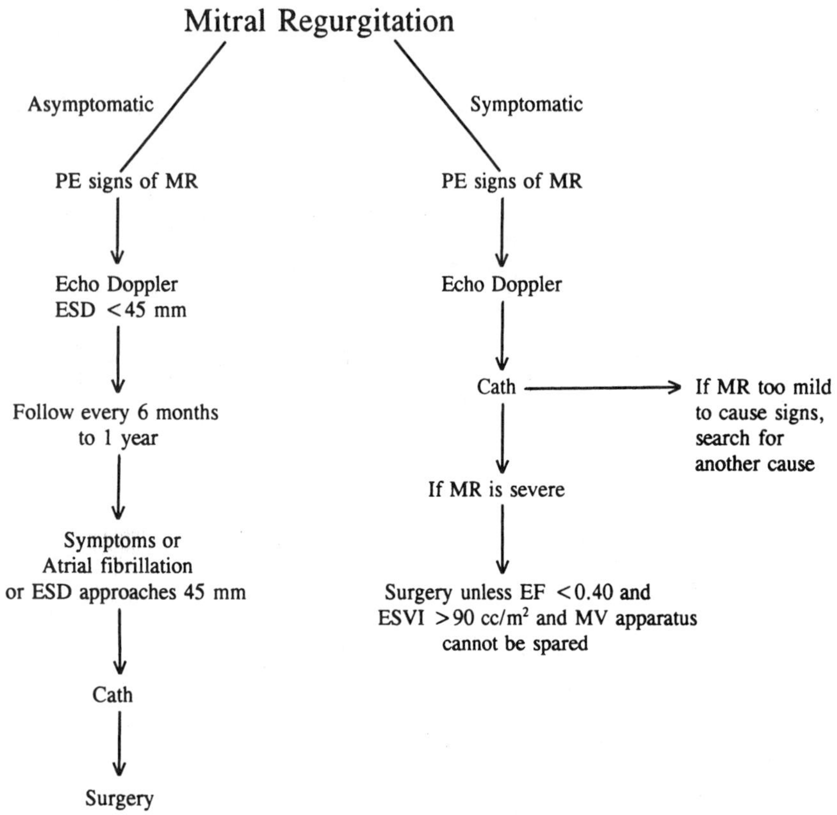

Figure 47–14. Algorithm for the treatment of chronic mitral regurgitation. *Abbreviations*: PE, physical examination; MR, mitral regurgitation; ESD, end-systolic dimension; EF, ejection fraction; ESVI, end-systolic volume index; MV, mitral valve.

mitral regurgitation, mitral valve surgery with chordal preservation should be performed. If valve anatomy makes conservation of apparatus unlikely, surgery may not be advisable for patients with severe left ventricular dysfunction indicated by an ejection fraction of less than or equal to .40 or an end-systolic volume index of greater than 90 mL/m^2, in which the outcome is likely to be unfavorable. Likewise, surgery resulting in mitral valve replacement is not advisable for patients with atrial fibrillation and good ventricular function who are otherwise asymptomatic, because the risk of surgery is not justified. Conservation of valve apparatus is more likely when pathology is confined to the posterior leaflet but is less successful in rheumatic valve disease or when the anterior leaflet is involved.

AORTIC REGURGITATION

Assessment of Severity

As with mitral regurgitation, the most helpful information obtained during the invasive assessment of the severity of aortic regurgitation is provided by qualitative and quantitative angiography. During qualitative angiography, a catheter is placed in the aorta, and the severity of regurgitation is judged by opacification of the left ventricle. A grading scale similar to that for opacification of the left atrium in mitral regurgitation is used. The method for calculating regurgitant fraction is also identical to that used in mitral regurgitation.

Other Hemodynamic Clues to the Severity of Aortic Regurgitation

Besides aortography and quantitative cineangiography, other hemodynamic clues that aortic regurgitation is severe include a widened pulse pressure, Hill's sign, and a rapid increase in left ventricular diastolic pressure during left ventricular filling. Pulse pressure increases as stroke volume increases. The wide pulse pressure usually present in aortic regurgitation is created by the very large stroke volume ejected into the aorta, which compensates the patient for the volume that is regurgitated into the left ventricle during diastole. This large stroke volume is responsible for many of the physical signs of aortic regurgitation, such as Hill's sign, the Quincke pulse, the Duroziez sign, and the Corrigan pulse. Hill's sign is an augmen-

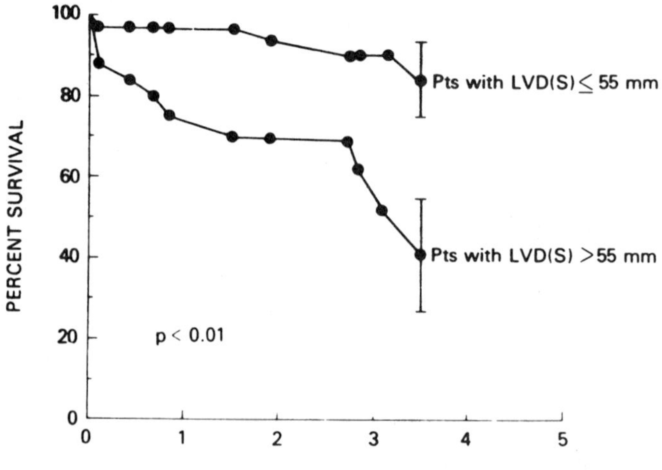

Figure 47–15. Postoperative survival for patients with aortic regurgitation is plotted according to preoperative left ventricular end-systolic dimension (LVD [S]). Among patients with preoperative left ventricular dysfunction, as indicated by a systolic internal dimension of greater than 55 mm, the 3-year survival was only 40%, whereas among patients with smaller ventricles, it was greater than 80%. (From Bonow RO, Rosing DR, Kent KM, Epstein SE: Timing of operation for chronic aortic regurgitation. Am J Cardiol 1982; 50[2]:325. Reprinted with permission from American Journal of Cardiology.)

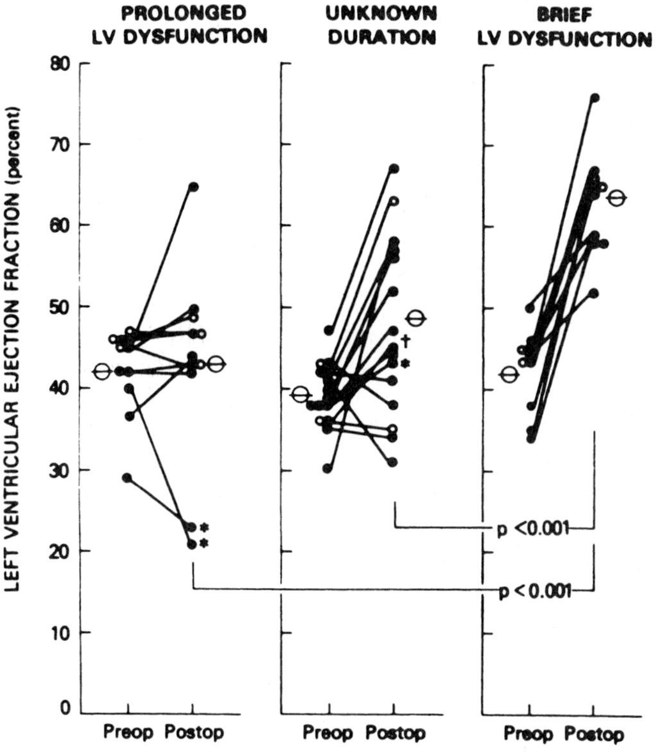

Figure 47–16. Improvement in ejection fraction before (Preop) and after (Postop) aortic valve replacement is plotted according to the duration of preoperative left ventricular (LV) dysfunction. When dysfunction was present for less than 15 months, there was almost universal improvement in postoperative left ventricular ejection performance. (From Bonow RO, Rosing DR, Maron BJ, et al: Reversal of left ventricular dysfunction after aortic valve replacement for chronic aortic regurgitation: influence of duration of preoperative left ventricular dysfunction. Circulation 1984; 70[4]:570.)

tation of systolic femoral artery pressure by more than 20 mm Hg over left ventricular systolic pressure. This augmentation probably occurs as standing waves along the aortic root reinforce the enlarged pulse as it travels down the aorta. When Hill's sign is present, the aortic regurgitation is almost always severe. It should be emphasized that in acute aortic regurgitation, before eccentric hypertrophy has had time to occur, total stroke volume will not be increased, pulse pressure will not be increased, and thus most of the physical signs of aortic regurgitation will be absent.[72]

Another hemodynamic clue to the severity of aortic regurgitation is the rapid rise in diastolic left ventricular pressure. In aortic regurgitation, left ventricular filling is rapid because it occurs both as blood enters the ventricle from the left atrium and also as blood is regurgitated through the incompetent aortic valve into the left ventricle. Finally, in *acute* aortic regurgitation, the very high left ventricular filling pressure generated by double-filling of the ventricle closes the mitral valve before mechanical systole occurs. Mitral valve preclosure is an ominous sign in acute aortic regurgitation that usually indicates that aortic valve replacement will be necessary. Preclosure is detected on physical examination as a soft S_1, can be confirmed visually during echocardiography, or can be confirmed hemodynamically as left ventricular pressure rises above simultaneously recorded left atrial (wedge) pressure in mid-diastole.

Timing of Surgery

Noninvasive parameters for the timing of surgery for chronic aortic regurgitation have been well developed. When symptoms develop, when left ventricular end-systolic dimension approaches 55 mm, or when shortening fraction becomes less than 0.27, surgery should be performed to prevent irreversible left ventricular dysfunction.[73, 74] As shown in Figure 47–15, survival after aortic valve replacement is enhanced if surgery is performed before the end-systolic dimension exceeds 55 mm.[74] These data, which were obtained in the late 1970s, have been confirmed by more recent longitudinal studies.[75, 76]

These noninvasive parameters have their invasive counterparts. Although the patient with aortic regurgitation should not be monitored by periodic cardiac catheterizations, confirmation of the noninvasive findings can be made during the invasive study that is usually performed just before surgery. An end-systolic volume index of less than 100 mL/m^2 is a satisfactory cutoff for predicting a good postoperative outcome.[69, 77, 78] When the end-systolic volume index exceeds 200 mL/m^2, surgical outcome is usually poor and attended by a high mortality rate.[79] This cutoff is at a much larger volume for aortic regurgitation than it is for mitral regurgitation, in which the cut-off is 60 mL/m^2.

After aortic valve replacement for aortic regurgitation, afterload that is increased preoperatively almost always decreases postoperatively, and thus ejection performance increases.[76, 78] This finding is in contrast to mitral regurgitation, in which a conventional mitral valve replacement increases afterload, causing ejection fraction to fall. Because the loading effects of restoring aortic valve competence in chronic aortic regurgitation are beneficial to ventricular performance, a good outcome can occur with a preoperative left ventricle that has larger volume and probably poorer function than it can in mitral regurgitation, in which conventional surgery is detrimental to ejection performance. As shown in Figure 47–16, the duration of left ventricular dysfunction in aortic regurgitation is also important in affecting outcome. A depressed ejection fraction can be expected to return to normal after surgery if surgery occurs within 15 months of the onset of ventricular dysfunction.[80]

Although surgery is the definitive therapy for aortic regurgitation, there is solid evidence to support the use of vasodilators in asymptomatic patients with aortic regurgitation who have well-preserved ventricular function. Scognamiglio and colleagues compared the use of the vasodilator nifedipine with that of digoxin with regard to the need for subsequent aortic valve replacement (Fig. 47–17).[55] As can be seen, the use of nifedipine substantially delayed or reduced the need for surgery. After surgery, the patients treated with nifedipine had normal left ventricular function, which indicates that the use of the drug had not delayed surgery at the cost of muscle dysfunction.

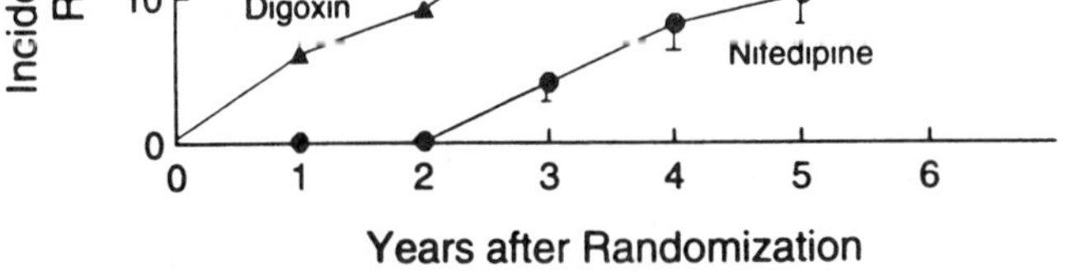

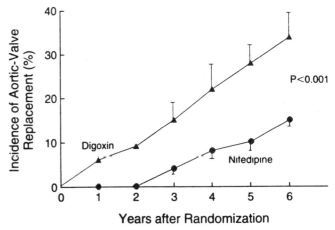

Figure 47–17. The need for aortic valve replacement is plotted for initially asymptomatic patients with aortic regurgitation treated either with digoxin or nifedipine. Nifedipine substantially delayed the need for aortic valve replacement. (From Scognamiglio R, Rahimtoola SH, Fasoli G, et al: Nifedipine in asymptomatic patients with severe aortic regurgitation and normal left ventricular function. N Engl J Med 1994; 331[11]:689.)

An algorithm for the treatment of patients with aortic regurgitation is shown in Figure 47–18. The algorithm indicates that asymptomatic patients with aortic regurgitation should undergo an initial echocardiographic Doppler study to assess the severity of the lesion and to assess left ventricular size and function. Asymptomatic patients with severe regurgitation should begin therapy with a vasodilator and be observed at an interval predicated on left ventricular end-systolic dimension. When symptoms develop or when left ventricular end-systolic dimension approaches 55 mm, aortic valve repair or replacement should be performed. Symptomatic patients with severe aortic regurgitation should undergo aortic valve replacement unless ventricular function has deteriorated to the point that it precludes the likelihood of an acceptable outcome.

TRICUSPID REGURGITATION

The invasive assessment of the severity of tricuspid regurgitation provides only limited information. Passage of a catheter across the tricuspid valve to enter the right ventricle can cause artifactual tricuspid regurgitation, which complicates the interpretation of a subsequent right ventriculogram. It is fair to point out that in most cases, the passage of the catheter alone causes only mild tricuspid regurgitation. Severe angiographic tricuspid regurgitation is usually caused by significant tricuspid valve disease. Nonetheless, right ventriculography to assess tricuspid regurgitation is not commonly practiced. On the other hand, hemodynamic measurements may be helpful in the assessment of tricuspid regurgitation severity. In most cases of severe tricuspid regurgitation, the right atrial pressure tracing shows a large V wave. As tricuspid regurgitation worsens further, the right atrial pressure tracing begins to resemble the right ventricular pressure tracing.

One important feature that can be assessed invasively in patients with tricuspid regurgitation is the severity of pulmonary hypertension that may coexist with the regurgitation. A coexisting condition, such as mitral stenosis, that causes pulmonary hypertension may also cause right ventricular dilatation and tricuspid regurgitation. Correction of the coexisting condition usually reduces pulmonary artery pressure and almost invariably leads to some improvement in the amount of tricuspid regurgitation.[81] The higher the antecedent pulmonary pressure is, the greater is the improvement in tricuspid regurgitation.

TRICUSPID STENOSIS

Not only is tricuspid stenosis a rare disease in industrialized countries, inasmuch as it is caused by repeated episodes of rheumatic fever, but it is also a rarity in nonindustrialized countries. Severity may be assessed by simultaneous measurement of right atrial and right ventricular pressure, allowing the clinician to measure the gradient across the tricuspid valve. As with aortic stenosis, discharge coefficients have never been developed for the estimation of valve area from the Gorlin formula. In general relatively small tricuspid valve gradients (5 mm Hg) may be consistent with severe tricuspid stenosis. As with mitral stenosis, if the resting hemodynamics cast doubt on the severity of the stenosis, exercise hemodynamics should be obtained.

PULMONIC STENOSIS IN ADULTS

Pulmonic stenosis is a congenital disease that is usually diagnosed and treated in childhood. Occasionally, the disease is diagnosed for the first time in adulthood. In adults, severity has been traditionally inferred by gradient alone.[82] A gradient of less than 40 mm Hg is assessed as mild and does not necessitate therapy. A gradient of more than 80 mm Hg is considered severe, indicating a need for mechanical correction. Therapy for the patient with a gradient in the midrange between 40 and 80 mm Hg is guided by whether the patient is symptomatic. There has been substantial success in the treatment of adults and children with balloon valvotomy (see Chapter 49).[83]

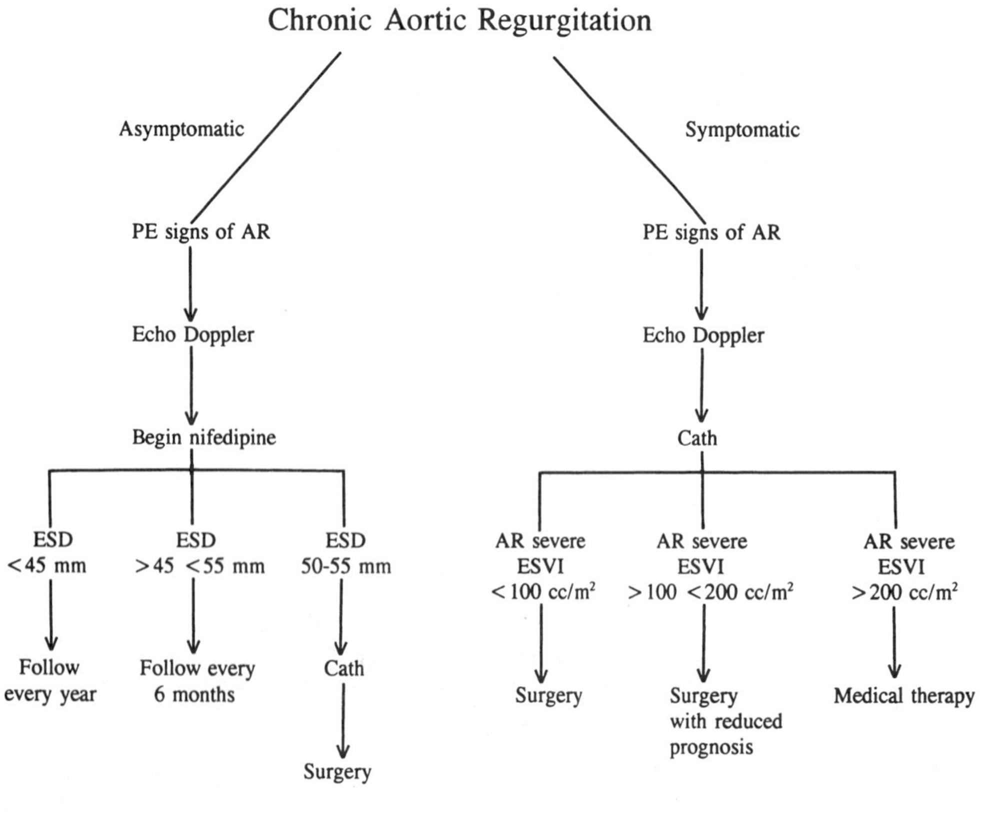

Figure 47–18. Algorithm for the therapy of chronic aortic regurgitation. *Abbreviations*: PE, physical examination; AR, aortic regurgitation; ESD, end-systolic dimension; ESVI, end-systolic volume index.

PROSTHETIC VALVES

The noninvasive evaluation of prosthetic valves to assess stenosis is usually satisfactory, and a "normal" Doppler gradient has been established for each type of valve. An exception is the St. Jude valve, in which high-velocity flow through the central orifice may overestimate the total gradient present when the two side orifices and central orifice are taken as a whole. Noninvasive assessment of prosthetic valve regurgitation may be hindered by acoustic shadowing.

Invasive evaluation of regurgitant prosthetic valves in the aortic and mitral positions is performed identically as for native valves. Both qualitative and quantitative angiography are employed. An evaluation of stenosis of a prosthesis in the mitral position is also performed in the same way as for native valves. The pulmonary capillary wedge pressure is recorded simultaneously with the left ventricular pressure, and the gradient is obtained.

Invasive evaluation of stenotic prostheses in the aortic position is more difficult. Although porcine valves can usually be crossed in a retrograde manner without difficulty, retrograde passage of catheters across mechanical valves is more problematic. Ball valves (e.g., the Starr-Edwards valve) can usually be crossed with a small straight catheter without interfering excessively with ball motion. However, retrograde passage of a catheter across a single tilting-disk valve must enter the major orifice. A catheter passed into the minor orifice can become entrapped, resulting in a catastrophe. In some Bjork-Shiley valves, a radiopaque hemicircle marks the major orifice. If the patient can be positioned so that the valve is projected en face, the major orifice can usually be entered successfully, but even then there is some risk of entering the minor orifice. The St. Jude valve is a bileaflet mechanical prosthesis for which retrograde passage is avoided because of potential catheter entrapment and also because of possible catheter damage to the valve. Invasive evaluation in such cases requires transthoracic ventricular puncture.

CONCLUSION

In summary, noninvasive and invasive techniques provide complementary data in the assessment of the severity of valvular heart disease and in the timing of surgery. Although noninvasive studies may be adequate to provide all the information needed, invasive evaluation of patients with valvular heart disease often adds important information that affects management even after a thorough noninvasive evaluation. Apart from knowledge gained by way of coronary arteriography, a hemodynamic evaluation is especially important in patients with aortic stenosis with low output and low gradient and also for most patients with valvular regurgitation.

REFERENCES

1. Ross J Jr, Braunwald E: Aortic stenosis. Circulation 1968; 38(1, suppl V):61.
2. Lombard JT, Selzer A: Valvular aortic stenosis: a clinical and hemodynamic profile of patients. Ann Intern Med 1987; 106(2):292.
3. Kelly TA, Rothbart RM, Cooper CM, et al: Comparison of outcome of asymptomatic to symptomatic patients older than 20 years of age with valvular aortic stenosis. Am J Cardiol 1988; 61(1):123.
4. Pellikka PA, Nishimura RA, Bailey KR, et al: The natural history of adults with asymptomatic, hemodynamically significant aortic stenosis. J Am Coll Cardiol 1990; 15(5):1012.
5. Currie PJ, Seward JB, Reeder GS, et al: Continuous-wave Doppler echocardiographic assessment of severity of calcific aortic stenosis: a simultaneous Doppler-catheter correlative study in 100 adult patients. Circulation 1985; 71(6):1162.
6. Lindblom D, Lindblom U, Qvist J, Lundström H: Long-term relative survival rates after heart valve replacement. J Am Coll Cardiol 1990; 15(3):566.
7. Schlant RC, Friesinger GC, Leonard JJ: ACP/ACC/AHA Task Force Statement: clinical competence in exercise testing. J Am Coll Cardiol 1990; 16(5):1061.
8. Atwood JE, Kawanishi S, Myers J, Froelicher VF: Exercise testing in patients with aortic stenosis. Chest 1988; 93(5):1083.
9. Areskog NH: Exercise testing in the evaluation of patients with valvular aortic stenosis. Clin Physiol 1984; 4(3):201.
10. Linderholm H, Osterman G, Teien D: Detection of coronary artery disease by means of exercise ECG in patients with aortic stenosis. Acta Med Scand 1985; 218(2):181.
11. Passik CS, Ackermann DM, Pluth JR, et al: Temporal changes in the causes of aortic stenosis: a surgical pathologic study of 646 cases. Mayo Clin Proc 1987; 62(2):119.
12. Miller DC, Stinson EB, Oyer PE, et al: Surgical implications and results of combined aortic valve replacement and myocardial revascularization. Am J Cardiol 1979; 43(3):494.
13. Bonow RO, Kent KM, Rosing DR, et al: Aortic valve replacement without myocardial revascularization in patients with combined aortic valvular and coronary artery disease. Circulation 1981; 63(2):243.
14. Czer LSC, Gray RJ, Stewart ME, et al: Reduction in sudden late death by concomitant revascularization with aortic valve replacement. J Thorac Cardiovasc Surg 1988; 95(3):390.
15. Mullany CJ, Elveback LR, Frye RL, et al: Coronary artery disease and its management: influence on survival in patients undergoing aortic valve replacement. J Am Coll Cardiol 1987; 10(1):66.
16. Lund O, Nielsen TT, Pilegaard HK, et al: The influence of coronary artery disease and bypass grafting on early and late survival after valve replacement for aortic stenosis. J Thorac Cardiovasc Surg 1990; 100(3):327.
17. Lytle BW, Cosgrove DM, Gill CC, et al: Aortic valve replacement combined with myocardial revascularization: late results and determinants of risk for 471 in-hospital survivors. J Thorac Cardiovasc Surg 1988; 95(3):402.
18. Gorlin R, Gorlin SG: Hydraulic formula for calculation of the area of the stenotic mitral valve, other cardiac valves, and central circulatory shunts: I. Am Heart J 1951; 41(1):1.
19. Marcus R, Bednarz J, Abruzzo J, et al: Mechanism underlying flow-dependency of valve orifice area determined by the Gorlin formula in patients with aortic valve obstruction [Abstract]. Circulation 1993; 88(4, pt 2, suppl I):103.
20. Voelker W, Raczynsky A, Schmitz B, et al: Effect of flow on valve area calculations in mitral stenosis—an in-vitro study in a pulsatile flow model [Abstract]. Circulation 1993; 88(4, pt 2, suppl I):207.
21. Wyman RM, Diver DJ, Lorell BH: The effects of increasing inotropy and transvalvular flow on Gorlin formula aortic valve area calculations in aortic stenosis [Abstract]. Circulation 1988; 78(4, suppl II):124.
22. Cannon SR, Richards KL, Crawford M: Hydraulic estimation of stenotic orifice area: a correction of the Gorlin formula. Circulation 1985; 71(6):1170.
23. Ford LE, Feldman T, Chiu YC, et al: Hemodynamic resistance as a measure of functional impairment in aortic valvular stenosis. Circ Res 1990; 66(1):1.
24. Cannon JD Jr, Zile MR, Crawford FA Jr, Carabello BA: Aortic valve resistance as an adjunct to the Gorlin formula in assessing the severity of aortic stenosis in symptomatic patients. J Am Coll Cardiol 1992; 20(7):1517.
25. Dehmer GJ, Firth BG, Hillis LD: Oxygen consumption in adult patients during cardiac catheterization. Clin Cardiol 1982; 5(8):436.
26. Kendrick AH, West J, Papouchado M, et al: Direct Fick cardiac output: are assumed values of oxygen consumption acceptable? Eur Heart J 1988; 9(3):337.
27. van Grondelle A, Ditchey RV, Groves DM, et al: Thermodilution method overestimates low cardiac output in humans. Am J Physiol 1983; 245(4, Heart Circ Physiol 14):H690.
28. Hillis LD, Firth BG, Winniford MD: Analysis of factors affecting the variability of Fick versus indicator dilution measurements of cardiac output. Am J Cardiol 1985; 56(12):764.
29. Carabello BA: Advances in hemodynamic assessment of stenotic cardiac valves. J Am Coll Cardiol 1987; 10(4):912.
30. Assey ME, Zile MR, Usher BW, et al: Effect of catheter positioning on the variability of measured gradient in aortic stenosis. Cathet Cardiovasc Diagn 1993; 30(4):287.
31. Pasipoularides A: Clinical assessment of ventricular ejection dynamics with and without outflow obstruction. J Am Coll Cardiol 1990; 15(4):859.
32. Folland ED, Parisi AF, Carbone C: Is peripheral arterial pressure a satisfactory substitute for ascending aortic pressure when measuring aortic valve gradients? J Am Coll Cardiol 1984; 4(6):1207.
33. Carabello BA, Green LH, Grossman W, et al: Hemodynamic determinants

of prognosis of aortic valve replacement in critical aortic stenosis and advanced congestive heart failure. Circulation 1980; 62(1):42.
34. Smith N, McAnulty JH, Rahimtoola SH: Severe aortic stenosis with impaired left ventricular function and clinical heart failure: results of valve replacement. Circulation 1978; 58(2):255.
35. Lund O: Preoperative risk evaluation and stratification of long-term survival after valve replacement for aortic stenosis: reasons for earlier operative intervention. Circulation 1990; 82(1):124.
36. Brogan WC III, Grayburn PA, Lange RA, et al: Prognosis after valve replacement in patients with severe aortic stenosis and a low transvalvular pressure gradient. J Am Coll Cardiol 1993; 21(7):1657.
37. Keelan ET, McBane RD, Higano ST, et al: Does dobutamine infusion during cardiac catheterization help in the assessment of the patient with low output/low gradient aortic stenosis? [Abstract]. Circulation 1994; 90(suppl I):52.
38. Greenberg BH, Massie BM: Beneficial effects of afterload reduction therapy in patients with congestive heart failure and moderate aortic stenosis. Circulation 1980; 61(6):1212.
39. Lange RA, Moore DM, Cigarroa RG, et al: Use of pulmonary capillary wedge pressure to assess severity of mitral stenosis: is true left atrial pressure needed in this condition? J Am Coll Cardiol 1989; 13(4):825.
40. Roy SB, Gopinath N: Mitral stenosis. Circulation 1968; 38(1, suppl V):68.
41. Reyes VP, Raju BS, Wynne J, et al: Percutaneous balloon valvuloplasty compared with open surgical commissurotomy for mitral stenosis. N Engl J Med 1994; 331(15):961.
42. Carabello BA, Crawford FA: Therapy for mitral stenosis comes full circle [Editorial]. N Engl J Med 1994; 331(15):1014.
43. Wilkins GT, Weyman AE, Abascal VM, et al: Percutaneous balloon dilatation of the mitral valve: an analysis of echocardiographic variables related to outcome and the mechanism of dilatation. Br Heart J 1988; 60(4):299.
44. Dalen JE, Matloff JM, Evans GL, et al: Early reduction of pulmonary vascular resistance after mitral valve replacement. N Engl J Med 1967; 277(8):387.
45. Quinones MA, Young JB, Waggoner AD, et al: Assessment of pulsed Doppler echocardiography in detection and quantification of aortic and mitral regurgitation. Br Heart J 1980; 44(6):612.
46. Slater J, Gindea AJ, Freedberg RS, et al: Comparison of cardiac catheterization and Doppler echocardiography in the decision to operate in aortic and mitral valve disease. J Am Coll Cardiol 1991; 17(5):1026.
47. Carabello BA: What exactly is 2–3+ mitral regurgitation? [Editorial]. J Am Coll Cardiol 1992; 19(2):339.
48. Kennedy JW, Doces JG, Stewart DK: Left ventricular function before and following surgical treatment of mitral valve disease. Am Heart J 1979; 97(5):592.
49. Corin WJ, Murakami T, Monrad ES, et al: Left ventricular passive diastolic properties in chronic mitral regurgitation. Circulation 1991; 83(3):797.
50. Nagatsu M, Ishihara K, Zile MR, et al: The effects of complete versus incomplete mitral valve repair in experimental mitral regurgitation. J Thorac Cardiovasc Surg 1994; 107(2):416.
51. Croft CH, Lipscomb K, Mathis K, et al: Limitations of qualitative angiographic grading in aortic or mitral regurgitation. Am J Cardiol 1984; 53(11):1593.
52. Carabello BA: Mitral regurgitation. Part 1: Basic pathophysiologic principles. Mod Concepts Cardiovasc Dis 1988; 57(10):53.
53. Braunwald E, Awe WC: The syndrome of severe mitral regurgitation with normal left atrial pressure. Circulation 1963; 27:29.
54. Fuchs RM, Heuser RR, Yin FCP, et al: Limitations of pulmonary wedge V waves in diagnosing mitral regurgitation. Am J Cardiol 1982; 49(4):849.
55. Scognamiglio R, Rahimtoola SH, Fasoli G, et al: Nifedipine in asymptomatic patients with severe aortic regurgitation and normal left ventricular function. N Engl J Med 1994; 331(11):689.
56. Carabello BA: Mitral valve disease. Curr Probl Cardiol 1993; 18(7):423.
57. Rushmer RF: Initial phase of ventricular systole: asynchronous contraction. Am J Physiol 1956; 184(1):188.
58. Hansen DE, Sarris GE, Niczyporuk MA, et al: Physiologic role of the mitral apparatus in left ventricular regional mechanics, contraction synergy, and global systolic performance. J Thorac Cardiovasc Surg 1989; 97(4):521.
59. Goldman ME, Mora F, Guarino T, et al: Mitral valvuloplasty is superior to valve replacement for preservation of left ventricular function: an intraoperative two-dimensional echocardiographic study. J Am Coll Cardiol 1987; 10(3):568.
60. David TE, Burns RJ, Bacchus CM, et al: Mitral valve replacement for mitral regurgitation with and without preservation of chordae tendineae. J Thorac Cardiovasc Surg 1984; 88(5, pt 1):718.
61. Rozich JD, Carabello BA, Usher BW, et al: Mitral valve replacement with and without chordal preservation in patients with chronic mitral regurgitation: mechanisms for differences in postoperative ejection performance. Circulation 1992; 86(6):1718.
62. Zile MR, Gaasch WH, Carroll JD, et al: Chronic mitral regurgitation: predictive value of preoperative echocardiographic indexes of left ventricular function and wall stress. J Am Coll Cardiol 1984; 3(2, pt 1):235.
63. Wisenbaugh T, Skudicky D, Sareli P: Prediction of outcome after valve replacement for rheumatic mitral regurgitation in the era of chordal preservation. Circulation 1994; 89(1):191.
64. Wisenbaugh T: Does normal pump function belie muscle dysfunction in patients with chronic severe mitral regurgitation? Circulation 1988; 77(3):515.
65. Enriquez-Sarano M, Tajik AJ, Schaff HV, et al: Echocardiographic prediction of survival after surgical correction of organic mitral regurgitation. Circulation 1994; 90(2):830.
66. Carabello BA, Nolan SP, McGuire LB: Assessment of preoperative left ventricular function in patients with mitral regurgitation: value of the end-systolic wall stress–end-systolic volume ratio. Circulation 1981; 64(6):1212.
67. Borow KM, Green LH, Mann T, et al: End-systolic volume as a predictor of postoperative left ventricular performance in volume overload from valvular regurgitation. Am J Med 1980; 68(5):655.
68. Crawford MH, Souchek J, Oprian CA, et al: Determinants of survival and left ventricular performance after mitral valve replacement. Department of Veterans Affairs Cooperative Study on Valvular Heart Disease. Circulation 1990; 81(4):1173.
69. Carabello BA, Williams H, Gash AK, et al: Hemodynamic predictors of outcome in patients undergoing valve replacement. Circulation 1986; 74(6):1309.
70. Horstkotte D, Schulte HD, Bircks W, et al: The effect of chordal preservation on late outcome after mitral valve replacement: a randomized study. J Heart Valve Dis 1993; 2:150.
71. Nakano K, Swindle MM, Spinale F, et al: Depressed contractile function due to canine mitral regurgitation improves after correction of the volume overload. J Clin Invest 1991; 87(6):2077.
72. Mann T, McLaurin L, Grossman W, et al: Assessing the hemodynamic severity of acute aortic regurgitation due to infective endocarditis. N Engl J Med 1975; 293(3):108.
73. Henry WL, Bonow RO, Borer JS, et al: Observations on the optimum time for operative intervention for aortic regurgitation: I. Evaluation of the results of aortic valve replacement in symptomatic patients. Circulation 1980; 61(3):471.
74. Bonow RO, Rosing DR, Kent KM, Epstein SE: Timing of operation for chronic aortic regurgitation. Am J Cardiol 1982; 50(2):325.
75. Bonow RO, Lakatos E, Maron BJ, Epstein SE: Serial long-term assessment of the natural history of asymptomatic patients with chronic aortic regurgitation and normal left ventricular systolic function. Circulation 1991; 84(4):1625.
76. Gaasch WH: Chronic aortic regurgitation: echocardiographic indices of function and prognosis. Primary Cardiol 1987; 13(3):104.
77. Carabello BA, Usher BW, Hendrix GH, et al: Predictors of outcome for aortic valve replacement in patients with aortic regurgitation and left ventricular dysfunction: a change in the measuring stick. J Am Coll Cardiol 1987; 10(5):991.
78. Taniguchi K, Nakano S, Kawashima Y, et al: Left ventricular ejection performance, wall stress, and contractile state in aortic regurgitation before and after aortic valve replacement. Circulation 1990; 82(3):798.
79. Taniguchi K, Nakano S, Hirose H, et al: Preoperative left ventricular function: minimal requirement for successful late results of valve replacement for aortic regurgitation. J Am Coll Cardiol 1987; 10(3):510.
80. Bonow RO, Rosing DR, Maron BJ, et al: Reversal of left ventricular dysfunction after aortic valve replacement for chronic aortic regurgitation: influence of duration of preoperative left ventricular dysfunction. Circulation 1984; 70(4):570.
81. Skudicky D, Essop MR, Sareli P: Efficacy of mitral balloon valvotomy in reducing the severity of associated tricuspid valve regurgitation. Am J Cardiol 1994; 73(2):209.
82. Johnson LW, Grossman W, Dalen JE, et al: Pulmonic stenosis in the adult: long-term follow-up results. N Engl J Med 1972; 287(23):1159.
83. Sievert H, Kober G, Bussman W-D, et al: Long-term results of percutaneous pulmonary valvuloplasty in adults. Eur Heart J 1989; 10(8):712.

48 Surgical Therapy for Valvular Heart Disease

Lawrence H. Cohn, MD
Wayne Evan Lipson, MD

Important advances have been made in the surgical treatment of acquired and congenital valvular heart disease since the development of the first artificial heart valve in 1961 by Starr and Edwards.[1] As new reparative and replacement techniques have been developed and evaluated, indications for aortic valve, mitral valve, and tricuspid valve surgery have evolved. With the use of important statistical treatments and actuarial analyses, the long-term survival of a variety of valve prostheses and valve operations and their various morbidities have been well documented since 1975.[2–11]

This chapter summarizes current surgical therapy for aortic stenosis and regurgitation, mitral stenosis and regurgitation, and tricuspid valve disease in the adult patient. The various surgical options for each valve position and the interplay between valve reconstruction and replacement are also discussed.

AORTIC VALVE DISEASE

Aortic Stenosis

One of the major breakthroughs in therapy for valvular heart disease was the development of successful operative techniques for aortic stenosis. In the current era, the most common operation for patients, either young or old, with severe calcific aortic valve disease is replacement of the aortic valve. Although various debridement techniques have been applied over the years, no particular technique has been applied universally with satisfactory long-term results. Thus, complete valvar excision, annular debridement, and replacement with either a biologic or prosthetic heart valve is the current therapy of choice. The decision to use a particular type of valve is based on anatomic findings, the age of the patient, various medical conditions that may prevent the use of anticoagulation, and the socioeconomic lifestyle wishes of the patient.[12] Valves are of two main types: (1) biologic valves, which include porcine, pericardial, and homograft valves (Fig. 48–1) and (2) prosthetic valves (Fig. 48–2), which include the Starr-Edwards ball valve, bileaflet valves (St. Jude and CarboMedics), and tilting disc valves (Medtronic-Hall and Omniscience). Each valve type can be differentiated by its major morbidity.[7–11, 13, 14] With the prosthetic valve, lifetime anticoagulation is necessary because of thromboemboli formation, and anticoagulation may cause hemorrhagic complications. Biologic valves have a finite long-term durability and require replacement in a large percentage of cases. Homografts and, more recently, pulmonary autografts have been indicated as a longer term solution to the biologic valve problem, but the long-term durability, particularly of the cryopreserved homograft, is as yet uncertain.[16–18]

For the younger patient (20–40 years old), the options for aortic valve replacement include any of the prosthetic valves, particularly the tilting disc or bileaflet valve, rather than the homograft or the pulmonary autograft. The porcine or pericardial valve has limited durability. The pulmonary autograft operation involves a transfer of the patient's own pulmonary valve to the aortic position and then reconstruction of the patient's right ventricular outflow tract with a pulmonary homograft.[19] For the middle-aged patient (40–70 years old), more frequent use of the prosthetic valves is in order, with some use of the homograft when appropriate. In the elderly age group (70 years and older), biologic valves, particularly the Hancock porcine and Carpentier-Edwards pericardial valves,[20, 21] are preferred. Although there is a well-known attrition rate for biologic valves in the young, it is considerably less in the elderly because of less active calcium metabolism, and many of the patients do not outlive their own valves.[22, 23]

Obviously these generalizations will be modified according to local situations and various other conditions in the patient. For example, in the young woman who either is pregnant or wishes to become pregnant, the well-known difficulties of experiencing pregnancy and delivery while taking anticoagulation medication militate against a prosthetic valve. In this circumstance, a biologic valve such as a porcine valve might be indicated. Similarly, in a critically ill elderly woman with an extremely small aortic root and severe aortic stenosis, a St. Jude, CarboMedics, or Medtronic-Hall valve might be inserted rapidly rather than attempting a long operation and reconstruction of the left ventricular outflow tract in the aorta. With a mechanical valve implantation in an elderly patient, it is hoped that the patient will tolerate anticoagulation without difficulty.

A summary of the long-term morbidity of various valve types is shown in Tables 48–1 to 48–3. Anticoagulant hemorrhage is the greatest long-term morbidity of the prosthetic heart valve, whereas structural valve dysfunction requiring reoperation is the most serious long-term morbidity in patients having aortic valve replacement with a biologic valve.

Aortic Regurgitation

Aortic regurgitation in the adult is usually caused by calcified congenital bicuspid aortic valve disease or rheumatic valve disease with retraction of the leaflets and severe central aortic regurgitation. The various valve prostheses noted previously are used in the vast majority of patients. In some instances, when there is minor calcification, reparative procedures may be performed in a trileaflet valve. Resuspension of a prolapsed cusp, usually the noncoronary cusp, may be performed, which eliminates the regurgitation. Some surgeons have extended reparative techniques to the bicuspid valve,[24] although long-term data on reparative procedures of the aortic valve are still lacking. In the young adult with congenital aortic regurgitation, the pulmonary autograft (Ross operation) seems, at present, to be an excellent operation, but it is technically more difficult and should be performed only in centers that have expertise with root reconstruction using homografts and prosthetic devices.[25–28] Figure 48–3 demonstrates the pulmonary autograft operation. Long-term results with the Ross procedure have been good, with some positive results extending up to 27 years.[29, 30] The major morbid conditions that occur with this procedure appear to be (1) calcification of the right ventricular outflow tract reconstruction in the homograft inserted to take the place of the patient's own pulmonic autograft, and (2) injury to the septal coronary artery of the left anterior descending artery. The latter may occur during harvesting of the pulmonary

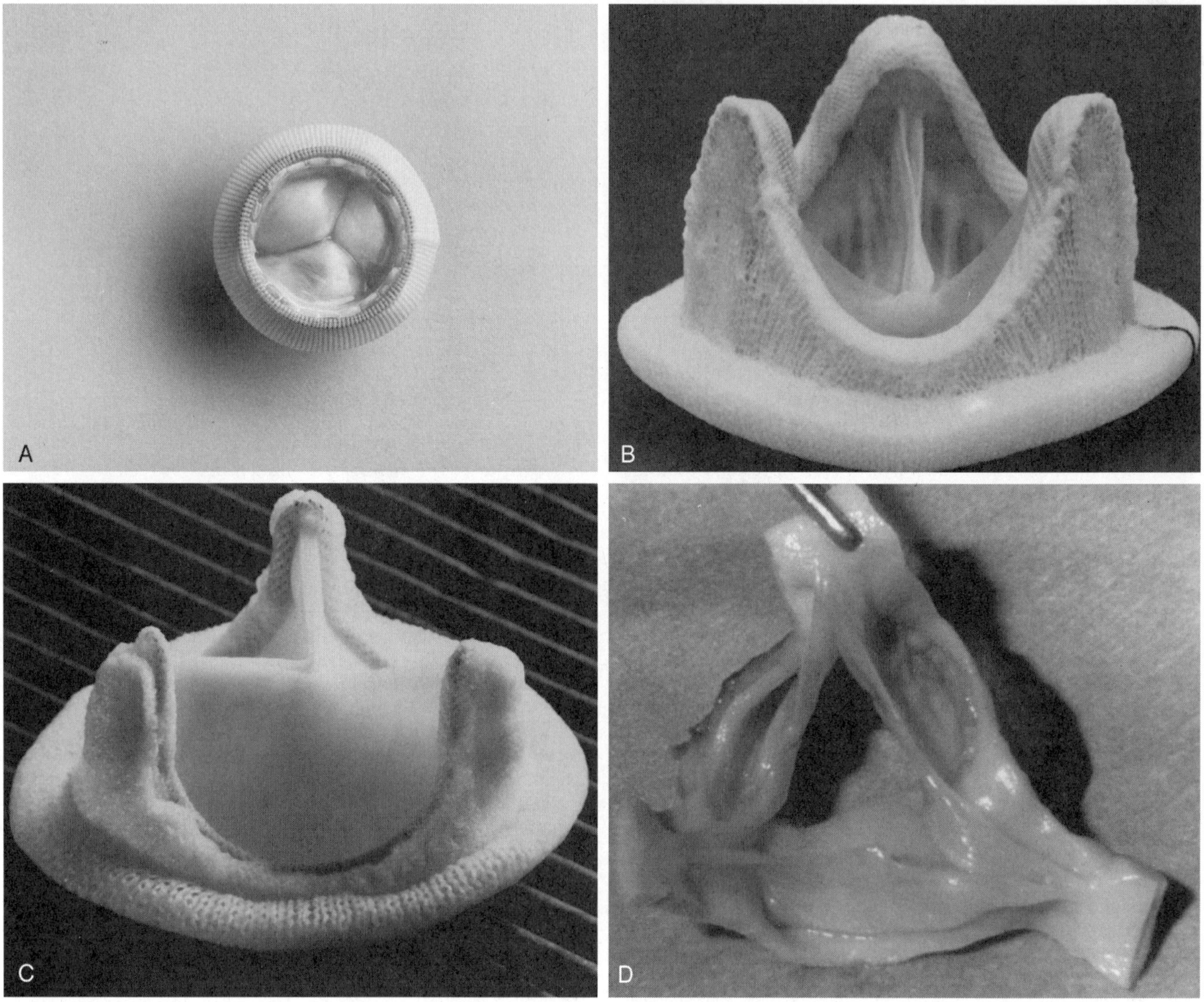

Figure 48–1. Commercially available bioprosthetic valves. *A,* Hancock MO (porcine). *B,* Carpentier-Edwards (porcine). *C,* Carpentier-Edwards pericardial (bovine). *D,* Cryolife homograft. (*A* courtesy of Medtronic; *B* and *C* courtesy of Baxter Healthcare Corp., Edwards CVS Division; *D* courtesy of Cryolife Cardiovascular.)

TABLE 48–1. COMPARISON OF VALVE-RELATED MORBIDITY

Event	Implant Site	Events Per Patient Year				
		Starr-Edwards	St. Jude Medical	Medtronic Hall	Omniscience	CarboMedics
Thromboembolism	Aortic valve	1.4–3.3	0.7–2.8	0.8–4.7	0–2.9	0.5–0.87
	Mitral valve	1.5–5.7	0.4–4.0	0.5–4.2	1.0–2.3	0.5–1.00
Anticoagulant–related hemorrhage	Aortic valve	0.8–3.1	0.2–7.9	0.7–2.6	0–1.6	1.55–1.58
	Mitral valve	1.0–3.7	0.3–2.9	0.5–4.8	0.6–2.7	1.56–1.70
Endocarditis	Aortic valve	0.4–1.1	0.1–2.1	0–1.2	0.2–1.3	0.4–0.6
	Mitral valve	0.3–0.8	0.1–2.2	0–1.7	0.5–0.8	0.35
Periprosthetic leak	Aortic valve		0–3.4	0–0.4	0–1.8	0.78
	Mitral valve		0.7–2.2	0.3–0.6	0–1.6	1.21

Data from references 3–15 and 28–32.

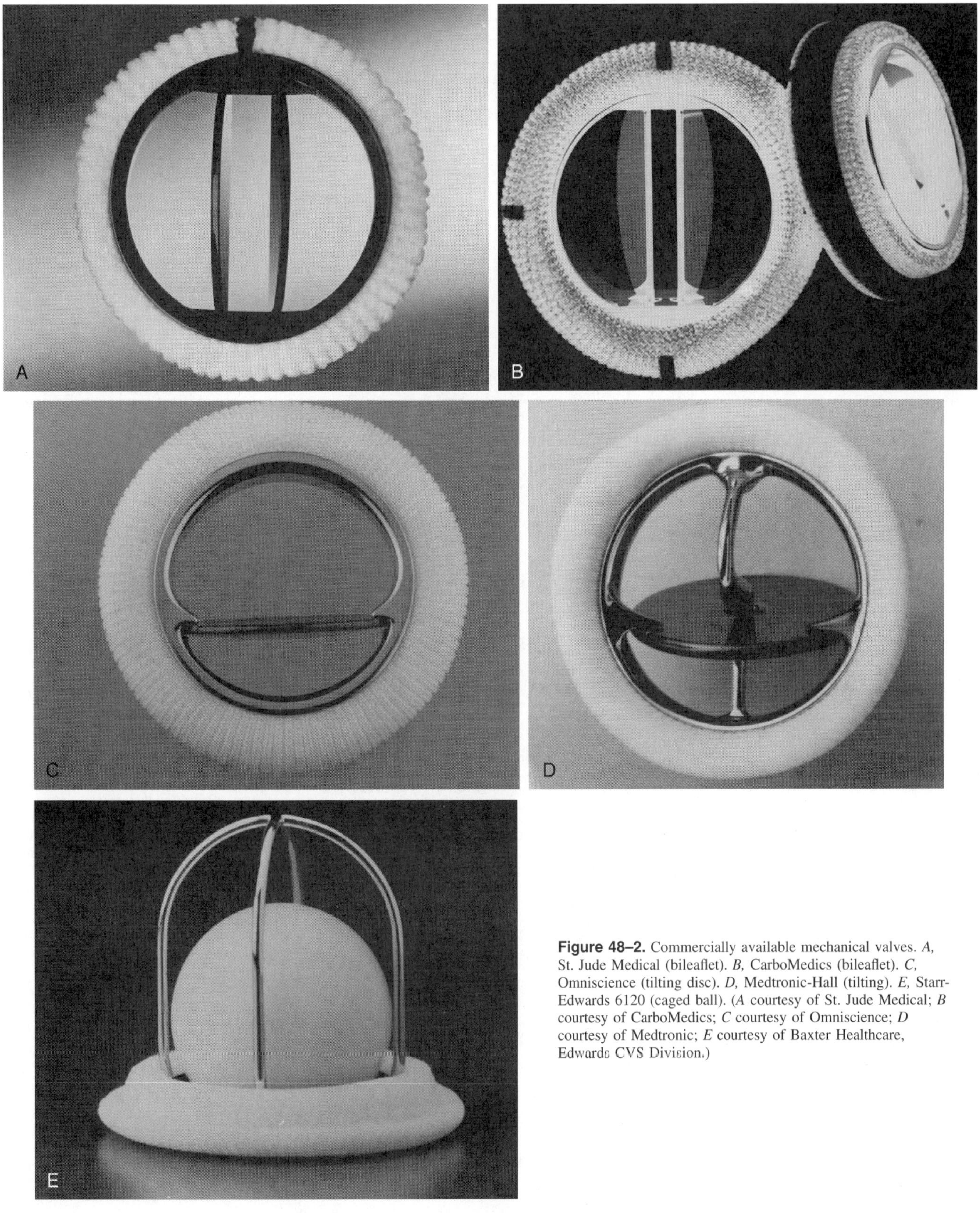

Figure 48–2. Commercially available mechanical valves. *A,* St. Jude Medical (bileaflet). *B,* CarboMedics (bileaflet). *C,* Omniscience (tilting disc). *D,* Medtronic-Hall (tilting). *E,* Starr-Edwards 6120 (caged ball). (*A* courtesy of St. Jude Medical; *B* courtesy of CarboMedics; *C* courtesy of Omniscience; *D* courtesy of Medtronic; *E* courtesy of Baxter Healthcare, Edwards CVS Division.)

TABLE 48–2. COMPARISON OF VALVE-RELATED MORBIDITY FOR PORCINE BIOPROSTHETIC VALVES

		Events Per Patient Year	
Event	**Implant Site**	**Medtronic Hancock**	**Carpentier-Edwards**
Thromboembolism	Aortic valve	0.7–0.97	1.0–1.2
	Mitral valve	1.7–1.93	1.4–1.7
Anticoagulant-related bleeding	Aortic valve	0.3–0.8	0.3–0.7
	Mitral valve	0.6–1.2	1.2–2.1
Endocarditis	Aortic valve	0.6–0.9	0.2–0.9
	Mitral valve	0.2–0.5	0.5–1.0
Structural valve deterioration	Aortic valve	0.4–1.11	0.4–1.0
	Mitral valve	1.1–1.93	1.1–2.6
Periprosthetic leak	Aortic valve	N/A	0–0.3
	Mitral valve		0.1–0.2

Abbreviation: N/A, not available.
Data pooled from references 6–10.

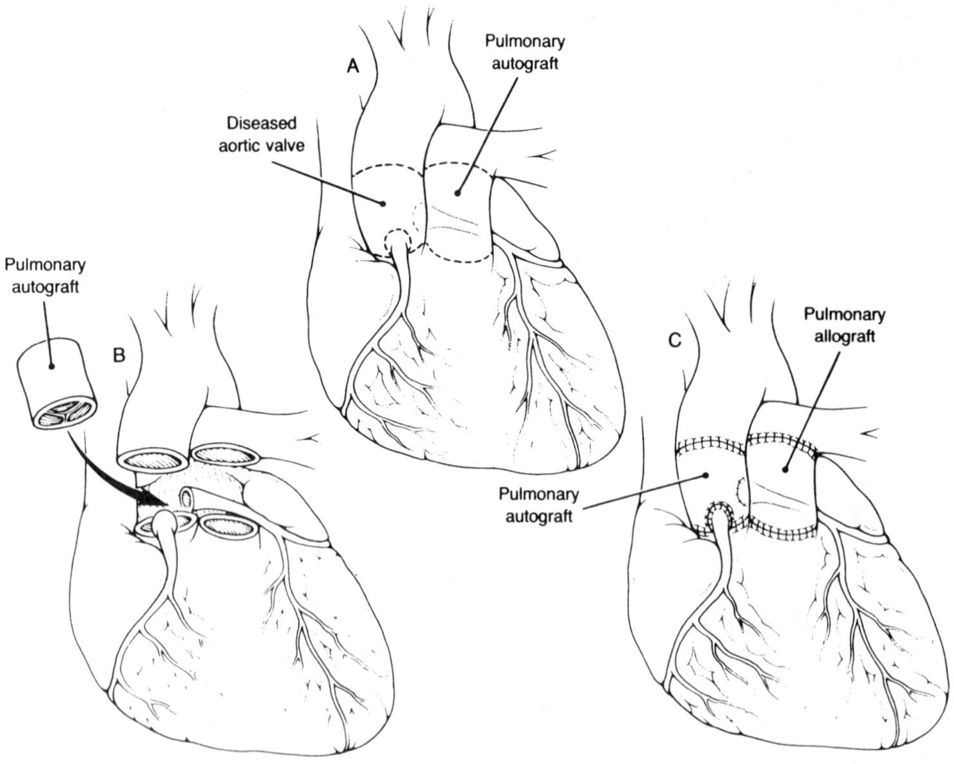

Figure 48–3. Schematic representation of the Ross operation. First, the aortic valve and the adjacent aorta are excised, leaving buttons of aortic tissue surrounding the coronary arteries *(A)*. The pulmonary valve, with a small rim of right ventricular muscle and the main pulmonary artery, is also excised. Next, the pulmonary autograft is sutured to the aortic annulus and to the distal aorta, and the coronary arteries are attached to openings in the pulmonary artery *(B)*. A pulmonary root allograft is then sutured into the right ventricular outflow tract *(C)*. (From Kouchoukos NT, Davila-Roman VG, Spray TL, et al: Replacement of the aortic root with a pulmonary autograft in children and young adults with aortic valve disease. N Engl J Med 1994; 330:1.)

TABLE 48–3. CRYOPRESERVED HOMOGRAFT VALVE PERCENT FREEDOM FROM EVENTS

Event	At 10 Years	At 14 Years
Structural deterioration	95%–98%	85%
Thromboembolism	95%–97%	94%
Endocarditis	92%–94%	94%

Data pooled from references 15–17.

autograft when it is removed from the ventricular septum.[30] In pediatric patients, the autograft has been shown to grow.[31]

Aortic regurgitation caused by severe endocarditis most often begins in an abnormal valve, either a congenital bicuspid valve or a calcific aortic stenotic valve.[32] Whatever the pathology, the result is severe aortic regurgitation that necessitates valve replacement. Extension of the infection into the annulus is a serious anatomic challenge in surgical reconstruction. Therefore, earlier operation in the presence of organisms such as *Staphylococcus aureus, S. epidermidis*, or fungi, which often produce this complication, is clearly indicated.[31] After aggressive antibiotic treatment is begun, indications for surgery include (1) persistent congestive heart failure, (2) persistent sepsis, (3) development of new arrhythmias suggesting extension into the annulus and the conduction system within the septum, (4) renal failure, and (5) the presence of a large vegetation that may give rise to embolization. Valve replacement is the treatment of choice for complicated endocarditis. The type of valve will depend on the anatomic damage and the ability of the surgeon to reconstruct the surrounding infected structures. The precepts of surgical repair are to eradicate the sepsis, repair all adjacent defects—such as ventricular septal defect and detachment of the mitral valve or subannular tissue—and secure fixation of an aortic valve device to the annulus. Recently, the use of the aortic homograft has been advocated as the valve of choice in endocarditis because no prosthetic material is placed in a septic field.[34, 35] Autologous pericardium is currently being used for lining the annulus and as pledgets when reinforcement of suture is required for closure of various defects. A tilting disc or bileaflet prosthetic valve may sometimes be necessary because of space limitations. Prosthetic valve endocarditis producing regurgitation is a difficult problem and must be dealt with aggressively by advanced valve replacement techniques. In this entity, infection almost always involves the annulus; a homograft would be desirable so that prosthetic material is not inserted into a septic field.[34, 36]

The long-term results of surgery for aortic regurgitation are generally good, although the survival rate for patients with severe aortic regurgitation is not as good as for patients with aortic stenosis.[37] Patients with aortic regurgitation have enlarged dysfunctional hearts, which may cause a chronic myopathic condition, predisposing the patient to chronic arrhythmia. This may occur despite a competent aortic valve operation. There is a higher operative mortality rate for prosthetic valve endocarditis than for native valve endocarditis, but once the operative period has passed, patients have a relatively normal life expectancy provided that there is no recurrence of infection.[33, 33, 36]

MITRAL VALVE DISEASE

Mitral Stenosis

The cause of mitral stenosis is rheumatic heart disease. The surgical treatment of mitral stenosis has been significantly altered by the introduction of percutaneous balloon mitral valve dilatation. This modality is currently the treatment of choice for noncalcific mitral stenosis.[38, 39] For calcific mitral stenosis, the therapy of choice is mitral valve replacement, although some have advocated aggressive debridement of these stenotic rheumatic mitral valves. Our experience at the Brigham and Women's Hospital has been that active debridement, although satisfactory in the short term, does not yield a good long-term result and freedom from reoperation.[40] Calcific mitral stenosis requires mitral valve replacement, unless there are superficial nodules on the valve. If a patient with noncalcific mitral stenosis is referred to the surgeon, the open mitral commissurotomy and valvulotomy is an extremely effective operation with low operative mortality (less than 2%) and a low risk of reoperation (<10%) at 10 years.[40, 41] Some patients with mitral valve stenosis have extreme pulmonary hypertension. With new advances in respiratory technology, cardiopulmonary bypass, and overall myocardial protection, even patients with severe pulmonary hypertension can be operated on with a risk only slightly higher than that in patients with lower pulmonary artery pressure.

Valves for mitral valve replacement are similarly biologic or prosthetic, but choices are fewer in this position than in the aortic position. The Federal Drug Administration (FDA)–approved biologic devices are the Carpentier-Edwards and the Hancock porcine valves, and approved prosthetic devices are the St. Jude, CarboMedics, Medtronic-Hall, and Omniscience valves. Valve type will again be determined by the patient's age, local anatomy to a certain extent, and pre-existing conditions, particularly the presence of chronic atrial fibrillation. In the United States, patients with chronic atrial fibrillation undergo chronic anticoagulation, thus obviating the advantage of a biologic valve, so most patients with atrial fibrillation receive a mechanical valve. Thus, a much higher percentage of patients receiving a mitral valve will have a mechanical valve placed. Current morbidity rates for mitral valve prosthetic and bioprosthetic valves are given in Tables 48–1 and 48–2.

Mitral Regurgitation

The causes of mitral regurgitation (MR) vary from rheumatic fever to a number of metabolic and degenerative diseases, endocarditis, and myocardial ischemia. The most important new advance in the treatment of MR has been the aggressive use of mitral valve reconstruction and repair for many causes of MR. Myxomatous degeneration is the most common cause of MR in North America. With the use of certain techniques, including partial leaflet resection, chordal shortening, and prosthetic ring annuloplasty, reconstruction preserves the annular chordal and papillary muscle interaction, which is important for preservation of left ventricular function. The technique of mitral valve repair for posterior leaflet prolapse with resection is shown in Figure 48–4. Prosthetic annuloplasty rings (Duran, Cosgrove, Carpentier) should be used to remodel the annulus, providing stability to repaired structures. A number of studies have summarized comparative results of mitral valve repair and replacement. These studies suggest that patients in the repair group have a shorter hospital stay, improved early and late myocardial function, and a lower incidence of thromboemboli than do patients undergoing valve replacement.[42] The improved survival over several years may be a result of preservation of the papillary muscle interaction. Reoperation is, of course, a possibility with reconstructive procedures from structural degeneration, but the incidence of this is between 5% and 8% over a 10-year period. The risk of repair operations appears to be lower than that of valve replacement.[43] At Brigham and Women's Hospital, in patients younger than 70 years, the risk was less than 1% for repair of myxomatous degenerative valves, whereas in the older than 70-year age group, the risk was 3% because of the increase in coronary artery disease. For mitral valve endocarditis producing regurgitation, the same principles as those mentioned previously for aortic valve endocarditis apply. Infection must be cleared, all associated defects must be repaired, and adequate fixation of the valve must be accomplished. The incidence of mitral valve endocarditis is considerably lower than that of aortic valve endocar-

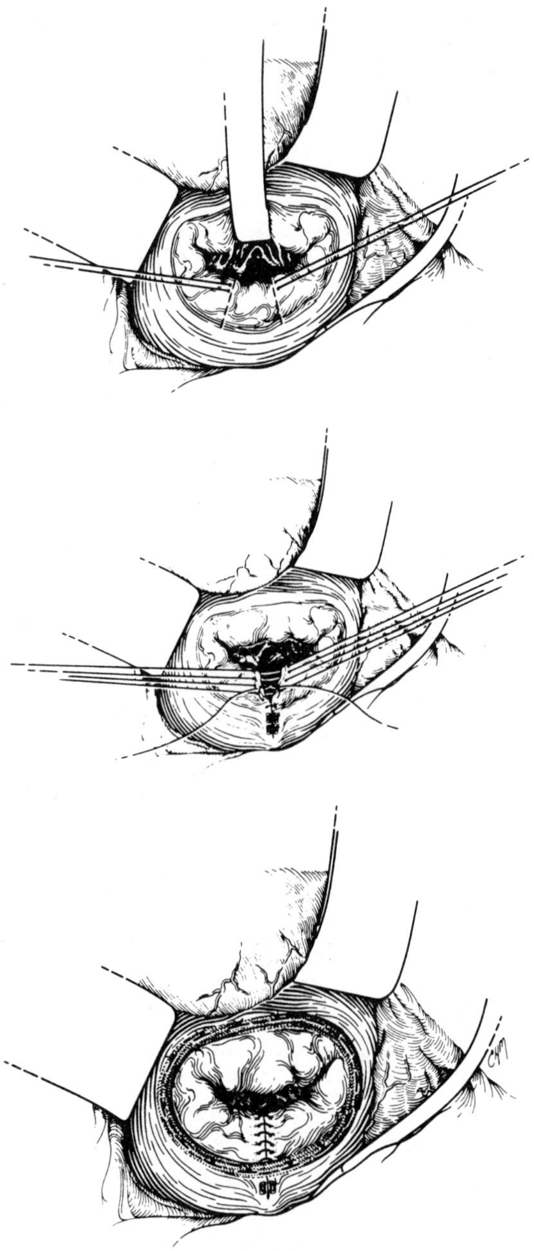

Figure 48–4. Schematic representation of resection of posterior leaflet of the mitral valve and ring annuloplasty. (From Cohn LH: Surgery for mitral regurgitation. JAMA 1988; 260:2885.)

ditis, but its results may be equally devastating. Autologous pericardial lining of the annulus, particularly if there is an abscess, is important and should occur before implanting the polyester (Dacron) sewing ring of any valve. Incidental vegetations are commonly found with mitral endocarditis. In general, if there is a loosely mobile, greater than 2-cm vegetation on the mitral valve (even in the asymptomatic patient), reparative mitral valve surgery is considered for evacuation of this potential source of thromboembolism.

Ischemic MR is a result of many pathophysiologic causes related to coronary artery disease. The general pathophysiologic classifications of ischemic MR include functional annular dilatation due to cardiomyopathy, constriction of chordae and papillary muscles because of ischemic scarification, and actual necrosis, either partial or total, of the papillary muscle head. The mortality rate for this diagnosis is the highest of any MR group because MR is superimposed on diffuse coronary artery disease. Operative mortality rates range from 6%–20% in some series but have improved as mitral reparative techniques have begun to play a role in the treatment of ischemic MR.[44, 45] There has been debate about the repair vs. replacement techniques for ischemic MR. We analyzed a group of 127 patients undergoing mitral valve surgery for ischemic MR and determined that operative and late mortality rates varied depending on the pathophysiologic cause of the regurgitation.[46] In patients who had functional annular dilatation only, usually secondary to decreased left ventricular function and ischemic cardiomyopathy, the long-term survival in this group (in whom repair was mostly by ring annuloplasties) was much worse than in patients who had undergone mitral valve replacement for other causes of ischemic MR. Thus, patients in this particular group who do not survive die because of the ravages of coronary artery disease rather than MR. In this group of patients, particularly those with ischemic cardiomyopathy, it is important to preserve as much of the normal annular chordal and papillary muscle interaction as possible. Valve replacement in this group often requires preservation of both the anterior and posterior mitral valve apparatus, which can be carried out by incising the anterior leaflet of the mitral valve and "reefing" it back along the annulus, thus preserving all the papillary muscle and chordal interaction with the annulus, both anteriorly and posteriorly. Cardiac output and ejection fraction are improved when these subvalvular structures are preserved.

TRICUSPID VALVE DISEASE

Tricuspid Stenosis

Tricuspid stenosis is an uncommon disease in the United States. It is primarily seen in Third World countries, with a high incidence of malignant rheumatic fever.[47] Should it be encountered, a simple tricuspid valvulotomy may be all that is required, but if there is extensive calcified disease of the tricuspid valve, valve replacement similar to that performed in the mitral area should be carried out. Preservation of papillary muscle and chordal interaction is important.

Tricuspid Regurgitation

In North Americans, the most common cause of tricuspid regurgitation (TR) is functional dilatation of the annulus, primarily from left-sided valve disease and pulmonary hypertension.[48] In the case of functional dilatation, annuloplasty techniques are very satisfactory. These techniques vary and include valve resections, annuloplasty rings, or posterior annulus suture annuloplasties as shown in Figure 48–5. Most of the functional dilatation that occurs is in the anterior and posterior leaflet annulus, and simple suture tightening by the Devega principle may be all that is necessary in patients with severe TR.[48] It is often debatable as to when to intervene with surgical techniques. In patients with severe (4+) TR, repair is mandatory. In patients with moderately severe (2 to 3+) TR, rapid suture annuloplasty techniques should be performed, which may prevent prolongation of the hospital stay because of retention of salt and fluid.

TR also results from severe endocarditis, usually seen in intravenous drug abuse or rarely as a finding in carcinoid disease. For the latter, valve replacement is usually indicated. For endocarditis, reparative techniques are most desirable because there is a high degree of septic foci in these areas. Reparative techniques include leaflet resections or suture annuloplasties. In some instances, it has been advocated that the entire tricuspid valve be removed in TR associated with endocarditis. This can be accomplished, but patients will have severe right-sided heart failure and disability until valve replacement is performed. This cannot be accomplished in patients with pulmonary hypertension. Delayed tricuspid valve replacement in these patients carries a high risk of bleeding because of liver decompensation. Thus, reparative techniques for TR are virtually

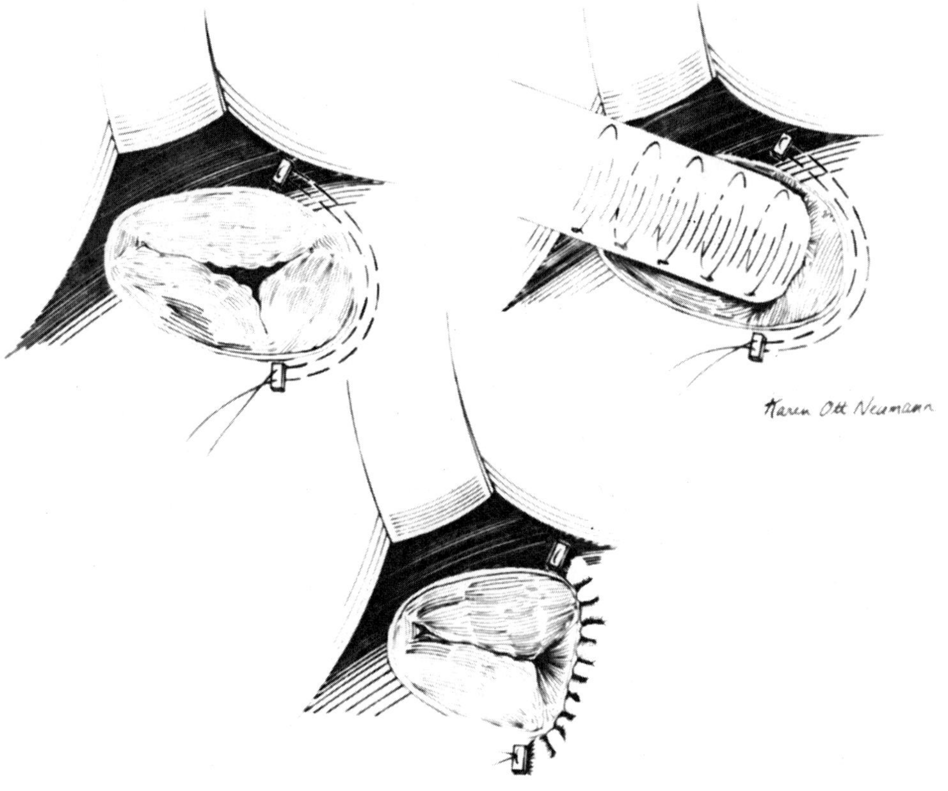

Figure 48–5. Posterior tricuspid suture annuloplasty tied over syringe barrel.

mandatory even if there is residual moderate TR. It is far preferable to repair the valve than to place a prosthetic device in this highly septic area.

In general, if valves are replaced in the tricuspid area, both prosthetic and bioprosthetic valves have performed well. In previous decades, biologic valves were less thrombogenic than the currently available prosthetic valves such as the Bjork-Shiley valve. In recent years, however, the St. Jude bileaflet valve has produced results similar to those of the porcine valve. Since most of these patients have chronic atrial fibrillation, prosthetic bileaflet disc valves are most commonly used.

REFERENCES

1. Starr A, Edwards ML: Mitral replacement: clinical experience with a ball valve prosthesis. Ann Surg 1961; 154:176.
2. Cohn LH: Aortic valve prostheses. Cardiol Rev 1994; 2:219.
3. O'Kane H, Cleland B, Gladstone D, et al: The St. Jude prosthesis. A thirteen year experience. J Thorac Cardiovasc Surg 1994; 108:221.
4. Czer LSC, Chaux A, Matloff JJ, et al: Ten year experience with the St. Jude medical valve for primary valve replacement. J Thorac Cardiovasc Surg 1990; 100:44.
5. Damle A, Coles H, Teijeira J, et al: A six year study of the Omniscience valve in five Canadian centers. Ann Thorac Surg 1987; 43:513.
6. Akins CW, Buckley MJ, Daggett WM, et al: Ten year follow-up of the Starr-Edwards prosthesis. *In* Rabago G, Cooley DA (eds): Heart valve replacement and future trends in cardiac surgery, p 137. New York: Futura, 1987.
7. Cohn LH, Collins JJ, DiSesa VJ, et al: Fifteen year experience with 1,678 Hancock porcine bioprosthetic heart valve replacements. Ann Surg 1989; 210:435.
8. Burdon TA, Miller DG, Oyer PE, et al: Durability of porcine valves at fifteen years in a representative North American patient population. J Thorac Cardiovasc Surg 1992; 103:738.
9. Akins CW, Carroll DC, Buckley JM, et al: Late results with Carpentier-Edwards porcine bioprosthesis. Circulation 1990; 82(suppl IV):65.
10. Hammermeister KE, Sethi G, Henderson WG, et al: A comparison of outcomes in men 11 years after heart-valve replacement with a mechanical valve or bioprosthesis. N Engl J Med 1993; 328:1290.
11. Jones EL, Weintraub WS, Craver JM, et al: Ten-year experience with porcine bioprosthetic valve: interrelationship of valve survival and patient survival in 1,050 valve replacements. Ann Thorac Surg 1990; 49:370.
12. Akins CW: Mechanical cardiac valvular prostheses. Ann Thorac Surg 1993; 52:161.
13. Peter M, Weiss P, Jenzer HR, et al: The omnicarbon tilting-disc heart valve prosthesis. J Thorac Cardiovasc Surg 1993; 106:599.
14. Dewall R, Pelletier U, Panebianco A, et al: Five-year experience with the Omniscience cardiac valve. Ann Thorac Surg 1994; 58:630.
15. Copeland JG, Sethi GK, and North American Team of Clinical Investigators for the CarboMedics Prosthetic Heart Valve: Four year experience with the CarboMedics valve: the North American experience. Ann Thorac Surg 1994; 58:630.
16. Kirklin JK, Smith D, Novick WS, et al: Long term function of cryopreserved aortic homograft: a ten year study. J Thorac Cardiovasc Surg 1993; 106:154.
17. Barratt-Boyes BG, Roche AHG, Subramanyan R, et al: Long-term follow-up of patients with the antibiotic sterilized aortic homograft valve inserted free hand in the aortic position. Circulation 1987; 75:768.
18. Mitsuki O, Robles A, Gibbs S, et al: Long term performance of 555 aortic homografts in the aortic position. Ann Thorac Surg 1988; 46:187.
19. Ross DW: Homograft replacement of the aortic valve. Lancet 1962; 2:487.
20. Pelletier LL, Leclerc Y, Bonon R, et al: The Carpentier-Edwards bovine pericardial prosthesis. Clinical experience with 301 valve replacements. *In* Bodnar E (ed): Surgery for Heart Disease, p 691. London: ICR Publishers, 1990.
21. Aupant M, Neville X, Dreyfus Y, et al: The Carpentier-Edwards pericardial aortic valve: intermediate results in 420 patients. Eur J Cardiothorac Surg 1994; 8:277.
22. Aranki SF, Rizzo, RJ, Couper GS, et al: Aortic valve replacement in the elderly: effect of gender and coronary artery disease on operative mortality. Circulation 1993; 88(part 2):17.
23. Cohn LH, Aranki SF, Rizzo RJ, et al: Decrease in operative risk of reoperative valve surgery. Ann Thorac Surg 1993; 56:15.
24. Fraser CD, Wang N, Mee RB, et al: Repair of insufficient bicuspid aortic valves. Ann Thorac Surg 1994; 58:386.

25. Ross DN: Aortic root replacement with a pulmonary autograft—current trends. J Heart Valve Dis 1994; 3:120.
26. Ross DN: Replacement of the aortic valve with a pulmonary autograft: "the switch operation." Ann Thorac Surg 1991; 52:1346.
27. Pacifico AD, Kirklin JK, McGiffin DC, et al: The Ross operation—early echocardiographic comparison of different operative techniques. J Heart Valve Dis 1994; 3:365.
28. Kouchoukos NT, Davila-Roman VG, Spray TL, et al: Replacement of the aortic root with a pulmonary autograft in children and young adults with aortic valve disease. N Engl J Med 1994; 330:1.
29. Gerosa G, Ross DN, Bauckle PE, et al: Aortic valve replacement with pulmonary homograft. J Thorac Cardiovasc Surg 1994; 107:424.
30. Robles A, Vaughan M, Lau JK, et al: Long-term assessment of aortic valve replacement with autologous pulmonary valve. Ann Thorac Surg 1985; 39:238.
31. Elkins RC, Knott-Craig CJ, Ward KE, et al: Pulmonary autografts in children: realized growth potential. Ann Thorac Surg 1994; 57:1387.
32. Cohn LH: Heart murmurs: acquired valvular heart disease. *In* Polk HC (ed): Basic Surgery, p 315. St. Louis: Quality Medical, 1994.
33. Larbalestier RI, Kinchla NM, Aranki SF, et al: Acute bacterial endocarditis. Circulation 1992; 86(suppl II):68.
34. Joyce F, Tingleff J, Aagaad J, et al: The Ross operation in the treatment of native and prosthetic aortic valve endocarditis. J Heart Valve Dis 1994; 3:371.
35. Haydock D, Barratt-Boyes B, Macedo T, et al: Aortic valve replacement for active endocarditis in 108 patients. J Thorac Cardiovasc Surg 1992; 103:130.
36. Jault F, Gandjbakch I, Chastre JC, et al: Prosthetic valve endocarditis. J Thorac Cardiovasc Surg 1993; 105:1106.
37. Cohn LH: The long term results of aortic valve replacement. Chest 1984; 85:387.
38. Reyes VP, Raju BS, Wynne J, et al: Percutaneous balloon valvuloplasty compared with open surgical commissurotomy for mitral stenosis. N Engl J Med 1994; 331:961.
39. Cohen JM, Glower DD, Harrison JK, et al: Comparison of balloon valvuloplasty with operative treatment for mitral stenosis. Ann Thorac Surg 1993; 56:1254.
40. Cohn LH, Allred EN, Cohn LA, et al: Long term results of open mitral valve reconstruction for mitral stenosis. Am J Cardiol 1985; 55:731.
41. Laschinger JC, Cunningham JN, Bauman M, et al: Early open radical commissurotomy: surgical treatment of choice for mitral stenosis. Ann Thorac Surg 1982; 34:287.
42. Cohn LH: Surgery for mitral regurgitation. JAMA 1988; 260:2885.
43. Cohn LH, Aranki SF, Rizzo RJ, et al: Decrease in operative risk of reoperative valve surgery. Ann Thorac Surg 1993; 56:15.
44. Rankin JS, Feneley MP, Hickey MSJ, et al: A clinical comparison of mitral valve repair versus valve replacement in ischemic mitral regurgitation. J Thorac Cardiovasc Surg 1988; 95:165.
45. Akins CW, Hilgenberg AD, Buckley MJ, et al: Mitral valve reconstruction versus replacement for degenerative or ischemic mitral valve regurgitation. Ann Thorac Surg 1994; 58:668.
46. Cohn LH, Couper GS, Kinchla NM, et al: Decreased operative risk of surgical treatment of mitral regurgitation with or without coronary artery disease. J Am Coll Cardiol 1990; 16:1575.
47. Duran CMG: Tricuspid valve surgery revisted. J Cardiovasc Surg 1994; 9(suppl):242.
48. Cohn LH: Tricuspid regurgitation secondary to mitral valve disease: when and how to repair. J Cardiovasc Surg 1994; 9(suppl):237.

49 Interventional Approaches to Congenital Heart Disease and Intracardiac Shunts

Michael J. Landzberg, MD
James E. Lock, MD

Adult patients with congenital heart disease who present with symptoms often have undergone multiple prior corrective surgeries or have suffered long-standing volume or pressure effects on the cardiac chambers or vascular beds. Surgical correction of residual defects may therefore carry unacceptable risks. Advances in the catheter-based approaches to intracardiac structures, coupled with mechanical innovations that have occurred over the past decade, have led to marked changes in the treatment strategies for these patients. Transcatheter therapies are offered to more than 50% of adult patients with congenital heart disease currently referred to the catheterization laboratory at our hospital.

In this chapter we review the practice of balloon and balloon-guided stent dilatations of cardiac and vascular stenoses (including those of aortic and pulmonary valves and peripheral pulmonary arteries) as well as the practice of transcatheter closure of cardiac defects (including occlusion of a patent ductus arteriosus [PDA], atrial and ventricular septal defects, and postoperative residual defects) in adult patients with congenital heart disease.

CATHETER-BASED DILATATION TECHNIQUES

Valvular Pulmonic Stenosis

Neonates and infants with valvular pulmonic stenosis (PS) associated with cyanosis, low cardiac output, or congestion benefit from relief of obstruction. However, the natural history of valvular PS in the older patient is less well defined. The natural history and treatment of PS have been summarized by the First and Second Natural History of Congenital Heart Defects Studies:[1]

1. Obstruction is unlikely to progress in patients with mild valvular PS associated with a peak systolic ejection gradient of less than 40 mm Hg. They are therefore unlikely to benefit from gradient relief if they are, in fact, asymptomatic. Unlike children with mild PS, however, many adults with "mild" PS can have symptoms.
2. Patients with severe valvular PS (peak systolic ejection gradient greater than 80 mm Hg) or "critical PS" (suprasystemic right

ventricular pressure) are likely to have progressive cardiovascular deterioration and therefore should undergo prompt relief of obstruction, regardless of symptoms.

3. Patients with moderate valvular PS (between 40 and 80 mm Hg) have a variable clinical course. The timing and need for intervention is unclear, especially if no symptoms are present. If intervention is chosen, goals include the relief and prevention of symptoms, changes in right ventricular and pulmonary arterial morphology, and progression to more severe levels of obstruction. If relief can be accomplished with minimal morbidity, therapy appears warranted.

The transcatheter approach was developed to replace surgical valvotomy (which was associated with a 1.5%–2% risk of mortality)[2] and was soon found to be both safe and effective.[3] Balloon valvuloplasty of the pulmonic valve is currently the procedure of choice for treatment of moderate to severe valvular PS in children.

Transcatheter Technique

Right-sided hemodynamic measurements are obtained and biplane right ventricular angiography is performed to confirm both the nature and level of the obstruction to right ventricular outflow and the size of the pulmonary annulus. A balloon-tipped end-hole catheter provides passage to the distal pulmonary vasculature for an 0.035- to 0.038-inch stiff exchange wire while avoiding catheter passage through the tricuspid valve tensor apparatus. A valvuloplasty balloon, chosen to be 120%–140% of the annulus diameter and 2–5 cm in length (depending on the age and size of the patient), is placed across the site of obstruction and is rapidly inflated and deflated. Concomitant inflation of two adjacent balloons, chosen to achieve a joint effective diameter of about 120%–140% of the diameter of the pulmonary annulus, may be necessary in older patients with a valve annulus larger than 20 mm. Although longer balloons seat more securely, they may carry an increased risk of right-sided cardiac injury during inflation. After adequate catheter positioning during inflation, the dilatation catheter is removed (over the guide wire) and replaced with a monitoring catheter to measure hemodynamics and cardiac output results. One must be careful to differentiate postprocedural dynamic infundibular obstruction from residual valvular PS. We consider a residual transvalvular peak systolic ejection gradient of less than 36 mm to be a successful result. Repeat dilatations are performed, as necessary, and hemodynamic measurements are obtained after each set of dilatations.

Results of Transcatheter Technique in Children and Adults

The pooled analysis of results for balloon pulmonic valvuloplasty demonstrates excellent hemodynamic benefit, with a mean reduction in gradient from 85 to 33 mm Hg (mean transvalvular peak systolic ejection gradient of 60 mm Hg with a mean transinfundibular peak systolic ejection gradient of 18 mm Hg). Immediate success has been achieved in 98% of 784 procedures in the Valvuloplasty and Angioplasty of Congenital Anomalies Registry.[4] McCrindle and Kan[5] combined results from multiple trials and found an overall success rate of 80% (immediate and long-term success was significantly lower with dysplastic valves). Nonthreatening complications occurred in approximately 4% of patients, and there was a procedure-related mortality rate of less than 0.5%. Pulmonary insufficiency and hyperdynamic infundibular stenosis of no hemodynamic significance were seen in approximately 20% of patients after valvuloplasty. No change in mean gradient was noted over a 33-month follow-up evaluation,[6] and the maximal gradient estimated by echocardiography remained less than 36 mm Hg in 75% of patients. At follow-up evaluation, surgical valvotomy, valvectomy with or without right ventricular outflow enlargement, or repeat balloon pulmonic valvuloplasty was performed in 8% of patients. Of note, nearly 7% of patients with immediate postvalvuloplasty gradient reduction to less than 36 mm Hg went on to require additional treatment during the follow-up period. During this time, no patient experienced severe pulmonic regurgitation and only 7% of patients had a moderate transvalvular leak. The long-term success of balloon pulmonic valvuloplasty has been shown by multivariable analysis to correlate with valve morphology, valve annulus size, the balloon-to-annulus dimension ratio, and immediate hemodynamic results.[6]

The role of balloon pulmonic valvuloplasty in the young and middle-aged adult with severe valvular PS has been less well defined. The previously described combined registry data included dilatations of stenotic pulmonary valves from 20 different centers in only 35 patients older than 20 years of age.[7, 8] Similar acute and short-term success has recently been demonstrated by Kaul and colleagues in 40 adult patients undergoing balloon pulmonic valvuloplasty in New Delhi.[9] At Boston Children's Hospital, we dilated stenotic pulmonary valves in 23 adults (aged 18–70 years) from March, 1984 to March, 1994.[10] Most patients had hemodynamic evidence of right ventricular dysfunction. A double-balloon technique was used in 75% of patients and a mean balloon-to-annulus ratio of 1.36 was achieved (Fig. 49–1). Successful valvular gradient reduction occurred in all but one patient in whom the pulmonary valve was dilated with an undersized balloon. In a mean follow-up of 64 months, one patient underwent surgical valvotomy performed at subsequent aortic valve replacement. Three patients had evidence of dynamic infundibular stenosis immediately after valvuloplasty without sequelae or the need for intervention. There has been no significant periprocedural or long-term morbidity. Symptomatic improvement has been sustained at most recent follow-up in all patients.

Balloon pulmonic valvuloplasty has proved to be a safe, efficient, and effective therapy for relief of obstruction in neonates and children and is the procedure of choice for patients with severe or symptomatic valvular PS. Although there are fewer data on the efficacy of balloon valvuloplasty in the adult patient with congenital valvular PS, results are promising. Given the low attendant morbidity of this procedure, we currently recommend pulmonary pulmonic valvular dilatation in any adult patient with symptomatic moderate or severe unoperated or recurrent valvular PS.

Valvular Aortic Stenosis

Balloon aortic valvuloplasty has become an accepted therapy for children with congenital valvular stenosis. This is in contrast to its role in the treatment of elderly patients with calcific aortic valvular disease. The Natural History of Heart Defects Study revealed that the peak systolic ejection gradient across the aortic valve is the strongest determinant of fatal outcome for the patient with congenital aortic stenosis.[11] The success of balloon dilatation in the treatment of valvular PS was the impetus for the development of techniques for transcatheter balloon aortic valve dilatation for congenital AS. As is true with surgical valvotomy, the goal of balloon aortic valvuloplasty is palliation and prolongation of time to surgical valve replacement, rather than cure.

Results of Balloon Aortic Valvuloplasty

The role of balloon aortic valvuloplasty in the young and intermediate-aged adult has been reported recently. At Boston Children's Hospital, 18 adult patients (aged 17–40 years) with congenital valvular AS underwent balloon valvuloplasty (using balloons chosen to be 90%–100% of the diameter of the aortic annulus) between March, 1986 and January, 1992.[12] Bicuspid valves were present in 12 of 15 patients with known valvular dysmorphology; three valves were unicuspid. Immediate procedural success was achieved in 16 of 18 patients, with a mean decrease in the peak systolic ejection gradient from 85 to 38 mm Hg. Although 11 patients had an increase in the degree of aortic insufficiency after dilatation, in all but one case it was mild to moderate. No periprocedural deaths, myocardial infarc-

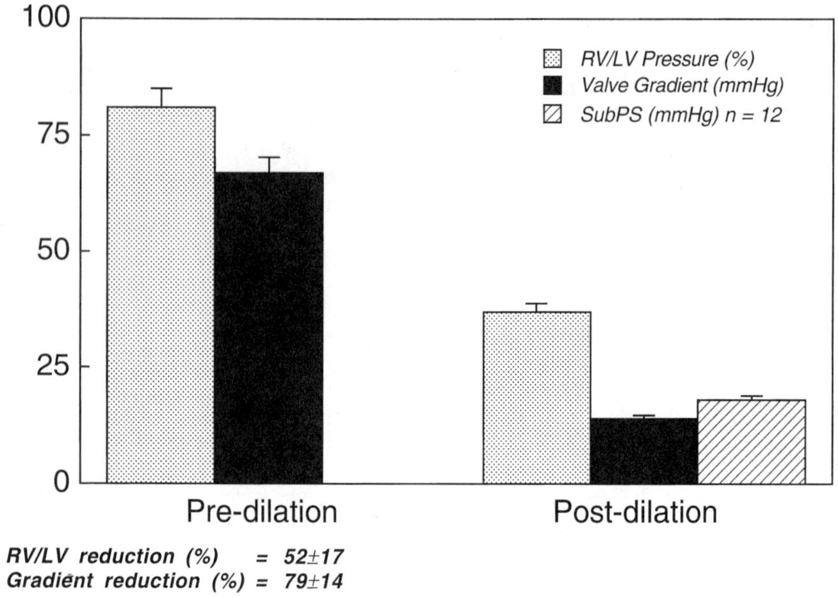

Figure 49–1. Acute reduction in peak systolic ejection gradient and RV hypertension after balloon pulmonic valvuloplasty. *Abbreviations:* RV, right ventricular; LV, left ventricular; SubPS, subpulmonic stensosis.

tions, or embolic events occurred. Local groin complications or transfusion requirements occurred in five patients. During a mean follow-up of 38 months, five patients required aortic valve surgery (two for initially ineffective dilatation, two for increasing peak instantaneous gradient measured by Doppler echocardiography, and one for bacterial endocarditis occurring 22 months after dilatation). Doppler echocardiographic measurements of peak instantaneous gradient at most recent follow-up revealed persistent improvement, but the mean gradient increased to 55 mm Hg. Patients having valvular calcification demonstrated a trend toward higher gradients both before and after dilatation, elevated peak instantaneous gradient at follow-up, and decreased incident-free survival compared with patients without calcified valves (Fig. 49–2).

Our preliminary findings support the concept that balloon valvuloplasty for noncalcified congenital AS in the young and adult patient can provide effective palliation and prolong the interval to surgical intervention without significantly increasing cardiac morbidity or serious complications. We currently recommend an attempt at valvuloplasty before valve replacement for symptomatic patients less than 40 years old with a bicuspid valve associated with gradients greater than 60 mm Hg.

Peripheral Pulmonary Arterial Stenoses

Application of balloon catheter dilatation and balloon-assisted stent placement in primary and postoperative narrowings in the distal pulmonary vasculature now offers a chance for improved survival

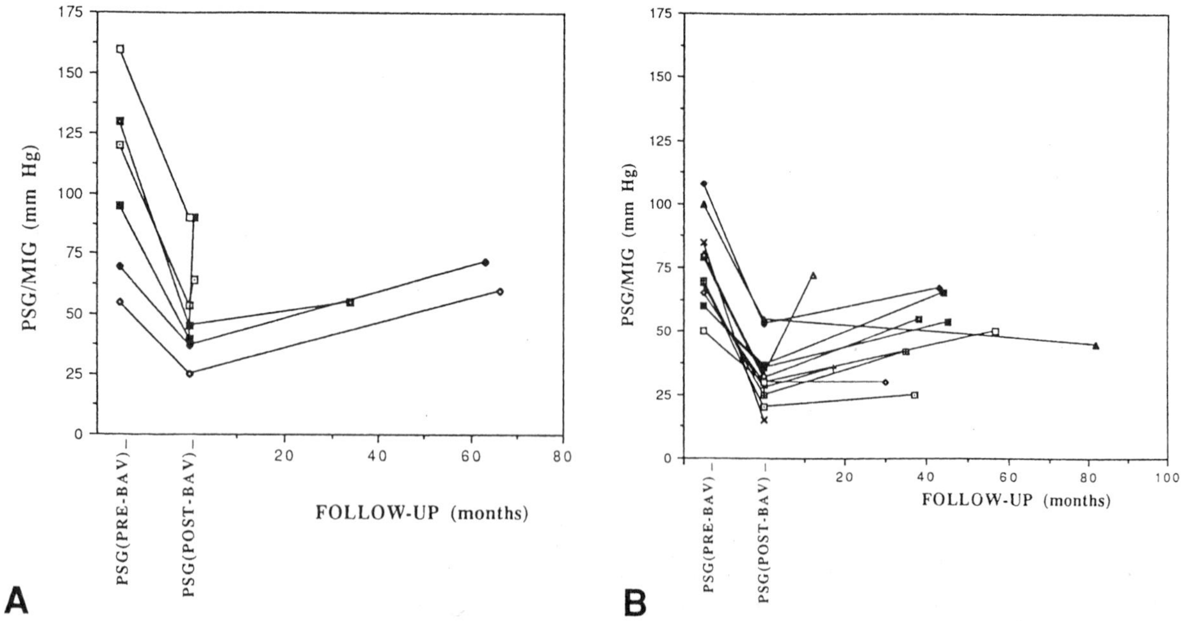

Figure 49–2. Peak systolic ejection gradient (PSG) before and after aortic valvuloplasty (catheterization) and maximal instantaneous gradient (MIG) at most recent follow-up (seen by echocardiography) in patients with calcified *(A)* and noncalcified *(B)* aortic valves. Abbreviation: BAV, balloon aortic valvuloplasty. (From Rosenfeld M, Landzberg M, Perry S, et al: Balloon aortic valvuloplasty in the young adult with congenital aortic stenosis. Am J Cardiol 1994; 73:1112–1117.)

and decreased morbidity in a large population of patients with diseases such as tetralogy of Fallot. Pulmonary arterial dilatations are currently the most commonly performed interventional procedures in our catheterization laboratory. A strategy combining dilatations with either low- or high-pressure balloons may achieve up to 75% procedural success in relief of obstruction in peripheral pulmonary arteries in patients of all age groups.[13] Dilatation of vessels with kinking or significant recoil can be further improved with placement of intraluminal iliac or renal stents (Johnson & Johnson, New Brunswick, NJ), achieving a greater than 90% initial procedural success.[14, 15] We consider balloon dilatation or balloon-assisted stent placement via a transcatheter approach to be the procedure of choice for palliation and relief of proximal and distal peripheral pulmonary artery stenosis.

TRANSCATHETER CLOSURE TECHNIQUES

Patent Ductus Arteriosus (PDA)

The ductus arteriosus remains patent in approximately 0.07% of live births, connecting the descending aorta and the junction of the main and left pulmonary arteries. Anatomically, it varies in size and shape and may be calcified or aneurysmal. PDA is usually asymptomatic, although it may produce symptoms caused by an increased volume load on the left ventricle. Endocarditis remains a constant risk (approximately 0.5–1% per year). The risk of the development of left ventricular dysfunction increases with age. Although operative closure in infancy is both safe and relatively straightforward, surgical repair requires general anesthesia, thoracotomy, and postoperative recuperation. In adults, surgical closure may be more complicated because of the anatomic features of the PDA (calcification, increased friability, and aneurysmal dilatation), as well as increased incidence of multiple organ system comorbidity.

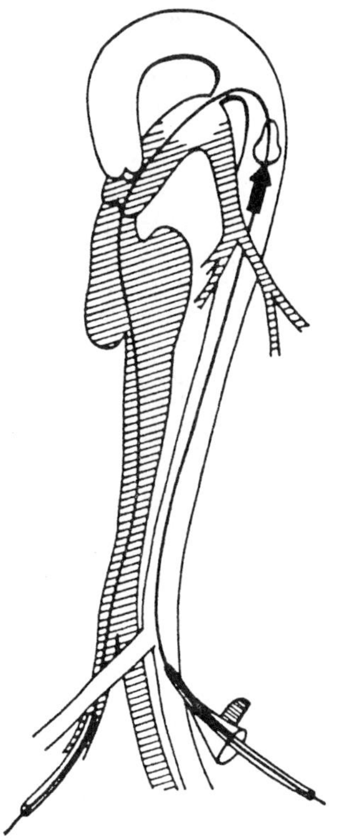

Figure 49–3. Portsmann's transarterial Ivalon plug method of PDA closure. (From Portsmann W, Wierny L, Warnke H, et al: Catheter closure of patent ductus arteriosus—62 cases treated without thoracotomy. Radiol Clin North Am 1971; 9:203–218.)

Ivalon Plug

A transarterial approach devised by Portsmann and colleagues[16] uses an 18-French arterial sheath and a catheter placed from the femoral artery retrograde across the PDA to gain access for transcatheter closure (Fig. 49–3). A guide wire is snared in the pulmonary artery and is pulled down the inferior vena cava and out the opposite femoral vein. A radiopaque polyvinyl alcohol (Ivalon) plug is hand-shaped to match the patient's ductal anatomy. Introduced via the femoral artery, the Ivalon plug is pushed along the guide wire tract and rammed into position within the ductus. Successful plugging of the PDA has been achieved in 197 of 208 primarily adult patients (94.7%).[17] This series included 49 patients with elevated pulmonary artery systolic pressures. Procedural time averaged 25 to 35 minutes; however, bed rest was mandated for 48 hours and length of hospitalization averaged 6 to 7 days because of the large sheath in the femoral artery. General anesthesia was required in 35% of patients and surgical arteriotomy/venotomy in 24% of patients. Vascular entry complications occurred in 8% of patients. Device embolizations at the time of implantation occurred in 16% of patients, although surgical retrieval of the device was uncommon. All symptomatic patients improved. More recent studies have shown complete PDA closure in 98.6% of 144 patients undergoing Ivalon plug PDA closure at 2 months to 8.3 years of follow-up.[18] In Europe and Japan, this technique is still used for transcatheter closure of PDA in adults.

Double Umbrella

The use of a multiarmed spring-loaded single- or double-umbrella prosthesis was pioneered by Rashkind. The currently available Rashkind device (Bard, Billerica, MA) is a polyurethane double disc, or umbrella, with a centrally welded elliptic loop mounted on two attached three-arm assemblies spring-loaded to create opposing tension (Fig. 49–4).

On collapse, the device is fitted into the distal casing of an 85-cm-long delivery system. The implantation technique, as modified by Mullins, employs an 8- or 11-French sheath passed via the right side of the heart through the ductus arteriosus and into the descending aorta. The delivery system and device are advanced through the sheath to the level of the tricuspid valve. The compacted device is then delivered out the thin metal casing and into the more pliable sheath by advancing the delivery system's internal guide wire and keeping the guide sheath and delivery catheter stationary. The guide wire–device system is advanced to the tip of the guiding sheath in the aorta. The entire delivery system and device is held stationary, and the sheath is retracted, allowing opening of the distal umbrella arms within the aorta. The entire system is retracted as a unit until the device flexes slightly against the aortic end of the PDA. With a

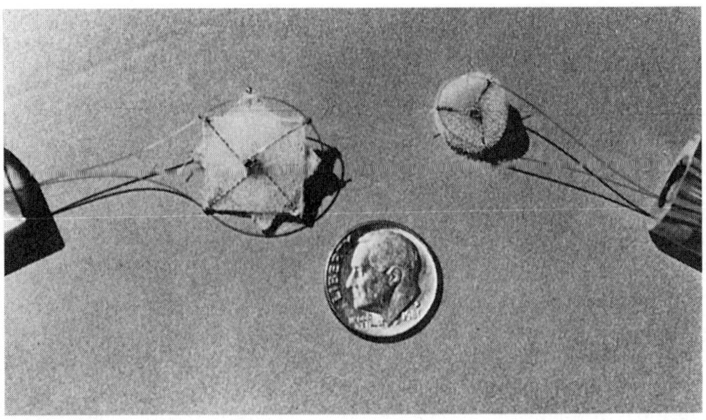

Figure 49–4. Rashkind double umbrellas are currently available in 12- and 17-mm-diameter sizes.

central guide wire held in constant position, the guide sheath is then further withdrawn, allowing the proximal umbrella arms to spring open to a fixed position against the pulmonary artery side of the PDA. After angiographic confirmation, the device is released from the delivery system. Occluding devices for the Rashkind double umbrella are currently available in 12- and 17-mm sizes.

With the use of Rashkind occluders, Clamshell devices, and coils, 100 consecutive patients treated for transcatheter closure of PDAs between July, 1988 and April, 1989 at Boston Children's Hospital had uniform, successful placement of prostheses.[19] Ninety-four patients had no subsequent murmur. Doppler echocardiographic evidence of residual ductal flow was present in 43 patients immediately after device placement. Of five patients with both residual murmur and persistent residual flow, all had a large PDA closed with a Rashkind device. The late incidence in minimal residual flow seen on color flow echocardiography has been less than 15%. There have been no episodes of endocarditis.

We have recently reported that transcatheter closure of a PDA with the double-umbrella or Clamshell device is safe in adult patients with large, small, or calcified PDAs in the presence of pulmonary hypertension or congestive heart failure.[20] In 21 consecutive adult patients with PDAs, successful device implantation was achieved, although most closures were achieved with a Clamshell occluder (see further on). Embolization after release of the device occurred in one patient, and the prosthesis was retrieved and replaced with a second occluder. Twenty of 21 patients had no residual murmur, whereas moderate residual shunting was present in one patient who had a long, wide PDA closed with a Rashkind device; this patient subsequently underwent surgical closure. Doppler echocardiography revealed a small amount of residual ductal flow in 11 of 17 patients immediately after implantation. All five patients with preclosure symptoms of congestive heart failure have become asymptomatic after device implantation.

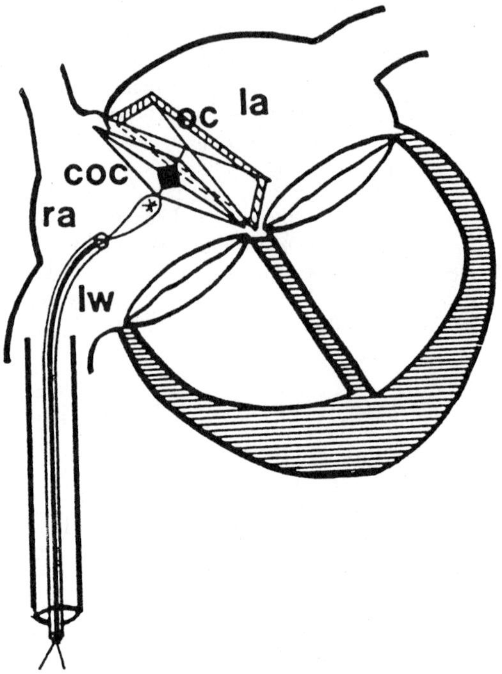

Figure 49–5. The "buttoned" double-disc prosthesis. *Abbreviations:* oc, occluder disc; coc, counteroccluder disc; la, left atrium; ra, right atrium; lw, loading wire. (From Sideris EB, Sideris SE, Fowlkes JP, et al: Transvenous atrial septal defect occlusion with a "buttoned" double-disk device. Circulation 1990; 81:312–318. Copyright 1990 by the American Heart Association; reprinted with permission.)

Buttoned Device

In 1990, Sideris and colleagues introduced a closure device consisting of an X-shaped wire-skeleton occluder, covered with polyurethane foam, and a second rhomboid wire-skeleton counteroccluder (Fig. 49–5).[21] These two pieces are attached by means of "push-pull" manipulation of a knotted, looped string (center of the occluder) through a rubber piece in the center of the counteroccluder. Preliminary short-term results in 20 adolescents and adults with small PDAs appear promising.[22]

Botallo Occluder

The Botallo occluder, a device similar to the Portsmann plug, has been deployed with a greater than 95% initial success rate in 273 patients in the First Moscow Hospital.[23] Late residual shunting was seen in 3% of patients and was corrected by surgical repair in all. Widespread clinical trials have not been performed with this device to date.

Coils

Since initial attempts in 1992,[24] growing experience has been achieved with transcatheter occlusion of PDAs less than 3 mm in minimal diameter with Gianturco embolization coils. Coils have been chosen to provide a helical diameter that is twice the minimal duct diameter or more as well as to achieve a length of three or more loops. Limited series report a successful placement of one or more coils in greater than 95% of patients, with abolishment of ductal murmurs in all patients.[25] Occasional coil embolization was noted; embolized coils have been successfully retrieved via a transcatheter approach. The incidence of flow abnormalities detected by Doppler echocardiography without associated murmurs has been less than 10% in the early follow-up period, but the late incidence of residual flow abnormalities is unknown. Widespread application to adults with PDA is unlikely given the larger size of PDAs in this population. However, we have successfully occluded PDAs with coils in selected adults up to 60 years of age at Boston Children's Hospital.

Recommendations

Currently, given the relative ease, limited risks, and excellent short- and long-term results of transcatheter closures, we recommend catheter closure in all adult patients with PDA and an associated murmur. Most patients with a small or moderate-sized ductus can undergo this procedure on an outpatient basis. We now prefer to close defects greater than 4 mm in adult patients with the larger Bard Clamshell device, although the availability of Clamshells for such procedures is limited. Although the merits of transcatheter closure of PDA in children and adolescents remain unclear, given the successful use of thoracoscopic clipping of PDAs in children, we speculate that transcatheter closure will become the treatment of choice for adult patients with PDA, especially those with evidence of ductal calcification.

Secundum-Type Atrial Septal Defects

Secundum-type atrial septal defects (ASDs) are among the most common congenital cardiac defects, occurring in approximately 7% of patients with congenital heart defects.[26] Most adult patients with significant ASDs of the secundum type (a ratio of pulmonary-to-systemic blood flow of greater than 1.5:1) have symptoms of dyspnea, congestive heart failure, or pulmonary hypertension. These patients may also experience atrial arrhythmias or paradoxical emboli if they do not undergo treatment until middle age. Surgical suture and patch closure of secundum-type ASDs remains one of the safest and most effective cardiac surgical procedures.[27] Significant perioperative morbidity occurs, however, and may include atrial arrhythmias, thromboembolism, hemorrhage, and pericardial inflammation.[28] Increasing age and the presence of pulmonary hypertension are independent risk factors for increased surgical mortality. Postoperative residual shunting may be detected. The incidence of persistent shunting detected by Doppler echocardiography after surgery is 7%–8%.[29] The incidence of major or minor neuropsychiatric complications of cardiopulmonary bypass has refocused attention on the indications for open heart surgery. Innovations from transcatheter closure techniques have therefore been extended to closure of ASDs.

Clamshell Occluder

Initial studies by King and colleagues[30] led Rashkind[31] and Lock[32] to develop umbrella devices that would clamp, in a stable fashion, onto the interatrial wall. The Clamshell prosthesis (Bard, US Catheter Instruments, Billerica, MA) has four spring-loaded, hinged arms on each side of the device, which fold back on each other by means of a second spring in the center of the arms (Fig. 49–6). With manual eversion, these arms take the shape of two cones, joined at their peaks. Animal studies revealed complete closure and device endothelialization within a few weeks of implantation. Clamshell devices are manufactured in 17-, 23-, 28-, 33-, and 40-mm diameters and are deployed via an 11-French system in adults. Accurate sizing of the ASD is achieved by imaging the atrial septum while dragging an inflated, compliant balloon from the left to the right atrium. A ratio of the device length to the "balloon-stretched" ASD diameter of greater than 1.8:1 is optimal when choosing the device size. Recent transesophageal studies suggest that approximately 50% of pediatric patients with secundum-type ASDs referred for surgical closure had defects sufficiently small and appropriately located to allow potential correction via a transcatheter approach.[8] The proportion of adult patients with secundum-type ASDs suitable for transcatheter closure is unknown.

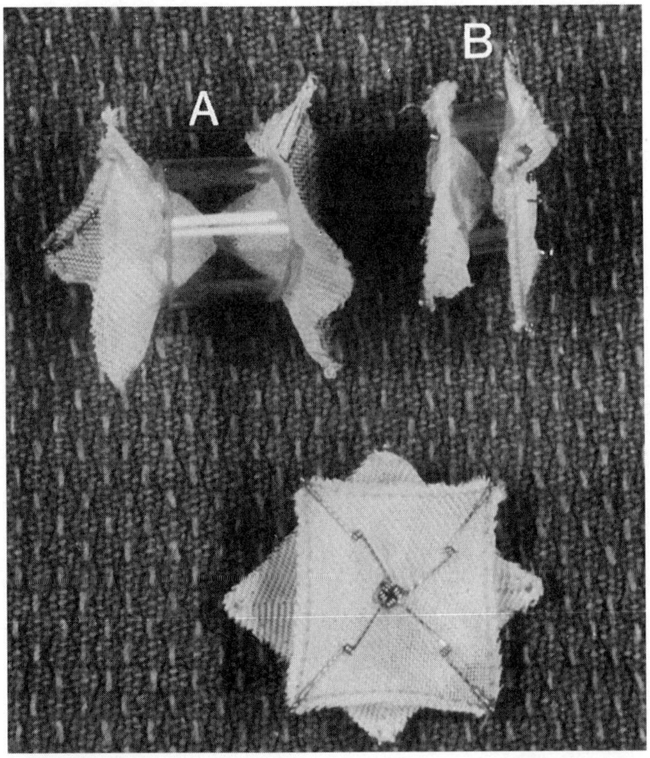

Figure 49–6. With manual eversion *(A)*, the device arms of the Clamshell occluder fold back to enable passage through the guiding catheter. Spring-loaded, hinged arms facilitate device "clamping" onto the atrial septum after extrusion *(B)*.

The first step in the transcatheter closure of ASDs involves placing a guiding sheath across the atrial septum via a right-sided approach (Fig. 49–7*A*). A device delivery system is inserted within the guide until the distal casement approaches the right atrium. With the delivery system held fixed, the central core guide wire–device unit is then advanced, allowing smooth passage of the device through the heart. With the guide wire–device unit kept stationary, the sheath is retracted over the distal arms of the device. This permits opening of the distal umbrella within the left atrium (see Fig. 49–7*B*). Next, the guiding sheath–delivery system–device unit is retracted until the distal umbrella arms flex against the left atrial side of the intra-atrial septum. The delivery system is held stationary and the guiding sheath is retracted further, allowing delivery of the proximal umbrella arms within the right atrium (see Fig. 49–7*C*). The device is released after confirmation of appropriate positioning (see Fig. 49–7*D*). Daily low-dose aspirin and prophylaxis for infective endocarditis are recommended for a 6-month period. Intraprocedural transesophageal echocardiography (TEE) has aided in the accuracy of device placement.[10] Temporary airway protection may be necessary if TEE is employed.

The multicenter experience of more than 400 patients who underwent transcatheter closure of ASDs with a Clamshell occluder revealed a 95% procedural success rate.[33] Follow-up has included chest radiography immediately after device deployment and physical examination, radiography, and transthoracic echocardiography at 1 day, 1 month, 6 months, and 1 year after deployment. In the multicenter experience, device embolization occurred immediately after device deployment in 11 patients and occurred 12 to 48 hours later in an additional 6 patients. No episodes of embolization have caused hemodynamic instability. Femoral vascular complications occurred in two patients. Systemic emboli were noted at the time of device placement in one patient. Echocardiographic follow-up revealed insignificant or small residual atrial septal leaks in approximately one third of patients.

Of 35 adult patients (aged 18–76 years) undergoing transcatheter ASD closure in Boston, 21 (60%) had either a significant increased risk of operative morbidity or mortality.[34] Clamshell deployment was attempted in 33 patients (2 patients had ASDs that were too large for closure). One patient with a 27-mm defect underwent attempted implantation of a 40-mm device that was believed to be unstable, and the occluder was withdrawn without release. All remaining 32 adult patients had stable deployment of a Clamshell on the atrial septum. Five patients had significant residual leaks. In three patients, this was caused by herniation of a device arm across the atrial septum at the time of deployment. In two additional patients, an inappropriately small device was implanted, causing significant residual transatrial shunting. Four of these patients had defects closed either by repeat transcatheter procedures (two patients) or subsequent operation (two patients). No embolic events or bouts of bacterial endocarditis have occurred in 18 to 43 months of follow-up. Three patients with either preprocedural palpitations or a history of supraventricular tachycardia have had new, nonsustained atrial arrhythmias occurring in the period after implantation. Minimal residual interatrial shunting detected by Doppler echocardiography was present in 32% of patients at 1 year of follow-up. A large residual shunt was detected in one patient.

Clinical trials of transcatheter closure of ASDs with the Clamshell occluder were suspended in 1991 when radiographic follow-up revealed a high incidence of occult device arm fractures. These strut breaks, typically occurring at the spring-loaded hinge point of a device arm, were most commonly noted as migration of the distal portion of a device arm along its attachment to its proximal portion (Fig. 49–8). An increasing incidence of arm fractures has been noted with increasing device size (greater than 50% incidence with devices 28 mm in diameter or larger). Device arm fractures contribute to residual shunting or the development of granulation tissue in areas

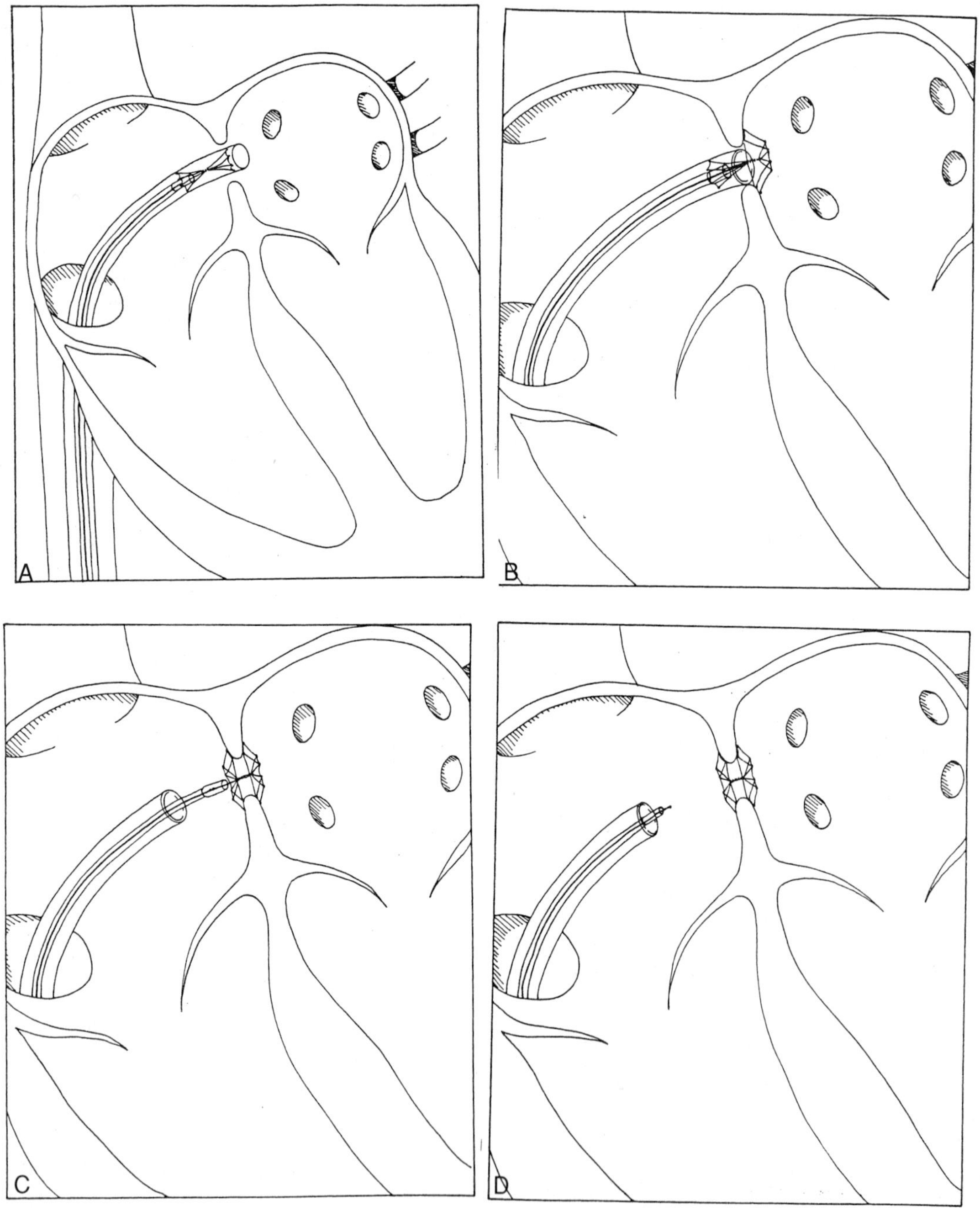

Figure 49–7. Technique of transcatheter deployment of a Clamshell occluder for secundum-type atrial septal defect closure.

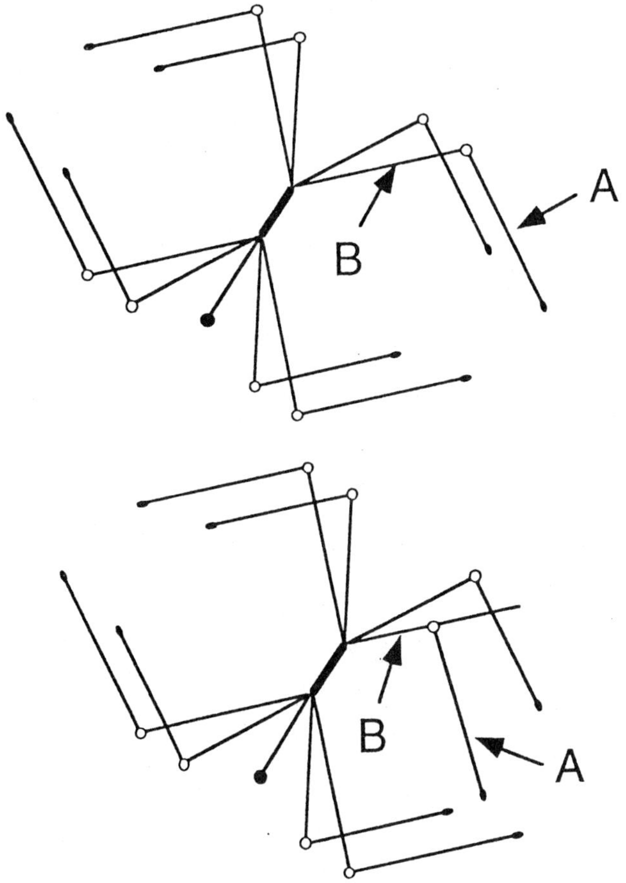

Figure 49–8. Device arm fracture, commonly at the hinge site, allows flotation of the distal arm (A) down the proximal arm (B) within the constraints of the covering polyester (Dacron) meshwork.

of contact between the device arm and the atrial wall in fewer than 1% of patients. Structural modification of the Clamshell occluder will presumably allow resumption of clinical trials for the use of this device for transcatheter closure of ASDs of the secundum type.

Buttoned Device

The Sideris double-disc buttoned device, available in diameters of 25 to 50 mm, has been deployed via 7-, 8-, and 9-French systems in an attempt to close ASDs of the secundum type with a diameter of less than 25 mm in 190 patients (aged 6 months to 70 years).[35] Stable device delivery on the atrial septum was achieved in 83% of patients. Immediate surgical removal of the prosthesis was required in four patients with inadequate deployment. Atrial perforation occurred in two patients. Device embolization to the pulmonary artery, without hemodynamic sequelae, occurred in one patient. Late device unbuttoning, without clinical consequence, occurred during follow-up in four patients. Twelve-month actuarial event-free survival was 89%. Twenty patients underwent subsequent surgery (14 cases because of device dislodgment, 3 because of residual shunts or atrial perforations, 2 for device inspection after wire abnormalities were noted on radiographs, and 1 because of paradoxical embolism). Minimal residual interatrial shunting was detected by Doppler echocardiography in 26% of patients at 12-month follow-up.

Other Devices

Preliminary experience with Nitinol and "screw-together" ASD occlusion systems appears promising, although investigation with these devices remains limited to date.[36]

Summary of ASD Treatments

Although surgical repair of ASDs is effective, transcatheter approaches remain appealing because they avoid the complications of cardiopulmonary bypass and thoracotomy. Closure of secundum-type ASDs with transcatheter techniques may be a suitable alternative to surgical therapy, especially in the adult with significant associated medical conditions. Defects should be less than 22 mm in maximal stretched diameter, producing a pulmonary-to-systemic blood flow ratio greater than 1.5:1 or significant right ventricular volume overload. An adequate rim of tissue surrounding the defect should be available to support the device arms. The incidence and late effects of small residual leaks occurring after transcatheter closure with all the noted devices requires further study, although they appear benign at this time. Although the clinical sequelae of Clamshell arm fractures are unclear, use of this device in low-risk patients has been suspended. Some of the current limitations of transcatheter Clamshell closures of routine ASDs of the secundum-type may be eliminated by reliable prosthesis manufacturing, although closure in high-risk patients continues to be performed in selected centers.

Patent Foramen Ovale

Pressure overload of the right atrium may lead to right-to-left shunting in patients with a patent foramen ovale (PFO). Right-to-left shunting may accompany chronic elevations of right-sided cardiac filling pressures (right ventricular infarction, pulmonary embolism, Ebstein anomaly) or transient increases in right atrial pressure after Valsalva maneuvers (normal individuals) or changing from a supine to an upright position (orthodeoxia-platypnea syndrome). We have closed PFOs with a Clamshell device in 25 adults with right ventricular infarctions, Ebstein anomaly, and the orthodeoxia-platypnea syndrome (Fig. 49–9).[37] In all but two patients with Ebstein anomaly, catheter closure has relieved cyanosis and symptoms and eliminated the need for open heart surgery.

Therapeutic closure of PFOs in patients with stroke and presumed paradoxical embolism remains controversial given that the causes and natural history of these embolic events are unknown. Although anticoagulant therapy has been recommended as a primary treatment in these patients, the natural history of treated patients and the duration of therapy remain unclear. Closure of PFOs, either surgically or via a transcatheter approach, has been suggested as a primary therapy for presumed paradoxical embolism. For these reasons, we instituted a pilot study in 1989 using Clamshell catheter closure of PFO in patients with prior strokes.[38] To date, 38 of 38 patients with PFOs and presumed paradoxical emboli have successfully undergone transcatheter closure of the defect with a Clamshell occluder. Systemic anticoagulation with warfarin was maintained in two patients (5%).[39] Small 1- to 2-mm residual right-to-left shunting around the device was noted in eight patients (21%) at most recent follow-up. No strokes have occurred during a mean follow-up period of 37 months, although two patients (5%) had recurrent transient ischemic attacks. One patient had a residual right-to-left shunt, and the other had left atrial granulation tissue near a broken device arm. Both patients underwent surgical device removal without complication or recurrent stroke. Trials with a fracture-resistant Clamshell II device are pending.

A recent pilot study of PFO closure using the "buttoned" device in patients with presumed paradoxical embolism reported successful closure in six of six patients.[40] Warfarin administration was maintained in three of six patients for an initial 3-month period. In a mean follow-up of 24 months, there were no recurrent strokes. Minimal right-to-left shunting around the device was noted in two of six patients at 3-month follow-up but subsequently disappeared. One patient experienced a thrombus near the device.

Ventricular Septal Defects

We have applied transcatheter closure techniques for the treatment of congenital and acquired forms of ventricular septal defects (VSDs) in an attempt to eliminate the need for, or to reduce the risk and complexity of, surgical repair.[41, 42] To date, the majority of closures

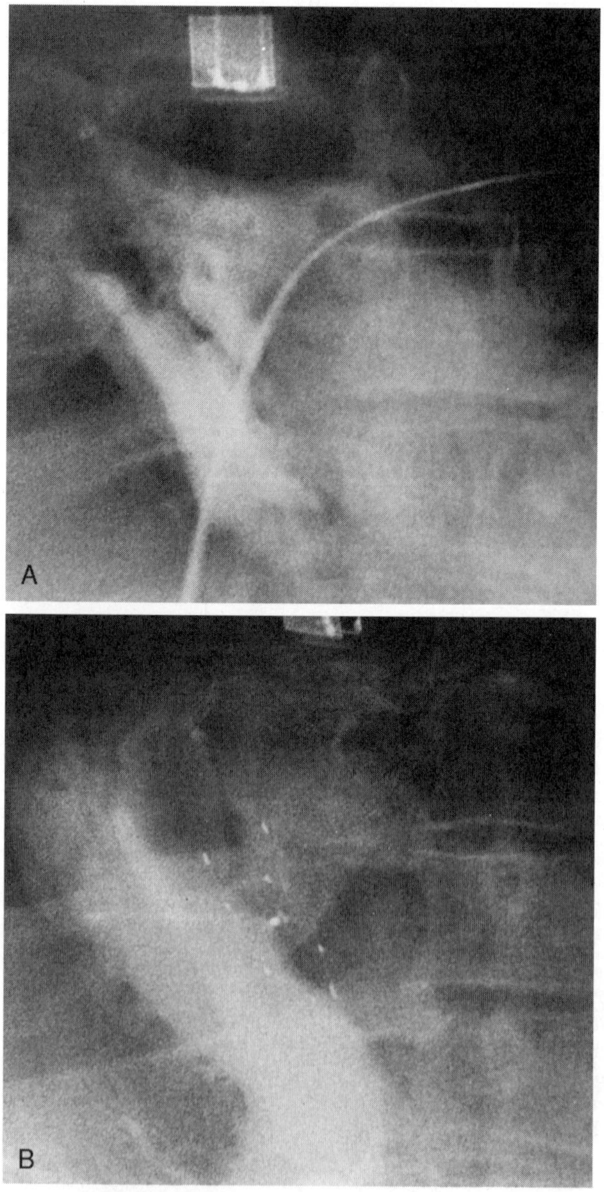

Figure 49–9. Right-to-left atrial passage *(A)* of contrast across a PFO in orthodeoxia-platypnea syndrome is eliminated *(B)* after transcatheter PFO closure with Clamshell occluder.

have been in patients with VSDs due to myocardial infarction and in those with congenital muscular VSDs anatomically distant from the aortic valve (not the commonly encountered congenital perimembranous VSDs). Although the procedure has been successful in more than 100 patients, it is technically the most demanding interventional catheter procedure performed in our laboratory.

Transcatheter Technique

A guide wire is placed via the transseptal approach into the left atrium and ventricle and across the VSD (Fig. 49–10). A left ventricular to right ventricular approach facilitates subsequent passage of a balloon flotation catheter through the widest portion of the defect. The guide wire is snared and delivered from either the contralateral femoral vein or a jugular vein, depending on the location of the defect. Balloon stretch sizing of the central portion of the defect facilitates choosing the umbrella size, which should be 2.5 to 3.0 times the size of the defect. A guiding sheath follows the guide wire through the right or left side of the heart and across the central channel of the defect. A device system is delivered in a fashion similar to the technique described for ASD closure. The guiding sheath frequently traverses the interventricular septum at an acute angle, making fluoroscopic confirmation of arm positioning difficult during deployment. We have therefore used TEE to assist in accurate visualization during most prosthesis placements.[43] This closure technique requires significant operator experience to reduce procedural morbidity.

We have recently applied this technique with Clamshell occluders to closure of VSDs occurring after myocardial infarction in adults.[34] Between February, 1990 and March, 1994, 11 patients 5 to 79 years of age presented with ventricular septal rupture after myocardial infarction. Five patients presented acutely with VSDs after myocardial infarction without surgical intervention (all required hemodynamic support and had multiple organ system failure). The location of ventricular septal ruptures was anterior in two patients (apical in one patient) and posterior in three patients (inferior in one patient). The size of the defects ranged between 18 and 20 mm in balloon-stretched diameter. Location of rupture on one side of the ventricular septum did not predict location on the contralateral side given the serpiginous course of these defects through the interventricular septum. Cavity formation within the ventricular septum was present angiographically in four patients. Six other patients survived attempted surgical repair of a VSD but had significant postoperative residual "patch-margin" defects of 8 to 19 mm in balloon-stretched size. All the patients had stable placement of one or more devices on the ventricular septum (Fig. 49–11). Of patients presenting acutely with a VSD after myocardial infarction, only one survived longer than 1 year after device implantation. It is likely that ongoing reabsorption of necrotic myocardium limits the success of early primary closure of post–myocardial infarction VSDs by available transcatheter devices. All the patients with postoperative residual defects who underwent closure are currently alive, however, with both hemodynamic and symptomatic improvement (8 to 58 months follow-up). It therefore appears that transcatheter VSD closure is most appropriate for patients with significant postoperative residual patch-margin defects.

In contrast to the limited success of umbrella closure of post–myocardial infarction VSDs, more than 100 congenital muscular and postoperative defects have been closed successfully with no in-hospital mortality.[41] These multiple devices have eliminated the need for operation in many patients with complex defects.

Radiographic follow-up has revealed device arm fractures in approximately 33% of patients who have undergone Clamshell closure of VSDs, but the significance of this finding is unknown at this time.

TABLE 49–1. CATHETER-BASED INTERVENTIONS FOR THE ADULT WITH CONGENITAL HEART DISEASE

Procedure of Choice	Effective Alternative to Surgery	Unproven Effect
Device closure PDA VSD—postoperative residual VSD—congenital muscular Fenestrated Fontan baffle PFO (cyanosis)	Device closure ASD secundum Paravalvular leaks VSD (post MI)	Device closure PFO (stroke)
Balloon/stent dilatation PPA stenosis Recurrent aortic coarctation	Balloon/stent dilatation Native aortic coarctation Conduit/baffle obstruction	Balloon/stent dilatation Subvalvular AS TOF Coarctation Pulmonary vein
Balloon valvulotomy Valvular PS Valvular AS		
Coil embolization Thoracic collaterals	Coil embolization Coronary artery fistulas	

Abbreviations: PDA, patent ductus arteriosus; VSD, ventricular septal defect; PFO, patent foramen ovale; PPA, peripheral pulmonary arterial; PS, pulmonic stenosis; AS, aortic stenosis; ASD, atrial septal defect; MI, myocardial infarct; TOF, tetralogy of Fallot.

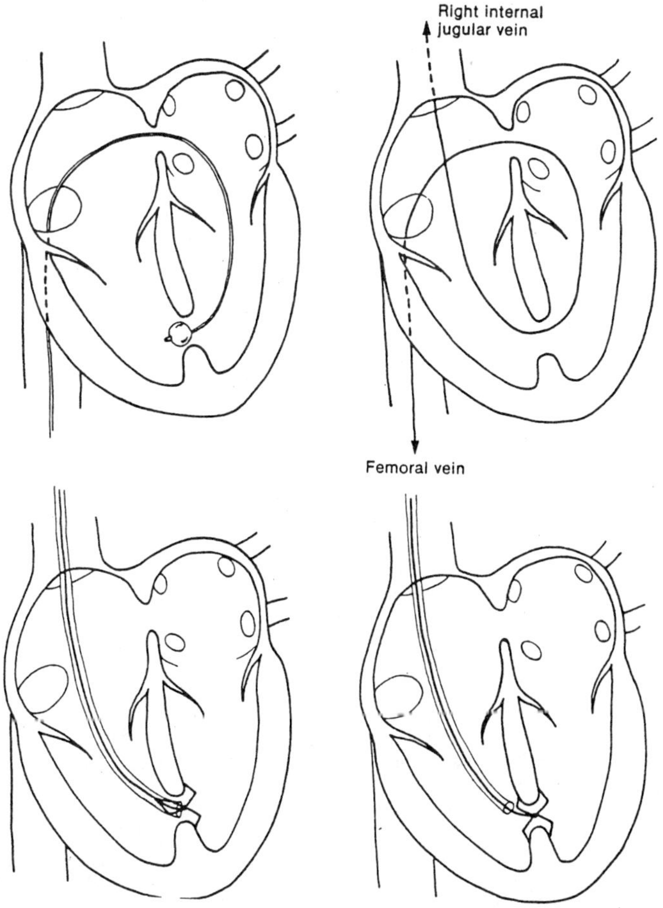

Figure 49–10. The Clamshell method of VSD closure. (From Bridges N, Perry S, Keane J, et al: Preoperative transcatheter closure of congenital muscular ventricular septal defects. N Engl J Med 1991; 324:1312–1317.)

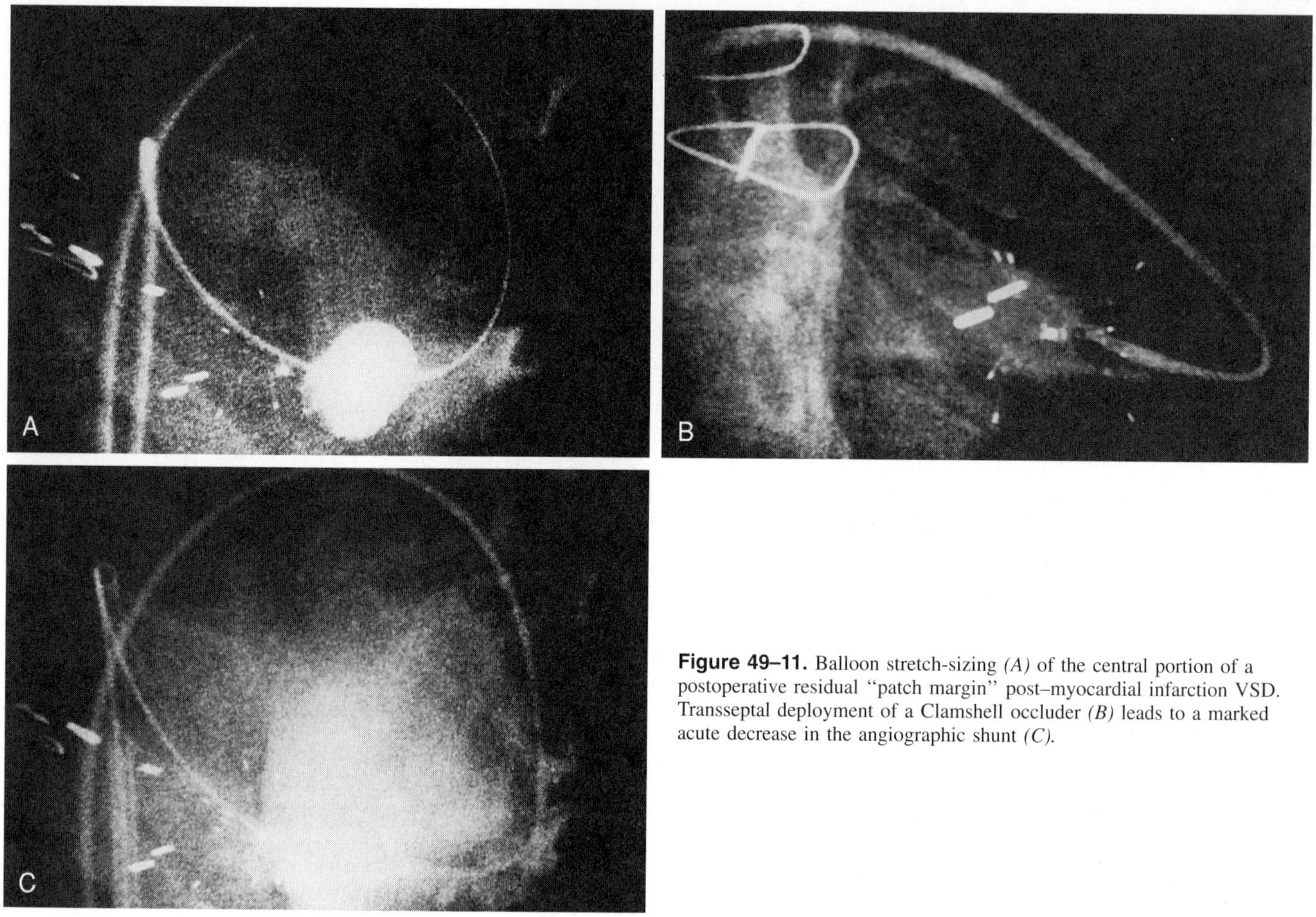

Figure 49–11. Balloon stretch-sizing *(A)* of the central portion of a postoperative residual "patch margin" post–myocardial infarction VSD. Transseptal deployment of a Clamshell occluder *(B)* leads to a marked acute decrease in the angiographic shunt *(C)*.

CONCLUSIONS

Although angioplasty and valvuloplasty techniques have become approved therapies, most closure techniques we have described remain investigational. Clinical trials of catheter-based technologies for adult patients with congenital heart disease have consisted of uncontrolled case series with a lack of standardized follow-up. As described earlier, however, adult patients with congenital heart disease may be at increased risk when undergoing surgical defect correction because of concomitant heart failure, pulmonary vascular disease, multiple prior operations, and comorbid illness. We therefore advocate continued investigation and use of catheter-based therapies to either support or supplant further surgical procedures in these patients. Currently, we consider the applications of these techniques as (1) procedures of choice, (2) effective alternatives to surgical therapy, or (3) treatments with unproved effects (Table 49–1). Additional prospective large-scale clinical trials of these therapies are necessary before they can be widely endorsed.

Acknowledgment

The authors thank Ms. Gretchen Lieb for her secretarial support in preparation of the manuscript.

REFERENCES

1. Nugent EW, Freedom RM, Nora JJ, et al: Clinical course in pulmonary stenosis. Circulation 1977; 56(suppl I):38–47.
2. Kirklin JN, Barratt-Boyes BG: Cardiac Surgery, pp 61–128. New York: Churchill-Livingstone, 1993.
3. Kan JS, White RJ, Mitchell SE, et al: Percutaneous balloon valvuloplasty: a new method for treating congenital pulmonary valve stenosis. N Engl J Med 1982; 307:540.
4. Stanger P, Cassidy SC, Girod DA, et al: Balloon pulmonary valvuloplasty: results of the Valvuloplasty and Angioplasty of Congenital Anomalies Registry. Am J Cardiol 1990; 65:775–783.
5. McCrindle BW, Kan JS: Long-term results after balloon pulmonary valvuloplasty. Circulation 1991; 83:1915–1922.
6. McCrindle BW: Independent predictors of long-term results after balloon pulmonary valvuloplasty. Circulation 1994; 89:1751–1759.
7. Cambier PA, Kirby WC, Wortham DC, et al: Percutaneous closure of the small (<2.5 mm) patent ductus arteriosus using coil embolization. Am J Cardiol 1992; 69:815–816.
8. Chan KC, Goodman MJ: Morphologic variations of fossa ovalis atrial septal defects (secundum): feasibility for transcutaneous closure with the clam-shell device. Br Heart J 1993; 69:52–55.
9. Kaul VA, Singh B, Tyagi S, et al: Long-term results after balloon pulmonary valvuloplasty in adults. Am Heart J 1993; 126:1152–1155.
10. Landzberg MJ, Keane JF, Lock JE: Balloon pulmonic valvuloplasty in the young and intermediate aged adult [Abstract]. Circulation 1993; 88(suppl I):341.
11. Wagner HR, Ellison RC, Keane JF, et al: Clinical course in aortic stenosis. Circulation 1977; 56(suppl I):47–56.
12. Rosenfeld HM, Landzberg MJ, Perry SB, et al: Balloon aortic valvuloplasty in the young adult with congenital aortic stenosis. Am J Cardiol 1994; 73:1112–1117.
13. Gentles TL, Lock JE, Perry SB: High-pressure angioplasty of pulmonary artery stenosis [Abstract]. J Am Coll Cardiol 1992; 19:24A.
14. O'Laughlin MP, Perry SB, Lock JE, et al: Use of endovascular stents in congenital heart disease. Circulation 1991; 83:1923–1939.
15. O'Laughlin MP, Slack MC, Perry SB, et al: Stent results and follow-up: an improved outlook for pulmonary arterial and systemic venous stenoses [Abstract]. Circulation 1992; 86(suppl I):632.
16. Portsmann W, Wierny L, Warnke H, et al: Catheter closure of patent

ductus arteriosus—62 cases treated without thoracotomy. Radiol Clin North Am 1971; 9:203–218.
17. Wierny L, Plass R, Portsmann W: Transluminal closure of patent ductus arteriosus: long-term results of 208 cases treated without thoracotomy. Cardiovasc Intervent Radiol 1986; 9:279–285.
18. Shrader R, Burger W, Dirk-Bussman W, et al: Residual ductal flow is uncommon after non-operative closure of persistent ductus arteriosus with Ivalon plugs (Portsmann technique). Circulation 1994; 90(suppl I):387.
19. Roth SJ, Perry SB, Keane JF, et al: Residual ductal flow after trascatheter occlusion of patent ductus arteriosus [Abstract]. Circulation 1991; 84(suppl II):545.
20. Landzberg MJ, Bridges ND, Perry SB, et al: Transcatheter occlusion—the treatment of choice for the adult with a patent ductus arteriosus [Abstract]. Circulation 1991; 84(suppl II):67.
21. Sideris EB, Sideris SE, Fowlkes JP, et al: Transvenous atrial septal defect occlusion with a "button" double-disk device. Circulation 1990; 81:312–318.
22. Rao PS, Onorato E, Kaul V, et al: Transvenous occlusion of patent ductus arteriosus with the adjustable button device in adults: initial clinic experience. Circulation 1994; 90(suppl I):387.
23. Verin VE, Saveliev SV, Kolody SM, et al: Results of transcatheter closure of the patent ductus arteriosus with the Botallo occluder. J Am Coll Cardiol 1993; 22:1509–1514.
24. Lloyd TR, Fedderly R, Mendelsohn AM, et al: Transcatheter occlusion of patent ductus arteriosus with Gianturco coils. Circulation 1993; 88:1412–1420.
25. Moore JW, George L, Kirkpatrick SE, et al: Percutaneous closure of the small patent ductus arteriosus using occluding spring coils. J Am Coll Cardiol 1994; 23:759–765.
26. Feldt RH, Co-Burn JP, Edwards SD, et al: Defects of the atrial septum and the atrioventricular canal. *In* Adams FH, Emmanouilides GC, Reimenschneider TA (eds): Heart Disease in Infants, Children and Adolescents, pp 170–189. Baltimore: Williams & Wilkins, 1989.
27. Murphy JG, Gersh BJ, McGoon MD, et al: Long-term outcome after surgical repair of isolated atrial septal defect. N Engl J Med 1990; 323:1645–1650.
28. Horvath KA, Burke RP, Collins JJ, et al: Surgical treatment of adult atrial septal defect: early and long-term results. J Am Coll Cardiol 1992; 20:1156–1159.
29. Pastorek JS, Allen HD, Davis JT: Current outcomes of surgical closure of secundum atrial septal defect. Am J Cardiol 1994; 74:75–77.
30. King TD, Thompson SL, Steiner C, et al: Secundum atrial septal defect—nonoperative closure during cardiac catheterization. JAMA 1976; 235:2506–2509.
31. Rashkind WJ: Interventional cardiac catheterization in congenital heart disease. Int J Cardiol 1985; 7:1–11.
32. Lock JE, Rome JJ, Davis R, et al: Transcatheter closure of ventricular septal defects—experimental studies. Circulation 1989; 779:1091–1099.
33. Latson LA, Benson LN, Hellenbrand WE, et al: Transcatheter closure of ASD—early results of multicenter trial of the Bard Clamshell septal occluder [Abstract]. Circulation 1991; 84(suppl II):544.
34. Landzberg MJ, Bridges ND, van der Velde M, et al: Double umbrella closure of atrial septal defects in adults [Abstract]. Circulation 1991; 84(suppl II):68.
35. Rao PS, Sideris EB, Hausdorg G, et al: International experience with secundum atrial septal defect occlusion by the buttoned device. Am Heart J 1994; 128:1022–1035.
36. Sievert H, Babic UU, Scherer D: Transcatheter closure of large atrial septal defects. Circulation 1994; 90(suppl I):387.
37. Landzberg MJ, Bridges ND, Bittl JA, et al: Transcatheter closure of atrial septal defects in adults with orthodeoxia-platypnea syndrome [Abstract]. J Am Coll Cardiol 1992; 19:289A.
38. Bridges ND, Hellenbrand W, Latson L, et al: Transcatheter closure of patent foramen ovale after presumed paradoxical embolism. Circulation 1992; 86:1902–1908.
39. Morrison BJ, Landzberg MJ, Newburger JW, et al: Infrequent occurrence of recurrent paradoxical embolism at intermediate follow-up after transcatheter closure of patent foramen ovale. Circulation 1994; 90(suppl I):237.
40. Ende DJ, Rao PS: Transcatheter occlusion of patent foramen ovales with Sideris' buttoned device to prevent recurrence of paradoxical embolism. Circulation 1994; 90(suppl I):387.
41. Bridges ND, Perry SB, Keane JF, et al: Preoperative transcatheter closure of congenital muscular ventricular septal defects. N Engl J Med 1991; 324:1312–1317.
42. Lock JE, Block PC, McKay RG, et al: Transcatheter closure of ventricular septal defects. Circulation 1988; 78:361–368.
43. Van der Velde ME, Sanders SP, Perry SB, et al: Transesophageal echocardiographic guidance for transcatheter device closure of ventricular septal defects [Abstract]. J Am Coll Cardiol 1991; 17:19A.

SECTION

EIGHT Miscellaneous Conditions

50 Gene Therapy for Cardiovascular Disease

Jonathan C. Fox, MD, PhD
Judith L. Swain, MD

Gene therapy for cardiovascular diseases is a new area of therapeutics under development. The greatest challenge of therapeutics in general has been to achieve progressively greater efficacy and specificity in how diseases are treated based on their biologic, biochemical, and, more recently, molecular mechanisms. The increasing recognition of the molecular mechanisms of disease has allowed the improved identification of specific genes or their products as targets for intervention. The techniques of molecular biology that have allowed this level of detail to be acquired have for the first time been adapted or applied to actually treating disease mechanisms at the gene level. Considered as a pharmacologic strategy, such a molecular therapeutic approach holds the promise of unprecedented specificity, potency, lack of toxicity, and, potentially, permanence when compared with conventional chemotherapeutics. The challenge of this field, now in its infancy, is to understand enough of the basic biology of disease to identify the correct targets and to develop the technology sufficiently to ensure safety and efficacy. The goals of this chapter are to identify cardiovascular disease processes amenable to gene therapy, describe methods for accomplishing gene therapy, and review the current studies under way that are using gene therapy to treat cardiovascular diseases.

The field of gene therapy owes its very existence and great potential to the major advances in basic biology made since the early 1970s. During that period, researchers have acquired the technology to isolate and purify to homogeneity individual stretches of DNA, allowing the determination of primary structure and opening the door to defining function at a molecular level. This has led to the development of methods to manipulate the expression of individual genes in a regulated and tissue-specific fashion. This capability is demonstrated perhaps most dramatically by the introduction or deletion of genes in the germ line of transgenic animals. Although the concept of germ line gene therapy should, in principle, be applicable to human disease, modifying the germ line of affected individuals or unaffected carriers to alter the genotype of subsequent offspring generates a host of technical and ethical issues that remain unresolved. Somatic cell gene therapy, however, is technically more feasible, targets specific cells or tissues involved in a disease process, and has fewer side effects. Because of our current state of knowledge of the molecular basis for disease, both congenital and acquired cardiovascular diseases make attractive targets for gene therapy.

Rational approaches to considering gene therapy for cardiovascular diseases require the identification of specific (or likely) molecular targets for intervention. These can include (but are not limited to)

- Replacing a missing or defective gene product
- Enhancing native functions through increased expression of a normal gene or a mutated gene with improved function
- Expressing a native function in a novel physiologic environment to take advantage of a unique biochemical or biophysical feature of a gene product
- Interfering with the expression or function of deleterious gene products by antisense, dominant negative, or competitive antagonist ("decoy") approaches

Once appropriate molecular targets have been identified, the cellular target of a proposed genetic manipulation must be chosen. Although this usually means the cell type most intimately involved in the disease process under consideration, it can also include a neighboring cell type or an organ distantly removed from the site of disease. Such distant sites might be related pathophysiologically or simply through the sharing of circulating blood. Once a cellular target has been chosen, the genetic information must be delivered in an efficient, selective fashion and must function in a physiologically relevant manner. Devising the efficient and effective means of packaging and delivering genetic information has posed one of the most significant technical challenges of developing gene therapy. Various approaches have been devised or are under development and generally rely on delivering genetic information (such as DNA or RNA) packaged as synthetic (chemical complexes), natural (viruses), or semisynthetic (biochemical conjugates) gene transfer vehicles delivered by a variety of mechanical means. These include genetic modification of cells or tissue ex vivo, with subsequent reimplantation, and gene delivery to target cells in situ. These approaches and techniques and their relative advantages, disadvantages, and current status of development will be set forth in more detail further on in the context of specific disease mechanisms or therapeutic goals.

IDENTIFYING TARGETS FOR GENE THERAPY

Despite the enormous pharmacopoeia currently available to the physician treating cardiovascular diseases, the treatment or prevention of many syndromes remains incomplete or inadequate. A variety of inherited or acquired metabolic and structural disorders, including dyslipidemias, cardiomyopathies, and vasculopathies, may be amenable to gene therapy–based treatment. A full discussion of the particular molecular defects of these varied disorders is beyond the scope of this chapter; however, when relevant to understanding the development of gene therapy, the molecular basis of a particular disease will be discussed. Despite the lack of a complete understanding of the precise molecular basis of many diseases, it may still be feasible to apply gene therapy to their treatment. For example, establishing the identity of a particular gene product (e.g., growth factors or cytokines) and its requirement for a particular disease process (e.g., restenosis) may provide enough information for an application of gene therapy even though the mechanism of its action remains undefined. Identifying gene products involved in disease processes is therefore an essential component of a sucessful gene therapy strategy for the treatment of any disease.

Functional Cloning

Identifying molecular targets for gene therapy depends on understanding the molecular pathophysiology of disease. This is often achieved in the case of inherited metabolic defects through the process of "forward genetics," or functional cloning of the gene for a recognized biochemical or structural defect. This approach takes advantage of a pre-existing knowledge of the specific biochemical defect, and at least some knowledge of the structure or immunoreactivity of the responsible gene product, to screen a collection of recombinant DNA molecules prepared from a source likely to contain copies of the gene of interest. The pre-existing structural or functional information is used to identify the cloned gene, which then yields the specific DNA sequence information describing the primary structure of the gene product. This genetic structural information can then be used to predict novel features of the gene product, its chromosomal location, the normal pattern of expression of the gene in normal individuals and those with disease, and the specific molecular mechanisms of disease by manipulating the expression or function of the gene in either in vitro or in vivo models of the disease. Based on this body of knowledge, some form of the information contained in the cloned gene may be used in devising gene therapy strategies according to the general principles outlined previously.

Functional Cloning: Low-Density Lipoprotein Receptor

A prime example of functional cloning is the characterization of the gene encoding the low-density lipoprotein, or LDL, receptor. Mutations in the LDL receptor are responsible for familial hypercholesterolemia. This syndrome was recognized for many years by its clinical hallmarks of markedly elevated LDL cholesterol and the consequences of accelerated atherogenesis resulting in premature coronary artery disease, myocardial infarctions, and death. Several years of basic laboratory research defined the biochemical identity of the cell surface receptor molecule responsible for the hepatic removal of the LDL particle. Taking advantage of some limited protein sequence data obtained from purified fragments of the receptor molecule, a set of oligodeoxynucleotides corresponding to the protein sequence was synthesized and used to screen a cDNA library. With the use of this strategy based on structural knowledge gained through study of the purified protein, the gene was isolated in 1983.[1] In this way, a known metabolic defect was used to identify the responsible gene product, and the purified gene product was used to identify the gene.

Positional Cloning

Although functional cloning has been successfully applied to isolating the genes involved in a variety of cardiovascular disorders, this approach is often not possible, as the nature of the precise structural or functional defect for a great many diseases simply is not known. To clone the genes involved in heritable diseases, many groups have successfully applied positional cloning or so-called reverse genetics.

The strategy of positional cloning relies on the identification of kindreds of patients with heritable diseases and their first-degree relatives. The process also depends on the existence of a rapidly expanding panel of cloned fragments of human chromosomal DNA for which the chromosomal location is precisely known and that exist in a number of divergent or polymorphic forms in the general population. Through the pattern of linked inheritance of the disease trait, coupled with the cosegregation of a series of these polymorphic chromosomal markers, the chromosomal location of the disease gene can be established. However, even tightly linked markers often localize the disease gene only to relatively large segments of DNA, forcing researchers to clone and sequence long stretches of DNA before positively identifying the disease gene. Since by definition, the nature of the gene is unknown from the outset, the identification by such positional cloning is often tentative and requires detailed study of the putative gene structure to infer that it is indeed the gene that was sought. Such identification can sometimes be facilitated by the evaluation of candidate genes whose function and approximate location may already be known. This latter approach has been used successfully for a number of disease genes, including several that have been shown to be responsible for some inherited forms of hypertrophic cardiomyopathy (HCM).

Positional Cloning: Familial Hypertrophic Cardiomyopathy

Several genes responsible for HCM have been identified by positional cloning.[2, 3] This approach used standard clinical criteria to establish the diagnosis of HCM, and DNA samples were prepared from collected blood samples from patients and their unaffected first-degree relatives. With the use of a panel of cloned polymorphic markers, the approximate chromosomal location was established for several different kindreds. It became clear at this point that familial HCM was a genetically heterogeneous disease caused by more than one gene.[4] As this work progressed, it was noted that the gene for at least one form of the disease shared the approximate chromosomal location as the beta-myosin heavy chain gene (β-MHC). This accelerated the study of the disease in at least some affected kindreds, as it was subsequently shown that these families carried mutations in the β-MHC gene.[5] Recent work has now identified other kindreds carrying mutations in both alpha-tropomyosin and cardiac troponin T,[6] demonstrating that HCM can be caused by the abnormal structure or function of any of several sarcomeric proteins. This work has also been used to construct survival analyses according to the specific mutation present in a particular family, and this has revealed that the prognosis in this disease can vary widely according to the nature of the mutation.[7, 8] This information can potentially be of great value in helping patients and their physicians weigh the risks and benefits of particular treatment options. The identification of the mutations causing this disease has now begun to shed light on its molecular pathogenesis. Such studies of how sarcomere dysfunction and myofiber disarray are produced by the expression of abnormal sarcomeric proteins[9, 10] may provide the necessary insights for designing gene replacement or augmentation therapies for this disease.

Despite these accomplishments in identifying single gene defects responsible for cardiovascular diseases, the vast majority of molecular disease mechanisms are more complex. Many syndromes are either multigenic in origin or depend on complex interactions between native mechanisms and environmental factors that conspire to overwhelm or subvert homeostasis. This applies to the most common acquired cardiovascular diseases represented within the patient population, especially atherosclerosis, hypertension, and heart failure. It also includes the sequelae of some important cardiovascular treatment modalities, including restenosis after mechanical revascularization, early graft failure after surgical revascularization, and cardiac allograft rejection and vasculopathy after transplantation. Despite the complex nature of these disorders, major advances have been made with respect to understanding their molecular pathogenesis, a necessary first step in identifying molecular targets for gene therapy. A long and rapidly growing list of cytokines, growth factors, hormones, adhesion molecules, enzymes, and cofactors has been implicated in many of these disorders, suggesting many potential targets for gene therapy of cardiovascular diseases. Besides the obvious cellular targets contained in the myocardium and the vascular wall, the liver (source of many coagulation factors, lipoproteins, and hormones) and skeletal muscle (as a "factory" for therapeutic recombinant proteins) are other potential targets for treating different cardiovascular diseases. The possibilities are limited only by our knowledge of specific molecular mechanisms of disease, the gene transfer technology at hand, and our imagination.

GENE TRANSFER TECHNOLOGY

Gene transfer technology was developed originally as a means of introducing cloned genes into cultured cells for the purposes of defining the function of that gene in the setting of the living cell. As the techniques for achieving gene transfer in vitro became more efficient, they could be applied to gene transfer in vivo. The development of transgenic mice demonstrated that foreign genes could be stably expressed and tolerated in a host animal. Although this technology depends on achieving gene transfer to the germ line through microinjection of DNA into single cells, the result that high-level expression of cloned genes could be achieved in a potentially regulated and tissue-specific fashion generated great excitement over the possibility that this could be carried out in the somatic cells of fully developed organisms. It was with this aim that the techniques of in vivo gene transfer have been progressively developed and refined, including techniques based on naked or chemically modified DNA, RNA tumor viruses, DNA tumor viruses, and hybrid technologies derived from combinations of these approaches. These techniques are summarized in Table 50–1, and will be discussed in detail in the following sections.

Plasmid DNA–Based Methods

Initial efforts to achieve in vivo gene transfer relied on techniques that had been developed for genetically manipulating cultured cells in vitro. The classic approach to in vitro gene transfer by nonviral means relies on applying purified preparations of cloned plasmid DNA, mixed with an appropriate vehicle, directly to cultured cells. This leads to a nonspecific uptake of the DNA and so-called transfection of the cells. In transient transfection, most of the recipient cells maintain the foreign DNA in an extrachromosomal state, which is not retained over time. A small fraction of cells incorporate the DNA at random sites in their chromosomes and therefore transmit the transfected DNA to their progeny. Although relatively inefficient, this technique is simple, and the introduction of a selectable marker gene (e.g., for resistance to a cytotoxic drug) can subsequently be used to genetically select for the progeny of transfected cells, resulting in homogeneous populations of genetically modified cells. Plasmid DNA transfection in vitro can be achieved by a variety of biochemical and mechanical means. Of these nonviral in vitro gene transfer methods, the use of a complex of plasmid DNA and synthetic cationic liposomes[11] has been most often applied to in vivo gene transfer. Cationic liposomes form a noncovalent complex with DNA through electrostatic interactions, and the hydrophobic portion of the liposome components is able to interact with cell membranes, promoting either fusion or endocytosis. Plasmid DNA transfection has been used to transfer genes to somatic cells or tissues in vivo with the use of either surgical or percutaneous approaches. These latter methods include liposomal DNA delivery, direct injection of naked DNA into recipient tissues, and ballistic delivery of DNA-coated microprojectiles. In general, plasmid DNA–based methods are less efficient than viral methods. (This will be discussed in further detail in the context of gene transfer to the cardiovascular system in a discussion later in this chapter.)

The greatest advantage of the methods relying on delivering naked DNA is their simplicity and relative technical ease. The greatest disadvantage is low efficiency, and to achieve stable expression, the DNA must be integrated into the host cell genome. This requires host cell replication, which limits the applicability of these methods in terms of appropriate target cells. In addition, integration occurs largely at random with respect to chromosomal location, theoretically risking insertional mutagenesis or inactivation of a normal host gene.

Recombinant Retrovirus

The field of in vivo gene transfer took a major step forward with the development of genetically engineered viral vectors. The rationale behind this development was that viruses, in general, have evolved an efficient mechanism for delivering their genetic material to target cells, and this mechanism could be enlisted for the purpose of delivering foreign DNA to target cells in an efficient fashion. The first such application came in the adaptation of RNA tumor viruses, or retroviruses, as gene transfer vectors.[12, 13] Originally described for their ability to transform host cells into malignant tumor cells, these viruses are relatively simple in their structure and biology. They consist of a linear, double-stranded RNA genome containing three structural genes. These genes are flanked by an inverted, duplicated region called the long terminal repeat (LTR) that directs high-level expression of the viral genes (or heterologous genes). The viral particle consists of the viral RNA and several associated proteins surrounded by an envelope made of host cell membrane and viral coat glycoprotein. This glycoprotein is recognized by specific cell surface proteins and promotes fusion of the viral particle with the cell. After entry of the viral particle into the cell, the RNA genome is copied by viral RNA-dependent DNA polymerase (reverse transcriptase) into a DNA copy, which then integrates stably into the host genome as a provirus, a process mediated by the LTR. This process requires host cell division at the time of infection.[14] Subsequent viral replication (and transformation to a malignant phenotype) requires the presence and proper expression of the three viral genes.

The great advantage of retroviruses as gene transfer vectors is that all three of the viral genes can be deleted and replaced with foreign DNA (the transgene). For the recombinant retrovirus to function as a gene transfer vector, only the preservation of the flanking LTRs, to drive constitutive expression of the transgene and integration of the provirus, and the packaging signal, for proper assembly of the recombinant virion, are required. This renders the recombinant virus replication-defective. Propagation of the recombinant retrovirus as infectious virions in vitro then requires provision of the missing viral genes in trans, either by coinfection with a helper virus (able to provide the viral gene products but lacking a packaging signal) or by transfection of the recombinant viral genome into a cell line expressing the viral genes (packaging cell line).

Recombinant retroviruses present several disadvantages as a gene transfer vector. Because of the obligatory requirement of vector integration into the host cell genome for expression of the transgene, retroviral vectors can transfer genetic material only to dividing cells. This may well confer some advantages for targeting gene transfer to rapidly dividing cells as in the treatment of cancer, but many other potential targets of interest divide slowly or not at all in the adult (e.g., cardiomyocytes, neurons). Stable integration can lead to persistent, high-level expression of the transgene, but as with naked DNA, integration at random locations may lead to insertional mutagenesis events. Efficient gene transfer requires the application of recombinant virus in high concentrations (titer), and the production of high-titer recombinant retrovirus is technically challenging. The retroviral particle is inherently unstable and easily inactivated. Recently, hybrid or so-called pseudotyped retroviral vectors have been designed that overcome some of these stability problems, allowing concentration

TABLE 50–1. GENE TRANSFER TECHNOLOGIES

Vector/Method	Target Cell	Efficiency	Integrates	Duration of Expression	Advantages	Disadvantages
Plasmid DNA-Based Methods						
Plasmid DNA transfection (naked DNA)	Proliferating or quiescent*	Low	Occasionally (stable transfection)	Long if integrates (stable transfection)	Vectors easily constructed and manipulated in vitro Technically less challenging than many viral methods Very pure recombinant DNA can be prepared in high concentrations Easily adapted to a variety of delivery methods Low toxicity	Efficiency very low, can vary widely Transfection vehicles can be toxic Long-term expression requires stable chromosomal integration that is not site-specific Requires target cell division Transgene expression may exert negative selective pressure
Plasmid DNA transfection (DNA/cationic liposome complex)	Proliferating or quiescent*	Low	Occasionally	Long if integrates	Same as above	Same as above
Recombinant retrovirus (replication-defective MMuLV or similar retrovirus	Proliferating; requires cell surface molecules recognizing viral coat glycoprotein (host range determinant)	Medium to high	Yes	Long	All three viral genes can be deleted and replaced with recombinant DNA sequences, rendering virus replication/transformation defective Stable chromosomal integration leads to persistent transgene expression Does not provoke significant immune response	Technically difficult to prepare Target cell must be actively dividing (may be an advantage) Chromosomal integration largely at random Potential rescue by helper virus in vivo could result in productive infection/ transformation
Recombinant adenovirus (replication-defective human Ad5 or Ad2 serotypes)	Proliferating or quiescent; requires expression of an as yet unidentified receptor (nearly ubiquitous)	High	No	<3 weeks in vivo	Large capacity for foreign DNA (>8 kb pairs) Infects a broad variety of cell types across species Does not require target cell proliferation Can be concentrated to very high titer Low toxicity at gene transfer doses	Technically difficult Immunogenic as currently used, limits duration of expression
Recombinant herpes simplex virus	Proliferating or quiescent; only cell types specified by host range (especially neurons)	Medium to high	Yes	Long	Neurotropic; can be prepared in high titer	Narrow host range Technically difficult
Recombinant adeno-associated virus	Proliferating or quiescent; must be infectable by adenovirus	High	Yes	Long?	Persistent expression mediated by site-specific chromosomal integration independent of cell division Large transgene capacity	Technically difficult Requires adenovirus for successful infection
Other viruses (vaccinia, Sindbis, others)					Different viruses may provide application-specific advantages, e.g., tissue tropism as with HSV	Vector development requires thorough characterization and ability to manipulate viral genome
Semisynthetic Conjugates						
Adenoviral-based (plasmid DNA complexed with poly-L-lysine conjugated, inactivated adenovirus)	Same as adenovirus	Medium to high	Depends on nature of genetic material	Depends on nature of genetic material	Technically simpler than recombinant virus Similar broad host range, proliferating or quiescent cells	Same as plasmid DNA or oligos
Adenoviral-based (same as above, but also containing targeting ligand [e.g, transferrin])	Specified by incorporated targeting ligand	Medium to high	Depends on nature of genetic material	Depends on nature of genetic material	Technically simpler than recombinant virus Specific host range, proliferating or quiescent cells	Same as plasmid DNA or oligos
Sendai virus (HVJ)–liposomes (plasmid DNA in complex with cationic liposomes and inactivated Sendai virus)	Proliferating or quiescent, infectable by Sendai virus	Medium to high	Depends on nature of genetic material	Depends on nature of genetic material	Technically simpler than recombinant virus	Same as plasmid DNA or oligos
Synthetic virus–like (synthetic liposomes containing fusigenic, endosomolytic viral peptide and plasmid DNA)	Proliferating or quiescent	Medium to high	Depends on nature of genetic material	Depends on nature of genetic material	Technically simpler than recombinant virus	Same as plasmid DNA or oligos

*Quiescent cells can be genetically modified, but not in a stable manner (transiently only). Stable modification requires chromosomal integration, which in turn requires cell division.
Abbreviations: MMuLV, Moloney murine leukemia virus; HVJ, hemagglutinating virus of Japan; HSV, herpes simplex virus.

of the viral preparation by ultracentrifugation, and the host range has been extended by packaging the recombinant virus with a pantropic envelope protein (vesicular stomatitis virus G protein).[15, 16] In addition to their successful use in mammalian cells, pantropic pseudotyped retroviruses have been used to achieve gene transfer to amphibians in vivo[17] and to generate transgenic zebra fish, an experimental model at the forefront of cardiovascular developmental biology.[18]

Malignant transformation resulting from retroviral infection in the host remains a concern, since productive retroviral infection could theoretically transform host cells into tumor cells.[19, 20] In addition, viral preparations can theoretically be contaminated with replication-competent virus, generated through recombination between recombinant viral sequences and helper or pre-existing proviral sequences to regenerate replication-competent virus, either during preparation or later after successful gene transfer to a host cell. The development of improved packaging cell lines that avoid containing the necessary viral genes in a contiguous segment of DNA has lowered the probability of a productive recombination event.[19, 20]

The advantages of recombinant retrovirus vectors for in vivo gene transfer stimulated many investigators to develop models for gene therapy, even bringing this technology to clinical trials (see further on). It became clear to many, however, that the potential of viral vectors in general was only partially fulfilled by retroviral vectors, and much effort has been invested in developing alternatives. Perhaps the vectors enjoying the most popularity currently are derived from the human adenovirus, a common DNA virus responsible for mild infections in the general population.

Recombinant Adenovirus

The development of recombinant adenovirus vectors for in vitro and in vivo gene transfer represents the culmination of many years of basic virology research.[21] The main advantages of recombinant adenoviruses are their broad host range, their ability to infect either replicating or quiescent cells, the ability to prepare the virus in very high titer (10^{12}–10^{13}/mL), and the lack of an association between adenoviruses and any human disease other than largely mild, self-limited respiratory and gastrointestinal infections. Human adenoviruses are a family of nonenveloped, icosahedral viruses containing a linear, 36-kb double-stranded DNA genome. The genome is divided into early (E) and late (L) regions in reference to when they are expressed in relation to viral DNA replication. Recombinant adenoviruses have the ability to carry 8 kb or more of foreign DNA. This large capacity is generated by deleting segments of the viral genome (portions of E3 or E4) that are not required for viral replication, packaging, or infection. Viral replication requires expression of the E1A and E1B genes, and these genes are also deleted from recombinant adenovirus vectors, rendering the virus replication defective. The deleted mutant viruses are propagated in the human embryonal kidney cell line 293, which is stably transfected with the deleted E1 genes, providing the required gene products in trans.[22] Several different strategies have been developed for inserting a foreign transgene into the adenoviral genome. Different strategies take advantage of the ability of transfected, naked viral DNA to initiate productive infection, resulting in accumulation of infectious virus particles in cells of the 293 cell line. One popular approach uses a shuttle plasmid, derived from a typical bacterial plasmid, containing the foreign transgene driven by an appropriate expression cassette, and flanked by segments of the adenoviral genome. Truncating the E1/E3 deleted mutant virus at the 5′ end deletes the viral packaging signal, generating an adenoviral genome that may replicate but cannot be packaged into virions in cells of the 293 cell line. The shuttle plasmid cannot itself replicate in cells of the 293 cell line, but it contains the packaging signal missing from the truncated viral DNA. These two purified DNAs are cotransfected into cells of the 293 cell line with the use of calcium phosphate coprecipitation, and the adenoviral sequences flanking the transgene in the shuttle vector are able to mediate a homologous recombination event with the truncated adenoviral DNA. The recombination product has the capability of both replicating and being packaged into infectious virions in the cells of the 293 cell line. Other approaches rely on preparing the entire recombinant viral genome as a single, large plasmid DNA molecule, propagating the plasmid for in vitro manipulation either in *Escherichia coli*[23] or in yeast.[24] The final recombinant vector is still prepared as infectious virions by transfecting the purified DNA into cells of the 293 cell line.

There are several distinct advantages that recombinant adenovirus vectors provide when compared with retroviral vectors. Perhaps most importantly, adenovirus will infect a very broad range of cell types and species, and infection with subsequent expression of the transgene does not depend on replication of the target cell. The recombinant adenovirus remains episomal in most cases, largely avoiding the concerns regarding chromosomal integration, although integration can occur if the target cell is infected with a very large number of virus particles (high multiplicity of infection). Recombinant adenovirus can be prepared in very high titer stocks, permitting its use in a variety of in vivo testing situations not amenable to other methods of gene transfer. The adenovirus strains that have been developed as gene transfer vectors are not associated with any naturally occurring diseases other than a variety of usually mild, self-limiting respiratory or gastrointestinal syndromes, and evidence of humoral immunity against these viruses, indicating prior infection, is evident in the great majority of people. Although tumorigenicity of this class of viruses cannot be rigorously excluded, it has not been observed to date.

The disadvantages of recombinant adenovirus primarily relate to its immunogenicity, which limits persistence of expression secondary to elimination of the virus via immune clearance of infected cells.[25–27] Evidence of the mechanisms responsible for this limitation has come from experiments using immunocompetent versus immunodeficient or immunosuppressed hosts and identification of activation of specific components of the immune response directed at viral antigens. Virally infected cells may in fact be capable of producing viral proteins in addition to the transgene as a result of "leaky" expression of delayed early genes despite deletion of the immediate early genes. It has been postulated that such expression is mediated by the activity of host genes that are able to complement the missing viral genes. Various approaches are currently being used in an attempt to circumvent this problem, including generating new adenoviral vectors containing further deletions or conditional (temperature-sensitive) mutations in the delayed early genes.[28] Another limitation that has emerged is based on the observation that adenovirus can infect many but not all target cells of interest with high efficiency. Adenoviral infection relies on the expression of a specific membrane surface receptor for the virus, which has not yet been identified. It is believed that certain cells express the receptor at very low levels or not at all, rendering them relatively or absolutely resistant to infection.

Other Viruses

Viruses other than adenovirus are also being developed as gene transfer vectors. For gene transfer into the central nervous system, the neurotropic herpes simplex virus (HSV) is particularly well suited,[29] and similar tissue tropism could conceivably be taken advantage of in cardiovascular gene transfer. Adeno-associated virus (AAV) is a small, defective DNA virus (parvovirus) that requires helper adenovirus to achieve infection but can achieve persistent expression of inserted transgenes.[30] The AAV genome is established as a provirus secondary to predominantly site-specific chromosomal integration[31] that is independent of cell division, although it occurs preferentially during the S phase of the cell cycle.[32] These vectors are currently under development for a variety of applications,[33, 34] and recent success in gene transfer to airway epithelium in vivo[35] and the phenotypic correction of Fanconi anemia cells in vitro[36] has helped spur further development of this class of viral vectors. The development of gene transfer vectors based on other viruses such as vaccinia[37, 38] and Sindbis[39] viruses is limited only by our knowledge of how to manipulate the genomes of these viruses to permit carriage of transgenes while eliminating the disease-related activities of the wild-type virus.

Semisynthetic Conjugates

The current generation of recombinant viral vectors offers unparalleled efficiency of gene transfer to a broad range of cellular targets. The general theme of using a specific molecule (in this case the viral coat protein) as a means of receptor-mediated entry into the cell has been approached in some alternative ways.[40] Semisynthetic conjugates based on adenovirus-mediated cellular entry and escape from lysosomal degradation have been prepared from both human[41] and avian[42] adenoviruses. These gene transfer vehicles use an inactivated or replication-defective adenovirus covalently modified with poly-L-lysine to incorporate naked DNA into a complex that is recognized by the viral receptor, thus permitting uptake and subsequent expression of the DNA. The high efficiency of adenoviral infection is in large part due to the ability of the viral capsid protein to disrupt the endosome before formation of the endolysosome, thus releasing the viral particle into the cytoplasm and avoiding degradation. The semisynthetic complexes take advantage of this endosomolytic activity. The polylysine moiety serves as a DNA-binding polycation, forming an electrostatic condensate with the DNA (plasmid or other form). A similar approach takes advantage of the ability of the Sendai virus (hemagglutinating virus of Japan) to mediate membrane fusion, and complexes of inactivated Sendai virus, DNA, and liposomes have been used successfully to transfer genes in vivo.[43] Other approaches have used semisynthetic virus–polylysine–DNA complexes that also incorporate natural ligands to target gene transfer via a specific receptor. For example, complexes containing transferrin[44] or asialo-orosomucoid[45] have demonstrated such receptor-specific targeting of adenovirus-assisted gene transfer. Newer approaches are being developed that use purified viral peptides that mediate endocytosis and endosomolysis incorporated into a completely synthetic complex with naked DNA.[46, 47] Such synthetic complexes may someday replace recombinant virions as gene transfer vectors.

Antisense Oligodeoxynucleotides and Other Approaches to Gene Inhibition

A variant on the naked DNA approach to gene modification is the use of short synthetic DNA or RNA molecules to inhibit rather than enhance gene function. These molecules rely principally on their ability to recognize their targets in a sequence-specific manner. Oligodeoxynucleotides have enjoyed the most attention because of their relative ease of preparation and dose-dependent activity in a variety of applications. The most common use of oligonucleotides in the setting of gene therapy is to use the antisense, or minus strand, to form base pairs with mRNA. Base pairing of the antisense oligonucleotide may act to inhibit the expression of the gene by a variety of mechanisms, including interference with processing of pre-mRNA to mature mRNA, premature degradation of the partially double-stranded RNA-DNA duplex, or inhibiting translation by preventing the proper interaction of the mRNA with the protein synthetic apparatus of the cell.[48] Antisense oligonucleotides can be delivered in solution without modification, applied as a biocompatible gel that slowly dissolves,[49] added to liposomes to form a complex conjugated with inactivated viruses,[43] or carried with other enhancing chemical modifications such as covalent linkage to cholesterol.[50] Although an attractive concept, the successful application of antisense oligonucleotides to inhibit gene expression can be problematic. The natural structure of the phosphodiester backbone makes the synthetic oligonucleotides sensitive to destruction by cellular nucleases, a problem partially overcome by the use of chemical modifications (phosphorothioate, methylphosphonate, or phosphorodithioate oligonucleotides). One novel approach substitutes the phosphodiester linkages of the backbone with amide bonds, creating so-called peptide nucleic acids that are nuclease-resistant.[51] Efficacy and specificity are often difficult to achieve; many cell systems respond to seemingly unrelated sequences in a fashion similar to the way they respond to the antisense sequence. In addition to oligonucleotides potentially interacting with unintended DNA or RNA targets, they may also interact with important nucleic acid–binding proteins (if intended, this can represent an effective gene targeting strategy). Oligonucleotides can also interact with proteins that normally do not bind nucleic acid simply by virtue of chance complementarity in their tertiary structure (so-called aptamers).[52] The specificity of this interaction can be quite precise and can be exploited as an alternative approach to drug development. For example, RNA aptamers that inhibit a specific isoform of the signal transduction molecule protein kinase C have been identified through functional screening.[50] In fact, phosphorothioate modification of oligonucleotides, simply intended to render these molecules resistant to degradation, may hamper their specificity and efficacy. Compared with minimally modified or unmodified oligonucleotides, phosphorothioate-modified oligonucleotides bind more avidly to a variety of cytoplasmic and nuclear proteins and may bind nuclear transcription factors in a nonspecific fashion.[53] Despite these caveats that may compromise the usual intended use of oligonucleotides, many studies have successfully applied antisense oligonucleotides to models of gene therapy, including cardiovascular problems such as inhibiting restenosis after angioplasty (see further on).

Triplex DNA–Forming Oligodeoxynucleotides

Another application of oligonucleotides is to form a triple-stranded DNA complex between the chromosomal DNA of the gene and the single-stranded oligonucleotide, thereby preventing the synthesis of the primary RNA transcript.[54, 55] Although an attractive concept, development of this approach is in the early stages.

Ribozymes

Single-stranded RNA molecules may also be used as therapeutic agents, especially if they are designed to possess catalytic activity (ribozymes). The structure and activity of ribozymes are based on the model of naturally occurring, autocatalytic RNAs that possess both self-recognition and catalytic domains targeted to another portion of the molecule (substrate) that requires hydrolytic cleavage for maturation of the entire molecule. Engineered ribozymes are designed to possess recognition domains that target a heterologous transcript (target gene activity to be altered), rather than recognizing another portion of the same molecule.[56, 57] Ribozymes have been developed mainly with the intention of destroying their intended target, especially in the case of human immunodeficiency virus–1 (HIV-1) RNA. These catalytic RNA molecules can also be engineered to replace stretches of RNA by a trans-splicing mechanism, however, suggesting a unique approach to gene therapy of defective mRNA molecules.[58] Although not applicable to a wide variety of problems amenable to gene therapy, this approach may well find problems for which it is particularly well suited.

Skeletal Myoblasts and Muscle Fibers as Gene Therapy Vehicles

Skeletal myoblasts can be removed from adult animals, cultured, and genetically modified in vitro. Gene transfer has been accomplished in cultured myoblasts by many of the naked DNA and viral vector methods discussed earlier and then reimplanted, where they fuse with the skeletal myofibers and continue to express the transgene.[59, 60] The transgene can be therapeutic for the target muscle, as in the heritable muscular dystrophies,[61, 62] or it can be a gene whose product (e.g., growth hormone) is targeted to other tissues.[63, 64] More recently, both naked DNA[65, 66] and recombinant adenovirus methods have been used to achieve direct in vivo gene transfer to skeletal muscle. Some investigators have found that naked DNA may be superior to currently available viral methods because of either low infectivity of viral vectors for terminally differentiated muscle[67, 68] or the now well recognized immune response that often limits the persistence of virally mediated gene transfer.[67] Despite these caveats, both approaches have been used to genetically modify skeletal muscle in vivo for therapeutic purposes—both in muscular dystrophy[69, 70] and in the systemic delivery of erythropoietin[71] and factor IX.[72] Although none of these experiments has targeted cardiovascular diseases, it has been recognized that skeletal muscle could be used in such an approach to deliver gene products that would benefit individuals with cardiovascular or thrombotic diseases and that such an approach may be applied to the myocardium (see further on).

GENE THERAPY OF THE CARDIOVASCULAR SYSTEM

Vascular Gene Transfer

Ex Vivo Modification and Reimplantation of Vascular Cells

As in vivo gene transfer technology was developed, several groups applied some of the approaches described earlier to achieve gene transfer to cells of the vasculature. Initial efforts concentrated on ex vivo genetic modification of endothelial and vascular smooth muscle cells followed by reimplantation of the cells on prosthetic graft material or onto the luminal surface of native vessels. It had been shown earlier that cultured rabbit endothelial cells could be genetically modified in vitro with the use of recombinant retrovirus vectors that contained a selectable drug resistance marker.[73] These same investigators subsequently used vectors encoding either a cytoplasmic protein (adenosine deaminase) or a secreted protein (growth hormone) and demonstrated high-level expression of these genes in vitro. The genetically modified cells could be seeded onto prosthetic graft material, where they proliferated in vitro and continued to express the transgene. A similar experiment showed that sheep endothelial cells genetically modified by recombinant retrovirus encoding either the marker gene beta-galactosidase (*lacZ*) or tissue plasminogen activator (t-PA) could be seeded onto metallic endovascular stents in vitro, where they continued to express the transgenes even after the stents were expanded with a balloon catheter and exposed to flow conditions.[74, 75] These important in vitro experiments were subsequently extended to in vivo models of gene therapy with the use of ex vivo modified vascular cells. Retrovirally modified endothelial cells could be seeded onto polyester (Dacron) grafts and then implanted into the arterial circulation of dogs[76] or could be seeded directly onto the luminal surface of porcine arteries from which the native endothelial cells had been removed.[77] Similar experiments showed that vascular smooth muscle cells modified ex vivo could also be seeded onto a previously balloon-injured arterial surface in vivo[78] and that such genetically modified implants could persist and continue to express foreign transgenes for at least 1 year.[79] Despite showing generally low numbers of modified cells relative to the treated vascular area, these studies demonstrated the important principle that vascular cells could be genetically modified ex vivo and reimplanted at a selected vascular site to achieve either local or systemic delivery of an expressed transgene. As a potential therapeutic approach, however, ex vivo vascular cell gene transfer poses several disadvantages. In order to produce a sufficient number of genetically modified cells, the cells must be harvested from the intended recipient (or a syngeneic donor), expanded in vitro, and then reimplanted. This would entail two invasive procedures (harvest and reimplantation) with a delay of up to several weeks between them. This approach will clearly not be practical for many of the applications that might be desirable for local gene delivery for the cardiovascular system, for example, the delivery of genes to the vasculature at the time of angioplasty to ameliorate or prevent restenosis (see further on). As a means of delivering recombinant proteins for systemic distribution, the effective number of modified cells exposed to the circulation in a treated vessel segment is much lower than can probably be achieved by gene transfer to skeletal muscle or liver. Still, these experiments established that genetic modification of vascular cells was feasible and did not disrupt the ability of the modified cells to be incorporated into implantable graft material or vascular tissue in situ and led to the further development of vascular gene transfer in vivo.

Vascular Gene Transfer In Vivo

Plasmid DNA and Retrovirus. Early attempts at in vivo vascular gene transfer used plasmid DNA/liposome transfer vehicles. These experiments demonstrated that marker genes (*lacZ* or the firefly luciferase genes) could be transferred to coronary or peripheral arteries of the dog, first with the use of surgical exposure of the vessels[80] and later a percutaneous catheter-based approach[81] to achieve delivery of the genetic material. Subsequent work demonstrated that plasmid DNA/liposomal gene transfer by a percutaneous approach was applicable to atherosclerotic as well as normal arteries in a rabbit model.[82] More recent work has shown that the efficiency of transfection with plasmid DNA can be improved through its delivery as a gel coating on an intravascular balloon catheter.[83] Although considered safe from the perspective of toxicity and side effects, gene transfer with the use of DNA/liposomes is of generally low efficiency. In an effort to improve on these results and extend the experience gained with vascular cells ex vivo, protocols using recombinant retrovirus have been developed. As discussed earlier, retrovirus-mediated gene transfer requires host cell division at the time of infection, limiting this approach to actively dividing cells. In addition, in vivo gene transfer requires very high titer solutions of recombinant retrovirus, which are rapidly inactivated by serum. Despite these technical hurdles, recombinant retrovirus expressing *lacZ* has been used to demonstrate direct in vivo gene transfer to the iliofemoral artery of pigs.[84] These investigators used a double-balloon catheter to create an isolated luminal segment of a surgically exposed vessel, which could then be emptied of blood and serum before the instillation of the viral solution. The same objective of exposing the arterial wall to recombinant retrovirus while avoiding exposure to serum was achieved in the rabbit aorta with the use of an angioplasty balloon containing microscopic perforations (Wolinsky balloon) that allowed delivery of the viral solution as high-pressure jets directed orthogonal to the vessel wall.[85] Despite variable and generally low efficiency of gene transfer, these results demonstrated the feasibility of retroviral gene transfer in vivo and were followed by a series of experiments designed to show that specific genes transferred with the use of retrovirus could play a pathogenetic role in the response to vascular injury. These will be discussed in detail in a subsequent section describing gene transfer specifically targeted to the problem of vascular injury.

Recombinant Adenovirus. The most efficient means of achieving in vivo gene transfer developed to date is the recombinant adenovirus. As reviewed earlier, these vectors can be prepared in very high titer (suitable for in vivo applications) and infect a broad range of both dividing and nondividing cells. Experiments have demonstrated efficient adenovirus-mediated gene transfer to the vasculature with the use of *lacZ*, alkaline phosphatase, and luciferase marker genes.[86–90] These studies have shown that gene transfer mediated by recombinant adenovirus is more efficient than recombinant retrovirus or DNA/liposomes, but it is transient, peaking at 7 to 14 days, declining by 21 days, and becoming undetectable by 28 days. Infection and gene transfer appear to be limited to endothelium if the virus is delivered to uninjured arteries, and infection of medial smooth muscle cells requires denudation of the endothelium and either balloon overstretch or hydrostatic pressure distention. There is evidence that the internal elastic lamina presents a physical barrier to the delivery of viral particles to the media,[91] which may explain the need for mechanical disruption (if only transient) of normal tissue architecture. The lack of persistence of transgene expression is thought to be mediated by the same or similar immune clearance mechanisms as those discussed earlier, and at least one group of investigators has reported finding a perivascular mononuclear infiltrate after successful adenoviral gene transfer to porcine coronary arteries.[89] Interestingly, these same authors found that intracoronary gene transfer of recombinant adenovirus delivered intramurally by the Wolinsky balloon was equally efficient in normal, balloon overstretch–injured, atherosclerotic, and oversized stent–injured arteries.

Vascular Gene Therapy and Restenosis

Over the past several years, the techniques of in vivo gene transfer and gene manipulation have been used to probe the mechanisms mediating vascular disease and to explore the potential for gene therapy of vascular diseases. Many of the targets chosen for manipulation have been based on previous work implicating specific growth factors, cytokines, nuclear factors, and other molecules in the control of vascular cell biology both in vitro and in vivo. Of particular interest has been the identification of the factors that are responsible for the often exuberant response of the vessel wall to mechanical injury that constitutes the process of restenosis after angioplasty. Postangioplasty restenosis remains the primary limitation of the success of this technique, resulting in considerably more morbidity, mortality, and expense than would be expected if the rate of restenosis were less than the current value of 30%–40%. Many clinical trials of drugs and devices for limiting restenosis have been disappointing in their failure to reveal an effective preventive strategy. Studies of humans and of current available animal models of restenosis have identified many important molecules that participate in the activation of quiescent medial smooth muscle cells, their migration from the media to the intima, and their concomitant or subsequent proliferation and elaboration of abundant extracellular matrix that characterize the process. A complete review of our state of knowledge regarding the molecular mechanisms of the response to vascular injury is beyond the scope of this discussion;[92–94] however, a great deal of experimental evidence supports important roles for products derived from the circulation, including humoral factors (e.g., thrombin), platelets and their products (e.g., platelet-derived growth factor, or PDGF), and locally produced inflammatory cytokines (e.g., interleukin-1), in addition to cellular elements (mononuclear cells). In response to as yet incompletely defined mechanical and exogenous biochemical signals, smooth muscle–derived growth factors (fibroblast growth factor [FGF], PDGF, transforming growth factor–beta [TGF-β], and others) are known to play an essential role through autocrine or paracrine signaling pathways. Although there appears to be redundancy in some of the pathways leading to smooth muscle cell activation, migration, proliferation, and extracellular matrix production, gene transfer or antisense experiments have shown many of these factors to be potentially useful targets in a gene therapy approach to restenosis. Much of this work has been performed in peripheral arteries of the rat, rabbit, and pig models, although some data exist with respect to the coronary circulation.

The study of gene therapy approaches for restenosis (beyond demonstrating the feasibility of vascular gene transfer or genetic manipulation in vivo) has followed a number of distinct strategies. One strategy is to target growth factors and cytokines that are known to stimulate smooth muscle cell migration or proliferation in vitro and that have been shown to play a role in vivo. Several studies have demonstrated a pathophysiologic role for growth factors in restenosis.[95] To extend these observations, and as proof of the principle of efficient gene delivery, investigators have overexpressed some of these genes, using in vivo gene transfer techniques. The local expression of acidic FGF,[96] PDGF-B,[97] TGF-β_1,[98] and angiotensin converting enzyme[99] have all produced neointimal hyperplasia or hypertrophy (either de novo or in response to vascular injury) in animal models. As of this writing, no studies have been published describing the inhibition of any of these factors by gene transfer, although antisense basic FGF oligonucleotides have been shown to inhibit the proliferation of Kaposi sarcoma cells in vivo in nude mice.[100] Another approach has been to target nuclear factors that are expressed or are required for progression through the cell cycle in all cells as a means of targeting a central pathway common to the actions of many growth factors and cytokines. A number of previously recognized proto-oncogenes such as c-*myc* and c-*myb* are expressed by many cell types in response to mitogens, including smooth muscle cells, and participate in normal progression through the cell cycle. Antisense oligodeoxynucleotides directed against these genes are effective in inhibiting smooth muscle cell proliferation in vitro. Delivered either to the luminal or adventitial surface, antisense oligodeoxynucleotides directed against c-*myb*[49] or c-*myc*[101, 102] have attenuated the neointimal response to vascular injury in animal models. Other genes known to be expressed by actively dividing cells include proliferating cell nuclear antigen (PCNA) and nonmuscle myosin heavy chain (nmMHC) isoforms. Both nmMHC[103] and PCNA[104] have been targeted with antisense oligodeoxynucleotides, resulting in an attenuation of neointimal hyperplasia. Recent progress in our understanding of genes that control progression through the cell cycle has identified cyclins and their associated cyclin-dependent kinases (cdks) whose activities in concert are required for proper cell cycling. These genes have been targeted by antisense oligodeoxynucleotides as well, and it was recently demonstrated that inhibition of at least two of these essential (although potentially redundant) components was required to achieve nearly complete inhibition of proliferation, whereas each oligodeoxynucleotide alone was partially effective.[105, 106] All of these oligodeoxynucleotide approaches are subject to the technical caveats and limitations discussed in an earlier section on the use of these agents to modify gene expression.

More recently, recombinant adenovirus has been used successfully to demonstrate efficient gene transfer to the vasculature (as reviewed previously). In a recent exciting development, two groups applied the HSV–thymidine kinase (HSV-tk)/ganciclovir system for achieving effective local killing of infected smooth muscle cells and their near neighbors. Initially developed in the context of gene therapy for a variety of neoplastic diseases,[107–117] this approach is based on transfer of the HSV-tk gene to target cells. The HSV-tk gene encodes a viral-specific enzyme of the pyrimidine salvage pathway that phosphorylates thymidine, rendering it available for incorporation into DNA. Ganciclovir, a DNA chain–terminating nucleoside analog, is useful as an antiviral drug because it is taken up by cells as a prodrug. The prodrug is phosphorylated efficiently by the virally encoded tk enzyme but only poorly by normal cellular enzymes, resulting in relative selectivity of its activity in cells harboring the viral enzyme. Incorporation of the active drug into DNA in cells expressing tk leads to DNA chain termination, effectively killing the cell. Adenoviral-mediated gene transfer to porcine iliofemoral[118] or rat carotid[119] arteries followed by systemic ganciclovir administration effectively attenuated neointimal thickening in these models.

Two other gene transfer experiments have recently been reported that also demonstrate effective inhibition of neointimal thickening in the rat carotid model. In the first, a nonphosphorylatable analog of the cell cycle regulatory protein Rb (the retinoblastoma gene product) was used to inhibit smooth muscle cell proliferation and neointimal thickening.[120] Phosphorylation of Rb is required for normal cell cycle progression, and the presence of the nonphosphorylatable analog serves as a dominant negative regulator preventing cell cycle progression. Adenoviral gene transfer of this analog was shown to prevent the typical neointimal accumulation of smooth muscle cells after vascular injury.

In the other recent study, endothelial cell nitric oxide synthase (ec-NOS) was transferred to carotid smooth muscle cells after injury as a means of inhibiting neointimal thickening.[121] Before this study, a number of observations suggested that local production of nitric oxide served to generate a negative growth regulatory signal for vascular smooth muscle cells. It was postulated that the loss of endothelium after vascular injury, in addition to exposing the vascular smooth muscle cells directly to the circulation, led to the loss of this negative growth regulatory influence. This gene transfer experiment suggests that the loss of local nitric oxide production contributes to the hyperplastic response after injury and that restoration of nitric oxide production to physiologic levels may partially ameliorate this response.

In summary, all these strategies targeting growth factors, proto-oncogenes, and cell cycle proteins that are common to many if not all cells signify that specificity is generated strictly by delivery techniques or the use of tissue-restricted expression in the case of gene transfer vectors. Further refinements in the design and delivery of gene therapy vectors suggest that several of these experimental approaches may well turn out to be practical for routine clinical use. These experiments also demonstrate the important principle that the delivery and expression of gene-enhancing or gene-inhibiting vectors may be efficient enough at the present stage of development to be physiologically meaningful. Further efforts to continue to improve the technology for vascular cell gene transfer and drug delivery are under way, and research on the molecular mechanisms controlling smooth muscle cell behavior continues in order to provide the rationale for choosing appropriate molecular targets for future intervention.

Myocardial Gene Therapy

The development of gene transfer methods for use in the heart has followed a track parallel to that of gene transfer to the vasculature. Approaches have included direct application of naked DNA, DNA in complex with liposomes, recombinant adenovirus, and genetically modified myoblast implantation. Each of these approaches has its advantages and disadvantages, but many of the experiments conducted to date have represented important contributions in terms of proof of principle, technologic development, or definition of pathophysiologic mechanisms of normal function and dysfunction. For example, transgenic mice have already demonstrated the potential of transferred genes to alter myocardial mass, proliferative capacity, and contractile function. Transgenic mice overexpressing the cellular proto-oncogene c-*myc* in their cardiomyocytes exhibit myocyte hyperplasia during normal development[122] and display an exaggerated hypertrophic response to certain stimuli.[123] Similarly, mice overexpressing the calcium-binding regulatory gene calmodulin also show altered proliferative capacity during development, with atrial enlargement.[124] When the viral oncogene SV40 large T-antigen is constitutively expressed in mouse heart, the hearts form giant atria, and derived atrial cardiomyocytes can be passaged to a limited extent in vitro as well as propagated indefinitely as subcutaneous tumors in syngeneic hosts in vivo.[125, 126] In a recent set of experiments that are perhaps more physiologically relevant, it was shown that transgenic overexpression of a beta-adrenergic receptor gene could confer enhanced contractile function even in the absence of receptor agonists.[127] This experiment complements previous observations of decreased beta-adrenergic receptor expression in human cardiac failure.[128] A similar transgenic experiment demonstrated the complexities of adrenergic receptor function and specificity of action in the heart in vivo: mice overexpressing an alpha-adrenergic receptor were shown to develop cardiac hypertrophy spontaneously.[129] These elegant studies give a glimpse of the potential for gene therapy of the heart to treat congestive or hypertrophic cardiomyopathies. As the fields of disease gene identification, molecular pathophysiology, and in vivo gene transfer continue to converge, the potential to intervene in the diseases of the heart continues to grow.

Direct Myocardial Injection of Plasmid DNA

Although direct injection of DNA into the myocardium is generally of much lower efficiency than in skeletal muscle, it has led to measurable gene expression.[130] In this study, plasmid DNA encoding the marker gene beta-galactosidase was injected directly into the rat ventricular myocardium in vivo. Expression of the marker gene was detected in rat hearts up to 4 weeks after the gene transfer procedure. Histochemical detection of gene expression was focal and patchy in distribution and limited to cardiomyocytes at the injection site of those animals receiving DNA. The distribution of gene expression suggested that the uptake and expression of the foreign DNA was a low-frequency event despite exposure of a large number of cells to many copies of the DNA. In addition, it was noted by these authors that there was evidence of acute inflammatory cell infiltrate along the needle track at the early time point as well as occasional foci of fibrosis noted at the injection site at the later time point. Similar results were obtained by another group,[131] although expression was detected for only 2 weeks after DNA injection. As in the previous study, an inflammatory response appeared to be involved in the host reaction to gene transfer. These issues of efficiency and host tissue responses to the gene transfer vehicle are the main limitations of many current approaches to gene transfer in vivo, but this early attempt at gene transfer in the beating heart in situ showed that such an approach was feasible and that nondividing functioning cardiomyocytes could be programmed to express a transgene.

As further proof of the principle using direct DNA injection into myocardium in vivo, this approach has been used to study tissue-specific[132, 133] or hormone-responsive[134] expression of transferred genes in the myocardium. In the first of these studies,[132] plasmid DNA vectors containing different promoters driving the expression of marker genes (either chloramphenicol acetyltransferase or firefly luciferase) were injected into the apex of the left ventricle of rats after surgical exposure of the beating heart. This study compared the tissue-specific expression of a viral LTR promoter (Rous sarcoma virus [RSV]), a heart-specific promoter (α-MHC), and a liver-specific promoter (α_1-antitrypsin). As predicted by the behavior of these promoter elements in their native environments and from in vitro studies in cultured cardiomyocytes, both the RSV and α-MHC promoters drove expression of the marker genes in rat heart in vivo, whereas the liver-specific promoter was silent. Furthermore, the viral promoter was about 20-fold more efficient at driving transgene expression than the α-MHC promoter. As in the earlier studies, expression was mainly restricted to the area immediately surrounding the injection site. With either promoter, expression peaked at 7 days and fell off fairly steeply after 2 weeks. This method was then used to demonstrate that the α-MHC promoter, known to confer thyroid hormone responsiveness of the native α-MHC gene in vivo, could be used to confer both tissue-specific expression and hormonal responsiveness on a heterologous reporter gene injected as plasmid DNA into rat heart in vivo.[134]

The study of tissue-specific gene expression in myocardium was later extended to a large animal model.[135] This study used plasmid DNA vectors containing marker genes (either chloramphenicol acetyltransferase or firefly luciferase) with expression driven by either a promiscuous (murine sarcoma virus) or a tissue-specific (β-MHC) promoter. These studies demonstrated several important observations. First, the use of the tissue-specific promoter, although not able to direct exclusive cardiac expression of the marker gene, could produce selective expression of the transgene that was two orders of magnitude greater in heart than in skeletal muscle. Second, this study carefully charted the time course of expression over a 3-week period and showed that in the dog heart, plasmid DNA-mediated gene transfer was detectable at 3 days, peaked at 7 days, and declined up to 21 days after gene transfer. Third, by using a series of plasmids containing deletions of the β-MHC promoter, these authors demonstrated the location within the promoter of regulatory sequences required for directing tissue-specific expression of the transgene in vivo. In addition, they showed that a plasmid containing the α-MHC promoter was about sixfold less active than the β-MHC promoter in canine myocardium, which is consistent with the relative levels of expression of the endogenous alpha and beta isoforms in canine ventricle.

An important study validated the in vivo gene transfer method as a means to define the hormone-responsive regulation of gene expression in a manner that is perhaps more relevant than transferring genes to cultured cardiomyocytes.[133] Previous studies showed that transgenic mice bearing the entire regulatory region between the α- and β-MHC genes coupled to a reporter gene displayed appropriate tissue-specific and hormone-responsive expression of the reporter gene.[136] Subsequently, the regulatory elements of the α-MHC gene thought to be responsible for thyroid hormone responsiveness in vivo were mapped within this large region through transfection of a series of reporter gene constructs into cultured fetal cardiomyocytes in vitro. These in vitro studies defined a region, called the thyroid hormone response element (TRE), located on a stretch of DNA only 20 base pairs long upstream of the α-MHC gene that can bind the thyroid hormone receptor, resulting in enhanced gene expression.[137, 138] The main contribution of the in vivo gene transfer studies of this regulatory element, as studied by direct injection of plasmid DNA into rat hearts in vivo, was that the TRE as defined by the in vitro studies was not sufficient to confer either positive or negative thyroid hormone responsiveness in vivo.[133] Mutating the TRE in the context of the entire regulatory region abolished positive thyroid hormone responsiveness in vivo, thus showing that the TRE was necessary, but not sufficient, to control hormonal responsiveness in the adult rat heart. This demonstration of important differences between studying the regulation of tissue-specific gene expression in vivo and studying it in vitro illustrates a major contribution of in vivo gene transfer to the study of molecular pathophysiology. Such an approach could conceivably be used to define the molecular mechanisms whereby altered gene expression or mutated gene products contribute to cardiac disease, such as in hypertrophic cardiomyopathy or cardiac failure. Direct myocardial injection of DNA is, therefore, potentially useful for such analytic approaches. Because of low efficiency and lack of persistent expression, however, this technique is probably not of any significant therapeutic value. It has been largely superceded by other approaches, chiefly the use of viral gene transfer vectors such as recombinant adenovirus.

Myocardial Gene Transfer With the Use of Recombinant Adenovirus

The use of recombinant adenovirus as an in vivo gene transfer vector for the heart has been under intensive investigation over the past few years. One of the first reports of myocardial transgene expression mediated by recombinant adenovirus actually used intravenous delivery, resulting in gene transfer to a variety of tissues, including the heart.[139] Subsequent reports have attempted to localize gene delivery through the use of intramyocardial delivery of virus.[140, 141] Perhaps the most exciting development in this area combines the more efficient adenoviral vector with a percutaneous, catheter-based approach targeting either the coronary vasculature[89] or the myocardium (or both).[142] This technique hints at the great therapeutic potential of vascular and myocardial gene therapy.

In the intravenous injection study,[139] several important observations were made. First, a single intravenous injection in neonatal mice of up to 4×10^9 plaque-forming units (pfu) of a recombinant virus expressing beta-galactosidase driven by the RSV LTR resulted in readily detectable expression in selected organs throughout the body, including heart, skeletal muscle, liver, lungs, and intestine, at 2 weeks after injection. Similar results were obtained with intravenous injection in adult mice with respect to tissue distribution of expression, but in general expression was less readily detectable in the larger, adult mice. Second, direct intramuscular injections in adult mice were effective in transferring the marker gene to the site of injection, but expression was not detected elsewhere in the body, in contrast to the intravenous delivery method. Third, and most intriguing, expression in the heart and skeletal muscle of the mice injected as neonates showed relatively stable expression for up to 1 year after gene transfer. Although not specifically discussed in this report, it has been speculated that the ability of the adenovirus to remain stable in the mouse tissues for many months reflects the lack of complete immune competence in neonates, especially of cell-mediated immunity. More recent studies designed to specifically address the lack of persistence of adenoviral gene transfer in immune-competent animals have documented a cell-mediated immune response directed against adenovirally infected cells,[25–27] which could account for these results. Although not necessarily applicable to the use of adenovirus for gene transfer in immunocompetent adults, these studies have helped develop a better understanding of the biology of the recombinant adenovirus as used for gene transfer and the associated host response. This host response is common to all of the so-called first-generation recombinant adenovirus vectors regardless of route of administration (see earlier discussion) and represents one of the ongoing challenges to those involved in vector development.

Intramyocardial delivery of recombinant adenovirus has been reported in the rat[140] and the pig.[141] These studies were useful in that they compared recombinant adenovirus in a head-to-head fashion with plasmid DNA–based gene transfer in the context of direct injection into the heart. The rat study compared the delivery by direct injection of either 5×10^8 pfu of adenovirus or 200 μg (about 2.5×10^{13} copies) of a plasmid DNA expression vector encoding beta-galactosidase. The pig study similarly compared the direct injection of either 1.4×10^9 pfu of virus per injection or 200 μg of a similar reporter plasmid encoding firefly luciferase. By measuring the production of reporter gene enzymatic activity in extracts of myocardium, a quantitative analysis could be performed to compare the functional end point of gene transfer, that is, the production of active gene product. These analyses showed in both cases that adenoviral delivery of the reporter gene was more efficient (on a molar basis or per gene copy delivered) than plasmid DNA by a factor of about 10^5. Despite this improved efficiency, both these studies noted that gene transfer was limited to the area of the injection site, and the duration of expression after adenovirus-mediated gene transfer was similar in duration (2–3 weeks) to gene transfer with the use of plasmid DNA. A local inflammatory cell infiltrate was noted at the injection site in both studies, which is consistent with the experience of other groups using plasmid DNA–mediated gene transfer. Although part of this inflammatory response may be due to a nonspecific reaction to the mechanical trauma of direct injection, in the pig heart study a significant component was associated with the immunohistochemical identification of $CD8^+$ lymphocytes in addition to $CD44^+$ leukocytes characteristic of the nonspecific response to mechanical trauma. These findings are again consistent with the more detailed studies of the immune response to adenoviral antigens characteristic of gene transfer with the first generation of replication-defective recombinant adenovirus vectors, as discussed in an earlier section. It is anticipated that advances in vector design based on the results of improved knowledge of the biology of the virus in the context of in vivo gene transfer will reduce the impact of the immune response on the survival of genetically modified host cells and persistence of transgene expression. More pertinent to the discussion at this point is the observation made in both of these studies that local delivery of recombinant adenovirus results in much more efficient transgene expression in cardiomyocytes than was previously observed with the use of other methods. As these studies used either direct (via thoracotomy) or indirect (transdiaphragmatic) surgical exposure of the heart to achieve in vivo gene transfer, the next major advance was the ability to deliver recombinant adenovirus percutaneously via intracoronary catheter to the myocardium.

Percutaneous delivery of gene therapy agents is generally regarded as the approach most likely to prove clinically useful in the long run. A nonsurgical, percutaneous approach that does not require general anesthesia and can take advantage of the catheter-based systems of the interventional cardiologist and radiologist presents obvious advantages over open surgical alternatives. It is therefore important that any gene therapy approach not only demonstrate high efficiency per se but also be adaptable to a catheter-based approach.

Catheter-based application has been shown to be effective in the delivery of gene transfer vectors other than recombinant adenovirus, although the efficiency was low and comparable to other means of delivering these vectors. Catheter-based delivery has now been used with recombinant adenovirus as well, and the efficiency of gene transfer was shown to be at least as high as with local injection and more widely distributed. With the use of an intracoronary catheter introduced percutaneously via the carotid artery in the rabbit, a recombinant adenovirus expressing beta-galactosidase was used to examine the extent and time course of gene transfer to the coronary vasculature and myocardium.[142] In sharp contrast to the results obtained with direct injection, percutaneous catheter delivery of the recombinant adenovirus to the coronary artery resulted in widespread expression along the length of the coronary artery and throughout the territory of myocardium perfused by the injected artery. Arterial gene transfer was somewhat patchy, involving predominantly endothelial cells of both large and small coronary arteries and of myocardial capillaries, but it also included occasional spindle-shaped cells in the media of large- and medium-sized arteries consistent with gene transfer to medial smooth muscle cells. Gene transfer to the myocardium was very efficient and resulted in detection of beta-galactosidase activity in an average of one third of the virus-perfused cardiomyocytes in animals receiving the highest dose of recombinant adenovirus (10^{10} pfu). Interestingly, gene transfer was also detected in nonmyocytic connective tissue cells, a result not observed in the direct injection experiments. As with delivery of recombinant adenovirus by direct injection, the duration of expression was limited to 2–4 weeks. Despite complete loss of expression by 4 weeks, which correlated with physical loss of the vector DNA as assessed by polymerase chain reaction (PCR) of tissue samples, the lack of transgene expression was not associated with an inflammatory infiltrate or any evidence of scarring or fibrosis of the target tissue. The basis for this observation, although of no obvious consequence in terms of persistence of expression, is unclear. Confirmation of these observations by other groups or in other species has not been reported and will undoubtedly be required for further development in this important area. In any event, the ability to deliver potentially therapeutic transgenes percutaneously to the myocardium in an efficient manner represents an important advance in the area of myocardial gene therapy. Although promising, this approach is not the only one that holds great potential for therapeutic intervention in a variety of myocardial diseases. Another area that has exciting therapeutic potential is that of implanting (grafting) genetically modified myoblasts into the myocardium.

Myocardial Implantation of Genetically Modified Myoblasts

The transfer of genetically modified skeletal myoblasts to host tissues could potentially offer solutions to clinical problems characterized by absent or defective muscular tissues. As discussed in the section on gene transfer to skeletal muscle, adult skeletal myofibers contain a population of satellite cells that represent a reservoir of quiescent myoblasts that can be harvested, expanded in vitro, and genetically modified before autologous grafting. One advantage of this ex vivo genetic modification is that a relatively homogeneous population of muscle cells can be modified and expanded in vitro before implantation, resulting in a significant mass of genetically modified cells that could potentially persist in the host. Although presenting its own disadvantages (surgical harvest, extensive ex vivo manipulation), this approach may be more appropriate than direct in vivo gene transfer to skeletal muscle, depending on the circumstances. What has now become apparent is that these skeletal myoblasts may be returned not only to the host skeletal myofibers, where they fuse and contribute genetic information to the mature myofibers, but also to the host heart, where they can take up residence and express transgenes. Preliminary experiments using a cultured mouse myoblast cell line (C2C12) showed that unmodified (wild-type) myoblasts could be implanted in the myocardium of syngeneic hosts, where they ceased proliferation, differentiated into mature skeletal myotubes, and were shown to have no apparent deleterious effect on cardiac function.[143] Subsequently, in an exciting application of the ex vivo modified myoblast approach, this group subjected C2C12 myoblasts to in vitro gene transfer with a constitutively active isoform of TGF-β_1 under the control of the heavy metal–inducible metallothionein promoter. The genetically modified myoblasts were transferred to the ventricular myocardium of syngeneic mice by direct injection after surgical exposure. After allowing the animals to recover for 1 month, expression of the transgene was induced by adding zinc sulfate to the drinking water. Expression of the transgene in the differentiated, intramyocardial grafts was easily detected by immunohistochemical studies. Remarkably, the animals receiving the genetically modified myoblasts (but not control transfected myoblasts) displayed an angiogenic response to the TGF-β_1 transgene. This response was assessed by a subjective increase in the density of immunohistochemical staining for the endothelial cell marker von Willebrand factor, as well as autoradiographic evidence of increased endothelial cell DNA synthesis after injection of the mice with tritiated thymidine. Another important observation was that the syngeneic grafts did not promote any identifiable rejection response.[144] Although not necessarily of physiologic importance to the function of the host tissue in this example, this study demonstrated that genetically modified myoblasts could be used as an intracardiac graft to deliver biologically important amounts of recombinant proteins to the heart in vivo.

One of the important caveats of these intracardiac myoblast graft experiments is the potential that the altered tissue architecture of an intracardiac mass of skeletal muscle would produce deleterious mechanical or electrical consequences. Although not apparent from these initial experiments in mice, the small size of the grafts and the high native heart rate of these animals may have masked important electrical abnormalities. Even if they are not arrhythmogenic, it is unclear whether intracardiac grafts of skeletal muscle cells would be capable of contributing any physiologically useful contractile force to the host myocardium. If this could be accomplished, the potential for the treatment of various cardiomyopathies would be tremendous. As an alternative approach to this question, the same group has shown that neonatal cardiomyocytes (derived from a transgenic strain expressing beta-galactosidase driven by the cardiac α-MHC promoter) could be harvested and transplanted to a syngeneic host. The engrafted cardiomyocytes were shown to survive for at least 2 months and formed intercalated disc structures between grafted cardiomyocytes and host myocardium. Again, no immunologic response suggesting rejection was seen with these syngeneic grafts.[145] Although not definitive proof of electromechanical coupling of the engrafted cells, this exciting result at least suggests the potential for this approach.

In a novel approach to using skeletal myoblasts as intracardiac grafts, another group has taken advantage of the ability of members of a family of myogenic regulatory genes to produce a skeletal muscle phenotype when constitutively expressed in a variety of heterologous cell types. By retrovirally mediated gene transfer of a myogenic regulatory gene to cardiac fibroblasts participating in the formation of scar after experimental myocardial infarction, a proportion of these fibroblasts were converted into myoblasts. Although reported in abstract form only,[146] this approach could potentially fill a unique niche in the developing field of myocardial gene therapy.

GENE THERAPY OF LIPID DISORDERS

The discussion of gene therapy for cardiovascular diseases would be incomplete without consideration of the approaches being developed to alter noncardiac diseases with serious cardiovascular consequences. The dyslipidemias are a heterogeneous group of syndromes caused by a complex array of genetic and environmental factors. Many of the important functions of individual components of lipoproteins, their synthetic and catabolic pathways, and the cells responsible for their production and clearance have been well defined over the past decades. Both the existence of naturally occurring mutations (such as those causing familial hypercholesterolemia) and the generation of transgenic or knockout mice corresponding to individual components of lipid metabolism have helped identify potential targets for gene therapy of lipid disorders.

The liver is one of the major sites of both synthesis and catabolism of lipoproteins and is responsible for many of the important pathways having an impact on cardiovascular consequences. Most of the current efforts in the area of gene therapy for lipid disorders are therefore focused on liver-directed gene therapy. The liver is also important to a wide spectrum of other disorders; therefore, a full discussion of liver-directed gene therapy is beyond the scope of this chapter. Interested readers are referred to recent reviews of this important area of gene therapy research.[147, 148] Several important concepts are worth mentioning. First, hepatocytes, unlike many other differentiated cell types, retain the capacity to proliferate in vivo and in vitro, and this can be taken advantage of in different ways. For example, this property makes recombinant retroviral vectors suitable for gene transfer. Second, this capacity to proliferate in vivo results in the well-known property of the liver to fully regenerate from as little as 10% of its original mass after injury or hepatectomy. This provides a ready source of autologous hepatocytes for schemes using ex vivo genetic modification and reimplantation. Third, hepatocytes have the ability, like bone marrow cells, to "home in" on their organ of origin when reinfused into the circulation,[149] which is another advantage for ex vivo modification and reimplantation strategies. Fourth, the liver is a natural site of filtration of the circulation, with a fenestrated endothelium that permits direct contact between the circulation and a large surface area of hepatic parenchyma, rendering the liver perhaps more susceptible than many other organs to gene therapy vectors. In fact, many studies of adenoviral gene transfer targeted to other organs have noted variable amounts of gene transfer to the liver (see previous discussion).

The area of liver-directed gene therapy for lipid disorders has been helped immensely by the prior existence of both a heritable disorder (familial hypercholesterolemia [FH]) known to be caused by mutations in a single gene (the LDL receptor) and a naturally occurring animal model of the same disease (the WHHL rabbit). The notion that replacement of the defective gene could potentially cure this progressive, fatal disease is based on the observation that the metabolic defect is completely corrected by orthotopic liver transplantation.[150] Furthermore, overexpression of the gene in transgenic mice leads to an almost complete absence of circulating LDL.[151] The WHHL rabbit model was used to demonstrate that autologous hepatocytes could be harvested, modified ex vivo with a recombinant retrovirus encoding a functional LDL receptor, and reimplanted, resulting in at least temporary improvement in hyperlipidemia.[152] This approach was eventually developed for one of the first clinical applications of gene therapy, and the initial experience with an FH patient has been reported.[153] Although an important milestone, this approach still requires surgical harvest (partial hepatectomy), considerable ex vivo manipulation of the patient's hepatocytes, and the use of recombinant retroviral vectors (with the caveats discussed in the earlier section on retroviruses). For these reasons, future approaches to gene therapy for FH will likely rely on strategies that can achieve gene transfer in vivo, such as recombinant adenovirus.

The principle of adenoviral gene transfer to the liver in vivo has been well demonstrated.[147, 148] With respect to gene therapy of FH, a recombinant adenovirus encoding the LDL receptor was shown to accelerate the clearance of circulating LDL acutely when delivered to normal mice.[154] In a murine model of gene therapy for the human disease, adenovirally mediated transfer of the LDL receptor gene to the liver of LDL receptor knockout mice was shown to correct the hypercholesterolemia associated with a complete lack of functional LDL receptors.[155] This same approach has been successful when applied to the WHHL rabbit[156] and has been applied to hepatocytes from FH patients in vitro.[157] Although the usefulness of the current generation of adenoviral gene transfer vectors in the setting of liver-directed gene therapy will likely be limited by the lack of persistence resulting from immunologic clearance mechanisms, improvements in vector design will eventually make in vivo gene transfer the method of choice for genetic correction of FH. In addition, this entire effort provides an instructive paradigm for the treatment of a range of disorders of hepatic origin or those amenable to the hepatogenous synthesis and delivery of therapeutic proteins to the circulation.

GENE THERAPY TO ALTER HEMOSTASIS

The final area to be considered in this discussion of gene therapy for cardiovascular diseases is that of gene therapy for hemostasis and thrombosis. Although most patients with cardiovascular diseases do not have intrinsic defects in hemostasis, a number of drugs designed to alter hemostasis make a significant contribution to our ability to treat common syndromes. The advent of widespread thrombolytic therapy has been credited with making a significant contribution to the progressive fall in mortality from acute myocardial infarction, and both heparin and aspirin make an important difference in outcome of unstable angina. Despite these recent improvements in the use of therapeutic agents and our understanding of pathophysiology, many cardiologists feel that there is more ground to be gained. For example, there has been little improvement in our ability to prolong the average life span of the saphenous vein coronary bypass graft, and thromboembolic complications remain a much feared aspect of life for those with endovascular prostheses such as mechanical valves. As our knowledge of fibrinolysis and hemostasis (including platelet function and vasomotor reactivity) has become more refined, the identification of individual molecular components has suggested potential targets for gene therapy of selected disorders. For example, it has become apparent that the natural anticoagulant and platelet-resistant surface of the normal endothelium might provide a model for the development of an engineered anticoagulant surface for use in endovascular prostheses. Specific knowledge of the activation cascade of platelets and the molecules that participate in their adhesion, aggregation, and degranulation might permit the local application of molecules designed to thwart these events. The ability of newer antithrombins to inhibit potently and specifically both the procoagulant and growth-promoting (thrombin receptor–dependent) effects of thrombin has generated strategies to deliver these agents to local sites to achieve greater efficacy and increase their therapeutic index.

CONCLUSIONS

The field of gene therapy and its application to cardiovascular diseases will continue to develop, and the specific approaches discussed in this chapter will likely be considered largely of historical interest. The principles behind these approaches, however, form the basis for future developments and therefore constitute the most important feature of this chapter. Improved viral and nonviral vectors are under development, and improved mechanical delivery systems will also enhance our future ability to modify basic disease mechanisms. Continued labratory research into the basic mechanisms contributing to cardiovascular diseases will help define the specific targets most appropriate for intervention and provide the highest likelihood of sustained therapeutic benefit. In concert with more traditional modes of drug therapy, gene therapy will permit an unprecedented ability to intervene in the treatment of a variety of cardiovascular diseases.

REFERENCES

1. Russell DW, Yamamoto T, Schneider WJ, et al: cDNA cloning of the bovine low density lipoprotein receptor: feedback regulation of a receptor mRNA. Proc Natl Acad Sci USA 1983; 80:7501–7505.
2. Fananapazir L, Epstein ND: Genotype-phenotype correlations in hypertrophic cardiomyopathy. Insights provided by comparisons of kindreds with distinct and identical beta-MHC gene mutations. Circulation 1994; 89:22–32.
3. Hengstenberg C, Schwartz K: Molecular genetics of familial hypertrophic cardiomyopathy [Review]. J Mol Cell Cardiol 1994; 26:3–10. [Published errata appear in J Mol Cell Cardiol 1994; 26(2):276 and 1994; 26(3):277.]
4. Solomon SD, Jarcho JA, McKenna W, et al: Familial hypertrophic cardiomyopathy is a genetically heterogeneous disease. J Clin Invest 1990; 86:993–999.
5. Geisterfer LA, Kass S, Tanigawa G, et al: A molecular basis for familial hypertrophic cardiomyopathy: a beta cardiac MHC gene missense mutation. Cell 1990; 62:999–1006.
6. Thierfelder L, Watkins H, MacRae C, et al: Alpha-tropomyosin and cardiac troponin T mutations cause familial hypertrophic cardiomyopathy: a disease of the sarcomere. Cell 1994; 77:701–712.
7. Watkins H, Rosenzweig A, Hwang DS, et al: Characteristics and prognostic implications of myosin missense mutations in familial hypertrophic cardiomyopathy. N Engl J Med 1992; 326:1108–1114.
8. Anan R, Greve G, Thierfelder L, et al: Prognostic implications of novel beta cardiac MHC gene mutations that cause familial hypertrophic cardiomyopathy. J Clin Invest 1994; 93:280–285.
9. Sweeney HL, Straceski AJ, Leinwand LA, et al: Heterologous expression of a cardiomyopathic myosin that is defective in its actin interaction. J Biol Chem 1994; 269:1603–1605.
10. Straceski AJ, Geisterfer LA, Seidman CE, et al: Functional analysis of myosin missense mutations in familial hypertrophic cardiomyopathy. Proc Natl Acad Sci USA 1994; 91:589–593.
11. Felgner PL, Gadek TR, Holm M, et al: Lipofection: a highly efficient, lipid-mediated DNA-transfection procedure. Proc Natl Acad Sci USA 1987; 84:7413.
12. Miller AD, Miller DG, Garcia JV, Lynch CM: Use of retroviral vectors for gene transfer and expression. Methods Enzymol 1993; 217:581–599.
13. Boris LK, Temin HM: Recent advances in retrovirus vector technology [Review]. Curr Opin Genet Dev 1993; 3:102–109.
14. Miller DG, Adam MA, Miller AD: Gene transfer by retrovirus vectors occurs only in cells that are actively replicating at the time of infection. Mol Cell Biol 1990; 10:4239–4242. [Published erratum appears in Mol Cell Biol 1992; 12(1):433.]
15. Burns JC, Friedmann T, Driever W, et al: Vesicular stomatitis virus G glycoprotein pseudotyped retroviral vectors: concentration to very high titer and efficient gene transfer into mammalian and nonmammalian cells. Proc Natl Acad Sci USA 1993; 90:8033–8037.
16. Yee JK, Miyanohara A, Laporte P, et al: A general method for the generation of high-titer, pantropic retroviral vectors—highly efficient infection of primary hepatocytes. Proc Natl Acad Sci USA 1994; 91:9564–9568.
17. Burns JC, Matsubara T, Lozinski G, et al: Pantropic retroviral vector-mediated gene transfer, integration, and expression in cultured newt limb cells. Dev Biol 1994; 165:285–289.
18. Lin S, Gaiano N, Culp P, et al: Integration and germ-line transmission of a pseudotyped retroviral vector in zebrafish. Science 1994; 265:666–669.
19. Cornetta K, Morgan RA, Anderson WF: Safety issues related to retroviral-mediated gene transfer in humans [Review]. Hum Gene Ther 1991; 2:5–14.
20. Boris LK, Temin HM: The retroviral vector. Replication cycle and safety considerations for retrovirus-mediated gene therapy [Review]. Ann NY Acad Sci 1994; 716:59–70.
21. Graham FL, Prevec L: Adenovirus-based expression vectors and recombinant vaccines [Review]. Biotechnology 1992; 20:363–390.
22. Haj AY, Graham FL: Development of a helper-independent human adenovirus vector and its use in the transfer of the herpes simplex virus thymidine kinase gene. J Virol 1986; 57:267–274.
23. Ghosh CG, Haj AJ, Brinkley P, et al: Human adenovirus cloning vectors based on infectious bacterial plasmids. Gene 1986; 50:161–171.
24. Ketner G, Spencer F, Tugendreich S, et al: Efficient manipulation of the human adenovirus genome as an infectious yeast artificial chromosome clone. Proc Natl Acad Sci USA 1994; 91:6186–6190.
25. Engelhardt JF, Litzky L, Wilson JM: Prolonged transgene expression in cotton rat lung with recombinant adenoviruses defective in E2a. Hum Gene Ther 1994; 5:1217–1229.
26. Kass-Eisler A, Falck-Pedersen E, Elfenbein DH, et al: The impact of developmental stage, route of administration and the immune system on adenovirus-mediated gene transfer. Gene Ther 1994; 1:395–402.
27. Yang Y, Nunes FA, Berencsi K, et al: Cellular immunity to viral antigens limits E1-deleted adenoviruses for gene therapy. Proc Natl Acad Sci USA 1994; 91:4407–4411.
28. Engelhardt JF, Ye X, Doranz B, Wilson JM: Ablation of E2A in recombinant adenoviruses improves transgene persistence and decreases inflammatory response in mouse liver. Proc Natl Acad Sci USA 1994; 91:6196–6200.
29. Geller AI, Keyomarsi K, Bryan J, Pardee AB: An efficient deletion mutant packaging system for defective herpes simplex virus vectors: potential applications to human gene therapy and neuronal physiology. Proc Natl Acad Sci USA 1990; 87:8950–8954.
30. Nahreini P, Larsen SH, Srivastava A: Cloning and integration of DNA fragments in human cells via the inverted terminal repeats of the adeno-associated virus 2 genome. Gene 1992; 119:265–272.
31. Samulski RJ: Adeno-associated virus: integration at a specific chromosomal locus [Review]. Curr Opin Genet Dev 1993; 3:74–80.
32. Russell DW, Miller AD, Alexander IE: Adeno-associated virus vectors preferentially transduce cells in S phase. Proc Natl Acad Sci USA 1994; 91:8915–8919.
33. Nahreini P, Woody MJ, Zhou SZ, Srivastava A: Versatile adeno-associated virus 2-based vectors for constructing recombinant virions. Gene 1993; 124:257–262.
34. Podsakoff G, Wong KF, Chatterjee S: Efficient gene transfer into non-dividing cells by adeno-associated virus-based vectors. J Virol 1994; 68:5656–5666.
35. Flotte TR, Afione SA, Conrad C, et al: Stable in vivo expression of the cystic fibrosis transmembrane conductance regulator with an adeno-associated virus vector. Proc Natl Acad Sci USA 1993; 90:10613–10617.
36. Walsh CE, Nienhuis AW, Samulski RJ, et al: Phenotypic correction of Fanconi anemia in human hematopoietic cells with a recombinant adeno-associated virus vector. J Clin Invest 1994; 94:1440–1448.
37. Pincus S, Mason PW, Konishi E, et al: Recombinant vaccinia virus producing the prM and E proteins of yellow fever virus protects mice from lethal yellow fever encephalitis. Virology 1992; 187:290–297.
38. Stein CA: Anti-sense oligodeoxynucleotides—promises and pitfalls. Leukemia 1992; 6:967–974.
39. Bredenbeek PJ, Frolov I, Rice CM, Schlesinger S: Sindbis virus expression vectors: packaging of RNA replicons by using defective helper RNAs. J Virol 1993; 67:6439–6446.
40. Michael SI, Curiel DT: Strategies to achieve targeted gene delivery via the receptor mediated endocytosis pathway. Gene Ther 1994; 1:223–232.
41. Cotten M, Wagner E, Zatloukal K, et al: High-efficiency receptor-mediated delivery of small and large 48 kilobase gene constructs using the endosome-disruption activity of defective or chemically inactivated adenovirus particles. Proc Natl Acad Sci USA 1992; 89:6094–6098.
42. Cotten M, Wagner E, Zatloukal K, Birnstiel ML: Chicken adenovirus (CELO virus) particles augment receptor-mediated DNA delivery to mammalian cells and yield exceptional levels of stable transformants. J Virol 1993; 67:3777–3785.
43. Morishita R, Gibbons GH, Kaneda Y, et al: Novel and effective gene transfer technique for study of vascular renin angiotensin system. J Clin Invest 1993; 91:2580–2585.

44. Wagner E, Zatloukal K, Cotten M, et al: Coupling of adenovirus to transferrin-polylysine/DNA complexes greatly enhances receptor-mediated gene delivery and expression of transfected genes. Proc Natl Acad Sci USA 1992; 89:6099–6103.
45. Fisher KJ, Wilson JM: Biochemical and functional analysis of an adenovirus-based ligand complex for gene transfer. Biochem J 1994; 299:49–58.
46. Plank C, Zatloukal K, Cotten M, et al: Gene transfer into hepatocytes using a sialoglycoprotein receptor mediated endocytosis of DNA complexed with an artificial tetra-antennary galactose ligand. Bioconjugate Chemistry 1992; 3:533–539.
47. Wagner E, Plank C, Zatloukal K, et al: Influenza virus hemagglutinin HA-2 N-terminal fusogenic peptides augment gene transfer by transferrin-polylysine-DNA complexes: toward a synthetic virus-like gene-transfer vehicle. Proc Natl Acad Sci USA 1992; 89:7934–7938.
48. Stein CA, Cheng YC: Antisense oligonucleotides as therapeutic agents—is the bullet really magical? [Review]. Science 1993; 261:1004–1012.
49. Simons M, Edelman ER, DeKeyser J-L, et al: Antisense c-*myb* oligonucleotides inhibit intimal arterial smooth muscle cell accumulation in vivo. Nature 1992; 359:67–70.
50. Conrad R, Keranen LM, Ellington AD, Newton AC: Isozyme-specific inhibition of protein kinase C by RNA aptamers. J Biol Chem 1994; 269:32051–32054.
51. Hanvey JC, Peffer NJ, Bisi JE, et al: Antisense and antigene properties of peptide nucleic acids. Science 1992; 258:1481–1485.
52. Bock LC, Griffin LC, Latham JA, et al: Selection of single-stranded DNA molecules that bind and inhibit human thrombin. Nature 1992; 355:564–566.
53. Stein CA, Cleary AM, Yakubov L, Lederman S: Phosphorothioate oligodeoxynucleotides bind to the third variable loop domain (v3) of human immunodeficiency virus type 1 gp120. Antisense Res Dev 1993; 3:19–31.
54. Reynolds MA, Arnold LJ, Almazan MT, et al: Triple-strand-forming methylphosphonate oligodeoxynucleotides targeted to messenger-RNA efficiently block protein synthesis. Proc Natl Acad Sci USA 1994; 91:12433–12437.
55. Kinniburgh AJ, Firulli AB, Kolluri R: DNA triplexes and regulation of the *c-myc* gene. Gene 1994; 149:93–100.
56. Altman S: RNA enzyme-directed gene therapy [Comment]. Proc Natl Acad Sci USA 1993; 90:10898–10900.
57. Sullivan SM: Development of ribozymes for gene therapy. J Invest Dermatol 1994; 103:85S–89S.
58. Krieg AM, Tonkinson J, Matson S, et al: Modification of antisense phosphodiester oligodeoxynucleotides by a 5′ cholesteryl moiety increases cellular association and improves efficacy. Proc Natl Acad Sci USA 1993; 90:1048–1052.
59. Blau HM, Dhawan J, Pavlath GK: Myoblasts in pattern formation and gene therapy [Review]. Trends Genet 1993; 9:269–274.
60. Rando TA, Blau HM: Primary mouse myoblast purification, characterization, and transplantation for cell-mediated gene therapy. J Cell Biol 1994; 125:1275–1287.
61. Gussoni E, Pavlath GK, Lanctot AM, et al: Normal dystrophin transcripts detected in Duchenne muscular dystrophy patients after myoblast transplantation. Nature 1992; 356:435–438.
62. Morgan JE, Moore SE, Walsh FS, Partridge TA: Formation of skeletal muscle in vivo from the mouse C2 cell line. J Cell Sci 1992; 102:779–787.
63. Barr E, Leiden JM: Systemic delivery of recombinant proteins by genetically modified myoblasts. Science 1991; 254:1507–1509.
64. Dhawan J, Pan LC, Pavlath GK, et al: Systemic delivery of human growth hormone by injection of genetically engineered myoblasts. Science 1991; 254:1509–1512.
65. Jiao S, Williams P, Berg RK, et al: Direct gene transfer into nonhuman primate myofibers in vivo. Hum Gene Ther 1992; 3:21–33.
66. Wolff JA, Ludtke JJ, Acsadi G, et al: Long-term persistence of plasmid DNA and foreign gene expression in mouse muscle. Hum Mol Genet 1992; 1:363–369.
67. Davis HL, Demeneix BA, Quantin B, et al: Plasmid DNA is superior to viral vectors for direct gene transfer into adult mouse skeletal muscle. Hum Gene Ther 1993; 4:733–740.
68. Acsadi G, Jani A, Huard J, et al: Cultured human myoblasts and myotubes show markedly different transducibility by replication-defective adenovirus recombinants. Gene Ther 1994; 1:338–340.
69. Quantin B, Perricaudet LD, Tajbakhsh S, Mandel JL: Adenovirus as an expression vector in muscle cells in vivo. Proc Natl Acad Sci USA 1992; 89:2581–2584.
70. Ragot T, Vincent N, Chafey P, et al: Efficient adenovirus-mediated transfer of a human minidystrophin gene to skeletal muscle of mdx mice. Nature 1993; 361:647–650.
71. Tripathy SK, Goldwasser E, Lu MM, et al: Stable delivery of physiologic levels of recombinant erythropoietin to the systemic circulation by intramuscular injection of replication-defective adenovirus. Proc Natl Acad Sci USA 1994; 91:11557–11561.
72. Yao S-N, Smith KJ, Kurachi K: Primary myoblast-mediated gene transfer: persistent expression of human factor IX in mice. Gene Ther 1994; 1:99–107.
73. Zwiebel JA, Freeman SM, Kantoff PW, et al: High-level recombinant gene expression in rabbit endothelial cells transduced by retroviral vectors. Science 1989; 243:220–222.
74. Dichek DA, Neville RF, Zwiebel JA, et al: Seeding of intravascular stents with genetically engineered endothelial cells. Circulation 1989; 80:1347–1353.
75. Flugelman MY, Virmani R, Leon MB, et al: Genetically engineered endothelial cells remain adherent and viable after stent deployment and exposure to flow in vitro. Circ Res 1992; 70:348–354.
76. Wilson JM, Birinyi LK, Salomon RN, et al: Implantation of vascular grafts lined with genetically modified endothelial cells. Science 1989; 244:1344–1346.
77. Nabel EG, Plautz G, Boyce FM, et al: Recombinant gene expression in vivo within endothelial cells of the arterial wall. Science 1989; 244:1342–1344.
78. Plautz G, Nabel EG, Nabel GJ: Introduction of vascular smooth muscle cells expressing recombinant genes in vivo. Circulation 1991; 83:578–583.
79. Clowes MM, Lynch CM, Miller AD, et al: Long-term biological response of injured rat carotid artery seeded with smooth muscle cells expressing retrovirally introduced human genes. J Clin Invest 1994; 93:644–651.
80. Lim CS, Chapman GD, Gammon RS, et al: Direct in vivo gene transfer into the coronary and peripheral vasculatures of the intact dog. Circulation 1991; 83:2007–2011.
81. Chapman GD, Lim CS, Gammon RS, et al: Gene transfer into coronary arteries of intact animals with a percutaneous balloon catheter. Circ Res 1992; 71:27–33.
82. Leclerc G, Gal D, Takeshita S, et al: Percutaneous arterial gene transfer in a rabbit model. Efficiency in normal and balloon-dilated atherosclerotic arteries. J Clin Invest 1992; 90:936–944.
83. Riessen R, Rahimizadeh H, Blessing E, et al: Arterial gene transfer using pure DNA applied directly to a hydrogel-coated angioplasty balloon. Hum Gene Ther 1993; 4:749–758.
84. Nabel EG, Plautz G, Nabel GJ: Site-specific gene expression in vivo by direct gene transfer into the arterial wall. Science 1990; 249:1285–1288.
85. Flugelman MY, Jaklitsch MT, Newman KD, et al: Low level in vivo gene transfer into the arterial wall through a perforated balloon catheter. Circulation 1992; 85:1110–1117.
86. Lee SW, Trapnell BC, Rade JJ, et al: In vivo adenoviral vector-mediated gene transfer into balloon-injured rat carotid arteries. Circ Res 1993; 73:797–807.
87. Guzman RJ, Lemarchand P, Crystal RG, et al: Efficient and selective adenovirus-mediated gene transfer into vascular neointima. Circulation 1993; 88:2838–2848.
88. Lemarchand P, Jones M, Yamada I, Crystal RG: In vivo gene transfer and expression in normal uninjured blood vessels using replication-deficient recombinant adenovirus vectors. Circ Res 1993; 72:1132–1138.
89. French BA, Mazur W, Ali NM, et al: Percutaneous transluminal in vivo gene transfer by recombinant adenovirus in normal porcine coronary arteries, atherosclerotic arteries, and two models of coronary restenosis. Circulation 1994; 90:2402–2413.
90. Steg PG, Feldman LJ, Scoazec JY, et al: Arterial gene transfer to rabbit endothelial and smooth-muscle cells using percutaneous delivery of an adenoviral vector. Circulation 1994; 90:1648–1656.
91. Rome JJ, Shayani V, Flugelman MY, et al: Anatomic barriers influence the distribution of in vivo gene transfer into the arterial wall. Modeling with microscopic tracer particles and verification with a recombinant adenoviral vector. Arterioscler Thromb 1994; 14:148–161.
92. Casscells W: Migration of smooth muscle and endothelial cells. Critical events in restenosis [Review]. Circulation 1992; 86:723–729.
93. Libby P, Schwartz D, Brogi E, et al: A cascade model for restenosis. A special case of atherosclerosis progression. Circulation 1992; 86(suppl III):47–52.

94. Casscells W, Engler D, Willerson JT: Mechanisms of restenosis. Tex Heart Inst J 1994; 21:68–77.
95. Casscells W: Smooth muscle cell growth factors [Review]. Prog Growth Factor Res 1991; 3:177–206.
96. Nabel EG, Yang ZY, Plautz G, et al: Recombinant fibroblast growth factor-1 promotes intimal hyperplasia and angiogenesis in arteries in vivo. Nature 1993; 362:844–846.
97. Nabel EG, Yang Z, Liptay S, et al: Recombinant platelet-derived growth factor B gene expression in porcine arteries induce intimal hyperplasia in vivo. J Clin Invest 1993; 91:1822–1829.
98. Nabel EG, Shum L, Pompili VJ, et al: Direct transfer of transforming growth factor beta 1 gene into arteries stimulates fibrocellular hyperplasia. Proc Natl Acad Sci USA 1993; 90:10759–10763.
99. Morishita R, Gibbons GH, Ellison KE, et al: Evidence for direct local effect of angiotensin in vascular hypertrophy. In vivo gene transfer of angiotensin converting enzyme. J Clin Invest 1994; 94:978–984.
100. Ensoli B, Markham P, Kao V, et al: Block of AIDS Kaposi's sarcoma (KS) cell growth, angiogenesis, and lesion formation in nude mice by antisense oligonucleotide targeting basic fibroblast growth factor—a novel strategy for the therapy of KS. J Clin Invest 1994; 94:1736–1746.
101. Bennett MR, Anglin S, McEwan JR, et al: Inhibition of vascular smooth muscle cell proliferation in vitro and in vivo by *c-myc* antisense oligodeoxynucleotides. J Clin Invest 1994; 93:820–828.
102. Shi Y, Fard A, Galeo A, et al: Transcatheter delivery of *c-myc* antisense oligomers reduces neointimal formation in a porcine model of coronary artery balloon injury. Circulation 1994; 90:944–951.
103. Simons M, Rosenberg RD: Antisense nonmuscle myosin heavy chain and c-myb oligonucleotides suppress smooth muscle cell proliferation in vitro. Circulation Res 1992; 70:835–843.
104. Simons M, Edelman ER, Rosenberg RD: Antisense proliferating cell nuclear antigen oligonucleotides inhibit intimal hyperplasia in a rat carotid artery injury model. J Clin Invest 1994; 93:2351–2356.
105. Morishita R, Gibbons GH, Ellison KE, et al: Single intraluminal delivery of antisense cdc2 kinase and proliferating-cell nuclear antigen oligonucleotides results in chronic inhibition of neointimal hyperplasia. Proc Natl Acad Sci USA 1993; 90:8474–8478.
106. Morishita R, Gibbons GH, Ellison KE, et al: Intimal hyperplasia after vascular injury is inhibited by antisense cdk 2 kinase oligonucleotides. J Clin Invest 1994; 93:1458–1464.
107. Moolten FL, Wells JM, Heyman RA, Evans RM: Lymphoma regression induced by ganciclovir in mice bearing a herpes thymidine kinase transgene. Hum Gene Ther 1990; 1:125–134.
108. Plautz G, Nabel EG, Nabel GJ: Selective elimination of recombinant genes in vivo with a suicide retroviral vector. New Biologist 1991; 3:709–715.
109. Culver KW, Ram Z, Wallbridge S, et al: In vivo gene transfer with retroviral vector-producer cells for treatment of experimental brain tumors. Science 1992; 256:1550–1552.
110. Barba D, Hardin J, Ray J, Gage FH: Thymidine kinase–mediated killing of rat brain tumors. J Neurosurg 1993; 79:729–735.
111. Caruso M, Panis Y, Gagandeep S, et al: Regression of established macroscopic liver metastases after in situ transduction of a suicide gene. Proc Natl Acad Sci USA 1993; 90:7024–7028.
112. Oldfield EH, Ram Z, Culver KW, et al: Gene therapy for the treatment of brain tumors using intra-tumoral transduction with the thymidine kinase gene and intravenous ganciclovir. Hum Gene Ther 1993; 4:39–69.
113. Culver KW, Van GJ, Link CJ, et al: Gene therapy for the treatment of malignant brain tumors with in vivo tumor transduction with the herpes simplex thymidine kinase gene/ganciclovir system. Hum Gene Ther 1994; 5:343–379.
114. DiMaio JM, Clary BM, Via DF, et al: Directed enzyme pro-drug gene therapy for pancreatic cancer in vivo. Surgery 1994; 116:205–213.
115. Ram Z, Walbridge S, Shawker T, et al: The effect of thymidine kinase transduction and ganciclovir therapy on tumor vasculature and growth of 9L gliomas in rats. J Neurosurg 1994; 81:256–260.
116. Smythe WR, Hwang HC, Amin KM, et al: Use of recombinant adenovirus to transfer the herpes simplex virus thymidine kinase (HSVtk) gene to thoracic neoplasms: an effective in vitro drug sensitization system. Cancer Res 1994; 54:2055–2059.
117. Vile RG, Nelson JA, Castleden S, et al: Systemic gene therapy of murine melanoma using tissue specific expression of the HSVtk gene involves an immune component. Cancer Res 1994; 54:6228–6234.
118. Ohno T, Gordon D, San H, et al: Gene therapy for vascular smooth muscle cell proliferation after arterial injury. Science 1994; 265:781–784.
119. Guzman RJ, Hirschowitz EA, Brody SL, et al: In vivo suppression of injury-induced vascular smooth muscle cell accumulation using adenovirus-mediated transfer of the herpes simplex virus thymidine kinase gene. Proc Natl Acad Sci USA 1994; 91:10732–10736.
120. Chang MW, Barr E, Seltzer J, et al: Cytostatic gene therapy for vascular proliferative disorders with a constitutively active form of the retinoblastoma gene product. Science 1995; 267:518–522.
121. Von der Leyen HE, Gibbons GH, Morishita R, et al: Gene-therapy inhibiting neointimal vascular lesion—in vivo transfer of endothelial-cell nitric-oxide synthase gene. Proc Natl Acad Sci USA 1995; 92:1137–1141.
122. Yakubov L, Khaled Z, Zhang LM, et al: Oligodeoxynucleotides interact with recombinant CD4 at multiple sites. J Biol Chem 1993; 268:18818–18823.
123. Tonkinson JL, Stein CA: Patterns of intracellular compartmentalization, trafficking and acidification of 5′-fluorescein labeled phosphodiester and phosphorothioate oligodeoxynucleotides in HL60 cells. Nucleic Acids Res 1994; 22:4268–4275.
124. Gruver CL, DeMayo F, Goldstein MA, Means AR: Targeted developmental overexpression of calmodulin induces proliferative and hypertrophic growth of cardiomyocytes in transgenic mice. Endocrinology 1993; 133:376–388.
125. Field LJ: Atrial natriuretic factor-SV40 T antigen transgenes produce tumors and cardiac arrhythmias in mice. Science 1988; 239:1029–1033.
126. Steinhelper ME, Lanson NA Jr, Dresdner KP, et al: Proliferation in vivo and in culture of differentiated adult atrial cardiomyocytes from transgenic mice. Am J Physiol 1990; 259:H1826–H1834.
127. Milano CA, Allen LF, Rockman HA, et al: Enhanced myocardial function in transgenic mice overexpressing the beta 2-adrenergic receptor. Science 1994; 264:582–586.
128. Bristow MR, Minobe WA, Raynolds MV, et al: Reduced beta 1 receptor messenger RNA abundance in the failing human heart. J Clin Invest 1993; 92:2737–2745.
129. Milano CA, Dolber PC, Rockman HA, et al: Myocardial expression of a constitutively active alpha(1b)- adrenergic receptor in transgenic mice induces cardiac hypertrophy. Proc Natl Acad Sci USA 1994; 91:10109–10113.
130. Lin H, Parmacek MS, Morle G, et al: Expression of recombinant genes in myocardium in vivo after direct injection of DNA. Circulation 1990; 82:2217–2221.
131. Acsadi G, Jiao SS, Jani A, et al: Direct gene transfer and expression into rat heart in vivo. New Biologist 1991; 3:71–81.
132. Buttrick PM, Kass A, Kitsis RN, et al: Behavior of genes directly injected into the rat heart in vivo. Circ Res 1992; 70:193–198.
133. Buttrick PM, Kaplan ML, Kitsis RN, Leinwand LA: Distinct behavior of cardiac myosin heavy chain gene constructs in vivo. Discordance with in vitro results. Circ Res 1993; 72:1211–1217.
134. Kitsis RN, Buttrick PM, McNally EM, et al: Hormonal modulation of a gene injected into rat heart in vivo. Proc Natl Acad Sci USA 1991; 88:4138–4142.
135. von Harsdorf R, Schott RJ, Shen YT, et al: Gene injection into canine myocardium as a useful model for studying gene expression in the heart of large mammals. Circ Res 1993; 72:688–695.
136. Subrimaniam A, Jones WK, Gulick J, et al: Tissue specific regulation of a myosin heavy chain promoter in transgenic mice. J Biol Chem 1991; 266:24613–24620.
137. Flink IL, Morkin E: Interaction of thyroid hormone with strong and weak cis-acting elements in the human alpha myosin heavy chain gene promoter. J Biol Chem 1990; 265:11233–11237.
138. Umesono K, Murakami KK, Thompson CC, Evans RM: Direct repeats as selective response elements for the thyroid hormone, retinoic acid, and vitamin D3 receptors. Cell 1991; 65:1255–1266.
139. Stratford-Perricaudet LD, Makeh I, Perricaudet M, Briand P: Widespread long-term gene transfer to mouse skeletal muscles and heart. J Clin Invest 1992; 90:626–630.
140. Guzman RJ, Lemarchand P, Crystal RG, et al: Efficient gene transfer into myocardium by direct injection of adenovirus vectors. Circ Res 1993; 73:1202–1207.
141. French BA, Mazur W, Geske RS, Bolli R: Direct in vivo gene transfer into porcine myocardium using replication-deficient adenoviral vectors. Circulation 1994; 90:2414–2424.
142. Barr E, Carroll J, Kalynych AM, et al: Efficient catheter-mediated gene transfer into the heart using replication-defective adenovirus. Gene Ther 1994; 1:51–58.
143. Koh GY, Klug MG, Soonpaa MH, Field LJ: Differentiation and long-

term survival of C2C12 myoblast grafts in heart. J Clin Invest 1993; 92:1548–1554.
144. Koh GY, Field LJ: Targeted expression of transforming growth factor-e1 in intracardiac grafts promotes vascular endothelial cell DNA synthesis. J Clin Invest 1995; 95:114–121.
145. Soonpaa MH, Koh GY, Klug MG, Field LJ: Formation of nascent intercalated disks between grafted fetal cardiomyocytes and host myocardium. Science 1994; 264:98–101.
146. Kedes L, Prentice H, Sartorelli V, Kloner RA: Conversion of myocardial infarct to skeletal muscle by retroviral gene transfer [Abstract]. J Cell Biochem 1994; S18A:233.
147. Wilson JM, Grossman M: Therapeutic strategies for familial hypercholesterolemia based on somatic gene transfer [Review]. Am J Cardiol 1993; 72:59D–63D.
148. Strauss M: Liver-directed gene therapy: prospects and problems. Gene Ther 1994; 1:156–164.
149. Ponder KP, Gupta S, Leland F, et al: Mouse hepatocytes migrate to liver parenchyma and function indefinitely after intrasplenic transplantation. Proc Natl Acad Sci USA 1991; 88:1217–1221.
150. Bilheimer DW, Goldstein JL, Grundy SM, et al: Liver transplantation to provide low-density-lipoprotein receptors and lower plasma cholesterol in a child with homozygous familial hypercholesterolemia. N Engl J Med 1984; 311:1658–1664.
151. Hofmann SL, Russell DW, Brown MS, et al: Overexpression of low density lipoprotein (LDL) receptor eliminates LDL from plasma in transgenic mice. Science 1988; 239:1277–1281.
152. Wilson JM, Chowdhury NR, Grossman M, et al: Temporary amelioration of hyperlipidemia in low density lipoprotein receptor-deficient rabbits transplanted with genetically modified hepatocytes. Proc Natl Acad Sci USA 1990; 87:8437–8441.
153. Grossman M, Raper SE, Kozarsky K, et al: Successful ex vivo gene therapy directed to liver in a patient with familial hypercholesterolemia. Nat Genet 1994; 6:335–341.
154. Herz J, Gerard RD: Adenovirus-mediated transfer of low density lipoprotein receptor gene acutely accelerates cholesterol clearance in normal mice. Proc Natl Acad Sci USA 1993; 90:2812–2816.
155. Ishibashi S, Brown MS, Goldstein JL, et al: Hypercholesterolemia in low density lipoprotein receptor knockout mice and its reversal by adenovirus-mediated gene delivery. J Clin Invest 1993; 92:883–893.
156. Kozarsky KF, McKinley DR, Austin LL, et al: In vivo correction of low density lipoprotein receptor deficiency in the Watanabe heritable hyperlipidemic rabbit with recombinant adenoviruses. J Biol Chem 1994; 269:13695–13702.
157. Kozarsky K, Grossman M, Wilson JM: Adenovirus-mediated correction of the genetic defect in hepatocytes from patients with familial hypercholesterolemia. Somat Cell Mol Genet 1993; 19:449–458.

51 Clinical Trials and Meta-Analysis

Elliott M. Antman, MD
Robert M. Califf, MD

Therapeutic recommendations for various cardiovascular diseases discussed in this text have been formulated after intensive clinical investigation. Uncontrolled observational studies of populations such as those cited in Chapter 1 provide valuable insight into pathophysiology and serve as the source for important hypotheses regarding the potential value of particular interventions. However, it is a rare therapy in medicine that has the dramatic effectiveness of penicillin for pneumococcal pneumonia so that epidemiologic data alone are sufficient for scientific acceptance and adoption into clinical practice. In view of the variability of the natural history of cardiovascular illnesses and wide range of individual responses to interventions, clinical investigators, representatives of regulatory agencies, and practicing physicians all have come to recognize the value of a control group and a rigorously performed clinical trial before widespread acceptance of a treatment.[1] The sequence of phases for evaluation of new therapies is seen in Table 51–1.

The practice of medicine is making a transition from patterns driven by pathophysiologic reasoning and nonquantitative reasoning to a broad belief in "evidence-based medicine." The importance of this concept has been reinforced more in cardiovascular disease treatment than in any other field by the demonstration in clinical trials that concepts that seemed to be quite rational and widely accepted have been associated with a substantial adverse effect on mortality. Type I antiarrhythmic drugs were often prescribed because of frequent premature beats until the Cardiac Arrhythmia Suppression Trial (CAST) demonstrated that such treatment increases the risk of death. Similarly, calcium channel blockers have been associated with a higher mortality in patients with left ventricular dysfunction despite their widespread use for many years, even in patients with symptomatic heart failure. Despite the recognized importance of empirical evidence in guiding therapeutic decision-making, only with the advent of powerful computers has computational and organizational capability begun to meet researchers' needs. The methods of aggregating and interpreting clinical trials and observational databases are in their infancy.

Despite limitations, demands for evidence-based therapeutic recommendations involving drugs, devices, and procedures are likely to be voiced even more stridently in the near future as managed care, cost-saving measures, and guidelines published by authoritative bodies become established as part of the fabric of clinical medicine.[2] With the increasing number of elderly patients in the population, there is also a clear need for improved information on their response to therapeutic interventions.[3] Thus, the proper design, conduct, analysis, interpretation, and presentation of a clinical trial is an "indispensable ordeal" for investigators.[4] Practitioners must also acquire the tools to read reports of clinical trials critically and, when appropriate, to translate the findings into clinical practice without the lengthy delays seen in the past.[5–7] This is an especially important task for generalist physicians because of the increased emphasis on primary care physicians in controlling healthcare costs and evidence that they are less aware or less certain about the results of clinical trials than specialists.[8]

TABLE 51–1. PHASES OF EVALUATION OF NEW THERAPIES

Phase	Features	Purpose
I	First administration of a new therapy to patients	Exploratory clinical research to determine if further investigation is appropriate
II	Early trials of new therapy in patients	To acquire information on dose-response relationship, estimate incidence of adverse reactions, and provide additional insight into pathophysiology of disease and potential impact of new therapy
III	Large-scale comparative trial of new therapy versus standard of practice	Definitive evaluation of new therapy to determine if it should replace current standard of practice; randomized controlled trials required by regulatory agencies for registration of new therapeutic modalities
IV	Monitoring of use of therapy in clinical practice	Post-"marketing" surveillance to gather additional information on impact of new therapy on treatment of disease, rate of use of new therapy and more robust estimate of incidence of adverse reactions established from registries

The sheer volume and broad range[9, 10] of clinical trials in cardiology is too large for even the most conscientious individual to digest on a regular basis. This has stimulated increased interest in biostatistical techniques for combining the findings from randomized controlled trials of the same intervention in the form of a meta-analysis or overview.

The goals of this chapter are to review the fundamental features of various types of clinical trials and the advantages and limitations of meta-analyses. The reader is referred to several excellent sources for additional information that fall outside the scope of this chapter.[11–13]

CLINICAL TRIAL DESIGN

Because of the importance of clinical trial findings, it is essential that investigators carefully formulate the scientific question to be answered and have realistic estimates of the sample size required to show the expected difference in treatments. Trials that conclude there is no statistically significant difference between treatment A and treatment B are often undersized and lack sufficient power to detect a difference when one truly exists. A well-coordinated organizational structure consisting of experienced trialists, biostatisticians, and data analysts is important to prevent these pitfalls in trial design as well as others such as unrealistic assessments of the ease of patient recruitment and timetable for completion of the trial.

The stages of a clinical trial are summarized in Table 51–2. These stages should be viewed as a rough guide to the orderly sequence of events that characterizes the clinical trial process. The dividing lines between stages are often indistinct. For example, sites that are randomizing patients may be brought into the trial in a rolling fashion so that some of the features of the protocol development stage may overlap with the patient recruitment phase. It is possible that some of the early sites enrolling patients may gain sufficient experience

TABLE 51–2. STAGES OF A CLINICAL TRIAL

Stage	Activities During Stage	Event Marking End of Stage
Initial design	Formulation of scientific question; outcome measures established; sample size calculated	Initiation of funding
Protocol development	Trial protocol and manual of operations written; case report forms developed; data management systems and monitoring procedures established; training of clinical sites completed	Initiation of patient recruitment
Patient recruitment	Channels for patient referrals established; development of regular monitoring procedures of trial data for accuracy, patient eligibility, and site performance; preparation of periodic reports to DSMB for review of adverse or beneficial treatment effects	Completion of patient recruitment
Treatment and follow-up	Continued monitoring of patient recruitment, adverse effects and site performance; updated trial materials sent to enrolling sites; reports sent to DSMB and recommendations reviewed; adverse event reports filed with regulatory agency; timetable for trial close-out procedures established	Initiation of close-out procedures
Patient/trial close-out	Identify final data items that require clarification so database can be "cleaned and locked"; initiate procedures for unblinding of treatment assignment, termination of study therapy, and monitoring of adverse events following discontinuation of treatment; preparation of final reports to DSMB; preparation of draft of final trial report	Completion of close-out procedures
Termination	Verify that all sites have completed close-out procedures, including disposal of unused study drugs; review final trial findings and submit manuscript for publication; submit final report to regulatory agency	Termination of funding for original trial
Posttrial follow-up (optional)	Recontact enrolling sites to acquire long-term follow-up data on patients in trial; link follow-up data with initial trial data and prepare manuscript summarizing results	Termination of all follow-up

Abbreviation: DSMB, data safety monitoring board.
Adapted from Meinert C: Clinical Trials. Design, Conduct, and Analysis. New York: Oxford University Press, 1986.

with the protocol to achieve different results from those sites joining the trial later. Evidence of this phenomenon is typically sought by performing a test for interaction between enrolling site and treatment effect when the data are analyzed.

Controlled Trials

The term control group refers to those subjects in a clinical trial who receive the treatment against which the test intervention is being compared. Requirements for the control and test treatments are outlined in Table 51–3. The randomized controlled trial that typically incorporates both test and control treatments is considered the gold standard for evaluating new therapies. However, the previously noted definition of a control does not require that the treatment be a placebo, although frequently this is the case, because new treatments may need to be compared with the current standard of practice to determine if they are more efficacious (e.g., direct antithrombins versus heparin; see Chaps. 7 and 30) or equally effective (e.g., new beta blocker versus propranolol for hypertension; see Chap. 34). Nor does this definition require that the control group be a collection of subjects distinct from the treatment group studied contemporaneously and allocated by random assignment (e.g., randomized controlled trial). Other possibilities considered less scientifically rigorous include nonrandomized concurrent and historic controls, crossover designs and withdrawal trials with each patient serving as a member of both the treatment and control groups, and group allocations, in which groups of subjects or a treatment site are assigned as a block to either test or control.

Two broad types of controlled trials exist: the fixed sample size design, in which the investigator specifies the necessary sample size before patient recruitment, and the open or closed sequential design, in which sequential pairs of patients are enrolled, one to test and one to control, only if the cumulative test-control difference from previous pairs of patients remains within prespecified boundaries.[11, 12] The sequential trial design is usually less efficient than the fixed sample size design and is practical only in those situations in which the outcome of interest can be ascertained shortly after enrollment.

Case-control studies that involve a comparison of persons with a disease of interest (cases) to a suitable group of subjects without the disease (matched controls) are integral to epidemiologic research but are not strictly clinical trials and are not discussed in this chapter (see Chap. 1).

Randomized Controlled Trials

The randomized controlled trial is the standard against which all other designs are compared for several reasons. In addition to the advantage of incorporating a control group, this type of trial centers around the process of randomization, which has three important influences: (1) it reduces the likelihood of patient selection bias that may occur either consciously or unconsciously[14]; (2) it enhances the likelihood that comparable groups of subjects are compared, especially if the sample size is sufficiently large; and (3) it validates the use of common statistical tests such as the chi-square test for comparison of proportions and Student's t test for comparison of means.[11] Randomization may be fixed over the course of the trial or may be adaptive based on the distribution of prior randomization assignments, baseline characteristic frequencies, or observed outcomes. Fixed randomization schemes are more common and are specified further by the allocation ratio (uniform or nonuniform assignment to study groups), stratification levels, and block size (i.e., constraining the randomization of patients to ensure a balanced number of assignments to the study groups, especially if stratification is used in the trial). Ethical considerations related to randomization have been the subject of considerable discussion in the clinical trial literature.[15–17]

Clinicians usually participate in a randomized controlled trial if they feel sufficiently uncertain about the potential advantages of the test treatment and can confidently convey this uncertainty to the patient who must provide informed consent. It is important that physicians realize that in the absence of rigorously obtained data, many well-intentioned therapeutic decisions thought to be in the best interest of the patient (e.g., suppression of ventricular premature beats after myocardial infarction) may be ineffective or even harmful.[18] To identify the appropriate therapeutic strategies from a societal perspective, randomized controlled trials are needed.

A difficult philosophical dilemma arises when one considers that as patients are enrolled in a trial, evidence is accumulating that tends to favor one study group over the other, and the degree of uncertainty about the likelihood of benefit or harm is constantly being updated. Because clinicians may feel uneasy about enrolling a patient who may be randomized to a treatment that the accumulating data suggest might be inferior but has not yet been proven statistically to be so with a conventional level of significance, the outcome data from the trial are not revealed to the investigators during the patient recruitment stage. The responsibility of safeguarding the welfare of patients enrolled in the trial rests with an external monitoring team referred to as a Data Safety Monitoring Board (DSMB) or Committee (DSMC).[19] Several prominent examples over the last decade of early termination of large randomized trials because of compelling evidence of benefit or harm from one of the treatments under investigation are evidence that the DSMB has become an integral element of clinical trial research.[19–21]

When both the patient and the investigator are aware of the treatment assignment, the trial is said to be unblinded. Trials of this nature have the potential for bias, particularly during the process of data collection and patient assessment, if subjective measures such as presence or absence of congestive heart failure are tabulated. In an effort to reduce bias, progressively stricter degrees of blinding may be introduced. Single-blind trials mask the treatment from the patient but permit it to be known by the investigator; double-blind trials mask the treatment assignment from both the patient and investigator; triple-blind trials mask the actual treatment assignment from the DSMB and provide data only in the form of group A and group B.

The specialty of cardiology is replete with examples of randomized controlled trials. An area particularly rich in this regard is the study of treatments for acute myocardial infarction (see Chap. 7), in which several types of randomized controlled trials have been performed over the past three decades. These types of randomized controlled trials have been broadly classified into mini-trials and mega-trials according to the features shown in Table 51–4. A further subdivision of the mini-trials into those that are of limited sample size and focus almost exclusively on mechanistic data and those with a sample size an order of magnitude larger and hybrid goals focusing on mechanistic data as it relates to mortality is illustrated in Figure

TABLE 51–3. REQUIREMENTS FOR TEST AND CONTROL TREATMENTS

They must be distinguishable from one another
They must be medically justifiable
There must be an ethical base for use of either treatment
Use of the treatments must be compatible with the health care needs of study patients
Either treatment must be acceptable to study patients and to treating physicians
There must be a reasonable doubt regarding the efficacy of the test treatment
There should be reason to believe that the benefits will outweigh the risks of treatment
The method of treatment administration must be compatible with the design needs of the trial (e.g., method of administration must be the same for all the treatments in a double-blind trial) and should be as similar to real-world as is practical

From Meinert C: Clinical Trials. Design, Conduct, and Analysis, p 469. New York: Oxford University Press, 1986.

TABLE 51–4. MAJOR FEATURES DISTINGUISHING TYPES OF RANDOMIZED CONTROLLED TRIALS OF TREATMENTS FOR ACUTE MYOCARDIAL INFARCTION

Feature	Mini-Trial	Mega-Trial
Patient population	<3000	>10,000
Clinical sites	4–30	200–2000
Data collected per patient	Maximal	Minimal
Protocol algorithm	More complex	Simple
Entry criteria	More restricted	Wide
Control of ancillary treatments	Complete protocolization of care possible	Cannot control ancillary treatments
Quality assurance of data	Full quality assurance possible	Very limited quality assurance of data
Ability to assess advanced technologies or high-risk therapies	Possible	Not possible
Ability to provide mechanistic information about disease process	Possible	Generally not possible
Monitoring of safety data during conduct of trial	Occurs "on-line"	Lag in reporting of safety information
Endpoint	In addition to mortality, focuses on nonfatal end points such as stroke, reinfarction, need for revascularization, quality of life, and ecnonomics	Major focus is on mortality
Ability to establish drug dosing	Possible	Not possible
Logistics of running the trial	Fewer enrolling sites but more data fields collected per patient	Much larger number of sites but fewer data fields collected per patient

Modified from Topol EJ, Califf RM: Answers to complex questions cannot be derived from "simple" trials. Br Heart J 1992; 68:348–351.

51–1. Because of the practical limitations of the very large sample size required when mortality is used as the primary endpoint in trials of new cardiovascular therapies, the majority of which are expected to have a treatment effect of 15%–20%, interest has arisen in the use of composite endpoints such as the sum of mortality, recurrent nonfatal myocardial infarction, and clinical congestive heart failure or surrogates for mortality as the primary endpoint.[22, 23] Trials using composite or surrogate endpoints are more likely to suffer from missing data than those using mortality as the primary endpoint. This ascertainment bias or noninformative censoring of the data necessitates statistical adjustments to compensate for the missing data.[23]

Nonrandomized Concurrent Control Studies

Trials in which the investigator selects the subjects to be allocated to the control and treatment groups are nonrandomized concurrent control studies. The advantages of this simpler trial design are that clinicians do not leave to chance the assignment of treatment in each patient, and there is no need for patients to accept the concept of randomization. Implicit in this design type is the assumption that the investigator can appropriately match subjects in the test and control groups for all relevant baseline characteristics. This is a difficult task and can produce a selection bias that may result in conclusions

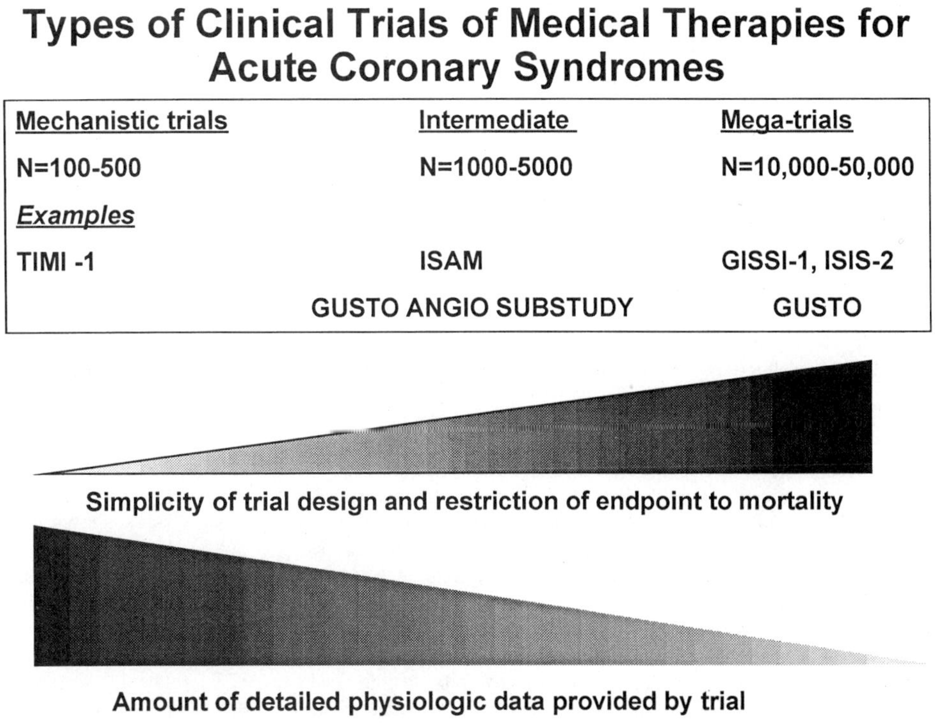

Figure 51–1. Types of clinical trials of thrombolytic therapy for acute myocardial infarction. Mechanistic trials study fewer than 500 patients but do so in considerable detail so as to provide important physiologic information, whereas mega-trials study tens of thousands of patients in a simpler format which, of necessity, provides much less detailed physiologic information. Typically, mega-trials have mortality as their primary endpoint, rather than intermediate or composite endpoints such as the combination of mortality, current infarction, and left ventricular dysfunction. Between the two extremes are intermediate trials that enroll several thousand patients either as part of the primary trial design or as a substudy within a larger trial (e.g., GUSTO Angiographic Substudy within the larger GUSTO Trial). (From Antman E: Overview of medical therapy. *In* Califf R [ed]: Acute Myocardial Infarction and Other Acute Ischemic Syndromes, pp 10.5. Philadelphia: Current Medicine, 1996.)

differing considerably from those obtained from randomized controlled trials.[24, 25]

Despite the difficult issues involved in observational studies, criteria for performance of adequate observational studies are being developed.[26] Well-done observational analyses contain many of the same structural characteristics as randomized trials except that the treatment is not randomized. These studies should have prospectively collected data with uniform definitions managed by a multidisciplinary group of investigators including clinicians, biostatisticians, and data analysts. Outcomes must be collected in a rigorous and unbiased fashion, just as in the randomized trial. The same issues of power and multiple comparisons are perhaps even more commonly ignored in observational analyses than in randomized controlled trials. Because observational analyses are particularly prone to bias, representation of investigators outside of the particular specialty being addressed can be useful.[26] In view of unbiased ascertainment of data through the use of the same methods as the randomized trial, statistical adjustments must be used to attempt to compensate for differences in baseline characteristics between patients receiving different treatments. These methods, predominantly multivariable regression techniques and survival analysis, require expert methodology, because failure to recognize the detailed relations among baseline characteristics as they relate to outcome can lead to insufficient adjustment for differences.

Historical Controls

Clinical trials using historical controls compare a test intervention to data obtained earlier in a nonconcurrent, nonrandomized control group. Potential sources for historical controls include previously published medical literature and unpublished databanks of clinic populations. The use of historical controls allows clinicians to offer potentially beneficial therapies to all subjects, thereby reducing the sample size for the study. The major drawbacks are bias in the selection of the control population and failure of the historical controls to reflect contemporary diagnostic criteria and concurrent treatment regimens for the disease under study.

It should be noted, however, that prospectively recorded registry data may be more representative of actual clinical practice than the control groups in randomized controlled trials. A recent illustration of this fact is the National Registry of Myocardial Infarction (NRMI), which catalogued data on 240,989 patients treated at 1073 hospitals in the United States between 1990 and 1993.[27] Whereas randomized controlled trials of thrombolytic therapy for acute myocardial infarction have shown a progressive decline in the in-hospital mortality rate to 6%–7%, the NRMI data on 156,512 patients not receiving thrombolytics revealed a mortality rate of 13.1%, indicating a need for additional research efforts to expand the use of thrombolytics and develop mortality-reducing strategies for patients who are not considered suitable candidates for thrombolysis.

Crossover Design

Crossover design is a special case of the randomized controlled trial, in that each subject serves as his own control. A simple, two-period, crossover design randomly assigns each subject to either the test or control group in the first period and to the alternative group in the second period. The appeal of this design is the ability to use the same subject for both test and control treatments, thereby diminishing the influence of interindividual variability and allowing a smaller sample size. However, important limitations to crossover design are the assumptions that the effects of the treatment assigned during the first period have no residual effect on the treatment assigned during the second period and that the patient's condition remains stable during both periods. The validity of these assumptions is often difficult to verify either clinically or statistically (e.g., testing for an interaction between period and intervention), leading some authorities to discourage the use of crossover designs.[28] One possible use of the crossover trial design is the preliminary evaluation of new antianginal agents for patients with chronic, stable exertional angina.[24]

Withdrawal Studies

In withdrawal studies, patients with a chronic cardiovascular condition are taken off therapy or undergo a reduction in dosage. The goal is to evaluate the response to discontinuation of treatment or reduction in its intensity. An important limitation is that only patients who have tolerated the test intervention for a period of time are eligible for enrollment, because those with incapacitating side effects would have been taken off the test intervention and are therefore not available for "withdrawal." This selection bias can overestimate benefit and underestimate toxicity associated with the test intervention.[11] Also, changes in the natural history of the disease may influence the response to withdrawal of therapy. For example, if a therapeutic intervention is beneficial early after the onset of the disease but loses its benefit over time, the withdrawal of therapy late in the course of treatment might not result in deterioration of the patient's condition. A conclusion that the intervention was not helpful because its withdrawal during the chronic phase of treatment did not result in a worsening of the patient's condition provides no information about the potential benefit of treatment in the acute or subacute phase of the illness. Nevertheless, withdrawal trials can provide clinically useful information, but they should be conducted with the same standards that are applied to controlled trials of prospective treatment, including randomization and blinding, if possible.[11]

The following withdrawal trial in cardiology illustrates many of the features discussed previously. Although digitalis has been used by physicians for more than 200 years, its benefits for the treatment of chronic congestive heart failure, particularly in the patient with normal sinus rhythm, remain controversial. To assess the consequences of withdrawing digoxin from clinically stable patients with New York Heart Association class II or III congestive heart failure who are receiving angiotensin converting enzyme inhibitors, the Randomized Assessment of [the effect of] Digoxin [in patients] on Inhibitors of the Angiotensin-Converting Enzyme (RADIANCE) investigators randomly allocated 178 patients in a double-blind fashion to continue receiving digoxin or switch to a matched placebo (see Chaps. 9 and 11).[29] Worsening heart failure necessitating discontinuation from the study occurred in 23 patients switched to placebo but in only 4 patients who continued to receive digoxin ($p < .001$). The results of the RADIANCE trial seem to indicate that withdrawal of digoxin in patients with mild-to-moderate congestive heart failure as a result of systolic dysfunction is associated with adverse consequences, but it does not provide information on the potential mortality benefit of digoxin when *added* to a regimen of diuretics and angiotensin converting enzyme inhibitors.[30] Information in the Digitalis Investigators' Group (DIG) Trial, a classic randomized controlled trial that will be reported in 1996,[31] suggests that consistent results are forthcoming in groups of patients for whom digoxin was added and those for whom the drug was withdrawn.

Factorial Design

When two or more therapies are to be tested in a clinical trial, investigators typically consider a factorial design, in which multiple treatments can be compared with control by independent randomization within a single trial. A schematic example of a 2 × 2 factorial design trial is shown in Figure 51–2. In this example, 10,000 patients are randomized to receive two interventions (Drug A and Drug B). There are four categories of patients: Active A/Active B, Placebo A/Active B, Active A/Placebo B, Placebo A/Placebo B. These groups of patients allow assessment of the treatment effect of Drug A in the absence of Drug B (Difference 1) and in the presence of Drug B (Difference 2). A grand summary (pooled) statement of the treatment effect of Drug A can be made, along with a measure of the interaction of coadministration of Drug B and Drug A. A similar and

BIOSTATISTICAL TOOLS FOR COMPARING THERAPIES FOR ACUTE CORONARY SYNDROMES

Use of Factorial Design to Evaluate Drug Interactions

Total Enrollment = 10,000 patients

	***Active A* 5000**	***Placebo A* 5000**
***Active B* 5000**	Active A Active B 2500	Placebo A Active B 2500
***Placebo B* 5000**	Active A Placebo B 2500	Placebo A Placebo B 2500

Evaluation of Drug A alone and in combination with Drug B :

Active A/ Placebo B vs Placebo A/ Placebo B = $\text{Difference}_1 = D_1$

Active A/ Active B vs Placebo A/ Active B = $\text{Difference}_2 = D_2$

Treatment Effect of Drug A in the absence of Drug B = D_1

Treatment Effect of Drug A in the presence of Drug B = D_2

Grand Summary of Treatment Effect of Drug A = $D_1 + D_2$

Interaction of Drug B on Treatment Effect of Drug A = $D_2 - D_1$

Figure 51–2. Factorial-design clinical trial. In this example, 10,000 patients are randomized to receive or not receive two interventions (Drug A and Drug B). Each patient will fall into one of four categories: Active A/Active B, Placebo A/Active B, Active A/Placebo B, or Placebo A/Placebo B. The differences in event rates for the comparisons shown at the bottom permit an assessment of the treatment effect of Drug A in the presence and absence of Drug B. (From Antman E: Overview of medical therapy. *In* Califf R [ed]: Acute Myocardial Infarction and Other Acute Ischemic Syndromes, pp 10.6. Philadelphia: Current Medicine, 1995.)

symmetric analysis could be performed for Drug B.[32] This line of reasoning can be extended to more than two test treatments, as was the case in the fourth International Study of Infarct Survival (ISIS-4), in which three interventions (i.e., captopril, nitrates, and magnesium) were evaluated in a 2 × 2 × 2 factorial design, and patients fell into one of eight separate categories.[33]

Factorial design trials are most appropriate when there is thought to be no interaction between the various test treatments, as is often the case when drugs have unrelated mechanisms of action.[34] If no interactions exist, multiple drug comparisons can be efficiently performed in a single large trial that is smaller than the sum of two independent clinical trials.[11] When interactions are detected, each intervention must be evaluated individually against a control and each of the other interventions in which an interaction exists.

The factorial design trial has an important place in cardiology, in which multiple therapies are typically given to the same patient for important conditions such as myocardial infarction and therefore in practical terms is more reflective of actual clinical practice than trials in which only a single intervention is randomized. Clinicians need to know how much incremental value comes from administering one more drug to the patient and whether any drug interactions exist. It is worth noting that it is probably an insurmountable task to rule out the possibility of a drug interaction because of the imprecision with which interaction effects are estimated (i.e., wide confidence intervals), the poor power of tests for statistical significance of interactions between the test interventions, and the vast number of non–protocol-related drugs a patient may receive.[32, 34] For example, in addition to the eight patient groups in the main design of ISIS-4, the type of thrombolytic prescribed, the presence or absence of intravenous beta blockers, and the use of nontrial nitrates such as intravenous nitroglycerin, among other factors, rapidly escalates the number of patient cells to nearly 100.

Trials Testing Equivalence of Therapies

Advances in cardiovascular therapeutics have dramatically improved the treatment of various diseases, such that several therapies of proven efficacy may coexist for the same treatment. However, it may still be desirable to develop new therapies that are equally efficacious but have an important advantage such as reduced toxicity, improved patient tolerability, more favorable pharmacokinetic profile, fewer drug interactions, or lower cost.[35, 36] For example, a new angiotensin II receptor antagonist might be compared with a standard angiotensin converting enzyme inhibitor for reducing mortality in patients with congestive heart failure, with the expectation that the former would have better tolerability because of its more specific activity.[37] Testing new therapies with placebo-controlled trials poses problems on ethical grounds, because one half of the patients would be denied treatment when an accepted therapy of proven effectiveness exists. This has led to a shift in clinical trial design to demonstrate therapeutic equivalence of two treatments rather than superiority of one of the treatments. The concept of equivalence trials has a precedent in the study of bioequivalence, where, for example, two drug preparations are considered equivalent if they produce similar areas under the curve (AUC) in plots of blood levels versus time.

It is not possible to show two active therapies to be completely equivalent without a trial of infinite sample size. Instead, investigators resort to specifying a value (delta) and consider the test therapy said to be equivalent to the standard therapy if, with a high degree of confidence, the true difference in treatment effects is less than delta.[11]

Sample Size Estimations and Sequential Stopping Boundaries

Estimating the sample size for trials involves a statement of the scientific question in the form of a null hypothesis (H_0) and an alternative hypothesis (H_A). For example, in the case of dichotomous variables (e.g., presence or absence of a primary outcome variable such as mortality), the null hypothesis states that the proportion of patients dying in the test group (P_{Test}) is equal to that in the control group ($P_{Control}$), such that

$$H_0: P_{Test} - P_{Control} = 0.$$

The alternative hypothesis is

$$H_A: P_{Test} - P_{Control} \neq 0.$$

False-Positive and False-Negative Error Rates and Power of Clinical Trial

To determine if the null hypothesis may be rejected, before initiation of the trial, the researcher must specify the type I (alpha) and type II (beta) errors, sometimes referred to as the false-positive and false-negative rates. The conventional alpha of 5% indicates that the investigator is willing to accept a 5% likelihood that an observed difference occurred by chance and proceeds to reject the null hypothesis. The beta value reflects the likelihood that a specified difference might be missed or not found to be statistically significant because an insufficient number of subjects were enrolled. The quantity (1-beta) is referred to as the power of the trial and quantifies the ability of the trial to find true differences of a given magnitude between the groups. The relations among estimated event rates, the prespecified alpha level, and desired power of the trial determines the number of patients that must be randomized to detect the anticipated difference in outcomes according to standard formulas.[11, 38] Similar concepts are applied to response variables that are not dichotomous but are measured on a continuous scale (e.g., blood pressure) or represent time to failure (e.g., Kaplan-Meier survival curves).[11]

Statistical methods are also available for monitoring a trial during the patient recruitment phase at certain prespecified intervals to ascertain whether the accumulated evidence strongly suggests an advantage of one treatment in the trial.[39] During such interim looks at the data, the differences between treatment groups expressed as a standardized normal statistic (Z_i) is compared with boundaries such as those shown in Figure 51–3. If the Z_i statistic falls outside the boundaries at an *i*th interim look, the DSMB may give serious consideration to recommending termination of the trial. Typically, the data are arranged as test:control, so that crossing of the upper boundary denotes statistically significant superiority of the test therapy over control, and crossing the lower boundary denotes superiority of the control therapy over the test therapy. Because of the considerable expense of large clinical trials, in some cases it may be desirable to discontinue a trial at an interim analysis if the accumulated data suggest the probability of a positive result should the trial proceed to completion is quite low. A "futility index" that describes the likelihood of a positive result based on accumulated data has been developed, allowing investigators to discontinue a nonproductive trial and concentrate limited resources on alternative trial options.[40]

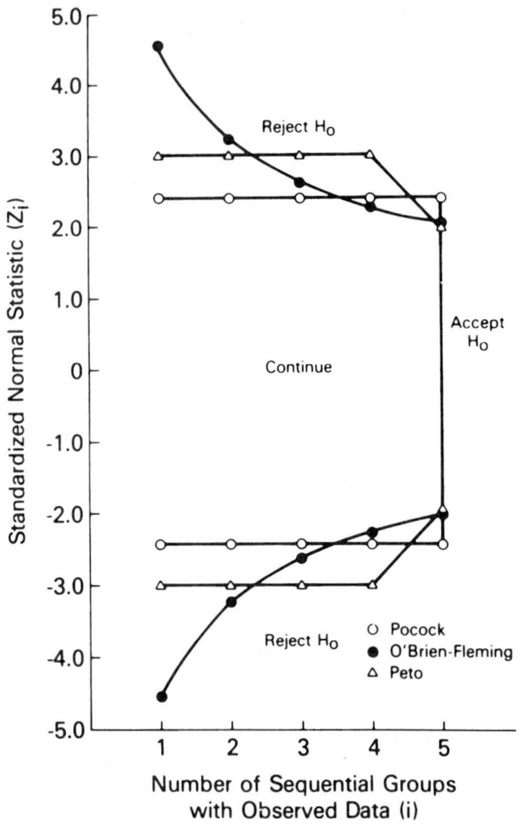

Figure 51–3. Sequential stopping boundaries are used in monitoring a clinical trial. In this example, three sequential stopping boundaries (Pocock, O'Brien-Fleming, and Peto) are used for the standardized normal statistic (Z_i) for up to five sequential groups of patients enrolled in trial by the *i*th analysis with a final two-sided significance level of .05. *Other abbreviation:* H_o, null hypothesis. (From Friedman L, Furberg C, DeMets D: Fundamentals of Clinical Trials, 2nd ed. Littleton, MA: PSG Publishing, 1985.)

Considerable clinical and statistical wisdom is required of DSMB members, because they must consider and integrate the consistency and timeliness of the trial data reviewed at each interim analysis, random variation in event rates during the course of the trial, the type and severity of the disease under study, the magnitude of the benefit versus the risks of the therapy being investigated, and emerging data from other trials and clinical experience. Although it may occasionally appear that an extreme treatment effect is present in a particular subgroup, this must be interpreted cautiously to be certain that this effect is consistent with a prior hypothesis and remains significant after adjusting for multiple comparisons, interactions, and the interim nature of the analysis.[41] Formal statistical stopping guidelines, ethical obligations to patients, common sense, and the obligation to the clinical community to ensure that willingness of patients to consent to participation in the trial leads to an advance in the state of knowledge about the optimum therapeutic strategy must be balanced.[19] For example, in 1989, the Beta-Blocker Heart Attack Trial was stopped early because of strong evidence of benefit from propranolol, especially in view of the previously published Norwegian Timolol Study.[19] In contrast, CAST was terminated early after the DSMB felt that compelling evidence had accumulated indicating that, contrary to the prevailing clinical impression at the time, suppression of ventricular premature beats with encainide or flecainide after myocardial infarction was associated with increased mortality.[18]

HOW TO READ AND INTERPRET A CLINICAL TRIAL

To properly interpret a clinical trial report and apply it in their practice, clinicians must have a working knowledge of the statistical and epidemiologic terms used to describe the results. To assist readers of clinical trial literature, the Evidence-Based Medicine Working Group at McMaster University has published a helpful series of "Users' Guides to the Medical Literature."[42, 43] By asking three main sets of questions, such as those in Table 51–5 adapted from the McMaster Group, and summarizing the trial findings as per the example in Figure 51–4, physicians will be equipped to integrate the information in reports of clinical trials into their own practice.

After ascertaining that the study was of sufficient caliber to provide valid results, the essential trial data can be extracted and entered into a 2 × 2 table. In the example shown in Figure 51–4, 10,000 patients who met the enrollment criteria for a clinical trial were randomized with an allocation ratio of 1:1, so that 5000 patients received treatment A and 5000 received treatment B. Because only 600 primary outcome events occurred in group A (12% event rate) and 750 occurred in group B (15% event rate) it would appear that treatment A is more effective than treatment B. Is this difference statistically significant, and is it clinically meaningful? When the data are arranged in a 2 × 2 table (see Fig. 51–4), a chi-square test or Fisher exact test can be readily performed according to standard formulas.[38, 44]

Although the investigators of the trial will likely have analyzed the results by using one of the methods illustrated in Figure 51–4, it is useful to have a measure of the precision of the findings and an impression of the potential impact of the results on clinical practice. Even a well-designed clinical trial can only give an estimate of the treatment effect of the test intervention because of random variations

TABLE 51–5. QUESTIONS TO ASK WHEN READING AND INTERPRETING THE RESULTS OF A CLINICAL TRIAL

Are the Results of the Study Valid?
Primary guides
- Was the assignment of patients to treatment randomized?
- Were all patients who entered the trial properly accounted for at its conclusion?
- Was follow-up complete?
- Were patients analyzed in the groups to which they were randomized?

Secondary guides
- Were patients, their clinicians, and study personnel blinded to treatment?
- Were the groups similar at the start of the trial?
- Aside from the experimental intervention, were the groups treated equally?

What Were the Results?
How large was the treatment effect?
How precise was the treatment effect (confidence intervals)?

Will the Results Help Me in Caring for My Patients?
Does my patient fulfill the enrollment criteria for the trial? If not, how close is my patient to the enrollment criteria?
Does my patient fit the features of a subgroup in the trial report? If so, are the results of the subgroup analysis in the trial valid?
Were all the clinically important outcomes considered?
Are the likely treatment benefits worth the potential harm and costs?

Adapted from material in Guyatt GH, Sackett DL, Cook DJ: The medical literature: users' guides to the medical literature. II. How to use an article about therapy or prevention. A. Are the results of the study valid? JAMA 1993; 270:2598–2601; and Guyatt GH, Sackett DL, Cook DJ. The medical literature: users' guides to the medical literature. II. How to use an article about therapy or prevention. B. What were the results and will they help me in caring for my patients? JAMA. 1994; 271:59–63.

in the sample of subjects studied, who are selected from the entire population of patients with the same disease. The imprecision of the statement regarding treatment effect can be estimated and incorporated into the presentation of the trial results by calculating the 95% confidence intervals around the observed treatment effect.[45] If the 95% confidence intervals are not reported in the trial, inspection of the p value may be useful to indicate whether the confidence interval spans a null effect. Alternatively, the 95% confidence intervals may be estimated as the treatment effect plus or minus twice the standard error of the treatment effect (if reported) or they may be calculated directly.[45]

Measures of Treatment Effect

When the outcome is undesirable and the data are arranged as test group:control group, a relative risk (RR) or odds ratio (OR) of less than 1 indicates the benefit of the test treatment. The relative risk of .80 (range, .72–.88) and odds ratio of .77 (range, .69–.87) in Figure 51–4 are indicative of benefit associated with treatment A. When the control rate is low, the OR will approximate the RR, and the OR may be thought of as an estimator of the RR. As the control rate increases, the OR deviates farther from the RR, and clinicians should rely more on the latter. The treatment effect, expressed as a relative risk reduction of 20% in this example, is similar to that reported in recent trials (e.g., reduction in mortality associated with captopril after myocardial infarction in the Survival and Ventricular Enlargement [SAVE] trial[46]), but its 95% confidence intervals range from 12% to 28%. Such statements should be interpreted in the context of the absolute risk of the adverse outcome it is designed to prevent (absolute risk reduction [ARR]; absolute risk difference [ARD]) and are even more meaningful if expressed as the number of patients that must be treated (= 1/ARD) to observe the beneficial effect if it is as large as reported in the trial.[43, 47, 48]

If practitioners are given clinical trial results only in the form of relative risk reduction, they tend to perceive a greater effectiveness of the test intervention than if a more comprehensive statement, including ARR or ARD and the number needed to treat, is provided.[49, 50] Thus, in view of the baseline risk of 15% in the control group (a value that might represent the 1-month mortality of contemporary patients with myocardial infarction not treated with thrombolytics), the 12% event rate in the test group represents an ARD of 3%, which corresponds to 1/.03 or approximately 33 patients requiring treatment to prevent one adverse event from occurring. This

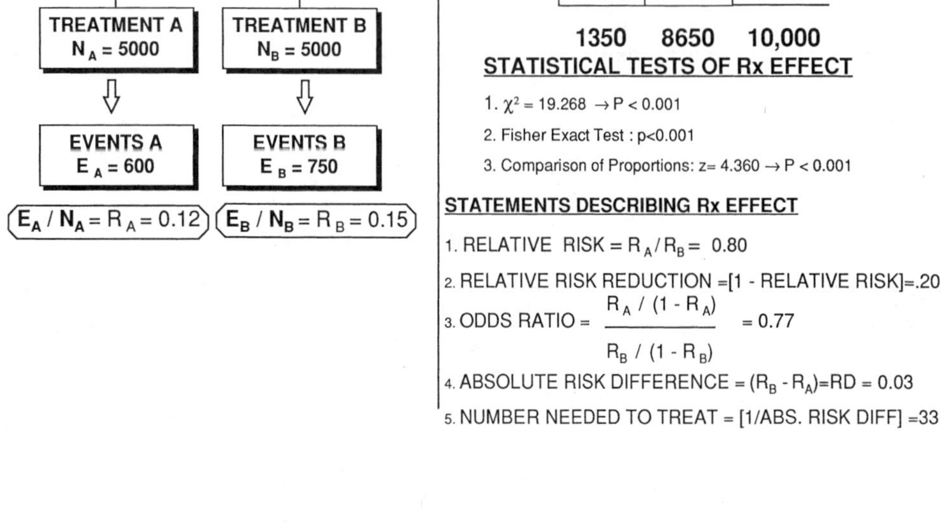

Randomized Controlled Trials
Summary Measures of Treatment Effect
Patients meeting enrollment criteria N=10,000
RANDOMIZE
TREATMENT A N A = 5000
TREATMENT B N B = 5000
EVENTS A E A = 600
EVENTS B E B = 750
E A / N A = R A = 0.12
E B / N B = R B = 0.15
EVENT
NO EVENT
A E A =600 4400 5000
B E B =750 4250 5000
1350 8650 10,000
STATISTICAL TESTS OF Rx EFFECT
1. χ2 = 19.268 → P < 0.001
2. Fisher Exact Test : p<0.001
3. Comparison of Proportions: z= 4.360 → P < 0.001
STATEMENTS DESCRIBING Rx EFFECT
1. RELATIVE RISK = R A / R B = 0.80
2. RELATIVE RISK REDUCTION =[1 - RELATIVE RISK]=.20
3. ODDS RATIO = R A / (1 - R A) / R B / (1 - R B) = 0.77
4. ABSOLUTE RISK DIFFERENCE = (R B - R A)=RD = 0.03
5. NUMBER NEEDED TO TREAT = [1/ABS. RISK DIFF] =33

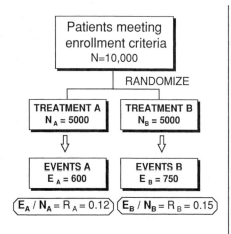

Figure 51–4. Evaluation of a clinical trial. In this example, 10,000 patients who meet enrollment criteria for the randomized controlled trial are randomized such that 5000 patients receive treatment A and 5000 patients receive treatment B. Six hundred patients in the treatment A group experience an event (e.g., mortality), yielding an event rate of 12%, compared with 750 patients in treatment B, yielding an event rate of 15%. The 2 × 2 table on the right is then constructed, and various statistical tests are performed to evaluate the significance of the difference in event rates between group A and group B. Common statements describing the treatment effect are the relative risk (of events in treatment A versus treatment B), the odds ratio (for development of events in treatment A versus treatment B), or the absolute risk difference (of events in treatment A versus treatment B) using the formulas shown. A clinically useful method of expressing the results is to calculate the number of patients that need to be treated to prevent one event. (From Antman E: Overview of medical therapy. *In* Califf R [ed]: Acute Myocardial Infarction and Other Acute Ischemic Syndromes, pp 10.6. Philadelphia: Current Medicine, 1995.)

statement is sometimes given as the number of lives saved per 1000 patients treated, corresponding to 30 lives in this example. Against this benefit must be weighed the risks associated with treatment (e.g., hemorrhagic stroke with thrombolytic therapy for myocardial infarction, proarrhythmia when antiarrhythmic drugs are prescribed) to obtain the net clinical benefit. In this example, if treatment A is associated with a 0.5% excess risk of an adverse outcome such as stroke compared with treatment B, then for every 1000 patients receiving treatment A, 30 lives would be saved at the expense of 5 strokes, for a net clinical benefit of 25 stroke-free lives saved.

These types of comparisons require the clinical community to make a judgment regarding the relative importance of various outcomes. How many deaths would have to be prevented to offset the causation of one stroke? Another example of recent interest is the possibility that some therapies (inotropic agents) may improve symptoms but at the same time may increase mortality, a scenario that may be acceptable to patients incapacitated by severe symptoms but not to patients with mild symptoms. This issue can be explicitly addressed with the use of decision analysis.

Number needed to treat is a complex concept that becomes even more difficult when the impact of therapies for chronic disease are considered. For acute therapies with only a short-term effect, such as thrombolytic therapy, the simple version of number needed to treat is adequate. However, saving 10 lives per 100 patients treated in the first 30 days is quite different from the same effect over 5 years. In some therapies, the concept of number needed to treat is even more complex, because the more effective treatment may have an early hazard, leading to a reversal of the treatment effect over time. For thrombolytic therapy, this early hazard lasts only for the first day, whereas for coronary bypass surgery, mortality with surgery is higher than with medical treatment until the survival curves cross more than 1 year after randomization.[51]

When weighing the evidence from clinical trials for a treatment decision in an individual patient, physicians must consider more than the level of significance of the findings. In addition to the rationale for a given treatment, practitioners need to know which patients to treat, what drug and dose to use, and when and where therapy should be initiated.[52] Not all clinical trial reports provide all information required to form a complete assessment of the validity, precision, and implications of the results and answer the questions noted previously. In an attempt to introduce consistency in the reporting of clinical trials in the biomedical literature, a checklist of information for trialists, journal editors, peer-review panels, and the general medical audience has been proposed (Table 51–6).[53, 54] Presentation of a minimal set of uniform information in clinical trial reports should assist clinicians in making treatment decisions.

TABLE 51–6. CHECKLIST OF INFORMATION FOR INCLUSION IN REPORTS OF CLINCAL TRIALS

Introduction
A priori hypothesis, specific protocol objectives

Methods
Study as designed, including
- Planned study population, including controls
- Inclusion and exclusion criteria
- Planned subgroup analyses
- Prognostic factors that may affect study results
- Outcome measures and minimum difference(s) to be considered clinically important
- Planned treatment interventions
- Method of assignment of subjects to treatments (e.g., randomization method, blinding or masking procedure, matching criteria)
- Planned sample size and power calculations
- Rules for stopping the study
- Methods of statistical analysis in sufficient detail to permit replication

Results
Study as conducted, including
- Inclusive dates of accrual of study population
- Sample size achieved
- How many subjects were excluded or withdrew and the reasons for exclusion or withdrawal
- Demographics and clinical characteristics of the study population, including controls
- How the study as conducted deviated from the study as planned and the reasons for deviation (e.g., compliance)

Study findings including
- Estimates of treatment effects, stated as comparisons among treatment groups (e.g., differences in risks, rates, or means of outcome measures, as well as exact p values, not just $p<.05$)
- Measures of precision for outcome measures and for estimates of treatment effects (e.g., confidence intervals, standard errors)
- Summary data and appropriate descriptive statistics
- Complications of treatment
- Repository where original data can be obtained

Discussion
Interpretation of study findings
Results considered in the context of results in other trials reported in the literature

Modified from Working Group on Recommendations for Reporting of Clinical Trials in Biomedical Literature: Call for comments on a proposal to improve reporting of clinical trials in the biomedical literature. Ann Intern Med 1994; 121:894–895.

META-ANALYSIS

Frequently, clinicians are faced with many trials of a given treatment, some of which provide seemingly conflicting results. A method of summarizing the data is needed. Meta-analysis is a systematic, quantitative synthesis of data from multiple clinical sources addressing a related question.[13, 55, 56] Meta-analysis is a well-defined, scientific, statistical discipline with established methods and standards.[13, 57–63] Synonymous terms encountered in the literature include overview, pooling, data pooling, literature synthesis, research synthesis, and quantitative review.[13, 44] Although the concept of data pooling has existed for nearly a century, its introduction into the clinical literature has met with mixed reactions, ranging from exuberant support and in-depth analysis[64, 65] to overt skepticism.[66–68] The large number of meta-analyses published in the field of cardiovascular medicine suggest that the technique is gaining in popularity and is likely to play an important role in the complex process of therapeutic decision making in the future.[5, 57, 69–80]

When pooling studies, it is important that all available trials are located and considered for inclusion. Because investigators are more likely to report only positive findings, the issue of publication bias must be considered when searching for trials to include in a meta-analysis. Statistical techniques have been proposed to screen for publication bias, although this appears to be more of a concern for observational and laboratory-based experimental studies than for randomized controlled trials.[81, 82]

The fundamental principle of a meta-analysis is that the statistical power to estimate a treatment effect is enhanced because of an increase in sample size. An inherent assumption is that the available studies are sufficiently similar that pooling is appropriate. The various techniques of pooling construct a weighted average of the study outcomes; the selection of weighting techniques and approach to handling between-study variability distinguishes the different analytic methodologies.[63, 83] Some authorities have proposed incorporating an adjustment for variations in the quality of individual trials when performing a meta-analysis, but this requires further research before formal recommendations can be made.[55, 84]

Principles of Pooling Studies: Fixed-Effects Model vs. Random-Effects Model

The fixed-effects model (Fig. 51–5) assumes that the trials are sampled from a homogenous group. Under the homogeneity assump-

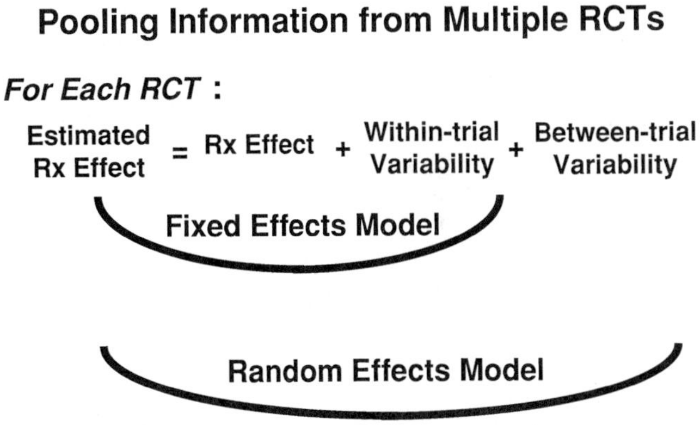

Figure 51–5. Fixed-effects and random-effects models for pooling results of randomized controlled trials (RCTs) in a meta-analysis. The fixed-effects model assumes that the trials are homogeneous and differences between their estimates of the true treatment effect are due only to experimental error (within-trial variability). The random-effects model assumes the trials are heterogeneous and that differences between estimates of the treatment effect are due to experimental error (within-trial variability) and differences among the trials (between-trial variability). *Abbreviation:* Rx, treatment.

tion, each trial provides an estimate of the single true treatment effect, and differences between the estimates from the various trials are the result only of experimental error (within-trial variability).[56, 57, 61] The random-effects model assumes the trials are heterogeneous and that differences among the various estimates of the treatment effect are the result of both experimental error (within-trial variability) and differences among the trials such as trial design and characteristics of the patients enrolled (between-trial variability).[62] The random-effects model is generally favored by most authorities, because heterogeneity that cannot be explained by experimental error often exists among trials, and this model takes such heterogeneity into account in estimation and hypothesis testing.[85] Unless extreme heterogeneity is present among the trials, the point estimate of the treatment effect is similar with the use of fixed- and random-effects models, but the 95% confidence intervals are generally wider with the random-effects method because they incorporate the uncertainty present in the among-trial variation (see Fig. 51–5).

Cumulative Meta-Analysis

In an effort to shorten the time delay between identification of an effective or ineffective therapy in clinical trials and translation of the findings into clinical practice, a technique of continuously updating meta-analyses has been developed.[55] This methodology, referred to as cumulative meta-analysis, updates the pooled estimate of the treatment effect each time the results of a new trial are published (Figs. 51–6 and 51–7). When cumulative meta-analyses on randomized controlled trials of acute and secondary therapies for acute myocardial infarction were compared with textbook chapters and review articles, discrepancies were detected between the meta-analytic patterns of effectiveness and the recommendations of clinical experts.[5] The reasons for these discrepancies may be complex and include a limited ability of authors of review articles to keep abreast of all the randomized controlled trials in a particular area, failure to recognize the limited power of small "negative" trials, unfamiliarity with or uncertainty about meta-analyses, and a natural conservatism about recommending new therapies until extensive, large-scale clinical trials are completed. The use of cumulative meta-analysis in formulating therapeutic guidelines in the future requires additional methodologic study before its role can be properly defined. Simulation studies suggest that there may be considerable sampling variation in the time when a cumulative meta-analysis is first significant.[86] Simulation methods can also estimate the type I error and power of a meta-analysis.[86] Because of the possibility in certain collections of trials of increasing risks of a type I error when multiple looks are taken at the accumulating data, more stringent statistical standards for declaration of significance may be required.[56]

Meta-Regression

The majority of meta-analyses in the cardiovascular literature report an average treatment effect estimated from the available studies. To move beyond the current methodology, several investigators have proposed that estimates of the treatment effect be expressed as a function of study-specific features such as years of study, drug dose, characteristics of patients enrolled (e.g., age, gender, race), or average mortality in the control group.[87–89] Adjustments for covariates in clinical trials can be accomplished with the use of regression techniques, and thus the term meta-regression has been introduced.[79, 90, 91] Meta-regression is useful for identifying sources of heterogeneity among clinical trials and establishing clinically important relations such as dose-response[88, 92] and changes in the incidence of outcome variables (e.g., primary ventricular fibrillation in acute myocardial infarction) between studies conducted in the distant past and those conducted more recently.[93]

When Clinical Trials and Meta-Analyses Disagree

Just as two randomized controlled trials of the same treatment for a cardiovascular illness may arrive at opposite conclusions, it is possible for meta-analyses that pool the results from trials up to a given point in time to arrive at conclusions that are discrepant from those seen in subsequent trials of the same therapy. The findings of individual trials may vary because of differences in the profile of patients enrolled, subtle variations in the treatment regimen (e.g., subcutaneous versus intravenous heparin with thrombolytic agents), differences in design or definition of endpoints, or simply by random variation. Although statistical tests do exist for detecting heterogeneity among trials when they are pooled in a meta-analysis, these tests are not very potent and may fail to identify heterogeneity when it truly exists. Meta-analyses performed with a fixed-effects model tend to obscure differences among trials more than those performed with a random-effects model.[13, 63, 85] However, neither model can correct for bias in the selection of studies to be pooled or the pooling of studies that have marked differences in important covariates such as patient characteristics and therapeutic regimens. Thus, a meta-analysis of trials may arrive at a conclusion that is different from that of a subsequent trial that enrolls a different patient population or incorporates an important modification of the treatment regimen. Evidence exists that the meta-analytic estimate of the magnitude of a treatment effect is closely linked to the underlying level of risk in the trials being pooled.[94]

Although it is tempting to believe that randomized controlled megatrials enrolling tens of thousands of patients provide definitive information about the efficacy or lack of efficacy of therapies and should supersede the findings of meta-analyses of smaller trials, this perspective may not always be correct.[95] A recent example of this problem is the controversy surrounding possible benefits of supplemental magnesium in patients with acute myocardial infarction.

Meta-analysis of seven small randomized controlled trials published between 1984 and 1991 and collectively enrolling about 1300 patients from the prethrombolytic era yielded an OR of .45 (.23, .86), indicating a significant benefit of magnesium in reducing mor-

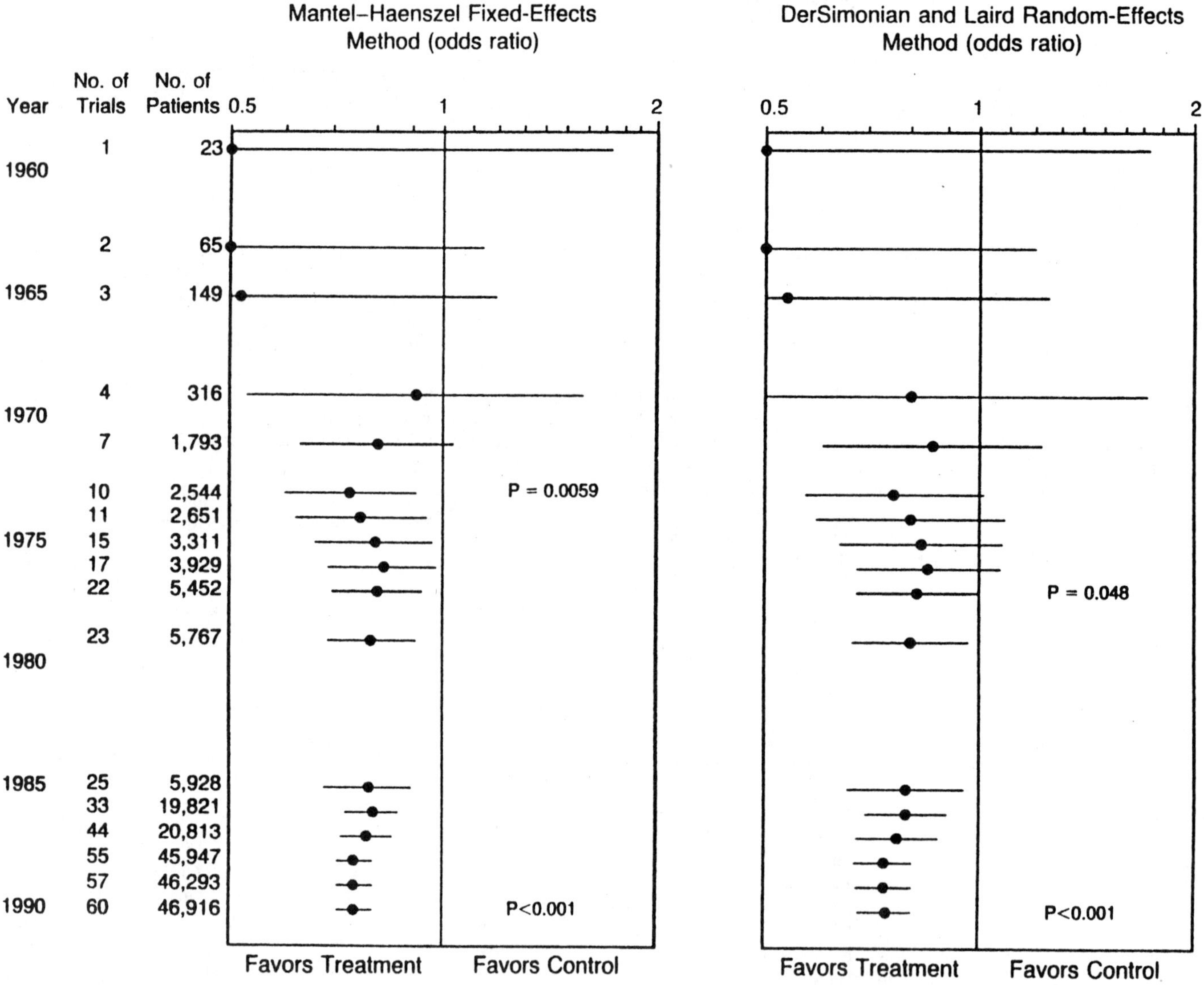

Figure 51–6. Cumulative meta-analyses of 60 trials of intravenous thrombolytic agents for myocardial infarction by the Mantel-Haenszel fixed-effects method and DerSimonian and Laird random-effects method. The odds ratios and 95% confidence intervals for an effect of treatment on mortality are shown on a logarithmic scale. The statistical significance reaches less than .05 in 1973 with the fixed-effects method and in 1977 with the random-effects method. (From Lau J, Antman EM, Jimenez-Silva J, et al: Cumulative meta-analysis of therapeutic trials for myocardial infarction. N Engl J Med 1992; 327:248–254.)

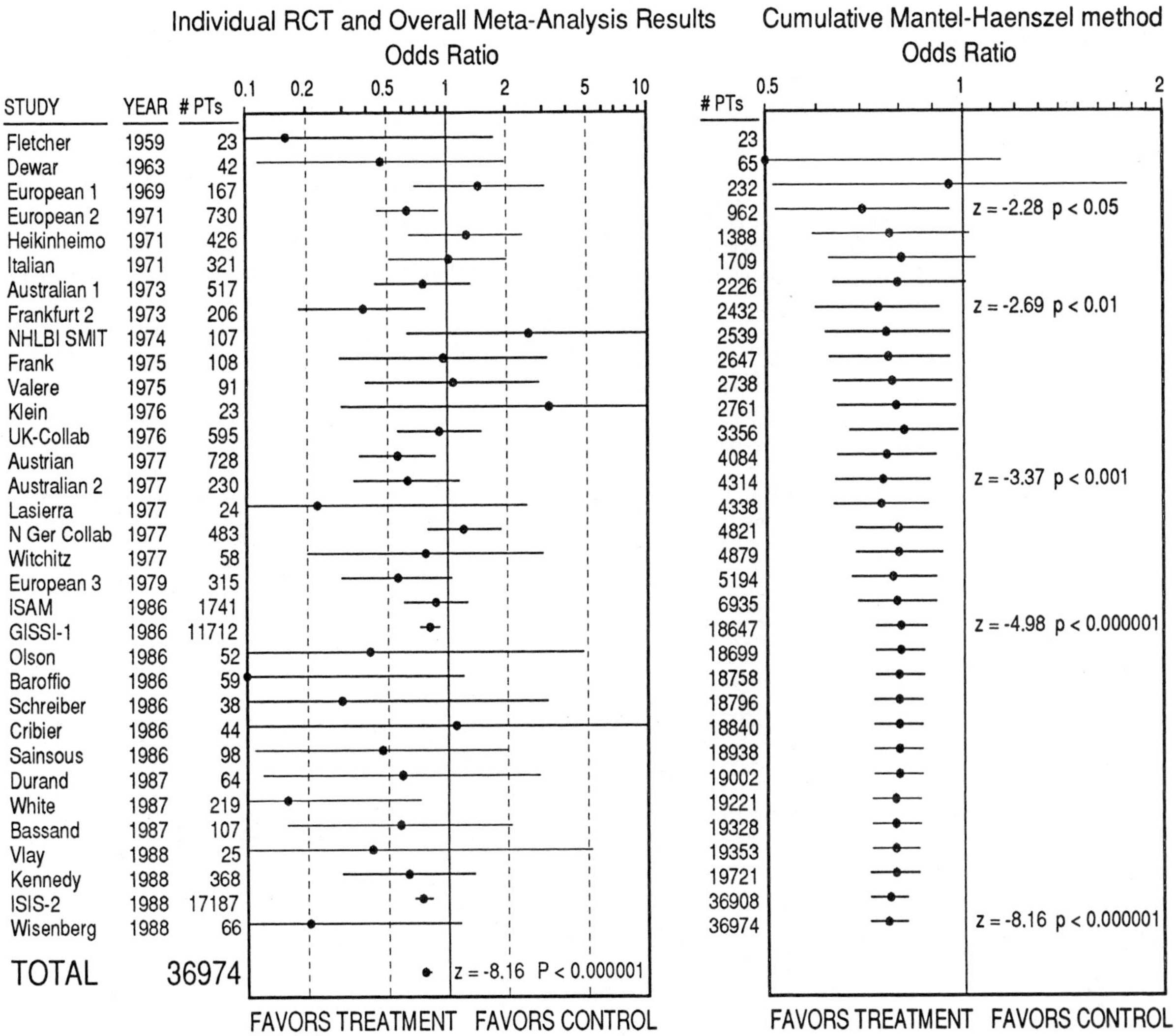

Figure 51–7. Conventional and cumulative meta-analyses for 33 trials of intravenous streptokinase for acute myocardial infarction. The odds ratios and 95% confidence intervals for an effect of treatment on mortality are shown on a logarithmic scale. Cumulative meta-analyses update the estimate of the treatment effect each time a new randomized controlled trial is published and makes it possible to study trends in potentially beneficial or harmful effects of therapies. *Abbreviation:* RCT, randomized controlled trial. (From Lau J, Antman EM, Jimenez-Silva J, et al: Cumulative meta-analysis of therapeutic trials for myocardial infarction. N Engl J Med 1992; 327:248–254.)

tality.[5, 55, 96] The Second Leicester Intravenous Magnesium Intervention Trial (LIMIT-2) published in 1992 reported a 24% reduction in mortality in accordance with the prior meta-analysis. The ISIS-4 mega-trial, however, reported no mortality benefit and even the possibility of slight harm with magnesium (OR = 1.06; .99–1.13).[97] Although it is possible that publication bias and an inadequate sample size per number of events in the trials that preceded ISIS-4 made the estimates of magnesium's effect biased, less robust, or both, several medical issues must also be considered.[56, 98] One of the leading hypotheses of the mechanism of magnesium's treatment effect is its ability to minimize reperfusion injury and myocardial stunning at the time of restoration of coronary perfusion. The relatively late administration of magnesium in ISIS-4 (after rather than before thrombolysis in the patients who received lytics and at a median of 12 h in the patients not receiving thrombolytics) coupled with a low control group mortality rate of 7.2% may have prevented the mortality-reducing potential of magnesium from being detected.[95, 98] In support of this hypothesis is a report from a more recent trial of a significant reduction in mortality when magnesium was administered early in patients not receiving thrombolytics.[99] Meta-regression techniques suggest that the benefit of magnesium is seen most prominently in patients at highest risk of mortality (e.g., elderly with contraindications to thrombolysis), inspiring clinical investigators to explore the potential role of magnesium more fully before casting aside such an inexpensive and easily administered medication.[95, 98]

Future Trends in Meta-Analysis

The previous discussion on meta-analysis treats the individual randomized controlled trial as the unit of analysis. The difference between the aggregate result for the test and control groups for each trial is calculated and then pooled with the observed differences in other trials. Ideally, the individual patients in each trial should be the unit of analysis to assess whether the treatment effect is modified by certain patient characteristics. Recent collaborative efforts of trialists studying antiplatelet therapy for a wide range of cardiovascular conditions, thrombolytic therapy for suspected myocardial infarction, and coronary artery bypass surgery versus medical therapy for coronary heart disease illustrate the power of pooling individual patient data to provide estimates of the treatment effect stratified by various clinical profiles (e.g., age, gender, ventricular function, history of infarction or stroke)[51, 69–71, 77] (Figs. 51–8 and 51–9). The success of these efforts is likely to inspire other investigators to plan prospectively for pooling of case report from information across related trials.

HOW TO READ AND INTERPRET A META-ANALYSIS

A series of practical questions that readers should ask when assessing a meta-analysis are shown in Table 51–7. The same standards should apply whether the physician is reading an overview of

Presentation features	Percent of patients dead: Fibrinolytic	Percent of patients dead: Control	Stratified statistics: O-E	Stratified statistics: Variance	Chi-square test of odds ratios in different patient categories: Heterogeneity	Trend
ECG					21.28 on 6 df (P < .01)	
BBB	18.7%	23.6%	-24.5	83.3		
ST elev, anterior	13.2%	16.9%	-122.0	420.6		
ST elev, inferior	7.5%	8.4%	-27.1	237.4		
ST elev, other	10.6%	13.4%	-42.1	159.6		
ST depression	15.2%	13.8%	12.9	108.7		
Other abnormality	5.2%	5.8%	-9.6	103.2		
Normal	3.0%	2.3%	3.4	12.9		
Hours from onset					9.69 on 4 df (P < .05)	9.55 on 1 df (2P = 0.002)
0- 1	9.5%	13.0%	-29.3	83.3		
2- 3	8.2%	10.7%	-100.2	354.8		
4- 6	9.7%	11.5%	-78.5	387.6		
7-12	11.1%	12.7%	-51.5	336.7		
13-24	10.0%	10.5%	-11.1	212.6		
Age (years)					8.27 on 3 df (P < .05)	6.58 on 1 df (2P = 0.01)
< 55	3.4%	4.6%	-45.9	155.6		
55-64	7.2%	8.9%	-86.3	360.0		
65-74	13.5%	16.1%	-113.7	533.0		
75 +	24.3%	25.3%	-12.6	266.6		
Gender					1.99 on 1 df (NS)	
Male	8.2%	10.1%	-208.1	928.0		
Female	14.1%	16.0%	-62.2	436.8		
Systolic BP (mm Hg)					1.31 on 3 df (NS)	0.68 on 1 df (NS)
< 100	28.9%	35.1%	-38.7	132.2		
100-149	9.6%	11.5%	-168.9	850.0		
150-174	7.2%	8.7%	-59.2	290.0		
175 +	7.2%	8.2%	-10.8	74.1		
Heart rate					0.51 on 2 df (NS)	0.31 on 1 df (NS)
< 80	7.2%	8.5%	-83.2	464.9		
80-99	9.2%	11.3%	-65.8	287.2		
100 +	17.4%	20.7%	-51.7	238.6		
Prior MI					2.09 on 1 df (NS)	
Yes	12.5%	14.1%	-43.7	322.4		
No	8.9%	10.9%	-228.5	1001.9		
Diabetes					1.57 on 1 df (NS)	
Yes	13.6%	17.3%	-41.4	145.7		
No	8.7%	10.2%	-142.6	830.4		
ALL PATIENTS	2820/29315 9.6%	3357/29285 11.5%	-269.5	1377.4		

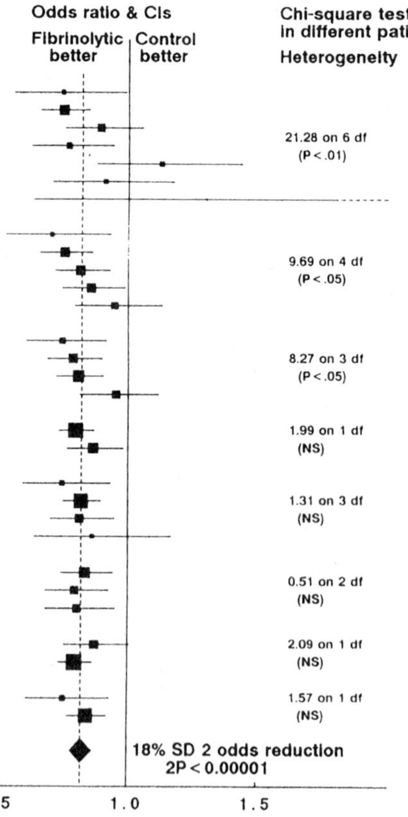

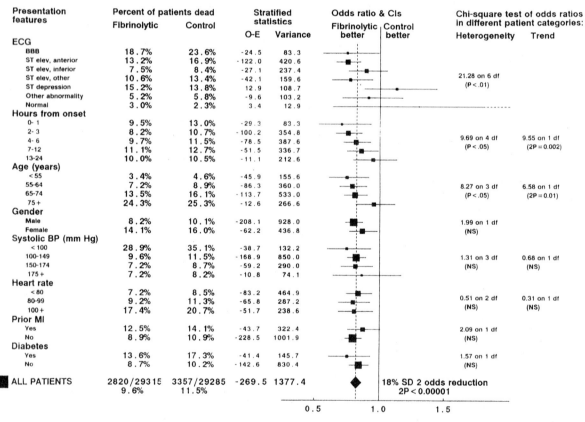

Figure 51–8. Proportional effects of fibrinolytic therapy on mortality during days 0–35, subdivided by presentation features. The "observed minus expected" (O-E) number of events among fibrinolytic-allocated patients and its variance is given for subdivisions of presentation features stratified by trial. The O-E is used to calculate odds ratios (ORs) of death among patients allocated to fibrinolytic therapy to that among those allocated to control. ORs (*black squares* with areas proportional to amount of "statistical information" contributed by the trials) are plotted with their 99% confidence intervals (CI; *horizontal lines*). Squares to left of the solid vertical line indicate benefit, which is significant at $2p < .01$ only when the entire CI is to the left of the vertical line. Overall result and 95% CI are represented by a diamond, with overall proportional reduction in the odds of death and statistical significance given beside the diamond. Chi-square tests for evidence of heterogeneity or trends in size of ORs in subdivisions of each presentation feature are also given. *Abbreviations:* BP, blood pressure; ECG, electrocardiogram; MI, myocardial infarction; SD, standard deviation. (From Fibrinolytic Therapy Trialists' [FTT] Collaborative Group: Indications for fibrinolytic therapy. Lancet 1994; 343:311.)

Category of trial	No of trials with data	MI, STROKE, OR VASCULAR DEATH: Anti-platelet	MI, STROKE, OR VASCULAR DEATH: Adjusted controls†	STRATIFIED STATISTICS: O–E	STRATIFIED STATISTICS: Variance	% odds reduction (SD)
Prior MI	11	1331/9877 (13.5%)	1693/9914 (17.1%)	−158·5	561·6	25% (4)
Acute MI	9	992/9388 (10.6%)	1348/9385 (14.4%)	−177·9	510·3	29% (4)
Prior stroke/TIA	18	1076/5837 (18.4%)	1301/5870 (22.2%)	−98·5	386·5	22% (4)
Other high risk	104	784/11 434 (6.9%)	1058/11 542 (9.2%)	−134·0	352·5	32% (4)
ALL HIGH RISK (four main categories)	**142**	**4183/36 536 (11.4%)**	**5400/36 711 (14.7%)**	**−568·8**	**1810·9**	27% (2)
ALL LOW RISK (primary prevention)	**3**	**652/14 608 (4.46%)**	**708/14 604 (4.85%)**	**−28·5**	**273·5**	10% (6)
ALL TRIALS† (high or low risk)	**145**	**4835/51 144 (9.5%)**	**6108/51 315 (11.9%)**	**−597·3**	**2084·4**	25% (2)

Heterogeneity of odds reductions:
– between four high risk categories χ^2_3 = 4.1; NS
– between high risk and low risk χ^2_1 = 10.5; P=0.001

†Crude, unadjusted control total = 5274/45 172.

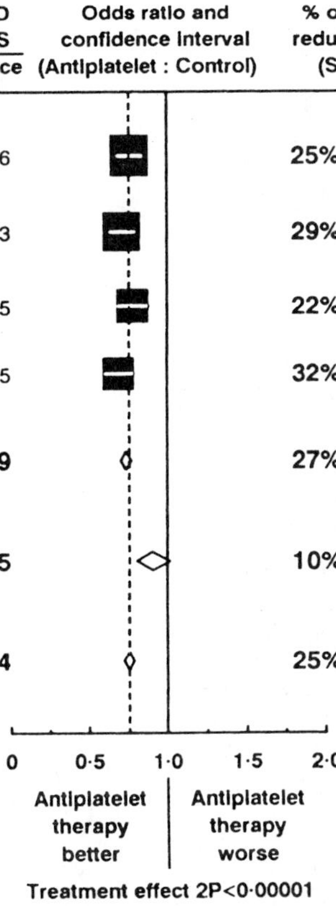

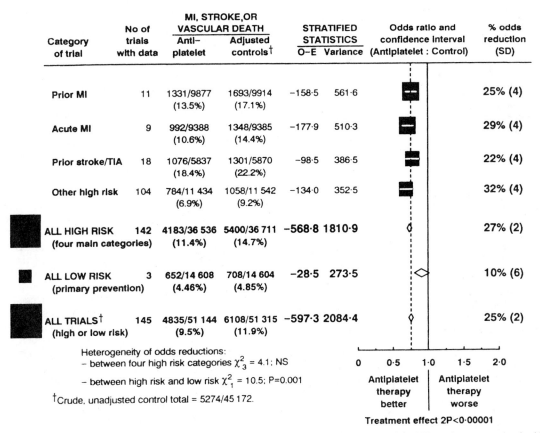

Figure 51–9. Proportional effects of antiplatelet therapy (145 trials) on vascular events (myocardial infarction [MI], stroke, or vascular death) in four main high-risk and low-risk (primary prevention) categories. Stratified ratio of odds of an event in treatment groups to that in control groups is plotted for each group of trials (*black squares*) along with its 99% confidence interval (*horizontal lines*). Overviews of results for certain subtotals and their 95% confidence intervals are represented by diamonds. Odds reductions observed in particular groups of trials are given to the right of the solid vertical line. *Abbreviations:* O-E, observed minus expected; SD, standard deviation; TIA, transient ischemic attack. (From Antiplatelet Trialist's Collaboration: Collaborative overview of randomised trials of antiplatelet therapy. I. Prevention of death, myocardial infarction, and stroke by prolonged antiplatelet therapy in various categories of patients. Br Med J 1994; 308:81–106.)

TABLE 51–7. HOW TO READ AND INTERPRET A META-ANALYSIS

Are the Results of the Study Valid?
Primary guides
- Does the overview address a focused clinical question?
- Are the criteria used to select articles for inclusion appropriate?

Secondary guides
- Is it unlikely that important, relevant studies were missed?
- Is the validity of the included studies appraised?
- Are the assessments of studies reproducible?
- Are the results similar from study to study?

What Are the Results?
What are the overall results of the review?
How precise are the results?

Will the Results Help Me in Caring for My Patients?
Can the results be applied to my patient?
Are all clinically important outcomes considered?
Are the benefits worth the risks and costs?

Modified from Oxman A, Cook D, Guyatt G, et al: Users' guides to the medical literature. VI. How to use an overview. JAMA 1994; 272:1367–1375.

a therapeutic modality or the results of a diagnostic test for a medical condition.[100, 101] Readers must be convinced that the authors attempted to answer a focused question of clinical importance, all relevant studies were included, and an attempt was made to assess the data for evidence of heterogeneity and to explain between-trial variability if it is present. As with individual clinical trial reports, an overview should include a statement of the pooled treatment effect that incorporates both relative risk reduction and ARD and conveys the information in a clinically practical fashion (e.g., number to treat, number of lives saved per 1000 patients treated).

When attempting to apply the findings of an overview to an individual patient, clinicians must ascertain whether their patient is similar to those enrolled in the trials included in the meta-analysis. Although there may be a temptation to focus on subgroup information from the meta-analysis to determine if a given patient is likely to experience more or less than the average benefit of the treatment, this must be done cautiously. Subgroup analyses are more reliable if there is a highly significant treatment difference, if they represent hypotheses established before trial initiation, if they are consistent across studies, and if they are biologically plausible.[100] The potential risks of the therapeutic intervention should be considered and discussed with the patient to ensure that the treatment decision is consistent with their concerns about quality of life.[102]

THERAPEUTIC DECISION MAKING: DECISION ANALYSIS AND COST-EFFECTIVENESS ANALYSIS

When weighing therapeutic alternatives for an individual patient, clinicians must integrate a complex array of data. Even the most rigorously conducted randomized controlled trial may only serve as a rough guide, because the patient in question may differ from those in the study in important ways (e.g., age, severity of illness, comorbid illnesses). Furthermore, simultaneously weighing the competing benefits and risks of the various alternatives frequently is difficult and involves too many variables for clinical intuition alone.[103, 104] Decision analysis is a semiquantitative method that applies probability and utility theory for assessing the relative value of one treatment decision versus another.[83] The process involves a statement of the problem followed by construction of a decision tree that outlines the various alternatives. The probabilities of each outcome are then assigned at all decision nodes by gathering data from clinical trials and meta-analyses such as those discussed in this chapter. The decision tree is formally analyzed to provide a quantitative statement about the probability of various outcomes if different courses of treatment are followed.

Because many of the processes in cardiovascular medicine involve transitions in and out of various states of health (e.g., unstable angina versus chronic stable angina) a technique that is frequently used in analyzing decision trees is the development of a Markov model that estimates the probabilities of various outcomes as the patient cycles through changing health states. After the decision tree is analyzed, its stability is tested by a sensitivity analysis that varies the assumptions made and helps identify those that are most critical to the decision-making process.[83]

It is important to involve the patient in the therapeutic decision-making process whenever possible. Individuals may vary in their preferences for certain outcomes or willingness to accept certain levels of risk to attain those outcomes (e.g., sinus rhythm versus proarrhythmia in patients contemplating suppressive antiarrhythmic therapy for atrial fibrillation). By employing a weighting factor, called a "utility," in the decision analysis process, utility analysis attempts to adjust for the patient's (or society's) preferences for quality of life; the results are commonly expressed as quality-adjusted life years (QALYs). Finally, by comparing the costs of various medical approaches with the QALYs for each approach, a cost-effectiveness analysis can be performed, allowing clinicians to appreciate the incremental (or marginal) costs of one therapeutic alternative versus another.[83]

An example that compared the relative risks and benefits of several clinical strategies for management of patients with chronic atrial fibrillation illustrates these principles quite effectively.[104] The authors used a Markov decision analysis to assess the outcomes in large, hypothetical cohorts of patients with chronic atrial fibrillation treated with four possible strategies: no treatment, warfarin, electrical cardioversion by quinidine to maintain sinus rhythm, and electrical cardioversion followed by low-dose amiodarone to maintain sinus rhythm (Fig. 51–10). The probabilities for various outcomes (e.g., well in sinus rhythm, disabled in sinus rhythm) after each Markov cycle were obtained from the literature, when available, and utilities were assigned for important events such as a disabling stroke or major amiodarone pulmonary toxicity. Amiodarone appeared to emerge as the preferred strategy, because it was associated with the lowest probability of a disabling event or mortality and had the highest net benefit in QALYs compared with the base case of no treatment.

Analyses of complex clinical decisions, such as the one performed by Disch and colleagues[104] for chronic atrial fibrillation, also illustrate how the foundation for future clinical trials is formed. Greater precision in the estimated probabilities for outcomes such as maintenance of sinus rhythm or development of disabling stroke or major hemorrhage in contemporary clinical practice with improved monitoring practices and new pharmacologic regimens (e.g., less aggressive use of warfarin) is needed, as is an assessment of the role of new therapeutic strategies such as catheter ablation and "Maze" surgery (see Chapter 17). Several randomized trials are presently under development to answer these questions and will undoubtedly be the subject of future reports in the evolving field of cardiovascular therapeutics.

Cost-effectiveness analysis has become increasingly important as the financial backing of the health care system has become constrained. Cost effectiveness is not an absolute term; rather, one therapy must be compared with another. To calculate a cost-effectiveness ratio, the difference in cost and the difference in effectiveness between the two therapies being compared must be considered. Effectiveness is usually expressed in terms of number of life years saved or number of QALYs saved, although other measures of efficacy, such as the prevention of complications, have been used. In general, therapies costing less than $50,000 per year of life saved are considered to be in the range of acceptable based on the societal norm that renal dialysis is considered to be worthwhile. It is important for the clinician to realize that directly comparing cost-effectiveness ratios for different therapies may be misleading. Simple

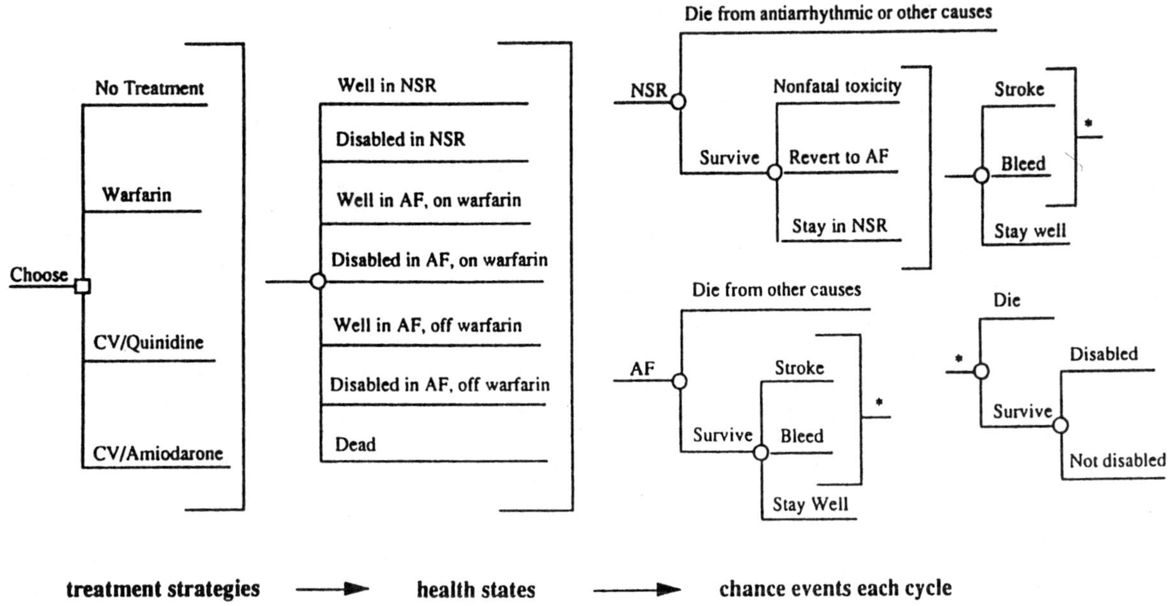

Figure 51–10. Schematic of a decision model for management of patients with chronic atrial fibrillation (AF). The square is a "decision node" of which treatment strategy to use. The circles are "chance nodes," at which each patient faces several chance events. Each "disabled" state represents several states in the actual model (e.g., disabled from stroke, disabled from bleeding event). Asterisks indicate that the model was not sensitive to the corresponding variable when its value was varied over a clinically plausible range of values. *Abbreviations:* CV, cardioversion; NSR, normal sinus rhythm. (From Disch DL, Greenberg ML, Holzberger PT, et al: Managing chronic atrial fibrillation: a Markov decision analysis comparing warfarin, quinidine, and low-dose amiodarone. Ann Intern Med 1994; 120:449–457.)

therapies such as aspirin or streptokinase are very effective and have a low cost-effectiveness ratio. Newer therapies may even be more effective, but they will almost certainly have a higher cost-effectiveness ratio. The major issue is the *incremental* cost-effectiveness ratio comparing the treatments of interest.

REFERENCES

1. U.S. Food and Drug Administration: Hearing regulations and regulations describing scientific content of adequate and well-controlled clinical investigations. Federal Register 1970, May 8; 35:7250–7253.
2. Naylor CD: Grey zones of clinical practice: some limits to evidence-based medicine. Lancet 1995; 345:840–842.
3. Wenger N: Inclusion of elderly individuals in clinical trials. Cardiovascular disease and cardiovascular therapy as a model. Kansas City: Marion Merrell Dow, 1993.
4. Fredrickson D: The field trial: some thoughts on the indispensable ordeal. Bull NY Acad Med 1968; 44:985–993.
5. Antman E, Lau J, Kupelnick B, et al: A comparison of results of meta-analyses of randomized control trials and recommendations of clinical experts. JAMA 1992; 268:240–248.
6. Lamas G, Pfeffer M, Hamm P, et al: Do the results of randomized clinical trials of cardiovascular drugs influence medical practice? N Engl J Med 1992; 327:241–247.
7. Kassirer J: Clinical trials and meta-analysis. What do they do for us? N Engl J Med 1992; 327:273–274.
8. Ayanian J, Hauptman P, Guadagnoli E, et al: Knowledge and practices of generalist and specialist physicians regarding drug therapy for acute myocardial infarction. N Engl J Med 1994; 331:1136–1142.
9. Scandinavian Simvistatin Survival Study Group: Randomised trial of cholesterol lowering in 4444 patients with coronary heart disease: the Scandinavian Simvastatin Survival Study (4S). Lancet 1994; 344:1383–1389.
10. The Writing Group for the PEPI Trial: Effects of estrogen or estrogen/progestin regimens on heart disease risk factors in postmenopausal women. The postmenopausal estrogen/progestin interventions (PEPI) trial. JAMA 1995; 273:199–208.
11. Friedman L, Furberg C, DeMets D: Fundamentals of Clinical Trials, 2nd ed. Littleton: PSG Publishing, 1985.
12. Meinert C: Clinical Trials. Design, conduct, and analysis. New York: Oxford University Press, 1986.
13. Dickersin K, Berlin J: Meta-analysis: state-of-the-science. Epidemiol Rev 1992; 14:154–176.
14. Schulz K, Chalmers I, Hayes R, et al: Empirical evidence of bias. Dimensions of methodological quality associated with estimates of treatment effects in controlled trials. JAMA 1995; 273:408–412.
15. Kraemer H, Fendt K: Random assignment in clinical trials: issues in planning (infant health and development program). J Clin Epidemiol 1990; 43:1157–1167.
16. Passamani E: Clinical trials—are they ethical? N Engl J Med 1991; 324:1589–1592.
17. Hellman S, Hellman D: Of mice but not men: problems of the randomized clinical trial. N Engl J Med 1991; 324:1585–1589.
18. Task Force of the Working Group on Arrhythmias of the European Society of Cardiology, Akhtar M, Breithardt G, et al: CAST and beyond. Implications of the Cardiac Arrhythmia Suppression Trial. Circulation 1990; 81:1123–1127.
19. Armstrong P, Furberg C: Clinical trial data and safety monitoring boards. The search for a constitution. Circulation 1995; 91:901–904.
20. Antman EM, for the TIMI 9A Investigators: Hirudin in acute myocardial infarction: safety report from the Thrombolysis and Thrombin Inhibition in Myocardial Infarction (TIMI) 9A trial. Circulation 1994; 90:1624–1630.
21. The Global Use of Strategies to Open Occluded Coronary Arteries (GUSTO) IIa Investigators: Randomized trial of intravenous heparin versus recombinant Hirudin for acute coronary syndromes. Circulation 1994; 90:1631–1637.
22. Braunwald E, Cannon CP, McCabe CH: Use of composite endpoints in thrombolysis trials of acute myocardial infarction. Am J Cardiol 1993; 72:3G–12G.
23. Wittes J, Lakatos E, Probstfield J: Surrogate endpoints in clinical trials: cardiovascular diseases. Stat Med 1989; 8:415–425.
24. Cole P, Beamer A, McGowan N, et al: Efficacy and safety of perhexiline maleate in refractory angina. A double-blind placebo-controlled clinical trial of a novel antianginal agent. Circulation 1990; 81:1260–1270.
25. Hlatky MA, Califf RM, Harrell FEJ, et al: Clinical judgment and therapeutic decision making. J Am Coll Cardiol 1990; 15:1–14.

26. Hlatky MA, Lee KL, Harrell FEJ, et al: Tying clinical research to patient care by use of an observational database. Stat Med 1984; 3:375–384.
27. Rogers W, Bowlby L, Chandra N, et al: Treatment of myocardial infarction in the United States (1990–1993). Observations from the National Registry of Myocardial Infarction. Circulation 1994; 90:2103–2114.
28. Brown BJ: The crossover experiment for clinical trials. Biometrics 1980; 36:69–80.
29. Packer M, Gheorghiade M, Young JB, et al: Withdrawal of digoxin from patients with chronic heart failure treated with angiotensin-converting-enzyme inhibitors. RADIANCE Study. N Engl J Med 1993; 329:1–7.
30. Smith T: Digoxin in heart failure. N Engl J Med 1993; 329:51–53.
31. Yusuf S, Garg R, Held P, et al: Need for a large randomized trial to evaluate the effects of digitalis on morbidity and mortality in congestive heart failure. Am J Cardiol 1992; 69:64G–70G.
32. Fleiss JL: The Design and Analysis of Clinical Experiments. New York: Wiley 1986.
33. ISIS–4 Collaborative Group: Fourth International Study of Infarct Survival: protocol for a large simple study of the effects of oral mononitrate, of oral captopril, and of intravenous magnesium. Am J Cardiol 1991; 68:87D–100D.
34. Hampton JR, Skene AM: Beyond the mega-trial: certainty and uncertainty. Br Heart J 1992; 68:352–355.
35. Durrleman S, Simon R: Planning and monitoring of equivalence studies. Biometrics 1990; 46:329–336.
36. Garbe E, Rohmel J, Gundert-Remy U: Clinical and statistical issues in therapeutic equivalence trials. Eur J Clin Pharmacol 1993; 45:1–7.
37. Gould AL: Sample sizes for event rate equivalence trials using prior information. Stat Med 1993; 12:2009–2023.
38. Glantz S: Primer of Biostatistics, 3rd ed. New York: McGraw–Hill, 1992.
39. Kim K, DeMets D: Design and analysis of group sequential tests based on the type I error spending rate function. Biometrika 1987; 74:149–154.
40. Ware J, Muller J, Braunwald E: The futility index. An approach to the cost-effective termination of randomized clinical trials. Am J Med 1985; 78:635–643.
41. Yusuf S, Wittes J, Probstfield J, et al: Analysis and interpretation of treatment effects in subgroups of patients in randomized clinical trials. JAMA 1991; 266:93–98.
42. Guyatt GH, Sackett DL, Cook DJ: The medical literature: users' guides to the medical literature. II. How to use an article about therapy or prevention. A. Are the results of the study valid? JAMA 1993; 270:2598–2601.
43. Guyatt GH, Sackett DL, Cook DJ: The medical literature: users' guides to the medical literature. II. How to use an article about therapy or prevention. B. What were the results and will they help me in caring for my patients? JAMA 1994; 271:59–63.
44. Ingelfinger J, Mosteller F, Thibodeau L, et al: Biostatistics in Clinical Medicine, 3rd ed. New York: McGraw-Hill, 1994.
45. Gardner M, Altman D: Statistics With Confidence. Confidence Intervals and Statistical Guidelines. London: British Medical Journal, 1989.
46. Pfeffer M, Braunwald E, Moyé L, et al: Effect of captopril on mortality and morbidity in patients with left ventricular dysfunction after myocardial infarction. N Engl J Med 1992; 327:669–677.
47. Sinclair J, Bracken M: Clinically useful measures of effect in binary analyses of randomized trials. J Clin Epidemiol 1994; 94:881–889.
48. Guyatt G, Cook D, Jaeschke R: How should clinicians use the results of randomized trials? ACP Journal Club 1995; 122:A12–A14.
49. Naylor C, Chen E, Strauss B: Measures of enthusiasm: does the method of reporting trial results alter perceptions of therapeutic effectiveness? Ann Intern Med 1992; 117:916–921.
50. Bucher H, Weinbacher M, Gyr K: Influence of method of reporting study results on decision of physicians to prescribe drugs to lower cholesterol concentration. Br Med J 1994; 309:761–764.
51. Yusuf S, Zucker D, Peduzzi P, et al: Effect of coronary artery bypass graft surgery on survival: an overview of 10-year results from randomised trials by the Coronary Artery Bypass Graft Surgery Trialists Collaboration. Lancet 1994; 344:563–570.
52. Pfeffer M: ACE Inhibition in acute myocardial infarction. N Engl J Med 1995; 332:118–120.
53. Working Group on Recommendations for Reporting of Clinical Trials in Biomedical Literature: Call for comments on a proposal to improve reporting of clinical trials in the biomedical literature. Ann Intern Med 1994; 121:894–895.
54. The Standards of Reporting Trials Group: A proposal for structured reporting of randomized controlled trials. JAMA 1994; 272:1926–1931.
55. Lau J, Antman EM, Jimenez-Silva J, et al: Cumulative meta-analysis of therapeutic trials for myocardial infarction. N Engl J Med 1992; 327:248–254.
56. Flather M, Farkouh M, Yusuf S: Meta-analysis in the evaluation of therapies. *In* Julian D, Braunwald E (eds): Management of Acute Myocardial Infarction, pp 393–406. London: WB Saunders, 1994.
57. Yusuf S, Peto R, Lewis J, et al: Beta blockade during and after myocardial infarction: an overview of the randomized trials. Prog Cardiovasc Dis 1985; 27:335–371.
58. Sacks H, Berrier J, Reitman D, et al: Meta-analyses of randomized controlled trials. N Engl J Med 1987; 316:450–455.
59. L'Abbe K, Detsky A, O'Rourke K: Meta-analysis in clinical research. Ann Intern Med 1987; 107:224–233.
60. Thacker S: Meta-analysis: a quantitative approach to research integration. JAMA 1988; 259:1685–1689.
61. Mantel N, Haenszel W: Statistical aspects of the analysis of data from retrospective studies of disease. J Natl Cancer Inst 1959; 22:719–748.
62. DerSimonian R, Laird N: Meta-analysis in clinical trials. Control Clin Trials 1986; 7:177–188.
63. Berlin J, Laird N, Sacks H, et al: A comparison of statistical methods for combining event rates from clinical trials. Stat Med 1989; 8:141–151.
64. Chalmers T, Levin H, Sacks H, et al: Meta-analysis of clinical trials as a scientific discipline: I. Control of bias and comparison with large cooperative trials. Stat Med 1987; 6:315–325.
65. Chalmers T, Berrier J, Sacks H, et al: Meta-analysis of clinical trials as a scientific discipline: II. Replicate variability and comparison of studies that agree and disagree. Stat Med 1987; 6:733–744.
66. Goldman L, Feinstein A: Anticoagulants and myocardial infarction. The problems of pooling, drowning, and floating. Ann Intern Med 1979; 90:92–94.
67. Spitzer W: Meta-meta-analysis: unanswered questions about aggregating data (editorial). J Clin Epidemiol 1991; 44:103–107.
68. Domanski MJ, Friedman LM: Relative role of meta-analysis and randomized controlled trials in the assessment of medical therapies. Am J Cardiol 1994; 74:395–396.
69. Antiplatelet Trialists' Collaboration: Collaborative overview of randomized trials of antiplatelet therapy: I. Prevention of death, myocardial infarction, and stroke by prolonged antiplatelet therapy in various categories of patients. Br Med J 1994; 308:81–106.
70. Antiplatelet Trialists' Collaboration: Collaborative overview of randomised trials of antiplatelet therapy: II. Maintenance of vascular graft or arterial patency by antiplatelet therapy. Br Med J 1994; 308:159–168.
71. Antiplatelet Trialists' Collaboration: Collaborative overview of randomised trials of antiplatelet therapy: III. Reduction in venous thrombosis and pulmonary embolism by antiplatelet prophylaxis among surgical and medical patients. Br Med J 1994; 308:235–246.
72. Yusuf S, Wittes J, Friedman L: Overview of results of randomized clinical trials in heart disease. I. Treatments following myocardial infarction. JAMA 1988; 260:2088–2093.
73. Yusuf S, Wittes J, Friedman L: Overview of results of randomized clinical trials in heart disease. II. Unstable angina, heart failure, primary prevention with aspirin, and risk factor modification. JAMA 1988; 260:2259–2263.
74. Teo K, Held P, Collins R, et al: Effect of intravenous magnesium on mortality in myocardial infarction. Circulation 1990; 82(suppl III):393.
75. Teo K, Yusuf S, Furberg C: Effects of prophylactic antiarrhythmic drug therapy in acute myocardial infarction. An overview of results from randomized controlled trials. JAMA 1993; 270:1589–1595.
76. Coplen S, Antman E, Berlin J, et al: Efficacy and safety of quinidine therapy for maintenance of sinus rhythm after cardioversion. A meta-analysis of randomized control trials. Circulation 1990; 82:1106–1116.
77. Fibrinolytic Therapy Trialists' (FTT) Collaborative Group: Indications for fibrinolytic therapy in suspected acute myocardial infarction: collaborative overview of mortality and major morbidity results from all randomised trials of more than 1000 patients. Lancet 1994; 343:311–322.
78. Henderson W, Goldman S, Copeland J, et al: Antiplatelet or anticoagulant therapy after coronary artery bypass surgery. Ann Intern Med 1989; 111:743–750.
79. Insua J, Sacks H, Lau T, et al: Drug treatment of hypertension in the elderly: a meta-analysis. Ann Intern Med 1994; 121:355–362.
80. Roux S, Christeller S, Ludin E: Effects of aspirin on coronary reocclusion and recurrent ischemia after thrombolysis: a meta-analysis. J Am Coll Cardiol 1992; 19:671–677.
81. Begg C, Berlin J: Publication bias: a problem in interpreting medical data. J R Stat Soc A 1988; 151:419–445.

82. Easterbrook P, Berlin J, Gopalan R, et al: Publication bias in clinical research. Lancet 1991; 337:867–872.
83. Petitti D: Meta-Analysis, Decision Analysis, and Cost-Effectiveness Analysis. New York: Oxford University Press, 1994.
84. Detsky A, Naylor C, O'Rourke K, et al: Incorporating variations in the quality of individual randomized trials into meta-analysis. J Clin Epidemiol 1992; 45:255–265.
85. National Research Council: Combining Information. Statistical Issues and Opportunities for Research. Washington, DC: National Academy Press, 1992.
86. Berkey C, Mosteller F, Lau J, et al: Uncertainty of the first instance of significance in random-effects cumulative meta-analysis. Control Clin Trials, in press.
87. Tukey J: Use of many covariates in clinical trials. Int Stat Rev 1991; 59:123–137.
88. Berlin J, Longnecker M, Greenland S: Meta-analysis of epidemiologic dose-response data. Epidemiology 1993; 4:218–228.
89. Berkey C, Hoaglin D, Mosteller F, et al: A random-effects regression model for meta-analysis. Stat Med 1995; 14:395–411.
90. Greenland S: Quantitative methods in the review of the epidemiologic literature. Epidemiol Rev 1987; 9:1–30.
91. Kasike B, Kalil R, Ma J, et al: Reviews: effect of antihypertensive therapy of the kidney in patients with diabetes: a meta-regression analysis. Ann Intern Med 1993; 118:129–138.
92. Galløe A, Graudal N: Magnesium and myocardial infarction (letter). Lancet 1994; 343:1286–1287.
93. Antman E, Berlin J: Declining incidence of ventricular fibrillation in myocardial infarction. Implications for the prophylactic use of lidocaine. Circulation 1992; 86:764–773.
94. Smith GD, Song F, Sheldon TA: Cholesterol lowering and mortality: the importance of considering the initial level of risk. Br Med J 1993; 306:1367–1373.
95. Antman E: Randomized trials of magnesium for acute myocardial infarction: big numbers do not tell the whole story. Am J Cardiol 1995; 75:391–393.
96. Teo KK, Yusuf S: Role of magnesium in reducing mortality in acute myocardial infarction. A review of the evidence. Drugs 1993; 46:347–359.
97. ISIS-4 (Fourth International Study of Infarct Survival) Collaborative Group: ISIS–4: A randomised factorial trial assessing early oral captopril, oral mononitrate, and intravenous magnesium sulphate in 58,050 patients with suspected myocardial infarction. Lancet 1995; 345:669–685.
98. Antman EM: Magnesium in acute MI. Timing is critical. Circulation 1995; 92:2367–2372.
99. Shechter M, Hod H, Kaplinsky E, et al: Magnesium therapy in acute myocardial infarction when patients are not candidates for thrombolytic therapy. Am J Cardiol 1995; 75:321–323.
100. Oxman A, Cook D, Guyatt G, et al: Users' guides to the medical literature. VI. How to use an overview. JAMA 1994; 272:1367–1375.
101. Irwig L, Tosteson A, Gatsonis C, et al: Guidelines for meta-analyses evaluating diagnostic tests. Ann Intern Med 1994; 120:667–676.
102. Wenger N, Mattson M, Furberg C, Elinson J: Assessment of Quality of Life in Clinical Trials of Cardiovascular Therapies. New York: Le Jacq, 1984, 374.
103. Kassirer JP, Kopelman RI: Learning Clinical Reasoning. Baltimore: Williams & Wilkins, 1991.
104. Disch DL, Greenberg ML, Holzberger PT, et al: Managing chronic atrial fibrillation: a Markov decision analysis comparing warfarin, quinidine, and low-dose amiodarone. Ann Intern Med 1994; 120:449–457.

52 Management of Cardiovascular Disease During Pregnancy

John D. Rutherford, MB, ChB

Circulatory changes occurring during pregnancy alter the clinical manifestations of cardiac disease, the therapeutic options, and the pharmacokinetics of administered drugs. Obviously, the influence of therapy on both the mother and the fetus needs to be considered in any given situation. To manage patients with cardiac disease during pregnancy, cardiologists, obstetricians, and anesthesiologists have to communicate well and coordinate therapy.

Cardiac output increases by 30%–50% during pregnancy, an increase that is well established by the end of the first trimester and is usually maintained until term. Under the influence of the hormones of pregnancy, peripheral vascular resistance and mean arterial pressure are lowest when cardiac output is maximal. Total maternal blood volume increases during normal pregnancy by 40%–50%. Whereas total red blood cell volume increases steadily, the plasma volume rises rapidly early in pregnancy and then more slowly until term.[1] During the first trimester, the increases in cardiac output, plasma volume, and extracellular fluid volume are associated with increases in renal plasma flow and glomerular filtration rate and an increase in total body water and exchangeable sodium. These changes in total body water and exchangeable sodium are associated with activation of the renin-angiotensin system and lowering of osmotic thresholds for vasopressin release and thirst stimulation. Thus, there is a fall in plasma sodium concentration and plasma osmolality, and clinical edema is found in up to 80% of healthy pregnant women.

These maternal physiologic changes occurring during pregnancy result in differences in pharmacokinetics of administered drugs. The volume of distribution for some drugs increases during pregnancy as a result of increases in maternal total body water and gain in fatty tissue between the 10th and 30th weeks. The increase in maternal glomerular filtration rate that occurs during pregnancy increases the rate of elimination of drugs excreted by the kidneys. Concomitantly, maternal hepatic enzyme activity appears to decrease. Last, delayed gastric motility and emptying may enhance or delay maternal drug absorption from the gastrointestinal tract. Prediction of the alteration in drug dosing required during pregnancy is difficult, and the clinician needs to carefully titrate the dose of administered drugs to the patient's pharmacologic response and at times to serum drug levels. Furthermore, any drug entering the maternal blood stream should be considered capable of crossing the placenta, and therefore reaching the fetus, unless information to the contrary exists. After implantation, most drugs pass freely to the embryo in concentrations generally lower than those measured simultaneously in the mother. Because the blood-brain barrier to diffusion is not developed in the fetus until the last half of pregnancy, the fetal central nervous system may be particularly susceptible to pharmacologic agents. Some pharmacologic agents can cause growth retardation, death, malformations, and functional deficits or impairments (i.e., they can be responsible for developmental toxicity). A valuable resource for the clinician seeking information concerning a particular drug is *Drugs in Pregnancy and Lactation: A Reference Guide to Fetal and Neonatal Risk.*[2]

VALVULAR HEART DISEASE[1]

In patients with mild cardiac symptoms, the mild or moderate regurgitant valvular lesions, such as mitral regurgitation and aortic regurgitation, are usually well tolerated if the patient maintains sinus rhythm, because the reduced peripheral vascular resistance (or afterload) of pregnancy tends to diminish the degree of regurgitation. Obviously, in patients with significant symptoms or major degrees of valvular regurgitation, the hemodynamic changes of pregnancy may impose an excessive load.

In contrast, the stenotic aortic and mitral valvular lesions tend to be poorly tolerated during pregnancy. The severity of the fixed stenosis is accentuated by the increase in both cardiac output and heart rate during pregnancy.

Mitral stenosis is the most common, and important, rheumatic cardiac lesion encountered during pregnancy. Indeed, pregnancy may be the first time that such patients have symptoms of breathlessness or the onset of atrial fibrillation. The onset of atrial fibrillation in a pregnant patient with mitral stenosis should be considered a medical emergency because acute pulmonary edema and cardiac decompensation can rapidly ensue. If a patient who is in sinus rhythm with mitral stenosis has symptoms, despite diuretic therapy, in the first trimester of pregnancy, it is unlikely that the patient and/or fetus will tolerate the lesion hemodynamically through pregnancy, labor, delivery, and the puerperium.

Routine use of diuretics for edema of pregnancy is not advised. If diuretic therapy is needed, a loop diuretic such as furosemide is often used. Loop diuretics suppress reabsorption of sodium chloride in the ascending limb of the nephron. Furosemide crosses the placenta, resulting in similar maternal and fetal levels, and increased fetal urine production has been observed.[3] After the first trimester, furosemide has been used for treatment of edema, hypertension, and toxemia during pregnancy without causing fetal or newborn adverse effects[3, 4] (Table 52–1). Neonatal thrombocytopenia has not been reported for furosemide. Furosemide is excreted into breast milk, and no adverse effects in nursing infants have been reported. Thiazide diuretics are not thought to be teratogenic, but they do cross the placenta, and neonatal thrombocytopenia, jaundice, and bradycardia have all been documented. (Many investigators now consider treatment of toxemia of pregnancy with diuretics inappropriate because they do not seem to prevent or alter the course of toxemia and they may decrease placental perfusion.)

The new onset of arrhythmias, such as atrial fibrillation or supraventricular tachycardia, should be regarded as a medical emergency in pregnant patients with significant mitral stenosis. Although digitalis may be appropriate for controlling the ventricular response, the onset of acute pulmonary edema may ensue rapidly if the ventricular rate is not controlled promptly or the sinus rhythm regained. Therefore, for rapid atrial fibrillation associated with symptoms, prompt cardioversion is recommended. The efficacy and safety of such an approach have been demonstrated.[5]

Digoxin has been used for both maternal and fetal indications during all stages of gestation without causing fetal harm. Pregnancy may be associated with increased levels of digoxin-like substances in the blood, which can cause errors in measurement of serum levels by radioimmunoassay.[6] There have been no reports linking digitalis glycosides with congenital defects. However, fetal intoxication resulting in neonatal death has been reported after maternal overdose.[7] The fetal/maternal serum digoxin concentration ratio varies from 0.5 to 1.0. Digoxin is excreted into breast milk, and the digoxin milk/plasma ratios have varied from 0.6 to 0.9.[8] Although these amounts in breast milk seem high, they represent small amounts of digoxin as a result of maternal protein binding. No adverse effects in nursing infants have been reported, and the American Academy of Pediatrics considers digoxin to be compatible with breastfeeding.[9]

Procainamide has been used for the termination and prophylaxis of atrial (and ventricular) tachyarrhythmias. Use of procainamide during pregnancy has not been linked to congenital abnormalities or other adverse fetal effects.[10, 11] Procainamide and its metabolite, *N*-acetylprocainamide, accumulate in breast milk,[12] but procainamide is considered to be compatible with breastfeeding.[9] The long-term effects of exposure of the nursing infant to procainamide are unknown with regard to development of antinuclear antibodies and lupus-like syndrome.

Quinidine has been used in pregnancy for more than 50 years. Quinidine crosses the placenta and achieves fetal serum levels similar to maternal levels. Neonatal thrombocytopenia has been reported after maternal use of quinidine.[9] In reviews of cardiovascular drugs, the use of quinidine during pregnancy has been classified as relatively safe for the fetus.[13, 14] In therapeutic doses, the oxytocic properties of quinidine have been rarely observed, but high doses can produce this effect and may result in abortion. Quinidine is excreted into breast milk but is considered to be compatible with breastfeeding.[9]

PROSTHETIC HEART VALVES

A mother with a prosthetic heart valve is exposed to the risks of thromboembolism and infective endocarditis. Antiplatelet agents (aspirin, dipyridamole) do not protect the mother sufficiently from thromboembolism to make their use advisable in pregnant women with prosthetic heart valves,[15, 16] and low-dose heparin does not protect against prosthetic valve thrombosis. Both coumarin derivatives and heparin given in full dosage provide effective protection against maternal thromboembolism, but both anticoagulants increase the risk for the mother and fetus. Whereas some authors favor treating patients with warfarin therapy except for the first 12 weeks of gestation (to avoid embryopathy) or close to term (to avoid commencement of labor with an anticoagulated fetus),[17] many physicians favor managing patients with high-dose, self-administered, subcutaneous heparin throughout pregnancy rather than using a regimen of heparin in the first and third trimesters and warfarin in the middle of pregnancy. One of the reasons for this is the difficulty of maintaining full anticoagulation during the conversion from one regimen to the other. In patients with prosthetic heart valves, the target International Normalized Ratio (INR) for warfarin should be 3.0–4.5, and the activated partial thromboplastin time (aPTT) should be at least twice the control value. Careful consultation between obstetricians and cardiologists as to the timing of delivery (or induction of labor) is required in order to ensure that the mother is not fully anticoagulated at the time of delivery.

ANTICOAGULANTS

In patients with rheumatic mitral valve disease (and associated paroxysmal or chronic atrial fibrillation), women with heart valve prostheses, and women who need prophylaxis to prevent recurrent pulmonary thromboembolism,[18] anticoagulant therapy may be needed during pregnancy.[1]

Warfarin is a typical example of a coumarin derivative. These drugs act by blocking vitamin K regeneration during enzymatic modification of several clotting proteins: factors II (prothrombin),

TABLE 52–1. RISK OF CARDIAC DRUGS TO FETUS AND NEWBORN

	Placental Transfer	Risk Factor*	Fetal Effects	Breast Feed
Adenosine	?	C_M	No adverse effects reported	No data
Amiodarone	Yes	C	Hypothyroidism, premature birth, hypotonia, large fontanelle	No
Atenolol	Yes	C_M	Low birth weight	Yes
Captopril	Yes	D_M	Teratogenic when used in second and third trimesters, producing renal defects and hypocalvaria (perhaps due to fetal hypotension and decreased renal blood flow)	Yes
Digitalis	Yes	C	Low birth weight	Yes
Diltiazem	Yes	C_M	No adequate human studies	Yes
Enalapril	Yes	D_M	Teratogenic when used in second and third trimesters, producing renal defects and hypocalvaria (perhaps due to fetal hypotension and decreased renal blood flow)	Yes
Furosemide	Yes	C_M	Decreased Na^+, K^+ glucose	Yes
Heparin	No	C	Abortion	Yes
Hydralazine	Yes	C_M	Thrombocytopenia, acute distress	Yes
Hydrochlorothiazide	Yes	D	Decreased Na^+, K^+, glucose	Yes; can suppress lactation
Isoproterenol	?	C	Tachycardia; no adequate human studies	No data
Labetalol	Yes	C_M	No adequate human studies	Yes
Lidocaine	Yes	C	Bradycardia and central nervous system toxic effects (keep maternal blood levels < 4 μg/mL)	No data
Metoprolol	Yes	B_M	No obvious risk—no long-term data	Yes
Mexiletine	Yes	C_M	Bradycardia, small infants, low Apgar score, hypoglycemia	Yes
Nifedipine	Yes	C_M	No adequate human studies; use with care	Yes
Nitroglycerin	?	C_M	No adequate human studies	No data
Procainamide	Yes	C_M	None	Yes
Propranolol	Yes	C_M	Growth retardation, prematurity, hypoglycemia, bradycardia, respiratory depression	Yes
Quinidine	Yes	C	Thrombocytopenia	Yes
Sodium nitroprusside	Yes	C	Potentially toxic; no adequate human studies	No
Streptokinase	Yes	C	No adequate human studies	No data
Verapamil	Yes	C_M	No adequate human studies	Yes
Warfarin	Yes	D	Abortion, hemorrhage	Yes

*Risk factors: *Category B:* Either animal reproduction studies have not demonstrated a fetal risk but there are no controlled studies in pregnant women, or animal reproduction studies have shown an adverse effect (other than a decrease in fertility) that was not confirmed in controlled studies in women in the first trimester (and there is no evidence of a risk in later trimesters). *Category C:* Either studies in animals have revealed adverse effects on the fetus and there are no controlled studies in pregnant women, or studies in women and animals are not available. Drugs should be given only if the potential benefit justifies the potential risk to the fetus. *Category D:* There is positive evidence of human fetal risk, but the benefits from use in pregnant women may be acceptable despite the risk (e.g., if the drug is needed in a life-threatening situation for a serious disease for which safer drugs cannot be used or are ineffective). If the manufacturer has rated the risk of the drug in the professional literature, the subscript M is used (e.g., C_M).

Data mainly from Briggs GG, Freeman RK, Yaffe SJ: Drugs in Pregnancy and Lactation. A Reference Guide to Fetal and Neonatal Risk, 4th ed. Baltimore: Williams & Wilkins, 1994.

VII, IX, and X and proteins C and S. Whereas coumarins inhibit the synthesis of functional clotting factors, they have no direct effect on factors already synthesized, and so there is a time delay before the clinical anticoagulant effect is observed. Warfarin crosses the placenta and is teratogenic; its use during the first trimester of pregnancy carries a significant risk to the fetus. Exposure in the sixth to ninth weeks of gestation may produce the fetal warfarin syndrome (nasal hypoplasia due to failure of development of the nasal septum and stippled epiphyses), resulting in depression of the bridge of the nose and neonatal respiratory distress resulting from upper airway obstruction. In addition, central nervous system abnormalities, including microcephaly, optic atrophy, and hydrocephalus, can occur.[19] Spontaneous abortions, stillbirths, and neonatal deaths may also occur. In general, the use of warfarin is to be avoided, especially between the 6th and 12th gestational weeks.

Mothers taking full-dose warfarin therapy can breastfeed without affecting the clotting mechanisms of their infants.[20] The American Academy of Pediatrics classified warfarin and dicumarol as compatible with breastfeeding[9]; however, it considers phenindione to be contraindicated because of the risk of hemorrhage in the infant. If the patient is fully anticoagulated with warfarin at the onset of labor, fresh-frozen plasma is usually administered. Warfarin can be restarted on the first postpartum day, and usually both heparin and warfarin are overlapped for 3–5 days when full-dose anticoagulation is required.

The complications of heparin therapy during pregnancy include hemorrhage, thrombocytopenia, and symptomless bone loss (osteopenia) that has been reported in more than one third of heparin-treated pregnant women.[21] Transient heparin-induced thrombocytopenia may occur in up to 10% of patients.[22] In rare instances, antiplatelet immunoglobulin antibodies are associated with heparin-induced thrombocytopenia-thrombosis. This serious complication can be associated with significant mortality and appears to occur more frequently with beef lung–derived heparin.) Clinically important thrombocytopenia, with or without associated thrombosis, is unusual. Most authors believe that heparin appears to have major advantages over oral anticoagulants as the treatment of choice during pregnancy. The administration of heparin on an ambulatory basis is feasible.[23]

Subcutaneous heparin is usually initiated in doses between 10,000 and 20,000 U every 12 h and is regulated by obtaining a 6-h postinjection aPTT, which should be 1.5 to 2.0 times higher than the control value for most patients. However, if patients have prosthetic heart valves, some authors suggest a minimal level of twice the control value.[17] Monitoring of high-dose subcutaneous heparin therapy can be achieved on an outpatient basis with a fingerstick PTT machine.

In addition to intermittent subcutaneous administration of heparin, other options for administration include long-term ambulatory subcutaneous infusion[24] and permanent venous access via a Hickman catheter.[25] Heparin injections are discontinued at the onset of labor and are usually resumed 12 h after a normal vaginal delivery.

There is interest in the use of heparin fragments of low molecular weight that are produced by enzymatic or chemical hydrolysis of longer chains of natural heparin and appear to exert a significant anticoagulant action with possibly reduced risk of bleeding and osteoporosis. Their role (if any) in pregnancy has not yet been clearly defined.

Heparin is not excreted into breast milk owing to its high molecular weight (15,000). Therefore, the mother may breastfeed her child safely while receiving full-dose heparin therapy.

ACUTE MYOCARDIAL INFARCTION

Acute myocardial infarction occurring during pregnancy is a rare but potentially lethal event for both mother and fetus, particularly when it occurs in the third trimester or peripartum period.[1, 26] The overall maternal mortality rate is approximately 30%; the greatest mortality occurs in those patients sustaining acute myocardial infarction late in pregnancy. Most maternal deaths occur either at the time of infarction (usually resulting in death of the fetus) or within 2 weeks of infarction, usually in relation to the onset of labor and delivery. Postpartum acute myocardial infarction is also associated with a high mortality rate.[27] Fetal outcome is generally dependent on maternal outcome; two thirds of fetal deaths occur simultaneously with demise of the mother. The possibility of cocaine use should always be considered as an etiologic factor. The particularly poor prognosis of patients suffering a myocardial infarction late in pregnancy is attributable to the increased hemodynamic demands on the heart in the latter half of pregnancy and during labor, delivery, and the puerperium. Any management plan requires close consultation among the cardiologist, the obstetric service, and the anesthesiologist to coordinate and plan an elective labor or provide optimal management of an unexpected premature labor and develop a strategy to provide a greater chance of prompt and effective rescue of the fetus in the event of sudden maternal demise. Because the course of events can change dramatically and rapidly, it is important that the goals of therapy and the alternatives be explained simply and clearly to the patient and her relatives.

The patient should be cared for in an intensive care unit capable of providing continuous maternal and fetal monitoring along with a complete obstetric service. Initial therapy should include complete rest, oxygen therapy, pain relief with intravenous morphine, and prophylactic use of subcutaneous low-dose heparin to prevent the formation of deep venous thrombosis (i.e., 10,000–15,000 units/day). If two-dimensional echocardiography demonstrates a significant area of left ventricular anterior dyskinesia and/or a definite left ventricular mural thrombus, high-dose anticoagulation is indicated to prevent thrombus formation or propagation and subsequent systemic embolization. Heparin is discontinued at the onset of labor, and reversal of its effects may be required before delivery with either protamine sulfate or, more usually, fresh-frozen plasma.

Thrombolytic agents such as streptokinase and urokinase have been used in pregnancy but have been associated with significant bleeding, premature labor, and incoordinate uterine contractions.[28, 29] Such risks may outweigh any potential benefits. Streptokinase has been used in the treatment of deep venous thrombosis during pregnancy in the second and third trimesters without fetal complications.[30] Urokinase has also been used in a pregnant woman (28 weeks' gestation) for treatment of hemodynamically significant pulmonary emboli; a healthy term infant was delivered 2 months after initiation of therapy.[31] Minimal amounts of streptokinase cross the placenta, and although fibrinolytic effects in the fetus do not ensue, streptokinase antibodies do cross to the fetus. No association between the use of streptokinase and the development of congenital defects has been reported.

Successful percutaneous transluminal coronary angioplasty has been achieved during pregnancy.[26, 32] If operative revascularization on an elective basis is deemed necessary, it seems that the rate of maternal mortality from present-day cardiopulmonary bypass during pregnancy is similar to that of the overall population undergoing cardiopulmonary bypass (2%–4%) and that fetal loss is relatively low (7%–9%).[33] Antianginal therapy with nitrates and beta blockers can be used. Nitroglycerin has been used during pregnancy in hypertensive patients without adverse effects on the fetus.[34] Use of calcium channel antagonists in pregnant women is relatively common, and these drugs may be useful in patients in whom changes in coronary vasomotor tone are thought to contribute to the pathogenesis of their condition. Nifedipine has been used as an antihypertensive agent and for tocolysis in pregnant women. Severe adverse reactions (muscle weakness and hypotension) have been reported when nifedipine has been combined with intravenous magnesium sulfate. (In nonhuman primates, intravenous magnesium has been associated with fetal hypoxemia and acidosis.[2, 9]) Therefore, nifedipine should be reserved for emergent situations in women with severe hypertension who are unresponsive to standard therapy.

Diltiazem has been used to treat myocardial ischemia during human pregnancy[35] without adverse effects, but some toxic effects in the embryo and fetus have been observed in experimental animals. The American Academy of Pediatrics considers the use of diltiazem, which is excreted in breast milk, to be compatible with breastfeeding.[9] Verapamil has been used successfully as an antiarrhythmic agent for fetal and maternal supraventricular arrhythmias. As in nonpregnant patients, intravenous verapamil can result in hypotension.[13] There have been no reports linking the use of verapamil with congenital defects. Verapamil is excreted in breast milk, but the American Academy of Pediatrics considers maternal verapamil use to be compatible with breastfeeding. In experimental studies, nicardipine is effective in abolishing uterine contractions, but fetal hypoxia, possibly resulting from a decrease in maternal uterine blood flow, has been observed.[36] This agent has been used for treating hypertension in women without perinatal deaths, adverse fetal effects, or neonatal outcomes.[37]

Sodium nitroprusside, an intravenous agent that reduces afterload and preload, should be reserved for life-threatening situations.[38] It should be given only for a short period because of the possible accumulation of the metabolites thiocyanate and cyanide in the fetus.[39] Recommendations for its use include monitoring of maternal serum pH, plasma cyanide, red blood cell cyanide, and methemoglobin levels.

PERIPARTUM CARDIOMYOPATHY

Peripartum cardiomyopathy is a poorly understood condition that manifests as a dilated cardiomyopathy in the last month of pregnancy or in the first 6 months post partum.[1] Echocardiography usually reveals generalized cardiac dilatation often involving the left ventricle and the left atrium more than the right-sided chambers. Ventricular thrombi may be seen. After the diagnosis, the mortality can be as high as 25%–50% with an initial high-risk period. Longitudinal studies have suggested that some patients can rapidly return to normal and that the initial severity of left ventricular dysfunction is not necessarily predictive of long-term functional outcome.[40] Persistence of cardiac dysfunction beyond 6–12 months often indicates a long-term problem, although recovery of left ventricular function can be seen later than this.

Prolonged bed rest has been thought by some authors to facilitate recovery.[41] In addition, routine therapy for dilated cardiomyopathy, including digitalization, diuretics, sodium restriction, and anticoagulation, is recommended. Afterload reduction with agents such as hydralazine and captopril is suggested. Hydralazine hydrochloride has been used widely for many years in pregnancy without adverse maternal or fetal effects.[42] Its use has not been linked to congenital defects, although it readily crosses the placenta. A number of studies using hydralazine, alone or in combination with other antihypertensive agents, have shown that it is relatively safe for the fetus.[43] Its use in pregnancy has been linked to a lupus-like syndrome.[44] It is excreted in breast milk, in which it appears in low concentration, but the American Academy of Pediatrics considers hydralazine to be compatible with breastfeeding.[9]

Because of toxicity identified in animal studies, the National Institutes of Health recommended (1984) that captopril be avoided during pregnancy.[45–47] However, the use of captopril limited to the first trimester does not appear to represent a significant risk to the fetus. Exposure after this time has been associated with teratogenicity and toxic effects in the fetus and newborn animals. Although captopril is excreted in breast milk in low concentrations, the American Academy of Pediatrics considers captopril compatible with breastfeeding.[9]

In patients with peripartum cardiomyopathy who continue to have refractory heart failure despite aggressive medical management including intra-aortic balloon counterpulsation, orthotopic cardiac transplantation remains an option in qualified patients.

PRIMARY OR SECONDARY PULMONARY HYPERTENSION

Patients with primary pulmonary hypertension or pulmonary hypertension secondary to other causes (e.g., Eisenmenger syndrome: patients with large intracardiac defects that allow free communication between the systemic and pulmonary circulations and who have predominantly right-to-left shunting secondary to fixed and markedly elevated pulmonary vascular resistance)[1] should avoid pregnancy because of the high maternal and fetal mortality rates and the apparent deleterious effect of pregnancy on a patient with the disease. With pregnancy and the usual maternal hemodynamic alterations (including an increased cardiac output and a fall in systemic vascular resistance), patients with Eisenmenger syndrome have more right-to-left shunting and experience deeper cyanosis and a reduced systemic arterial oxygen saturation with a rise in hematocrit. This is one of the few cardiac conditions for which sterilization is usually recommended because pregnancy is poorly tolerated[48] and the maternal mortality rate is high.

If termination of pregnancy is not feasible or is declined, supportive measures must include avoidance of operative procedures and hypotension, hypovolemia, and thromboembolic phenomena. Gleicher and colleagues[48] recommended hospitalization and prolonged bed rest, anticoagulation of patients from midpregnancy to term, noninduced labor, administration of high concentrations of oxygen during labor, epidural anesthesia, and vaginal delivery (noninduced) with elective low forceps delivery used to shorten the second stage of labor. Despite these active measures, the maternal mortality rate still remains substantial in the first week after delivery.

Primary pulmonary hypertension is also associated with a high maternal mortality rate, and the frequency of spontaneous abortions and of neonatal deaths is high.[1] Both tubal ligation and pregnancy terminations are indicated. If the patient elects to continue with pregnancy, bed rest should be enforced, anticoagulation instituted,[49] and adequate oxygenation with careful hemodynamic monitoring undertaken during labor and delivery. In primary pulmonary hypertension, oral calcium channel blockers have been shown to have a modest effect in patients with some preservation of pulmonary vasoreactivity.[50]

THE MARFAN SYNDROME

In patients with the Marfan syndrome and minimal cardiovascular involvement, pregnancy may be tolerated without serious problems.[1, 51, 52] Women with mild aortic dilation and no evidence of valvular regurgitation have a small risk of dissection, and monitoring every 8–12 weeks with echocardiograms is appropriate.[52] However, women who have moderate or severe cardiovascular dysfunction may be at considerable risk during pregnancy. Aortic dissection during pregnancy occurs most frequently during the third trimester and first postpartum month, and most dissections have occurred in women with aortic regurgitation or evidence of marked aortic root enlargement.[51] It is recommended that women with the Marfan syndrome who are considering pregnancy have expert genetic counseling, and a clinical cardiac assessment, including echocardiography, should be performed to determine whether aortic root dilation or valvular dysfunction exists. There is a relatively small risk of aortic dissection during pregnancy, provided that the patient is asymptomatic, the aortic root diameter is less than 40 mm, and there is no significant valvular dysfunction.[51] Nevertheless, patients should be observed at a "high-risk" clinic.

Beta blockers are given to virtually all patients with the Marfan syndrome, even during pregnancy, because it is thought that they will reduce the rate of aortic dilation and the risk of complications.[53] Certainly, it is thought that the maternal advantages of beta blockers far outweigh their potential adverse effects on the fetus. It should be understood that even in patients with a normal aortic root and no evidence of valvular dysfunction, the presence of the Marfan syndrome alone can predispose a patient to a poor outcome with morbid or fatal events.[54]

CARDIAC ARRHYTHMIAS

The principles of antiarrhythmic therapy during pregnancy have been carefully documented.[13] The most common arrhythmias during pregnancy include premature atrial ventricular beats, reentrant supraventricular tachyarrhythmias, and occasional tachyarrhythmias associated with Wolff-Parkinson-White syndrome. In patients with normal cardiac function, there is usually no need to treat asymptomatic or mildly symptomatic patients with ventricular or supraventricular premature beats. A history of caffeine use, alcohol use, or other precipitants of arrhythmias should be sought (e.g., sympathomimetic amine inhalers for asthma). Interestingly, there are reports of paroxysmal supraventricular tachyarrhythmias that occur only during pregnancy. Vagal maneuvers are always taught to the patient and should be attempted initially in all patients with such arrhythmias. If vagal maneuvers are ineffective, patients may be treated with digitalis, beta blocking agents, adenosine, or intravenous verapamil. Adenosine was first used in human pregnancy in a patient with a recurrent narrow complex tachycardia and reported in 1991.[55] Other reports have since described the use of adenosine to treat maternal supraventricular tachycardia.[56–58] No adverse effects attributable to adenosine in the fetus or newborn have been reported in any of these cases. Occasionally, cardioversion may be needed to achieve sinus rhythm.

Ventricular tachycardia can occur in pregnant patients and has been reported in the absence of detectable organic disease. Therapy with lidocaine is used acutely, and subsequent recurrence is prevented with beta blocking drugs, procainamide, or quinidine. The majority of the information on lidocaine in pregnancy comes from its use as a local anesthetic during labor and delivery. The drug rapidly crosses the placenta to the fetus, appearing in the fetal circulation within minutes after administration to the mother. It may produce central nervous system depression in the newborn with high serum levels. However, lidocaine is the treatment of choice for

TABLE 52–2. PROPHYLACTIC REGIMENS FOR GENITOURINARY PROCEDURES

Drug	Adult Dosage Regimen
Standard Regimen	
Ampicillin, gentamicin, and amoxicillin	Intravenous or intramuscular ampicillin, 2.0 g, plus gentamicin 1.5 mg/kg (not to exceed 80 mg), 30 min before procedure followed by amoxicillin 1.5 g orally 6 h after initial dose; alternatively, the parenteral regimen may be repeated once, 8 h after initial dose
Ampicillin/Amoxicillin/Penicillin–Allergic Patient Regimen	
Vancomycin and gentamicin	Intravenous administration of vancomycin 1.0 g in 1 h plus intravenous or intramuscular administration of gentamicin 1.5 mg/kg (not to exceed 80 mg) 1 h before procedure; may be repeated once, 8 h after initial dose
Alternative Low-Risk Patient Regimen	
Amoxicillin	3.0 g orally 1 h before procedure; then 1.5 g 6 h after initial dose

ventricular arrhythmias. Small amounts of lidocaine are excreted in breast milk, but the American Academy of Pediatrics considers lidocaine to be compatible with breastfeeding.[9]

In the event of cardiopulmonary resuscitation during pregnancy, the main objective before the onset of fetal viability (approximately the 24th week of gestation) is to resuscitate the mother. After this stage of pregnancy, consideration has to be given to delivery of the fetus, which is usually expedited by emergency cesarean section if 15 min or more or cardiopulmonary resuscitation is unsuccessful.[59]

ANTIBIOTIC PROPHYLAXIS

The American Heart Association Committee on Prevention of Bacterial Endocarditis recommends prophylaxis for patients with certain cardiac conditions (mitral valve prolapse with valvular regurgitation, prosthetic cardiac valves, rheumatic and other acquired valvular dysfunction even after cardiac surgery, most congenital cardiac malformations, previous bacterial endocarditis [even in the absence of heart disease], and hypertrophic cardiomyopathy) who are delivering vaginally, undergoing vaginal hysterectomy, or undergoing urethral catheterization if urinary tract infection is present. Endocarditis prophylaxis is not recommended for cesarian section or in the absence of infection for urethral catheterization, uncomplicated vaginal delivery, therapeutic abortion, dilatation and curettage, sterilization procedures, or insertion or removal of intrauterine devices[60] (Table 52–2).

REFERENCES

1. Elkayam U: Pregnancy and cardiovascular disease. *In* Braunwald E (ed): Heart Disease. A Textbook of Cardiovascular Medicine, 4th ed, pp 1790–1809. Philadelphia: WB Saunders, 1992.
2. Briggs GG, Freeman RK, Yaffe SJ: Drugs in Pregnancy and Lactation. A Reference Guide to Fetal and Neonatal Risk, 4th ed. Baltimore: Williams & Wilkins, 1994.
3. Beerman B, Groschinsky-Grind M, Fahraeus L, Lindstroem B: Placental transfer of furosemide. Clin Pharmacol Ther 1978; 24:560.
4. Lindheimer MD, Katz AI: Sodium and diuretics in pregnancy. N Engl J Med 1973; 288:891.
5. Metcalfe J, McNulty JH, Ueland K: Burwell and Metcalfe's Heart Disease and Pregnancy: Physiology and Management. Boston: Little, Brown, 1986.
6. Valdes R: Endogenous digoxin-like immunoreactive factors: impact on digoxin measurements and potential physiologic implications. Clin Chem 1985; 31:1525.
7. Sherman JL, Locke RV: Transplacental neonatal digitalis intoxication. Am J Cardiol 1960; 6:834.
8. Finley JP, Waxman MB, Wong PY, Lickrish GM: Digoxin excretion in human milk. J Pediatr 1979; 94:339.
9. Committee on Drugs, American Academy of Pediatrics: The transfer of drugs and other chemicals into human milk. Pediatrics 1994; 93:137.
10. Allen NM, Page RL: Procainamide administration during pregnancy. Clin Pharm 1993; 12:58.
11. Little BB, Gilstrap LC: Cardiovascular drugs during pregnancy. Clin Obstet Gynecol 1989; 32:13.
12. Pittard WB, Glazier H: Procainamide excretion in human milk. J Pediatr 1983; 102:631.
13. Rotmensch HH, Rotmensch S, Elkayam U: Management of cardiac arrhythmias during pregnancy: current concepts. Drugs 1987; 33:623.
14. Ward RM: Maternal drug therapy for fetal disorders. Semin Perinatol 1992; 16:12.
15. Salazar E, Zajarias A, Gutierrez N, et al: The problem of cardiac valve prosthesis, anticoagulants and pregnancy. Circulation 1984; 70(suppl I):I-169.
16. Iturbe-Alessio I, Fonseca M, Mutchinik O, et al: Risks of anticoagulant therapy in pregnant women with artificial heart valves. N Engl J Med 1986; 315:1390.
17. Ginsberg JS, Barron WM: Pregnancy and prosthetic heart valves. Lancet 1994; 344:1170.
18. de Swiet M: Prescribing in pregnancy: anticoagulants. Br Med J 1987; 294:428.
19. Pettifor JM, Benson R: Congenital malformations associated with administration of oral anticoagulants during pregnancy. J Pediatr 1975; 86:459.
20. McKenna R, Cole ER, Vasan U, et al: Is warfarin sodium contraindicated in the lactating mother? Clinical and laboratory observation. J Pediatr 1983; 103:325.
21. Barbour LA, Kick SD, Steiner JF, et al: A prospective study of heparin-induced osteoporosis in pregnancy using bone densitometry. Am J Obstet Gynecol 1994; 170:862.
22. Calhoun BC, Hesser JW: Heparin associated antibody with pregnancy. Discussion of two cases. Am J Obstet Gynecol 1987; 156:964.
23. Henny CP, Ten Cate MT, Buller HR, et al: Ambulatory heparin treatment. Lancet 1982; 1:615.
24. Rabinovici J, Mani A, Barkai G, et al: Long-term ambulatory anticoagulation by constant subcutaneous infusion in pregnancy. Br J Obstet Gynaecol 1987; 94:89.
25. Nelson DM, Stempel LE, Fabri PJ, et al: Hickman catheter use in a pregnant patient requiring anticoagulation. Am J Obstet Gynecol 1984; 149:461.
26. Hands ME, Johnson MD, Saltzman DH, Rutherford JD: The cardiac, obstetric, and anesthetic management of pregnancy complicated by acute myocardial infarction. J Clin Anesth 1990; 2:258.
27. Hankins GDV, Wendall GD, Leveno KJ, Stoneham J: Myocardial infarction during pregnancy. A review. Obstet Gynecol 1985; 65:139.
28. Hall RJC, Young C, Sutton GC, Campbell S: Treatment of acute massive pulmonary embolism by streptokinase during labor and delivery. Br Med J 1972; 4:647.
29. Pfeifer GW: The use of thrombolytic therapy in obstetrics and gynaecology. Aust Ann Med 1970; 19(suppl 1):28.
30. Ludwig H: Results of streptokinase therapy in deep venous thrombosis during pregnancy. Postgrad Med J 1973; 49(suppl 5):65.
31. Delclos GL, Davila F: Thrombolytic therapy for pulmonary embolism in pregnancy; a case report. Am J Obstet Gynecol 1986; 155:375.
32. Cowan NC, de Belder MA, Rothman MT: Coronary angioplasty in pregnancy. Br Heart J 1988; 59:588.
33. Bernal JM, Miralles PJ: Cardiac surgery with cardiopulmonary bypass during pregnancy. Obstet Gynaecol Surg 1986; 41:1.
34. Cotton DB, Jones M, Longmire S, et al: Role of intravenous nitroglycerin in the treatment of severe pregnancy-induced hypertension complicated by pulmonary edema. Am J Obstet Gynecol 1986; 154:91.
35. Lubbe WF: Use of diltiazem during pregnancy. N Z Med J 1987; 100:121.
36. Holbrook RH, Lirette M, Katz M: Cardiovascular and tocolytic effects of nicardipine HCl in the pregnant rabbit: comparison with ritodrine HCl. Obstet Gynecol 1987; 69:83.

37. Carbonne B, Jannet D, Touboul C, et al: Nicardipine measurement of hypertension during pregnancy. Obstet Gynecol 1993; 81:908.
38. Stempel JE, O'Grady JP, Morton MJ, Johnson KA: Use of sodium nitroprusside in complications of a gestational hypertension. Obstet Gynecol 1982; 60:533.
39. Shoemaker CT, Myers M: Sodium nitroprusside for control of severe hypertensive disease of pregnancy: a case report and discussion of potential toxicity. Am J Obstet Gynecol 1984; 149:171.
40. Cole P, Cook F, Plappert T, et al: Longitudinal changes in left ventricular architecture and function in peripartum cardiomyopathy. Am J Cardiol 1987; 60:871.
41. Julian DG, Slzekely P: Peripartum cardiomyopathy. Prog Cardiovasc Dis 1985; 27:223.
42. Teramo K, Elder M, Rabinowitz B, Neufeld HN: Medical treatment of cardiovascular disorders during pregnancy. Am Heart J 1982; 104:1357.
43. de Swiet M: Antihypertensive drugs in pregnancy. Br Med J 1985; 291:365.
44. Yemini M, Shoham (Schwartz) Z, Dgani R, et al: Lupus-like syndrome in a mother and newborn following administration of hydralazine: a case report. Eur J Obstet Gynecol Reprod Biol 1989; 30:193.
45. The 1984 report of the Joint National Committee on Detection, Evaluation, and Treatment of High Blood Pressure. Arch Intern Med 1984; 144:1045.
46. Duminy PC, Burger PT: Fetal abnormality associated with the use of captopril during pregnancy. S Afr Med J 1981; 60:805.
47. Ferris TK, Weir EK: The effect of captopril on uterine blood flow and prostaglandin synthesis in the rabbit. J Clin Invest 1983; 71:80.
48. Gleicher N, Midwall J, Hochberger D, et al: Eisenmenger's syndrome and pregnancy. Obstet Gynecol Surv 1979; 34:721.
49. Fuster V, Steele PM, Edwards WD, et al: Primary pulmonary hypertension: natural history and importance of thrombosis. Circulation 1984; 70:580.
50. Rich S, Brundage BH, Levy PS: The effect of vasodilator therapy on the clinical outcome of patients with primary pulmonary hypertension. Circulation 1985; 71:1195.
51. Pyeritz RE: Maternal and fetal complications of pregnancy in the Marfan syndrome. Am J Med 1981; 71:784.
52. Pyeritz RE: The Marfan syndrome. Am Fam Physician 1986; 34:83.
53. Zahka KG, Hensley C, Glesby M, et al: The impact of medical therapy on the cardiovascular prognosis of the Marfan syndrome in early childhood [Abstract]. J Am Coll Cardiol 1989; 13:119.
54. Rosenblum NG, Grossman AR, Mennuti MT, et al: Failure of serial echocardiographic studies to predict aortic dissection in the pregnant patient with Marfan's syndrome. Am J Obstet Gynecol 1983; 146:470.
55. Podolsky SM, Varon J: Adenosine use during pregnancy. Ann Emerg Med 1991; 20:1027.
56. Afridi I, Moise KJ, Rokey R: Termination of supraventricular tachycardia with intravenous adenosine in a pregnant woman with Wolff-Parkinson-White syndrome. Obstet Gynecol 1992; 80:481.
57. Harrison JK, Greenfield RA, Wharton JM: Acute termination of supraventricular tachycardia by adenosine during pregnancy. Am Heart J 1992; 123:1386.
58. Mason BA, Ricci-Goodman J, Koos BJ: Adenosine in the treatment of maternal supraventricular tachycardia. Obstet Gynecol 1992; 80:478.
59. Lee RV, Rodgers BD, White LM, et al: Cardiopulmonary resuscitation of pregnant women. Am J Med 1986; 81:311.
60. Dajani AS, Bisno AL, Kyung KJ, et al: Prevention of bacterial endocarditis. Recommendations by the American Heart Association. JAMA 1990; 264:2919.

53 Medical Management of Adults With Congenital Heart Disease

Joseph K. Perloff, MD

Advances in diagnostic techniques and in surgical and medical management of patients with congenital heart disease have appreciably extended their age range.[1] *Natural history* is a term that is applied when cardiac surgery has not been performed, but the term is a misnomer, because advances in medical management of unoperated patients have materially improved survival. This chapter focuses on medical management of adults with unoperated and postoperative congenital heart disease, dealing with the topics listed in Table 53–1. A broad assessment of congenital heart disease in adults can be found elsewhere.[1]

PSYCHOSOCIAL CONCERNS

Fundamental to an understanding of the psychological problems in adults with congenital heart disease is a comprehension of how their childhood experience differed from that of normal, healthy persons.[2] A significant percentage of these adult patients have experienced dramatic and sometimes psychologically traumatic diagnostic and therapeutic procedures during key developmental phases of their childhood. The lives of patients with serious chronic illnesses, especially chronically ill children or adolescents who reach adulthood, are often punctuated with reminders of their fragility and mortality. Unconscious denial may take the form of medical noncompliance, missed appointments, and physical exercise that is deliberately extended beyond capacity. Immature patients may passively follow the instructions of parents and physicians and resist moving toward independence and adult responsibility. Nevertheless, many if not most adults with congenital heart disease perform at high levels, often in demanding occupations, especially if they were encouraged as children to strive to reach their maximum capabilities and to view their illness as a surmountable obstacle rather than as a limiting handicap.[2, 3] Cardiologists responsible for the care of adults with congenital heart disease may become adept at dealing with the psychosocial concerns of their patients, but most major centers enjoy the collaboration of psychiatrists whose counsel and psychopharmacologic expertise can be pivotal.[3]

NEUROLOGIC COMPLICATIONS

Neurologic disorders found in adults with congenital heart disease are listed in Table 53–2. Brain abscess may first occur in adulthood

TABLE 53–1. MEDICAL MANAGEMENT IN ADULTS WITH CONGENITAL HEART DISEASE

Psychosocial
Neurologic
Electrophysiological
Ventricular function
Exercise and athletics
Infective endocarditis
Pregnancy, genetics, contraception
Coexisting acquired cardiac and vascular disease
Noncardiac surgery
Hematologic disorders, renal involvement, and urate metabolism

(Fig. 53–1*A*), or a healed abscess that occurred during childhood may express itself as a seizure disorder in adulthood. Susceptibility to abscess formation depends on bacteremia, venoarterial mixing (cyanotic congenital heart disease), and focal brain injury (vulnerability of the tissue substrate).[4, 5] Often, a primary source of hematogenous infection cannot be identified, but clinical management focuses on potential sources such as septic emboli, ear or oral infection, or tooth extraction. Proper management of a new brain abscess requires an expeditious diagnosis prompted by symptoms of headache, focal neurologic signs, seizures, and fever. The diagnosis can be established by computed axial tomography, setting the stage for neurosurgical drainage, antibiotics, and administration of Dilantin or Tegretol to suppress seizure activity. Seizures that accompany an abscess may persist or recur years later as a result of focal brain injury. Patients may require Tegretol or Dilantin indefinitely.

Mycotic aneurysms (better termed *septic aneurysms;* Fig. 53–2) result from inflammatory weakening of the wall of a cerebral artery caused by septic microemboli to vasa vasora or to impaction of an infected embolus in the lumen of the artery.[5] A cerebral septic aneurysm may progressively enlarge and rupture despite antibiotic eradication of the offending organism. Headaches or seizures announce an enlarging or perforating aneurysm, which can be diagnosed by computed tomography and cerebral angiography. Aneurysms approaching 1 cm in diameter are treated by surgical excision to prevent catastrophic rupture.[5]

Ischemic neurologic disorders are caused by cerebral emboli; cerebral venous or arterial thrombosis; subclavian steal after a Blalock-Taussig shunt; in rare instances, a congenital subclavian steal; and syncope associated with aortic stenosis.[4] Of most importance statistically are bland or infected cerebral emboli (discussed previously) that originate in either the systemic circulation or in peripheral or pelvic veins (paradoxical embolization). Management depends on the source of the embolus, which may be a left-sided prosthetic cardiac valve, the left atrial appendage (atrial fibrillation), left-sided infective endocarditis, or left ventricular endocardium (mural thrombus). Transesophageal echocardiography has been a major step in establishing the diagnosis of emboli and setting the stage for specific treatment.[6] Emboli from a rigid prosthesis require diagnostic confirmation by transesophageal echocardiography and adjustment of anticoagulants. Emboli from a bioprosthetic valve require echocardiographic investigation for confirmation of the embolic source and for detection of degeneration.

TABLE 53–2. PRINCIPAL NEUROLOGIC DISORDERS IN ADULTS WITH CONGENITAL HEART DISEASE

Infectious
Brain abscess
Mycotic aneurysm
Ischemic
Cerebral paradoxical or systemic emboli
Subclavian steal
After Blalock-Taussig shunt
Congenital subclavian steal
Syncope associated with aortic stenosis or cyanotic congenital heart disease
Hemorrhagic
Intracerebral hemorrhage
Subarachnoid hemorrhage
Seizures

More unique to congenital heart disease—usually but not necessarily cyanotic—are paradoxical emboli that originate in the lower extremities or pelvic veins and reach the brain because peripheral venous blood has direct access to the systemic arterial circulation via a right-to-left shunt. Paradoxical cerebral emboli in adults with cyanotic congenital heart disease pose a therapeutic dilemma, because anticoagulants that seem intuitively appropriate reinforce hemostatic defects inherent in cyanotic patients, increasing the risk of

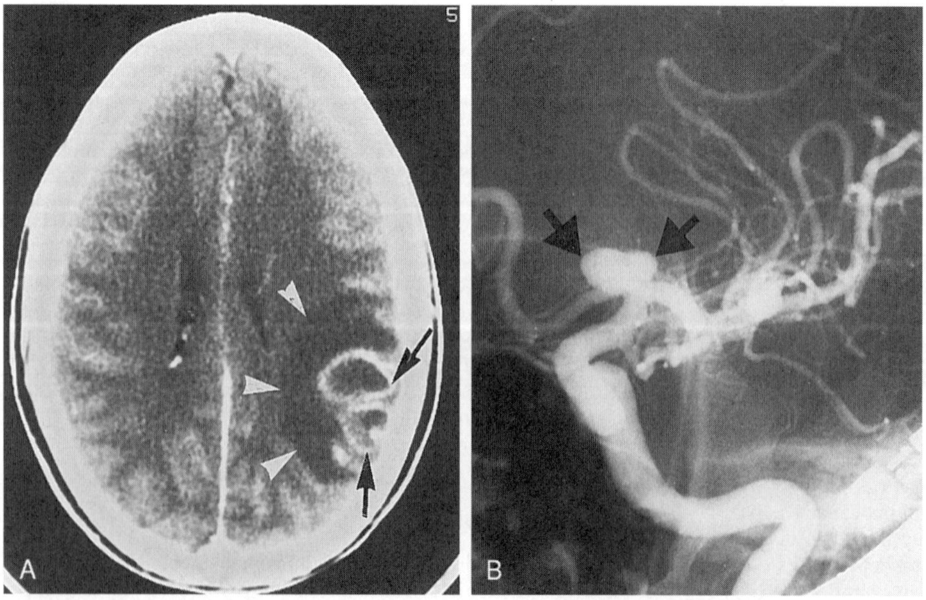

Figure 53–1. *A,* Fresh brain abscess in a 37-year-old cyanotic woman with double-outlet right ventricle, ventricular septal defect, and pulmonary stenosis. Black arrows identify ring enhancement around the abscess. White arrowheads identify surrounding edema. The abscess was surgically drained. *B,* Arrows point to a congenital berry aneurysm in a 28-year-old woman with tetralogy of Fallot and pulmonary atresia. The aneurysm, which is the type usually found with coarctation of the aorta, was surgically excised.

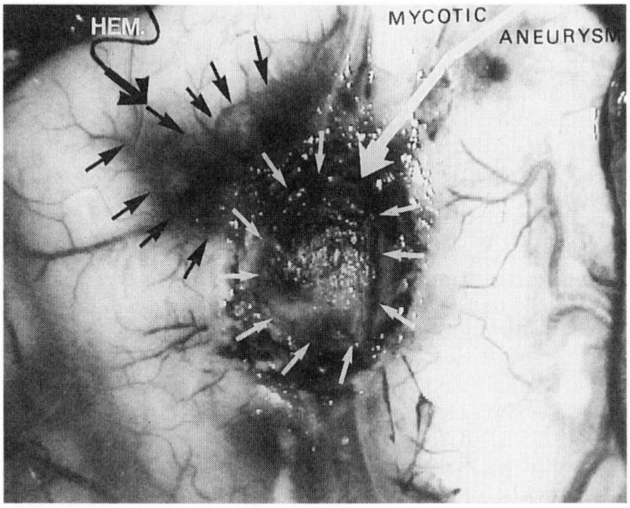

Figure 53–2. Surgical view of a septic aneurysm with surrounding hemorrhage (HEM.) in a 27-year-old man with infective endocarditis (*Streptococcus viridans*). Years before, the patient had undergone intracardiac repair of pulmonary stenosis and ventricular septal defect in the context of congenitally corrected transposition of the great arteries.

hemorrhage (discussed later). A preventable source of paradoxical embolization in hospitalized cyanotic patients is the improper use of intravenous lines for infusions or drugs. Insertion of an air or particle filter (Fig. 53–3) eliminates the risk of introducing air or particles into an intravenous line and should be routine. Paradoxical emboli in acyanotic patients occur when an ostium secundum atrial septal defect or a patent foramen ovale permits inferior caval blood to stream across the atrial septum into the left atrium and systemic circulation. Women with an ostium secundum atrial septal defect who are pregnant or who have recently given birth are at special risk, particularly during the puerperium; therefore, meticulous leg care and early ambulation after delivery are advisable. Surgical closure of the atrial septal defect prevents paradoxical emboli.

More controversial is the management of strokes caused by paradoxic emboli through a patent foramen ovale, a pathway analogous to that of an ostium secundum atrial septal defect but otherwise functionally unimportant. Management should take into account the provocative role of straining (Valsalva maneuver) or vigorous coughing, which serve to initiate transient venoarterial mixing that provides the physiologic substrate for a paradoxical embolus. An atrial septal aneurysm may be responsible for transient ischemic attacks in acyanotic patients because of fibrin platelet thrombi attached to the aneurysm at the site of a patent or nonpatent foramen ovale.[4] Treatment of normal young adults with strokes caused by paradoxical emboli via a patent foramen ovale or emboli from an atrial septal aneurysm is controversial. Therapeutic options for the former include administration of antiplatelet or anticoagulant agents and closure of the patent foramen ovale, either surgically or with a catheter-delivered umbrella device. If the cerebral event is characterized by a single mild transient ischemic attack, and if there is a convincing provoking cause (discussed previously), risk can be reduced if not eliminated by avoiding vigorous coughing or straining. When there is a peripheral source of venous embolus, anticoagulants should be used, at least temporarily. If the initial stroke is more than a mild transient ischemic attack, if there is a recurrence, or if a right-to-left shunt through the foramen ovale occurs without provocation, closure using surgery or a catheter-delivered device is recommended. For cerebral emboli that are thought to originate from a large, mobile atrial septal aneurysm, especially if the emboli are recurrent, surgical correction is warranted.

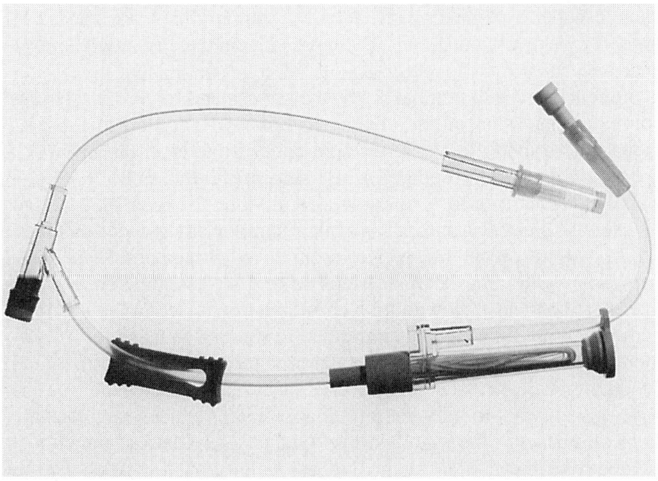

Figure 53–3. An air-particle filter is inserted at the distal end of an intravenous line to prevent paradoxical air or particle emboli in patients with cyanotic congenital heart disease.

The subclavian steal is an occasional complication of a Blalock-Taussig anastomosis that can create an anatomic and physiologic substrate identical to that of the atherosclerotic subclavian steal.[7] Symptoms may appear decades after the shunt was created, depending on the development of cervical and intrathoracic collateral arteries. The subclavian steal is not necessarily corrected by ligation of the anastomosis, with or without intracardiac repair. Congenital subclavian steal is rare.

In patients with congenital aortic stenosis, cerebral symptoms may consist of nothing more than giddiness, faintness, or lightheadedness with effort, but syncopal episodes are sometimes recurrent and potentially dangerous. Sudden death is a feared sequela, but in young adults with normal coronary arterial circulations, the risk is small in comparison with the risk in adults with aortic stenosis and coexisting coronary artery disease.[8] Syncope associated with aortic stenosis is the result of an inappropriate exercise-induced fall in systemic vascular resistance mediated by left ventricular baroreceptors. Patients should be advised to avoid abrupt, strenuous, and isometric exercise. Malignant ventricular arrhythmias seldom initiate syncope but are the chief cause of death after a faint. Syncope-induced hypotension is more likely to provoke ventricular arrhythmias and sudden death in adults with calcific aortic stenosis and coexisting atherosclerotic coronary disease than in young adults with hemodynamically equivalent congenital aortic valve stenosis and normal coronary arteries.[8] Surgical relief of aortic stenosis, with or without coronary bypass surgery, obviates recurrences of syncope and eliminates the attendant risk.

A preventable cause of syncope in cyanotic patients is the fall in systemic vascular resistance and increase in the right-to-left shunt provoked by the vasodilatation that occurs with a hot bath or a hot shower. The risk of syncope associated with standing in a hot shower or rising from a sitting position after immersion in a hot bath can be avoided by following appropriate practical advice.

Cerebral hemorrhage in adults with congenital heart disease tends to occur under three circumstances: (1) the injudicious use of anticoagulants in cyanotic patients with intrinsic hemostatic defects, (2) rupture of an aneurysm of the circle of Willis in patients with coarctation of the aorta, and (3) rupture of a septic aneurysm (discussed previously). A berry aneurysm (see Fig. 53–1*B*) can rupture in a normotensive patient long after successful coarctation repair. Cerebral angiography sets the stage for neurosurgical intervention (see Fig. 53–2).

ELECTROPHYSIOLOGIC ABNORMALITIES

There are three general categories of electrophysiologic abnormalities in adults with congenital heart disease: (1) rhythm and conduction disturbances that are inherent components of certain unoperated malformations and that persist as obligatory residua after reparative surgery; (2) electrophysiologic abnormalities that develop as a result of the hemodynamic or hypoxic stress imposed on the heart by the basic unoperated malformation and that may or may not persist as postoperative residua; and (3) electrophysiologic abnormalities that are sequelae of reparative surgery. Electrophysiologic abnormalities—principally but not exclusively postoperative—constitute one of the most prevalent medical problems in adults with congenital heart disease.[9] The following are selective but representative examples of electrophysiologic abnormalities in these patients.

In unoperated patients with ostium secundum atrial septal defect, the incidence of supraventricular arrhythmias, usually atrial fibrillation or flutter, increases with increasing age.[8] An age-related augmentation of left-to-right shunt in response to a reduction in left ventricular compliance is partly responsible for this increase. Surgical closure of the atrial septal defect removes the mechanical stimulus of volume overload and may permit spontaneous return to sinus rhythm or preservation of sinus rhythm in response to pharmacologic interventions that previously were unsuccessful. Spontaneous reversion to sinus rhythm can occur months after surgery in patients who experience early postoperative atrial fibrillation, or atrial flutter or fibrillation may occur or recur decades after successful closure of an ostium secundum atrial septal defect, unless closure is achieved in early childhood.

In Ebstein anomaly of the tricuspid valve, supraventricular tachyarrhythmias—re-entrant supraventricular tachycardia, atrial fibrillation, atrial flutter—occur in 25%–30% of patients, and patterns of pre-excitation are present in 5%–25% of surface electrocardiograms.[8] An accessory pathway with a short anterograde refractory period permits an excessively rapid ventricular response to atrial flutter or atrial fibrillation (Fig. 53–4), setting the stage for ventricular fibrillation, which is responsible for syncope or sudden death. A rapidly conducting accessory pathway requires antiarrhythmic medications that slow conduction and prolong refractoriness in the pathway (e.g., procainamide, lidocaine). Digoxin and verapamil reinforce conduction via accessory pathways and are contraindicated. It is usually wise to promptly cardiovert patients with Ebstein anomaly and atrial fibrillation or flutter when there is a rapid ventricular response. Surgical reconstruction of the malformed right atrioventricular orifice permits division of accessory pathways, the presence of which is a weight in the balance that favors intracardiac repair (see Fig. 53–4). In the occasional patient with a mild form of Ebstein anomaly that does not warrant repair, or if the anterior tricuspid leaflet does not lend itself to tricuspid reconstruction, catheter ablation of accessory pathways should be attempted.

In congenitally corrected transposition of the great arteries (i.e., ventricular inversion), a normally located posterior atrioventricular node is either absent or does not connect with infranodal conduction tissue. If the latter is the case, atrioventricular block exists from birth. More commonly, prolonged atrioventricular conduction expresses itself initially as an increase in PR interval followed by second-degree atrioventricular block (almost always 2 to 1 conduction), and ultimately by complete heart block, which should be anticipated by insertion of a dual-chamber pacemaker.[9] Repair of the ventricular septal defect is accompanied by complete heart block in about 25% of patients, because the nonpenetrating atrioventricular conduction bundle runs along the superior margin of the defect.

Three major postoperative settings for disturbances in rhythm and conduction are tetralogy of Fallot, atrial switch repairs for complete transposition of the great arteries, and Fontan repairs for univentricular heart or tricuspid atresia.[9] After operation for tetralogy of Fallot, bifascicular block indicates damage to the anterior fascicle of the left bundle branch and to the contiguous proximal portion of the right bundle branch, setting the stage for high-degree heart block, the management of which is similar to that of analogous conduction defects in other settings. The choice of dual-chamber vs. right ventricular pacing is a matter of clinical judgment.

More important and more prevalent than conduction defects after repair of tetralogy of Fallot are disturbances in ventricular rhythm, especially those originating in the incised right ventricle.[10] Alternatively, disturbances in rhythm may be provoked by decades of volume overload of the left heart via an aortopulmonary shunt. Sudden death can result from late postoperative complete heart block, but ventricular tachyarrhythmias are the major causes of sudden death. The first necessity is to determine the probability of electrical ventricular instability. The older the patient at the time of intracardiac repair, the longer the time that has elapsed after repair, the greater the loading conditions imposed on the incised right ventricle, and the poorer the right ventricular function, the greater the risk of right ventricular arrhythmias.

An exercise stress test tends to be more useful than a 24-h ambulatory electrocardiogram in uncovering clinically occult ventricular arrhythmias. Electrophysiologic management falls into three categories. First, if disturbances in ventricular rhythm occur in the context of hemodynamically significant postoperative obstruction to right ventricular outflow or appreciable pulmonary valve regurgitation (transannular patch), control of the ventricular tachyarrhythmia requires re-repair, especially if an outflow aneurysm is a residuum of prior operation. Second, if exercise electrocardiography or Holter monitor reading identifies ventricular tachycardia or an unacceptable frequency of ventricular ectopic beats in patients who do not otherwise need reoperation, intracardiac electrophysiologic studies can establish the focus of electrical instability and set the stage for catheter ablation. The third therapeutic option is pharmacologic, which serves as an adjunct to re-repair or catheter ablation or can be employed if disturbances in ventricular rhythm persist after other therapeutic options have been tested.

Because of the widespread use of intra-atrial baffle operations since the 1960s, appreciable numbers of adults with complete transposition of the great arteries are presenting with atrial arrhythmias, sinus node injury, and damage to the atrioventricular node.[11] The majority of these electrophysiologic disorders express themselves as sinus bradycardia, junctional escape rhythms, atrioventricular block, and supraventricular tachycardia, chiefly atrial flutter, atrial fibrillation, or junctional tachycardia. Atrial tachyarrhythmias may coexist with sinus bradycardia (bradycardia/tachycardia). Impaired atrioventricular conduction decreases the ventricular response to atrial fibrillation or flutter, but risk exists even if the ventricular rate is not rapid. These concerns argue for aggressive suppression of atrial tachyarrhythmias, especially atrial flutter (cardioversion), in conjunction with evaluation of sinus node function and atrioventricular conduction, abnormalities of which may warrant an implanted pacemaker.

Although patients with complete atrioventricular block and adequate escape rhythms may remain asymptomatic for long periods of time, the risk of syncope and sudden death persists. A dual-chamber pacemaker is generally required (Fig. 53–5). A permanent pacemaker is often necessary to control bradyarrhythmias and to permit pharmacologic suppression of the tachyarrhythmia. In addition to the previously described electrophysiologic concerns after an atrial switch operation, depressed function of the subaortic right ventricle predisposes that chamber to disturbances in rhythm that can be detected by exercise electrocardiography, Holter monitor, or an event recorder.

The Fontan procedure, which is employed principally in patients with a univentricular heart or tricuspid atresia, has undergone many modifications and is now employed in a variety of complex cyanotic malformations in which biventricular repair is not feasible.[12] Common to all modifications is a circulation in series without a functional subpulmonary ventricle. Earlier types of atriopulmonary connections have given way to the lateral tunnel repair, which excludes the right atrium from the systemic-to-pulmonary circulation. Functional adequacy of the Fontan repair depends chiefly on low resistance to flow through the pulmonary vascular bed, which, in the absence of increased pulmonary vascular resistance, depends on left ventricular filling pressure. Sinus rhythm is therefore important, if not crucial.

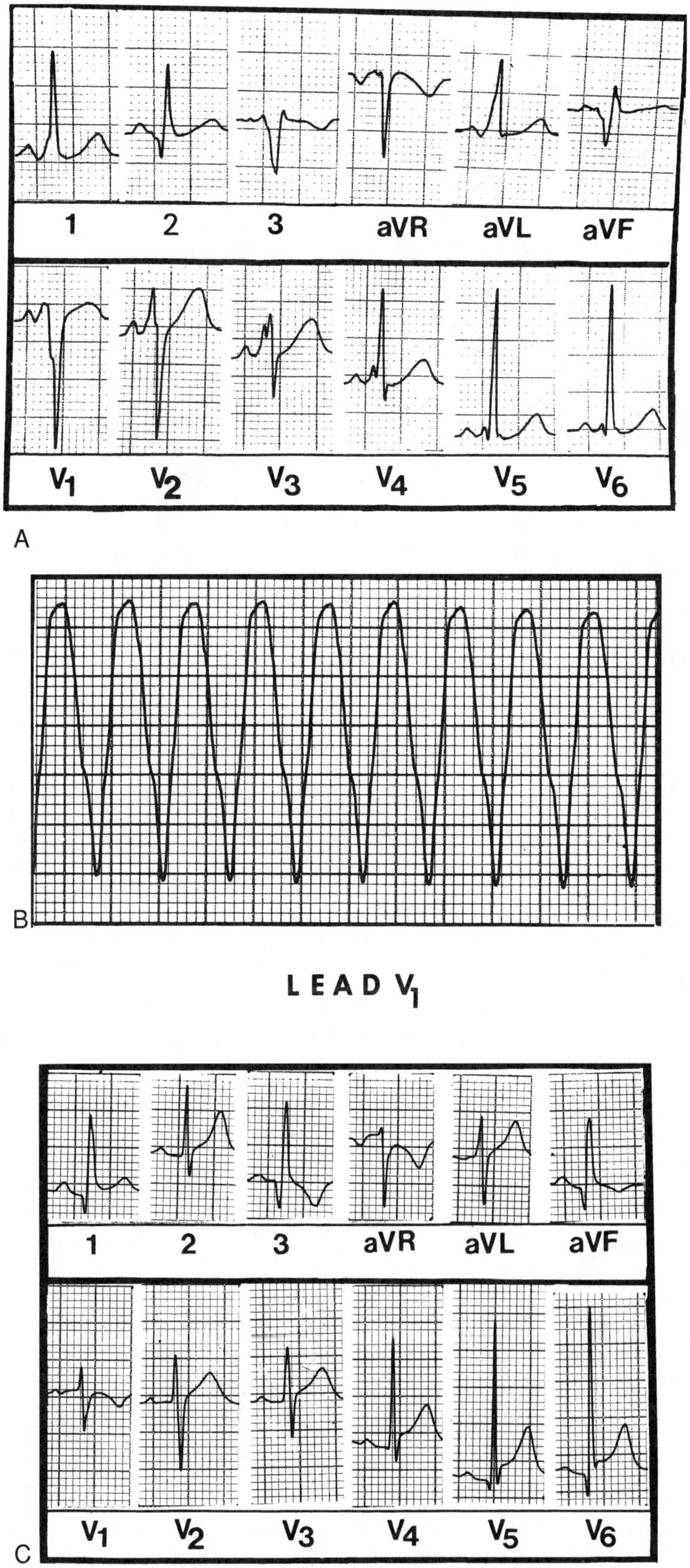

Figure 53–4. *A,* A 12-lead scalar electrocardiogram from a 32-year-old man with Ebstein anomaly of the tricuspid valve and the typical accessory pathway delta wave directed to the left, superior, and posterior. *B,* Atrial fibrillation with rapid, wide, QRS tachycardia via the accessory pathway. *C,* A 12-lead scalar electrocardiogram after surgical dissociation of the right atrium from the right ventricle during tricuspid reconstruction. The delta wave is no longer present.

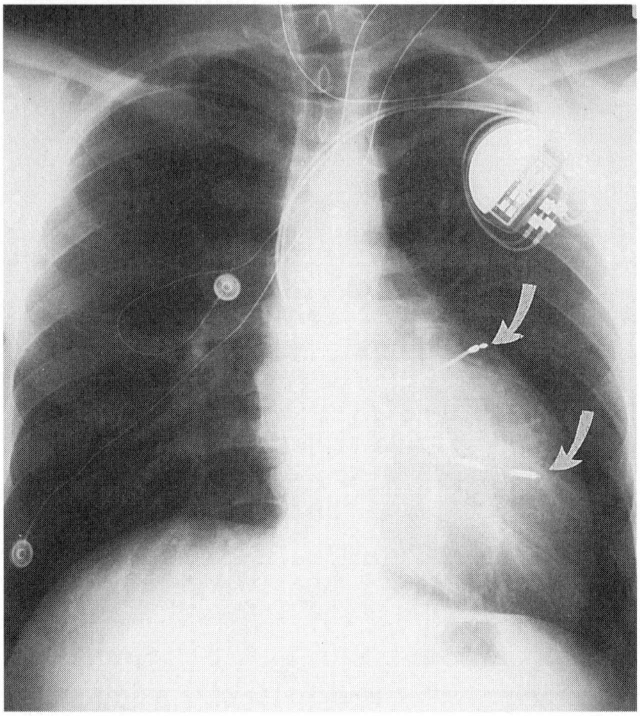

Figure 53–5. Chest radiograph from a 21-year-old man who at age 3 years had undergone a Mustard atrial switch operation for complete transposition of the great arteries. High-degree atrioventricular block necessitated a dual-chamber pacemaker with one lead in the left atrial appendage (*upper arrow*) and the other lead in the left ventricular endocardium (*lower arrow*). Access was from the superior vena cava, which had been baffled into the left atrium.

Atrial tachyarrhythmias adversely affect left ventricular function, initiating a rise in end-diastolic pressure that is transferred through the lungs into the right atrium and venae cavae, compromising anterograde flow into the pulmonary circulation.[12] Atrial fibrillation or flutter can be accompanied by rapid hemodynamic deterioration and death, although some patients tolerate atrial arrhythmias surprisingly well. Nevertheless, every attempt should be made to restore sinus rhythm, including the use of amiodarone. The complexity of the Fontan repair lends itself poorly to catheter ablation of an arrhythmogenic focus. Because of the importance of the functional adequacy of the systemic ventricle after a Fontan repair, there is strong consensus that patients should be treated with afterload reduction that entails the use of angiotensin converting enzyme inhibitors, preferably captopril.

VENTRICULAR FUNCTION

Because ventricular function depends on a number of variables peculiar to congenital cardiac malformations, the settings are more complex than those in acquired heart disease. The malformed heart may be equipped with two ventricles; the two ventricles may be inverted or noninverted; the great arteries may be transposed or normally related; or there may be a single ventricle that is either morphologically left, right, or indeterminate. In hearts equipped with two noninverted ventricles, ventricular function—right or left—is determined by the response to loading conditions or hypoxemia. In Eisenmenger complex (nonrestrictive ventricular septal defect, pulmonary vascular disease, and reversed shunt), right ventricular afterload is determined by systemic vascular resistance via the ventricular septal defect. The deleterious effect of systemic hypertension on right ventricular function should be addressed, but control must be meticulous because an inappropriate reduction in systemic vascular resistance augments the right-to-left shunt. Pharmacologic management should be monitored by a home blood pressure record.

In the presence of ventricular inversion (i.e., congenitally corrected transposition of the great arteries), the morphologic right ventricle is subaortic.[8] The long-term durability of a morphologic right ventricle in this systemic location continues to be a matter of lively interest. The inverted right ventricle maintains a normal stroke volume at a lower ejection fraction than does a systemic left ventricle without implying abnormal systolic function,[8] a point that must be recognized when afterload reduction is considered. If congenitally corrected transposition of the great arteries is accompanied by incompetence of the left atrioventricular valve, the volume load imposed on the subaortic ventricle is an additional argument for afterload reduction.

Single ventricle of the left ventricular type is the commonest variety of univentricular heart (about 65% of cases).[8] Univentricular hearts of the right ventricular type represent about 25% of cases.[8] The least common variety, representing fewer than 10% of cases, is characterized by a single ventricle with an indeterminate trabecular pattern.[8] The single ventricle serves as the only effective pump for both the systemic and pulmonary circulations. Ventricular volume is necessarily increased, and there is an adaptive increase in ventricular mass. In relation to a normal systemic ventricle, the single ventricular chamber, regardless of its morphology, usually exhibits abnormal systolic function with a relatively low ejection fraction. Indices of ventricular mass are significantly lower in patients with univentricular hearts of the right ventricular type, implying a comparatively poor adaptive response indicated by inadequate mass relative to ventricular volume.[8] The inherent functional limitations of univentricular hearts argue for the relatively routine use of afterload reduction with angiotensin converting enzyme inhibitors after a Fontan repair, especially, but not exclusively, when there is left atrioventricular valve regurgitation.

In complete transposition of the great arteries, left ventricular function is normal at birth and during the first few weeks of life, but left ventricular mass does not increase in proportion to volume. The inadequate mass-to-volume ratio is reflected in decreased systolic function. With the passage of time, the subpulmonary left ventricle assumes the characteristics of a volume pump. The ventricular septum tends to encroach on the left ventricular cavity, impairing diastolic filling. Afterload reduction of the systemic right ventricle is not likely to influence the position of the ventricular septum or the filling properties of the left ventricle. In simple complete transposition, the right ventricle functions normally at birth. When an interatrial communication is established by balloon septotomy, there is an increase in right ventricular volume, contractility, and ejection fraction. In adult survivors of atrial switch repairs, right ventricular function is usually depressed but is responsive to afterload reduction, especially when aortic regurgitation is present.

In congenital aortic valve stenosis, systolic performance of the afterloaded left ventricle is typically supernormal.[13] An increase in left ventricular mass caused by myocyte hyperplasia and a parallel (proportionate) growth in the microvascular bed are believed to be responsible for low left ventricular systolic wall stress and supernormal ejection performance. Enhanced systolic function is likely to persist after successful surgical or balloon dilatation of the stenotic aortic valve. The anticipated supernormal ejection performance of the left ventricle should be taken into account when patients are selected for relief of aortic stenosis by direct repair or interventional catheterization. Response of the left ventricle in coarctation of the aorta is similar to but lesser in magnitude than that of the afterloaded left ventricle in aortic valve stenosis, as just described.

When ventricular function and physiologic reserve in patients with cyanotic congenital heart disease are judged, the fact that exercise may significantly increase the right-to-left shunt and materially influence the dynamics of oxygen uptake and ventilation must be taken into account.[14] An increase in ventilatory drive is the result of the response of the respiratory center to the sudden changes in blood

TABLE 53–3. CONGENITAL HEART DISEASE FUNCTIONAL CLASSES BY PRESENCE AND DEGREE OF SYMPTOMS

Class 1:	Asymptomatic
Class 2:	Symptoms are present but do not interfere with normal activities
Class 3:	Symptoms interfere with some but not most activities
Class 4:	Symptoms interfere with most if not all activities

gas composition and pH that are induced by the increased venoarterial mixing that is provoked by the fall in systemic vascular resistance that accompanies isotonic exercise. Breathlessness during isotonic exercise in patients with cyanotic congenital heart disease is more likely to be related to hyperventilation rather than depressed ventricular function. Accordingly, therapeutic decisions based on the New York Heart Association functional classification may not apply. The functional classification in Table 53–3 is more relevant to congenital heart disease.

EXERCISE AND ATHLETICS

It is intuitively recognized that individuals with certain types of congenital disorders of the heart or circulation—unoperated or postoperative—are at risk when engaging in strenuous exercise or competitive sports.[15] Although athletic activities can be regarded as either competitive or recreational, the distinction is less than categoric, and overlap is common. In competitive athletics, physical and emotional efforts are unfettered, permitting little or no latitude for the patient-athlete to judge when it is prudent to desist. Many individuals are temperamentally ill-equipped to engage in recreational athletics without being competitive. In advising patients, consideration must be given to (1) the type, intensity, and duration of exercise; (2) the risk of body collision inherent in contact sports; (3) the training program (conditioning) required for a given sport; (4) the emotional response (stress) that the participant experiences in anticipation of or during a sport event; and (5) the risk of bodily injury to the participant, to spectators, or to bystanders if the patient-athlete loses consciousness. Low- to moderate-intensity isotonic exercise of limited duration may be not only permissible but desirable, whereas performance of high-intensity isotonic exercise of prolonged duration requires physician approval. Similarly, isometric exercise of low to medium intensity and brief duration is likely to be tolerated without ill effect, but strenuous isometric exercise is seldom desirable, although occasionally permissible. In advising patients, the physician must take into account their ventricular function (discussed previously), as well as the potential for exercise-induced disturbances in rhythm, particularly ventricular ectopic rhythms.

INFECTIVE ENDOCARDITIS: RISKS AND PROPHYLAXIS

The number and age range of patients susceptible to infective endocarditis have increased with the increase in adult survival.[16] Surgical interventions and prosthetic materials have had a significant impact on the risk of infection. Certain operations (e.g., ligation of a patent ductus arteriosus) eliminate that risk, whereas other operations (e.g., rigid prosthetic valves or conduits) heighten the risk. There are two major predisposing causes of infective endocarditis: a susceptible cardiac or vascular substrate and a source of bacteremia. Susceptible lesions are those with high-velocity flow, jet impact, and focal increases in the rate of shear; however, there are unexplained exceptions. High-velocity regurgitant flow across a systemic semilunar valve (aortic regurgitation) represents a relatively high-risk substrate for infective endocarditis, whereas high-velocity regurgitant flow across a pulmonary semilunar valve (Graham Steell regurgitation) represents a relatively low risk.

Prophylaxis for infective endocarditis includes day-to-day nonchemotherapeutic measures in addition to antibiotic prophylaxis for bacteremia anticipated during planned interventions.[16] In general, the rationale for prophylaxis is the presence and degree of risk (susceptibility) associated with a given cardiac abnormality. Lesions have been categorized as unoperated low or intermediate risk and postoperative no risk, low risk, intermediate risk, or high risk.[16] High-risk settings include rigid prosthetic valves (especially left-sided), external valved conduits, and aortopulmonary shunts, especially those employing synthetic materials such as Gortex.

Nonchemotherapeutic day-to-day prophylaxis includes oral hygiene, skin care, nail care, and female contraception. Patients are advised to brush their teeth twice a day with a soft-bristle tooth brush and focus on gum care, especially when gums are spongy and fragile as a result of cyanotic congenital heart disease. Dental floss must be used cautiously to avoid gum injury. Food that predisposes to cavities (e.g., hard candy) should be avoided. Skin care, especially in adolescents and young adults with acne or pustules, must be meticulous because of the risk of staphylococcal bacteremia. Gentle, nonabrasive cleansing of the skin is advised to avoid inadvertent injury to skin lesions, particularly pustules, which should never be squeezed or otherwise manipulated. Biting of nails or picking of fingers risks injury to contiguous skin and predisposes to paronychial staphylococcal infection. Nail biting can be especially difficult to manage, because it is often a manifestation of compulsive behavior. Intrauterine contraceptive devices are best avoided because of the risk of bacteremia. Bleeding hemorrhoids are potential sources of bacteremia and should be treated.

Chemotherapeutic prophylaxis is based on the cardiac lesion, the source of potential bacteremia, and the presence or absence of antibiotic sensitivity. To increase compliance, the regimen for a given patient should be the most effective as well as the simplest, least costly, least painful, and lowest risk for side effects. The American Heart Association guidelines have been incorporated into convenient, wallet-sized instructions that can be given to patients. The American Heart Association Special Report on Prevention of Infective Endocarditis[17] and the Working Party of the British Society for Antimicrobial Chemotherapy[18] also provide the necessary recommendations and deserve careful study. Chemotherapeutic prophylaxis focuses on dental work and on procedures involving the upper respiratory, genitourinary, and gastrointestinal tracts. Genitourinary procedures in males include prostatic massage as well as instrumentation. Dilatation and curettage are potential causes of bacteremia, and transient bacteremia occurs relatively frequently in women undergoing suction abortions.

PREGNANCY AND GENETICS

An understanding of the circulatory and respiratory physiology of the normal gravid state serves as a backdrop against which the physiologic derangements caused by heart disease can be assessed.[19, 20] Peripheral edema occurs in 50%–80% of normal gravidas, chiefly as a result of an increase in total body water and exchangeable sodium and elevation in lower extremity venous stasis in response to compression of the inferior vena cava by the gravid uterus. Spontaneous diuresis after delivery restores blood volume to pregravid levels within 4–6 weeks, assuming the patient has normal renal function. Diuretics should be used for the edema of cardiac failure but not for the edema of normal pregnancy. Progesterone stimulation of the respiratory center during normal gestation provokes an increase in minute ventilation beginning in the first trimester, anticipating a progressive rise in oxygen consumption that reaches its peak near term. This normal hyperventilatory response should not be mistaken for cardiac dyspnea. Easy fatigability, a decrease in exercise tolerance, and basal rales (high diaphragm) that disappear with cough or deep breathing must not be misconstrued.

The objectives of reparative surgery are to increase the safety and success of pregnancy, to preserve the health of the mother, and to reduce fetal risk.[19, 20] The following are some important principles in the management of the unoperated or operated gravida with congenital heart disease (Table 53–4).

A major goal is to minimize the factors that encroach on limited circulatory reserve of the gravida with congenital heart disease: anxiety; sodium and water retention; sudden, strenuous, or isometric exercise; heat and humidity; anemia; infection; disturbances in cardiac rhythm and conduction; and thromboembolic predispositions. Anxiety is a special concern for the primigravida. The expectant mother should be told what to anticipate during pregnancy, labor, delivery, and the puerperium to minimize fear of the unknown. Exercise adds to the physiologic burden of pregnancy; therefore, the gravida should limit herself to moderate isotonic exercise. Heat and humidity add to the pregnant woman's hemodynamic burden; a dry, cool atmosphere is therapeutic. The physiologic anemia of pregnancy must be distinguished from pathologic anemia and the latter assiduously addressed. Meticulous leg care reduces the gestational tendency for lower extremity venous stasis and the attendant risk of thromboembolism, points of special concern because of the risk of paradoxical embolization. The supine position should be avoided because of compression of the inferior vena cava by the gravid uterus. The woman should minimize or avoid passive standing or sitting with her knees flexed and legs dependent. Oxygen administration during gestation in cyanotic women may or may not be indicated; there is little or no evidence of benefit to the mother, and less than convincing evidence of a favorable effect on growth retardation in the fetus.

Maternal mortality among gravidas with cardiac disease has been related to functional class, but the symptoms associated with congenital malformations of the heart, especially cyanosis, have prompted the use of the functional classification shown in Table 53–3. In addition to and apart from symptoms and functional limitations, certain congenital cardiac malformations impose such a formidable threat to maternal survival that pregnancy is proscribed or should be terminated. Of the two major maternal cardiac risks—pulmonary vascular disease and pulmonary edema—the former is more relevant to congenital heart disease. Pulmonary vascular disease in any context is a major hazard limiting or precluding rapid adaptive responses to the circulatory changes of pregnancy and the volatile hemodynamic changes during labor, delivery, and the puerperium. Maternal risk can sometimes be appreciably reduced even late in gestation by balloon dilatation of congenitally stenotic aortic or pulmonary valves (Fig. 53–6).

In women with functionally mild, unoperated lesions, and in patients who have undergone successful cardiac surgery, the management of labor and delivery is the same as for normal gravidas, except for selective risk of infective endocarditis. The need for antibiotic prophylaxis during routine delivery has been questioned because of the low incidence of bacteremia that accompanies a normal uncomplicated vaginal delivery. However, it should not be assumed that a given delivery will be uncomplicated, and episiotomy is, strictly speaking, not normal. Accordingly, pregnant women with cardiac lesions susceptible to infective endocarditis should receive antibiotic prophylaxis from the onset of labor through the third or fourth postpartum day. The incidence of bacteremia increases appreciably with premature rupture of membranes and with prolonged, difficult labor.

For gravidas with functionally important, unoperated or postoperative congenital cardiac disease, the anticipation and management of labor, delivery, and the puerperium are crucial if risk is to be minimized.[20] The first necessity is to underscore the benefits of vaginal delivery. Cesarean section should be reserved for cephalopelvic disproportion or preterm labor in gravidas receiving warfarin (Coumadin) anticoagulation. Spontaneous onset of labor should be avoided by planned induction. Amniocentesis around the 37th week of gestation determines whether fetal lung maturity has been achieved and whether delivery can proceed safely. The gravida is then admitted for induction of labor.

Delivery is planned as much as possible to occur during the working day so an experienced high-risk obstetrician, a neonatologist, and a cardiologist can be in attendance. Intracervical and intravaginal topical prostaglandin softens and dilates the cervix and, after absorption, usually initiates uterine contractions, which can be augmented by oxytocin.[20] Labor should take place with the patient in the lateral decubitus position to attenuate the hemodynamic fluctuations associated with major uterine contractions in the supine position. Meperidine relieves pain and the patient's apprehension. A lumbar epidural anesthetic controls pain without reducing the strength of uterine contractions, which are monitored along with fetal heart rate (see Fig. 53–2). The fetus should be allowed to pass through the pelvis in response to the force of uterine contractions unassisted by straining to avoid the undesirable circulatory effects of the Valsalva maneuver. Delivery is assisted by vacuum extraction and low forceps. Oxygen is often administered during labor, especially in cyanotic women, although its efficacy is unproven (discussed previously).

During the postpartum period, meticulous leg care, elastic stockings, and early ambulation are important preventive measures that reduce the risk of thromboembolism. Breast feeding may encroach on cardiac reserve by interfering with the mother's sleep and by increasing the risk of mastitis and bacteremia. Breast feeding should therefore be selective and its duration minimized. Maternal congenital heart disease exposes the fetus to risks that threaten its intrauterine viability and to risks that are manifest as congenital and developmental malformations. Intrauterine viability is influenced by maternal functional class (with qualifications noted previously), maternal cyanosis, and oral anticoagulants.[20] Cyanosis threatens fetal growth, development, and viability and materially increases the incidence of fetal wastage, dysmaturity, and prematurity. The fetal risk of maternal oral anticoagulant administration cannot be satisfactorily resolved. The need for anticoagulants should therefore be minimized.

Valve reconstruction is recommended in women of childbearing age unless anticoagulants are obligatory for other reasons. A bioprosthetic valve obviates the need for anticoagulants but confronts the patient with the need for reoperation at a higher risk. In addition, there is concern that pregnancy may accelerate degeneration of tissue valves. There is no consensus on how best to administer anticoagulants to pregnant women. It is currently believed that the risk of fetal wastage from heparin is less than that for warfarin (Coumadin). Whatever regimen of heparin or warfarin is employed, the patient and her partner should be so advised before conception. Warfarin should be replaced by heparin prior to conception to avoid its teratogenic risk in early gestation. Heparin can be continued throughout gestation, provided that the anticoagulant response is meticulously controlled, or it can be replaced with warfarin in the second trimester and reinstituted in the 36th week of gestation. In light of the concern that the risk of embryopathy varies with the level of oral anticoagulation, warfarin dosage should be monitored according to the International Normalized Ratio (INR) to achieve a therapeutic response at the lowest dose. There are four concerns

TABLE 53–4. COMMON MALFORMATIONS WITH EXPECTED ADULT SURVIVAL BY ORDER OF FEMALE PREVALENCE

Acyanotic
Atrial septal defect (secundum)
Patent ductus arteriosus
Pulmonary valve stenosis
Coarctation of the aorta
Aortic valve disease
Cyanotic
Tetralogy of Fallot

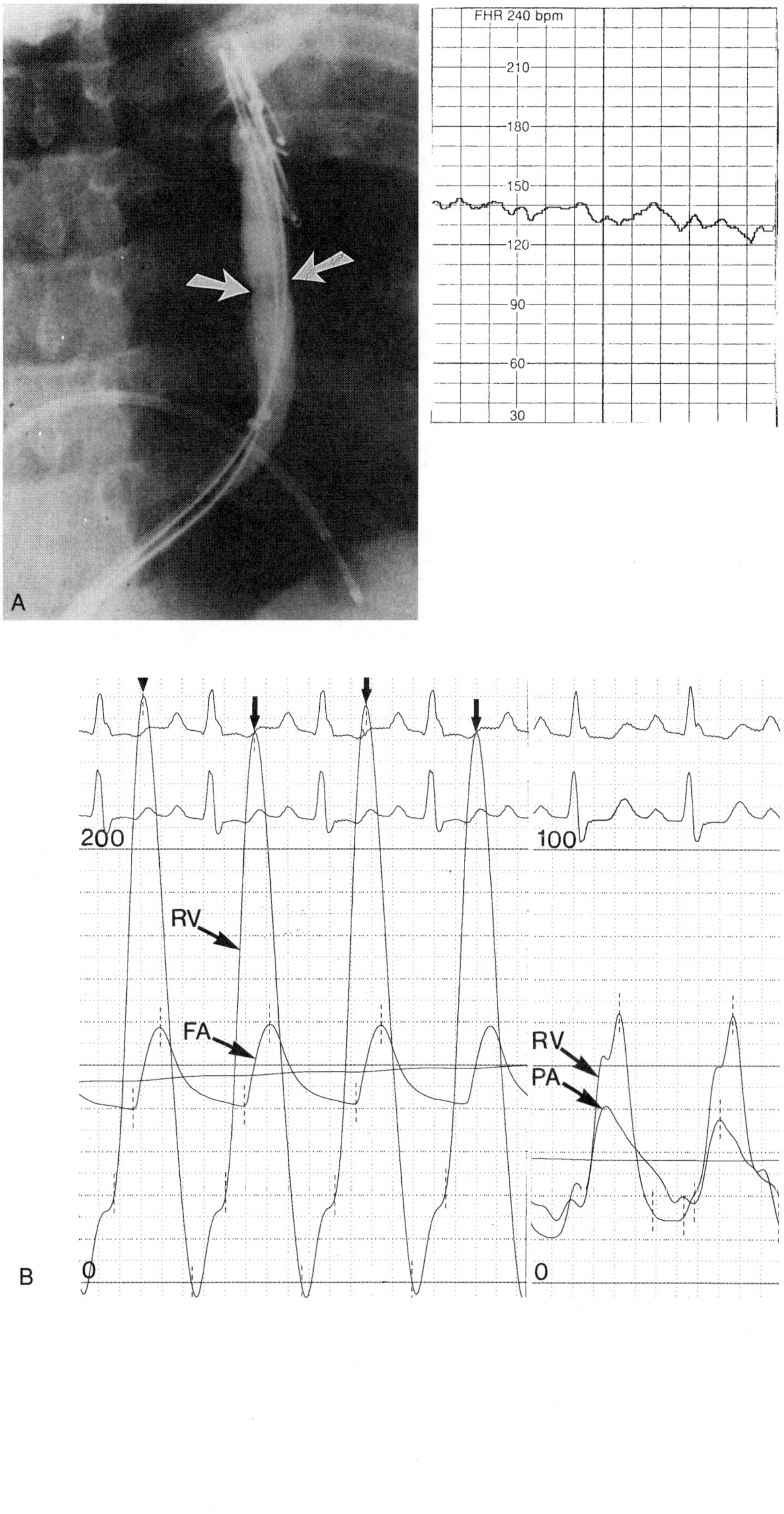

Figure 53–6. *A*, A single balloon across a severely stenotic mobile pulmonary valve of an 18-year-old pregnant woman who was near term. The balloon is indented (*arrow*) by the stenotic valve. The fetal heart rate (FHR) is shown in the panel on the right. *B*, Pressure pulses before (*left*) and after (*right*) balloon dilatation of the stenotic pulmonary valve. Right ventricular (RV) pressure fell from 280 to 60 mm Hg. The right ventricular-to-pulmonary arterial gradient fell to 40 mm Hg. Right ventricular pulsus alternans was present before dilatation, indicating right ventricular failure. Three days after balloon dilatation, the patient experienced an uncomplicated vaginal delivery. *Abbreviations:* FA, femoral arteries; PA, pulmonary artery.

regarding the administration of heparin throughout pregnancy: greater difficulty in achieving a therapeutic response; inconvenience of parenteral administration; risk of heparin-induced thrombocytopenia; and risk of bone demineralization.

Management of the gravida includes counseling regarding potential genetic transmission of maternal congenital cardiac disease. The risk of occurrence of cardiac disease in offspring is believed to be greater if the mother rather than the father is the affected parent.[20] Certain congenital cardiac malformations incur a higher probability of genetic transmission than do others. The risk to offspring varies from as low as 2.5% to as high as 15%. Although individual risks cannot be ignored, it is prudent to provide parental reassurance by stating that the probability of having a normal offspring is about 90%.

CONTRACEPTION

Apart from barrier methods and tubal ligation, Norplant is the safest and most efficacious method of contraception for patients with cyanotic congenital heart disease and pulmonary vascular disease, but installation and supervision must be meticulous.[21] Fluid retention with Norplant is modest and does not preclude the use of the implant provided that heart failure is controlled. Depo-Provera is not recommended in patients with heart failure because of the greater tendency to retain fluid. Low-estrin contraception is considered safe and nonthrombogenic, with a high level of efficacy unless a dose is missed. An intrauterine device in a monogamous relationship probably does not increase the risk of infection and infective endocarditis, but endometrial irritation with bleeding is a potential complication. Intrauterine devices are therefore not recommended, especially in women with cyanotic congenital heart disease, because of the intrinsic hemostatic defects.

ACQUIRED CARDIAC AND VASCULAR DISEASE

Pediatric patients with congenital heart disease usually have one illness. The adult with unoperated or postoperative congenital heart disease may have additional illnesses inherent in the aging process. The two commonest of these are ischemic heart disease (atherosclerotic coronary artery disease) and systemic hypertension. Adults undergoing operation or reoperation for congenital heart disease may require study of the coronary circulation because of the potential need for bypass grafting. Ischemic heart disease and systemic hypertension adversely affect left ventricular filling and increase the left-to-right shunt through an ostium secundum atrial septal defect. Systemic hypertension augments the left-to-right shunt through a ventricular septal defect and imposes additional afterload on the high-pressure right ventricle in the presence of a nonrestrictive ventricular septal defect and pulmonary vascular disease (Eisenmenger complex; discussed previously).

MEDICAL MANAGEMENT DURING NONCARDIAC SURGERY

When adults with unoperated or postoperative congenital heart disease require noncardiac surgery, perioperative safety can be increased, often appreciably, if risks inherent in this patient population are anticipated.[22] The most important factor in reducing risk is the anesthesiologist.[23] Every attempt should be made to secure the collaboration of a cardiac anesthesiologist with experience in congenital heart disease. Hospitals with cardiothoracic surgical services can usually meet this need. Specific malformations necessitate specific attention, although certain generalities merit emphasis. In patients with pulmonary vascular disease, noncardiac surgery, even minor procedures, can be hazardous. Preoperative sedation and reassurance are obligatory. The risks inherent in cyanosis compound the risks of pulmonary vascular disease. In Eisenmenger complex, for example, meticulous monitoring of blood pressure is crucial. A sudden fall in systemic resistance may precipitate intense cyanosis and death, or a sudden rise in systemic resistance may abruptly and dangerously depress systemic blood flow. Insertion of a flotation catheter incurs risks that outweigh the potential benefits. An experienced anesthesiologist can monitor systemic vascular resistance using nothing more than pulse oximeter oxygen saturation levels, which reflect moment-to-moment changes in systemic vascular resistance by rising and falling in parallel. Postural hypotension tends to occur during early convalescence, especially after general anesthesia. Because the attendant drop in systemic vascular resistance serves to augment a right-to-left shunt, cyanotic patients with pulmonary vascular disease should change position slowly until the risk of postoperative postural hypotension has abated.

Oral anticoagulants in patients with rigid prosthetic valves complicate the management of noncardiac surgery.[22] Perioperative decisions depend chiefly on the type and location of the prosthesis. If noncardiac surgery is elective, and if the prosthesis carries a high thromboembolic risk, warfarin should be replaced with an in-hospital continuous infusion of heparin until the INR is close to normal. Intravenous heparin is discontinued 4–6 h before the elective operation, restarted 48 h after operation, and replaced by warfarin as soon as safety permits, generally between the second and fifth postoperative days. For a lower risk prosthetic valve in the aortic location, it is relatively safe to discontinue warfarin 2–3 days before noncardiac surgery and restart the drug 2–3 days postoperatively. For emergency noncardiac surgery, hemostasis is best achieved by infusion of fresh-frozen plasma. Vitamin K does not result in prompt reversal of the hemostatic defects and appreciably blunts the response to readministration of warfarin after operation.

Depressed ventricular function poses a perioperative risk that varies with the degree to which ejection fraction is reduced. Of particular concern are depressed ventricular function in patients with Fontan repairs and depressed function of the subaortic morphologic right ventricle in complete transposition of the great arteries after an atrial switch operation. The development of perioperative atrial fibrillation or atrial flutter may suddenly further reduce already poor ventricular function, with catastrophic consequences. Maintenance of sinus rhythm is therefore crucial. Patients with disturbances in atrial or ventricular rhythm require careful monitoring, and those who have or are at risk of high-degree heart block should have a temporary pacing wire inserted, provided the morphologic substrate permits, which, in the setting of complex postoperative cyanotic congenital heart disease, may not be the case.

Perioperative improvement of hemostasis in cyanotic patients can be achieved if surgery is elective. When the hematocrit level is above 65% (measured by Coulter electronics), reduction by isovolumetric phlebotomy to just below 65% is believed to improve hemostasis. Phlebotomized units can be reserved for potential autologous transfusion.

Cyanotic adults have an increased incidence of calcium bilirubinate gallstones that express themselves overtly as acute cholecystitis (Fig. 53–7).[22] Biliary colic may become clinically manifest years after intracardiac surgery has eliminated the cyanosis and reduced the risk of noncardiac surgery. An additional hazard of acute cholecystitis is bacteremia and infective endocarditis. Management of cyanotic patients in this situation therefore includes antibiotic therapy.

Intravenous lines, infusions, and drugs must be managed cautiously in cyanotic patients. Air or particles introduced into peripheral veins may be delivered into the systemic circulation because of the right-to-left shunt. All such patients should have air-particle filters inserted into the distal end of their intravenous lines[22] (see Fig. 53–3).

Administration of high levels of oxygen by mask may raise arterial oxygen saturation (dissolved oxygen) in cyanotic patients, but there is little or no evidence that routine perioperative use of oxygen is beneficial. Oxygen exerts a drying effect on nasal mucous mem-

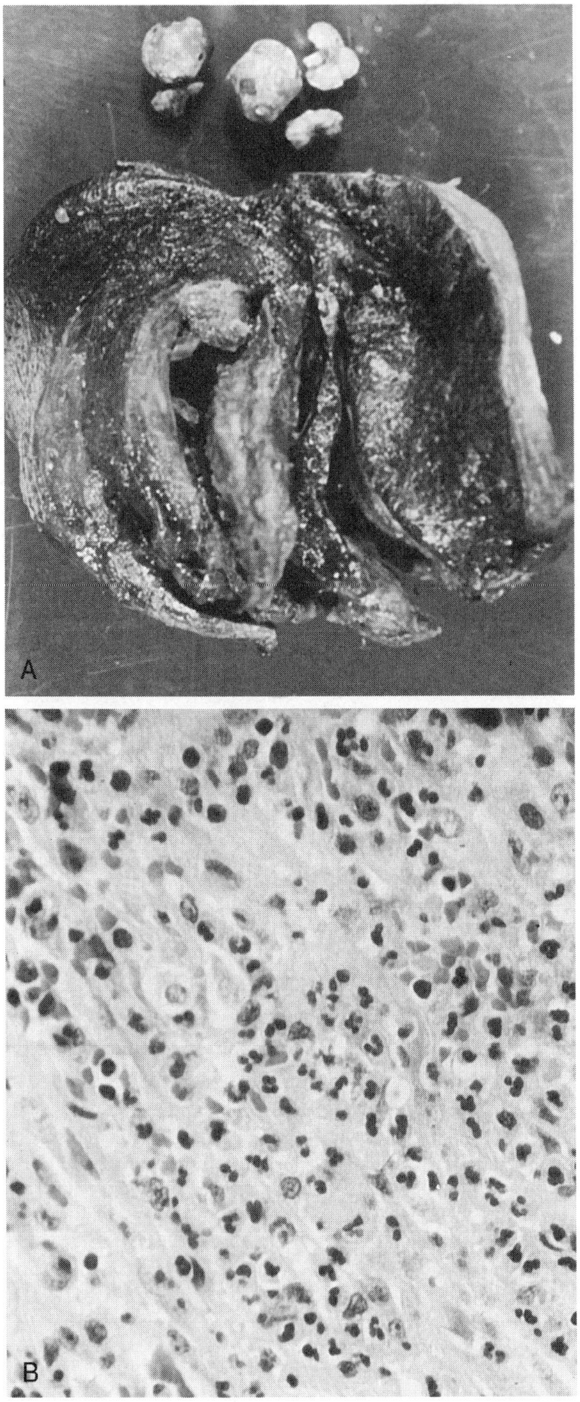

Figure 53–7. *A*, A surgical specimen shows calcium bilirubinate gallstones and the thick-walled gallbladder from a 43-year-old man with Eisenmenger complex. *B*, Histologic examination of the gallbladder wall shows acute inflammation.

branes and increases the risk of epistaxis because of the hemostatic defects in cyanotic patients.

Prophylaxis for infective endocarditis is an important aspect of perioperative management of patients with congenital heart disease undergoing noncardiac surgery. The guidelines were dealt with previously, and individual judgment determines the relative risks and the antibiotic of choice. A highly susceptible substrate argues for prophylaxis even if the risk of bacteremia is comparatively small.

The risk of a postoperative paradoxical embolus is of particular concern in patients with unoperated ostium secundum atrial septal defect or cyanotic congenital heart disease. Postoperative thrombophlebitis provides the source of emboli that are carried by the inferior vena cava and stream across an atrial septal defect or through a right-to-left shunt. Meticulous leg care and early ambulation minimize venous stasis. An additional postoperative concern in patients with ostium secundum atrial septal defect is hemorrhage, which can provoke a rise in systemic vascular resistance and a decrease in venous return, a combination that augments the left-to-right interatrial shunt, sometimes appreciably.

CYANOTIC CONGENITAL HEART DISEASE, HEMATOLOGIC DISORDERS, RENAL INVOLVEMENT, AND URATE METABOLISM

In adults with cyanotic congenital heart disease and erythrocytosis, routine employment of phlebotomy presupposes an increase in the risk of stroke as a result of cerebral arterial thrombotic infarction; this presupposition has not withstood scrutiny.[24] Apart from its potential value in improving perioperative hemostasis (discussed previously), the firmest indication for phlebotomy is for temporary relief of marked to severe hyperviscosity symptoms in patients with hematocrit levels exceeding 65%, provided dehydration is not the cause.[25] Heat and humidity result in a decrease in plasma volume, an increase in hematocrit level, and an increase in hyperviscosity symptoms, which should be treated by volume repletion, not by phlebotomy. Significant symptomatic hyperviscosity in an iron-replete state seldom occurs with hematocrit levels lower than 65%. Hyperviscosity symptoms in this setting are almost always the result of iron deficiency. Phlebotomy further depletes iron stores and aggravates rather than alleviates the symptoms, which respond instead to iron repletion. The dose of iron should be small (325 mg of ferrous sulfate or 65 mg of elemental iron once daily, or 150 mg bid of Niferex, a highly water-soluble complex of iron with a low-molecular-weight polysaccharide that minimizes gastrointestinal side effects). Iron is discontinued at the first discernible rise in hematocrit level, which usually occurs within 1 week.

The amount of blood removed should be the minimum required to achieve short-term relief of hyperviscosity symptoms while avoiding the cycle of phlebotomy-induced iron depletion, administration of iron followed by an excessive erythrocytic response, recurrence of hyperviscosity symptoms, and additional phlebotomy provoking further iron deficiency. The following simple, safe outpatient method of phlebotomy usually suffices. Five hundred milliliters of blood are withdrawn over 30–45 min, followed by quantitative replacement of volume with isotonic saline. If saline is clinically undesirable, isovolumetric replacement can be achieved with dextran 40 (5% dextrose in water), which is salt free. Cuff blood pressure is recorded with the patient in the supine position, sitting and standing before phlebotomy, and at 15-min intervals after the procedure. Beneficial effects of phlebotomy are usually evident within 24 h and reflect an increase in systemic blood flow induced by isovolumetric reduction in red blood cell mass.

Carboxyhemoglobinemia that accompanies tobacco smoking impairs oxygen capacity and augments erythrocytosis. Smoking is therefore proscribed, especially in patients with cyanotic congenital heart disease.

Clinically overt hemostatic defects in cyanotic congenital heart disease tend to be mild; therefore, specific treatment is usually not required.[25] Serious spontaneous bleeding sometimes occurs, however. There is the risk of accidental trauma, and perioperative bleeding may pose a significant hazard (discussed previously). Aspirin reinforces the hemostatic defects in cyanotic patients and should be avoided. Nonsteroidal anti-inflammatory drugs and anticoagulants also reinforce the hemostatic abnormalities and increase the risk of bleeding. Epistaxis and hemoptysis are the principal sources of copious spontaneous hemorrhage, whereas oral surgery is the principal cause of excessive traumatic bleeding. Copious bleeding may respond to administration of an intravenous cryoprecipitate. Bronchoscopy for the investigation of hemoptysis should be avoided, with rare exceptions.

Hyperuricemia is common in adults with cyanotic congenital heart disease. Both increased production and decreased renal clearance of uric acid are important in the pathogenesis of hyperuricemia.[26] The low incidence of acute gouty arthritis in patients with cyanotic congenital heart disease and hyperuricemia is of the same order as the low incidence of gout in other forms of secondary hyperuricemia. When acute gouty arthritis occurs in adults with cyanotic congenital heart disease, the treatment of choice is intravenous colchicine (1–2 mg over 5 min), which produces a rapid clinical response while minimizing the undesirable dehydrating gastrointestinal side effects of oral colchicine. The initial intravenous dose can be followed by 1-mg doses 6 and 12 h later, with the total not to exceed 4 mg in 24 h. Prophylaxis after resolution of acute gouty arthritis can often be achieved with low-dose oral colchicine (0.6 mg once or twice per day), a schedule that prevents recurrences in a substantial majority of patients and is usually well tolerated. Nonsteroidal anti-inflammatory drugs (e.g., indomethacin) are less efficacious, and even in low doses reinforce the intrinsic hemostatic defects. Hyperuricemia appears to have little or no deleterious effect on renal function and need not be treated. In hyperuricemic patients with recurrent gouty arthritis, probenecid or sulfinpyrazone (uricosuric agents), allopurinol (decrease in synthesis of uric acid), or combined therapy is employed.

Renal involvement is a common feature of cyanotic congenital heart disease and is characterized initially by enlarged hypervascular glomeruli with subsequent development of increased cellularity, basement membrane thickening, focal interstitial fibrosis, and late hyalinization of the glomerular tuft.[25] Abnormal renal function may adversely influence risk during cardiac or noncardiac surgery, and an occasional older cyanotic adult experiences chronic renal failure.

REFERENCES

1. Perloff JK, Child JS (eds): Congenital Heart Disease in Adults. Philadelphia: WB Saunders, 1991.
2. Sillanpaa M: Social adjustment and functioning of chronically ill and impaired children and adolescents. Acta Paediatr Scand 1987; 340(suppl):1.
3. Hamburgen ME: Psychosocial concerns and life-style. 22nd Bethesda conference: Congenital Heart Disease After Childhood: an Expanding Patient Population. J Am Coll Cardiol 1990; 18:333.
4. Perloff JK, Marelli AJ: Neurological and psychosocial disorders in adults with congenital heart disease. Heart Stroke 1992; 1:218.
5. Tunkel AR, Kaye D: Neurologic complications of infective endocarditis. Neurol Clin 1993; 11:419.
6. Marelli AJ, Child JS, Perloff JK: Transesophageal echocardiography in congenital heart disease in the adult. Cardiol Clin 1993; 11:505.
7. Kurlan R, Krall RL, Deweese JA: Vertebrobasilar ischemia after repair of tetralogy of Fallot: significance of subclavian steal created by Blalock-Taussig anastomosis. Stroke 1984; 15:359.
8. Perloff JK: Clinical Recognition of Congenital Heart Disease, pp 91, 247, 293. Philadelphia: WB Saunders, 1994.
9. Stevenson WG, Klitzner TS, Perloff JK: Electrophysiologic abnormalities: natural occurrence and postoperative residua and sequelae. *In* Perloff JK, Child JS (eds): Congenital Heart Disease in Adults, p 259. Philadelphia: WB Saunders, 1991.
10. Chandar JS, Wolff GS, Garson A, et al: Ventricular arrhythmias in postoperative tetralogy of Fallot. Am J Cardiol 1990; 65:655.
11. Flinn CJ, Wolff GS, Dick M, et al: Cardiac rhythm after Mustard operation for complete transposition of the great arteries. N Engl J Med 1984; 310:1635.
12. Weber HS, Hellenbrand WE, Kleinman CS, et al: Predictors of rhythm disturbances and subsequent morbidity after Fontan operation. Am J Cardiol 1989; 64:762.
13. Assey ME, Wisenbaugh T, Spann JF, et al: Unexpected persistence into adulthood of low wall stress in patients with congenital aortic stenosis. Circulation 1987; 75:973.
14. Sietsema KE, Cooper DM, Perloff JK, et al: Control of ventilation during exercise in patients with central venous-to-systemic arterial shunts. J Appl Physiol 1988; 64:234.
15. Kaplan S, Perloff JK: Exercise and athletics before and after surgery or interventional catheterization. *In* Perloff JK, Child JS (eds): Congenital Heart Disease in Adults, p 166. Philadelphia: WB Saunders, 1991.
16. Child JS, Perloff JK: Infective endocarditis, risks and prophylaxis. *In* Perloff JK, Child JS (eds): Congenital Heart Disease in Adults, p 111. Philadelphia: WB Saunders, 1991.
17. Shulman ST, Amren DP, Bisno AL, et al: Prevention of bacterial endocarditis: a statement for health professionals by the Committee on Rheumatic Fever and Infective Endocarditis of the Council on Cardiovascular Disease in the Young. Circulation 1984; 70:1123A.
18. Working party of the British Society for Antimicrobial Chemotherapy: The antibiotic prophylaxis of infective endocarditis. Lancet 1982; 2:1323.
19. Pitkin RM, Perloff JK, Koos BJ, Beall MH: Pregnancy and congenital heart disease. Ann Intern Med 1990; 112:445.
20. Perloff JK: Congenital heart disease and pregnancy. Clin Cardiol 1994; 17:579.
21. Sciscione A, Callan NA: Pregnancy and contraception. Cardiol Clin 1993; 11:701.
22. Perloff JK: Noncardiac surgery in adults with congenital heart disease. *In* Perloff JK, Child JS (eds): Congenital Heart Disease in Adults, p 239. Philadelphia: WB Saunders, 1991.
23. Baum VC, Perloff JK: Anesthetic implications of adults with congenital heart disease. Anesth Analg 1993; 76:1342.
24. Perloff JK, Marelli AJ, Miner PD: Risk of stroke in adults with cyanotic congenital heart disease. Circulation 1993; 87:1954.
25. Perloff JK: Systemic complications of cyanosis on adults with congenital heart disease: hematologic derangements, renal function and urate metabolism. Cardiol Clin 1993; 11:689.
26. Ross EA, Perloff JK, Danovitch GM, et al: Renal function and urate metabolism in late survivors with cyanotic congenital heart disease. Circulation 1986; 73:396.

54 Treatment of Primary Pulmonary Hypertension: Lessons Learned

Bruce H. Brundage, MD

Primary pulmonary hypertension (PPH) is a rare disease that occurs mainly in young women and carries a very poor prognosis. Until the 1970s, little was known regarding how to effectively treat the disease. The tragic outcome usually associated with PPH has focused physicians' interest on the search for better forms of treatment.

A major drawback to the effective treatment of any disease is a lack of knowledge regarding pathogenesis. This is certainly true for PPH, which may be several diseases and is probably better labeled *unexplained pulmonary hypertension.* The diagnosis of PPH is made by excluding all known causes of pulmonary hypertension. The assumption that what remains should be a single disease is probably unrealistic. Pulmonary hypertension may well be the final common pathway for several diseases. This chapter describes the past and current forms of therapy for PPH. Furthermore, lessons learned from treating PPH are discussed as they relate to other forms of pulmonary hypertension. As might be expected, when the etiology of a disease is unknown, there is considerable overlap, from a diagnostic point of view, with other, similar disorders. Therefore, treatments demonstrating some effectiveness in patients with PPH have been tried in patients with other diseases that cause pulmonary hypertension, such as collagen vascular disease.

Before the treatment of PPH is discussed, it is important to understand the meaning of this diagnosis, because the depth of understanding influences the approach to treatment. The diagnosis of PPH is made by ruling out all known causes of pulmonary hypertension with a careful and detailed diagnostic evaluation.[1] Congenital heart disease, parenchymal lung disease, chronic pulmonary thromboembolism, left-sided heart disease, and connective tissue disorders must all be meticulously excluded. The remaining group of patients has unexplained pulmonary hypertension and thus is said to have PPH. Any treatment strategy must recognize that it is likely that several diseases are being treated in the same way. Consequently, it is unlikely that all patients will respond in the same manner. Until the pathogenesis of unexplained forms of pulmonary hypertension is more thoroughly understood, therapy will probably be suboptimal.

An understanding of the natural history of PPH is also essential when therapy is planned.[2] The disease is most prevalent among young adults between the ages of 20 and 40 years. Three times as many women as men are affected. The disease also occurs in younger and older individuals. In people over 40 years of age, the greater prevalence among women is no longer seen, which suggests that the etiology may be different in this age group from that in the younger age group. The onset of the disease is usually insidious and is marked by the advent of dyspnea. Symptoms progress in severity quite rapidly in most patients; the average time to diagnosis from

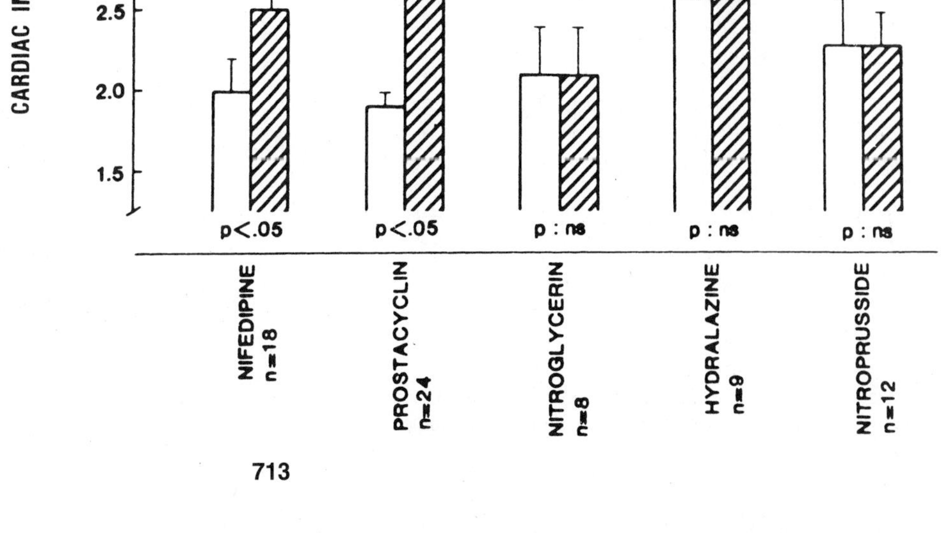

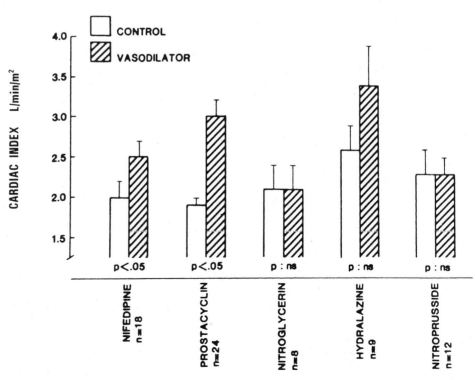

Figure 54–1. Nifedipine and prostacyclin were the only vasodilators tried in National Institutes of Health Primary Pulmonary Hypertension Registry patients that produced a significant increase in cardiac index. (From Weir EK, Rubin LJ, Ayers SM, et al: The acute administration of vasodilators in primary pulmonary hypertension: experience from the National Institutes of Health Registry on Primary Pulmonary Hypertension. Am Rev Respir Dis 1989; 140:1623–1630.)

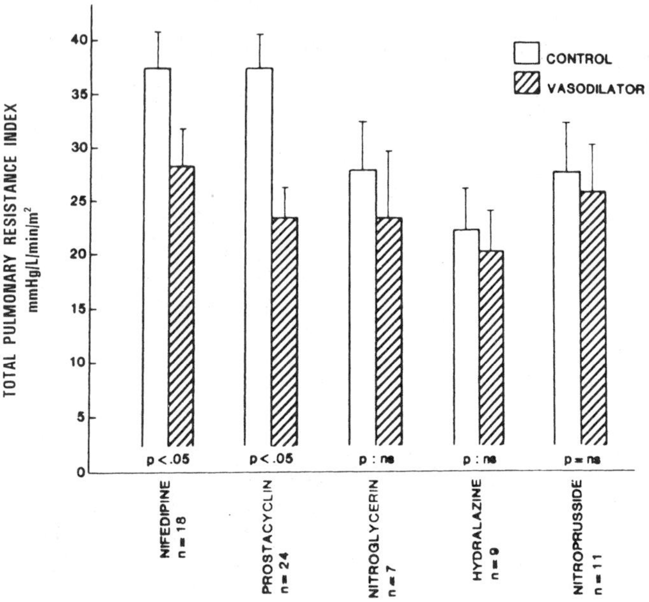

Figure 54–2. Nifedipine and prostacyclin were the only vasodilators tried in National Institutes of Health Primary Pulmonary Hypertension Registry patients that produced a significant decrease in total pulmonary vascular resistance index. (From Weir EK, Rubin LJ, Ayers SM, et al: The acute administration of vasodilators in primary pulmonary hypertension: experience from the National Institutes of Health Registry on Primary Pulmonary Hypertension. Am Rev Respir Dis 1989; 140:1623–1630.)

the onset of symptoms averages less than 2 years. Symptoms continue their relentless course in the majority of patients until right-sided heart failure occurs, followed rapidly by death. The median life expectancy is 2.8 years from diagnosis.[3] After overt right-sided heart failure occurs, median survival is less than 6 months. The most common cause of death is right-sided heart failure; the second most common cause is usually presumed to be an arrhythmia. The ominous prognosis of PPH dictates the need for aggressive forms of therapy.

For many years, clinicians approached treatment of the patient with PPH with great trepidation, because the prognosis was abysmal and no effective forms of therapy existed. In the 1970s, the increasing availability of a number of vasodilators encouraged physicians to try these drugs in patients with PPH because of their effectiveness in treating systemic hypertension. In the late 1970s and early 1980s, virtually every known vasodilator was tried on an anecdotal basis in patients with PPH. In 1981, the National Institutes of Health (NIH) started a patient registry for PPH and requested that all participants carefully record the hemodynamic effects of any drugs tried in the treatment of their patients.[4] Analysis of the registry patients for beneficial drug effects indicated that no therapy produced dramatic hemodynamic results, but nifedipine and prostacyclin did demonstrate promising trends by increasing cardiac output and reducing pulmonary vascular resistance (Figs. 54–1 and 54–2). No drug produced a consistent drop in pulmonary artery pressure. Until the advent of the NIH registry, all testing of drugs' hemodynamic effects was done in the acute setting. However, some investigators wondered whether acute hemodynamic effects could be relied on to predict long-term effects and whether or not they were beneficial.

In 1984, Fuster and colleagues[5] performed a retrospective analysis of 100 patients with PPH treated at the Mayo Clinic over the previous 25 years that indicated that those who received anticoagulation therapy with warfarin had a better survival rate than those who did not. Since this report was published, most clinicians have treated their PPH patients with chronic warfarin anticoagulation. Unfortunately, data on patients in this series were collected from as far back as the 1950s, when the diagnostic evaluation of patients suspected of having PPH was limited; thus it is likely that some patients with secondary pulmonary hypertension were included in the study.

CALCIUM CHANNEL BLOCKERS

Another outcome of early therapeutic investigations, particularly from the NIH registry experience, was further evaluation of calcium channel blockers in the treatment of PPH. Rich and Brundage[6] gave nifedipine or diltiazem in hourly doses until the pulmonary artery pressure was decreased by 20%, systemic hypotension occurred, or side effects (usually nausea and vomiting) developed. The patients who could tolerate the drug and demonstrated a 20% fall in pulmonary artery pressure were called responders and were continued on large doses of the calcium channel blocker to which they responded (Fig. 54–3). Nifedipine doses averaged 172 ± 41 mg/day (range, 120–240 mg/day), and diltiazem doses averaged 720 ± 208 mg/day (range, 540–900 mg/day). One year later, many of these patients underwent repeat cardiac catheterization, which showed that the initial improvement in hemodynamics was maintained. Improved hemodynamics were associated with improved symptoms, regression of right ventricular hypertrophy as seen by electrocardiogram, and normalization of right ventricular architecture as seen by echocardiography. These patients were observed for 5 years and had a much better survival rate (94%) than similar patients in the NIH registry (38%)[7] (Fig. 54–4). The differences in survival were highly significant ($p < .003$). This cohort demonstrated that PPH patients who respond to high doses of calcium channel blockers can be markedly improved. However, only about 25% of PPH patients respond to and tolerate therapy with high doses of calcium channel blockers. Therefore, the search for other therapies continued.

PROSTACYCLIN

Prostacyclin, also known as epoprostenol, is another drug that was identified from the NIH registry experience as having potential value in treating PPH. Initially, prostacyclin was used only acutely in the cardiac catheterization laboratory to test pulmonary vascular reactivity.[8] Prostacyclin is a potent vasodilator with a very short half-

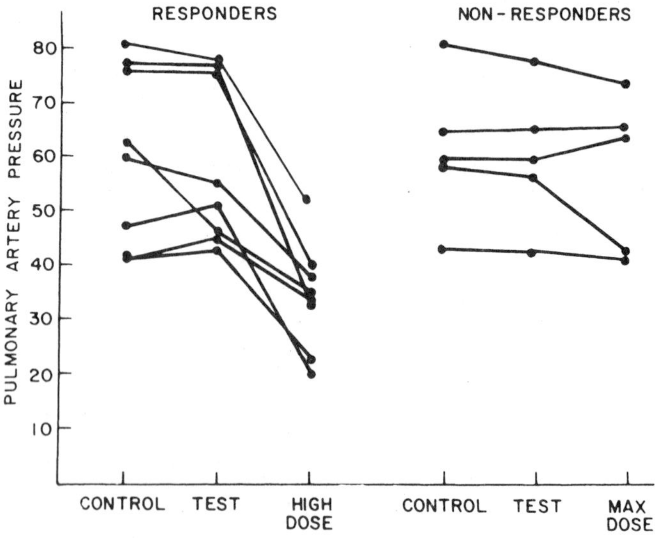

Figure 54–3. Nifedipine or diltiazem produces marked decreases in pulmonary artery pressure in some primary pulmonary hypertension patients. (From Rich S, Brundage BH: High dose calcium channel-blocking therapy for primary pulmonary hypertension: evidence for long-term reduction in pulmonary arterial pressure and regression in right ventricular hypertrophy. Circulation 1987; 76:135–141.)

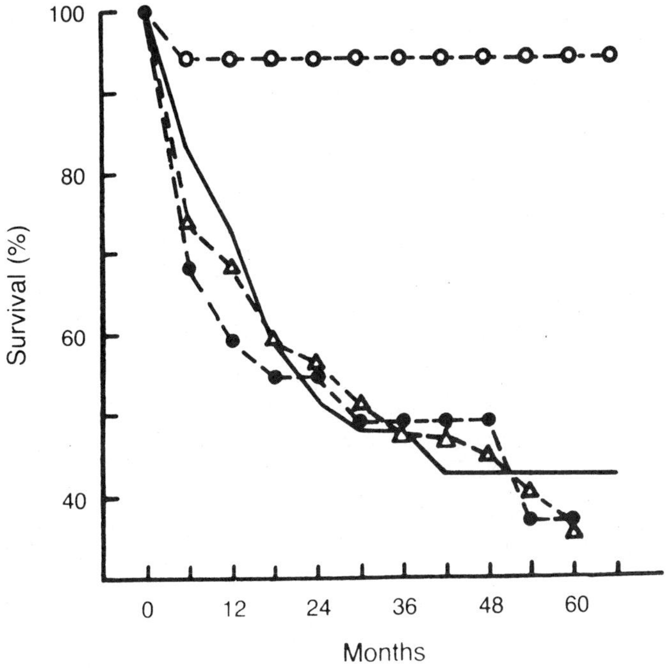

Figure 54–4. Survival was significantly improved ($p < .003$) in primary pulmonary hypertension patients who responded to high-dose calcium channel blockers (*open circles*), in comparison with nonresponders (*solid line*) and two National Institutes of Health Registry cohorts (*solid circles and open triangles).* (From Rich S, Kaufmann E, Levy PS: The effect of high doses of calcium-channel blockers on survival in primary pulmonary hypertension. N Engl J Med 1992; 327:76–81.)

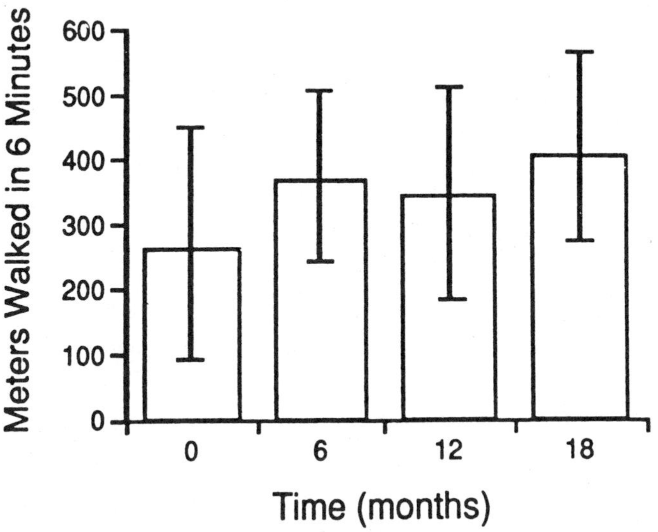

Figure 54–5. Exercise capacity increased progressively over 18 months in patients with primary pulmonary hypertension who were treated with continuous intravenous prostacyclin. (From Barst RJ, Rubin LJ, McGoon MD, et al: Survival in primary pulmonary hypertension with long-term continuous intravenous prostacyclin. Ann Intern Med 1994; 121:409–415.)

life (several minutes). Therefore, it requires continuous intravenous infusion to maintain its hemodynamic effects. Prostacyclin is also a potent platelet inhibitor, which may also be beneficial in preventing small pulmonary vessel thrombosis, a common feature of PPH. In 1982 and 1987, Rubin and colleagues in the United States[8] and Jones and colleagues in Great Britain[9] began to administer prostacyclin chronically to class III and class IV PPH patients by continuous infusion via a permanent intravenous line connected to a battery-powered infusion pump. Jones and colleagues demonstrated in a nonrandomized study that chronic infusions of prostacyclin produced improvement in exercise capacity.[9] Subsequently, in an 8-week randomized study, Rubin and associates[10] found a significant improvement in pulmonary hemodynamics (i.e., reduction in pulmonary artery pressure and increase in cardiac output) in patients treated with prostacyclin, and these improvements were maintained at 8 weeks by chronic infusion. Barst and colleagues[11] reported continued improvement in exercise capacity (Fig. 54–5) up to 18 months after instituting chronic prostacyclin infusion. They also documented that increases in cardiac output and reductions in pulmonary and right atrial pressure were maintained for 12 months. Furthermore, the improvement in exercise capacity correlated with the drop in pulmonary artery ($r = -.73$) and right atrial ($r = -0.75$) pressure. In comparison with historical controls from the NIH registry, class III and class IV patients on chronic prostacyclin infusions also had improved survival (Fig. 54–6).

The initial promising results from these studies led to another randomized trial of 81 class III and class IV PPH patients in the United States.[12] After 12 weeks, the patients on chronic prostacyclin infusion were able to walk farther and were symptomatically improved. There were no deaths in the prostacyclin-treated group and eight deaths in the control group. Because of these remarkable results, more than 300 patients in the United States are now on chronic prostacyclin therapy. Side effects from prostacyclin are frequent but usually mild, most commonly consisting of flushing, headache, jaw pain, nausea, and diarrhea, and are usually well controlled by decreasing the dose. The short half-life of the drug ensures that side effects will abate quickly. Tolerance does occur; therefore, the dose needs to be increased periodically. Most patients are started on 4–6 ng/kg/min, and the dose is increased about 1–2 ng/kg/min/month.

The most significant problems with chronic prostacyclin therapy are related to the risk of infection associated with the permanent intravenous line.[11] At least 20% of patients experience one infection per year. Most infections can be eliminated with antibiotics, but on occasion, the intravenous line must be replaced. A major benefit of prostacyclin in comparison with calcium channel blockers is that virtually all class III and class IV patients can tolerate the drug.

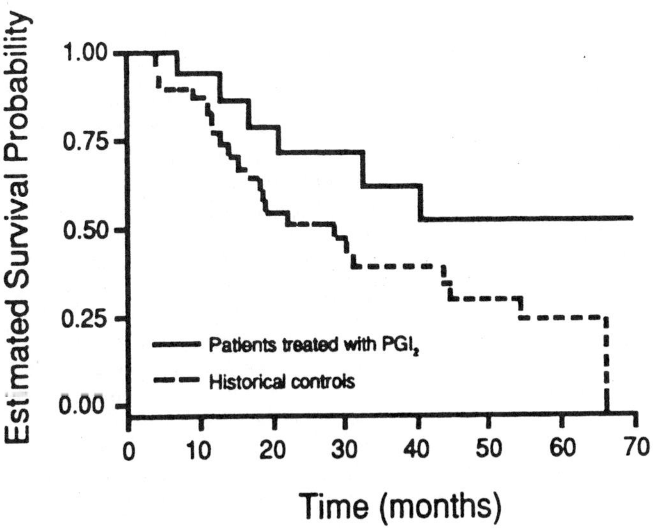

Figure 54–6. Survival was significantly ($p = .045$) improved in primary pulmonary hypertension patients treated with continuous intravenous prostacyclin (PGI_2), in comparison with National Institutes of Health Registry historic controls. (From Barst RJ, Rubin LJ, McGoon MD, et al: Survival in primary pulmonary hypertension with long-term continuous intravenous prostacyclin. Ann Intern Med 1994; 121:409–415.)

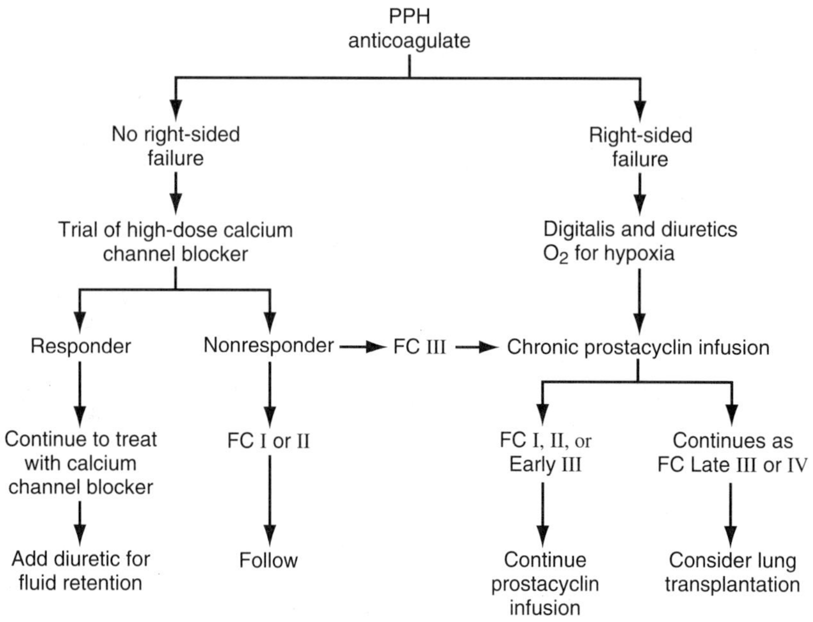

Figure 54–7. Treatment algorithm for primary pulmonary hypertension. *Abbreviation:* FC, functional class.

Many patients with severe right-sided heart failure do not tolerate calcium channel blockers, and these agents can even be dangerous, especially in patients with right atrial pressure higher than 15 mm Hg and cardiac output lower than 2.5 L/min. With prostacyclin, nearly all patients experience some improvement in symptoms. Prostacyclin is now the treatment of choice for functional class III and class IV patients, many of whom are awaiting lung transplantation (Fig. 54–7). Some patients may demonstrate such a dramatic improvement in symptoms and functional class that transplantation may be postponed indefinitely.[11] Chronic prostacyclin therapy is the most significant advance in the treatment of PPH since the first recognition of this nearly uniformly fatal disease.

ADJUNCTIVE THERAPIES

Warfarin Anticoagulation

As previously discussed, anticoagulants have been used frequently in the treatment of PPH, especially since the report by Fuster and colleagues.[5] More recently, Rich and associates[7] demonstrated improved survival in patients not responding to high-dose calcium channel blockers if they were receiving anticoagulants (Fig. 54–8). Although definitive evidence supporting the value of long-term anticoagulation is not available, currently, most clinicians with experience treating PPH administer anticoagulants to their patients. Histopathologic studies indicate that small pulmonary artery thrombosis is a common feature of PPH; therefore, there is some logic to recommending chronic anticoagulation in the hopes of preventing further vascular obstruction.[13] One study compared lung scan patterns with histologic findings.[14] A mottled-appearing lung scan correlated with the presence of small pulmonary vessel thrombosis. These findings suggest that lung scans may identify patients who will best benefit from anticoagulation. However, because no prospective study has confirmed this hypothesis, all PPH patients should receive anticoagulation therapy unless there are clear contraindications.

Digitalis

For many years, clinicians have cautioned against the use of digitalis in the treatment of cor pulmonale. The most common cause of pulmonary hypertension in the absence of left-sided heart disease is pulmonary parenchymal disease. These patients are usually very hypoxic and often suffer from CO_2 retention. These disorders of gas exchange often lead to electrolyte imbalance and therefore make the patient more susceptible to digitalis toxicity. However, PPH is less frequently associated with hypoxia than is pulmonary parenchymal disease and, when present, is usually only mild or moderate. Hypercarbia does not ordinarily accompany PPH. Therefore, electrolyte imbalance occurs much less frequently in PPH patients. There are no systematic studies of the value of digitalis in PPH, but clinical experience suggests that improvement in symptoms occurs if the patient is in overt right-sided heart failure.[6] The mild inotropic effect of digitalis appears to improve right ventricular function in such patients. Therefore, administration of digitalis is recommended when right-sided heart failure is present.

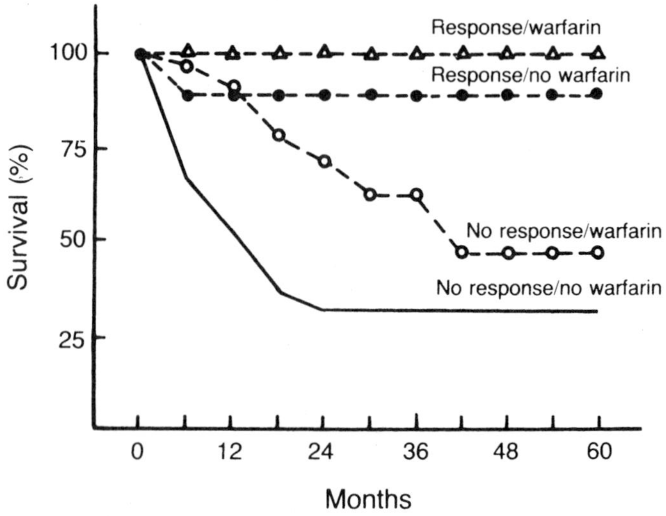

Figure 54–8. Survival was significantly (p = .025) improved for primary pulmonary hypertension patients receiving long-term warfarin, particularly if they did not respond to high-dose calcium channel blockers. (From Rich S, Kaufmann E, Levy PS: The effect of high doses of calcium-channel blockers on survival in primary pulmonary hypertension. N Engl J Med 1992; 327:76–81.)

Diuretics

Diuretics are helpful in improving symptoms related to systemic venous congestion such as peripheral edema and liver tenderness. Loop diuretics are required in most patients. As with all low cardiac output states, the benefits of diuresis must be balanced against the effects of further reduction in cardiac output. Overdiuresis can lead to renal insufficiency and worsened fatigue. Patients who respond well to chronic prostacyclin therapy may note a reduction in their diuretic requirements. Patients on high doses of calcium channel blockers who are not in right-sided heart failure may experience peripheral edema and benefit from diuretic therapy.

Oxygen

Mild to moderate hypoxia may occur in the course of PPH. Severe hypoxia is uncommon. In some cases, the hypoxia may be the result of right-to-left shunting via a patent foramen ovale. Such patients are usually in right-sided heart failure, with substantial elevation of right atrial pressure. In some patients, intrapulmonary shunting may play a role, although the mechanism is obscure. In any case, some PPH patients with hypoxia are symptomatically improved with oxygen therapy.[15] Chronic oxygen therapy should be offered if a trial improves oxygenation and symptoms and increases exercise capacity.

OTHER DRUGS

The recognition that endothelial cell–derived relaxing factor (EDRF) is nitric oxide or a related compound has led to experimental trials of inhaled nitric oxide in patients with PPH.[16] All experiments have been acute, and although some studies suggest a vasodilator effect in these patients, chronic studies have not yet been reported.

Angiotensin converting enzyme inhibitors are now being used to treat a wide variety of diseases, including systemic hypertension and coronary artery disease. This family of drugs has been tried in the treatment of PPH but has been uniformly ineffective. Although plasma renin levels may be elevated in patients with PPH, the renin-angiotensin system has not been demonstrated to play a role in the pathogenesis of the disease.

OTHER FORMS OF PULMONARY HYPERTENSION

Thus far, the discussion of treatment has been limited to patients with "pure" PPH. However there are several diseases that are similar to PPH. Some patients who initially present with PPH subsequently develop other features of collagen vascular disease and can be categorized as having systemic lupus erythematosus, scleroderma, CREST syndrome (*c*alcinosis, *R*aynaud phenomenon, *e*sophageal motility disorders, *s*clerodactyly, and *t*elangiectasia), or mixed connective tissue disease. Many patients with PPH have an elevated, albeit mild, antinuclear antibody titer but never develop other features of collagen vascular disease.[17] The question therefore arises: "Will therapies effective in the treatment of PPH work for patients with pulmonary hypertension and collagen vascular disease?" Systematic studies of calcium channel blocker therapy are lacking. Anecdotal experience occasionally suggests benefit, although in general, the results of calcium channel blocker therapy in related diseases are not as good as with PPH.

An association between pulmonary hypertension and liver disease has been known since 1951.[18] Closer evaluation of this relation indicates that shunting of the splanchnic venous effluent around the liver and directly into the pulmonary circulation seems to be the essential cause of the association. Patients who have portacaval shunts are at risk for developing pulmonary hypertension, and those with liver disease who do develop pulmonary hypertension almost always have evidence of esophageal varices. The splanchnic shunt association suggests that some substance in the splanchnic venous blood causes the pulmonary hypertension. The association is rare; therefore, there are no systematic studies of therapy in these patients. Anecdotal experience with chronic intravenous prostacyclin therapy suggests that these patients may obtain a beneficial lowering of pulmonary pressure.

Other causes of severe pulmonary hypertension, such as pulmonary fibrosis, chronic pulmonary embolism, and congenital heart disease (Eisenmenger reaction), do not respond well to any of the vasodilators that have shown some benefit in PPH.

Single- or double-lung transplantation, as well as heart-lung transplantation, is being used with increasing frequency to treat end-stage pulmonary hypertension.[19–21] The waiting period after a patient is placed on a transplant list is long, often exceeding 2 years. Therefore, patients with severe PPH and right-sided heart failure may not survive with conventional therapy until a donor organ is available. Continuous prostacyclin infusion may stabilize these patients, improve quality of life, and extend survival enough so that they have an increased chance of receiving an organ.

The therapy of PPH has changed dramatically since 1985. High-dose calcium channel blockers in some patients may result in marked improvement in hemodynamics and significantly improve survival. Chronic continuous infusion of prostacyclin is also demonstrating promising results and has an advantage over calcium channel blockers in that it is better tolerated and produces some improvement in nearly all patients. The development of lung transplantation offers yet another therapeutic option for end-stage patients. Lessons learned from treating patients with PPH may have some value when patients with secondary forms of severe pulmonary hypertension are treated; however, randomized clinical trials are lacking. Development of treatments for pulmonary hypertension of any type is a fertile area for further clinical and basic research.

REFERENCES

1. Rich S: Primary pulmonary hypertension. Prog Cardiovasc Dis 1988; 31:205–238.
2. Rich S, Dantzker DR, Ayers SM, et al: Primary pulmonary hypertension: a national prospective study. Ann Intern Med 1987; 107:216–223.
3. D'Alonzo GE, Barst RJ, Ayers SM, et al: Survival in patients with primary pulmonary hypertension: results from a National Prospective Registry. Ann Intern Med 1991; 115:343–349.
4. Weir EK, Rubin LJ, Ayers SM, et al: The acute administration of vasodilators in primary pulmonary hypertension: experience from the National Institutes of Health Registry on Primary Pulmonary Hypertension. Am Rev Respir Dis 1989; 140:1623–1630.
5. Fuster V, Steele PM, Edwards WD, et al: Primary pulmonary hypertension: natural history and the importance of thrombosis. Circulation 1984; 70:580–587.
6. Rich S, Brundage BH: High dose calcium channel-blocking therapy for primary pulmonary hypertension: evidence for long-term reduction in pulmonary arterial pressure and regression in right ventricular hypertrophy. Circulation 1987; 76:135–141.
7. Rich S, Kaufmann E, Levy PS: The effect of high doses of calcium-channel blockers on survival in primary pulmonary hypertension. N Engl J Med 1992; 327:76–81.
8. Rubin LJ, Groves BM, Reeves, JT, et al: Prostacyclin-induced pulmonary vasodilation in primary pulmonary hypertension. Circulation 1982; 66:334–338.
9. Jones DK, Higginbottam TW, Wolwork J: Treatment of primary pulmonary hypertension with intravenous epoprostenol (prostacyclin). Br Heart J 1987; 57:270–278.
10. Rubin LJ, Mendoza J, Hood M, et al: Treatment of primary pulmonary hypertension with continuous prostacyclin (epoprostenol). Results of a randomized trial. Ann Intern Med 1990; 112:485–491.
11. Barst RJ, Rubin LJ, McGoon MD, et al: Survival in primary pulmonary hypertension with long-term continuous intravenous prostacyclin. Ann Intern Med 1994; 121:409–415.

12. Long W, Rubin L, Barst R, et al: Randomized trial of conventional therapy alone [CT] vs. conventional therapy and continuous infusions of prostacyclin [CT + PGI_2] in primary pulmonary hypertension (PPH): a 12 week study [Abstract]. Am Rev Respir Dis 1993; 147:A538.
13. Pietra GG, Edwards WD, Kay JM, et al: Histopathology of primary pulmonary hypertension. A qualitative and quantitative study of pulmonary blood vessels from 59 patients in the National Heart, Lung and Blood Institute Primary Pulmonary Hypertension Registry. Circulation 1989; 80:1198–1206.
14. Rich S, Pietra GG, Kieras K, et al: Primary pulmonary hypertension: radiographic and scintigraphic patterns of histologic subtypes. Ann Intern Med 1986; 105:499–502.
15. Morgan JM, Griffiths M, du Bois RM, et al: Hypoxic pulmonary vasoconstriction in systemic sclerosis and primary pulmonary hypertension. Chest 1991; 99:551–556.
16. Ivy DD, Wiggins JW, Badesch DB, et al: Nitric oxide and prostacyclin treatment of an infant with primary pulmonary hypertension. Am J Cardiol 1994; 74:414–416.
17. Rich S, Kieras K, Hart K, et al: Antinuclear antibodies in primary pulmonary hypertension. J Am Coll Cardiol 1986; 8:1307–1311.
18. Groves BM, Brundage BH, Elliott CG, et al: Pulmonary hypertension associated with hepatic cirrhosis. *In* Fishman AP (ed): The Pulmonary Circulation: Normal and Abnormal, pp 359–369. Philadelphia: University of Pennsylvania Press, 1990.
19. Reitz BA, Wallwork JL, Hunt SA, et al: Heart-lung transplantation: successful therapy for patients with pulmonary vascular disease. N Engl J Med 1982; 306:557–564.
20. Pasque MK, Trulock EP, Kaiser LR, et al: Single lung transplantation for pulmonary hypertension. Three-month hemodynamic follow-up. Circulation 1991; 84:2275–2279.
21. Glanville AR, Burke CM, Theodore J, et al: Primary pulmonary hypertension. Length of survival in patients referred for heart-lung transplantation. Chest 1987; 91:675–681.

55 Treatment of Infective Endocarditis

Adolf W. Karchmer, MD

The treatment of infective endocarditis has two major objectives: to eradicate the infecting microorganism and to correct or at least limit the potential morbidity resulting from either the intracardiac or extracardiac complications of infection. The first objective is achieved largely through judicious antimicrobial therapy. The second objective often exceeds the capacity of effective antimicrobial therapy, however, and requires cardiac or other surgical intervention.

The principles that guide current treatment of endocarditis are derived from relatively simple observations. The endocardial-based platelet-fibrin vegetations in which infecting microorganisms proliferate are relatively devoid of phagocytic cells and thus are areas of impaired host defenses. Bacteria in the vegetations are able to multiply to population densities approaching 10^9 organisms per gram of tissue. Under these conditions, bacteria become metabolically dormant and less vulnerable to the killing action of antimicrobial agents. These observations, supplemented by clinical experience, suggest that optimal therapy should use bactericidal antibiotics or antibiotic combinations rather than bacteriostatic agents, should be administered parenterally to avoid potentially erratic absorption after oral administration, and should be continued for prolonged periods to ensure eradication of dormant microorganisms. In addition, endocarditis is occasionally complicated by abscesses or disruption of structures. These events are not amenable to antimicrobial therapy alone but require surgical intervention for drainage or to repair (or replace) the disrupted structures and restore function. Thus, for example, myocardial and splenic abscesses or cardiac valve disruption with hemodynamic decompensation commonly require surgical therapy. This chapter focuses on the details of antimicrobial therapy for specific microbial causes of endocarditis as well as the treatment of intracardiac and extracardiac complications of these infections.

INFECTIVE ENDOCARDITIS SYNDROMES

To develop therapeutic strategies for endocarditis, it is useful to consider not only the general features of the syndrome but also the microbiologic and clinical aspects of several subtypes of endocarditis: native valve endocarditis (NVE), nosocomial endocarditis, prosthetic valve endocarditis (PVE), and endocarditis occurring in intravenous drug abusers. Although virtually any bacterial or fungal species can cause endocarditis, in fact, a relatively small number of bacterial species cause the majority of cases of endocarditis. This observation is helpful when selecting antimicrobial regimens for empirical therapy and also when considering the need to pursue the diagnosis of endocarditis in bacteremic patients. In patients with community-acquired NVE unrelated to intravenous drug abuse, gram-positive cocci—primarily streptococci (non–group A streptococci and non-*Streptococcus pneumoniae)* and *Staphylococcus aureus*—cause 80% of the infections (Table 55–1).[1–4] NVE caused by *S. aureus* is likely to present as a brief illness with striking constitutional symptoms, so-called acute bacterial endocarditis. In contrast, streptococcal, enterococcal, coagulase-negative staphylococcal, and fastidious gram-negative coccobacillary infection is more likely to present as an indolent subacute syndrome. Nosocomial endocarditis is caused primarily by *S. aureus*, coagulase-negative staphylococci, and enterococci and is often the consequence of bacteremia associated with intravascular devices or manipulation of the genitourinary tract.[1, 4, 5] Nosocomial bacteremia due to these organisms that persists for 3 days or more with the patient receiving therapy or that relapses after abbreviated antimicrobial therapy suggests endocarditis. Although the spectrum of organisms causing en-

TABLE 55–1. MICROBIOLOGY OF NATIVE VALVE ENDOCARDITIS IN URBAN AND COMMUNITY HOSPITALS, 1975–1992*

	Number of Cases (%)	
Organism	**Community-Acquired N = 603**	**Nosocomial N = 82**
Streptococci	186 (31)	6 (7)
Pneumococci	8 (1)	—
Enterococci	53 (9)	13 (16)
Staphylococcus aureus	217 (36)	45 (55)
Coagulase-negative staphylococci	28 (5)	8 (10)
Gram-negative bacilli	21 (3)	4 (5)
Fastidious gram-negative coccobacilli†	18 (3)	—
Fungi	5 (1)	3 (4)
Polymicrobial/miscellaneous	36 (6)	1 (1)
Culture-negative	31 (5)	2 (2)

*When possible, cases of endocarditis associated with intravenous drug abuse or involving prosthetic valves have been deleted.

†*Haemophilus* species, *Actinobacillus actinomycetemcomitans, Cardiobacterium hominis, Eikenella* species, *Kingella* species (called HACEK group).

Data from references 1–5.

docarditis associated with intravenous drug abuse is similar to that causing community-acquired NVE, *S. aureus* is the predominant pathogen (Table 55–2). Furthermore, almost 50% of drug abuse–associated cases involve the tricuspid valve; almost 80% of these infections are caused by *S. aureus*.[6, 7] Polymicrobial and *Candida* endocarditis occur with increased frequency among intravenous drug abusers.[6, 8] The microbiologic features of PVE are best viewed in terms of the time elapsed between valve implantation and the onset of symptoms (Table 55–3).[9–11] Infections that are apparent within 2 months after surgery are caused primarily by coagulase-negative staphylococci and other organisms associated with nosocomial infections, including *S. aureus*, gram-negative bacilli, diphtheroids, and fungi. In contrast, the organisms causing infection beginning a year or more after surgery resemble those that cause community-acquired NVE. Infections occurring between 2 months and 12 months after surgery are caused primarily by coagulase-negative staphylococci, but occasional infections are caused by streptococci, enterococci, and fastidious gram-negative coccobacilli, organisms more typical of

TABLE 55–2. MICROBIOLOGY OF ENDOCARDITIS ASSOCIATED WITH INTRAVENOUS DRUG ABUSE

	Number of Cases (%)		
Organism	**Right-Sided N = 157**	**Left-Sided N = 179**	**All Cases N = 336**
Staphylococcus aureus	121 (77)	41 (23)	162 (48)
Streptococci	4 (2)	24 (13)	28 (8)
Enterococci	3 (2)	47 (26)	50 (15)
Gram-negative bacilli*	10 (6)	17 (9)	27 (8)
Fungi (predominantly *Candida* species)	0 (0)	25 (14)	25 (7)
Polymicrobial	7 (4)	12 (6)	19 (6)
Culture-negative	9 (6)	7 (4)	16 (5)
Miscellaneous	3 (2)	6 (4)	9 (3)

**Pseudomonas aeruginosa, Serratia marcescens,* and Enterobacteriaceae.

Data from Sande MA, Lee BL, Mills J, et al: Endocarditis in intravenous drug users. *In* Kaye D (ed): Infective Endocarditis, 2nd ed, p 345. New York: Raven Press, 1992.

TABLE 55–3. MICROBIOLOGY OF PROSTHETIC VALVE ENDOCARDITIS, 1975–1989

	Number of Cases (%) and Time of Onset After Cardiac Surgery		
Organism	**<2 Mo N = 50**	**2–12 Mo N = 34**	**>12 Mo N = 79**
Coagulase-negative staphylococci	27 (54)	19 (56)	12 (15)
Staphylococcus aureus	4 (8)	3 (9)	10 (13)
Gram-negative bacilli	6 (12)	1 (3)	1 (1)
Streptococci	0	1 (3)	27 (34)
Enterococci	0	2 (6)	9 (11)
Diphtheroids	4 (8)	0	1 (1)
Fastidious gram-negative coccobacilli	0	1 (3)	11 (14)
Fungi	3 (6)	2 (6)	2 (3)
Miscellaneous	3 (6)	2 (6)	1 (1)
Culture-negative	3 (6)	3 (9)	5 (6)

Data from references 9–11.

the later onset episodes. Importantly, 85% of coagulase-negative staphylococci causing infection within a year after surgery are methicillin-resistant. In contrast, methicillin resistance is noted in only 30% of coagulase-negative staphylococci causing PVE more than a year after surgery.[9]

Community-acquired NVE that is not associated with intravenous drug abuse primarily involves the mitral or aortic valve and occasionally extends beyond the valve leaflet into the adjacent perivalvular tissue, causing abscess formation or fistulas.[12, 13] Perivalvular extension is suggested by persistence of unexplained fever in spite of appropriate antimicrobial therapy, the development of new and persistent electrocardiographic conduction abnormalities, new murmurs suggesting intracardiac fistulas, and pericarditis in patients with aortic valve endocarditis.[2, 13, 14] Two-dimensional transesophageal echocardiography with Doppler is significantly more sensitive than transthoracic echocardiography for the detection of perivalvular infection in patients with NVE or PVE.[13, 15] Invasion of the annulus or myocardial abscess formation complicates almost 45% of infections involving mechanical prostheses and occurs with similar frequency when endocarditis involving bioprosthetic valves, particularly those in the aortic position, presents during the initial year after valve surgery.[9] The risk of perivalvular extension of infection is increased when endocarditis is associated with intravenous drug abuse or involves the aortic valve.[12]

In addition to perivalvular extension of infection in patients with mitral or aortic valve endocarditis, other complications require specific therapy or affect the outcome of endocarditis (Table 55–4). Intracardiac structural damage, often resulting in clinically significant hemodynamic deterioration, and neurologic events, including cerebral embolism, intracranial mycotic aneurysm, and intracranial hemorrhage, are the most commonly encountered complications.[16] Focal extracardiac infection, for example, septic arthritis, splenic abscess, and vertebral osteomyelitis, are not restricted to episodes caused by *S. aureus* and other virulent organisms. Septic pulmonary emboli occur in 75% of episodes of tricuspid valve endocarditis in intravenous drug users.[6, 7] These septic infarcts may subsequently undergo necrosis and cavitation and ultimately result in a pyopneumothorax. To prevent these complications or to minimize their morbidity, patients with active endocarditis require careful monitoring.

DIAGNOSIS OF INFECTIVE ENDOCARDITIS

Endocarditis is obvious in the bacteremic patient with fever, classic peripheral signs, and a murmur of valvular dysfunction. In many

TABLE 55–4. COMPLICATIONS OF INFECTIVE ENDOCARDITIS

Event	Frequency (%)
Perivalvular extension of infection	
Native valve endocarditis	10–14
Prosthetic valve endocarditis	45–60
Neurologic events	
Embolism	20–30
Intracranial hemorrhage	5–7
Mycotic aneurysm (with/without hemorrhage)	1–5
Extracranial arterial emboli (noncutaneous)	10–20
Extracranial mycotic aneurysm	1–5
Immune complex nephritis	10–15
Splenic abscess (clinical)	3–5

patients, however, particularly early in the evaluation process, the diagnosis of endocarditis is complex. Criteria for such a diagnosis have been developed (Tables 55–5 and 55–6).[17–19] Although these criteria were designed primarily to facilitate clinical and epidemiologic research, when applied judiciously and over the entire evaluation sequence—that is, not limited to initial findings—this schema provides a highly sensitive and specific approach to the diagnosis of endocarditis for patient management. Erroneous rejection of the diagnosis of endocarditis is unlikely. When these diagnostic criteria are used as a guide for therapy, conditions that are categorized as possible endocarditis should be treated accordingly. Using bacteremia caused by coagulase-negative staphylococci or diphtheroids (organisms that often contaminate blood cultures) to support the diagnosis of endocarditis requires persistently positive blood culture results or a demonstration of clonality among multiple, sporadically positive culture results.[17, 20] Inclusion of echocardiographic evidence of endocardial infection in these criteria recognizes the high sensitivity of two-dimensional echocardiography with color Doppler, especially if the transesophageal approach is used, and the relative infrequency of false-positive studies when experienced operators apply specific criteria.[15, 21–24] Although the sensitivity of transesophageal echocardiographic evaluation for the diagnosis of infective endocarditis is 89%–94% (or higher if a follow-up study is performed), negative findings do not exclude the diagnosis and need for therapy if the clinical suspicion is high.[22, 23] Conversely, the false-negative rate is 6%–11% (or lower if the study is repeated). With repeat examinations, the likelihood of false-negative transesophageal studies is 4%–6%, and thus these studies help exclude the diagnosis when the clinical suspicion is low.[22, 23] These criteria are vulnerable to misidentifying nonbacterial thrombotic endocarditis complicating marasmus, cryptic collagen-vascular disease, or antiphospholipid antibodies as culture-negative infective endocarditis. To select optimal antimicrobial therapy, the organism causing endocarditis must be isolated and its susceptibility to antimicrobial agents carefully assessed. The minimal inhibitory concentration (MIC) and minimal bactericidal concentration (MBC) of candidate therapeutic agents must be determined. When prior clinical experience suggests that synergistic combination antimicrobial therapy is necessary, in vitro tests to evaluate this synergistic effect should be performed.

A microbial cause for infective endocarditis is commonly established by recovering the infecting agent from the blood stream. In some instances, however, the causative agent is recovered from surgically removed endocardial vegetations or embolic material in peripheral arteries. Because endocarditis is characterized by a continuous low-level bacteremia, the first two blood cultures will yield the causative agent in more than 95% of patients. Three separate sets of blood cultures, each from a separate venipuncture and obtained

TABLE 55–5. CRITERIA FOR DIAGNOSIS OF INFECTIVE ENDOCARDITIS

Definitive infective endocarditis
- Pathologic criteria
  - Microorganisms: demonstrated by culture or histologic examination in a vegetation *or* in a vegetation that has embolized *or* in an intracardiac abscess *or*
  - Pathologic lesions: vegetation or intracardiac abscess present, confirmed by histologic studies showing active endocarditis
- Clinical criteria, using specific definitions listed in Table 55–6
  - Two major criteria *or*
  - One major and three minor criteria *or*
  - Five minor criteria

Possible infective endocarditis
- Findings consistent with infective endocarditis that fall short of definite endocarditis but are not rejected
- Rejected
  - Firm alternative diagnosis for manifestations of endocarditis *or*
  - Sustained resolution of manifestations of endocarditis with antibiotic therapy for 4 days or less *or*
  - No pathologic evidence of infective endocarditis at surgery or autopsy after antibiotic therapy for 4 days or less

Adapted from Durack DT, Lukes AS, Bright DK, Duke Endocarditis Service: New criteria for diagnosis of infective endocarditis: utilization of specific echocardiographic findings. Am J Med 1994; 96:200–209.

TABLE 55–6. TERMINOLOGY USED IN CRITERIA FOR THE DIAGNOSIS OF INFECTIVE ENDOCARDITIS

Major Criteria

Positive blood culture
- Typical microorganism for infective endocarditis from two separate blood cultures
  - viridans streptococci, *Streptococcus bovis,* HACEK group, *or*
  - community-acquired *Staphylococcus aureus* or enterococci, in the absence of a primary focus, *or*
- Persistently positive blood culture, defined as recovery of a microorganism consistent with infective endocarditis from:
  - Blood cultures drawn more than 12 hours apart *or*
  - All of three or a majority of four or more separate blood cultures, with first and last drawn at least 1 h apart

Evidence of endocardial involvement
- Abnormal echocardiogram
  - Oscillating intracardiac mass on valve or supporting structures *or* in the path of regurgitant jets *or* on implanted material in the absence of an alternative anatomic explanation *or*
  - Abscess *or*
  - New partial dehiscence of prosthetic valve *or*
- New valvular regurgitation (increase or change in pre-existing murmur not sufficient)

Minor Criteria

- Predisposition: predisposing heart condition *or* intravenous drug use
- Fever ≥ 38°C (100.4°F)
- Vascular phenomena: major arterial emboli, septic pulmonary infarcts, mycotic aneurysm, intracranial hemorrhage, conjunctival hemorrhages, Janeway lesions
- Immunologic phenomena: glomerulonephritis, Osler nodes, Roth spots, rheumatoid factor
- Microbiologic evidence: positive blood culture result but not meeting major criteria as noted previously* *or* serologic evidence of active infection with organism consistent with infective endocarditis
- Echocardiogram: consistent with infective endocarditis but not meeting major criteria

*Excluding single positive cultures for coagulase-negative staphylococci and organisms that do not cause endocarditis.

Adapted from Durack DT, Lukes AS, Bright DK, Duke Endocarditis Service: New criteria for diagnosis of infective endocarditis: utilization of specific echocardiographic findings. Am J Med 1994; 96:200–209.

over 24 h, are recommended to evaluate patients with suspected endocarditis. Each set should include two flasks, one containing an aerobic medium and the other containing thioglycollate broth (anaerobic medium). At least 10 mL of blood should be placed in each flask, and the laboratory should be advised that endocarditis is a possible diagnosis and also which, if any, unusual organisms are suspected (*Legionella* species, *Bartonella* species, *Chlamydia trachomatis* as well as *Haemophilus parainfluenzae, Haemophilus aphrophilus, Actinobacillus actinomycetemcomitans, Cardiobacterium hominis, Eikenella corrodens, and Kingella kingae* [HACEK] organisms). If alerted, the laboratory can both hold the culture for a prolonged period (3–4 weeks) and use special isolation techniques. Administration of antimicrobial agents during the several weeks before obtaining blood culture specimens significantly reduces the frequency of positive culture results. If fungal endocarditis is suspected (patients with negative blood culture results and bulky vegetations, patients with embolic occlusion of large arteries, and patients with negative blood culture results and nosocomial or intravenous drug abuse–associated endocarditis), blood culture specimens should be obtained with the use of the lysis-centrifugation method. The laboratory should be asked to save the organism causing endocarditis until successful therapy has been completed. Occasionally, serologic tests are used to make the presumptive etiologic diagnosis of endocarditis caused by *Brucella* species, *Legionella* species, *Bartonella* species, *Coxiella burnetii*, or *Chlamydia* species.

ANTIMICROBIAL THERAPY FOR SPECIFIC AGENTS

The antimicrobial therapy for endocarditis is based on the precise susceptibility of the causative agent, the reported experience with endocarditis caused by the organism, the efficacy of antimicrobial agents in the treatment of experimental endocarditis, and clinical considerations that limit therapeutic options in a given patient, including end organ dysfunction, existing allergies, and other anticipated toxicities. With the exception of staphylococcal endocarditis, the antimicrobial regimens recommended for the treatment of patients with NVE and PVE are similar, although more prolonged treatment is often advised for patients with PVE (Table 55–7).

Penicillin-Susceptible Viridans Streptococci or *Streptococcus Bovis*

Approximately 85% of viridans streptococci, other streptococci, and *Streptococcus bovis* isolated from patients with endocarditis are highly susceptible to penicillin (MIC $\leq$ 0.1 μg/mL). Streptococci that require pyridoxal or thiol supplementation of media for growth, so-called nutritionally variant streptococci, are generally more resistant to penicillin; patients with endocarditis caused by these streptococci are treated with regimens recommended for enterococcal endocarditis (see Table 55–7, 3*A-C*). Four regimens provide highly effective, comparable therapy for patients with endocarditis caused by penicillin-susceptible streptococci (see Table 55–7, 1*A-D*).[25, 26] These regimens yield bacteriologic cure rates of 98% in patients who complete therapy. The synergistic killing of streptococci by penicillin plus streptomycin or gentamicin permits comparable therapeutic efficacy with the use of a 2-week regimen of combination therapy with penicillin plus an aminoglycoside. This regimen (see Table 55–7, 1*C*) is recommended for patients with uncomplicated NVE who are not at increased risk for aminoglycoside toxicity. Patients with endocarditis caused by nutritionally variant streptococci, endocarditis involving a prosthetic valve, or endocarditis complicated by mycotic aneurysm, myocardial abscess, perivalvular infection, or extracardiac foci of infection should not be treated with this short-course regimen. From 2%–8% of viridans streptococci and *S. bovis* causing endocarditis are highly resistant to streptomycin and are not killed synergistically by penicillin plus streptomycin. These highly streptomycin-resistant strains are, however, killed synergistically by penicillin plus gentamicin. Consequently, unless a causative streptococcus can be evaluated to exclude high-level resistance to streptomycin, gentamicin is recommended for use in the short-course combination regimen.

Vancomycin is recommended for treatment of streptococcal endocarditis in patients with a history of immediate allergic reactions (urticarial or anaphylactic reactions) to a penicillin or cephalosporin antibiotic (see Table 55–7, 1*E*). Patients with other forms of penicillin allergy (delayed maculopapular skin rash) may be treated with the ceftriaxone regimen or with cefazolin, 2 g intravenously every 8 h for 4 weeks.

For patients with PVE caused by penicillin-susceptible streptococci, treatment with 6 weeks of penicillin is recommended, with gentamicin given during the initial 2 weeks.[9]

Relatively Penicillin-Resistant Streptococci

Approximately 15% of streptococci that cause endocarditis are relatively resistant to penicillin (MIC $\geq$ 0.2 μg/mL). Four weeks of high-dose parenteral penicillin plus an aminoglycoside (primarily gentamicin for the reasons noted previously) during the initial 2 weeks is recommended for treatment of patients with endocarditis caused by streptococci with an MIC for penicillin between 0.2 and 0.5 μg/mL (see Table 55–7, 2*A*). Patients with endocarditis caused by one of the moderately resistant streptococci, who cannot tolerate penicillin because of immediate hypersensitivity reactions, can be treated with vancomycin alone (see Table 55–7, 1*E*). For those with nonimmediate penicillin hypersensitivity, effective treatment can be accomplished with vancomycin alone (Table 55–7, 1*E*) or by adding gentamicin to the initial 2 weeks of the ceftriaxone regimen (see Table 55–7, 1*D*). For endocarditis caused by streptococci that are highly resistant to penicillin (MIC $>$ 0.5 μg/mL), treatment with one of the regimens for enterococcal endocarditis is recommended (see Table 55–7, 3*A-C*).

Streptococcus Pyogenes, Streptococcus Pneumoniae, and Groups B, C, and G Streptococci

Although endocarditis is uncommonly caused by *S. pyogenes, S. pneumoniae,* and groups B, C, and G streptococci, such occurrences have been refractory to antibiotic therapy or associated with extensive valvular damage. Intravenous penicillin G in a dose of 20 million units/day for 4 weeks is recommended for the treatment of group A streptococcal and pneumococcal endocarditis. Pneumococci that are relatively resistant (MIC range, >0.1–1 μg/mL) and highly resistant (MIC $>$ 1 μg/mL) to penicillin are widely distributed and frequently encountered as causes of respiratory tract infection. Many of the highly resistant strains are also resistant to erythromycin, trimethoprim-sulfamethoxazole, and cephalosporins, including ceftriaxone. These strains remain susceptible to vancomycin. Although serum concentrations of penicillin G or ceftriaxone (with the use of doses recommended for treatment of endocarditis) will markedly exceed the MICs of these penicillin-resistant pneumococci, the efficacy of treatment with penicillin or ceftriaxone for the very uncommon episode of endocarditis caused by penicillin-resistant pneumococci is not established. Treatment with vancomycin may prove preferable. In contrast to endocarditis caused by penicillin susceptible viridans streptococci, cases caused by Group G, C, or B streptococci are considered more difficult to treat. Consequently, the addition of gentamicin to the first 2 weeks of a 4-week regimen with the use of high doses of penicillin is often advocated (see Table 55–7, 2*A*).

Enterococci

Enterococcus faecalis and *E. faecium*, which cause 85% and 10% of the cases of enterococcal endocarditis, respectively, are relatively

TABLE 55–7. RECOMMENDED ANTIBIOTIC THERAPY FOR INFECTIVE ENDOCARDITIS

Infecting Organism	Antibiotic	Dose and Route*	Duration (wk)	Comments
1. Penicillin-susceptible viridans streptococci, *Streptococcus bovis,* and other streptococci, penicillin MIC ≤ 0.1 μg/mL	A. Penicillin G	12–18 million units IV daily in divided doses q4h	4	
	B. Penicillin G plus gentamicin	12–18 million units IV daily in divided doses q4h 1 mg/kg IM or IV q8h	4 2	Avoid aminoglycoside-containing regimens when potential for nephrotoxicity or ototoxicity is increased
	C. Penicillin G plus gentamicin	Same doses as noted previously	2 2	See text
	D. Ceftriaxone	2 g IV or IM daily as single dose	4	Can be used in patients with nonimmediate penicillin allergy, intramuscular administration of ceftriaxone is painful
	E. Vancomycin†	30 mg/kg IV daily in divided doses q12h	4	Use for patients with immediate or severe penicillin or cephalosporin allergy. Infuse doses over 1 h to avoid histamine release reaction (red man syndrome)
2. Relatively penicillin-resistant streptococci Penicillin MIC 0.2–0.5 μg/mL	A. Penicillin G plus gentamicin	18–24 million units IV daily in divided doses q4h 1 mg/kg IM or IV q8h	4 2	
Penicillin MIC >0.5 μm/mL	B. Penicillin G plus gentamicin	See regimens recommended for enterococcal endocarditis	4	Preferred for nutritionally variant (pyridoxal- or cysteine-requiring) streptococci
3. Enterococci (in vitro evaluation for MIC to penicillin and vancomycin, beta-lactamae production, and high-level resistance to gentamicin and streptomycin required)	A. Penicillin G plus gentamicin	18–30 million units IV daily in divided doses q4h	4–6	See text for use of streptomycin instead of gentamicin in these regimens. Four weeks of therapy recommended for patients with shorter history of illness (>3 mo) who respond promptly to treatment.
	B. Ampicillin plus gentamicin	12 g IV daily in divided doses q4h Same dose as noted previously	4–6 4–6	
	C. Vancomycin† plus gentamicin	30 mg/kg IV daily in divided doses q12h Same dose as noted previously	4–6 4–6	Use for patients with penicillin allergy. Do not use cephalosporins.

4. Staphylococci infecting native valves (assume penicillin resistance) Methicillin-susceptible	A. Nafcillin or oxacillin plus	12 g IV daily in divided doses q4h	3–5 days	Penicillin—18–24 million units daily in divided doses q4h can be used instead of nafcillin, oxacillin, or cefazolin if strains do not produce beta-lactamase
	optional addition of gentamicin	Same dose as previously		
	B. Cefazolin plus	2 g IV q8h	6	Cephalothin or other first-generation cephalosporin in equivalent doses can be used
	optional addition of gentamicin	Same dose as previously	3–5 days	
	C. Vancomycin†	30 mg/kg IV in divided doses q12h	6	Use for patients with immediate penicillin allergy
5. Staphylococci infecting native valves, methicillin-resistant	A. Vancomycin†	30 mg/kg IV in divided doses q12h	6	
6. Staphylococci infecting prosthetic valves Methicillin-susceptible (assume penicillin-resistance)	A. Nafcillin or oxacillin	12 g IV daily in divided doses q4h	6	First-generation cephalosporin or vancomycin could be used in penicillin-allergic patients. Use gentamicin during initial 2 weeks. See text for alternatives to gentamicin. For patients with immediate penicillin allergy, use regimen 7.
	plus gentamicin	1 mg/kg IV or IM q8h	2	
	plus rifampin§	300 mg orally q8h	6	
7. Staphylococci infecting prosthetic valves Methicillin-resistant	A. Vancomycin†	30 mg/kg IV in divided doses q12h	6	Use gentamicin during the initial 2 weeks of therapy. See text for alternatives to gentamicin. Do not substitute a cephalosporin or imipenem for vancomycin.
	plus gentamicin	1 mg/kg IV or IM q8h	2	
	plus rifampin§	300 mg orally q8h	6	
8. HACEK organisms‡	A. Ceftriaxone	2 g IV or IM daily as a single dose	4	Cefotaxime or other third-generation cephalosporin in comparable doses may be used
	B. Ampicillin	12 g IV daily in divided doses q4h	4	Test organism for beta-lactamase production. Do not use this regimen if beta-lactamase is produced.
	plus gentamicin	1 mg/kg IV or IM q8h	4	

*Recommended doses are for adults with normal renal and hepatic function. Doses of gentamicin, streptomycin, and vancomycin must be adjusted in patients with renal dysfunction. Use ideal body weight to calculate doses (men = 50 kg + 2.3 kg per inch over 5 feet; women = 45.5 kg plus 2.3 kg per inch over 5 feet).

†Peak levels obtained 1 hour after completion of the infusion should be 30 to 45 μg/mL.

‡HACEK organisms include *Haemophilus parainfluenzae, Haemophilus aphrophilus, Actinobacillus actinomycetemcomitans, Cardiobacterium hominis, Eikenella corrodens, Kingella kingae.*

§Rifampin increases the dose of warfarin or dicumarol required for effective anticoagulation.

Abbreviations: IV, intravenously; IM, intramuscularly; MIC, minimal inhibitory concentration.

resistant to penicillin, ampicillin, and vancomycin and, in fact, are at best inhibited rather than killed by these antibiotics. Moreover, these organisms are overtly resistant to cephalosporins and semisynthetic penicillinase-resistant penicillins (nafcillin, oxacillin), as well as to therapeutic concentrations of aminoglycosides. Optimal therapy for enterococcal endocarditis is contingent on the synergistic bactericidal interaction of an antimicrobial agent targeted against the bacterial cell wall (penicillin, ampicillin, or vancomycin) and an aminoglycoside that is able to exert a lethal effect (primarily streptomycin or gentamicin). High-level resistance, defined as the inability of high concentrations of streptomycin (2000 μg/mL) or gentamicin (500–2000 μg/mL) to inhibit the growth of an enterococcal organism, is predictive of the agent's inability to exert this lethal effect and participate in the bactericidal synergistic interaction in vitro and in vivo.

Standard regimens for the treatment of enterococcal endocarditis (see Table 55–7, 3*A*–*C*) are based on these observations regarding antimicrobial susceptibility and bactericidal synergy as well as the clinical observation that synergistic combination therapy has resulted in a cure rate of 85% compared with 40% for single-agent nonbactericidal treatment.[27] Some authorities prefer gentamicin doses of 1.5 mg/kg every 8 h. Because this dose may be associated with an increased frequency of nephrotoxicity, others advocate doses of 1 mg/kg every 8 h. Peak serum gentamicin concentrations of approximately 5 μg/mL and 3.5 μg/mL, respectively, are sought with these doses. Previously, 40% of enterococci demonstrated high-level resistance to streptomycin, whereas none was highly resistant to gentamicin. Furthermore, penicillin, ampicillin, and vancomycin inhibited all enterococci at concentrations achieved in the serum with standard intravenous doses. Accordingly, one of the standard regimens could be selected for treatment with confidence that bactericidal synergy would be achieved. In the absence of high-level resistance to streptomycin in the causative strain, streptomycin, 9.5 mg/kg intramuscularly or intravenously every 12 h to achieve a peak serum concentration of approximately 20 μg/mL, can be substituted for gentamicin in the standard regimens. For patients allergic to penicillin, the vancomycin regimen (see Table 55–7, 3*C*) is recommended; alternatively, patients can be desensitized to penicillin. Cephalosporins are not effective in the treatment of enterococcal endocarditis.

Currently, antimicrobial resistance among enterococci is complex and cannot be predicted without in vitro testing. High-level resistance to gentamicin has been noted in 10%–25% of *E. faecalis* and 45%–50% of *E. faecium*, and resistance to penicillin, ampicillin, and vancomycin has become commonplace, especially in *E. faecium*. To determine whether a standard regimen for enterococcal endocarditis will provide optimal therapy, the strain causing endocarditis must be tested for high-level resistance to streptomycin and gentamicin, as well as for its MIC to penicillin or ampicillin or vancomycin. In addition, the strain, especially if it is an *E. faecalis*, must be screened for beta-lactamase production with nitrocefin to identify resistance to penicillin and ampicillin that may not be detected by MIC determination. If the strain is either resistant to achievable serum concentrations of the cell wall–active agent or highly resistant to the aminoglycosides, synergy and optimal therapy cannot be obtained with a standard regimen that includes the inactive antimicrobial agent. Furthermore, high-level resistance to gentamicin predicts resistance to all other aminoglycosides except streptomycin, which must be tested individually. These susceptibility data allow the selection of a bactericidal synergistic regimen, if one is possible.[28] If synergistic therapy is not feasible because of high-level resistance to both streptomycin and gentamicin, treatment with large doses of one of the cell wall–active agents for 8–12 weeks is recommended. If this approach fails, surgery to excise the infected valve should be considered.

Staphylococci

The overwhelming majority of coagulase-positive and coagulase-negative staphylococci produce penicillinase; consequently, these organisms should be considered penicillin-resistant unless specifically demonstrated not to elaborate penicillinase. Methicillin resistance is commonly noted among coagulase-negative staphylococci and is a less frequent but important characteristic in *S. aureus*. Methicillin-resistant strains are resistant to all beta-lactam antibiotics but remain susceptible to vancomycin. Although staphylococci are killed by cell wall–active antibiotics, the bactericidal effects of these agents can be enhanced by aminoglycosides. Combinations of semisynthetic penicillinase-resistant penicillins or vancomycin with rifampin does not result in predictable bactericidal synergism; nevertheless, rifampin uniquely enhances antibiotic activity against staphylococcal infections that involve foreign material. Staphylococcal infections involving prosthetic heart valves are treated differently from NVE caused by the same species.[9, 29]

Staphylococcal Native Valve Endocarditis

The treatment of endocarditis caused by methicillin-susceptible staphylococci is built around semisynthetic penicillinase-resistant penicillins or, when patients have nonimmediate penicillin allergy, a first-generation cephalosporin (see Table 55–7, 4*A*-*B*). Although the synergistic interaction of beta-lactam antibiotics combined with an aminoglycoside has not increased the cure rates for staphylococcal endocarditis, these combinations increase the rate of eradication of staphylococci in vegetations and from the blood. To achieve this potential benefit, gentamicin may be added to beta-lactam antibiotic therapy for *S. aureus* during the initial 3–5 days of treatment.[25] The role for combination therapy is less clear in NVE caused by coagulase-negative staphylococci.[29] Patients with endocarditis caused by penicillin-susceptible staphylococci can be treated with penicillin G, 18–24 million units intravenously divided into six daily doses, in lieu of nafcillin or oxacillin.[25] Methicillin-susceptible *S. aureus* endocarditis that is apparently uncomplicated and limited to the right-sided heart valves in intravenous drug addicts has been treated with 2 weeks of a semisynthetic penicillinase-resistant penicillin (but not vancomycin) plus an aminoglycoside (doses as noted in Table 55–7, 4*A*).[30, 31] Although this abbreviated course of therapy has been reported to be highly effective, a significant proportion of patients with right-sided *S. aureus* endocarditis remain febrile and toxic after completing 2 weeks of combination therapy.[32] Hence, this regimen must be used with caution; therapy should be extended in those patients who remain febrile after 2 weeks of treatment. Endocarditis caused by methicillin-resistant staphylococci requires treatment with vancomycin (see Table 55–7, 5*A*). Suitable alternatives to vancomycin are not available. Teicoplanin, a glycopeptide antibiotic similar to vancomycin, holds promise but is not available in the United States. If the strain is not resistant, gentamicin can be used in combination with vancomycin to enhance activity against these organisms; however, the frequency of renal toxicity may also be increased by this combination. The addition of rifampin to vancomycin for treatment of methicillin-resistant *S. aureus* endocarditis has not been beneficial.[33] Right-sided endocarditis caused by methicillin-resistant *S. aureus* is not treated with a 2-week regimen.

Staphylococcal Prosthetic Valve Endocarditis

Evidence from in vitro studies, experimental animal models of infection, and clinical studies suggest that staphylococcal infections involving foreign bodies, such as prosthetic heart valves, should be treated with two or three antibiotics in combination. Rifampin provides unique antistaphylococcal activity when infection involves foreign bodies. However, staphylococcal resistance to rifampin emerges rapidly when rifampin is used alone and when rifampin has been used in combination with vancomycin to treat staphylococcal PVE. Consequently, staphylococcal PVE is treated with two antimicrobials plus rifampin.[9] Rifampin therapy is delayed briefly until known effective antistaphylococcal therapy is in place. For PVE caused by methicillin-resistant staphylococci, treatment is initiated with vancomycin plus gentamicin with rifampin added if the organism is susceptible to gentamicin. The three-drug regimen is continued for 2 weeks, at which time gentamicin is discontinued and therapy with vancomycin and rifampin continued to complete a 6-week course (see Table 55–7, item 7).[9] If the organism is resistant to gentamicin, an alternative aminoglycoside to which the organism is susceptible should be sought. If the organism is resistant to all aminoglycosides, a quinolone to which it is susceptible may be used in lieu of the aminoglycoside.[9] For treatment of PVE caused by methicillin-susceptible staphylococci, a semisynthetic penicillinase-resistant penicillin should be substituted for vancomycin in this combination regimen (see Table 55–7, item 6). For treatment of patients with a nonimmediate penicillin allergy, a first-generation cephalosporin may be used in lieu of the semisynthetic penicillin. PVE caused by coagulase-negative staphylococci that occurs within the initial year after valve placement is often complicated by perivalvular extension of infection, and valve replacement surgery is often required to eradicate infection and maintain suitable valve function.[9] Similarly, *S. aureus* PVE is associated with intracardiac complications and exceptionally high mortality rates. Patients with this infection should be considered for early surgical intervention if the response to antimicrobial therapy is not prompt.[9, 34]

Haemophilus parainfluenzae, Haemophilus aphrophilus, Actinobacillus actinomycetemcomitans, Cardiobacterium hominis, Eikenella corrodens, and *Kingella kingae* (HACEK Organisms)

Endocarditis caused by the HACEK group has in the past been treated with ampicillin administered alone or in combination with gentamicin. As a result of the identification of occasional beta-lactamase–producing HACEK organisms (ampicillin-resistant) and the marked susceptibility of both beta-lactamase–producing and non-beta-lactamase–producing HACEK strains to third-generation cephalosporins, ceftriaxone or a comparable third-generation cephalosporin is recommended for treatment of NVE or PVE caused by these organisms (see Table 55–7, 8*A*).[25] For endocarditis caused by strains that do not produce beta-lactamase, ampicillin combined with gentamicin can be used in lieu of ceftriaxone (see Table 55–7, 8*B*).

Other Pathogens

Sporadic cases of this infection are caused by a broad variety of bacteria and fungi. The antimicrobial therapy for many of these infections is based on limited clinical experience and data from animal models and in vitro studies. Therapeutic regimens for most of these are beyond the scope of this chapter; in fact, physicians are urged to review the published experience with a specific etiologic agent as well as seek assistance from experienced infectious disease consultants when treating these patients. Among the more common of the unusual agents causing endocarditis are *Pseudomonas aeruginosa* and *Candida* species, both of which are seen with increased frequency among intravenous drug abusers. The preferred treatment for patients with endocarditis caused by *P. aeruginosa* is an antipseudomonal penicillin (ticarcillin or piperacillin) plus high doses of tobramycin (8 mg/kg/d intramuscularly or intravenously in divided doses every 8 h to achieve peak serum concentrations of 15 μg/mL). Amphotericin at full doses is recommended for treatment of *Candida* endocarditis. It has been reported that several patients with *Candida* endocarditis have been cured by prolonged treatment with fluconazole.[35] Endocarditis caused by *P. aeruginosa* is often both destructive and poorly responsive to antibiotic therapy. As a result, many patients with *P. aeruginosa* endocarditis will require cardiac surgery; similarly, early surgical intervention is a component of standard treatment for *Candida* endocarditis.

Culture-Negative Endocarditis

Standard blood culture results are negative in 2.5%–14% of patients having a clinical diagnosis consistent with infective endocarditis.[36, 37] Approximately 50% of those with negative blood culture results have recently received antibiotics, which accounts for the inability to recover pathogens from their blood. By using prolonged incubation times for blood cultures (3 or 4 weeks) and special culturing and subculturing techniques, fastidious organisms such as those of the HACEK group, *Brucella* species, corynebacteria, *Legionella* species, *Bartonella* species, *Chlamydia* species, and fungi can be recovered from the blood when standard culture results would be negative.[36, 38–40] In addition, *Coxiella burnetii*, chlamydiae, and some of these fastidious organisms can be implicated serologically. Occasionally a vegetation is not infective but rather thrombotic (Libman-Sacks endocarditis, marantic endocarditis, antiphospholipid antibody syndrome), or even a myxoma.

Unless clinical or epidemiologic clues suggest an etiologic diagnosis, the recommended treatment for culture-negative NVE is ampicillin plus gentamicin (see regimen for enterococcal endocarditis, Table 55–7, 3*B*); for analogous patients with PVE, vancomycin is added to this regimen.[9, 36] Mortality rates are lower for patients with culture-negative endocarditis who had received antibiotics before obtaining blood cultures and those who become afebrile during the initial week of antimicrobial treatment.[36, 37] Patients with culture-negative endocarditis who do not fully respond to empirical antimicrobial therapy may be candidates for surgical intervention, particularly those with prosthetic valves in whom persistent fever may represent perivalvular invasion by infection as well as ineffective antimicrobial therapy.[9] If surgical intervention is undertaken, a detailed microbiologic and pathologic examination of excised material, or extracted arterial emboli if available, must be performed to establish an etiologic diagnosis.

TIMING THE INITIATION OF ANTIMICROBIAL THERAPY

Current cost containment pressures often prompt initiation of antimicrobial therapy for suspected endocarditis immediately after blood culture specimens have been obtained. This practice is appropriate in the management of patients with highly destructive, rapidly progressive acute bacterial endocarditis or those presenting with hemodynamic decompensation requiring urgent or emergent surgical intervention. In these settings, immediate therapy may forestall further tissue damage or prepare patients for imminent surgery. In contrast, precipitous initiation of therapy in hemodynamically stable patients with suspected subacute endocarditis will not prevent early complications and may, by compromising subsequent blood cultures, obscure the etiologic diagnosis of endocarditis. In these latter patients, it is prudent to delay antibiotic therapy briefly pending the results of blood cultures. If initial cultures are not positive promptly, this delay provides an important opportunity to obtain additional blood culture specimens without the confounding effect of empirical treatment. This opportunity is particularly important when patients have received antibiotics within the preceding several weeks.

MONITORING THERAPY FOR ENDOCARDITIS

Patients with endocarditis require careful clinical monitoring during therapy and for several months thereafter. Clinical evaluation for complications of endocarditis (see further on) is essential. Failure of antimicrobial therapy, myocardial or metastatic abscess, emboli, hypersensitivity to antimicrobial agents, and other complications of therapy (catheter-related infection, thrombophlebitis) or intercurrent illness may be manifested by persistent or recurrent fever. Clinical events may indicate a need for potentially life-saving revision of antimicrobial therapy or adjunctive surgical therapy.

Measurement of the serum bactericidal titer (SBT)—the highest dilution of the patient's serum during therapy that in vitro kills 99.9% of a standard inoculum of the patient's infecting organism—as a method of assessing the adequacy of antimicrobial therapy is controversial. Because the test has often been performed in a nonstandardized manner and because complications of endocarditis have a marked impact on outcome, the SBT has correlated poorly with outcome of therapy. Several studies have suggested, however, that when a standardized SBT method, including the presence of 50% human serum in the test system, is used, peak and trough titers of at least 1:64 or 1:32 and 1:32, respectively, correlate with bacteriologic cure.[41, 42] When regimens with predictably high SBTs are used and considered optimal on the basis of clinical experience (see Table 55–7), monitoring therapy with the SBT is not recommended.[25] The SBT may be useful when treating patients with endocarditis caused by organisms for which optimal therapy is not established or when unconventional antimicrobial regimens are used.

Measurement of the serum concentration of vancomycin and aminoglycosides allows dose adjustment to ensure optimal therapy and avoid adverse events. In addition, renal function should be monitored in patients receiving these two antimicrobials, and the complete blood count should be checked at least weekly in patients receiving high-dose beta-lactam antibiotics or vancomycin.

Repeat blood cultures should be performed early during therapy to document that the bacteremia has been controlled. Blood cultures to assess breakthrough bacteremia are essential when patients are febrile during therapy. It is common practice to confirm the eradication of infection by obtaining several blood culture specimens 2–8 weeks after completion of therapy. In patients with recrudescent fever after treatment, however, prompt cultures are essential to assess the possible recurrence of endocarditis.

OUTPATIENT ANTIMICROBIAL THERAPY

Technical advances allowing the safe administration of single- and multiple-dose daily antimicrobial regimens, including treatment with the use of two antibiotics, combined with a well-developed home care system that provides supplies and monitors outpatient treatment, makes it feasible to treat endocarditis on an outpatient basis. Doing so can reduce the cost of therapy significantly. However, only those patients who are not experiencing threatening complications, whose compliance is assured, and whose home situation is physically suitable should be considered for treatment in this setting. Furthermore, patients being treated at home must be apprised of the potential complications of endocarditis, instructed to seek advice promptly when encountering unexpected or untoward clinical events, and undergo assiduous clinical and laboratory monitoring. Lastly, outpatient therapy must not result in compromises of antimicrobial therapy, leading to suboptimal regimens.

SURGICAL TREATMENT OF INTRACARDIAC COMPLICATIONS

Some intracardiac complications of NVE and PVE are not responsive to antimicrobial therapy. As a result, cardiac surgery plays an essential role in the treatment of endocarditis. Although the efficacy of cardiac surgery in these situations has not been evaluated in prospective trials, retrospective data suggest that mortality is unacceptably high when patients with these complications are treated with antibiotics alone, whereas mortality is reduced when treatment combines antibiotics and surgical intervention.[43–45] Accordingly, these complications have become indications for cardiac surgery (Table 55–8).

TABLE 55–8. INDICATIONS FOR CARDIAC SURGERY IN PATIENTS WITH NATIVE OR PROSTHETIC VALVE ENDOCARDITIS

Absolute Indications
Moderate to severe congestive heart failure due to valve dysfunction
Unstable prosthesis
Uncontrolled infection: Persistent bacteremia, ineffective antimicrobial therapy, fungal endocarditis
Relative Indications
Perivalvular extension of infection
Staphylococcus aureus endocarditis (aortic, mitral, prosthetic valves)
Relapse after optimal antimicrobial therapy (prosthetic valves)
Large (>10 mm) hypermobile vegetations
Persistent unexplained fever (≥10 days) in culture-negative endocarditis

Valvular Dysfunction

When treated with medical therapy alone, NVE that is complicated by moderate to severe (New York Heart Association Class III and IV) congestive heart failure due to new or worsening valvular dysfunction (primarily incompetence) results in mortality rates of 50%–90%. In contrast, among a similar group of patients treated with antibiotics and cardiac surgery, survival rates of 60%–80% are noted.[43–48] Although survival rates with surgical intervention for patients with PVE complicated by valvular dysfunction and congestive heart failure are somewhat lower (45%–64%), few patients are alive at 6 months when treated with antibiotics alone.[9] New or worsening aortic valve incompetence is associated with more severe and more rapidly progressive congestive heart failure than is mitral valve incompetence. Hence, patients with aortic valve endocarditis not only account for the majority of surgically treated patients but also require surgery on a more urgent basis when cardiac failure supervenes. Nevertheless, progressive cardiac failure due to severe mitral valve insufficiency will be inexorable and requires surgical intervention. Doppler echocardiography and color flow mapping indicating significant valvular regurgitation during the initial week of endocarditis treatment does not reliably identify patients with progressive valvular dysfunction who will require valve replacement during active endocarditis. Alternatively, despite the absence of significant valvular regurgitation on early echocardiography, marked congestive heart failure may still develop. Decisions regarding surgical intervention should not be made solely on the basis of echocardiographic findings but rather by integrating clinical data during careful monitoring.[49] On occasion, very large vegetations on the mitral valve, particularly mitral valve prostheses, result in significant obstruction and require surgery.

Unstable Prostheses

Dehiscence of prosthetic valves from the annulus is a manifestation of perivalvular infection and often results in hemodynamically significant valvular dysfunction. As a consequence, this finding identifies patients with PVE for whom surgical intervention is recommended.[9, 45] Patients with PVE who are at increased risk for these complications are those with onset of endocarditis within the year after valve implantation and those with infection of an aortic valve prosthesis.[50] Endocarditis in these patients is often caused by organisms that are either more invasive or antimicrobial-resistant, for example, *S. aureus*, gram-negative bacilli, *Candida* species, or coagulase-negative staphylococci. Consequently, the benefit of combined medical-surgical therapy is enhanced further. Patients who are clinically stable but have overtly unstable and hypermobile prostheses, a finding indicative of dehiscence in excess of 40% of the circumference, are likely to have further valve instability for mechanical reasons and warrant surgical treatment. There are occasional patients with PVE caused by noninvasive, highly antibiotic-susceptible organisms—for example, streptococci—who, despite a favorable clinical course during antibiotic therapy, late in treatment experience minor valve dehiscence without prosthesis instability or hemodynamic deterioration. These patients can be treated medically and surgery deferred unless clear indications arise.

Perivalvular Invasive Infection

NVE at the aortic site and PVE are most commonly associated with perivalvular invasion by infection with abscess or intracardiac fistula formation.[2, 9, 12, 13, 50] In patients with NVE, invasive infection occurs in 10%–14%, whereas in patients with PVE, 45%–60% experience this complication.[2, 9, 13] Persistent, otherwise unexplained fever in spite of appropriate antimicrobial therapy or pericarditis in patients with aortic valve endocarditis suggests infection extending beyond the valve leaflet. New-onset and persistent electrocardiographic conduction defects, although not a sensitive indicator of perivalvular infection (28%), are relatively specific (85%–90%).[2, 13]

Although transthoracic echocardiography has a sensitivity of 28%, a specificity of 98%, and a negative predictive value of 69%, transesophageal echocardiography is a superior test for detecting invasive infection in patients with NVE and PVE. The transesophageal approach yields a sensitivity of 87%, specificity of 95%, and positive and negative predictive values of 91% and 92%, respectively.[15] Doppler and color flow Doppler or contrast two-dimensional echocardiography may further elucidate invasive infection that has formed fistulas.[13] Magnetic resonance imaging (MRI) may be used to diagnose invasive infection; however, studies comparing this technique to echocardiography are not available.[13] Patients with endocarditis should be assessed routinely by transthoracic echocardiography and serial electrocardiography. Those in whom an abscess is suspected but not detected by these studies, particularly if there is mitral or prosthetic valve infection, should be evaluated with the use of transesophageal echocardiography with Doppler. If the studies remain inconclusive, MRI including magnetic resonance angiography should be performed. Cardiac catheterization may add little to these imaging studies and is not recommended unless coronary angiography is needed for patients suspected of having significant coronary artery disease.[13, 48]

Convention suggests that patients with endocarditis complicated by perivalvular extension of infection should undergo cardiac surgery to debride invasive infection, ablate abscesses, and reconstruct anatomic damage. Surgery is warranted in patients with invasive disease that significantly disrupts cardiac structures or disease that is associated with congestive heart failure, results in instability of a prosthetic valve, or renders infection uncontrolled (persistent fever). However, it is likely that increasingly sensitive imaging techniques will elucidate invasive infection that does not require surgery. Patients with perivalvular infection detected by MRI have been effectively treated with antibiotics alone.[13] Similarly, recent experience indicates that conservative medical management can be effective for selected patients with perivalvular infection detected by transesophageal echocardiography.[51]

Uncontrolled Infection

Surgical intervention has improved the outcome of several forms of endocarditis in which maximal antimicrobial regimens fail to eradicate infection and, in some instances, even to suppress bacteremia. It is generally conceded that amphotericin B is inadequate therapy for fungal endocarditis and that surgical intervention is indicated shortly after initiation of full doses of antifungal therapy. Although isolated instances of successful medical therapy of *Candida* endocarditis with the use of prolonged medical therapy with fluconazole have been noted,[35] this approach is not recommended currently. Endocarditis caused by some gram-negative bacilli, for example, *P. aeruginosa* and *Achromobacter xylosoxidans*, may not be eradicated by maximal tolerable antibiotic therapy and require surgical excision of the infected tissue to achieve cure. Similarly, surgery is incorporated into the standard therapy of endocarditis caused by *Brucella* species, since medical therapy is rarely successful.[52] Surgical intervention is recommended when enterococcal endocarditis caused by a strain that is resistant to synergistic bactericidal therapy (see discussion of antimicrobial therapy) does not respond to initial therapy or relapses. Perivalvular invasive infection is in some instances a form of ineradicable infection. Relapse of PVE after optimal antimicrobial therapy in most instances represents this phenomenon, and patients with relapse of PVE are treated by surgical intervention.[9, 50] In contrast, relapse of NVE, unless associated with a highly resistant microorganism or demonstrable perivalvular infection, often is treated by intensifying and prolonging another course of antimicrobial therapy.

Endocarditis caused by *S. aureus* and involving the aortic or mitral valve has been considered a form of uncontrolled infection or perhaps more correctly endocarditis that is poorly controlled, highly destructive, and associated with unacceptable mortality. For this reason, some authors have suggested that patients with left-sided *S. aureus* endocarditis should be considered for surgical treatment when the response to antimicrobial therapy is not prompt and complete.[46, 53, 54] PVE caused by *S. aureus* is associated with mortality rates exceeding 80% and thus is an even stronger indication for surgical treatment.[9, 34] Although *S. aureus* endocarditis limited to the tricuspid or pulmonary valves in intravenous drug abusers is often associated with prolonged fever during antimicrobial therapy, which suggests uncontrolled infection, the vast majority of these patients respond to prolonged courses of antimicrobial therapy and do not require surgery.[7, 32]

Patients with culture-negative endocarditis who experience unexplained persistent fever during empirical antimicrobial therapy, particularly those with PVE, should be considered for surgical intervention. In these patients, it is likely that persistent fever represents either unrecognized perivalvular infection or ineffective antimicrobial therapy.

Large Vegetations (>10 mm) and the Prevention of Systemic Emboli

Patients with clinical evidence of endocarditis and echocardiographically detectable vegetations appear to have an increased frequency of systemic emboli, congestive heart failure, requirement for cardiac surgery, and death. Not all studies, however, confirm these associations.[55, 56] In a meta-analysis, the risk of systemic embolization was increased in patients with vegetations greater than 10 mm (greatest diameter) versus those with smaller or no detectable vegetations, 33% versus 19%.[55] The association of larger vegetations (>10 mm) with systemic emboli (all emboli as well as those occurring after echocardiography) was confirmed when vegetations were sized by transesophageal imaging and was particularly correlated with mitral valve lesions. In this study, however, vegetation size was not related to the development of congestive heart failure or increased mortality.[21] Although there may be a relationship between vegetation characteristics—including size, mobility, and extent (number of leaflets involved) —and complications, the implications for surgical intervention are not clear. Multivariate analyses examining the relationship between both the need for surgical intervention and the outcome and variables—including not only vegetation characteristics but also valve dysfunction, perivalvular invasion by infection, organism, and infection site—have not been performed. Nevertheless, some authors have concluded that vegetation characteristics alone might warrant surgery.[48] For example, vegetations greater than 10 mm on the mitral valve have been considered an independent indication for surgery.[21] This recommendation, as well as the practice of using all vegetations greater than 10 mm as an indication for surgery to prevent systemic emboli, can be questioned. Several studies indicate a significant decrease in the rate of systemic or cerebral emboli in patients with NVE and PVE during the course of effective antibiotic therapy.[56–60] In addition, it is not clear that surgical intervention reduces the frequency of systemic emboli.[43, 45] Finally, the hazards of cerebral and coronary emboli (those causing major morbidity and mortality) are rarely compared with the immediate and long-term risks of valve replacement surgery. The latter include perioperative mortality, recrudescent endocarditis on the prosthesis, thromboembolic complications, early and late valve dysfunction requiring repeat valve replacement, the hazards of warfarin anticoagulation therapy (including its contraindication during pregnancy), and the risk and morbidity of late-onset PVE.[45] These considerations suggest that vegetation size alone is not an indication for surgery but rather that the clinical findings, evidence of other intracardiac complications, and echocardiographic findings must be weighed against the immediate and remote hazards of cardiac surgery when recommending therapy.[55, 61] Thus, the risk of systemic embolization as related to vegetation size is only one of many factors to be considered when planning treatment. Prior systemic embolization should be considered in a manner analogous to vegetation size and not as an independent indication for surgical intervention.[56–60]

Techniques for Repair of Intracardiac Defects

The early replacement of infected malfunctioning native and prosthetic valves during active endocarditis has become a standard element of optimal therapy for selected patients.[34, 44–48, 50, 53, 54] New surgical techniques to address severe tissue destruction in NVE and PVE have been developed. Although these are beyond the scope of this discussion, examples include valve composite graft replacement of the aortic root, use of sewing skirts attached to the prostheses, and homograft replacement of the aortic valve and root with coronary artery reimplantation.[62–67] Furthermore, with less severe perivalvular destruction but significant hemodynamic dysfunction, repair of the mitral valve in patients with acute or healed endocarditis avoids insertion of prosthetic materials and the associated hazards.[68, 69] Although tricuspid valvulectomy without valve replacement has been advocated for treatment of uncontrolled tricuspid valve infection in intravenous drug abusers at high risk of recidivism and recurrent endocarditis,[70] the likelihood of refractory right-sided heart failure after valvulectomy makes tricuspid valve repair preferable if possible.[48] On rare occasion, heart transplantation has been used to salvage patients with refractory endocarditis.[71]

Timing of Surgical Intervention

When endocarditis is complicated by valvular regurgitation and significant impairment of cardiac function, early surgical intervention before the development of severe intractable hemodynamic dysfunction is recommended, regardless of the duration of prior antimicrobial therapy.[44, 45, 72] This approach recognizes that postoperative mortality correlates with the severity of preoperative hemodynamic dysfunction. In patients who have sustained severe valvular damage but in whom infection is controlled and cardiac function is fully compensated, surgery may be delayed until antimicrobial therapy has been completed. If infection is not controlled, however, surgery should be performed promptly. Similarly, if a large vegetation is present indicating a high risk for systemic embolization, early cardiac surgery is appropriate. In order to avoid intracranial hemorrhagic complications in patients who have sustained recent neurologic injury, the timing of surgical intervention may require modification. When cardiac function permits, surgery should be delayed for patients who have had prior embolic infarcts until at least 4 and ideally 10 days have elapsed[73–77] and for those who have sustained an intracranial hemorrhagic event until at least 21 days have elapsed.[75, 77] Before cardiac surgery, it is prudent to evaluate the cerebral vasculature in patients who have sustained an embolic infarct or who have persistent headaches. Finding a mycotic aneurysm should cause a reconsideration of the timing of cardiac surgery as well as avoidance of a prosthesis that requires postoperative anticoagulant therapy.

Duration of Antimicrobial Therapy After Surgical Intervention

Inflammatory changes and bacteria are commonly seen in culture-negative vegetations removed from patients who have received most or all of the standard antibiotic therapy recommended for endocarditis caused by the specific microorganism.[78] This is not indicative of failed antimicrobial therapy and the need for a full course of antibiotic therapy postoperatively. The duration of antimicrobial therapy after surgery depends on the length of preoperative therapy, the causative organism (whether it is highly antibiotic-susceptible or more resistant), whether infection is limited to the excised valve leaflet or has invaded myocardial tissue, and whether intraoperative culture results are positive (Table 55–9). In general, for endocarditis caused by relatively antibiotic-resistant organisms with negative culture results of operative specimens, preoperative plus postoperative therapy should at least equal a full course of recommended therapy; for those patients with positive intraoperative culture results, a full course of therapy should be given postoperatively. Patients with PVE should be treated conservatively and receive a full course of antimicrobial therapy postoperatively when organisms are seen in resected material.[9]

TREATMENT OF EXTRACARDIAC COMPLICATIONS

Patients with endocarditis caused by pyogenic organisms may experience focal septic complications that require modification of therapy to ensure penetration of antibiotics to a specific site, drainage of loculated infection, or sufficient duration of therapy to eradicate metastatic infection. Examples of such complications include meningitis, septic arthritis, and vertebral osteomyelitis. Several extracardiac complications require particular attention.

Splenic Abscess

Three to five percent of patients with endocarditis experience splenic abscess; *S. aureus*, streptococci, and gram-negative bacilli are the organisms commonly associated with endocarditis and concurrent splenic abscess.[16, 79] Ultrasonography and computed tomography identify splenic defects but cannot discriminate between abscess and infarct. Although progressive enlargement of the lesion during antimicrobial therapy suggests an abscess, confirmation requires percutaneous needle aspiration. Therapy of splenic abscess is rarely successful without drainage; percutaneous placement of a catheter

TABLE 55–9. ANTIBIOTIC THERAPY AFTER CARDIAC SURGERY FOR NATIVE VALVE ENDOCARDITIS

	Weeks of Postoperative Therapy			
	Sterile		Culture-Positive	
Organism	*Valve*	*Abscess*	*Valve*	*Abscess*
Streptococci	1–1.5	2*	2	4
HACEK organisms	1–1.5	2*	2	4
Staphylococci	≥2*	3–4*	3–4*	4–6
Gram-negative rods	≥2*	3–4*	3–4*	4–6

*Total preoperative and postoperative course at least a full recommended course of therapy.

for drainage has allowed successful treatment.[79] In patients with endocarditis complicated by multiple splenic abscesses or in whom percutaneous drainage is unsuccessful, splenectomy is required.[79] Splenic abscesses should be effectively treated before valve replacement surgery to avoid recrudescent infection and seeding of the valve prosthesis.

Mycotic Aneurysms and Septic Arteritis

From 2%–10% of patients with endocarditis have mycotic aneurysms, including the 1%–5% who have cerebral mycotic aneurysms.[60, 73] Cerebral mycotic aneurysms occur at the branch points in cerebral vessels, are located distally over the cerebral cortex, and most commonly affect branches of the middle cerebral artery. These lesions arise either from occlusion of vessels by septic emboli with secondary arteritis and vessel wall destruction or by bacteremic seeding of the vessel wall through the vasa vasorum; *S. aureus* is commonly implicated in the former and streptococci in the latter.[80, 81] Although many patients with mycotic aneurysms or septic arteritis present with devastating intracranial hemorrhage, focal deficits from embolic events and persistent focal headache may be premonitory symptoms. In patients with subarachnoid hemorrhage, cerebral angiography is required. Others suggest angiography to detect cryptic aneurysms in patients experiencing focal neurologic deficits or persistent severe headache or those in whom anticoagulant therapy is planned.[73, 82] Mycotic aneurysms may resolve during antimicrobial therapy[82]; however, aneurysms that have ruptured should be repaired surgically, when possible. Aneurysms that have not leaked should be followed angiographically during antimicrobial therapy. Surgery should be considered for a single lesion that enlarges during or after antimicrobial therapy. Anticoagulant therapy should be avoided in patients with a persistent mycotic aneurysm. Although persistent stable aneurysms may rupture after completion of standard antimicrobial therapy, there is no accurate estimation of risk for late rupture, and recommendations for surgical intervention are arbitrary. The potential existence of occult aneurysms in patients without neurologic symptoms or in those who have had a normal angiographic evaluation is not considered a contraindication to anticoagulant therapy after completion of antimicrobial therapy.[82]

ANTICOAGULANT THERAPY

Patients with PVE involving devices that would usually warrant maintenance anticoagulation are continued on anticoagulant therapy.[9] Prothrombin times should be maintained at 1.5 times the control (International Normalized Ratio [INR] = 3). Anticoagulation is not advised for patients with PVE involving devices that do not usually require this therapy. There is no evidence that anticoagulant therapy will prevent embolization in patients with NVE, and in some instances it may contribute to intracranial hemorrhage, particularly in the presence of a recent cerebral infarct or a mycotic aneurysm.[73, 80, 82] Accordingly, anticoagulant therapy in patients with NVE should be restricted to those in whom there is a clear indication for this therapy and in whom there is not a known increased risk for intracranial hemorrhage. If central nervous system complications occur, particularly hemorrhage, anticoagulation should be reversed immediately.

REFERENCES

1. Watanakunakorn C, Burkert T: Infective endocarditis at a large community teaching hospital, 1980–1990: a review of 210 episodes. Medicine 1993; 72:90–102.
2. DiNubile MJ, Calderwood SB, Steinhaus DM, et al: Cardiac conduction abnormalities complicating native valve active infective endocarditis. Am J Cardiol 1986; 58:1213–1217.
3. Kazanjian P: Infective endocarditis: review of 60 cases treated in community hospitals. Infect Dis Clin Pract 1993; 2:41–46.
4. Terpenning MS, Buggy BP, Kauffman CA: Hospital-acquired infective endocarditis. Arch Intern Med 1988; 148:1601–1603.
5. Fernandez-Guerrero ML, Verdejo C, Azofra J, et al: Hospital-acquired infectious endocarditis not associated with cardiac surgery: an emerging problem. Clin Infect Dis 1995; 20:16–23.
6. Sande MA, Lee BL, Mills J, et al: Endocarditis in intravenous drug users. *In* Kaye D (ed): Infective Endocarditis, 2nd ed, p 345. New York: Raven Press, 1992.
7. Hecht SR, Berger M: Right-sided endocarditis in intravenous drug users: prognostic features in 102 episodes. Ann Intern Med 1992; 117:560–566.
8. Baddour LM: Polymicrobial infective endocarditis in the 1980's. Rev Infect Dis 1991; 13:963–970.
9. Karchmer AW, Gibbons GW: Infections of prosthetic heart valves and vascular grafts. *In* Bisno AL, Waldvogel FA (eds): Infections Associated with Indwelling Devices, 2nd ed, pp 213–249. Washington, DC: American Society for Microbiology, 1994.
10. Tornos P, Sanz E, Permanyer-Miralda G, et al: Late prosthetic valve endocarditis: immediate and long-term prognosis. Chest 1992; 101:37–41.
11. Grover FL, Cohen DJ, Oprian C, et al: Determinants of the occurrence of and survival from prosthetic valve endocarditis. J Thorac Cardiovasc Surg 1994; 108:207–214.
12. Omari B, Shapiro S, Ginzton L, et al: Predictive risk factors for periannular extension of native valve endocarditis: clinical and echocardiographic analyses. Chest 1989; 96:1273–1279.
13. Carpenter JL: Perivalvular extension of infection in patients with infective endocarditis. Rev Infect Dis 1991; 13:127–138.
14. Blumberg EA, Robbins N, Adimora A, et al: Persistent fever in association with infective endocarditis. Clin Infect Dis 1992; 15:983–990.
15. Daniel WG, Mugge A, Martin RP, et al: Improvement in the diagnosis of abscesses associated with endocarditis by transesophageal echocardiography. N Engl J Med 1991; 324:795–800.
16. Mansur AJ, Grinberg M, Lemos da Luz P, et al: The complications of infective endocarditis: a reappraisal in the 1980's. Arch Intern Med 1992; 152:2428–2432.
17. Durack DT, Lukes AS, Bright DK: New criteria for diagnosis of infective endocarditis: utilization of specific echocardiographic findings. Am J Med 1994; 96:200–209.
18. Bayer AS, Ward JI, Ginzton LE, et al: Evaluation of new clinical criteria for the diagnosis of infective endocarditis. Am J Med 1994; 96:211–219.
19. von Reyn CF, Arbeit RD: Case definitions for infective endocarditis. Am J Med 1994; 96:220–222.
20. Breen JD, Karchmer AW: Usefulness of pulsed-field gel electrophoresis in confirming endocarditis due to *Staphylococcus lugdunensis*. Clin Infect Dis 1994; 19:985–986.
21. Mugge A, Daniel WC, Frank G, et al: Echocardiography in infective endocarditis: reassessment of prognostic implications of vegetation size determined by the transthoracic and transesophageal approach. J Am Coll Cardiol 1989; 14:631–638.
22. Shively BK, Gurule FT, Roldan CA, et al: Diagnostic value of transesophageal compared with transthoracic echocardiography in infective endocarditis. J Am Coll Cardiol 1991; 18:391–397.
23. Sochowski RA, Chan KL: Implication of negative results on a monoplane transesophageal echocardiographic study in patients with suspected infective endocarditis. J Am Coll Cardiol 1993; 21:216–221.
24. Mugge A: Echocardiographic detection of cardiac valve vegetations and prognostic implications. Infect Dis Clin North Am 1993; 7:877–898.
25. Wilson WR, Karchmer AW, Bisno AL, et al: Antibiotic treatment of adults with infective endocarditis due to viridans streptococci, enterococci, other streptococci, staphylococci, and HACEK microorganisms. JAMA, in press.
26. Francioli P, Etienne J, Hoigne R, et al: Treatment of streptococcal endocarditis with a single daily dose of ceftriaxone sodium for 4 weeks. JAMA 1992; 267:264–267.
27. Eliopoulos GM: Enterococcal endocarditis. *In* Kaye D (ed): Infective Endocarditis, 2nd ed, pp 209–223. New York: Raven Press, 1992.
28. Eliopoulos GM: Aminoglycoside resistant enterococcal endocarditis. Infect Dis Clin North Am 1993; 7:117–133.
29. Whitener C, Caputo GM, Weitekamp MR, et al: Endocarditis due to coagulase-negative staphylococci: microbiologic, epidemiologic, and clinical considerations. Infect Dis Clin North Am 1993; 7:81–96.
30. Chambers HF, Miller T, Newman MD: Right-sided *Staphylococcus aureus* endocarditis in intravenous drug abusers: two-week combination therapy. Ann Intern Med 1988; 109:619–624.

31. Torres-Tortosa M, de Cueto M, Vergara A, et al: Prospective evaluation of a two-week course of intravenous antibiotics in intravenous drug addicts with infective endocarditis. Eur J Clin Microbiol Infect Dis 1994; 13:559–564.
32. Bayer AS, Blomquist IK, Bello E, et al: Tricuspid valve endocarditis due to *Staphylococcus aureus*: correlation of two-dimensional echocardiography with clinical outcome. Chest 1988; 93:247–253.
33. Levine DP, Fromm BS, Reddy BR: Slow response to vancomycin or vancomycin plus rifampin in methicillin-resistant *Staphylococcus aureus* endocarditis. Ann Intern Med 1991; 115:674–680.
34. Sett SS, Hudon MPJ, Jamieson WRE, et al: Prosthetic valve endocarditis: experience with porcine bioprostheses. J Thorac Cardiovasc Surg 1993; 105:428–434.
35. Venditti M, DeBernardis F, Micozzi A, et al: Fluconazole treatment of catheter-related right-sided endocarditis caused by *Candida albicans* and associated endophthalmitis and folliculitis. Clin Infect Dis 1992; 14:422–426.
36. Tunkel AR, Kaye D: Endocarditis with negative blood cultures. N Engl J Med 1992; 326:1215–1217.
37. Hoen B, Selton-Suty C, Lacassin F, et al: Infective endocarditis in patients with negative blood cultures: analysis of 88 cases from a one-year nationwide survey in France. Clin Infect Dis 1995; 20:501–506.
38. Daly JS, Worthington MG, Brenner DJ, et al: *Rochalimaea elizabethae* sp. nov. isolated from a patient with endocarditis. J Clin Microbiol 1993; 31:872–881.
39. Drancourt M, Mainardi JL, Brouqui P, et al: *Bartonella (Rochalimaea) quintana* endocarditis in three homeless men. N Engl J Med 1995; 332:419–423.
40. Shapiro DS, Kenney SC, Johnson M, et al: Brief report: *Chlamydia psittaci* endocarditis diagnosed by blood culture. N Engl J Med 1992; 326:1192–1195.
41. Weinstein MP, Stratton CW, Ackley A, et al: Multicenter collaborative evaluation of a standardized serum bactericidal test as a prognostic indicator in infective endocarditis. Am J Med 1985; 78:262–269.
42. Stratton CW: The role of the microbiology laboratory in the treatment of infective endocarditis. J Antimicrob Chemother 1987; 20(suppl A):41–49.
43. Croft CH, Woodward W, Elliott A, et al: Analysis of surgical versus medical therapy in active complicated native valve infective endocarditis. Am J Cardiol 1983; 51:1650–1655.
44. DiNubile MJ: Surgery in active endocarditis. Ann Intern Med 1982; 96:650–659.
45. Alsip SG, Blackstone EH, Kirklin JW, et al: Indications for cardiac surgery in patients with active infective endocarditis. Am J Med 1985; 78(suppl 6B):138-148.
46. Mullany CJ, McIsaacs AI, Rowe MH, et al: The surgical treatment of infective endocarditis. World J Surg 1989; 13:132–136.
47. Al Jubair K, Al Fagih M, Ashmeg A, et al: Cardiac operations during active endocarditis. J Thorac Cardiovasc Surg 1992; 104:487–490.
48. Larbalestier RI, Kinchla NM, Aranki SF, et al: Acute bacterial endocarditis: optimizing surgical results. Circulation 1992; 86(suppl II):II68-II74.
49. Karalis DG, Blumberg EA, Vilaro JF, et al: Prognostic significance of valvular regurgitation in patients with infective endocarditis. Am J Med 1991; 90:193–197.
50. Calderwood SB, Swinski LA, Karchmer AW, et al: Prosthetic valve endocarditis: analysis of factors affecting outcome of therapy. J Thorac Cardiovasc Surg 1986; 92:776–783.
51. Chan KL, Sochowski RA: Conservative medical treatment can be appropriate in the management of perivalvular abscess: diagnosis and follow-up by transesophageal echocardiography [Abstract No. 931-50]. J Am Coll Cardiol 1994; p 322A
52. Jacobs F, Abramowicz D, Vereerstraeten P, et al: Brucella endocarditis: the role of combined medical and surgical treatment. Rev Infect Dis 1990; 12:740–744.
53. Richardson JV, Karp RB, Kirklin JW, et al: Treatment of infective endocarditis: a 10-year comparative analysis. Circulation 1978; 58:589–597.
54. D'Agostino RS, Miller C, Stinson EB, et al: Valve replacement in patients with native valve endocarditis: what really determines operative outcome?. Ann Thorac Surg 1985; 40:429–438.
55. Aragam JR, Weyman AE: Echocardiographic findings in infective endocarditis. *In* Weyman AE (ed): Principles and Practice of Echocardiography, 2nd ed, pp 1178–1197. Philadelphia: Lea & Febiger, 1994.
56. Steckelberg JM, Murphy JG, Ballard D, et al: Emboli in infective endocarditis: the prognostic value of echocardiography. Ann Intern Med 1991; 114:635–640.
57. Davenport J, Hart RG: Prosthetic valve endocarditis 1976–1987: antibiotics, anticoagulation, and stroke. Stroke 1990; 21:993–999.
58. Hart RG, Foster JW, Luther MF, et al: Stroke in infective endocarditis. Stroke 1990; 21:695–700.
59. Paschalis C, Pugsley W, John R, et al: Rate of cerebral embolic events in relation to antibiotic and anticoagulant therapy in patients with bacterial endocarditis. Eur Neurol 1990; 30:87–89.
60. Salgado AV, Furlan AJ, Keys TF, et al: Neurologic complications of endocarditis: a 12-year experience. Neurology 1989; 39:173–178.
61. Jaffe WM, Morgan DE, Pearlman AS, et al: Infective endocarditis, 1983–1988: echocardiographic findings and factors influencing morbidity and mortality. J Am Coll Cardiol 1990; 15:1227–1233.
62. Ergin MA, Raissi S, Follis F, et al: Annular destruction in acute bacterial endocarditis: surgical techniques to meet the challenge. J Thorac Cardiovasc Surg 1989; 97:755–763.
63. Miller DC: Predictors of outcome in patients with prosthetic valve endocarditis (PVE) and potential advantages of homograft aortic root replacement for prosthetic ascending aortic valve-graft infections. J Cardiac Surg 1990; 5:53–62.
64. Ross D: Allograft root replacement for prosthetic endocarditis. J Cardiac Surg 1990; 5:68–72.
65. McGiffin DC, Galbraith AJ, McLachian GJ, et al: Aortic valve infection: risk factors for death and recurrent endocarditis after aortic valve replacement. J Thorac Cardiovasc Surg 1992; 104:511–520.
66. Jault F, Gandjbakheh I, Chastre JC, et al: Prosthetic valve endocarditis with ring abscesses: surgical management and long-term results. J Thorac Cardiovasc Surg 1993; 105:1106–1113.
67. Pagano D, Allen SM, Bonser RS: Homograft aortic valve and root replacement for severe destructive native or prosthetic endocarditis. Eur J Cardiothorac Surg 1994; 8:173–176.
68. Dreyfus C, Serraf A, Jebara VA, et al: Valve repair in acute endocarditis. Ann Thorac Surg 1990; 49:706–713.
69. Hendren WG, Morris AS, Rosenkranz ER, et al: Mitral valve repair for bacterial endocarditis. J Thorac Cardiovasc Surg 1992; 103:124–129.
70. Arbulu A, Holmes RJ, Asfaw I: Tricuspid valvulectomy without replacement: Twenty years' experience. J Thorac Cardiovasc Surg 1991; 102:917–922.
71. DiSesa VJ, Sloss LJ, Cohn LH: Heart transplantation for intractable prosthetic valve endocarditis. J Heart Transplant 1990; 9:142–143.
72. Middlemost S, Wisenbaugh T, Meyerowitz C, et al: A case for early surgery in native left-sided endocarditis complicated by heart failure: results in 203 patients. J Am Coll Cardiol 1991; 18:663–667.
73. Kanter MC, Hart RG: Neurologic complications of infective endocarditis. Neurology 1991; 41:1015–1020.
74. Maruyama M, Kuriyama Y, Sawada T, et al: Brain damage after open heart surgery in patients with acute cardioembolic stroke. Stroke 1989; 20:1305–1310.
75. Ting W, Silverman N, Levitsky S: Valve replacement in patients with endocarditis and cerebral septic emboli. Ann Thorac Surg 1991; 51:18–22.
76. Zisbrod Z, Rose DM, Jacobowitz IJ, et al: Results of open heart surgery in patients with recent cardiogenic embolic stroke and central nervous system dysfunction. Circulation 1987; 76(suppl V):109–112.
77. Matsushita K, Kuriyama Y, Sawada T, et al: Hemorrhagic and ischemic cerebrovascular complications of active infective endocarditis of native valve. Eur Neurol 1993; 33:267–274.
78. Morris A, Strickett A, MacCulloch D: Gram stain culture and histology results of heart valves removed during active bacterial endocarditis (Abstract 1174). Programs of the 31st Interscience Conference on Antimicrobial Agents and Chemotherapy 1991; p 294.
79. Allan JD Jr: Splenic abscess: pathophysiology, diagnosis and management. *In* Remington JS, Swartz MN (eds): Current Clinical Topics in Infectious Diseases, vol. 14, pp 23–51. Boston: Blackwell Scientific, 1994.
80. Hart RG, Kagan-Hallet K, Joerns SE: Mechanisms of intracranial hemorrhage in infective endocarditis. Stroke 1987; 18:1048–1056.
81. Masuda J, Yutani C, Waki R, et al: Histopathological analysis of the mechanisms of intracranial hemorrhage complicating infective endocarditis. Stroke 1992; 23:843–850.
82. Salgado AV, Furlan AJ, Keys TF: Mycotic aneurysm, subarachnoid hemorrhage, and indications for cerebral angiography in infective endocarditis. Stroke 1987; 18:1057–1060.

56 Rehabilitation of the Patient With Cardiovascular Disease

Jonathan N. Myers, PhD
Victor F. Froelicher, MD

Before the 1970s, patients were completely immobilized after a myocardial infarction for 6 weeks or longer; the prevailing view was that this period of time was necessary for complete healing of the myocardium to occur. The post–myocardial infarction patient was generally not expected to ever return to normal occupational or recreational activities. The process known as cardiac rehabilitation evolved to restore the patient to optimal physical, psychologic, and social function. Substantial data have documented the benefits of early ambulation as well as the numerous detrimental effects of strict bed rest. The action of merely sitting in the upright position has been shown to reduce the detrimental effects of remaining supine.[1, 2] In the 1960s and 1970s, the recovery and return to work of popular public figures did a great deal to change the public's attitude with regard to having a heart attack. In more recent years, cardiac rehabilitation has evolved even further with changes in health care policy. For example, phase I has become almost superfluous with the shortening of hospital stays. Approximately 50% of patients undergo cardiac catheterization; this factor has had a significant impact on the approach to the patient who has sustained a myocardial infarction.

Once limited to supervised exercise in the post–myocardial infarction patient, both the indications for and scope of cardiac rehabilitation services have broadened. Advances in the treatment of cardiovascular disease and data supporting the value of secondary prevention have greatly increased the spectrum of patients who may benefit from cardiac rehabilitation. This spectrum of patients now includes not only post–myocardial infarction patients but also post-bypass patients, post–cardiac transplantation patients, post–percutaneous transluminal coronary angioplasty (PTCA) patients, patients with chronic heart failure, and patients with implantable pacemakers. Interestingly, of the roughly one million people in the United States annually who survive an acute myocardial infarction, only 10%–15% undergo formal outpatient rehabilitation.[3] The reasons why most eligible patients do not receive these services vary; however, a wider application of rehabilitation services has the potential for reducing morbidity and mortality from cardiovascular disease even further.

In addition, it is now widely recognized that exercise is only one component of cardiac rehabilitation. Patient objectives include not only preventing the effects of deconditioning but also improving functional capacity, relieving symptoms, and providing education, risk factor reduction, assistance in returning to normal activities, and psychosocial support. Societal objectives include decreasing health care costs by reduction in treatment time, reduction of medications, and prevention of premature disability, thus maintaining individual productivity and lessening the need for societal support. It is noteworthy in this context that exercise trials, when combined, have shown that the rate of mortality from cardiovascular causes (defined as fatal reinfarction or sudden cardiac death) is reduced 20%–25% among patients participating in rehabilitation.[4, 5]

A critical issue is whether cardiac rehabilitation is going to become superfluous with the application of new interventions, such as PTCA and thrombolysis for acute myocardial infarction. Multicenter trials have confirmed that the rate of mortality from acute myocardial infarction can be decreased by approximately 25% with thrombolysis. Depending on population selection, approximately 20% of patients presenting with an acute myocardial infarction meet the indications for thrombolysis. Thrombolysis is most effective in patients with large anterior infarcts who are admitted to the hospital within 3 h after the onset of symptoms. The place for acute PTCA during myocardial infarction appears to be rather limited. The need for PTCA after thrombolysis appears to be best determined by exercise testing, because early attempts at PTCA carry a high complication rate. Data are lacking with regard to the effectiveness of PTCA in prolonging life or averting myocardial infarction, although it is highly effective in the treatment of angina pectoris. Thus, despite these advances in therapy, a large number of patients nonetheless benefit from cardiac rehabilitation.

PHYSIOLOGIC RESPONSES TO EXERCISE

The acute response to exercise essentially involves the transformation of chemical energy bound in the muscle into mechanical energy, which permits the individual to perform work. The transformation of chemical energy into mechanical energy requires the complex integration of the cardiovascular and pulmonary systems, which provide gas exchange between the muscle cells and the atmosphere. Although virtually all of the body's physiologic and metabolic systems function in a coordinated manner to provide this energy to the exercising muscle, the cardiopulmonary system has a particularly crucial role in the acute response to exercise. The cardiovascular system responds to exercise with a series of adjustments that ensure (1) that active muscles receive blood supply that is appropriate to their metabolic needs, (2) that heat generated by the muscles is dissipated, and (3) that blood supply to the brain and the heart is maintained. These adjustments require a major redistribution of cardiac output along with a number of local metabolic changes.

The magnitude by which the basic hemodynamic and metabolic variables change from rest to a moderately high level of exercise is illustrated in Figure 56–1. Note that oxygen uptake, heart rate, arteriovenous oxygen difference, and cardiac output increase linearly with increasing work. Stroke volume increases to a level corresponding to approximately 50% of maximal capacity, after which stroke volume reaches a plateau. Oxygen uptake increases from its resting value to a degree ranging from 5 to 20 times. This is accomplished by a two- to threefold increase in heart rate and a 50% increase in stroke volume, resulting in an increase in cardiac output ranging from two to five times. Increases in cardiac output are paralleled by increases in ventilation, in such a way that ventilation and perfusion are appropriately matched in the lung. The increase in cardiac output is also balanced by a reduction in total peripheral resistance with the result that mean arterial pressure increases only slightly.

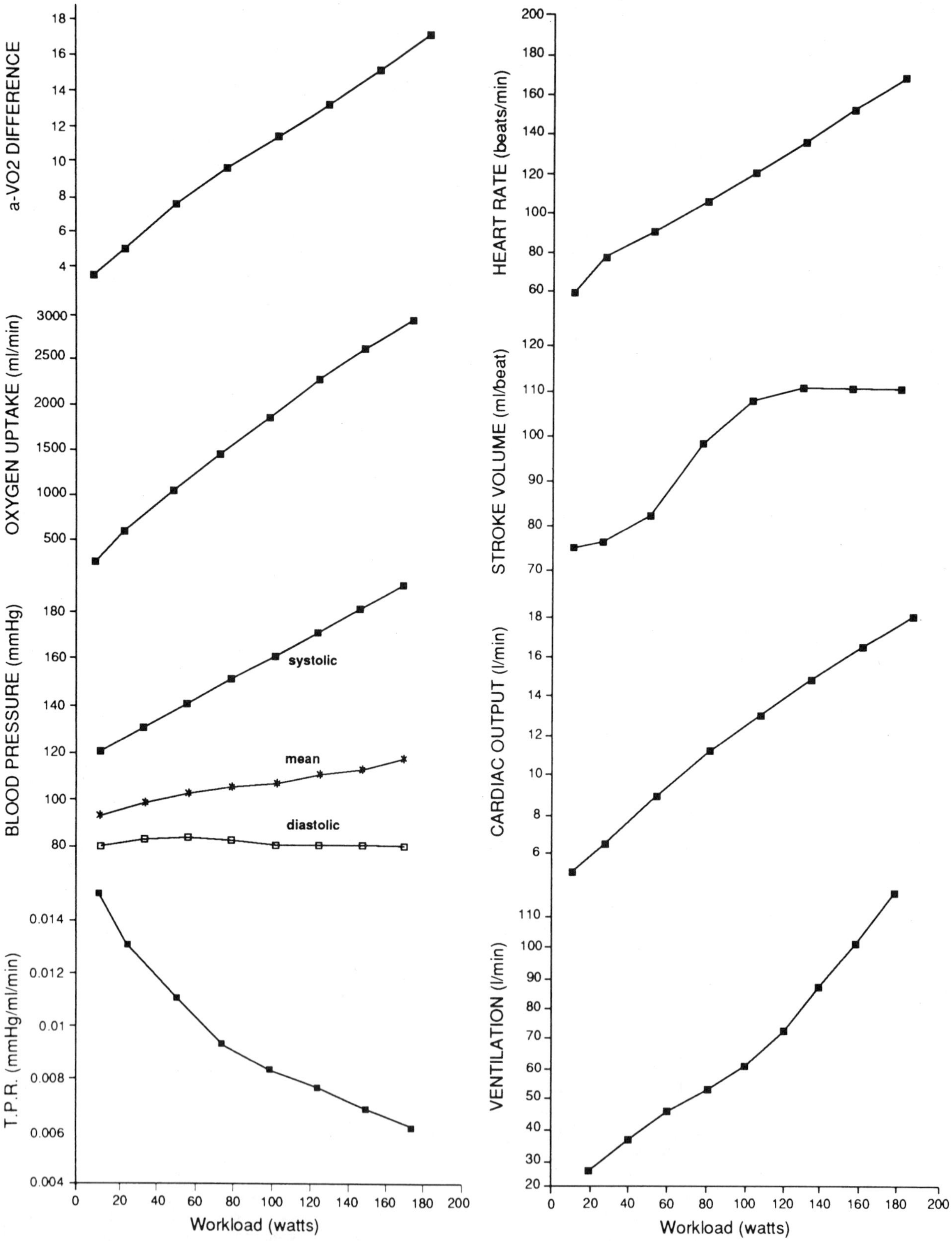

Figure 56–1. Basic hemodynamic and metabolic variables and the magnitude of the response from rest to a moderately high level of exercise. Units for a-VO_2 difference are mL of O_2/100 mL of blood. *Abbreviation*: a-VO_2, arteriovenous oxygen; TPR, total peripheral resistance. (From Myers JN: The physiology behind exercise testing. Prim Care 1994; 21:415–437.)

The usual measure of the capacity of the body to deliver and utilize oxygen is the maximal oxygen uptake (Vo_2 max), which can be expressed by the Fick principle:

$$Vo_2 \text{ max} = \text{maximal cardiac output} \times \text{maximal arteriovenous oxygen difference}$$

The cardiopulmonary limits (Vo_2 max) are therefore defined by a central component (cardiac output) that describes the capacity of the heart to function as a pump and peripheral factors (arteriovenous oxygen difference) that describe the capacity of the lung to oxygenate the blood delivered to it and the capacity of the working muscle to extract this oxygen from the blood. Figure 56–2 outlines the factors that affect cardiac output and arteriovenous oxygen difference. Exercise capacity can be limited in patients with cardiovascular or pulmonary disease by one or several of these links in the chain that determine blood flow to the tissues.

With exercise, blood flow is directed away from the inactive tissues to the active skeletal muscle. In the skeletal muscle, oxygen uptake depends on capillary density, diffusion, muscle fiber distribution, and the total oxidative potential of the muscle fibers. Cardiac output must closely match ventilation in the lung in order to deliver oxygenated blood to the working muscle. The matching of ventilation and cardiac output is determined by the ratio of alveolar ventilation to lung perfusion. Some patients with abnormal cardiac output responses to exercise (e.g., patients with chronic heart failure) or abnormal diffusion in the pulmonary vasculature (e.g., patients with chronic lung disease) have a mismatching of ventilation to perfusion, breathe inefficiently, and demonstrate exercise intolerance due to shortness of breath.

It is important to recognize that total body oxygen uptake and myocardial oxygen uptake are distinct in their determinants and in the way that they are measured or estimated (Table 56–1). Total body or ventilatory oxygen uptake is the amount of oxygen that is extracted from the inspired air as the body performs work. Myocardial oxygen uptake is the amount of oxygen consumed by the heart muscle. This distinction is important because patients with coronary artery disease are frequently limited in activity by myocardial oxygen demand and not by total body oxygen uptake. The determinants of myocardial oxygen uptake include intramyocardial wall tension (left ventricular pressure × end-diastolic volume), contractility, and heart rate. It has been shown that myocardial oxygen uptake is estimated accurately by the product of heart rate and systolic blood pressure (double product).[6] This relationship between myocardial oxygen demand and double product is valuable clinically because stable exercise-induced angina often occurs at the same myocardial oxygen demand (double product) and thus is one physiologic variable useful when therapy is evaluated.

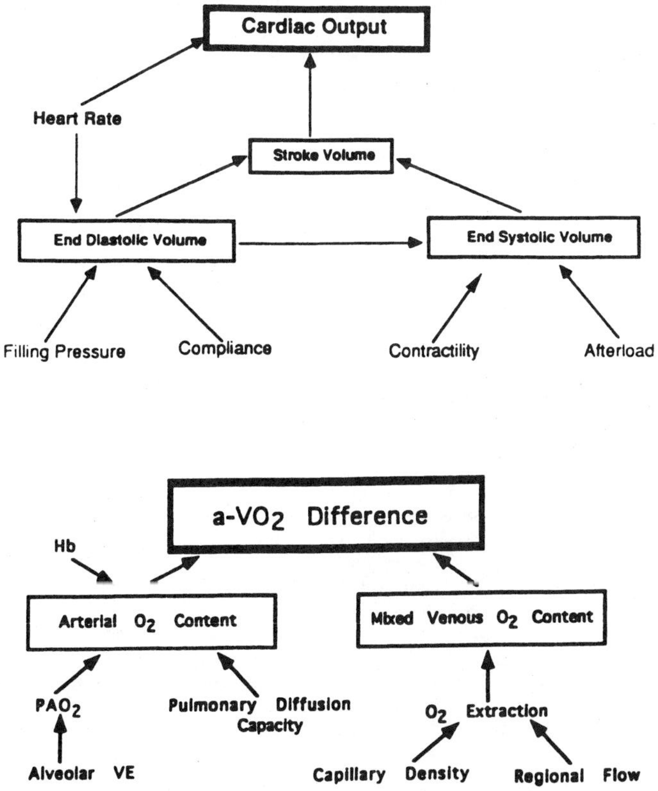

Figure 56–2. Central and peripheral determinants of maximal oxygen uptake. *Abbreviations*: a-VO_2, arteriovenous oxygen; Hb, hemoglobin; PAO_2, alveolar oxygen tension; VE, minute ventilation.

TABLE 56–1. TWO BASIC PRINCIPLES OF EXERCISE PHYSIOLOGY

Myocardial oxygen consumption	= Heart rate × systolic blood pressure (determinants include wall tension = left ventricular pressure × volume; contractility; and heart rate)
Ventilatory oxygen consumption (VO_2)	= External work performed, or cardiac output × a-VO_2 difference*

*The arteriovenous O_2 difference is approximately 15–17 mL O_2/100 mL at maximal exercise; therefore, VO_2 max is a noninvasive method for estimating cardiac output.
Abbreviations: a-VO_2, arteriovenous oxygen; VO_2, oxygen consumption.

PHYSICAL TRAINING

Regular exercise increases work capacity; hundreds of studies have documented greater exercise capacity among active persons than among sedentary individuals cross-sectionally or in comparisons of groups after a period of training. In general, patients with cardiovascular disease are equally able to benefit from exercise training. The magnitude of the improvement in exercise capacity with training varies widely, generally ranging from 5% to 25%, but increases as large as 50% have been reported. The degree of change in Vo_2 max depends primarily on the patient's initial state of fitness, but it is also affected by age and the type, frequency, and intensity of training. Vo_2 max may range as low as 10–15 mL/kg/min in patients with severe cardiovascular disease, and values as high as 80–90 mL/kg/min have been observed among élite endurance athletes.

The physiologic benefits of a training program can be classified as morphologic, hemodynamic, and metabolic (Table 56–2). Many animal studies have demonstrated significant morphologic changes with training, including myocardial hypertrophy with improved myocardial function, increases in coronary artery size, and increases in the myocardial capillary:fiber ratio. However, such changes have been difficult to demonstrate in humans.[7, 8] The major morphologic outcome of a training program in humans is probably an increase in cardiac size. Hemodynamic changes after training include reductions in heart rate at rest and any matched submaximal work load. For the patient with coronary artery disease, this is beneficial in that it results in a reduction in myocardial oxygen demand during activities of daily living. Other hemodynamic changes that have been demonstrated after training include reductions in blood pressure, increases in blood volume, and increases in maximal cardiac output; the latter underlies an increase in maximal oxygen uptake. In patients with heart disease, the major physiologic effects of training occur in the skeletal muscle. The metabolic capacity of the skeletal muscle is

TABLE 56–2. PHYSIOLOGIC ADAPTATIONS TO PHYSICAL TRAINING IN HUMANS

Morphologic Adaptations
Myocardial hypertrophy

Hemodynamic Adaptations
Increased blood volume
Increased end-diastolic volume
Increased stroke volume
Increased cardiac output
Reduced heart rate for any submaximal workload

Metabolic Adaptations
Increased mitochondrial volume and number
Greater muscle glycogen stores
Enhanced fat utilization
Enhanced lactate removal
Increased enzymes for aerobic metabolism
Increased maximal oxygen uptake

enhanced through increases in mitochondrial volume and number, capillary density, and oxidative enzyme content. These adaptations enhance perfusion and the efficiency of oxygen extraction.[9]

CARDIOVASCULAR EFFECTS OF IMMOBILITY

Data published since 1970 on the deleterious physiologic effects of bed rest (Table 56–3) have been an important stimulus for the benefits for cardiac rehabilitation. In contrast to the past, patients hospitalized for cardiac events today are encouraged to begin physical activities as soon as possible. Simply exposing the patient to orthostatic stress has a major influence on counteracting the negative physiologic effects of prolonged bed rest. Properly supervised early ambulation not only counteracts the numerous adverse effects of bed rest but also provides the patient with tangible affirmation of improvement, increases self-confidence, and provides hope for reasonable restoration of function. The following discussion outlines the physiologic effects of bed rest on the major systems.

Hemodynamic Effects

Most of the studies in this area have been performed among normal individuals subjected to 10–30 days of controlled bed rest. Reductions in maximal oxygen uptake, maximal cardiac output, stroke volume, and plasma volume after bed rest have been extensively described.[2, 10] Because of the rapid cardiovascular deconditioning, all levels of activity are accompanied by a greater myocardial oxygen demand. Considerable increases in heart rate at rest and for matched submaximal work levels (35–40 beats per minute during exercise) have been observed after various durations of bed rest.[2, 11]

Maximal heart rate is unaffected by bed rest.[12] Thus the reduction in cardiac output is due to a reduction in stroke volume, which occurs in proportion to the reduction in V_{O_2} max.[9, 12] Because of considerable reductions in muscle fiber size, the capillary:fiber ratio may actually increase after prolonged bed rest.[9] Oxygen extraction (a-V_{O_2} difference) therefore remains relatively normal despite marked reductions in oxidative enzyme capacity. Mean arterial pressure and systemic vascular resistance generally do not change significantly at rest or during submaximal levels of exercise after bed rest, although maximal systolic pressure is reduced.[2]

Cardiac Size and Function

Echocardiographic and radionuclide techniques have demonstrated reductions in resting end-diastolic volume after periods of bed rest in the order of 11%–16%.[1, 9, 13] Both heart rate and ejection fraction appear to increase in order to compensate for the reduction in ventricular filling. However, these mechanisms are inadequate for maintaining normal cardiac output during upright exercise.[1] From these observations, it has been suggested that no major changes in intrinsic myocardial contractility occur as a result of bed rest; rather, stroke volume is reduced because of reduced ventricular filling.

Orthostatic Intolerance

A frequent finding after a period of immobilization is orthostatic intolerance, or a transient decrease in blood pressure when the patient moves from the supine to the standing position, resulting in syncope. The cause of orthostatic intolerance is most likely a reduction in venous return due to some combination of (1) altered venous compliance; (2) loss of extracellular fluid volume; and possibly (3) a degree of autonomic dysfunction. Normally, heart rate increases and systemic vascular resistance decreases reflexively on standing, but after bed rest the balance between these two is often not adequate to maintain mean arterial pressure.

Thrombus Formation

Prolonged bed rest is thought to cause an increase in the risk of thrombus formation. With bed rest, the normal skeletal muscle "pump" that enhances venous return is absent; circulation is comparatively stagnant. Venous tone in the leg is diminished, and fluid loss increases blood viscosity. All of these factors are thought to account for a greater incidence of thrombus formation with prolonged bed rest.

Fluid Changes

In the supine position, there is an initial shift in the distribution of blood flow. A greater fraction of the blood volume is distributed to the thorax, which causes an increase in ventricular filling pressure. Among the hormonal manifestations of a greater filling pressure is diuresis. Greenleaf and associates reported losses of 500–1000 mL of fluid within 48 h of bed rest.[10] Other studies have reported significant though less drastic fluid losses.[1] Red blood cell volume remains relatively constant during bed rest[14]; thus, hematocrit and hemoglobin rise slightly and remain elevated for up to 30 days.[15] Although the functional significance of changes in blood volume among normal people after training has been well described,[16] less is known about the changes associated with bed rest in patients with cardiovascular disease who are exposed to bed rest.

TABLE 56–3. PHYSIOLOGIC CONSEQUENCES OF PROLONGED BED REST

1. Loss of muscle mass, strength, and endurance
2. Decreased plasma and blood volume
3. Decreased ventricular volume
4. Increased hematocrit and hemoglobin
5. Diuresis and natriuresis
6. Venous stasis
7. Bone demineralization
8. Increased heart rate at rest and submaximal levels of activity
9. Decreased resting and maximum stroke volume
10. Decreased maximum cardiac output
11. Decreased maximal oxygen uptake
12. Increased venous compliance
13. Increased risk of venous thrombosis and thromboembolism
14. Decreased orthostatic tolerance
15. Increased risk of atelectasis, pulmonary emboli

PHASES OF CARDIOVASCULAR REHABILITATION AFTER MYOCARDIAL INFARCTION

The typical phases included in rehabilitation are phase I, which includes the coronary care unit and inpatient care during the first few days after the event; phase II, which involves convalescence, an outpatient program, or a home program; and phase III, which is usually a longer term community-based or home program. The precise course of each program naturally depends on the individual's needs and clinical status. In addition, changes in health care economics have drastically altered the way in which cardiac rehabilitation is implemented. Hospital stays are shorter; progression through the program is more rapid; and much of "cardiac rehabilitation" as it was traditionally known has changed. Reimbursement patterns differ considerably from one state to another and from one program to another. With shorter periods of time for physicians to interact with and monitor patients, as well as cover educational materials adequately, there is a greater need for structured outpatient programs in the home or community.

Phase I: In-Hospital After a Myocardial Event

The purpose of the in-hospital phase is to counteract the negative effects of deconditioning rather than to promote training adaptations. It also provides an ideal time to begin education and psychosocial support. These first 3–5 days after a myocardial infarction or bypass surgery are critical for beginning these processes. The literature is replete with studies documenting the efficacy and safety of beginning activities and education soon after a coronary event in stable patients.[17] Initially, it is worthwhile for the primary physician to assess the patient's stability and the severity of the myocardial infarction.

Severity of the Myocardial Infarction. Increases in risk are generally associated with postinfarction ischemia and/or a history of prior myocardial infarction. In addition to ischemia, postinfarction chest pain can also be caused by anxiety and pericarditis. These factors can usually be distinguished by a careful history and an electrocardiogram (ECG). The ECG pattern predicts the clinical course and outcome surprisingly well. The greater the number of areas with Q waves and the greater the R-wave loss, the larger will be the myocardial infarct. Non–Q wave myocardial infarctions are usually less frequently associated with congestive heart failure or shock but they can also be complicated, particularly when a prior myocardial infarction has occurred. The concept that an initial subendocardial myocardial infarction is "incomplete" and poses an increased risk has not been substantiated. Inferior infarcts are usually smaller, result in less of a decline in ejection fraction, and are less likely to be associated with shock or congestive heart failure. Anterior infarcts are more likely to cause aneurysms and a greater decrease in ejection fraction.

The size of a myocardial infarction can be judged by the creatine kinase (CK) levels, particularly by the MB fraction released. CK has improved the laboratory diagnosis of myocardial infarction because it is highly specific for the myocardium. In general, the higher the amount of CK-MB released and the longer the CK level stays elevated, the larger will be the myocardial infarction. The occurrence of congestive heart failure, shock, or pericarditis is also an indicator of a relatively large myocardial infarct.

Complicated Vs. Uncomplicated Myocardial Infarctions. The rates of morbidity and mortality among post-infarction patients who have complicated courses are much higher than among those with uncomplicated myocardial infarctions. The criteria for a complicated myocardial infarction are presented in Table 56–4. The most important clinical predictors have been prior myocardial infarction and the presence of congestive heart failure and/or cardiogenic shock.

It is possible to assess risk at different temporal points from presentation in the emergency department, through the coronary care unit and pre-discharge time, and during later follow-up. However, the clinical picture changes over time, and a low-risk patient can become a high-risk patient and vice versa. These changes in risk are partially due to the vicissitudes of the atherosclerosis process, reformation of thrombus, interventions, and disease-host interactions. For instance, a patient may present with premature ventricular contractions that then can disappear or worsen; chest pain may come and go; the ECG may change; or the enzymes may have a late peak. This makes it difficult to classify a patient strictly as high or low risk; risk stratification often requires good judgment on the part of the patient's physician along with the nursing staff. In addition, changes signifying progress or regression of the patient's condition can change quickly during hospitalization after an event. The progressive steps very often must be adjusted for a particular patient.

TABLE 56–4. CRITERIA FOR CLASSIFICATION OF A COMPLICATED MYOCARDIAL INFARCTION*

1. Continued cardiac ischemia (e.g., angina, late enzyme rise, ST shifts)
2. Left ventricular failure (e.g., congestive heart failure, new murmurs, roentgenographic changes)
3. Cardiogenic shock
4. Important cardiac dysrhythmias (frequent premature ventricular contractions or atrial fibrillation)
5. Conduction disturbances (e.g., bundle branch block, atrioventricular block, hemiblock)
6. Severe pleurisy or pericarditis
7. Complicating illnesses
8. Marked creatine kinase rise without a noncardiac explanation or after thrombolysis
9. Cerebrovascular accident or transient ischemic attacks

*One or more criteria classify a myocardial infarction as complicated.

Patient Education. Education should be initiated before physical activities are begun; the patient may lack self-confidence and need affirmation that the activities are safe. Patient education during the acute phase usually consists of explanations about the coronary care unit, the cardiac rehabilitation program, symptoms, and the delivery of routine diagnostic and therapeutic modalities. The patient should be educated as to the limitations imposed by the disease, potential for improvement, and precautions to be observed. The program must be individualized for the patient depending on his or her psychosocial and medical status. The medical status is determined largely by the severity of the myocardial infarction, but the medical history must also be considered.

Early Ambulation. After stability is established, including the absence of congestive heart failure, dangerous arrhythmias, or unstable angina, formal ambulation may begin. Table 56–5 outlines one of the progressive approaches used for early ambulation after a complicated myocardial infarction. The protocol should begin with range-of-motion exercises and sitting with legs dangling and progress to ambulation and calisthenics. Blood pressure should remain within 20 mm Hg of the resting level during exercise, and heart rate should stay within 20 beats per minute (bpm) of the resting level. If complications arise, the activity should be stopped and later restarted at a lower level. The patient should be able to walk stairs before discharge, and by the time of discharge the patient should be able to perform activities of daily living independently (three to four metabolic equivalents [METs]). Because the effects of prolonged exercise on myocardial remodeling during the acute phase have not been carefully studied, it is prudent to avoid causing fatigue and to limit the duration of exercise by symptoms of fatigue and perceived effort.

Exercise Testing Before Hospital Discharge. The exercise test

TABLE 56–5. POST–COMPLICATED MYOCARDIAL INFARCTION PROTOCOL: EIGHT LEVELS OF ACTIVITY

Level	Activities	Nursing	Exceptions
I-CCU	<2 METs Strict bed rest Commode vs. bedpan Feed self if can sit up	Complete bed bath (patient may wash genitalia) *Exercise:* 5 × each b.i.d.: exercises 1–4 (see below)	Chest pain DOE Frequent PVCs HR greater than 100 Dizziness Diaphoresis
Teaching: Simple explanations of equipment and procedures. Reassurance!			
II-CCU	<2 METs Bed rest, up in chair 1× vs. dangle Bedside commode Feed self	Bed bath: Patient may wash hands, face, genitalia *Exercises:* Passive ROM b.i.d. 5 × each b.i.d.: exercises 1–5	Chest pain DOE Frequent PVCs HR greater than 100 Dizziness Diaphoresis
Teaching: If diagnosis known—simple explanation. "You had a heart attack," and the role that the cardiac rehabilitation team will play in education and increasing the patient's activity.			
III-CCU or Ward	2 METs Bed rest, up in chair 20 min t.i.d. Bedside commode Meals in chair	Bed bath: Patient may wash hands, face, genitalia *Exercises:* Active ROM all extremities 5 × each b.i.d.: exercises 1–6	Chest pain DOE Frequent PVCs HR greater than 100 Dizziness Diaphoresis
Teaching: Restate diagnosis with healing time: 3 months. Activity progression to be slow and steady with attention to pacing convalescence. Stress: Report any cardiac symptoms (e.g., chest, neck, jaw, arm, or abdominal discomfort).			
IV-Ward	3 METs Partial bath (in bed or at sink) Bed rest—bathroom privileges Up in chair as desired Walk about room	Patient not to wash back, legs, or feet *Exercises:* Active ROM b.i.d. 10 × each b.i.d.: exercises 1–6 Add 5 × each b.i.d.: exercise 7	Chest pain DOE Frequent PVCs HR greater than 110 Dizziness Diaphoresis
Teaching: Rehabilitation group discussion—family invited. 1. Anatomy and physiology of heart in relation to MI. 2. Convalescent care, activity progression, and risk factor management—HBP, diet, activity, smoking, stress reduction. 3. Diet class: low sodium and low cholesterol. Re-explain class information on one-to-one level. Begin medication teaching including use of nitroglycerin.			

after an acute myocardial infarction has been shown to be safe. When performed before discharge, it should be submaximal (five METs or less and not to exceed a Borg Scale level of 16). In many hospitals, a submaximal target heart rate is used (e.g., 110 bpm for patients taking beta blockers). The protocol should be modified, in view of the reduced exercise tolerance of most patients recovering from a myocardial infarction; individualized ramp or Naughton protocols are preferable.[18] Later, when return to full activities is intended, the test can be symptom and sign-limited. The predischarge test has many benefits, including clarification of the response to exercise, development of an exercise prescription, and recognition of the need for medications or interventions. It can have a beneficial psychologic impact on recovery and begins the rehabilitation process. The test is considered the first step in the outpatient cardiac rehabilitation exercise program.

The prognostic value of the predischarge test has been debated. Meta-analysis has shown that an abnormal exercise capacity or abnormal systolic blood pressure responses are better predictors of increased risk than is ST segment depression.[19] However, ST segment depression probably indicates increased risk in men who do not take digoxin and whose resting ECGs do not show extensive damage. The criterion of 2 mm or more of ST segment depression along with symptoms or abnormal hemodynamic responses appears to be useful for identifying high-risk patients who should be considered for cardiac catheterization and revascularization.

Return to Work and Recreational Activities. The economic burden of cardiovascular disability has been enormous, and a great deal of effort has been directed toward vocational rehabilitation. Postdischarge activity recommendations, including determination of disability, are among the biggest challenges facing the primary physician. Historically, the patient's return to work, ability to drive, and sexual activity have been based on clinical judgments rather than on physiologic assessments. These decisions should be based on the consequence of the coronary event (e.g., ischemia, symptoms of congestive failure, or dysrhythmias), the nature of the patient's occupational or recreational activities, and the response to the predischarge exercise test. In general, if patients do not exhibit any untoward responses to submaximal exercise testing and achieve five or more METs, it is unlikely that they will encounter difficulties during activities of daily living. More strenuous job or recreational requirements should not be initiated until a symptom-limited exercise test can be performed and exercise capacity can be determined and related to the desired physical activities of the patient.

Factors that influence a patient's return to work include age, work history, severity of cardiac damage, financial compensation for illness, employer's ignorance about the patient's abilities, termination of employment, and, most important, the patient's perception of his or her health status. Efforts of the rehabilitation team to develop a positive attitude and a sense of well-being for the patient may facilitate appropriate vocational adjustments. The physician's attitude

TABLE 56–5. POST–COMPLICATED MYOCARDIAL INFARCTION PROTOCOL: EIGHT LEVELS OF ACTIVITY *Continued*

Level	Activities	Nursing	Exceptions
V-Ward	4 METs Up in room Walk to TV room and back after warm-up exercises Up in chair 5 × each b.i.d.: exercise 8	Chair shower *Exercises:* Active ROM b.i.d. 10 × each b.i.d.: exercises 1–7	Chest pain DOE Frequent PVCs HR greater than 110 Dizziness Diaphoresis
Teaching: Taking pulse. Explain medications, beta blockers and digitalis (if applicable), action of medications. Reasons for slow, steady activity increase over 3-month period. Report any problems noted as activity increases (e.g., [1] chest, neck, jaw, arm, abdominal pain, and/or pressure or discomfort; and [2] shortness of breath).			
VI-Ward	<5 METs Ward ambulation Work toward walking around floor square nonstop (1/6 mile) Start with 1 leg of square—gradually increase pace before distance 12 × around = mile)	Chair shower *Exercises:* 10 × each b.i.d.: exercises 1–8	Chest pain DOE Frequent PVCs HR greater than 110 Dizziness Diaphoresis
Teaching: Reinforce activity progression. Do not leave ward unless pushed in a wheelchair (needs ward nurse knowledge and aid to leave ward). No patient with a cardiac problem is to push another patient!			
VII-Ward	5 METs Ambulate off ward Walk up one flight of stairs with team member	Shower *Exercises:* 10 × each b.i.d.: exercises 1–9 Frequent PVCs Dizziness Diaphoresis	Chest pain DOE HR greater than 120

Exercises for post-MI protocols (numbers used above in "Nursing" column)

1. Foot circles
2. Ankle pumps
3. Toe flexion and extension
4. Neck exercises
   a. Head nod, chin on chest, then look to sky
   b. Head tilt: lean left ear on left shoulder, then right ear to right shoulder
   c. Head turn: look to left, then right with chin over shoulder
   d. Five complete head circles, both right and left
5. Quadriceps setting, thigh press and knee locked
6. Shoulder exercises
   a. Shrug both shoulders up toward ears
   b. Move each shoulder in a circle forward and then backward
   c. Lift arms straight up over head until elbow is straight; alternate arms
7. Bring alternate knee to chest
8. Straight leg lifts, alternate legs
9. Side bends

Abbreviations: ROM, range of motion; DOE, dyspnea on exertion; PVC, premature ventricular contraction; MI, myocardial infarction; HR, heart rate; MET, metabolic equivalent. The physician is to draw a line down through levels, date, and initial order. The patient may be held at any level.

also greatly affects the patient's return to work; encouragement can be very beneficial.

MEDICAL EVALUATION FOR EXERCISE

Hospital admission for an acute myocardial infarction is a stressful experience with a powerful impact. However, hospital discharge can be equally stressful after the patient has relied on the highly protective hospital support systems. Discharge into an uncertain future and to a home and work setting in which the patient may be considered a helpless invalid can be as damaging to the patient's self-esteem as the acute event itself. The physician is faced with the difficult tasks of not only supervising the physical recovery of the patient but also maintaining morale, providing education, helping the family cope and provide support, and facilitating the return to a gratifying lifestyle.

Not all patients need a formal exercise program, but most patients can benefit in some way from it. Some patients benefit from exercising with a group, whereas others do better by themselves. The approach to each patient must be individualized because each patient's reaction to problems and needs differs. The following section outlines one approach to assess patients, placing them in a "niche" so one knows how to react to their symptoms and to their test results. For every clinical situation there are exceptions: the high-risk patient who outlives his or her physician, the patient with minimal myocardium remaining who can run a marathon, and the low-risk patient who dies. Biologic systems are complex, and all physicians continue to learn with each patient they treat.

History and Physical Examination

The tools for assessment begin with the history and physical examination. The first step in evaluating patients for cardiac rehabilitation is to determine whether the coronary heart disease is stable. "Stability" is determined primarily by the presence or absence of myocardial ischemia, congestive heart failure, and dysrhythmias. The hallmark symptom of ischemia is chest pain. Most patients have chest pains of some type; they are frequently ignored. Once told about heart disease, the patient's routine pains can become frightening. It is important to separate nonischemic from ischemic chest pains. Chest pain that occurs only at rest, only after exercise, or is sharp is usually not attributable to ischemia, and not all chest pains should be called angina pectoris. Angina becomes unstable when it changes in pattern (i.e., occurs more frequently, at rest, or at lower workloads). Increasing symptoms of congestive heart failure include sudden weight gain, edema in the lower extremities, dyspnea on exertion, and paroxysmal nocturnal dyspnea. Combinations of both ischemia and congestive heart failure are difficult to manage. Ischemia can cause transient congestive heart failure.

If the patient is stable, further assessment can proceed. In general, patients can be categorized as those with myocardial damage, those with myocardial ischemia, or those with both. Initially, the ischemic threshold should be determined by the onset of angina pectoris or ST segment depression at a particular heart rate, double product, or workload. Once this threshold is clarified, the amount of mechanical damage should be determined. Clinical clues that suggest that the patient has myocardial damage include a history of congestive heart failure, cardiogenic shock, a previous myocardial infarction, a large anterior myocardial infarction, cardiomegaly, a large CK elevation, multiple Q waves, or underlying problems such as cardiomyopathy or valvular heart disease. These patients must be watched for signs and symptoms of congestive heart failure, whereas patients with ischemia usually do not require such observation. Patients with myocardial damage are limited by reduced maximal cardiac output, which leads to early fatigue and pulmonary symptoms, rather than chest pain. A strong effort should be made to explain the symptoms related to congestive heart failure. In the patient with myocardial infarction, the symptoms could be caused by mitral valve insufficiency secondary either to papillary muscle dysfunction or rupture or to a dilated mitral annulus. Secondary processes include cardiomyopathy or valvular defect. A rare explanation is ventricular septal defect resulting from septal infarction.

In addition to myocardial ischemia and dysfunction, the other key features of heart disease to consider are arrhythmias, valvular function, and exercise capacity. These five features are important because they determine the prognosis as well as the manifestation of symptoms. Patients should be evaluated for these features for optimal management, including individualization of the rehabilitation program.

The ECG, chest roentgenogram, and exercise test are next in importance. The exercise test is the key to prescribing exercise. Specialized tests, including echocardiography and nuclear and cardiac catheterization, can be used to confirm impressions, clarify incongruous clinical situations, or identify coronary pathoanatomic patterns that necessitate revascularization. Table 56–6 provides an assessment of the key features of heart disease and the relative value of the various means of assessment.

Rehabilitation in Patients With Chronic Heart Failure

In the mid-1980s and earlier, stable chronic heart failure (CHF) was considered by many authorities to be a contraindication to participation in an exercise program. Today it is known that selected patients with CHF derive considerable benefits from cardiac rehabilitation. With improvements in therapy (i.e., thrombolytics, ACE inhibitors), survival among patients with CHF has improved considerably, and more of these patients are available as candidates for rehabilitation. The incidence of CHF is currently about 500,000 per year in the United States. Studies performed at Duke University and in Europe suggest that the major physiologic benefit from training in CHF occurs in the skeletal muscles rather than in the heart itself.[20, 21]

The clinical approach to the patient with CHF who is considered for a rehabilitation program is similar to that for the post–myocardial infarction patient described earlier, although several important differences are worth noting. The risk for sudden cardiac death is higher in patients with CHF relative to patients with normal left ventricular function. This is the population in whom sudden, fatal arrhythmia occurs most often. There are a greater number of medications to be considered that can influence exercise responses, including vasoactive, antiarrhythmic, inotropic, and, in recent years, beta blocking agents. Exercise capacity tends to be significantly lower than in the typical patient with coronary disease. Numerous hemodynamic abnormalities underlie the reduced exercise capacity commonly observed in CHF, including impaired heart rate responses, inability to distribute cardiac output normally, abnormal arterial vasodilatory capacity, abnormal cellular metabolism in the skeletal muscle, higher-than-normal systemic vascular resistance, higher-than-normal pulmonary pressures, and ventilatory abnormalities that increase the work of breathing and cause exertional dyspnea.[22, 23] Studies using magnetic resonance imaging suggest that some of these abnormalities can be improved by exercise training.[21]

Many patients with reduced left ventricular function who are clinically stable and have reduced exercise tolerance are candidates for exercise programs. It is often necessary to exclude patients with signs and symptoms of right-sided failure or to treat them judiciously before entry into a program. An exercise test is particularly important before initiating the program to ensure safety of participation. Rhythm abnormalities, exertional hypotension, or other signs of instability should be ruled out. Expired gas exchange measurements are particularly informative in this group because they provide an improvement in accuracy and permit an assessment of ventilatory abnormalities that are common in this condition.[22, 23] ECG monitoring

TABLE 56–6. EVALUATION OF THE KEY FEATURES OF HEART DISEASE

Key Features	History	Physical Examination	Chest Radiograph	ECG	Exercise Test	Echo-cardiogram	Nuclear Cardiology Thallium/RNV		Holter Monitoring	Cardiac Catheterization
Myocardial dysfunction	++++	+++	+++	++	++	+++	++	+++	+	++++
Myocardial ischemia	++++	++	+	+++	++++	+	+++ (with exercise)	++	+	++++
Functional capacity	+++	+++	++	+	++++	++	+	+	+	++
Atrial fibrillation and ventricular dysrhythmias	+++	+++	+	+++	++	+++	+	+	++++	+ (EP for VT+++)
Valvular function	++++	++++	++	+++	++	++++	+	+	+	++++
Cost	*	*	*	*	**	***	***	**	**	****
Risk	*	*	**	*	***	*	**	*	*	****

Abbreviations: ECG, electrocardiogram; EP, electrophysiology studies; VT, sustained ventricular tachycardia; RNV, radionuclide ventriculography. *Symbols:* ++++, very helpful part of assessment (high yield of information) or high benefit; +, least helpful (low yield of information) or low benefit; *, low cost or risk; ****, high cost or risk.

Need for test determined by a physician's assessment of the ratio of benefit to cost and risk.

Adapted from Froelicher VF, Atwood JE: Cardiac Disease: A Logical Approach Considering DRGS. Chicago: Year Book Medical, 1986.

during exercise is more often indicated in this group. Attention should be paid to daily changes in body weight, rhythm status, and symptoms.

There are increasing numbers of patients who have undergone cardiac transplantation for end-stage heart failure, and today approximately three quarters of these patients remain alive after 5 years.[24, 25] The question has been raised as to whether these patients can also benefit from exercise training. Because the transplant patient's heart is denervated, some intriguing hemodynamic responses to exercise are observed. The heart is not responsive to the normal actions of the parasympathetic and sympathetic systems. The absence of vagal tone explains the high resting heart rates in these patients (100–110 bpm) and the relatively slow adaptation of the heart to a given amount of submaximal work.[26] This slows the delivery of oxygen to the working tissue, contributing to an earlier-than-normal metabolic acidosis and hyperventilation during exercise. Maximal heart rate is lower in transplant patients than in normal persons, which contributes to a reduction in cardiac output and exercise capacity. Only a few reports in the literature discuss the effects of training after cardiac transplantation. These studies have demonstrated increases in peak oxygen uptake, reductions in resting and submaximal heart rates, and improved ventilatory responses to exercise.[27] Whether the major physiologic adaptation to exercise is improved cardiac function, changes in skeletal muscle metabolism, or simply an improvement in strength remains to be determined.[27] Psychosocial studies of rehabilitation in transplant patients are lacking, as are the effects of regular exercise on survival.

Contraindications to Exercise Training

Absolute contraindications are those known or suspected conditions that prevent the patient from participating in an exercise program. Absolute contraindications include unstable angina pectoris, dissecting aortic aneurysm, complete heart block, uncontrolled hypertension, decompensated congestive heart failure, uncontrolled dysrhythmias, thrombophlebitis, and other complicating illnesses. In some conditions, contraindications are relative; that is, the benefits outweigh the risks involved if the patient exercises with proper supervision. Relative contraindications include frequent premature ventricular contractions, controlled dysrhythmias, intermittent claudication, metabolic disorders, and moderate anemia or pulmonary disease. Studies show that if these contraindications are considered, the incidence of exertion-related cardiac arrest in cardiac rehabilitation programs is extremely low and, because of the availability of rapid defibrillation, death rarely occurs.

Outpatient Cardiac Rehabilitation (Phase II)

There have been multiple approaches to outpatient rehabilitation. Typically, this phase begins 1–2 weeks after discharge from the hospital and may last from 1 to 4 months. Most commonly, patients attend group exercise sessions three times per week; however, in practice, frequency of exercise is often modified by the individual patient's overall goals, functional capabilities, reimbursement, proximity to the hospital or clinic, and personal commitment. The first few exercise sessions after hospital discharge usually emphasize warm-up and cool-down activities with only a modest aerobic component; some programs use direct electrocardiographic telemetry for approximately six sessions in all patients to ensure safety. There is less emphasis today on the need for direct ECG monitoring than in the past (see later discussion). A symptom-limited maximal exercise test is usually recommended approximately 6 weeks after hospitalization to determine appropriate activity limitations.

Changes in reimbursement patterns have changed phase II programs more than other components of cardiac rehabilitation. In some states, only a few exercise or educational sessions are reimbursed. The transition from an outpatient to a home-based maintenance program occurs more rapidly. Randomized trials have demonstrated that patients can return to work quickly and safely during the rehabilitation and that participation in rehabilitation facilitates this process.[28] Debusk and colleagues at Stanford University have advocated home exercise that is either unmonitored or monitored via telephone or microprocessor. Safety and efficacy in these home programs have been shown to be similar to more conventional programs.[29]

Safety. The safety of outpatient cardiac rehabilitation has been well documented in both the United States and Europe. In 1986, Van Camp and Peterson sent questionnaires to 167 randomly selected cardiac rehabilitation centers.[30] Data were gathered on more than 51,000 patients who exercised more than 2 million hours from January 1980 to December 1984. During this time there were only 21 cardiac resuscitations (3 of which failed) and eight myocardial infarctions. This amounts to 8.9 cardiac arrests, 3.4 myocardial infarctions, and 1.3 fatalities per million hours of patient exercise. Surprisingly, ECG monitoring had little influence on complications, which suggests that the additional expense of telemetry may not be necessary. However, appropriate medical personnel must be available to resuscitate patients who do suffer an untoward event.

Monitoring in Outpatient Rehabilitation. It is now recognized that only a small percentage of patients require continuous ECG monitoring during exercise. Efforts to reduce the cost of rehabilitation in addition to the recognition that most patients can exercise quite safely without continuous telemetry have brought about this change. Table 56–7 lists the criteria for ECG monitoring outlined in the American College of Cardiology's Position Statement on Cardiac Rehabilitation.[31]

Phase III: Maintenance Program

Progression to an out-of-hospital maintenance program is desirable after patients have participated in a phase II program for a suitable period. The period of time required before patients move to a maintenance program can vary considerably, depending on reimbursement, patient stability, exercise capacity, and individual patient needs, but it rarely exceeds 12 weeks. The purpose of phase III is to maintain training adaptations, to prevent recurrence of events or symptoms, and to maintain progress. It is important that the patient understand how to monitor his or her own exercise intensity, understand how to recognize symptoms, and have a basic knowledge of the particular disease and medications.

It is useful to perform an exercise test before the maintenance program in order to provide an outgoing exercise prescription, confirm the safety of exercise for a given patient, and assess risk for future cardiac events. Funding for this phase must often be borne by the patient because most types of health insurance do not cover it; however, mechanisms for follow-up should be in place.

TABLE 56–7. AMERICAN COLLEGE OF CARDIOLOGY CRITERIA FOR ELECTROCARDIOGRAPHIC MONITORING DURING CARDIAC REHABILITATION

1. Severely depressed left ventricular function (ejection fraction under 30)
2. Resting complex ventricular arrhythmia (Lown type 4 or 5)
3. Ventricular arrhythmias appearing or increasing with exercise
4. Decrease in systolic blood pressure with exercise
5. Survivors of sudden cardiac death
6. Patients following myocardial infarction complicated by congestive heart failure, cardiogenic shock, and/or serious ventricular arrhythmias
7. Patients with severe coronary artery disease and marked exercise-induced ischemia
8. Inability to self-monitor intensity due to physical or intellectual impairment

Exercise Prescription for Phase II and Phase III Patients

The American College of Sports Medicine defines exercise prescription as ". . . the process whereby a person's recommended regimen of physical activity is designed in a systematic and individualized manner."[32] An "individualized manner" implies specific strategies to optimize return to work or activities of daily living, reduction of risk factors for future cardiac events, and maximization of the patient's capacity to maintain an active lifestyle. The development of an appropriate exercise prescription to meet the individual patient's needs has a sound scientific foundation,[17, 32] but there is also an art to effective exercise programming. The "art" of exercise prescription has become increasingly important in this era of cost containment (shorter rehabilitation), surgical and technologic advances (larger numbers of transplant, pacemaker, or CHF participants than ever before), and the multitude of new medicines available. There is no single program that is best for all patients or even one patient over time; capabilities, vocational needs, and expectations differ among patients and can change with the passing of time. Thus the art of exercise prescription relies on the physician's or exercise physiologist's abilities to synthesize the patient's pathophysiologic, psychosocial, and vocational factors and to tailor them to the patient's needs and realistic goals. A final but important consideration is the selection of activities that the individual enjoys and that will provide the best chance that he or she will continue to perform safely after the formal rehabilitation program ends.

Principles of Exercise Prescription. *Training* implies adaptations of the body to the demands placed on it. A training effect is best measured as an increase in maximal ventilatory oxygen uptake, but not all institutions have gas exchange equipment, and there are many other ways of quantifying functional outcomes of rehabilitation. For example, some patients after rehabilitation may be better suited to carry out submaximal levels of activity for longer periods, remain independent, continue working, or rejoin their friends on the golf course. All of these can be important goals for a given patient and may occur even with a minimal change in maximal oxygen uptake.

The major ingredients of the exercise prescription are the frequency, intensity, duration, mode, and rate of progression. In general, these principles apply for both the patient with heart disease and the healthy adult; however, the ways in which they are applied differ. On the basis of numerous studies performed since the 1950s, it is generally accepted that increases in maximal oxygen uptake are achieved if a person exercises dynamically for a period ranging from 15–60 minutes, three to five times per week, at an intensity equivalent to 50%–80% of the maximum capacity. "Dynamic" exercises are those that employ large muscle groups in a rhythmic manner, such as treadmill walking, cycle ergometry, rowing, stepping, and arm ergometry. Short warm-up and cool-down periods are strongly encouraged for participants in cardiac rehabilitation programs. Again, however, an effective exercise prescription must consider the patient's goals, health status, and availability of time, in addition to practical considerations such as cost, availability of equipment, and facilities.

Much of the art of exercise prescription clearly involves individualizing the exercise intensity. Typically, exercise intensity is expressed as a percentage of maximal capacity, either in absolute terms (i.e., workload or watts) or in relation to the maximal heart rate, maximal oxygen uptake, or perceived effort. Training benefits have been shown to occur with the use of exercise intensities ranging from 40% to 85% of maximal oxygen uptake, which are generally equivalent to 50%–90% of the maximal heart rate. However, the intensity that a given individual can maintain for a specified period of time varies widely. In general, the most appropriate intensity for most patients in phase II and III rehabilitation programs is 50%–70% of maximal capacity. The actual prescribed exercise intensity for the patient should naturally depend on goals, on health status, on length of time since infarction or surgery, on symptoms, and on initial state of fitness.

Training is a general phenomenon; there is no true threshold beyond which patients achieve benefits. Thus as long as patients exercise safely, setting the exercise intensity is a less rigid practice than it was years ago. In addition, the patient's ability to tolerate activities can change daily. Other factors, such as time of day, environment, and time since medications were taken can influence the patient's response to exercise, and the exercise prescription must be adjusted accordingly. It is also useful to employ a window of intensity that ranges approximately 10% above and 10% below the desired level.

The graded exercise test is the foundation on which a safe and effective exercise prescription is based. To achieve a desired training intensity, oxygen uptake or some estimation of it must be quantified during a maximal or symptom-limited exercise test. Because heart rate is easily measured and is linearly related to oxygen uptake, it has become a standard by which training intensity is estimated during training sessions. The most useful method is known as the *heart rate reserve*. This method uses a percentage of the difference between maximal heart rate and resting heart rate and adds this value to the resting heart rate. For example, for a patient who achieves a maximal heart rate of 150 bpm, has a resting heart rate of 70 bpm, and wishes to exercise at an intensity equivalent to 60% of maximum,

Maximal heart rate	=	150 bpm
− Resting heart rate	=	70
= Heart rate range		80
× desired intensity	=	60%
		48
+ Resting heart rate	=	70
= Training heart rate		118

A reasonable training heart rate range for this individual would be 115–125 bpm. This is also referred to as the Karvonen formula and is reliable in patients with normal sinus rhythm whose measurements of resting and maximal heart rates are accurate.[33] An estimated target heart rate for exercise should be supplemented by considering the patient's MET level relative to his or her maximum, the perceived exertion, and symptoms.

CLOSING COMMENT

Early and progressive ambulation of patients after a myocardial infarction is now considered routine care. Despite the advent of new therapies in cardiovascular medicine, cardiac rehabilitation maintains an important place in reducing morbidity and mortality.[4, 5] The controlled trials, when combined, demonstrate that the efficacy of rehabilitation in reducing mortality is similar to the best medical interventions.[34] Moreover, cardiac rehabilitation has redirected interest to humanistic concerns, providing a balance to the emphasis on complex technology. It also provides an ideal environment for patient supervision and for ensuring stability after an interventional procedure. Data suggest that cardiac rehabilitation is economically sound.[35, 36]

Medicine is presently experiencing an evolution toward technologfical efficacy and outcomes assessment. Health economists and legislators are reexamining the value placed on all forms of medical care. Although this movement has changed the way that cardiac rehabilitation is implemented, studies have confirmed its value. Some of the ways in which the current economic environment has changed cardiac rehabilitation include a lessening of direct ECG monitoring, shorter hospital stays, and a more rapid progression to home programs. The frequency of interventions has lessened the morbidity associated with myocardial infarction. Modifications in cardiac rehabilitation have prompted maximal participation by the greatest number of patients possible. Data on efficacy, safety, and technologic advances in the treatment of cardiovascular disease have changed cardiac rehabilitation in such a way that a wider range of patients can benefit from these services than in the past. For example, patients with stable CHF, once excluded from cardiac rehabilitation programs, are now thought to be among those who benefit the most. Pacemaker, post-transplantation, post-bypass, post-valvular surgery, and claudicant patients now make up a significant fraction of the patients in many programs. Despite this fact, most eligible patients (as many as 90%) fail to receive these services. It is clear that not all patients need cardiac rehabilitation, but directing these services to patients who need them the most remains one of the important challenges for the field.

Lastly, there has been a change in the public health care message toward physical "activity" as inherently beneficial regardless of objective measurements of "fitness."[37] This has caused a shift in focus from morbidity, mortality, and exercise capacity to issues related to maintaining an active lifestyle and optimizing the patient's capacity to perform the physical challenges offered by occupational or recreational activities. Further studies on costs, benefits, and other outcomes should solidify the role of cardiac rehabilitation in the clinical management of patients with cardiovascular disease.

REFERENCES

1. Hung J, Goldwater D, Convertino VA, et al: Mechanisms for decreased exercise capacity after bed rest in normal middle-aged men. Am J Cardiol 1983; 51:344–348.
2. Saltin B, Blomqvist G, Mitchell JH, et al: Response to exercise after bed rest and after training. Circulation 1968; 38(suppl 7):1–78.
3. Wittels EH, Hay JW, Gotto AJ: Medical costs of coronary artery disease in the United States. Am J Cardiol 1990; 65:432–440.
4. Oldridge NB, Guyatt GH, Fischer ME, Rimm A: Cardiac rehabilitation after myocardial infarction: combined experience of randomized clinical trials. JAMA 1988; 260:945–950.
5. O'Connor GT, Buring JE, Yusuf S, et al: An overview of randomized trials of rehabilitation with exercise after myocardial infarction. Circulation 1989; 80:234–244.
6. Nelson RR, Gobel FL, Jorgensen CR, et al: Hemodynamic predictors of myocardial oxygen consumption during static and dynamic exercise. Circulation 1974; 50:1179–1189.
7. Froelicher VF, Myers J, Follansbee WP, Labovitz AJ: Exercise and the Heart. St. Louis: CV Mosby, 1993.
8. Froelicher VF, Jensen D, Genter F, et al: A randomized trial of exercise training in patients with coronary heart disease. JAMA 1984; 252:1291–1297.
9. Rowell LB: Human Circulation: Regulation During Physical Stress, pp 257–286. New York: Oxford University Press, 1986.
10. Greenleaf JE, Bernauer EM, Juhos LT, et al: Effects of exercise on fluid exchange and body composition in man during 14-day bed rest. J Appl Physiol 1977; 43:126–132.
11. Taylor HL, Henschel A, Brozek J, et al: Effects of bed rest on cardiovascular function and work performance. J Appl Physiol 1949; 2(5):223–239.
12. Saltin B, Rowell LB: Functional adaptations to physical activity and inactivity. Fed Proc 1980; 39:1506–1516.
13. Blomqvist CG, Stone HL: Cardiovascular adjustments to gravitational stress. *In* Shepherd JT, Abbound FM (eds): Handbook of Physiology: The Cardiovascular System, pp 1025–1063. Bethesda, MD: American Physiological Society, 1983.
14. Greenleaf JE, Brock PJ, Haines RF, et al: Effect of hypovolemia, infusion, and oral rehydration on plasma electrolytes, ADH, renin activity, and $+G_z$ tolerance. Aviat Space Environ Med 1977; 48:693–700.
15. Morse BS: Erythrokinetic changes in man associated with bed rest. Lectures in Aerospace Medicine, 6th series. National Technical Information Service No. AD-665. 1967; 107:240–254. Cited in Sandler H: Effects of bed rest and weightlessness on the heart. *In* Bourne GH (ed): Hearts and Heart-Like Organs, vol 2, pp 120–126. New York: Academic Press, 1980.
16. Covertino VA: Blood volume: its adaptation to endurance training. Med Sci Sports Exerc 1991; 23:1338–1348.
17. American Association of Cardiovascular and Pulmonary Rehabilitation: Guidelines for Cardiac Rehabilitation Programs, pp 77–104. Champaign, IL: Human Kinetics, 1991.
18. Myers J, Froelicher VF: Optimizing the exercise test for pharmacological investigations. Circulation 1990; 82:1839–1846.
19. Chang JA, Froelicher VF: Clinical and exercise test markers of prognosis in patients with stable coronary artery disease. Curr Probl Cardiol 1994; 19:533–588.
20. Sullivan MJ, Higgenbotham MB, Cobb FR: Exercise training in patients with severe left ventricular dysfunction: hemodynamic and metabolic effects. Circulation 1988; 78:506–515.
21. Adamopoulos S, Coats AJS, Brunotte F, et al: Physical training improves skeletal muscle metabolism in patients with chronic heart failure. J Am Coll Cardiol 1993; 21:1101–1106.
22. Myers J, Froelicher VF: Hemodynamic determinants of exercise capacity in chronic heart failure. Ann Intern Med 1991; 115:377–386.
23. Myers J: Ventilatory mechanisms of exercise intolerance in chronic heart failure. Am Heart J 1992; 124:710–719.
24. Fragomeni LS, Kaye MP: The Registry of the International Society of Heart Transplantation: fifth official report—1988. J Heart Transplant 1988; 7:249–252.
25. Kriett JM, Kaye MP: The Registry of the International Society of Heart and Lung Transplantation: eighth official report—1991. J Heart Lung Transplant 1991; 10:491–498.
26. Stinson EB, Griepp RL, Schroeder JS, et al: Hemodynamic observations one and two years after cardiac transplantation in man. Circulation 1972; 14:1181–1193.
27. Shephard RJ: Responses of the cardiac transplant patient to exercise and training. Exerc Sport Sci Rev 1992; 20:297–320.
28. Dennis C, Houston-Miller N, Schwartz RG, et al: Early return to work after complicated myocardial infarction: results of a randomized trial. JAMA 1988; 260:214–220.
29. DeBusk RF, Haskell WL, Miller NH, et al: Medically directed at-home rehabilitation soon after clinically uncomplicated acute myocardial infarction: a new model for patient care. Am J Cardiol 1985; 55:251.
30. Van Camp SP, Peterson RA: Cardiovascular complications of outpatient cardiac rehabilitation programs. JAMA 1986; 256:1160–1163.
31. American College of Cardiology: Position report on cardiac rehabilitation. J Am Coll Cardiol 1986; 7:451–453.
32. American College of Sports Medicine: Guidelines for Exercise Testing and Exercise Prescription, 5th ed. Philadelphia: Lea & Febiger, 1995.
33. Karvonen M, Kentala K, Musta O: The effects of training heart rate: a longitudinal study. Ann Med Exp Biol Fenn 1957; 35:307–315.
34. May GS, Eberlein KA, Furberg CD, et al: Secondary prevention after myocardial infarction: a review of long-term trials. Prog Cardiovasc Dis 1982; 24:331–352.
35. Oldridge N, Furlong W, Feeny D, et al: Economic evaluation of cardiac rehabilitation soon after acute myocardial infarction. Am J Cardiol 1993; 72:154–161.
36. Ades PA, Huang D, Weaver SO: Cardiac rehabilitation predicts lower rehospitalization costs. Am Heart J 1992; 123:916–921.
37. Blair SN: Physical activity, fitness, and coronary artery disease. *In* Bouchard C, Shephard RJ, Stephens T (eds): Physical Activity, Fitness, and Health, pp 579–590. Champaign, IL: Human Kinetics, 1994.

57 Treatment of Pericardial Disease

Ralph Shabetai, MD

Treatment of pericardial disease and pericardial heart disease can be simple and rewarding, as in the case of acute fibrinous pericarditis with a nonsteroidal anti-inflammatory agent, or difficult and frustrating, requiring numerous modifications depending upon the clinical response, as in the case of an intractable course of recurrent pericarditis. The clinician responsible for treating pericardial disease is handicapped by the paucity of data based on large placebo-controlled multicenter trials, which forces a considerable degree of reliance on the clinician's own judgment. The correct decision between treatment with prednisone and a nonsteroidal agent for severe acute or recurrent pericarditis is one upon which not only the response of the disease but the general well-being of the patient may depend.

Physicians lack authoritative data upon which to base a decision of whether to evacuate a large asymptomatic pericardial effusion of unknown etiology. In the treatment of cardiac tamponade or removal of pericardial fluid for other indications, the decision of whether to perform pericardiocentesis or subxiphoid pericardiotomy is often best based on local experience. Likewise, pericardiocentesis can be performed with the use of fluoroscopy or echocardiographic visualization. Consensus exists among clinicians with regard to the need for pericardiectomy for severe constrictive pericarditis, but the role for this operation is far from clear in the instances of recurrent pericarditis, milder constrictive pericarditis, and end-stage pericarditis. Limitation of exercise capacity may be modest or unnoticed in patients with moderately severe constrictive pericarditis, and liver function may remain normal in spite of raised hepatic venous pressure. There remains the question, however, of whether the operation will become more difficult and dangerous the longer it is postponed. Similarly, many internists, if not surgeons, recognize that pericardiectomy for very late-stage constrictive pericarditis is not only dangerous but futile. Exact guidelines regarding these and other therapeutic dilemmas have not been published. This chapter is therefore an attempt to summarize what has generally been agreed upon but is also heavily colored by the author's experience, preferences, and perhaps prejudices. This chapter also emphasizes aspects of treatment that are not readily found in standard texts.

ACUTE PERICARDITIS

By *acute pericarditis,* most clinicians mean the syndrome of chest pain, pericardial friction rub, and widespread ST segment elevation of probable viral or idiopathic etiology; this is the entity discussed in this section. Other forms of acute pericarditis and pericardial heart disease are discussed under their respective headings.

The diagnosis of acute idiopathic or viral pericarditis is usually straightforward. When the diagnosis is in doubt, pericardial effusion should be sought by echocardiography; its absence by no means rules out the diagnosis, but the presence of a small effusion can be strong confirmatory evidence. Treatment can be initiated with an anti-inflammatory agent, with the recognition that if another specific etiology is uncovered by the rapid clinical and laboratory investigation that ensues, the treatment may need to be changed. The disease is often self-limiting and should respond promptly to aspirin, up to 650 mg every 3 or 4 h, or indomethacin, 25–50 mg three or four times per day.[1] Some patients respond more promptly to ibuprofen, 400–800 mg four times per day. Pain should resolve or be significantly ameliorated by 24–48 h. Resolution of the friction rub and ST segment deviation soon follows. Failure of this resolution to occur strongly suggests that the etiologic diagnosis is in error and should prompt further investigation. In a minority of patients, pericarditis cannot be suppressed by these simple means. Recourse then has to be prednisone; usually a short course starting with 60–80 mg/day for about a week and followed by a rapid taper suffices. Sometimes, failure to respond to anti-inflammatory treatment is a first signal that the patient will develop recurrent pericarditis (vide infra).

RECURRENT OR RELAPSING PERICARDITIS

In a small proportion of patients with acute viral or idiopathic pericarditis, as well as in a minority of patients with acute pericarditis after myocardial infarction (Dressler syndrome) and after pericardiectomy or after traumatic pericarditis, the disease takes on a recurrent or relapsing form.[2, 3] Recurrences after an apparent cure usually manifest several weeks or months after the initial episode and may continue for many years. The pain is severe; thus the syndrome is extremely troublesome to patient and physician alike. The pain responds to high-dose steroid therapy in most cases, but once prednisone therapy has been started, it may be difficult or impossible to manage this and subsequent recurrences without it. These patients may become dependent upon steroids, which makes weaning difficult or impossible. It has therefore been argued that steroid treatment should never be given for fear of initiating this deleterious train of events. However, although most clinicians strive to avoid the use of prednisone, most would agree that prednisone treatment is inevitable in some of the cases. The physician should attempt to use nonsteroidal anti-inflammatory drugs such as ibuprofen. The dose can be pushed to 800 mg or more, three or four times a day, but these agents also have significant toxic effects. The patient must be monitored carefully for peptic ulceration, renal dysfunction, and fluid retention. Colchicine can be useful in lessening or abolishing the need for prednisone treatment.[4] Two milligrams per day are given for the first day or two; the dosage thereafter is 1 mg/day.

When nonsteroidal treatment fails, the clinician may decide that there is no alternative to prednisone. In this case, 60 or 80 mg/day should be given. Usually, pain, friction rub, and electrocardiographic (ECG) changes resolve promptly. High-dose treatment should be maintained for 1 or 2 weeks. If all manifestations of acute pericarditis are then absent, rapid weaning (e.g., 10 mg every other day) can begin. When the dosage approaches 20 mg/day, the clinician should be on the alert for early signs of recurrence. Should these appear, the dosage should be adjusted upward to the last one that left the patient entirely free from manifestations of pericarditis. This dosage should be maintained for 1 or 2 weeks and then weaning recommenced. When weaning ceases to be successful (e.g., at a dosage of approximately 20 mg/day), combination treatment of colchicine with prednisone, ibuprofen, or indomethacin can be instituted in an attempt to further reduce the prednisone dosage. If possible, prednisone should be given only on alternate days.

Subsequent relapses should be treated in a similar way. With each one, a determined attempt to avoid prednisone is mandatory. If prednisone is necessary, it should be in a dosage that is clearly enough to fully suppress the syndrome, and that dosage should be maintained for 2 and sometimes 3 weeks before tapering is begun.

In difficult cases, 100–200 mg/day of azathioprine can be added in an attempt to reduce or abolish steroid dependency. To the author's knowledge, cyclosporine has not been used.

Treatment of these patients is often challenging. Patients who have received significant doses of prednisone for prolonged periods on many occasions often have marked Cushingoid features. Unfortunately, this is often the situation when the patient is first referred to a cardiologist; thus the cardiologist may never have the opportunity to avoid the initiation of treatment with prednisone. In younger women in particular, it is advisable to establish the bone density and to monitor for compression fractures.

Atypical Manifestations

Difficulty may arise in interpretation of the pain. A patient may begin complaining of pain or dysphagia or other manifestations of recurrence, and yet no abnormality may be found on clinical examination. Sometimes after reassurance, the patient returns a day or two later, reporting that the pain is worse, and then exhibits fever, pericardial friction rub, ST segment elevation, and a raised erythrocyte sedimentation rate. An even more difficult problem arises when symptoms are not followed by clinical and laboratory signs of pericarditis. In some of these patients, the pain results from drug-induced peptic ulceration; in others, no apparent cause is found. Many of these patients have already learned to recognize the symptoms of pericarditis and resume treatment, often with high doses of prednisone or other anti-inflammatory agents, before consulting the physician. Frequently, the therapeutic response is minimal or absent; this is strong evidence against a true recurrence. This situation calls for infinite tact and patience on the part of the physician and understanding on the part of the patient. The evidence against acute pericarditis should be clearly explained to the patient, who should be encouraged to endure the pain without anti-inflammatory treatment. Patients can be told that if objective evidence appears, treatment will be reinstituted, but that if it does not, they should make every effort not to restart treatment. With strong support and encouragement of the patient, sometimes with the help of simple analgesics, the pain may eventually disappear.

Pericardiectomy is sometimes suggested when the response to medical treatment is inadequate.[2, 3, 5, 6] However, there are a number of limitations to this approach. First, because recurrent pericarditis is an autoimmune process, it would be desirable to remove every last vestige of the pericardium, but this is not surgically feasible. Although pericardiectomy cures some patients, it has no effect on others,[3] and in some, it shortens the course and lessens the severity but is not curative. Pericardiectomy should be considered when the patient has severe unwanted effects from prednisone, such as severe osteoporosis or necrosis of the femoral head, often with obesity and hypertension, especially when pericardial pain persists in spite of medical treatment. Even then, it is extremely important to manage the patient without prednisone therapy for a prolonged period before sternotomy if wound infection and sternal dehiscence are to be avoided.

PERICARDIAL EFFUSION

Virtually any disease that affects the pericardium may be associated with pericardial effusion. Therefore, an important component of treatment is that directed against the underlying cause.

The usual indications for removal of pericardial fluid are cardiac tamponade and suspected purulent pericarditis.[7] Less commonly, pericardial fluid is removed to help establish the etiologic diagnosis, particularly tuberculosis,[8] in patients undergoing chronic dialysis and, as a last resort, during cardiopulmonary resuscitation. Pericardiocentesis or pericardiotomy suffices for purulent pericarditis only when the fluid is thin, not loculated, or associated with thickening of or constriction by the pericardium.[9] In the absence of these favorable conditions, pericardiectomy is required, should be as complete as possible, and often must include the visceral pericardium.[5, 10]

The increase in intrapericardial pressure caused by a large *chronic* pericardial effusion is modest, for which reason patients may be asymptomatic.[11] Authorities differ in opinion about the need to evacuate these effusions, because in some cases a treatable cause such as tuberculosis or severe cardiac tamponade is discovered late in the course. Pericardiectomy has been advocated if the effusion persists for 6 months.[12] However, most chronic effusions are idiopathic. This author believes that when evidence of compression of mediastinal structures is absent and regular follow-up is ensured, removal of pericardial fluid has a low diagnostic yield, produces no therapeutic benefit, and therefore should not be performed. However, if follow-up findings are likely to be unsatisfactory, the fluid should be removed. When pericardiocentesis or pericardiotomy is selected for this purpose, the effusion may recur, and therefore pericardiectomy is the preferred procedure because it may disclose the etiology and should be definitive. Pericardial effusion, sometimes large enough to cause tamponade or need aspiration, is encountered in acquired immunodeficiency syndrome (AIDS)[13] and after cardiac transplantation.[14]

CARDIAC TAMPONADE

Very mild cardiac tamponade, especially when secondary to acute viral or idiopathic pericarditis that should respond quickly to anti-inflammatory treatment, does not mandate removal of pericardial fluid. Anti-inflammatory treatment should be begun promptly, and the patient should be observed in the hospital for regression of the clinical signs of cardiac tamponade and echocardiographic degree of pericardial effusion. Patients to be treated in this way should not have symptoms of tamponade, the blood pressure should be normal without pulsus paradoxus, and the jugular venous pressure should not be above 8–10 cm H_2O. At the opposite extreme are patients with hyperacute cardiac tamponade, often secondary to blunt or sharp trauma or rupture of the heart or aorta. Here, immediate pericardiocentesis or subxiphoid pericardiotomy should be performed as a triage procedure. Because of the steep nature of the pericardial pressure-volume curve (Fig. 57–1), the patient may be dramatically improved and saved from death by removal of only a small portion of the effusion or blood.

Pericardiocentesis for acute, especially hemorrhagic, effusion can present difficulties because the relatively small effusion significantly reduces the margin of safety. Also, when bleeding is rapid, the rule that intrapericardial blood does not clot does not apply. Finally, in these cases, time may not permit the operator to observe many of the precautions customary in elective pericardiocentesis, such as performing the procedure in a cardiac catheterization laboratory and using a catheter rather than a needle to remove pericardial fluid.

In most patients, the condition is between the extremes of the life-threatening hyperacute syndrome and mild, subtle asymptomatic tamponade. In the following discussion, this large group is divided into those who have recently undergone cardiac operation and medical patients[15]—that is, patients with cardiac tamponade caused by such entities as neoplasm, viral or idiopathic pericarditis, uremia, prior radiation, and collagen vascular disease.

Postoperative Patients

In patients who have recently undergone a cardiac operation, the effusion may be localized or clotted, and numerous other causes

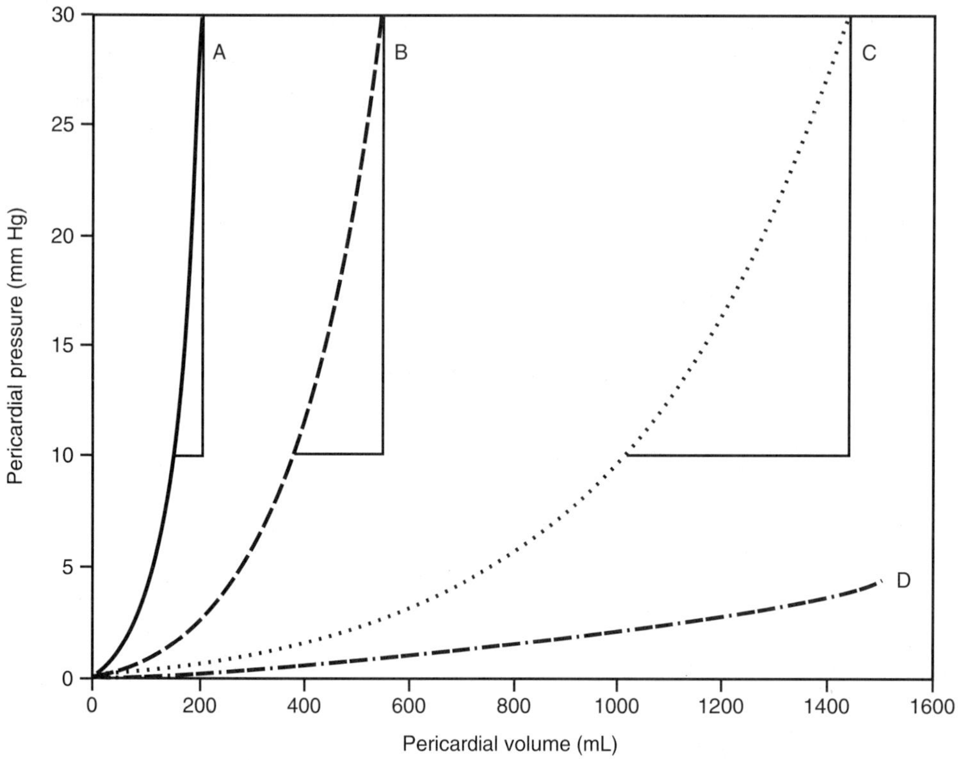

Figure 57–1. Schematic to illustrate the pressure-volume relation of the pericardium in the presence of pericardial effusion. *A,* Hyperacute cardiac tamponade, as often seen in surgical patients, such as those with gunshot or stab wounds of the heart. *B,* Subacute cardiac tamponade, such as may be seen in surgical or medical patients with effusion that has developed over a period of a few days. *C,* The relationship in medical patients with effusion that has developed over a period of several weeks to a few months. *D,* The relationship in patients with chronic effusive pericarditis in whom pericardial pressure is slightly elevated but does not cause major hemodynamic impairment. When tamponade is relatively acute, aspiration of a small volume of pericardial fluid dramatically lowers pericardial pressure (i.e., decreases the severity of cardiac tamponade).

may contribute to elevation of venous pressure, low cardiac output, hypotension, and pulsus paradoxus. When bleeding is still active, the treatment is surgical removal of the effusion with control of hemorrhage.[16] Later in the postoperative course,[17] pericardial effusion may occur and treatment can be the same as for medical patients, although most surgeons explore the chest even when bleeding is no longer active.[18]

Medical Patients

Cardiac tamponade may be acute or subacute. The more rapidly the pericardial effusion accumulates, the less is the volume required for elevating pericardial pressure to a given level, because pericardial compliance is highly time dependent (see Fig. 57–1). In less acute tamponade, the effusion is larger, but pericardial pressure elevation can nonetheless cause severe hemodynamic compromise that necessitates urgent, although seldom emergency, relief. Time almost always allows for preceding echocardiography and for transfer to a hemodynamic suite or operating room—precautions that sometimes have to be forgone in hyperacute cases if the patients are to be saved.

Treatment

Pericardiocentesis

The procedure of pericardiocentesis and the hemodynamic and electrocardiographic monitoring accompanying it were described in detail by Lorell and Braunwald[18] and are not repeated here. Here, a few points are emphasized and some comments are added. Unless the patient is particularly obese, a very long needle should not be used, because if the pericardium is not reached by a needle 6 or 7 cm long, it is not because the needle is too short, but because it has been misdirected. A needle that is too long may injure mediastinal structures when advanced to the hilt in an attempt to seek the pericardial space. The bevel of a pericardiocentesis needle should always be short, to decrease the likelihood of lacerating the heart or a coronary vessel. Contrast injection is a highly reliable and safe technique for determining whether the needle or catheter tip is intracardiac or intrapericardial, but it should be done sparingly and with caution if fluid or blood cannot be aspirated. In addition, the local electrogram can be recorded from the pericardiocentesis needle[19] (Fig. 57–2).

Pericardiocentesis is almost always well tolerated hemodynamically, but pulmonary edema,[20, 21] circulatory collapse,[22] acute right-sided heart failure,[23] and transient left ventricular dysfunction[24] have been reported. The pressure signal recorded from the needle is helpful when it shows a ventricular contour, but atrial and pericardial pressures are indistinguishable.[25] When it is hard to decide whether red aspirate is blood or a sanguinous effusion, a few drops should be placed on a sponge because blood creates a far lighter stain. The total complication rate has been summarized.[26] Pericardiocentesis is especially hazardous in dissecting hematoma of the aorta because it may exacerbate bleeding. Ideally, these patients are treated surgically. Pericardiocentesis should be avoided unless the patient is in profound shock; in that case, the volume aspirated should be limited to the amount that restores a viable blood pressure.[27]

If the intrapericardial catheter is left in place for continued drainage, only a slightly negative pressure should be applied. Plugging of the catheter is often caused by fibrin, in which case, the catheter can be closed off periodically and filled with a lytic agent. Strict precautions against introducing small amounts of air into the pericardium during flushing or aspirating are not necessary.

Pericardiotomy or Pericardiocentesis?

Except in a dire emergency, pericardiocentesis should not be attempted if a physician experienced and skilled at the technique is not available to perform or at least supervise the procedure. In the era when pericardiocentesis was performed at the bedside by unsupervised house officers, the morbidity and mortality rates were appalling. In general, pericardiocentesis is not advisable when the echocardiogram shows less than 1 cm of effusion, a localized collec-

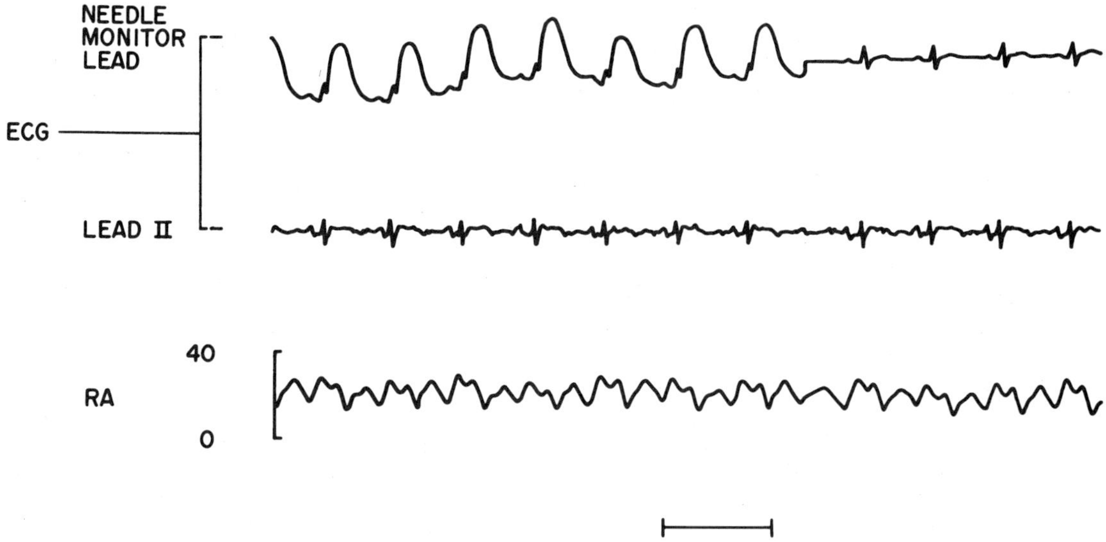

Figure 57–2. In an environment in which all electrical sockets are properly and equally grounded, the position of the tip of a pericardiocentesis needle can be monitored by an ECG lead connected to the needle. The top tracing shows the ECG recorded by this means. During the first eight beats, the needle tip was in contact with the heart, creating a large current of injury. Thereafter, the needle was withdrawn until the tracing became normal. In the second tracing, made through lead II of the ECG, the current of injury (ST segment elevation) was much too small to be easily appreciated by an operator observing the monitor. The bottom tracing shows the elevated central venous pressure. (From Shabetai R: The Pericardium. New York: Grune & Stratton, 1981.)

tion, fibrin, or adhesions. Subxiphoid pericardiotomy is then preferred, especially if a surgeon with experience and skill with the technique who is willing to use local anesthesia when indicated is available. Cardiologists who perform invasive procedures should be trained to perform or at least begin this procedure, because in some cases of catheter-induced tamponade, pericardiocentesis cannot adequately deal with circulatory collapse, and there is no guarantee that a surgeon will be immediately available.

Alternatives to Pericardiocentesis

When fluid recurs after pericardiocentesis or sometimes as the primary intervention, fluid can be removed and its reaccumulation prevented by a number of surgical approaches. The relative merits of pericardiocentesis vs. surgical drainage are summarized in Table 57–1. In general, subtotal pericardiectomy is preferred when the patient is expected to survive for 1 year or more and the patient is judged to be at low risk for complications from the operation. Persistent or recurrent symptomatic pericardial effusion can be treated by creation of a "window" between the pericardium and the

TABLE 57–1. RELATIVE MERITS OF PERICARDIOCENTESIS VS. OPEN SURGICAL DRAINAGE

	Pericardiocentesis	Surgical Drainage
Cost	Lower	High
Hospitalization	Shorter	Longer
Postoperative pain	Less	More
Biopsy	Difficult, small	Easy, adequate size
Pericardium examined	No	Yes
Hemodynamic data quality	Excellent	Usually poor
Effusive constrictive recognized	Very well	Not as well, more subjective
Coexistent heart disease	Clearly identified	May not be adequately assessed

left pleural cavity, an operation that requires left thoracotomy. The pleural cavity provides a much larger area for absorption of the fluid, and the pathophysiologic effects of pleural effusion are less than those of pericardial effusion.

Subxiphoid pericardiotomy should not be considered as a window between the pericardial and pleural or peritoneal cavities because the pericardiotomy usually closes spontaneously, unless a ring or another device is used to maintain patency.

Percutaneous Balloon Pericardiotomy

Palacios and associates were the first to perform and describe the treatment of pericardial effusion by means of percutaneous balloon pericardiotomy.[28] Subsequently, a multicenter registry was developed, and a description of the technique was published.[29] Subxiphoid pericardiocentesis is performed in the standard manner with the use of an 18-gauge needle, a 0.035-inch J-tipped guide wire, and an 8F catheter. A residual volume of 100–200 mL is left in the pericardial space in case repuncture of the pericardium is needed. Twenty milliliters of 50% radiographic contrast material is injected into the pericardial space, after which a 0.038-inch extra-stiff J-tipped guide wire is looped into the pericardial space. The catheter is removed and replaced with a 10F dilator, over which an 18- to 25-mm wide, 3-cm long Mansfield balloon containing 30% radiographic contrast material is advanced over the wire to straddle the border of the pericardium and is gently inflated to locate the margin of the pericardium (Fig. 57–3). In cases in which the pericardium is apposed to the chest wall, the proximal portion of the balloon fails to expand. When this occurs, the catheter is gently advanced while traction is applied to the skin. Thereafter, the balloon is manually inflated to create the window (see Fig. 57–3).

After dilatation, the balloon is removed and replaced with the catheter through which contrast material is slowly injected during continuous withdrawal until the side holes are just within the pericardial space. Once this location has been ascertained, 10 mL of diluted contrast material is rapidly injected into the pericardial space and should be seen to flow freely from it (see Fig. 57–3). The catheter is left in place until pericardial drainage ceases. When needed, two balloons can be used; alternatively, if preferred, the Inoue balloon[30] can be used, but it is more expensive. Recurrence of pericardial

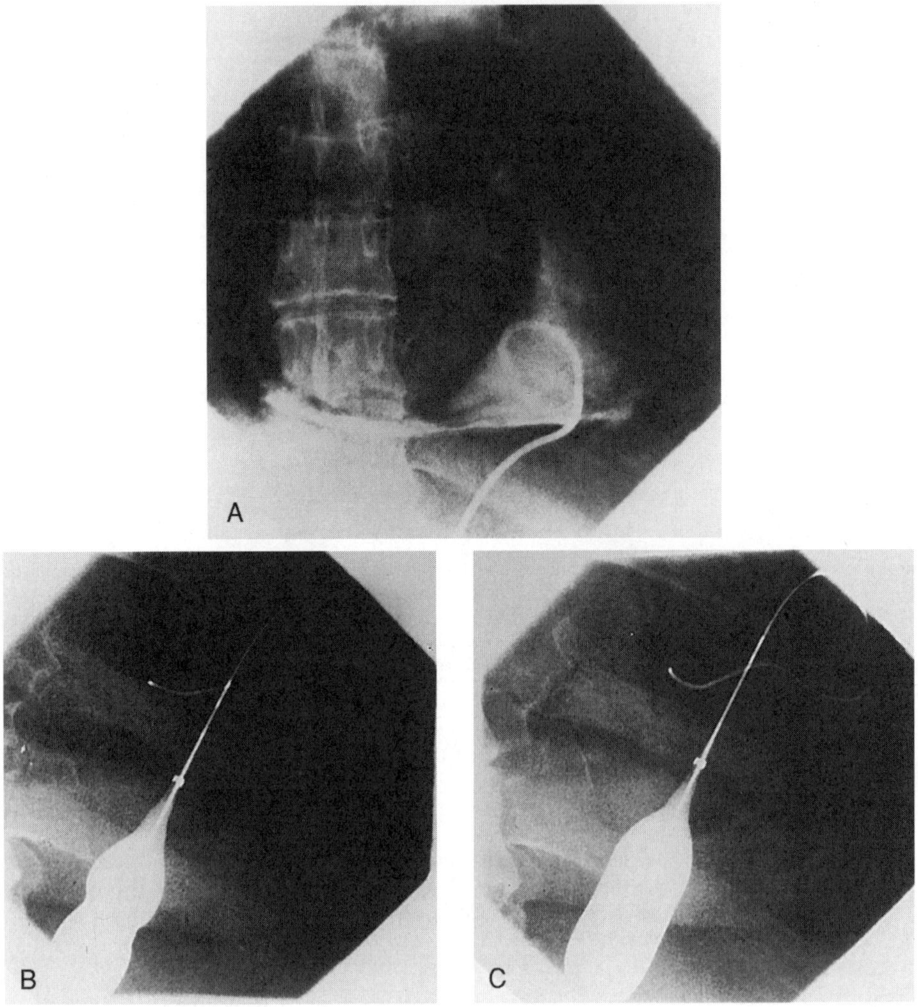

Figure 57–3. *A,* The parietal pericardium has been outlined by injection of contrast agent. *B,* The balloon has been gently partly inflated to visualize the waist to indicate the location of the parietal pericardium. *C,* The fully inflated balloon immediately after creation of the pericardiotomy. (From Palacios IF, Tuzcu EM, Ziskind AA, et al: Percutaneous balloon pericardial window for patients with malignant pericardial effusion and tamponade. Cathet Cardiovasc Diagn 1991; 22:244.)

effusion in the registry series[29] was uncommon, as was the need for postoperative treatment of procedural complications. Percutaneous balloon pericardiotomy may well become the procedure of choice for the treatment of pericardial effusion, particularly malignant effusion, in which the avoidance of radical treatment is extremely important.

CONSTRICTIVE PERICARDITIS

Atypical Cases: Medical Management

Once the diagnosis of constrictive pericarditis has been made, the usual treatment is pericardiectomy; however, the clinician should be aware of exceptions. One is that pericardial constriction is rarely transitory[31]; therefore, when the disease is not clearly chronic, the patient should be carefully observed before being committed to surgery. Transient constrictive pericarditis is uncommon, but when it occurs, it is in patients recently ill with acute effusive pericarditis. The effusion is usually moderate or large. As the signs of acute pericarditis and pericardial effusion subsist, a deep y descent of jugular venous pressure, a pericardial knock, or other signs of constriction develop. However, these are transitory, usually disappearing in a matter of days or weeks. The constriction tends not to be severe. In patients with subacute constrictive pericarditis, the operation should be deferred until the physician is confident that the constrictive process is not transitory.

Another exception concerns the fact that some patients with mild or moderate constrictive pericarditis have the typical findings, but no actual evidence, of hemodynamic compromise or hepatic insufficiency. In such patients, the jugular venous pressure is commonly elevated only modestly, but it may be as high as 12 cm H_2O. The patients deny symptoms, but before the physician decides to defer pericardiectomy, exercise tolerance should be estimated with a bicycle or treadmill test and, if the facilities are available, maximal oxygen consumption should be measured. In such patients, an advantage of pericardiectomy is that the operation is easy and safe and sometimes can be accomplished without the need for cardiopulmonary bypass. The obvious disadvantage is the potential for morbidity and mortality from surgery. The author's approach is to explain carefully the advantages and disadvantages, giving patients ample opportunity to express their own preferences. Most of them accept operative treatment, and the surgeons are pleased because of the low operative risk and the predictability of an excellent result. When the decision is against early operation, the patients are again reminded that pericardiectomy may well eventually be required. They should be observed by means of clinical evaluation and liver function testing every 6 months and by exercise testing annually. Indications for surgical treatment include increasing jugular venous pressure, early evidence of hepatic insufficiency, and decreased exercise tolerance.

Another exception to the rule that constrictive pericarditis should be treated by pericardiectomy is the patient with far advanced disease. In such a patient, jugular venous pressure often exceeds 20 cm H_2O, and fluid retention is manifest by pleural effusion, prominent ascites, and severe edema. Hepatic insufficiency is manifested not only on laboratory tests but by spider angiomata, massive ascites, severe edema, and sometimes obvious jaundice. Protein-losing enteropathy is common at this stage of the disease. Severe cachexia provides a striking contrast with the protuberant and swollen lower extremities. Atrial fibrillation has almost invariably supervened by this time. Many internists, although perhaps fewer surgeons, would argue that little benefit can accrue from pericardiectomy once the disease has progressed to this extent and that palliative medical treatment is preferable.

Preoperative Management

The issues concerning medical management differ for patients with milder asymptomatic pericarditis that does not mandate early operation, for patients being prepared for pericardiectomy, and for patients in whom the stage of disease is considered too late for pericardiectomy.

The author's policy for patients who do not require operation is not to administer diuretic treatment, because the need for a diuretic indicates the need for surgical intervention. Such patients may be free from edema and have no need for pharmacologic treatment for years, although many of them need pericardiectomy sooner or later. In patients who are being prepared for pericardiectomy, it is of great importance to use diuretics sparingly. Edema and ascites should be treated, not until they disappear, but until the patient is comfortable. Obviously, no attempt should be made to achieve a normal venous pressure, but moderate lowering to a value of approximately 15 cm H_2O or a little lower, if feasible, is desirable. During diuretic treatment, liver function should be monitored, and when possible, treatment should be continued until the test results plateau at an improved level. Patients who are treated too vigorously with diuretics have a higher operative risk and recover more slowly. Although restraint should be exercised in diuretic treatment of these patients, spontaneous diuresis is likely to occur postoperatively; if it does not, diuretics given at this time are effective and safe.

Pericardiectomy

Pericardiectomy for indications in which the pericardium is not thickened, calcified, or adherent to the heart is a safe operation but becomes increasingly less so as pericardial thickening increases and calcification develops. In the absence of calcification and dense fibrosis, pericardiectomy can often be accomplished without the need for cardiopulmonary bypass,[10] although the apparatus and perfusionist must be standing by. Because the pericardial layers are fused, parietal pericardiectomy is a far more straightforward procedure than visceral pericardiectomy, which is required in constrictive pericarditis.[10] Pericardial dissection can be aided by the use of an ultrasonic dissector.[32] The need for visceral pericardiectomy can also be anticipated in any patient who recently has had a large pericardial effusion, because in such patients the parietal pericardium has been stretched and cannot be the cause of constriction. This situation is particularly true after purulent pericarditis and in patients with effusive constrictive pericarditis. In a minority of patients, resection is not possible; in those cases, extensive meshing is applied.

It is of paramount importance to refer a candidate for pericardiectomy for constrictive pericarditis to a surgeon who is experienced with the treatment of this disease. A number of outstanding cardiac surgeons have had no or little experience with pericardiectomy for constrictive pericarditis because the disease, although important, is not common in the United States and Europe.

Postoperative Care

It is well known that the central venous pressure may take some weeks or even months to return to normal after successful pericardiectomy. This phenomenon has been ascribed to incomplete resection, especially of scar tissue around the atrioventricular junction and at the entrances of the great veins. However, this phenomenon is also seen in patients who have undergone a remarkably complete pericardiectomy. Pericardiectomy may exacerbate tricuspid regurgitation.[33] Thus, in many of the cases, raised central venous pressure is the manifestation of heart failure or tricuspid valve disease, not persisting constriction. It has been proposed that heart failure after pericardiectomy is caused by myocardial atrophy, but it is equally likely to be caused by the rapid expansion in ventricular volume that follows successful pericardiectomy. The left ventricular ejection fraction, characteristically normal in patients with constrictive pericarditis,[34] frequently falls to subnormal values in the postoperative period and remains low for some months. Therefore, digoxin, vasodilator, and diuretic therapy should be instituted postoperatively and maintained until the venous pressure and ventricular ejection fraction have returned to normal.

EFFUSIVE CONSTRICTIVE PERICARDITIS

As the name implies, this is a syndrome in which cardiac compression is caused in part by cardiac tamponade but also by pericardial constriction. As mentioned earlier, one of the advantages of pericardiocentesis over open surgical drainage of pericardial effusion is that the diagnosis of effusive constrictive pericarditis is easily established during cardiac catheterization. When hemodynamics and intrapericardial pressure are measured at the beginning of the procedure, the findings are those of cardiac tamponade. During pericardiocentesis, pericardial pressure falls to normal, but right atrial pressure and pulmonary wedge pressure remain elevated and equal to one another. The venous pressure develops the characteristic y descent that was absent before pericardiocentesis, when cardiac tamponade dominated the hemodynamics (Fig. 57–4). It stands to reason that constriction in these cases must be caused by the visceral pericardium and that the treatment is visceral, not just parietal, pericardiectomy.

PERICARDITIS OF SPECIFIC ETIOLOGY

Tuberculous Pericarditis

Pericardial involvement in pulmonary tuberculosis is distinctly rare; therefore, radiologic evidence of old pulmonary tuberculosis plays an insignificant role in the decision of whether to treat pericardial disease, assuming that the cause is tuberculosis. Mycobacterium tuberculosis cannot be grown from the sputum of most patients. Tuberculous pericardial effusion may thus be strictly analogous to primary pleural effusion. These primary pericardial effusions are often large and may cause cardiac tamponade. Effusive constrictive pericarditis is not a feature of primary pericardial effusion. The fluid should be removed and cultured, and the patient should begin antituberculous chemotherapy with three drugs (e.g., rifampin, ethambutol, and isoniazid). Treatment should be continued for 18 months or longer.

Although it has been suggested that the addition of prednisone to the regimen may prevent subsequent constrictive pericarditis as a sequel to primary pericardial effusion, supporting data have never been published. The author does not advocate its use in this context. The situation is different when clinical, ECG, and imaging data suggest pericarditis in addition to effusion. In that case, there is a strong possibility either that the patient already has effusive constrictive pericarditis that may presage severe constriction or that this sequence of events will soon develop. These patients, therefore, require aggressive chemotherapeutic and hemodynamic management. Ideally, the patients are managed by a cardiologist in cooperation with an infectious disease specialist who has expertise in the management of tuberculosis. A large effusion can be removed by pericardiocentesis; however, depending on the characteristics of the fluid and the appearance of the heart and pericardium on subsequent imaging, the procedure may need to be followed by subxiphoid surgical

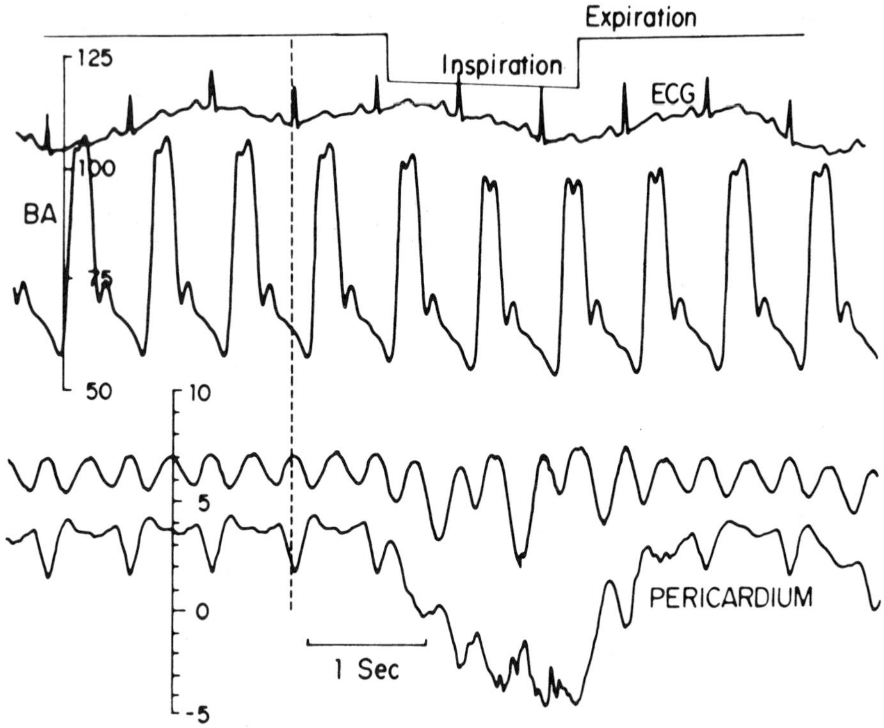

Figure 57–4. Recording made during pericardiocentesis in a patient with effusive constrictive pericarditis resulting from bronchogenic carcinoma. Pericardial pressure was lowered almost to normal, but the right atrial pressure remained elevated with prominent x and y descents and respiratory variation limited to the y descent; these findings are characteristic of constrictive pericarditis. (From Shabetai R: The Pericardium. New York: Grune & Stratton, 1981.)

drainage. If, during pericardiocentesis, the hemodynamics are consistent with significant effusive constrictive disease, a plan should be made for parietal and visceral pericardiectomy after a few weeks of chemotherapy. Should the venous pressure return to normal during this period, the operation becomes unnecessary.

The two consultants should agree on a longer term drug regimen and its duration. The cardiologist must monitor the patient regularly for evidence of constriction. When it is clear that constriction has occurred and is not transient, plans should be made for early pericardiectomy. In developed countries, chronic calcific tuberculous pericarditis should become a disease of the past.

The decision regarding antituberculous chemotherapy for patients in whom tuberculosis is suspected but not proven is more difficult. Many patients are subjected to this form of treatment on indirect evidence such as a positive result of a skin tuberculin test, especially if they have had contact with a patient with tuberculosis. There can be little doubt, however, that many of the patients so treated had viral or some other nontuberculous pericarditis. Probes for mRNA of *Mycobacterium tuberculosis* and polymerase chain reaction promise to help to identify the true cases of tuberculous pericarditis.[35] When the physician is confident that the patient can be observed serially for the next few years with periodic echocardiography, the danger that constrictive pericarditis will develop is minimal and antituberculous chemotherapy need not be given. Patients in whom good follow-up findings are improbable should be placed on long-term triple antituberculous chemotherapy, but some of these patients may fail to comply with the regimen. Treatment for the presumptive diagnosis is justified if the patient has had contact with a person who produces sputum from which *M. tuberculosis* has been identified.

Bacterial (Purulent) Pericarditis

The management of this important disease has been covered by Lorell and Braunwald.[18] This section emphasizes the critical importance of exploring the pericardial space whenever a bacterial pericardial effusion is suspected. The need for a high index of suspicion is apparent. The use of echocardiography to explore the possibility of pus in the pericardium is too often postponed or omitted in the evaluation of septic patients. The importance of these considerations cannot be overemphasized because the antibiotic era has had much less impact on purulent pericarditis than on most of the infectious diseases.[36] For the same reasons, persistence with pericardiocentesis for evacuating the fluid is not advisable. Affected patients require formal pericardiectomy to guarantee complete drainage of the infected pericardial space. Antibiotic treatment, although important, is adjuvant.[37]

Uremic Pericarditis

Until the late 1970s, cardiac tamponade was the scourge of dialysis units. For reasons that are not entirely apparent but that may be related to the material used for dialysis membranes, symptomatic pericardial effusion in dialysis patients is now quite rare. When pericardial effusion does not respond to more intensive dialysis, the fluid should be removed either by pericardiocentesis or by subxiphoid drainage.[38] If pericardiocentesis needs to be repeated, especially more than once, subxiphoid drainage is indicated. Instillation of nonabsorbable steroid preparations was quite common in the past[39] but is now seldom performed, and the author does not recommend this treatment modality. In these patients, before it is decided to remove pericardial effusion, it is critically important to be certain that raised jugular venous pressure and hypotension are in fact caused by cardiac tamponade and not by fluid disturbances related to renal failure or the associated heart disease. When any doubt exists, pericardiocentesis with measurement of pericardial, central venous, and aortic pressures, along with cardiac output before and after pericardiocentesis, is the preferred management.

Neoplastic Pericarditis

Cardiac tamponade almost always calls for removal of fluid from the pericardium, although in a few cases with terminal disease and hopeless prognosis, even this intervention may not be appropriate. The patient should be managed jointly by an oncologist and a cardiologist. When the prognosis is judged to be relatively good and other medical considerations are favorable, a partial pericardiectomy via sternotomy or thoracotomy provides the best chance for one-time effective treatment. In other patients, balloon pericardiotomy will most likely replace subxiphoid surgical pericardiotomy.

In the 1970s and 1980s, an extensive literature appeared concerning the intrapericardial instillation of a variety of cytotoxic or sclerosing agents to slow the advance of pericardial neoplastic disease and the rate of accumulation of malignant pericardial effusion.[40] At present, the general consensus is that adequate fluid drainage or pericardiectomy, depending on the nature of the case, achieves equally satisfactory results and that there is little advantage in intrapericardial chemotherapy.[41]

Ischemic Heart Disease

Acute pericarditis manifested by a pericardial friction rub necessitates either no treatment or simple analgesics. Thrombolytic therapy is given early (i.e., before pericarditis is expected to manifest) and thus is not linked to an increased risk of pericardial hemorrhage or cardiac tamponade,[42] although the latter has been reported with thrombolysis.[43] Thrombolysis is associated with less, not more, frequent acute pericarditis in the first few days after myocardial infarction.[44] In spite of earlier studies to the contrary,[45] pericardial effusion is frequently present with myocardial infarction, is generally mild, and does not necessitate the withholding of anticoagulant therapy.[46] Dressler syndrome is treated in the same manner as episodes of acute effusive pericarditis of other etiology.

Chylopericardium

Patients who fail to respond to a diet rich in medium-chain triglycerides or to ligation of the thoracic duct with partial pericardiectomy can be treated by means of a valved conduit from the pericardial space to the peritoneal space.[47]

Cardiac Transplantation

Pericardial effusion, often quite large and occasionally causing cardiac tamponade, may occur after orthotopic cardiac transplantation. This appears to be more common among patients who have not had prior median sternotomy and in those with mismatch between body size and the size of the transplanted heart.[14] Therapy is not usually required, and the immunosuppressive regimen usually does not need to be modified, because these effusions are not related to acute rejection. In rare instances, cardiac tamponade does develop and necessitates pericardiocentesis.

Acquired Immunodeficiency Syndrome

Pericardial effusion is the most common manifestation of AIDS, being detectable by echocardiography in about 15 percent of human immunodeficiency virus (HIV)–infected persons.[13] Cardiac tamponade is rare but may occur.[48, 49] Therapeutic pericardiocentesis often results in discovery of the etiology of the effusion. Infecting organisms include *Staphylococcus aureus, Mycobacterium avium–intracellulare*, cytomegalovirus (CMV), and *M. tuberculosis,* which may necessitate specific treatment, depending on the patient's general condition. In other patients, pericardial effusion is a marker of lymphoma or Kaposi sarcoma.

REFERENCES

1. Lorell B, Braunwald E: Pericardial disease. *In* Braunwald E (ed): Heart Disease: A Textbook of Cardiovascular Medicine, 4th ed, p 1471. Philadelphia: WB Saunders, 1992.
2. Fowler NO, Harbin AD III: Recurrent acute pericarditis: follow-up study of 31 patients. J Am Coll Cardiol 1986; 7:300.
3. Fowler NO: Recurrent pericarditis. Cardiol Clin 1990; 8:621.
4. Guindo J, de la Serna AR, Ramio J, et al: Recurrent pericarditis: relief with colchicine. Circulation 1990; 82:1117.
5. Tuna IC, Danielson GK: Surgical management of pericardial diseases. Cardiol Clin 1990; 8:683.
6. DeValeria PA, Baumgartner WA, Casale AS, et al: Current indications, risks and outcome after pericardiectomy. Ann Thorac Surg 1991; 52:219.
7. Permanyer-Miralda G, Sagrista-Sauleda J, Soler-Soler J: Primary acute pericardial disease: a prospective series of 231 consecutive patients. Am J Cardiol 1985; 56:623.
8. Sagrista-Sauleda J, Permanyer-Miralda G, Soler-Soler J: Tuberculous pericarditis: ten year experience with a prospective protocol for diagnosis and treatment. J Am Coll Cardiol 1988; 11:724.
9. Rubin RH, Moellering RC Jr: Clinical, microbiologic and therapeutic aspects of purulent pericarditis. Am J Med 1975; 59:68.
10. Nataf P, Cacoub P, Dorent R, et al: Results of subtotal pericardiectomy for constrictive pericarditis. Eur J Cardiothorac Surg 1993; 7:252.
11. Reddy PS, Curtiss EI, Uretsky BF: Spectrum of hemodynamic changes in cardiac tamponade. Am J Cardiol 1990; 66:1487.
12. Soler-Soler J: Massive chronic ideopathic pericardial effusion. *In* Soler-Soler J, Permanyor-Miralda G, Sagrista-Sauleda J (eds): Pericardial Disease: New Insights and Old Dilemmas, p 153. Boston: Kluwer, 1990.
13. Hsia J, Ross AM: Pericardial effusion and pericardiocentesis in human immunodeficiency virus infection. Am J Cardiol 1994; 74:94.
14. Hauptman PJ, Couper GS, Aranki SF, et al: Pericardial effusion after cardiac transplantation. J Am Coll Cardiol 1994; 23:1625.
15. Guberman BA, Fowler NO, Engel PJ, et al: Cardiac tamponade in medical patients. Circulation 1981; 64:633.
16. Engleman RM, Spencer FC, Reed GE, et al: Cardiac tamponade following open heart surgery. Circulation 1970; 41(suppl II):165.
17. Borkan MA, Schaff H, Gardner TJ: Diagnosis and management of postoperative pericardial effusions and late cardiac tamponade following open heart surgery. Ann Thorac Surg 1981; 31:512.
18. Lorell B, Braunwald E: Pericardial disease. *In* Braunwald E (ed): Heart Disease: A Textbook of Cardiovascular Medicine, 4th ed, pp 1479–1481. Philadelphia: WB Saunders, 1992.
19. Bishop LH, Estes EH, McIntosh HD: The electrocardiogram as a safeguard in pericardiocentesis. JAMA 1956; 62:264.
20. Vandyke WH Jr, Cure J, Chakko CS, et al: Pulmonary edema after pericardiocentesis for cardiac tamponade. N Engl J Med 1983; 309:595.
21. Shenoy MM, Dhar S, Gittin R, et al: Pulmonary edema following pericardiotomy for cardiac tamponade. Chest 1984; 86:647.
22. Hamaya Y, Dohi S, Ueda N, et al: Severe circulatory collapse immediately after pericardiocentesis in a patient with chronic cardiac tamponade. Anesth Analg 1993; 77:1278.
23. Armstrong WF, Feigenbaum H, Dillon JC: Acute right ventricular dilation and echocardiographic volume overload following pericardiocentesis for relief of cardiac tamponade. Am Heart J 1984; 107:1266.
24. Wolfe MW, Edelman ER: Transient systolic dysfunction after relief of cardiac tamponade. Ann Intern Med 1993; 119:42.
25. Shabetai R: Pericardiocentesis. *In* Shabetai R (ed): The Pericardium, p 325. New York: Grune & Stratton, 1981.
26. Duvernoy O, Borowiec J, Helmius G, et al: Complications of percutaneous pericardiocentesis under fluoroscopic guidance. Acta Radiologica 1992; 33:309.
27. Isselbacher EM, Cigarroa JE, Eagle KA: Cardiac tamponade complicating proximal aortic dissection: is pericardiocentesis harmful? Circulation 1994; 90:2375.
28. Palacios IF, Tuzcu EM, Ziskind AA, et al: Percutaneous balloon pericardial window for patients with malignant pericardial effusion and tamponade. Cathet Cardiovasc Diagn 1991; 22:244.
29. Ziskind AA, Pearce AC, Lemmon CC, et al: Percutaneous balloon pericardiotomy for the treatment of cardiac tamponade and large pericardial effusions: description of technique and report of the first 50 cases. J Am Coll Cardiol 1993; 21:1.
30. Chow W-H, Chow T-C, Cheung K-L: Nonsurgical creation of a pericardial window using the Inoue balloon catheter. Am Heart J 1992; 124:1100.
31. Sagrista-Sauleda J, Permanyer-Miralda G, Candell-Riera J, et al: Transient cardiac constriction: an unrecognized pattern of evolution in effusive acute idiopathic pericarditis. Am J Cardiol 1987; 59:961.
32. Ninan M, Treasure T: Pericardiectomy using an ultrasonic dissector. Ann Thorac Surg 1994; 58:233.

33. Johnson TL, Bauman WB, Josephson RA: Worsening tricuspid regurgitation following pericardiectomy for constrictive pericarditis. Chest 1993; 104:79.
34. Gaasch WH, Peterson KL, Shabetai R: Left ventricular function in chronic constrictive pericarditis. Am J Cardiol 1974; 34:107.
35. Seino Y, Ikeda U, Kawaguchi K, et al: Tuberculous pericarditis presumably diagnosed by polymerase chain reaction analysis. Am Heart J 1993; 126:249.
36. Kauffman CA, Watanakunakorn C, Phair JP: Purulent pneumococcal pericarditis. A continuing problem in the antibiotic era. Am J Med 1973; 54:743.
37. Boyle JD, Pearce ML, Guze LB: Purulent pericarditis: review of literature and report of eleven cases. Medicine 1961; 40:119.
38. Rutsky EA, Rostand SG: Treatment of uremic pericarditis and pericardial effusion. Am J Kidney Dis 1987; 10:2.
39. Buselmeier TJ, Simmons RL, Najarian JS, et al: Uremic pericardial effusion. Nephron 1976; 16:371.
40. Wilding G, Green HL, Longo DL, et al: Tumors of the heart and pericardium. Cancer Treat Rev 1988; 15:165.
41. Hancock EW: Neoplastic pericardial disease. Cardiol Clin 1990; 8:673.
42. Gregoratos G: Pericardial involvement in acute myocardial infarction. Cardiol Clin 1990 8:601.
43. Heymann TD, Culling W: Cardiac tamponade after thrombolysis. Postgrad Med J 1994; 70:455.
44. Correale E, Maggioni AP, Romano S, et al: Comparison of frequency, diagnostic and prognostic significance of pericardial involvement in acute myocardial infarction treated with and without thrombolytics. Am J Cardiol 1993; 71:1377.
45. Goldstein R, Wolff L: Hemorrhagic pericarditis in acute myocardial infarction treated with bis-hydroxycoumarin. JAMA 1951; 146:616.
46. Galve E, Garcia-del-Castillo H, Evangelista A, et al: Pericardial effusion in the course of myocardial infarction: incidence, natural history, and clinical relevance. Circulation 1986; 73:294.
47. Molnar F, Jeyasingham K: Pericardioperitoneal shunt for persistent pericardial effusions: a new drainage procedure. Ann Thorac Surg 1992; 54:569.
48. Turco M, Seneff M, McGrath BJ, et al: Cardiac tamponade in the acquired immunodeficiency syndrome. Am Heart J 1990; 120:1467.
49. Nathan PE, Arsura EL, Zappi M: Pericarditis with tamponade due to cytomegalovirus in the acquired immunodeficiency syndrome. Chest 1991; 99:765.

Index

Note: Page numbers in italics *refer to illustrations; page numbers followed by t refer to tables.*

B

C

D

E

I

N

O

P

U

V

W

Z

SMITH

5660-9

ISBN 0-7216-5660-9

90038

9 780721 656601

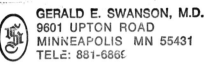